Comprehensive Textbook of Thoracic Oncology

Editors

JOSEPH AISNER, M.D.
Cancer Institute of New Jersey
Chief, Medical Oncology
Professor of Medicine & Environmental &
Community Medicine
Associate Director of Clinical Sciences
New Brunswick, New Jersey

RODRIGO ARRIAGADA, M.D.
Department of Radiation Oncology
Institut Gustave-Roussy
Villejuif, France

MARK R. GREEN, M.D.
Professor of Medicine
Edwin and Evelyn Tasch Professor in Cancer Research
Division of Hematology/Oncology
University of California-San Diego Cancer Center
San Diego, California

NAEL MARTINI, M.D.
Attending Thoracic Surgeon
Memorial Sloan-Kettering Cancer Center
Professor of Surgery
Cornell University Medical College
New York, New York

MICHAEL C. PERRY, M.D., M.S., F.A.C.P.
Professor of Medicine
Nellie B. Smith Chair of Oncology
Director, Division of Hematology/Medical Oncology
University of Missouri/Ellis Fischel Cancer Center
Columbia, Missouri

COMPREHENSIVE TEXTBOOK OF THORACIC ONCOLOGY

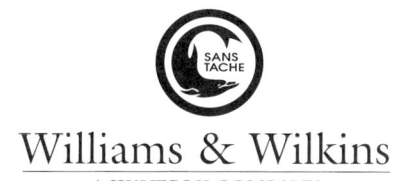

Williams & Wilkins
A WAVERLY COMPANY

BALTIMORE • PHILADELPHIA • LONDON • PARIS • BANGKOK
BUENOS AIRES • HONG KONG • MUNICH • SYDNEY • TOKYO • WROCLAW

1996

Editor: Jonathan W. Pine, Jr.
Managing Editor: Molly L. Mullen
Production Coordinator: Barbara J. Felton
Copy Editor: Lois Shipway
Designer: Dan Pfisterer
Illustration Planner: Ray Lowman
Cover Designer: Tom Scheuerman
Typesetter: University Graphics
Printer/Binder: Maple Press
Digitized Illustrations: Publicity Engravers

Copyright ©1996 Williams & Wilkins

351 West Camden Street
Baltimore, Maryland 21201-2436 USA

Rose Tree Corporate Center
1400 North Providence Road
Building II, Suite 5025
Media, Pennsylvania 19063-2043 USA

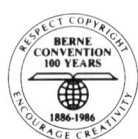

All rights reserved. This book is protected by copyright. No part of this book may be reproduced in any form or by any means, including photocopying, or utilized by any information storage and retrieval system without written permission from the copyright owner.

Accurate indications, adverse reactions and dosage schedules for drugs are provided in this book, but it is possible that they may change. The reader is urged to review the package information data of the manufacturers of the medications mentioned.

Printed in the United States of America

Library of Congress Cataloging-in-Publication Data

Comprehensive textbook of thoracic oncology / edited by Joseph Aisner . . . [et al.].
    p. cm.
   Includes index
   ISBN 0-683-00062-4
   1. Chest—Cancer. I. Aisner, Joseph.
   [DNLM: 1. Neoplasms. WF 970 C737 1995]
RC280.C5C66   1995
616.99' 494—dc20
DNLM/DLC
   for Library of Congress   95-2030
                                                                        CIP

The publishers have made every effort to trace the copyright holders for borrowed material. If they have inadvertently overlooked any, they will be pleased to make the necessary arrangements at the first opportunity.

                                                              96 97 98 99 00
                                                          1 2 3 4 5 6 7 8 9 10

Reprints of chapters may be purchased from Williams & Wilkins in quantities of 100 or more. Call our Special Sales Department at (800)358-3583.

To my wife, Seena, and our children, Dara and Leon: May the understanding of these diseases reduce the burden they impose on all our lives.—J.A.

To my wife and children.—R. A..

For my father, H. Howard Green, M.D., whose professional standards are worthy of striving hard to emulate, and for my wife and daughters, with much love.—M.R.G.

To my wife, Robin, and my children, John, Suzanne, and Jinan, for their moral support in pleasant and hard times.—N.M.

To my parents, who taught me compassion; to my teachers, colleagues, and students, who provided knowledge; and to my patients, who taught me courage. Special thanks are due to Nancy, Becca, and Katie Perry, who generously let me abandon them to contribute to this effort, and to my administrative assistant, Patty Moore, who helped me juggle patient care, teaching, administration, and this book.—M.C.P.

Foreword

The task of diagnosing and managing the therapy for patients with malignant thoracic disease remains the greatest challenge for all physicians who are involved, whatever their specialty, in the overall care of these patients. Such physicians include radiologists, pulmonary and gastroenterologic physicians, oncologists, radiotherapists, and general thoracic surgeons. This *comprehensive* textbook is directed especially to them but will be of interest also to anatomists, pathologists, epidemiologists, occupational health experts, and even some basic laboratory scientists. It will be of enormous benefit to the student and resident becoming interested in the developing field of thoracic oncology.

It is intriguing to reflect on my fifty years in medicine, an interval that has included much of the progress in the management of thoracic malignant disease. The mid-1940s was only a decade beyond the first successful pneumonectomy for lung cancer (Graham, 1933). In those years there were no imaging techniques to define the extent of disease. Endoscopy was limited to the use of open, rigid bronchoscopes and esophagoscopes. Staging of lung cancer was unknown. Even the relationship of smoking to cancer of the lung had not been totally accepted. Indeed, the specialty of oncology had not yet been born. Yet, despite these limitations, surgical resection for lung and esophageal cancer was already producing reasonable salvage of patients.

It is also sobering to assess just where we are today in the cure of patients with lung and esophageal cancer. Imaging techniques, thoroughly presented in Chapter 6, and invasive diagnostic measures (needle aspiration biopsy, mediastinoscopy, video-assisted thoracoscopy) provide the means for establishing the diagnosis and staging the disease. Staging techniques have helped identify candidates for surgical resection, thus largely eliminating unnecessary thoracotomies. Operative mortalities have dropped remarkably. Improved radiotherapeutic measures and the coming of age of chemotherapy provide useful adjuvant treatment. However, the *overall* cure rates for lung and esophageal cancer have not shown a dramatic rise. For example, in an early report on esophageal cancer patients treated by resection, the three-year survival was 22% (Sweet, 1952); this rate is not that different from the survival of patients undergoing either modern transhiatal or radical en bloc esophageal resection. The challenge of improving therapy remains.

My personal experience is in the field of general thoracic surgery, a specialty which the scholarly Leo Eloesser in his honored speaker's address before the fiftieth annual meeting of the American Association for Thoracic Surgery in 1970 described as having "become a purposely intended and scientifically directed art." The scientific direction of general thoracic surgery now must include other modes of oncologic therapy. It seems perfectly clear that surgical resection alone, except perhaps in patients with Stage I disease, is inadequate total therapy for the majority of thoracic oncology patients. Radiation therapy is routine for patients with regional lymph node metastases. There are tantalizing, if not yet totally substantiated, reports of improved survival in esophageal cancer patients undergoing combined modality therapy.

This is where the *Comprehensive Textbook of Thoracic Oncology* will be an essential tool for the thoracic oncologist, medical or surgical. The adjective *comprehensive* provides a remarkably accurate description of the book. It covers the entire breadth of the spectrum of subjects and subspecialties related to thoracic oncology, from Basic Concepts to Therapeutic Approaches. It provides a basis for a comprehensive understanding for all thoracic oncology.

It has been a great privilege that Nael Martini has asked a thoracic surgical colleague to contribute the Foreword for this superb book. I look forward to therapeutic results matching the advances in imaging and diagnosis.

Earle W. Wilkins, Jr., M.D.
Clinical Professor of Surgery, Emeritus
Harvard Medical School
Senior Surgeon
Massachusetts General Hospital
Boston, Massachusetts

Preface

Thoracic neoplasms, especially those associated with tobacco use and environmental pollution, pose a rapidly growing international problem that requires global cooperation. Lung cancer remains the leading cancer killer in the United States, and is still increasing in both developed and emerging nations. It is estimated that there are more than 600,000 deaths this year from lung cancer alone. As recently as the turn of the 20th century, these tumors were rare, and except for a few rare mediastinal tumors and lymphomas, the overall approach was essentially nihilistic.

Today, there has been a virtual explosion of both basic and clinical scientific information in the area of thoracic neoplasms as evidenced by the huge number of articles and monographs dealing with these cancers. This wealth of information is evident in all specialties and subspecialties dealing with thoracic tumors. Many publications have organized these tumors along specialty orientations, and some have viewed the area from a multispecialty approach. Do we need yet another comprehensive textbook?

Together with the increasing knowledge of the biology and therapy of thoracic tumors, there has been an improvement in treatment options and outcome, suggesting that the prior pessimism may no longer be appropriate. Many of the improvements arose from the cooperative interaction of multiple specialties working in tandem, including epidemiologists, chest physicians, thoracic radiologists, pathologists, thoracic surgeons, and radiation and medical oncologists. This is reflected at many institutions by the formation of thoracic oncology conferences or tumor boards.

This evolution into a team approach is further facilitated by the ongoing worldwide changes in health care. The major reason for this team effort, however, arises from the recent changes in diagnostic techniques such as fine needle aspiration and thoracoscopic staging, new treatment techniques such as video-assisted thoracoscopic surgery, and the rapidly expanding use of multimodality therapies. The opportunity now exists to take advantage of the increasing understanding of the biology of these diseases. In many ways, thoracic oncology has become a subspecialty of its own, built on the principles of basic oncology.

Our approach in this textbook mirrors the multispecialty nature of the various institutional thoracic tumor conferences. We brought together an experienced international group of thoracic cancer specialists as editors and invited authors who are focused across the broad range of the specialties. The resulting work is a comprehensive overview of thoracic oncology, and one which can add insight into these diseases for the thoracic specialties, and physicians at large.

The Editors

Contributors

JOSEPH AISNER, M.D.
Cancer Institute of New Jersey
Chief, Medical Oncology
Professor of Medicine & Environmental & Community Medicine
Associate Director of Clinical Sciences
New Brunswick, New Jersey

NASSER K. ALTORKI, M.D.
Associate Professor
Department of Cardiothoracic Surgery
Cornell University Medical College
Associate Attending Surgeon
Department of Cardiothoracic Surgery
New York Hospital
New York, New York

YUTAKA ARIYOSHI, M.D.
Chief
Department of Hematology and Chemotherapy
Aichi Cancer Center
Nagoya City, Aichi, Japan

RODRIGO ARRIAGADA, M.D.
Department of Radiation Oncology
Institut Gustave-Roussy
Villejuif, France

JOSEPH S. BAILES, M.D., F.A.C.P.
Executive Vice President and National Medical Director
Physician Reliance Network, Inc.
Dallas, Texas

CHANDRA P. BELANI, M.D.
Associate Professor of Medicine
Division of Medical Oncology
Department of Medicine
University of Pittsburgh Medical Center
Co-Director, Experimental Therapeutics Program
Pittsburgh Cancer Institute
Pittsburgh, Pennsylvania

JEAN BIGNON, M.D.
Director
Unit 139, INSERM
Hôpital Henri Mondor
Creteil, France

GEORGE J. BOSL, M.D.
Head, Division of Solid Tumor Oncology
Memorial Sloan-Kettering Cancer Center
Professor of Medicine
Cornell University Medical College
New York Hospital-Cornell Medical Center
New York, New York

P. BROCHARD, M.D.
Professor of Occupational Health
Université Bordeaux II
Bordeaux, France

DAVID M. BURNS, M.D.
Professor of Medicine
Department of Pulmonary and Critical Care
University of California, San Diego
San Diego, California

MICHAEL E. BURT, M.D., PH.D.
Attending Thoracic Surgeon
Memorial Sloan-Kettering Cancer Center
Professor of Surgery
Cornell University Medical College
New York, New York

DAVID P. CARBONE, M.D., PH.D.
Associate Professor of Internal Medicine
Simmons Cancer Center
University of Texas Southwestern Medical Center
Dallas, Texas

NEIL COLMAN, M.D.
Senior Physician
Respiratory Department
Montreal General Hospital
Montreal, Canada

HENRI G. COLT, M.D., F.C.C.P.
Assistant Professor, Pulmonary and Critical Care
    Division
University of California, San Diego Medical Center
San Diego, California

JOSEPH M. CORSON, M.D.
Director, Surgical Pathology Division
Department of Pathology
Brigham & Women's Hospital
Professor of Pathology
Department of Pathology
Harvard Medical School
Boston, Massachusetts

TIMOTHY R. COTÉ, M.D., M.P.H.
Division of Cancer Etiology
Viral Epidemiology Branch
National Cancer Institute
Bethesda, Maryland

ANN CULL, PH.D.
Consultant Clinical Psychologist
Imperial Cancer Research Fund
Medical Oncology Unit
Western General Hospital
Edinburgh, United Kingdom

MICHAEL DAVIS, M.S., J.D.
Senior Medical Physicist
Department of Radiation Physics
University of Texas M.D. Anderson Cancer Center
Houston, Texas

DAPHNE M. deMELLO, M.D.
Professor of Pathology and Pediatrics
Department of Pathology
St. Louis University School of Medicine
St. Louis, Missouri

TODD L. DEMMY, M.D., F.A.C.S., F.C.C.P.
Assistant Professor
Department of Surgery
University of Missouri Hospital and Clinics
Chief, Thoracic Oncology
University of Missouri/Ellis Fischel Cancer Center
Columbia, Missouri

MANISH DHAWAN, M.D.
Clinical Associate
Division of Medical Oncology and Hematology
University of Pittsburgh Medical Center
Pittsburgh, Pennsylvania

LEE C. DRINKARD, M.D.
Associate
Inland Hematology-Oncology Medical Group, Inc.
San Bernardino, California

M. JOSEPH FEDORUK, M.D., C.I.H.
Assistant Clinical Professor
Department of Medicine
University of California, Irvine
Irvine, California

ELLEN G. FEIGAL, M.D.
Division of Cancer Treatment
Cancer Treatment Evaluation Program
National Cancer Institute
Bethesda, Maryland

MARK K. FERGUSON, M.D.
Associate Professor of Surgery
Chief, Section of Thoracic Surgery
University of Chicago
Chicago, Illinois

PETER F. FERSON, M.D.
University of Pittsburgh
Veterans Administration Medical Center
Pittsburgh, Pennsylvania

ARMANDO E. FRAIRE, M.D.
Associate Professor of Pathology
Department of Pathology
University of Massachusetts Medical Center
Worcester, Massachusetts

MASAHIRO FUKUOKA, M.D.
Chief, Department of Pulmonary Medicine
Osaka City General Hospital
Osaka City, Osaka
Chief, Department of Internal Medicine
Osaka Prefectural Habikino Hospital
Habikino, Osaka, Japan

ADAM S. GARDEN, M.D.
Assistant Radiotherapist and Assistant
Professor of Radiotherapy
University of Texas M.D. Anderson Cancer Center
Houston, Texas

YEVGENIY GINCHERMAN, M.D.
Resident in Internal Medicine
University of Pennsylvania
School of Medicine
Philadelphia, Pennsylvania

ROBERT J. GINSBERG, M.D.
Chief of Thoracic Service
Department of Surgery
Memorial Sloan-Kettering Cancer Center
Professor of Surgery
Cornell University Medical College
New York, New York

GEOFFREY M. GRAEBER, M.D.
Professor of Surgery
Thoracic and Cardiovascular Surgery
West Virginia University
Director, Department of Surgery
Section of Surgical Research
Morgantown, West Virginia

MARK R. GREEN, M.D.
Professor of Medicine
Edwin and Evelyn Tasch Professor in Cancer Research
Division of Hematology/Oncology
University of California, San Diego Cancer Center
San Diego, California

ANNA GREGOR, F.R.C.P., F.R.C.R.
Department of Clinical Oncology
University of Edinburgh
Edinburgh, Scotland

STEPHEN R. HAZELRIGG, M.D.
Associate Professor
Chairman, Division of Cardiothoracic Surgery
Southern Illinois University School of Medicine
Springfield, Illinois

STEPHEN S. HECHT, PH.D.
Director of Research
American Health Foundation
Valhalla, New York

ROBERT T. HEELAN, M.D.
Attending Radiologist
Department of Radiology
Memorial-Sloan Kettering Cancer Center
Professor
Department of Radiology
Cornell University Medical College
New York, New York

DENISE M. HICKEY, M.D.
Instructor Medicine
Dartmouth-Hitchcock Medical Center
Norris Cotton Cancer Center
Lebanon, New Hampshire

JANE C. HUANG, M.D.
Fellow in Surgical Pathology
Department of Pathology
Washington University
St. Louis, Missouri

WILLIAM G. HUGHSON, M.D.
Director, Occupational Health Center
University of California, San Diego
San Diego, California

DAVID H. ILSON, M.D., PH.D.
Clinical Assistant Attending Physician
Gastrointestinal Oncology Service
Department of Medicine
Memorial Sloan-Kettering Cancer Center
New York, New York

JAMES R. JETT, M.D.
Professor of Medicine
University of Pittsburgh
Division of Pulmonary Medicine and Medical Oncology
Pittsburgh, Pennsylvania

DAVID R. JONES, M.D.
Division of Cardiothoracic Surgery
University of North Carolina
Chapel Hill, North Carolina

HARUBUMI KATO, M.D., PH.D.
Professor and Chairman
Department of Surgery
Tokyo Medical College
Tokyo, Japan

ROBERT J. KEENAN, M.D.
Assistant Professor
Section of Thoracic Surgery
University of Pittsburgh Medical Center
Pittsburgh, Pennsylvania

DAVID P. KELSEN, M.D.
Chief, Gastrointestinal Oncology Service
Memorial Sloan-Kettering Cancer Center
Professor of Medicine
Cornell University Medical College
New York, New York

JEAN KLASTERSKY, M.D., PH.D.
Professor and Chief of Medicine
Department of Medicine
Institut Jules-Bordet
Brussels, Belgium

RITSUKO KOMAKI, M.D., F.A.C.R.
Associate Professor of Radiotherapy
Department of Radiotherapy
University of Texas M.D. Anderson Cancer Center
Houston, Texas

MARK J. KRASNA, M.D.
Director, General Thoracic Surgery
Department of Surgery
University of Maryland Medical Center
Baltimore, Maryland

KEVIN LACHAPELLE, M.D., F.R.C.S.C.
Clinical Fellow
Department of Cardiothoracic Surgery
McGill University
Montreal, Canada

RODNEY J. LANDRENEAU, M.D.
Head, Section of Thoracic Surgery
Assistant Professor of Surgery
Department of Thoracic Surgery
University of Pittsburgh
Pittsburgh, Pennsylvania

STEVEN LARSON, M.D.
Chief, Nuclear Medicine Service
Memorial Sloan-Kettering Cancer Center
Professor of Radiology
Cornell University Medical College
New York, New York

TERESA MURRAY LAW, M.D.
Fellow
Section of Medical Oncology
Memorial Sloan-Kettering Cancer Center
New York, New York

THIERRY LE CHEVALIER, M.D.
Medical Oncologist (Chief of Service)
Department of Medicine
Institut Gustave Roussy
Villejuif, France

CYNTHIA C. LEMMON, M.S.
Research Coordinator
Division of Cardiology
Department of Medicine
University of Maryland
Baltimore, Maryland

DR. PHILIPPE LEVASSEUR
Head of Department
Thoracic and Vascular Surgery
Hôpital Marie Lannelongue
Le Plessis Robinson, France

ROGERIO C. LILENBAUM, M.D.
Assistant Professor
Department of Medicine
Division of Hematology/Oncology
University of Maryland and Veterans Affairs Medical Center
Baltimore, Maryland

MICHAEL J. LIPTAY, M.D.
Fellow in Thoracic Surgery
Division of Thoracic Surgery
Brigham & Women's Hospital
Boston, Massachusetts

MICHAEL J. MACK, M.D.
Clinical Assistant Professor
Department of Cardiothoracic Surgery
University of Texas Southwestern Medical School
Dallas, Texas

NAEL MARTINI, M.D.
Attending Thoracic Surgeon
Memorial Sloan-Kettering Cancer Center
Professor of Surgery
Cornell University Medical College
New York, New York

NORIYUKI MASUDA, M.D., PH.D.
Chief
IInd Department of Internal Medicine
Osaka Prefectural Habikino Hospital
Habikino City, Osaka, Japan

DOUGLAS J. MATHISEN, M.D.
Visiting Surgeon
Department of Thoracic Surgery
Massachusetts General Hospital
Associate Professor of Surgery
Harvard Medical School
Boston, Massachusetts

L. HERBERT MAURER, M.D.
Professor of Oncology
Department of Medicine
Dartmouth Medical School
Lebanon, New Hampshire

PATRICIA M. MCCORMACK, M.D.
Attending Thoracic Surgeon
Department of Surgery
Memorial Sloan-Kettering Cancer Center
Professor of Surgery
Cornell University School of Medicine
New York Hospital
New York, New York

SI-CHUN MING, M.D.
Emeritus Professor
Department of Pathology & Laboratory Medicine
Temple University School of Medicine
Philadelphia, Pennsylvania

RODOLFO C. MORICE, M.D., F.C.C.P.
Associate Professor and Internist
Chief, Section of Pulmonary and Critical Care
    Medicine
University of Texas M.D. Anderson Cancer Center
Houston, Texas

JAMES L. MULSHINE, M.D.
Chief
Biomarkers & Prevention Research Branch
National Cancer Institute
Bethesda, Maryland

ARNO J. MUNDT, M.D.
Assistant Professor
Department of Radiation and Cellular Oncology
University of Chicago Hospitals
Chicago, Illinois

KEITH S. NAUNHEIM, M.D.
Professor of Surgery
Division of Cardiothoracic Surgery
St. Louis University Health Sciences Center
St. Louis, Missouri

TETSUYA OKUNAKA, M.D., PH.D., F.C.C.P.
Senior Lecturer
Department of Surgery
Tokyo Medical College
Tokyo, Japan

SIN-TIONG ONG, M.A., M.R.C.P.
Department of Medicine
Section of Hematology/Oncology
University of Chicago Medical Center
Chicago, Illinois

KELL ØSTERLIND, M.D., DR.MED.
Medical Dept. F.
Hillerod Sygehus
Hillerod, Denmark

J.C. PAIRON, M.D.
Service de Pneumologie et de Pathologie
    Professionnelle
Centre Hôpitalier Intercommunal de Creteil
Creteil, France

HARVEY I. PASS, M.D.
Head, Thoracic Oncology Section
Surgery Branch
National Cancer Intitute/National Institutes of Health
Bethesda, Maryland

UGO PASTORINO, M.D.
Consultant Thoracic Surgeon
Royal Brompton Hospital
London, United Kingdom

ASHOKAKUMAR M. PATEL, M.D.
Senior Associate Consultant
Division of Pulmonary & Critical Care Medicine
Mayo Clinic
Rochester, Minnesota

DAVID G. PAYNE, M.D.
Assistant Professor
Department of Surgery
University of Toronto
Staff Radiation Oncologist
Ontario Cancer Institute-Princess Margaret Hospital
Toronto, Ontario, Canada

MICHAEL C. PERRY, M.D., M.S., F.A.C.P.
Professor of Internal Medicine
Nellie B. Smith Chair of Oncology
Director, Division of Hematology/Medical Oncology
University of Missouri/Ellis Fischel Cancer Center
Columbia, Missouri

JEAN-PIERRE PIGNON, M.D., PH.D.
Doctor
Departement de Biostatistique et d'Epidemiologie
Institut Gustave-Roussy
Villejuif Cedex, France

RENÉ REGNIER, M.D.
Professor
Department of Radiotherapy
Institut Jules-Bordet
Brussels, Belgium

LYNNE M. REID, M.D.
Simeon Burt Wolbach Professor of Pathology
Harvard Medical School
Pathologist-in-Chief, Emeritus
Children's Hospital
Boston, Massachusetts

ANDREW A. RENSHAW, M.D.
Staff Pathologist
Brigham & Women's Hospital
Instructor, Department of Pathology
Harvard Medical School
Boston, Massachusetts

ANDREW L. RIES, M.D., M.P.H.
Professor
Department of Medicine
University of California, San Diego
San Diego, California

JON H. RITTER, M.D.
Assistant Professor
Department of Pathology
Washington University School of Medicine
St. Louis, Missouri

VALERIE W. RUSCH, M.D.
Attending Surgeon and Member
Thoracic Service, Department of Surgery
Memorial Sloan-Kettering Cancer Center
Professor of Surgery
Department of Surgery
Cornell University Medical College
New York, New York

FARID M. SHAMJI, M.D.
Associate Professor
University of Ottawa Faculty of Medicine
Head, Division of Thoracic Surgery
Ottawa Civic Hospital
Ottawa, Ontario, Canada

HANI SHENNIB, M.D., F.R.C.S.C., F.A.C.S.
Associate Professor
Department of Surgery and Oncology
McGill University
Montreal, Canada

FRANCES A. SHEPHERD, M.D.
Director, Medical Oncology
Department of Medicine, The Toronto Hospital
Associate Professor, Faculty of Medicine
University of Toronto
Toronto, Ontario

Chairman, Lung Cancer Committee
National Cancer Institute of Canada
Kingston, Ontario, Canada

STÉPHANE SIMON
Engineer in Physics
Head of Physics Department
Institut Jules-Bordet
Brussels, Belgium

JENS BENN SØRENSEN, M.D.
Chief
Finsen Center
Department of Oncology
The National University Hospital
Copenhagen, Denmark

GARY D. STONER, PH.D.
Professor
Department of Preventive Medicine
Ohio State University
Columbus, Ohio

DAVID J. SUGARBAKER, M.D.
Chief, Division of Thoracic Surgery
Department of Surgery
Brigham & Women's Hospital
Boston, Massachusetts

EVA SZABO, M.D.
Senior Investigator
Biomarkers & Prevention Research Branch
National Cancer Institute
Rockville, Maryland

BARBARA K. TEMECK, M.D.
Senior Investigator
Thoracic Oncology Section
National Cancer Institute/National Institutes of Health
Bethesda, Maryland

MELVYN S. TOCKMAN, M.D.
Associate Professor
Department of Environmental Health Sciences
The Johns Hopkins University School of Hygiene and
    Public Health
Baltimore, Maryland

VICTOR F. TRASTEK, M.D.
Associate Professor of Surgery
Department of Surgery
Mayo Clinic & Mayo Foundation
Rochester, Minnesota

PAUL VAN HOUTTE, M.D.
Professor
Department of Radiation Oncology
Institut Jules-Bordet
Brussels, Belgium

NICHOLAS J. VOGELZANG, M.D.
Professor of Medicine
Director, Genitourinary Oncology
Section of Hematology/Oncology
University of Chicago Medical Center
Chicago, Illinois

EVERETT E. VOKES, M.D.
Professor of Medicine and Radiation Oncology
Director for Clinical Affairs
Cancer Research Center
University of Chicago Medical Center
Chicago, Illinois

GARRETT L. WALSH, M.D.
Assistant Professor of Surgery
Department of Thoracic & Cardiovascular Surgery
University of Texas M.D. Anderson Cancer Center
Houston, Texas

STEVEN J. WESTGATE, M.D.
Director, Radiation Oncology
Radiation Oncology Department
University of Missouri/Ellis Fischel Cancer Center
Columbia, Missouri

MARK R. WICK, M.D.
Professor of Pathology
Department of Pathology
Washington University School of Medicine
St. Louis, Missouri

REBECCA S. WOLFER, M.D.
Chief Resident
Department of Surgery
University of Maryland Medical System
Baltimore, Maryland

ANDREW A. ZISKIND, M.D.
Assistant Professor of Medicine
Division of Cardiology
Department of Medicine
University of Maryland Medical System
Director, Cardiac Catheterization Laboratory
Baltimore, Maryland

Contents

Dedication   *v*
Foreword   *vii*
Preface   *ix*
Contributors   *xi*

Section I
Basic Concepts

1. Anatomic Development of Intrathoracic Structures   3
   Daphne E. deMello, Lynne M. Reid

2. Lung and Esophageal Carcinogenesis   25
   Stephen S. Hecht, Gary D. Stoner

3. Cigarette Smoking   51
   David M. Burns

4. Occupational and Environmental Causes of Lung Cancer and Esophageal Cancer   66
   William G. Hughson, M. Joseph Fedoruk

5. Screening/Secondary Prevention

   5A. Screening & Secondary Prevention of Lung Cancer   90
   Eva Szabo, James L. Mulshine

   5B. Progress in the Early Detection of Lung Cancer   105
   Melvyn S. Tockman

6. Imaging of Thoracic Neoplasms   112
   Robet T. Heelan, Steven Larson

7. Pulmonary Function Evaluation vis à vis Tumor Treatment   169
   Hani Shennib, Kevin Lachapelle, Neil Colman

8. Treatment Evaluation   188
   Jean-Pierre Pignon, Rodrigo Arriagada

9. Modern Principles of Radiation Therapy   215
   Paul Van Houtte, Stéphane Simon, René Regnier

Section II.
Lung Cancer: General

10. Pathology of Lung Cancer Armando E. Fraire	245
11. Molecular Biology in the Diagnosis, Prognosis, and Therapy of Lung Cancer David P. Carbone	276
12. Clinical Presentation and Staging of Lung Cancer Ashokakumar M. Patel, James R. Jett	293
13. Prognostic Factors Kell Østerlind, Jens Benn Sørensen	319

Section III.
Therapeutic Approaches to Non–Small Cell Lung Cancer

14. Treatment of Stage I and II Disease Nael Martini, Robert J. Ginsberg	338
15. Surgical Management of Stage IIIA Non–Small Cell Lung Cancer Valery W. Rusch, Yevgeniy Gincherman	351
16. Superior Sulcus Tumors Robert J. Ginsburg, David G. Payne, Farid Shamji	375
17. Therapeutic Options in Locally Advanced Non–Small Cell Lung Cancer (Stage IIIB) Thierry Le Chevalier, Rodrigo Arriagada	388
18. Role of Surgery in the Treatment of Patients with Solitary Metastasis from Non–Small Cell Lung Cancer Michael E. Burt	416
19. Management of Disseminated Non–Small Cell Lung Cancer Rogerio C. Lilenbaum, Mark R. Green	426

Section IV.
Therapeutic Approaches to Small Cell Lung Cancer

20. Role of Surgery in the Management of Small Cell Lung Cancer Frances A. Shepherd	439

21. REGIONAL DISEASE *Rodrigo Arriagada, Thierry Le Chevalier*	456
22. THERAPEUTIC APPROACH TO DISSEMINATED SMALL-CELL LUNG CANCER *Masahiro Fukuoka, Noriyuki Masuda, Yutaka Ariyoshi*	496
23. PROPHYLACTIC CRANIAL IRRADIATION *Anna Gregor, Ann Cull*	512
24. ISOLATED EXTENSIVE DISEASE *Denise M. Hickey, L. Herbert Maurer*	525

SECTION V.
ESOPHAGEAL CANCER

25. PATHOLOGY OF ESOPHAGEAL CANCER *Si-Chun Ming*	533
26. ESOPHAGEAL CARCINOMA: DIAGNOSIS, EVALUATION, AND STAGING *Mark J. Krasna, Rebecca S. Wolfer*	563
27. BARRETT'S ESOPHAGUS (AND OTHER PREMALIGNANT LESIONS) AND MANAGEMENT OF LOCALIZED ESOPHAGEAL CANCER *Nasser K. Altorki*	585
28. THERAPY OF ESOPHAGEAL CANCER *Lee C. Drinkard, Mark K. Ferguson, Arno J. Mundt, Everett E. Vokes*	606
29. SYSTEMIC THERAPY IN ESOPHAGEAL CANCER *David H. Ilson, David P. Kelson*	630

SECTION VI.
MEDIASTINAL TUMORS

30. THYMOMAS *Philippe Levasseur*	653
31. MEDIASTINAL GERM CELL TUMORS *George J. Bosl, Teresa Murray Law*	668
32. TUMORS OF THE HEART AND PERICARDIUM *Todd L. Demmy*	681
33. POSTERIOR MEDIASTINAL TUMORS *David R. Jones, Geoffrey M. Graeber*	711

Section VII.
Mesothelioma

34. Mesothelioma: Causes and Fiber-Related Mechanisms   735
Jean Bignon, Patrick Brochard, Jean-Claude Pairon

35. Pathology of Mesothelioma   757
Joseph M. Corson, Andrew A. Renshaw

36. Diagnosis, Staging, and Natural History of Pleural Mesothelioma   779
Joseph Aisner

37. Therapeutic Approaches in Malignant Mesothelioma   786
David J. Sugarbaker, Michael J. Liptay

38. Current Therapeutic Approaches to Unresectable (Primary and Recurrent) Disease   799
Sin-Tiong Ong, Nicholas J. Vogelzang

Section VIII.
Other Malignancies

39. Malignant Nonepithelial Neoplasms of the Lungs and Pleural Surfaces   815
Jane C. Huang, Jon H. Ritter, Mark R. Wick

40. Bronchial Carcinoids   850
Victor F. Trastek

41. Tracheal Tumors   855
Douglas J. Mathisen

42. Tumors of the Chest Wall   870
Patricia M. McCormack

43. Management of Malignant Pleural and Pericardial Effusions   880
Chandra P. Belani, Andrew A. Ziskind, Manish Dhawan, Cynthia C. Lemmon

44. Intrathoracic Metastases   906
Barbara K. Temeck, Harvey I. Pass

Section IX.
Special Topics

45. Endoscopic Techniques

    45A. Bronchoscopic Laser Resection in Patients with Thoracic Neoplasia — 925
Henri G. Colt

    45B. High-Dose–Rate Remote Afterloading Endobronchial Brachytherapy — 940
Ritsuko Komaki, Rodolfo C. Morice, Garrett L. Walsh, Adam S. Garden, Michael Davis

46. Endobronchial Photodynamic Therapy — 947
Harubumi Kato, Tetsuya Okunaka

47. Video-Assisted Thoracic Surgery — 965
Rodney J. Landreneau, Stephen R. Hazelrigg, Michael J. Mack, Keith S. Naunheim, Robert J. Keenan, Peter F. Ferson

48. Supportive Care in Cancer Patients — 980
Jean Klastersky

49. Complications

    49A. Complications of Combined Modality Therapy — 1002
Steven J. Westgate, Michael C. Perry

    49B. Pulmonary Rehabilitation in Patients with Thoracic Neoplasm — 1019
Andrew L. Ries

50. Thoracic Neoplasms Associated with Human Immunodeficiency Virus Infection — 1030
Ellen G. Feigal, Timothy R. Coté

51. Chemoprevention of Lung Cancer in High-Risk Individuals — 1053
Ugo Pastorino

52. Government Regulation of Tobacco and Tobacco Products — 1080
Joseph S. Bailes

Index — 1091

SECTION I

BASIC CONCEPTS

1

ANATOMIC DEVELOPMENT OF INTRATHORACIC STRUCTURES

Daphne E. deMello and Lynne M. Reid

INTRODUCTION

Oncology, the study of human tumors and their treatment, draws on our understanding of structure and function and their development at all ages. Advances in molecular genetics increasingly reveal an internet of communication and control that links oncology to ontogeny, not only through the fertilized germ cell, but through the subsequent development of genes and their mutations. Molecular biology is compiling the chemical dictionary of signals and moderators that provides the language of genetic control of normal and disordered growth, including tumorigenesis. Although the revelations and connections are startling, they have only highlighted the gaps in our understanding of the dialogue involved in patterns of interaction and control. The field is expanding so rapidly that these mechanisms are only alluded to in this chapter. In the chapters dealing with particular tumors, the latest knowledge of the genetic and molecular etiology and sequelae are discussed in detail.

Structure reveals the basis of function. Aspects of structure are therefore important in understanding the nature and clinical manifestations of tumors and their modification by treatment. For example, the circulation of pleural fluid and lymph movement, as well as collateral air drift in the lung, are features requiring an understanding of function and structure during diagnosis and treatment.

Such features of lung anatomy are important regardless of the tumor or its site because virtually every patient presenting for diagnosis or treatment has a chest radiograph or some other record of the chest and lungs. Understanding the anatomic arrangement of lung constituents, particularly of the various vascular, lymphatic, and aerating systems, as well as the connective tissue framework, is essential to their interpretation.

Growth, with increase in mass and differentiation of structure, uses pathways perverted in tumor formation. During childhood, tumors and their treatment produce secondary effects on growth. Postnatally, the lung shows a striking change in its template for growth, thus organ growth of lung is also included in this discussion.

EMBRYOLOGY: GROWTH

The earliest stages of growth, those of the simplest and most basic differentiation, are emphasized. In recent decades research has concentrated particularly in this area. Molecular biology is used to identify unsuspected combinations of markers in cells: differentiated and tumor cells carry unsuspected baggage. Increasingly, it is in the earliest stages of development that we find reasons for seemingly "unreasonable" baggage and connections between cell types and tumors.

FETAL GROWTH: CELLS, GERM LAYERS, TISSUES, AND ORGANS

After fertilization, cell multiplication occurs. It is within the morula or mulberry, a compact ball of cells, that polarization is established—cephalad and caudad, dorsal and ventral, and lateralization to right and left (1). The homeobox genes are critical to these developments (2–4). In addition, there are transcription factors that modulate these basic genes to determine specific temporospatial events, such as a limb bud, that are essential for appropriate regional development.

The outer cells differentiate to form the trophoblast that invades the endometrium, whereas the inner cells represent the future embryo. Within this cell mass, a cavity forms to produce the blastocyst, which implants in the uterine cavity (Fig. 1.1). Ovula-

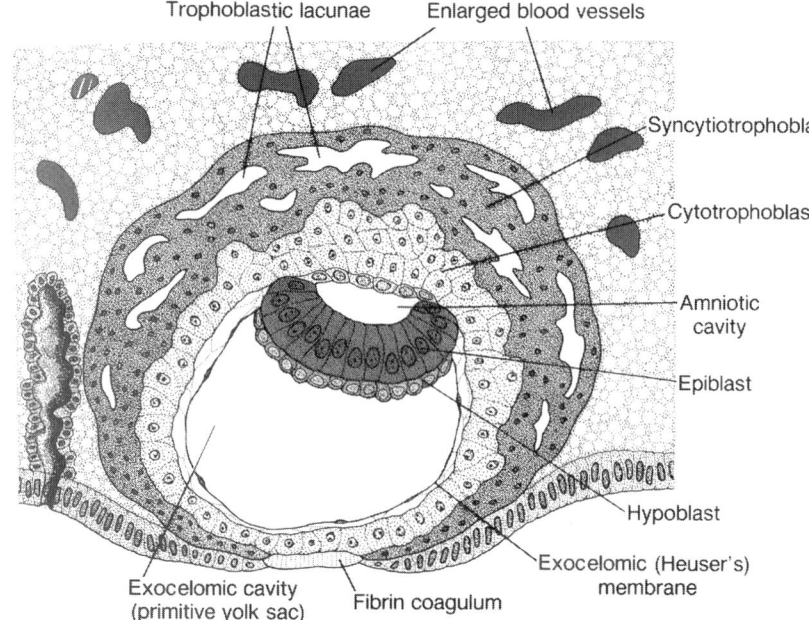

FIGURE 1.1. Drawing of a 9-day human blastocyst. The syncytiotrophoblast shows a large number of lacunae. Note the flat cells that form the exocelomic membrane. The bilaminar germ disc consists of a layer of columnar epiblast cells and a layer of cuboidal hypoblast cells. The original uterine surface defect is closed by a fibrin coagulum. (From Sadler TW. Langman's medical embryology. 6th ed. Baltimore: Williams & Wilkins, 1990:41.)

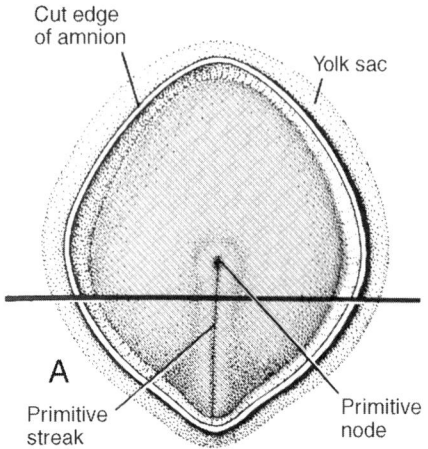
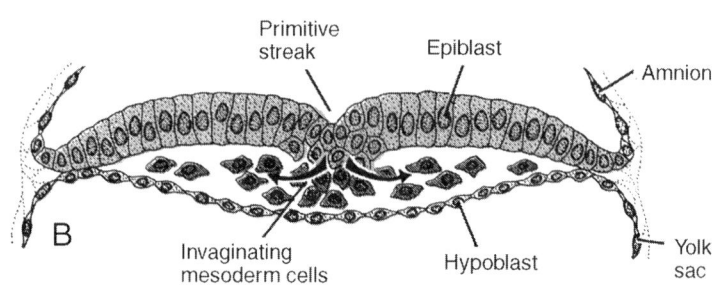

FIGURE 1.2. A. Schematic drawing of the dorsal side of a 16-day presomite embryo. The primitive streak and node are clearly visible. B. Transverse section through the region of the primitive streak as indicated in Fig. 1.1A showing the invagination and subsequent lateral migration of the epiblast cells that will form the embryonic mesoderm and endoderm. (From Sadler TW. Langman's medical embryology. 6th ed. Baltimore: Williams & Wilkins, 1990:51.)

tion to implantation finishes the 1st week of development.

During the 2nd week, the bilaminar germ disc separates the amniotic cavity from the exocelomic cavity or primitive yolk sac (Fig. 1.2). The epiblast, one cell layer thick, faces the amniotic cavity; the hypoblast, the other layer, faces the yolk sac. From each, cells migrate to line the adjacent cavity. Mesoderm develops between the trophoblast and these lining cells. Extraembryonic somatopleuric mesoderm cells line the cytotrophoblast and amnion, and the extraembryonic splanchnopleuric mesoderm lines the yolk sac.

During the 3rd week, the trilaminar germ disc or gastrula develops; it is at this time that the three germ layers form (Figs. 1.2 and 1.3). The primitive streak lies at the caudal end, from which the epiblast cells grow down and spread to form endoderm by replacing the hypoblast; between these two layers epiblast cells form the mesoderm. All three definitive germ layers arise from the epiblast.

Cephalad, the mesoderm passes under the prochordal plate to form the cardiogenic plate. Cells invaginate to form a tube that passes in the cephalad direction to form the notochordal or head process. The small central canal is considered an extension of the

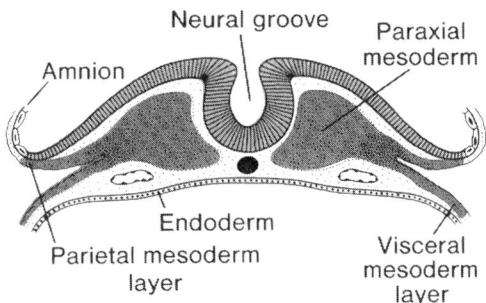 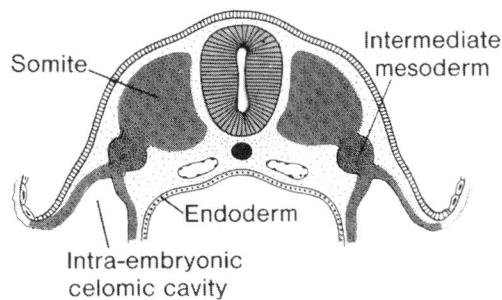

FIGURE 1.3. Transverse sections showing the development of the mesodermal germ layer. A. Day 20. B. Day 21. A mesodermal sheet gives rise to the paraxial mesoderm (the future somites), the intermediate mesoderm (the future excretory units), and the lateral plate, which is split into the parietal and visceral mesoderm layers lining the intraembryonic coelomic cavity. (From Sadler TW. Langman's medical embryology. 6th ed. Baltimore: Williams & Wilkins, 1990:68.)

primitive pit that lies at the cranial end of the primitive streak.

By 17 days' gestation mesoderm and the notochordal process separate the endoderm and ectoderm. The notochord fuses with the endoderm, at which point the two layers disintegrate. What remains of the notochord forms a narrow plate of cells intercalated into the endodermal germ layer. These cells proliferate and form a solid and definitive notochord, which detaches from the endoderm. The notochord gives rise to the midline structures that are the basis of the skeleton.

The neural tube is formed by infolding of the surface ectoderm to form a neural groove (Fig. 1.3). Cells at the dorsal and lateral edges of this groove differentiate and then separate, constituting the neural crest cell population. These cells start a migratory life that includes their transformation from epithelial to mesenchymal as they move to the underlying mesoderm (5, 6). (Mesoderm refers to cells derived from epiblast and extraembryonic tissues. Mesenchyme refers to loosely organized embryonic connective tissue, regardless of origin [1].)

These cells give rise to a heterogeneous array of tissues—spinal (1, 7–12) and autonomic ganglia and parts of the cranial nerve ganglia, specifically melanocytes. These melanocytes synthesize melanin and through dendritic processes transfer it to other cells in the skin, cells of the trunco-conal endocardial cushion (13, 14), and the chromaffin cells of the paraganglia, carotid body, and medulla of the suprarenal. From the neural crest cells arise that migrate into the future airway epithelium to differentiate into neuroendocrine cells, which sometimes are basal, sometimes reach the surface, or sometimes are concentrated into neuroepithelial bodies (15).

Cell multiplication leads to an increase in size, but as sculpting of tissues and organs proceeds, multiplication is also balanced by apoptosis or programmed cell death (16, 17). Not only do cells differentiate, they also migrate relatively great distances throughout the developing fetus. This process leads to mixing of cells within tissues. Such differentiation of function within a germ layer, followed by migration, is exemplified by the behavior of the neural crest cells. Invasion and migration of cells is reminiscent of the "autonomous" growth and metastasis of tumors. Differential growth rates lead to changes in body shape that also are an essential feature of development.

In the early fetus it is the cervical region that is critical to the development of the thorax. The diaphragm first appears in this region. As it descends to its final site, it takes with it the phrenic or nerve of respiration: pain referred from the diaphragm to the shoulder recalls this origin.

The thoracic cage develops in the territory of 12 somites between the cervical and lumbar groups. The development of vertebral bodies, ribs, and sternum in the thorax preserves the segmental pattern typical of early development in the fetus.

The first nutrient or bronchial artery to the lung arises from the aorta in the neck, adjacent to the celiac axis (18, 19). Normally, these arteries disappear at about the 6th week, several weeks before the definitive bronchial arteries arise from the descending aorta. If the primitive bronchial arteries persist, they migrate with the celiac axis to the region of the diaphragm, entering the lung through the inferior pulmonary ligament.

Lymphatics do not appear until the 5th week of gestation, after the central connections of the cardiovascular system are established and the respiratory system has begun formation (1, 20, 21). It is still unclear whether the lymphatics develop in situ as lakes or whether they originate as directed branching from the endothelium of veins (20). This discussion is reminiscent of the doubt that has long surrounded the pat-

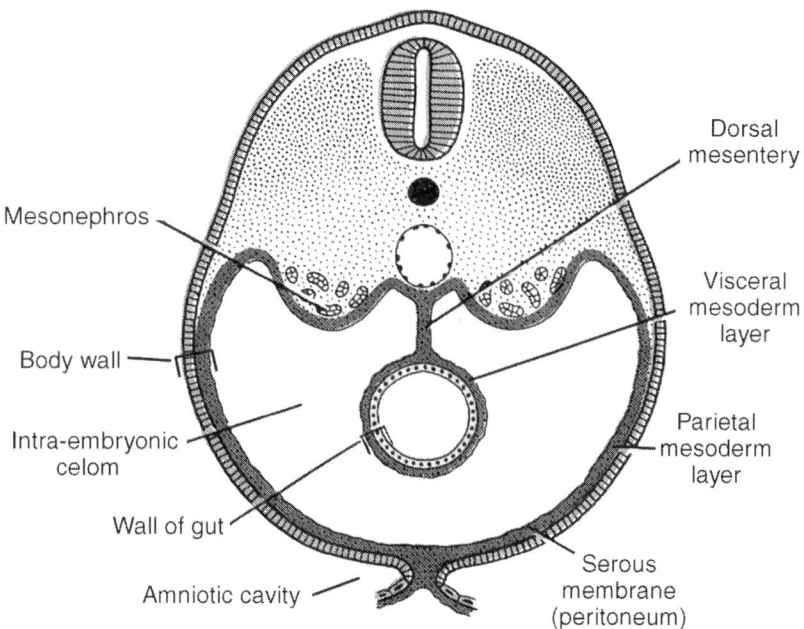

FIGURE 1.4. A. Transverse section through an embryo in the region of the mesonephros at the end of the 4th week. Note the parietal and visceral mesoderm layers. The intraembryonic and extraembryonic coelomic cavities no longer communicate. The parietal mesoderm and the overlying ectoderm form the ventral and lateral body wall. Note the peritoneal (serous) membrane. (From Sadler TW. Langman's medical embryology. 6th ed. Baltimore: Williams & Wilkins, 1990:71.)

tern of arterial branching, although increasingly it seems that both methods contribute (22). Peripheral lakes form within the mesenchyme, but the central connections are made between these lakes and channels that have, in fact, grown out from the appropriate sites to which the system will ultimately drain (23).

Whatever the detail the development of the six primary sacs can be identified early in gestation (1): the right and left jugular, right and left iliac, a retroperitoneal sac near the base of the mesentry, and another retroperitoneal sac, the cisternachyli, dorsal to this. Thoracic ducts, which are paired right and left, are important channels that join the cisterna chyli to the jugular sacs. These channels rearrange themselves so that ultimately the thoracic duct, which will drain into the left subclavian at its junction with the jugular, is formed from the cranial part of the left thoracic channel, an anastomosis and the distal part of the right duct. This thoracic duct has passed upward on the right side of the midline, but then crosses to drain into the veins on the left. The right lymphatic duct represents the cranial end of the right channel and drains into the jugular and subclavian junction on the right. The route taken by these two systems and their drainages contributes to the crossover that can occur between apparent metastases and the site of origin of tumor.

EMBRYONIC GROWTH

From the 3rd to the 8th week, during the embryonic period, each germ layer gives rise to appropriate

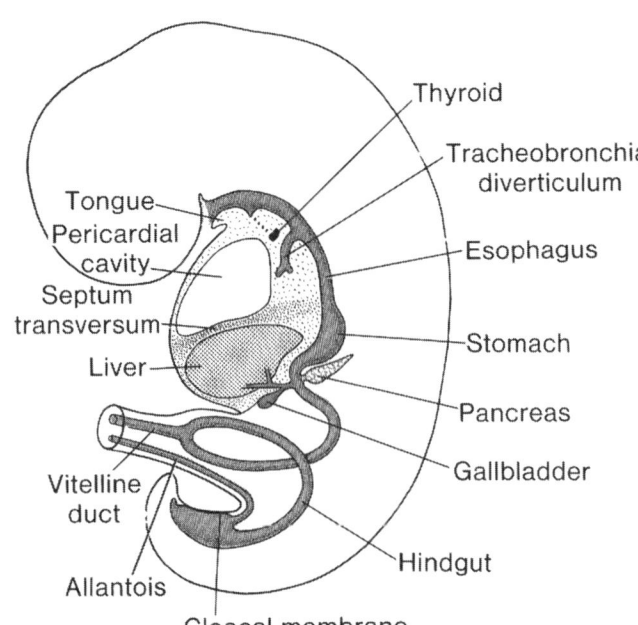

FIGURE 1.5. Drawing of a 9-mm embryo (approximately 36 days). The liver expands caudally into the abdominal cavity. Note the condensation of mesenchyme in the area between the liver and the pericardial cavity, foreshadowing the formation of the diaphragm. The tracheobronchial diverticulum has separated from the esophagus. (From Sadler TW. Langman's medical embryology. 6th ed. Baltimore: Williams & Wilkins, 1990:243.)

tissues, and organ patterns appear (Fig. 1.4). The mesoderm can be identified as including three parts—the paraxial, intermediate, and lateral plate—located progressively further from the midline (Fig. 1.3). The paraxial mesoderm forms the somites from which skeletal muscle develops. Cardiac muscle and smooth muscle develops from splanchnic mesoderm.

Endoderm gives rise to the epithelium of the esophagus and trachea and the airway bronchial and bronchiolar and alveolar lining (Fig. 1.5). The endothelium, vascular smooth muscle, vascular adventitia, vertebral bodies and ribs, sternum, intercostal muscle, diaphragm, and cardiac muscle develop from the mesoderm. From the ectoderm develop the spinal cord, sympathetic nerve chain, intercostal nerves, and neuroendocrine cells. A special contribution is made by the neural crest cells.

PERICARDIUM AND DIAPHRAGM

The cavities of the body, specifically the two pleural cavities, the pericardium and peritoneum, are formed from body wall and from a series of folds and tissue that arise from it (Fig. 1.6). The mesothelium of the parietal lining of the cavities derives from the somatic mesoderm that lines the intraembryonic celomic cavity. It is from the splanchnic mesoderm that the visceral layer of the serous membranes forms.

The diaphragm is the great divide between the thorax and abdomen and represents an interface between different blood and lymphatic arrangements.

The transverse septum, a thick plate of mesoderm, arises at about the 4th week of gestation from the anterolateral abdominal wall and starts the separation of the thorax from the abdomen. The liver bud develops by branching within this septum (Fig. 1.5). Posteromedially, the septum leaves open the large pleuro-pericardio-peritoneal canals (Fig. 1.7).

At its beginning the diaphragm, as septum transversum, lies opposite the cervical somites. Nerves and muscle cells from the third, fourth, and fifth cervical segments enter the septum: the phrenic nerve is formed from these nerves (Fig. 1.7). As the heart descends and the esophagus lengthens, so does the diaphragm. The phrenic nerve passes through the pleuropericardial folds and is localized in the fibrous pericardium. This descent occurs mostly because of rapid growth in the thorax, particularly its dorsal part. By the beginning of the 3rd month, the diaphragm originates from the first lumbar vertebra. Some lower intercostal nerves contribute to the nerve supply of the most peripheral muscular part of the diaphragm.

The parietal pericardium is derived from the body wall (Fig. 1.7). As the lungs in their pleural cavity grow into and along the body wall, the parietal pericardium is separated, and the pericardial fold passes to the midline and fuses behind the heart. Failure of this differentiation occurs most often on the left, causing perhaps a small defect or sometimes a complete absence of the pericardium.

The pleuropericardial folds appear as small ridges in front of the developing lungs as the lung expands

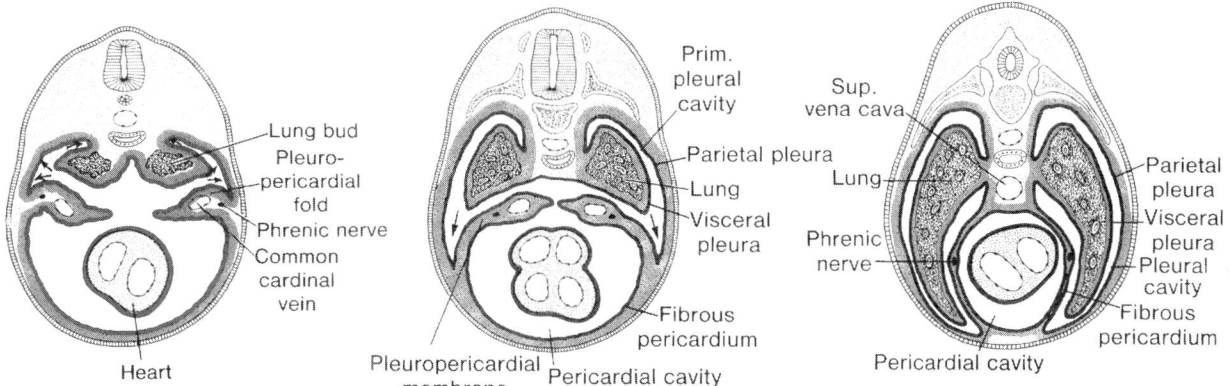

FIGURE 1.6. A. Schematic drawing of a transverse section of embryo (about the 4th week of gestation) to show the growth of the lung buds into the pericardioperitoneal canals. Note the pleuropericardial folds. Note the direction of expansion of the lung buds (*arrows*). B. Schematic drawing showing the transformation of the pericardioperitoneal canals into the pleural cavities and the formation of the pleuropericardial membranes. Note the pleuropericardial membranes with the common cardinal vein and phrenic nerve. The mesenchyme of the body wall is split into the pleuropericardial membranes and the definitive body wall. Note the direction of expansion of the primitive pleural cavity (*arrows*). C. Drawing through the thorax after fusion of the pleuropericardial folds with each other and with the root of the lungs. Note the position of the phrenic nerve, which is now located in the fibrous pericardium. The right common cardinal vein has developed into the superior vena cava. (From Sadler TW. Langman's medical embryology. 6th ed. Baltimore: Williams & Wilkins, 1990:166, 167.)

FIGURE 1.7. Schematic drawings illustrating the development of the diaphragm. **A.** The pleuroperitoneal folds appear at the beginning of the 5th week. They fuse with the septum transversum and the mesentery of the esophagus in the 7th week, thus separating the thoracic cavity from the abdominal cavity. **B.** Transverse section at the 4th month of development. An additional rim derived from the body wall forms the most peripheral part of the diaphragm. (From Sadler TW. Langman's medical embryology. 6th ed. Baltimore: Williams & Wilkins, 1990:168.)

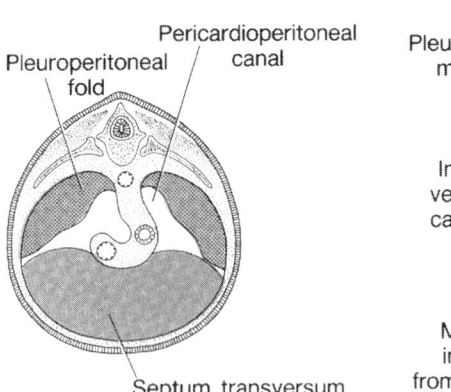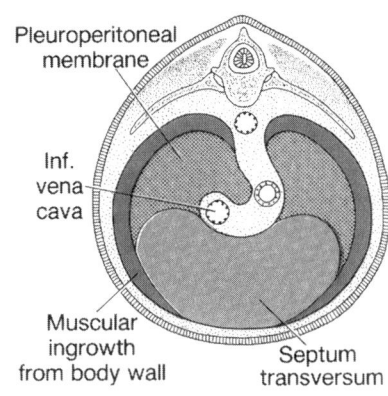

caudally and posteriorly. This fold fuses behind the heart, forming the fibrous pericardium. Mesothelium lines the pericardial sac on both its parietal and visceral surfaces. The visceral, sometimes called epicardium, is closely applied to the myocardium. A pleuroperitoneal fold develops predominantly horizontally from the posterolateral part of the thoracic cage and fuses with the septum transversum. It extends medially and ventrally and by the 7th week fuses with the mesentery of the esophagus and septum transversum. The anterolateral rim of the diaphragm is completed by pleuroperitoneal membranes (Fig. 1.7). Myoblasts pass from the body wall and penetrate the membranes to form the muscular part of the diaphragm. The crura of the diaphragm develop in the mesentery of the esophagus. It is through the space between the crura that the esophagus enters the abdomen.

LUNG GROWTH

There is sufficient change in the lung template, and increase in the number and size of micro units after birth, that childhood disease, or its treatment, often produces significant secondary effects on lung growth and thus on function and reserve (18, 24).

The lungs of the newborn are not adult lungs in miniature, and the premature infant is not the term infant in miniature. Airways, alveoli, and blood vessels dance to a different tune (18, 24–26). For example, whereas all airways of the lung are formed in the first half of intrauterine life (27–30), the alveolar region is virtually a postnatal development. At birth the future alveoli are represented by "saccules" (31–34). The premature lung has its full complement of airways, but not of alveoli.

LAWS OF LUNG DEVELOPMENT

The "program" of intrauterine development, as well as of postnatal development, proceeds by a series of steps or stages that can start or stop quickly and, at different times, focus on multiplication or differentiation of the various structures. For example, airways form before differentiation of alveoli proceeds, but complete fulfillment of the airway multiplication program is not necessary for the switch to alveolar development to occur (18, 24). A signal can be turned off before its part of the program is completed. This fact is important in understanding normal lung growth and its developmental anomalies. The intrauterine developmental timetables for airways, alveoli, and blood vessels are linked, but also are dissociated. The following laws of lung development conveniently summarize the pattern of growth through intrauterine and postnatal development. They also offer a way to determine the critical time that developmental anomalies occur and to predict the long-term effect of certain injuries.

LAW I: AIRWAYS

All airways are present by week 16 of intrauterine life (vide infra) (27–30).

LAW II: ALVEOLI

At birth, the alveoli are represented by primitive saccules (33, 34). There are about 20 million of these in total. Mature alveoli form and multiply, so that by about 8 years of age, 300 million are found, which is within the adult range (33, 35–39). The fastest rate of growth occurs during the 1st year, slows to year 4, and subsequently slows at an even faster rate. There is no agreement regarding the duration and rate of multiplication in these later years, but certainly there is considerable individual variation.

LAW III: BLOOD VESSELS

The development of blood vessels reflects both law I and law II (36, 40–45). The pulmonary artery, which branches with the airways, develops before birth, i.e., all preacinar branches appear as the accompanying airways appear. The intraacinar arteries develop only as alveoli appear, and their density increases in the early years after birth (41, 42, 46, 47). Muscularization lags behind the appearance of new arteries; as a result, relatively larger arteries in the child are more free of muscle than in either the fetus or adult (48).

The lung develops first at about week 4 of intrauterine life, when the trachea forms as a pouch from the foregut. It separates from the esophagus by infolding of the esophageal lateral walls, and divides into right and left main bronchi (Fig. 1.5). These future airway tubes, like the esophagus, are invested with mesenchyme.

The interaction of epithelium and mesenchyme is essential to the branching by each lung bud to form lobar and segmental airways (49), and then to form the more than 25 intrasegmental generations or branches from an axial airway as it passes to alveoli beneath the distal segmental pleural surface (50, 51). The more proximal regions are supplied by shorter pathways with fewer branches.

In cross-section the microscopic appearance of the lung changes during development (24). It is first described as pseudoglandular, a stage that continues until week 16: hollow tubes lined by epithelium branch to produce bronchi and then bronchioli, and the last few generations represent the future alveolar region. Cartilage and submucosal glands now appear in the trachea and bronchi (29, 30).

Between weeks 16 and 24, the lung is in its canalicular stage. In the distal several generations along any airway, the epithelium thins and the future alveolar region is recognizable, although Boyden preferred to call these primitive alveoli, which are present at birth, saccules. Until term, during the saccular stage, increased differentiation occurs, and the number of saccules increases. On average, at birth, a radian across an acinus transects the walls of four or five such saccules. In the 28-week fetus, it would transect only about 2.6 (35, 37, 38).

DISTURBED LUNG GROWTH INCLUDING BRONCHIOLITIS OBLITERANS

Certain antenatal conditions disturb the program of lung development resulting in fewer airway branches than normal (18, 52–58)—such as occurs in idiopathic hypoplasia (59, 60) and aplasia of lung (61). Congenital diaphragmatic hernia, which reduces the intrathoracic space, typically reduces airway number (52, 53), indicating that herniation occurred before the 16th week of intrauterine life. In all infants in a series of fatal cases of rhesus isoimmunization, airway number was reduced, regardless of whether lung volumes were low (62). This finding suggests that the antibody circulates early enough and in a high enough concentration to interfere with airway branching. Reduction in airway number is usually, but not always, associated with impaired alveolar development (18). In Down's syndrome the airway number can be normal or reduced (63, 64). Alveolar number is either normal, reduced, or even increased, i.e., a polyalveolar acinus, illustrating the dissociation of airway from alveoli. The disturbed pattern of alveolar multiplication does not correlate with the airway disturbance.

Both before and after birth, dissociation among the various tissues can be identified. For example, after birth in cases of congenital heart disease with high flow, alveolar development may be appropriate, but the density of the small arteries is too low (65, 66). This interference with growth in congenital heart disease is an important early disturbance of structure and function (48, 65–69) that supplements the original signs of pulmonary vascular obstructive disease (24, 46).

Bronchiolitis obliterans is an example of disturbed growth after birth: the functional effects of airway injury interfere with the postnatal multiplication of the alveoli and appropriate vascularization (70–72). This condition is commonly associated with a hyperlucent lung, such as in McLeod's syndrome (73). Obliteration of the bronchiolus, although permitting distal aeration, is associated with reduced blood flow to the distal lung. The relatively avascular airspaces do not multiply normally. Inspiration is favored by collateral ventilation, which accentuates the reduced blood flow because alveolar wall flow occurs particularly during expiration, not inspiration. The airspaces expand as the thoracic cage expands, becoming abnormally large, i.e., emphysematous; however, the development of blood vessels and subsequent blood flow is reduced. The lung is still aerated because of the phenomenon of collateral ventilation (74, 75). Bronchiolitis obliterans causes an important acquired hypoplasia in which postnatal lung growth has not occurred normally because of the bronchiolar disease.

Bronchiolitis obliterans is important to the oncologist because it is a troubling sequela of airway damage during graft versus host disease following transplantation (76–79). This damage occurs in the immune-suppressed patient, whether the transplant is of heart, lung, or bone marrow.

COMPENSATORY GROWTH

Surgical resection of the lung or a part thereof, or local lung damage such as that caused by radiation, raises questions for the clinician about the nature, at various ages, of compensatory growth in residual lung after such resection or injury. The experimental results reported in the literature seem to conflict: in some instances, after pneumonectomy the residual lung increases its alveolar number in the weeks after resection, although such an increase above control values was not found in other studies. These results can be reconciled if the age at which the pneumonectomy was performed is considered (80–82). If the resection is performed before alveolar multiplication is complete, resection temporarily causes a faster than normal multiplication of alveoli, but the final total number achieved is not above the normal adult total. The faster growth temporarily gives a number above that of age-matched controls, but not above that of adult controls. Lobectomy or pneumonectomy in adults is associated with some adaptive increase in lung mass and surface area, but not with the multiplication of new units.

In one series the behavior of the residual lung, after lobectomy for lobar emphysema, suggested that the larger the amount of lung excised, the greater the stimulus to compensatory adaptation of lung function (83).

INTRATHORACIC STRUCTURES AND CHEST WALL

Lung

LOBAR AND SEGMENTAL ARRANGEMENT

Topographically, each lung is divided into 10 segments, usually arranged in two lobes on the left and three lobes on the right. On each side the lower lobe is caudal to the oblique fissure (84).

The left upper lobe includes three apical segments as well as two (superior and inferior) segments in the lingula, a tonguelike region that dips down over the heart. The left lower lobes include an apical and three basal segments. The right lung is similar except that the two segments analogous to the lingula are distributed in the middle lobe, as medial and lateral lobes. On the right side an additional basal segment, the cardiac, is found medially; it fills the space occupied on the left by the heart. Sometimes, on the left, a corresponding segment is identified. The oblique fissures run from the second thoracic vertebra posteriorly to the diaphragm anteriorly, and the lesser fissure separates the upper from the middle lobe and passes anteriorly from the hilum. Typically, each lobe is surrounded by pleura, which isolates a lobe as an end unit. Often the pleural isolation is incomplete, thus collateral ventilation (see below) can even occur between lobes. A bronchopulmonary segment is a topographical unit as well as a functional one. Resection of a segment can be performed surgically, respecting anatomic boundaries.

AIRWAYS: BRANCHING AND STRUCTURE

Bronchi and bronchioli are defined based on the distribution of cartilage in their walls. Bronchi are airways proximal to the last piece of cartilage along any pathway, and bronchioli are those located distally to this cartilage. In the trachea and main bronchi, cartilage is found only in the anterior and lateral walls, whereas muscle is found only in the posterior wall (28, 29) (sometimes described as membranous). The muscle inserts into the posterior ends of the C-shaped plates of cartilage. As the main bronchus enters the lung, the plates of cartilage approximate posteriorly and surround the whole circumference. The muscle is also rearranged so that it no longer inserts into cartilage but is distributed as a complete muscular coat internal to the cartilage plates. It is arranged as interlacing bands forming a geodesic network (85). Whereas muscle constriction in the trachea does not occlude the lumen, constriction within the lung can completely occlude it. The density of the cartilage is greater in the more proximal airways and sparser in the more peripheral, before finally disappearing. The submucosal glands have a distribution similar to that of the cartilage: in the trachea and large bronchi, they are numerous, and they are not found in bronchioli (28, 30).

The respiratory unit of the lung, the acinus, is about 1 cm^3 in volume. Each is supplied by a terminal bronchiolus (approximately 2 mm in diameter). Acini near the hilum are separated from the trachea by fewer airway branches than those against the diaphragm. Less than 10 generations of airway can reach an acinus near the hilum, whereas upwards of 25 arise along an axial pathway from the segmental hilum to the diaphragm. The lateral pathways supplying the intermediate regions have intermediate numbers of preacinar branchings (27, 29, 51). The terminal bronchiolus has a complete epithelial lining. Beyond the terminal bronchiolus are respiratory bronchioli, part of whose walls are lined by airway epithelium with alveoli arising from other parts. Several generations of respiratory bronchioli branch before alveolar ducts and then alveoli.

The airways are lined by respiratory epithelium—so-called pseudostratified ciliated columnar—in which at least eight cell types can be identified (86, 87). All cells are attached to the basement membrane, and all but two reach the lumen. The ciliated cell, undifferentiated columnar cell, and several types of secretory cell (mucous, serous, and Clara) reach the lumen surface. The basal cell and the Kulchitsky cells do not reach the lumen; the Kulchitsky cells contain neuroendocrine granules containing a variety of bioactive agents, many of which are still "in search of a function."

Including these airway cells, the quota of fixed and migratory cells within the lung is well over 40 (87). Whereas the basal cell once was considered the precursor cell for the rest of the epithelium, it is now apparent that the goblet cell is a universal progenitor for the columnar epithelium. It is known that a serous cell can convert quickly to a mucous or goblet cell. Presumably, with discharge of its secretory granules, the cell can stay a serous cell or develop into a mucous cell, or even a ciliated cell, depending on environmental stimuli. Where there is denudation of epithelium, it may be that the basal cell plays the role of progenitor and multiplies to cover the surface (88–90).

Brush cells are rare and essentially have a structure similar to that seen in the gut (86, 91). The position of the brush cells in relation to the mucociliary escalator suggests that they have an absorptive role in regulating the intraairway liquid. The Kulchitsky cells are part of the disperse neuroendocrine system; they occur singly or in clusters as neuroepithelial bodies. Their innervation is cholinergic, adrenergic, or purinergic fibers, and the products of the cells contribute to the regulation of airway and blood vessel diameter (15).

In the smaller airways, the bronchioli, the mucous cells, and the serous cells are replaced by the Clara cell. The Clara cell secretes surfactant proteins SPA and SPB, in addition to the secretory protein CC10. At this level the Clara cell is thought to be a progenitor of ciliated cells. The Clara cell can quickly transform into a mucous cell. The transformation of a serous or Clara cell to a mucous cell arises from a number of stimuli that include irritation, drugs, and infection (92).

Alveolar cell carcinoma usually arises from the Clara cell. An important feature is the characteristic pattern of growth in which the tumor grows along and lines the alveolar wall. This tumor can be large and involve a great deal of lung with relatively little involvement of central structures or lymph nodes, the hallmark of tumors of similar size arising in large airways. Ultimately, these tumors do metastasize to lymph nodes.

The collecting ducts of the submucosal gland are lined by tall, mitochondria-rich cells (93): from this duct coiled secretory tubules open that, in cross-section, are described as acini. Mucous cells are distributed along the central part of each tubule, whereas serous cells line its distal part. Myoepithelial cells and clear cells of the lymphocyte series are also present in these ducts. Inflammatory mediators and nerve transmitters can empty the ducts without necessarily stimulating the secretory cells.

ALVEOLI: SPACES, LINING, AND INTERSTITIUM

In the lung the diameter of the distal air spaces, i.e., of the alveoli, is more than 250 μm. The alveoli represent such fine subdivisions that the surface available for the exchange of gases is about the size of a singles tennis court. At its thinnest, the blood-gas barrier consists of an epithelial cell lining the alveoli and an endothelial cell lining the capillary, fused through their basement membranes (94, 95). Albumin and immunoglobulins, as well as gases, are transported across these membranes. This blood-gas barrier is part of the capillary circumference; over the rest, the endothelium is separated from the epithelium by an interstitial space that contains extracellular proteoglycan, and in which fibers, notably elastin, collagen, and reticulin, provide a framework that confers strength and form on the lung. Migratory cells and fluid accumulate in this location. The fused basement membrane is sometimes separated by injury, such as occurs in hyperoxia (96).

The alveolar epithelium includes three types of pneumocytes. The type I pneumocyte is a cell that looks like a fried egg—a small nucleus, the "yolk," is surrounded by a spread out and thin cell process, the "white." These cells are only just more than 5%, by number, of the epithelial lining cells, but they cover 95% of the alveolar surface area. Denudation of the alveolar surface follows injury to this cell (97–99).

The type II pneumocyte, making up more than 90% of the population, covers only the small residual area and is regarded as the alveolar progenitor. It produces surfactant lipid and the proteins SPA, SPB, SPC, and SPD, in addition to the components of membrane, complement, and class II proteins of the major histocompatibility complex. The three layers of any of the blood vessels include the endothelium for the intima, the smooth muscle cell or its precursors (the intermediate cell or pericyte) for the media, and the fibroblast for the adventitia (41). The interstitial cells include resident populations of cells, such as fibroblasts, smooth muscle, and myofibroblasts, as well as typically migratory cells, such as lymphocytes, monocytes, and the rarer blood cells. The resident alveolar macrophages are believed to be derived from blood monocytes. Their normal turnover time is 25 days, but injury dramatically increases replication. The macrophage contributes to surfactant catabolism, an essential stage in normal surfactant metabolism.

The type II pneumocyte secretes a compound of lecithin and sphingomyelin that reduces surface tension: it is a "detergent" known as surfactant (101–102). To know how it was discovered makes it easier to understand and to recall its function. The first story is like that of Newton, the apple, and gravity: if it is not true, it well should be. Pattle, during a study of pulmonary edema produced by toxic gases, collected a beaker full of frothy fluid from the lungs of sheep (103). He left the beaker on his desk while attending a committee meeting. Upon his return, he was struck by the stability of the froth. "If that had been beer," he mused, "it would have gone flat. Something is stabilizing those bubbles," he deduced.

The other story is of Mead calculating the work needed to expand the myriad air spaces of the lung during breathing (104). "This demands we all have chest muscles like a wrestler. Something must reduce the surface tension of the alveolar surface." Surfactant, a protein-lipid complex produced mainly by the type II pneumocyte, is the answer to both questions. The infant born prematurely, in whom this system has not yet matured, is at risk of hyaline membrane disease or respiratory distress of the newborn.

The type III pneumocyte is a rare cell whose structure resembles that of the brush cell in the gut or trachea and large airways. Its detailed function is not known (91).

Surfactant

The treatment of tumors in the thorax, either by chemotherapy or radiation, often disturbs the production and function of the surfactant lining. With increased research and understanding of the composition and function of surfactant, its complexity is increasingly apparent (105–108). The final molecular assembly includes lipids and at least three proteins—surfactant apoproteins A, B, and C (109–113). A surfactant effect by apoprotein D has not yet been shown. The type II pneumocyte is responsible for the synthesis of the constituents (111–113). The alveolar macrophage takes part in the intraalveolar space catabolism. The intracellular and extracellular events include synthesis of the constituent molecules, their assembly into the lipid-protein complex, migration, and apical polarization of the final product with secretion, then catabolism or breakdown and, finally, reabsorption (114–120). Recently, an inherited deficiency of surfactant protein B has been identified as a cause of congenital alveolar proteinosis (119).

Cell Types and Tumors

A variety of benign and malignant tumors have been described in the lung. This finding is not surprising because of the large number of fixed and migratory cell types contained in the lung. Saldana (121) has proposed a simple histologic classification of the primary epithelial malignant tumors based on their frequency: (*a*) usual epithelial tumors, 90%—including adenocarcinoma, 40%; squamous cell, 25%; small cell, 15%; and large cell carcinoma, 10%; and (*b*) rare epithelial tumors, 4%—including carcinoid and other neuroendocrine cancers, 3%; bronchiogland tumors, 0.7%; and the papillary tumors of surface epithelium, 0.3%.

Double Blood Supply and Drainage

Important functional interactions occur between the right and left side of the heart within the lung, because of the lung's double arterial supply and a double venous drainage—the pulmonary and bronchial arteries and the pulmonary and true bronchial veins (Fig. 1.8). The arterial and venous distributions do not correspond precisely (122–124).

The pulmonary artery runs with the airways and divides as the airways divide, but it does not supply a capillary bed until it reaches the alveolar region, i.e., within the respiratory region, the acinus beyond the terminal bronchiolus. The pulmonary artery gives rise to 3 to 4 times as many branches as the airway; these branches are of two types—the conventional type, which runs with the airway, and the supernumerary type, which runs a short course to supply the alveoli adjacent to the artery (125, 126). The veins receive two similar types of tributaries.

The pulmonary artery supplies the alveolar region and virtually all of the pleura, except for a small region at the hilum of the airway walls, lymph nodes, and pleura, which are supplied by the bronchial arteries. The bronchial arteries arise from the aorta and join the trachea and main bronchi outside the lung; they run within the wall of the bronchi and supply a capillary bed that lies both internal and external to the cartilage.

The blood from all intrapulmonary structures drains into the pulmonary veins, which receive blood from the airway wall as well as from the alveolar region. The blood that comes from the bronchial artery thus represents a small degree of systemic venous admixture to the pulmonary venous blood as it returns to the left ventricle. The small region around the hilum of the lung drains into the azygos system, that is, to the right side of the heart, through the so-called "true" bronchial veins.

With congestion of the pulmonary veins or an increase in pressure of the left atrium, pressure is transmitted not only to the alveoli but to the intrapulmonary airway walls. Wheezing and airway hypersecretion reflect the secondary congestion of airways. The territory supplied by the bronchial artery includes a watershed: the central part drains to the right atrium, the distal to the left. Pressure differences can result in diversion between these two parts.

The effluent that drains to the azygos vein and thus to the right side of the heart recirculates through the lung before passing into the systemic system. It is a feedback between the large airway and respiratory region. The fact that bronchial products are cleared to the lung suggests pathway of feedback between the central airway walls and the alveolar or respiratory region.

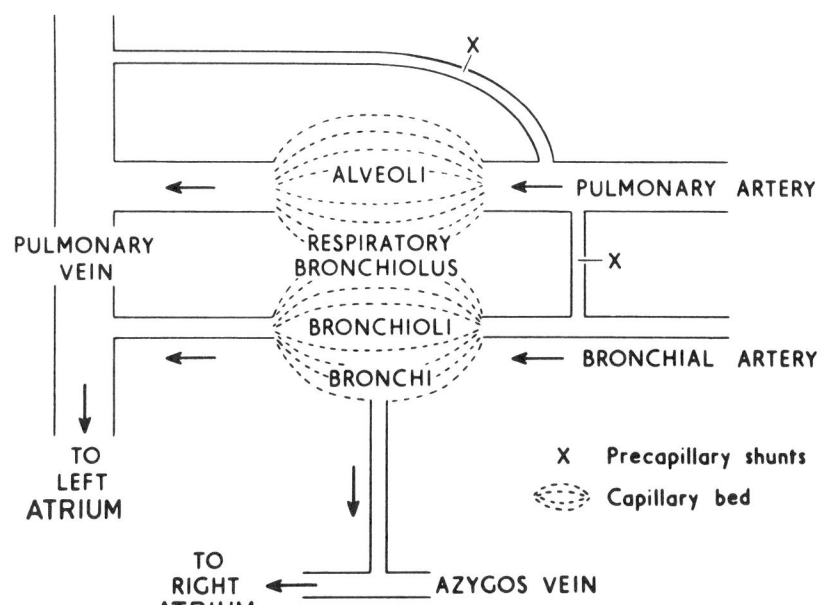

FIGURE 1.8. Diagrammatic representation of the double arterial and venous systems of the lung. The capillary bed of the bronchi and bronchioli is supplied by the bronchial artery; the capillary bed of the respiratory bronchiolus and alveoli is supplied by the pulmonary artery. All intrapulmonary structures drain to the pulmonary veins. Only the bronchi at the hilum drain into the true bronchial veins, to the azygos system. Precapillary shunts, i.e., precapillary in position and size, connect the pulmonary to bronchial artery systems in the airway walls. In the normal, these are structurally present but functionally closed. In many diseases they open. The precapillary anastomoses between the pulmonary artery and vein are not reliably demonstrated. (From Bergofsky HE, ed. Contemporary issues in pulmonary disease: abnormal pulmonary circulation. New York: Churchill Livingstone, 1986;4:223.)

There is another important way in which bronchial and pulmonary arteries interact, i.e., through the presence of so-called precapillary anastomoses between the two arterial systems (123, 127, 128). These are precapillary in position and size, and are present in the wall of the airways. Such anastomoses are found in the normal lung but are functionally closed. If there is occlusion of either of the arterial systems, vessels of the other open to divert blood to the occluded system beyond the block. For example, if the pulmonary artery is blocked, the bronchial artery takes over and supplies the lung distal to the block.

In the presence of inflammation or with the growth of a tumor, bronchial artery flow is increased and, particularly when inflammation involves the airway wall, these anastomoses open. Virtually any pathologic condition affecting the airways leads to an increase in bronchial artery supply. This increase is seen particularly where infection is associated with bronchitis, bronchiolitis, or lung abscess. It explains why, typically, hemoptysis produces bright red blood because such hemorrhage is usually from the bronchial artery. Anastomoses also develop in granulation tissue, such as in the wall of an abscess in which pulmonary artery and bronchial artery systems come together.

Any lesion that impinges on an airway wall or is bigger than the acinus automatically impinges on the bronchial artery vascular bed. The bronchial system is thus stimulated to produce new or increased flow.

The bronchoarterial bundle includes, within the same connective tissue sheath, the airway, with the bronchial artery in its wall, and the pulmonary artery and lymphatics. The pulmonary veins run at the periphery of any unit in the lung; they are at the edge of an acinus, lobule, or segment. Whereas centrally the pulmonary artery runs with the main airway, at the hilum veins leave the lung at a distance above and below the hilum to enter the left atrium. On a chest radiograph, the veins are identified separately from the arteries by their position and direction.

CONNECTIVE TISSUE SEPTA AND COLLATERAL VENTILATION

Connective tissue septa in the various regions of the lung have a widely different distribution (82, 129, 130). They are numerous at the sharp edges of the lung and, at this position, partly subdivide the lung into units, the acini and the lobules. Even in this location no unit is isolated from its neighbor. Thickened connective tissue septa are often identified in the radiograph. This finding is based either on edema of the connective tissue septa or dilation of the lymph channels that run into them: tumor can occupy either the lymphatic lumen or infiltrate the connective tissue. If macrophages containing electron-dense material, such as industrial dust or iron, accumulate in the alveoli adjacent to the septa, the effect is etching of the septa. Macrophages accumulate either centrally in the acinus on their way to the mucociliary escalator and clearance, or at the acinar periphery, sequestered in the peripheral alveoli.

Collateral ventilation is an important function that describes the phenomenon of air drift between alveoli, acini, and even segments; the air passes across the alveolar wall without needing to pass along the main airways (74, 75). This means that an airway can be obstructed, even obliterated, and yet the distal lung that it supplies is still aerated. It is important to remember this fact when interpreting a radiograph or in pathologic examination of lung. Aerated lung does not guarantee that its supplying airway is patent. For example, in McLeod's syndrome (73), the lung, distal to patchy bronchiolitis obliterans, is commonly aerated. Such lung is usually pink, although, if supplied by patent airways, it would contain dust and soot, giving the typical gray or black color of the city dweller's lung (123). An airway can be completely blocked by tumor even with a mucocele distending the airway it subtends, and yet the radiograph may show completely and satisfactorily aerated lung in the region subtended by the blocked bronchus.

The anatomic basis of collateral ventilation is partly provided by the pores of Kohn (131). Located in the alveolar wall, these pores are holes through which air or cells, including macrophages, can migrate or through which transudate or exudate can flow. Another shortcut from the airway to the alveoli is seen in the distal few generations of airways—the so-called bronchoalveolar communications of Lambert (132). These communications are small channels lined by respiratory epithelium that open from small bronchioli into the adjacent alveoli. The drift of air from segment to segment underlines the anatomic fact that the units of the lung, i.e., the acini, lobules, or segments, are not isolated by continuous connective tissue sheets. Where pleura is complete, as is usually the case around a lobe, it creates an end unit. Collateral ventilation does not cross a pleural boundary. Collateral ventilation operates in a newborn lung, but less effectively than in the adult lung.

Collateral ventilation is protective to minimize both collapse or airlessness of lung beyond a block, as well as overinflation or air trapping, such as when a check valve operates within an airway lumen. Inflammatory exudate can block the channels for air drift and render it ineffective. In certain sites in the lung, such as the tip of the lingula and right middle lobe, the relatively large number of septa puts the lung at risk either for blow-up through a check-valve effect or for collapse (133). Inspiration favors collateral air drift, just as collateral air drift favors the inspiratory state. Lung that relies on collateral ventilation for aeration is usually in the inspiratory phase with relative reduction in blood flow—encouraging and perpetuating hypoperfusion as well as a relative increase in the size of the airspaces.

The lymph nodes that lie at the hilum of the right middle lobe have a special clinical importance because of their arrangement in relation to the right middle lobe bronchus and the small number of segments this lobe contains. Enlargement of the lymph nodes at the hilum of the middle lobe easily causes compression of this bronchus (133). The isolation of the two segments within the typically complete pleural sac of the middle lobe means that airway obstruction in this location is more likely to be followed by airlessness than by a similar degree of blockage of two segments in any of the other lobes. Thus, it is the arrangement of lymph nodes and airways at the lobar hilum that determines the frequency of obstruction of this airway; however, it is the isolation of the two segments and the septa within the right middle lobe that determines the frequency with which the lobe becomes airless.

PLEURA AND DIAPHRAGM: STRUCTURE AND BLOOD SUPPLY

The primary nerve supply of the diaphragm is the phrenic; the lower six or seven intercostal nerves contribute to its periphery. The internal mammary artery supplies the diaphragm, pleura, and pericardium. One of its branches, the pericardiophrenic, accompanies the phrenic nerve between the pleura and pericardium to supply the adjacent diaphragm (134). The internal mammary artery arises from the subclavian laterally to the sternum and descends behind the upper six ribs. At the sixth intercostal space, it divides into the musculophrenic and superior epigastric arteries. It is the musculophrenic that passes caudally and laterally behind rib cartilages seven and eight and, like the internal mammary, gives branches to the anterior end of the adjacent intercostal spaces. The phrenic arteries, sometimes called the inferior phrenic, are two small arteries arising from the aorta or celiac axis, or even the nearby renal artery, that supply the adjacent diaphragm.

The posterior part of the chest wall is supplied mainly from aortic branches—the bronchial, esophageal, and intercostal arteries. Branches from these are distributed as parietal, mediastinal, or phrenic. Whereas the intercostal nerve runs along the inferior margin of a rib, the intercostal space has two arteries, a superior and an inferior. The veins and lymphatics have a regional distribution similar to that of the arteries.

Structure of Parietal and Visceral Pleura

The lung surface is covered by visceral pleura, a continuous layer of mesothelium lying on loose connective tissue that contains a layer of elastin following the contour of the lobe. Deep to this lies more loose connective tissue containing lymphatics and vascular capillaries (85). In the subjacent alveolar walls lies another elastin layer that represents the inner margin of the pleura and is part of the alveolar wall. Where a connective tissue septum abuts the pleura, this elastic lamina follows the alveolar wall, the connective tissue of the septum being continuous with that of the pleura (123).

The parietal pleura also is lined by mesothelium, but it has different structural features than the visceral (135). The parietal pleura is interrupted by pores or stomata, several micra in diameter, demarcated by mesothelial cells and opening directly into dilated and terminal lymphatic lacunae, lying close to the pleural surface in loose connective tissue (Fig. 1.9A). The stomata are located particularly in the most mobile portions of the chest wall—close to the sternum, near the vertebral column, and along the retrocardiac pleural folds.

The human visceral pleura is supplied by the pulmonary artery except for a small region—about the size of a hand palm—around the hilum (see Bronchial Artery) (113). The small branch of the pulmonary artery that runs centrally in an acinus continues to the overlying pleura and breaks into an array of capillaries radiating from the central artery like the crown of a palm tree. From the intrapleural capillary bed, venous channels form, providing venous tributaries draining into the periphery of the acinus, and then back centrally into the main pulmonary vein. The veins always lie peripherally in a unit, be it acinus, lobule, or segment. The parietal pleura receives its blood supply from the intercostal circulation.

Esophagus

The esophagus is a foregut derivative. Its three layers can be identified by the 3rd month of gestation (1, 136). The esophagus is lined by stratified squamous epithelium but has submucosal glands. It extends from the pharynx at the level of the larynx to the level at which the tube passes through the diaphragm between its two crura (134). The cricopharyngeus is considered the upper esophageal sphincter. The upper part of the esophagus includes striated and smooth muscle, the lower part only smooth muscle. The lower end is identified as the lower esophageal sphincter, but although it acts functionally in this way, structurally it is not a well-defined sphincter (15, 137).

The upper, mid, and lower third each has a characteristic venous drainage. The upper third drains into the superior vena cava, the middle into the azygos system, and the lower into the portal vein by way of the gastric vein. Thus, in liver disease the varices of portal hypertension affect the lower third of the esophagus.

Esophagitis is a predisposing factor to carcinoma, with a variety of conditions causing irritation and thus esophagitis. Reflux is common with hiatal hernia and achalasia, strictures, and webs, whether they follow an identified cause or are spontaneous (138). Irradiation or chemotherapy often causes esophagitis, particularly when immunosuppression and infection are present. Esophagitis is part of graft versus host disease. Atrophy of esophageal smooth muscle with periesophageal and submucosal fibrosis occurs in scleroderma. The so-called esophageal ring involves the lower part of the esophagus close to the esophagogastric junction. Its cause is unclear, but it consists of a fold whose core includes vascular fibrous tissue, with the upper surface covered by esophageal epithelium and the lower by gastric-type mucosa.

In neonates and older subjects, heterotopic gastric-type mucosa is sometimes identified, usually with patchy distribution, in the upper third of the esophagus. This condition is different from Barrett's esophagitis, which affects the lower end of the esophagus and is associated with reflux (139).

Barrett's esophagitis was long thought to be a developmental anomaly (139–144), but these changes are now considered metaplastic and precancerous, especially for adenocarcinoma. Barrett's esophagitis refers to replacement of the normal stratified squamous epithelium of the lower esophagus by columnar epithelium, either in patchy or diffuse distribution. When diffuse, its upper edge is usually an ulcerated, inflamed region of stratified epithelium. The metaplastic columnar epithelium is identified as gastric when chief or parietal cells are present, or as intestinal by the presence of Paneth cells. Correction of the reflux is reported to be associated with reversal.

Approximately 90% of esophageal carcinomas are squamous cell in type; about 5% are adenocarcinomas. The submucosal glands as well as Barrett's metaplastic epithelium are the source of the latter. Given the lymph and venous drainage of the esophagus, it is not surprising that the liver and lung are the common sites of metastasis from its tumors.

Thymus

The thymus is a lymphoepithelial organ derived bilaterally in the neck from the third pharyngeal pouch and groove (1, 12, 137, 145); it contains both endodermal and ectodermal derivatives. Its bilateral origin is reflected in its two lobes connected by an isthmus across the midline. The dorsal wing of the third pouch gives rise to the inferior parathyroid gland, and the ventral, to the thymus. Sometimes the

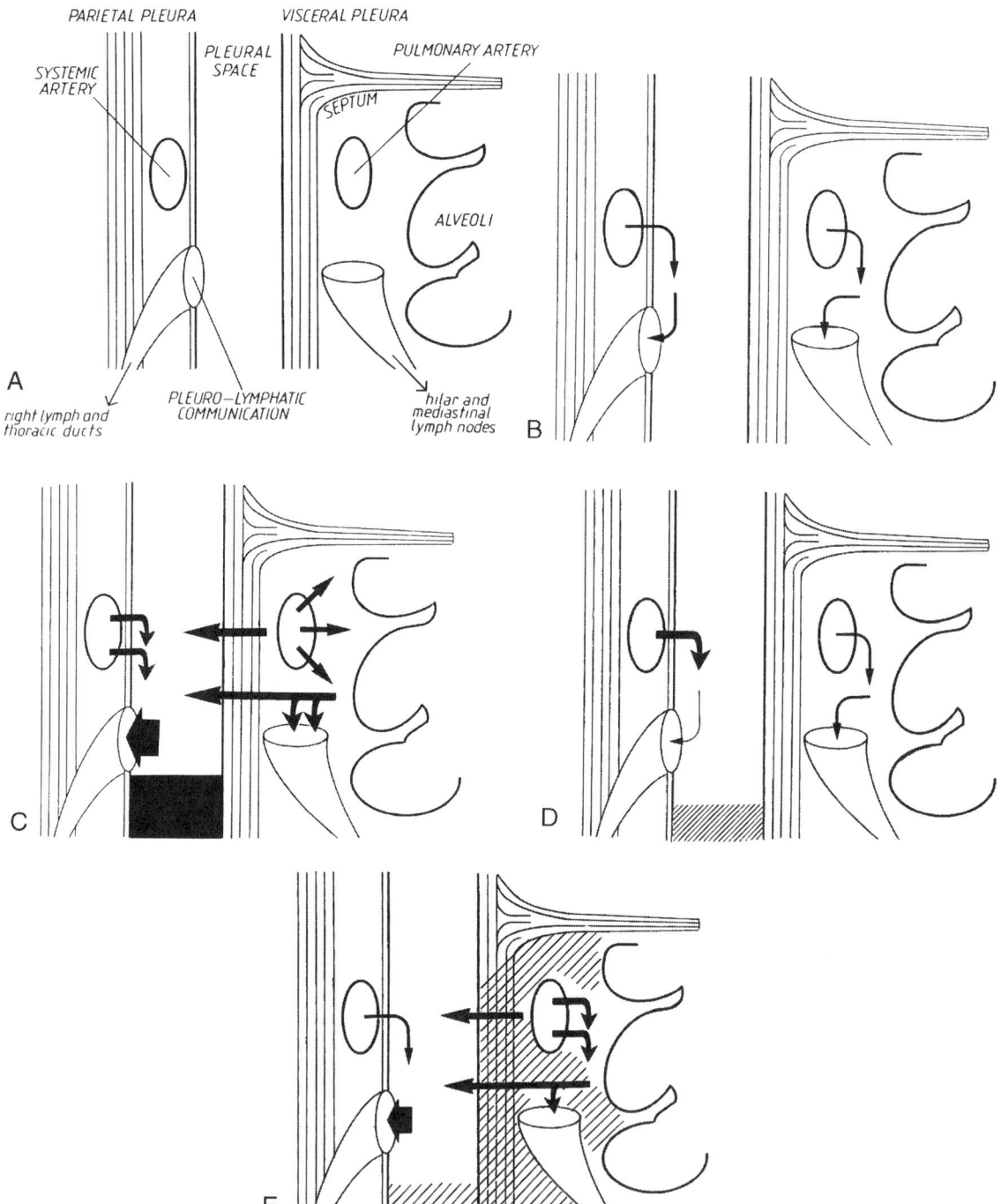

FIGURE 1.9. **A.** Schematic representation of the anatomic features of the pleura relevant to liquid and solute exchange. **B.** Schematic representation of pleural liquid and solute exchange under physiologic conditions. Note the filtration or absorption (*curved arrows*) according to their direction. **C.** Schematic representation of the mechanisms of pleural effusion in the course of diseases primarily affecting the permeability of the pleura and its microcirculation. Liquid and protein leak from the microvessels supplying the visceral and parietal pleura and enter the pleural space through damaged pleural membranes (*thick straight arrow* and *curved arrows*). The marked increase in lymphatic outflow (*large arrowhead*) is exceeded by liquid inflow; a pleural effusion with the characteristics of an exudate develops (*dark area*) in the pleural space. The pleural effusion is larger whenever lymphatics are involved in the pathologic process. **D.** Schematic representation of the mechanisms of pleural effusion in the course of systemic venous hypertension. Increased systemic venous pressure can cause increased filtration from parietal pleural microvessels (*thick curved arrow*), which drain into the right atrium and hinder reabsorption from the parietal pleural lymphatics (*thin curved arrow*) that drain into the neck veins. A pleural effusion with the characteristics of a transudate can develop, especially in conditions of acute elevation of systemic venous pressure. Chronic adaptation of the lymphatics can reduce or prevent the effusion. **E.** Schematic representation of the mechanisms of pleural effusion in the course of pulmonary venous hypertension. Subpleural interstitial edema liquid leaks directly into the pleural space (*thick straight arrows*). Under these circumstances hyperventilation hastens lymph flow from the pleura (*large arrowhead*). Pleural effusion with the characteristics of a transudate (*hatched area*) can develop, especially in conditions of acute elevation of pulmonary venous pressure. Chronic adaptation of the lymphatics can reduce or prevent the effusion. (From Potchen EJ, Grainger RG, Greene R, eds. Pulmonary radiology: the Fleischner Society. Philadelphia: WB Saunders, 1993:152.)

fourth pair of parathyroid glands is found within the thymus and descends with it to its final location in the anterior mediastinum.

The thymic cortex consists mainly of immature T lymphocytes that express terminal deoxynucleotidyl transferase (Tdt) and OKT6 and OKT10 antigens. The medulla contains T lymphocytes, which in this microenvironment develop into mature T lymphocytes; with this phenotype they are released into the peripheral circulation. This maturation is brought about by secreted humoral factors such as thymosin, thymin, and thymopoietin. Also in the medulla are concentric aggregates of keratinized epithelial cells, the Hassall's corpuscles, as well as macrophages, neuroendocrine cells, and myoid cells. The latter three have ultrastructural and antigenic similarities to skeletal muscle. It is intriguing to assume a link between these cells and the skeletal muscle dysfunction of myasthenia gravis to which thymic dysfunction contributes.

The normal thymus rarely includes lymphoid follicles with germinal centers. Their presence is a marker of thymic hyperplasia, a common accompaniment of myasthenia gravis and usual in a number of autoimmune disorders. Congenital thymic aplasia or hypoplasia is associated with a variety of immunodeficiency states: reticular dysgenesis, combined immunodeficiency disease, ataxia-telangiectasia, and DiGeorge or Nezelof syndromes. In all these disorders, there are severe T-cell and variable B-cell defects.

At birth the thymus weighs 10 to 35 g, increasing in size until puberty, when it may weigh up to 50 g. Thereafter it undergoes progressive age-involution and is replaced by fatty tissue. Involution is sometimes produced suddenly by severe stress, steroid therapy, malnutrition, or irradiation. The result is cytolysis and fibrosis.

Among the neoplastic conditions to involve the thymus are thymomas, thymolipomas, carcinoid tumors, germ cell tumors, lymphomas, leukemias, and vascular tumors. Most thymomas are benign: it is the epithelial component that is neoplastic, not the lymphocytes. (For further discussion of thymomas, see Chapter 29, and for mediastinal germ cell tumors, Chapter 31.) Thymolipomas are uncommon; they grow to be quite large and are composed of thymic tissue embedded in mature adipose tissue. Carcinoid tumors of the thymus are rare, arising from thymic neuroendocrine cells; because of active secretion they are sometimes associated with Cushing's syndrome.

CHROMAFFIN SYSTEM: PARAGANGLIA INCLUDING THE SYMPATHETIC CHAIN

Paraganglia refer to the chromaffin cells of the adrenal medulla and carotid body, and in the thorax to the clumps of these cells associated with the parasympathetic nervous system (15, 134, 145). The primitive neuroectoderm (neural crest) differentiates to form these paravertebral paraganglia. Because these cells are able to take up and decarboxylate simple amine precursors such as dihydroxyphenylalanine (DOPA) and 5-dihydroxytryptamine (5-HT) to form biogenic amines, they were described as part of an amine precursor uptake and decarboxylation (APUD) system (146, 147). It is now recognized that these cells make neurotransmitters and peptide hormones, thus they are now labeled neuroendocrine cells. Not all are derived from the neural crest. This cell type is scattered throughout many organs in collections described as the dispersed neuroendocrine system. All contain neuron specific enolase, chromogranin, a part of the granule structure, and synaptophysin, a membrane component of presynaptic vesicles, that serve as immunohistochemical markers. An ultrastructural marker is a cytoplasmic electron-dense granule bound by a single membrane. Epinephrine and norepinephrine are the most common neurotransmitters in this granule, and their chief metabolites are metanephrine, normetanephrine, vanillylmandelic acid (VMA), and homo-vanillic acid (HVA). Any of these metabolites may be produced by tumors arising from these cells.

A range of tumors arise from this tissue, differing in their degree of differentiation. Neuroblastoma, the least differentiated, is one of the most common solid tumors of childhood. The paravertebral sympathetic chain in the posterior mediastinum is the second most common site of their origin: they are most common intraabdominally arising from the adrenal medulla or the retroperitoneal collections of cells. Partly differentiated tumors are termed ganglioneuroblastomas, and completely differentiated tumors, ganglioneuromas (see Chapter 32) (148–150). A behavior unique to this group is that as tumor differentiates from malignant or immature to the mature histologic type, i.e., from neuroblastoma to ganglioneuroma, it transforms from a malignant to a benign tumor. This progressive differentiation is a feature unique to this system. Genetic abnormalities are associated with this differentiation. It seems that a chromosomal abnormality is found on the short arm of chromosome 1. When this abnormality is associated with amplification of N-*myc*, the prognosis and subsequent behavior follow the malignant pattern.

HEART AND PERICARDIUM

The neural crest cells are uniquely important to the development of the heart and great vessels (11, 13, 14, 151–155). Whereas the heart is a common site for metastases, particularly to the pericardium—tumors from the lung, breast, and gastrointestinal tract being the most common source—it is rarely the site of primary tumors, although these do affect the myocardium, pericardium, or endocardium.

About 80% of primary cardiac tumors are benign, and half of these are myxomas (156–158). Of these, 90% arise in the atrium and 80% of these on the left side, where the common origin is the fossa ovalis. This tumor is found even in infants. In the past the view that this tumor was an organized thrombus was favored. The general consensus is that it is a benign neoplasm originating from primitive mesenchyme.

The special embryonic properties of the cardiac endothelial cell and its infra layer of cardiac jelly at these sites suggests a link to histogenesis. It is the combination of the endothelium and the cardiac jelly that is responsible for a special feature of cardiac development—the endocardial cushions from which the heart valves and the large central arteries develop. Production of an extracellular matrix as well as cell proliferation are important in the formation of valve cusps and the membranous portion of the atrial and ventricular septa. The two sites at which endothelial cushions are present are the atrioventricular and the trunco-conal region. The cells populating the latter are of neural crest origin. Constitutional symptoms are common with this tumor. Myxomas sometimes present dramatically because of fever: they evidently elaborate a pyrogenic cytokine that has recently been identified as interleukin 6 (159, 160).

Rhabdomyomas are rare but are the most common cardiac tumor seen in infants. They are often seen with tuberous sclerosis, suggesting they are phakomas or malformations.

The rarer mesothelioma arises particularly from the interatrial septum, at the site of the atrioventricular node. In this site it is more likely that cells are endodermal in origin, rather than mesodermal like the pleural or pericardial tumors of the same name.

The heart is susceptible to drug damage, and cardiomyopathy occurs as a complication of treatment, particularly after doxorubicin therapy. The reason for its interaction with the contractile cells of the heart is not clear.

Approximately 150 million milliliters of blood can suffice to cause death from tamponade if it accumulates rapidly in the pericardium. However, many times this amount of fluid can be relatively asymptomatic if it accumulates slowly and includes cytokines and mediators of inflammation that allow an increase in compliance without an increase in intrapericardial pressure to embarrass cardiac function.

CELL MARKERS

With new molecular biology techniques, it is possible to detect in many tumor cells markers that indicate their cell of origin, although morphologically they look very different from their origin (161). Cells can be identified either by their products, secreted or within granules, or by their cell or surface markers. For example, the macrophage has as its products lysozyme or α-1 antitrypsin; the eosinophil, granule content; the fibroblast, intracellular procollagen; the mesothelial cell, cytokeratin; the Clara cell, intracellular CC10, a 10Kd protein; the endothelial cell, factor VIII; migrating cells such as lymphocytes of thymic origin; the surface markers CD4 and CD8; and the smooth, cardiac, and skeletal muscles, myosin of the isoform appropriate to each.

PLEURAL FLUID FORMATION AND LYMPHATIC CIRCULATION

NORMAL PLEURAL FLUID

It is increasingly clear that normally the parietal pleura is the site of the formation of pleural fluid and of its absorption. The "circulation" of normal pleural fluid depends on the parietal pleura through its pores or stomata (135, 162, 163) (Fig. 1.9A). This conclusion is a major change in the long-held dogma that the lung makes a major contribution to normal pleural fluid formation (164–167). This theory of parietal pleural function reflects studies of Courtice and his colleagues (20, 21, 163), their first studies being reported just over 40 years ago.

Differences in the structure of the parietal and visceral pleura are important to the homeostatic mechanisms that operate normally and are key to the understanding of response in disease (Figs. 1.9A through E). It is also the parietal pleura that is responsible for the clearance of particulate matter, including red cells and large molecules, from the pleural space. Dyed proteins or particulate matter injected into the pleural space stain the parictal pleural lymphatics intensely, although no trace of the marker is demonstrated in the lymphatics of the visceral pleura (168). Cells such as erythrocytes introduced into the pleural space are recovered in the blood stream. Stoma that are several micra in diameter increase up to 10 times that diameter on respiration.

Pleural fluid is produced from systemic microvessels. It is the interstitial liquid of the parietal pleura that is filtered from microvessels according to hydrostatic and colloid osmotic gradients described by Starling's model. The fluid, if excessive, is absorbed into the chest wall through the parietal pleural stomata. For a given hydrostatic pressure, the accumulated volume of pleural liquid is greater during isolated systemic hypertension than during isolated pulmonary venous hypertension (Fig. 1.9B). A pleural effusion represents either a transudate, such as when there is an imbalance of the hydrostatic forces, or an exudate, when leakage of liquid and proteins occurs from a change in the permeability of the pleura (Fig. 1.9C). Obstructed lymphatic drainage centrally modifies pleural behavior (164). Peritoneal liquid transfers to the thorax via pores and transdiaphragmatic lymphatic channels (169).

LYMPHATIC DRAINAGE

THE LUNG

The lung is concerned with the intrapulmonary balance of the fluid produced in the lung and absorbed or drained through its lymphatics. Under conditions of lung disease with inflammation and exudation, permeability through the visceral pleura is increased, and the lung becomes a source of pleural fluid. The parietal pleura is still significant for its absorption. Lung circulation, in addition to the double arterial supply and venous drainage, includes the lymphatic system. The lung includes two main sets of lymphatics, the superficial or pleural, and the deep or central (170, 171). The superficial or subpleural set drains the outer rim of the lung, primarily following the lung's contour to reach the hilar lymph nodes. These lie internally to the external elastic pleural lamina. The deep lymphatics radiate to the hilum, and drainage in them is directed to the hilum.

The alveolar spaces are free of lymphatic channels. The smallest appear centrally in the acinus in the region of the terminal and respiratory bronchioli. These channels also appear at the periphery of the acinus; where connective tissue septa are present, the lymphatics run in these structures (172). These are the basis of the Kerley B lines seen on radiographs. This lymphatic system in the peribronchoarterial bundle, and in the perivenous sheath and connective tissue septa, represents the broad anatomic pattern of drainage. The lymphatics, like the veins, receive drainage from adjacent regions of adjacent units: the lymphatics are not confined to a single unit, be it acinus or segment. Occasional large channels arise near the periphery of a lobe and, by a meandering path, pass through to the hilum. These are the basis of Kerley C lines seen on radiographs.

The arterial supply and venous drainage represent directed flow, although within the capillary bed, flow is often slow, even sluggish, and retrograde flow occurs. The lymphatic system represents lower pressure and slower flow with meandering channels that accept a higher protein than the tissue fluid, which under normal conditions returns to capillaries. The geographic catchment is represented by a group of lymphatics and does not correspond precisely to that of an artery or vein. Because of this and the slower flow, there is an opportunity for the mixing of fluid and cells, be they migratory or tumor. The intrathoracic organs share extracellular tissue fluid through lymphatic ebb and flow. The slow flow of the intercommunicating channels connects the intrathoracic channels to the cervical, abdominal, and peritoneal cavities.

The lung is a metabolic organ that filters the blood that drains from the rest of the body. It has a special relation to the gut in that the lacteals, the term given to gut lymphatics, bypass the liver, enter the thoracic duct and azygos vein, and thus proceed to the pulmonary artery and lung. The presence of fat in gut lymph probably accounts for fat increases in lung macrophages under certain conditions, such as airway obstruction with stasis. The pulmonary artery and capillary bed represent the first relay station for gut drainage. In liver disease the failure of the liver to detoxify also means that blood returning from the portal system to the lung needs additional metabolic treatment.

COLLECTION OF LYMPHOCYTES

The lymph nodes within the thoracic cavity are described below. Hilar lymph nodes, i.e., those around the main airways, are still intrapulmonary and lie within the connective tissue sheath of the large bronchi. Within the lung, lymphocytes are seen as poorly organized collections in the alveolar region, connective tissue septa, and airway wall. Bronchial-associated lymphoid tissue (BALT) is the name given to the collections of lymphocytes often seen in a bronchial wall, but not defined by a capsule. The number of such cell collections increases with age (173–175).

A distinction is made between the connective tissue sheaths that always surround lymphatics, veins, or airways of moderate or large size and connective tissue septa. Connective tissue septa are flat sheets of connective tissue of limited distribution. A septum, when present, provides demarcation of acini and includes the veins and lymphatics that run in this position. The lymphatics and veins are present, however, at sites where connective tissue septa, i.e., flat sheets of connective tissue, are not seen; at these points the connective tissue sheath is circumscribed.

There are three primary groups of mediastinal nodes: (*a*) the right paratracheal, (*b*) the aortopulmonary, and (*c*) the subcarinal. Their importance is that the subcarinal nodes receive drainage particularly from the lower lobes, and that the left lobe often drains to the right via these nodes. The importance of this left to right flow, particularly in the pericarinal region, means that lymph nodes in the right paratracheal or cervical group do not necessarily indicate a right-sided tumor, because in many subjects left lower lobe drainage commonly crosses the pleura.

TNM (tumor, node, and metastasis) cancer staging indicates that the right paratracheal nodes are those most often apparent radiographically. This visualization results partly because the left group is harder to see. CT scanning shows that the left paratracheal nodes are enlarged less often. The so-called aortopulmonary nodes are actually found in the fat pad laterally to the aorta, and lie between the left pulmonary artery and aorta, and the right pulmonary artery.

The development of pleural effusion, perhaps with adhesions and spread of metastases to the thoracic wall, means that chest wall lymphatics can also be implicated.

There are four other important groups of nodes: (*a*) the intercostal nodes, which lie close to the vertebral bodies and are small; and (*b*) the internal mammary nodes, which lie near the edge of the sternum at the anterior extremity of each rib and follow the line of the internal mammary artery (and are continuous with the cervical and abdominal systems). The lymphatics lie in the intercostal space rather than with the intercostal vessels and drain mainly to the thoracic duct. The internal mammary lymphatics are joined by the anterior end of the intercostal channels. On the right they ultimately drain into the right lymphatic duct and on the left, into the thoracic duct. The internal mammary lymphatics communicate with the epigastric lymphatics. (*c*) The anterior and (*d*) posterior mediastinal nodes lie in the loose areolar tissue of the mediastinum. The anterior group includes those that lie against the diaphragm in front of the pericardium. The posterior mediastinal group includes those lying around the great vessels at the base of the heart. These connect easily so that thoracic lymph mixes with cervical and lumbar lymph, both through lymphatics and lymph nodes as well as through openings in the diaphragm.

Secretions of the airways and bronchoalveolar lavage are important in the search for tumor cells as a screening procedure for lung cancer. In such cases a tumor may not be visible within the bronchoscopic field (176).

OTHER ORGANS

PERICARDIUM

Two sets of lymphatics, the superficial or parietal pericardium, as well as the visceral lymphatics that drain the deep tissues of the heart, are identified here. The latter drain with the coronary vessels to the root of the aorta. Both systems join the cardiac glands and pass particularly into the right lymphatic duct (134).

THYMUS

The lymphatics from the thymus are typically paired and arise from the posterior or deep surface. These vessels pass to the superior mediastinum and join the right lymphatic duct and thoracic duct (134).

ESOPHAGUS

The esophagus is well supplied with lymphatics: the upper third drains into cervical lymph nodes; the middle to the mediastinum, into the paratracheal and carinal lymph nodes; and the lower third to below the diaphragm into gastric and celiac nodes (15).

REFERENCES

1. Sadler TW. Langman's medical embryology. 6th ed. Baltimore: Williams & Wilkins, 1990.
2. Edelman GM, Jones FS. Outside and downstream of the homeobox. J Biol Chem 1993;20683–20686.
3. Redline RW, Neish A, Holmes LB, Collins T. Biology of disease. Lab Invest 1992;66:659–670.
4. Wewer UM, Mercurio AM, Chung SY, Albrechtsen R. Deoxyribonucleic-binding homeobox proteins are augmented in human cancer. Lab Invest 1990;63:447–454.
5. Kirby ML, Bockman DE. Neural crest and normal development: a new perspective. Anat Rec 1984;209(Suppl 1):1–6.
6. Bockman DE, Redmond ME, Kirby ML. Altered development of pharyngeal arch vessels after neural crest ablation. Ann N Y Acad Sci 1990;588:296–304.
7. Sulik AA. Dr. Beverly R. Rollnick memorial lecture. Normal and abnormal craniofacial embryogenesis. Birth defects: Original Article Series, 1990;26(Suppl 3):1–18.
8. Miyagawa-Tomita S, Waldo K, Tomita H, Kirby ML. Temporospatial study of the migration and distribution of cardiac neural crest in quail-chick chimeras. Am J Anat 1991;192(Suppl 1):79–88.
9. Kuratani SC, Kirby ML. Initial migration and distribution of the cardiac neural crest in the avian embryo: an introduction to the concept of the circumpharyngeal crest. Am J Anat 1991;191(Suppl 3):215–227.
10. Kuratani SC, Miyagawa-Tomita S, Kirby ML. Development of cranial nerves in the chick embryo with special reference of the alterations of cardiac branches after ablation of the cardiac neural crest. Anat Embryol (Berl) 1991;183(Suppl 5):501–514.
11. Kirby ML. Overview of problems and approaches in heart development. Ann N Y Acad Sci 1990;588:1–7.

12. Bockman DE, Kirby ML. Neural crest function in thymus development. Immunol Ser 1989;45:451–467.
13. Waldo KL, Kirby ML. Cardiac neural crest contribution to the pulmonary artery and sixth aortic arch artery complex in chick embryos aged 6 to 18 days. Anat Rec 1993;237:385–399.
14. Waldo KL, Kumiski DH, Kirby ML. Association of the cardiac neural crest with development of the coronary arteries in the chick embryo. Anat Rec 1994;239:315–31.
15. Rubin E, Farber JL, eds. Pathology. 1st ed. Philadelphia: JB Lippincott, 1988.
16. Majno G, Joris I. Apoptosis, oncosis and necrosis: an overview of cell death. Am J Pathol 1995;146:3–15.
17. Hockenbery D. Defining apoptosis. Am J Pathol 1995;146:16–19.
18. Reid LM. The lung: its growth and remodeling in health and disease. Edward B. D. Neuhauser lecture. AJR Am J Roentgenol 1977;129:777–788.
19. Boyden EA. The developing bronchial arteries in a fetus of the 12th week. Am J Anat 1970;129(a):357–368.
20. Yoffey JM, Courtice FC. Lymphatics, lymph and the lymphomyeloid complex. London: Academic Press, 1970.
21. Courtice FC. Milestones in lymphology. Lymphology 1989;22:154–156.
22. Noden DM. Embryonic origins and assembly of blood vessels. Am Rev Respir Dis 1989;140:1097–1103.
23. Sawyer D, Galvin N, Lagunoff D, deMello, DE. Fetal development of pulmonary vasculature in the mouse (abstract). Mod Pathol 1994;7(Suppl 1):9P,47.
24. deMello DE, Davies P, Reid LM. Lung growth and development. In: Simmons D, ed. Current pulmonology. Chicago: Year Book Medical Publishers, 1989;10:159–208.
25. Hislop A, Reid L. Formation of the pulmonary vasculature. In: Hodson WA, ed. Development of the lung. In: Lenfant C, exec ed. Lung biology in health and disease. New York: Marcel Dekker, 1977;6:37–86.
26. Hislop A, Reid L. Growth and development of the respiratory system: anatomical development. In: Davis JA, Dobbing J, eds. Scientific foundations of paediatrics. 2nd ed. London: Heinemann Medical Publications, 1981:390–431.
27. Hayward J, Reid L. Observations on the anatomy of the intrasegmental-bronchial tree. Thorax 1952;7:89–97.
28. Hayward J, Reid L. The cartilage of the intrapulmonary bronchi in normal lungs, in bronchiectasis, and in massive collapse. Thorax 1952;7:98–110.
29. Bucher UG, Reid L. Development of the intrasegmental bronchial tree: the pattern of branching and development of cartilage at various stages of intra-uterine life. Thorax 1961;16:207–218.
30. Bucher UG, Reid L. Development of the mucus-secreting elements in human lung. Thorax 1961;16:219–225.
31. Dunnill MS. Postnatal growth of the lung. Thorax 1962;17:329.
32. Davies G, Reid L. Growth of the alveoli and pulmonary arteries in childhood. Thorax 1970;25:669–681.
33. Hislop A, Reid L. Development of the acinus in the human lung. Thorax 1974;29:90–94.
34. Boyden EA. The mode of origin of pulmonary acini and respiratory bronchioles in the fetal lung. Am J Anat 1974;141:317–328.
35. Emery JL, Mithal A. The number of alveoli in the terminal respiratory unit of man during late intrauterine life and childhood. Arch Dis Child 1960;35:544–547.
36. Davies GM, Reid L. Growth of the alveoli and pulmonary arteries in childhood. Thorax 1970;25:669–681.
37. Cooney TP, Thurlbeck WM. The radial alveolar count method of Emery and Mithal: a reappraisal 1—postnatal lung growth. Thorax 1982;37:572–579.
38. Cooney TP, Thurlbeck WM. The radial alveolar count method of Emery and Mithal: a reappraisal 2—intrauterine and early postnatal lung growth. Thorax 1982;37:580–583.
39. Wigglesworth JS, Desai R. Use of DNA estimation for growth assessment in normal and hypoplastic fetal lungs. Arch Dis Child 1981;56:601–605.
40. Reid LM. Structural remodelling of the pulmonary vasculature by environmental change and disease. In: Wagner WW, Weir EK, eds. The pulmonary circulation and gas exchange. Armonk, NY: Futura, 1994;77–110.
41. Reid L. The pulmonary circulation: remodeling in growth and disease. The 1978 J. Burns Amberson lecture. Am Rev Respir Dis 1979;119:531–546.
42. deMello DE, Reid LM. Respiratory tract and lungs. In: Reed G, Claireaux AE, Cockburn F, eds. Diseases of fetus and newborn, pathology, imaging, genetics and management. 2nd ed. London: Chapman & Hall, 1995:I:523–560.
43. Hislop A, Reid L. Intrapulmonary arterial development during fetal life: branching pattern and structure. J Anat 1972;113:35–48.
44. Davies P, deMello D, Reid L. Structural methods in the study of development of the lung. In: Gil J, ed. Models of lung disease: microscopy and structural methods. In: Lenfant C, exec ed, Lung biology in health and disease. New York: Marcel Dekker, 1990; 47:409–472.
45. Davies P, deMello D, Reid L. Methods in experimental pathology of pulmonary vasculature. In: Gil J, ed. Models of lung disease: microscopy and structural methods. In: Lenfant C, exec ed. Lung biology in health and disease. New York: Marcel Dekker, 1990;47:843–904.
46. Rabinovitch M, Reid L. Quantitative structural analysis of the pulmonary vascular bed in congenital heart defects. Cardiovasc Clin Pediatr Cardiovasc Dis 1980;11:149–169.
47. Meyrick B, Reid L. Pulmonary arterial and alveolar development in normal postnatal rat lung. Am Rev Respir Dis 1982;125:468–473.
48. Hislop A, Reid L. Pulmonary arterial development during childhood: branching pattern and structure. Thorax 1973;28(a): 129–135.
49. Alescio T. Effect of a proline analogue, azatadine-2-carboxylic acid, on the morphogenesis in vitro of mouse embryonic lung. J Embryol Exper Morphol 1973;29:439–451.
50. Reid L. The secondary lobule in the adult human lung, with special reference to its appearance in bronchograms. Thorax 1958;13:110–114.
51. Reid L, Simon G. The peripheral pattern in the normal bronchogram and its relation to peripheral pulmonary anatomy. Thorax 1958;13:103–109.
52. Areechon W, Reid L. Hypoplasia of lung with congenital diaphragmatic hernia. Br Med J 1963;I:230–233.
53. Kitagawa M, Hislop A, Boyden EA, Reid L. Lung hypoplasia in congenital diaphragmatic hernia. A quantitative study of airway, artery, and alveolar development. Br J Surg 1971;58:342–346.
54. deMello DE, Reid L. Patterns of disturbed lung growth in newborns with skeletal dysplasia (abstract). Mod Pathol 1990;3 (Suppl 1):2P.
55. Sanford W, deMello D, Reid L. Patterns of pulmonary arterial growth in hypoplastic lungs of skeletal dysplasia (abstract 44). J Lab Invest 1993;68(Suppl 1):8P.

56. Shapiro JR, Burn JE, Chipman SD, et al. Pulmonary hypoplasia and osteogenesis imperfecta type II with defective synthesis of alpha-1 I pro-collagen. Bone 1989;10:165–179.
57. Williams AJ, Vawter G, Reid L. Lung structure in asphyxiating thoracic dystrophy. Arch Pathol Lab Med 1984;108:658–661.
58. Goldstein JD, Reid L. Pulmonary hypoplasia resulting from phrenic nerve agenesis and diaphragmatic amyoplasia. J Pediatr 1980;97:282–287.
59. Thibeault DW, Beatty EC, Hall RT, et al. Neonatal pulmonary hypoplasia with premature rupture of fetal membranes and oligohydramnios. J Pediatr 1985;107:273–277.
60. Askenazi SS, Perlman M. Pulmonary hypoplasia: lung weight and radial alveolar count as criteria of diagnosis. Arch Dis Child 1979;54:614–618.
61. Ryland D, Reid L. Pulmonary aplasia—a quantitative analysis of the development of the single lung. Thorax 1971;26:602–609.
62. Chamberlain D, Hislop A, Hey E, Reid L. Pulmonary hypoplasia in babies with severe rhesus isoimmunization: a quantitative study. J Pathol 1977;122:43–52.
63. Schloo BL, Vawter F, Reid L. Down syndrome: patterns of disturbed lung growth. Hum Pathol 1991;22:919–923.
64. Kirby ML. Neural crest and the morphogenesis of Down syndrome with special emphasis on cardiovascular development. Prog Clin Biol Res 1991;373:215–225.
65. Rabinovitch M, Castaneda A, Reid L. Lung biopsy with frozen section as a diagnostic aid in patients with congenital heart defects. Am J Cardiol 1981;47:77–84.
66. Fried R, Falkovsky G, Newburger J, Gorchakova AI, Rabinovitch M, Gordonova MI, Fyler D, et al. Pulmonary arterial changes in patients with ventricular septal defects and severe pulmonary hypertension. Pediatr Cardiol 1986;7:147–154.
67. Haworth SG, Sauer U, Buhlmeyer K, Reid L. Development of the pulmonary circulation in ventricular septal defect: a quantitative structural study. Am J Cardiol 1977;40:781–788.
68. Rabinovitch M, Herrera-deLeon V, Castaneda AR, Reid L. Growth and development of the pulmonary vascular bed in patients with tetralogy of Fallot with or without pulmonary atresia. Circulation 1981;64:1234–1249.
69. Rabinovitch M, Keane JF, Fellows KE, et al. Quantitative analysis of the pulmonary wedge angiogram in congenital heart defects: correlation with hemodynamic data and morphometric findings in lung biopsy tissue. Circulation 1981;63:152–164.
70. Reid L, Simon G. Unilateral lung transradiancy. Thorax 1962;17:230–239.
71. Reid L, Simon G. The role of alveolar hypoplasia in some types of emphysema. Br J Dis Chest 1964;58:158–168.
72. Reid L, Simon G, Zorab PA, Seidelin R. The development of unilateral hypertransradiancy of the lung. Br J Dis Chest 1967;61:190–192.
73. Mcleod WM. Abnormal transradiancy of one lung. Thorax 1954,9.147–153.
74. Van Allen CM, Jung TS. Postoperative atelectasis and collateral respiration. J Thorac Surg 1931;1:3–14.
75. Van Allen CM, Lindskog GE, Richter HG. Collateral respiration. Transfer of air collaterally between pulmonary lobules. J Clin Invest 1931;10:559–590.
76. Yousem SA, Burke CM, Billingham ME. Pathologic pulmonary alterations in long term human heart-lung transplantation. Hum Pathol 1985;16:911.
77. Yousem SA, Dauber JH, Griffith BP. Bronchial cartilage alterations in lung transplantation. Chest 1990;98:1121–1124.
78. Veith F, Sinha S, Blumcke S, Norm AJ, Montefusco CM, Kamholz SL, et al. Nature and evolution of lung allograft rejection with and without immunosuppression. J Thorac Cardiovasc Surg 1972;63:509–520.
79. Marchevsky A, Hartman G, Walts A, Ross D, Koerner S, Waters P. Lung transplantation: the pathologic diagnosis of pulmonary complications. Mod Pathol 1991;4:133–138.
80. Davies P, McBride J, Murray GF, Wilcox BR, Shallal JA, Reid LR. Structural changes in the canine lung and pulmonary arteries after pneumonectomy. J Appl Physiol Respir Environ Exerc Physiol 1982;53(Suppl 4):859–864.
81. McBride JT, Kirchner KK, Russ G, Finkelstein J. Role of pulmonary blood flow in postpneumonectomy lung growth. J Appl Physiol 1992;73:2448–2451.
82. Davies P, Reid L. Developmental constraints in compensatory postnatal growth of the lung. J Dev Physiol 1982;4:265–272.
83. McBride JT, Wohl MEB, Streider DJ, et al. Lung growth and airway function after lobectomy in infancy for congenital lobar emphysema. J Clin Invest 1980;66:962–970.
84. Boyden EA. Segmental anatomy of the lungs. New York: McGraw-Hill, 1955.
85. Miller WS. The lung. 2nd ed. Springfield, IL: CC Thomas, 1947.
86. Jeffrey PK, Reid L. The respiratory mucous membrane. In: Brain JD, Proctor DF, Reid L, eds. Respiratory defense mechanisms. In: Lenfant C, exec ed. Lung biology in health and disease. New York: Marcel Dekker, 1977;5:193–245.
87. Coalson JJ. The adult lung: structure and function. In: Saldana MJ, ed. Pathology of pulmonary disease. Philadelphia: JB Lippincott, 1994:3–14.
88. Johnson NF, Hubbs AF. Epithelial progenitor cells in the rat trachea. Am J Respir Cell Mol Biol 1990;3:579–585.
89. Shimizu T, Nettesheim P, Ramaekers FCS, Randell SH. Expression of "cell-type-specific" markers during rat tracheal epithelial regeneration. Am J Respir Cell Mol Biol 1992;7:30–41.
90. Shimizu T, Mishihara M, Kawaguchi S, Sakakura Y. Expression of phenotypic markers during regeneration of rat tracheal epithelium following mechanical injury. Am J Respir Cell Mol Biol 1994;11:85–94.
91. Meyrick B, Reid L. The alveolar brush cell in rat lung: a third pneumocyte. J Ultrastruct Res 1968;23:71–80.
92. Reid L, Jones R. Experimental chronic bronchitis. Int Rev Exper Pathol 1983;24:335–382.
93. Meyrick B, Sturgess JM, Reid L. A reconstruction of the duct system and secretory tubules of the human bronchial submucosal gland. Thorax 1969;24:729–736.
94. Brody JS, Williams MC. Pulmonary alveolar epithelial cell differentiation. Ann Rev Physiol 1992;54:351–371.
95. Weibel ER. Morphological basis of alveolar capillary gas exchange. Physiol Rev 1973;53:419–495.
96. Jones RC. Ultrastructural analysis of contractile cell development on lung microvessels in hyperoxic pulmonary hypertension. Fibroblasts and intermediate cells selectively reorganize nonmuscular segments. Am J Pathol 1992;141:1491–1505.
97. Dimaio M, Gil J, Ciurea D, Katten M. Structural maturation of the human fetal lung: a morphometric study of the development of air-blood barriers. Pediatr Res 1989;26(Suppl 2):88–93.
98. Campiche MA, Gautier A, Hernandez EI, Reymond A. An electron microscopic study of the fetal development of human lung. Pediatrics 1963;329–334.
99. Meyrick B, Reid L. The blood/gas barrier including its ultrastructure. In: Hatzfeld C, ed. Distribution of pulmonary gas exchange. Les colloques de INSERM/SEPCR, 1975. Paris: INSERM, 1976;145–154.
100. Clements JA. Surface tension of lung extracts. Proc Soc Exp Biol Med 1975;95:170–172.

101. Klaus MH, Clements JA, Havel RJ. Composition of surface active material isolated from beef lung. Proc Natl Acad Sci U S A 1961;47:1858–1859.
102. Shelley SA, Paciga JE, Balis JU. Lung surfactant phospholipids in different animal species. Lipids 1984;19:857–862.
103. Pattle RE. Properties, function and origin of the alveolar lining layer. Nature Lond, 1955;175:1125–1126.
104. Avery M E, Mead J. Surface properties in relation to atelectasis and hyaline membrane disease. Am J Dis Child 1959;97:517–523.
105. King RJ. Isolation and chemical composition of pulmonary surfactant. In: Robertson B, van Golde LMG, Batenburg JJ, eds. Pulmonary surfactant. Elsevier: Amsterdam, 1984;1–15.
106. King, RJ. Pulmonary surfactant. J Appl Physiol 1982;53:1–8.
107. Rooney SA. The surfactant system and lung phospholipid biochemistry. Am Rev Respir Dis 1985;131:439–460.
108. Sanders RL. The composition of pulmonary surfactant. In: Farrell PM, ed. Lung development: biological and clinical perspectives. New York: Academic, 1982;193–210.
109. Sueishi K, Turnaca K, Oda T. Immunoultrastructural study of surfactant system. Distribution of specific protein of surface active material in rabbit lung. Lab Invest 1977;37:136–142.
110. Voorhout WF, Veenedaal T, Haagsman HP, et al. Surfactant protein A is localized at the corners of the pulmonary tubular myelin lattice. J Histochem Cytochem 1991;39:1331–1336.
111. deMello DE, Heyman S, Phelps DS, Floros J. Immunogold localization of SP-A in lungs of infants dying from respiratory distress syndrome. Am J Pathol 1993;142:1631–1640.
112. Suzuki Y, Fujita Y, Kogishi K. Reconstitution of tubular myelin from synthetic lipids and proteins associated with pig pulmonary surfactant. Am Rev Respir Dis 1989;140:75–81.
113. Weaver T, Whitsett JA. Function and regulation of expression of pulmonary surfactant proteins. Biochem J 1991;273:249–264.
114. Rice WR, Ross GF, Singleton FM, et al. Surfactant-associated protein inhibits phospholipid secretion from type II cells. J Appl Physiol 1987;63:692–698.
115. Dobbs LG, Wright JR, Hawgood S, et al. Pulmonary surfactant and its components inhibit secretion of phosphatidylcholine from cultured rat alveolar type II cells. Proc Natl Acad Sci U S A 1987;84:1010–1014.
116. Tenner AJ, Robinson SL, Borchelt J, et al. Human pulmonary surfactant protein (SP-A), a protein structurally homologous to C1q, can enhance FcR- and CR1-mediated phagocytosis. J Biol Chem 1989;264:13923–13928.
117. deMello DE, Chi EY, Doo E, et al. Absence of tubular myelin in lungs of infants dying with hyaline membrane disease. Am J Pathol 1987;127:131–139.
118. deMello DE, Phelps DS, Patel G, et al. Expression of the 35kDa and low molecular weight surfactant associated proteins in the lungs of infants dying with respiratory distress syndrome. Am J Pathol 1989;134:1285–1293.
119. Nogee LM, deMello DE, Dehner LP, et al. Deficiency of pulmonary surfactant protein B in congenital alveolar proteinosis. N Engl J Med 1993;406–410.
120. deMello DE, Nogee LM, Heyman S, Krous H, Hussain M, Merritt TA, Hseuh W, et al. Molecular and phenotypic variability in congenital alveolar proteinosis (CAP) caused by inherited surfactant protein B (SP-B) deficiency. J Pediatr 1994;125:43–50.
121. Saldana MJ. Pathology of pulmonary disease. Philadelphia: JB Lippincott, 1994.
122. Jones R, Reid L. Vascular remodeling in the clinical and experimental pulmonary hypertensions. In: Bishop J, Reeves J, Laurent G, eds. Pulmonary vascular remodelling. London: Portland Press, 1995:47–115.
123. Reid L. The pathology of emphysema. London: Lloyd-Luke (Medical Books), 1967.
124. deMello, DE, Reid, LM. Arteries and veins. In: Crystal RG, West JB, Barnes PJ, Cherniak NS, Weibel ER, eds. The lung: scientific foundations. New York: Raven Press, 1991;1:767–777.
125. Elliott FM, Reid L. Some new facts about the pulmonary artery and its branching pattern. Clin Radiol 1965;16:193–198.
126. Reid L. Structure and function in pulmonary hypertension. New perceptions. Seventh Simon Rodbard memorial lecture. Chest 1986;89:279–288.
127. Verloop MC. The arteriae bronchiales and their anastomoses with the arteria pulmonalis in the human lung; a microanatomical study. Acta Anat (Basel) 1948;5:171–205.
128. Verloop MC. On the arteriae bronchiales and their anastomosing with the arteria pulmonalis in some rodents; a microanatomical study. Acta Anat (Basel) 1949;7:1–32.
129. Reid L, Rubino M. The connective tissue septa in the fetal lung. Thorax 1959;14:3–13.
130. Reid L. The connective tissue septa in the adult human lung. Thorax 1959;138–145.
131. Kohn HM. Zur Histologie der fibrinosen Pneumonie. Munch Med Wochenschr 1983;40:42.
132. Lambert MW. Accessory bronchiole-alveolar communications. J Pathol Bacteriol 1955;70:311–314.
133. Brock, RC, ed. The anatomy of the bronchial tree. 2nd ed. London: Oxford University Press, 1954.
134. Williams PL, Warwick R, Dyson M, Bannister LH, eds. Gray's anatomy. 37th ed. Edinburgh: Churchill Livingstone, 1989.
135. Pistolesi M, Miniati M, Milne ENC. Formation and absorption of pleural liquid: physiologic and pathophysiologic aspects and radiologic significance. In: Potchen EJ, Grainger RG, Green R, eds. Pulmonary radiology: the Fleischner Society. Philadelphia: WB Saunders, 1993; IV:141–154.
136. Peters-van der Sanden MJ, Kirby ML, Gittenberger-de Groot A, Tibboel D, Mulder MP, Meijers C. Ablation of various regions within the avian vagal neural crest has differential effects on ganglion formation in the fore-, mid- and hindgut. Dev Dyn 1993;196(Suppl 3):183–194.
137. Cotran RS, Kumar V, Robbins SL, eds. Pathologic basis of disease. 5th ed. Philadelphia: WB Saunders, 1994.
138. Behar J, Sheahan DC. Histologic abnormalities in reflux esophagitis. Arch Pathol 1975;99:387.
139. Jamieson GG, Duranceau A. The pathology of gastroesophageal reflux. In: Duranceau A, Jamieson GG, eds. Gastroesophageal reflux. Philadelphia, WB Saunders, 1988:46.
140. Barrett NK. The lower esophagus lined by columnar epithelium. Surgery 1957;41:881–894.
141. Spechler SJ, Goyal RK. Barrett's esophagus. N Engl J Med 1986;315:362.
142. Reid BJ, Haggitt RC, Rubin CE, Roth G, Surawicz CM, Van Belle G, Lewin K, et al. Observer variation in the diagnosis of dysplasia in Barrett's esophagus. Hum Pathol 1988;19:166.
143. Thomson JJ. Barrett's metaplasia and adenocarcinoma of the esophagus and gastroesophageal junction. Hum Pathol 1983; 14:42.
144. Naef AP, Savary M, Ozzello L. Columnar-lined lower esophagus, an acquired lesion with malignant predisposition. Report on 140 cases of Barrett's esophagus with 12 adenocarcinoma. J Thorac Cardiovasc Surg 1975;70:826.
145. Bockman DE, Kirby ML. Dependence of thymus development on derivatives of the neural crest. Science 1984;223(Suppl 4635):498–500.
146. Gould VE, Sommers SC. Adrenal medulla and paraganglia. In:

Bloodworth JMB, ed. Endocrine pathology. 2nd ed. Baltimore: Williams & Wilkins, 1982;473–511.
147. Fontaine J, LeDouarin NM. Analysis of endoderm formation in the avian blastoderm by the use of quail-chick chimeras. J Embryol Exp Morphol 1977;4:209.
148. Brodeur GM, Pritchard J, Berthold F, Carlsen NLT, Castel V, Castleberry RP, De Bernardi B, et al. Revisions of the international criteria for neuroblastoma diagnosis, staging and response to treatment. J Clin Oncol 1993;11: 1466–1477.
149. Brodeur GM, Castleberry RP. Neuroblastoma. In: Pizzo PA, Poplack DG, eds. Principles and practice of pediatric oncology. 2nd ed. Philadelphia: JB Lippincott, 1993;739–767.
150. Nakagawara A, Arima-Nakagawara M, Scavarda NJ, Azar CG, Cantor AB, Brodeur GM. Association between high levels of expression of the TRK gene and favorable outcome in human neuroblastoma. N Engl J Med 1993;328:847–854.
151. Kirby ML. Nodose placode contributes autonomic neurons to the heart in the absence of cardiac neural crest. J Neurosci 1988;8(Suppl 4):1089–1095.
152. Kirby ML. Role of extracardiac factors in heart development. Experientia 1988;44(Suppl 11–12):944–951.
153. Leatherbury L, Connuck DM, Kirby ML. Neural crest ablation versus sham surgical effects in a chick embryo model of defective cardiovascular development. Pediatr Res 1993;33(Suppl 6):628–631.
154. Kirby ML, Kumiski DH, Myers T, Cerjan C, Mishima N. Back-transplantation of chick cardiac neural crest cells cultured in LIF rescues heart development. Dev Dyn 1993;198(Suppl 4):296–311.
155. Kirby ML, Waldo KL. Role of neural crest in congenital heart disease. Circulation 1990;82(Suppl 2):332–340.
156. Scully RE, Mark EJ, McNeely WF, McNeely BU. Case records of the Massachusetts General Hospital. N Engl J Med 1994; 330:1143–1149.
157. Gertner E, Learhsrman JW. Intracardiac mural thrombus mimicking atrial myxoma in the antiphospholipid syndrome. J Rheumatol 1992;19:1293–1298.
158. Goodwin JF. Diagnosis of left atrial myxoma. Lancet 1963; 1:464–468.
159. Osada T, Cho M, Fukushima H, Kudo T, Sakamoto M, Furukawa K. Changes in plasma interleukin 6 in a surgical case of left atrial myxoma. Kyobu Geka Japan J Thorac Surg 1994;47:405–407.
160. Wiedermann CJ, Reinisch N, Fischer-Colbrie R, Vollmar AM, Herold M, Knapp E. Proinflammatory cytokines in cardiac myxomas. J Intern Med 1992;232:263–265.
161. Rosai J. Ackerman's surgical pathology. 7th ed. St. Louis: CV Mosby, 1989:1.
162. Bernaudin JF, Jaurand MC, Fleury J, Bignon J. Mesothelial cells. In: Crystal RG, West JB, et al, eds. The lung: scientific foundations. New York: Raven Press, 1991:631–638.
163. Courtice FC, Simmonds WJ. Absorption of fluids from the pleural cavities of rabbits and cats. J Physiol (Lond) 1949;109: 117–130.
164. Turton CW. Pleural effusions (review). Br J Hosp Med 1980;23: 239–240.
165. Black LF. The pleural space and pleural fluid (review). Mayo Clin Proc 1972;47:493–506.
166. Agostini E, D'Angelo E. Pleural liquid pressure. J Appl Physiol 1991;71:393–403.
167. Von Neergaard K. Neue Auffassungen uber einen Grundbegriff der Atemmechanik. Die Retraktionskraft der Lunge, abhangig von der Oberflachenspannung in den Alveolen. Z Gesamte Exp Med 1929;66:373–394.
168. Takada K, Otsuki Y, Magari S. Lymphatics and pre-lymphatics of the rabbit pericardium and epicardium with special emphasis on particulate absorption and milky spot-like structures. Lymphology 1991;24(Suppl 3):116–124.
169. Devaney K, Snyder R, Norris HJ, Tavassoli FA. Proliferative and histologically malignant struma ovarii: a clinicopathologic study of 54 cases. Int J Gynecol Pathol 1993;12: 333–343.
170. Trapnell DH. The peripheral lymphatics of the lung. Br J Radiol NS 1963;36:660–672.
171. Trapnell DH. Recognition and incidence of intrapulmonary lymph nodes. Thorax 1964a;19:44–50.
172. Trapnell DH. Radiological appearances of lymphangitis carcinomatosa of the lung. Thorax 1964b;19:251–260.
173. Bienenstock J, Johnston N, Perey DVE. Bronchial lymphoid tissue. I. Morphologic characteristics. Lab Invest 1973;28:686–892.
174. Bienenstock J, Befus O. Gut and bronchus-associated lymphoid tissue. Am J Anat 1984;170:437–445.
175. Otsuki Y, Ito Y, Magari S. Lymphocyte subpopulations high endothelial venules and lymphoid capillaries of bronchus associated lymphoid tissue (BALT) in the rat. Am J Anat 1989;184: 139–146.
176. Cordonnier C, Escudier E, Verra F, Brochard L, Bernaudin JF, Fleury-Feith J. Bronchoalveolar lavage during neutropenic episodes: diagnostic yield and cellular pattern. Eur Respir J 1994;7:114–120.

2

Lung and Esophageal Carcinogenesis

Stephen S. Hecht and Gary D. Stoner

This chapter considers some of the etiologic factors associated with the development of cancers of the lung and esophagus, as well as some possible approaches to the chemoprevention of these cancers. The principal carcinogens for the lung and esophagus, pathways for their metabolic activation and detoxification, types of DNA damage they can elicit, and mechanisms for DNA repair are important considerations. The roles of activated oncogenes and inactivated tumor suppressor genes in the development of lung and esophageal tumors are also considered in the context of dysregulated cell growth. Results from chemoprevention studies of lung and esophageal cancer in animals and humans are highlighted. Finally, animal models in common use for experimental studies of the etiology, development, and chemoprevention of lung and esophageal cancer are summarized.

LUNG CANCER

CAUSATIVE FACTORS

Cigarette smoking is the overwhelming cause of lung cancer in the United States and worldwide. Of the more than 172,000 new cases of lung cancer anticipated in the United States in 1994, at least 80% will have been caused by cigarette smoking (1, 2). Smoking is the major cause of all four major types of lung cancer: squamous cell carcinoma (SCC), adenocarcinoma, large cell carcinoma, and small cell carcinoma. In the past two decades, the incidence of adenocarcinoma has increased substantially in the United States. The ratio of adenocarcinoma to SCC was 1:2.3 among white males in 1969–1971, whereas it was 1:1.4 in 1984–1986 (3). The dramatic increase in adenocarcinoma is thought to result from the changing design of cigarettes (4).

Extensive epidemiologic studies have shown that there is a direct relationship between the daily dose of cigarette smoke and the excess risk of lung cancer in both men and women. The incidence of lung cancer also depends on the duration of smoking. The greatest risk is among those who start smoking in adolescence and continue throughout their lives. Cessation of smoking gradually decreases the risk for lung cancer. The risk for lung cancer is much greater in cigarette smokers than in pipe or cigar smokers (1).

Whereas the relative risk for lung cancer development in cigarette smokers is typically 10 to 15 times that of controls who did not smoke, the relative risk for lung cancer in nonsmokers exposed to environmental tobacco smoke is typically 1 to 2 times that of nonexposed individuals. The U.S. Environmental Protection Agency has estimated that more than 3000 lung cancer deaths per year are caused by environmental tobacco smoke, but this estimate is controversial (5).

Epidemiologic studies of underground miners have shown that exposure to high levels of radon gas, specifically radon 222 (^{222}Rn) and its decay products, can cause lung cancer. ^{222}Rn, a decay product of uranium 238 (^{238}U), can enter homes from subsoils and accumulate; however, the levels in homes are far lower than those in mines. Based on models developed from studies of lung cancer in underground miners, it is estimated that 11% to 13% of lung cancer deaths among residents of single-family dwellings in the United States could be attributable to indoor radon exposure, thus accounting for 9% of all lung cancer deaths in the United States, i.e., approximately 13,000 deaths per year. However, the role of indoor radon exposure in lung cancer has not been confirmed in epidemiologic studies designed for that purpose (6).

Among the carcinogens in cigarette smoke, polynuclear aromatic hydrocarbons (PAHs) and nitrosamines are strongly implicated as causative agents for lung cancer in smokers. PAHs, which are products of the incomplete combustion of organic matter, are present in certain occupational settings in which excess risk of lung cancer has been documented. These include aluminum production, coal gasification, and coke production. Exposure to soots also is associated with an increased risk for lung cancer. PAHs are present in polluted urban air, but the role of air pollution as a cause of lung cancer is uncertain (7).

Exposure to metals in occupational settings is a documented cause of lung cancer, particularly for hexavalent chromium, arsenic, nickel, and, to a lesser extent, cadmium. People diagnosed with silicosis after occupational exposure to dusts containing crystalline silica also are thought to be at increased risk for lung cancer (7).

Asbestos exposure, mainly in occupational settings, is a cause of mesothelioma. Some nonoccupational exposures leading to mesothelioma also have been documented. The risk of mesothelioma appears to be independent of smoking. Smoking exerts a strong synergistic effect with asbestos in the induction of lung cancer (7).

TOBACCO SMOKE CARCINOGENS AND LUNG CANCER

Because smoking is by far the major cause of lung cancer, carcinogenesis of the lung is best understood by considering the cancer-causing agents in cigarette smoke. Cigarette smoke contains at least 3500 identified chemical compounds, of which more than 40 are established carcinogens (1, 8). The role of specific carcinogens of tobacco and tobacco smoke in human cancers of various types can be assessed. Relevant factors include the amounts of the carcinogens in tobacco products, their target tissues and carcinogenic potency in laboratory animals, and biochemical evidence that humans respond in similar ways to laboratory animals. Likely causative agents for lung cancer are summarized in Table 2.1 (8).

PAHs such as benzo(a)pyrene (BaP), which are formed by the incomplete combustion of tobacco during smoking, are well-recognized carcinogens that have been shown to induce tumors of the lung in laboratory animals exposed by inhalation, instillation in the trachea, or implantation in the lung. SCCs of the lung generally are induced by carcinogenic PAHs such as BaP. Considering the amounts of these compounds in cigarette smoke and their carcinogenic potency, one can plausibly argue that they play some role in lung cancer induction. This argument is bolstered by biochemical studies showing that human lung tissue can metabolize PAHs by pathways that lead to covalent modification of DNA (adduct formation) and by the detection of the relevant DNA adducts in lung tissue of smokers.

TABLE 2.1. Smoking and Lung Cancer: Causative Agents

CARCINOGENS	MODIFYING AGENTS
Strong evidence[a]	Co-carcinogens (catechols)
PAH: benzo(a)pyrene	Tumor promoters (phenols and others)
benzo(b, j, and k) fluoranthenes	Toxic aldehydes (acrolein)
5-methylchrysene	Diet
dibenz(a,h)anthrocene	
indeno(1,2,3-cd)pyrene	
NNK	
Weak evidence	
^{210}Po, Cr, Cd, Ni	
Aldehydes, butadiene	
Free radicals	

From Hoffmann D, Hecht SS. Advances in tobacco carcinogenesis. In: Cooper CS, Grover PL, eds. Handbook of experimental pharmacology. Berlin: Springer-Verlag, 1990; 94(I): 63–107.

Abbreviations. PAH, polynuclear aromatic hydrocarbons; NNK, 4-(methylnitrosamino)-1-(3-pyridyl)-1-butanone.

[a]Criteria: animal carcinogenicity, presence in smoke, biochemical studies (animal and human lung).

4-(Methylnitrosamino)-1-(3-pyridyl)-1-butanone (NNK), a nitrosamine formed from the major tobacco constituent nicotine during the processing of tobacco and during smoking, is a powerful lung carcinogen in laboratory animals, independent of the route of administration. NNK is one of a family of nicotine-derived nitrosamines that collectively are called tobacco specific nitrosamines. Adenocarcinoma of the lung is the main type of lung cancer induced by NNK. The total amount of NNK required to produce lung cancer in rats is similar to that to which a smoker would be exposed in a lifetime of smoking. These data support the role of NNK in the induction of lung cancer, particularly adenocarcinoma. Human lung tissue has been shown to activate NNK metabolically, although not as efficiently as rodent lung tissue. DNA adducts specific to NNK and the related compound N'-nitrosonornicotine (NNN) have been detected in smokers' lungs, and metabolites of NNK are present in smokers' urine. Interestingly, the ratio of adenocarcinoma to SCC in smokers has been increasing in the past three decades. Changes in cigarettes have been such that the levels of NNK have been increasing during this period, whereas levels of BaP have been decreasing (4). The increase in human exposure to NNK, which induces adenocarcinoma, and the decrease in exposure to BaP, which induces SCC, may account in part for the increase in adenocarcinoma of the lung being observed in smokers.

Table 2.1 lists some other tobacco smoke constituents that could be involved in lung cancer induction; the evidence suggesting a role for these compounds is weaker than that noted for PAH and NNK. Several modifying agents in tobacco smoke are likely to enhance the carcinogenicity of PAHs and possibly NNK. These include catechol, a well-known cocarcinogenic compound, and weakly acidic tumor promoters found in tobacco smoke. Animal studies as well as epidemiologic evidence indicate that a high-fat diet may also enhance susceptibility to lung cancer.

METABOLIC ACTIVATION AND DETOXIFICATION OF CARCINOGENS

Most known respiratory carcinogens to which humans are exposed require metabolism before exerting their carcinogenic effects. This process, referred to as metabolic activation, is part of the general response of an organism to exposure to foreign compounds (9). It is summarized in Figure 2.1.

Upon uptake, the carcinogen is first metabolized by so-called phase I enzymes that carry out oxygenation reactions designed to make it more polar and more readily excretable. The phase I enzymes that catalyze these transformations are frequently members of the cytochrome *P450* enzyme superfamily (10). The oxygenated polar metabolites formed can be further transformed to conjugates by phase II enzymes, which include *UDP*-glucuronosyltransferases, sulfotransferases, and glutathione *S*-transferases. These conjugates are readily excreted and often can be considered detoxification products.

The initially formed oxygenated polar metabolites are in some cases electrophilic, or they may undergo further metabolism or spontaneous reactions, producing electrophiles. Electrophiles react with nucleophilic centers in cellular macromolecules such as DNA, RNA, and protein. The reaction of these electrophiles with cellular macromolecules produces covalently bound products called adducts. DNA adducts are particularly important in the initiation of the carcinogenic process. The activation of oncogenes and inactivation of tumor suppressor genes, discussed in detail below, are both major events in the multistep carcinogenic process. These events are most likely caused by mutations in DNA that result from miscoding during replication of DNA adducts.

METABOLISM OF LUNG CARCINOGENS TO DNA REACTIVE PRODUCTS

Metabolism is the key to understanding the mechanisms by which carcinogens interact with DNA. Metabolic activation and detoxification reactions of representative lung carcinogens can serve as a good example of this process. Figure 2.2 summarizes several known metabolism reactions of BaP, a representative PAH. Metabolism reactions of PAHs are complex (11). The initial reactions involve formation of a series of arene oxides, catalyzed by cytochrome *P450* enzymes. There is great selectivity in the formation of these arene oxides; depending on the PAH, only certain ones are formed and then generally with a high degree of stereoselectivity (e.g., one optical isomer of each arene oxide generally predominates). The arene oxide may rearrange spontaneously to form phenols in a reaction termed the National Institutes of Health (NIH) shift. Some phenols, such as 6-hydroxybenzo(*a*)pyrene, are formed by direct hydroxylation. Competing with the rearrangement of arene oxides to phenols is their hydration to *trans*-dihydrodiols, catalyzed by the enzyme epoxide hydrolase, as well as by the conjugation with glutathione catalyzed by glutathione *S*-transferases. Arene oxides are electrophiles and react with DNA in vitro. Thus, it was widely thought that they were ultimate carcinogens of PAH, but DNA binding studies carried out in vivo did not support this hypothesis and it has been discredited.

The *trans*-dihydrodiols formed by hydration of arene oxides can be conjugated as glucuronides or, in some cases, can undergo further oxidation to form diol epoxides. The epoxide ring can be added to the molecule on the same side as the benzylic hydroxyl group, producing a *syn*-diol epoxide, or on the opposite side, producing an *anti*-diol epoxide. Each *syn*-diol or *anti*-diol epoxide can exist in two optically isomeric (enantiomeric) forms. Thus, a racemic *trans*-dihydrodiol can be oxidized to four possible diol epoxides. Diol epoxides in which the epoxide ring is in the bay region of a PAH are major ultimate carcinogens of a number of PAHs. The three-sided bay regions of some PAHs,

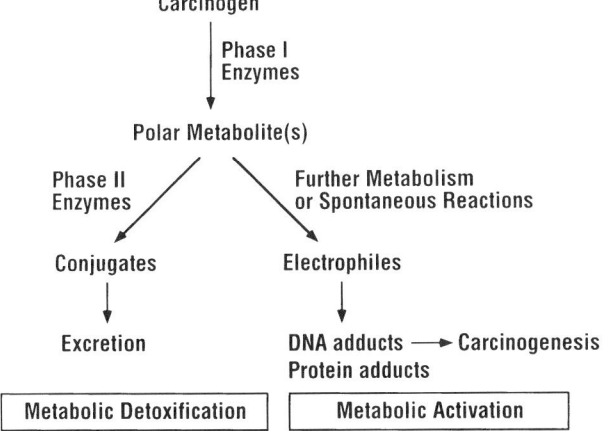

FIGURE 2.1. Metabolic activation and detoxification of carcinogens.

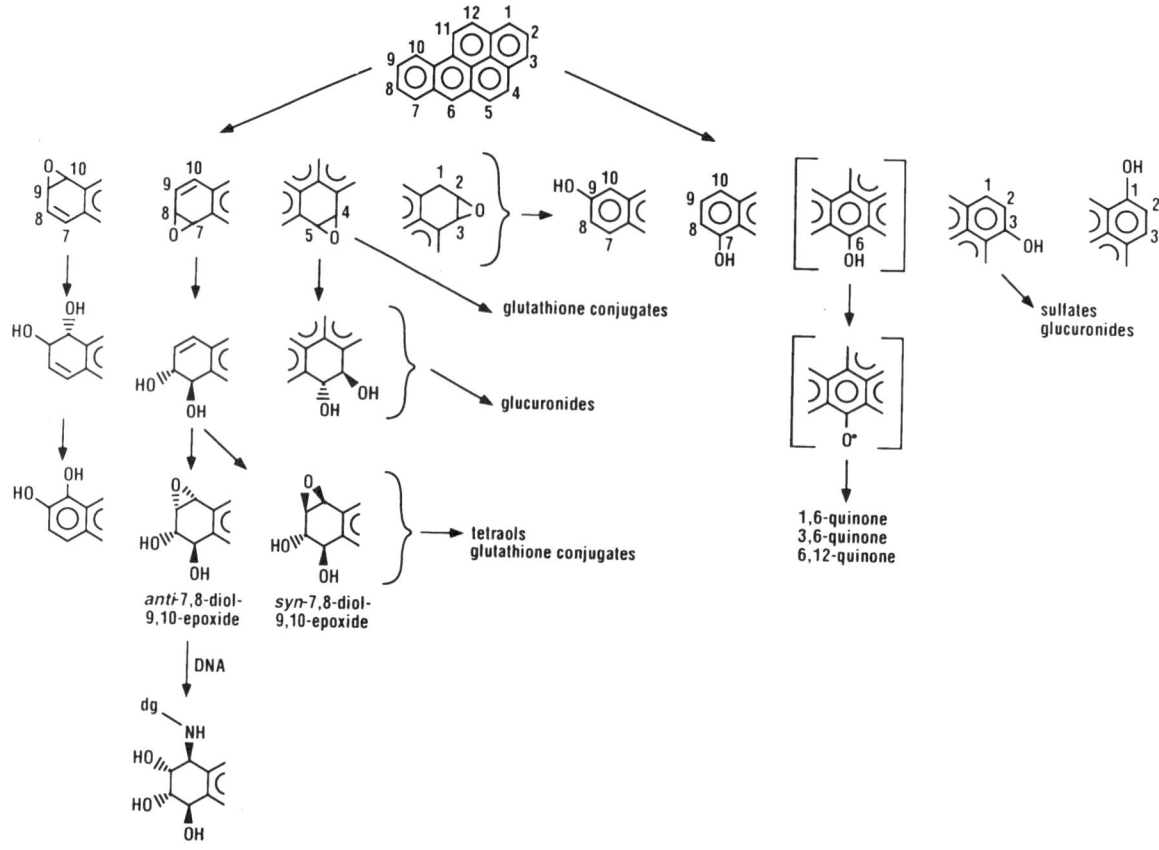

FIGURE 2.2. Metabolism of benzo(*a*)pyrene.

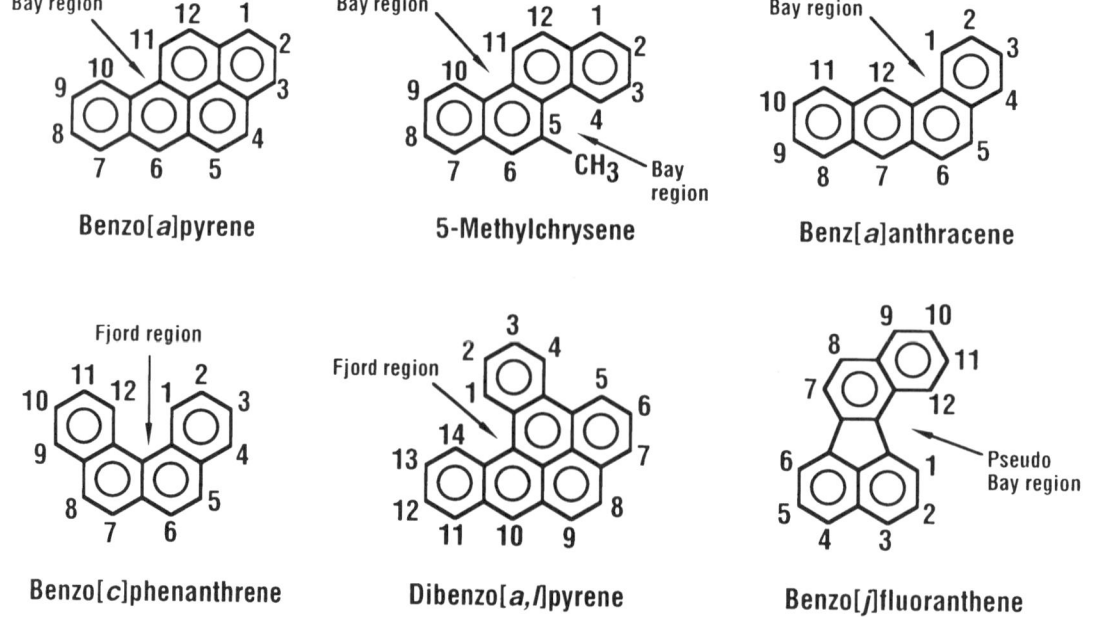

FIGURE 2.3. Bay regions and fjord regions of some PAHs.

formed by three adjoining rings, are illustrated in Figure 2.3. Some PAHs have sterically crowded bay regions that contain a methyl group, fjord regions formed by four adjoining rings, or pseudo-bay regions formed by four adjoining rings, one of which is saturated. Diol epoxides with their epoxide rings in one of these regions often are highly reactive with DNA and frequently have high mutagenic and carcinogenic properties. Steric factors play a major role in the reactivity of diol epoxides with DNA, influencing the extent of the reaction, the types of adducts formed, and the mutagenicity and carcinogenicity of adducts. In general, the *anti*-diol epoxides are more effective carcinogens; among these, the *R,S,S,R*-diol epoxide enantiomers are the most effective. DNA adducts formed from the *R,S,S,R*-diol epoxide enantiomers result predominantly from *trans*-addition of the exocyclic amino groups of deoxyguanosine or deoxyadenosine to the benzylic position of the epoxide ring.

Of the many reactions illustrated in Figure 2.2, only formation of the *R,S,S,R*-enantiomer of the *anti*-7,8-diol-9,10-epoxide has been shown conclusively to be a metabolic activation pathway. All other reactions represent probable detoxification pathways. Quantitatively, the metabolic activation pathway resulting in the formation of a diol epoxide–ultimate carcinogen is a minor one; however, the diol epoxide is highly carcinogenic and mutagenic, and the DNA adducts formed cause somatic mutations. It thus is plausible that these DNA adducts are responsible for many of the carcinogenic effects of BaP.

Figure 2.4 summarizes some major pathways of the metabolism of NNK (12). Reduction of the carbonyl group, catalyzed by carbonyl reductase enzymes, is a major metabolic pathway. This process produces 4-(methylnitrosamino)-1-(3-pyridyl)-1-butanol (NNAL), which is another potent pulmonary carcinogen. NNAL can be conjugated as its *O*-glucuronide, NNAL-Gluc. The latter is thought to be a detoxification product of NNK. Oxidation of the pyridine ring at nitrogen produces NNK-*N*-oxide, which generally is regarded as a detoxification pathway. In laboratory animals the major metabolic activation pathways result from cytochrome *P450* catalyzed oxidation at the methylene carbon adjacent to the *N*-nitroso group, leading to intermediate 1, and the corresponding oxidation at the methyl carbon, leading to intermediate 2. These reactions are called α-hydroxylation, which is thought to be the main metabolic activation pathway for most nitrosamines. The α-hydroxy compounds 1 and 2 are un-

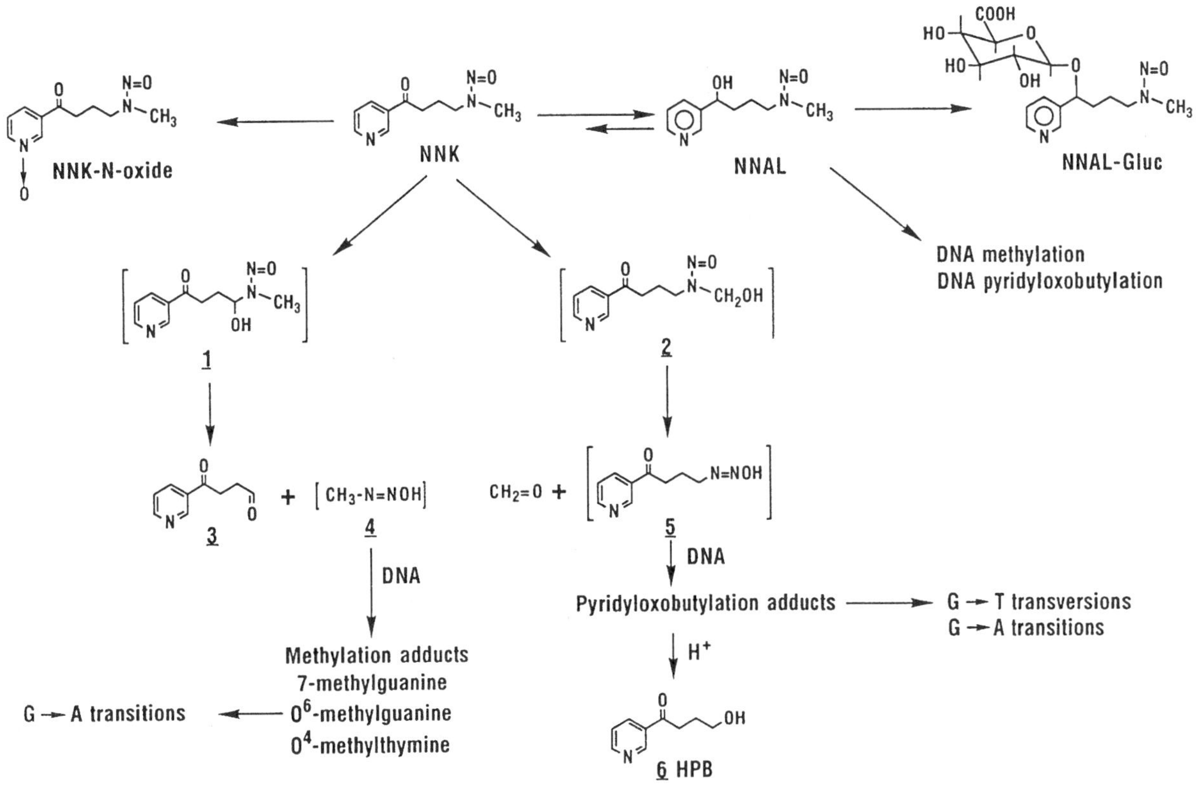

FIGURE 2.4. Metabolism of 4-(methylnitrosamino)-1-(3-pyridyl)-1-butanone (NNK).

stable and spontaneously decompose to produce aldehydes, such as 3 and formaldehyde, together with diazohydroxides, such as 4 and 5. The diazohydroxides are electrophiles with very high reactivity toward DNA. Methanediazohydroxide compound 4 methylates DNA forming at least 13 different adducts, among which 7-methylguanine, O^6-methylguanine, and O^4-methylthymidine have been detected in the DNA isolated from tissues of animals treated with NNK. O^6-Methylguanine is known to cause miscoding, leading to a G to A transition (purine to purine) mutation. The other diazohydroxide, compound 5, also reacts with cellular macromolecules such as DNA and globin, giving adducts that can be hydrolyzed to 4-hydroxy-1-(3-pyridyl)-1-butanone (HPB). The adducts formed in DNA from compound 5 are structurally uncharacterized but are present in the DNA of animals treated with NNK. These adducts have been shown to cause both G to A transition mutations and G to T transversion (purine to pyrimidine) mutations in DNA. Both pathways are regarded as metabolic activation modes for NNK, and both are important in the induction of tumors by this compound. Quantitatively, the α-hydroxylation pathways and conversion to NNAL are generally the major metabolic routes seen for NNK in rodents. NNAL also undergoes further activation by α-hydroxylation, leading to DNA methylation and pyridoxobutylation.

Comparing the metabolic activation pathways of PAH and nitrosamines, an interesting difference is that metabolic activation of the latter involves only one enzymatic step, α-hydroxylation. The diol epoxide metabolites of PAH are generally more stable than the α-hydroxy and diazohydroxide metabolites of nitrosamines. The latter react mainly at their site of formation, although evidence exists for their transport. Diol epoxides of PAHs can be transported to sites other than those at which they are formed. Although α-hydroxylation of nitrosamines generally exceeds diol epoxide formation from PAHs, both types of compounds modify DNA to similar extents in laboratory animals.

Chromium IV (Cr[VI]) is one of the most extensively studied metals known to induce lung cancer (13, 14). Cr(VI) is taken up by cells via passive anion transport channels and is reduced intracellularly, resulting ultimately in Cr(III). Various forms of DNA damage result from this process, including the formation of Cr-DNA adducts, DNA-protein cross-links, and DNA strand breaks. The mechanisms by which these effects occur are the subject of some controversy, but it seems clear that reductive metabolism of Cr(VI) is necessary. Some studies in vitro have demonstrated the formation of 8-oxodeoxyguanosine in DNA upon exposure to Cr(VI) and reducing agents. This action presumably results from the generation of reactive oxygen species, such as the hydroxyl radical associated with Cr(VI) metabolism, but the relevance of this process in vivo in the lung is not clear.

DNA Adduct Formation and Repair

Figure 2.5 illustrates representative structures of several deoxyguanosine adducts that could be formed

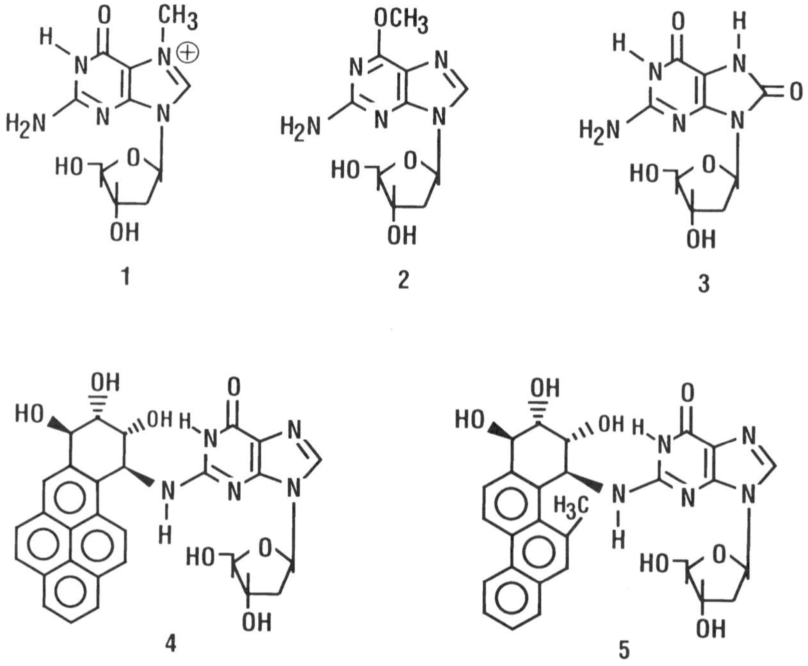

FIGURE 2.5. Some DNA adducts that would form in lung upon inhalation of tobacco smoke.

in lung DNA upon exposure to tobacco smoke. Deoxyguanosine is the base in DNA that generally is the most reactive with metabolically activated carcinogens, although reactions at this site are never exclusive. As noted previously, 7-methyldeoxyguanosine (1) or O^6-methyldeoxyguanosine (2) would typically be formed, among other methylated adducts, by nitrosamines such as NNK. 8-Oxodeoxyguanosine (3) is formed as a result of the reaction with active oxygen species often associated with carcinogen metabolism. A large number of DNA adducts are formed from the PAHs of tobacco smoke. Only two of these (4, 5), which are derived from BaP and 5-methylchrysene, are illustrated.

Techniques have been developed to assess individually the miscoding consequences of specific DNA adducts, such as those illustrated in Figure 2.5. The most extensive information of this type is available for O^6-methyldeoxyguanosine (2). During DNA replication, this adduct is recognized by the DNA polymerase as deoxyadenosine, resulting in the incorporation of thymidine into the newly synthesized strand. In the next round of replication, this thymidine is paired with deoxyadenosine, resulting in the permanent conversion of what was originally a G-C base pair to an A-T base pair. In contrast to O^6-methyldeoxyguanosine, the most common point mutation associated with adducts such as 3-5 (Fig. 2.5) is a G-C to T-A transversion. G to T transversions also are associated with some types of structurally uncharacterized DNA damage, e.g., the pyridyloxobutylation of DNA by NNK.

Tobacco smoke is a complex mixture containing carcinogens likely to produce a mixture of adducts that in simplified form may resemble those illustrated in Figure 2.5. Because most of the adducts in Figure 2.5 produce G to T transversions, it might be assumed that G to T transversions would be the most common mutations found in genes of tumors taken from smokers. This transversion is in fact observed. This simplified view of tobacco carcinogenesis assumes that all adducts would be formed and would persist in DNA to equal extents. However, the formation of different adducts depends on the metabolic activation and detoxification processes for the carcinogens of tobacco smoke, whereas the persistence of the adducts depends on DNA repair and the extent of cell replication, which in turn can be influenced by toxic constituents of tobacco smoke.

Two relevant DNA repair processes involved in lung carcinogenesis are the alkyltransferase pathway, which removes alkyl groups from the O^6 position of deoxyguanosine, and the excision repair pathway, which removes sterically bulky adducts and alkyl adducts formed at the 7 position of guanine or 3 position of adenine from DNA (16–18). Repair of mutagenic O^6-alkylguanines is carried out by the repair protein O^6-alkylguanine DNA-alkyltransferase. This protein removes the alkyl group from the O^6 position of guanine and transfers it to a cysteine acceptor site in the protein, regenerating the original DNA structure in a single step. The cysteine site of the protein is not regenerated, and the new protein must be synthesized to continue repair. Thus, in this stoichiometric process, the cellular levels of protein and O^6-alkylguanine adduct are critical. DNA methylation by NNK has been studied in this regard in various cell types of the lung. Clara cells, which are highly efficient in activating NNK to a DNA methylating species because of their specific cytochromes $P450$, are readily depleted in O^6-alkylguanine-DNA-alkyltransferase activity upon exposure to NNK, thus leading to persistence of O^6-methylguanine in this cell type. DNA pyridyloxobutylation by NNK also has been shown to inhibit the alkyltransferase activity.

Excision repair can be classified broadly into nucleotide excision repair and base excision repair. In nucleotide excision repair, sterically bulky adducts, such as those formed from PAHs, are removed from DNA. A section of the damaged DNA strand is excised, probably in reactions involving several proteins, and a new strand is synthesized by DNA polymerase using the undamaged strand as a template. Adducts such as 7-methylguanine frequently are removed by base excision repair. The damaged base is removed by a glycosylase, leaving an abasic site in DNA (a substrate for an endonuclease), before resynthesis of the DNA and ligation occur.

Many studies have indicated that certain types of adducts are removed preferentially from the transcribed strand of DNA. This process leads to a bias in favor of mutations resulting from unrepaired adducts in the nontranscribed strand.

ONCOGENES AND TUMOR SUPPRESSOR GENES

It has been known for many years that the development of cancer is a multistep process. Insight into the nature of the process has been gained through advances in molecular and cellular biology, and it now is apparent that mutations in a limited number of genes controlling cell proliferation, and differentiation are a key feature of this process. Two particular catagories of genes have been implicated: protooncogenes and tumor suppressor genes. Protooncogenes become activated to oncogenes through mutation or gene amplification, so that either a mutant protein is produced or the normal protein is overexpressed. Expression of tumor suppressor genes is thought to restrain cells from unregulated proliferation and inactivation of both homologues of the gene releases cells from these controls.

Molecular studies of lung cancers have been conducted with both small cell lung cancer (SCLC) and non–small cell lung cancers (NSCLC). SCLC, an extremely aggressive neoplasm, accounts for approximately 25% of all lung tumors and has the poorest prognosis of all lung cancers. NSCLCs account for the remaining 75% of lung cancers. There are several subtypes of NSCLC including adenocarcinomas, which exhibit mucous differentiation; SCCs, which produce keratins; mixed adenosquamous carcinomas, which contain both mucus and keratins; and large cell carcinomas, which are largely undifferentiated tumors. The following section discusses the role of oncogenes and tumor suppressor genes in the development of SCLCs and NSCLCs.

ONCOGENE ACTIVATION

ONCOGENES IN SMALL CELL LUNG CANCER

The *myc* protooncogene family (c-*myc*, N-*myc*, and L-*myc*) encodes three highly related, cell cycle specific, nuclear phosphoproteins of molecular weights 62 to 68 kilodaltons (kd). These phosphoproteins are located in the nucleus, bind to DNA, and associate with at least one other protein, Max (19). Expression of c-*myc* is closely linked to the action of growth factors and with cell cycle progression, suggesting that c-*myc* expression may be a major component of the regulatory networks associated with normal cell proliferation. The c-*myc* product also has been implicated in cell differentiation and programmed cell death (apoptosis). Activation of *myc* is thought to occur by gene amplification or overexpression of the protein, not by point mutation.

Initial studies of *myc* expression in SCLC were performed on cell lines, and evidence of c-*myc* or N-*myc* gene amplification was found in approximately 30%. Gene amplification of all three members of the *myc* family has been observed in primary SCLC, and *myc* amplification appears to be an early event in tumor development. There does not appear to be a correlation between the degree of *myc* gene amplification in primary tumors and survival time.

The *raf*-1 protooncogene encodes a 74-kd phosphoprotein with serine/threonine kinase activity that is located on the internal side of the plasma membrane (20). This phosphoprotein contains a C-terminal kinase domain and an N-terminal regulatory domain that normally suppress kinase activity. Deletion of the N-terminal domain leads to high levels of *raf* kinase activity and converts c-*raf* into a potent oncogene. Although the substrates of *raf* proteins have not been identified fully, it is evident that *raf* proteins can induce expression of the promoter for the c-*fos* protooncogene and thus stimulate the expression of genes required for mitogenesis. The *raf*-1 oncogene may be of special importance in the development of SCLC because of its location on the short arm of chromosome 3 at locus 3p25. Cytogenetic and restriction fragment length polymorphism (RFLP) studies have shown that interstitial or terminal deletions of 3p occur in all SCLCs, and these deletions frequently involve the *raf*-1 locus.

The role of the *ras* protooncogene family in the development of lung cancer is discussed in more detail under NSCLC. Mutations in *ras* genes are essentially absent in SCLC, and elevation of *ras* protein expression is rare.

ONCOGENES IN NON–SMALL CELL LUNG CANCER

Amplification of the c-*myc* gene is found in approximately 10% and overexpression in about 50% of all types of NSCLCs. L-*myc* and N-*myc* appear not to be activated in NSCLC.

The H-*ras*, N-*ras*, and K-*ras* protooncogenes encode highly homologous protein monomers, p21 *ras*, that are located on the cytoplasmic side of the plasma membrane. Their similarity in sequence to G proteins suggests that they may play a role in transmitting proliferation signals from receptors on the cell surface to the nucleus. They bind guanosine triphosphate (GTP) and display an intrinsic GTPase activity that is enhanced by interaction with the GTPase-activating protein (GAP). *ras* Proteins are in an active state for signalling when bound to GTP and are inactive when the GTP has been hydrolyzed to GDP. Overexpression of the normal gene is activating in vitro, as are point mutations in codons 12, 13, or 61, which prevent intrinsic GTP hydrolysis by trapping the protein in the active form.

Activating mutations in H-*ras* and N-*ras* genes are rare in NSCLCs. K-*ras* is mutated in approximately 30% of adenocarcinomas, but this activation is rare in other types of NSCLC (21). There is a correlation between K-*ras* mutations in adenocarcinomas and a history of smoking with approximately 30% of smokers, compared with 2% of nonsmokers, having G-C to T-A transversions at codon 12. This type of mutation is consistent with exposure to carcinogens in tobacco smoke. There is no correlation between K-*ras* mutations and age, sex, age at diagnosis, or tumor stage, but mutations in K-*ras* are associated with a poor prognosis. A recent study showed the feasibility of detecting

K-*ras* mutations in sputum specimens taken from individuals with lung cancer and in asymptomatic individuals with a history of tobacco use (22). This approach could result in the development of a test for the early detection of lung cancer. In addition, a recent report on the inhibition of tumor growth by antisense constructs directed against the mutated K-*ras* oncogene may offer a novel therapeutic strategy in patients with NSCLC as well as those with preneoplastic endobronchial disease (23). Amplification of the *ras* genes is relatively uncommon in NSCLC.

The *erb*B-1 protooncogene encodes the epidermal growth factor receptor (EGFR), a transmembrane glycoprotein of molecular weight 170 kd that possesses intrinsic tyrosine kinase activity and is thought to play a role in signal transduction (24). Activation is commonly by overexpression of the protein, not by mutation. Approximately 25% of SCCs overexpress *erb*B-1 protein (25).

The c-*erb*B-2 (HER2*neu*) protooncogene encodes a *p185* transmembrane receptor with tyrosine kinase activity (26). It is a putative growth factor receptor, related in sequence and structure to the EGFR. Amplification of the c-*erb*B-2 oncogene is an infrequent event in lung cancer; however, overexpression of *p185neu*, as detected immunohistochemically, is found in both adenocarcinomas and SCCs. In adenocarcinomas *p185neu* overexpression is more frequent in older patients, and there is an association with short survival times. In SCCs, *p185neu* expression does not correlate with these parameters.

The c-*fos* and c-*jun* protooncogenes encode nuclear proteins that form a complex, activating protein–1 (AP-1), which acts as a transcription factor (27). The level of AP-1 activity in nuclear extracts of adenocarcinomas and SCCs is higher than in adjacent normal lung tissues. AP-1 is involved in signal transduction, and elevated levels of AP-1 may lead to the development of these types of NSCLC.

RFLP analysis of NSCLCs showed that there was a loss of heterozygosity in a chromosomal region containing the c-*raf*-1 protooncogene. These results suggest that this gene might play a role in the pathogenesis of both NSCLC and SCLC.

The protein product of the *bcl*-2 protooncogene protects cells from programmed cell death (apoptosis). Thus, the inappropriate expression of *bcl*-2 may permit neoplastic proliferation. The *bcl*-2 protein was detected in 20% of NSCLCs and in the basal cells of normal respiratory epithelium. Interestingly, patients with *bcl*-2 positive SCCs had significantly better survival that did those with *bcl*-2 negative tumors, suggesting a prognostic role for dysregulated *bcl*-2 expression (28).

The c-*myb* protooncogene encodes a nuclear protein of 75 kd that serves as a regulator of transcription (29). Analysis of several NSCLCs has shown defects in RNA transcription such that no c-*myb* transcripts were detected. These results suggest that aberrant c-*myb* expression may play a role in the generation of NSCLCs.

Other protooncogenes associated with human lung cancer include c-*fur*, c-*src*, c-*sis*, c-*fes*, and c-*kit*. The importance of these genes to the development of specific types of human lung cancer has not been determined fully, although in most cases the cellular function of the genes is known. One approach to determining the role of these and other protooncogenes in lung cancer development is to transfect the genes, either alone or in combination, into immortalized human bronchial epithelial cells in vitro and assess the ability of the genes to transform the cells. For example, Pfeifer et al. (30) found that the combination of transfected c-*myc* and c-*raf*-1 genes transforms cultured human bronchial epithelial cells into neoplastic cells that exhibit some phenotypic traits found in SCLCs. These results provide direct evidence that protooncogenes dysregulate the pathways of growth and differentiation of human lung epithelial cells and play an important role in human lung carcinogenesis.

A summary of oncogene changes in SCLC and NSCLC is given in Table 2.2.

TABLE 2.2. Oncogenes in Human Lung Cancer

	MECHANISM	HISTOLOGY
Protooncogenes		
Nuclear transcription factors		
c-*myc*	A, OE	S, N
N-*myc*	A, OE	S
L-*myc*	A, OE	S
c-*jun*	IE	S, N
c-*myb*	IE	S
G protein		
K-*ras*	M	N
Receptor protein kinases		
c-*erb*B-2 (HER2*neu*)	OE	N
c-*fms*	IE	N
c-*kit*	IE	S, N
c-*met*	OE	S, N
Cytoplasmic serine kinase		
c-*raf*-1	LOH	S
Apoptosis inhibitor		
bcl-2	IE	N

From Kalemkerian GP. Biology of lung cancer. Curr Opin Oncol 1994; 6:147–155.

Abbreviations. A, amplification; IE, inappropriate expression; LOH, loss of heterozygosity; M, mutation; N, non–small cell lung cancer; OE, overexpression; S, small cell lung cancer.

Tumor Suppressor Gene Inactivation

TUMOR SUPPRESSOR GENES IN SMALL CELL LUNG CANCER

The *p53* gene encodes a 53-kd nuclear phosphoprotein that serves as a transcription factor in cell cycle regulation (31). Elevated levels of the wild-type gene product inhibit growth, possibly through action as a checkpoint for DNA damage at the G0-G1 transition of cell division. Several mutant alleles of *p53* with particular single base substitutions encode proteins that confer altered cell growth regulatory properties.

Mutations in *p53* are the most common genetic aberrations in different types of cancers and are present in more than 75% of SCLCs. In one study loss of one *p53* allele and mutation of the other was found in 16 of 16 stage III-IV tumors and 3 of 6 stage I-II tumors (32). The allelic loss and/or mutation found in primary tumors also was observed in metastases, suggesting that alterations in *p53* are early events in the development of SCLC.

The first tumor suppressor gene discovered was retinoblastoma-1 (*Rb*-1), which predisposes to familial retinoblastoma (33). The *Rb*-1 gene encodes a DNA binding protein of 110 kd that is important in controlling cell division. Inactivation of the *Rb*-1 gene by deletion and loss of heterozygosity has been found in several cancers. Structural abnormalities within the *Rb* gene have been detected in approximately 15% of primary SCLC tumors and cell lines. Absence of *Rb* mRNA and p105 *Rb* protein, however, is common in SCLC cell lines.

Loss of heterozygosity in the tumor suppressor genes *MCC* (mutated in colon cancer) and *APC* (adenomatous polyposis coli) have been implicated in the pathogenesis of several cancers. Both genes are located on the long arm of chromosome 5 (5q21), a region often deleted in SCLC (34). More than 80% of SCLCs show allelic deletion of these genes, suggesting that they play a role in the pathogenesis of SCLC.

Deletions in the short arm of chromosome 3 are frequent events in SCLC with three regions between 3p21 and 3p25 being involved (35). Four genes—*D8*, *APEH*, *PTPG*, and *ACY1*—have been cloned from this region and their expression in SCLC cell lines compared with that in normal lung tissue. All are underexpressed to varying degrees, but the data are insufficient to establish them as tumor suppressor genes in SCLC.

TUMOR SUPPRESSOR GENES IN NON–SMALL CELL LUNG CANCER

Mutations in the *p53* gene are common molecular events in NSCLC (36). The frequency of mutation varies with the type of cancer: approximately 70% of SCCs and 40% of adenocarcinomas have *p53* mutations. Large cell lung carcinomas also carry *p53* mutations. The mutations have been found at many positions along the gene. Approximately 50% of the NSCLCs have been shown to carry G-C to T-A transversions in the *p53* gene (37). This mutation in *p53* is uncommon in other types of human cancer. Because various carcinogens in tobacco smoke, including the PAHs, have been shown to produce this mutation in DNA, it is likely that it is associated with the use of tobacco.

The prognostic significance of *p53* mutations in patients with NSCLC remains controversial. Immunohistochemical detection of p53 protein in tissues and cells is considered a marker for *p53* mutation because the half-life of the mutant protein is much longer than that of the wild-type protein. The immunohistochemical accumulation of p53 protein in tissues appears to be predictive of poor prognosis in patients with both early-stage and late-stage NSCLC.

p53 Mutations have been detected in preneoplastic lesions of the lung, suggesting that they occur in the early stages of lung carcinogenesis (38). This raises the possibility that screening for *p53* mutations could be a feasible approach to the early detection of lung cancer, and that transfection of a normal *p53* gene into these lesions might inhibit their progression.

The role, if any, of the *Rb*-1 gene in the development of NSCLC is unknown, but no abnormalities in *Rb*-1 were found in several NSCLC-derived cell lines (39). Anti–*Rb*-1 peptide antibodies precipitated *Rb*-1 protein in eight of nine NSCLC-derived cell lines; thus, at least in cell lines, the *Rb*-1 protein is expressed.

The *nm23* gene located on the long arm of chromosome 17 encodes a nucleoside diphosphate kinase (40). Relatively low amounts of *nm23* mRNA and the kinase have been found to correlate with high metasta-

TABLE 2.3. Tumor Suppressor Genes in Human Lung Cancer

Gene	Mechanism	Histology
p53	I, M	S, N
Rb	I	S
APC	LOH, ?	S, N
MCC	LOH, ?	S, N
nm23	LOH, LE	N
MST-1	LOH	N
MST-2	LOH	N
3p	?	S, N

From Kalemkerian GP. Biology of lung cancer. Curr Opin Oncol 1994; 6:147–155.

Abbreviations. I, inactivation; LE, low expression; LOH, loss of heterozygosity; M, mutation; N, non–small cell lung cancer; S, small cell lung cancer.

tic potential in numerous tumors. Somatic deletion of an allele of *nm23* has been detected in adenocarcinomas of the lung, but there appears to be no correlation between the presence of nm23 protein and survival rates.

A putative tumor suppressor gene or genes has been localized to human chromosome 9p21, based on its frequent deletion in many cancer types. The gene, *MTS-1* (multiple tumor suppressor–1), encodes p16, an inhibitor of cyclin dependent kinase 4 (41). *MTS-1* is frequently deleted in NSCLC and in cell lines derived from NSCLC but not in SCLC (42, 43).

A summary of tumor suppressor gene changes in SCLC and NSCLC is presented in Table 2.3.

ANIMAL MODELS FOR STUDYING LUNG CANCER

STRAIN A MICE

Strain A mice show a high incidence of spontaneous lung tumors. These tumors may be found in animals as young as 3 to 4 months of age with a steady increase to nearly 100% by 24 months of age (44). Most animals develop at least one tumor in their lungs by the age of 24 months, and some have two to three tumors. Male and female mice are equally susceptible to lung tumor development. Other inbred mouse strains are relatively less susceptible to the development of spontaneous lung tumors with the order of susceptibility of strain A being greater, in descending order, than SWR ("Swiss"), BALB/c, C3H, and C57BL.

Lung tumors in strain A mice arise in the peripheral lung, and most tumors are situated just below the visceral pleura. Grossly, or after fixation, the tumors are yellowish-white, discreet nodules that can be enumerated easily with the naked eye or under a dissecting microscope. Histologically, the tumors appear as solid, papillary, or mixed lesions, and they resemble bronchoalveolar carcinomas in the human lung. The tumors are devoid of a connective tissue capsule and infiltrate and compress the surrounding pulmonary tissue. Ultrastructural and immunohistochemical studies indicate that most lung tumors in mice, including those in strain A mice, are derived from type II cells of the alveolar epithelium (45–47). Some tumors, however, appear to arise from pulmonary Clara cells (48). Recent histopathologic studies in chemically treated mice indicate that lung tumor development is a multistage process that proceeds, in order of occurrence, from hyperplasia to adenoma to carcinoma arising within adenoma to carcinoma (49). Approximately one third of carcinomas metastasize to other organ sites, most commonly the mediastinal lymph nodes, liver, kidney, and heart.

Activation of the K-*ras* protooncogene is an early and frequent event in the development of both spontaneous and chemically induced lung tumors in strain A mice (50). Early lesions with as few as 50 to 100 cells, and more than 90% of adenomas and carcinomas, contain an activated K-*ras* gene. In spontaneous tumors, point mutations in codons 12 and 61 of the gene occur randomly. In chemically induced tumors, the site of mutation in codons 12 and 61 tends to correlate with the formation of a specific carcinogen to DNA adduct (50–55). For example, BaP and 5-methylchrysene induce predominantly G-C to T-A transversions in the first nucleotide of codon 12, which correlates with the formation of diol epoxide adducts in DNA. Methylating agents such as methylnitrosourea, *N*-nitrosodimethylamine (NDMA), and NNK induce predominately G-C to A-T transitions in the second nucleotide of codon 12, which correlates with the formation of O^6-methylguanine adducts in DNA. In contrast, most mutations induced by ethylating agents such as *N*-ethyl-*N*-nitrosourea and *N*-nitrosodiethylamine (NDEA) occur in codon 61. These mutations may result from the formation of thymidine adducts in DNA.

Interestingly, the high susceptibility of strain A mice to lung tumor development appears to result, at least in part, from the presence of an RFLP in the K-*ras* gene (56). Polymerase chain reaction (PCR)–DNA sequence analysis revealed a 37 base pair (bp) deletion in the second intron of the K-*ras* gene in normal lung and in lung tumors of strain A mice (57). This deletion appears to be the binding site of one or more proteins that control expression of the gene (58). Other lung tumor susceptible mouse strains have the deletion, but resistant strains do not. Molecular studies of spontaneous and chemically induced lung tumors in F1 hybrid mice produced by crossing strain A mice (high lung tumor susceptible) with C3H mice (low lung tumor susceptible) revealed that mutations in codons 12 or 61 were restricted to the K-*ras* allele derived from the strain A parent (57, 59). The K-*ras* allele from the strain A parent is expressed at much higher levels than that from the C3H parent, indicating that tumor development may involve selection of cells containing the activated strain A allele. These data indicate that in mouse lung tumorigenesis, the K-*ras* gene is a tumor susceptibility gene as well as an oncogene.

Other molecular alterations detected in strain A mouse lung tumors include c-*myc* overexpression without amplification, and decreased expression of the *Rb* and growth arrest specific–3 (*gas-3*) genes (60). Mutations in the *p53* gene are uncommon and tend to occur only in carcinomas. A recent study revealed a region on chromosome 4 of mouse lung tumors immediately distal to the alpha interferon locus as the likely domain of a novel tumor suppressor gene (61). This region is syntenic to the location of the *MST-1* gene on human chromosome 9p21-22, suggesting the involvement of the mouse homologue of *MTS-1* in the development of mouse lung tumors.

The strain A mouse, compared with other inbred mouse strains, also is highly susceptible to the induction of lung tumors by chemical carcinogens; it has been used extensively as a mouse lung tumor bioassay for assessing the carcinogenic activity of more than 400 environmental chemicals (44, 62, 63). The lung tumor bioassay is of 6 months' duration and can distinguish twofold differences in the carcinogenic potential of compounds from several chemical classes. Specifically, the assay is sensitive to PAHs, nitrosamines, nitrosoureas, carbamates, aflatoxin, certain metals, hydrazines, and others, but it is relatively insensitive to aromatic amines, aliphatic halides, and other compounds that are carcinogenic in the rodent liver.

Many carcinogens in tobacco smoke, such as NNK and BaP, are potent inducers of lung tumors in strain A mice with amounts as low as 1 to 20 μmol per mouse required to produce a positive carcinogenic response. Most strong carcinogens induce tumors in a single intraperitoneal injection, whereas weaker agents are given repeatedly over a period of 8 weeks.

In addition to its use in carcinogen detection, the strain A mouse lung tumor model has been employed extensively for the identification of inhibitors of chemical carcinogenesis (64). A number of chemopreventive agents have been shown to inhibit chemically induced lung tumors in strain A mice. In most instances inhibition of lung tumorigenesis has been correlated with effects of the chemopreventive agent on the metabolic activation/detoxification of carcinogens. To date, few chemopreventive agents have been shown to inhibit lung tumorigenesis in strain A mice when administered after the carcinogen, i.e., during the promotion and progression stages of tumor development.

SYRIAN GOLDEN HAMSTER

The Syrian golden hamster is resistant to respiratory infections and inflammation and has a low incidence of spontaneous pulmonary tumors. Therefore, it has been used fairly extensively as a model for induction of respiratory tract tumors (65–67). Bioassays of cigarette smoke in the Syrian golden hamster have predominantly produced tumors and other changes in the larynx with relatively few lung tumors (68). This result occurs partially because of a lack of inhalation of the smoke. Smoke inhalation is not a practical method for induction of lung tumors in rodents.

Among the carcinogenic components of cigarette smoke, nitrosamines and PAHs have been employed most widely for lung and tracheal tumor induction in Syrian golden hamsters. NDEA has been used frequently. Regardless of the route of administration, tumors develop in the trachea, oral cavity, nasal cavity, and larynx, with a lower incidence in the stem bronchi and peripheral lung. Tracheal tumors are induced readily with relatively low doses of NDEA given subcutaneously. Higher doses can be employed to induce not only tracheal tumors but also a relatively high incidence of lung tumors. The spectrum of tumors induced by nitrosamines in Syrian golden hamsters generally consists of papillomas, papillary polyps, and SCCs in the trachea, whereas adenomas, adenocarcinomas, and SCCs have been reported in the lungs. Two cell types—Clara cells and amine precursor uptake and decarboxylation cells—have been identified as targets for carcinogenesis by nitrosamines in the Syrian golden hamster. Invasive cancers in a localized area of the trachea also have been induced by direct catheter application of *N*-methyl-*N*-nitrosourea, a synthetic carcinogen not known to occur in tobacco smoke or the human environment.

Intratracheal instillation of BaP and Fe_2O_3 has been used to induce tumors of the lung in Syrian golden hamsters. Fe_2O_3 enhances the carcinogenicity of BaP by delaying its clearance and by inducing some cell injury, proliferation, and hyperplasia. Single or multiple intratracheal instillations of BaP and Fe_2O_3 caused bronchogenic adenomas, adenocarcinomas, and SCCs of the lung. Papillary polyps, papillomas, and SCCs were produced in the trachea. Dose-response relationships have been established. Other PAHs have also been shown to be tumorigenic in the respiratory tract of Syrian golden hamsters after intratracheal administration. Because of its complexity, this model is not used widely at present.

RAT

The induction of lung tumors in the F344 rat can be accomplished readily by treatment with NNK (69–71). All routes of administration tested thus far, including subcutaneous injection, administration in the drinking water, swabbing in the oral cavity, and instillation into the bladder, result predominantly in tumors of the lung. The subcutaneous route has been used most widely. Injections of NNK in trioctanoin are given 3 times weekly for 20 weeks, and the animals are killed 2 years after the start of injections. At higher doses tumors of the nasal cavity and liver are also observed. Lower doses that cumulatively approach the lifetime exposure of cigarette smokers to NNK induce predominantly lung tumors. The tumors are mainly adenomas and adenocarcinomas, with the latter predominating at the higher doses. When NNK is given to rats in the drinking water for life, pancreatic acinar and ductal tumors are observed in addition to lung tumors.

Dose-response studies have shown a correlation between O^6-methylguanine formation in Clara cells and lung tumor incidence, suggesting a cause and effect relationship. However, pathologic evaluation of the tumors indicates that they arise predominantly from the type II cells. DNA pyridyloxobutylation by NNK in Clara cells and type II cells has not been studied extensively, but various lines of evidence indicate that this process is also important in the induction of lung tumors by NNK in the rat.

The rat NNK lung tumor induction model has several advantages, including a well-characterized dose-response relationship, ease of tumor induction by subcutaneous injection or drinking water routes, and relevance to humans because of extensive NNK exposure, specifically in smokers.

Induction of lung tumors in rats by PAHs requires direct application either by intratracheal instillation or lung implantation of the PAH dissolved in a mixture of beeswax and trioctanoin (66, 72). A variety of PAHs have been tested using the latter protocol, with BaP showing the highest activity of those commonly encountered in respiratory environments. These studies have produced predominantly SCC.

BIOMARKERS SPECIFICALLY RELATED TO LUNG CARCINOGENS

The metabolic activation and detoxification of lung carcinogens vary in different people. Both higher extents of metabolic activation and lower extents of detoxification presumably are associated with a higher risk for lung cancer. Biomarkers, which are quantitative measures of parameters reflecting carcinogen metabolic activation or detoxification, are now becoming available (73–76).

Biomarkers related to the uptake and metabolic activation of PAHs and nitrosamines, the major lung carcinogens to which humans are exposed, have been developed. These include urinary metabolites, DNA adducts, and hemoglobin adducts. Urinary metabolites can provide a profile of metabolic activation and detoxification of a carcinogen. Adducts are a measure of the internal dose of the carcinogen. Although DNA is considered the important target in carcinogenesis, proteins such as hemoglobin, because of their availability, have been employed as surrogates for adduct measurement.

PAH-DNA adducts in human tissues have been determined by a variety of methods, including immunoassay, ^{32}P-postlabeling, synchronous fluorescence spectroscopy, and other fluorescence techniques, as well as gas chromatography–mass spectrometry. Among these, immunoassay and ^{32}P-postlabeling have been applied most widely; however, they lack specificity to individual PAH carcinogens, which makes results difficult to evaluate. The more specific methods have been employed less extensively but have resulted in the identification of a BaP DNA adduct in lung tissue from smokers. Gas chromatography–mass spectrometry also has been applied for characterization of PAH-hemoglobin adducts, but quantitation is lacking at present. Presently available data on PAH-DNA adducts suggest that their levels are higher in smokers than in nonsmokers. Biomarkers of NNK uptake and metabolism have the advantage of being specific to tobacco smoke, because NNK is formed from nicotine, whereas PAHs are present in any mixture resulting from incomplete combustion of organic matter. Presently available biomarkers for NNK include hemoglobin adducts, DNA adducts, and urinary metabolites. The hemoglobin adducts and DNA adducts are formed by metabolic activation of NNK and are not entirely specific to this carcinogen because they also are produced by activation of NNN; the latter is not a strong lung carcinogen. The hemoglobin and DNA adducts are determined by gas chromatography–mass spectrometry of 4-hydroxy-1-(3-pyridyl)-1-butanone, which is released upon hydrolysis. DNA adduct levels are higher in the lungs of smokers than nonsmokers. Hemoglobin adducts are higher in some smokers than in nonsmokers, and they are elevated in most snuff users. Because the hemoglobin adducts of NNK and NNN result from metabolic activation, they could be biomarkers of risk.

Urinary metabolites of NNK are readily quantifiable and provide important information about the dose and metabolic activation of this lung carcinogen. In rodents and primates, NNK is metabolized extensively, and virtually all the metabolites are excreted in the urine within 24 hours. The major metabolite of NNK in almost all animal and human tissues is its carbonyl reduction product NNAL, which also is a potent lung carcinogen in rodents. NNAL and its glucuronide diastereomers (NNAL-Gluc) account for approximately 25% of the dose of NNK in primates. In humans NNAL and NNAL-Gluc are excreted in urine, with the latter generally predominating. NNAL and NNAL-Gluc have been quantified in human urine using gas chromatography with a nitrosamine selective detector. The total levels of NNAL and NNAL-Gluc provide an estimate of NNK exposure in humans. An interesting and potentially useful parameter is the ratio of NNAL-Gluc to NNAL, which has been shown to vary at least 10-fold in smokers. NNAL-Gluc is presumed to be a detoxification product of NNAL; consequently, this ratio might provide a measure of detoxification potential upon exposure to NNK.

NNAL and NNAL-Gluc in urine can provide information on the exposure of nonsmokers to environmental tobacco smoke. Subjects exposed to sidestream tobacco smoke have increased levels of NNAL and NNAL-Gluc in their urine, providing evidence that nonsmokers exposed to sidestream smoke take up and metabolize a lung carcinogen (77). It is interesting to note that NNK and NNAL induce primarily pulmonary adenocarcinoma in rodents, the prevalent tumor type observed in nonsmokers exposed to environmental tobacco smoke.

Although biomarkers of carcinogen uptake, metabolic activation, and detoxification have not yet been applied in large epidemiologic studies of lung cancer, the presently available results from pilot and transitional studies indicate that they will be important in understanding the mechanisms of lung cancer induction. These biomarkers are based on metabolic transformations of established lung carcinogens and thus can potentially provide essential specific information relevant to lung cancer etiology.

Another approach to assessing risk upon exposure to lung carcinogens is consideration of the enzymes that metabolically activate and detoxify them (75, 76). Cytochrome *P450* enzymes are most commonly involved in the metabolic activation of carcinogens. Cytochrome *P450 1A1* is involved in the activation of BaP and perhaps other PAHs, whereas cytochrome *P450 1A2* is involved in the activation of aromatic amines. Cytochrome *P450 2E1* is important in the metabolic activation of NDMA but not of NNK. Cytochrome *P450 1A1* is inducible by exposure to tobacco smoke, and correlations have been observed between the activity of this enzyme and PAH-DNA adducts in smokers' lungs. Polymorphisms in the cytochrome *P450 1A1* and *2E1* genes have been associated with lung cancer in certain populations, presumably reflecting increased carcinogen metabolic activation by some genotypes. Another cytochrome *P450* enzyme that has been studied in connection with lung cancer risk is cytochrome *P450 2D6*, which metabolizes the drug debrisoquine. Extensive metabolizers of debrisoquine are at higher risk for lung cancer according to some epidemiologic studies, whereas others have found no relationship. Currently, the relationship of these findings to metabolism of lung carcinogens is obscure. GSTs are involved in the detoxification of metabolites of BaP and other PAHs. Human GSTs can be classified into at least three genetically distinct groups: μ, α, and π. *GST1* is a mu class enzyme. The deficient phenotype of *GST1* has been associated with increased risk for lung cancer, presumably because of less facile detoxification of PAHs in tobacco smoke. Collectively, these biomarkers may have great promise for assessing individual risk for cancer development upon exposure to carcinogens. This approach has become known as molecular epidemiology.

CHEMOPREVENTION OF LUNG CANCER

Chemoprevention is the use of naturally occurring or synthetic compounds to arrest or reverse the carcinogenic process. Intervention with chemopreventive agents at an early stage in carcinogenesis is theoretically more appealing than attempting to eradicate fully developed tumors with chemotherapeutic drugs. Thus, carcinogenesis can be viewed as a continuum from early molecular changes to the appearance and metastasis of tumors. Chemoprevention and chemotherapy merge when viewed along this continuum, with chemoprevention being the more attractive option in high-risk groups.

Intervention with chemopreventive agents may be a plausible way to lengthen life or prevent lung cancer in smokers who are addicted to nicotine. The use of chemopreventive approaches in smokers would be limited to those who had failed smoking cessation programs with nicotine therapy as an adjunct but who were still highly motivated to decrease their cancer risk. Chemoprevention would have the most promise in individuals who had been smoking for a relatively short time, e.g., less than 15 years. Chemopreventive agents must necessarily be nontoxic. Because there are no known chemopreventive agents with lengthy persistent effects, they would need to be consumed regularly, probably for life, unless an individual's risk pattern had changed markedly.

Numerous chemopreventive agents have been identified in animal studies, and there presently are naturally occurring and synthetic compounds of multiple structural types that can inhibit cancer development in various organs. Wattenberg (78) and others (79) classify chemopreventive agents generally into two categories: blocking agents and suppressing agents. Blocking agents interfere with the metabolic activation process or enhance detoxification of carcinogens such that the overall result is diminished DNA damage. Examples of blocking agents include terpenes, organo-sulfides, aromatic isothiocyanates, indoles, dithiole-thiones, phenols, flavones, tannins, ellagic acid, curcumin, coumarins, conjugated dienoic linoleic acids, antioxidants, organoselenium compounds, and various nucleophiles. Suppressing agents are compounds that can delay or reverse the carcinogenic process once genetic damage has occurred, essentially by interfering with the promotion and progression stages. Examples of suppressing agents include retinoids, beta carotene, vitamin A, protease inhibitors, inhibitors of the arachidonic acid cascade, difluoromethylornithine, dehydroepiandrosterone, monoterpenes, aromatic isothiocyanates, sodium cyanate, organoselenium compounds, inorganic selenium compounds, and inositol hexaphosphate.

Many of the these compounds are naturally occurring plant constituents. The ability of these structurally diverse compounds to inhibit cancer in animal studies is consistent with epidemiologic evidence that has shown that people who consume diets rich in vegetables are at lower risk for cancer than those who do not (80). Thus, an attractive approach to chemoprevention is isolation and identification of specific chemopreventive compounds from vegetables. It is essential that such compounds have low toxicity because they would be consumed daily.

Chemoprevention of lung cancer in humans would necessarily entail inhibition of carcinogenesis by NNK and PAHs. There are already a substantial number of compounds that have been shown to inhibit lung carcinogenesis induced by NNK and BaP in rats and mice. Phenethyl isothiocyanate (PEITC) is a relatively nontoxic compound that occurs in watercress as a thioglucoside conjugate. It is released upon chewing. PEITC is an effective inhibitor of lung cancer induced by NNK in both rats and mice (81, 82). Its mode of action is inhibition of metabolic activation of NNK by selectively inhibiting cytochrome *P450* enzymes. It also induces *UDP*-glucuronosyltransferase activity, resulting in increased conjugation of NNAL. PEITC does not inhibit carcinogenesis by BaP, but a related naturally occurring isothiocyanate, benzyl isothiocyanate, is a good inhibitor of BaP-induced lung tumorigenesis in mice (83). A combination of PEITC and benzyl isothiocyanate inhibits lung tumorigenesis by a combination of NNK and BaP. Other isothiocyanates are known inhibitors of tumor development at other sites. Notable among them is sulforaphane, a constituent of broccoli (84).

Some of the other compounds shown to inhibit lung carcinogenesis by NNK include butylated hydroxyanisole, an antioxidant used in food preservation; d-limonene, a constituent of orange juice and other citrus products; and diallyl sulfide, a constituent of garlic. Inhibition of NNK carcinogenesis also has been observed in animals treated with green and black teas, as well as with their major polyphenolic constituents. Inhibitors of lung tumorigenesis induced by BaP include β-naphthoflavone, butylated hydroxyanisole, ethoxyquin, diallyl sulfide, and *myo*-inositol. It seems likely that properly designed combinations of some of these inhibitors will be effective chemopreventive agents against lung cancer in humans.

A number of human trials are already in progress, and several of these have centered on beta carotene as a potential chemopreventive agent for lung cancer. The initial results from a study in Finland are not encouraging, however; beta carotene actually was found to have some enhancing effect on lung cancer, whereas vitamin E and a combination of beta carotene and vitamin E had no inhibitory effect (85). However, the results of this trial were consistent with animal studies, which have not shown efficacy against lung cancer for these two agents.

ESOPHAGEAL CANCER

Esophageal cancer in humans occurs worldwide with a variable geographic distribution. A recent estimate has placed it seventh in order of cancer occurrence in both sexes (86). There is a higher incidence of the disease in males, with a male to female ratio of 2:1 or higher. The highest incidence rates are found in China, Iran, parts of Central Asia, and the Transkei region of South Africa (87). The disease occurs consistently among the poor in most areas of the world where the diet is restricted and nutritional imbalance is common.

Worldwide, more than 90% of esophageal cancers are SCCs. The characteristics of this neoplasm include keratinization, with occasional keratin pearl formation, and intracellular bridges. About 5% of esophageal cancers are adenocarcinomas. Adenocarcinomas usually arise from Barrett's esophagus, a condition in which the normal squamous epithelium of the esophagus is replaced by a glandular epithelium. The remaining 5% of esophageal neoplasms represent metastases from other organs.

CAUSATIVE FACTORS

Excessive use of tobacco has been implicated repeatedly as a principal factor in the etiology of SCC of the esophagus (88, 89). The presence in tobacco tars and cigarette smoke of chemical carcinogens such as PAHs, nitrosamines, aromatic amines, and others, as well as promoting agents such as various aldehydes, phenols, and related compounds, all undoubtedly contribute to the disease. Extensive histologic studies of esophageal specimens taken from tobacco smokers and nonsmokers have revealed smoking-related histopathologic changes in the esophagus similar to those observed in the trachea and bronchus (90).

The chewing of tobacco, betel, or combinations of these substances with lime is common is some regions of the world, especially in India, Sri Lanka, Burma, and other Southeast Asian countries. They probably are responsible for the high incidence in these regions of cancer in the oral cavity and, possibly, the esophagus. Chronic irritation of the mucosa by constituents of tobacco, betel, or lime damages the epithelium and stimulates preneoplastic and neoplastic changes in the epithelium (87, 91).

Epidemiologic studies provide strong evidence that alcohol consumption increases the risk of SCC in the esophagus of tobacco smokers (92). Ethanol is an effective solvent, especially for fat soluble compounds, and may increase the penetration of tobacco carcinogens into esophageal epithelial cells. It has been shown to modify the metabolic activation and detoxification of carcinogens. Ethanol also increases cellular exposure to oxidants, thus increasing the risk of DNA damage and neoplastic transformation. Finally, individuals who consume significant quantities of alcohol tend to be nutritionally deficient and may lack cancer inhibitory substances in their diet. In addition to the ethanol, various congeners and contaminants in alcoholic beverages may be carcinogenic; these substances include certain nitrosamines, mycotoxins, urethane, and various tannins.

Contaminants in foods and water also have been indicted as causative agents in the etiology of SCC of the esophagus. Grains and other foods are frequently contaminated with fungi in areas where esophageal cancer is common. Some of the more common fungal species, e.g., *Fusarium* and *Alternaria*, produce toxins that are both mutagenic and carcinogenic. These and other fungal species may also promote the formation of nitrosamines in the stomach by their ability to reduce nitrates to nitrites and to degrade proteins into amines. Fungal infection and invasion in esophageal tissue is another type of local irritation that may contribute to neoplastic changes in the esophagus. Finally, the drinking of hot beverages such as tea is thought to contribute to the occurrence of esophageal cancer.

Extensive research in China and South Africa has suggested that N-nitroso compounds and their precursors are probable etiologic factors of esophageal cancer in these high-incidence areas (93). Trace amounts of nitrosamines, especially NDMA, NDEA, N-nitrosomethylbenzylamine (NMBA), and N-(1-methylacetonyl-N-3-methylbutyl)nitrosamine, have been identified in the cornbread and pickled vegetables consumed in high-incidence regions of China. Although the levels of these nitrosamines in food are usually less that 10 parts per billion (ppb), their precursors, specifically nitrates, nitrites, and secondary or tertiary amines, are widely distributed in foodstuffs and in the environment. Under acidic conditions, N-nitroso compounds can easily be formed in the stomach by the reaction of nitrates and amines. The potential role of N-nitroso compounds in the etiology of esophageal SCC is discussed below.

Other factors associated with an increased risk of SCC of the esophagus include vitamin and trace mineral deficiencies. With respect to vitamins, an increased risk of esophageal cancer has been associated with deficiencies in vitamin A (or its precursor, beta carotene), vitamin C, folic acid, vitamin E, vitamin B_{12}, and riboflavin. Plasma levels of these vitamins tend to be lower in patients with esophageal cancer than in noncancer patients, and/or in patients from areas of high esophageal cancer risk. Comparative studies of trace elements between areas of high and low incidence of esophageal carcinoma revealed an inverse relationship between mortality caused by esophageal cancer and the levels of zinc, selenium, molybdenum, and other trace elements in crops, soil, and foodstuffs (93).

There is an emerging body of literature that suggests a role for the human papilloma virus (HPV) in the etiology of SCC of the esophagus. Early studies found either no HPV or a low frequency of HPV involvement in esophageal carcinomas. However, recent studies that used more sensitive molecular techniques have detected either HPV-16 or HPV-18 in approximately 15% of esophageal tumor samples, and 10% of tumors harbored a novel HPV genotype (94). The exact mechanism by which HPV contributes to carcinogenesis of the esophagus has yet to be elucidated.

NITROSAMINES AND ESOPHAGEAL CANCER

In rats, nitrosamines are the most powerful and versatile esophageal carcinogens known (95–97). Among all carcinogens tested, only nitrosamines can readily induce high incidences of esophageal tumors. This result can frequently be achieved with relatively low doses and is often independent of the route of administration. The high sensitivity of the rat esophagus to tumor induction by nitrosamines has been confirmed repeatedly in hundreds of experiments from various laboratories worldwide. In extensive studies by Lijinsky (96), 51% of 130 nitrosamines tested induced esophageal tumors in rats, and the esophagus was the most common target organ for tumor induction in these compounds. Curiously, in Syrian golden hamsters, esophageal tumors are not induced by nitrosamines. Some representative structures of nitrosamines that induce esophageal tumors in rats are shown in Figure 2.6.

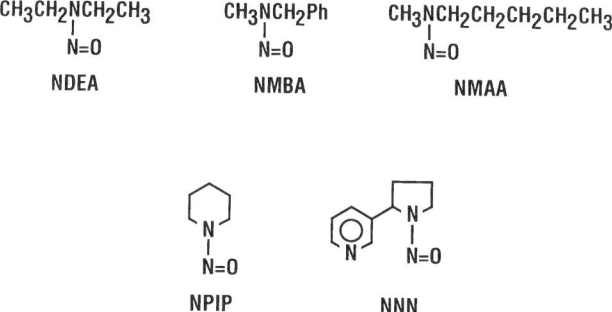

FIGURE 2.6. Structures of some esophageal carcinogens.

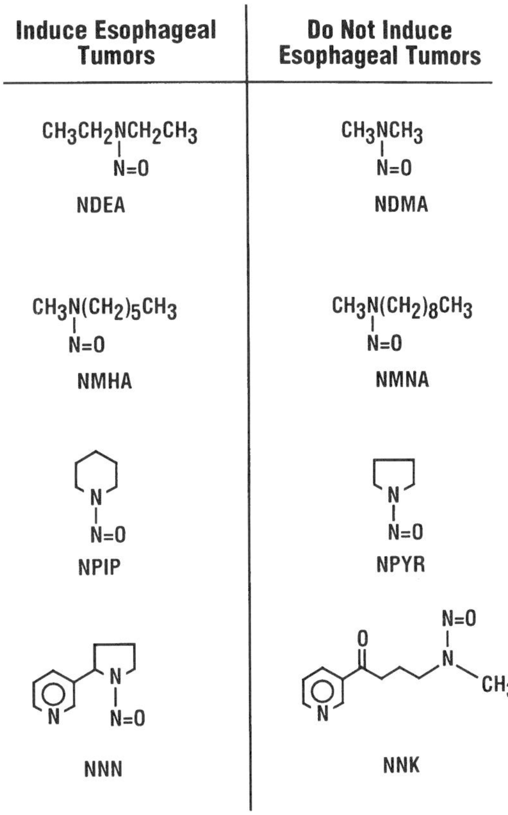

FIGURE 2.7. Some nitrosamines with contrasting carcinogenic activities toward the rat esophagus.

The structure-activity relationships among nitrosamine esophageal carcinogens are interesting. Some pairs of nitrosamines with differing organoselectivities in the rat are illustrated in Figure 2.7. Whereas NDEA causes tumors of both the esophagus and liver in rats, the lower homologue, NDMA, causes only liver tumors in chronic dosing experiments and never affects the esophagus. Among unsymmetrical methylalkylnitrosamines, the lower homologues with alkyl chain lengths up to six, such as N-nitrosomethylhexylamine (NMHA), all induce esophageal tumors in rats, whereas members of the series with seven or more carbons, such as N-nitrosomethylnonylamine (NMNA), do not. The latter compounds, which have an even number of carbons in the alkyl chain, are frequently bladder carcinogens, whereas the odd-numbered members induce liver and lung tumors. The cyclic nitrosamine N-nitrosopiperidine (NPIP) produces tumors of both the esophagus and liver, whereas the lower homologue N-nitrosopyrrolidine (NPYR) causes only liver tumors in rats. Higher cyclic homologues such as N-nitroso-hexamethyleneimine are effective esophageal carcinogens. The tobacco specific nitrosamine NNN causes esophageal tumors in rats, whereas the related compound NNK never produces tumors of the esophagus.

The high carcinogenicity of nitrosamines toward the rat esophagus has led to the plausible hypothesis that these compounds could be involved as etiologic agents in cancer of the esophagus in humans (98–100). Studies carried out in northern China, which has the highest incidence of esophageal cancer in the world, have demonstrated the presence of low levels of several nitrosamines in food consumed in Linxian County, one of the highest incidence areas. However, the presence of substantial amounts of known esophageal carcinogens has not been confirmed. Other investigations in this high-risk area have indicated that there is elevated endogenous nitrosation of amines, as measured by the presence in urine of nitrosoproline, a noncarcinogenic nitrosamine. These results suggest that carcinogenic nitrosamines may be formed to a higher extent in people living in the areas of China having higher incidences of esophageal cancer, compared with those living in the lower risk areas. Further studies showed that esophageal cancer mortality rates in 69 counties of China were positively and significantly associated with urinary levels of nitrosamino acids. Analysis of esophageal tissue indicated elevated levels of O^6-methylguanine in people from the high-risk area. Collectively, the results indicate that nitrosamines play a role as etiologic factors in cancer of the esophagus in China.

One of the major causes of esophageal cancer worldwide is smoking, especially in combination with heavy alcohol consumption. Nitrosamines are the most prevalent esophageal carcinogens in cigarette smoke, and NNN, an established esophageal carcinogen in the rat, occurs in the highest concentration. The levels of NNN in cigarettes (usually 100 to 200 ng per cigarette) are such that the dose in a lifetime of smoking is significant (approximately 60 mg). NDEA is another potent esophageal carcinogen in cigarette smoke, but its levels are much lower than those of NNN (101).

Metabolism and DNA Adduct Formation of Esophageal Carcinogens

All presently available data indicate that α-hydroxylation is the major metabolic activation pathway of nitrosamines, which are carcinogenic to the esophagus. This process for NMBA is illustrated in Figure 2.8. Microsomes isolated from the epithelium of the esophagus contain cytochrome *P450* enzymes that can catalyze the α-hydroxylation of NMBA (102). Hydroxylation of the methylene carbon produces the α-hydroxy derivative 1, which spontaneously decomposes to the electrophile methanediazohydroxide (Fig. 2.8, *3*) and benzaldehyde (Fig. 2.8, *4*). Methanediazohydroxide methylates DNA to form the methylation adducts 7-methylguanine and O^6-methylguanine. Hydroxylation of the methyl carbon of NMBA produces formaldehyde (Fig. 2.8, *5*) and benzyldiazohydroxide (Fig. 2.8, *6*). Benzylation of DNA has not been reported. Both pathways of NMBA metabolism have been detected in esophageal epithelial microsomes. The methylene hydroxylation pathway far exceeds methyl hydroxylation. Metabolism of NMBA by esophageal epithelial microsomes was more extensive than metabolism of the non–esophageal carcinogen NDMA. In rats treated intravenously with NMBA, levels of 7-methylguanine and O^6-methylguanine were higher in the esophagus than in any other tissue (103). Treatment with NMBA depletes O^6-alkylguanine-DNA alkyltransferase activity in the esophagus, which presumably leads to the accumulation of O^6-methylguanine (104). Although limited studies have been carried out on adduct persistence in the esophagus, the available data indicate that preferential metabolic activation of NMBA in the esophagus plays a role in its high carcinogenicity toward this tissue.

The metabolism of NMAA by rat and human esophageal microsomes results in α-hydroxylation at both the methyl and methylene carbons; rat esophagus also can hydroxylate the other four carbons of the alkyl group (105, 106). Methylation of esophageal DNA, but not pentylation, has been detected. Structure-activity studies of methylalkyl nitrosamines have shown that formation of 7-methylguanine and O^6-methylguanine in the rat esophagus closely follows carcinogenic activity and is greatest for methylalkylnitrosamines with alkyl chains of four to six carbons (107). Together with investigations of NMBA, the studies of methylalkyl nitrosamines suggest that formation of O^6-methylguanine in the rat esophagus is closely associated with tumor induction.

The metabolism of NNN by the rat esophagus proceeds as illustrated in Figure 2.9 (108–110). *N*-oxidation to produce NNN-*N*-oxide is a detoxification pathway whose extent is minor. The major metabolic pathway is α-hydroxylation at the 2′ position, which leads to the unstable intermediates 1 and 3, and ultimately to pyridyloxobutylation of DNA as well as production of metabolites 5, 8, and 9. α-Hydroxylation at the 5′ position also occurs, leading to hydroxy acid 10, but it is not known to result in DNA adduct formation. The ratio of 2′ hydroxylation to 5′ hydroxylation is ap-

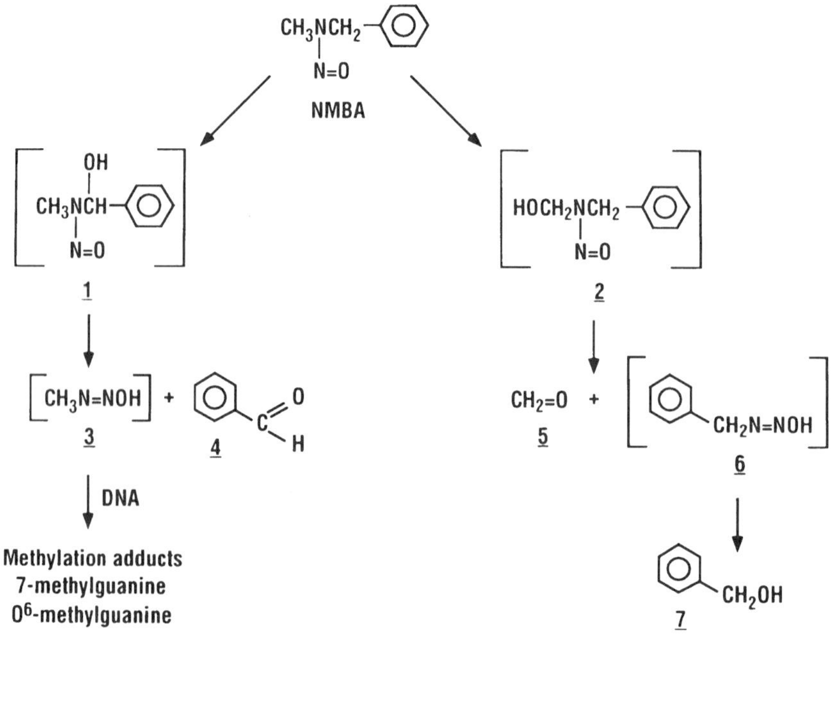

FIGURE 2.8. Metabolism of *N*-nitrosomethylbenzylamine.

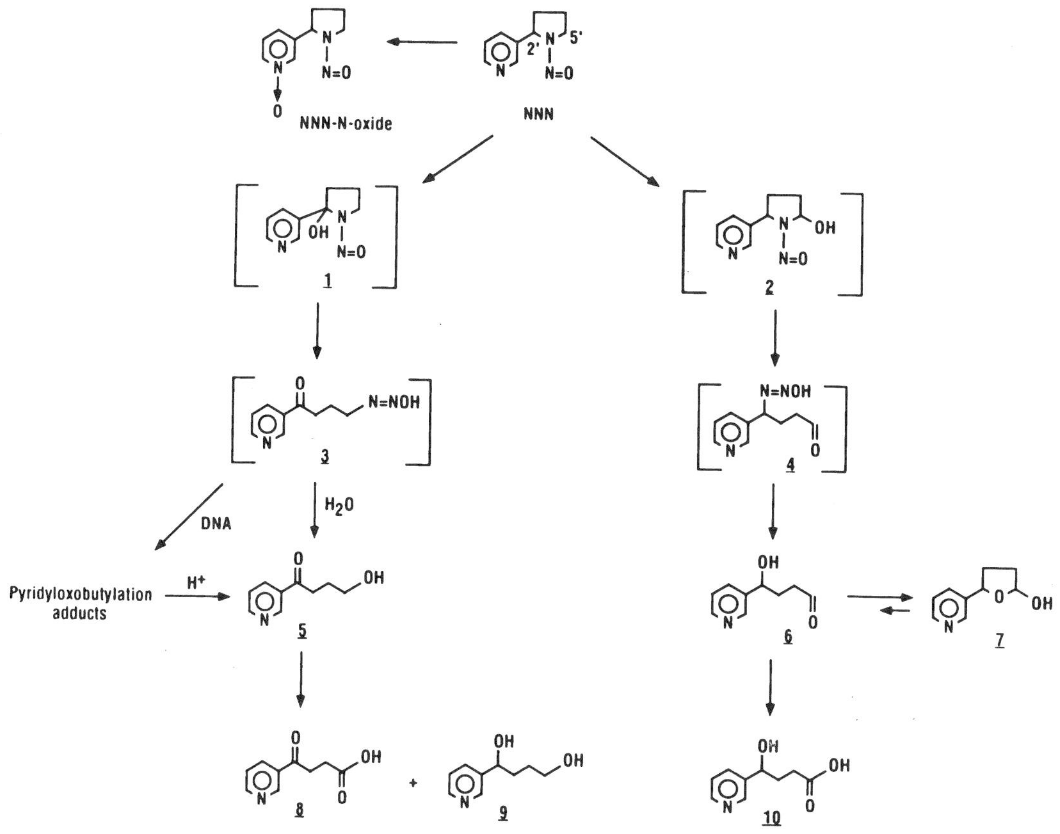

FIGURE 2.9. Metabolism of N'-nitrosonornicotine.

proximately 3 in the rat esophagus. Per gram of tissue, α-hydroxylation of NNN in the rat esophagus exceeds that in the liver, as does the ratio of 2′ hydroxylation to 5′ hydroxylation. Thus, efficient metabolic activation of NNN by 2′ hydroxylation appears to be important in its esophageal carcinogenicity. Interestingly, NNK, which does not induce esophageal tumors in the rat, is detoxified extensively by N-oxidation in the rat esophagus and is metabolically activated to a lesser extent than NNN in this tissue.

ONCOGENE ACTIVATION IN ESOPHAGEAL CANCER

Cyclin D1, a protooncogene that maps to the 11q13 region, is critical in the mid G1 phase of the cell cycle and contributes to the transition from the G1 to the S phase. The cyclin D1 protein interacts with cyclin dependent kinases, and this complex regulates key substrates, e.g., the retinoblastoma gene product. Importantly, cyclin D1 is amplified (DNA level) and overexpressed (RNA and protein levels) in a subset of esophagus SCCs (111, 112). The hst-1 and int-2 oncogenes in the same chromosomal region of cyclin D1 are amplified as well in SCC of the esophagus, but there is no RNA expression of hst-1 or int-2 (113). The overexpression of cyclin D1 probably accelerates transversion of cells from the G1 to the S phase and thus contributes to progression of SCC of the esophagus.

Overexpression of epidermal growth factor (EGF), transforming growth factor-α (TGF-α), and EGFR by tumor cells is closely correlated with tumor invasion and prognosis. The EGFR is encoded by the erb-1 protooncogene. EGF and TGF-α act as autocrine growth factors and induce the expression of mRNAs for multiple growth factors and their receptors. It seems likely that both EGF and TGF-α bind to EGFR, and that coexpression of EGF or TGF-α and EGFR results in autocrine growth stimulation of tumor cells. In addition, EGF and TGF-α exert oncogenic effects by induction of the intranuclear c-fos and c-myc genes (114). Amplification and overexpression of EGF has been detected in nearly 25% of esophagus SCCs (115). Furthermore, the number of EGFRs, as well as the EGF content in esophagus SCCs, are at least 10 times higher than those in gastric carcinoma cells (116). TGF-α is overexpressed in SCC of the head and neck and in numerous other malignancies; however, its potential overexpression in SCC of the esophagus has not been reported.

Overexpression of TGF-α and EGFR has been observed in a small proportion of patients with Barrett's esophagus and esophageal adenocarcinomas (117). Recent studies have provided evidence of both EGFR and *erb*B-2 gene amplification in these lesions (118).

The c-*myc* gene product has been implicated in cell cycle progression, transformation, differentiation, and programmed cell death. Expression of c-*myc* is closely linked to the action of growth factors and with cell cycle progression, suggesting that c-*myc* expression may be a major component of the regulatory networks associated with normal cell proliferation. In cancer, c-*myc* becomes activated by several different mechanisms, including proviral insertion, chromosomal translocation, and gene amplification. The c-*myc* gene has been shown to be amplified in 15% of esophageal SCCs from China (115).

There is no evidence of mutational activation of any members of the *ras* gene family in esophageal SCC (119). This finding contrasts with SCC of the rat esophagus in which mutation of the H-*ras* oncogene is a common molecular event.

TUMOR SUPPRESSOR GENE INACTIVATION IN ESOPHAGEAL CANCER

Loss of heterozygosity involving different chromosomal regions has been observed in esophageal cancers. Huang et al. (120) examined 72 esophageal cancers (46 SCCs and 26 adenocarcinomas) for loss of heterozygosity at the *p53*, *Rb*, *APC*, *MCC*, and *DCC* loci. Loss of heterozygosity occurred in 55% of informative cases at *p53*, 48% at *Rb*, nearly two thirds at *APC/MCC*, and 24% at *DCC*. Interestingly, 93% of tumors informative at all loci had loss of heterozygosity of at least one locus. These observations have in large measure been substantiated in other studies (121). Loss of heterozygosity also has been noted in other loci in esophageal SCC (122), suggesting that yet-to-be-identified tumor suppressor genes may be involved. Although loss of heterozygosity implies inactivation of a known or candidate tumor suppressor gene, mutational analysis of the gene furnishes more definitive proof of its involvement in the cancer. In this respect *p53* point mutations are found in 40% to 50% of esophageal SCCs from different regions of the world (123–125). In one study of 14 human esophageal SCCs, 5 tumors contained a mutated *p53* allele (123). Several were missense mutations occurring at the G-C base pairs in codons at or near mutations previously reported in other cancers. Point mutations in the *p53* gene also have been observed in dysplastic Barrett's mucosa and in adenocarcinomas of the esophagus (126).

TABLE 2.4. Oncogenes and Tumor Suppressor Genes in Human Esophageal Cancer

	MECHANISM	HISTOLOGY
Protooncogenes		
Nuclear transcription factor		
c-*myc*	A, OE	SCC
Kinase activator		
cyclin D1	A, OE	SCC
Receptor protein kinase		
c-*erb*B-1	A, OE	SCC, Ad, B
c-*erb*B-2	A, OE	Ad, B
Fibroblast growth factor (FGF)		
hst-1	A	SCC
int-2	A	SCC
Tumor suppressor genes		
p53	I, M	SCC, Ad, B
Rb	I	SCC
APC	LOH	SCC
MCC	LOH	SCC
DCC	LOH	SCC
MST-1	LOH	SCC

Abbreviations. A, amplification; OE, overexpression; I, inactivation; M, mutation; LOH, loss of heterozygosity; SCC, squamous cell carcinoma; Ad, adenocarcinoma; B, Barrett's esophagus.

Point mutations or microdeletions in the *MTS*-1 gene exon 2 coding sequence were found in 14 of 27 primary esophageal SCCs (127). Furthermore, 10 of 15 esophagus SCCs had deletions of *MTS*-1 exons 1 and 2 (128). Finally, the *DCC* gene locus is deleted frequently. In one study 23% of esophageal SCCs had loss of heterozygosity of the *DCC* locus, but only 2 of the 51 tumors had point mutations (129). Oncogene and tumor suppressor gene alterations in esophageal cancer are summarized in Table 2.4.

RAT ESOPHAGEAL TUMOR MODEL

The rat has been used almost exclusively as an animal model for studies of esophageal cancer. Many asymmetric nitrosamines—including NNN, *N*-nitrosomethylamylamine (NMAA), and NMBA—act as fairly specific inducers of tumorigenesis in the rat esophagus. NMBA is by far the most potent inducer of esophageal tumors in rats; tumors can be induced in 15 weeks or less (130). A number of readily discernible preneoplastic lesions are produced as well, including simple hyperplasias, leukoplakias, and dysplastic lesions (131). In general, most tumors induced by NMBA are squamous cell papillomas, although a small incidence of basal or SCCs may also be detected (131). Because of occlusion of the esophagus and/or induction of respiratory distress, a large esophageal papilloma can be life threatening. Thus, many NMBA-treated animals cannot survive long enough to develop carcinomas.

Although a sufficient dose of NMBA must be given to induce tumors, the duration of NMBA administration appears to be crucial in esophageal tumorigenesis. Single NMBA doses of 7.5 mg/kg or higher are lethal to rats (132). Cumulative NMBA doses of 7.5 mg/kg or more administered over 1 or 2 weeks fail to induce esophageal tumors by 30 weeks, whereas a cumulative NMBA dose of 7.5 mg/kg administered as 15 individual doses 3 times weekly for 5 weeks or once weekly for 15 weeks results in a 100% tumor incidence by 20 weeks (132, 133).

NMBA is principally a methylating agent, although preliminary data have indicated that benzylation of DNA does indeed occur after NMBA administration (102, 134). O^6-Methylguanine and 7-methylguanine adducts have been detected in target and nontarget tissues. A characteristic feature of methylating agents is the induction of point mutations such as G to A transitions, mutations that can be attributed to the formation of O^6-methylguanine and subsequent mispairing of O^6-methylguanine with thymine. Using the 15-week, 0.5 mg/kg dosing regimen, G to A transitions in the second base of codon 12 of H-*ras* are found in more than 90% of rats (135). Although p53 mutations appear in a minority of tumors, at least some of the mutations induced by NMBA are G to A transitions (136).

A variety of dosing regimens have been devised for NMBA. One method involves weekly injections of 3.5 mg/kg for 5 weeks (130), with quantitation of tumors at 15 weeks; this regimen yields an 80% tumor incidence. In general, lower doses of NMBA are preferred to avoid toxicity; a common means of inducing tumors in rats with a 100% incidence and a multiplicity of approximately 10 tumors per rat is the administration of NMBA once weekly subcutaneously for 15 weeks, with evaluation of tumors at 25 weeks (133). This latter regimen has proven quite useful as a model to test various chemopreventive agents. One disadvantage is that it does not allow one to distinguish between potential blocking activity (e.g., antiinitiating activity) and potential suppressing activity (e.g., antipromotional activity) because the carcinogen is administered over most of the duration of the experiment, making it difficult to discern the point at which initiation ended and promotion began. In this regard a convenient regimen for assessing mechanisms of chemoprevention of rat esophageal tumorigenesis involves 3-times-weekly administration of NMBA subcutaneously at a dose of 0.5 mg/kg for 5 weeks (132). Tumor incidence and multiplicity are evaluated at 25 weeks. This regimen yields a 100% tumor incidence and approximately two to three tumors per animal. Most of the duration of this protocol (approximately 80%) encompasses the presumed postinitiation period.

CHEMOPREVENTION OF ESOPHAGEAL CANCER

Several compounds that function as blocking agents have inhibitory activity against NMBA-induced esophageal tumorigenesis in rats. Diallyl sulfide (200 mg/kg) administered orally 3 hours before NMBA administration (3.5 mg/kg, once weekly for 5 weeks) completely inhibited NMBA-induced preneoplastic lesions and tumors (130). Diallyl sulfide is known to inhibit the metabolism of a number of nitrosamines, including NMBA (137). Ellagic acid, when given in the diet for the duration of the experiment at concentrations of 0.4 and 4.0 g/kg, significantly inhibits NMBA-induced esophageal tumors (131). This effect appears to be antagonized by coadministration of 13-*cis*-retinoic acid (133). At least a portion of the effect of ellagic acid in this situation appears to result from a blocking effect. Dietary ellagic acid also inhibits NMBA activation in the esophagus of rats (138), whereas ellagic acid added to in vitro cultures of rat esophagus inhibits both NMBA activation and NMBA-induced DNA adduct formation (139).

One of the most interesting groups of compounds evaluated in the rat esophagus is the arylalkyl isothiocyanates. Dietary PEITC completely inhibits NMBA-induced esophageal tumorigenesis when administered at concentrations of 3.0 μmol/g or greater (140, 141). This effect seems to be related to inhibition of NMBA activation, because PEITC inhibits NMBA-induced DNA adduct formation in vivo (141) and has no effects on NMBA tumorigenesis if administered post initiation (132). 3-Phenylpropyl isothiocyanate is a considerably more potent inhibitor than PEITC, whereas benzyl isothiocyanate and 4-phenylbutyl isothiocyanate are decidedly less potent than PEITC (142). Interestingly, 6-phenylhexyl isothiocyanate (PHITC) actually enhances NMBA-induced tumorigenesis (G. D. Stoner, unpublished observations).

Ellagic acid fed post initiation at a dietary concentration of 4 g/kg has a modest inhibitory effect on NMBA esophageal tumorigenesis (132). Green tea inhibits NMBA tumorigenesis when either intact NMBA or its precursors, sodium nitrite and methylbenzylamine, is administered (143, 144). Tea and tea components are known to possess both blocking and suppressing activities (145); thus, it is not surprising that decaffeinated green tea and decaffeinated black tea inhibit NMBA-induced esophageal tumors when administered during or after NMBA administration (146). Both dietary sulindac (125 parts per million [ppm]) and supplemental dietary calcium (2%) fail to inhibit NMBA-induced tumorigenesis when administered during or after NMBA administration (132). Dietary selenium has no inhibitory effects on

NMBA-induced esophageal tumorigenicity, DNA adduct formation, or oncogene expression (147).

A number of human trials, designed principally to address known nutritional deficiencies in high-risk international populations, are in progress (148). They involve an assessment of beta carotene, retinol and related synthetic retinoids, calcium, and several vitamin and mineral combinations for their ability to inhibit the progression of preneoplastic conditions, such as chronic esophagitis, basal cell hyperplasia, and dysplasia. In some studies the effect of the chemopreventive agents on surrogate endpoint biomarkers, such as the proliferation index (measured as the number of proliferating cell nuclear antigen (PCNA) or Ki67-positive cells), and on DNA ploidy and nuclear/nucleolar morphology is being assessed (149). To date, only limited results have been obtained from these studies, and they have been negative or marginally suggestive of positive effects. For example, in one study in which a combination of retinol, beta carotene, and vitamin E was administered to male subjects for a period of 20 months, the risk of progression of chronic esophagitis was reduced in subjects with a high blood concentration of either beta carotene or vitamin E; however, the data were not significant (150). In another study of 200 subjects with esophageal hyperplasia or dysplasia, the oral administration of 1200 mg of calcium daily for 11 months did not alleviate the lesions or reduce abnormal cell proliferation patterns (151). In a recent study in which four combinations of vitamins and minerals were administered to subjects in Linxian County, China, for a period of 5 years, a reduction in esophageal cancer incidence was suggested among those receiving the combined treatment of beta carotene, vitamin E, and selenium, as well as riboflavin and niacin (152). These results are encouraging in that they suggest that longer term treatments may result in even greater inhibitory effects.

To date, none of the chemopreventive agents that have demonstrated efficacy in the rat esophagus tumor model has been evaluated in human clinical trials. Because several of these agents inhibit tumor initiation by nitrosamines and other classes of carcinogens found in high-risk areas, their evaluation as preventive agents for human esophageal cancer seems warranted.

References

1. International Agency for Research on Cancer. IARC monographs on the evaluation of the carcinogenic risk of chemicals to humans: tobacco smoking. Lyon, France: IARC, 1986:38.
2. Shopland DR, Eyre HJ, Pechachek TF. Smoking-attributable cancer mortality in 1991: is lung cancer now the leading cause of death among smokers in the United States? J Natl Cancer Inst 1991;83:1142–1148.
3. Devesa SS, Shaw GL, Blot WJ. Changing patterns of lung cancer incidence by histological type. Cancer Epidemiol Biomarkers Prev 1991;1:29–34.
4. Hoffmann D, Rivenson A, Murphy SE, Chung FL, Amin S, Hecht SS. Cigarette smoking and adenocarcinoma of the lung: the relevance of nicotine-derived N-nitrosamines. J Smoking Related Dis 1993;4:165–189.
5. U.S. Environmental Protection Agency (EPA). Respiratory health effects of passive smoking: lung cancer and other disorders. Washington, DC: EPA, 1992.
6. U.S. Department of Health and Human Services (DHHS). Radon and lung cancer risk: a joint analysis of 11 underground miner studies. Bethesda, MD: National Institutes of Health, Publication No. 1994;94:3644.
7. International Agency for Research on Cancer. IARC monographs on the evaluation of carcinogenic risks to humans: overall evaluation of carcinogenicity: an updating of IARC monographs volumes 1 to 42. Lyon, France: IARC, 1987;Suppl 7.
8. Hoffmann D, Hecht SS. Advances in tobacco carcinogenesis. In: Cooper CS, Grover PL, eds. Handbook of experimental pharmacology. Berlin, Germany: Springer-Verlag, 1990;94/I: 63–107.
9. Miller EC, Miller, JA. Searches for ultimate chemical carcinogens and their reaction with cellular macromolecules. Cancer 1981;47: 2327–2345.
10. Guengerich FP, Shimada T. Oxidation of toxic and carcinogenic chemicals by human cytochrome P450 enzymes. Chem Res Toxicol 1991;4:391–407.
11. Thakker DR, Yagi H, Levin W, Wood AW, Conney AH, Jerina DM. Polycyclic aromatic hydrocarbons: metabolic activation to ultimate carcinogens. In: Anders MW, ed. Bioactivation of foreign compounds. New York: Academic Press, 1985:177–242.
12. Hecht SS. Metabolic activation and detoxification of tobacco-specific nitrosamines—a model for cancer prevention strategies. Drug Metab Rev 1994;26:373–390.
13. Klein CB, Frenkel K, Costa M. The role of oxidative processes in metal carcinogenesis. Chem Res Toxicol 1991;4:592–604.
14. Standeven AM, Wetterhahn KE. Is there a role for reactive oxygen species in the mechanism of chromium (VI) carcinogenesis? Chem Res Toxicol 1991;4:616–625.
15. Basu AK, Essigmann JM. Site-specifically modified oligodeoxynucleotides as probes for the structural and biological effects of DNA-damaging agents. Chem Res Toxicol 1988;1: 1–18.
16. Scicchitano DA, Hanawalt PC. Intragenomic repair heterogeneity of DNA damage. Environ Health Perspect 1992;98:45–51.
17. Belinsky SA, Dolan ME, White CM, Maronpot RR, Pegg AE, Anderson MW. Cell specific differences in O^6-methylguanine-DNA methyltransferase activity and removal of O^6-methylguanine in rat pulmonary cells. Carcinogenesis 1988;9:2053–2058.
18. Peterson LA, Liu X-K, Hecht, SS. Pyridyloxobutyl DNA adducts inhibit the repair of O^6-methylguanine. Cancer Res. 1993;53: 2780–2785.
19. Cole MD. *myc* Meets its *Max*. Cell 1991;65:715–716.
20. Morrison DK, Kaplan DR, Rapp U, Roberts TM. Signal transduction from membrane to cytoplasm: growth factors and membrane-bound oncogene products increase *raf*-1 phosphorylation and associated protein kinase activity. Proc Natl Acad Sci U S A 1988;85:8855–8859.
21. Rodenhuis S, Slebos RJC. Clinical significance of *ras* oncogene activation in human lung cancer. Anticancer Res 1992;52: 2665–2669.

22. Takeda S, Ichii S, Nakamura Y. Detection of K-*ras* mutation in sputum by mutant-allele-specific amplification (MASA). Human Mutation 1993;2:112–117.
23. Kalemkerian GP. Biology of lung cancer. Curr Opin Oncol 1994;6:147–155.
24. Hunter T. The epidermal growth factor receptor gene and its product. Nature 1984;311:414–424.
25. Gorgoulis V, Aninos D, Mikou P, et al. Expression of EGF, TGF-α and EGFR in squamous cell lung carcinomas. Anticancer Res 1992;12:1183–1187.
26. Schechter AL, Stern DF, Vaidyanathan L, et al. The NEU oncogene: an *erb*B related gene encoding a 185,000 *Mr* tumour antigen. Nature 1984;312:513–516.
27. Ransome LJ, Verma IM. Nuclear proto-oncogenes *FOS* and *JUN*. Ann Rev Cell Biol 1990;60:539–557.
28. Pezzella F, Turley H, Kuzu I, et al. *bcl*-2 Protein in non–small-cell lung carcinoma. N Engl J Med 1993;329:690–694.
29. Sakura H, Kanei-Ishii C, Nagase T, Nakagoshi H, Gonda TJ, Ishii S. Delineation of three functional domains of the transcriptional activator encoded by the c-*myb* proto-oncogene. Proc Natl Acad Sci U S A 1989;86:5758–5762.
30. Pfeifer AMA, Mark GE, Malan-Shibley L, Graziano S, Amstad P, Harris CC. Cooperation of c-*raf*-1 and c-*myc* protooncogenes in the neoplastic transformation of SV40 T antigen immortalized human bronchial epithelial cells. Proc Natl Acad Sci U S A 1989;86:10075–10079.
31. Farmer G, Bargonetti J, Zhu H, Friedman P, Prywes R, and Prives C. Wild-type *p53* activates transcription in vitro. Nature 1992;358:83–86.
32. Sameshima Y, Matsuno Y, Hirohashi S, et al. Alterations of the *p53* gene are common and critical events for the maintenance of malignant phenotypes in small-cell lung carcinoma. Oncogene 1992;7:451–457.
33. Friend SH, Bernardo R, Rogely S, et al. A human DNA segment with properties of the gene that predisposes to retinoblastoma and osteosarcoma. Nature 1986;323:643–646.
34. D'Amico D, Carbone DP, Johnson BE, Meltzer SJ, Minna JD. Polymorphic sites within the *MCC* and *APC* loci reveal very frequent loss of heterozygosity in human small cell lung cancer. Cancer Res 1992;52:1996–1999.
35. Hibi K, Takahashi T, Yamakawa K, et al. Three distinct regions involved in *3p* deletions in human lung cancer. Oncogene 1992;7:445–449.
36. Hollstein M, Sidransky D, Vogelstein B, Harris CC. *p53* Mutations in human cancers. Science 1991;253:49–53.
37. Suzuki H, Takahashi T, Kuroishi T, et al. *p53* Mutations in non–small cell lung cancer in Japan: association between mutations and smoking. Cancer Res 1992;52:734–736.
38. Sundaresan V, Ganly P, Hasleton P, et al. *p53* And chromosome 3 abnormalities, characteristic of malignant lung tumors, are detectable in preinvasive lesions of the bronchus. Oncogene 1992;7:1989–1997.
39. Yokota J, Akiyama T, Fung Y-KT, et al. Altered expression of the retinoblastoma (*Rb*) gene in small cell carcinoma of the lung. Oncogene 1988;3:471–475.
40. Wallet V, Mutzel R, Troll H, et al. *Dictyostelium* nucleotide diphosphate kinase highly homologous to nm23 and Awd proteins involved in mammalian tumor metastasis and *Drosophila* development. J Natl Cancer Inst 1990;82:1199–1202.
41. Serrano M, Hannon GJ, Beach D. A new regulatory motif in cell-cycle control causing specific inhibition of cyclin D/CDK4. Nature 1993;36:704–707.
42. Marlo A, Gabrielson E, Askin F, Sidransky D. Frequent loss of chromosome 9 in human primary non–small cell lung cancer. Cancer Res 1994;54:640–642.
43. Washimi O, Nagatake M, Osada H, et al. In vivo occurrence of p16 (*MTS1*) and p15 (*MTS2*) alterations preferentially in non–small cell lung cancers. Cancer Res 1995;55:514–517.
44. Shimkin MB, Stoner GD. Lung tumors in mice: application to carcinogenesis bioassay. Adv Cancer Res 1975;21:1–58.
45. Brooks RE. Pulmonary adenoma of strain A mice: an electron microscopic study. J Natl Cancer Inst 1968;47:719–742.
46. Rehm S, Ward JM, Ten Have-Opbroek AAW, et al. Mouse papillary lung tumors transplacentally induced by *N*-nitrosoethylurea: evidence for alveolar type II cell origin by comparative light microscopic, ultrastructural, and immunohistochemical studies. Cancer Res 1988;48:148–160.
47. Belinsky, SA, Devereux TR, Foley JF, Maronpot RR, Anderson MW. Role of the alveolar type II cell in the development and progression of pulmonary tumors induced by 4-(methylnitrosamino)-1-(3-pyridyl)-1-butanone in the A/J mouse. Cancer Res 1992;52:3164–3173.
48. Kauffman SL. Histogenesis of the papillary Clara cell adenoma. Am J Pathol 1981;103:174–180.
49. Foley JF, Anderson MW, Stoner GD, Gaul BW, Hardisty JF, Maronpot RR. Proliferative lesions of the mouse lung: progression studies in strain A mice. Exp Lung Res 1991;17:157–168.
50. You M, Maronpot RR, Stoner GD, Anderson MW. Activation of the K-*ras* protooncogene in chemically induced lung tumors of the strain A mouse. Proc Natl Acad Sci U S A 1989;86:3070–3074.
51. Belinsky SA, Devereux TR, Maronpot RR, Stoner GD, Anderson MW. The relationship between the formation of promutagenic adducts and the activation of the K-*ras* proto-oncogene in lung tumors from A/J mice treated with nitrosamines. Cancer Res 1989;49:5305–5311.
52. You M, Wang Y, Lineen A, et al. Activation of protooncogenes in mouse lung tumors. Exp Lung Res 1991;17:389–400.
53. You M, Wang Y, Lineen AM, Gunning W, Stoner GD, Anderson MW. Mutagenesis of the *ras* protooncogene in mouse lung tumors induced by *N*-ethyl-*N*-nitrosourea and *N*-nitrosodiethylamine. Carcinogenesis 1992;13:1583–1586.
54. Mass MJ, Jeffers AJ, Ross JA, Nelson G, Galati AJ, Stoner GD, Nesnow S. K-*ras* oncogene mutations in tumors and DNA-adducts formed by benz(*j*)aceanthrylene and benzo(*a*)pyrene in the lungs of strain A/J mice. Mol Carcinog 1993;8:186–192.
55. You L, Wang D, Galati AJ, et al. Tumor multiplicity, DNA adducts, and K-*ras* mutation pattern of 5-methylchrysene in strain A/J mouse lung. Carcinogenesis 1994;15:2613–2618.
56. Ryan J, Barker PE, Ruddle FH. An *Eco*RI restriction fragment length polymorphism at the K-*ras* locus on mouse chromosome 6. Nucleic Acids Res 1986;14:9222.
57. You M, Wang Y, Maronpot RR, Stoner GD, Anderson MW. Parental bias of K-*ras* oncogenes detected in lung tumors from mouse hybrids. Proc Natl Acad Sci U S A 1992;89:5804–5808.
58. Chen B, Wang Y, You M. Characterization of two protein-binding sites in the second intron of the mouse K-*ras* gene. Cancer Res 1995;55: in press.
59. You M, You L, Chen B, Wang Y, Stoner GD. Allele-specific activation of the K-*ras* gene in hybrid mouse lung tumors induced by chemical carcinogens. Carcinogenesis 1994;15:2031–2035.
60. Re FC, Manenti G, Borrello MG, et al. Multiple molecular alterations in mouse lung tumors. Mol Carcinog 1992;5:155–160.
61. Herzog CR, Wiseman RW, You M. Deletion mapping of a putative tumor suppressor gene on chromosome 4 in mouse lung tumors. Cancer Res 1994;54:4007–4010.

62. Stoner GD, Shimkin MB. Strain A mouse lung tumor bioassay. J Am Coll Toxicol 1982;1:145–169.
63. Stoner GD. Lung tumors in strain A mice as a bioassay for carcinogenicity of environmental chemicals. Exp Lung Res 1991;17:405–423.
64. Stoner GD, Adam-Rodwell G, and Morse MA. Lung tumors in strain A mice: application for studies in cancer chemoprevention. J Cell Biochem 1993;17F:5–103.
65. Wynder EL, Hecht SS, eds. Lung cancer. UICC technical report series. Geneva: International Union Against Cancer, 1976;25:95–101.
66. Reznik-Schuller HM. Comparative respiratory tract carcinogenesis. Volume II. Boca Raton FL: CRC Press, 1983;II:75–93, 109–134.
67. Moon RC, Rao KVN, Detrisac CJ, Kelloff GJ. Retinoid chemoprevention of lung cancer. In: Wattenberg LW, Lipkin M, Boone CW, Kelloff GJ, eds. Cancer chemoprevention. Boca Raton, FL: CRC Press, 1992:83–93.
68. Dontenwill W, Chevalier H-J, Harke H-P, Lafrenz U, Reckzeh G, Schneider B. Investigations on the effects of chronic cigarette-smoke inhalation in Syrian golden hamsters. J Natl Cancer Inst 1973;51:1781–1832.
69. Hecht SS, Hoffmann D. Tobacco-specific nitrosamines, an important group of carcinogens in tobacco and tobacco smoke. Carcinogenesis 1988;9:875–884.
70. Rivenson A, Hoffmann D, Prokopczyk B, Amin S, Hecht SS. Induction of lung and exocrine pancreas tumors in F344 rats by tobacco-specific and Areca-derived N-nitrosamines. Cancer Res 1988;48:6912–6917.
71. Belinsky SA, Foley JF, White CM, Anderson MW, Maronpot RR. Dose-response relationship between O^6-methylguanine formation in Clara cells and induction of pulmonary neoplasia in the rat by 4-(methylnitrosamino)-1-(3-pyridyl)-1-butanone. Cancer Res 1990;50:3772–3780.
72. Deutsch-Wenzel R, Brune H, Grimmer G. Experimental studies in rat lungs on the carcinogenicity and dose-response relationship of eight frequently occurring environmental aromatic hydrocarbons. J Natl Cancer Inst 1983;71:539–544.
73. Hecht SS, Carmella SG, Murphy SE, Foiles PG, Chung FL. Carcinogen biomarkers related to smoking and upper aerodigestive tract cancer. J Cell Biochem. 1983;17F(Suppl):27–35.
74. Hecht SS, Carmella SG, Foiles PG, Murphy SE. Biomarkers for human uptake and metabolic activation of tobacco-specific nitrosamines. Cancer Res 1994;54:1912S–1917S.
75. U.S. Department of Health and Human Services. Biomarkers in human cancer, part I. Environ Health Perspect 1992;98:5–286.
76. U.S. Department of Health and Human Services. Biomarkers in human cancer, part II. Environ Health Perspect 1993;99:5–390.
77. Hecht SS, Carmella SG, Murphy SE, Akerkar S, Brunnemann KD, and Hoffmann D. A tobacco-specific lung carcinogen in the urine of men exposed to cigarette smoke. N Engl J Med 1993;329:1543–1546.
78. Wattenberg LW. Chemoprevention of cancer by naturally occurring and synthetic compounds. In: Wattenberg LW, Lipkin M, Boone CW, Kelloff GJ, eds. Cancer chemoprevention. Boca Raton, FL: CRC Press, 1992:19–39.
79. Morse MA, Stoner GD. Cancer chemoprevention: principles and prospects. Carcinogenesis 1993;14:1737–1746.
80. Steinmetz KA, Potter JD. Vegetables, fruit, and cancer. Journal of Epidemiology, Cancer Causes and Control 1991;2:325–357.
81. Morse MA, Wang C-X, Stoner GD, et al. Inhibition of 4-(methyl-nitrosamino)-1-(3-pyridyl)-1-butanone–induced DNA adduct formation and tumorigenicity in lung of F344 rats by dietary phenethyl isothiocyanate. Cancer Res 1989;49:549–553.
82. Morse MA, Amin SG, Hecht SS, Chung F-L. Effects of aromatic isothiocyanates on tumorigenicity, O^6-methylguanine formation, and metabolism of the tobacco-specific nitrosamine 4-(methylnitrosamino)-1-(3-pyridyl)-1-butanone in A/J mouse lung. Cancer Res 1989;49:2894–2897.
83. Lin J-M, Amin S, Trushin N, Hecht SS. Effects of isothiocyanates on tumorigenesis by benzo[a]pyrene in murine tumor models. Cancer Lett 1993;74:151–159.
84. Zhang Y, Talalay P, Cho CG, Posner GH. A major inducer of anticarcinogenic protective enzymes from broccoli: isolation and elucidation of structure. Proc Natl Sci U S A 1992;89:2399–2403.
85. Heinonen OP, Albanes D. The effect of vitamin E and beta carotene on the incidence of lung cancer and other cancers in male smokers. N Engl J Med 1994;330:1029–1035.
86. Parkin DM, Stjernsward J, Muir CS. Estimates of the worldwide frequency of twelve major cancers. Bull World Health Org 1984;62:163–182.
87. Warwick GP, Harington JS. Some aspects of the epidemiology and etiology of esophageal cancer with particular emphasis on the Transkei, South Africa. Adv Cancer Res 1973;17:81.
88. Wynder EL, Bross IJ. A study of etiological factors in cancer of the esophagus. Cancer 1961;14:389.
89. Tuyns AJ. Epidemiology of esophageal cancer in France. In: Pfeifer CJ, ed. Cancer of the esophagus. Boca Raton, FL: CRC Press, 1982;1:3.
90. Auerbach O, Stout AP, Hammond EC, Garfinkel L. Histologic changes in esophagus in relation to smoking habits. Arch Environ Health 1965;11:4–15.
91. Malhotra SL. Geographic distribution of gastrointestinal cancers in India with special reference to causation. Gut 1967;8:361–372.
92. Tuyns AJ. Recherches concernant les facteurs etiologiques du cancer de l'oesophage dans l'ouest de la France. Bull Cancer (Paris) 1980;67:15–28.
93. Li MN, Cheng SJ. Etiology of carcinoma of the esophagus. In: Huang GJ, Kai W Y, eds. Carcinoma of the esophagus and gastric cardia. Berlin: Springer-Verlag, 1984:26–51.
94. Togawa K, Jaskiewicz K, Takahashi H, Meltzer SJ, Rustigi AK. Human papillomavirus DNA sequences in esophagus squamous cell carcinoma. Gastroenterology 1994;107:128–136.
95. Druckrey H, Preussmann R, Ivankovic S, Schmahl D. Organotrope carcinogen wirkungen bei 65 verschiedenen N-nitrosoverbindungen an BD-ratten. Zeitschrift Krebsforschungen 1967;69;103–201.
96. Lijinsky W. Chemistry and biology of N-nitroso compounds: Cambridge monographs on cancer research. Cambridge: Cambridge University Press, 1992:251–403.
97. Craddock VM. Cancer of the esophagus—approaches to the etiology: Cambridge monographs on cancer research. Cambridge: Cambridge University Press, 1993:69–116.
98. Magee PN. The experimental basis for the role of nitroso compounds in human cancer. Cancer Surv 1989;8:207–239.
99. Bartsch H, Ohshima H, Pignatelli B, Calmels S. Human exposure to endogenous N-nitroso compounds: quantitative estimates in subjects at high risk for cancer of the oral cavity, oesophagus, stomach and urinary bladder. Cancer Surv 1989;8:335–362.
100. Wu Y, Chen J, Ohshima H, et al. Geographic association between urinary excretion of N-nitroso compounds and oesophageal cancer mortality in China. Int J Cancer 1993;54:713–719.

101. Hecht SS, Hoffmann D. The relevance of tobacco-specific nitrosamines to human cancer. Cancer Surv 1989;8:273–294.
102. Labuc GE, Archer MC. Esophageal and hepatic microsomal metabolism of N-nitrosomethylbenzylamine and N-nitrosodimethylamine in the rat. Cancer Res 1982;42:3181–3186.
103. Hodgson M, Wiessler M, Kleihues P. Preferential methylation of target organ DNA by the oesophageal carcinogen N-nitrosomethylbenzylamine. Carcinogenesis 1980;1:861–866.
104. Craddock VM, Henderson AR. Effect of N-nitrosamines carcinogenic for the oesphagus on O^6-alkyl-guanine-DNA-methyl transferase in rat oesophagus and liver. J Cancer Res Clin Oncol 1986;111:229–236.
105. Huang Q, Stoner G, Resau J, Nickols J, Mirvish SS. Metabolism of N-nitrosomethyl-n-amylamine by microsomes from human and rat esophagus. Cancer Res 1992;52:3547–3551.
106. Mirvish SS, Ji C, Rosinsky S. Hydroxy metabolites of methyl-n-amylnitrosamine produced by esophagus, stomach, liver, and other tissues of the neonatal to adult rat and hamster. Cancer Res 1988;48:5663–5668.
107. von Hofe E, Schmerold I, Lijinsky W, Jeltsch W, Kleihues P. DNA methylation in rat tissues by a series of homologous aliphatic nitrosamines ranging from N-nitrosodimethylamine to N-nitrosomethyldodecylamine. Carcinogenesis 1987;8:1337–1341.
108. Hecht SS, Reiss B, Lin D, Williams GM. Metabolism of N′-nitrosonornicotine by cultured rat esophagus. Carcinogenesis 1982;3:453–456.
109. Castonguay A, Rivenson A, Trushin N, et al. Effects of chronic ethanol consumption on the metabolism and carcinogenicity of N′-nitrosonornicotine in F344 rats. Cancer Res 1984;44:2285–2290.
110. Murphy SE, Heiblum R, Trushin N. Comparative metabolism of N′-nitrosonornicotine and 4-(methylnitrosamino)-1-(3-pyridyl)-1-butanone by cultured rat oral tissue and esophagus. Cancer Res 1990;50:4685–4691.
111. Jiang W, Kahn SM, Tomita N, et al. Cyclin D1 amplification and overexpression in human esophageal cancers. Cancer Res 1992;52:2980–2983.
112. Jiang W, Zhang YU, Kahn S, et al. Altered expression of the cyclin D1 and retinoblastoma gene in human esophageal cancer. Proc Natl Acad Sci U S A 1993;90:9026–9030.
113. Tsuda T, Tahara E, Kajiyama G, et al. High incidence of coamplification of hst-1 and int-2 genes in human esophageal carcinomas. Cancer Res 1989;49:505–508.
114. Cutry AF, Kinniburgh AJ, Krabak MJ, Hui S-W, Wenner CE. Induction of c-fos and c-myc proto-oncogene expression by epidermal growth factor and transforming growth factor alpha is calcium independent. J Biol Chem 1989;264:19700–19705.
115. Lu SH, Hsieh LL, Luo FC, Weinstein IB. Amplification of the EGF receptor and c-myc genes in human esophageal cancers. Int J Cancer 1988;42:502–505.
116. Yamamoto T, Kamata N, Kawano H, et al. High incidence of amplification of the epidermal growth factor receptor gene in human squamous carcinoma cell lines. Cancer Res 1986;46:414–416.
117. Yoshida, Kyo E, Tsuda T, et al. EGF and TGF-alpha, the ligands of hyperproduced EGFR in human esophageal carcinoma cells, act as autocrine growth factors. Int J Cancer 1990;45:131–135.
118. Al-Kasspooles M, Moore JH, Orringer MB, and Beer DG. Amplification and over-expression of the EGFR and erbB-2 genes in human esophageal adenocarcinomas. Int J Cancer 1993;54:213–219.
119. Hollstein MC, Peri L, Mandard AM, et al. Genetic analysis of human esophageal tumors from two high incidence geographic areas: frequent p53 base substitutions and absence of ras mutations. Cancer Res 1991;51:4102–4106.
120. Huang Y, Boynton RF, Blount PL, et al. Loss of heterozygosity involves multiple tumor suppressor genes in human esophageal cancers. Cancer Res 1992;52:6525–6530.
121. Maesawa C, Tamura G, Suzuki Y, et al. Aberrations of tumor suppressor genes (p53, ape, mcc, Rb) in esophageal squamous cell carcinoma. Int J Cancer 1994;57:21–25.
122. Shibagaki I, Shimada Y, Wagata T, et al. Allelotype analysis of esophageal squamous cell carcinoma. Cancer Res 1994;54:2996–3001.
123. Hollstein MC, Metcalf RA, Walsh JA, Montesano R, and Harris CC. Frequent mutation of the p53 gene in human esophageal cancer. Proc Natl Acad Sci U S A 1990;87:9958–9961.
124. Hollstein MC, Mandard AM, Walsh JA, et al. Genetic analysis of human esophageal tumors from two high incidence geographic areas: frequent p53 base substitutions and absence of ras mutations. Cancer Res 1991;51:4102–4106.
125. Bennett WP, Hollstein MC, Metcalf RA, et al. p53 Mutation and protein accumulation during multistage human esophageal carcinogenesis. Cancer Res 1992;52:6092–6097.
126. Moore JH, Lesser EJ, Erdody DH, Natale RB, Orringer MB, and Beer DG. Intestinal differentiation and p53 gene alterations in Barrett's esophagus and esophageal adenocarcinoma. Int J Cancer 1994;56:487–493.
127. Mori T, Miura K, Aoki T, Nishihira T, Mori S, Nakamura Y. Frequent somatic mutation of the MTS1/CDK4I (multiple tumor suppressor/cyclin-dependent kinase 4 inhibitor) gene in esophageal squamous cell carcinoma. Cancer Res 1994;54:3396–3397.
128. Liu Q, Yan YX, McClure M, Nakagawa H, Fujimura F, Rustigi AK. MTS-1 (CDKN2) tumor suppressor gene deletions are a frequent event in esophagus squamous cancer and pancreatic adenocarcinoma cell lines. Oncogene 1995;10:619–622.
129. Miyake S, Nagai K, Kunihide Y, Oto M, Endo M, Yuasa Y. Point mutations and allelic deletion of tumor suppressor gene DCC in human esophageal squamous cell carcinomas and their relation to metastasis. Cancer Res 1994;54:3007–3011.
130. Wargovich MJ, Woods C, Eng VWS, Stephens LC, and Gray K. Chemoprevention of N-nitrosomethylbenzylamine–induced esophageal cancer in rats by the naturally-occurring thioether, diallyl sulfide. Cancer Res 1988;48:6872–6875.
131. Mandal S, Stoner GD. Inhibition of N-nitrosobenzylmethylamine–induced esophageal tumorigenesis in rats by ellagic acid. Carcinogenesis 1990;11:55–61.
132. Siglin JC, Khare L, Stoner GD. Evaluation of dose and treatment duration on the esophageal tumorigenicity of N-nitrosomethylbenzylamine in rats. Carcinogenesis 1995;16:259–265.
133. Daniel EM, Stoner GD. The effects of ellagic acid and 13-cis-retinoic acid on N-nitrosobenzylmethylamine–induced esophageal tumorigenesis in rats. Cancer Lett 1991;56:117–124.
134. Peterson LA. Detection of benzylated DNA adducts in livers from N-nitrosomethylbenzylamine (NMBzA) treated rats. Proc Am Assoc Cancer Res 1995;36:829.
135. Wang Y, You M, Reynolds SH, Stoner GD, Anderson MW. Mutational activity of the cellular Harvey ras oncogene in rat esophageal papillomas induced by methylbenzylnitrosamine. Cancer Res 1990;50:1591–1595.
136. Lozano JC, Nakazawa H, Cros MP, Cabral R, Yamasaki H. G-A transitions in p53 and Ha-ras genes in esophageal papillomas induced by N-nitrosomethylbenzylamine in two strains of rats. Mol Carcinog 1994;9:33–39.

137. Brady JF, Li DC, Ishizaki H, Yang CS. Effect of diallyl sulfide on rat liver microsomal nitrosamine metabolism and other monooxygenase activities. Cancer Res 1988;48:5937–5940.
138. Barch DH, Fox CC. Dietary ellagic acid reduces the esophageal microsomal metabolism of methylbenzylnitrosamine. Cancer Lett 1989;44:39–44.
139. Mandal S, Shivapurkar NM, Galati AJ, Stoner GD. Inhibition of N-nitrosomethylbenzylamine metabolism and DNA binding in cultured rat esophagus by ellagic acid. Carcinogenesis 1988;9:1313–1316.
140. Stoner GD, Morissey DT, Heur YH, Daniel EM, Galati AJ, Wagner SA. Inhibitory effects of phenethyl isothiocyanate on N-nitrosobenzylmethylamine carcinogenesis in the rat esophagus. Cancer Res 1991;51:2063–2068.
141. Morse MA, Zu H, Galati AJ, Schmidt CJ, Stoner GD. Dose-related inhibition by dietary phenethyl isothiocyanate of esophageal tumorigenesis and DNA methylation induced by N-nitrosomethylbenzylamine in rats. Cancer Lett 1993;72:103–110.
142. Wilkinson JT, Morse MA, Kresty LA, Stoner GD. Effect of alkyl chain length on inhibition of N-nitrosomethylbenzylamine–induced esophageal tumorigenesis and DNA methylation by isothiocyanates. Carcinogenesis 1995;16:1011–1015.
143. Xu Y, Han C. The effect of Chinese tea on occurrence of esophageal tumor induced by N-nitrosomethylbenzylamine in rats. Biomed Environ Sci 1990;3:35–42.
144. Xu Y, Chi H. The effect of Chinese tea on occurrence of esophageal tumor induced by N-nitrosomethylbenzylamine formed in vivo. Biomed Environ Sci 1990;3:406–412.
145. Yang CS, Wang ZY. Tea and cancer. J Natl Cancer Inst 1993;85:1038–1049.
146. Wang ZY, Wang LD, Chen WF, et al. Inhibition of N-nitrosomethylbenzylamine (NMBzA)–induced esophageal tumorigenesis in rats by decaffeinated green tea and black tea. Proc Am Assoc Cancer Res 1993;34:A746.
147. Hu G, Han C, Wild CP, Hall J, Chen J. Lack of effects of selenium on N-nitrosomethylbenzylamine–induced tumorigenesis, DNA methylation, and oncogene expression in rats and mice. Nutr Cancer 1992;18:287–295.
148. Greenwald P, Stern HR. Role of biology and prevention in aerodigestive tract cancers. Monogr Natl Cancer Inst 1992;13:3–14.
149. Lipkin M. Gastrointestinal cancer: pathogenesis, risk factors and the development of intermediate biomarkers for chemoprevention studies. J Cell Biochem 1992;16G (Suppl):1–13.
150. Zaridze D, Evstifeeva T, Boyle P. Chemoprevention of oral leukoplakia and chronic esophagitis in an area of high incidence of oral and esophageal cancer. Ann Epidemiol 1993;3:225–234.
151. Wang L-D, Qiu S-L, Yang G-R, Lipkin M, Newmark HL, Yang CS. A randomized double-blind intervention study on the effect of calcium supplementation on esophageal precancerous lesions in a high-risk population in China. Cancer Epidemiol Biomarkers Prev 1993;2:71–78.
152. Blot WJ, Li JY, Taylor PR, et al. Nutrition intervention trials in Linxian, China: supplementation with specific vitamin/mineral combinations, cancer incidence, and disease-specific mortality in the general population. J Natl Cancer Inst 1993;85:1483–1492.

3

CIGARETTE SMOKING

David M. Burns

INTRODUCTION

At the start of the 20th century (1), lung cancer was a rare disease, but it has become the largest cause of cancer death in the United States for both males and females. Cigarette smoking is responsible for approximately 90% of lung cancers in this country (2). Other agents, most notably asbestos and radon, also cause lung cancer. Their more limited contribution to lung cancer deaths in the United States is the result of smaller numbers of individuals exposed to these agents and of the success our society has had in eliminating these agents from occupational and other environments. Differences in intensity of exposure and the fraction of the population exposed result in the high proportion of lung cancers attributed to cigarette smoke exposure, rather than the potency or uniqueness of cigarette smoke as a pulmonary carcinogen.

Exposure to cigarette smoke, either through active smoking or as environmental tobacco smoke (ETS), is a nearly universal experience in our society. Eliminating or reducing low-dose exposure to cigarette smoke as ETS has been much less successful than the reduction in exposure to other occupational or environmental carcinogens. If exposure to cigarette smoke can be elimited, lung cancer may once again return to a rare and unusual disease.

CIGARETTE SMOKE CHEMISTRY

Cigarette smoke is a complex aerosol of distillation and combustion products produced when tobacco is burned. Mainstream smoke is produced when air is drawn through the column of tobacco; it is generated at a higher temperature (up to 950°C) than is sidestream smoke (3) and is the predominant source of smoke exposure for the smoker. Sidestream smoke is produced at lower temperatures (350°C)(4) during the smoldering of the cigarette between puffs and is the major source of ETS. Tar is the total particulate matter of the smoke after nicotine and water have been removed.

The chemical composition of mainstream smoke, and the concentrations of constituents in mainstream compared with sidestream smoke, can vary substantially from one cigarette to another (5) and with different patterns of smoking (6). One measure of this variability, the machine-measured tar yield of American cigarettes, had been declining from a sales-weighted average of 35 mg in 1957 to the current yield of approximately 13 mg (2). This decline has resulted from both a reduction in tar yields of the same brand of cigarettes over time and a shift in the market share of individual brands, which favors those with lower tar yield. Changes in tar yield during the mid-1950s and early 1960s were often the result of putting less tobacco leaf in each cigarette by "puffing" the tobacco and using reconstituted tobacco sheets to manufacture cigarettes. These changes may have actually reduced the tar exposure of individuals smoking these cigarettes. However, more recent changes lowered the machine-measured yields without actually reducing the tar received by the smoker. Cigarettes with machine-measured yields of 0.01 mg of tar (essentially no mainstream smoke) have been manufactured using holes and channels in the filter that allow air to be entrained during machine smoking but that occluded when smoked by the smoker. When these cigarettes are machine smoked, very little smoke is drawn through the filter, and the volume of smoke used to measure tar is composed largely of air. Because the smoker smokes to obtain the tobacco smoke, not simply air, the smoker inhales more deeply and more rapidly. This pattern of inhalation generates a substantially higher yield of tar from the cigarette.

More than 4000 individual chemical constituents of cigarette smoke have been identified (2). Unadulterated tobacco contributes 2550 of these with the remainder representing additives, pesticides, and other organic and metallic compounds (7, 8). Table 3.1 lists

TABLE 3.1. Toxic and Tumorigenic Agents of Cigarette Smoke; Ratio of Sidestream Smoke (SS) to Mainstream Smoke (MS)

A. Gas phase	Amount/cigarette				SS/MS
Carbon dioxide	10	–	80	mg	8.1[1]
Carbon monoxide	0.5	–	26	mg	2.5[1]
Nitrogen oxides (NO_2)	16	–	600	g	4.7–5.8
Ammonia	10	–	130	g	44–73
Hydrogen cyanide	280	–	550	g	0.17–0.37
Hydrazine			32	g	3
Formaldehyde	20	–	90	g	51
Acetone	100	–	940	g	2.5–3.2
Acrolein	10	–	140	g	12
Acetonitrile	60	–	160	g	10
Pyridine			32	g	10
3-Vinylpyridine			23	g	28
N-Nitrosodimethylamine	4	–	180	ng	10–830
N-Nitrosoethylmethylamine	1.0	–	40	ng	5–12
N-Nitrosodiethylamine	0.1	–	28	ng	4–25
N-Nitrosopyrrolidine	0	–	110	ng	3–76

B. Particulate phase	Amount/cigarette				SS/MS
Total particulate phase	0.1	–	40	mg	1.3–1.9[1]
Nicotine	0.06	–	2.3	mg	2.6–3.3[1]
Toluene			108	g	5.6
Phenol	20	–	150	g	2.6
Catechol	40	–	280	g	0.7
Stigmasterol			53	g	0.8
Total phytosterols			130	g	0.8
Naphthalene			2.8	g	16
1-Methylnaphthalene			1.2	g	26
2-Methylnaphthalene			1.0	g	29
Phenanthrene	2.0	–	80	ng	2.1
Benz(a)anthracene	10	–	70	ng	2.7
Pyrene	15	–	90	ng	1.9–3.6
Benzo(a)pyrene	8	–	40	ng	2.7–3.4
Quinoline			1.7	g	11
Methylquinoline			6.7	g	11
Harmane	1.1	–	3.1	g	0.7–2.7
Norharmane	3.2	–	8.1	g	1.4–4.3
Aniline	100	–	1,200	ng	30
o-Toluidine			32	ng	19
1-Naphthylamine	1.0	–	22	ng	39
2-Naphthylamine	4.3	–	27	ng	39
4-Aminobiphenyl	2.4	–	4.6	ng	31
N'-Nitrosonornicotine	0.2	–	3.7	g	1–5
NNK[2]	0.12	–	0.44	g	1–8
N'-Nitrosoanatabine	0.15	–	4.6	g	1–7
N-Nitrosodiethanolamine	0	–	40	ng	1.2

[1] In cigarettes with perforated filter tips the SS/MS ratio rises with increasing air dilution. In the case of smoke dilution with air to 17%, the SS/MS ratios for TPM rise to 2.14, CO_2 36.5, CO 23.5, and nicotine to 13.1.
[2] NNK, 4-(Methylnitrosamino)-1-(3-pyridyl)-1-butanone.
SOURCE: 1982 Surgeon General's Report.

some constituents of the particulate and vapor phases of mainstream smoke. The chemical composition of smoke and the distribution of the constituents between the particulate and vapor phases of the smoke change as the smoke cools, ages, and mixes with air. Nicotine, which is contained largely in the particulate phase in fresh smoke, volatilizes into the gas phase as smoke ages and is a major vapor phase constituent in ETS (9).

The water content of smoke particles changes with the relative humidity of the environment, with a resultant change in particle size.

Radioactive constituents are present in both tobacco and tobacco smoke. They include radon and its decay products, as well as lead (^{210}Pb), bismuth (^{210}Bi), and polonium (^{210}Po) (10). These radioisotopes may contribute to the carcinogenicity of cigarette smoke (11–14). The absorption of ^{210}Po from the lung into the bloodstream has been shown (15). The radiation dose from ^{210}Po in cigarettes has been estimated variously at 1 rad per year (16), 8 rem per year (17), and 80 to 100 rad per lifetime (18).

DEPOSITION AND ABSORPTION OF SMOKE

Mainstream cigarette smoke emerges from the cigarette with approximately 109 to 1010 particles per milliter. The particles range in size from 0.1 to 1.0 μm with a mean of 0.2 μm (19). After being inhaled, the particle size may change with the increased humidity in the airway and with aggregation of the particles because of their high concentration (20). The aerodynamic diameter of the particle influences the sites of deposition in the airways and alveolar regions of the lung (21). The fraction of smoke retained by the smoker also varies markedly with the pattern of inhalation. Smokers who hold smoke in their mouth and do not inhale retain only a small fraction of the smoke, whereas smokers who inhale deeply and hold their inhalation may retain up to 90% of the smoke (22, 23). Once deposited, smoke particles are cleared through the normal pulmonary clearance mechanisms: alveolar macrophages and mucociliary transport. However, acute and chronic inhalation of smoke may alter these clearance mechanisms. Acute inhalation of cigarette smoke results in ciliostasis (24–26) and reduced mucociliary clearance (25, 26). Chronic inhalation of smoke alters clearance by converting ciliated epithelium to nonciliated epithelium by altering the amount and character of the mucus produced and by inflammatory and emphysematous narrowing of the airway (27). The result is longer retention of carcinogens and higher concentrations of carcinogens reaching the basal cell layer.

Absorption of constituents from the gas phase of smoke varies markedly with solubility and other characteristics of the constituent. Highly soluble compounds are absorbed in the upper airway and reach the alveoli in much lower concentrations than exist as the smoke leaves the cigarette.

Exfoliative cytology in populations of smokers at high risk of developing lung cancer shows progression of changes over time from dysplasia through metaplasia to carcinoma in situ. With cessation, these changes revert toward normal. Pathologic studies in smokers show that the extent of these changes is closely correlated with the number of cigarettes smoked per day and the duration of smoking (28).

EPIDEMIOLOGY OF CIGARETTE SMOKING AND LUNG CANCER

The enormous body of epidemiologic literature defining the relationship between cigarette smoking and lung cancer precludes its presentation here. It has been presented in reports of the U.S. Surgeon General (2, 6, 10, 27, 29–35) and elsewhere (3, 36, 37, 38). The relationships of dose and duration of exposure are summarized using examples drawn largely from the American Cancer Society Cancer Prevention Study I, a 12-year prospective epidemiologic study of more than 1 million men and women (39).

CHANGES IN THE RISK OF SMOKING WITH AGE

Lung cancer mortality rates increase with age among both smokers and nonsmokers. The risk of dying from lung cancer for cigarette smokers is commonly expressed as a ratio of the mortality rate in smokers compared with that of people who have never smoked (relative risk), and a single summary relative risk for smoking often is derived across all age groups. This unitary experience of risk is based in part on the concept that lung cancer occurs as a function of aging and that exposure to carcinogens in cigarette smoke acts as a multiplier of the effect of aging. However, relative risks for lung cancer are not constant across age groups, and current models of lung carcinogenesis suggest that lung cancer is well modeled by functions of cumulative carcinogenic exposures rather than as a function of aging (39, 40). These models suggest that smoking risks are better expressed as excess risk (the difference between the mortality rates in smokers and those in nonsmokers). Understanding changes in smoking risk with age requires an appreciation both of change in relative risk with age and changes in excess mortality rates with age.

Figure 3.1 presents age specific relative risks and excess mortality rates for lung cancer among cigarette smokers. An increased risk for lung cancer is first evident in the mid-40s to late 40s. Relative risk peaks rapidly at younger ages and then declines with increas-

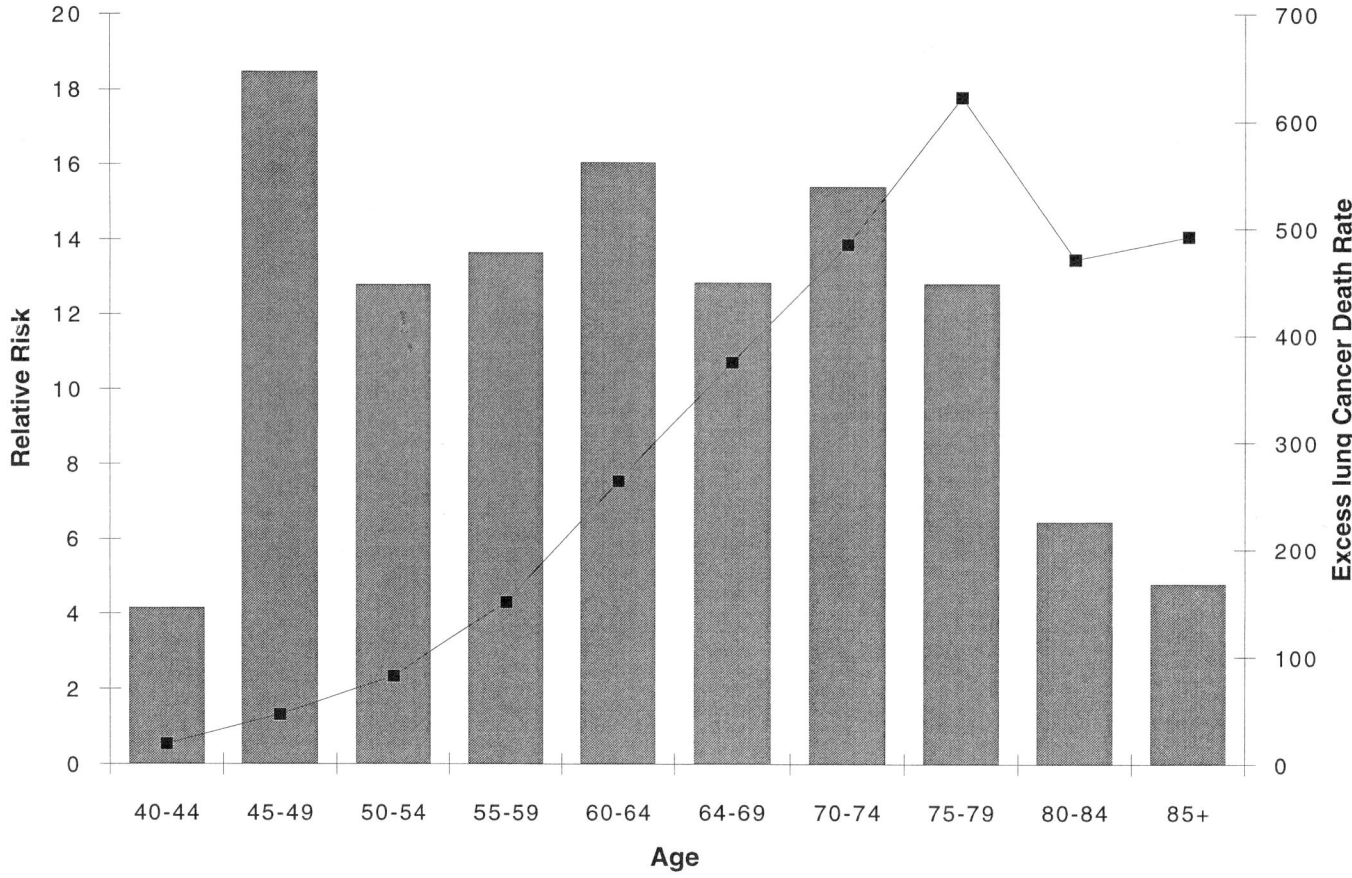

FIGURE 3.1. Age specific relative risk of developing lung cancer among smokers compared with nonsmokers. (Figures 3.1 through 3.11 reproduced and data derived with permission from Burns D, Shanks T, Choi W, Thun M, Heath C, Garfinkel L. The American Cancer Society cancer prevention study #1: 12-year follow up on one million men and women. Washington, DC: U.S. Department of Health and Human Services, National Institutes of Health, National Cancer Institute, Prospective Mortality Studies on Smoking and Disease, Smoking and Tobacco Control Monograph No 6, 1995; in press.)

ing age. This decline in relative risk with age is somewhat misleading, because the excess mortality rate attributable to smoking increases rather than decreases with age. High relative risks at younger ages reflect a very low mortality rate from lung cancer among younger nonsmokers, rather than a large mortality effect from smoking at these younger ages.

NUMBER OF CIGARETTES SMOKED PER DAY AND DURATION OF EXPOSURE

The risk of lung cancer because of smoking is produced by prolonged exposure to the carcinogens in tobacco smoke. This exposure can be defined by two measures of smoking behavior: number of cigarettes smoked per day (a measure of intensity of exposure) and duration of smoking. Relative risks for lung cancer mortality increase roughly proportionally to the number of cigarettes smoked per day (Fig. 3.2). This dose-response relationship suggests that there is no safe level of smoking because even low numbers of cigarettes smoked per day result in substantial increased risk. It also indicates that there is no ceiling to the carcinogenic effect evident for numbers of cigarettes commonly smoked.

Risks of smoking cigarettes are traditionally expressed in relation to the age of the smoker, using age specific rates for those who have never smoked as a comparison group. However, individuals begin smoking at different ages, and a given age group of smokers may contain individuals with markedly different durations of exposure. Therefore, categorizing disease risks by duration of smoking, rather than by age, may be a more useful method of examining this exposure. Figure 3.3 presents relative risks of cigarette smoking by duration of smoking. The comparison rate of those who have never smoked is a weighted average of this

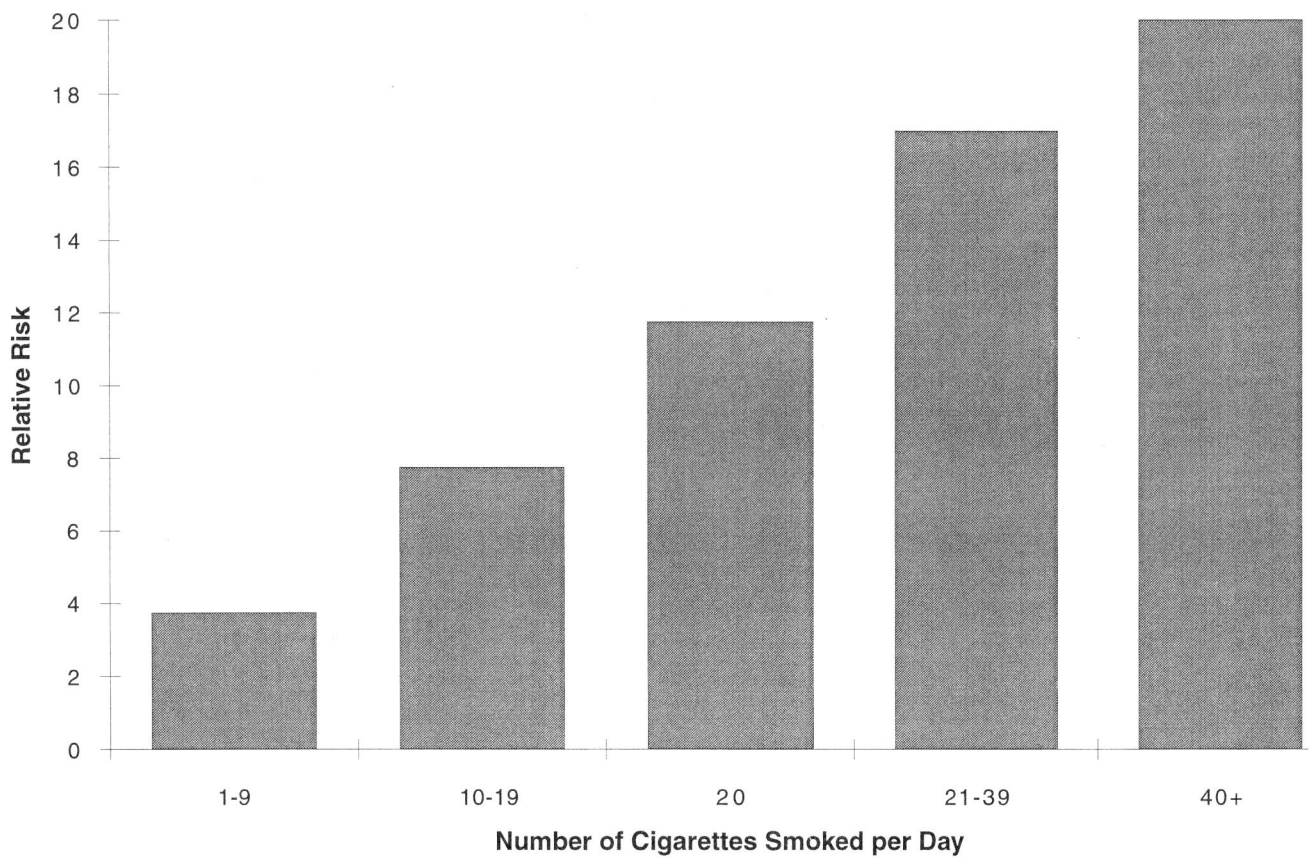

FIGURE 3.2. Relative risks of developing lung cancer among smokers of different numbers of cigarettes per day compared with nonsmokers.

group's age specific rates, corresponding to those age groups of smokers present within each duration category.

In contrast to age specific relative risks that increase, peak, and then decline with advancing age, duration specific risks increase steadily with increasing duration. There is a time lag between the initiation of smoking and the onset of an increased risk. Relative risks for lung cancer are low, and there is no clear dose-response relationship with number of cigarettes smoked per day, until the 20- to 24-year–duration category (41).

Lung cancer mortality rates and relative risks are lower for white females than for white males. Excess mortality rates among smokers are also lower. The general pattern of dose-response relationships and changes in risk with age are similar for males and females, once differences in the magnitude of risks are considered. Part of the difference between males and females in relative and excess mortality relates to differences in duration of smoking between males and females of the same age, particularly among the older age groups in which the majority of lung cancer deaths occur. Males began smoking cigarettes in large numbers in the early part of this century, whereas females began smoking during the 1930s and 1940s. Female smokers also smoked fewer cigarettes per day than male smokers, contributing to their lower age specific relative risks. Figure 3.4 presents duration specific lung cancer relative risks for males and females who smoke 20 cigarettes per day and for all levels of consumption combined. The lung cancer risks for males are higher than those for females for all levels of consumption combined and for a specific dose (20 cigarettes per day). The risk ratios for 20 cigarettes per day are similar to those of all levels for males, but the combined risk ratios are lower than the 20 cigarettes per day level for females. This suggests that there are additional reductions in combined relative risks in females produced by the relative distribution of female smokers into strata with lower numbers of cigarettes smoked per day. Past differences in the number of cigarettes smoked per day, tar yield of the cigarettes smoked, depth of inhalation, or other factors may explain these gender-based differences in lung cancer risks.

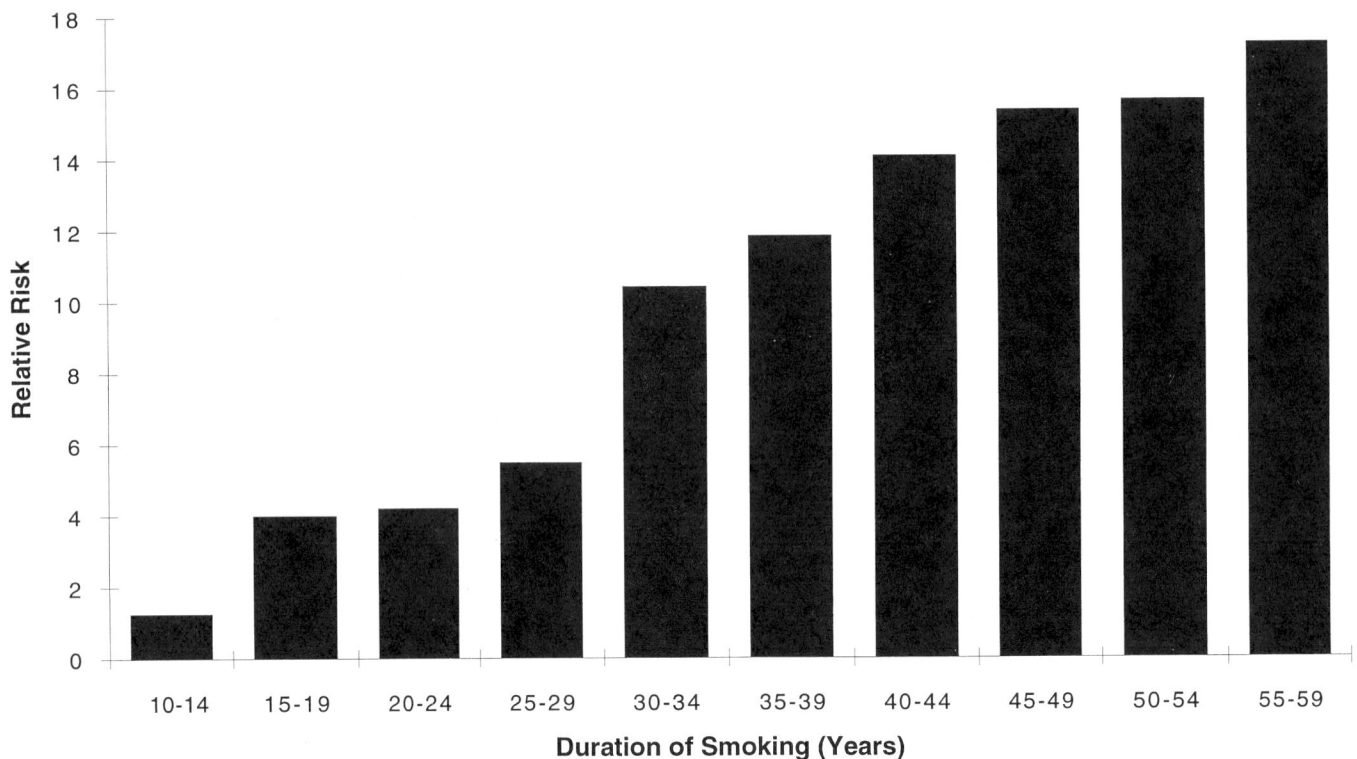

FIGURE 3.3. Relative risk of developing lung cancer among smokers of different durations compared with nonsmokers. The comparison rate of those who have never smoked is a weighted average of never smoker age specific rates corresponding to those age groups of smokers present within each duration category. The age specific rates of those who have never smoked are weighted by the person-months of follow-up in each age group of smokers within the duration category.

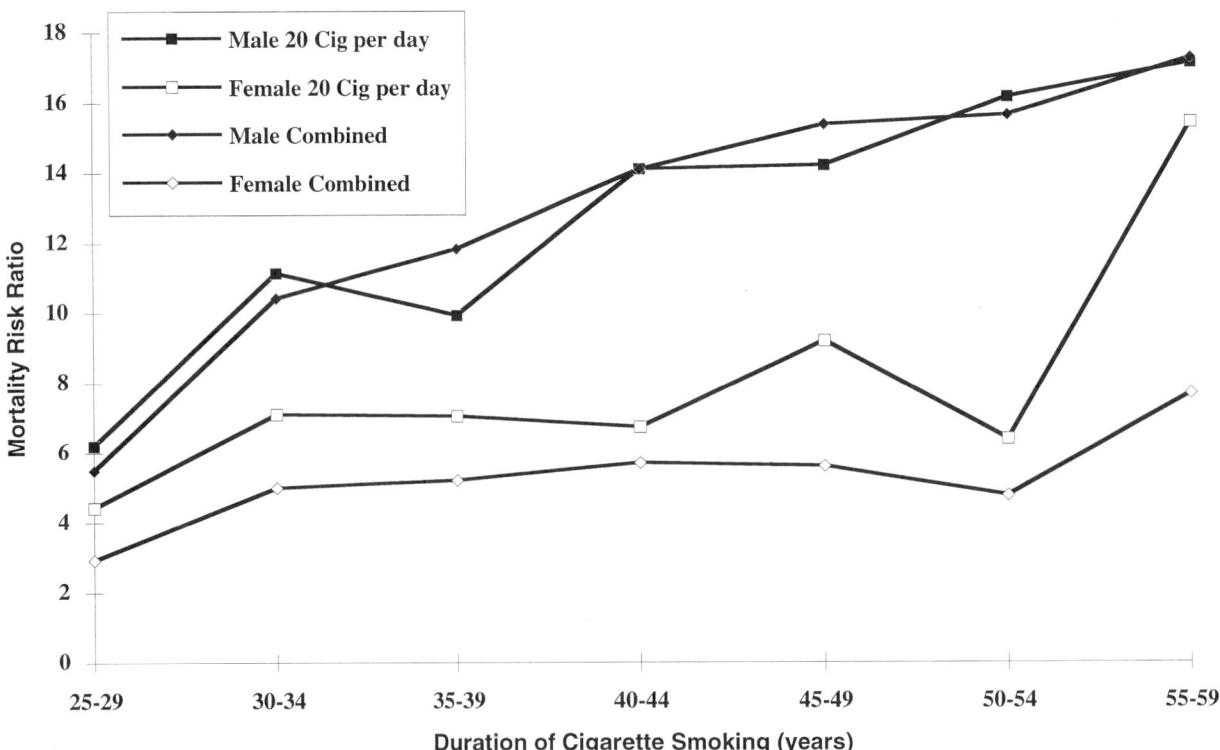

FIGURE 3.4. Duration and number of cigarettes per day—specific relative risks of developing lung cancer among male smokers compared with female smokers. The comparison rate of those who have never smoked is a weighted average of never smoker age specific rates corresponding to those age groups of smokers present within each duration category. The age specific rates of those who have never smoked are weighted by the person-months of follow-up in each age group of smokers within the duration category.

CHANGES IN THE RISK OF SMOKING WITH DURATION OF CESSATION

Relative risks for lung cancer decline with the cessation of cigarette smoking (Fig. 3.5). Mortality risks within the first year of cessation often are reported to be higher than those for continuing smokers because many individuals quit after the diagnosis of disease. For this reason, relative risks, beginning after the second year of cessation and excluding those deaths and person-years of follow-up that occurred during the first 24 months of cessation, are presented. The relative risks for lung cancer decline with continuing cessation but seem to plateau once 20 years of cessation has been reached. Relative risk remains elevated at approximately 1.5 to 2 times that of those who have never smoked even after long durations of cessation.

ENVIRONMENTAL TOBACCO SMOKE

Concentrations of smoke constituents are far lower in ETS than those inhaled by the smoker, and the total quantity of smoke constituents inhaled over time also is much lower. This difference in exposure dose explains the lower disease risks experienced by nonsmokers compared with smokers. However, exposure to ETS commonly begins earlier in life than does active smoking, particularly for children of smokers, and the duration of carcinogenic exposure is a powerful determinant of lung cancer risk.

Levels of ETS in air are determined by the number of smokers, the size of the room, and the amount of air brought in from the outside by the ventilation system. The small particle size of the smoke aerosol makes most conventional air filters ineffective for removing smoke. Therefore, in buildings that recirculate air, smoke generated in one part of the building is dispersed rapidly throughout the entire structure. As a result, separating smokers and nonsmokers within the same ventilated space is not an effective approach to eliminating exposure.

High levels of ETS exposure occur in smokey environments (e.g., taverns), when one is in close proximity to the smoker (e.g., infants of a nursing mother), and when one is exposed to smokers both at work and at home. Bans on smoking at work that include all work areas are effective in reducing exposure (42).

Given the steep dose-response relationship between the number of cigarettes smoked per day by ac-

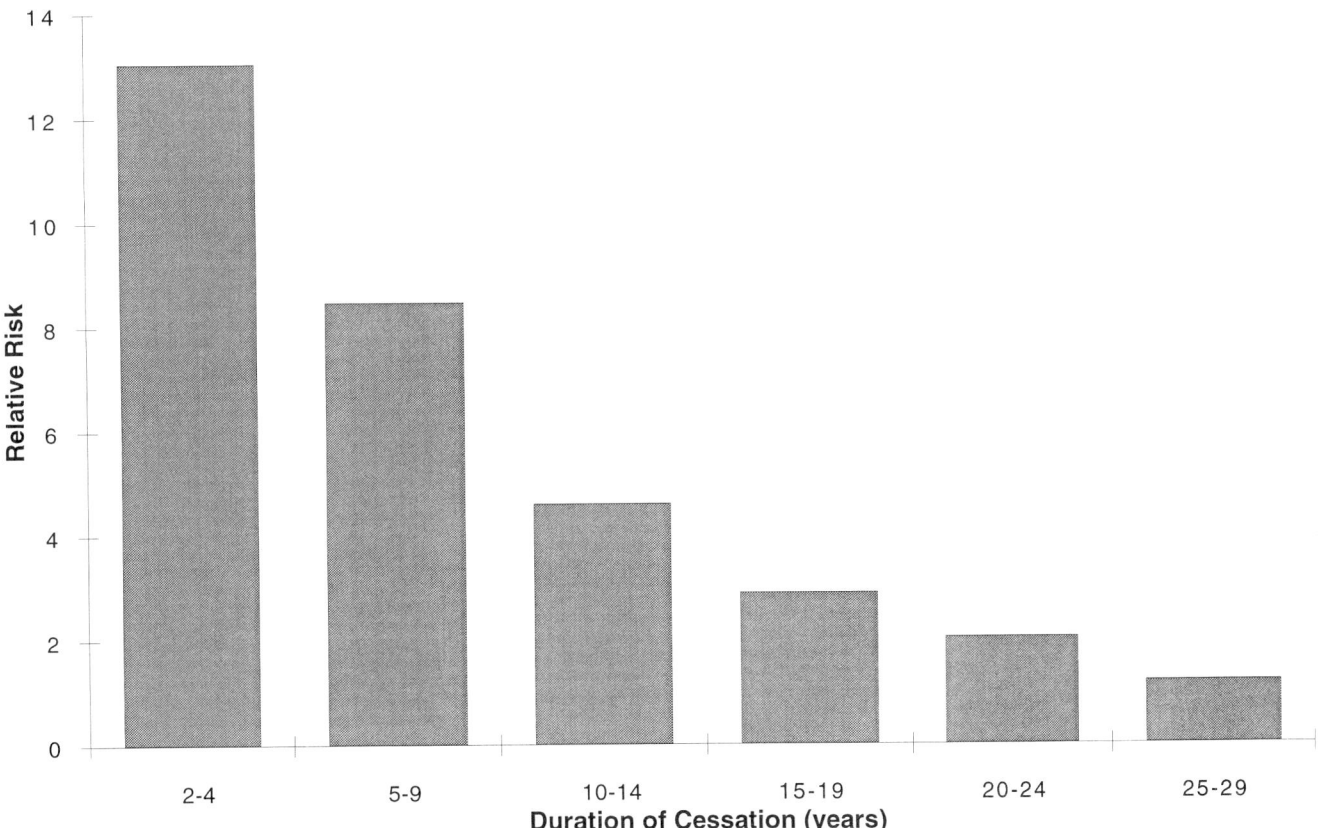

FIGURE 3.5. Relative risk of developing lung cancer among former smokers with different durations since cessation compared with nonsmokers.

tive smokers and the risk of developing lung cancer, one could predict that the levels of exposure measured in the general environment and the amount of smoke absorption found among nonsmokers would result in an increased risk of lung cancer. Epidemiologic studies of nonsmokers exposed to higher doses of ETS compared with those with lower dose exposures, usually the spouses of smokers compared with spouses of nonsmokers, show an increased risk of lung cancer and a dose-response relationship between intensity of exposure and relative risk.

SMOKING BEHAVIOR

Tobacco was used by Native American populations before the arrival of Columbus in the Americas. Tobacco was used commonly in the American colonies, and subsequently in the United States, as chewing tobacco and snuff and in pipes and cigars during the 18th and 19th centuries. However, widespread use of tobacco as cigarettes is more recent, occurring largely during the 20th century. Figure 3.6 presents the quantity of tobacco used in the United States as different product types during the last 100 years. Figure 3.7 shows per capita and total consumption of cigarettes from 1900 to the present. There have been substantial changes in the use of tobacco products over time, with a shift toward cigarettes and away from other forms of tobacco. A dramatic increase and decrease in the per capita and total number of cigarettes smoked also has occurred over the last century.

Smoking behavior has been influenced profoundly by events and trends in the larger social environment within which smoking occurs (1), as well as by the dependence-producing properties of cigarettes acting within the psychologic and physiologic structure of the individual (34). Interpretation of data on smoking behavior requires an understanding of the social and political contexts within which smoking developed and which have prompted smokers to quit.

Cigarette smoking as a form of tobacco use was uncommon before 1900 (Fig. 3.6). Per capita consumption of cigarettes in the United States was 54 in 1900 (2), in contrast to its peak of 4345 in 1963 (Fig. 3.7). Conversion of tobacco use from pipes, cigars, and chewing tobacco to cigarettes was enabled by the in-

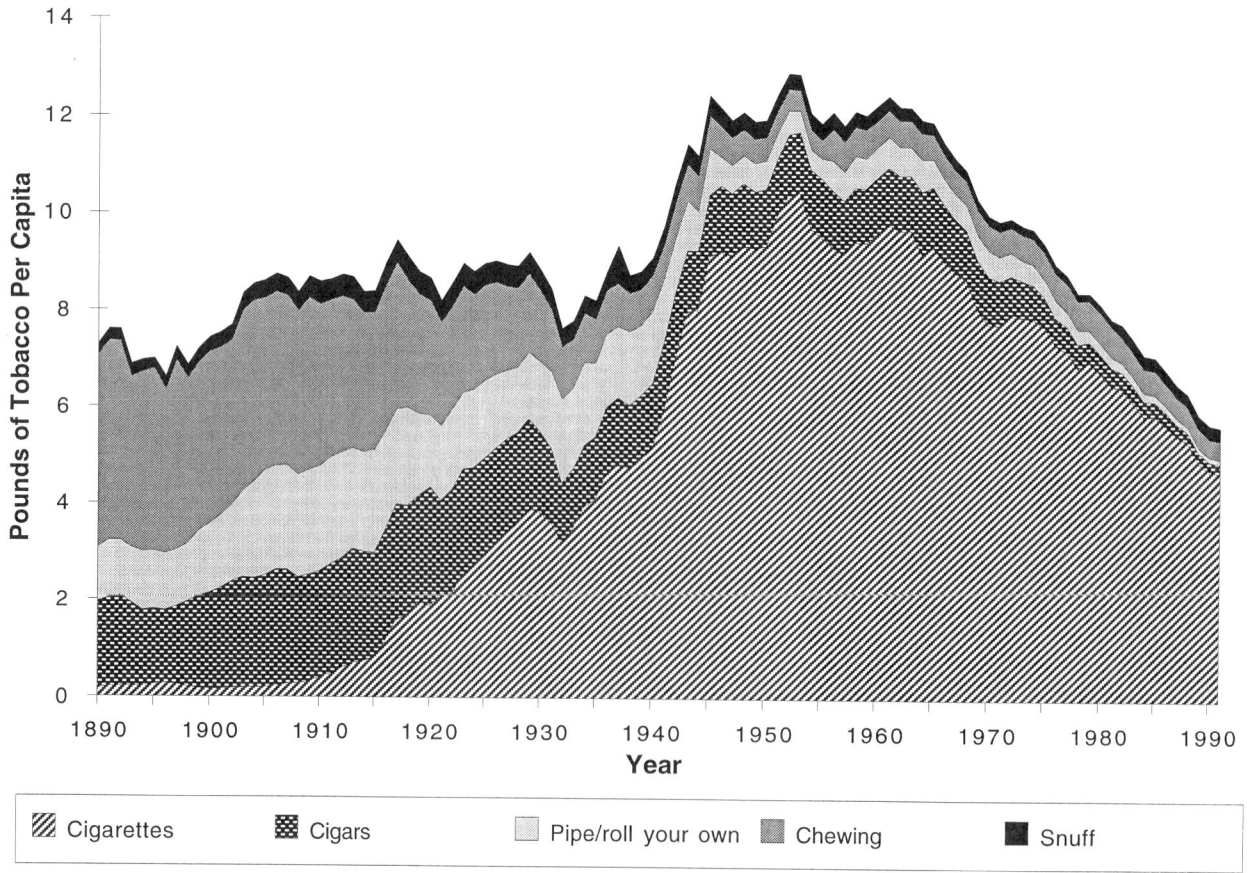

FIGURE 3.6. Per capita consumption of different forms of tobacco in the United States from 1890 to 1990.

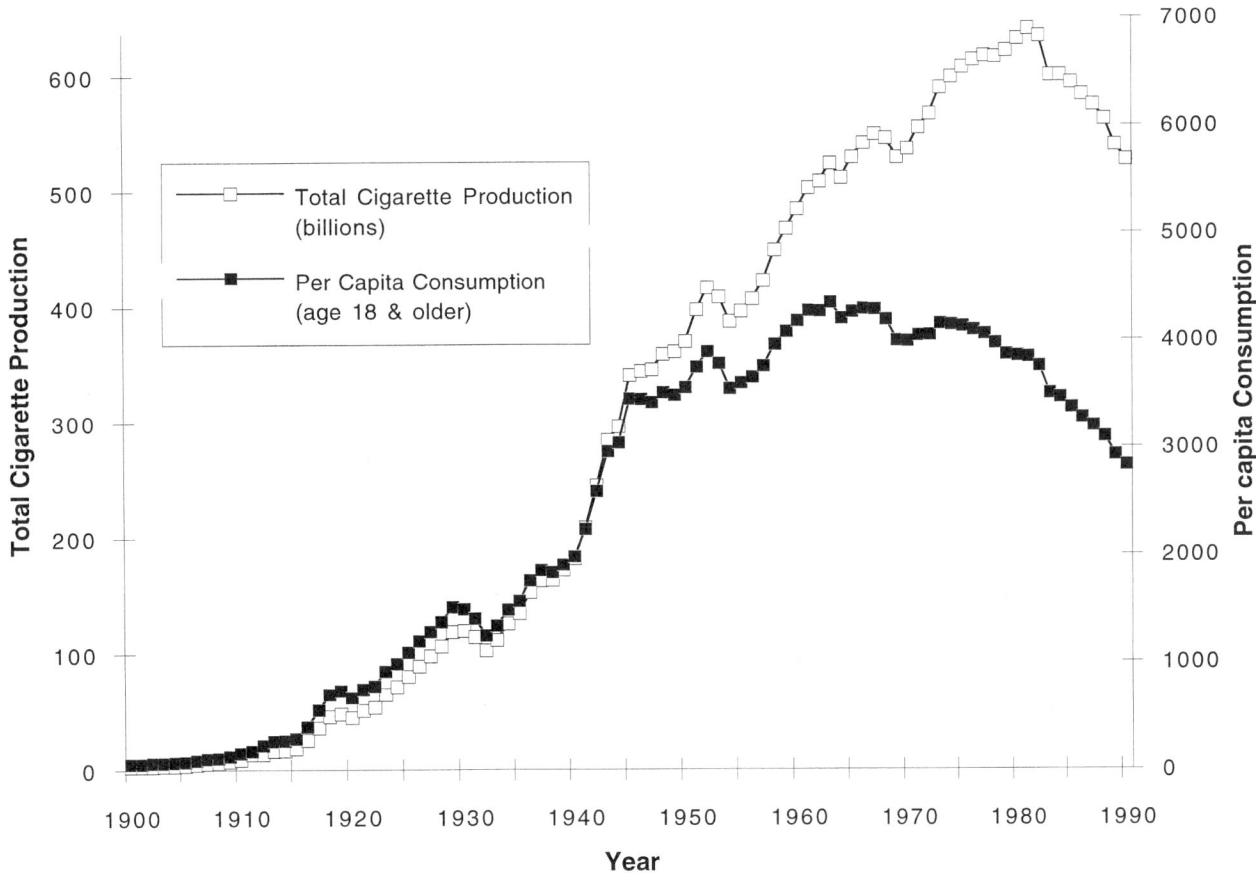

FIGURE 3.7. Total and per capita cigarette consumption in the United States from 1900 to 1992.

vention of machines that could mass produce cigarettes, eliminating the need to hand roll cigarettes, and by the development of safety matches that allowed a convenient, portable means of lighting cigarettes (43). However, the real growth in cigarette sales occurred after the application of advertising and mass marketing techniques to the sale of cigarettes during the second decade of this century. The remarkable growth in sales of Camel cigarettes following a national promotional campaign in 1913 established the power of advertising in promoting sales (44). It set the stage for mass marketing of other brands of cigarettes and for a dramatic jump in cigarette use during the next several decades (44). Initially, cigarette marketing targeted males, but beginning in the late 1920s and 1930s, advertising campaigns directed toward women began to appear (45). The most notorious of these campaigns was the Reach for a Lucky—instead of a sweet—series of advertisements that began a marketing theme linking cigarette smoking to weight control; this theme continues with other brands of cigarettes to this day (45, 46).

Dramatic changes have occurred in per capita consumption of cigarettes during each of the world wars with the mobilization of large numbers of males into the military and, during the second world war, of women into the workforce. Marketing and free distribution of cigarettes to military personnel during the second world war is likely to have played a prominent role in generating the very high prevalence (approximately 80%) of smoking among cohorts of males who were of the correct ages to have served in the military during the second world war (41).

Concern among members of the scientific community that cigarette smoking caused disease grew with the publication of retrospective epidemiologic studies of lung cancer in the late 1940s and early 1950s. Publication, and widespread dissemination in the lay press, of the first major prospective mortality studies defining the disease risks of smoking cigarettes occurred during the mid-1950s (2). Initial response to this knowledge included a public information campaign and development of smoking cessation interventions for individuals (1). The tobacco industry's response was the creation of the Council for Tobacco Research (47), which legitimized the tobacco industry's media campaign to confuse the public about the strength of the scientific evidence linking cigarette smoking and disease (43, 46). At the same time, cigarette companies introduced and marketed filtered cigarettes and low tar and low nicotine yield cigarettes in an effort to counter growing health concerns among smokers (6, 46).

On June 2, 1967, the U.S. Federal Communications Commission ruled that significant amounts of free time be made available for antismoking commercials to balance the cigarette advertisements on television and radio (2). During the period between 1967 and 1970, a large number of antismoking television announcements were broadcast free by the major television networks. The time donated for these public service announcements was worth approximately $75 million per year in 1970 dollars (48). Substantial tobacco control efforts also were made by voluntary health agencies and other concerned groups during these years (1, 2). Cigarette advertising was banned from television and radio in 1970, and the number of antismoking announcements broadcast declined by an estimated 80% (49). Effectiveness of this antitobacco advertising is supported by changes in per capita consumption in the United States during the period of intense broadcast activity (50–56) occurring between 1967 and 1970 (Fig. 3.7). Per capita consumption declined 6.9% between 1967 and 1970, in contrast to a 2% increase during the years immediately preceding the media campaign (1965–1967). When cigarette advertising was banned from broadcast media after 1970, antismoking spots also were removed, and per capita consumption increased 4.1% from 1971 to 1973 (50, 57, 58).

Concerns about exposure to ETS and the social acceptability of smoking surfaced around 1970 (59) and grew rapidly in the 1970s and early 1980s (10). These concerns were confirmed by the demonstration of a causal link between ETS and lung cancer in the mid-1980s (10, 60).

DIFFERENCES IN SMOKING BEHAVIOR AMONG POPULATION SUBGROUPS

Cross-sectional surveys of the American population show differences in smoking prevalence among various demographic categories (2, 61). Males have a higher prevalence of smoking than females (61, 62). There are differences in smoking prevalence among different age and racial groupings (62) with peak smoking prevalence occurring in young adulthood. Blacks of both genders have higher smoking prevalences than whites (61). Hispanic smokers, particularly Hispanic women, have lower rates of smoking, as do Asian women (42).

Men took up smoking in large numbers earlier in the century (30, 63) than women, and differences among racial groups also have varied over time (10, 63, 64). Patterns of smoking prevalence, initiation, and cessation vary across age, gender, and racial categories, and are different for individuals born in different years.

The prevalence of smoking varies with a variety of measures of socioeconomic status, including income and job classification, but one of the strongest relationships is with the number of years of formal education achieved (62). Individuals with higher levels of education are less likely to begin smoking and are more likely to have quit. Because most of the initiation of cigarette smoking occurs before the age at which education is complete, this correlation with education reflects the environmental factors that predict both educational achievement and nonsmoking status. The gradient in smoking status with socioeconomic status shown for adults is even more evident for adolescents. College freshman have smoking prevalence rates of less than 10%, whereas Job Corps applicants of the same age have smoking prevalence rates of more than 60%.

PREVALENCE OF CURRENT SMOKING

Differences in smoking behaviors by year of birth make interpretation of age specific estimates from multiple cross-sectional samples over time difficult and often confusing. A given age group in cross-sectional surveys done at different points in time will contain individuals who were born in different years. Changes in smoking behaviors within the specified age group over time may be produced by either temporal (calendar year) or cohort (year of birth) effects. Analyses in this chapter are presented by race specific and gender specific 5-year birth cohorts. A birth cohort is comprised of individuals born during specific calendar years—5-year groups in this presentation. Birth cohort analyses describe changes in smoking behavior among individuals born during the same calendar years as they age. This format presents a more accurate picture of the life history of smoking than can be derived from examining the differences in smoking behavior among different age groups in single or multiple, independent, cross-sectional samples of the population. The description is based on a pooling of data from the National Health Interview Surveys (NHIS) conducted between 1965 and 1991 (41). Current smoker prevalence is presented by calendar year, rather than age, to examine changes in smoking behavior in relation to temporal events occurring over the last century.

Initiation of regular smoking within each birth cohort is manifested as a rapid increase in prevalence during adolescence and early adulthood. Examination of Figures 3.8 through 3.11 shows that initiation is largely confined to adolescence and very early adulthood. With the exception of older cohorts of women, most smokers become regular smokers before achieving adulthood. Two descriptors are of interest in relation to the initiation of cigarette smoking: the percentage of the cohort that becomes cigarette smokers and the age distribution of initiation within the cohort.

A rapid increase in smoking prevalence occurring during adolescence is evident in all of the male cohorts (Figs. 3.8 and 3.9) and is manifest in these figures as a rapid increase in prevalence occurring 5 calendar years apart for each succeeding cohort. The percentage of the cohort who ultimately become smokers increases for the first several cohorts of white males. Increasing rates of initiation occurred between 1910 and 1920, coinciding with a rise in per capita consumption after 1910 (Fig. 3.7). Change across male cohorts coincides with mass marketing of machine-manufactured cigarettes around 1913 (44). Older male cohorts were in early adulthood when tobacco manufacturers began using mass marketing approaches to induce males to become cigarette smokers and, therefore, may have been less vulnerable to advertising approaches than younger cohorts. Those cohorts born after 1900 were subjected to tobacco advertising and promotion throughout adolescence, took up smoking in large numbers (more than 80%), and began smoking predominantly before age 25.

Male cohorts born after 1900 and before 1934 have relatively similar patterns of uptake and rates of peak cohort smoking prevalence. The major difference in the pattern of current smoking among these cohorts, and between these cohorts and the more recent cohorts, is the width of the plateau that occurs around peak prevalence and the rate of decline in current smoking prevalence over time. Older cohorts have very broad plateaus, indicating that very little cessation occurred during the years before 1950. More recent cohorts have a narrower plateau, with a rapid decline in prevalence occurring almost as soon as the peak prevalence is achieved. A rapid decline in smoking prevalence occurs across all of the older male cohorts beginning in 1955, and the rate of decline accelerates in the

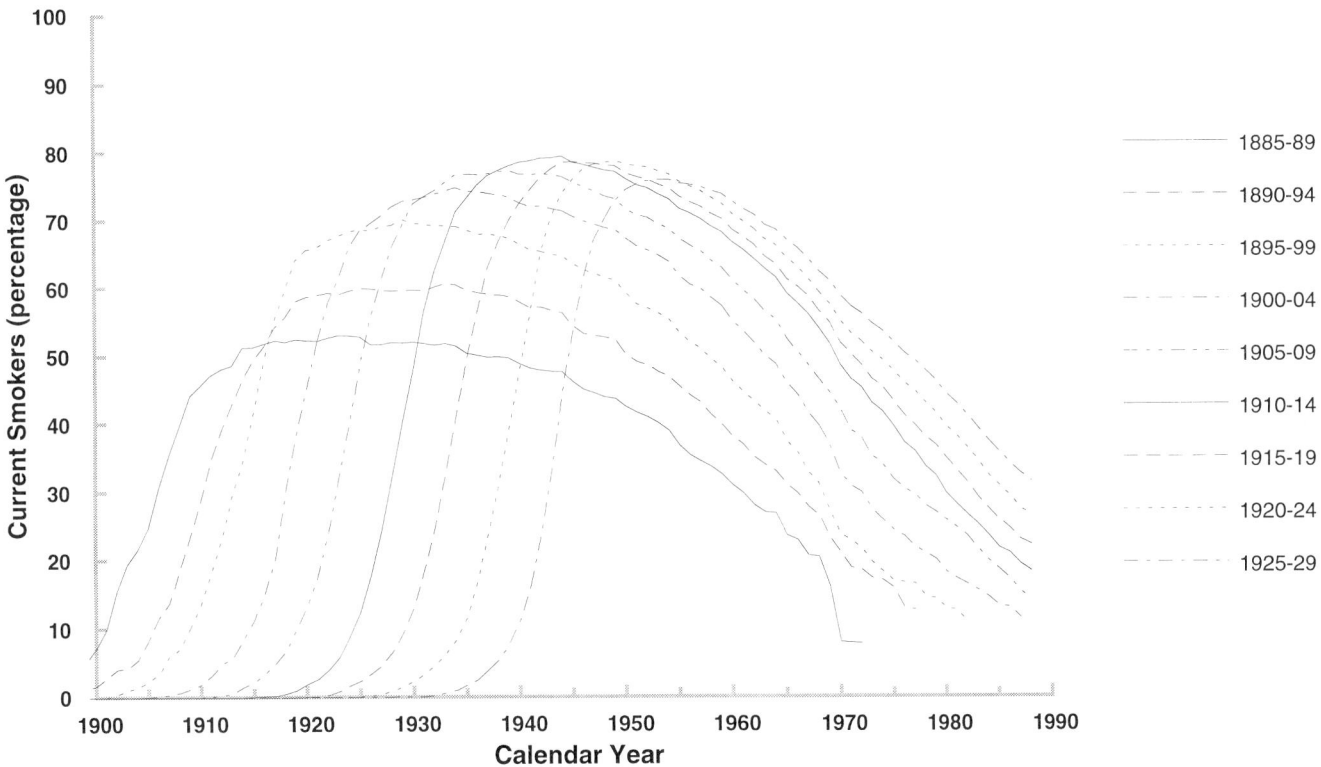

FIGURE 3.8. Current smoking prevalence by calendar year for 5-year birth cohorts of white males born between 1885 and 1929.

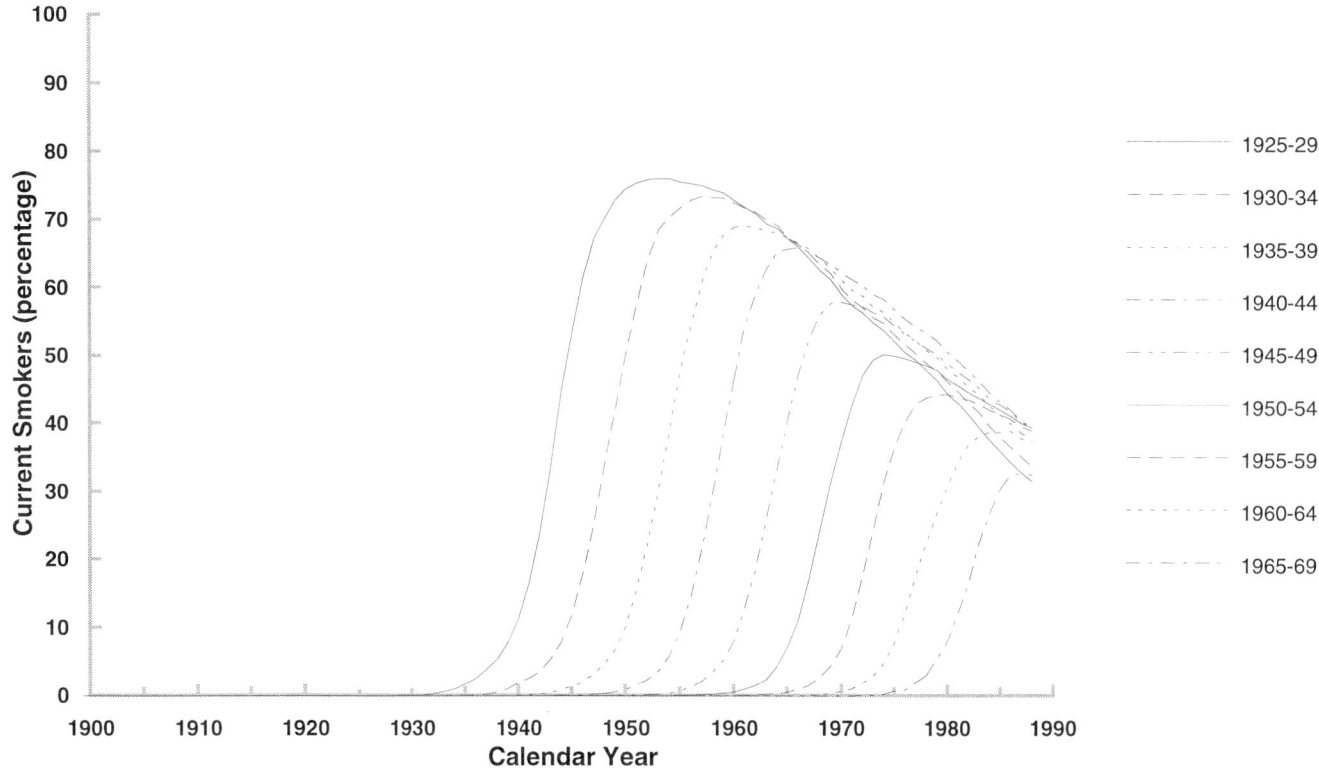

FIGURE 3.9. Current smoking prevalence by calendar year for 5-year birth cohorts of white males born between 1925 and 1969.

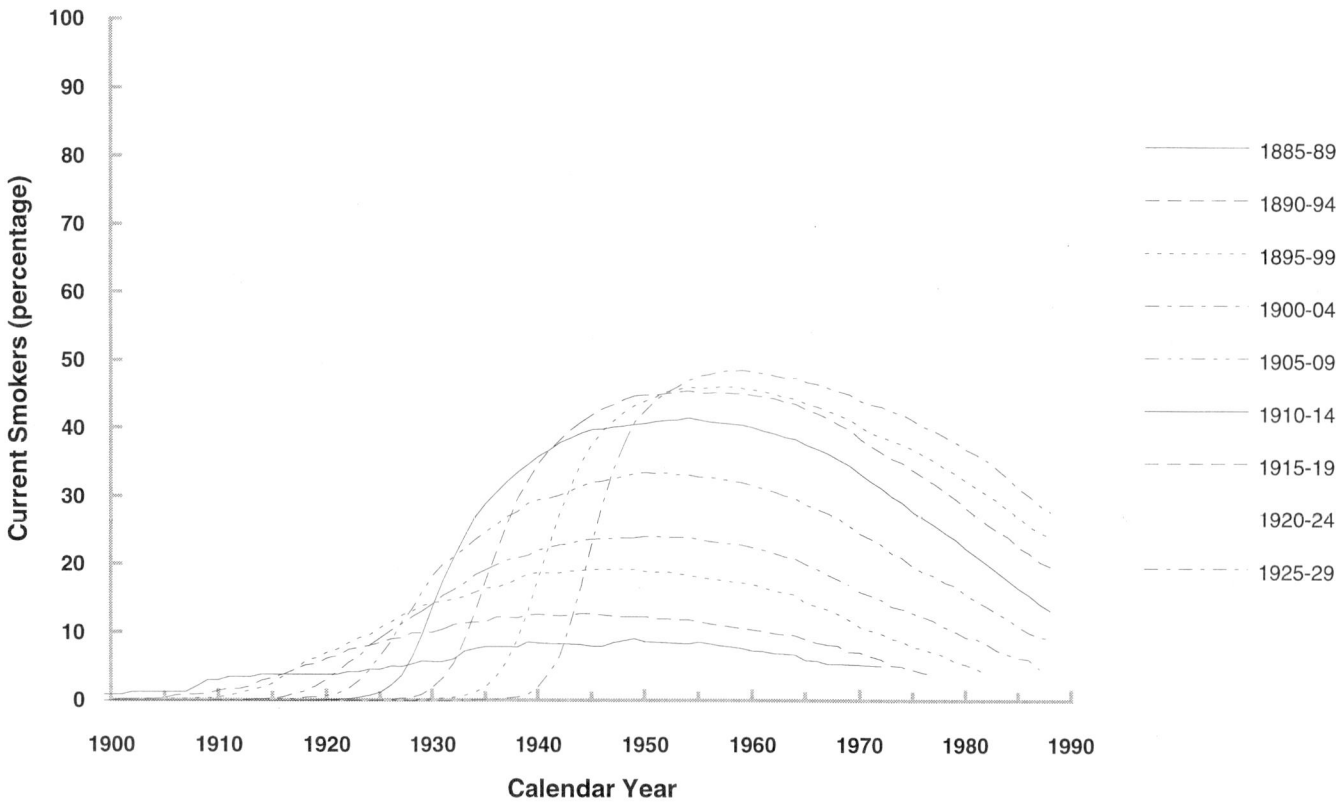

FIGURE 3.10. Current smoking prevalence by calendar year for 5-year birth cohorts of white females born between 1885 and 1929.

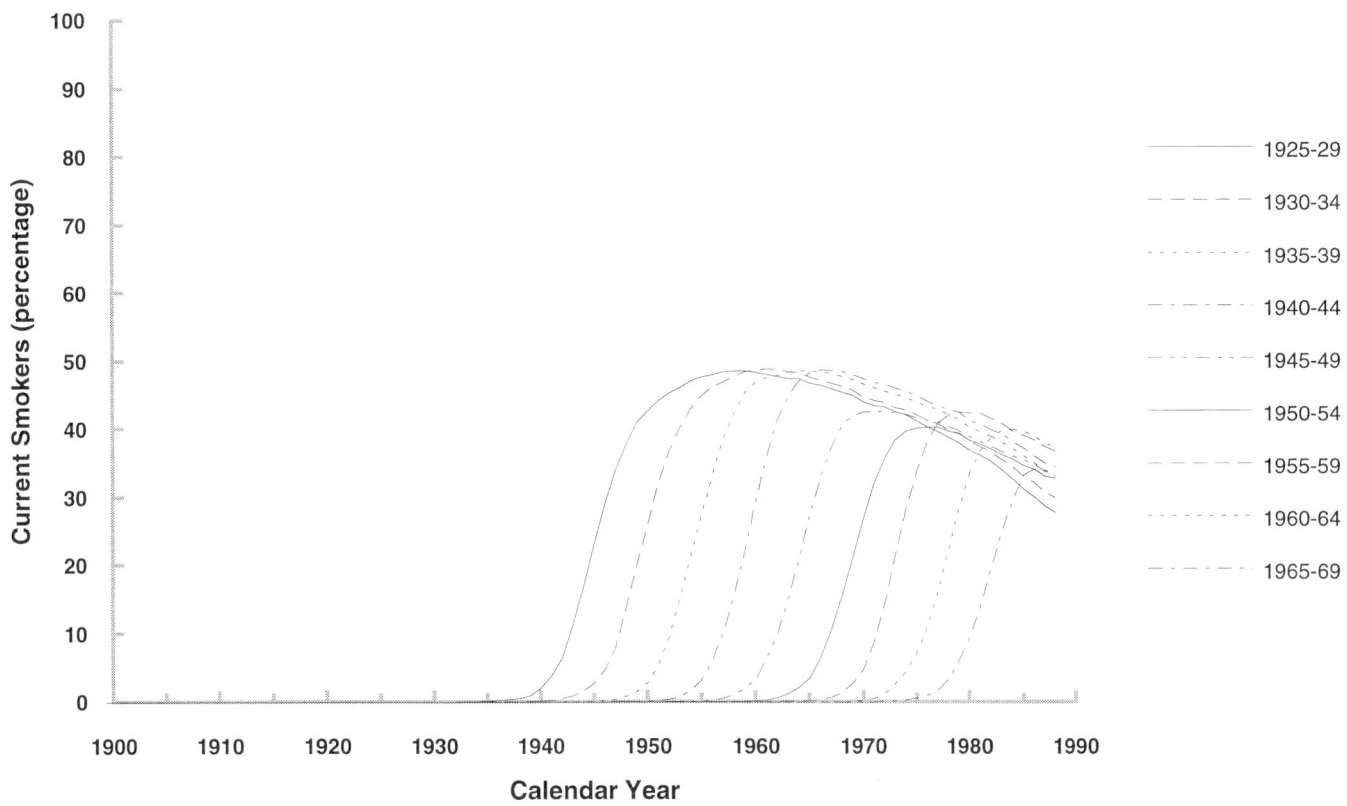

FIGURE 3.11. Current smoking prevalence by calendar year for 5-year birth cohorts of white females born between 1925 and 1969

late 1960s. The first major prospective mortality studies linking cigarettes to disease were published in the mid-1950s, and there was a concerted tobacco control effort, including a highly visible television antismoking campaign, between 1967 and 1970. Data for white males suggest that the effects of these tobacco control influences were felt across all cohorts of adult smokers and resulted in substantial changes in smoking behavior among white males of all ages.

The pattern of current smoking prevalence observed among those male cohorts born after 1930 (Fig. 3.9) is one of declining peak prevalences with each succeeding cohort. The prevalence of smoking in any given calendar year is very similar across all recent cohorts, again suggesting that temporal events may have a more powerful influence on smoking prevalence than does age.

Smoking initiation among older cohorts of white females shows a clear relationship with calendar year (Fig. 3.10). Very few women smoked before 1925, and a rapid increase in smoking prevalence is evident during the 1930s across several cohorts. This dramatic change in smoking behavior among women coincides with the tobacco industry's efforts to target women through tobacco advertising during the 1930s and 1940s (45). The pattern of initiation among white females is strikingly different from that for white males among those cohorts born before 1930. Differences are evident both in the highest prevalence achieved by the cohort and by the age range over which initiation occurred. The percentage of women who took up smoking increases with each sequential cohort from 1895 to 1940–1944, but the most dramatic differences between white males and white females are in the age distribution over which initiation occurs. In more recent cohorts, initiation is confined to adolescence and very early adulthood for both genders. However, earlier cohorts of females had substantial initiation during the third, fourth, and fifth decades of life. Before 1930, cigarette smoking was largely a male behavior, but initiation occurred across all birth cohorts of women during the 1930s and 1940s. Initiation was, therefore, spread across all age groups and not confined to adolescence and early adulthood. The peak prevalence of smoking among females is lower than that of comparable cohorts of white males for all but the two most recent cohorts.

SUMMARY

Lung cancer is a preventable disease process. The vast majority of lung cancers occurring in the United

States could be eliminated if cigarette smoking disappeared as a human behavior. Risks of smoking are proportional to the number of cigarettes smoked per day, and they increase exponentially with the duration of smoking. Lung cancer relative risks are evident after 20 years of smoking, and they decline with cessation.

Cigarette smoking is a form of tobacco use largely confined to the 20th century. The onset of cigarette smoking in the early 1900s resulted from the successful application of mass marketing techniques directed to males, with the targeting of females resulting in a rapid increase in smoking among women in the 1930s. Currently, initiation of cigarette smoking occurs almost exclusively during adolescence and before adulthood.

References

1. U.S. National Cancer Institute (NCI). Strategies to control tobacco use in the United States: a blueprint for public health action in the 1990s. Washington, DC: Department of Health and Human Services, National Institutes of Health/NCI, Smoking and Tobacco Control Monograph No 1, 1992;1:3–31.
2. U.S. Department of Health and Human Services (DHHS). The health consequences of smoking: 25 years of progress. Washington, DC: DHSS, Public Health Service, Centers for Disease Control and Prevention, Office on Smoking and Health, DHHS Publication No (CDC) 89-8411, 1989.
3. International Agency for Research on Cancer (IARC). Tobacco smoking. Lyon, France: IARC, IARC Monographs on the Evaluation od Carcinogenic Risk of Chemicals to Humans, 1986.
4. Baker RR. The effect of ventilation on cigarette combustion mechanisms. Recent Advances in Tobacco Science 1984;10:88–150.
5. Adams JD, O'Mara-Adams KJ, Hoffmann D. On the mainstream-sidestream distribution of cigarette smoke components. Paper presented at the 39th Tobacco Chemists' Research Conference, Montreal, Canada, Oct. 2–5, 1985.
6. U.S. Department of Health and Human Services (DHHS). The health consequences of smoking: the changing cigarette. Washington, DC: DHHS, Public Health Service, Office of the Assistant Secretary for Health, Office on Smoking and Health, DHHS Publication No (PHS) 81-50156, 1981.
7. Dube MF, Green CR. Methods of collection of smoke for analytical purposes. Recent Advances in Tobacco Science: Formation, Analysis and Composition of Tobacco Smoke 1982;8:42–102.
8. Wynder EL, Hoffman D. Tobacco and tobacco smoke. Studies in experimental carcinogenesis. New York: Academic Press, 1967.
9. Eudy LW, Green CR, Heavor DL, Ingebrethsen BJ, Thorne FA. Studies on the vapor-particulate phase distribution of environmental nicotine by selective trapping and detection methods. Presented at the 39th Tobacco Chemists' Research Conference, Montreal, Canada, Oct 2–5, 1985.
10. U.S. Department of Health and Human Services (DHHS). The health consequences of smoking: involuntary smoking. Washington, DC: DHHS, Public Health Service, Office of the Assistant Secretary for Health, Office on Smoking and Health, DHHS Publication No (PHS) 87-8398, 1986.
11. Radford EP, Hunt VR. Polonium-210: a volatile radioelement in cigarettes. Science 1964;14:247–249.
12. Black SC, Bretthaauer EW. Polonium-210 in tobacco. Radiological Health Data and Reports 1968;9:145–152.
13. Radford EP. Radioactivity in cigarette smoke (letter). N Engl J Med 1982;307:1449–1450.
14. Cross FT. Radioactivity in cigarette smoke issue. Health Phys 1984;46:205–208.
15. Little JB, McGandy RB. Systemic absorption of polonium-210 inhaled in cigarette smoke. Arch Environ Health 1968;17:693–696.
16. Cohen BS, Eisenbud M, Harley NH. Alpha radioactivity in cigarette smoke. Radiat Res 1980;83:190–196.
17. Steinfeld AD. Environmental radiation hazards. Am Fam Physician 1980;22:95–99.
18. Martell EA. Alpha radiation dose at bronchial bifurcations of smokers from indoor exposure to radon progeny. Proc Natl Acad Sci 1983;80:1285–1289.
19. Ingebrethsen BJ. Aerosol studies of cigarette smoke. Recent Advances in Tobacco Science 1986;12:54–142.
20. Hinds WC. Aerosol technology. New York: John Wiley, 1982.
21. International Committee on Radiation Protection, Task Group on Lung Dynamics. Deposition and retention models for internal dosimetry of the human respiratory tract. Health Phys 1966;12:173–207.
22. Mitchell RI. Controlled measurement of smoke-particle retention in the respiratory tract. Am Rev Respir Dis 1962;85:526–533.
23. Hinds WC, First MW, Huber GL, Shea JW. A method for measuring respiratory deposition of cigarette smoke during smoking. Am Ind Hyg Assoc J 1983;44:113–118.
24. Donnelly GM, McKean HE, Heird CS, Green J. Bioassay of a cigarette smoke fraction. I. Examination of dose-response relations and dilution bioassay assumptions in a ciliostasis system. J Toxicol Environ Health 1981;7:405–417.
25. Hilding AC. On cigarette smoking, bronchial carcinoma and ciliary action. II. Experimental study on the filtering action of cow's lungs, the deposition of tar in the bronchial tree and removal by ciliary action. N Engl J Med 1956;254:1150–1160.
26. Dalhamn T. The effect of cigarette smoke in the ciliary activity of the upper respiratory tract. Arch Otolaryngol 1959;70:166–168.
27. U.S. Department of Health and Human Services (DHHS). The health consequences of smoking: chronic obstructive lung disease. Washington, DC: DHHS, Public Health Service, Office of the Assistant Secretary for Health, Office on Smoking and Health, DHHS Publication No (PHS) 84-50205, 1984.
28. Auerbach O, Hammond EC, Garfinkel L. Changes in the bronchial epithelium in relation to cigarette smoking, 1955–1960 vs 1970–1977. N Engl J Med 1979;300:381–386.
29. U.S. Department of Health, Education, and Welfare (DHEW). The health consequences of smoking: a report of the surgeon general. Washington, DC: DHEW, Public Health Service, Office of the Assistant Secretary for Health, Office on Smoking and Health, DHEW Publication No (PHS) 79-50066, 1979.
30. U.S. Department of Health and Human Services (DHHS). The health consequences of smoking for women. Washington, DC: DHHS, Public Health Service, Office of the Assistant Secretary for Health, Office on Smoking and Health, 1980.
31. U.S. Department of Health and Human Services (DHHS). The health consequences of smoking: cancer. Washington, DC: DHHS, Public Health Service, Office of the Assistant Secretary for Health, Office on Smoking and Health, DHHS Publication No (PHS) 82-50179, 1982.
32. U.S. Department of Health and Human Services (DHHS). The health consequences of smoking: cardiovascular disease. Washington, DC: DHHS, Public Health Service, Office of the Assistant

Secretary for Health, Office on Smoking and Health, DHHS Publication No (PHS) 84-50204, 1983.
33. U.S. Department of Health and Human Services (DHHS). The health consequences of smoking: cancer and chronic lung disease in the workplace. Washington, DC: DHHS, Public Health Service, Office of the Assistant Secretary for Health, Office on Smoking and Health, DHHS Publication No (PHS) 85-50207, 1985.
34. U.S. Department of Health and Human Services (DHHS). The health consequences of smoking: nicotine addiction. Washington, DC: Department of Health and Human Services, Public Health Service, Centers for Disease Control and Prevention, Office on Smoking and Health, DHHS Publication No (CDC) 88-8406, 1988.
35. U.S. Department of Health and Human Services (DHHS). The health benefits of smoking cessation. Washington, DC: DHHS, Public Health Service, Centers for Disease Control and Prevention, Office on Smoking and Health, DHHS Publication No (CDC) 90-8416, 1990.
36. Doll R, Peto R. Cigarette smoking and bronchial carcinoma: dose and time relationships among regular smokers and lifelong non-smokers. J Epidemiol Community Health 1978;32:303–313.
37. Hammond EC, Garfinkel L, Seidman H, Lew EA. Some recent findings concerning cigarette smoking. In: Hiatt HH, Watson JD, Winsten JA, eds. Origins of human cancer. Book A: incidence of cancer in humans. Cold Spring Harbor Conference on Cell Proliferation. Cold Spring Harbor, NY: Cold Spring Harbor Laboratory, 1977;4:101–122.
38. Kahn HA. The Dorn study of smoking and mortality among US veterans: report on eight and one-half years of observation. In: Haenszel W, ed. Epidemiological approaches to the study of cancer and other chronic diseases. J Natl Cancer Inst Monograph 1966;19:7–11.
39. Burns D, Shanks T, Choi W, Thun M, Heath C, Garfinkel L. The American Cancer Society Cancer prevention study #1: 12-year follow up on one million men and women. Washington, DC: US Department of Health and Human Services, National Institutes of Health, National Cancer Institute, Prospective Mortality Studies on Smoking and Disease, Smoking and Tobacco Control Monograph No 6, 1995; in press.
40. Moolgavkar SH, Dewanji A, Luebeck G. Cigarette smoking and lung cancer: reanalysis of the British doctor's data. J Natl Cancer Inst 1989;81:415–420.
41. Burns D, Lee L, Shen Z, Gilpin B, Tolley D, Vaughn J, Shanks T. Cigarette smoking behavior in the United States. Washington, DC: US Department of Health and Human Services, National Institutes of Health, National Cancer Institute, Prospective Mortality Studies of Smoking and Disease, Smoking and Tobacco Control Monograph No 6, 1995; in press.
42. Burns D, Pierce J. Tobacco use in California 1990–1991. Sacramento: California Department of Health Services, 1992.
43. Whelan EW. A smoking gun: how the tobacco industry gets away with murder. Philadelphia: George Stickley, 1984.
44. Burrough B, Helyar J. Barbarians at the gate. New York: Harper Perennial Publishers, 1990.
45. Health Advocacy Center. Sixty years of deception: an analysis and compilation of cigarette ads in Time magazine, 1925–1985. Palo Alto, CA: Health Advocacy Center, 1986;1:1925–1939.
46. U.S. National Cancer Institute. Tobacco and the clinician, interventions for medical and dental practice, smoking and tobacco control. Monograph No. 5, Washington, DC: Department of Health and Human Services, National Institutes of Health, NCI, 1994:3–12.
47. Freedman AM, Cohen LP. Smoke and mirrors. Wall Street Journal 1993(Feb 11):A1.
48. Lydon C. Ban of TV cigarette ads could halt free spots against smoking. New York Times 1970(Aug 16):63.
49. Lewit EM, Coate D, Grossman M. The effect of government regulation on teenage smoking. Journal of Law and Economics 1981;24:545–569.
50. Warner KE. The effect of the anti-smoking campaign on cigarette consumption. Am J Public Health 1977;67:645–650.
51. Warner KE. Effects of the antismoking campaign: an update. Am J Public Health 1989;79:144–51.
52. Baltagi BH, Levin D. Estimating dynamic demand for cigarettes using panel data: the effects of bootlegging, taxation and advertising reconsidered. Review of Economic and Statistics 1986;68:148.
53. Schneider L, Klein B, Murphy KM. Government regulation of cigarette health information. Journal of Law and Economics 1981;24:575–612.
54. Fugii ET. The demand for cigarettes: further empirical evidence and its implication for public policy. Applied Economics 1980;12:479–489.
55. Hamilton JL, Gori GB, Benowitz NL, Lynch CJ. Mouth verses deep airways absorption of nicotine. The demand for cigarettes: advertising, the health scare, and the cigarette advertising ban. Review of Economics and Statistics 1972;54:401–411.
56. Doron G. The smoking paradox: public regulation in the tobacco industry. Cambridge, MA: Abt Books, 1979.
57. U.S. Department of Agriculture. Tobacco situation and outlook report. Washington, DC: Department of Agriculture, Economic Research Service, Publication No TS-199, June 1987.
58. Warner KE. Cigarette smoking in the 1970s: the impact of the antismoking campaign on consumption. Science 1981;211:729–731.
59. Steinfeld JL. The public's responsibility: a bill of rights for the non-smoker. R I Med J 1972;55:124–126.
60. US Environmental Protection Agency (EPA). Respiratory health effects of passive smoking: lung cancer and other disorders. Washington, DC: US EPA, Publication No 600/6-90/006F, December 1992.
61. Fiore MF, Novotny TE, Pierce JP, Hatziandreu E, Patel K, Davis R. Trends in cigarette smoking in the United States: the changing influence of gender and race. JAMA 1989;261:49–55.
62. Pierce J, Hatziandreu E. Report of the 1986 adult use of tobacco survey. Washington, DC: U.S. Department of Health and Human Services, Public Health Service, Centers for Disease Control and Prevention, Office on Smoking and Health, Government Printing Office Publication No 10491, 1989:625–512.
63. Harris J. Cigarette smoking among successive birth cohorts of men and women in the United States during 1900–80. J Natl Cancer Inst 1983;71:473–479.
64. Crane L, Herman-Shipley N, Tolley D. Smoking prevalences and lung cancer mortality rates. In: Burns D, Samet J, Gritz E, eds. Comprehensive approaches to tobacco control. Washington, DC: U.S. Department of Health and Human Services, Public Health Service, National Cancer Institute, Tobacco Control Monograph No 1, 1992.

4

Occupational and Environmental Causes of Lung Cancer and Esophageal Cancer

William G. Hughson and M. Joseph Fedoruk

INTRODUCTION

This chapter describes occupational and environmental causes of lung cancer and esophageal cancer. The emphasis is placed on occupational risk factors rather than environmental carcinogens, because most data come from studies of industrially exposed populations.

Lung cancer was rare until the 1920s when increased incidence was noted in Europe and North America. Initially, the increase was attributed to greater life expectancy, allowing survival to an age when cancer might be expected. It also was thought that improved methods of diagnosis with radiography and bronchography allowed identification of cases previously missed. However, the more rapid increase occurring in men compared with women, and autopsy records documenting greater frequency of primary bronchogenic tumors, convinced many experts that research was needed. Two major causal agents were suspected: tobacco smoking and increased atmospheric pollution. By the 1950s, epidemiologic investigations had established cigarette smoking as the major risk factor for lung cancer. Unanswered was the degree to which environmental and occupational factors were responsible (1).

Even before the epidemic caused by smoking, there was concern that industrial activities such as cobalt mining (radon), coal gas production (polycyclic aromatic hydrocarbons), manufacture of chromates (hexavalent chromium), and refining of nickel could cause lung cancer. Research in the ensuing decades established these and other agents as occupational lung carcinogens. In 1981, Doll and Peto (2) reported that occupational exposures caused approximately 15% of lung cancers in American men and 5% of lung cancers in American women; these figures remain the most widely quoted estimate today. Subsequent reviews have concluded that between 0.6% and 40% of lung cancers are occupational (3–5). This wide range is explained by the degree of risk associated with specific agents, the population studied and selection of comparison groups, the nature and intensity of exposure, and the study methods.

In general, when a particular occupational exposure causes an increased frequency of lung cancer, all cell types are increased to about the same extent. Exceptions are bis(chloromethyl) ether and radon, which cause a disproportionate increase in small cell cancer (6).

SOURCES OF INFORMATION CONCERNING OCCUPATIONAL CARCINOGENS

IN VITRO AND IN VIVO METHODS

In vitro assays have been developed to test for carcinogenesis. These include bacterial and mammalian mutation assays, measurement of unscheduled DNA synthesis, cell transformation assays, and cytogenetic assays (7). One problem with in vitro assays occurs when an inactive procarcinogen must undergo metabolic transformation in an intact animal to produce an active carcinogen. Multiple techniques must be used, because false-negative results can occur, e.g., asbestos tests being negative using mutation assays but positive with cell transformation.

Animal studies provide important information concerning the potential for an agent to cause cancer in humans. Regulatory agencies must often rely on animal data in assessing hazards to the public from chemical exposures because human epidemiologic data are not available or do not have sufficient statistical power to detect small risks. Animal data are used by the International Agency for Research on Cancer (IARC), the

U.S. Environmental Protection Agency (EPA), the U.S. National Institute for Occupational Safety and Health (NIOSH), and other regulatory bodies to classify carcinogens. IARC has taken the position that, "in the absence of adequate data on humans, it is biologically plausible and prudent to regard agents for which there is sufficient evidence of carcinogenicity in experimental animals as if they present a carcinogenic risk to humans" (8). This approach is consistent with the philosophy of most regulatory agencies and is supported by the fact that all known or suspected human carcinogens that have been adequately tested experimentally have been shown to cause cancer in at least one species of animal.

There are difficulties in extrapolating the results of animal studies to risks in humans. Among these are interspecies differences in the activation (or detoxification) of carcinogens, rate of DNA repair, and biochemical activity in target organs (9). Within species, some strains have very high rates of certain tumors, which appear to arise spontaneously.

There are well-defined protocols for animal testing of carcinogens (10, 11). In addition to choosing the species and route of administration, a range of doses is given, including the maximum tolerated dose. At the maximum tolerated dose, systemic toxicity frequently occurs. This toxicity is manifest by lethargy, poor appetite, and weight loss in the animals. Concern has been expressed by some experts that this degree of toxicity may cause cellular injury and mitogenesis, leading to increased rates of mutagenesis and carcinogenesis (12, 13). Because toxic cellular damage would occur rarely under exposure conditions in the normal human environment, inferences drawn from high-dose animal studies may be imprecise concerning hazards for the general population.

Similarly, intratracheal instillation or inhalation experiments of agents at very high levels can cause fibrotic lesions in the lungs of experimental animals. These may be interpreted pathologically as neoplastic, although their relevance to the human condition is debatable.

Role of Epidemiology

Historically, the development of information concerning cancer risks in humans often has begun with the publication of one or more case reports. An example would be the 1935 article by Lynch and Smith (14), which described lung cancer in a patient with asbestosis. However, case reports cannot be used to prove a causal relationship, because they do not provide information concerning the number of people exposed to the agent, the rate of disease in exposed or control populations, or quantitative information concerning risk. In essence, case reports are numerators without denominators.

After an accumulation of case reports, the next step in the evolution of scientific information is the publication of formal epidemiologic studies. The first are usually retrospective, using either case control or cohort design to provide a comparison group. The major difficulty with retrospective studies is the avoidance of bias, because the epidemiologist must make a number of assumptions concerning conditions that existed previously.

Selection bias occurs when there is noncomparable admission of diseased (or nondiseased) persons into the exposed (or nonexposed) groups. It can be avoided in case control studies if knowledge of exposure is masked in selection of diseased and nondiseased groups. This task is complex, because the criteria used in making a diagnosis often include knowledge of exposure. For cohort studies it is necessary to mask information concerning the disease when selecting entrants. Only exposure criteria are used in defining the exposed and comparison groups; information about disease is collected after the two study groups have been defined.

Observation bias (information bias) occurs when information about disease outcome is obtained in a noncomparable manner. A frequent cause is the use of different techniques for obtaining information about employees who are still at work, have left work, have developed the disease of interest, or have died.

Confounding bias occurs when there is a third variable that is a cause of the disease and also is associated with exposure. A common example is the greater frequency of smoking in blue collar workers compared with the general population. Any analysis of lung cancer frequency in blue collar workers exposed to a particular agent is potentially confounded if the control group smokes at a lower rate.

The most powerful data come from prospective cohort studies. Because the investigator is present when exposed and nonexposed populations are defined and is able to observe the groups over time, the prospective study should (at least in theory) minimize the risk of bias. However, because of the time required to observe the exposed and control populations, and the considerable expense involved, prospective data are usually the last to be developed.

It is always possible that an increased risk of cancer in a single study may have occurred by chance. This finding requires repetition of the study on another population or observation for a further period. When data from several studies have been published, it is necessary to evaluate the information to determine whether a causal relationship exists between a suspected agent and an increased risk of cancer, or if there is simply an association because of bias or chance. The principles used to prove causation were described by Sir Austin Bradford Hill in 1965 and have been reviewed and revised by Doll and others (Table 4.1) (15–19).

The *strength of the association* is the degree of risk demonstrated by the data. Commonly used statistical concepts are the relative risk (RR), odds ratio (OR), and standardized mortality ratio (SMR). From these it is possible to calculate the attributable risk and the attributable proportion, which describe the excess of cancer in the exposed population compared with the control group (Table 4.2). Strong associations, such as smoking one pack of cigarettes per day (RR, 10), are unlikely to be caused by chance or bias. If the lower confidence limit of the RR is greater than two after appropriate standardization for age, there is seldom any difficulty in recognizing an occupational hazard (17). For lesser risks, it can be extremely difficult to draw conclusions. Unfortunately, for many suspected occupational carcinogens, the RR is less than 2, and the lower 95% confidence limit includes 1.

Physicians and scientists are sometimes asked to provide expert opinions in legal cases regarding whether a particular exposure caused a patient's cancer. The usual legal standard is that it is medically probable that the occupational exposure was a substantial contributing factor. This definition means that the physician thinks it is more probable (i.e., a greater than 50% likelihood) that the occupational exposure was responsible. To express this opinion, data should demonstrate that the attributable proportion of cancer in exposed populations exceeded 50%. Considering the definition of attributable proportion (Table 4.2), this conclusion would require relative risks greater than the 2:1 ratio shown consistently in the medical literature.

Consistency of the association is extremely important. If studies indicating a positive association are contradicted by others showing no risk, and they are of comparable size and scientific merit, it is impossible to conclude that a risk exists. More studies are needed to decide the issue.

Specificity of the association refers to the degree of linkage between an exposure and a particular type of cancer. If an occupational agent causes many types of diseases (including cancer), or if a malignancy is caused by a variety of different exposures, it is difficult to recognize a causal relationship. Perhaps the best example of specificity is mesothelioma in men, for which approximately 75% of patients have a history of occupational exposure to asbestos.

Biologic plausibility means that the postulated effect in humans should be supported by known biologic mechanisms and animal studies, assuming that such data are available. *Biologic gradient* (dose response) refers to the expectation that the incidence of disease increases as the level or duration of exposure to the suspected agent rises. Assuming that the study design allows analysis, failure to demonstrate dose response is a significant argument against a causal relationship, and it suggests that any observed risk may be the result of bias.

Temporal relationship at its most simplistic means that the exposure to an agent must precede the disease for a causal relationship to exist. For cancer, this concept is extended to include the expected latency period, which is at least 10 years for most carcinogens and may exceed 20 years (e.g., asbestos). *Statistical significance of the association* requires that the observed excess of cancer would not have occurred because of chance. To exhibit some degree of stability, this decision should be based on sufficient data and requires analysis of repeated studies.

TABLE 4.1. Epidemiologic Criteria for a Causal Association Between a Risk Factor and a Disease

Strength
Consistency
Specificity
Biologic plausibility
Biologic gradient
Temporal relationship
Statistical significance

TABLE 4.2. Definitions of Relative Risk, Odds Ratio, and Attributable Proportion

	CASES	CONTROLS	TOTAL
Exposed	a	b	a + b
Not exposed	c	d	c + d
Total	a + c	b + d	a + b + c + d

Relative risk (RR), $\dfrac{a}{a+b} \div \dfrac{c}{c+d}$

Odds ratio, $\dfrac{a \times d}{b \times c}$

Attributable risk, $\left(\dfrac{a}{a+b} - \dfrac{c}{c+d}\right) \times 100$

Attributable proportion in exposed, $\dfrac{RR - 1}{RR} \times 100$

This discussion illustrates the considerable time required to develop information sufficient to allow scientifically valid decisions concerning causal relationships. Because complete consistency has virtually never occurred, the accumulation of data from studies with contradictory results may delay rather than speed the decision-making process. For occupational and environmental carcinogens, the time from initial case reports to the completion of formal epidemiologic studies often has been several decades. An unfortunate (and unavoidable) consequence is that workers have continued to be exposed to carcinogens at times when, with the benefit of hindsight, there was some (inconclusive) evidence of risk.

TOBACCO SMOKING AND OCCUPATIONAL LUNG CANCER

Tobacco smoking is responsible for 80% to 90% of lung cancers. This subject is discussed in detail in Chapter 3. The prevalence of smoking is greater among blue collar workers compared with the general population. For the period between 1987 and 1990, 39.2% of blue collar workers smoked compared with 34.5% of service workers, 24.2% of white collar workers, and 27.4% of all adults (20). The higher prevalence of smoking among blue collar workers, coupled with the greatest potential for exposures to carcinogens, is an important confounding variable that can lead to spurious conclusions. For example, assuming a 10-fold risk for current smokers versus nonsmokers and the rates of smoking given above, a blue collar work force would have a relative risk of lung cancer of 1.3 compared with the general population. Risks of this magnitude are reported commonly in industrial studies. Conversely, the large relative risk because of smoking may obscure the effects of occupational carcinogens. Accurate smoking histories often are not available, and many published studies are flawed by the absence of this crucial information.

Combined exposure to tobacco smoke and occupational carcinogens can greatly increase the risk of lung cancer. The best example is the synergistic (i.e., multiplicative) interaction between the risk of smoking (10-fold) and the presence of asbestosis (fivefold), causing a lung cancer risk of 50-fold to 90-fold among smoking insulators (21, 22). Data also suggest that smokers who were exposed at work to radon, arsenic, or chloromethyl ethers have a lung cancer risk greater than the additive effect of both risk factors (23, 24). When there is a multiplicative interaction between risk factors, elimination of one factor has a disproportionate effect in reducing risk. It is worth noting that lung cancer risk caused by smoking alone exceeds that of any individual occupational carcinogen with the exception of chloromethyl ethers and chromium. Smoking cessation is by far the most effective method of preventing lung cancer in populations also exposed to occupational carcinogens.

CLASSIFICATION OF OCCUPATIONAL CARCINOGENS

For the purposes of this review, the individual agents described below have been classified using the criteria of the IARC (8). Group 1 (known carcinogens) includes agents for which there is sufficient evidence of carcinogenicity in humans from epidemiologic studies in which chance, bias, and confounding could be ruled out with reasonable confidence.

Group 2A (probable carcinogens) includes agents for which there is limited evidence of carcinogenicity in humans and sufficient evidence in experimental animals. Limited evidence exists when a positive association between exposure to the agent and human cancer exists, but when the data are inadequate to rule out bias, confounding, or chance with reasonable confidence.

Group 2B (possible carcinogens) consists of agents for which there is limited evidence in humans in the absence of sufficient evidence in experimental animals. This classification also may be used when there is inadequate or nonexistent data in humans but sufficient evidence in animals. Some agents that are proven carcinogens in one body system may only be probable or possible carcinogens for lung or esophageal cancer (e.g., vinyl chloride).

KNOWN CARCINOGENS (GROUP 1)

ARSENIC

Arsenic is a naturally occurring metal routinely found in the earth's crust. The major sources of atmospheric inorganic arsenic include smelting of sulfidic ores (including copper, nickel, and cobalt), and combustion of fossil fuels and wood (boilers, auto engines, wood stoves, fireplaces). Arsenic also is released from mining, lead smelting operations, agricultural use of arsenical pesticides, agricultural burning, waste incineration, and manufacturing processes involving arsenic compounds. Organoarsenicals present in marine organisms are a source of organic arsenic exposure in humans.

The general population is exposed to arsenic in air, water, soil, and foods. Atmospheric arsenic concentrations vary. In rural areas they are less than 3 ng/m^3; urban concentrations are typically 20 to 30 ng/m^3 (25, 26). Residents of neighborhoods near copper smelters are reported to have an increased incidence of lung cancer, although the results have not always been statistically significant (27, 28). One epidemiologic study of residents surrounding a pesticide manufacturing plant found a significantly increased risk of lung cancer (29). Risks from lower level exposures found in many environments are less certain. Using conservative extrapolation models, exposure 24 hours a day for a lifetime of 70 years to an atmosphere containing 20 ng/m^3 would result in an excess cancer risk of 1 in 10,000 (30).

Ingestion of water containing high concentrations of arsenic has been associated with an increased risk of skin cancer in Taiwan, Chile, Argentina, and Mexico (31–34). Limited data suggest that drinking contaminated well water may increase the risk of lung cancer, but further research needs to be done (35, 36). Although skin cancer has been linked with chronic arsenic poisoning from the medicinal use of arsenite (Fowler's solution), there is no clear association with lung cancer (37). Epidemiologic studies of workers exposed to inorganic arsenic have shown dose dependent associations between lung cancer and arsenic exposure. Copper smelter workers exposed to arsenic trioxide in Tacoma, Washington, have an excess lung cancer mortality of nearly six-fold (SMR, 578) for those with the greatest intensity and longest duration of exposure (38, 39). A three-fold to five-fold increase in lung cancer also has been observed among copper smelter workers exposed to arsenic trioxide in Magna, Utah (40). Studies involving more than 8000 copper smelter workers in Anaconda, Montana, showed a significantly increased risk of lung cancer, even among those classified with low exposures (SMR, 183) (41–43). Risk was greater for men starting at a young age compared with workers experiencing similar exposures who began employment later in life. Studies of Swedish and Japanese copper smelter workers and Chinese tin miners also have demonstrated an increased risk of developing lung cancer (44–46). Exposure to lead and calcium arsenate during manufacture of arsenical pesticides caused an excess of lung cancer (47, 48). All types of lung cancer were increased in these cohorts, but adenocarcinoma has been noted more often in some studies (49).

The increased lung cancer risk observed in these epidemiologic studies was not caused by a confounding factor or tobacco use. It was present after controlling for smoking, and it has been observed in nonsmokers. There is evidence of an interactive effect between smoking and arsenic exposure that is intermediate between additive and synergistic (multiplicative) (38, 46, 50).

Inorganic arsenic is a recognized human carcinogen (26, 51). In the United States, Occupational Safety and Health Administration (OSHA) regulations require that workers exposed to significant concentrations of inorganic arsenic receive medical surveillance or monitoring. Mandated tests include periodic physical examinations, sputum cytology, and chest radiographs. The frequency of examinations is dependent on the age of the individual and the duration of occupational exposure. The exposure limit for inorganic arsenic compounds is 0.10 mg/m^3 averaged over 8 hours for a working lifetime. The concentration of serum and urine total arsenic varies greatly in the general population depending on the intake of seafood, and it should be considered in determining whether a person is exposed excessively (52).

ASBESTOS

The word asbestos refers to a group of naturally occurring mineral silicates. Although different in chemical composition and physical properties, they share characteristics of heat and chemical resistance. Asbestos has been used for multiple purposes including textiles, asbestos cement, thermal insulation, building materials, and friction products such as brake linings. There have been hundreds of commercial applications of asbestos since the expansion of this industry began in the late 1800s.

Unfortunately, the adverse health effects of asbestos were not widely appreciated at first. There was confusion regarding whether asbestos caused pulmonary fibrosis distinct from silicosis, and whether pulmonary disease seen in asbestos workers actually was caused by tuberculosis. The term asbestosis did not appear in the medical literature until 1927 (53). The first case report of asbestosis in which tuberculosis was excluded was published in 1928 (54). This report led to an extensive study of the asbestos textile industry in England by Merewether (55, 56), who reported that asbestosis could be prevented if dust levels were kept below the level of the spinners. A similar study in the United States by Dreessen and colleagues (57) resulted in the recommendation of 5 million particles per cubic foot (mppcf) as a safe level of asbestos dust. The 5-mppcf level was adopted in 1946 by the American Conference of Governmental Hygienists as the threshold limit value for asbestos, and it remained in force until 1968. Since then, a succession of regulations has lowered asbestos exposure to the current permissible level of 0.1 fibers per milliliter of air.

Asbestos exposure in mines and textile plants during the first part of this century was very high, in the range of 10 to 100 fibers per milliliter. This caused the rapid development of pulmonary fibrosis and early death because of respiratory failure. For example, the patients in the first two published reports of asbestosis died at age 33 (53). Asbestos workers lived longer after dust levels were reduced, allowing survival into later years when malignancies could develop. The first description of lung cancer in a patient with asbestosis was published in 1935 (14). In 1949 Merewether (58) reported that lung cancer was found more often in autopsies of patients with asbestosis than of those with silicosis. The first epidemiologic study was published by Doll in 1955 (59). He reported a 10-fold increased risk of lung cancer in asbestos textile workers. In 1964, a major conference was held in New York to examine the health effects of asbestos; of particular interest was the increased risk of lung cancer and other malignancies seen in insulation workers (60). Subsequent studies indicated that the risk of lung cancer because of heavy asbestos exposure (fivefold), combined with the risk from cigarette smoking (10-fold), acted synergistically to increase the risk of lung cancer 50- to 90-fold in insulation workers (21, 22, 61). This alarming result led to multiple studies that examined other trades such as shipyard and factory workers. Although there was a consistent increase in lung cancer, none matched the risk of insulation workers.

An important defect in the insulation worker studies was failure to separate lung cancers in patients with asbestosis from those without pulmonary fibrosis. This point was resolved finally in 1987 when clinical, radiographic, and pathologic findings were correlated (62). All of the insulation workers who died from lung cancer had pathologic evidence of asbestosis. The majority had radiographic evidence of pulmonary fibrosis, and a rating of 1/1, using the International Labor Office system for interpreting radiographs, was an accurate predictor of the excess lung cancer rate (63). These and other observations have led to the conclusion that increased lung cancer risk in people exposed to asbestos is confined to those with asbestosis (64). This point is very important, because pulmonary fibrosis does not occur without substantial exposure to asbestos.

Although the previous exposure levels seen in insulation workers (approximately 10 fibers per milliliter) are a thing of the past, the widespread use of asbestos-containing construction materials has led to concern that occupants of public buildings and schools may be at risk of asbestos-related malignancies. Asbestos fibers are present in the air of many buildings. However, the levels are very low, typically in the range of 0.001 to 0.0001 fibers per milliliter. It is generally agreed that asbestosis does not occur below a cumulative exposure of 25 fibers per milliliter-years (a fiber per milliliter-year is the amount of asbestos breathed by working in an environment with an average concentration 1 fiber per milliliter for 1 year) (65, 66). Considering the low levels, it would not be possible to accumulate a dose sufficient to cause asbestosis or lung cancer simply by living or working in buildings that contain asbestos (67).

BIS(CHLOROMETHYL) ETHER

Bis(chloromethyl) ether (BCME) is a chemical used in the synthesis of anionic exchange resins and as an alkylating agent in the manufacture of polymers. Bioassay data from rats and mice provide sufficient evidence of carcinogenicity. Inhalation of BCME produced a marked increase in the incidence of several types of respiratory tract tumors in male Sprague-Dawley rats (68).

There is sufficient human epidemiologic evidence to demonstrate that BCME is a cause of lung cancer. This association was first observed in 1964 and 1965, when two young men who worked in a BCME cholormethylation processing plant died of lung cancer. During the next 7 years, four other cases were detected, including a 39-year-old male research laboratory chemist (69). Subsequent epidemiologic studies have demonstrated a statistically significant increase in lung tumors, particularly small cell (oat cell) carcinoma. This increase could not be explained by cigarette smoking (8). The relative risk for lung cancer can be up to 10-fold among those most heavily exposed to BCME, although precise quantitative exposure information is lacking in past studies. Those developing lung cancer ranged in age from 35 to 54, and latency periods as short as 8 years were reported.

There has been some controversy regarding whether BCME can be formed at significant concentrations in work environments that contain formaldehyde and hydrogen chloride. BCME has been detected at very low concentrations in textile operations and other processes. Concentrations are thought to be significantly affected by temperature and humidity (70).

Technical-grade chloromethyl methyl ether (CMME), an agent used for chloromethylation, usually contains BCME, and use of this product can be a source of potential exposure. Mice exposed to CMME vapors at either 1 ppm or 2 ppm contaminated with 0.3 to 2.6% BCME had an increased incidence of lung tumors (71). An increase in lung cancer risk has been shown among workers exposed to technical-grade

CMME (8, 72) As for BCME, oat cell cancer was the predominant tumor.

BCME is no longer produced in the United States, and its use is limited to small laboratories. It is regulated as a generic carcinogen by OSHA, and extensive measures to protect exposed workers must be employed for all uses. The current 8-hour exposure limit is 1 part per billion (ppb). There is no specific CMME exposure limit, although any atmospheric BCME that would be generated by operations involving this chemical would be covered by the BCME standard.

CHROMIUM

Chromium is a metal most often found in three chemical forms: chromium (0), trivalent (III), and hexavalent (VI). Chromium III occurs in nature and is an essential element, whereas chromium VI and chromium 0 are produced from industrial activities. Chromium is used in many products and processes including metal alloys, stainless steel, chrome plating, leather tanning, wood preserving, chemicals, and dye and paint manufacture. Exposure can occur in a variety of industrial operations including electroplating, welding, cutting and grinding of chromium alloys, and mining. Sources of atmospheric inorganic chromium include combustion of coal, natural gas, and oil, and industrial processes such as cement production, municipal waste incineration, and emissions from cooling towers containing chromate rust inhibitors (73). Chromium also is found in food and water.

The three forms of chromium have different biologic properties. In vitro genetic toxicology assays have shown that chromium VI is mutagenic in bacteria, whereas chromium III is not (74–76). Animal studies involving chromium VI have revealed evidence of carcinogenicity, and inhalation has produced lung neoplasms. Animal studies of chromium III generally have been negative (77). Water soluble chromium VI salts have greater carcinogenic potential than those with low solubility.

Human evidence of the carcinogenicity of chromium compounds was identified initially in chromate production workers. Case reports of lung and nasal cancers were published in the early 1900s. A study of 1445 workers employed in seven chromate production plants from 1930 to 1947 showed that respiratory cancer accounted for 21.8% of the deaths, and that the SMR was 2889 (78). Subsequent studies in several countries confirmed a significantly increased lung cancer risk. A cohort study of 1212 male workers at three chromate plants in the United States showed an SMR of 942.6 for lung cancer (79). A study of 2101 Baltimore chromate workers employed for at least 90 days showed a twofold increased risk of lung cancer (SMR, 202) (80). Italian (81) and Japanese (82) chromate production workers also have demonstrated an increased risk. Production of chromium pigments, primarily zinc chromate, has been associated with an increased lung cancer risk in several countries (83). During the last several decades, the introduction of control measures to limit industrial chromium exposures has decreased the risk of lung cancer (84).

Studies of electroplating operations generally showed an increased risk of lung cancer (85–88), although not all have been positive (89). Studies of ferrochromium workers (90–92) have been inconclusive with respect to lung cancer risk. Tannery workers exposed to trivalent chromium in the United States (93), the United Kingdom (94), and Germany (95) have not shown an excess risk of cancer.

Human studies of workers exposed to both chromium III and VI indicate that only hexavalent compounds are carcinogenic (96). Hexavalent chromium is a recognized human carcinogen, and atmospheric concentration in workplaces is regulated by OSHA. The allowable limit for chromates and chromic acid is a ceiling concentration of 0.1 mg/m^3. The concentration for soluble metal salts is 0.5 mg/m^3, whereas the limit for insoluble salts is 1 mg/m^3. These levels may be lowered with the issuance of a new OSHA standard. The extent of chromium exposure can be assessed by monitoring blood and urine. Because urinary chromium concentrations reflect past and current exposure, differences between the beginning-of-shift and end-of-shift values reflect current exposure (97). Other factors, such as beer drinking and diabetes, can affect urinary chromium levels (98).

NICKEL

Nickel is a white silvery metal that occurs in several oxidation states and forms complexes with a wide variety of compounds. Physical properties including hardness, strength, and corrosion resistance make it desirable for metal alloys. More than 80% of nickel is used to manufacture copper-nickel, nickel-chromium, nickel-cadmium, and steel. Stainless steel can contain up to 25% nickel. Nickel alloys are used in a many products including industrial plumbing, heat exchangers, pumps, welding electrodes, gas turbine engines, marine and petrochemical equipment, and metal coins. Nickel salts are widely used in electroplating, paint pigments, and ceramics.

The general population is exposed to nickel in air, water, and food. Nickel is released into the general atmosphere from mining, combustion of coal and oil, industrial emissions, and dispersion of nickel-containing soils. The atmospheric concentration of nickel in rural and urban areas ranges from 1 to 328 mg/cm^3 (99).

The significance of environmental nickel exposure is unclear.

Several forms of nickel are human carcinogens. Epidemiologic studies of nickel refinery workers have consistently shown increased lung cancer, with relative risks in the fivefold to ninefold range (100–103). There is a dose-response relationship, because workers in the dustiest areas with the longest duration of employment have the greatest risk. Nasal cancer also is increased from ninefold to 26-fold. The increased risk of nasal and lung cancers from exposure to nickel refinery dust has been attributed in part to nickel subsulfide. The EPA has classified nickel refinery dust and nickel subsulfide as recognized human carcinogens (104).

The carcinogenicity of other nickel compounds is less clear. Nickel carbonyl is considered a probable human carcinogen. It is used as a catalyst in the petroleum, plastic, and rubber industries. A study of Welch workers exposed to nickel carbonyl did not show an increased risk of lung cancer (101). However, inhalation of nickel carbonyl produced lung tumors in animals (105). Studies of persons exposed to soluble nickel salts and some nickel oxides suggest an association with lung cancer. Metallic nickel has not been shown to cause lung or nasal cancer (106).

Possible confounding from other agents, such as polycyclic aromatic hydrocarbons, chromium, and asbestos, has not been evaluated in many studies (107). For example, polycyclic aromatic hydrocarbons may be the cause of lung cancer mortality among copper-nickel smelter and refinery workers. Exposure to cigarette smoke (which also contains nickel) is not controlled adequately in many studies.

Analysis of lung tissue for nickel content has revealed considerable variability among lung segments in the same individual, and among persons with no apparent occupational or environmental exposure (108). Therefore, interpretation of only a single lung specimen must made cautiously. The nickel concentration in lung in 224 cases of lung cancer did not differ from those in a control group, and tissue analysis generally has not distinguished between lung cancer patients and control subjects (109)

NIOSH recommends an exposure limit of 0.015 mg/m^3 for nickel. The OSHA exposure limit is 0.1 mg/m^3 for soluble nickel compounds, and 1.0 mg/m^3 for nickel metal and insoluble compounds. OSHA regulations do not mandate medical monitoring of exposed workers.

POLYCYCLIC AROMATIC HYDROCARBONS

Polycyclic aromatic hydrocarbons (PAHs) are a group of chemicals formed from incomplete combustion of organic matter. They are ubiquitous in the environment. The greatest source of general population exposure is the diet, followed by air and water. Cigarette smoke is certainly the most potent (and harmful) lifestyle factor causing PAH exposure. The primary source of manmade atmospheric PAHs is combustion of organic materials including wood burning, automobile exhaust from diesel and gasoline engines, and emissions from industrial facilities (110). Natural sources include forest fires and volcanoes. PAHs also are found in coal tars, creosote, shale oil, soot, and roofing tar.

Animal studies have shown that several of the PAHs are carcinogenic after inhalation, dermal contact, and oral ingestion. Benzo(a)pyrene, one of the most studied PAHs, is carcinogenic in laboratory animals by all three routes of exposure. The mechanism of carcinogenicity is thought to be its metabolism to a reactive diolepoxide derivative that can interact with DNA (110).

Animal toxicology studies have shown that steam-refined petroleum bitumens can initiate skin tumors in mice at the site of contact. Air-refined (oxidized) bitumens in general are negative in skin-painting studies. There is insufficient evidence that bitumens alone are carcinogenic in humans, and there are no regulations that mandate medical monitoring of workers exposed to bitumens, including asphalt products. Coal tars also have been shown to cause skin cancer in animals (111).

The association between PAHs and human cancer was demonstrated initially in 1775 by Pott, who observed cancer of the scrotum in chimney sweeps exposed to soot. Following the institution of control measures, the incidence of scrotal cancer among chimney sweeps diminished (112). Occupational exposure to complex mixtures of PAHs has been associated with an increased risk of lung cancer. A study of 5939 roofers employed more than 20 years showed a 1.5 to 2 times greater lung cancer risk (113). Other studies of roofers also have shown an increased risk of lung cancer (114). Roofers are exposed to asphalt and other materials, including coal tars.

Studies of coke oven workers also have shown a significant lung cancer risk because of coke oven emissions. This finding was initially reported in 1937 among Japanese workers at a coking operation in a steel company (115). Subsequent studies in the United States, England, and Japan have shown a threefold to sevenfold lung cancer risk (116). Those who work on top of the ovens, with the highest exposure to PAHs, are at greatest risk. OSHA regulations mandate medical monitoring of workers employed in coke oven work. Testing requirements include chest roentgenograms, and sputum and urine cytology. Studies of aluminum production, which involves exposure to airborne PAHs, have shown a significantly increased risk of lung cancer (114, 117, 118). Some studies of workers in iron and steel foundries and coal gassification plants also suggest an excess of lung cancer.

Although epidemiologic studies have shown an association between exposure to PAHs and lung cancer, they have not identified the specific agent(s) responsible. Typically, industrial processes are complex and include multiple possible carcinogens. Changes in industrial methods, and enactment of exposure control measures, also make it difficult to assess dose-response relationships. Estimates of previous exposures may not be accurate, and many studies have no quantitative information. The significance of low-level PAH exposures to the general population is unclear. Atmospheric levels in the United States and other areas of the world are declining because of the lessened use of coal for heating and enhanced air pollution control measures (119).

RADON

Radon is a colorless and odorless gas formed from the decay of naturally occurring uranium 238 and radium 226, which exist in soil, rocks, and groundwater. Radon is found in the ambient atmosphere and often is present at higher concentrations inside homes and buildings. Radon decays to produce several radioisotopes, called radon daughters. They include two α-emitters, polonium 214, and polonium 218, that can produce local radiation to tissues (120, 121).

The radioactivity from radon can be measured in several ways. Occupational studies have reported exposure in working levels (WLs). A WL represents a release of 1.3×10^5 MeV of α-energy in 1 L of air resulting from any combination of radon progeny. Occupational studies of miners have used a unit called a working level month (WLM), which is exposure to 1 WL for 170 hours. Radon exposure can be expressed in becquerels (Bq), which represent the number of radioactive transformations of a radionuclide over time. A becquerel is equivalent to one disintegration per second, and radon activity is reported as becquerels per cubic meter of air (Bq/m^3). One WL corresponds to 3.7×10^3 Bq/m^3. Radon concentration also can be expressed as picocuries per liter (pCi/L). A concentration of 1 pCi/L is equivalent to approximately 0.005 WL, or 37 Bq/m^3.

Radon gas is a recognized human carcinogen. Numerous studies of uranium and hard rock miners have demonstrated an increased risk of lung cancer (122). Factors influencing mortality include age at first exposure, total cumulative dose, and rate of exposure. Lower exposure rates lead to higher risks per unit dose (123–128). Studies of United States and Canadian miners showed an excess of lung cancer after exposure to 100 WLM (129, 130). Cumulative exposures of less than 50 WLMs had the same effect in Czechoslovakian miners (127). Studies have generally shown a greater proportion of small cell cancer, although all histologic types are increased (131–133).

There is considerable concern that radon may cause lung cancer in the general population, because it can accumulate in homes. Levels in buildings are related primarily to the concentration in soils and to the ventilation rate. Radon typically enters homes through cracks in the floors or walls, drains, pipes, electrical outlets, and other openings (134). Building materials, water used inside the home, and natural gas used for cooking and heating also may contribute (135–138). Concentrations can vary by several orders of magnitude and are higher in poorly ventilated basements. The average occurring inside most houses in the United States is 1.5 pCi/L, but 1% to 3% of homes (approximately 1 million in the United States) exceed 8 pCi/L (139). Levels in excess of 80 pCi have been measured in regions with geologic formations favoring radon accumulation (140). These approach concentrations measured inside mines.

At the present time there are only limited data concerning lung cancer risk from radon caused by nonoccupational exposure. Ecologic studies have correlated lung cancer incidence to radon concentration in different geographic areas. Results have been mixed, with about half showing a positive relationship. Early case control studies were small and often did not evaluate smoking. More recent studies have shown lung cancer risks approximately doubled among those living in homes with higher radon concentrations compared with those in houses having lower concentrations (141–143). However, other studies involving larger numbers of subjects have had both positive (144) and negative results (145). Many prospective studies are in progress, but the results will not be known for several years. Existing evidence suggests that radon in homes causes some lung cancer, but at present it is difficult to draw precise conclusions about the size of the risk.

Various agencies have developed risk projection models from the studies of miners. For example, the Committee on Biological Effects of Ionizing Radiation has estimated that about 10% of lung cancers in the United States and 6% in the United Kingdom are caused by radon in the general environment. This fact would make radon the second most important cause of lung cancer, exceeded only by cigarette smoking. There appears to be an interaction between radon and smoking. The combined risk of lung cancer from both exposures is intermediate between additive and multiplicative (120, 121, 128).

VINYL CHLORIDE

Vinyl chloride is a colorless, sweet-smelling chemical used in the manufacture of polyvinyl chloride (PVC), a plastic employed extensively in many applications. Vinyl chloride also has been used as a propellant in spray cans and as a constituent of some cosmetic products. The general public is potentially exposed to vinyl chloride from emissions at hazardous waste sites and landfills, by residing near plastics industries that discharge vinyl chloride, and through contact with contaminated drinking water.

Animal toxicology studies provide supportive evidence for a carcinogenic effect on lung tissue. Inhalation studies involving mice have demonstrated an increased risk of lung tumors. Dose-related increases in lung cancer were observed at concentrations ranging up to 600 ppm for periods of 4 weeks (146). Acute exposures of 5000 ppm for 1 hour, and intermittent 1-hour exposures of 50 ppm, produced an increased risk of bronchoalveolar adenomas (147).

Vinyl chloride's potential for human carcinogenicity was first noted in 1974 after the detection of four cases of hepatic angiosarcoma in BF Goodrich plant workers (148). Subsequent studies of occupationally exposed workers in the United States, Great Britain, Italy, and Canada also have shown an increased risk of developing this rare liver cancer (149). Some studies suggested an increased risk of other types of malignancies, including lung cancer, brain tumors, and leukemia (150).

The role of occupational vinyl chloride exposure in producing lung cancer is not clear, and studies of exposed workers have shown differing results. Small increases in lung cancer risk have been reported by several investigators (151–153). A study of 464 employees at a vinyl chloride plant showed an SMR for lung cancer of 289, but four of the five cases were in smokers (154). The SMR for lung cancer was 149 in a study of 4806 men employed at a synthetic plastics plant, and polyvinyl chloride dust was determined to be the most likely cause (155). In other investigations, although an increase of respiratory cancer was observed, there was no relationship between dose or cumulative exposure to vinyl chloride, in contrast with a demonstrated dose-response relationship between exposure and the incidence of angiosarcoma (156). Excess lung cancer risk has not been observed in other studies (157, 158), including a European multicentric cohort study coordinated by the IARC (159).

Epidemiologic studies do not provide consistent evidence of an increased cancer risk. However, animal toxicology studies and existing data on humans have led to the conclusion that occupational exposure to vinyl chloride is probably a small risk factor for the development of lung cancer (149).

PROBABLE CARCINOGENS (GROUP 2A)

ACRYLONITRILE

Acrylonitrile is a volatile, flammable liquid used for the production of acrylic fibers, resins, rubbers, and plastics. Oral and inhalation studies of rats have demonstrated an increased incidence of gastrointestinal, central nervous system, Zymbal gland, and mammary gland tumors (160, 161). An association between exposure to acrylonitrile and lung cancer was first reported in a study of DuPont textile fiber workers, and subsequent reports have also shown an increased risk (162–165). The relative risks have been consistently less than 2, and confounding factors such as smoking and other occupational carcinogens have not been excluded. Other studies have been negative (166). The general consensus is that human data are suggestive but limited.

BERYLLIUM

Beryllium is a metal with a unique combination of light weight, extreme stiffness, and high heat absorption. Its commercial value as a precipitation hardener in copper and nickel alloys was first appreciated in 1926, and production was greatly expanded during World War II. Occupational exposures to beryllium and its compounds occur in mining, extraction refining, alloy and ceramics manufacture, and industrial uses. The electronics industry uses beryllium for transistors, heat sinks, and cathode tubes. The aerospace industry consumes beryllium alloys for high-performance brakes, and beryllium is used as a neutron moderator in the nuclear industry (167).

In experimental animal studies, beryllium compounds have been shown to cause osteosarcomas and pulmonary cancers (168–172). Beryllium appears to be the most potent inorganic pulmonary carcinogen tested in rats, 1000 times more active than chrysotile asbestos (173).

Unfortunately, the convincing and consistent data on animals are not matched in the literature on humans, and the issue of whether beryllium is carcinogenic in humans under realistic conditions of exposure is controversial. Studies of companies in Ohio and Pennsylvania, and of the U.S. Beryllium Case Registry, indicated an excess of lung cancer of approximately 50% (174–181). The risk was greatest in those with a history of acute berylliosis, suggesting a dose-response gradient in those with high levels of exposure. However, chronic beryllium disease, also a marker of exposure, did not appear to increase risk, nor was there a consistently increased risk with duration of employment. Criticism of published studies has included failure to control properly for smoking, absent or incorrect statistical analysis, and a tendency to exaggerate the risk of lung cancer while ignoring shortcomings of study design (182). The IARC has listed beryllium as a class 2A carcinogen based on the animal studies and limited human data. The EPA considers the epidemiologic data inadequate to support or refute a carcinogenic hazard for humans. In any case, the very high levels of exposure to beryllium experienced in the past (100 to 1000 $\mu g/m^3$) are unlikely to occur under current conditions, when the permissible exposure limit is 2 $\mu g/m^3$.

CADMIUM

Cadmium is used for electroplating of metals, pigment manufacture, stabilization of plastics, and other products such as nickel-cadmium batteries and metal alloys. Cadmium was established as a carcinogen in rodents in the early 1960s; it causes sarcomas at sites of injection, and testicular tumors after oral or parenteral exposure. Inhalation studies produced lung neoplasms in rats but not in mice and hamsters (183–185). Initial data for carcinogenesis in humans indicated an increased risk of prostate cancer; most subsequent studies have been negative, and lung cancer has become the major concern (186, 187).

Studies of workers exposed to cadmium have shown an increased lung cancer risk of 25% to 50% (188, 189). Several have demonstrated a dose-response relationship (190–192). However, the exposure data were often imprecise, leading to semiquantitative estimates based on job title and duration of employment (189, 193, 194). Most epidemiologic studies did not classify workers according to a quantitative index of cumulative exposure. A major problem with the data is concomitant exposure to nickel during battery manufacture and to arsenic during smelting operations. These confounding exposures make it very difficult to assess the effect of cadmium (195, 196). Detailed smoking data are not available for most studies. In addition to the multiple carcinogens present in tobacco, cigarettes also are a major source of exposure to cadmium (189, 197, 198). At present, the question of whether cadmium is a pulmonary carcinogen, and determination of a safe level of occupational exposure, remains debatable (199–204).

FORMALDEHYDE

Formaldehyde is a highly reactive molecule used in a variety of applications including adhesives for particle board and plywood, insulating materials, rubber manufacture, clothing, photographic film, cosmetics, and embalming fluids. Concern for carcinogenicity arose when inhalation experiments produced squamous cell carcinomas in the nasal cavity of rats (205, 206). This research led to a number of epidemiologic studies of exposed populations including pathologists, anatomists, morticians, and workers in the chemical and garment industries. These data did not show a consistently increased risk of lung cancer (207). In one of the largest studies, 26,561 workers employed in 10 formaldehyde-producing or formaldehyde-using facilities demonstrated a standardized mortality ratio for lung cancer of 111. However, the risk was not significantly correlated with intensity or duration of exposure to formaldehyde (208). Reanalysis of these and other data led to controversy over whether lung cancer risk was caused by formaldehyde or by coincidental exposure to other agents such as wood dust and phenols (209–216). At present, the evidence indicates that formaldehyde is a cause of cancer in the nasal cavities and nasopharynx but probably not the lung (217, 218).

POSSIBLE CARCINOGENS (GROUP 2B)

ACETALDEHYDE

Acetaldehyde is a chemical used in the manufacture of many products including plastics, synthetic rubbers, resins, dyes, and other substances. Animal toxicology studies provide sufficient evidence of respiratory carcinogenicity. Hamsters exposed to average concentrations of 2000 ppm for 1 year showed a significantly increased incidence of laryngeal tumors and a slight increase in nasal tumors (219). Studies of rats exposed to a range of concentrations up to 3000 ppm showed a dose-related increase in the incidence of respiratory tract tumors (220). Increases in adenocarcinomas were observed at all exposure levels, whereas squamous cell carcinomas were seen at high doses. Acetaldehyde significantly increased the number of laryngeal tumors produced by benzo(a)pyrene when the two agents were administered together (221).

Human epidemiologic information concerning the carcinogenicity of acetaldehyde is very limited. The only epidemiologic study involving acetaldehyde exposure concerned workers in the German Democratic Republic and showed an increase in the crude incidence rate of total cancer when compared with the national population (8). There were only five lung cancer cases, and all were smokers. The study is inconclusive because of the small number of cases, exposures to other possible carcinogens, and poor definition of the exposed population.

The IARC and EPA conclude that there is sufficient evidence of carcinogenicity in animals but insufficient evidence in humans (8, 222). The current OSHA exposure limit for acetaldehyde is 100 ppm averaged over 8 hours. There are no specific medical monitoring provisions required by law for workers exposed to acetaldehyde.

MANMADE MINERAL FIBERS

Manmade mineral fibers (MMMF), also referred to as manmade vitreous fibers, are divided into three main groups: mineral wools (rock and slag), fibrous glass, and refractory ceramic fibers (RCF). Rock and slag wools were first produced in Europe in 1840, and production in the United States began in 1897. They are made by melting raw materials and centrifuging, drawing, or blowing the molten material into the desired fibrous form. Rock wool is made by melting igneous rock containing high levels of calcium and magnesium. Slag wool is produced from the waste material of metal smelting, and composition varies with the source of the slag. It is usually a calcium aluminum silicate with varying amounts of iron and magnesium. The production methods for mineral wools produce a wide distribution of fiber diameters, with a significant proportion in the respirable range (diameter of less than 3 μm) (223).

Fibrous glass production began in the 1930s, with materials generally manufactured in two basic forms: wool-type fibers and textile fibers. Wool-type glass fibers are produced by spinning or blowing molten glass containing oxides of silicon, aluminum, boron, calcium sodium, and other metals. Most are 3 to 8 μm in diameter, but fine glass wool fibers (less than 1 μm) are produced for certain applications. Textile glass fibers are drawn or extruded in a continuous process. Fiber diameters are much more uniform, typically 6 to 15 μm, with very few in the respirable range. Those fibers, which do penetrate the lung, are subject to transverse fracture and dissolution (224).

Refractory ceramic fibers are the third general category of MMMF. Production began in the 1950s. They are made by blowing molten kaolin clay or metal oxides, and a large proportion of the fibers is respirable.

Discovery of the fibrogenic and tumorigenic effects of asbestos led to concern that MMMF would have the same consequences. Numerous animal studies have been performed using intrapleural or intraperitoneal injection, intratracheal instillation, or inhalation techniques of exposure (224–228). The size and shape of the fibers are critical in causing tumors after intrapleural or intraperitoneal injection; those longer than 8 μm and with diameters no more than 0.25 μm are the most potent (229). It has become apparent that this method of carcinogenicity testing is extremely sensitive. Most fiber samples, including MMMF, have been carcinogenic. Although effective in determining the biologic potential for carcinogenesis in animals, this route of exposure has limited relevance for humans (230).

Intratracheal injection of glass microfibers was reported to cause lung carcinomas and mesotheliomas (231, 232). However, this observation has not been confirmed in other laboratories, and some investigators have attributed the findings to the instillation protocol (227, 228). Inhalation exposures, which would be more relevant to humans, have generally been negative for lung tumors or mesotheliomas when rock wool, slag wool, or glass fibers were studied. High concentrations of RCF caused lung tumors and mesothelioma in rats exposed by inhalation (226). This difference may result from the greater persistence of RCF in lung tissue compared with other types of MMMF, which are subject to transverse fracture and dissolution.

Human data concerning MMMF come primarily from three studies. The first examined 16,661 workers employed at 17 manufacturing plants in the United States (233, 234). The second was a study of 24,609 employees of 13 MMMF plants in Europe (235, 236). The third examined 2,557 men employed in a Canadian plant manufacturing glass wool insulation (237). Combining these studies, there was an excess of lung cancer of approximately 20%. However, there was no consistent correlation between duration of employment and lung cancer incidence. In fact, workers with short-term exposure appeared to have the greatest risk, a finding not consistent with a causal relationship. The strongest evidence of lung cancer risk was for slag wool, particularly during the early technical phases of production. Some plants used copper slag contaminated with arsenic, and others manufactured asbestos products; these exposures may account for the lung cancer excess (224, 238–240). Existing data indicate that MMMFs are not a risk factor for mesothelioma.

Based on the animal and human evidence, the IARC has classified rock and slag wool, fibrous glass, and RCF as possible human carcinogens (group 2B). Continuous glass filaments were found to be not classifiable (group 3).

SILICA

Silica, or silicon dioxide (SiO_2), is a principal constituent of the earth's crust and exists in crystalline and amorphous states. There are three principal forms of crystalline silica: quartz, tridymite, and cristobalite. Quartz is the preponderant form and is a major constituent of commercial sands.

Occupational exposure to crystalline silica causes silicosis, a pneumoconiosis characterized by parenchymal fibrosis and calcification of thoracic lymph nodes (241). NIOSH has estimated that approximately 3.2 million workers in the United States are exposed to crystalline silica during industrial processes such as mining and quarrying, metal foundry work, glass and ceramic manufacturing, sandblasting, and other operations involving cutting, polishing, and grinding of rocks (242). Agricultural operations involving soil disturbance and manufacture of silica-containing products can cause exposure.

Silicosis also had been described occasionally among persons with heavy environmental exposures. Residents of communities with significant exposure to sand storms, including Himalayan village residents and Bedouins of the Nigerian desert, have developed silicosis (243). Crystalline silica is also a constituent of ambient particulate matter in the general atmosphere, although there is little published information regarding background concentrations.

Animal studies provide supportive data that crystalline silica exposure can produce lung cancer (244). Inhalation studies using rats have shown that quartz is carcinogenic, producing adenocarcinomas and epidermoid carcinomas of the lung (245, 246). Most of the rats also developed pulmonary fibrosis. The animal studies show species specificity. Whereas rat studies have been positive for fibrosis and lung tumors, experiments in mice, hamsters, and guinea pigs have been negative (244, 247, 248). The IARC has concluded that there is sufficient evidence of carcinogenicity in animal studies, but this response appears to occur in the context of lung fibrosis.

Whether silica causes lung cancer in humans has been debated since the early part of this century. Conventional wisdom during much of this time has been that silica exposure and silicosis are not risk factors for lung cancer in humans. However, the issue has been reevaluated in recent years, and there is now a growing body of evidence that workers with a history of significant silica exposure are at increased risk (249, 250). Studies of miners exposed to free silica have generally have shown increased lung cancer incidence. These include miners of metal ore, lead-zinc, mercury, chromium, copper-iron, and tin. Some of these studies are confounded by concomitant exposures to other known carcinogens. For example, gold miners were also exposed to radon, arsenic, chromium, and nickel (251, 252). Smoking has not been adequately controlled in many studies. Trades other than mining have silica exposures and have demonstrated increased lung cancer rates. These include stonemasons, sandblasters, brick kiln workers, foundry workers, and potters in the ceramic industry (250, 253) For silica-exposed workers, the relative risk levels are consistently elevated across studies, usually in the range of 1.3 to 1.7.

A dose-response relationship for silica exposure and lung cancer risk has been shown in a number of studies. In particular, the risk is greatest for those workers with silicosis, leading some to conclude that parenchymal fibrosis is a necessary intermediate step in carcinogenesis, an observation supported by the animal studies. This would be analogous to the requirement for asbestosis in causing asbestos-related lung cancer. It is also consistent with the observation that lung cancer often arises in areas of parenchymal scarring (scar cancer) and is a complication of idiopathic pulmonary fibrosis (254–256).

Autopsy studies of patients with silicosis have generally not shown an increased incidence of lung cancer compared with nonsilicosis cases and general autopsy series (250). These results contrast with epidemiologic studies, which show a consistent increase in lung cancer rates among silicotics, with risks ranging from 1.4 in Austria (257) to 6.5 in Japan (258). A study of 68,000 Chinese workers with silica exposure showed a greater than 30-fold excess rate of death from pneumoconiosis. The risk of lung cancer was 22% greater among workers who had silicosis (259). The risk of lung cancer is increased among persons with silicosis regardless of the industry in which they were exposed. Case control studies based on silicosis registries generally shown an increased risk of lung cancer (253, 260).

The overall human epidemiologic evidence supports an association between silica exposure and lung cancer risk. Most studies have reported an SMR between 1.2 and 2.0. The mechanism for silica-induced carcinogenicity is not well understood, and it is not certain whether parenchymal fibrosis is a necessary intermediate step. NIOSH regards silica exposure as potentially carcinogenic, but OSHA does not regulate silica as a carcinogen. The OSHA permissible exposure limit is 0.1 mg/m^3 for silica, and 0.05 mg/m^3 for tridymite and cristobalite. Respirable crystalline silica is considered carcinogenic in California, and a cancer warning label is required on some silica-containing products. Risks to the general public from low-level environmental silica exposure are controversial. Risk estimates based on animal studies have been calculated using worst case assumptions and no-threshold models (250). There is no direct evidence that lung cancer is a significant problem among persons with typical environmental exposure. Certainly, silicosis is not a risk for the general public.

WELDING

Welding has been an important industrial process since World War I, when armament manufacture increased rapidly. Later, the automobile industry and World War II led to further expansion and to the development of modern welding technology. It has been estimated that approximately 185,000 workers in the United States are employed as welders, braziers, or thermal cutters, and up to 700,000 workers in the United States perform some welding. Welding fumes are a complex mixture of gases, vapors, and particulates. Concern for carcinogenesis has been centered on the presence of nickel and hexavalent chromium in fumes, particularly with stainless steel welding (261).

Animal data concerning carcinogenicity are limited. Instillation and implantation of welding fume particulate in hamsters and rats failed to induce significant numbers of tumors (262, 263). Human data include a large number of case control and cohort studies. These show a fairly consistent excess of about 30% to 40% for lung cancer among welders (261, 264–267). However, the data are difficult to interpret because of inadequate smoking information and the presence of asbestos in the welding environment. Those confounding exposures may explain most, or all, of the lung cancer excess in published studies (268–271). The IARC has concluded that there is limited evidence in humans for the carcinogenicity of welding fumes and gases, and that they are possibly carcinogenic to humans (group 2B) (261).

AIR POLLUTION AND LUNG CANCER

The apparent epidemic of lung cancer in the middle part of this century led to concern that pollution of outdoor air by residential fires, automobiles, industry, and power plants might be responsible. By the mid-1950s it was demonstrated that cigarette smoking caused the vast majority of lung cancers (272). However, recognition that air pollution contains a number of known carcinogens, and the involuntary nature of the exposure sustained by the general public, have kept the issue of outdoor air pollution as a cause of lung cancer as a public health concern. Urban air contains a number of known or suspected lung carcinogens, almost always at higher concentrations than in rural air. These include arsenic, asbestos, cadmium, chromium, nickel, uranium and radioactive nuclides, and a variety of gaseous and particulate organic compounds such as benzo(a)pyrene (273). There are approximately 3000 chemicals in ambient air; only a small fraction has been tested for carcinogenesis in animals. Fewer still have been studied in human populations. Data that exist usually describe the effects of a single agent, in contrast to the complex mixtures present in air pollution (274–276). Another problem is the lack of objective data concerning the nature and levels of air pollution in the past. Many studies have relied on surrogate measures, such as coal consumption, number of vehicles registered, and population density (277).

The lack of basic information concerning the components of air pollution is compounded by the limitations of epidemiology. Because most lung cancers are caused by smoking, it is difficult to detect lesser risks. Passive smoking, which is now recognized as a lung carcinogen, must be considered as a confounding factor in assessing air pollution risks among nonsmokers (278). Descriptive studies of the geographic distribution of lung cancer support the hypothesis that air pollution causes lung cancer. The presence of an urban-rural gradient for lung cancer was demonstrated in the 1950s and 1960s, with relative risks up to twofold (279, 280). Part of this risk was probably because of differences in smoking habits. Urban dwellers typically start smoking at an earlier age, and they smoke more than their rural counterparts (2). Access to medical facilities and diagnostic testing in the cities, as well as more frequent autopsies, may have contributed to a higher rate of diagnosis. It also is likely that urban dwellers have been exposed more often to occupational carcinogens such as asbestos.

More recent epidemiologic studies have attempted to control for the effect of smoking and, to some extent, for social and occupational factors. Although it was estimated previously that air pollution doubled the risk of lung cancer and caused 10% of cases, there has been a downward assessment in recent years. Generally, the urban-rural gradient for relative risk in nonsmokers is in the range of 1.1 to 1.4, which in most studies is not statistically significant (281–287). The risk is greater in urban smokers, suggesting that the combination of air pollution and tobacco smoke causes a risk that is greater than additive. The EPA now estimates that fewer than 1% of lung cancers are caused by air pollution (288).

Air inside residences and buildings also contains known or suspected lung carcinogens, often at higher concentrations than in outside air. These include formaldehyde, polycyclic aromatic hydrocarbons from kerosene and wood combustion, and secondhand tobacco smoke (289). Whether indoor air pollution contributes to lung cancer in the general population, and the degree of any possible risk, is unknown at this time (290).

OCCUPATIONAL AND ENVIRONMENTAL CAUSES OF ESOPHAGEAL CANCER

It is estimated that there were 11,000 new cases of esophageal cancer in the United States in 1994 and 10,400 deaths (291). This disease accounts for approximately 1% of new cancer cases and for 2% of cancer deaths. The incidence is approximately 3 times greater in men compared with women, and about 3 times greater in blacks than whites. Mortality rates in whites have been quite stable, but mortality in black males has been rising since 1940 (292, 293). The reason for the racial difference is not known, but it may be caused by tobacco and alcohol consumption, or diet (294, 295).

There are distinct regional differences in the frequency of esophageal cancer. In most parts of the world, incidence rates per 100,000 are 2.5 to 5.0 for males and 1.5 to 2.5 for females. But they may exceed 100 per 100,000 in parts of Asia, India, and Africa (292, 296). In France the rate is very high among males. No single explanation for the regional variation has been found. Researchers have postulated that cultural differences such as consuming hot liquids, pickled vegetables, seeds containing large quantities of silica fibers, foods containing high concentrations of nitrosamines, or a diet deficient in certain vitamins might be responsible (292, 296–300). Others have suggested that infectious agents, such as fungi found in certain foods or viruses known to infect esophageal epithelium, might be responsible (301).

Tobacco and alcohol are the major risk factors for esophageal cancer, accounting for 80% to 90% of cases in the United States and western Europe (292, 302). Smoking cigarettes, pipes, or cigars increases the risk of esophageal cancer by fourfold to fivefold (303). Alcohol, even moderate social use, increases the risk of esophageal cancer by about twofold to threefold (304–306). There is a positive dose response for tobacco or alcohol viewed individually as risk factors; the incidence of esophageal cancer increases with the amount of alcohol or tobacco consumed. The combination of tobacco and alcohol acts synergistically to increase the risk of esophageal cancer (307, 308).

Considering the predominant effects of tobacco and alcohol in causing esophageal cancer, occupational exposures have a relatively minor effect on risk for developing this tumor. Studies of insulation workers exposed to asbestos have described an increased risk of esophageal cancer. The most recent report of this cohort indicated a relative risk of 1.68 (309, 310). However, there was no information concerning tobacco and alcohol consumption, and these studies have been criticized for the different methods used to confirm the diagnosis among insulation workers compared with the control group (311). Workers with a lower level of asbestos exposure, such as pipefitters and shipyard workers, have not shown an increased risk (312–319). Many studies are hampered by a lack of specific data for esophageal tumors and have no information concerning tobacco and alcohol use. Existing data suggest that heavy exposure to asbestos may cause a slightly increased risk of esophageal cancer (311, 320).

Studies of workers in the rubber industry have indicated an increased risk of esophageal cancer (321, 322). A study of Swedish vulcanization workers showed an SMR of 10 compared with other employed men (323). Workers in the American rubber industry do not consistently show an excess risk (324–326).

Other groups for which an increased risk of esophageal cancer has been reported include cement workers (327), metal polishers and platers (328), wood workers (329, 330), chimney sweeps (331), and workers exposed to combustion products (332). However, these studies generally have shown no relationship between the degree of risk and duration of employment or level of exposure, and they lack information concerning smoking and alcohol use.

PREVENTION OF OCCUPATIONAL AND ENVIRONMENTAL THORACIC NEOPLASMS

Programs designed to prevent occupational and environmental thoracic neoplasms can be characterized by the timing of the interventions used. Primary prevention programs are intended to stop the occurrence of disease. The goal of secondary prevention programs is the detection of illness at an early stage, hopefully when there is the potential for reversibility. Tertiary prevention programs detect the condition when it is fully established, usually for the purpose of providing medical benefits and disability rating (333). Although secondary and tertiary programs have been useful in preventing morbidity and mortality from some occupational diseases (e.g., byssinosis, occupational asthma), they have not been effective for lung and esophageal neoplasms. The natural history of those conditions is that, with few exceptions, diagnosis is followed inexorably by death. Despite the improved sensitivity and specificity of screening techniques (e.g., chest radiographs, computed tomography, sputum cytology, monoclonal antibodies, flexible endoscopy), most lung and esophageal cancers are incurable when identified (334, 335). Although screening programs have demonstrated the ability to detect more cancers at an earlier stage, long-term survival of screened patients has not differed significantly from unscreened populations (335–338). Secondary programs may be useful in early identification of conditions that may predispose to the development of lung cancer (e.g., asbestosis, silicosis). Because there is some evidence that the risk of lung cancer is related to the degree of pulmonary fibrosis, removal of the worker from further exposure may have some efficacy. Tertiary programs may be useful in identifying high-risk groups who might benefit from intensive screening, although the results to date are not promising (339).

Primary prevention obviously should be the main focus of attention. The single most effective measure for preventing lung cancer is to stop nonsmokers from starting, and to persuade smokers to quit. This also is true for esophageal cancer, along with reducing alcohol consumption. Other interventions pale in comparison; indeed, they will have little effect if smoking persists.

Industrial hygiene and safety programs in the workplace are useful in recognizing the presence and magnitude of hazardous agents and processes, and implementing measures to reduce risk (340). Strategies include substitution of a hazardous material with a less dangerous one, local exhaust and general dilution ventilation, and use of respirators or other personal equipment.

Education plays a fundamental role in cancer prevention. In addition to smoking avoidance and cessation, education programs allow individual workers and their employers to participate effectively in reducing risks. Compliance with safety programs is much better in an educated workforce (341). Education programs should provide information concerning hazard recognition, health effects, methods of preventing exposure, and legal issues such as right-to-know laws. Workers should be aware of material safety data sheets, which contain information about the health effects of products and recommended safe practices. The employer is obliged legally to maintain a material safety data sheet for each chemical or agent used in the workplace and must provide a copy to the worker upon request. Company-sponsored education programs are mandated for workers engaged in certain activities, such as hazardous waste management and asbestos abatement. Many unions also provide education programs. Clearly, the best situation is for management and labor to cooperate in a combined effort to promote hazard awareness and risk reduction.

REFERENCES

1. Doll R. Introduction and overview. In: Samet JM, ed. Epidemiology of lung cancer. New York: Marcel Dekker, 1994:1–14.
2. Doll R, Peto R. The causes of cancer: quantitative estimates of the avoidable risks of cancer in the United States today. J Natl Cancer Inst 1981;66:1191–1308.
3. Simonato L, Vineis P, Fletcher AC. Estimates of the proportion of lung cancer attributable to occupational exposure. Carcinogenesis 1988;9:1159–1165.
4. Vineis P, Thomas T, Hayes RB, et al. Proportion of lung cancers in males, due to occupation, in different areas of the USA. Int J Cancer 1988;42:851–866.
5. Vineis P, Simonato L. Proportion of lung and bladder cancers in males resulting from occupation: a systematic approach. Arch Environ Health 1991;46:6–15.
6. Churg A. Lung cancer cell type and occupational exposure. In: Samet JM, ed. Epidemiology of lung cancer. New York: Marcel Dekker, 1994:413–436.
7. Santella RM. In vitro testing for carcinogens and mutagens. Occup Med 1987;2:39–46.
8. International Agency for Research on Cancer (IARC). IARC monographs on the evaluation of carcinogenic risks to humans. Overall evaluations of carcinogenicity: an updating of IARC monographs volumes 1 to 42 (Suppl 7). Lyon: IARC, 1987.
9. Squire RA. Carcinogenicity testing and safety assessment. Fundam Appl Toxicol 1984;4:S326–S334.
10. Goodman DG. Animal testing of carcinogens. Occup Med 1987;2:47–59.
11. Hallenbeck WH, Cunningham KM. Quantitative risk assessment for environmental and occupational health. Chelsea, MI: Lewis Publishers, 1986.
12. Ames BN, Gold LS. Chemical carcinogenesis: too many rodent carcinogens. Proc Natl Acad Sci U S A. 1990;87:7772–7776.
13. Carr CJ, Kolbye AC. A critique of the maximum tolerated dose in bioassays to assess cancer risk from chemicals. Regul Toxicol Pharmacol 1991;14:78–87.
14. Lynch KM, Smith WA. Pulmonary asbestosis III: carcinoma of lung in asbesto-silicosis. Am J Cancer 1935;24:56–64.
15. Hill AB. The environment and disease: association and causation. Proc R Soc Med 1965;58:295–300.
16. Lilienfeld AM, Lilienfeld DE. Foundations of epidemiology. Oxford: Oxford University Press, 1980.
17. Doll R. Occupational cancer: problems of interpreting human evidence. Ann Occup Hyg 1984;28:291–305.
18. Elwood JM. Causal relationships in medicine: a practical system for critical appraisal. Oxford: Oxford University Press, 1988.
19. Monson RR. Occupational epidemiology. 2nd ed. Boca Raton, FL: CRC Press, 1990.
20. Nelson DE, Emont SL, Brackbill RM, et al. Cigarette smoking prevalence by occupation in the United States: a comparison between 1978 to 1980 and 1987 to 1990. J Occup Med 1994; 36:516–525.

21. Selikoff IJ, Hammond EC, Churg J. Asbestos, smoking and neoplasia. JAMA 1968;204:104–110.
22. Hammond EC, Selikoff IJ, Seidman H. Asbestos exposure, cigarette smoking and death rates. Ann NY Acad Sci 1979;330:473–490.123.
23. Steenland K, Thun M. Interaction between tobacco smoking and occupational exposures in the causation of lung cancer. J Occup Med 1986;28:110–118.
24. Saracci R, Boffeta P. Interactions of tobacco smoking with other causes of lung cancer. In: Samet JM, ed. Epidemiology of lung cancer. New York: Marcel Dekker, 1994:465–493.
25. Davidson CI, Goold WD, Mathison TP, et al. Airborne trace elements in Great Smoky Mountains, Olympic, and Glacier National Parks. Environ Sci Technol 1985;19:27–35.
26. International Agency for Research on Cancer (IARC). IARC monographs on the evaluation of carcinogenic risk of chemicals to man: some metals and metallic compounds. Lyon: IARC, 1980:23.
27. Blot WJ, Fraumeni JF. Arsenical air pollution and lung cancer. Lancet 1975;2:142–144.
28. Frost F, Harter L, Milham S, et al. Lung cancer among women residing close to an arsenic emitting copper smelter. Arch Environ Health 1987;42:148–152.
29. Matanoski GE, Landau J, Tonascia C, et al. Cancer mortality in an industrial area of Baltimore. Environ Res 1981;25:8–28.
30. U.S. Environmental Protection Agency (EPA). Integrated risk information system (IRIS) online data base, Washington, D.C. Washington, DC: U.S. EPA.
31. Tseng WP. Effects and dose response relationships of skin cancer and blackfoot disease with arsenic. Environ Health Perspect 1977;19:109–119.
32. Borgono JM. Epidemiologic study of arsenic poisoning in the city of Antofagasta. Rev Med Chil 1971;99:702–707.
33. Bergoglio RM. Mortality from cancer in regions of arsenical waters of the province of Cordoba Argentine Republic. Prensa Medica Argentina 1964;51:994–998.
34. Cebrian ME, Albores A, Aguilar M, Blakely E. Chronic arsenic poisoning in the north of Mexico. Hum Toxicol 1983;2:121–133.
35. Wu M, Kuo T, Huang Y, Chen C. Dose-response relation between arsenic concentration in well water and mortality from cancers and vascular diseases. Am J Epidemiol 1989;130:1123–1132.
36. Chen C, Wang C. Ecological correlation between arsenic level in well water and age-adjusted mortality from malignant neoplasms. Cancer Res 1990;50:5470–5474.
37. Robson AO, Jelliffe AM. Medicinal arsenic poisoning and lung cancer. BMJ 1963;2:207–209.
38. Enterline PE, Marsh GM, Esmen NA, et al. Some effects of cigarette smoking, arsenic and SO_2 on mortality among US copper smelter workers. J Occup Med 1987;29:831–838.
39. Enterline PE, Marsh GM. Cancer mortality among workers exposed to arsenic and other substances in a copper smelter. Am J Epidemiol 1982;116:895–911.
40. Rencher AC, Carter MW, McKee DW. A retrospective epidemiological study of mortality at a large western copper smelter. J Occup Med 1978;19:754–758.
41. Lee-Feldstein A. Arsenic and respiratory cancer in man: follow-up of an occupational study. In: Lederer W, Fensterheim R, eds. Arsenic: industrial, biomedical, and environmental perspectives. New York: Van Nostrand Reinhold, 1983:245–265.
42. Lee-Feldstein A. Cumulative exposure to arsenic and its relationship to respiratory cancer among copper smelter employees. J Occup Med 1986;28:296–302.
43. Lee-Feldstein A. A comparison of several measures of exposure to arsenic. Matched case-control study of copper smelter employees. Am J Epidemiol 1989;129:112–124.
44. Axelson OE, Dahlgren CD, Jansson CD, Rehnlund SO. Arsenic exposure and mortality: a case referent study from a Swedish copper smelter. Br J Ind Med 1978;35:8–15.
45. Tokudome S, Kuratsune A. A cohort study on mortality from cancer and other causes among workers at a metal refinery. Int J Cancer 1976;17:310–317.
46. Taylor PR, Qiao YL, Schatzkin A, et al. Relation of arsenic exposure to lung cancer among tin miners in Yunnan Province, China. Br J Ind Med 1989;46:881–886.
47. Ott MG, Holder BB, Gordon HL. Respiratory cancer and occupational exposure to arsenicals. Arch Environ Health 1974;29:250–255.
48. Mabuchi KA, Lilienfeld A, Snell L. Lung cancer among pesticide workers exposed to inorganic arsenicals. Arch Environ Health 1979;34:312–319.
49. Pershagen G, Bergman F, Klominek J, et al. Histological types of lung cancer among smelter workers exposed to arsenic. Br J Ind Med 1987;44:454–458.
50. Welch K, Higgins I, Oh M, Burchfield C. Arsenic exposure, smoking, and respiratory cancer in copper smelter workers. Arch Environ Health 1982;37:325–335.
51. U.S. Environmental Protection Agency. Health assessment document for inorganic arsenic. Research Triangle Park, NC: Environmental Criteria and Assessment Office, 1984: EPA/600/8-83/021F.
52. Lauwreys RR, Hoet P. Industrial chemical exposure: guidelines for biological monitoring. Boca Raton, FL: Lewis Publishers, 1993:21–31.
53. Cooke WE. Pulmonary asbestosis. BMJ 1927;2:1024–1025.
54. Seiler HE. A case of pneumoconiosis: result of the inhalation of asbestos dust. BMJ 1928;2:982.
55. Merewether ERA. The occurrence of pulmonary fibrosis and other pulmonary affections in asbestos workers. J Ind Hyg 1930;12:198–222.
56. Merewether ERA. The occurrence of pulmonary fibrosis and other pulmonary affections in asbestos workers (concluded). J Ind Hyg 1930;12:239–257.
57. Dreessen WC, Dallavalle JM, Edwards TI, et al. A study of asbestosis in the asbestos textile industry. Public health bulletin no. 241. Washington, DC: U.S. Government Printing Office, 1938:91.
58. Merewether ERA. Annual report of the chief inspector of factories for the year 1947. London: Her Majesty's Stationery Office, 1949.
59. Doll R. Mortality from lung cancer in asbestos workers. Br J Ind Med 1955;12:81–86.
60. Hammond EC, Selikoff IJ. Neoplasia among insulation workers in the United States with special reference to intra-abdominal neoplasia. Ann NY Acad Sci 1965,132:519–525.
61. Hammond EC, Selikoff IJ. Relation of cigarette smoking to risk of death of asbestos-associated disease among insulation workers in the United States. IARC Sci Publ 1973;8:312–317.
62. Kipen HM, Lilis R, Suzuki Y, et al. Pulmonary fibrosis in asbestos workers with lung cancer. Br J Ind Med 1987;44:96–100.
63. Weiss W. Pulmonary fibrosis in asbestos workers with lung cancer. Br J Ind Med 1989;46:430.
64. Churg A. Asbestos-related disease in the workplace and the environment: controversial issues. In: Churg A, Katzenstein AA, eds. The lung: current concepts. Baltimore: Williams & Wilkins, 1993:54–77.

65. Report of the Royal Commission on Matters of Health and Safety Arising from the Use of Asbestos in Ontario. Toronto: Queen's Printer for Ontario, 1984:281.
66. Browne K. Asbestos-related disorders. In: Parkes WR, ed. Occupational lung disorders. 3rd ed. Oxford: Butterworth-Heinemann, 1994:411–485.
67. Gaensler EA. Asbestos exposure in buildings. Clin Chest Med 1992;13:231–242.
68. Kuschner M, Laskin S, Drew RT, et al. Inhalation carcinogenicity of alpha halo ethers. III. Lifetime and limited period inhalation studies with bis(chloromethyl)ether at 0.1 ppm. Arch Environ Health 1975;30:73–77.
69. American Conference of Governmental Industrial Hygienists (ACGIH). Documentation of the threshold limit values and biological exposure indices, 6th ed. Cincinnati, OH: ACGIH, 1991:192–293.
70. Travenius SZ. Formation and occurrence of bis(chloromethyl) ether and its prevention in the chemical industry. Scand J Work Environ Health 1982;8:1–86.
71. Leong BKJ, MacFarland HN, Reese WH. Induction of lung adenomas by chronic inhalation of bis(chloromethyl)ether. Arch Environ Health 1971;22:663–666
72. Gowers DS, Schaffer P, Karli A, et al. Incidence of respiratory cancer among workers exposed to chloromethyl-ethers. Am J Epidemiol 1993;137:31–42
73. U.S. Environmental Protection Agency. Noncarcinogenic effects of chromium; update to a health effects document. Research Triangle Park, NC: Environmental Criteria and Assessment Office, 1990:EPA 600/8-87/048F.
74. Lofroth G. The mutagenicity of hexavalent chromium is decreased by microsomal metabolism. Naturvissenschaften 1978;65:207–208.
75. Petrilli FL, DeFlora S. Toxicity and mutagenicity of hexavalent chromium on salmonella typhimurium. Appl Environ Microbiol 1977;33:805–809.
76. Petrilli FL, DeFlora S. Oxidation of inactive trivalent chromium to the mutagenic hexavalent form. Mutat Res 1978;58:167–178.
77. U.S. Department of Health and Human Services. Toxicological profile for chromium. Atlanta: Agency for Toxic Substances and Disease Registry, 1993:ATSDR/TP-92/08.
78. Machle W, Gregorius F. Cancer of the respiratory system in the United States chromate-producing industry. Public Health Rep 1948;63:1114–1127.
79. Enterline PE. Respiratory cancer among chromate workers. J Occup Med 1974;16:523–526
80. Hayes RB, Lilienfeld AM, Snell LM. Mortality in chromium chemical production workers: a prospective study. Int J Epidemiol 1979;4:365–374.
81. DeMarco R, Bernardinelli L, Mangione MP. Death risk due to cancer of the respiratory apparatus in chromate production workers. La Medicina del Lavoro 1988;79:368–376.
82. Satoh KY, Fukuda K, Tori I, Katsuno N. Epidemiologic study of workers engaged in the manufacture of chromium compounds. J Occup Med 1981;23:835–838.
83. Langard S, Norseth T. A cohort study of bronchial carcinomas in workers producing chromate pigments. Br J Ind Med 1975;32:62–65.
84. Hill WJ, Ferguson WS. Statistical analysis of epidemiological data from a chromium chemical manufacturing plant. J Occup Med 1979;21:103–106.
85. International Agency for Research on Cancer (IARC). IARC monographs on the evaluation of carcinogenic risk of chemicals to man. Chromium, nickel and welding. Lyon: IARC, 1990;49.
86. Silverstein M, Mirer F, Kotelchuck D, et al. Mortality among workers in a die-casting and electroplating plant. Scand J Work Environ Health 1981;4:156–165.
87. Franchini I, Magnani F, Mutti A. Mortality experience among chromeplating workers. Scand J Work Environ Health 1983;9:247–252.
88. Sorhan T, Burgess DC, Waterhouse JA. A mortality study of nickel/chromium platers. Br J Ind Med 1987;44:250–258.
89. Okubo T, Tsuchiya K. An epidemiological study of chromium platers in Japan. Biol Trace Elem Res 1979;1:35–44.
90. Pokrovskaya LV, Shabynina NK. Carcinogenic hazards in the production of chromium ferroalloys. Gig Tr Prof Zabol 1973;10:23–26.
91. Langard S, Anderson A, Gylseth B. Incidence of cancer among ferrochromium and ferrosilicon workers. Br J Ind Med 1980;37:114–120.
92. Axelsson G, Rylander R, Schmidt A. Mortality and incidence of tumours among ferrochromium workers. Br J Ind Med 1980;37:121–127.
93. Stern FB, Beaumont JJ, Halperin WE, et al. Mortality of chrome leather tannery workers and chemical exposures in tanneries. Scand J Work Environ Health 1987;3:108–117.
94. Pippard EC, Acheson ED, Winter PD. Mortality of tanners. Br J Ind Med 1985;42:2385–2387.
95. Korallus U, Ehrlicher H, Wustefeld E. Trivalent chromium compounds: results of a study in occupational medicine. Arbeitsmedizin Sozialmedizin Praventiv Medizin 1974;9:76–79.
96. Langard S. One hundred years of chromium and cancer: a review of epidemiological evidence and selected case reports. Am J Ind Med 1990;17:189–215.
97. Lauwerys RR, Hoet P. Industrial chemical exposure: guidelines for biological monitoring. Boca Raton, FL: Lewis Publishers, 1993.
98. Bukowski J, Goldstein M, Johnson BB. Biological markers in chromium exposure assessment: confounding variables. Arch Environ Health 1991;46:230–236.
99. Schroeder WH, Dobson M, Jane DM. Toxic trace elements associated with airborne particulate matter: a review. Air Pollution Control Association Journal 1987;11:1267–1287.
100. Roberts RS, Julian JA, Muir DC, Shannon HS. Cancer mortality associated with the high-temperature oxidation of nickel subsulfide. IARC Sci Publ 1984;53:23–35.
101. Peto J, Cuckle H, Doll R, et al. Respiratory cancer mortality of Welsh nickel refinery workers. IARC Sci Publ 1984;53:36–46.
102. Roberts RS, Julian JA, Muir DC, Shannon HS. A study of mortality in workers engaged in mining, smelting, and refining of nickel. II: mortality from cancer of the respiratory tract and kidney. Toxicol Ind Health 1989;5:975–993.
103. Magnus K, Andersen A, Hogetveit A. Cancer of respiratory organs among workers at a nickel refinery in Norway. Int J Cancer 1982;30:681–685.
104. U.S. Environmental Protection Agency (EPA). Integrated risk information system (IRIS) online data base, Washington, DC: U.S. EPA.
105. Sunderman FW, Donnelly AJ. Studies of nickel carcinogenesis. Metastasizing pulmonary tumors in rats induced by the inhalation of nickel carbonyl. Am J Pathol 1965;46:1027–1041.
106. International Committee on Nickel Carcinogenesis in Man. Report of the International Committee on Nickel Carcinogenesis in Man. Scand J Work Environ Health 1990;16:1–82.
107. Verma DK, Julian JA, Roberts RS, et al. Polycyclic aromatic hydrocarbons (PAHs). A possible cause of lung cancer mortal-

108. Raithel HJ, Ebner G, Schaller KH, et al. Problems in establishing normal values for nickel and chromium concentrations in human pulmonary tissue. Am J Ind Med 1987;12:55–70.
109. Adachi S, Takemoto K, Ohshima S, et al. Metal concentrations in lung tissue of subjects suffering from lung cancer. Int Arch Occup Environ Health 1991;63:193–7.
110. International Agency for Research on Cancer (IARC). IARC monographs on the evaluation of carcinogenic risk of chemicals to humans. Polynuclear aromatic compounds, part 1, chemical, environmental and experimental data. Lyon: IARC, 1983;32.
111. International Agency for Research on Cancer (IARC). IARC monographs on the evaluation of carcinogenic risk of chemicals to humans. Polynuclear aromatic hydrocarbons, part 4, bitumens, coal-tars and derived products, shale-oils and soots. Lyon: IARC, 1985:35.
112. Schamberg JF. Cancer in tar workers. Journal of Cutaneous Diseases 1910;28:644–662.
113. Hammond EC, Selikoff IJ, Lawther PL, Seidman H. Inhalation of benzpyrene and cancer in man. Ann NY Acad Sci 1976;271:116–124.
114. Andersen A, Dahlberg BE, Magnus K, Wanning A. Risk of cancer in the Norwegian aluminum industry. Int J Cancer 1982;29:295–298.
115. Kuroda S. Occupational pulmonary cancer of generator gas workers. Ind Med 1937;6:304–306.
116. International Agency for Research on Cancer (IARC). IARC monographs on the evaluation of carcinogenic risk of chemicals to humans. Polynuclear aromatic hydrocarbons, part 3, industrial exposure to aluminum production, coal gasification, coke production, and iron and steel founding. Lyon: IARC, 1984;34.
117. Rockette HE, Arena VC. Mortality studies of aluminum reduction plant workers: potroom and carbon department. J Occup Med 1983;25:549–557.
118. Gibbs GW, Horowitz I. Lung cancer mortality in aluminum reduction plant workers. J Occup Med 1979;21:347–353.
119. Menichini E. Urban air pollution by polycyclic aromatic hydrocarbons: levels and sources of variability. Sci Total Environ 1992;116:109–35.
120. Samet JM. Radon and lung cancer. J Natl Cancer Inst 1989;81:745–757.
121. Samet JM. Review of radon and lung cancer risk. Risk Anal 1990;10:65–75.
122. National Research Council Committee on the Biological Effects of Ionizing Radiation. Health risks of radon and other internally deposited alpha-emitters: BEIR IV. Washington, DC: National Academy Press, 1988.
123. Howe GR, Nair RC, Newcombe HB, et al. Lung cancer mortality (1950–80) in relation to radon daughter exposure in a cohort of workers at the Eldorado Beaverlodge uranium mine. J Natl Cancer Inst 1986;77:357–362.
124. Howe GR, Nair RC, Newcombe HB, et al. Lung cancer mortality (1950–80) in relation to radon daughter exposure in a cohort of workers at the Eldorado Port radium uranium mine: possible modification of risk by exposure rate. J Natl Cancer Inst 1987;79:1255–1260.
125. Hornung RW, Meinhardt TJ. Quantitative risk assessment of lung cancer in U.S. uranium miners. Health Phys 1987;52:417–430.
126. Lubin JH, Qiao YL, Taylor PR, et al. Quantitative evaluation of the radon and lung cancer association in a case control study of Chinese tin miners. Cancer Res 1990;50:174–180.
127. Sevc J, Kunz E, Tomasek L, et al. Cancer in man after exposure to radon daughters. Health Phys 1988;54:27–46.
128. Samet JM. Radon. In: Samet JM, ed. Epidemiology of lung cancer. New York: Marcel Dekker, 1994:219–243.
129. Samet JM, Pathak DR, Morgan MV, et al. Radon progeny exposure and lung cancer risk in New Mexico uranium miners: a case-control study. Health Phys 1989;56:415–421.
130. Waxweiler R, Roscoe R, Archer V, et al. Mortality follow-up through 1977 of the white underground uranium miners cohort examined by the United States Public Health Service. In: Gomez M, ed. Radiation hazards in mining: control, measurement, and medical aspects. New York: Society of Mining Engineers of the American Institute of Mining, Metallurgical, and Petroleum Engineers, 1981:823–830.
131. Saccommanno GS, Huth GC, Auerbach O, Kuschner M. Relationship of radioactive radon daughters and cigarette smoking in the genesis of lung cancer in uranium miners. Cancer 1988;62:1402–1408.
132. Butler C, Samet JM, Kutvirt DM, et al. Histopathologic findings of lung cancer in Navajo men: relation to uranium mining. Health Phys 1986;51:365–368.
133. Kunz E, Sevc J, Placek V, Horacek J. Lung cancer in man in relation to different time distribution of radiation exposure. Health Phys 1979;36:699–706.
134. United States Environmental Protection Agency. A citizen's guide to radon. What it is and what to do about it. Washington, DC: Government Printing Office, 1986:EPA-86-004.
135. Nero AV, Nazaroff WW. Characterizing the source of radon indoors. Radiation Protection Dosimetry 1984;7:23–29.
136. Nazaroff WW, Moed BA, Sextro RG. Soil as a source of indoor radon: generation, migration, and entry. In: Nazaroff WW, Nero AV, eds. Radon and its decay products in indoor air. New York: Wiley, 1988:57–112.
137. Stranden E. Building materials as a source of indoor radon. In: Nazaroff WW, Nero AV, eds. Radon and its decay products in indoor air. New York: Wiley, 1988:113–130.
138. Nazaroff WW, Doyle SM, Nero AV, et al. Radon entry via potable water. In: Nazaroff WW, Nero AV, eds. Radon and its decay products in indoor air. New York: Wiley, 1988:131–157.
139. Nero AV, Schwehr MB, Nazaroff WW, Revzan KL. Distribution of airborne radon-222 concentrations in US homes. Science 1986;234:992–997.
140. Fleischer RL. A possible association between lung cancer and a geological outcrop. Health Phys 1986;50:823–827.
141. Edling C, Wingren G, Axelson O. Quantification of the lung cancer risk from radon daughter exposure in dwellings—an epidemiological approach. Environment International 1986;12:55–60.
142. Axelson O, Andersson K, Desai G, et al. Indoor radon exposure and active and passive smoking in relation to the occurrence of lung cancer. Scand J Work Environ Health 1988;14:286–292.
143. Schoenberg JB, Klotz JB, Wilcox HB, et al. Case-control study of residential radon and lung cancer among New Jersey women. Cancer Res 1990;50:6520–6524.
144. Pershagen G, Akerblom G, Axelson O, et al. Residential radon exposure and lung cancer in Sweden. N Engl J Med 1994;330:159–164.
145. Letourneau EG, Krewski D, Choi NW, et al. Case-control study of residential radon and lung cancer in Winnipeg, Manitoba, Canada. Am J Epidemiol 1994;140:310–322.

146. Suzuki Y. Neoplastic effect of vinyl chloride in mouse lung—lower doses and short-term exposure. Environ Res 1983;32:91–103.
147. Hehir RM, McNamara BP, McLaughlin J, et al. Cancer induction following single and multiple exposures to a constant amount of vinyl chloride monomer. Environ Health Perspect 1981;41:63–72.
148. Creech JL, Johnson MN. Angiosarcoma of liver in the manufacture of polyvinyl chloride. J Occup Med 1974;16:150–151.
149. Doll R. Effects of exposure to vinyl chloride—an assessment of the evidence. Scand J Work Environ Health 1988;14:61–78.
150. Infante PF. Observations of the site-specific carcinogenicity of vinyl chloride to humans. Environ Health Perspect 1981;41:89–94.
151. Monson RR, Peters JM, Johnson MN. Proportional mortality among vinyl chloride workers. Environ Health Perspect 1975;11:75–77.
152. Storetvedt-Heldaas S, Langard SL, Andersen A. Incidence of cancer among vinyl chloride and polyvinyl chloride workers. Br J Ind Med 1984;41:25–30.
153. Hagmar L, Akesson B, Nielsen J, et al. Mortality and cancer morbidity in workers exposed to low levels of vinyl chloride monomer at a polyvinyl chloride processing plant. Am J Ind Med 1990;17:553–565.
154. Buffler PA, Wood S, Eifler C, et al. Mortality experience of workers in a vinyl chloride monomer production plant. J Occup Med 1979;21:195–203.
155. Waxweiler RJ, Smith AH, Falk H, Tyroler HA. Excess lung cancer risk in a synthetic chemicals plant. Environ Health Perspect 1981;41:159–165.
156. Wu W, Steenland K, Brown D, et al. Cohort and case-control analyses of workers exposed to vinyl chloride: an update. J Occup Med 1989;31:518–523.
157. Wong O, Whorton MD, Foliart DE, Rogland D. An industry wide epidemiologic study of vinyl chloride workers, 1942–1982. Am J Ind Med 1991;20:317–34.
158. Jones RD, Smith DM, Thomas PG. A mortality study of vinyl chloride monomer workers employed in the United Kingdom in 1940–1974. Scand J Work Environ Health 1988;14:153–60.
159. Simonato L, L'Abbe KA, Andersen A, et al. A collaborative study of cancer incidence and mortality among vinyl chloride workers. Scand J Work Environ Health 1991;17:159–160.
160. Koerselman W, van der Graaf M. Acrylonitrile: a suspected human carcinogen. Int Arch Occup Environ Health 1984;54:317–324.
161. Strother DE, Mast RW, Kraska RC, Frankos V. Acrylonitrile as a carcinogen: research needs for better risk assessment. Ann NY Acad Sci 1988;534:169–178.
162. O'Berg MT. Epidemiologic study of workers exposed to acrylonitrile. J Occup Med 1980;22:245–252.
163. Werner JB, Carter JT. Mortality of United Kingdom acrylonitrile polymerization workers. Br J Ind Med 1981;38:247–253.
164. Delzell E, Monson RR. Mortality among rubber workers: VI. Men with potential exposure to acrylonitrile. J Occup Med 1982;24:767–771.
165. O'Berg MT, Chen JL, Burke CA, et al. Epidemiologic study of workers exposed to acrylonitrile: an update. J Occup Med 1985;27:835–840.
166. Swaen GMH, Bloemen LJN, Twisk J, et al. Mortality of workers exposed acrylonitrile. J Occup Med 1992;34:801–809.
167. Stonehouse AJ, Zenczak S. Properties, production processes and applications. In: Rossman MD, Preuss OP, Powers MB, eds. Beryllium: biomedical and environmental aspects. Baltimore: Williams & Wilkins, 1991:27–55.
168. Groth DH. Carcinogenicity of beryllium: review of the literature. Environ Res 1980;21:56–62.
169. Kuschner M. The carcinogenicity of beryllium. Environ Health Perspect 1981;40:101–105.
170. Flamm WG. Beryllium: laboratory evidence. IARC Sci Publ 1985;65:199–201.
171. Reeves AL, Deitch D, Vorwald AJ. Beryllium carcinogenesis: I. Inhalation exposure of rats to beryllium sulfate aerosol. Cancer Res 1967;27:439–445.
172. Reeves AL. Experimental pathology. In: Rossman MD, Preuss OP, Powers MB, eds. Beryllium: biomedical and environmental aspects. Baltimore: Williams & Wilkins, 1991:59–75.
173. Saracci R. Beryllium and lung cancer: adding another piece to the puzzle of epidemiologic evidence. J Natl Cancer Inst 1991;83:1362–1363.
174. Mancuso TF, El-Attar AA. Epidemiologic study of the beryllium industry. Cohort methodology and mortality studies. J Occup Med 1969;11:422–434.
175. Mancuso TF. Relation of duration of employment and prior respiratory disease among beryllium workers. Environ Res 1970;3:251–275.
176. Mancuso TF. Mortality study of beryllium industry workers' occupational lung cancer. Environ Res 1980;21:48–55.
177. Infante PF, Wagoner JK, Sprince JL. Mortality patterns from lung cancer and nonneoplastic respiratory disease among white males in the Beryllium Case Registry. Environ Res 1980;21:35–43.
178. Wagoner JK, Infante PF, Bayliss DL. Beryllium: an etiologic agent in the induction of lung cancer, nonneoplastic respiratory disease, and heart disease among industrially exposed workers. Environ Res 1980;21:15–34.
179. Steenland K, Ward E. Lung cancer incidence among patients with beryllium disease: a cohort mortality study. J Natl Cancer Inst 1991;83:1380–1385.
180. Ward E, Okun A, Ruder A, et al. A mortality study of workers at seven beryllium processing plants. Am J Ind Med 1992;22:885–904.
181. Meyer KC. Beryllium and lung disease. Chest 1994;106:942–946.
182. MacMahon B. The epidemiological evidence on the carcinogenicity of beryllium in humans. J Occup Med 1994;36:15–26.
183. Waalkes MP, Coogan TP, Barter RA. Toxicological principles of metal carcinogenesis with special emphasis on cadmium. Crit Rev Toxicol 1991;22:175–201.
184. Maximilien R, Poncy JL, Monchaux G, et al. Validity and limitations of animal experiments in assessing lung carcinogenicity of cadmium. IARC Sci Publ 1992;118:415–424.
185. Heinrich U. Pulmonary carcinogenicity of cadmium by inhalation in animals. IARC Sci Publ 1992;118:405–413.
186. Kipling MD, Waterhouse JAH. Cadmium and prostatic carcinoma. Lancet 1967;1:730–731.
187. Doll R. Is cadmium a human carcinogen? Ann Epidemiol 1992;2:336–337.
188. Elinder CG, Kjellstrom T, Hogstedt C, et al. Cancer mortality of cadmium workers. Br J Ind Med 1985;42:651–655.
189. Boffetta P. Methodological aspects of the epidemiological association between cadmium and cancer in humans. IARC Sci Publ 1992;118:425–433.
190. Thun MJ, Schnorr TM, Smith AB, et al. Mortality among a cohort of U.S. cadmium production workers—an update. J Natl Cancer Inst 1985;74:325–333.

191. Kazantzis G, Lam TH, Sullivan KR. Mortality of cadmium-exposed workers. A five-year update. Scand J Work Environ Health 1988;14:220–223.
192. Stayner L, Smith R, Thun M, et al. A quantitative assessment of lung cancer risk and occupational cadmium exposure. IARC Sci Publ 1992;118:447–455.
193. Sorahan T. Mortality from lung cancer among a cohort of nickel cadmium battery workers: 1946–84. Br J Ind Med 1987;44:803–809.
194. Sorahan T, Lancashire R. Lung cancer findings from the NIOSH study of United States cadmium recovery workers: a cautionary note. Occup Environ Med 1994;51:139–140.
195. Ades AE, Kazantzis G. Lung cancer in a non-ferrous smelter: the role of cadmium. Br J Ind Med 1988;45:435–442.
196. Lamm SH, Parkinson M, Anderson M, Taylor W. Determinants of lung cancer risk among cadmium-exposed workers. Ann Epidemiol 1992;2:195–211.
197. Kazantzis G. Cadmium: sources, exposure and possible carcinogenicity. IARC Sci Publ 1986;71:93–101.
198. Kollmeier H, Seemann J, Rothe G, Muller KM. Cadmium in human lung tissue. Int Arch Occup Environ Health 1990;62:373–377.
199. Doll R. Cadmium in the human environment: closing remarks. IARC Sci Publ 1992;118:459–464.
200. Kazantzis G. Cadmium mortality assessment. Am J Ind Med 1991;20:701–704.
201. Thun MJ, Elinder CG, Friberg L. Scientific basis for an occupational standard for cadmium. Am J Ind Med 1991;20:629–642.
202. Masse R. Occupational standards are controversial. Am J Ind Med 1991;20:705–706.
203. Crump KS, Gentry R. A response to OMB's comments regarding OSHA's approach to risk assessment in support of OSHA's final rule on cadmium. Risk Anal 1993;13:487–489.
204. Chettle DR, Ellis KJ. Further scientific issues in determining an occupational standard for cadmium. Am J Ind Med 1992;22:117–124.
205. Albert RE, Sellakumar AR, Laskin S, et al. Nasal cancer in the rat induced by gaseous formaldehyde and hydrogen chloride. J Natl Cancer Inst 1982;68:597–603.
206. Kerns WD, Pavkov KL, Donofrio DJ, et al. Carcinogenicity of formaldehyde in rats and mice after long-term inhalation exposure. Cancer Res 1983;43:4382–4392.
207. Nelson N, Levine RJ, Albert RE, et al. Contribution of formaldehyde to respiratory cancer. Environ Health Perspect 1986;70:23–35.
208. Blair A, Stewart P, O'Berg M, et al. Mortality among industrial workers exposed to formaldehyde. J Natl Cancer Inst 1986;76:1071–1084.
209. Sterling TD, Weinkam JJ. Reanalysis of lung cancer mortality in a National Cancer Institute study on mortality among industrial workers exposed to formaldehyde. J Occup Med 1988;30:895–901.
210. Sterling TD, Weinkam JJ. Reanalysis of lung cancer mortality in a National Cancer Institute study on "Mortality among industrial workers exposed to formaldehyde." Exp Pathol 1989;37:128–132.
211. Blair A, Steward PA. Formaldehyde revisited. J Occup Med 1989;31:881.
212. Sterling TD, Weinkam JJ. Reanalysis of lung cancer mortality in a National Cancer Institute study of "Mortality among industrial workers exposed to formaldehyde": additional discussion. J Occup Med 1989;31:881–884.
213. Buncher CR. Did formaldehyde cause lung cancer? J Occup Med 1989;31:885.
214. Blair A, Stewart PA, Hoover RN. Mortality from lung cancer among workers employed in formaldehyde industries. Am J Ind Med 1990;17:683–689.
215. Marsh GM, Stone RA, Henderson VL. A reanalysis of the National Cancer Institute study on lung cancer mortality among industrial workers exposed to formaldehyde. J Occup Med 1992;34:42–44.
216. Marsh GM, Stone RA, Henderson VL. Lung cancer mortality among industrial workers exposed to formaldehyde: a poisson regression analysis of the National Cancer Institute study. Am Ind Hyg Assoc J 1992;53:681–691.
217. Blair A, Saracci R, Stewart PA, et al. Epidemiologic evidence on the relationship between formaldehyde exposure and cancer. Scand J Work Environ Health 1990;16:381–393.
218. Partanen T. Formaldehyde exposure and respiratory cancer—a meta-analysis of the epidemiologic evidence. Scand J Work Environ Health 1993;19:8–15.
219. Feron VJ, Kruysse A, Woutersen RA. Respiratory tract tumors in hamsters exposed to acetaldehyde vapour alone or simultaneously to benzo(a)pyrene or diethylnitrosamine. Eur J Cancer Clin Oncol 1982;18:13–31.
220. Woutersen RA, Appelman LM, Van Garderen-Hoetmer A, Feron VJ. Inhalation toxicity of acetaldehyde in rats. III. Carcinogenicity study. Toxicology 1986;41:213–231.
221. Feron VJ. Effects of exposure to acetaldehyde in Syrian hamsters simultaneously treated with benzo(a)pyrene or diethylnitrosamine. Prog Exp Tumor Res 1979;24:162–176.
222. U.S. Environmental Protection Agency. Health assessment document for acetaldehyde. Research Triangle Park, NC: Office of Health and Environmental Assessment, 1987: EPA/600/8-86/015A.
223. Young J. Properties, applications, and manufacture of man-made mineral fibers. In: Liddell D, Miller K, eds. Mineral fibers and health. Boca Raton, FL: CRC Press, 1991:37–53.
224. Lippmann M. Man-made mineral fibers (MMMF): human exposures and health risk assessment. Toxicol Ind Health 1990;6:225–246.
225. Wheeler CS. Exposure to man-made mineral fibers: a summary of current animal data. Toxicol Ind Health 1990;6:293–307.
226. Bunn WB, Bender JR, Hesterberg TW, et al. Recent studies of man-made vitreous fibers. J Occup Med 1993;35:101–113.
227. Kuschner M. The effects of MMMF on animal systems: some reflections on their pathogenesis. Ann Occup Hyg 1987;31:791–797.
228. Meek ME. Lung cancer and mesothelioma related to man-made mineral fibers: the toxicological evidence. In: Liddell D, Miller K, eds. Mineral fibers and health. Boca Raton, FL: CRC Press, 1991:265–281.
229. Stanton MF, Layard M, Tegeris A, et al. Relation of particle dimension to carcinogenicity in amphibole asbestos and other fibrous minerals. J Natl Cancer Inst 1981;67:965–975.
230. Davis JMG. Information obtained from fiber-induced lesions in animals. In: Liddell D, Miller K, eds. Mineral fibers and health. Boca Raton, FL: CRC Press, 1991:249–263.
231. Mohr U, Pott F, Vonnahme FJ. Morphological aspects of mesotheliomas after intratracheal instillation of fibrous dusts in Syrian golden hamsters. Exp Pathol 1984;26:179–183.
232. Pott F, Ziem U, Reiffer FJ, et al. Carcinogenicity studies on fibres, metal compounds and some other dusts in rats. Exp Pathol 1987;32:129–152.
233. Enterline PE, Marsh GM, Henderson V, Callahan C. Mortality update of a cohort of U.S. man-made mineral fibre workers. Ann Occup Hyg 1987;31:625–656.

234. Marsh GM, Enterline PE, Stone RA, Henderson VL. Mortality among a cohort of U.S. man-made mineral fiber workers: 1985 follow-up. J Occup Med 1990;32:594–604.
235. Simonato L, Fletcher AC, Cherrie J, et al. The man-made mineral fiber European historical cohort study. Scand J Work Environ Health 1986;12(Suppl 1):34–47.
236. Simonato L, Fletcher AC, Cherrie JW, et al. The international agency for research on cancer historical cohort study of MMMF production workers in seven European countries: extension of the follow-up. Ann Occup Hyg 1987;31:603–623.
237. Shannon HS, Jamieson E, Julian JA, Muir DCF, Walsh C. Mortality experience of Ontario glass fibre workers—extended follow-up. Ann Occup Hyg 1987;31:657–662.
238. Miettinen OS, Rossiter CE. Man-made mineral fibers and lung cancer: epidemiologic evidence regarding the causal hypothesis. Scand J Work Environ Health 1990;16:221–231.
239. Musselman RP. Respiratory cancer among mineral workers. J Occup Med 1991;33:585.
240. Enterline PE. Role of manmade mineral fibres in the causation of cancer. Br J Ind Med 1990;47:145–146.
241. Weill H, Jones RN, Parkes WR. Silicosis and related diseases. In: Parkes WR, ed. Occupational lung disorders. 3rd ed. Oxford: Butterworth-Heinemann, 1994:285–339.
242. National Institute for Occupational Safety and Health. Criteria document for occupational exposure to crystalline silica. Cincinnati, OH: U.S. Department of Health, Education and Welfare, 1974:HEW (NIOSH)Publ No 75-120.
243. Franco G, Massola A. Nonoccupational pneumoconiosis at high altitude villages in central Ladakh. Br J Ind Med 1992;49:452–453.
244. Saffiotti U. Lung cancer induction by crystalline silica. Prog Clin Biol Res 1992;374:51–69.
245. Holland LM, Wilson JS, Tillery MI, Smith DM. Lung cancer in rats exposed to fibrogenic dusts. In: Goldsmith DF, Winn DM, Shy CM, eds. Silica, silicosis, and cancer: controversy in occupational medicine. New York: Praeger, 1986:267–279.
246. Dagle GE, Wehner AP, Clark ML, Buschbom RL. Chronic inhalation exposure of rats to quartz. In: Goldsmith DF, Winn DM, Shy CM, eds. Silica, silicosis, and cancer: controversy in occupational medicine. New York: Praeger, 1986:255–266.
247. Wilson T, Scheuchenzuber WJ, Eskew ML, Zarkower A. Comparative pathological aspects of chronic olivine and silica inhalation in mice. Environ Res 1986;39:331–344.
248. International Agency for Research on Cancer (IARC). IARC monographs on the evaluation of the carcinogenic risk of chemicals to humans. Silica and some silicates. Lyon: IARC, 1987;42.
249. Simonato L, Fletcher AC, Saracci R, Thomas TL. Occupational exposure to silica and cancer risk. IARC Sci Publ 1990;97:55–64.
250. Goldsmith DF. Silica exposure and pulmonary cancer. In: Samet JM, ed. Epidemiology of lung cancer. New York: Marcel Dekker, 1994:245–298.
251. Checkoway H, Heyer NJ, Demers PA, Breslow NE. Mortality among workers in the diatomaceous earth industry. Br J Ind Med 1993;50:586–593.
252. McLaughlin JK, Chen JQ, Dosemeci M, et al. A nested case-control study of lung cancer among silica exposed workers in China. Br J Ind Med 1992;49:167–171.
253. Chia SE, Chia KS, Phoon WH, Lee HP. Silicosis and lung cancer among Chinese granite workers. Scand J Work Environ Health 1991;17:170–174.
254. Auerbach O, Garfinkel L, Parks VR. Scar cancer of the lung: increase over a 21 year period. Cancer 1979;43:636–642.
255. Bakris GL, Mulopulo GP, Korchik R, et al. Pulmonary scar carcinoma: a clinicopathologic analysis. Cancer 1983;52:493–497.
256. Turner-Warwick M, Lebowitz M, Burrows B, Johnson A. Cryptogenic fibrosing alveolitis and lung cancer. Thorax 1980;35:496–499.
257. Neuberger M, Kundi M, Westphal G, Brundorfer W. The Viennese dusty worker study. In: Goldsmith DF, Winn DM, Shy CM, eds. Silica, silicosis and cancer: controversy in occupational medicine. New York: Praeger, 1986:415–422.
258. Chiyotani K, Saito K, Okubo T, Takahashi K. Lung cancer risk among pneumoconiosis patients in Japan, with special reference to silicotics. IARC Sci Publ 1990;97:95–104.
259. Chen J, McLaughlin JK, Zhang JY, et al. Mortality among dust-exposed Chinese mine and pottery workers. J Occup Med 1992;34:311–316.
260. Partanen T, Pukkala E, Vainio H, et al. Increased incidence of lung and skin cancer in Finnish silicotic patients. J Occup Med 1994;36:616–622.
261. International Agency for Research on Cancer (IARC). IARC monographs on the evaluation of carcinogenic risks to humans. Chromium, nickel and welding fumes. Lyon: IARC, 1990;49:447–525.
262. Reuzel PGJ, Beems RB, de Raat WK, Lohman PHM. Carcinogenicity and in vitro genotoxicity of the particulate fraction of two stainless steel welding fumes. In: Stern RM, Berlin A, Fletcher AC, Jarvisalo J, eds. Health hazards and biological effects of welding fumes and gases. Amsterdam: Excerpta Medica, 1986:329–332.
263. Berg NO, Berlin M, Bohgard M, et al. Bronchocarcinogenic properties of welding and thermal spraying fumes containing chromium in the rat. Am J Ind Med 1987;11:39–54.
264. Beaumont JJ, Weiss NS. Lung cancer among welders. J Occup Med 1981;23:839–844.
265. Simonato L, Fletcher AC, Andersen A, et al. A historical prospective study of European stainless steel, mild steel, and shipyard welders. Br J Ind Med 1991;48:145–154.
266. Moulin JJ, Wild P, Haguenoer JM, et al. A mortality study among mild steel and stainless steel welders. Br J Ind Med 1993;50:234–243.
267. Danielsen TE, Langard S, Andersen A, Knudsen O. Incidence of cancer among welders of mild steel and other shipyard workers. Br J Ind Med 1993;50:1097–1103.
268. Rinsky RA, Melius JM, Hornung RW, et al. Case-control study of lung cancer in civilian employees at the Portsmouth naval shipyard, Kittery, Maine. Am J Epidemiol 1988;127:55–64.
269. Hull CJ, Doyle E, Peters JM, et al. Case-control study of lung cancer in Los Angeles county welders. Am J Ind Med 1989;16:103–112.
270. Morgan WKC. On welding, wheezing and whimsy. Am Ind Hyg Assoc J 1989;50:59–69.
271. Sjogren B, Hansen KS, Kjuus H, Persson PG. Exposure to stainless steel welding fumes and lung cancer: a meta-analysis. Occup Environ Med 1994;51:335–336.
272. Doll R, Hill AB. Lung cancer and other causes of death in relation to smoking. Br Med J 1956;2:1071–1076.
273. Natusch DFS. Potentially carcinogenic species emitted to the atmosphere by fossil-fueled power plants. Environ Health Perspect 1978;22:79–90.
274. Lewtas J. Complex mixtures of air pollutants: characterizing the cancer risk of polycyclic organic matter. Environ Health Perspect 1993;100:211–218.
275. Lewtas J. Airborne carcinogens. Pharmacol Toxicol 1993;72 (Suppl 1):55–63.

276. Lewtas J. Human exposures to complex mixtures of air pollutants. Toxicol Lett 1994;72:163–169.
277. Speizer FE, Samet JM. Air pollution and lung cancer. In: Samet JM, ed. Epidemiology of lung cancer. New York: Marcel Dekker, 1994:131–150.
278. Burns DM, ed. The health consequences of involuntary smoking: a report of the Surgeon General. Rockville, MD: U.S. Department of Health and Human Services, 1986.
279. Shy C. Lung cancer and the urban environment; a review. In: Finkel AJ, Duel WC, eds. Clinical implications of air pollution research. Acton, MA: Publishing Science Group, 1976:3–38.
280. Doll R. Atmospheric pollution and lung cancer. Environ Health Perspect 1978;22:23–31.
281. Stocks P, Campbell J. Lung cancer death rates among non-smokers and pipe and cigarette smokers. BMJ 1955;2:923–929.
282. Dean G. Lung cancer and bronchitis in Northern Ireland. BMJ 1966;1:1506–1514.
283. Vena JE. Air pollution as a risk factor in lung cancer. Am J Epidemiol 1982;116:42–56.
284. Samet JM, Humble CG, Skipper BE, Pathak DR. History of residence and lung cancer risk in New Mexico. Am J Epidemiol 1987;125:800–811.
285. Hitosugi M. Epidemiological study of lung cancer with special reference to the effect of air pollution and smoking habit. Bull Inst Publ Health 1968;17:236–255.
286. Jedrychowski W, Becher H, Waherndorf J, Basa-Cierpialed Z. A case-control study of lung cancer with special reference to the effect of air pollution in Poland. J Epidemiol Community Health 199;44:114–120.
287. Xu Z, Blot WJ, Xiao HP, et al. Smoking, air pollution, and the high rates of lung cancer in Shenyang, China. J Natl Cancer Inst 1989;81:1800–1806.
288. U.S. Environmental Protection Agency. Cancer risk from outdoor exposure to air toxics, vol. 1, final report. Research Triangle Park, NC: Environmental Criteria and Assessment Office, 1990:EPA/450/1-90/004A.
289. Cooke TF. Indoor air pollutants: a literature review. Rev Environ Health 1991;9:137–160.
290. Samet J. Environmental controls and lung disease. Am Rev Respir Dis 1990;142:915–939.
291. Boring CC, Squires TS, Tong T, Montgomery S. Cancer Statistics, 1994. CA Cancer J Clin 1994;44:7–26.
292. Schottenfeld D. Epidemiology of cancer of the esophagus. Semin Oncol 1984;11:92–100.
293. Devesa SS, Blot WJ, Fraumeni JF. Cohort trends in mortality from oral, esophageal, and laryngeal cancers in the United States. Epidemiology 1990;1:116–121.
294. Pottern LM, Morris LE, Blot WJ, et al. Esophageal cancer among black men in Washington, D.C. I. Alcohol, tobacco, and other risk factors. J Natl Cancer Inst 1981;67:777–783.
295. Keller AZ. The epidemiology of esophageal cancer in the west. Prev Med 1980;9:607–612.
296. Sons HU. Etiologic and epidemiologic factors of carcinoma of the esophagus. Surg Gynecol Obstet 1987;165:183–190.
297. Ghadirian P, Vobecky J, Vobecky JS. Factors associated with cancer of the oesophagus; an overview. Cancer Detect Prev 1988;11:225–234.
298. Newman R. Association of biogenic silica with disease. Nutr Cancer 1986;8:217–222.
299. Decarli A, Liati P, Negri E, Franceschi S, La Vecchia C. Vitamin A and other dietary factors in the etiology of esophageal cancer. Nutr Cancer 1987;10:29–37.
300. Taylor PR, Li B, Dawsey SM, et al. Prevention of esophageal cancer: the nutrition intervention trials in Linxian, China. Cancer Res 1994;54(Suppl):2029S–2031S.
301. Chang F, Syrjanen S, Wang L, Syrjanen K. Infectious agents in the etiology of esophageal cancer. Gastroenterology 1992;103:1336–1348.
302. Tuyns AJ, Pequignot G, Gignous M, Valla A. Cancers of the digestive tract, alcohol and tobacco. Int J Cancer 1982;30:9–11.
303. Luoto J, ed. The health consequences of smoking: cancer. A report of the surgeon general. Rockville, MD: U.S. Department of Health and Human Services, 1982:90–101.
304. La Vecchia CL, Negri E. The role of alcohol in oesophageal cancer in non-smokers, and of tobacco in non-drinkers. Int J Cancer 1989;43:784–785.
305. Yu MC, Garabrant DH, Peters JM, Mack TM. Tobacco, alcohol, diet, occupation, and carcinoma of the esophagus. Cancer Res 1988;48:3843–3848.
306. Tuyns AJ, Pequignot G, Abbatucci JS. Oesophageal cancer and alcohol consumption; importance of type of beverage. Int J Cancer 1979;23:443–447.
307. Tuyns AJ. Epidemiology of alcohol and cancer. Cancer Res 1979;39:2840–2843.
308. Notani PN. Role of alcohol in cancers of the upper alimentary tract: use of models in risk assessment. J Epidemiol Community Health 1988;42:187–192.
309. Selikoff IJ, Hammond EC. Mortality experience of insulation workers in the United States and Canada, 1943–1976. Ann NY Acad Sci 1979;330:91–116.
310. Selikoff IJ, Seidman H. Asbestos-associated deaths among insulation workers in the United States and Canada, 1967–1987. Ann NY Acad Sci 1991;643:1–14.
311. Doll R, Peto J. Other asbestos-related neoplasms. In: Antman K, Aisner J, eds. Asbestos-related malignancy. New York: Grune & Stratton, 1987:81–96.
312. Lumley KPS. A proportional study of cancer registrations of dockyard workers. BMJ 1976;33:108–114.
313. Puntoni R, Vercelli M, Merlo F, et al. Mortality among shipyard workers in Genoa, Italy. Ann NY Acad Sci 1979;330:353–377.
314. Kolonel LN, Hirohata T, Chappell BV, et al. Cancer mortality in a cohort of naval shipyard workers in Hawaii: early findings. J Natl Cancer Inst 1980;64:739–743.
315. Kolonel LN, Yoshizawa CN, Hirohata T, Myers BC. Cancer occurrence in shipyard workers exposed to asbestos in Hawaii. Cancer Res 1985;45:3924–3928.
316. Beaumont JJ, Weiss NS. Mortality of welders, shipfitters and other metal trades workers in boilermakers local no. 104, AFL-CIO. Am J Epidemiol 1980;112:775–786.
317. Cantor KP, Sontag JM, Heid MF. Patterns of mortality among plumbers and pipefitters. Am J Ind Med 1986;10:73–89.
318. Tola S, Kalliomaki PL, Pukkala E, et al. Incidence of cancer among welders, platers, machinists, and pipe fitters in shipyards and machine shops. Br J Ind Med 1988;45.209–218.
319. Kaminski R, Stanislawczyk K, Geissert MPH, Dacy E. Mortality analysis of plumbers and pipefitters. J Occup Med 1980;22:183–189.
320. Morgan RW, Foliart DE, Wong O. Asbestos and gastrointestinal cancer: a review of the literature. West J Med 1985;143:60–65.
321. Delzell E, Monson RR. Mortality among rubber workers: X. Reclaim workers. Am J Ind Med 1985;7:307–313.
322. Sorahan T, Parkes HG, Veys CA, et al. Mortality in the British rubber industry 1946–85. Br J Ind Med 1989;46:1–11.
323. Norell S, Ahlbom A, Lipping H, Osterblom L. Oesophageal cancer and vulcanisation work. Lancet 1983;1:462–463.
324. Andjelkovic D, Taulbee J, Symons M. Mortality experience of a

cohort of rubber workers 1964–73. J Occup Med 1976;18:387–394.
325. Delzell E, Monson RR. Mortality among rubber workers: III. Cause-specific mortality. J Occup Med 1981;23:677–684.
326. Monson RR, Nakano KK. Mortality among rubber workers: I. White male union members in Akron, Ohio. Am J Epidemiol 1976;103:284–296.
327. Jakobsson K, Attewell R, Hultgren B, Sjoland K. Gastrointestinal cancer among cement workers: a case-referent study. Int Arch Occup Environ Health 1990;62:337–340.
328. Blair A. Mortality among workers in metal polishing and plating. J Occup Med 1980;22:158–162.
329. Acheson ED, Pippard EC, Winter PD. Mortality among English furniture makers. Scand J Work Environ Health 1984;10:211–217.
330. Stellman SD, Garfinkel L. Cancer mortality among wood workers. Am J Ind Med 1984;5:342–357.
331. Gustavsson P, Gustavsson A, Hogstedt C. Excess of cancer in Swedish chimney sweeps. Br J Ind Med 1988;45:777–781.
332. Gustavsson P, Evanoff B, Hogstedt C. Increased risk of esophageal cancer among workers exposed to combustion products. Arch Environ Health 1993;48:243–245.
333. Harber P. Pulmonary prevention: programmatic characterization. Occup Med 1991;6:133–143.
334. Fontana RS. Screening for lung cancer. In: Miller AB, ed. Screening for cancer. New York: Academic Press, 1985:378–395.
335. Berlin NI, Buncher CR, Fontana RS, et al. National Cancer Institute's cooperative early lung detection program: results of the initial screen (prevalence). Am Rev Respir Dis 1984;130:545–570.
336. Lilienfeld A, Archer PG, Burnett CH, et al. An evaluation of radiologic and cytologic screening for the early detection of lung cancer: a cooperative pilot study of the American Cancer Study and the Veterans Administration. Cancer Res 1966;26:2083–2121.
337. Boucot KR, Weiss W. Is curable lung cancer detected by semiannual screening? JAMA 1973;224:1361–1365.
338. Brett GZ. Earlier diagnosis and survival in lung cancer. BMJ 1969;4:260–262.
339. Marfin AA, Schenker M. Screening for lung cancer: effective tests awaiting effective treatment. Occup Med 1991;6:111–132.
340. Hinds WC. The role of industrial hygiene in preventing occupational lung disease. Occup Med 1991;6:29–42.
341. McQuiston TH, Coleman P, Wallerstein NB, et al. Hazardous waste worker education: long-term effects. J Occup Med 1994;36:1310–1323.

Screening/Secondary Prevention

5A

Lung Cancer Prevention: Historical and Future Considerations

Eva Szabo and James L. Mulshine

Despite major advances in our understanding of lung cancer biology and causation, lung cancer remains the leading cause of cancer death in the United States, with an estimated 157,400 deaths in 1995 alone (1). The potential approaches to reducing mortality are threefold: (*a*) cure existing disease, (*b*) prevent disease by eliminating causative factors such as smoking and environmental exposures, and (*c*) detect disease at a curable stage or prevent early disease from progressing to an incurable stage. The mortality associated with the diagnosis of lung cancer remains at 87% despite various attempts at treatment, demonstrating that most cancers are metastatic at presentation and that current therapies have little efficacy in all but the most localized settings (2). Even if all causes of lung cancer could be eliminated (a sociological challenge of vast magnitude and one that is unlikely to be accomplished in the near future), the existence of high-risk populations by virtue of genetic susceptibility and past exposures to tobacco ensures that lung cancer will remain a major public health problem for decades to come. Thus, the most reasonable approach to diminishing the lung cancer epidemic is the development of effective strategies that either detect cancer at an early, potentially curable stage (screening) or that prevent carcinogenic progression to invasive cancer (secondary prevention).

As discussed below, historical evidence suggests that the currently available noninvasive techniques used for lung cancer diagnosis are not sensitive enough for lung cancer detection. To develop effective screening modalities, two a priori conditions must be satisfied. First, evidence must exist that a detectable preclinical phase exists. This evidence could be either preneoplastic conditions with a high rate of progression to overt neoplasia or a locally confined fully neoplastic condition. The pioneering work of Saccomanno et al. (3) in 1974 showed that in lung carcinogenesis, progression exists from increasing atypia to carcinoma in situ and ultimately to invasive carcinoma over the course of many years. Secondly, successful intervention strategies during this preclinical phase must exist or at least be potentially possible. Clearly, if one can detect cancer but cannot alter the natural history of the disease, then detection is of no benefit. Long-term survival with stage I disease can be as high as 85%, suggesting that detection at this or earlier stages would be translated into prolonged survival; thus, successful early treatment strategies are known to exist (4). Furthermore, the newly developing field of secondary prevention using dietary and pharmacologic interventions intends to control the progression of even earlier forms of lung cancer The ultimate goal is to intervene during a preclinical precancerous phase to prevent the progression to invasive neoplasia.

HISTORY OF SCREENING
RETROSPECTIVE STUDIES

The initial studies of lung cancer early detection were retrospective analyses of outcomes from individuals participating in screening programs for tuberculosis using photofluorograms (Table 5A.1). Shimizu et al. (5) compared the survival of screen-detected versus symptom-detected cases and found a survival advantage for screening. Naruke et al. (6) compared survival among 1297 participants with screen-detected lung cancer and 1297 participants with symptom-detected lung cancer. Better survival for both resected and unresectable screen-detected cases was observed at 5 and 10 years. However, Sobue et al. (7) conducted a retrospective study of lung cancer screening using annual chest radiography and sputum cytology in 273 high-risk individuals (by virtue of smoking history) compared with 1269 controls and found no difference in

TABLE 5A.1. Results of Reported Studies of Lung Cancer Screening

STUDY	DIAGNOSTIC TOOL	RESULTS	REFERENCE NO.
Retrospective			
Japan	Chest radiograph, sputum cytology for high-risk patients	Increased survival, no change in mortality	(5–7)
GDR	Chest radiograph	No change in mortality	(8, 9)
Prospective nonrandomized			
Veterans Administration	Chest radiograph, sputum cytology	No change in mortality	(10)
South London	Chest radiograph	Increased survival	(11)
Philadelphia	Chest photofluorogram	No change in mortality	(12, 13)
GDR	Chest photofluorogram	Increased survival	(14)
United Kingdom	Chest radiograph	No change in mortality	(15)
Prospective randomized			
London	Chest photofluorogram	No change in mortality	(16)
NCI Early Lung Cancer Group	Chest radiograph, sputum cytology	No change in mortality	(20–24)
Czechoslovakia	Chest radiograph, sputum cytology	Increased survival, no change in mortality	(25)

Abbreviations. GDR, German Democratic Republic; NCI, (U.S) National Cancer Institute.

the relative risk of dying from lung cancer between the two groups (odds ratio, 0.72; 95% confidence interval, 0.5–1.03). Although chest radiography detected a greater proportion of resectable tumors, the overall incidence and mortality at 5 years was the same between the two populations.

Two German studies also took advantage of tuberculosis screening programs using biennial chest radiographs. Ebeling and Nischan (8) studied 130 cases of lung cancer from the German Democratic Republic between 1980 and 1985 and compared them with population-based and hospital-based control groups. There was no difference in the risk of dying from lung cancer between individuals screened within 2 years before cancer diagnosis and the two control groups (relative risk, 0.9 and 1.1, respectively, for the two control groups). These authors (9) then reported a similar study that limited the analysis to individuals under the age of 60, again using biennial chest radiography as the screening modality. From 1979 through 1987, 278 subjects dying of lung cancer were matched with 3 to 4 controls selected from the screening program files. Again, the risk of dying from lung cancer was not significantly different between the two groups (relative risk, 0.93; 95% confidence interval, 0.65–1.33).

PROSPECTIVE NONRANDOMIZED STUDIES

A number of nonrandomized prospective studies evaluating the role of radiographic screening for lung cancer detection have shown little benefit to screening (Table 5A.1). Lilienfeld et al. (10) screened 14,607 residents of Veterans Administration Retirement Homes from 1958 through 1961 with chest roentgenograms and sputum cytology every 6 months for 3 years. There was no unscreened comparison group. Of the 200 cases diagnosed, only 26 were considered resectable and only 3 survived for 3 years. Although sputum cytology was thought to improve the diagnostic yield of chest radiographs, there was no difference in outcome.

Nash et al. (11) screened 67,400 men older than 45 years in South London between 1959 and 1963 on a semiannual basis. In this uncontrolled study, 147 lung cancers were identified with a 4-year survival of 27%. When compared with registry data on lung cancers diagnosed in patients outside of the screening program, survival was better in the screen-detected cases.

The Philadelphia Neoplasm Research Project (12, 13) conducted from 1951 through 1961 was an uncontrolled study of 6136 male volunteers aged 45 and older screened every 6 months with check photofluorograms. Survival was compared for screen-detected cancers versus cancers diagnosed in the intervals between screens. The 5-year survival of 8% to 12% was not significantly different between the two groups.

Two more recent nonrandomized European studies also have shown similarly little benefit for radiographic screening. Wilde (14) reported a study involving 41,532 men born between 1907 and 1932 who were screened every 6 months with chest fluorography and compared them with 102,348 age-matched male controls screened every 18 months. Despite a higher detection rate and greater resectability, no significant reduction in overall mortality or lung cancer mortality was demonstrated. In a similar fashion, radiographic screening every 8 to 12 months of high-risk workers at three British chromates plants between 1955 and 1989 revealed no significant improvement in survival at 5 or 10 years (15).

PROSPECTIVE RANDOMIZED STUDIES

In contract to the retrospective and prospective nonrandomized trials, all of the published prospective randomized studies to date show no benefit for screening in terms of overall survival (Table 5A.1). The first such study, reported in 1969, compared 29,723 male factory workers in London aged more than 40 years who were offered semiannual chest photofluorography for 3 years and 25,000 similar male factory workers offered photofluorography only at the beginning and end of the 3-year period (16). Despite the detection of a greater number of resectable tumors in the group screened every 6 months, lung cancer incidence and 5-year survival were not significantly different between the two groups.

In 1974, Saccomanno et al. (3) showed that sputum cytology can be used to follow the progression from metaplasia to increasing atypia to carcinoma in situ and finally to invasive disease within the bronchial epithelium of uranium miners at high risk for developing lung cancer. This finding was of major importance for two reasons: the changes found occurred over the course of several years (i.e., suggesting a long preclinical phase) and the apparent ability to detect some early cancers by cytologic examination suggested that this technique could become a major screening tool. This work provided the impetus for the formation of the National Cancer Institute (NCI) Early Lung Cancer Group—consisting of the Johns Hopkins Medical Institutions, the Mayo Clinic, and the Memorial Sloan–Kettering Cancer Center—to address specifically the questions of whether detection of lung cancer could be improved by adding sputum cytology to chest radiography screening and whether mortality could be decreased by screening. Approximately 30,000 men older than 45 years who smoked at least one pack of cigarettes per day in the previous year were randomized (4, 17—19). In the Johns Hopkins and Memorial Sloan–Kettering studies, patients in the screened group received chest radiographs annually and sputum cytology every 4 months, whereas the control group received only an annual chest radiograph. In the Mayo Clinic study, the screened group received a chest radiograph and sputum cytology every 4 months, whereas the control group received the "standard Mayo advice" of the time, consisting of an annual chest radiograph and annual sputum cytology, but without reminders to comply after the first visit. There were no unscreened control arms in any of these studies, but the assumption underlying them was based on previously published information that chest radiography alone had an insufficient impact on lung cancer detection to warrant a totally unscreened control; thus, the addition of sputum cytology was the experimental variable for these studies. The conclusion from all three trials, however, was that screening with chest radiography and sputum cytology was of no benefit in reducing lung cancer mortality (20–24). Despite lower stage at presentation, increased resectability, and an apparently higher 5-year survival rate in lung cancer patients in the screened group (35% in the screened group versus 15% for the control group), the cumulative lung cancer mortality and overall survival were the same for both screened and control populations in all three trials.

Similar negative results were reported by Kubik et al. (25) from Czechoslovakia, who randomized 6364 male smokers aged between 40 and 64 years to semiannual screening by chest radiography and sputum cytology, versus a control arm with no asymptomatic investigations for 3 years after an initial chest radiograph and sputum cytology at study entry. After 3 years both groups underwent chest radiography and sputum cytology examinations, followed by an annual chest radiograph for another 3 years. Again, despite the detection of a greater number of earlier cancers with higher resectability rates in the screened group, there was no difference in mortality between the two groups.

PERSPECTIVES ON EVALUATING SCREENING STUDIES

The negative results from the prospective randomized trials described above illustrate several important points regarding screening studies. In the NCI Early Lung Cancer Group, nearly 50% of the cancers detected in the screened group were diagnosed by interval chest radiographs performed for other reasons or by symptoms rather than by the screen, suggesting the insensitivity of this modality for screening. The imprecision in interpreting chest radiographs was underscored by a review of the films from patients in the Mayo Clinic study (26), which concluded that 90% (45 of 50 subjects) of the peripheral lung cancers could be seen on the chest radiograph from the prior 4-month screening visit that had been read as negative by at least two physicians. In retrospect, 18 of the 45 tumors were visible for more than 1 year. Furthermore, cytology detected fewer additional cases than was expected. In the Memorial Sloan–Kettering study, more occult squamous cell carcinomas were detected initially in the screened group, but this increased incidence was compensated for by an increased incidence of such tumors within 3 years detectable by chest radiography in the control group, with no change in mortality (thereby demonstrating the more indolent nature of this subtype because these tumors remained confined locally even when radiologically evident). Thus, the combination of chest radiography and sputum cytology did not possess sufficient sensitivity to make any difference in mortality. It has been estimated that the sensitivity of screening was approximately 50% for chest radiography alone, 25% to 30% for sputum cytology alone, and approximately 65% for both (27).

Several potential biases need to be accounted for when evaluating results of any screening study. Overdiagnosis bias results from the inclusion of potentially indolent cases that would not have been diagnosed before death from competing causes of mortality. Sobue et al. (28) analyzed the survival of patients with stage I lung cancer not surgically treated and found that, given the uniformly high lethality of lung cancer, overdiagnosis is not likely to be a factor contributing to positive results. A second potential confounder in these studies is lead-time bias, resulting from the identification of disease at an earlier stage that previously would not have been recognized as being part of the clinical disease. By diagnosing earlier, survival appears to be prolonged but mortality does not change. Length-time bias is caused by the detection of indolent cancers with a more prolonged natural history. These cancers are detected more frequently, but overall survival does not change. Thus, screening programs need to be controlled carefully and to be lengthy enough to account for these potential biases.

NOVEL APPROACHES TO EARLY LUNG CANCER DETECTION

The recent advances in our understanding of the biology of lung cancer hold much promise in identifying targets for both the early detection of this disease and intervention to prevent full neoplastic conversion. It has been recognized increasingly over the past 50 years that neoplastic transformation is a multistage process occurring over decades (Fig. 5A.1) (29). The discrete stages of this process have been termed initiation, promotion, and progression. Initiators are substances that cause irreversible genetic damage to a cell and its progeny, whereas promoters cause reversible effects on cell growth that cease once the promoter is withdrawn. Because the entire process from initiation through progression appears to take many years, an understanding of the changes involved would identify targets both for screening and for intervention to halt the inexorable progression to invasive cancer. Although a particular sequence of events leading to the full expression of the neoplastic phenotype has not yet been determined for lung cancer, multiple changes occurring during carcinogenesis have been identified and have already begun to be applied toward both early detection and intervention.

IMMUNOCYTOCHEMICAL ANALYSIS OF SPUTUM

One approach to improving the sensitivity of sputum cytology is combining it with an analysis of cancer specific antigens (if, indeed, such exist), or with other antigens that are expressed abnormally by cancer cells. Tockman et al. (30) used two murine monoclonal antibodies reactive either with a glycolipid antigen of small cell lung cancer (SCLC) or a protein antigen of non–small cell lung cancer (NSCLC) to analyze 63 sputum specimens from subjects with moderate-to-severe atypical changes found during follow-up in the Johns Hopkins Lung Project. In specimens collected up to 6 years before the clinical diagnosis of cancer (average, approximately 2 years), immunostaining results predicted the subsequent development of cancer with a sensitivity of 91% and a specificity of 88%.

Analysis of these antibodies has shown subsequently that one (i.e., 624H12) recognizes difucosylated Lewis X, a blood group–like antigen akin to developmental markers expressed during fetal development (31). The reexpression of fetal markers on epithelial surfaces has long been recognized as a potential target for the identification of cancer cells (32, 33). Examination of such markers directly from the bronchial epithelium (in the form of shed cells in the sputum) allowed the differential expression of these markers in normal versus preneoplastic tissues to form the basis of an early detection assay. This immunocytochemical approach is currently being validated prospectively in a high-risk population of resected stage I lung cancer patients who have a 1%–3% per year risk of developing a second primary lung cancer (34, 35).

ROLE OF ONCOGENES IN THE EARLY DETECTION OF LUNG CANCER

Cytogenetic analyses of lung cancer have revealed multiple nonrandom abnormalities subsequently shown to involve a number of oncogenes (Table 5A.2), with multiple oncogenes often being involved in a single tumor (36, 37). Two broad categories of oncogenes exist: dominant oncogenes, whose in-

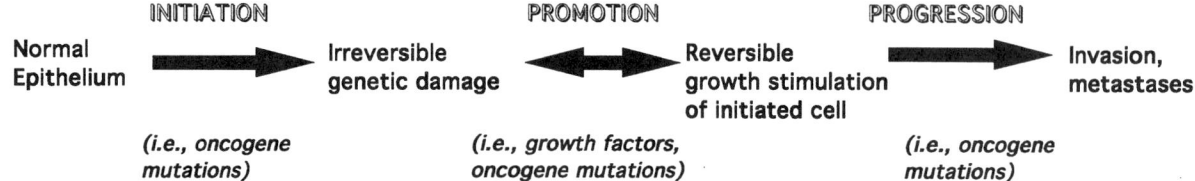

FIGURE 5A.1 Multistage process of lung carcinogenesis. The neoplastic transformation of epithelial cells can be divided into multiple phases occurring over a long time period. The earliest changes involve irreversible genetic alterations, termed initiation. These changes provide the cell with a growth advantage compared with noninitiated cells, allowing the expansion of this population under the influence of tumor promoters. The effects of tumor promoters are fully reversible upon their withdrawal, but the subsequent accumulation of further genetic alterations in the progression phase leads to acquisition of the invasive and metastatic phenotypes.

TABLE 5A.2. Oncogenes Abnormally Expressed in Lung Cancer

ONCOGENE	HISTOLOGY	FREQUENCY	REFERENCE NO.
Dominant			
Ki-*ras*[a]	NSCLC (adenocarcinoma)	30%	(42–47)
myc Family	SCLC/NSCLC	11%–44%/58%	(53, 61, 62)
HER2 *neu*	NSCLC	30%	(54, 55)
c-*myb*	SCLC	87%	(57)
c-*raf*-1	SCLC/NSCLC	Common	(56)
c-*jun*	SCLC/NSCLC	Common/43%	(58–60)
c-*fos*	NSCLC	60%	(59, 60)
Recessive			
Rb	SCLC/NSCLC	90%+/15%	(64, 65, 72)
p53[a]	SCLC/NSCLC	70%+/45%+	(67–69)
3p deletion	SCLC/NSCLC	90%+/25%–50%	(36, 70, 71)

Abbreviations. NSCLC, non–small cell lung cancer; SCLC, small cell lung cancer.
[a]Aberrantly expressed during early carcinogenesis

creased expression and function produce transformation and neoplasia, and recessive oncogenes (or tumor suppressor genes), whose absent or reduced expression permits the development of neoplasia. The protein products of oncogenes are involved in key cellular processes such as growth, differentiation, and cell death, and they may be involved in the process of carcinogenesis at numerous early and late stages. Ongoing efforts are directed at defining the range of significant genetic changes and assigning a chronology to these changes. The goal is the determination of which of these deregulated genes may be useful targets for early cancer detection and intervention.

Perhaps the best studied dominant oncogenes in lung carcinogenesis are the members of the *ras* family (38–41). The three members of this family (N-*ras*, Ha-*ras*, and Ki-*ras*) encode a 21-kilodalton (kd) protein involved in signal transduction. Point mutations in codons 12, 13, or 61 lead to constitutive activation of the protein with ensuing growth stimulation to the cell. Mutations in Ki-*ras* have been found in approximately one third of lung adenocarcinomas, particularly in patients with a history of smoking, and they confer a poorer prognosis to this group (42, 43). The exact role of *ras* in the pathogenesis of lung cancer is not clear. However, animal studies of carcinogen-exposed mice with a high rate of spontaneous lung tumors show Ki-*ras* mutations in both adenomas and carcinomas, suggesting an early occurrence of these mutations (44). Furthermore, Brandt-Rauf and colleagues (45) measured serum Ras levels in 46 patients with asbestosis or silicosis and found elevated Ras serum levels in 7 of 11 patients who developed lung cancer or mesothelioma. In 6 of the patients, these serum levels preceded the clinical diagnosis of cancer by an average of 16.3 months (range, 3 to 26 months). Because 2 of 28 noncancer controls also had elevated Ras levels, a follow-up of this study would be of great interest. In a similar vein, Mao et al. (46) recently used a polymerase chain reaction–based assay to examine oncogene mutations in stored sputum from patients originally entered on the Johns Hopkins Lung Project who later developed adenocarcinoma of the lung. Of the 10 patients whose tumors contained either Ki-*ras* or *p53* mutations, 8 of

10 demonstrated these mutations in sputum samples preceding the diagnosis of cancer (7 of 8 *ras* mutations were identified correctly in this assay). More recently, Sugio et al. (47) examined the occurrence of *ras* mutations in atypical, in situ, and invasive lung adenocarcinomas and found mutations in 80% of the in situ cancers in which the invasive component had a *ras* mutation, but in only 17% of atypical lesions examined. Although the authors concluded that *ras* mutations occur late in the pathogenesis of lung adenocarcinomas, for the purposes of early detection, the identification of lesions at the in situ state still would be early enough to alter the mortality associated with lung cancer (4).

Because the technology used to detect activating Ki-*ras* mutations in small tissue samples (and potentially in serum or other body fluids) has been well delineated, *ras* mutations represent an attractive target for early detection should their presence prove to be specific enough for early carcinogenesis (46, 47). In addition, available mevalonate inhibitors also are pharmacologic antagonists of Ras action and thus could theoretically be useful for abrogating Ras action (48). Preliminary studies show that a specific synthetic inhibitor of enzymes mediating post-translational modification of Ras (farnesylation) can block anchorage of the Ras molecule (49). The enzymatic inhibitor results in growth inhibition of *ras*-dependent tumors in nude mice (49). However, because *ras* mutations are present in only a small proportion of lung tumors (approximately 15%), screening for *ras* mutations would not be very efficient. Its main use would be limited to certain extremely high-risk subgroups with a known high frequency of *ras* mutations, such as the asbestosis patients referred to above (46).

Less is known about other dominant oncogenes implicated in lung carcinogenesis. These include the *myc* family, HER2*neu*, c-*raf*-1, c-*myb*, c-*jun*, and c-*fos* (50-60). The three *myc* family members (c-*myc*, N-*myc*, and L-*myc*) have been found to be amplified in 11% of SCLC from untreated patients and in 28% to 44% of tumors from treated patients (61, 62). Overexpression not associated with amplification is probably a much more common event, however. Using the sensitive RNA-RNA in situ hybridization technique, c-*myc* overexpression also has been found in 58% of NSCLCs, and c-*myc* expression has been found in nonneoplastic lung, with the highest levels in bronchial basal cells and, significantly, in hyperplastic type II cells (53). However, the roll of *myc* in early lung carcinogenesis is not yet clear.

The protein product of the HER2*neu* oncogene is thought to be a growth factor receptor by virtue of its homology to the epidermal growth factor receptor (55). Overexpression in adenocarcinoma of the lung is associated with shortened survival, and immunohistochemical staining provides a convenient tool for the detection of this oncogene in small amounts of tissue (54, 55).

The c-*jun* and c-*fos* oncogenes are part of the AP-1 nuclear transcription factor implicated in mediating the effects of tumor promoters (63). Both are expressed frequently in primary NSCLCs and are associated with shortened survival in patients with squamous cell carcinomas (59, 60). The role of all of these genes in early detection has not yet been elucidated.

Tumor suppressor genes implicated in lung carcinogenesis include the product of the retinoblastoma gene (*Rb*), *p53*, and the yet unidentified gene(s) on chromosome 3p (64–71). Abnormalities in Rb protein expression are present in approximately 90% of SCLCs but in only 15% of NSCLCs (72). With the advent of new immunohistochemical techniques for analysis, the technical difficulties in defining the structural and functional abnormalities of this large gene are beginning to be overcome, although commercially available antisera may recognize some mutant proteins that are nevertheless nonfunctional. However, the chronology of *Rb* mutations during lung carcinogenesis is not known. *p53* Abnormalities, in contrast, occur in more than 50% of both small cell and non–small cell lung cancers; they have been described recently in preneoplastic lesions in the lung as well (67–69, 73, 74). Furthermore, evidence from transgenic mouse models and from the observation that patients with the Li-Fraumeni syndrome, who have a germ line *p53* mutation and are at high risk of developing numerous malignancies including lung cancer, also suggests an early role for *p53* in lung carcinogenesis (75–77). Immunohistochemical analysis of *p53* affords a potential tool for evaluation as a screening marker. Nevertheless, although these various oncogenes and tumor suppressor genes present intriguing targets for early detection, more needs to be known about the molecular biology of lung cancer before rational use of these targets can be accomplished.

ROLE OF GROWTH FACTORS IN THE EARLY DETECTION OF LUNG CANCER

The identification of growth factor production by lung cancer cell lines that also possess receptors for the same growth factor, thus resulting in dysregulated growth (autocrine growth loops), has uncovered another potential class of molecules with implications for both early detection and intervention (78, 79). By virtue of their action (i.e., growth enhancement), growth factors most likely function during the promotion phase of carcinogenesis and provide an attractive target for early detection and intervention because of the long duration (2 years) of this phase (79). To date, multiple growth factors affecting lung cancer biology have been described, including gastrin-releasing peptide (GRP), insulinlike growth factor I, transferrin, and epidermal growth factor-α (78, 80–86). The best studied of these growth factors is GRP, and thus the following discussion uses this growth factor as an example.

GRP has been found to be an autocrine growth factor for SCLC, which frequently expresses both receptors for GRP and GRP itself (78). Thus, the components for uninterrupted growth without any dependence on growth stimulation from the tissue environment are potentially present for these cells. Studies have shown that GRP functions during fetal lung growth and maturation and that it is mitogenic for normal bronchial epithelial cells (87, 88)). It is expressed during lung injury and subsequent proliferation. In fact, GRP levels have been found to be increased in the bronchoalveolar lavage fluid of asymptomatic smokers, suggesting that its presence may be a general marker of tissue injury (89). GRP may also contribute to the pathogenesis of smoking-related diseases. GRP can be detected in urine, and a subgroup of smokers with elevated urine GRP levels (compared with controls) has been identified (90). Whether this finding will predict for subsequent lung neoplasia remains to be determined by clinical follow-up.

The actions of GRP can be antagonized by neutralizing antibodies and peptide antagonists (78, 91). In advanced disease, a recent clinical trial using monoclonal antibodies showed little efficacy (92). However, if growth factors function primarily to expand the initiated clone of cells with a differentially greater induction of growth in these cells compared with the uninitiated normal cells, then removing the growth signal after the cells have already established the invasive phenotype may have little effect. Intervention earlier during carcinogenesis when the cells are more dependent on a small number of specific growth factors may be more reasonable. Furthermore, because multiple growth factors are being identified as operational in lung cancer, perhaps a more reasonable strategy would be to target downstream signal transduction pathways shared by several growth factors (93). This kind of approach has the potential for systemic toxicity because normal cellular processes may depend on the same signal transduction pathways, but further basic science studies and clinical trials will help determine the correctness of this hypothesis.

SECONDARY PREVENTION OF LUNG CANCER

BIOLOGIC RATIONALE

The concept of secondary prevention of cancer is deeply rooted in two biologic models of carcinogenesis that are supported by the scientific data presented above. The first is the idea that cancer is a multistep process requiring the accumulation of multiple genetic abnormalities that eventually lead to the expression of the malignant phenotype (Fig. 5A.1). The identification of multiple genetic abnormalities (oncogene amplifications and mutations, and growth factor ligand and receptor expression) in any one tumor supports this hypothesis.

The second model is the concept of field cancerization, proposed by Slaughter et al. (94) during the 1950s in reference to oral cancer. Field cancerization refers to the fact that large areas of the epithelial surface frequently are exposed to the same carcinogenic insults. Thus, multiple premalignant foci form, each progressing independently to overt cancer. This progression is best illustrated by the very high rate of additional primary cancers after the onset of lung cancer and head and neck cancer (up to 7% per year) and the multifocal nature of bladder carcinoma (35, 95). These field cancerization changes are linked closely to carcinogenic exposures such as tobacco (35, 95). As one would expect, these multiple tumors, although linked to the same offending carcinogens, are not derived from the same cell and thus may have a somewhat different spectrum of genetic mutations. In fact, Chung et al. (96) examined *p53* expression in 31 patients with head and neck cancer and related second primary tumors and found discordance between tumors in the same patient. Of 21 patients with *p53* mutations in at least one tumor, 16 had mutations in only one primary tumor. Of the remaining 5 patients with *p53* mutations in both primary tumors, in 4 patients the mutations were in different exons, and in one patient the mutations were in the same exon but in different codons. Nevertheless, the majority of the tumor mutations were of the same class (transitions), reflecting the common origin from the same carcinogenic insult. These results show that the second primary tumors arise independently and support the notion that the entire epithelium is at risk because of exposure to the same carcinogens.

CLINICAL TRIALS ISSUES

Several issues unique to chemoprevention trials need recognition. Although the designs of phase I through III chemoprevention trials may use standard chemotherapeutic trial designs as a model, the nature of the population and of the desired result is very different for chemoprevention trials. Issues of long-term compliance and toxicity assume new importance because of the potentially lengthy duration of intervention for chemoprevention purposes in a population that is relatively healthy compared with the conventional cancer patient.

In chemoprevention trials, a number of potential study endpoints can be examined. The incidence of cancer and cancer-related mortality are the definitive endpoints. However, even when high-risk populations having an increased incidence of lung cancer are studied, the incidence of lung cancer is still very low (i.e., 3 to 5 per 1000 person-years for smokers with a 20 pack-year history) (97). Thus, large numbers of patients and lengthy (and costly) follow-up may be required to address particular trial issues definitively. An alternative to lengthy trials with definitive endpoints is the use of intermediate endpoint markers. The use of intermediate endpoints can shorten the duration of follow-up significantly, thereby reducing the cost of studies and significantly speeding the accrual of valuable information. To qualify as an appropriate intermediate biomarker, a marker must satisfy several important criteria, including: (*a*) it must be detectable in small tissue specimens to allow for repeated determinations in the same patient; (*b*) it should be expressed differently between normal and high-risk tissue, allowing for the measurement of changes in expression during carcinogenesis; (*c*) it should be modulated by chemoprevention agents; and (*d*) it should have a low rate of spontaneous fluctuations in the absence of treatment (95).

To date, no intermediate biomarker has been validated adequately for use in chemoprevention trials. The development of such biomarkers hinges on both the identification of a suitable target and on technical developments related to the ability to quantify these markers reliably from small amounts of tissue or body fluids in a manner that is as noninvasive as possible. Thus, the problem is identifying markers that satisfy the criteria described above and developing simple, widely applicable techniques to detect them noninvasively. Although several nonspecific markers such as micronuclei and proliferative indices have been proposed for intermediate endpoint analysis, none has yet proven to be useful. Current molecular biology research of lung cancer is beginning to identify key contributors to the process of lung carcinogenesis, thereby presenting potential specific targets for intermediate endpoint analysis such as frequent oncogene mutations or growth factor expression.

A second potential problem unique to chemoprevention trials relates to the size of the study populations. Because the goal is prevention of the development of a cancer (which is an infrequent occurrence in the general population), many subjects must be enrolled to ensure that a statistically meaningful number of cancers eventually develop in the study population. One reasonable means of decreasing the study size is to target a higher risk population. For lung cancer, multiple risk factors have been well documented, including extensive smoking history, especially with associated chronic obstructive pulmonary disease; various high-risk occupations such as roofers, asphalt workers, and shipyard workers; environmental exposures such as asbestos and radon; and family history (98–103). Patients with previously cured early-stage lung cancer or head and neck cancer also have a very high risk of developing second primary tumors (10-fold to 100-fold greater incidence than heavy smokers), and thus they represent another good study population.

Although enrichment for the development of cancer in the study population clearly enables a smaller population to be used, researchers must be careful about generalizing these results to the population at large. Certain high-risk subgroups may not be representative of the entire population. An example is the recent report of a 13% reduction in cancer deaths in malnourished tin miners treated for 5 years with beta carotene, vitamin E, and selenium in Linxian Province, China (104). A similar intervention in a population of male smokers in Finland (beta carotene and vitamin E therapy) who were not malnourished did not result in any reduction in lung cancer risk (105). Among the potential explanations for the discrepancy between the studies may well be the nutritional status of the study populations or a difference in the carcinogenic stimuli resulting in the cancers in each study. The complexity of cancer underscores the importance of cautious extrapolation of results from small studies. Similarly, one could postulate that the lung cancer in patients with particular environmental exposures such as asbestos may have a different spectrum of genetic mutations and thus may behave differently with respect to chemopreventive agents.

A third issue unique to chemoprevention trials relates to compliance and toxicity. Unlike chemotherapy for potentially terminal diseases, chemopreventive agents are administered to relatively healthy patients who may or may not develop cancer. These agents may need to be administered for long periods, perhaps even a lifetime. Investigators must be concerned with both acute and chronic toxicities. The acceptance of toxicity by the patient and physician often is directly proportional to the magnitude of the short-term threat from the underlying disease. Thus, agents with significant side effects or significant long-term risks such as secondary cancers or end organ damage are clearly inappropriate for the chemopreventive setting. The mode, frequency, and ease of delivery also are issues. Any infringement of a relatively healthy person's lifestyle frequently results in noncompliance. For this reason, it has been suggested that a 2- to 4-month "run-in" phase be used in chemoprevention clinical trials (95). Noncompliant individuals can be eliminated, and the expense associated with their randomization and long-term follow-up can be minimized.

These issues have been tested in two pilot studies that laid the groundwork for the ongoing Carotene and Retinol Efficacy Trial (CARET) (106, 107). These studies addressed the feasibility of a cancer prevention trial specifically for lung cancer. They determined that high-risk populations can be recruited through labor unions, occupational health clinics, and the major health insurance companies. The combination of agents used, retinyl palmitate at a dose of 25,000 units/day and beta carotene at 15 or 30 mg/day, resulted in the same toxicity as placebo or either agent alone, and compliance was greater than 80% at 3 years. These studies suggest that large-scale chemoprevention trials can overcome the obstacles inherent to their nature in dealing with at risk but otherwise healthy populations. Whether these interventions will lead to a decreased number of cancers remains to be determined by the ongoing CARET study.

CLINICAL CHEMOPREVENTION TRIALS: PREMALIGNANCY AND SECOND PRIMARY TUMORS

The development of chemoprevention agents has been guided by epidemiologic studies linking cancer development and dietary intake and by animal studies testing potential agents for their ability to prevent the development of carcinogen-induced cancers. These studies have led to the identification of dietary micronutrients such as beta carotene and vitamin A as potential chemopreventive agents. Although studies in lung cancer chemoprevention are currently ongoing, a growing body of evidence exists from studies of the tumors of the head and neck that retinoids (analogues of vitamin A) have significant chemopreventive potential. These strategies are applicable to lung cancer as well. The common exposure to tobacco specific carcinogens for both head and neck cancer and lung cancer suggests that the upper aerodigestive tract comprises a single cancer field.

Among the first placebo-controlled phase III chemoprevention trials for the upper aerodigestive tract was a 1986 report by Hong et al. (108) using high-dose 13-cis-retinoic acid (cRA) for the treatment of oral leukoplakia, a premalignant precursor of squamous cell carcinoma. This study was based on a number of earlier uncontrolled trials that noted the activity of topical or systemic vitamin A in reversing these oral lesions (109). Oral leukoplakia is a particularly attractive system to study because it has a known rate of progression to overt carcinoma, and the reversal of a premalignant lesion offers a reasonable short-term study endpoint. In the 1986 trial (108), 44 patients were randomized to receive 1 or 2 mg/kg/day of cRA or placebo for 3 months; they were then followed for an additional 6 months. The results showed a 67% major clinical response rate with cRA versus 10% with placebo, and a 54% major histologic response rate with cRA versus 10% with placebo. However, unacceptable toxicity and relapse were major problems in this study. More than 50% of responding patients relapsed within 2 to 3 months of stopping treatment.

A subsequent study of oral leukoplakia used a short, high-dose induction of cRA (1.5 mg/kg/day for 3 months) followed by randomization to maintenance for 9 months with either low-dose cRA (0.5 mg/kg/day) or beta carotene (30 mg/day) (110). The results of this trial reaffirmed the activity of cRA and demonstrated an 8% progression during or after low-dose cRA administration versus a 55% progression during or after beta carotene therapy. Importantly, toxicity was generally mild and acceptable with low-dose cRA. Whether this regimen will ultimately decrease the incidence of squamous cell carcinoma remains to be proven, but the ability to reverse known premalignant lesions suggests that there may be a long-term benefit for such a regimen.

Given the efficacy demonstrated for retinoids in oral premalignancy, a strong rationale exists for testing these compounds in other tumors affected by the same carcinogenic exposures in the aerodigestive tract. In head and neck tumors, one of the major causes of mortality after curative surgery is the development of second primary tumors (95). Hong et al. (111) demonstrated in a phase III trial using cRA or placebo for 1 year after definitive local therapy that the development of second primary tumors is significantly reduced with cRA whereas there is no significant impact on primary disease recurrence or metastasis or on overall survival after a median of 32 months of follow-up (111). Significantly, longer follow-up of these patients (median, 55 months) revealed that the protective effect against all second primary tumors decreased during the time interval, although it still remained significant (112). The protective effect against the subset of aerodigestive tract second primary tumors remained at the same statistical level of significance after 55 months as after 32 months (112). This long-term protective effect, in contrast to the results seen with oral leukoplakia, offers much promise for chemoprevention after head and neck cancer.

LUNG CANCER CHEMOPREVENTION TRIALS

Given the similar etiologic role of tobacco use in head and neck cancer and lung cancer, chemoprevention trials in lung cancer to date have followed the paradigm established in head and neck cancer trials. Several trials have been conducted that used premalignancy as an endpoint (Table 5A.3). In 1982, Saccomanno et al. (113) found that cRA treatment in 26 smokers with preexisting metaplasia had no effect on the degree of sputum atypia. In 1986, Misset et al. (114) reported in an uncontrolled study that etretinate (25 mg/day) treatment of heavy smokers for 6 months led to a reduction in squamous metaplasia as determined by biopsy. The mean metaplasia index decreased from 34.57% before treatment to 26.96% after treatment in 29 of 40 subjects studied. These results were interpreted to mean that retinoid therapy was highly effective in reversing squamous metaplasia.

Two subsequent randomized studies could not reproduce these positive results. Arnold et al. (115) administered etretinate to 138 patients and evaluated squamous metaplasia by sputum cytology. After 6 months of treatment, the reversal of metaplasia occurred with similar frequencies in both etretinate subjects (32.4%) and placebo subjects (29.8%). Similarly, Lee at al. (116) reported a placebo-controlled trial of isotretinoin in 87 subjects using bronchoscopic biopsy to evaluate squamous metaplasia. Reduction in the squamous metaplasia index occurred with similarly high frequencies in both isotretinoin subjects (54.3%) and placebo subjects (58.8%). Reduction in the metaplasia index was correlated mainly with the cessation of smoking.

The results of these three trials emphasize several important points. The paramount significance of placebo-controlled trials in confirming the results of preliminary single-arm chemoprevention studies is obvious. In this respect, chemoprevention trials must use the same strategy as chemotherapeutic agent trials to establish efficacy. The second point, however, emphasizes the difficulty in establishing intermediate endpoint markers for judging the efficacy of potential chemoprevention agents. Squamous metaplasia is thought to be a premalignant lesion for lung cancer, but clearly not all squamous metaplasias proceed to overt carcinoma, and the high rate of spontaneous conversion (or conversion in the absence of further smoking insult) suggests that it is not a good marker for these trials. The fact that these lesions are scattered throughout the epithelium, making sampling error a potential problem, and that they lack specificity for lung carcinogenesis (metaplasia may simply be a measure of airway irritation caused by a variety of insults) demonstrate a need for defining other more specific intermediate endpoint markers.

Two other studies using premalignancy as an endpoint have been reported. In 1988, Heimburger at al. (117) reported a placebo-controlled trial of the combination of folic acid and vitamin B_{12} for 4 months in 73 smokers with metaplasia determined by sputum cy-

TABLE 5A.3. Completed Chemoprevention Trials in Lung Cancer

TRIAL (YEAR)	ENDPOINT	INTERVENTION	OUTCOME	REFERENCE NO.
Saccomanno (1982)	Sputum atypia	13 cRA	Negative	(113)
Misset (1986)	Metaplasia (bx)	Etretinate	Positive[a]	(114)
Heimburger (1988)	Sputum atypia	Folate/vitamin B_{12}	Positive[b]	(117)
Arnold (1992)	Sputum atypia	Etretinate	Negative	(115)
van Poppel (1992)	Micronuclei	Beta carotene	Positive	(118)
Lee (1993)	Metaplasia (bx)	13 cRA	Negative	(116)
Pastorino (1993)	Second primary cancer	Retinyl palmitate	Positive	(119)
ATBC, Finland (1994)	Lung cancer	Vitamin E, beta carotene	Negative	(105)

Abbreviations. bx, biopsy; cRA, 13-cis-retinoic acid; ATBC, Alpha-Tocopherol, Beta Carotene Cancer Prevention Study.
[a]Uncontrolled study.
[b]Results were not significant when using standard statistical analysis.

tology. The folate vitamin B_{12} group was reported to have significant improvement in metaplasia compared with the placebo group. However, this analysis has been called into question because of assumptions made in the statistical analysis. Reanalysis using standard analytical methods revealed no significant difference between the two groups (95). The other randomized study reported by van Poppel et al. (118) was a placebo-controlled trial of beta carotene in smokers using micronuclei frequency as the study endpoint (118). A significant reduction in sputum micronuclei frequency was associated with the intervention, but the significance of this reduction is unclear because modulation of micronuclei frequency does not correlate well with carcinogenic progression (95).

To date, only two trials have addressed the development of lung cancer as an endpoint, either in the primary setting in a high-risk population of smokers or in the development of second primary tumors. Pastorino et al. (119) reported the first positive chemoprevention trial in lung cancer using retinyl palmitate as the intervention. In this study, 307 patients with completely resected stage I NSCLC were randomized to receive either retinyl palmitate at a dose of 30,000 IU/day, or to a no treatment control arm for 12 months. The endpoints were recurrence of the primary tumor or occurrence of a second primary tumor. After a median follow-up of 46 months, 56 (37%) of the treated patients and 75 (48%) of the control patients had either a recurrence or a second primary tumor. However, only 18 patients in the treated group, compared with 29 patients in the control group, developed second primary tumors. Furthermore, only patients in the control group developed more than one additional primary tumor. Subset analysis revealed that the time to development of tobacco-related secondary primary tumors was significantly longer in the vitamin A-treated group. The 5-year survival, however, was no different between the two groups, reflecting the effective salvage rates with current modalities in patients with second primary tumors. These results are encouraging with regard to the potential for chemoprevention in lung cancer, although such therapy is hardly standard clinical practice as yet (120).

The other large-scale trial of interest is the recently published Finnish study that examined the development of cancer in a cohort of 29,133 male smokers aged 50 to 69 years who were treated with vitamin E, beta carotene, both vitamin E and beta carotene, or placebo (105). Surprisingly, no reduction in the incidence of lung cancer was noted in the treated groups; in fact, there was a slight increase in lung cancer among the men treated with beta carotene. Overall, the mortality was 8% higher among the men treated with beta carotene, primarily because of the presence of lung cancer and ischemic heart disease in these subjects. There may be many reasons why no beneficial effect was noted in this study given the multiple prior epidemiologic studies documenting the inverse relationship between the consumption of carotene rich foods and the incidence of lung cancer. These range from the possibility that beta carotene is not the agent with the protective effect in these foods or that it is merely an indicator of other lifestyle issues that actually have the protective effect; the possibility also exists that the intervention was of too brief a duration and occurred too late in the progression toward carcinogenesis to alter the incidence of lung cancer. The study points out the complexity of determining which chemoprevention agents to study and raises the possibility that micronutrient supplementation may be associated with risks as well as benefits.

Multiple trials are currently underway to address chemoprevention in lung carcinogenesis (Table 5A.4) (95). These include studies analyzing lung cancer development and prevention of second primary tumors as endpoints. The Euroscan study (121) is the largest study to date of patients with previously treated early-stage lung cancer or head and neck cancer. The endpoints of the study are the development of second primary tumors, local or regional recurrence, distant metastases, and long-term survival. The 2000 subjects in this study were randomized to receive retinyl palmitate at a dose of 300,000 IU/day for 1 year followed by 150,000 IU/day for the second year versus N-acetylcysteine, 600 mg/day for 2 years, versus both drugs versus neither drug in a 2×2 factorial design. As of June 1992, nearly 1500 patients had been randomized. One significant difference between this study and the previous head and neck chemoprevention study by Hong et al. (108) using isotretinoin is the inclusion of only early-stage patients. The lack of effect on survival by chemoprevention efforts thus far may well reflect the need to administer these agents earlier in the course of the disease because they may not have any effect on recurrence or metastases.

CONCLUSIONS

Although the retinoids remain the most promising agents because of the results of prior clinical trials and basic science studies showing their important role in cell growth and differentiation, other agents are being developed and combinations of agents may be of value. These agents include N-acetylcysteine, difluoromethylornithine, oltipraz, organosulfur compounds

TABLE 5A.4. Ongoing Chemoprevention Trials in Lung Cancer

TRIAL	STUDY POPULATION	INTERVENTION	ENDPOINT
Physicians Health Study	Male physicians	Beta carotene, aspirin	Cancer, cardiovascular disease
Women's Health Study	Female nurses	Beta carotene, α-tocopherol, aspirin	Cancer, cardiovascular disease
CARET	Smokers, asbestos workers	Beta carotene, retinyl palmitate	Lung cancer
Radiation Therapy Oncology Group	Stage I and II head and neck cancers	13 cRA	Second primary tumors
U.S. Intergroup Study	Stage I NSCLC	13 cRA	Second primary tumors
Euroscan	Early stage NSCLC and head and neck cancers	Retinyl palmitate, N-acetylcysteine	Second primary tumors
Eastern Cooperative Oncology Group	Stage I and II head and neck cancers	13 cRA	Second primary tumors
Yale	Stage I and II head and neck cancers	Beta carotene	Second primary tumors
University of Texas	Asbestos workers	Retinol, beta carotene	Sputum atypia

From Lippmann SM, Benner SE, Hong WK. Cancer chemoprevention. J Clin Oncol 1994;12:851–873.

such as S-allyl-cysteine, isothiocyanates, and alternative synthetic retinoids such as fenretinide (95). Agents targeting various phases of carcinogenesis, ranging from initiation to promotion and progression, are being combined in an effort to prevent carcinogenesis at all phases of development. As more is learned about the biology of lung cancer, specific inhibitors of key processes underlying neoplastic transformation can be developed. Only the maturation of studies already accruing patients and the further development of promising new agents can show whether chemoprevention has a role as standard therapy in lung cancer.

The approach to eliminating lung cancer as a major public health nightmare must consist of multiple efforts. These begin with primary prevention in the form of the elimination of smoking. The current interest in understanding the molecular biology of lung cancer is exposing many potential targets for early detection of lung cancer and for intervention in the process of carcinogenesis. Future efforts in these fields can be planned rationally based on an understanding of biology rather than on circumstantial and historical evidence. A strong linkage between well-planned clinical trials and the basic science support guiding these trials offers hope for the development of strategies to reduce the mortality from lung cancer.

REFERENCES

1. Wingo PA, Tont T, Bolden S. Cancer statistics, 1995. CA Cancer J Clin 1995;45:8–30.
2. Mulshine JL, Tockman MS. Early detection of lung cancer: Where are we? In: DeVita VT, Hellman S, Rosenberg SA, eds. Cancer Prevention. Philadelphia: JB Lippincott, 1991:1–8.
3. Saccomanno G, Archer VE, Auerbach O, Saunders RP, Brennan, LM. Development of carcinoma of the lung as reflected in exfoliated cells. Cancer 1974;33:256–270.
4. Flehinger BJ, Melamed MR, Zaman MB, et al. Early lung cancer detection: Results of the initial (prevalence) radiologic and cytologic screening in the Memorial Sloan–Kettering study. Am Rev Respir Dis 1984;130:555–560.
5. Shimizu N, Ando A, Teramoto S, Moritani Y, Nishii K. Outcome of patients with lung cancer detected via mass screening as compared to those presenting with symptoms. J Surg Oncol 1992;50:7–11.
6. Naruke T, Kuroishi T, Suzuki T, Ikeda S, Japanese Lung-Cancer Screening Research Group. Comparative study of survival of screen-detected compared with symptom-detected lung cancer cases. Semin Surg Oncol 1993;9:80–84.
7. Sobue T, Suzuki T, Naruke T. A case-control study for evaluating lung-cancer screening in Japan. Int J Cancer 1992;50:230–237.
8. Ebeling K, Nischan P. Screening for lung cancer—results from a case-control study. Int J Cancer 1987;40:141–144.
9. Berndt R, Nischan P, Ebeling K. Screening for lung cancer in the middle aged. Int J Cancer 1990;45:229–230.
10. Lilienfeld A, Archer PG, Burnett CH, et al. An evaluation of radiologic and cytologic screening for the early detection of lung cancer: a cooperative pilot study of the American Cancer Study and the Veterans Administration. Cancer Res 1966;26:2083–2121.
11. Nash FA, Morgan JM, Tomkins JG. South London Cancer Study. BMJ 1968;2:715–721.
12. Boucot KR, Weiss W. Is curable lung cancer detected by semi-annual screening? JAMA 1973;224:1361–1365.
13. Weiss W, Seidman H, Boucot KR. The Philadelphia Pulmonary Neoplasm Research Project. Am Rev Respir Dis 1975;111:M289–297.
14. Wilde J. A 10-year follow-up of semi-annual screening for lung cancer in Erfurt County, GDR. Eur Respir J 1989;2:656–662.
15. Schilling CJ, Schilling JM. Chest X-ray screening for lung cancer at three British chromates plants from 1955-1989. Br J Indust Med 1991;48:476–479.
16. Brett GZ. Earlier diagnosis and survival in lung cancer. BMJ 1969;4:260–262.
17. Fontana RS, Sanderson DR, Taylor WF, et al. Early lung cancer detection: results from the initial (prevalence) radiologic and cytologic screening in the Mayo Clinic Study. Am Rev Respir Dis 1984;130:561–565.

18. Frost JK, Ball WC, Levin ML, et al. Early lung cancer detection: results of the initial (prevalence) radiologic and cytologic screening in the Johns Hopkins Study. Am Rev Respir Dis 1984;130:549–554.
19. Melamed MR, Flehinger BJ, Zaman MB, et al. Screening for early lung cancer. Results of the Memorial Sloan–Kettering Study in New York, Chest 1984;86:44–53.
20. Fontana RS, Sanderson DR, Woolner LB, et al. Lung cancer screening: the Mayo program. J Occup Med 1986;28:746–750.
21. Martini N. Results of the Memorial Sloan–Kettering study in screening for early lung cancer. Chest 1986;89(Suppl):325S.
22. Sanderson DR. Lung cancer screening. The Mayo study. Chest 1986;89(Suppl):324S.
23. Tockman MS. Survival and mortality from lung cancer in a screened population. The Johns Hopkins study. Chest 1986;89(Suppl):324S–325S.
24. Fontana RS, Sanderson DR, Woolner LB, et al. Screening for lung cancer. A critique of the Mayo Lung Project. Cancer 1991;67:1155–1164.d
25. Kubik A, Parkin DM, Khlat M. Erban L. Polak J, Adamec M. Lack of benefit from semi-annual screening for cancer of the lung: Follow-up report of a randomized controlled trial on a population of high-risk males in Czechoslovakia. Int J Cancer 1990;45:26–33.
26. Muhm JR, Miller WE, Fontana RS, Sanderson DR, Uhlenhopp MA. Lung cancer detected during a screening program using four-month chest radiographs. Radiology 1983;148:609–615.
27. Sobue T, Suzuki T, Matsuda M, et al. Sensitivity and specificity of lung cancer screening in Osaka, Japan. Jpn J Cancer Res 1991;82:1069–1076.
28. Sobue T, Suzuki T, Matsuda M, et al. Survival for clinical stage I lung cancer not surgically treated. Cancer 1992;69:685–692.
29. Birrer MJ, Alani, R, Cuttitta F, et al. Early events in the neoplastic transformation of respiratory epithelium. J Natl Cancer Inst Monogr 1992;13:31–37.
30. Tockman MS, Gupta PK, Myers JD, et al. Sensitive and specific monoclonal antibody recognition of human lung cancer antigen on preserved sputum cells. A new approach to early lung cancer detection. J Clin Oncol 1988;6:1685–1693.
31. Kyogashima M, Mulshine J, Linnoila RI, et al. Antibody 624H12, which detects lung cancer at early stages, recognizes a sugar sequence in the glycosphingolipid difucosylneolactonorhexaosyl-ceramide ($V_3FucIII_3FucnLc6Cer$). Arch Biochem Biophys 1989;275:309–314.
32. Hakomori S. Glycosphingolipids. Sci Am 1986;254:44–53.
33. Hakomori S. Biochemical basis and clinical application of tumor-associated carbohydrate antigens: Current trends and future perspectives. Jpn J Cancer Chemother 1989;16:715–731.
34. Mulshine JL, Linnoila RI, Jensen SM, et al. Rational targets for the early detection of lung cancer. J Natl Cancer Inst Monogr 1992;13:183–190.
35. Thomas P, Rubenstein L, Lung Cancer Study Group. Cancer recurrence after resection: T1N0 non–small-cell lung cancer. Ann Thorac Surg 1990;49:242–247.
36. Whang-Peng, J. 3p Deletions and small cell lung carcinoma. Mayo Clin Proc 1989;64:256–260.
37. Yokota J, Wada M, Shimosato Y, et al. Loss of heterozygosity on chromosomes 3, 13, and 17 in small-cell carcinoma and on chromosome 3 in adenocarcinoma of the lung. Proc Natl Acad Sci U S A 1987;84:9252–9256.
38. Kurzrock R, Gallick GE, Gutterman JU. Differential expression of p21 ras gene products among histologic subtypes of fresh primary human lung tumors. Cancer Res 1986;46:1530–1534.
39. Rodenhuis S, vande Wetering ML, Mooi WJ, et al. Mutational activation of the K-ras oncogene: A possible pathogenetic factor in adenocarcinoma of the lung. N Eng J Med 1987;317:929–935.
40. Rodenhuis S, Slebos RJC, Boot AJM, et al. Incidence and possible clinical significance of K-ras oncogene activation in adenocarcinoma of the human lung. Cancer Res 1988;48:5738–5741.
41. Bos JL. ras Oncogenes in human cancer: A review. Cancer Res 1989;49:4682–4689.
42. Slebos RJC, Kibbelaar RE, Dalesio O, et al. K-ras oncogene activation as a prognostic marker in adenocarcinoma of the lung. N Engl J Med 1990;323:561–565.
43. Slebos RJC, Rodenhuis S. The ras gene family in human non–small-cell lung cancer. J Natl Cancer Inst Monogr 1992;13:23–29.
44. You M, Candrian U, Maronpot RR, et al. Activation of the Ki-ras protooncogene in spontaneously occurring and chemically induced lung tumors of the strain A mouse. Proc Natl Acad Sci U S A 1989;86:3070–3074.
45. Brandt-Rauf PW, Smith S, Hemminski K, et al. Serum oncoproteins and growth factors in asbestosis and silicosis patients. Int J Cancer 1992;50:881–885.
46. Mao L, Hruban RH, Boyle JO, Tockman M, Sidransky D. Detection of oncogene mutations in sputum precedes diagnosis of lung cancer. Cancer Res 1994;54:1634–1637.
47. Sugio K, Kishimoto Y, Virmani AK, Hung JY, Gazdar AF. K-ras mutations are a relatively late event in the pathogenesis of lung carcinomas. Cancer Res 1994;54:5811–5815.
48. Schafer WR, Kim R, Sterne R, et al. Genetic and pharmacologic suppression of oncogenic mutations in ras genes of yeast and humans. Science 1989;245:379–385.
49. Kohn NE, Wilson FR, Mosser SD, et al. Protein farnesyltransferase inhibitors block the growth of ras-dependent tumors in nude mice. Proc Natl Acad Sci U S A 1994;91:9141–9145.
50. Wong AJ, Ruppert JM, Eggleston J, et al. Gene amplification of c-myc and N-myc in small cell carcinoma of the lung. Science 1986;233:461–464.
51. Kiefer PE, Bepler G, Kubasch M, et al. Amplification and expression of protooncogenes in human small cell lung cancer cell lines. Cancer Res 1987;47:6236–6242.
52. Yokota J, Wada M, Yoshida T, et al. Heterogeneity of lung cancer cells with respect to the amplification and rearrangement of myc family oncogenes. Oncogene 1988;2:607–611.
53. Broers JLV, Viallet J, Jensen SM, et al. Expression of c-myc in progenitor cells of the bronchopulmonary epithelium and in a large number of non–small cell lung cancers. Am J Respir Cell Mol Biol 1993;9:33–43.
54. Kern JA, Schwartz DA, Nordberg JE, et al. p185[neu] Expression in human lung adenocarcinomas predicts shortened survival. Cancer Res 1990;50:5184–5191.
55. Weiner DB, Nordberg J, Robinson R, et al. Expression of the neu gene-encoded protein (p185[neu]) in human non–small cell carcinomas of the lung. Cancer Res 1990;50:421–425.
56. Rapp U, Huleihel M, Pawson T, et al. Role of raf oncogenes in lung carcinogenesis. Lung Cancer 1988;4:162–167.
57. Griffin CA, Baylin SB. Expression of the c-myb oncogene in human small cell lung carcinoma. Cancer Res 1985;45:272–275.
58. Schutte J, Nau NM, Birrer M, et al. Constitutive expression of multiple mRNA forms of the c-jun oncogene in human lung cancer cell lines. Proc Am Assoc Cancer Res 1988;29:455.
59. Volm M, Drings P, Wodrich W. Prognostic significance of the expression of c-fos, c-jun and c-erbB1 oncogene products in

human squamous cell lung carcinomas. J Cancer Res Clin Oncol 1993;119:507–510.
60. Wodrich W, Volm M. Overexpression of oncoproteins in non–small cell lung carcinomas of smokers. Carcinogenesis 1993;14:1121–1124.
61. Johnson BE, Ihde DC, Makuch RW, et al. myc Family oncogene amplification in tumor cell lines established from small cell lung cancer patients and its relationship to clinical status and course. J Clin Invest 1987;79:1629–1634.
62. Brennan J, O'Connor T, Makuch RW, et al. myc Family DNA amplification in 107 tumors and tumor cell lines from patients with small cell lung cancer treated with different combination chemotherapy regimens. Cancer Res 1991;51:1708–1712.
63. Lee W, Mitchell P, Tjian R, Purified transcription factor AP-1 interacts with TPA-inducible enhancer elements. Cell 1987;49:741–752.
64. Harbour JW, Lai S-L, Whang-Peng J, et al. Abnormalities in structure and expression of the human retinoblastoma genes in SCLC. Science 1988;241:353–357.
65. Yokota J, Akiyama T, Fung Y-KT, et al. Altered expression of the retinoblastoma (RB) gene in small-cell carcinoma of the lung. Oncogene 1988;3:471–475.
66. Hensel CH, Hsieh CL, Gazdar AF, et al. Altered structure and expression of the human retinoblastoma susceptibility gene in small cell lung cancer. Cancer Res 1990;50:3067–3072.
67. Takahashi T, Nau NM, Chiba I, et al. p53: A frequent target for genetic abnormalities in lung cancer. Science 1989;246:491–494.
68. D'Amico D, Carbone D, Mitsudomi T, et al. High frequency of somatically acquired p53 mutations in small cell lung cancer cell lines and tumors. Oncogene 1992;7:339–348.
69. Chiba I, Takahashi T, Nau NM, et al. Mutations in the p53 gene are frequent in primary, resected non–small cell lung cancer. Oncogene 1990;5:1603–1610.
70. Whang-Peng J, Kao-Shan CS, Lee EC, et al. Specific chromosome defect associated with human small cell lung cancer: Deletion 3p(14-23) Science 1982;215:181–182.
71. Falor WH, Ward-Skinner R, Wegryn S. A 3p deletion in small cell lung cancer. Cancer Genet Cytogenet 1985;16:175–177.
72. Shimizu E, Coxon A, Otterson GA, et al. Rb protein status and clinical correlation from 171 cell lines representing lung cancer, extrapulmonary small cell carcinoma, and mesothelioma. Oncogene 1994;9:2441–2448.
73. Sozzi G, Miozzo M, Donghi R, et al. Deletions of 17p and p53 mutations in preneoplastic lesions of the lung. Cancer Res 1992;52:6079–6082.
74. Bennett WP, Colby TV, Travis WD, et al. p53 Protein accumulates frequently in early bronchial neoplasia. Cancer Res 1993;53:4817–4822.
75. Lavigueur A, Maltby V, Mock D, et al. High incidences of lung, bone and lymphoid tumors in transgenic mice overexpressing mutant alleles of the p53 oncogene. Mol Cell Biol 1989;9:3982–3991.
76. Malkin D, Li FP, Strong LC, et al. Germ line p53 mutations in a familial syndrome of breast cancer, sarcomas, and other neoplasms. Science 1990;250:1233–1238.
77. Srivastava S, Zou Z, Pirollo K, et al. Germ-line transmission of a mutated p53 gene in a cancer-prone family with Li-Fraumeni syndrome. Nature 1190;348:747–749.
78. Cuttitta F, Carney DN., Mulshine JL, et al. Bombesin-like peptides can function as autocrine growth factors in human small-cell lung cancer. Nature 1988;316:823–826.
79. Mulshine JL, Birrer MJ, Treston AM, et al. Growth factors and other targets for rational application as intervention agents. In: Newell GR, Hong WK, eds. The biology and prevention of Aerodigestive Tract Cancers. New York: Plenum, 1992:81–88.
80. Nakanishi Y, Mulshine JL, Kasprzyk PG, et al. Insulin-like growth factor-1 can mediate autocrine proliferation of human small cell lung cancer cell lines in vitro. J Clin Invest 1988;82:354–359.
81. Natale RB, Cuttitta F, Nakanishi Y, et al. IGF-1 can stimulate proliferation of non–small cell lung cancer cell lines in vitro. Proc Am Soc Clin Oncol 1988;7:197.
82. Nakanishi Y, Cuttitta F, Kasprzyk PG, et al. Growth factor effects on small cell lung cancer cell using a colorimetric assay: can a transferrin-like factor mediate autocrine growth? Expl Cell Biol 1988;56:74–85.
83. Vostrejs M, Moran PL, Seligman PA. Transferrin synthesis by small cell lung cancer cells acts as an autocrine regulator of cellular proliferation. J Clin Invest 1988;82:331–339.
84. Hendler FJ, Ozanne BW. Human squamous cell lung cancers express increased epidermal growth factor receptors. J Clin Invest 1984;74:M647–651.
85. Siegfried JM, Owens SM. Response of primary human lung carcinomas to autocrine growth factors produced by a lung carcinoma cell line. Cancer Res 1988;48:4976–4981.
86. Mendelsohn J. Epidermal growth factor receptor as a target for therapy with antireceptor monoclonal antibodies. J Natl Cancer Inst Monogr 1992;13:M125–131.
87. Willey J, Lechner J, Harris C. Bombesin and the C-terminal tetradecapeptide of gastrin-releasing peptide are growth factors for normal human bronchial epithelial cells. Exp Cell Res 1984;153:245–248.
88. Sunday ME, Hua J, Dai HB, et al. Bombesin increases fetal lung growth and maturation in utero and in organ culture. Am J Respir Cell Mol Biol 1990;3:199–205.
89. Aguayo SM, Kane M, King TE, et al. Increased levels of bombesin-like peptides in the lower respiratory tract of asymptomatic cigarette smokers. J Clin Invest 1989;84:1105–1113.
90. Aguayo SM, King TE, Kane MA, et al. Urinary levels of bombesin-like peptides in asymptomatic cigarette smokers: a potential risk marker for smoking-related diseases. Cancer Res 1992;52(Suppl):2727S–2731S.
91. Coy DH, Jensen RT, Jiang N-Y, et al. Systematic development of bombesin/gastrin-releasing peptide antagonists. J Natl Cancer Inst Monogr 1992;13:133–139.
92. Mulshine JL, Cuttita F, Scott, F, et al. Strategies for lung cancer chemoprevention. Lung Cancer 1993;9:357–360.
93. Sethi T, Langdon S, Smyth J, et al. Growth of small cell lung cancer cells: stimulation by multiple neuropeptides and inhibition by broad spectrum antagonists in vitro and in vivo. Cancer Res 1992;52(Suppl):2737S–2742S.
94. Slaughter DP, Southwick HW, Smejkal W. Field cancerization in oral stratified squamous epithelium: Clinical implications of multicentric origin. Cancer 1953;6:963–968.
95. Lippmann SM, Benner SE, Hong WK. Cancer chemoprevention. J Clin Oncol 1994;12:851–873.
96. Chung KY, Mukhopadhyay T, Kim J, et al. Discordant p53 gene mutations in primary head and neck cancers and corresponding second primary cancers of the upper aerodigestive tract. Cancer Res 1993;53:1676–1683.
97. Goodman GE. The prevention of primary lung cancer. In: Johnson BE, Johnson DH, eds. Lung cancer. New York: Wiley-Liss, 1994:41–53.
98. Skillrud DM, Offord KP, Miller RD. Higher risk of lung cancer in chronic obstructive pulmonary disease. Ann Intern Med 1986;105:503–507.

99. Tockman MS, Anthonisen NR, Wright EC, et al. Airways obstruction and the risk for lung cancer. Ann Intern Med 1987;106:512–518.
100. Vineis P, Thomas T, Hayes RB, et al. Proportion of lung cancers in males due to occupation in different areas of the U.S. Int J Cancer 1988;42:851–856.
101. Ooi WL, Elston RC, Chen VW, Bailey-Wilson JE, Rothschild H. Increased familial risk for lung cancer. J Natl Cancer Inst 1986;76:217–222.
102. Shaw GL, Falk RT, Pickle LW, Mason TJ, Buffler PA. Lung cancer risk associated with cancer in relatives. J Clin Epidemiol 1991;44:429–437.
103. Sellers TA, Bailey-Wilson JE, Elston RC, et al. Evidence for mendelian inheritance in the pathogenesis of lung cancer. J Natl Cancer Inst 1990;82:1271–1279.
104. Blot WJ, Li J-Y, Taylor PR, et al. Nutrition intervention trials in Linxian, China: supplementation with specific vitamin/mineral combinations, cancer incidence, and disease-specific mortality in the general population. J Natl Cancer Inst 1993;85:1483–1492.
105. The Alpha-Tocopherol, Beta Carotene Cancer Prevention Study Group. The effect of vitamin E and beta carotene on the incidence of lung cancer and other cancers in male smokers. N Engl J Med 1994;330:1029–1035.
106. Goodman GE, Omenn GS, Thornquist MD, Lund B, Metch B, Gylys-Colwell I. The Carotene and Retinol Efficacy Trial (CARET) to prevent lung cancer in high risk populations: pilot study with cigarette smokers. Cancer Epidemiol Biol Prev 1993;2:381–387.
107. Omenn GS, Goodman GE, Thornquist MD, et al. CARET, the Carotene and Retinol Efficacy Trial to prevent lung cancer in high risk populations: pilot study with asbestos-exposed workers. Cancer Epidemiol Biol Prev 1993;2:381–387.
108. Hong WK, Endicott J, Itri LM, et al. 13-*cis*-Retinoic acid in the treatment of oral leukoplakia. New Engl J Med 1986;315:1501–1505.
109. Lippman SM, Benner SE, Hong WK. Chemoprevention strategies in lung carcinogenesis. Chest 1993;103(Suppl)15S–19S.
110. Lippman SM, Batsakis JG, Toth BB, et al. Comparison of low-dose isotretinoin with beta carotene to prevent oral carcinogenesis. N Engl J Med 1993;328:15–20.
111. Hong WK, Lippman SM, Itri LM, et al. Prevention of second primary tumors with isotretinoin in squamous cell carcinoma of the head and neck. N Engl J Med 1990;323:795–801.
112. Benner SE, Pajak TF, Lippman SM. Prevention of second primary tumors with isotretinoin in squamous cell carcinoma of the head and neck: long term follow-up. J Natl Cancer Inst 1994;86:14–141.
113. Saccomanno G, Moran PG, Schmidt RD, et al. Effects of 13-*cis*-retinoids on premalignant and malignant cells of lung origin. Acta Cytol 1982;26:78–85.
114. Misset JL, Mathe G, Santelli G, et al. Regression of bronchial epidermoid metaplasia in heavy smokers with etretinate treatment. Cancer Detect Prev 1986;9:167–170.
115. Arnold AM, Browman GP, Levine MN, et al. The effect of the synthetic retinoid etretinate on sputum cytology: results from a randomized trial. Br J Cancer 1992;65:737–743.
116. Lee JS, Lippman SM, Benner SE, et al. Randomized placebo-controlled trial of isotretinoin in chemoprevention of bronchial squamous metaplasia. J Clin Oncol 1994;12:937–945.
117. Heimburger DC, Alexander, B, Birch R, et al. Improvement in bronchial squamous metaplasia in smokers treated with folate and vitamin B_{12}. Report of a preliminary randomized, double-blind intervention trial. JAMA 1988;259:1525–1530.
118. van Poppel G, Kok FJ, Hermus RJJ. beta carotene supplementation in smokers reduces the frequency of micronuclei in sputum. Br J Cancer 1992;66:1164–1168.
119. Pastorino U, Infante M, Maioli M, et al. Adjuvant treatment of stage I lung cancer with high-dose vitamin A. J Clin Oncol 1993;11:1216–1222.
120. Lippman SM, Hong WK. Not yet standard: retinoids versus second primary tumors. J Clin Oncol 1993;11:1204–1207.
121. DeVries M, van Zandwijk N, Pastorino U. The Euroscan study: a progress report. Am J Otolaryngol 1993;14:62–66.

5B

Progress in the Early Detection of Lung Cancer

Melvyn S. Tockman

The prognosis for patients with lung cancer is primarily dependent on the stage of the tumor at the time of clinical diagnosis. Currently, only one third (25% to 40%) of all lung tumors are considered resectable at the time of initial assessment, and only 20% are found to have limited disease at the time of surgery. However, patients diagnosed early with stage I tumors have a 40% to 70% survival after surgical resection (1–3). These data led to a substantial effort to detect lung cancer earlier, assuming that earlier detection would lead to diagnosis at an earlier stage that is more amenable to potentially curative surgical therapy.

Through the time of the National Cancer Institute (NCI) collaborative trials (4) (at Johns Hopkins University [5], Memorial Sloan–Kettering Hospital [6], and the Mayo Clinic [7]), only chest radiography and the recognition of dysplastic morphology in exfoliated epithelial cells by light microscopy were available to detect "early" pulmonary neoplastic changes (8). Fifteen years ago, as part of the NCI collaborative trials, researchers at the Johns Hopkins Lung Project (JHLP) recruited a volunteer, high-risk population consisting of men 45 years of age and older who smoked at least one pack of cigarettes per day to determine whether the addition of cytologic examination of sputum to screening by chest radiography would result in a reduction of lung cancer mortality compared with a similar group screened by radiography alone (9).

Volunteers in the JHLP were recruited from among licensed drivers in the Baltimore metropolitan area, where lung cancer mortality among men aged 60 to 64 years was 450 per 100,000 in 1980 (10, 11). All of the 10,387 middle-aged, cigarette-smoking men who entered the JHLP received annual chest radiographic screening. By random assignment, half also received cytologic examination of induced sputum. Routine sputum cell morphology was the only test that could detect 28% of the initial (prevalence) lung cancer cases, but with repeated annual screening, cytologic detection added only 13% to the number of lung cancers detected, particularly carcinoma of the squamous cell type (12–14). Chest radiography detected more than 70% of lung cancers at the initial screening, but radiographic detection fell to 43% on annual reexamination. The majority (51%) of the JHLP lung cancer cases presented clinically in the interval between annual screenings. The three NCI-sponsored clinical trials demonstrated, among 30,000 high-risk participants, that although chest radiography and sputum cell morphology can detect presymptomatic, earlier stage carcinoma, higher resectability and survival rates among the study groups did not translate into lowered (overall) lung cancer mortality, compared with the control population (5, 15). Length-biased sampling, lead-time bias, and misclassification, in addition to failures of detection and therapy, contributed to the lack of significant improvement in mortality rates (9, 16–18). A similar lack of mortality reduction was found in Czechoslovakia after 6346 male smokers were allocated randomly to receive either dual screening or usual care(19). These NCI collaborative studies along with the similar study in Czechoslovakia have become the lung cancer screening standards for comparison.

No current screening techniques employing radiologic studies, bronchoalveolar cytology, or direct biopsies have proven adequate for detecting lung cancer at an earlier, curable stage (15, 20). Our enhanced understanding of tumor biology now has focused current attention on the detection of individual cellular and genetic markers of the preclinical process of carcinogenesis (21). The focus on carcinogenesis shifts emphasis away from the detection of bulk malignancy, which for many epithelial organs (especially lung, breast, and colon) often is metastatic (uncurable) at the time of diagnosis.

The sequence of genetic events that underlie the

initiation and promotion of cancer is now becoming understood (22). Mutational events in four types of genes seem to underlie the process of epithelial carcinogenesis. Evidence of these mutational events in the airway has been detected in the sputum; finding this evidence has shaped recent progress in the development of lung cancer screening tests. These mutations presumably arise from the initiating action of a carcinogen and persist because of repair failure prior to cell division. First, translocations and point mutations within or adjacent to protooncogenes may alter the expression (amplify transcription or translation) or alter the biochemical function of oncogene products. For example, the K-*ras* point mutations in exon 1 (at codons 12 or 61) lead to an inability of the usual mechanism (guanosine triphosphate [GTP] hydrolysis) to regulate the mutant *ras* protein (23). Interference with signal transduction and transcription through oncogene alteration may shift the balance from cell differentiation (in G0 or interphase) toward proliferation (mitosis). Again, using the *ras* pathway as an example, the persistence of the activated *ras* protein may prolong the signal from cell surface tyrosine-kinase growth factor receptors that stimulate cell proliferation (23). For this reason oncogene activation has been likened to the "accelerator" for carcinogenesis.

The second type of gene mutated during carcinogenesis is the tumor suppressor gene, thought to be inactivated in cancer progression by the loss of one or more specific alleles. This follows from Knudson's hypothesis: after studying the kinetics of inherited childhood tumors, Knudson suggested that children afflicted with retinoblastoma inherited one of two mutations that were rate limiting for tumor development (24). Tumor suppressor genes are now incorporated into this theory through mutational inactivation of one copy during somatic tumor development followed by another mutation or loss of the second allele (25). Loss of both tumor suppressor gene alleles may remove the regulatory brakes holding the cell in interphase (G0) and allow progression through the checkpoints of the proliferation cycle: from G1, the gap before DNA synthesis; through S, the period of DNA synthesis; G2, the gap between synthesis and division; and mitosis, cell division from prophase through telophase. For example, the *p53* tumor suppressor gene was found to be mutated in a variety of cancers, including those of the lung (26), breast (27), esophagus (28), liver (29), bladder (30), ovary (31), and brain (32), as well as almost every other tumor type (33). The *p53* gene has been identified as one (along with *9p21*, another suppressor gene with cell cycle control function) of the most commonly mutated genes in human cancers (34).

The third type of gene mutated in carcinogenesis is the group of DNA repair genes (mismatch repair and excision repair). The regulation of cell division is tied closely to DNA repair. Evolution of normal cells into cancer cells is facilitated by loss of coordination between genome repair and the cyclin dependent kinases and checkpoint controls responsible for progression through the cell cycle (35). Failure to repair cellular DNA normally leads to instability of the genome and a more rapid evolution toward cancer, manifested by a "mutator phenotype" in some hereditary tumors (36). The human homologue of a mismatch repair gene critical to both yeast (37) and bacteria (38) was cloned (named *h-MSH-2*) and found to be subject to germline mutation as well as somatic inactivation in patients with hereditary nonpolyposis colorectal cancer (Lynch syndrome) (39, 40). The bacterial gene (*MUT-S*) recognizes single base pair mismatches and small displaced loops that can occur through slippage during replications of repeat regions (microsatellites). Mutation of the human mismatch repair homologue (*h-MSH-2*) leads to microsatellite instability because of frequent replication errors of these repeats. In bacteria the mismatch repair system utilizes three major gene products including *MUT-S*, *MUT-H*, and *MUT-L* (38). Mutations of the human *MUT-L* homologue on chromosome 3p may be recognized by similar microsatellite alterations in nonpolyposis colorectal cancer patients whose cancers are linked to this region (41, 42). Although similar widespread instability may be rare in human somatic tumors, occasional microsatellite alterations are common (43). Microsatellites occur between transcribed DNA sequences and therefore offer the cell no survival advantage. The appearance of microsatellite alterations in the polymerase chain reaction (PCR) product, accordingly, indicates the presence of multiple cells (a cell clone) bearing an identical allelic change. Microsatellites, which have been found to be altered in a tissue specific pattern, thus may have a role in detecting populations of neoplastic cells.

A fourth type of gene mutation also seems to play a major role in carcinogenesis. Recently, mutations in genes that encode components of cell cycle checkpoints have been found to increase genetic instability (35). Hartwell and Kastan (35) recently summarized the evidence for tight control of the passage of cells from one stage of the cell cycle to another. They described a model in which activation of cyclin–cyclin dependent kinase complexes are required for progression to the next step of the cell cycle. Mutation of genes that control the activation of these complexes may result in loss of checkpoint function. For example, progression from G1 into the S phase requires Rb protein and may be partially dependent on p53 and probably requires p16 (35).

Roth et al. (44) suggest that an informative marker of carcinogenesis should have several characteristics (Table 5B.1): (a) the presence of the marker should be associated with the subsequent development of the cancer; (b) expression of changes in the marker, i.e., mutations, should proceed frankly malignant morphology in the neoplastic cells; and (c) the mutations expressed in the premalignant specimens should be preserved clonally in the tumor. Validation of new markers of carcinogenesis thus requires recognition of those markers in premalignant specimens from individuals who later develop cancer, and the absence of the markers in premalignant specimens from those who remain cancer free (45). Several of these markers of carcinogenesis are now detectable in the premalignant sputum. Serial sputum specimens from high-risk populations followed by examination of subsequently resected tumor offer an ideal opportunity to detect whether molecular markers of carcinogenesis are indeed predictive of lung cancer.

The pertinent question remains whether the airway can be adequately sampled by examination of sputum for exfoliated epithelial cells. The surface area of the adult pulmonary epithelium is similar in size to that of a tennis court. The cellular monolayer examined on a glass slide covers only a few square centimeters. The concept of field carcinogenesis is particularly useful when considering sampling of the epithelium. In the early 1950s, Slaughter and coworkers (46) suggested that the common exposure of the (upper) airway to inhaled carcinogens led to multiple areas of neoplastic transformation. Evidence is now accumulating that, in individuals with lung cancer, extensive areas of airways epithelium without evidence of atypia (dysplasia) already manifest evidence of molecular transformation. Hung et al. (47) found deletions in the short arm of chromosome 3 (at 3p14, 3p21.3, and 3p25) in the cells of hyperplastic epithelium from cases of resected non–small cell lung cancer. Thus, although it may not always be possible to sample cells from the clone most advanced toward malignancy, exfoliative cytology clearly has the potential to recognize individuals with an at-risk airways epithelium.

TABLE 5B.1 Carcinogenesis Marker Criteria

Associated with subsequent cancer development.
Marker changes (e.g., mutations) precede malignant morphology in neoplastic cells.
Premalignant mutations are preserved clonally in the tumor.
Absent from those who remain cancer free.

Biologic specimens and data banks have been essential to the validation and refinement of potential markers of carcinogenesis (43, 48, 49). Many of the original JHLP alcohol-preserved sputum slurries and paraffin-embedded tumor blocks are still available for the development of novel lung cancer screening techniques. A second specimen archive was established recently at the Yunnan Tin Corporation in the Peoples Republic of China. This renewable lung cancer specimen bank is a collaborative project initiated among Yunnan tin miners by the NCI/Division of Cancer Prevention and Control (DCPC) Cancer Prevention Studies Branch, the Yunnan Tin Corporation, and the Johns Hopkins School of Hygiene and Public Health. It seems clear that these prospectively collected, banked specimens, and follow-up tumor specimens, represent rare resources that, like those from the JHLP, can be used to validate a variety of markers and develop optimal lung cancer screening strategies.

The importance of banking the carefully obtained, serial, premalignant specimens from a high-risk population along with specimens of subsequent tumors cannot be overstated. The genetic instability of cells undergoing malignant transformation leads to a plethora of mutational events preserved in the genome of neoplastic daughter cells. Those events, which arise early in carcinogenesis and are preserved in the final tumor, have the greatest potential as early biomarkers of neoplastic progression. In contrast, if only tumor tissue were available to provide mutational clues (as in comparisons of marker expression in cancer with that of nearby normal lung), arbitrary selection of possibly late-developing events could lead to misdirected screening efforts. Similarly, if only sputum were available (as in comparisons of marker expression in specimens from smokers and nonsmokers), markers of the genetic lesions that might later be repaired (for example, during the $p53$-directed G1 growth arrest [50]) would serve as a smoking dosimeter, not a measure of cancer risk. Several brief examples of lung cancer biomarkers validated through the JHLP archive serve as illustrations.

Applying two monoclonal antibodies (MABs) originally developed against small cell and non–small cell lung cancer (51, 52), investigators from the NCI–Johns Hopkins study (the JHLP) immunostained archived specimens and found that in subjects with moderate atypical metaplasia, these MABs(to a 31 kD tumor-associated cell surface antigen and a di-fucosylated Lewis-X differentiation antigen, respectively) can recognize epitope expression on banked sputum cells 2 years (on average) before clinical development of lung cancer (48). These antibodies could predict the later development of lung cancer with a sensitivity of 91% and a specificity of 88%. A follow-up study confirmed that dual-wavelength–transmitted light image cytometry with MAB staining can distinguish premalignant sputum cells from morphologically similar cells in normal individuals with an 87% accuracy in a blinded analysis (53). A prospective, collaborative, Eastern Cooperative Oncology Group (ECOG)/Southwest Oncology Group (SWOG) clinical trial is currently underway that tests the efficacy of these MABs compared with routine Papanicolaou staining of sputum in individuals at high risk for developing a second primary lung cancer after complete resection of their original primary (stage I non–small cell) lung cancer (54).

The revolution in molecular genetic techniques has made possible the identification of mutant genes in human tumors (55). Following the model provided by studies of colon cancer, most solid tumors are now thought to progress through successive well-defined clinical and histopathologic stages, wherein a series of genetic changes (carcinogenesis) including activation of protooncogenes and inactivation of several tumor suppressor genes, leads to tumor progression (56). With specific respect to lung cancer, the archived JHLP material was used to show that three complementary approaches to the detection of molecular lesions in lung tumors also can distinguish identical DNA alterations in associated premalignant sputum specimens (43, 48, 49). These studies first determined that DNA expressing specific mutations (*ras* and *p53*) from lung tumors can be shed into sputum (49). Secondly, loss of heterozygosity *p16* and *p53* has been found in premalignant tissue (57); and finally, a rapid, sensitive, and specific test for microsatellite alterations detects "clonal markers" indicating the presence of neoplasia in sputum (43).

Briefly, progress in tumor biology indicates that sampling the cells of the epithelium at risk is the appropriate strategy for the early detection of solid tissue (epithelial) tumors. Theoretically, even small early lung tumors can shed tumor cells into the airways. Presumably, these cells would be rare and degraded to some degree at expectoration. These factors might be more pronounced when the tumor arose in the small distal airways, and they may partly explain the low detection of these exfoliated epithelial cells by conventional methods. However, even degraded DNA can be amplified by recently developed, PCR-based techniques to identify one cell carrying a mutant gene among a large excess (greater than 10,000) of normal cells (30).

The specific mutations in p53 have been well characterized and are clustered in specific "hot spots" in lung cancer (58). Likewise, mutations of K-*ras* occur almost entirely in conserved codons 12 and 13, allowing rapid identification of these mutations. In a pilot study of archived JHLP material, researchers identified *p53* and *ras* gene mutations were identified in the sputum of patients who later manifested adenocarcinoma of the lung (48). Adenocarcinomas were chosen because these tumors have a higher incidence of K-*ras* mutations (30%) than other lung tumors (59). Sequence analysis of the PCR products from the two target genes in 15 patients identified 10 primary tumors that contained either a K-*ras* (codon 12) or a *p53* (codons 273 or 281) mutation. All of the available corresponding sputum samples from these patients were analyzed by a PCR-based assay that can detect one mutant-containing cell among an excess background of 10,000 normal cells (30). Using this assay neoplastic cells in previously "negative" cytologic sputum samples were detected from 8 of the 10 patients who had tumors containing oncogene mutations. None of the 5 cases without tumor mutation expressed mutant DNA in the sputum.

The pattern of allelic loss on chromosome 9 has been described recently in freshly resected tumor from 40 primary human non–small cell lung cancers including 16 squamous cell, 18 adenocarcinomas, and 6 large cell carcinomas (57). Using 24 polymorphic microsatellite markers spanning chromosome 9, 27 (67.5%) of 40 neoplasms displayed loss of heterozygosity. Five tumors delineated a minimal area of loss at 9p21-22, which includes the p16 tumor suppressor gene locus. The accuracy of the analysis for allelic loss depends critically on the quality of tumor specimens being analyzed. The identification, enrichment, and separation of exfoliated epithelial cells undergoing carcinogenesis from the heterogenous cellular and mucoid sputum have been a formidable challenge. Recently, this challenge has been met by mucus sulfhydryl bond disruption using dithiothreitol and microfiltration, which yields a separation of sputum cellular elements from mucus glycoprotein (60).

After screening 100 tumors with a panel of nine trinucleotide and tetranucleotide repeat markers (microsatellites), 26 (26%) were identified that displayed alterations in at least one locus (43). This high frequency of microsatellite alterations suggests that certain loci may be inherently more unstable than others (61) The mechanism producing the altered alleles is likely to differ from the mutated mismatch repair gene underlying nonpolyposis colorectal cancer tumors and remains unknown. However, monoclonality is a fundamental characteristic of all neoplasms, and the detection of a clonal cell population in archived premalignant JHLP cytologic samples indicates great biomarker potential for this technique. The ability to combine these microsatellite markers is a major advantage in the ability to eventually screen for cancer with one rapid PCR reaction (62). The current interpretation of gene marker and immunocytochemical data, which have shown detection of specific mutations, microsatellite alterations, and p31 antigen expression in premalignant sputum, is shown in the lung cancer progression model (Fig. 5B.1).

This model has been developed to test the expression and timing of several promising markers in prospectively collected, banked, population-based screening specimens. Preliminary (as yet unpublished) data have shown MAB recognition of p31 expression in the presence of no morphologic abnormality in exfoliated epithelial cells collected from 56 individuals at risk of developing a second primary lung cancer. This expression may be the earliest change detectable in an epithelium destined to become neoplastic. Hung et al. (47) have demonstrated dinucleotide repeat polymorphisms at three chromosome 3p loci (3p14, 3p21.3, and 3p25) at sites in uninvolved airways in which epithelial hyperplasia was the only morphologic abnormality in seven patients who underwent surgical resection for localized lung cancer. In moderately atypical sputum specimens preserved during the JHLP, K-*ras* and p53 mutations first identified in resected tumor were found after PCR amplification and hybridization. p16 Mutations, found with high frequency in lung cancer tumor specimens, have not yet been sought systematically in the premalignant sputum.

In summary, the advances of cellular and molecular biology have been applied to the banked premalignant sputum and paired tumor specimens collected and preserved during population screening of the JHLP. The value of such an archive has been demonstrated by the development of specific mutations, allelic loss, and microsatellite alterations that have been tested as early markers of lung carcinogenesis. Two prospective studies now underway will refine and improve the lung cancer progression model (Fig. 5B.1) as researchers draw nearer to the time when markers of lung carcinogenesis might become available for early lung cancer detection in high-risk individuals.

Acknowledgment

The author acknowledges the support provided by the National Cancer Institute (Grants N01-CN-25420 and 1P50-CA58184).

References

1. Boring CC, Squires TS, Tong T. Cancer statistics, 1993. CA Cancer J Clin 1993;43:7–26.
2. Mountain CF. Assessment of the role of surgery for control of lung cancer. Ann Thorac Surg 1977;24:365–373.
3. Epstein DM. The role of radiologic screening in lung cancer. Radiol Clin North Am 1990;28:489–495.
4. Berlin NI, Buncher CR, Fontana RS, Frost JK, Melamed MR. The National Cancer Institute cooperative early lung cancer detection program. Am Rev Respir Dis 1984;130:545–549.
5. Frost JK, Ball WC Jr, Levin ML, Tockman MS, Baker RR, Carter D, Eggleston JC, Erozan YS, et al. Early lung cancer detection: results of the initial (prevalence) radiologic and cytologic screening in the Johns Hopkins study. Am Rev Respir Dis 1984;130:549–554.
6. Flehinger BJ, Melamed MD, Zaman MB, et al. Early lung cancer detection: results of the initial (prevalence) radiologic and cytologic screen in the Memorial Sloan–Kettering study. Am Rev Respir Dis 1984;130:555–560.
7. Fontana RS, Sanderson DR, Taylor WF, et al. Early lung cancer detection: results of the initial (prevalence) radiologic and cytologic screening in the Mayo Clinic study. Am Rev Respir Dis 1984;130:561–565.
8. Saccomanno G, Archer VE, Auerbach O, Saunders RP, Brennan LM. Development of carcinoma of the lung as reflected in exfoliated cells. Cancer 1974;33:256–270.
9. Tockman MS. Survival and mortality from lung cancer in a screened population—the Johns Hopkins Study. Chest 1986;89:324S–325S.
10. Baltimore City Bureau of Biostatistics. Annual vital statistics report for Baltimore, Maryland—1980. Baltimore: Baltimore City Health Department, 1980.
11. U.S. Bureau of the Census. 1980 Census of population. Characteristics of the population. General population characteristics. Part 22, Maryland. US Department of Commerce. Washington, DC: U.S. Government Printing Office, Document PC80-1-B22, 1982;1.

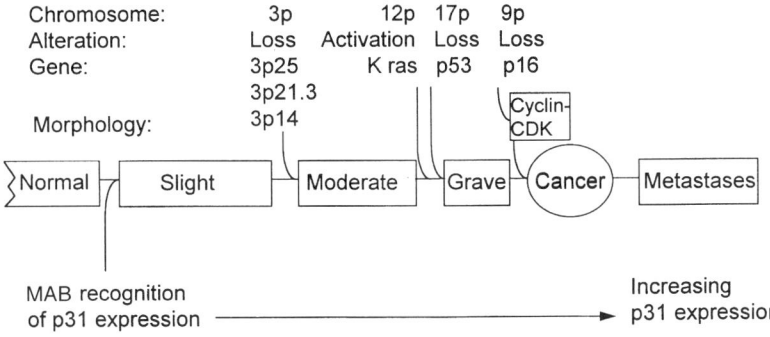

FIGURE 5B.1. This lung cancer progression model diagrams the current interpretation of gene markers and immunocytochemical data, which have shown detection of specific mutations, microsatellite alterations, and p31 antigen expression in premalignant sputum.

12. Frost JK, Ball WC Jr, Levin ML, Tockman MS. Final report: lung cancer control, detection and therapy, phase II. Washington, DC: National Cancer Institute, Publication No (PHS) N01-CN-45037, 1984.
13. Tockman MS, Levin ML, Frost JK, Ball WC Jr, Stitik FP, Marsh BR. Screening and detection of lung cancer. In: Aisner J, ed. Lung cancer. New York: Churchill Livingstone, 1985:25–40.
14. Stitik FP, Tockman, MS, Khoury NF. Chest radiology. In: Miller AB, ed. Screening for Cancer. San Diego: Academic Press, 1985: 163–199.
15. Frost JK, Fontana RS, Melamed MD, et al. Early lung cancer detection: summary and conclusions. Am Rev Respir Dis 1984;130: 565–570.
16. Frost JK, Ball WC Jr, Levin ML, Tockman MS, Erozan YS, Gupta PK, Eggleston JC, et al. Sputum cytopathology: use and potential in monitoring the workplace environment by screening for biological effects of exposure. J Occup Med 1986;28:692–703.
17. Mulshine JL, Tockman MS, Smart CR. Considerations in the development of lung cancer screening tools. J Natl Cancer Inst 1989;81:900–906.
18. Prorok PC, Connor RJ. Screening for the early detection of cancer. Cancer Invest 1986;4(3):225–238.
19. Kubik A, Parkin DM, Khlat M, Erban J, Polak J, Adamec M. Lack of benefit from semi-annual screening for cancer of the lung: follow-up report of a randomized controlled trial on a population of high-risk males in Czechoslovakia. Int J Cancer 1990;45:26–33.
20. Mulshine JL, Tockman MS. Early detection of lung cancer: Where are we? In: DeVita VT, Hellman S, Rosenberg SA, eds. Cancer prevention. Philadelphia: Lippincott, 1991:1–8.
21. Sporn MB. Carcinogenesis and cancer: different perspectives on the same disease. Cancer Res 1991;51:6215–6218.
22. Bishop JM. The molecular genetics of cancer. Science 1987;235: 305–311.
23. Feig LA. The many roads that lead to *ras*. Science 1993;260: 767–768.
24. Knudson AG. Mutation and cancer: statistical study of retinoblastoma. Proc Natl Acad Sci U S A 1971;68:820–828.
25. Stanbridge EJ. Human tumor suppressor genes. Ann Rev Genet 1990;24:615–657.
26. Takahashi T, Nau MM, Chiba I, Birrer MJ, Rosenberg RK, Vinocour M, Levitt M, et al. *p53*: A frequent target for genetic abnormalities in lung cancer. Science 1989;246:491–494.
27. Varley JM, Brammar WJ, Lane DP, Swallow JE, Dolan C, Walker RA. Loss of chromosome 17p13 sequences and mutation of *p53* in human breast carcinomas. Oncogene 1991;6:413–421.
28. Hollstein MC, Metalf RA, Welsh JA, Montesano R, Harris CC. Frequent mutation of the *p53* gene in human esophageal cancer. Proc Natl Acad Sci U S A 1990;87:9958–9961.
29. Bressac B, Kew M, Wands J, Ozturk M. Selective G to T mutations of p53 gene in hepatocellular carcinoma from Southern Africa. Nature 1991;350:429–431.
30. Sidransky D, Von Eschenbach A, Tsai YC, Jones P, Summerhaven I, Marshall F, Paul M, et al. Identification of *p53* gene mutations in bladder cancers and urine samples. Science 1991;252: 706–709.
31. Marks JR, Davidoff AM, Kerns BJ, Humphrey PA, Pence JC, Dodge RK, Clarke-Pearson DL, et al. Overexpression and mutation of *p53* in epithelial ovarian cancer. Cancer Res 1991;51: 2979–2984.
32. Sidransky D, Mikkelsen T, Schwechheimer K, Rosenblum ML, Cavanee W, Vogelstein B. Clonal expansion of *p53* mutant cells is associated with brain tumour progression. Nature 1992;355: 846–47.
33. Nigro JM, Baker S, Preisinger AC, Jessup JM, Hostetter R, Cleary K, Bigner SH, et al. Mutations in the *p53* gene occur in diverse human tumour types. Nature 1989;342:705–708.
34. Hollstein M, Sidransky D, Vogelstein B, Harris CC. *p53* Mutations in human cancers. Science 1991;253:49–53.
35. Hartwell LH, Kastan MB. Cell cycle control and cancer. Science 1994;266:1821–1828.
36. Loeb LA. Mutator phenotype may be required for multistage carcinogenesis. Cancer Res 1991;51:3075–3079.
37. Strand M, Prolla TA, Liskay RM, Petes T. Destabilization of tracts of simple repetitive DNA in yeast by mutations affecting DNA mismatch repair. Nature 1993;365:274–276.
38. Modrich P. Mismatch repair, genetic stability and cancer. Science 1994;266:1959–1960.
39. Leach FS, Nicolaides NC, Papadopoulos N, Kiu B, Jen J, Parsons R, Peltomaki P, et al. Mutations of a mutS homolog in hereditary nonpolyposis colorectal cancer. Cell 1993;75:1215–1225.
40. Fishel R, Lescoe MK, Rao MRS, Copeland NG, Jenkins NA, Garber J, Kane M, et al. The human mutator gene homolog MSH2 and its association with hereditary nonpolyposis colon cancer. Cell 1993;75:1027–1038.
41. Papadoppoulos N, Nicholaides NC, Wei YF, Ruben SM, Carter KC, Rosen CA, Haseltine WA, et al. Mutation of a mutL homolog in hereditary colon cancer. Science 1994;263:1825–1828.
42. Bronner CE, Baker SM, Morrison PT, Warren G, Smith LG, Loescoe MK, Kane M, et al. Mutation in the DNA mismatch repair gene homologue hMLH1 is associated with hereditary non-polyposis colon cancer. Nature 1994;368:258.
43. Mao L, Lee DJ, Tockman MS, Erozan YS, Askin F, Sidransky D. Microsatellite alterations as clonal markers in the detection of human cancer. Proc Natl Acad Sci U S A 1994;91:9871–9875.
44. Roth JA, Mukhopadhyay T, Casson AG, Chung KY. Molecular strategies for early detection, prevention, and therapy. In: Srivastava S, Lippman SM, Hong WK, Mulshine JL, eds. Early detection of cancer: molecular markers. Armonk: Futura, 1994:45–52.
45. Tockman MS, Gupta PK, Pressman NJ, Mulshine JL. Biomarkers of pulmonary disease. In: Schulte P, Perera F, eds. Molecular epidemiology: principles and practices.San Diego: Academic Press, 1992.
46. Slaughter DP, Southwick HW, Smejkal W. "Field cancerization" in oral stratified squamous epithelium. Cancer 1953;6:963–968.
47. Hung J, Kishimoto Y, Sugio K, Virmani A, McIntire, Minna JD, Gazdar AF. Allele-specific chromosome 3p deletions occur at an early stage in the pathogenesis of lung carcinoma. JAMA 1995;273:558–563.
48. Tockman MS, Gupta PK, Myers JD, Frost JK, Baylin SB, Gold EB, Chase AM, et al. Sensitive and specific monoclonal antibody recognition of human lung cancer antigen on preserved sputum cells: a new approach to early lung cancer detection. J Clin Oncol 1988;6:1685–1693.
49. Mao L, Hruban RH, Boyle JO, Tockman MS, Sidransky D. Detection of oncogene mutations in sputum precedes diagnosis of lung cancer. Cancer Res 1994;54:1634–1637.
50. Harris CC. *p53*: At the crossroads of molecular carcinogenesis and risk assessment. Science 1993;262:1980–1981.
51. Mulshine JL, Cuttitta F, Bibro M, Fedorko J, Fargion S, Little C, Carney DN, et al. Monoclonal antibodies that distinguish non–small cell from small cell lung cancer. J Immunol 1983;131:497–502.
52. Rosen ST, Mulshine JL, Cuttitta F, et al. Analysis of human small cell lung cancer differentiation antigens using a panel of rat monoclonal antibodies. Cancer Res 1984;44:2052–2061.
53. Tockman MS, Gupta PK, Pressman NJ, Mulshine JL. Cytometric

validation of immunocytochemical observations in developing lung cancer. Diagn Cytopathol 1993;9:615–622.
54. Tockman MS, Erozan YS, Gupta PK, Piantadosi S, Mulshine JL, Ruckdeschel JC, and the LCEDWG Investigators. The early detection of second primary lung cancers by sputum immunostaining. Chest 1994;106:385S–390S.
55. Bishop JM. Molecular themes in oncogenesis. Cell 1991;64(2): 235–248.
56. Vogelstein B, Fearon ER, Hamilton SR, Kern SE, Preisinger AC, Leppert M, Nakamura Y, et al. Genetic alterations during colorectal-tumor development. N Engl J Med 1988;319(9):525–532.
57. Merlo A, Gabrielson E, Askin F, Sidransky D. Frequent loss of chromosome 9 in human primary non–small cell lung cancer. Cancer Res 1994;54:640–642.
58. Chiba I, Takahashi T, Nau MM, D'Amico D, Curiel DT, Mitsudomi T, Buchhagen DL, et al. Mutations in the *p53* gene are frequent in primary, resected non–small cell lung cancer. Oncogene 1990;5:1603–1610.
59. Rodenhuis S, Slebos RJ, Boot AJ, Evers SG, Mooj WJ, Wagenaar SS, Van Bodegom PC, et al. Incidence and possible clinical significance of K-*ras* oncogene activation in adenocarcinoma of the human lung. Cancer Res 1988;48:5738–5741.
60. Tockman MS, Qiao YL, Li L, Zhao GZ, Sharma R, Cavenaugh L, et al. Safe separation of sputum cells from mucoid glycoprotein. Acta Cytol 1996: in press.
61. Weber JL, Wong C. Mutation of human short tandem repeats. Hum Mol Genet 1993;2:1123–1128.
62. Cairns P, Tokino K, Eby Y, Sidransky D. Homozygous deletions of 9p21 in primary human bladder tumors detected by comparative multiplex polymerase chain reaction. Cancer Res 1994;54: 1422–1424.

6

IMAGING OF THORACIC NEOPLASMS

Robert T. Heelan and Steven Larson

The ability to obtain accurate images of intrathoracic pathology, particularly neoplasms, has taken rapid strides in the past several decades. Chest radiography has been widely used since the beginning of the century. The gas density contained within the lung provides an optimal natural tissue contrast to pathologic processes, whether inflammatory or neoplastic, which tend to occupy air space. Abnormalities within the mediastinum and chest wall are more difficult to evaluate with plain chest radiography. The introduction of computed tomography (CT) in the mid-1970s permitted better differentiation of various soft tissue structures within the thorax, particularly with the use of intravenous contrast material. The slices or tomographic images were obtained by using computed reconstruction techniques. More recently, magnetic resonance imaging (MRI), which uses a completely different series of physical principles and interactions but similar computed reconstruction techniques, allowed imaging of the entire body including the thorax in various planes with great contrast sensitivity. Compared with CT whole body MRI, however, is more expensive and somewhat more cumbersome to perform. Also, MRI has the added disadvantage that 5% to 7% of patients are claustrophobic and thus unable to complete the scan. Ultrasonography, because of the large amount of air contained within the thorax, which acts as a barrier to the ultrasound beam, is largely limited to transthoracic evaluation of the heart and pericardium as well as to endoluminal ultrasonography studies.

Nuclear medicine uses radiotracers to study the function of specific human tissues. Medical applications within the thorax include detecting the presence of tumor and monitoring the effects of treatment. In addition, the physiology of normal tissue such as the heart and lungs may be studied. A list of radiopharmaceutical agents for the clinical study of intrathoracic organs is listed in Table 6.1. The test information is collected using radioactivity detectors that convert the radioactive decay detected into images of the function of specific organs or tissues. Advances in instrumentation permit high-resolution images that are usually collected as a digital image in a specialized computer. The workhorse clinical imaging instrument for nuclear medicine is the gamma camera; it is available virtually throughout the world. Single photon emission computed tomography (SPECT) is a technique in which the three-dimensional (3D) distribution of radioactivity in the body is imaged by rotating the standard gamma camera around the patient and reconstructing the images using techniques similar to those for CT.

Positron emission tomography (PET) is the highest resolution and most sensitive of all these nuclear medicine imaging methods. PET provides 3D images of in vivo radiotracer distribution that can be used to measure specific biochemical properties of living tissues, such as glycolysis. Technical advances in nuclear medicine instrumentation have been rapid in the last decade, and the interested reader is referred to more comprehensive reviews (1).

The issue of cost and efficacy has become increasingly important with the proliferation of available imaging studies creating some confusion concerning indications and utility in specific circumstances. This chapter addresses these issues in several neoplastic conditions. The goal of medical imaging is to achieve maximum diagnostic information, either for staging or for follow-up, at minimum cost. Needless duplication of imaging examinations offering identical or similar information should be avoided. However, some examinations provide important complementary information, such as CT and advanced nuclear medicine imaging studies designed to detect tumor metabolic activity; in specific instances there is adequate indication for obtaining several studies. Following is a broad outline of the appropriate use of imaging procedures and illustrative examples in the workup and follow-up of neoplasms involving the thorax. More comprehensive,

TABLE 6.1. Radiopharmaceuticals in Common Use for Imaging of Thorax

RADIONUCLIDE	DRUG FORM	PURPOSE	MECHANISM
^{99m}Tc	Phosphonate, e.g., methylene diphosphonate	Bone scanning	Taken up in hydroxyapatite crystal of bone hot spot where tumor involves bone
^{111}In	Octreotide	Lymphoma, SCLC, endocrine tumors	Targets somatostatin receptor
^{99m}Tc	Labeled red blood cells	Blood pool imaging and heart function	Vascular distribution
^{99m}Tc	Antitumor monoclonal antibody	Tumor detection and staging	Antigen binding to cell 43KD protein trapped in the capillaries
^{99m}Tc	Macroaggregated albumin	Lung perfusion scanning	Shows tissue perfusion
^{99m}Tc	Sulfur colloid (in food) citrate	Esophageal and gastric mobility	Transmechanical propulsion: (*a*) protein binding in area of ECF-inflammatory cell uptake; (*b*) *transferrin*-receptor uptake in proliferating tissue
Kr^{81m}	Noble gas	Ventilation studies	Ventilatory kinetics
T^{201}	Chloride	Tissue perfusion Tumor viability	K + analogue "chemical" microsphere glycolysis
^{18}F	2-Fluoro-2-deoxyglucose	Tumor viability Monitor response to treatment	Glycolysis is increased in tumors

technically oriented radiographic reviews are referenced (2–4).

LUNG CANCER

The incidence of lung cancer, a highly lethal malignancy, continues to increase, especially among women, in whom it has replaced breast cancer as the leading cause of cancer death. Cigarette smoking is closely related to lung cancer and other cancers of the aerodigestive tract as well as to an increased incidence of cardiovascular disease and hypertension. Passive smoking, i.e., exposure of family members living in the same house with a smoker or workers exposed to cigarette smoking in the work place, has also been shown to play a lesser role in the etiology of lung cancer (5). Other causative factors such as asbestos exposure and occupational exposure to heavy metals are statistically less important. The incidence of lung cancer in the absence of cigarette smoking would be much reduced, although not eliminated: the incidence of lung cancer would be 10% to 20% of current incidence, almost exclusively the adenocarcinoma cell type. In recent years there appears to have been a leveling or slight decline in male mortality rates from lung cancer that parallels, with a latency of approximately 20 years, a decrease in cigarette consumption beginning in the early 1970s (6).

The histologic classification of lung cancer is given in Chapter 10. From clinical and imaging viewpoints, the importance of the distinction of small cell lung cancer from the other histologic varieties (squamous cell carcinoma, adenocarcinoma, including bronchoalveolar carcinoma, and large cell carcinoma, many of which appear to represent a variety of adenocarcinoma) needs to be emphasized.

SMALL CELL LUNG CANCER

Small cell lung cancer (SCLC), which constitutes approximately 15% and 20% of primary lung neoplasms, is highly lethal and behaves in a manner distinctly different from the other varieties of lung cancer. At presentation the tumor is almost always large and diffuse with multiple regional sites of bulky metastatic disease (Fig. 6.1) as well as distant metastatic disease (e.g., brain, bone marrow). This presentation is not amenable to surgical therapy, and the first line of therapeutic intervention is by chemotherapy with radiation therapy for limited disease. Imaging studies are useful insofaras they permit the distinction of limited-stage SCLC (the entire clinically apparent tumor can be encompassed in a single radiation port) and diffuse SCLC (the involved region cannot be encompassed in a single radiation port) (7). The presence of limited SCLC suggests the possibility of treatment by radiation therapy in addition to chemotherapy because of the fact that the entire tumor volume can be encompassed in a single radiation port. The imaging workup includes CT of the chest, CT or MRI of the brain, and bone scanning. The purpose of these imaging studies is to uncover more extensive disease in a patient thought on plain chest radiography to have limited stage.

In patients with SCLC, the bone scan is a sensitive tool for distinguishing limited from extensive tumor involvement. For this reason, the technetium-

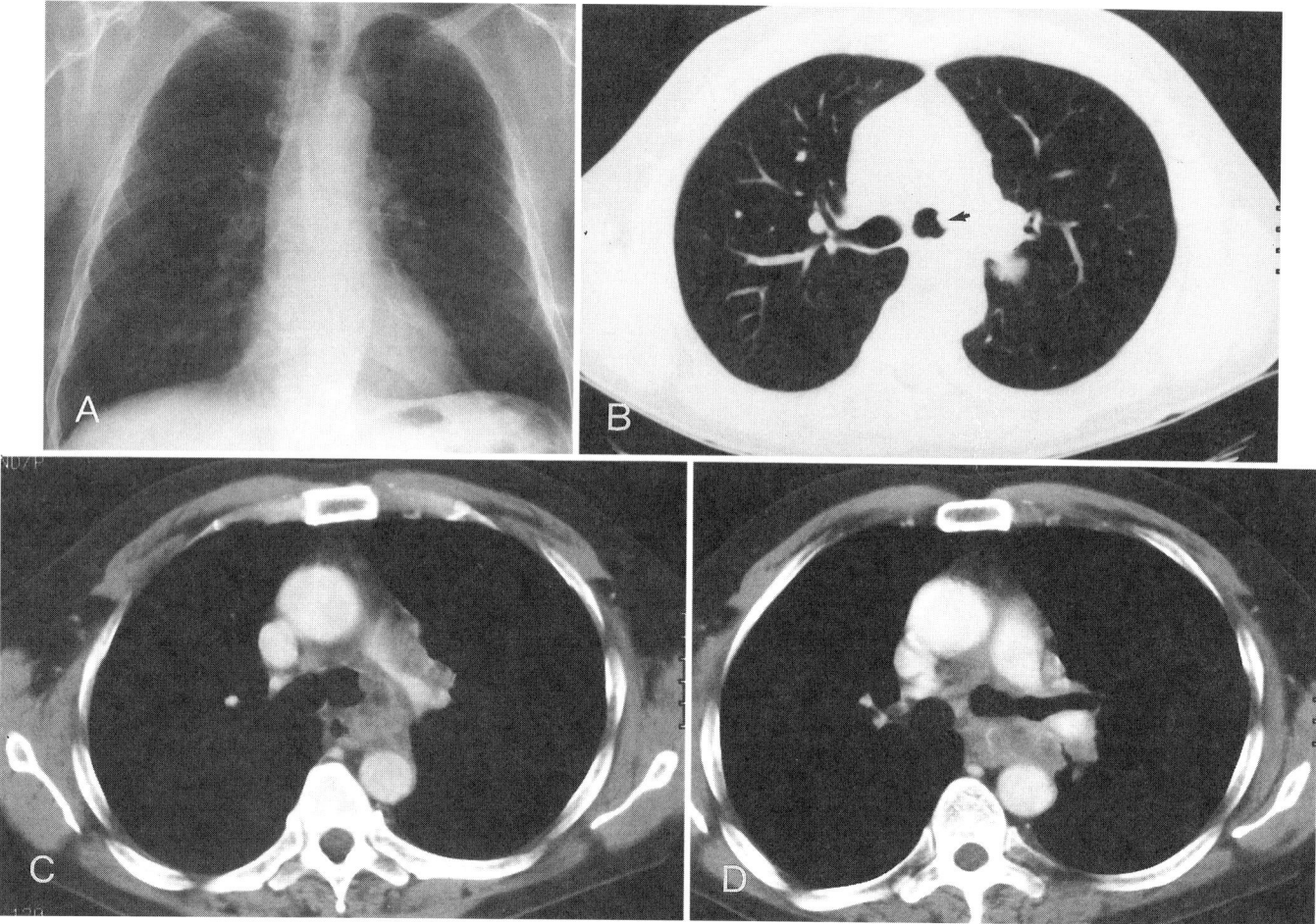

FIGURE 6.1. Small cell lung cancer. A. Posteroanterior (PA) chest radiograph. The peripheral lungs appear clear. The only abnormality that can be detected is a possible slight prominence of the left hilar region. B. CT scan through the tracheal carina region imaged with lung windows. Again, the peripheral lungs appear clear. The soft tissues of the mediastinum and hilar regions are not evaluated on this study. Note, however, the lobular mass density within the lateral aspect of the left main bronchus (*arrow*). This represents tumor invading the bronchial wall in this region. C. and D. CT scans obtained with soft-tissue windows just below the level of the tracheal carina. Note the extensive infiltrative mediastinal and hilar involvement by tumor in this small cell lung cancer. The lymph node involvement in the mediastinum is not bound by lymph node capsules but has extended beyond the capsules, infiltrating mediastinal adipose tissue. Multiple mediastinal structures are either partially or wholly encased by tumor, including the left main pulmonary artery, the carina, and left main stem bronchus. There may be partial encasement of the esophagus and the descending thoracic aorta. Note the absence of a fat plane between the mediastinal tumor and the descending thoracic aorta.

99m (^{99m}Tc) bone scan was included as one of the standard tests for staging SCLC patients in the U.S. Veterans Administration cooperative group study of lung cancer (8). The technique is generally considered comparable in sensitivity to MRI for detecting involvement of the bony skeleton in SCLC. Both bone scan and MRI can detect more lesions than iliac crest bone marrow biopsy. MRI can detect smaller lesions in the spine and pelvis, whereas bone scanning is more accurate in the ribs, skull, and extremities. For this reason, MRI may be used to confirm lesions in the spine or pelvis that are suspicious on bone scanning (9). Bone scans are also useful for monitoring patient response to therapy.

A variety of monoclonal antibodies have been proposed for imaging of lung cancer. The greatest success for the antibody ^{99m}Tc–NRLU-10 appears to be in SCLC. It was as effective in distinguishing limited from extensive disease as a standard workup, which included CT, bone scan, and laboratory testing (10).

Limited SCLC carries a better prognosis than the extensive stage. Although the imaging appearance of SCLC is grouped with that of non–SCLC, it should be noted that the imaging workup and follow-up may differ in important details, insofaras the staging system for SCLC is considerably simpler than that of non–SCLC. Treatment of limited SCLC is most frequently a combination of radiation and chemotherapy, and 5-year survival is approximately 20%. Occasionally, SCLC may present as a small peripheral lung nodule without hilar, mediastinal, or distant spread; these nodules are frequently resected. A number of cures have been reported with this unusual presentation of SCLC in which the disease has not yet spread to the regional lymph nodes.

NON–SMALL CELL LUNG CANCER

The remaining common histologic varieties of lung cancer—adenocarcinoma, squamous cell carcinoma, large cell carcinoma, including several subtypes—behave as a group in a biologically similar fashion and respond similarly to therapeutic intervention, whether surgery, chemotherapy, or radiation therapy. These tumors account for approximately 85% of all lung cancers. The newer staging system for non–small cell lung cancer (NSCLC) is presented in Chapter 12. The therapeutic approach to these tumors depends in large measure on the clinical stage at presentation. This, in turn, depends on the findings of a complete imaging workup, as well as on more invasive modalities as required, e.g., percutaneous lung biopsy, bronchoscopy, mediastinoscopy, and video-assisted thoracoscopic surgery.

In general, cure of NSCLC can be achieved only by complete surgical resection; the possibility of surgical resection, in turn, depends on the stage of the tumor at presentation. T1 and T2 as well as N1 tumors are considered resectable. T3 tumors extending into the mediastinal structures or chest wall are also considered potentially resectable. The resectability of these tumors depends on the extent of the T3 disease. For example, a peripheral lung cancer that extends through the parietal pleura into the superficial tissues of the chest wall may well be resectable (Figs. 6.2 and 6.3). A T3 lesion involving a large area of chest wall or extending through the entire thickness of the chest wall to the subcutaneous region even though representing T3 disease, is usually considered unresectable. Similarly, N2 disease, i.e., the presence of ipsilateral tumor containing lymph nodes, is considered potentially resectable. However, when there is extensive N2 disease with marked enlargement of mediastinal lymph nodes or extension of tumor beyond the lymph node capsules, resection, practically speaking, may well be impossible. In general, T4 primary tumors as well as N3 or M1 tumor involvement are considered unresectable; these patients are referred for primary chemotherapy and/or radiation therapy, or for investigational protocols.

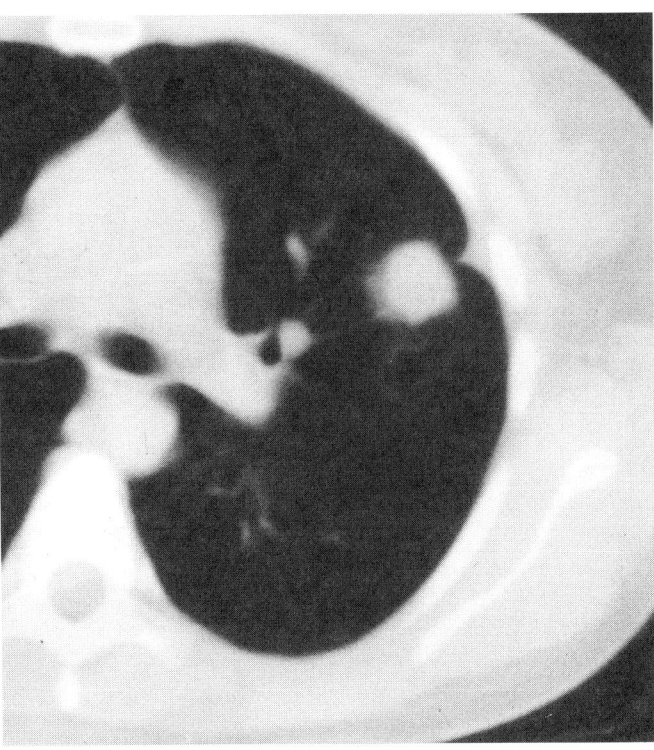

FIGURE 6.2. Non–small cell lung cancer. The CT scan shows a pulmonary nodule that has a well-defined peripheral border and a poorly defined medial border. The nodule was a peripheral adenocarcinoma. Note the triangular-shaped region of tenting extending from the periphery of the tumor to the pleural surface. This appearance frequently indicates a small focus of collapse peripheral to a tumor, or localized pleural reaction or fluid. It is not diagnostic for tumor involvement of the pleura, although this possibility cannot be ruled out.

IMAGING WORKUP OF LUNG CANCER

Imaging is important both in the initial assessment of lung cancer as well as in the follow-up of patients who have been treated with surgery, chemotherapy, or radiation therapy in order to assess response and detect recurrence. In the initial assessment of lung cancer, imaging studies provide a vital piece of information for overall staging management, which in turn determines therapeutic choices.

Lung cancer is a tumor that is generally suspected by the patient's symptoms, rather than initially detected by radiographic means. The latter serve to confirm the presence of a mass and indicate the extent of the disease. Unfortunately, symptomatic lung cancer is frequently a manifestation of advanced lung cancer with patients frequently having extensive regional or distant metastatic disease at the time of presentation. Lung cancer detected during its early, asymptomatic phase is generally an earlier stage cancer and is particularly amenable to effective treatment.

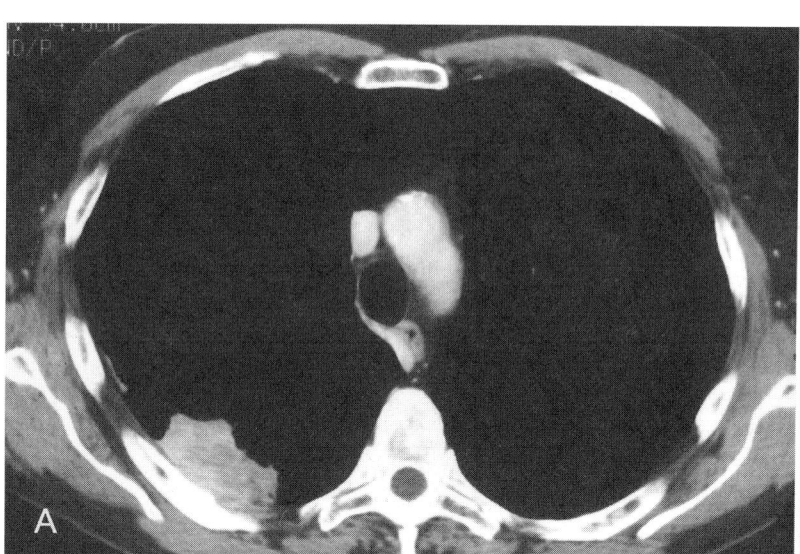 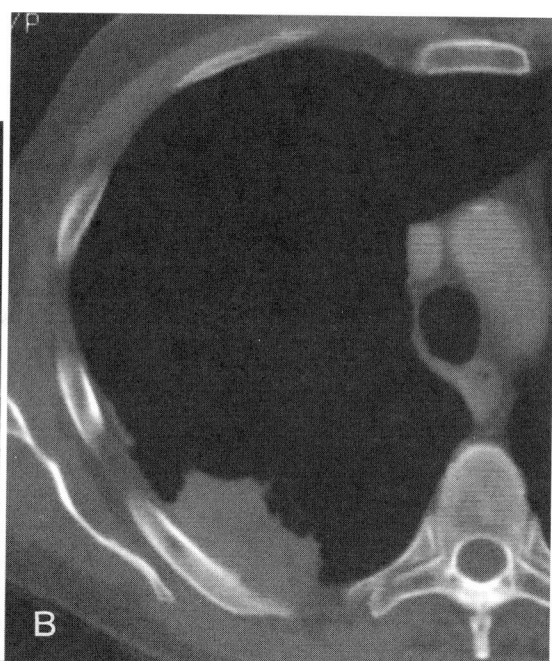

FIGURE 6.3. Non–small cell lung cancer. A. and B. CT scans of the chest at the level of the upper aortic arch. There is a pleural-based tumor situated posteriorly. Note the absence of extrapleural and intercostal adipose tissue that can normally be visualized in other regions (Fig. 6.7B). The tumor directly abuts the rib and, in Figure 6.7B (obtained with bone windows), there are some irregularity and interruption of the normal cortical margin at its interface with the tumor. In addition, in comparing the density of the medullary cavity of this rib to that of the other ribs on this scan, one notes a slight but definite increase in density, suggesting blastic reaction to local tumor infiltration. At surgery, the rib was found to be invaded. The pleural or subpleural linear density lateral to the main tumor mass is of indeterminate histology.

Several lung cancer screening programs, using various forms of periodic chest radiography (some of them accompanied by sputum cytology screening) have been done in the past. The justification for radiographic screening studies has been that detection of lung cancer when the tumor is small and has not yet metastasized regionally results in a greater number of cures if these tumors are treated aggressively (11–13). Comparison with previous normal radiographs also results in greater confidence in the diagnosis of peripheral nodules (14). In general, these studies, especially the most recent cooperative studies (15–17), did not show any advantage in the overall survival of lung cancer as a result of screening with yearly or quarterly chest radiography. Two points deserve mentioning, however: these programs did not compare patients who were screened radiographically with those who were not screened radiographically; also, the results of the screening programs did not disprove the value of chest radiography in early diagnosis of lung cancer but, rather, failed to show a benefit of chest radiography in lung cancer mortality.

Therefore, the utility of yearly screening by chest radiography in patients at high risk for the development of lung cancer has been neither proved nor disproved. However, many clinicians still feel justified in screening high-risk patients with yearly chest radiographs, both for the possibility of detecting early lung cancer and for the evaluation of a variety of other chest diseases to which this population is prone.

The plain chest radiograph is typically the first radiographic examination obtained in patients presenting with symptoms suggesting pulmonary pathology. These symptoms may include cough, shortness of breath, fever, chest pain, and hemoptysis. The threshold for ordering chest radiographs is, in general, considerably lower for cigarette smokers than for nonsmokers for the reasons outlined above. Many of the radiographic findings of lung cancer described originally have been known for many years, but it is helpful to review the most salient plain film features of lung cancer. It should be noted that many of these findings can be transposed to cross-sectional tomographic imaging techniques such as CT, MRI, or even nuclear medicine imaging procedures. The plain radiographic features, as well as the cross-sectional imaging features, reflect the growth of the local tumor as well as invasion of adjacent structures, including lymphatic vessels, lymph nodes, and hematogenous routes of spread (18). The plain radiographic features of lung cancer may be divided somewhat arbitrarily into peripheral and central tumors.

PERIPHERAL LUNG CANCER

Peripheral tumors may present as small, well-defined peripheral nodules or as large masses with irregular borders (Fig. 6.4). In general, the limit of detectability of small peripheral nodules in the lung on plain chest radiography is considered to be 8 to 10 mm. Lung cancers initially grow by local extension, which may be quite irregular, perhaps reflecting growth variations in different regions of the tumor (19). Notching along the tumor edge also is noted frequently. Tumor strands extending into the surrounding lung parenchyma are seen frequently but are shown better on CT (20). The borders of peripheral tumors may show poorly defined edges in as many as 25% of cases (19). In such cases difficulty can be encountered in differentiating the tumor from pneumonia. Peripheral tumors can be associated (to a lesser extent than central tumors) with distal pneumonia or atelectasis. Similarly, tumors in a subpleural location frequently have localized pleural thickening present. Although this thickening may indicate pleural invasion by tumor, just as frequently it is a reactive phenomenon (Fig. 6.2).

All lung cancers may potentially form cavities: overall, approximately 16% of peripheral cancers show cavitation (20–21). Squamous cell cancer cavitates most frequently, with adenocarcinoma and large cell carcinoma cavitating less so. Cavitation in small cell carcinoma is distinctly uncommon. Cavitation may be seen in any size tumor, including fairly small tumors; the walls of the cavitated tumor nodule are typically irregular, especially in larger tumors. The walls of the cavity are usually thick, approaching 1 cm or more (22).

Radiographically visible calcification in peripheral lung cancers is distinctly unusual (Fig. 6.4). Calcification is more frequently shown pathologically and occasionally on CT (22). Diffuse dense calcification or laminated calcification in the central portion of a lung cancer mass is not seen on plain films.

Peripheral nodules increase in size over time, and the rate of increase is highly variable. SCLCs in general grow with great rapidity, particularly in the hilar and mediastinal nodes. Some information about peripheral

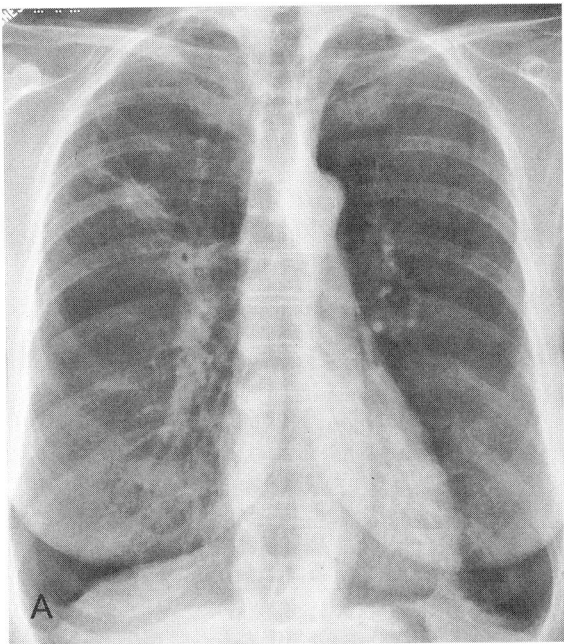
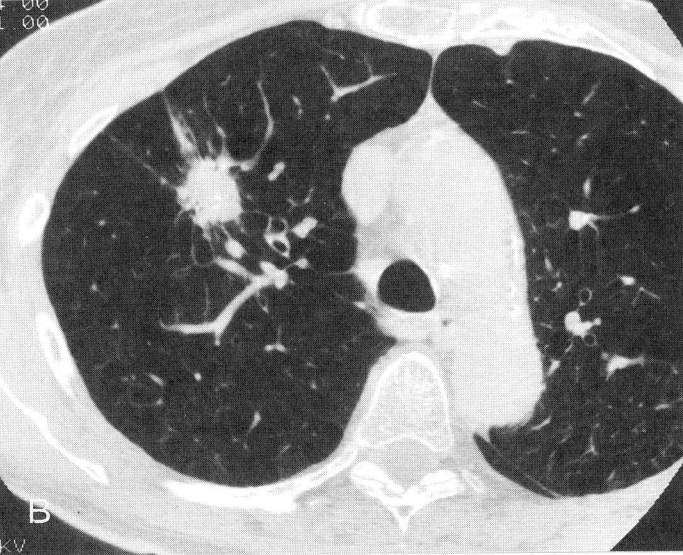

FIGURE 6.4. Malignant solitary pulmonary nodule (SPN). **A.** This chest radiograph shows several features suggesting that the solitary pulmonary nodule in the right upper lung zone is malignant: it is very poorly defined; has dendritic projections extending from its periphery toward the lateral pleura and centrally toward the hilum; and there is a suggestion of faint calcification along its periphery. Such faint calcification, however, does not suggest a diagnosis of benignity in this patient. Lung cancers may calcify, and particularly scar cancers may contain some small foci of eccentric calcification at the site of the original granuloma. **B.** CT scan. A CT scan through the center of the pulmonary nodule shows the small islands of eccentric calcification, the extremely poor definition of the nodule, and its infiltrative extension into surrounding lung parenchyma. There is no obvious mediastinal nodal disease on this scan. Note the extensive bullous change within the lung parenchyma.

tumor growth can be gleaned from the lung cancer screening studies. In several of these studies (23–25), a large percentage of small peripheral lung cancers were missed initially but diagnosed on subsequent screening examinations. When the lung cancer nodule was missed and then subsequently detected on follow-up screening chest radiography, survival was better, indicating that the rate of tumor growth, as well as local and regional spread, was considerably slower in these patients in whom the cancer had been present for a long period. Survival in this group, i.e., those in whom the lung cancer was present but missed on previous screening studies, was considerably better than in those in whom no tumor could be seen in retrospect. The preferred treatment of peripheral lung cancer is lobectomy and mediastinal lymph node dissection; lesser procedures such as wedge resection and segmentectomy result in an increased incidence of local recurrence (26) (Fig. 6.5).

CENTRAL LUNG CANCER

Centrally positioned lung tumors, because of the multiplicity of vital structures that may be involved, can frequently result in secondary imaging findings.

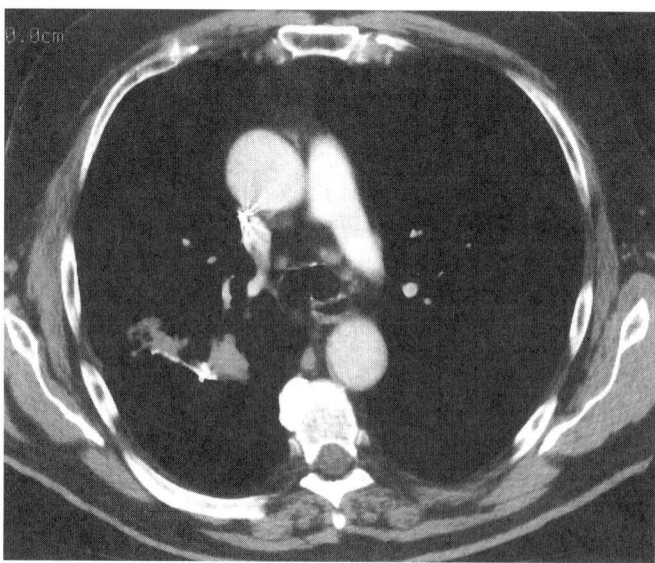

FIGURE 6.5. Lung cancer. CT scan of the mid thorax. This patient had a segmental resection of an adenocarcinoma performed 2 years before the scan. Segmental resection was performed because of poor pulmonary function. The current scan shows recurrent irregular lobular tumor recurrence along the suture line. Lymph nodes present in the mediastinum are not enlarged by measurement. There is artifact in the superior vena cava associated with the presence of a central venous catheter. Segmental resection for lung cancer is associated with an increased incidence of local tumor recurrence, compared with complete lobectomy.

They may, therefore, present a very different plain film radiographic and cross-sectional appearance.

Squamous cell tumors and SCLC commonly present as masses that enlarge the hilum, often to a considerable degree. In the case of a squamous cancer, the enlargement frequently is caused by the primary tumor mass, which slowly invades surrounding structures including multiple lymph nodes in the hilum (Fig. 6.6). In SCLC the hilar mass may be related more to the presence of enlarged hilar lymph nodes than to the primary mass, which may be situated more peripherally and may be quite small.

In a series of studies, the Mayo Clinic group (27–31) found that 38% of patients presenting with lung cancer had a hilar or perihilar mass on plain chest radiography, and in 12% the hilar mass was the only abnormality seen. Occasionally, the hilar mass may be quite small and either not visible on chest radiographs or visible only as a subtle increase in density of the hilus (32) (Fig. 6.1). Sometimes, a mass on posteroanterior chest view that is either anterior or posterior to the hilum may simulate a mass originating from the hilus; however, the normal hilar anatomy can usually be delineated through the mass (Fig. 6.7). The lateral chest view frequently also shows the anterior or posterior origin of the mass.

Lobulation of a hilar mass frequently indicates presence of lymphadenopathy. Frequently, poorly defined masses without lobulation are caused by extensive primary tumor involvement.

One of the more common features of central hilar masses is the presence of obstructing segmental or lobar atelectasis or consolidation (Fig. 6.6). This usually results from central bronchial occlusion by tumor. Occasionally, the irregular narrowing of a major bronchus may be seen on plain chest radiography. More frequently, the patient presents with obstruction of a bronchus and collapse or consolidation of the peripheral portion of the lung that is fed by the bronchus. As may be expected, the incidence of collapse or consolidation is highest with squamous cell carcinoma, being found in more than 50% of patients in one series (28). The incidence of collapse or consolidation with pneumonitis from adenocarcinoma or small cell cancer is considerably lower.

In the collapsed segment of lung, air bronchograms are not usually present, because the bronchi distal to the tumor fill with secretions and debris. The peripheral collapsed lung has a variable appearance: there may be some loss of volume and/or stranding, i.e., linear densities extending from the hilum to the periphery of the lung, resulting from partial collapse. Complete lobar collapse with loss of volume may result

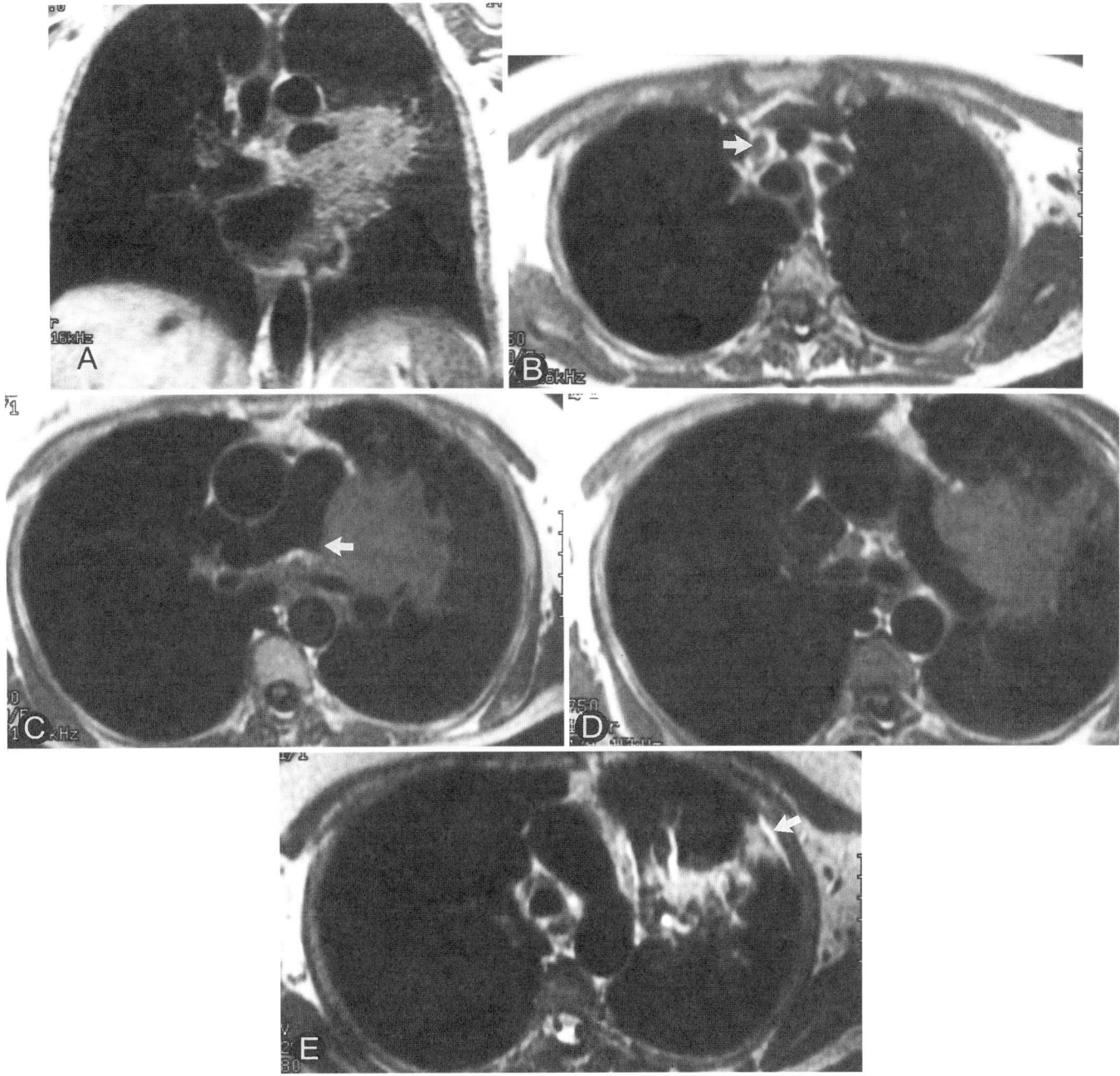

FIGURE 6.6. Squamous lung cancer. Cardiac-gated and respiratory-compensated MRI scans of the chest. **A.** The coronal T1-weighted scan shows an extensive left medial lung central tumor with peripheral infiltrate. The tumor encases the left main pulmonary artery and extensively invades the mediastinum, replacing mediastinal adipose tissue. **B.** Axial T1-weighted MR scan in the upper mediastinum. There is a moderately enlarged lymph node present on the opposite side of the mediastinum (*arrow*) potentially representing contralateral (N3) mediastinal adenopathy. This finding, however, must be confirmed by mediastinoscopy for staging purposes, insofar as lung cancer, particularly large cancers associated with peripheral infiltrate or pneumonia, may have enlarged hyperplastic nodes within the mediastinum that do not contain tumor. **C.** Axial T1-weighted scan through the main pulmonary artery. This large, bulky, hilar tumor is again seen to infiltrate the mediastinum. There is a suggestion on this scan of occlusion of the left main pulmonary artery by tumor (*arrow*). **D.** On a similar scan obtained at a slightly higher level, the left main pulmonary artery is seen to be patent, although encased. The apparent occlusion seen in *C* is an artifact of tomographic sectioning. **E.** T2-weighted scan through the upper lung zones shows some central tumor with peripheral lung infiltrate. The line of demarcation between the tumor and infiltrate is indistinct. In this T2-weighted scan, tumors and inflammatory conditions typically have a bright (*white*) signal. These scans, which have high contrast between normal tissues and tumor (or inflammatory tissue), are obtained at a cost of spatial resolution, resulting in some loss of anatomic detail. Note the bright signal peripheral to the lung infiltrate at the pleural surface (*white arrow*). Again, this appearance is nonspecific, possibly representing local pleural involvement by tumor or reactive change in the pleura without tumor involvement. It does not indicate chest wall invasion by tumor.

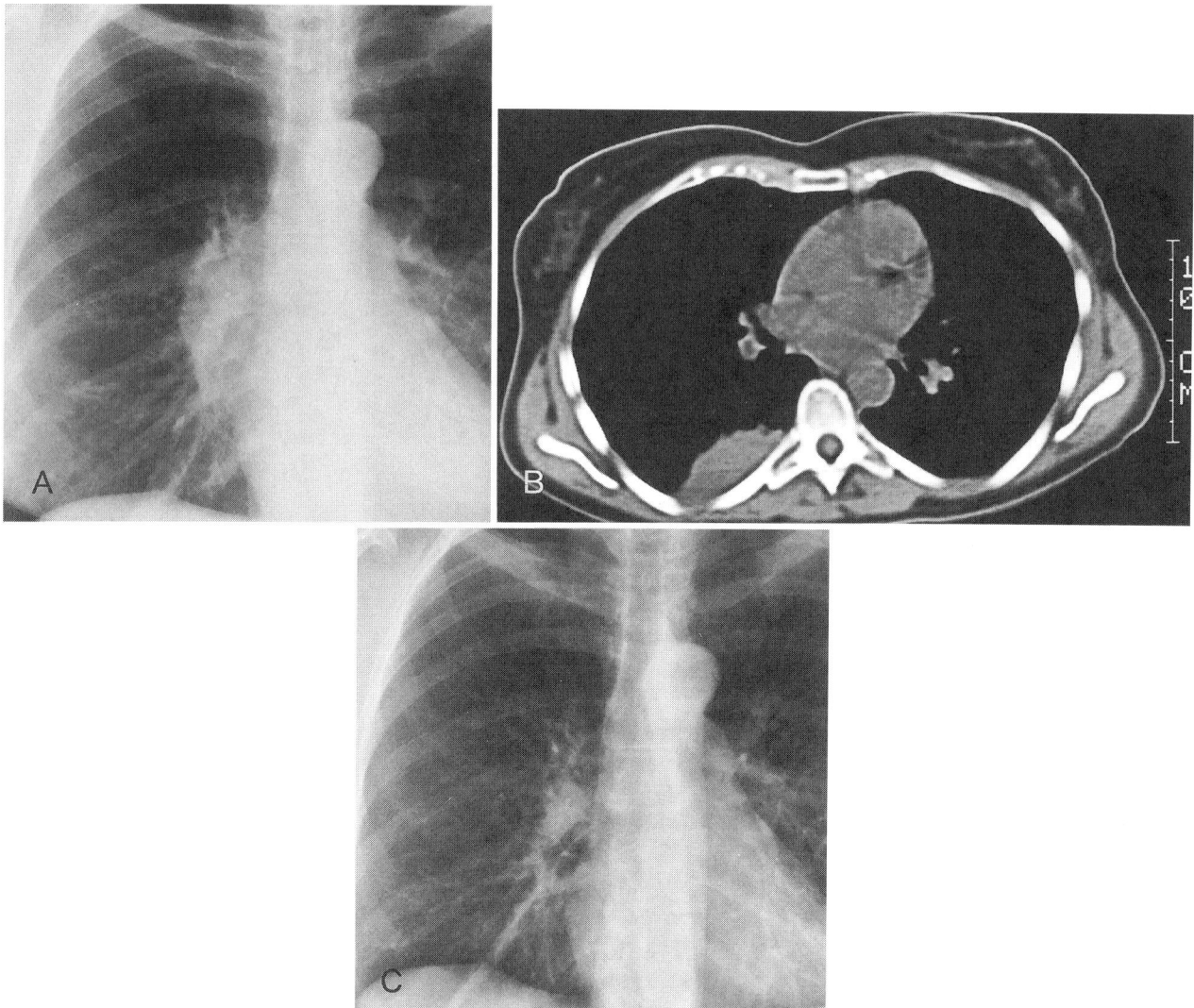

FIGURE 6.7. Non–small cell lung cancer (NSCLC). A. Chest radiograph, view of the right lung. The right hilum is apparently markedly enlarged, suspicious for lung cancer. Note, however, on this PA chest radiograph that the hilar structures can be visualized despite the presence of this mass. This finding indicates that the mass is not in the hilum but rather overlies the hilum on the PA view, either anteriorly or posteriorly. This is a biopsy-proven NSCLC. B. The CT scan obtained at the time of the chest radiograph confirms that this tumor is located in the posteromedial lung field, abutting the posterior pleura. Note the lucent line separating the tumor mass from the rib, suggesting that the tumor has not extended beyond the pleural surface. There is no bony erosion. (Compare this appearance to that shown in Figure 6.3A and B). C. After several courses of combination chemotherapy, the PA chest radiograph has assumed an essentially normal appearance with no evidence of residual mass on plain film. Follow-up CT scan showed minimal subpleural or pleural-based persistent thickening.

in some shift of the mediastinum toward the affected side. Occasionally, the distal lung may be consolidated, i.e., opacification without evident loss of volume, because of the presence of an infectious process distal to the bronchial obstruction. Rarely, this may result in an increase in the overall volume of the consolidated lung. A plain film radiographic sign considered quite typical for a central obstructing lesion in the hilus with a peripheral infiltrate or collapse is the so-called "S" sign of Golden (or reverse "S" sign in the right lung) (33). The lower portion of the S is caused by the central hilar tumor and the upper portion of the S, by the atelectasis with volume loss and retraction of the involved portion of upper lobe (Fig. 6.8).

The problem of an unexplained or persistent pneumonia in a patient, particularly one at high risk because of cigarette smoking or other exposure, should alert the clinician to the possibility of a small obstructing central lesion without a mass effect. In smokers, segmental or lobar pneumonias should be followed

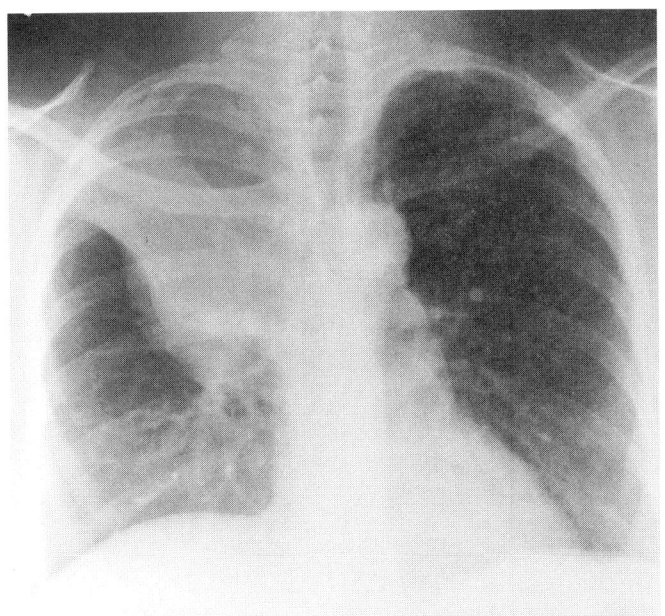

FIGURE 6.8. Central lung cancer. Posteroanterior chest radiograph. This radiograph illustrates the reverse S sign: there is a large right hilar mass with obstruction of the right upper lobe bronchus (not seen on this radiograph) and collapse of the right upper lobe. The lower portion of the reverse S is formed by the bulge of the hilar tumor mass. The upper portion of the reverse S is caused by the right upper lobe collapse and volume loss. (Courtesy of J. F. Caravelli, M.D., Memorial Sloan–Kettering Cancer Center.)

until complete resolution; they should then be followed periodically by radiography to be sure that there is no small central tumor causing partial or complete bronchial obstruction. Central carcinoid tumors, discussed below, are particularly prone to this presentation.

Spread of Tumor

The routes of permeation of lung cancer include direct extension as well as lymphatic and hematogenous spread. Tumors may be invasive locally and involve a variety of structures, many of which are only poorly visualized on plain chest radiography. Tumors may invade adjacent hilar and mediastinal or chest wall structures (Fig. 6.1); Pancoast (or superior sulcus) tumors may extend through the apex of the lung to involve the brachial plexus, ribs, vessels, and the stellate ganglion, producing the Pancoast syndrome. Direct tumor involvement by posterior lung masses of the vertebral bodies and the spinal canal can also be seen. Direct spread to the pleura and beyond is frequently associated with considerable pain.

Tumors also spread along the lymph channels of the lung, usually centrally to the hilar lymph nodes and then to the mediastinal nodes. This pattern is particularly true on the right side. Left upper lobe tumors may spread to ipsilateral superior hilar and aorticopulmonary window lymph nodes, whereas tumors of the left lower lobe more frequently drain into the left hilum. Lower lobe tumors may spread, via the inferior pulmonary ligament nodes, to the paraesophageal and paraphrenic regions.

The principal reason for unresectability of lung cancer is extensive regional spread either by lymphatics or by the hematogenous route. In resected specimens involvement of pulmonary veins by tumor carries a poor prognosis (34): tumor emboli from lung cancer permeate the systemic circulation and seed to various organs. Brain, bone, and adrenal glands are the most common site of metastatic disease; however, any organ may be involved by a metastatic lung cancer. Extensive experience with CT and more recently with MRI shows that the liver is less frequently a site of early distant metastatic disease. Frequently, liver masses uncovered on routine CT scans of the chest turn out, upon further examination, to represent hemangiomas or liver cysts. Nevertheless, metastatic disease to the liver from lung cancer is well known.

Computed Tomography and Magnetic Resonance Imaging

The introduction of CT and subsequent technical improvements and the ready availability of the modality after 1980, as well as the subsequent introduction of MRI, led to a dramatic change in the ability to visualize lung tumors accurately. The cross-sectional tomographic techniques allowed the radiologist to separate out adjacent layers of lung anatomy. Compared with plain chest radiography, there was a decrease in spatial resolution but greatly improved contrast resolution, which permits differential visualization of various soft tissue structures. This improved resolution resulted in a large increase in the ability to visualize lung pathology, particularly neoplasms, and their precise anatomic relationship to surrounding structures. Moreover, as opposed to bronchoscopy and mediastinoscopy, the new digital imaging procedures are noninvasive. During the early evolution of these new modalities, several articles suggested a high overall accuracy for CT in the staging of both the primary tumor (T disease); spread to regional lymph nodes (N disease), including hilar and ipsilateral and contralateral mediastinal lymph nodes as well as supraclavicular nodes (Fig. 6.9); and distant metastases (M disease), both within the thorax (e.g., chest wall, contralateral lung) and more distantly (e.g., head, liver, bone, adrenals).

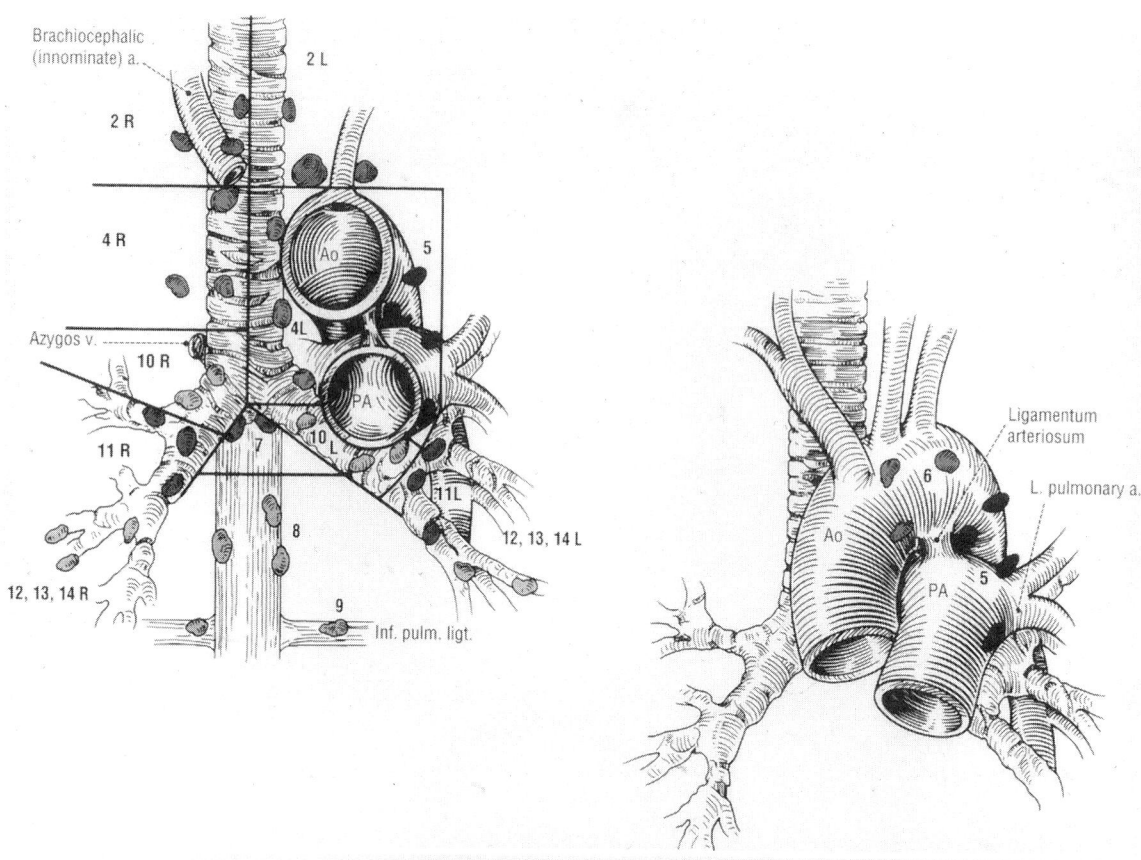

●	2R	Right upper paratracheal nodes	Between intersection of caudal margin of innominate artery with trachea and the apex of the lung (supra-innominate nodes).
●	2L	Upper left paratracheal nodes	Between top of aortic arch and apex of the lung (supra-aortic nodes).
●	4R	Right lower paratracheal nodes	Between intersection of caudal margin of innominate artery with trachea and cephalic border of azygos vein.
●	4L	Left lower paratracheal nodes	Between top of aortic arch and carina (medial to ligamentum arteriosum).
○	10R	Right tracheo-bronchial angle nodes	From cephalic border of azygos vein to origin of RUL bronchus.
○	10L	Left tracheo-bronchial angle nodes	Between carina and LUL (medial to ligamentum arteriosum).
●	5	Aorto-pulmonary nodes	Subaortic and para-aortic nodes lateral to the ligamentum arteriosum (proximal to first branch of left PA).
●	6	Anterior mediastinal nodes	Anterior to ligamentum arteriosum.
●	7	Subcarinal nodes	Caudal to the carina of the trachea.
●	8	Paraesophageal nodes	Dorsal to the posterior wall of the trachea and to the right or left of the midline of the esophagus.
○	9	Pulmonary ligament nodes	Nodes within the inferior pulmonary ligament.
●	11	Interlobar nodes	
○	12	Lobar nodes	
○	13	Segmental nodes	
○	14	Subsegmental nodes	

FIGURE 6.9. Regional nodal stations for lung cancer staging. See color plates.

The early reports indicating high overall accuracy (35–38) were tempered by subsequent articles in which improved methodologies were employed, including prospective blinded studies with a gold standard of surgical and pathologic verification (39–48). The availability of MRI in the mid- and late 1980s again provoked initial reports suggesting that MRI could be superior to CT in the evaluation and staging of lung cancer (49–52). Again, these early reports were hindered by methodological problems: as larger series were published, several tendencies began to emerge:

1. These larger series suggested that MRI, despite the availability of coronal and sagittal formats as well as its greater contrast sensitivity, was not more sensitive than CT in staging lung cancer; this finding is almost certainly related to the loss of tissue definition on MRI resulting from various kinds of thoracic movements including respiratory and cardiac motion as well as motion of blood within vessels.
2. It became apparent that the overall accuracy of both modalities was somewhat less than it had been indicated in earlier publications (53–58). Indeed, the lowest reported sensitivity for detection of mediastinal nodal metastases by CT scan was reported in a study in which total surgical nodal sampling was performed (47).

Nevertheless, despite the limitations of CT and MRI in staging lung cancer, the majority of clinicians surveyed thought that CT provided significant information in planning preoperative biopsy and surgical resection (59). Several recent studies, most notably a cooperative study involving several centers completed in 1991 by the Radiology Diagnostic Oncology Group (RDOG) (60), have assessed the relative accuracy of CT and MRI in staging lung cancer. This study, involving 250 patients from four centers, focused on assessment of the primary tumor including location and relationship to the bronchial tree; presence or absence of pleural, chest wall, and/or mediastinal invasion; and determination of the presence and location of lymph node metastases in the pulmonary hilum and the mediastinum.

IMAGING LOCAL TUMOR EXTENT (T STAGE)

Overall, CT and MRI were equally accurate in diagnosing both bronchial involvement (accuracy, .78–.84) and chest wall invasion (accuracy, .86–.87) (60). MRI was more accurate than CT, however, in the diagnosis of mediastinal invasion (accuracy, .83 for CT; .92 for MR), and the increased accuracy of MRI was statistically significant. The two modalities have similar overall accuracy in distinguishing T1-T2 tumors from T3-T4 tumors with acceptable accuracy in the 70% to 80% range. Unfortunately, this study did not address the important distinction between T3 disease (direct extension to chest wall, diaphragm, or mediastinum, including pericardial involvement but not involvement of the heart, great vessels, trachea, esophagus, or vertebral body, or tumor within a main bronchus located within 2 cm of the carina but not involving it) and T4 disease (i.e., tumor invasion of the heart, great vessels, trachea, esophagus, vertebral body, or carina, or associated with a malignant pleural effusion). T3 lesions are generally considered potentially resectable disease, whereas T4 lesions are considered unresectable. From a surgical point of view, differentiation of T3 from T4 disease would be important, but, unfortunately, there were only two verified T4 lesions in the study, and neither of them was correctly detected by imaging modalities. Other patients with suspected T4 disease were not admitted to the study, because they were not candidates for surgery and hence not eligible for inclusion. The evidence that MRI is more accurate than CT in the diagnosis of mediastinal invasion is of interest. In addition, the greater accuracy of MRI in evaluation of lung apex invasion in patients with superior sulcus tumors has been reported (61). In cases of suspected mediastinal invasion, there may be a role for high-resolution CT or thin-section MRI. However, the ability of these modalities to detect both chest wall and mediastinal invasion may be limited: areas of gross chest wall and mediastinal involvement with destruction of ribs or replacement (rather than displacement) of mediastinal adipose tissue and intradigitation of tumor between mediastinal structures are the usually accepted parameters for invasion. Subtle chest wall and mediastinal invasion present greater diagnostic challenges and resultant inaccuracies, e.g., whether there is involvement of the visceral and/or parietal pleura, or subtle extension beyond the pleura to involve chest wall or mediastinal structures.

IMAGING SPREAD OF LUNG CANCER TO HILAR AND MEDIASTINAL LYMPH NODES (N STAGE)

The accuracy of CT and MRI in detecting mediastinal (N2 or N3) lymph node metastases was not significantly different (65% for CT versus 61% for MRI) in the RDOG study. The overall accuracy was somewhat disappointing with both significant false-positive and false-negative diagnoses. Other reports had shown higher accuracy for CT and MRI than that reported by the RDOG group (60), with the exception of the report of Grenier et al. (58). The low overall sensitivities and accuracy of these two studies as well as that of McKenna et al. (47) may well have resulted from the extensive nodal sampling performed at surgery. Twenty patients in the RDOG study were excluded because of CT- or MRI-diagnosed advanced disease. Overall staging accuracy presumably would have increased if these patients had undergone surgery.

The conclusion based on this and several other studies is that CT remains the procedure of choice for staging lung cancer. Although MRI cannot be recommended routinely, there may well be specific indications for it in the following instances: (a) severe contrast allergy, (b) superior sulcus tumor, (c) tumors abutting the diaphragm, (d) possible chest wall or mediastinal invasion (including spine), or (e) CT with equivocal results. In other cases the equal accuracy and lower overall cost as well as the decreased time necessary to perform the examination make CT the clear choice in the routine assessment of lung cancer.

Given the somewhat disappointing accuracy of CT (and MRI) in the staging of lung cancer, especially hilar and mediastinal adenopathy, its value may be questioned. However, it is the firm opinion of a number of clinicians that CT is of great utility in determining treatment choices (59).

Furthermore, in addition to its limited utility in lung cancer staging, CT may be extremely useful in several other ways. It may be used to confirm abnormalities suspected on chest radiographs, such as chest wall or mediastinal invasion. In addition, unexpected findings are frequently noted as a result of a pretherapeutic CT examination. Included among these findings would be bone metastases, adrenal enlargement, or liver metastases. Furthermore, CT serves as an important indicator or road map in the overall management of patients and in determining subsequent diagnostic or therapeutic choices. For example, a patient with a presumed operable lung cancer on plain chest radiography may have a nodule in the opposite lung or an enlarged lymph node in the contralateral mediastinum that is not visible on the chest film but well seen on CT. Histologic confirmation by lung biopsy or mediastinoscopy could confirm more extensive disease than originally diagnosed, thus altering therapeutic options. In general, CT uncovers more disease than was previously suspected, resulting in upstaging and thus perhaps sparing the patient an unneeded surgical procedure. As previously noted, some abnormalities uncovered by cross-sectional imaging may be unrelated to the patient's lung cancer (e.g., hepatic hemangiomas and adrenal adenomas).

ADRENAL METASTASES VERSUS BENIGN ADRENAL ADENOMA

During the course of a standard CT staging workup for lung cancer, asymptomatic adrenal masses are frequently detected on scans of the upper abdomen. The majority of these (approximately 60%) represent benign adrenal adenomas. However, a significant minority represent metastatic disease, crucial information in determining therapeutic choices. There continues to be intense interest in the potential of MRI to distinguish, based on signal characteristics using a variety of pulsing sequences, benign adrenal adenomas from metastatic disease. Several of the more innovative studies have shown promising results, and it may well be true that in the near future an MRI diagnosis of benign adrenal adenoma may be made with sufficient certainty so as to exclude the need for histologic confirmation (62). However, at the present time it is our practice to obtain histologic confirmation of adrenal masses in patients with primary lung cancer whenever possible (63).

COMPUTED TOMOGRAPHIC TECHNIQUE

The chest radiograph remains the basic, relatively inexpensive, imaging modality used to detect a pulmonary abnormality in symptomatic patients. The current standard of care for further workup of suspected lung cancer always includes a carefully performed CT examination of the chest. The quality of the equipment used in many cases is of greater importance than the specific technical parameters employed. Use of obsolete equipment for staging of lung cancer significantly detracts from the diagnostic information.

Routine CT for staging of suspected lung cancer should include a scan of the entire chest and upper abdomen to the midlevel of the kidneys, being sure to include the entire adrenal glands. Ten-millimeter contiguous scans of the upper chest, lower chest, and upper abdomen are obtained, with 5-mm contiguous scans obtained through the central hilar regions. At our institution we routinely administer intravenous contrast for staging of lung cancer to more easily distinguish vessel structures in the mediastinum and hilar regions from involvement by tumor. It should be noted, however, that this practice is not universal.

RADIOGRAPHIC EVALUATION AND FOLLOW-UP OF PATIENTS TREATED WITH CHEMOTHERAPY AND RADIATION THERAPY

The initial evaluation of these patients includes chest radiography well as CT, the latter obtained to delineate the pretherapy baseline extent of disease precisely and to detect unexpected foci of regional or distant metastatic disease.

Patients undergoing chemotherapy for lung cancer are divided into those with measurable disease and those whose disease is not measurable but is evaluable. Patients with measurable disease have tumors that are almost completely surrounded by lung parenchyma. These tumors may abut mediastinum or chest wall but may not invade these structures extensively. The criterion for measurability is the ability to obtain perpendicular diameters of the tumor mass. On follow-up radiographs a partial response is designated in patients who have at least a 50% area decline in the product of the two measurable perpendicular diameters. A complete response is designated by radiographic disappearance of all tumor. A less than 50% area decrease in the products of the perpendicular diameters is considered nonsignificant.

The second category of patients undergoing chemotherapy are those whose tumors cannot be measured on plain chest radiography. However, these lesions are usually evaluable. Patients in this category usually have pleural effusions or associated infiltrates, or tumors extensively abutting or invading chest wall or mediastinum that effectively prohibit obtaining accurate perpendicular tumor diameters for area measurement. It has been our practice to categorize these nonmeasurable lung cancers on follow-up chest radiographs as either "not significantly improved," "significantly improved," or complete response, i.e., disappearance of all radiographic evidence of tumor. In a large clinical series, the significantly improved category has been shown to correspond in terms of survival to the partial-response group (i.e., in the lung cancers in which perpendicular tumor diameters could be measured). On plain chest radiography the evaluable category thus has proved to be a valuable and accurate estimate of tumor response or nonresponse.

More recently, with the ready availability of CT, there has been a tendency to follow patients undergoing chemotherapy for plain radiographic evaluable disease with CT. This is especially true in patients with large pleural effusions or infiltrates or in those with significant mediastinal disease. The CT scan allows a more precise delineation of tumor extent and response both before initiation of therapy and on posttherapy follow-up.

PREOPERATIVE NUCLEAR MEDICINE ASSESSMENT OF EXTENT OF DISEASE AND FUNCTIONAL STATUS

For patients with NSCLC, the bone scan is used as a standard preoperative tool to determine the extent of skeletal involvement (Fig. 6.10). This practice is

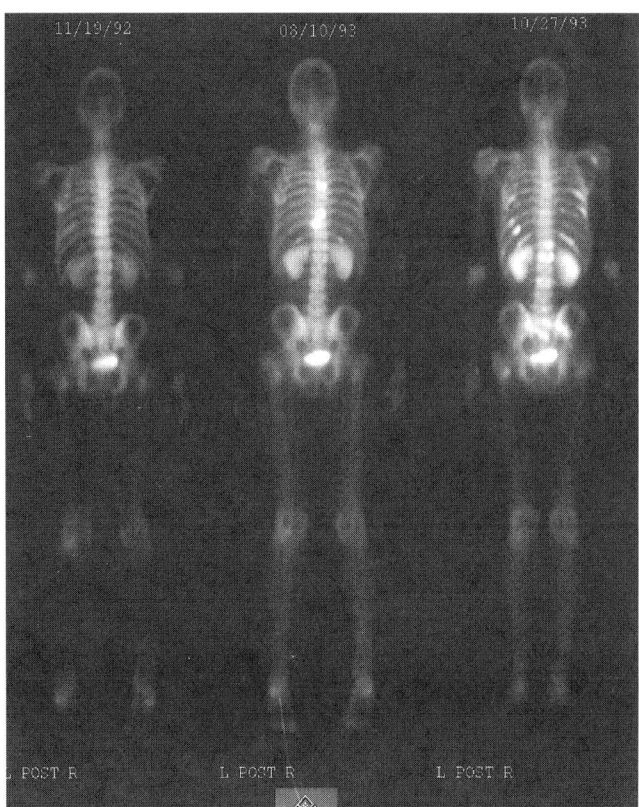

FIGURE 6.10. Nuclear medicine bone scan. ^{99m}Tc bone scan in a patient with NSCLC showing rapid progression of metastatic tumor to spine and ribs. The patient's baseline study (*left*) is normal, but 9 months later (*middle*) the thoracic spine is involved by tumor. The tumor progresses to involve the bones of the ribs and pelvis (*right*).

based on our experience that the incidence of unsuspected bone scan abnormality, which influences surgical management, is frequent: in a series of 117 consecutive bone scan patients reviewed, the incidence of abnormalities was 28%, i.e., about three fourths of the screened patients are found to show no evidence of bony involvement, thus clearing these patients for surgery (S. Larson, unpublished data). Of the one fourth with abnormalities caused by malignancy, three types were seen: (*a*) disseminated (or hematogenous) spread of tumor to the axial skeleton, (*b*) local invasion of the chest wall, and (*c*) distant metabolic effects on bone, most commonly hypertrophic pulmonary osteoarthropathy.

Based on this preliminary review, we estimate that preoperatively in NSCLC patients, about one fourth have bone scan abnormalities. Of these, about one third have benign conditions and two thirds, or 67% of the total population, have bone scan findings that are surgically relevant (16%–18% of the total). A significant fraction of these abnormalities (40%–50%) are actually caused by local involvement of bone by tumor, which may be resectable.

Functional perfusion and ventilation imaging with ^{99m}Tc macroaggregated albumin (MAA) and krypton 81m (^{81m}Kr), respectively, are used in preoperative evaluation of patients with NSCLC who have borderline pulmonary function to assess the impact of surgical resection. Postoperative complication rates rise very rapidly in patients with preoperative 1-second forced expiratory volume (FEV_1) measurement of less than 1 L. The quantitative perfusion imaging method determines the fractional perfusion to different parts of the lung. Postoperative lung function correlates extremely well with that predicted by considering that the lung function is reduced by surgical resection of the lung in direct correlation to the percentage of perfused lung removed (64).

Patients with risk factors for myocardial ischemia are screened with a thallium 201 chloride (^{201}Tl Cl) perfusion test. The size of an ischemic defect after exercise is a good predictor of the risks of perioperative infarct or other adverse cardiac event in the immediate postoperative period (65).

MONOCLONAL ANTIBODY IMAGING IN NON–SMALL CELL LUNG CANCER

^{99m}Tc–NRLU-10 scanning has been used to image NSCLC of the thorax. This antibody recognizes a 40 kilodalton (kd) glycoprotein on the surface of the cell. In a series of patients studied at our institution, 20 to 30 millicurie (mCi) of ^{99m}Tc-FAB was injected intravenously, and planar and SPECT imaging was performed. However, there were false-positive readings (4 of 5) for both CT scans and the SPECT scan. The most accurate diagnostic approach occurred when the CT scan and the functional ^{99m}Tc-FAB scan were combined into fusion images. The fused images showed that false-positive uptake on antibody imaging was caused by blood vessels. SPECT imaging was necessary to have sufficient contrast to perform the studies.

Epidermal growth factor receptor (EGFR) is present in NSCLC, and this receptor is thought to play an important role in autocrine stimulation of tumor growth. Antibodies to EGFR have been labeled with indium 111 (^{111}In) and used to evaluate patients with NSCLC. At antibody doses of more than 40 mg, all sites of metastatic and primary tumor were detected on the antibody scans.

Gallium 67 (^{67}Ga) citrate is taken up by lung cancer and avidly concentrated both in the primary lesion as well as in metastases. Before the advent of CT, ^{67}Ga citrate was proposed as a screening test for mediastinal involvement. A rule of thumb was developed, i.e., if the tumor uptake of ^{67}Ga was "hot" and there was no uptake in the mediastinum, then tumor involvement of the mediastinum was unlikely and the patient could proceed to thoracotomy. In contrast, if uptake was seen in the mediastinum, then these patients were candidates for mediastinoscopy to confirm the involvement of the lymph nodes with tumor. A recent small series performed at the author's center using SPECT technology confirmed that ^{67}Ga was avidly taken up in the primary tumor, with 100% sensitivity (S. Larson, published data). However, false-positive uptakes were also seen because of inflammatory involvement of mediastinal lymph nodes and the bronchial tree. Thus ^{67}Ga has a limited role in staging of lung tumor, because of the high likelihood of associated inflammatory changes in the mediastinum, which are detected as a positive uptake. As a measure of tumor viability, ^{67}GA may have a role in some clinical situations, but it is ordinarily not very helpful in NSCLC.

UNCOMMON BRONCHOPULMONARY MALIGNANCIES

BRONCHIAL CARCINOID

Carcinoids (as well as adenoid cystic carcinoma and mucoepidermoid carcinoma) formerly were grouped under the misleading term bronchial adenomas. Carcinoid is by far the most prevalent of the less common pulmonary tumors (Table 6.2), representing between 1% and 2.5% of all lung tumors (66–68). It has a considerably better prognosis than lung cancer be-

TABLE 6.2. Uncommon Bronchopulmonary Tumors

Carcinoid
Tumors of tracheobronchial gland origin
   Adenoid cystic carcinoma (cylindroma)
   Mucoepidermoid carcinoma
   Acinic cell tumor
   Oncocytoma (oxyphilic adenoma)
   Pleomorphic adenoma (mixed tumor)
   Mucus gland tumor (bronchial cyst adenoma)
True pulmonary adenoma
Primary tracheobronchial malignant melanoma
Pulmonary sarcoma
   Fibrosarcoma
   Leiomyosarcoma
   Chondrosarcoma
   Fibroleiomyosarcoma
   Rhabdomyosarcoma
   Neurofibrosarcoma
Pulmonary blastoma
Carcinosarcoma
Hemangiopericytoma
Plasmacytoma
Kaposi's sarcoma

cause it is typically slow growing and can frequently be fully resected at surgery. Most observers, but not all, think that the cell of origin is the neuroendocrine cell of the tracheobronchial tree. In this sense it is thought by some to represent a more benign counterpart of small cell cancer, despite the fact that it is not related to cigarette smoking.

There are two clinical and histologic varieties of this tumor, the so-called typical carcinoid, which is slow growing and metastasizes very late, and the less common atypical (69) form, which is considerably more aggressive with a higher incidence of metastatic disease and histologically increased mitotic activity.

Radiographically, these tumors are divided into those with a central presentation and those with a peripheral presentation. Central tumors, comprising approximately 80% of all bronchial carcinoids, frequently present with symptoms based on the central location (shortness of breath, wheezing, peripheral pneumonia, and/or atelectasis or radiographic hyperaeration from collateral air drift distal to an obstructed bronchus) or from its abundant vascularity (hemoptysis). Because of its associated symptomatology, diagnosis tends to be somewhat earlier for the central than for the peripheral variety (70). The degree of bronchial occlusion from these central tumors is highly variable. The tumor may be almost completely endobronchial, but more frequently the tip of the tumor presents within the bronchial lumen with the large bulk of it extending through the bronchial wall into surrounding lung parenchyma ("iceberg" presentation) (Fig. 6.11). These tumors do not typically metastasize early to regional lymph nodes but can grow aggressively along the bronchial tree to reach the mediastinum, rendering complete surgical removal technically more difficult. Occasional bronchial occlusion can be associated with peripheral mucus obstruction (mucocele) (71, 72). Occasionally, the chest radiograph can be normal in patients presenting with symptoms such as hemoptysis, and the diagnosis can only be made bronchoscopically (73, 74).

The less common peripheral carcinoid is usually diagnosed in an older age group and can remain asymptomatic for long periods. Not infrequently, at surgery multiple smaller foci of bronchial carcinoid (tumorlets) are noted scattered throughout the lung parenchyma (75).

CT is useful in showing the extent of disease of the primary tumor and also in excluding the less likely possibility of regional nodal metastases. Frequently, the workup for these tumors is performed assuming that they represent lung cancer. One common characteristic of carcinoid tumor of the lung is that it is hypervascular on CT after intravenous contrast administration, an appearance that is highly suggestive of the diagnosis.

Nuclear medicine methods may prove useful, particularly when other studies are negative and the patient is symptomatic. A somatostatin-receptor–binding tracer, ^{111}In concentrate has a high accuracy for detecting carcinoid, and bronchial carcinoid has been visualized. Uptake of this tracer also suggests that the patient's symptoms may be pharmacologically blocked by somatostatin analogues such as octreotide (76).

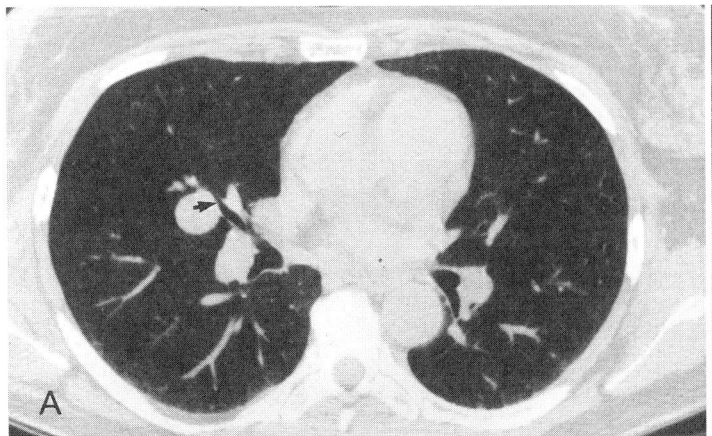
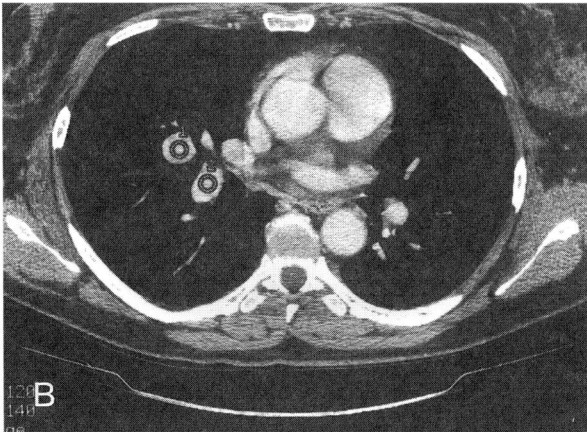

FIGURE 6.11. Central carcinoid. **A.** CT scan through the lower third of the chest with lung parenchymal windows. There is a well-defined central tumor in the right middle lobe that is causing some narrowing of the right middle lobe bronchus (*arrowhead*). This patient presented with hemoptysis. **B.** CT scan through the same region with soft-tissue windows obtained after intravenous contrast administration. The regions of interest are Hounsfield unit (HU) density measurements. The mass (region of interest [ROI]) (1) has a very high HU reading (101), similar to the HU density of the right main pulmonary artery (2), which is 118. This suggests that the mass is either a highly vascular tumor or an arteriovenous malformation. At surgery a carcinoid tumor was completely resected. These tumors are typically highly vascular.

ADENOID CYSTIC CARCINOMA

Adenoid cystic carcinoma and mucoepidermoid carcinoma are tumors of tracheobronchial gland origin, with adenoid cystic carcinoma representing approximately 80% of these tumors. The tumor typically arises in the trachea and main stem bronchi. On chest radiography (as well as CT), an endotracheal or endobronchial mass, which may be smooth or lobulated, is seen. CT is useful to show the mediastinal extent of tumor (77). The prognosis for these tumors is quite good if they are fully resected, and, even in patients with residual tumor, a prolonged course is quite common with survival of many years in patients with residual disease.

MUCOEPIDERMOID CANCER

This rare tumor of tracheobronchial gland origin can be found in all age groups, with a typically indolent behavior (78). It arises in the main stem or lobar bronchi and can block these structures with development of atelectasis and/or pneumonia (79). Mucoepidermoid tumors typically present both on CT and plain chest radiography as a polypoid mass.

PULMONARY KAPOSI'S SARCOMA

In the pre–acquired immunodeficiency syndrome (AIDS) era, this highly unusual tumor was found exclusively in the lower extremities of elderly people. A tumor of histologically identical appearance has been described commonly in AIDS patients in recent years and has become relatively common (80). Both a localized and a widespread form are described, with the widespread form being more common (80%) (81). The appearance typically presents in both central and peripheral lung fields with a nodular and linear appearance roughly conforming to the bronchovascular tree distribution. Plain radiographic as well as CT evaluation can be difficult because of the frequent concomitant presence of opportunistic infections such as *Pneumocystis carinii* pneumonia (PCP).

From the perspective of nuclear medicine imaging, this diagnosis is frequently one of exclusion. The lesions of Kaposi's sarcoma never concentrate ^{67}Ga citrate. However, they are relatively cellular, and lesions larger than a few centimeters concentrate ^{201}Tl-Cl readily (82, 83).

PULMONARY BLASTOMA

Among the rare pulmonary tumors are a variety of sarcomas, as well as unique tumors such as pulmonary blastoma, that histologically resembles embryonic bronchial architecture in a sarcomatous background. Approximately 20% to 25% of these tumors appear in children (84). The tumors present a nonspecific imaging appearance and present as peripheral solitary pulmonary nodules of any size, or as central masses. As with all central masses, complications such as atelectasis, pneumonia, or even hemoptysis may be seen with these lesions.

HAMARTOMA

Hamartoma is the most common benign pulmonary neoplasm (Table 6.3). Some consider it a malformation, rather than a neoplasm, consisting of normal pulmonary and bronchial elements, frequently containing calcium and/or adipose tissue, especially on high-resolution CT (85). Visualization of calcium in hamartomas is not particularly common, occurring in 10% to 15% of plain chest radiographs (86). The typical popcorn configuration, although practically diagnostic, is unusual. Although these tumors are not considered to have significant potential for malignancy, they frequently are removed surgically, the justification being that peripheral hamartomas frequently continue to grow slowly, and central hamartomas may cause the complications previously described in central tumors.

The very low incidence of uncommon malignant as well as benign pulmonary tumors prevents detailed discussion. The possible presence of these tumors on imaging examinations (in addition to the more common primary and metastatic pulmonary lesions) should be borne in mind: they emphasize the importance of histologic diagnosis of thoracic abnormalities prior to therapeutic intervention.

TABLE 6.3. Benign Pulmonary Neoplasms and Reactive Nonneoplastic Masses

Hamartoma
Amyloidoma
Granular cell myoblastoma
Benign neoplasms of connective tissue origin
    Fibroma
    Chondroma
    Lipoma
    Hemangioma
    Neurofibroma
    Neurilemoma
Leiomyoma (can be multiple)
Tumors usually found in other locations
    Chemodectomas
    Benign clear cell tumors
    Endometriosis
Plasma cell granuloma (reactive granulomatous inflammation)
Squamous papillomas (children)

SOLITARY PULMONARY NODULE

The patient presenting to a physician with the radiographic finding of a solitary pulmonary nodule (SPN), either on chest radiography or on CT, is fairly common. The problem is the determination of whether the nodule is benign or malignant. Malignant nodules require aggressive diagnostic workup and treatment. Benign nodules can usually be observed (87).

The use of radiographic methods in evaluating SPN is primarily directed to avoiding more invasive procedures such as biopsy, video-assisted thoracoscopic surgery, or thoracotomy, if possible. Evaluation by CT and chest radiography is usually augmented by sputum cytology evaluation. This diagnostic procedure, when positive, is highly specific for tumor. However, negative sputum cytology does not allow one to exclude malignancy as the cause of an SPN.

Of paramount importance in the initial evaluation of SPN is the patient's history and clinical presentation. Clinical findings suggesting a benign etiology would be age under 30 or 35 years (88) or nonsmoker status. Conversely, prior malignancy and age above 45 years, or a history of cigarette smoking raises the possibility of malignancy as an explanation for the presence of an SPN (89).

Although evaluation of the chest radiograph may yield valuable clues about the etiology of the pulmonary nodule, perhaps the most important single evaluation consists of the availability and evaluation of any prior chest radiographs. The presence of an SPN without demonstrable change for a period of 2 years or more strongly suggests a benign etiology. This finding would suggest that radiographic follow-up over a period of several years on a 4- to 6-month basis would be adequate for a stable pulmonary nodule. In this regard, the importance of uncovering and obtaining old films for comparison cannot be overestimated, and the demonstration of a stable nodule over a long period is the single most important criterion indicating a benign etiology.

Another extremely important plain film finding is the presence of calcification, particularly if the calcification is diffuse, central, popcorn, or laminar in appearance (Figs. 6.12 and 6.13). Stippled or eccentric calcification is indeterminate and could represent either a benign or a malignant nodule. In evaluating pulmonary nodules for the presence of calcium on plain chest radiography, relatively low kilovoltage brings out calcium best. It should be noted, however, that the presence of calcium on plain chest radiography, although highly suggestive of a benign lesion, is not seen frequently and is seem much more frequently on roentgenograms of pathology specimens following surgery (90).

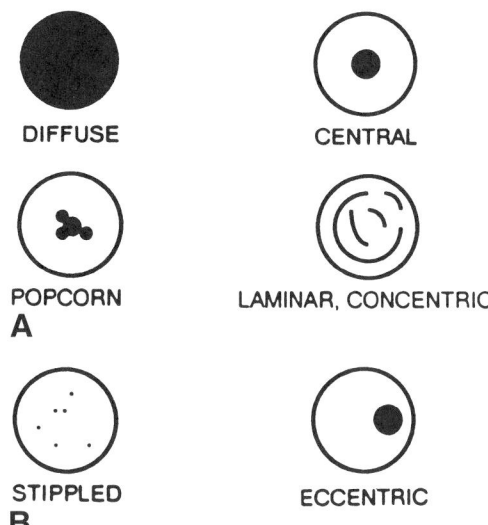

FIGURE 6.12. Benign pattern of SPN calcifications. **A.** This illustration shows the typical appearances of calcifications within pulmonary nodules caused by benign disease, such as granuloma or hamartoma. These signs include diffuse, central, popcorn, and concentric patterns. **B.** Nonspecific, possibly malignant patterns of SPN calcification. The two illustrations in *B* represent nonspecific patterns of calcification within the SPN that carry a potential diagnosis of either benign granuloma or malignant pulmonary nodule with calcification. (Reproduced with permission from Webb WR. Radiologic evaluation of the solitary pulmonary nodule. AJR Am J Roentgenol 1990;154:701–708.)

Other radiographic features of the SPN on plain chest radiography are of relative value and include small size, smooth or rounded contours, and a sharp edge (Fig. 6.14). Conversely, large or poorly defined nodules or pulmonary nodules with hilar or mediastinal adenopathy are suggestive of malignant origin. The availability of CT has had a dramatic effect on the overall evaluation of solitary pulmonary nodules, generally decreasing the need for more invasive procedures. Initially, a screening CT examination of the chest with 1-cm contiguous scans are obtained in a patient with an SPN. This is done to localize the pulmonary nodule and also to ensure that there are no multiple pulmonary nodules.

The screening procedure is followed by a series of high-resolution scans (1.5- or 1-mm slice thickness) with bone or edge enhancement reconstruction algorithm (91). The recent availability of spiral (or helical) CT scanners in which a large number of scans can be obtained during a single breath hold has resulted in more accurate delineation of the anatomy of the chest, without the anatomic misregistration resulting from variations in inspiratory effort. This procedure has a

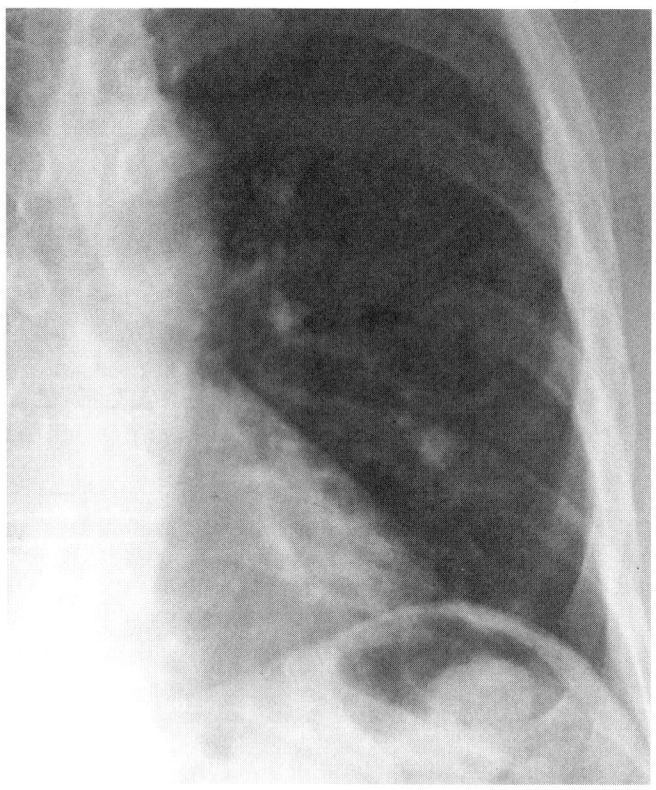

FIGURE 6.13. Solitary pulmonary nodule. Chest radiograph shows a well-defined dense nodule in the left lower lung zone containing calcium. The calcium distribution throughout the nodule is quite diffuse, resulting in a considerable overall increase in density of the nodule. This pattern of calcification is quite typical for a benign granuloma.

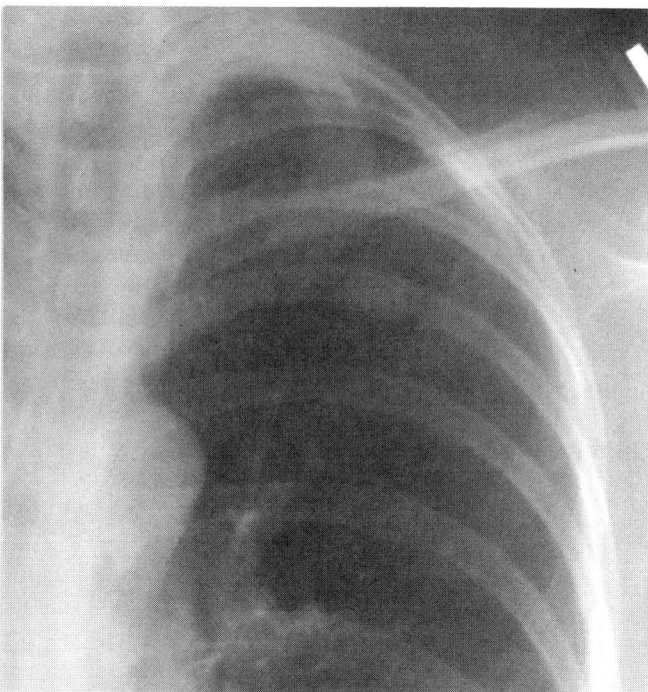

FIGURE 6.14. Solitary pulmonary nodule. Chest radiograph of the left upper lung zone shows a well-defined noncalcified pulmonary nodule overlying the right 5th posterior rib. A lung location was confirmed by oblique radiographs. CT scanning showed no evidence for calcification within the nodule. The possibility of lung cancer could not be excluded, particularly a small peripheral adenocarcinoma. At surgery this nodule proved to be a hamartoma. Its well-defined appearance is typical. Some hamartomas exhibit a typical popcorn calcification, but these are a minority.

number of advantages. The appearance and contour of a solitary pulmonary nodule may result in a highly specific diagnosis. Entities such as arteriovenous malformation, rounded atelectasis, fungus balls, and mucous plugs tend to have a highly individual appearance, and diagnosis of these entities can frequently be made with a high degree of certainty.

In addition, pulmonary nodules having an irregular or spiculated border would be more suggestive of a diagnosis of cancer than of other entities (92) (Fig. 6.2).

Two or more pulmonary nodules uncovered by CT suggest the presence of probable metastatic disease. It should be noted that the presence of two or more nodules poses an interesting diagnostic dilemma. Diagnosis of one of these nodules, for example, by percutaneous biopsy, suggests but does not indicate with certainty that the other nodule may have the same diagnosis. However, it is possible that there might be two concomitant nodules of differing histology present: one of the nodules may be a tumor and the other, a granuloma. In some cases it may be necessary to obtain histologic material from more than one of the pulmonary nodules (93, 94).

The most important advantage of high-resolution CT is in the detection of small areas of calcification within pulmonary nodules. Individual picture element readings (pixels) may be obtained through areas of a solitary pulmonary nodule in which the density of small regions can be mapped quantitatively with Hounsfield unit (HU) readings. Significantly large areas of central calcification with readings of 200 HU or more are highly suggestive of the presence of calcifications within a granuloma. In a minority of cases, there may be some utility in performing CT densitometry (95–98). Briefly, this procedure consists of comparison of the density of the patient's nodule on high-resolution CT with spheres of known density in an anthropomorphic phantom scanned on the same CT scanner. Significant areas of density above a threshold yields a diagnosis of microcalcification and, therefore, probable benignity. Failure to demonstrate such regions of high density within a nodule suggests that the nodule does not contain microcalcifications and is therefore histologically indeterminate, indicating further, more aggressive workup. This procedure probably has some utility as an adjunct to conventional high-resolution CT but is indicated in a minority of cases for two reasons: (a) in most cases, high-resolution CT can demonstrate areas of subtle calcification within a nodule; and (b) this procedure is somewhat complex and difficult to perform, requiring some experience. The CT phantom apparatus is also relatively expensive.

ROLE OF POSITRON EMISSION TOMOGRAPHY

Positron emission tomography (PET) is a powerful imaging method for assessing the metabolism of tumors noninvasively in vivo (99). A recent study evaluated PET-fluorodeoxyglucose (FDG), an indicator of metabolic activity, as a technique to distinguish malignant from benign SPNs (100). This study is particularly important because pulmonary nodules may not be diagnosed adequately regarding their potential for malignancy despite the use of sophisticated imaging procedures. In a study using PET-FDG scanning to assess the SPN, a group of 53 patients with SPN (nodule less than 4 cm in diameter) were studied after injection of 10 mCi of FDG. PET-FDG imaging was highly sensitive for malignancy. With all of the malignant tumors having a standardized uptake value (SUV) of more than 2.5 (defined as the ratio of the tumor region radioactivity to the radioactivity in a region of interest in the contralateral lung, normalized for the dose injected per body weight), the malignant lesion SUVs averaged 6.0 (Fig. 6.15). There were three benign lesions that also had SUVs of more than 2.5 that were proven to be granulomas. In this series the PET-FDG imaging had a sensitivity of 100% and a specificity of 95%. There is a multiinstitutional trial underway to corroborate these potentially important findings.

Additional benefits of PET-FDG imaging in lung cancer may be the more accurate staging of spread of tumor to mediastinum (101), and the detection of whether an abnormality seen on chest roentgenogram or CT in the posttreatment period is tumor recurrence (102). Initial results are promising but preliminary.

PERCUTANEOUS LUNG BIOPSY

Lung biopsy has become increasingly common for the diagnosis of tumor masses as well as solitary pulmonary nodules within lung (103, 104). The degree to which this procedure is used in diagnostic radiology departments is highly variable, depending on the experience and expertise of the individuals performing the biopsy. The procedures are usually performed by radiologists, but occasionally by pulmonologists or surgeons.

One advantage of this procedure is high specificity. The cytologic diagnosis of malignant disease is associated with an extremely small false-positive rate. Lung biopsy in general can be highly specific for the diagnosis of neoplasm, with a positive yield of up to 90%; in inflammatory disease there may be a positive yield of up to 70% in bacterial infection and even of other benign entities such as hamartoma, in which a highly specific diagnosis can be made. The diagnosis of benign entities, however, usually requires a somewhat more invasive technique involving the use of cutting biopsy instruments that allow histologic sections to be obtained; this procedure often permits specific diagnoses to be made, including entities such as sarcoid, granuloma, and hamartoma. However, sampling may be incomplete, e.g., an inflammatory region of a lung cancer (peripheral infiltrate) may be sampled with a cutting needle, and the region containing tumor not sampled, resulting in a false-negative diagnosis.

Clinically, the major advantage of percutaneous biopsy is in evaluating patients who are not candidates for surgery; this procedure helps to avoid more invasive procedures such as surgery or video-assisted thoracoscopic surgical procedures. However, a negative percutaneous biopsy does not indicate a benign process and suggests rather that either a repeat biopsy or more invasive definitive diagnostic procedure may be indicated.

Pneumothorax occurs in 20% to 30% of patients undergoing percutaneous lung biopsy and represents the most important complication. Fortunately, only between 4% and 7% of these pneumothoraces are symptomatic and require treatment. More commonly, a catheter is inserted percutaneously into the pleural space for treatment of symptomatic pneumothoraces. Formerly, chest tubes were used, but their use has decreased with the availability of flexible percutaneous catheters.

Dissemination of tumor through a needle tract is uncommon with the incidence being described in case reports rather than in series. There are anecdotal reports that melanoma is more prone to cause needle tract implantation of tumor.

Localization for percutaneous needle biopsy can be done either fluoroscopically or with CT. It appears that with easy access to fast CT scanning, this method of localization is becoming increasingly common. In addition, with CT smaller tumors may be localized accurately. CT has a relative disadvantage in that a finite period must elapse between the placement of the nee-

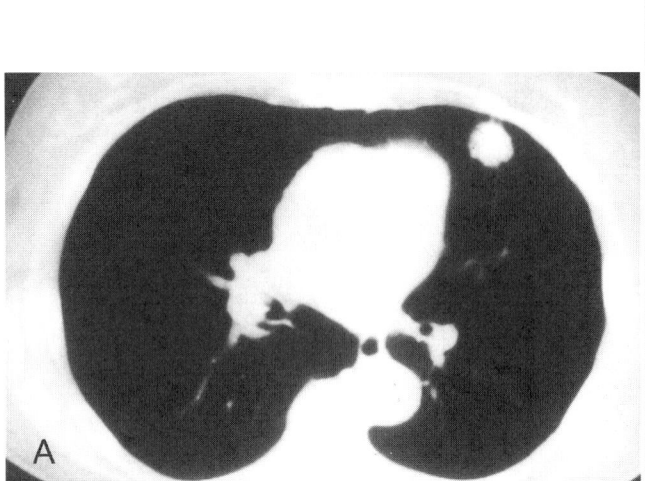
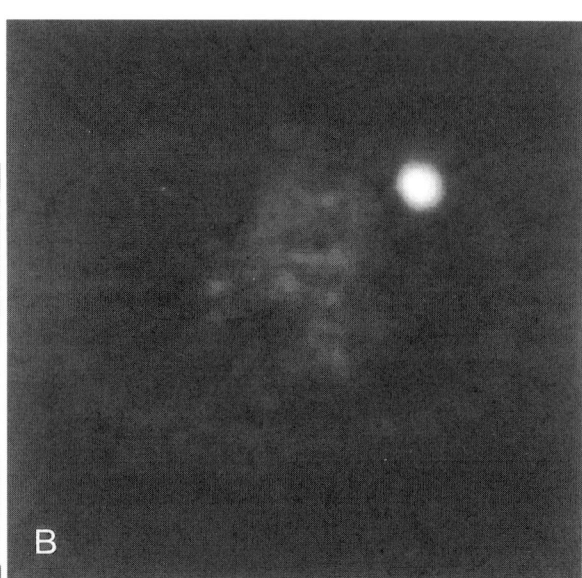

FIGURE 6.15. PET scan of an SPN. **A.** CT scan showing an SPN (*arrow*) in the left lung. **B.** Positron emission tomography (F-18)–2-fluoro-2-deoxy-D-glucose (PET-FDG) scans, showing intense localization in the SPN (*arrow*), which at surgery proved to be lung cancer. The FDG uptake reflects increased metabolic activity, most commonly lung cancer, although granulomas and other processes having metabolic activity may have increased activity on PET scan. (Courtesy of R. Edward Coleman, M.D., Duke University Medical School.) See color plates.

dle within the chest and the acquisition of the CT and reconstruction of the image to verify the position of the needle tip. However, CT appears to be used increasingly for biopsy localization, as well as for direct bronchoscopic procedures to areas of bronchial narrowing or other abnormalities (105, 106).

ESOPHAGEAL CANCER

Esophageal cancer, although less prevalent than lung cancer, is a highly lethal tumor because of its propensity to spread locally and regionally during its asymptomatic phase. It is etiologically related both to tobacco use and alcohol consumption. Imaging studies are particularly useful in the evaluation of esophageal cancer. Barium esophagrams have long been used to diagnose both cancer and other abnormalities within the esophagus, including disturbances of motility. In recent years this study has been supplemented by endoscopy with biopsy. The barium esophagram, however, remains important in delineating overall tumor extent and length of involvement, as well as in suspected cases of perforation and fistulization. In contrast, endoscopic procedures retain importance both for diagnosis and histologic confirmation of suspected abnormalities. In recent years these techniques have been supplemented by newer diagnostic staging procedures, such as CT, MRI, and endoscopic ultrasonography (EUS).

The pretherapeutic imaging staging of esophageal cancer using the tumor, node, metastasis (TNM) classification (see Chapter 26) has been facilitated by the clinical development and application of CT as well as magnetic resonance scanning and, more recently, EUS. Posttherapeutic evaluation of the esophagus by imaging means is largely limited to esophagram and CT.

Recent years have seen a proliferation of imaging modalities capable of visualizing the esophagus and surrounding structures in considerable detail—EUS, CT, MRI. This proliferation has resulted in a veritable menu of competing diagnostic examinations. Unlike lung cancer, in which the sequence of radiographic staging examinations is well established (chest radiography, CT, occasional MRI), the situation with esophageal cancer is considerably more fluid: for example, the routine use of CT for pretherapeutic esophageal cancer staging has been called into question. Whereas there is currently no general consensus concerning the optimal imaging workup for esophageal cancer, several tendencies have emerged.

T STAGE

The ability of CT to stage local tumor extent and penetration of the gastrointestinal tract lumen, initially thought to be highly accurate (107), was subsequently modified especially with regard to local penetration and extension to contiguous structures (trachea, main

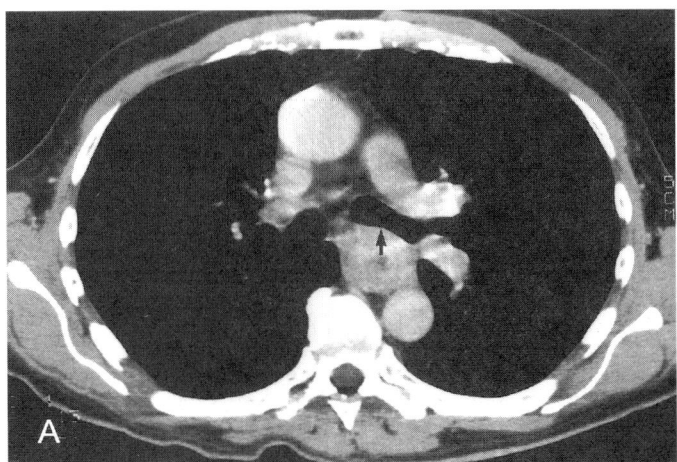 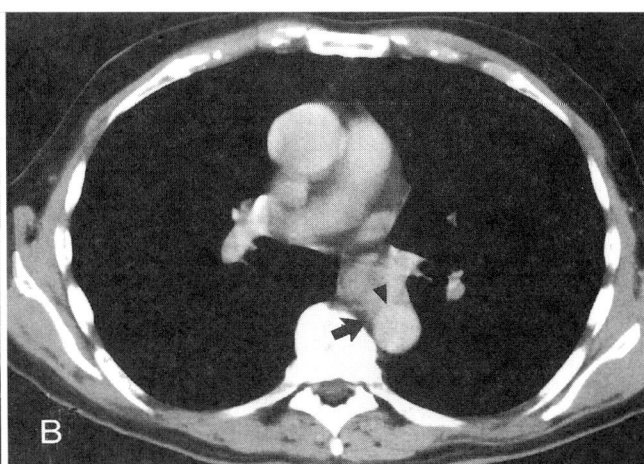

FIGURE 6.16. Esophageal cancer. **A.** CT scan in a patient with a tumor of the esophagus obtained just below the level of the tracheal carina. The large tumor produces marked thickening of the esophageal wall. There is virtual obliteration of the esophageal lumen; proximal obstruction to the flow of barium was noted on an esophagram. The outer margins of the tumor are poorly defined, suggesting local invasion of mediastinal structures. There is extrinsic pressure on the left main stem bronchus (*arrow*). Although bronchial invasion may be suspected from this finding, the radiographic appearance is nonspecific and may merely be related to extrinsic pressure resulting from tumor growth and expansion. **B.** At a level inferior to the tracheal carina, the bulky tumor mass producing irregular thickening of the esophageal wall is again noted. The normal fat plane between the descending thoracic aorta and mediastinal structures has been obliterated (*arrowhead*). This finding suggests the possibility of aortic invasion. Note also the partial obliteration of the normal fat space between the esophagus, vertebral body, and aorta (*arrow*).

stem bronchi, pericardium, aorta) (Fig. 6.16). However, a number of studies indicated overall accuracy in detecting local organ invasion in the 90% to 100% range, based on mass effect or loss of fat plane between tumor and adjacent structure (108–115). Studies comparing MRI and CT in local invasion reported similar high accuracy (115), with the recommendation that CT be employed routinely because of its lower cost and ease of performance.

The recent introduction and clinical use of EUS has added another dimension to the staging problem. This modality, which uses high frequency transducers (7.5–12.5 MHz) permits high-resolution imaging of the five layers (from inner to outer: [*a*] mucosa interface, [*b*] lamina propria, [*c*] submucosa, [*d*] muscularis, and [*e*] adventitia) of the esophageal (and gastric) wall as well as their disruption and invasion by tumor. Endoscopic ultrasonography potentially far surpasses the very limited abilities of CT (and MRI) to determine extent of esophageal wall invasion (Fig. 6.17). Tumors, as well as tumor-involved lymph nodes, are hypoechoic, i.e., appear quite dark or black with a few white speckles present. Initial reports indicated very high accuracy in the range of 90% for esophageal wall invasion (116).

Indeed, the ability of EUS to determine local esophageal wall invasion accurately has been confirmed by other studies (117, 118). However, there is an important caveat: between 17% and 50% of patients with esophageal cancer cannot be staged by EUS because the highly stenotic or obstructing lesions do not permit passage of the EUS instrument, thus preventing full evaluation. These patients, therefore, cannot be staged by this modality, and CT must be used as the next best staging modality. It is possible that, with the development of smaller diameter EUS probes, a much larger percentage of patients may be staged locally by EUS.

N STAGE

The overall accuracy of EUS in detecting N disease depends on two factors:

1. As with T-stage evaluation of esophageal cancer, adequate visualization of periesophageal tissues depends on the ability to pass the EUS probe beyond the tumor.
2. The high-frequency transducers, which allow highly accurate anatomic delineation, have a limited penetration of 2 to 5 cm or less; detection of metastases beyond this distance is therefore not possible with EUS.

In general, EUS is considered useful, and probably superior to CT, in the delineation of periesophageal metastases (118). Lymph nodes stations beyond the immediate periesophageal region (porta hepatis, gastrohepatic ligament, retroperitoneum) are best detected by carefully performed CT examination, al-

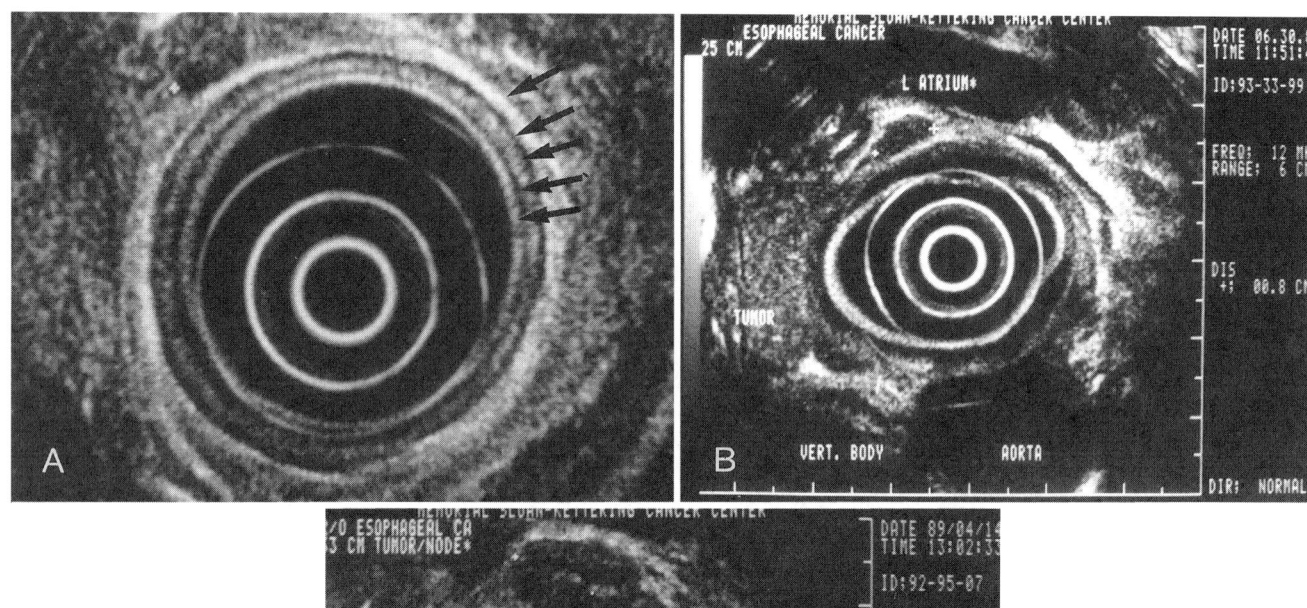

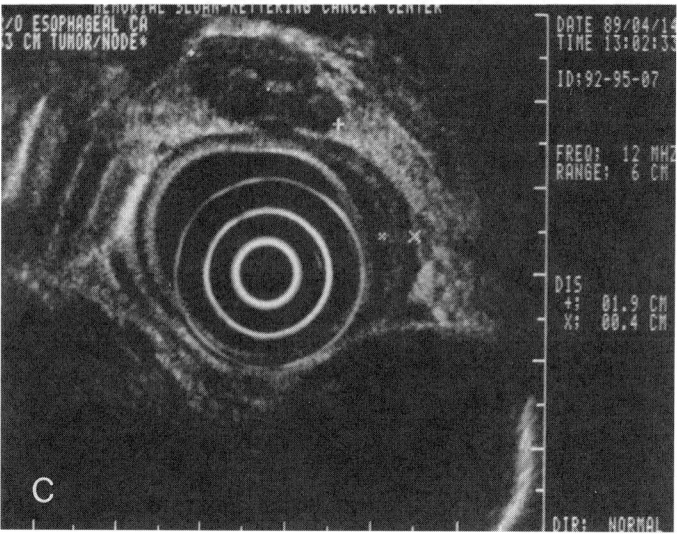

FIGURE 6.17. Endoscopic ultrasonography (EUS). A. EUS in a normal region of an esophagus using a 12-MHz transducer. The alternating layers of the esophageal wall are hyperechoic (*white*) and hypoechoic (*dark*). There are five layers bounded by the inner layer of (hyperechoic) (*white*) submucosal fat and the outer hyperechoic layer of serosal fat (*arrows*). The central circles are the sonographic transducer, which is present in the lumen of the esophagus. B. A large tumor is seen to obliterate the normal architecture of the wall of the esophagus. This tumor extends through the entire wall of the esophagus into the surrounding mediastinal adipose tissue. The normal architecture of the esophageal wall in other regions is also distorted, suggesting possible tumor infiltration. Anteriorly, just below the left atrium, there is a paraesophageal mediastinal abnormal lymph node marked by two cross hairs. C. This patient had a tumor infiltrating the wall of the esophagus that proved upon biopsy to represent an esophageal carcinoma shown between the two Xs. Because of the largely mural location of this tumor, findings on the esophagram were minimal. Despite the relatively small size of the this tumor, an enlarged paraesophageal metastatic lymph node is seen on the superior aspect of this scan, delimited by cross hairs. (Courtesy of Jose Botet, M.D., Memorial Sloan–Kettering Cancer Center.)

though the overall accuracy of CT, when correlated with surgery, is not as high as EUS in the immediate periesophageal region.

M STAGE

CT, with its accurate delineation of thoracic and upper abdominal anatomy, remains the procedure of choice for delineating lung, bone, adrenal, and liver metastases. A possible role exists for MRI in evaluating the liver: reports have suggested greater accuracy for MRI in detection and characterization of liver lesions. This may apply to esophageal cancer as well. It appears at present, however, that the role of MRI is as an adjunct to CT or as a problem-solving technique in specific patients in whom the CT findings in liver are questionable or nonspecific.

The utility of imaging examinations in the follow-up of patients treated either medically or surgically for esophageal cancer is well established. An upper gastrointestinal series, as well as endoscopy, is useful in detecting intraluminal abnormalities and tumor recurrence. Suspected tumor recurrence beyond the lumen of the esophagus (or intrathoracic gastric pull-up) is best evaluated with CT.

CONCLUSION

Endoscopic ultrasonography is an important diagnostic staging device for evaluation of the extent of tumor within the esophageal wall as well as involvement of periesophageal lymph nodes. The limitations of the modality (inability to pass through the stenotic segment of esophagus, limited penetration of the high-frequency probes, the relative complexity of performing this invasive study that is both operator dependent and operator intensive), combined with the possibility that the information obtained may not significantly change therapeutic approach, indicate that the ultimate role of EUS has not yet been determined. The development of narrow-diameter probes may further increase the utility of this procedure by allowing passage through the stenotic segment. The utility of EUS, however, is clear in the evaluation of local wall penetration by tumor and periesophageal lymph nodes.

CT, to a large extent, remains the method of choice for evaluation beyond the wall of the esophagus—lymph nodes beyond the immediate periesophageal region, local involvement of mediastinal contiguous structures, and distant nodal disease and organ involvement.

The role of MRI is currently being developed, and there may be a future role for this modality in routine evaluation for liver pathology, depending on further clinical investigation and the ultimate cost of the modality.

METASTATIC TUMOR TO THE LUNGS AND BRONCHI

Metastatic disease to the lungs and bronchi is more common than primary lung cancer. It is generally considered an ominous finding from a prognostic point of view, although treatment of metastatic disease in recent years has become both more aggressive and more effective. Most commonly, breast, kidney, and head and neck cancers metastasize to the lungs (119). Some less common tumors—such as germ cell tumors, bone and soft part sarcomas, melanoma, and thyroid cancer—frequently metastasize to the lungs but are encountered less commonly because of their lower incidence. Much of the information concerning metastatic disease to the thorax comes from the pre-CT era: autopsy series indicate a frequency of pulmonary metastases of between 20% and 54% in patients dying from cancer (120–122), at least partially depending on the technique of autopsy. As expected, autopsy series show a much greater percentage of pulmonary metastases than that seen at initial presentation (123).

MECHANISM OF SPREAD TO LUNG

The paths of metastatic spread to lung are quite variable. Most commonly, tumors grow locally, extending through the artery and compressing surrounding structures. These tumor emboli can also originate from the systemic lymph vessels flowing into the thoracic duct and eventually emptying into the systemic venous system. Unusual vascular routes to the pulmonary parenchyma are also possible, e.g., from bronchial arteries. Lymphangitic spread of cancer to the lungs represents a distinct entity with unique pathologic, radiographic, and clinical features. Extensive infiltration of the lymph channels of the lungs is present, with resultant thickening of the interlobular pulmonary septae by tumor cells and associated desmoplastic reaction. The mechanism of spread (121) is by extension of small peripheral pulmonary emboli through vessel walls into the lymphatic vessels, with subsequent extensive spread along these channels. Less commonly, upper abdominal tumors can spread via lymph vessels directly to hilar nodes and then in a retrograde fashion into the pulmonary lymph vessels.

RADIOGRAPHIC APPEARANCE OF PULMONARY METASTASES

Pulmonary metastases are most frequently seen on plain radiographs or on CT as well-defined pulmonary nodules, more frequently at the periphery of the lung and at the lung bases (Fig. 6.18) (122, 123). They usually compress but do not invade surrounding lung parenchyma and vary greatly in size from the limits of plain film visibility (2 to 3 mm) to huge masses. Less commonly, they can have irregular and poorly defined borders. Metastatic adenocarcinomas as well as choriocarcinomas (124) are prone to develop shaggy borders, which may reflect either local hemorrhage or invasion of surrounding lung parenchyma.

Cavitation can be seen in 4% to 6% of cases (125), more commonly with squamous cancer metastases from the head and neck region (126). There is a modest incidence of cavitation of adenocarcinomas, particularly from the gastrointestinal tract. Both small and large lesions may cavitate, perhaps reflecting internal tumor metabolism rather than lack of blood supply (125). When multiple nodules are present, usually no more than a few of them are cavitated (127).

Cavitation of subpleural metastatic deposits can result in communication of the tracheobronchial tree

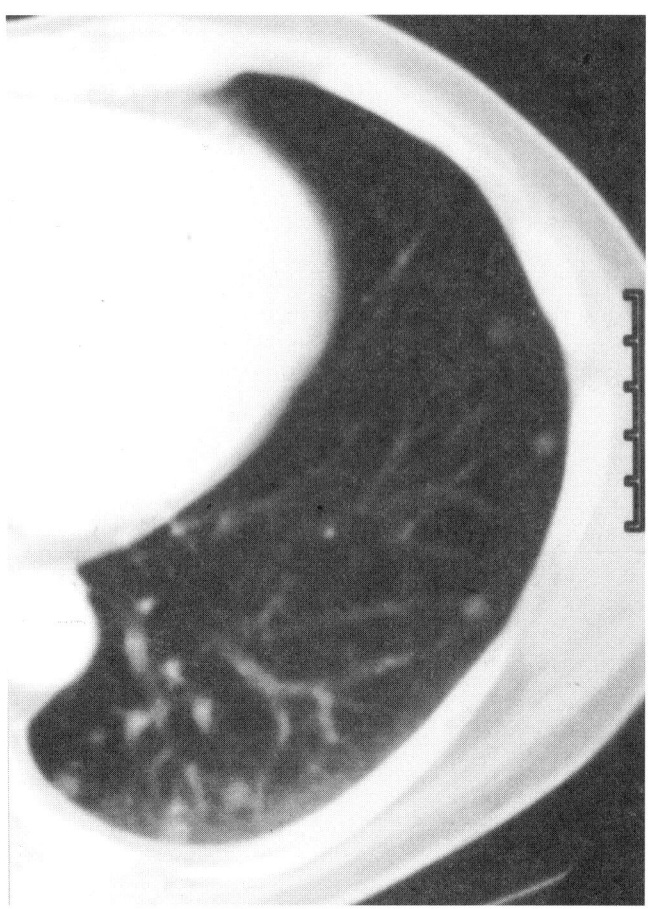

FIGURE 6.18. Metastatic disease. CT scan through the left lower lung zone. Multiple, small, peripheral, pulmonary nodules are present. Their hematogenous origin is indicated by their almost universal presence at the end of small vessels. Presumably the small blood-borne tumor emboli lodged at the ends of vessels and began to increase in size, gradually becoming visible on CT and chest radiography. There is no evidence of lymphangitic spread on this chest radiograph. Invasion and permeation of lymphatics from these foci of hematogenous disease could result in the CT appearance and the clinical manifestations of lymphangitic tumor spread.

and the pleural space with consequent pneumothorax (128–131). The nodule may be invisible on chest radiography or CT, with the appearance of an apparently spontaneous pneumothorax, most frequently seen in patients with sarcomas. Calcification is most frequently seen in metastatic osteosarcoma and chondrosarcoma, in which the osteoid or chondroid matrix of the tumor calcifies. Calcification in other forms of metastatic cancer is uncommon, usually representing calcification of a mucin-producing tumor matrix of breast, ovarian, colon, or thyroid origin (132).

The presence of calcified pulmonary nodules raises the possibility of the presence of granulomata. Appropriate history and previous imaging studies are helpful in the differential diagnosis, but in some cases histologic confirmation may be required, either by lung biopsy or by a video-assisted thoracoscopic procedure. (See Solitary Pulmonary Nodules, above).

Less common radiographic signs for metastatic disease include a miliary appearance occasionally seen in metastatic thyroid, renal carcinoma, osteosarcoma, trophoblastic disease, or melanoma. In addition, pulmonary infiltrates or consolidation, simulating infection or other nonneoplastic pulmonary processes, may be seen. This has been described in melanoma (133–135).

Uncommonly, residual stable pulmonary masses are seen in patients treated intensively for susceptible tumors such as germ cell tumors, particularly choriocarcinoma (124, 136, 137). Some of these tumors, when resected, have contained only residual fibrosis and some calcification with no evidence of the presence of viable tumor. In addition, residual masses from germ cell tumors may contain mature teratoma, representing a benign counterpart of the original malignant germ cell tumor. Unfortunately, one cannot differentiate this mass from residual viable tumor with current plain film or CT methods (138). The response of pulmonary metastases to chemotherapy depends on the tumor histology and the origin and extent of disease, and the chemotherapeutic regimen employed. The effectiveness of treatment of metastases is therefore highly variable. Some responsive tumors such as seminoma may disappear entirely. More commonly, however, metastatic nodules have a less dramatic response ranging from progression in size of the nodules during therapy to significant decrease in size of all nodules. Frequently, a mixed response occurs, with some nodules increasing in size while others diminish.

The appearance of pulmonary nodules in patients with known primary malignancy elsewhere, including lung, is highly suspicious. Histologic confirmation may be required when there is the possibility that the nodules may have another etiology. Granulomata (sarcoid, tuberculosis, fungus) may appear on the chest, especially in patients who had been immunocompromised as a result of therapy.

The appearance of a solitary pulmonary nodule in a patient with a known primary tumor raises the issue of metastatic disease versus a new primary lung tumor. Cahan (139) drew attention to the large proportion of new primary lung tumors appearing more than 1 year after treatment for a primary cancer elsewhere. Depending on the histology of the primary tumor, the likelihood of a solitary pulmonary nodule representing either metastatic disease or a new lung primary tumor is highly variable. Certain primary neoplasms are associated with a high incidence of synchronous or metachronous lung cancers, i.e., head and neck tumors (140). Others, such as gastrointestinal tract neoplasms, have a lower, although significant, incidence of synchronous or metachronous primary lung cancers (141). Others still, such as metastatic sarcoma, have a distinctly rare incidence of synchronous or metachronous lung cancers, often because these patients are younger and frequently do not share the risk factors for other lung cancer.

For these reasons, histologic confirmation assumes great importance. Frequently, the issue may be resolved by percutaneous lung biopsy, but occasionally more extensive sampling requiring a video-assisted thoracoscopic procedure or open thoracotomy may be necessary.

Characteristic findings of metastatic carcinoma on nuclear medicine studies are currently relatively uncommon, except in two instances: (a) ^{99m}Tc polyphosphate uptake in osteoid-forming neoplasms or large primary tumors, and (b) radioiodine uptake in metastatic thyroid cancer. Functioning osteoid matrix is common in osteosarcoma metastatic to lungs, with about 30% to 40% taking up and concentrating the ^{99m}Tc bone agent on bone scanning (142). Other lesions, including lung primary tumors, may have a small degree of soft-tissue uptake of ^{99m}Tc bone agent sufficient to cause a easily discerned diffuse uptake in the tumor. This tendency of large non–osteoid-forming tumors to take up the bone agent is thought to be related to regions of necrosis, in which hydroxyapatite crystals are precipitated in the mitochondria of the dying cells. Well-differentiated thyroid cancer metastatic to lungs concentrates radioiodine avidly, and uptake in the lungs may be seen even when the chest roentgenogram is negative (143). A miliary pattern on chest radiography should suggest the possibility of metastatic thyroid cancer; the disease is curable if treatment with high-dose radioiodine is begun at an early stage.

ENDOBRONCHIAL METASTASES

Endobronchial metastases are distinctly unusual, representing approximately 2% of all metastases in a large series (144). Attention is usually drawn to these endobronchial lesions by the symptoms the patient develops as a result of bronchial or tracheal obstruction (e.g., cough, wheezing, atelectasis) (145, 146). Kidney, breast, and colorectal tumors are the most common primary tumors causing tracheobronchial metastases. We have observed several instances of metastatic melanoma to the tracheobronchial tree. Endobronchial metastases may be difficult to diagnose on plain chest radiography and are frequently missed on CT if no related findings, such as atelectasis and/or obstructive pneumonia, are present.

LYMPHANGITIC SPREAD

The chest radiographic appearance reflects the pathologic changes with fine reticular and nodular shadows present and thickened septal lines, similar to the septal lines seen in pulmonary edema. Subpleural edema can result in pleural lines and thickening of the fissures (Fig. 6.19). Lymphangitic spread is most commonly seen in primary carcinomas of the lung, breast, stomach, and pancreas. Dyspnea is common, frequently severe, and out of proportion to the radiographic appearance.

ROLE OF COMPUTED TOMOGRAPHY AND MAGNETIC RESONANCE IMAGING IN METASTATIC DISEASE

The technique of resection of pulmonary metastases in patients with primary tumors has gained popularity in recent years (147–149) and appears to be of real efficacy, provided that resection criteria are adhered to rigorously: (a) all visible metastatic disease can be resected, and (b) no other known foci of metastatic disease can be detected. Chest radiography consistently underestimates the true number of nodules found at surgery. CT also frequently does not detect metastatic nodules, particularly if they are very small.

Plain chest radiographs in the 120–140 kV range are the standard imaging examination for detection of metastatic disease. The role of linear or complex motion tomography in the evaluation of lung parenchyma has been superseded by CT because of CT's improved visualization of lung parenchyma, particularly in the costophrenic angles and adjacent to the mediastinum, as well as improved visualization and differentiation of soft-tissue structures in the hilar region, mediastinum, and chest wall.

Nodules of 3-mm diameter can be detected on CT, compared with a threshold of 1 cm or slightly less for plain chest radiography. This increased sensitivity in detection of small nodules carries with it the possibility of reduced specificity, i.e., the detection of small nontumor nodules not related to the primary tumor. Several investigators have suggested that this is indeed the case (150), whereas others showed that more than 80% of nodules seen on CT not present on the chest radiograph are metastatic (151, 152). In the report of Peuchot and Libshitz (152), 87% of pulmonary resected nodules proved to be metastatic. Only 9% were benign, with 4% being unexpected primary lung cancer.

Surgeons operating on pulmonary nodules routinely report observing and resecting more nodules

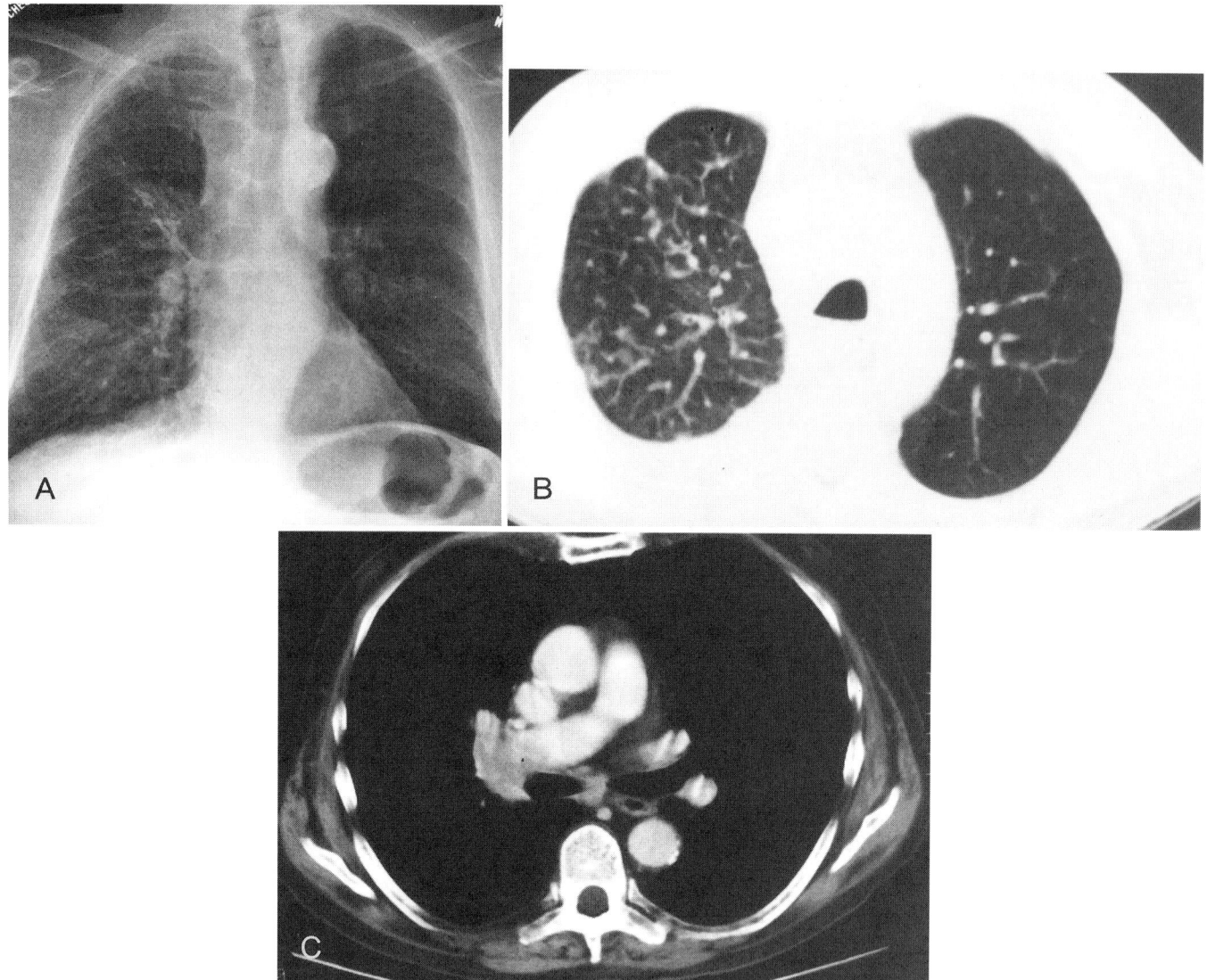

FIGURE 6.19. Metastatic disease. **A.** Chest radiograph shows extensive accentuation of interstitial lung markings throughout the right lung. Some small ill-defined nodules are also present. There is prominence of the right hilum as well as of the right paratracheal region. The left lung appears clear. The patient was short of breath. **B.** CT scan through the left upper lung field with lung parenchymal windows. The slice thickness was 5 mm. There is generalized accentuation of the interstitial markings that appear both more numerous, thicker, and more irregular than those observed in the opposite lung. A number of small nodules are present, and there are some areas of subpleural increased density. The finding is very typical for lymphangitic spread of tumor, although not pathognomonic. **C.** CT scan through the right hilar region with soft-tissue windows. There is prominent adenopathy in the right hilum. One of the explanations for lymphangitic spread of tumor is retrograde permeation of lymphatics, associated with a desmoplastic reaction, from central hilar and/or mediastinal disease.

than are confirmed by CT, suggesting that CT is not sensitive enough, although considerably more sensitive than chest radiography. This conclusion is borne out in the article by Peuchot and Libshitz (152), in which 27% of nodules resected at surgery were not detected on preoperative CT.

One potential serious pitfall in CT detection of pulmonary nodules should be mentioned: at the lung bases there can be considerable variability in inspiratory effort, resulting in horizontal bands of lung that are not visualized, with the potential of nonvisualization of significant portions of tumor-bearing lung. Recently, spiral, or helical, scanning has been introduced. It uses a series of 5 to 30 contiguous (or overlapping) scans obtained during a single breath hold, eliminating the likelihood of missing sections of lung.

There are two questions a clinician must ask in deciding whether to obtain a CT scan of the chest in patients with tumor and negative chest radiograph: (*a*) does the tumor frequently metastasize to lung, and (*b*) will the detection of pulmonary nodules significantly alter therapy?

CT should be obtained routinely in patients who are candidates for resection of pulmonary metastatic disease, both to confirm the presence of pulmonary nodules on plain radiographs and to detect additional nodules not seen on chest films. The resection of pulmonary nodules is advantageous if all visualized disease can be removed. Tumors most amenable to resection of pulmonary metastases include various sarcomas, head and neck tumors, and genitourinary tract, colon, and testicular cancers (147).

Patients in whom pulmonary metastases are common at the time of presentation should have routine (noncontrast enhanced) CT of the chest. These tumors include bone and soft-parts sarcomas, as well as germ cell tumors. CT detection of metastatic disease in these patients significantly alters therapy.

Obtaining routine CT scans in locally advanced melanoma (in patients with negative chest radiographs or with only one nodule visible) is controversial. It appears that in most cases detection of new or additional pulmonary nodules does not alter therapy (153).

CT scanning of lung for primary cancer in other sites (head and neck, kidney, bladder, gastrointestinal tract, breast, prostate) is not recommended routinely unless there is evidence of regional or other distant spread, e.g., bone or liver metastases, or unless there is plain radiographic evidence or clinical suspicion for the presence of metastatic lung disease (154).

High-resolution CT, using 1- or 1.5-mm cuts separated by 8- to 10-mm intervals, provides a detailed survey of the pulmonary parenchyma and has been useful in evaluating lymphangitic carcinoma. High-spatial-frequency reconstruction algorithms are used in obtaining images with finer detail. Lymphangitic carcinoma has numerous peripheral linear shadows or branching Y, U, or polygonal densities extending to the pleural surface (155–158). These densities, which represent thickened interlobular septa, may also contain fine discrete nodules not visible on plain chest radiographs. More centrally, thickening of the bronchovascular bundle may be evident.

Lastly, an SPN on a chest roentgenogram in a patient with a history of a primary tumor elsewhere may prove to be multiple lesions on CT. This finding increases the likelihood of metastatic disease in patients in whom a solitary lung lesion may have represented a new lung primary neoplasm (141).

The role of MRI in the detection of pulmonary nodules has received attention recently in an article indicating similar sensitivity to CT in detecting pulmonary nodules (155). MRI, however, had several important disadvantages compared with CT: requirements for relatively thick sections (to preserve signal to noise ratio), insensitivity to the presence of calcium within pulmonary nodules, long duration of the study, patient susceptibility to claustrophobia, and considerably greater expense (156). CT thus remains the gold standard for evaluating patients for pulmonary metastases.

Metastatic disease is seen less commonly in the mediastinal and hilar lymph nodes, with involvement of contiguous structures as a result of tumor growth. Melanoma and some sarcomas have a propensity to metastasize to the pericardium and heart (Fig. 6.20).

MEDIASTINUM

The mediastinum is a complex compartment containing multiple anatomic structures. In the predigital tomography era, visualization and differentiation of soft-tissue structures within the mediastinum were hampered by insensitive invasive imaging techniques (chest radiograph, esophagram, angiography). With the availability of CT, MRI, and newer nuclear medicine techniques, our ability to delineate the anatomy of this region has improved greatly, frequently permitting confident diagnoses as well as accurate extent of disease evaluations.

Mediastinal masses may be caused by a variety of congenital anomalies or other benign conditions such as bronchogenic cysts, aortic aneurysms, mediastinal lipomas and lipomatosis, and neurenteric cysts. It is important that these lesions, which frequently are unexpected findings on imaging studies obtained for other reasons, not be mistaken for thoracic malignancies. Their diagnosis is frequently apparent on imaging examinations because of their characteristic appearance (e.g., thoracic aortic aneurysm) or density (e.g., mediastinal lipomatosis); occasionally, however, the differential diagnosis from malignant tumors may be difficult, requiring biopsy or excision. Readers are referred to standard radiologic texts for comprehensive discussion of benign mediastinal disease (2–4).

The great value of the radiographic input is found in the close cooperation with clinicians and the integration of the image interpretation into the total clinical background. This integration necessitates a close dialogue with the clinician to optimize therapeutic decisions.

PLAIN CHEST RADIOGRAPHY

For chest radiographic analysis, the mediastinum is divided into three components—anterior, middle,

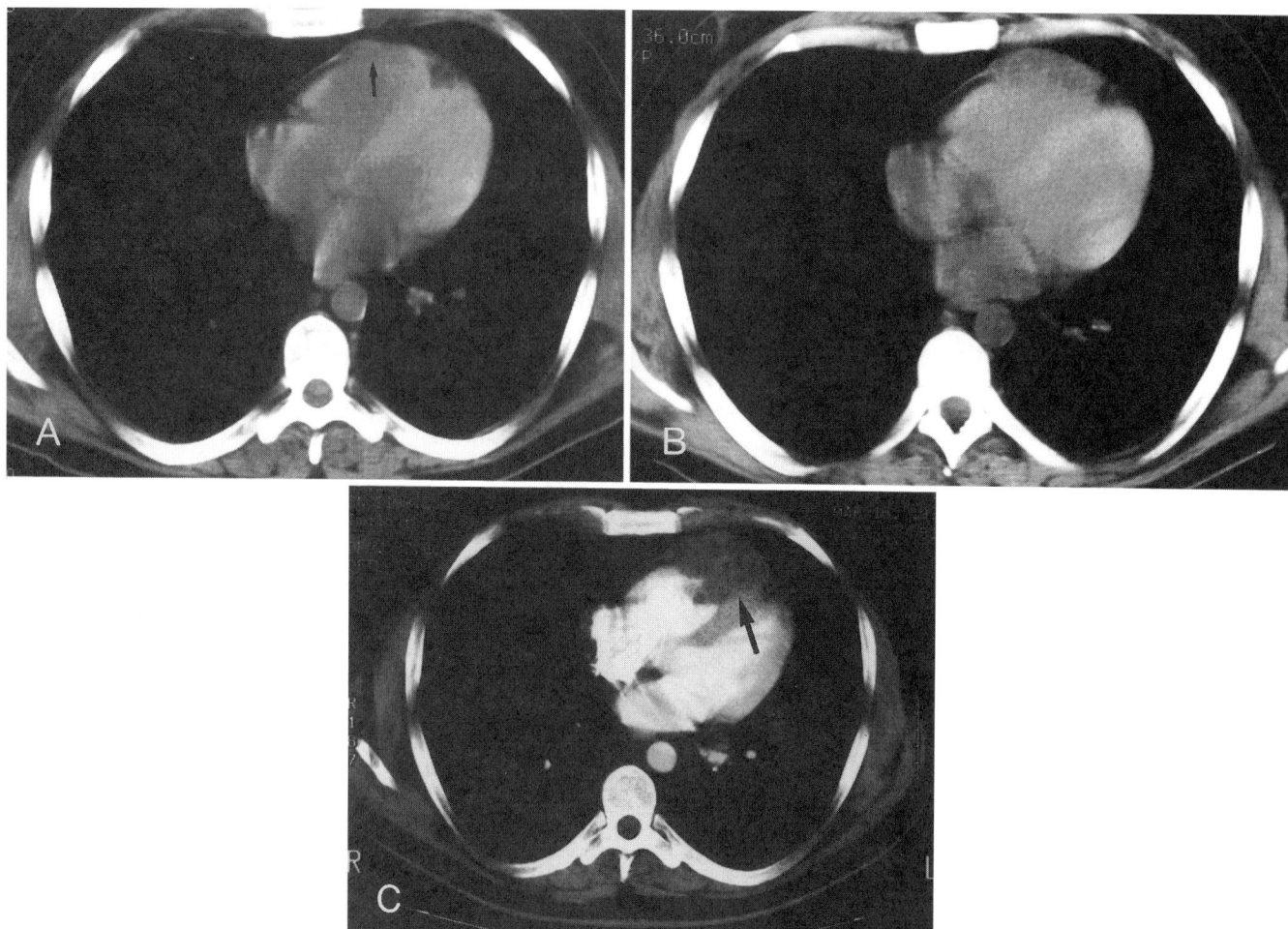

FIGURE 6.20. Metastatic disease to the heart. **A.** CT scan through the heart in a patient with a history of primitive neuroectodermal tumor. There is subtle localized thickening of the anterior pericardium with obliteration of the epicardial fat in this region. This finding was present on a single slice and was missed at the time of interpretation. **B.** A follow-up CT scan obtained 3 months later shows enlargement of the mass, rendering it considerably more visible on this scan. Intravenous contrast was not administered for these two scans. Note that it is not possible to determine the posterior extent of the mass, which blends imperceptibly with the myocardium and cardiac chambers. **C.** CT scan obtained 1 month after *B*, with intravenous contrast administration. Note that the cardiac chambers are well opacified. A large mass is seen to invade the myocardium and the chamber of the right ventricle. The mass extends posteriorly to involve the interventricular septum (*arrow*). The apparent large increase in tumor involvement in *C* may be partly spurious because of improved visualization resulting from intravenous contrast administration. In *B* the interface among tumor, myocardium, and cardiac chamber cannot be delineated because contrast was not administered. Thus the true posterior extent of tumor could not be determined.

and posterior mediastinum, based on lateral chest radiographs, which are characterized by differing groups of pathologic processes (with considerable overlap) in each compartment. For example, an anterior mediastinal mass would likely represent a thymic mass, lymphoma (especially Hodgkin's disease), or germ cell tumor, whereas a posterior mediastinal mass would most likely represent a neural tumor or aneurysm of the descending thoracic aorta. Plain film analysis of mediastinal disease is discussed comprehensively in the text by Reed (157).

COMPUTED TOMOGRAPHY AND MAGNETIC RESONANCE IMAGING OF THE MEDIASTINUM

Although adequate images of the mediastinum do not require intravenous contrast administration (158), most radiologists prefer contrast-enhanced scans using a power-injected bolus technique to opacify vessels and cardiac chambers and differentiate these structures from lymph node and nonvascular mediastinal abnormalities.

MRI is typically used when the CT scan does not provide adequate information or in patients with severe contrast allergy; cardiac gating and respiratory compensation are employed and T1-weighted images of the mediastinum are always obtained. T2-weighted images may be obtained in cases in which greater tissue specificity is desired. Gradient-echo images may be employed for evaluation of the vascular anatomy or for possible vascular thrombosis or tumor involvement.

LYMPHOMAS

The treatment and prognosis both of Hodgkin's disease and non-Hodgkin's lymphoma (NHL) depends on several factors, including the histology of these neoplasms and the extent of disease at presentation. The Ann Arbor staging classification is used for both Hodgkin's disease and NHL (159).

HODGKIN'S DISEASE

Involvement of the chest at presentation in Hodgkin's disease occurs in 85% of cases; it almost always involves the superior mediastinum, including both the prevascular and paratracheal nodes (160, 161). Hilar nodes are involved by Hodgkin's disease in 25% of patients. However, careful CT evaluation frequently shows involvement of subcarinal nodes (22%), posterior mediastinal nodes (5%), and cardiophrenic angle nodes (8%). Detection of nodal disease in these regions is particularly important for radiation therapy planning; recurrence may occur at the edge of a radiation port if the true extent of regional tumor involvement is not delineated by CT.

In approximately 10% of patients, pulmonary parenchyma is involved, almost always immediately adjacent to mediastinal and/or hilar nodal disease. This pulmonary parenchymal involvement is characterized both on chest radiography and CT by ill-defined peripheral margins indicating infiltration of lung tissue.

Pleural effusion is present in approximately 15% of cases, although most do not have tumor cells. The pericardium is involved in approximately 5% of patients. The chest wall and the spinal column may be involved by direct extension, but this occurrence is less common.

Involvement of the abdominal structures is less common than involvement of the mediastinum. The liver is involved only if there is preexisting splenic involvement.

For evaluation of intrathoracic Hodgkin's disease, chest radiography followed by carefully performed contrast-enhanced CT should be obtained (Fig. 6.21). The CT scan adds additional information and more accurately indicates the true extent of mediastinal nodal involvement, particularly cardiophrenic angle nodes and subcarinal nodal disease. Conventional chest tomography is no longer used.

The posttreatment radiographic follow-up of patients with Hodgkin's disease continues to evolve. It appears that CT scanning is becoming more common as a surveillance measure in the posttreatment period because of its ability to detect small recurrent masses. Currently, the acquisition of a baseline chest, abdomen, and pelvic CT scan is recommended. If these baseline studies show residual disease, further studies, such as MRI or gallium scanning, may be indicated.

NUCLEAR MEDICINE IN HODGKIN'S DISEASE

^{67}Ga citrate was recognized as a tumor-seeking agent when patients with Hodgkin's lymphoma were enrolled in a study evaluating ^{67}Ga citrate as a bone imaging agent. Tumor uptake was seen in a neck node (162). Since that time it has become apparent that ^{67}Ga is taken up by rapidly proliferating malignant tissues, particularly the lymphomas, as well as by inflammatory tissues. ^{67}Ga is used commonly to evaluate patients with Hodgkin's disease, both for initial staging and probably most importantly for follow-up (163) (Fig. 6.22).

Using ^{67}Ga with single proton emission CT (SPECT) has been shown to be 90% sensitive for Hodgkin's involvement of the mediastinum. It is thus much superior to planar gamma camera imaging alone (164).

A residual mass frequently is seen on CT in the mediastinum following response to therapy: it is not possible to determine by CT alone whether this mass contains viable tumor or merely masslike fibrosis. In a study of 27 biopsied patients with Hodgkin's disease and involvement of the mediastinum, ^{67}Ga SPECT was performed and the results compared with those from CT. In 25% of these patients, residual mass persisted on the CT scan. ^{67}Ga was accurate for predicting the presence or absence of disease in 25 of 27 biopsied tumor sites, even in patients for whom the CT was indeterminate. Thus, there appears to be a clear role for ^{67}Ga SPECT scanning in patients with residual mass on CT after treatment for Hodgkin's disease (165).

NON-HODGKIN'S LYMPHOMA

NHLs are somewhat less well-defined and more complex entities than Hodgkin's disease (166). In contrast to Hodgkin's disease, extra nodal tumor involvement is common in the nasopharynx, and gastrointestinal tract, liver, bone marrow, among other sites. Imaging examinations, although extremely important,

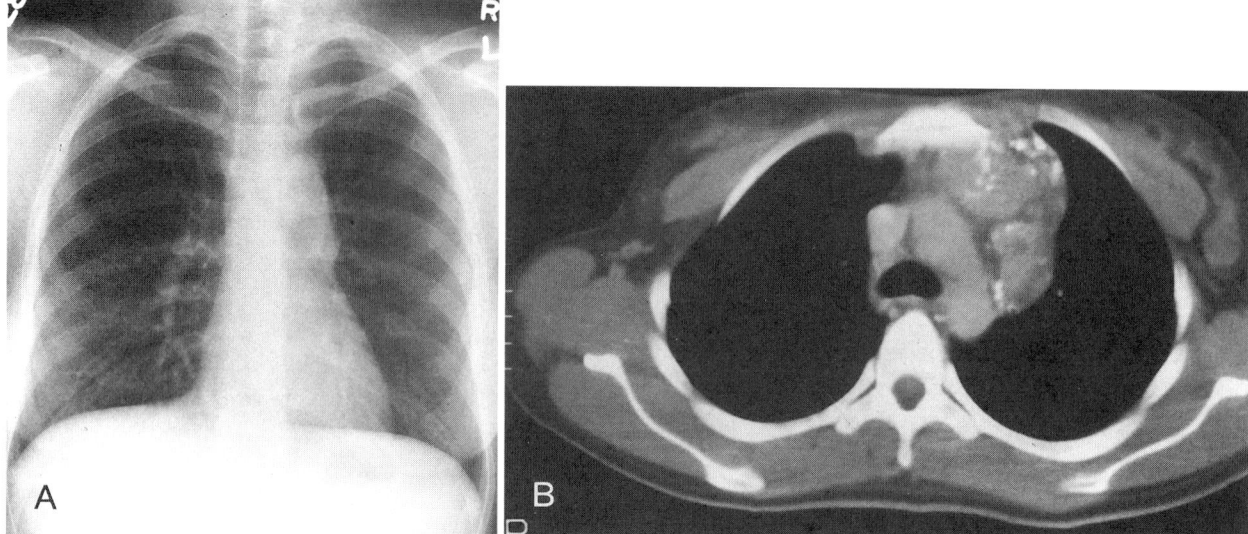

FIGURE 6.21. Hodgkin's disease. **A.** Chest. A PA chest radiograph demonstrates clear peripheral lung zones. The mediastinal contour is prominent at the level of the left hilum. **B.** CT scan at the level of the anterior mediastinum. This scan shows a bulky anterior mediastinal mass. The small speckled densities contained within this mass represent lymphangiographic dye, which has diffused into the tumor from a bipedal lymphangiogram (LAG). This appearance is atypical, in that usually the oil-based contrast for lymphangiography collects in the cisterna chyli and exits into the venous system at the left subclavian trunk through the thoracic duct. Occasionally, however, lymph nodes, and in this case anterior mediastinal tumor, may become opacified with LAG dye, representing anomalous lymphatic connections within the thorax. Treated Hodgkin's disease nodules may calcify, particularly in the anterior mediastinum, but these are typically small.

may be less specific for staging purposes than those used for Hodgkin's disease.

CT is the most useful examination for staging and follow-up of patients with NHL. Lymphography has gradually diminished in relative importance. In addition, the frequent extrapelvic and extraretroperitoneal nodal presentation renders lymphography relatively less important for this tumor. MRI can be useful for evaluating possible bone marrow involvement (167). Similarly, the spleen and liver may be evaluated effectively with MRI, using superparamagnetic contrast agents (iron oxide).

For NHL involving the chest, an initial contrast-enhanced CT scan is performed (Fig. 6.23). Forty percent to 50% of patients presenting with NHL have chest disease; in contrast, 85% of Hodgkin's disease presents in the mediastinum. NHL may involve all lymph node sites diffusely within the chest as well as lung parenchyma, pleura, and pericardium.

^{67}Ga citrate is effective in targeting tumor of intermediate and high-grade NHL (Fig. 6.24). The proper approach to the use of ^{67}Ga in lymphoma involves serial studies: a baseline assessment obtained before therapy and repeated at the time of restaging procedures. In many regimens this assessment often is obtained at 3- and 6-month intervals after beginning treatment. The persistence of ^{67}Ga uptake after initial treatment is a bad prognostic sign (168).

Thallium 201 (^{201}Th) has been used to image lymphoma and appears to have a role in distinguishing whether uptake of ^{67}Ga citrate is neoplastic or inflammatory in origin. It is normally concentrated in viable tumor, whereas inflammatory processes do not take up the radionuclide (169).

GERM CELL TUMORS

Eighty percent of mediastinal germ cell tumors are benign, the majority being composed of dermoid cysts (i.e., derived from the ectodermal layer of germ cell only) and benign teratomas (derived from all germ cell layers). The vast majority of these tumors present in the anterior mediastinum, but up to 5% are found in the posterior mediastinum (170, 171). The two benign varieties have a similar CT appearance: well-defined and encapsulated with as many as one third containing calcium. Fat density is considered highly specific (especially a fat fluid level) (172, 173). Calcium is frequently present, and teeth and other anatomic parts may be seen. Malignant teratomas are bulky, poorly defined, and invasive.

Seminomas and non–seminomatous germ cell tumors are less common. They are nonspecific on CT, with seminomas typically having a homogeneous appearance and non–seminomatous germ cell tumors having an inhomogeneous appearance resulting from extensive necrosis (174–177). CT is important not only

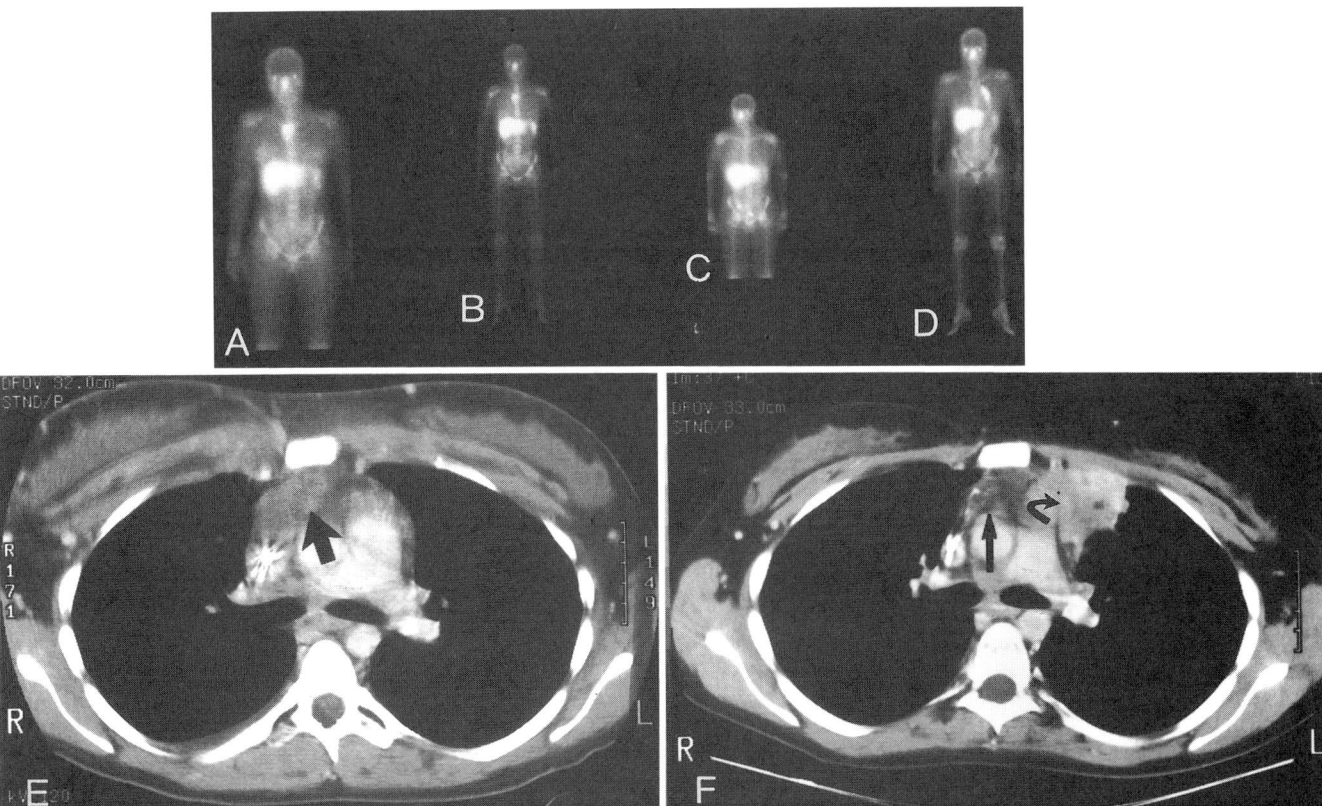

FIGURE 6.22. ^{67}Ga imaging of Hodgkin's disease. **A.** ^{67}Ga imaging in Hodgkin's lymphoma at presentation with abnormal area in upper mediastinum. **B.** The abnormal uptake area persists on ^{67}Ga-citrate scanning through the first 3 months post therapy. **C.** The lymphoma is no longer evident at the 1-year follow-up. **D.** The tumor recurs at a different site 2 years later. The original CT scan shows a large mass (*thick arrow*) in the upper mediastinum, just above the aortic arch. **E.** The follow-up image at 2 years post treatment. **F.** Small residual density which has no ^{67}Ga citrate activity in the right mediastinum (*arrow*). A recurrent mass is present in the left side of the mediastinum extending into the lung parenchyma (*curved arrow*), corresponding to the new abnormal ^{67}Ga citrate region present in *D*.

for determining extent of disease of the tumor for surgical removal but, in the case of malignancy, for evaluating regional and distant spread as well as follow-up after therapy. The role of MRI, if any, in evaluation of these lesions has not been defined: the modality does not visualize calcification with sensitivity, and its ability to diagnosis fat is inferior to that of CT (178).

THYMUS

The normal thymus involutes rapidly from puberty through early adulthood, with the gland becoming smaller and infiltrated by fat (179–182). It is located in the anterior mediastinum and extends down to the base of the heart. It is present at puberty as a bilobed structure with a maximum thickness of 1.8 cm before the age of 20 years, decreasing to 1.3 cm after age 20. Both increases in these dimensions and changes in the shape of the thymus (e.g., lobulation) are indications of thymic abnormality.

THYMIC HYPERPLASIA

Lymphoid follicular hyperplasia is the presence of an increased number of lymphoid germinal centers in the medulla of the thymus (183), frequently seen in patients with myasthenia gravis. Glands involved by lymphoid follicular hyperplasia may not be increased in overall size on CT (184, 185), although enlargement can be present. The CT appearance is not specific and should be correlated with the clinical findings. This condition is usually seen before the age of 20, when the presence of thymoma is extremely rare.

THYMIC REBOUND

Following involution resulting from stress, the thymus returns to its normal size after removal of the stress-inciting agent, commonly chemotherapy (186, 187) but also including recovery from burns (188) and treatment of Cushing's disease (189). One fourth of patients exhibit thymic rebound following stress, i.e., increase in thymic volume exceeding the original size by

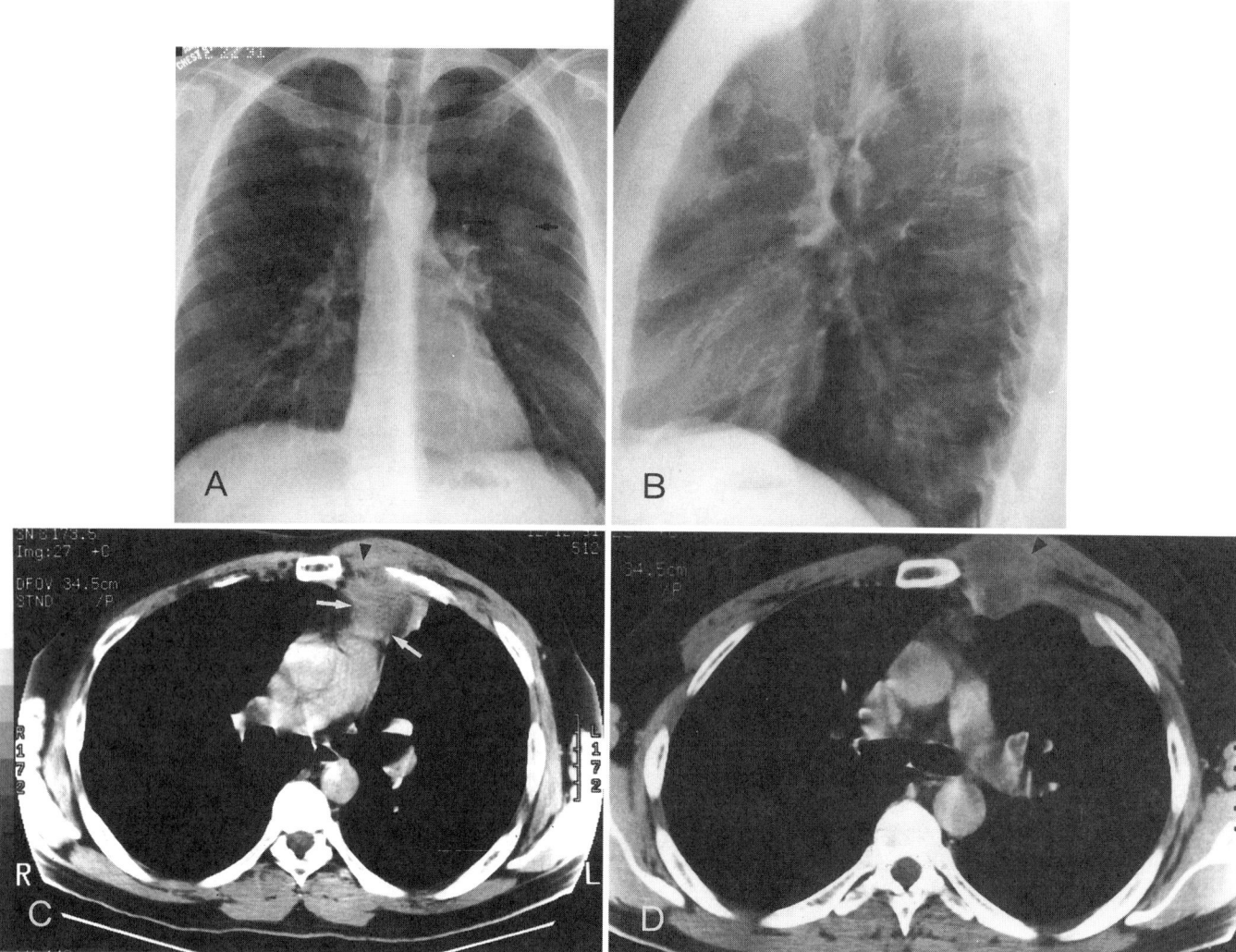

FIGURE 6.23. Non-Hodgkin's lymphoma. **A.** PA chest radiograph shows a prominence overlying the left hilum. There is also an ill-defined left midlung zone mass density that may be either pleural or parenchymal in origin (*arrow*). Its sharp medial border (*long arrow*) suggests the possibility of a pleural origin. **B.** The lateral chest radiograph shows the anterior mediastinal mass with pleural thickening. A second component is seen superior to this, and there appears to be some thickening of the pleura anteriorly, where the tumor abuts the anterior chest wall. **C.** CT scan through the lower anterior mediastinum. There is a bulky tumor mass anterior to the main pulmonary artery (*white arrows*). This mass extends anteriorly, and there is suggestion of infiltration into the anterior mediastinal soft tissues, with obliteration of fat planes in the region, in the vicinity of the internal mammary vessels (*black arrowhead*). **D.** CT scan at a slightly higher level shows a bulky chest wall mass in continuity with the anterior mediastinal mass infiltrating soft tissues, including the medial aspect of the pectoralis muscle (*arrowhead*). A second pleural-based mass nodule is seen in the anterior pleura of the left thorax, corresponding to the more peripheral mass present in *A*.

50% or more. It is important to be aware of this relatively common phenomenon and not to mistake it for mediastinal spread of tumor. In particular, in patients with lymphoma isolated thymic enlargement after chemotherapy almost always represents thymic rebound. Only when accompanied by lymphadenopathy elsewhere in the mediastinum should involvement of the thymus by recurrent lymphoma be considered.

Thymic rebound is also a common occurrence on ^{67}Ga scanning and may cause confusion regarding the differentiation of persistent uptake in a lymphomatous mass from a normal finding of uptake in the thymus recovering from chemotherapy. In children younger than 15 years, thymic rebound is the rule rather than the exception (Fig. 6.25). Biopsy-documented uptake in the thymus has occurred in adults as old as 22 years of age. The characteristic appearance and location of the uptake on ^{67}Ga SPECT imaging helps differentiate mediastinal mass or lymph node uptake from thymic uptake (190).

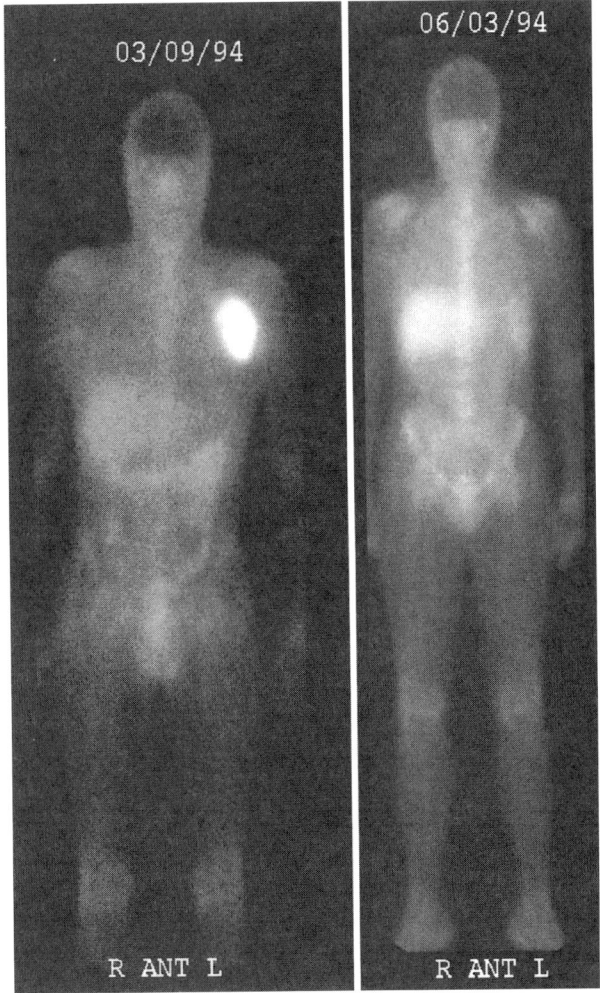

FIGURE 6.24. Gallium imaging of non-Hodgkin's lymphoma. ^{67}Ga citrate images in a patient with AIDS and non-Hodgkins lymphoma, intermediate grade. Images obtained before (*left*) and after (*right*) show beneficial effects of therapy for a lesion in the left axilla.

THYMOMA (AND MYASTHENIA GRAVIS)

Thymoma is the most common thymic neoplasm seen in patients over the age of 30 years. On CT (185, 191–195) the tumor may be in the midline, but most commonly it extends predominantly to one side of the mediastinum as a spherical or lobulated mass surrounded by mediastinal fat. Calcification is quite common. Most thymomas show soft-tissue density and relative homogeneity on CT but may rarely have cystic components. CT is capable of diagnosing thymoma with a high degree of accuracy (185).

Thymomas are histologically classified as epithelial, lymphocytic, or mixed lymphoepithelial. A more consistently aggressive variety is thymic carcinoma, which is capable of distant metastases. Thirty percent of thymomas behave aggressively, with local and regional spread to mediastinal structures (pericardium, superior vena cava and great vessels, and pleural surfaces, lung, and chest wall) spreading by contiguity. Distant metastases are unusual.

Three stages are recognized:

1. An intracapsular stage: no spread to surrounding structures is present. Surgery is usually curative at this stage.
2. Pericapsular and local mediastinal involvement by tumor: radiation therapy is usually administered as a supplement or in an adjuvant setting to surgery.
3. Local organ invasion and pleural implants: surgery and radiation therapy are supplemented with chemotherapy (196–198). Occasionally, at presentation the extent of local invasiveness, with involvement of multiple structures, precludes surgery. (Fig. 6.26). The presence of fat surrounding the circumference of tumor suggests resectability (195). CT may reveal unsuspected local and regional extension of thymoma, e.g., extension to the retrocrural space and retroperitoneum (199, 200).

Fifteen percent of all patients with myasthenia gravis have or develop thymoma. All myasthenia gravis patients with a discrete thymic mass, especially those over the age of 45 year, may have thymoma. Sixty-five percent of patients have thymic hyperplasia (i.e., no discrete mass may be present or the lobes may be enlarged diffusely and partially infiltrated by fat). A normal-sized thymic gland may be hyperplastic at pathology, because this diagnosis depends on the number of active germinal centers rather than on the gland size (201).

THYMIC TUMORS

The lymphomas, especially Hodgkin's disease, may involve the thymus but not as an isolated event. They are usually associated with involvement of mediastinal lymph nodes. The presence of thymic cysts is sometimes noted after radiation therapy for Hodgkin's disease (202, 203) or thoracotomy (204). Other rare tumors that may originate from the thymus include metastases (lung and breast), neuroendocrine tumors (205), and carcinoid, simple, or cavernous hemangiomas and lymphangiomas.

Thymolipoma is a rare thymic neoplasm manifested by an inhomogeneous fatty mass in the anterior mediastinum. It is frequently mistaken for other processes on plain films (206), but it has a characteristic appearance on CT: many strands or islands of soft-tissue density in a matrix of adipose tissue density that

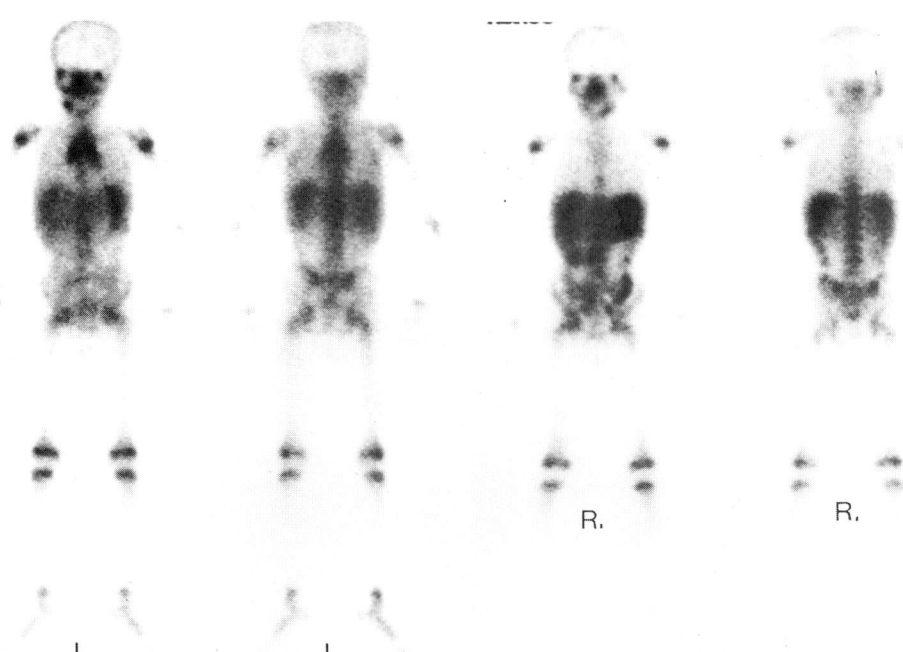

FIGURE 6.25. Thymic rebound on ^{67}Ga citrate scan. Avid thymic uptake post chemotherapy in a child. After treatment for lymphoma (*two left scans*) and 4 months later (*two right scans*). The characteristic butterfly shape of the thymus and its location in the mediastinum (*two left scans*) were helpful in making the appropriate diagnosis. Four months later the thymic rebound had resolved.

does not compress surrounding anatomic structures in the mediastinum.

THYROID MASSES

Thyroid masses within the neck are most frequently evaluated with ultrasound, which visualizes the anatomy in this region accurately separating cystic from solid masses, and radionuclide studies, which accurately depict anatomy and extent of thyroid enlargement as well as indicate function. Iodine 131 (^{131}I) scanning is performed in patients with well-differentiated thyroid cancer to determine the extent of tumor and the feasibility of treatment with radioactive ^{131}I treatment. Uptake is strongly dependent on the histology, with well-differentiated thyroid cancer of papillary or follicular histologies taking up radioactive iodine in the large majority of instances (close to 90%). Patients should have a thyroid-stimulating hormone of more than 25 μU/mL and be on a low-iodide diet prior to the scan. Thyroid cancer metastasizes first to regional lymph nodes of the neck, but also is capable of direct extension into the upper mediastinum, invading the musculature of the trachea and esophagus. Spread to the lymph nodes in the paratracheal and lower mediastinum nodes is also possible as well as direct spread to the lungs. Follicular cancers tend to spread early to lungs and also to vertebrae and ribs in the region of the bony thorax (207).

Nonneoplastic goiters are usually connected to the neck portion of the thyroid. The diagnosis of goiter versus neoplasm frequently is apparent clinically, e.g., in the case of substernal masses that exhibit little or no change over time. In this regard the availability of past imaging studies is frequently of great importance. CT is typically used to determine the morphology and extent of mediastinal thyroid tissue. Approximately 80% of thyroid extensions, which are almost always connected to the cervical portion of the thyroid, are prevascular, involving the anterior mediastinum in contiguity to the thymus gland. Twenty percent extend into the posterior mediastinum behind the brachiocephalic vessels on the right side and adjacent to the right border of the trachea (208). Other locations are extremely rare.

On CT mediastinal extension of the thyroid is identified by its shape, position, and high density on noncontrast scans (related to the high iodine content of this organ) (209–211). Mediastinal extension of thyroid on CT is characterized by: (*a*) anatomic continuity of the neck component of the gland, (*b*) prolonged and intense enhancement of intravenous contrast administration (209), and (*c*) inhomogeneity of cystic areas, foci of calcification, or of high density corresponding to regions of high iodine content.

The differential diagnosis of intrathoracic goiter from malignancy can be difficult because the radiographic findings are not specific: the patient's history and availability of prior chest radiographs and/or CT studies showing no change over time are most important. Malignant processes tend to have irregular contours with loss of soft-tissue planes, sometimes associ-

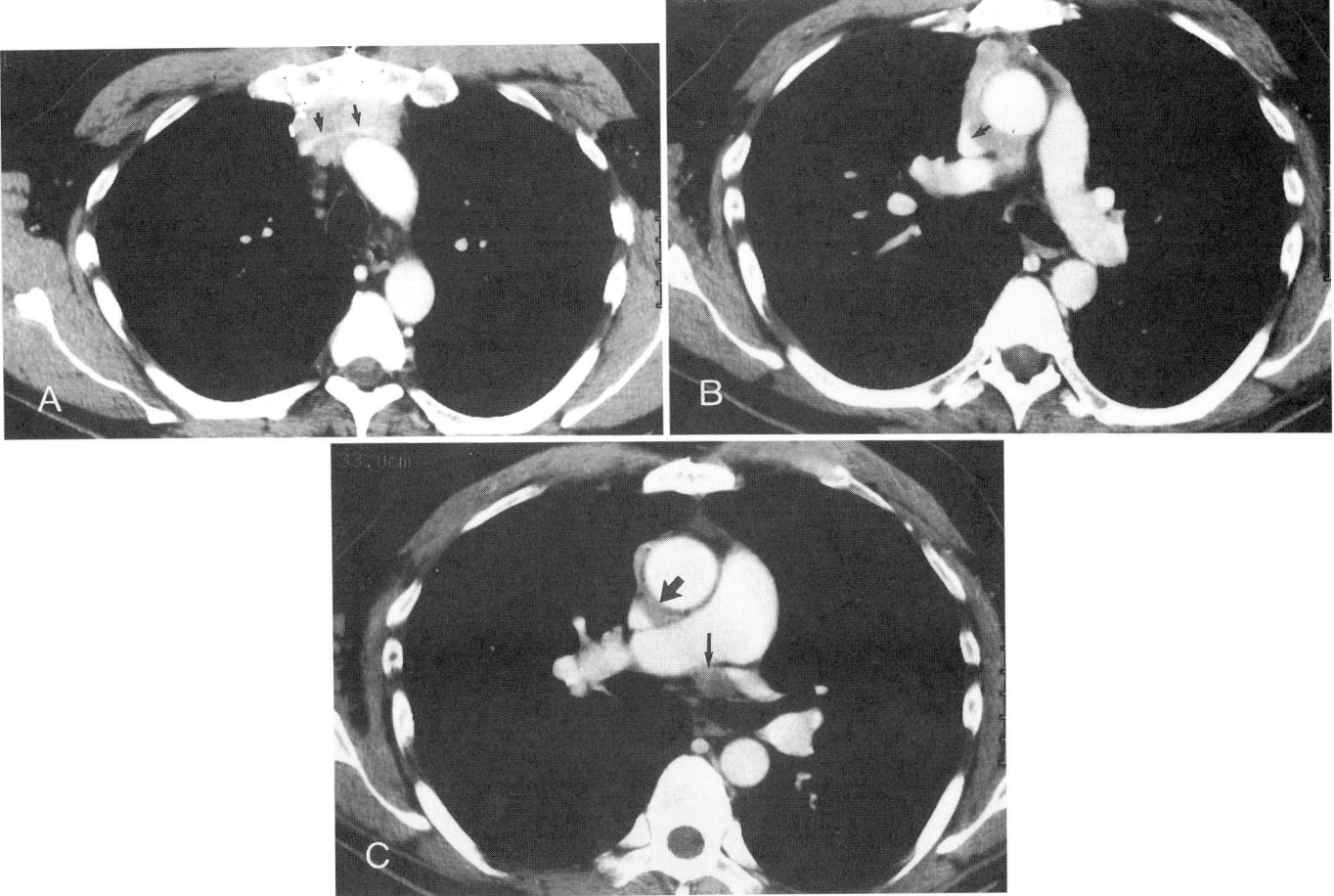

FIGURE 6.26. Recurrent thymoma. **A.** CT scan at the level of the aorticopulmonary window. There is recurrent tumor in the anterior mediastinum situated between the ascending aorta and the sternum, replacing mediastinal adipose tissue. The left innominate vein is encased and markedly narrowed by the recurrent tumor (*arrows*). **B.** At a level below *A*, the recurrent thymoma is seen to infiltrate posteriorly within the mediastinum, partially surrounding the ascending aorta and causing marked extrinsic compression along the medial surface of the superior vena cava (*arrow*). **C.** The tumor is seen to infiltrate the middle mediastinum at a more caudal level below the level of the tracheal carina. Tumor is situated between the ascending aorta, right pulmonary artery, and superior vena cava (*thick arrow*). Tumor has also infiltrated posterior to the right pulmonary artery and is situated anterior to the left main stem bronchus (*thin arrow*). Intravenous contrast was administered for these scans, aiding in separating recurrent tumor from normal vascular structures.

ated with mediastinal adenopathy. Unfortunately, CT and other imaging modalities are of limited specificity (212–214).

Because of the frequent nonspecificity of imaging examinations, especially in symptomatic patients or those with enlarging cervical or mediastinal masses, histologic confirmation may be necessary. In addition, large symptomatic mediastinal goiters should be removed because of potential impingement on other structures as well as the risk of hemorrhage. CT, especially high-resolution CT, is ideal for illustrating the extent of intrathoracic tumor and size in preoperative planning. MRI shows the same morphologic characteristics with the addition of potentially important T1- and T2-weighting signal characteristics. Patients with Graves' disease have increased T1- and T2-weighted signal reflecting the clinical hyperactivity of the gland (215) as well as dilated vessels within the organ (216). MRI also appears to be a sensitive indicator of recurrence of tumor in the neck and mediastinum following surgery.

PARATHYROID DISEASE

Parathyroid tumors within the mediastinum are uncommon: approximately 10% of parathyroid tumors are situated in an ectopic location. Sixty-two percent of these tumors are located in the anterior mediastinum situated close to the thymus. Thirty percent are located within the thyroid gland, and 8% are located in the posterior-superior mediastinum (217).

Solitary parathyroid adenomas cause approximately 85% of all cases of primary hyperparathyroidism. The remaining 15% are divided among diffuse hyperplasia (10%), multiple adenomas (5%), and carcinoma (1%). In the case of primary hyperparathyroidism, neck exploration is successful in detecting and removing more than 90% of these tumors (218). Therefore, the possibility of ectopic parathyroid tissue becomes important only in that small percentage of patients who have persistent or recurrent primary hyperparathyroidism after adequate neck exploration.

A variety of diagnostic techniques are available to evaluate for both abnormal and ectopic parathyroid tissue. These modalities include ultrasonography, thallium scanning, and scintigraphy, as well as magnetic resonance scanning and (high-resolution) CT. The latter modality has been described as having an 80% detection rate (219). Magnetic resonance scanning, however, may have some advantage because of the unusually high signal of abnormal parathyroid T2 signal of abnormal parathyroid tissue within both the neck and mediastinum (220–222). It is considered particularly valuable in this context for evaluation of recurrent or difficult to locate disease.

PARASPINAL TUMORS

A variety of tumors may involve the posterior mediastinum or paraspinal region. Additionally, nontumorous conditions may occur, such as extramedullary hematopoiesis or tuberculous involvement of the spine (Pott's disease) with development of a "cold" abscess in the paraspinal region. Neurogenic tumors, both benign and malignant, are most common in the paraspinal region; these tumors originate both from the peripheral nerves and from the sympathetic ganglia (Fig. 6.27). Other tumors found in this region include lymphoma, metastatic disease (frequently originating from spine or rib), and a variety of nonneurogenic benign neoplasms (223–225).

CT is accurate in delineating these tumors. Many of the neurogenic tumors are characterized by low density that is, however, well above the density of adipose tissue (226). MRI is considered the diagnostic modality of choice in this region for evaluation of osseous spinal, nerve root, and cord involvement. The multiplanar format of MRI is particularly suited to demarcation of these lesions (227–229).

PLEURAL AND CHEST WALL MASSES

Approximately 95% of all pleural masses (with or without effusion) are metastatic in origin. Primary pleural tumors therefore are rare but important clinical entities. Pleural metastases are a common manifestation of disseminated tumor and may present as masses, effusions, or both. However, not all effusions associated with tumor disease are malignant. Nonmalignant pleural effusions in patients with malignancies can be caused by lymphatic blockade, chemotherapy, (the recently introduced chemotherapeutic agent docetaxel [230] is associated with a high incidence of exudative nonneoplastic pleural effusions), radiation therapy, or the effects of widespread metastatic tumor (231). Malignant pleural effusions are most commonly associated with lung and breast cancer. A small percentage of patients present with pleural effusions from tumors of unknown origin, usually adenocarcinomas. Twenty-five percent of all pleural effusions in older patients are malignant (232) and represent the first indication of malignancy in 46% of the patients (233). The mechanism of formation of malignant pleural effusions includes spread of tumor along lymph channels from hilar or mediastinal nodes as well as small arterial tumor emboli (234). Bilateral effusions are occasionally associated with hematogenous spread of tumor from the liver. Hematogenous spread to the pleura from elsewhere in the body can occur, and, occasionally, malignant pleural effusions and/or masses may result from chest wall neoplasms. The diagnosis of malignant pleural effusion can be extremely difficult, and pleural taps are frequently negative, despite repeated attempts (235–237). The appearance of a malignant pleural effusion is associated with a very poor prognosis, i.e., on the order of months. The exception to this finding appears to be breast cancer, in which aggressive therapy can result in considerably longer survival.

Involvement of the pleura by solid tumor is most commonly found in association with lung cancer (especially adenocarcinoma) followed by breast cancer, and tumors of the gastrointestinal tract, kidney, and ovary (231, 233, 234). Thymoma, when the tumor has broken out its capsule, is associated with involvement of the pleura by solid tumor nodules representing contiguous invasion and direct pleural seeding by tumor (238, 239).

The radiographic appearance of involvement of the pleura by metastatic disease is quite variable, both on chest films and on digital cross-sectional imaging modalities such as CT and MRI. These include fine studding, or the presence of pleural nodules, large masses, or even diffuse pleural plaques simulating mesothelioma. This latter presentation is frequently caused by extensive involvement of the pleura by adenocarcinomas, usually lung in origin. In turn, the presence of studding or masses may be obscured by variable amounts of pleural fluid. CT is useful in

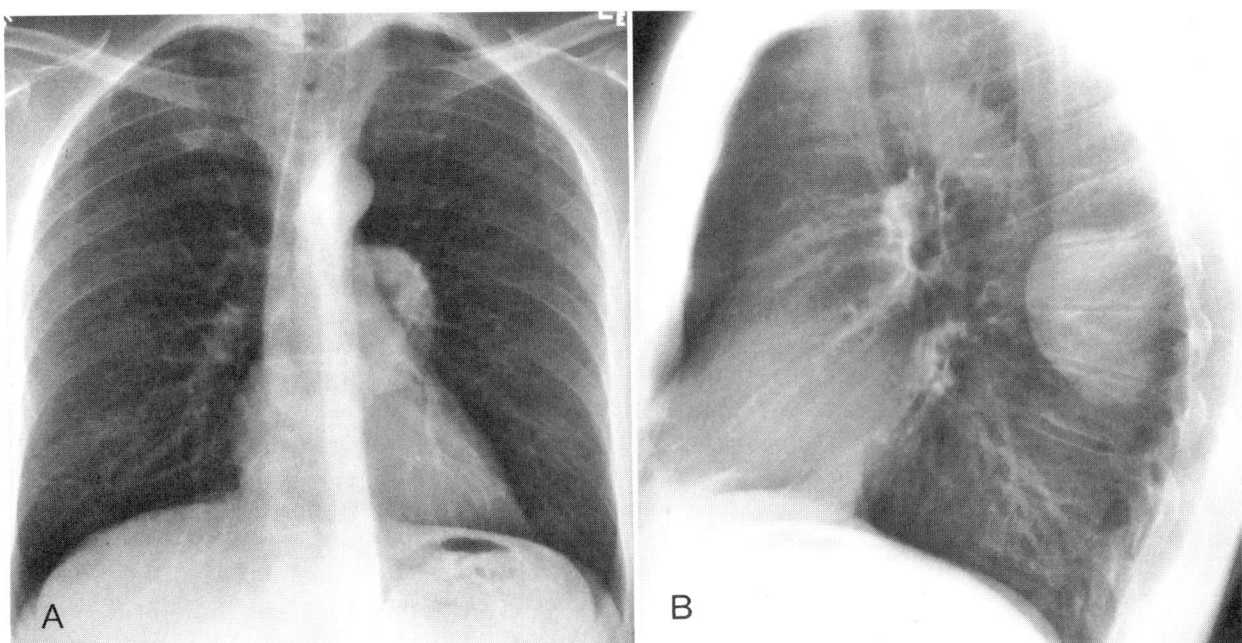

FIGURE 6.27. Pleural-based mass. **A.** PA view shows a large mass overlying the left hilum. Lateral view confirms a posterior location. **B.** This mass has a very well-defined anterior border on the lateral view and a poorly defined posterior contour with obtuse angles superiorly and inferiorly at the chest wall border, suggesting a pleural or extrapleural origin rather than a lung parenchymal origin. The well-defined appearance raised the possibility of a benign entity, and a diagnosis of a solitary fibrous tumor of the pleura was entertained. Alternatively, the mass may have originated from the extrapleural space and/or posterior mediastinum. At surgery a large benign schwannoma originating in the extrapleural nerve roots was resected.

delineating foci of solid disease in the context of a pleural effusion.

The presence of a peripheral lung mass abutting the pleura frequently raises the question of whether the pleura is involved by tumor. Both CT and MRI may be helpful in determining tumor extent, but a firm diagnosis of tumor involvement of the pleura may not be possible when the tumor only contacts the pleura on cross-sectional imaging. When the mass extends from the peripheral lung into the chest wall with direct invasion of soft-tissue structures and/or rib destruction, including invasion of intercostal muscles and obliteration of intercostal fat planes, a diagnosis of pleural involvement by a peripheral lung tumor may be made with some confidence. However, it is frequently the case that such extensive chest wall involvement is not present; and in such situations even when there is clear pleural thickening associated with peripheral lung mass, it may be impossible to tell whether actual invasion of pleura has occurred (240, 241). In these situations thin-section T1-weighted sagittal and coronal MRI (5-mm) scans may prove helpful, especially in the region of the lung apex and diaphragm (61, 242–244).

Primary tumors of the pleura, compared with metastatic disease, are quite rare. Primary pleural masses having a characteristic, although not pathognomonic, appearance include localized fibrous tumor of the pleura, the large majority of which are benign, and malignant pleural mesothelioma.

LOCALIZED FIBROUS TUMOR OF THE PLEURA

This uncommon tumor has a characteristic radiographic appearance, is usually asymptomatic, and is discovered incidentally on a chest radiograph obtained for other reasons. There can be difficulty in distinguishing pleural from extrapleural origin on chest films (Fig. 6.27). Surgical excision is usually curative. Uncommonly, the tumor can recur after surgery and behave in a malignant fashion. This usually benign pleural tumor, thought to originate from submesothelial connective tissue (245–249), is attached to the visceral pleural surface by a pedicle in 30% to 50% of cases (250). This latter finding is associated with a good prognosis after complete surgical removal. On CT the tumor presents as a well-defined pleural mass that, when attached to the pleural surface by a pedicle, may show changes in position on serial scans, a radiographic sign considered very characteristic (251). With intravenous contrast injection the tumor is highly vascular, containing areas of central necrosis with increased vascularity at the periphery. The CT findings are considered characteristic (252–254). The tumors may originate from the fissures simulating a lung parenchymal tumor and rarely may present as an intrapulmonary mass (255, 256). Occasionally, the tumor is detached from the pedicle and may move freely within the pleural cavity. A small percentage may contain calcium, and 17% have a pleural effusion associated with them (246). Large size may be associated with symptoms such as hypertrophic pulmonary osteoarthropathy, digital clubbing, hypoglycemia, or malignancy. Treatment consists of complete surgical removal. There is a 12% recurrence rate, usually associated with broad-based attachment to the pleural surface, delayed diagnosis, and/or large size. Malignant-appearing histology, however, does not appear to be associated with recurrence when the tumor has been excised completely (257).

Diffuse Malignant Mesothelioma

This rare tumor, which is related to previous exposure to asbestos, particularly Crocidolite fibers, appears to be increasing in frequency. Previously, industrial exposure to these fibers was notable in the shipbuilding industry and in the extensive use of asbestos insulation. Three histologic varieties of malignant mesothelioma are distinguished: epithelial, sarcomatous, and mixed (biphasic). There can be difficulty in distinguishing malignant mesothelioma from metastatic carcinoma diffusely involving the pleura. Radiographically, the appearance of these histologic varieties of malignant mesothelioma is identical.

The current modality of choice for evaluation of malignant mesothelioma is CT, which is superior to conventional chest radiography in evaluating these tumors (258). The CT appearance is quite variable, the common denominator being diffuse pleural involvement. In addition to the common finding of diffuse, irregular, pleural thickening with pleural effusion, malignant mesothelioma may occasionally present as a large well-defined solitary mass and may therefore simulate solitary fibrous tumors of the pleura. In addition, there may be diffuse involvement of the pleura with only a very slight amount of pleural thickening and no pleural effusion. This finding may simulate local pleural changes of asbestosis or other long-standing inflammatory disease involving the pleura. Metastatic disease, especially adenocarcinoma, can have CT findings identical to the radiographic appearance of malignant mesothelioma, but without the typical history of long-standing asbestos exposure. A history of asbestos exposure is not always present, however, in patients with mesothelioma.

Malignant mesothelioma spreads along the pleural surfaces involving both the parietal and visceral pleura, frequently surrounding and entrapping the lung. Growth along the pleural surfaces is characteristic, and thick pleural tumor plaques may be seen in the minor and major fissures, delineating the anatomy of the lungs. These tumors frequently invade the chest wall, diaphragm, mediastinum, and lung (Fig. 6.28). They may metastasize to mediastinal lymph nodes or to the opposite lung (259). In a review of the CT findings in 50 patients with proven malignant mesothelioma (260), pleural thickening was noted to be present in 92% and was quite variable in extent, thickness, and nodularity. In addition, intralobar pleural thickening was present in 86% and pleural effusion in 74%. Pleural calcification was seen in 20% of patients. The majority of these were plaquelike calcifications associated with the underlying asbestosis. Occasionally, tumor calcification within the mesothelioma mass itself was noted. Regional spread to chest wall, diaphragm, mediastinum, and mediastinal lymph nodes was noted in a total of 48% of patients.

CT tends to underestimate the true extent of disease, and failure to diagnose chest wall invasion, mediastinal lymph node involvement, or transdiaphragmatic tumor extension is quite common (259). Currently, magnetic resonance scanning of malignant mesothelioma is not recommended routinely. As noted in the discussion of CT scanning of apical and diaphragmatic lung cancer, thin-section T1-weighted sagittal and coronal scans may occasionally contribute important information concerning extent of disease, particularly in patients who are considered candidates for radical surgical procedures. Malignant mesothelioma has an intermediate signal on T1-weighted scans and a high signal on T2-weighted scans. Areas of pleural effusion have very high T2-weighted signal.

CHEMOTHERAPY-INDUCED CHEST DISEASE

This discussion of lung abnormalities induced by chemotherapeutic agents is limited to cytotoxic agents commonly used in oncologic practice. Both these agents and noncytologic agents that induce pulmonary disease have been reviewed previously (261–268). A list of the cytotoxic drugs that may produce pulmonary parenchymal injury is shown in Table 6.4.

Pulmonary injury caused by cytotoxic drugs produces a variety of clinical manifestations. These pulmonary injuries are for the most part only partially or

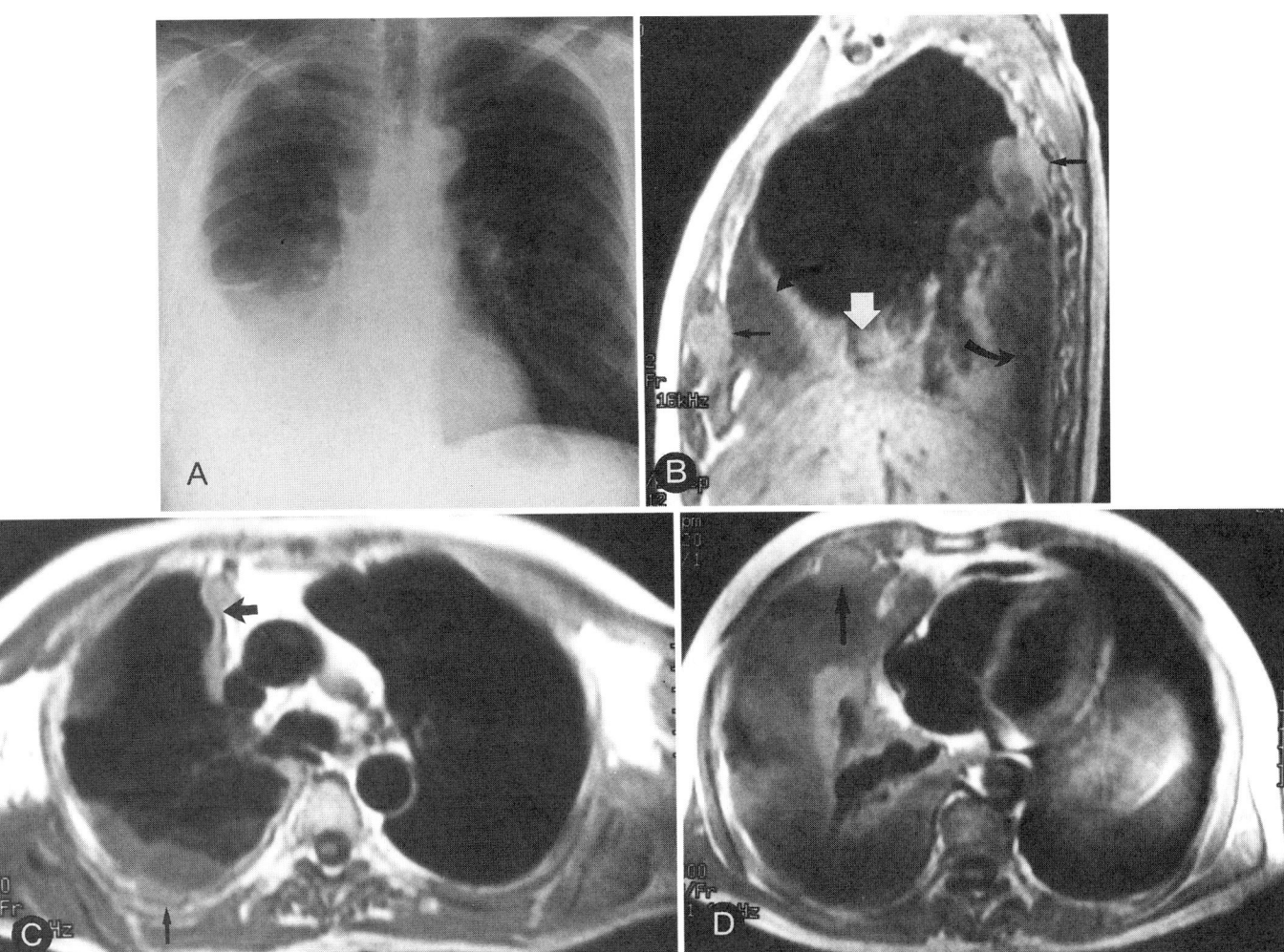

FIGURE 6.28. Malignant mesothelioma. A. Frontal chest radiograph shows pleural effusion and diffuse pleural thickening. This is a nonspecific appearance and is commonly found both in mesothelioma and in involvement of the pleura by metastatic disease. Benign causes of pleural effusion could not be excluded, although these become increasingly infrequent in an older age group. B. A sagittal T1-weighted MRI scan through the central portion of the right lung shows a combination of pleural effusion, mass, and secondary lung parenchymal changes. The pleural-based thickening largely represents tumor. In two locations, at the anterior lower chest wall and the posterior upper chest wall (*small arrows*), there appears to be invasion of the chest wall. Fairly large irregularly shaped pleural effusions (*curved arrows*) are interspersed with areas of pleural neoplasm. More centrally (*white arrow*) it is difficult to distinguish pleural-based tumor from lung parenchymal invasion or from secondary atelectasis. C. T1-weighted MRI scan through the upper thorax in axial projection shows considerable pleural-based tumor along the anterior mediastinal surface (*thick arrow*) with some superficial invasion of mediastinal adipose tissue. Posteriorly, superficial invasion of the chest wall is seen (*thin arrow*). D. At the right anterior lung base, there is definite evidence for tumor invasion of chest wall with disruption of fascial planes (*arrow*). Elsewhere there is considerable pleural effusion, interspersed with tumor. The irregular signal seen centrally may well represent either lung invasion or secondary lung collapse as a result of the expanding pleural disease.

poorly understood (262). A number of radiographic patterns are produced by these agents. In particular, several agents, such as bleomycin, can produce a variety of radiographic appearances, and some of the more common manifestations are summarized below. In most cases pulmonary symptoms as well as pulmonary function abnormalities precede radiographic manifestations of cytotoxic drug-induced disease. Several of the more common types of radiographic pattern are described in the following paragraphs with brief descriptions of the most common agents causing these patterns.

DIFFUSE INTERSTITIAL DISEASE

Early manifestations of this pattern include multifocal reticular, or linear lesions, or a fine nodular appearance. In general, CT has increased sensitivity in

TABLE 6.4. Cytotoxic Agents that Cause Pulmonary Parenchymal Injury

Antibiotics
  Bleomycin
  Mitomycin
  Neocarzinostatin
Alkylating agents
  Busulfan
  Cyclophosphamide
  Chlorambucil
  Melphalan
Nitrosoureas
  Bischloroethyl-nitrosourea (carmustine) (BCNU)
  Semustine (methyl-1-[2-chloroethyl]-3-cyclohexyl-1-nitrosourea (CCNU)
  Lomostine (1-[2-chloroethyl]-3-cyclohexyl-1-nitrosourea)
  Chlorozotocin
Antimetabolites
  Methotrexate
  Azathioprine
  Mercaptopurine
  Cytosine arabinoside hydrochloride
Miscellaneous
  Procarbazine
  Teniposide (VM-26)
  Vinblastine
  Vindesine
Taxanes
  Paclitaxel
  Docetaxel
Cytokines (biologic agents)
  Interleukin-2

Modified with permission from Twohig KJ, Matthay RA. Pulmonary effect of cytotoxic agents other than bleomycin. Clin Chest Med 1990;11:31–54.

detecting the pulmonary abnormalities, compared with plain chest radiography, demonstrating subpleural lines as well as multiple small nodules and reticulation. High-resolution CT may be particularly useful in showing early radiographic signs in patients developing interstitial disease with normal chest radiographs. ^{67}Ga citrate nuclear medicine scanning is also considered particularly sensitive in evaluation of the lung parenchyma, frequently showing positive findings when the chest radiograph is normal (269). A late manifestation of interstitial disease is represented by confluence of interstitial and nodular opacities with involvement of large areas of lung parenchyma.

Bleomycin is the most common agent implicated in the development of interstitial lung disease, with approximately 4% of patients developing this pattern of involvement. The incidence increases after cumulative doses of more than 400 mg. In addition, previous debilitation or multidrug therapy, or administration of concomitant radiotherapy further increases the incidence of bleomycin lung toxicity (270–273). Patients frequently improve with the administration of corticosteroids, especially those who have minimal pulmonary function, and radiographic abnormalities may resolve completely. However, a small percentage progress to pulmonary fibrosis. Mitomycin can produce similar interstitial disease and pulmonary function abnormalities (Fig. 6.29).

Another agent commonly implicated in the development of interstitial opacities is methotrexate, whose toxicity appears to be immunologically mediated and not dose related, based on findings of bronchoalveolar lavage. The overall incidence of interstitial disease related to methotrexate toxicity is approximately 7%. Plain chest radiographs show increased interstitial lung markings. Alveolar opacities are also noted with occasional pleural effusion. These findings typically regress with the cessation of therapy. It is uncommon for progression to pulmonary fibrosis to occur (274, 275).

Carmustine (BiCNU) (Bristol Myers Squibb, Princeton, NJ) is also related to the presence of interstitial pneumonitis; this condition appears to be dose related, developing in approximately 20% to 30% of patients. A typical appearance of bibasal interstitial disease and fibrosis without significant inflammatory reaction pathologically has been described. Less commonly, upper lobe opacities may occur. The overall mortality is as high as 90% (262).

ALVEOLAR INFILTRATES

Cytosine arabinoside hydrochloride (Cytosar-U; Upjohn Company, Kalamazoo, MI), interleukin-2, and, uncommonly, methotrexate can be responsible for the development of alveolar infiltrates (276–280). These infiltrates represent acute noncardiac pulmonary edema caused by capillary injury and increased permeability. These findings may be delayed in onset for a considerable period; in the case of cytosine arabinoside hydrochloride, up to 1 month after initiation of treatment. Early findings are represented by lower lobe alveolar or alveolar/interstitial infiltrates that can progress to a diffuse alveolar pattern. With cytosine arabinoside hydrochloride and interleukin, eventual resolution of these alveolar infiltrates after a period of time is the rule. Methotrexate alveolar densities, however, may progress to interstitial pulmonary disease.

PULMONARY NODULES

The appearance of pulmonary nodules represent a very unusual manifestation of bleomycin toxicity. Cyclosporine, used in the treatment of transplant rejection, can result in a multiorgan lymphoproliferative

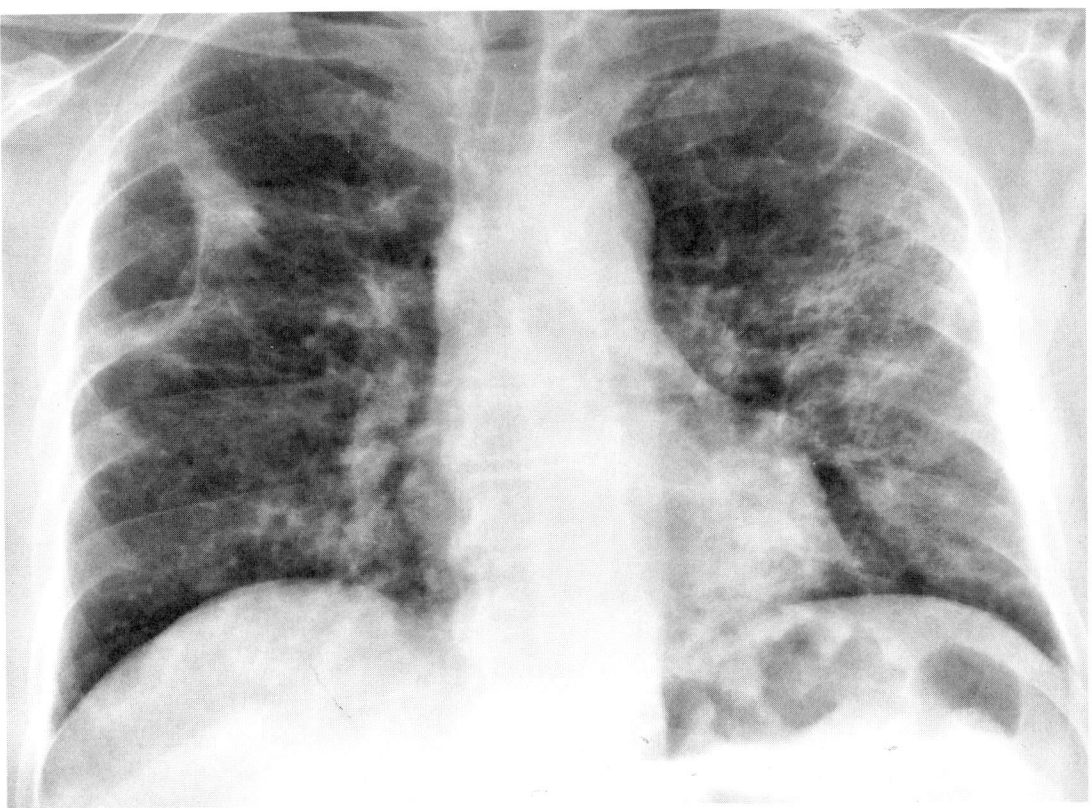

FIGURE 6.29. Mitomycin pulmonary toxicity. This patient developed progressive shortness of breath while undergoing combination chemotherapy, including mitomycin, for an NSCLC in the right upper lung. Aside from the tumor in the right upper lung, previous chest radiographs and CT scan showed normal lung parenchyma. The current chest radiograph shows diffuse interstitial lung disease, most prominently in the left mid and lower lung zones, but also involving the right mid and lower lung zones. The patient responded to withdrawal of mitomycin and to administration of corticosteroids. In this case the differential would include opportunistic infections that may be associated with administration of chemotherapy as well as with lymphangitic tumor spread.

disorder involving B cells, including the presence of pulmonary nodules, in patients with preexisting Ebstein-Barr infection. The mechanism (281, 282) and the radiographic features (283) have been described, and include both hilar and mediastinal lymphadenopathy as well as pulmonary nodules. Ultimately, malignant lymphoma may develop in a small percentage of these patients.

PLEURAL EFFUSION

The new chemotherapeutic agents paclitaxel (Taxol; Bristol Myers Squibb, Princeton, NJ) and docetaxel (Taxotere; Thone Poulenc Rorer, Inc., Collegeville, PA) have been associated with a significant incidence of pleural effusions. These effusions develop during therapy and usually stabilize with minimal symptomatology. Aspiration shows exudative fluid. These effusions are part of a general capillary injury syndrome that can also produce ascites, soft-tissue edema, and in several cases, pericardial effusions. These findings tend to regress or disappear after cessation of therapy (230).

CARDIAC ABNORMALITIES

Uncommonly, cyclophosphamide use may result in a serofibrinous pericarditis associated with myocardial hemorrhagic injury, especially when used in combination with other cytotoxic agents or radiation therapy in patients who have had marrow transplantation (283).

Severe progressive cardiomyopathy may be caused by doxorubicin hydrochloride (Adriamycin PFS; Adria Laboratories, Dublin, OH) and its analogue daunorubicin. In the case of doxorubicin, 30% of patients who receive more than 550 mg/m^2 of body surface develop cardiomyopathy. Previous radiation with fields including the heart potentiates this effect. The radiographic appearance is characterized by global cardiomegaly and, in later stages, by pulmonary vascular congestion (284).

The procedure of choice for assessing cardiac toxicity is the resting radionuclide-gated blood pool scan, which should be performed sequentially in patients who are undergoing high-dose adriamycin chemotherapy. Schwartz and Zaret (285) have proposed the following procedure for adults: (*a*) perform a baseline study at a total dose of 100 mg/m^2 or less of Adriamycin PFS, and (*b*) repeat at a dose of 350 to 400 mg/m^2, and (*c*) then at each dose above 450 mg/m^2. If possible, the dose should be repeated at least 3 weeks after the last dose of Adriamycin PFS. If there is a decline of resting ejection fraction of more than 10% or to a level below the normal range (50% in most centers), the Adriamycin PFS should be discontinued. In patients, who have ejection fractions below 50% before beginning anthracycline therapy, a drop of more than 10% or/and absolute value below 30% is cause for stopping the drug.

EFFECTS OF RADIATION THERAPY ON THE THORAX

Radiation therapy effects generally, but not always, are confined within the boundaries of the radiation port. In an effort to include the entire tumor volume in the radiation field, normal structures inevitably are included in the field. The most common organ in the chest to be damaged by radiation therapy is the lung. Both the acute and chronic pathologic and radiographic changes are discussed. Other structures in the chest may also be damaged. Bones become weakened and osteoporotic on a long-term basis, with frequent fractures and poor healing. Cardiac failure may result from myocardial damage. In addition, pericarditis (with effusion) may occur. Radiation-induced damage to the esophagus may result in dysphagia, dysmotility, and aspiration. The effects of radiation on all of these structures may be potentiated by chemotherapy.

Factors determining radiation injury to the lungs have been described (286). As with chemotherapy, considerable variation in individual susceptibility to the pathologic effects of radiation is noted. The effects of radiation therapy may be potentiated by underlying lung disease or previous or concomitant treatment with chemotherapy. Other important factors in determining lung damage by radiation therapy include:

1. Total dose: 30 gray (Gy) (1 Gy = 100 rad) total lung irradiation in a single dose destroys lung and results in tissue death.
2. Total volume of lung irradiated: smaller volumes of irradiated lung produce lesser effects. Usually up to one third of total lung volume may be included in the radiation therapy port without significant compromise of pulmonary function.
3. Fractionation, i.e., dividing the total dose into a series of smaller doses, administered over time, lessens the deleterious effects on normal tissue while maintaining the cytotoxic effects on tumor cells.

The pathologic changes that occur are complex and are described elsewhere in detail (287). Acutely, there is edema and hyperemia with white blood cell infiltration of the bronchial wall. Bronchial swelling occurs as a result of this process. Uncommonly, this swelling can result in significant narrowing of the bronchial lumen. In the following 1 to 6 months, acute radiation pneumonitis may ensue, with alveolar thickening, edema, membrane formation, and cell damage. These changes can be manifested clinically by cough with thickened sputum and shortness of breath. Low-grade fever may be present.

The acute phase gradually progresses to a regenerative healing phase, in which inflammatory changes gradually disappear, with a fibrotic phase occurring simultaneously with scar formation and bronchiectasis. These latter changes are frequently asymptomatic, but if the irradiated volume is sufficiently large, there may be global compromise of lung function with symptoms of chronic pulmonary disease or cough, shortness of breath, clubbing, and recurring infection.

The radiographic changes, both on plain films and on CT, are quite characteristic. When combined with the clinical history, they usually are sufficiently diagnostic to avert further workup. This is especially true in asymptomatic patients. The differential diagnosis includes both infectious processes and tumor recurrence. An acute superimposed infection usually allows diagnosis by the combination of clinical symptoms and the important finding that the pulmonary infiltrate does not conform to the radiation field, but rather extends beyond it, possibly even involving the opposite lung. Difficulty may be encountered in inflammatory processes confined to the radiation field. Plain radiographs and CT changes may be subtle and not well appreciated, with the presence of the superimposed acute radiation pneumonitis. Serial CT scans may be useful in these situations, uncovering subtle changes on successive scans not apparent on chest radiography.

The problem of tumor recurrence can be especially difficult in a lung field that has been irradiated, especially in the phase of acute radiation pneumonitis.

On chest radiography, subtle masses recurring in the irradiated lung can easily be missed, or be invisible on cross-sectional images because of the presence of patchy, radiation-induced infiltrates. Recurrence of tumor has many manifestations: lymphangitic spread (especially difficult to detect if only involving the irradiated field), lung mass (Fig. 6.28), and hilar or mediastinal adenopathy. MRI has been proposed as a test to distinguish recurrent tumor (dark T1-weighted signal; bright T2-weighted signal) from chronic fibrosis (dark T1- and T2-weighted signal) (288). This interesting work has not yet been confirmed by a large series; additionally, it would appear difficult to differentiate recurrent tumor from either an inflammatory process or acute radiation pneumonitis.

The acute changes of radiation pneumonitis (Fig. 6.30), first noted approximately 1 to 2 months after therapy, are manifested by hazy or patchy pulmonary infiltrates, progressing gradually into an appearance of fibrosis with interstitial stranding seen at 12 to 18 months. In both cases, the salient radiographic feature is noncorrespondence of the radiographic abnormality to normal lobar or segmental boundaries; instead, the infiltrate typically corresponds closely to the field of radiation. This is especially true in the acute phase; chronically, there may be some retraction and consequent shrinkage of the abnormal lung from the original irradiated field (Fig. 6.31).

CT allows more accurate delineation of postirradiation changes (289), including detection of bronchiectasis, pulmonary fibrotic contraction, vessel shrinkage, and hyperlucency in lung peripheral to the irradiated field (290, 291). To these long-term effects may be added eventual calcification of tumor-bearing lymph nodes in patients with Hodgkin's disease, commonly seen in the hilar regions and mediastinum (292).

The eventual development of malignant sarcoma, usually but not always originating in bone in the irradiated field, is a rare but highly lethal long-term complication of irradiation (293).

In conclusion, both chest radiography and CT are accurate in delineating the changes occurring as a result of thoracic irradiation. CT, in particular, is useful in detecting subtle radiation changes as well as for evaluating superimposed infections or the presence of tumor recurrence. After completion of radiation therapy and the resolution of the acute changes, it is useful to obtain a baseline CT scan of the chest. This scan provides a basis of comparison for evaluating future inflammatory changes or changes of tumor recurrence that may occur over time. The baseline CT obtained after resolution of acute changes allows more subtle abnormalities to be detected than a CT scan obtained during the acute phase.

PULMONARY INFECTION IN THE IMMUNOCOMPROMISED HOST

Both neoplastic processes and the chemotherapeutic agents used to combat them, including steroids and radiation therapy, result in impaired ability to

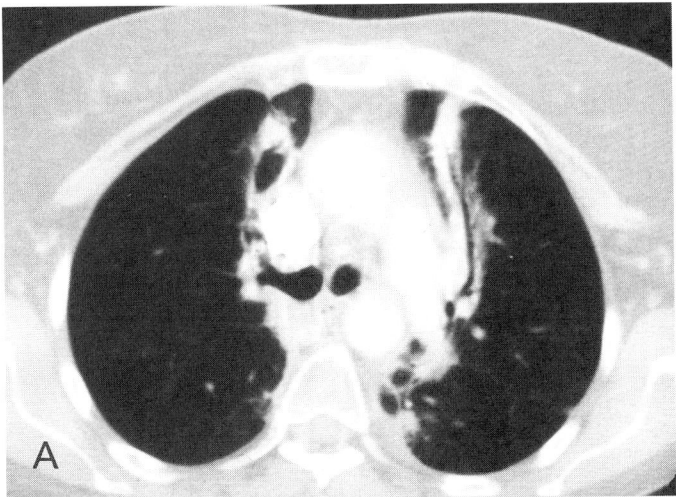
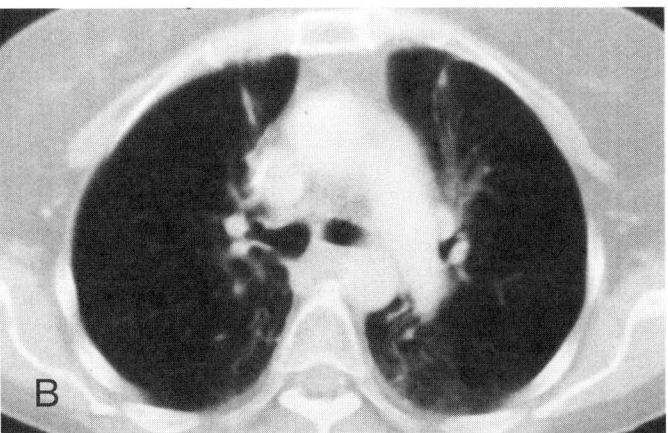

FIGURE 6.30. Radiation pneumonitis. **A.** CT scan through the central portion of the thorax. The patient had undergone a course of radiation therapy to the mediastinum that had concluded 3 weeks before the CT scan. The patient developed low-grade fever, dry cough, and some shortness of breath. The scan shows bilateral parahilar infiltrates that are fairly sharply demarcated and which correspond to the radiation field. Note that the paramediastinal infiltrates do not correspond to any lobar or segmental distribution. **B.** After a course of steroids, the patient's symptoms improved and a follow-up CT scan obtained 1 month later showed marked improvement in the paramediastinal infiltrates with a small amount of residual filtrate present.

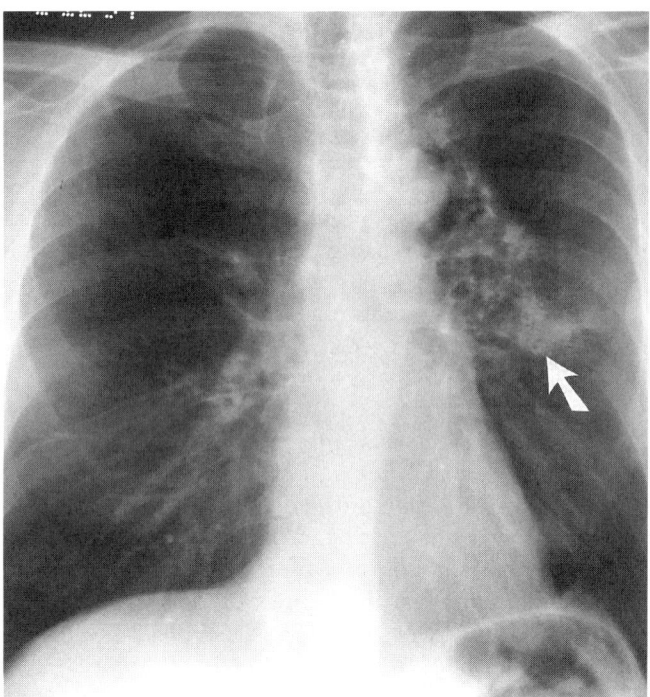

FIGURE 6.31. Postradiation change with tumor recurrence. PA chest radiograph. The patient had undergone radiation therapy for lung cancer involving the left hilum 3 years before this radiograph. There had been a good response. For the previous 2½ years, there had been stable infiltrative density in the left mid lung zone with a sharp exterior border roughly corresponding to the radiation port. During that time there had been slight retraction of the lateral margin of the chronic radiation pneumonitis as a result of fibrosis. On the current radiograph a new density was seen along the inferior border of the chronic radiation change, extending into previously unirradiated lung (*arrow*). This density was subsequently proved to represent local recurrence of tumor within the radiation port.

fight infection. Pulmonary infiltrates are the most common manifestation of infection in the immunocompromised host; the mechanism of action is complex and involves, in varying proportions, impaired granulocyte, and T- and B-cell lymphocyte function, resulting in increased susceptibility to bacterial, fungal, parasitic, and viral infectious agents. Depending on which autoimmune function is more severely compromised, there may be a consequent greater or lesser susceptibility to specific varieties of infectious agents. For example, defects in lymphocyte function render the individual more susceptible to viral or parasitic infections, than, for instance, an isolated defect in granulocyte function. However, there is considerable overlap, not only of the various forms of immunocompromise, some or all of which may coexist, but also in the susceptibility to specific agents to which they render the host prone.

The chest radiographic findings in immunocompromised patients are almost never specific, either as isolated findings or with the background of clinical information available. With appropriate clinical information, however, a reasonable differential diagnosis may be obtained, the pulmonary findings themselves providing indications for further workup (Fig. 6.32). In patients with immunocompromise accompanied by fever and pulmonary infiltrates, 75% of these infiltrates result from infection (294). In addition, pulmonary infiltrates frequently have more than one etiology, e.g., pulmonary neoplasm (or lymphangitic spread) and infection, or pulmonary edema and/or pulmonary infiltrates resulting from chemotoxicity plus infection.

Pulmonary infiltrates in an immunocompromised patient carry a mortality as high as 50%. In as many as 20% of patients, precise diagnosis is never established before death, despite open lung biopsy. Furthermore, knowledge of the etiologic agent frequently does not prevent death from overwhelming infection.

In this context it is not surprising that the chest radiograph is almost always a nonspecific finding. It serves to confirm the presence of a clinically suspected lung abnormality or to uncover an unsuspected infiltrate in immunocompromised patients with evidence for infection. In some situations the radiographic findings point to a specific diagnosis, which may be then confirmed: more than 70% of infiltrates in AIDS patients, for example, are associated with Pneumocystis carinii pneumonia (PCP) (295). Even in this case, however, PCP may be complicated by other concomitant inflammatory processes, for example cytomegalic virus pneumonia (CMV), *Mycobacterium avium* complex (MAC), or neoplasms such as Kaposi's sarcoma or lymphoma.

Pulmonary infiltrates in immunocompromised hosts can also be caused by a variety of noninfectious agents including nonspecific interstitial infiltrates; not infrequently after an exhaustive workup, including open lung biopsy, no cause for an acute air space or interstitial pneumonia can be diagnosed (295–298) in as many as 30% to 45% of patients. Nonspecific infiltrates are particularly common in AIDS patients (299).

Other causes of pulmonary infiltrates in this group of patients include tumor growth in the lung: recurrent lymphoma in particular can mimic opportunistic infections. Lymphangitic spread of neoplasm can also simulate inflammation, although the clinical presentation is frequently different. AIDS patients are also prone to develop lymphoid interstitial pneumonia (300), which is either an early form of lymphoma or may develop into it. Pulmonary hemorrhage is particularly common in leukemic patients with diminished clotting factors. Its incidence as a sole cause of pul-

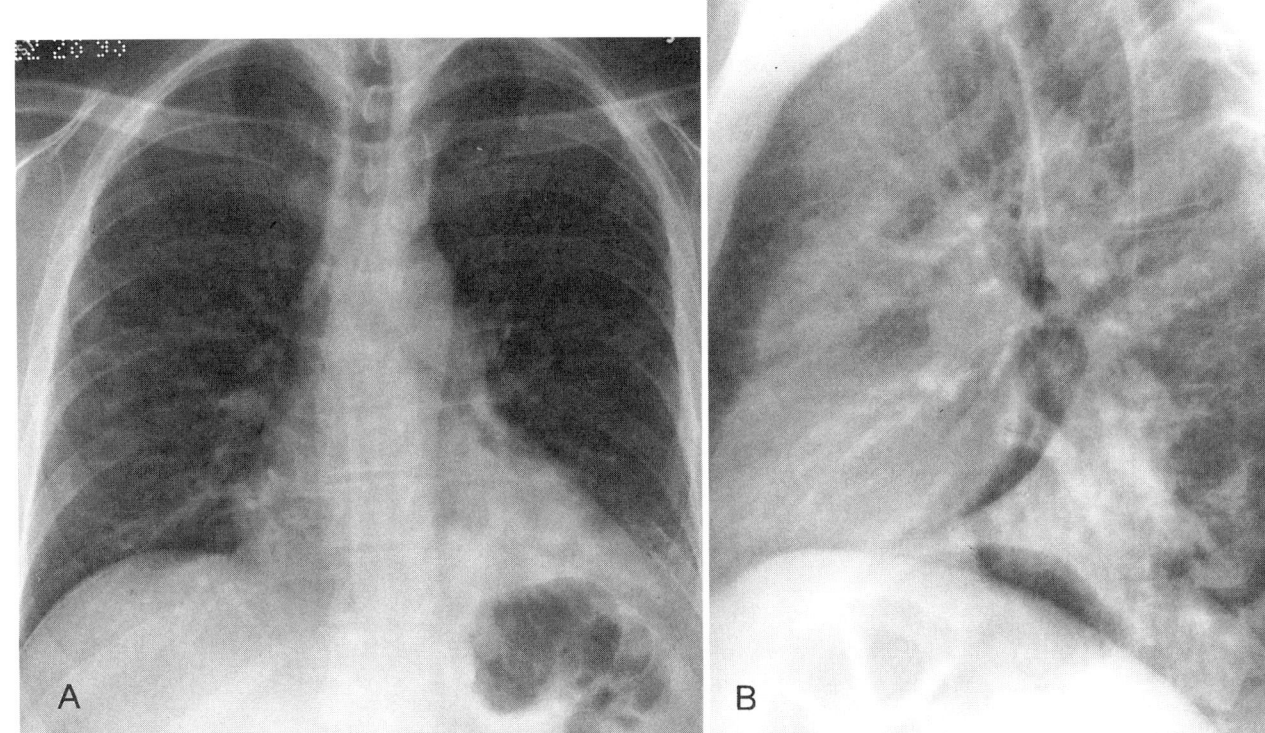

FIGURE 6.32. Opportunistic infection. A. This patient with AIDS was not under treatment. The patient developed shortness of breath with high fever and shaking chills. Chest radiography revealed a left lower lobe infiltrate involving several segments. Ill-defined fluffy infiltrate was also present in the right mid lung field. Clinically, the patient was thought to have a bacterial pneumonia. *Pneumococcus* infection was diagnosed from sputum cytology. B. The lateral view shows the segmental consolidation involving the lower lobe. The anterior border of the infiltrate is sharply demarcated by the lower portion of the major fissure.

monary infiltrate can be as high as 40% in these patients (301), but it usually is suspected clinically by the presence of a bleeding tendency or frequent hemoptysis, or a decrease in hematocrit.

Graft versus host disease of the lungs in bone marrow transplant patients may be manifested by pulmonary infiltrates (302). The appearance of patchy infiltrates bilaterally may indicate the development of bronchiolitis obliterans in patients with bronchopulmonary graft versus host disease (303). In addition, pulmonary infiltrates can result from transfusion, either as a result of fluid overload or antibody reactions involving transfusate and patient.

COMMON AGENTS OF OPPORTUNISTIC INFECTIONS

PNEUMOCYSTIS CARINII INFECTION

P. carinii infection is responsible for 70% of pulmonary complications in AIDS patients and is a major cause of death. This infection is a pulmonary alveolar filling process that only very infrequently becomes disseminated. Death from Pneumocystis infection is usually the result of respiratory insufficiency. The chest radiograph may be normal in the early phase (304, 305). At this stage ^{67}Ga citrate nuclear medicine imaging may be particularly sensitive to the presence of *P. carinii* infection (306, 307) (Fig. 6.33). This phase is followed by a stage of interstitial infiltrate that is first perihilar and symmetric, at a later stage becoming confluent, diffuse, and/or patchy with a combination of alveolar and interstitial infiltrates. Healing with appropriate therapy may be very slow, extending over a period of weeks or months.

Atypical appearances in Pneumocystis include focal and asymmetric interstitial appearances, occasionally limited to one lung. Cavitation has been described with *P. carinii* (308), particularly in patients undergoing azidothymidine (AZT) therapy. A nodular appearance has also been noted (309, 310).

PCP is frequently complicated by the presence of other pathogenic organisms, and an atypical radiographic appearance may indicate the concomitant presence of these organisms. In particular, the presence of adenopathy should alert the clinician to the

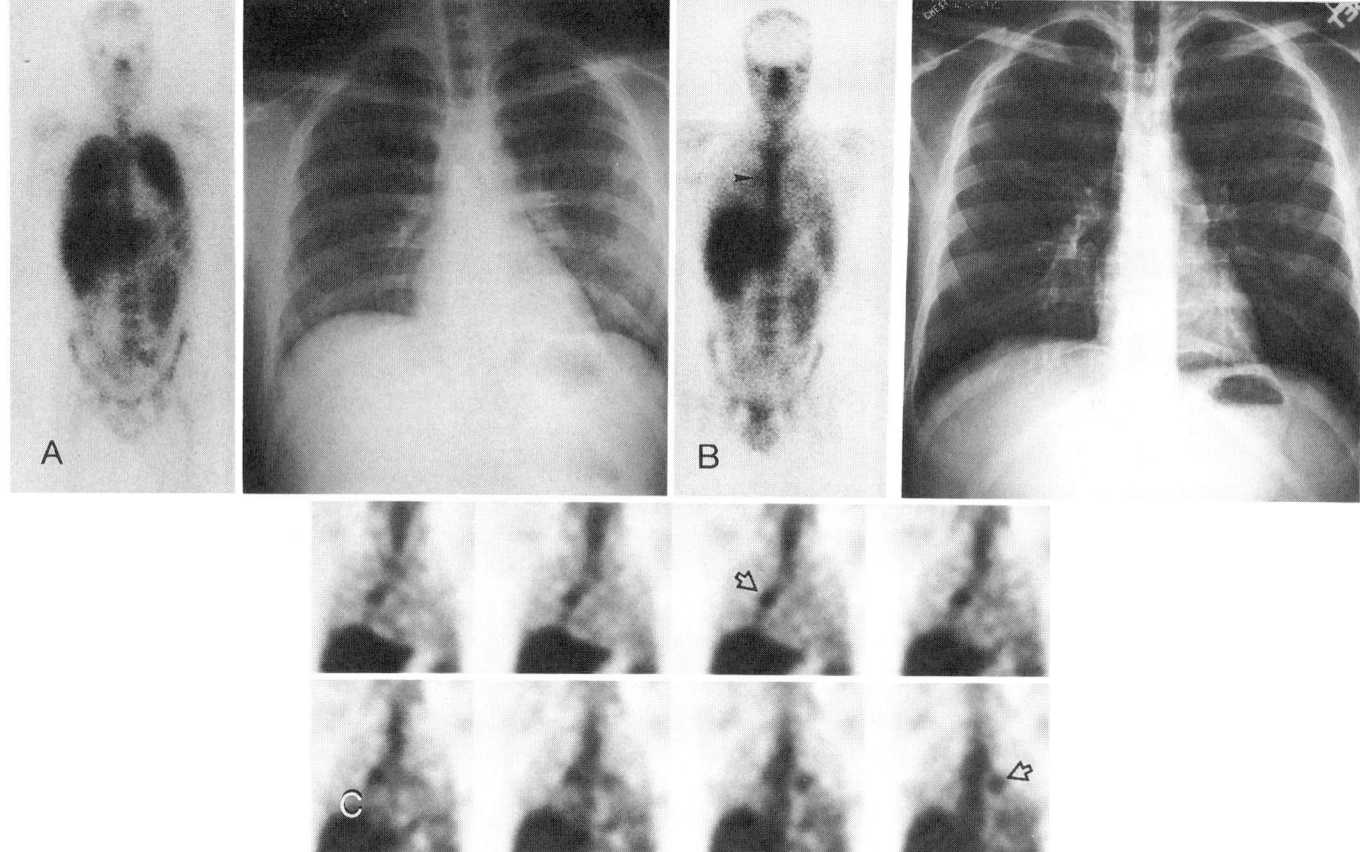

FIGURE 6.33. ^{67}Ga citrate in AIDS. **A.** ^{67}Ga-citrate in patient with AIDS and PCP. The chest radiograph shows basilar infiltrates, which are somewhat subtle, but the ^{67}Ga-citrate whole body scan shows the extensive nature of the pulmonary inflammation. **B.** One year later, the patient's fever and cough have returned. The chest radiograph is normal. ^{67}Ga whole body scan shows right hilar uptake (*arrowhead*). **C.** On coronal SPECT scan, this is clearly seen to be nodular involvement of lymph nodes on both sides of the mediastinum (*arrows*). CT-guided biopsy showed granuloma with the presence of *Mycobacterium avium–intracellulare*.

possibility of tuberculosis, MAI infection, or even lymphoma. Perihilar nodules may indicate the concomitant presence of Kaposi's sarcoma. Pleural effusion may indicate complicating inflammatory processes.

ASPERGILLUS FUMIGATUS INFECTION

The degree of immunologic compromise of the patient with *Aspergillus fumigatus* infection generally determines the invasiveness of the organism. Patients with intact immunity may demonstrate the presence of Aspergillus granulomas. Conversely, severe immune compromise results in manifestations of invasive pulmonary aspergillosis with the presence of infiltrates (Fig. 6.34). Intermediate degrees of immune compromise may result in the appearance of so-called semiinvasive (311) aspergillosis with the development of chronic cavitary disease.

Aspergillosis in its invasive stage is manifested by the presence of infiltrates with vessel invasion and infarction eventually resulting in cavitation. On chest radiography and, in particular, on CT (312), foci of rounded pneumonia with poorly defined edges indicating invasiveness are noted (313). Less commonly, a miliary or nodular appearance may be present.

During the recovery phase from invasive aspergillosis, cavitation may appear, representing a sign of recovery of immune function. During this phase the air crescent sign may be visible on CT or chest radiography, representing cavitation with a necrotic fungus ball contained within the cavity.

CANDIDA ALBICANS INFECTION

Infection by *Candida albicans* is noted with some frequency in patients with treated leukemia or lymphoma (314). Pulmonary findings are usually part of a disseminated picture of *C. albicans* (315) manifested by neutropenia, fever, and abundant *C. albicans* colonies present on mucus membranes. The pulmonary shadows present either a diffuse, bilateral, patchy infiltrative pattern or a miliary/nodular pattern

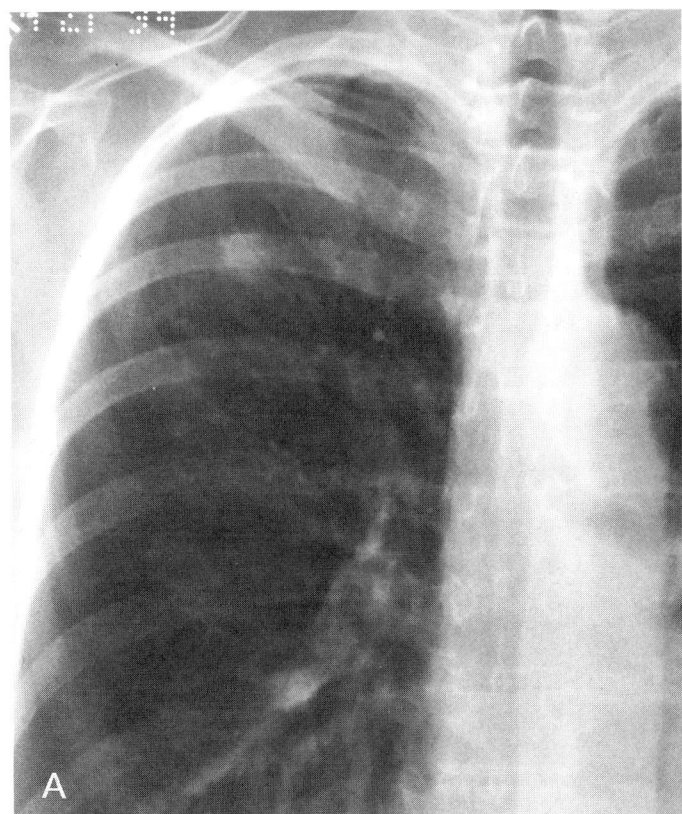
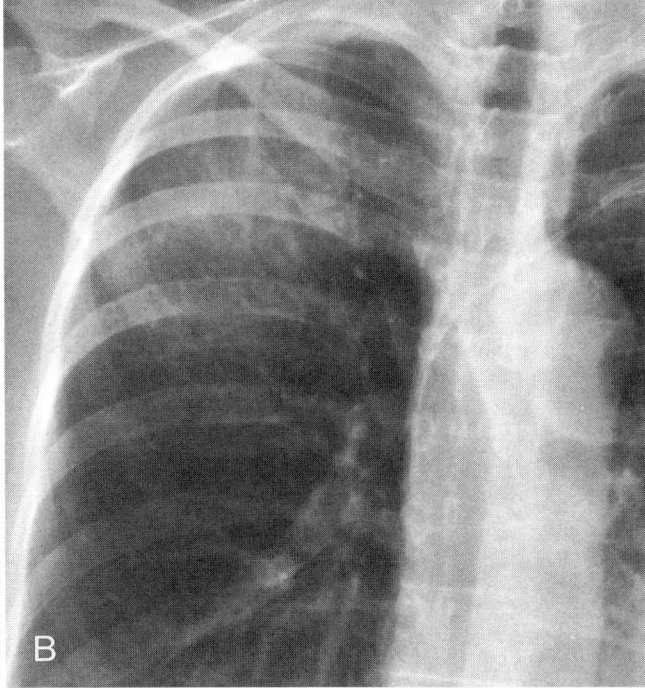

FIGURE 6.34. Opportunistic infection. A. This patient developed an ill-defined nodular density in the right upper lung zone while receiving chemotherapy for acute myelogenous leukemia. The patient's effective white blood cell counts were very low. B. On a chest radiograph obtained 10 days later, the ill-defined nodule had diffusely extended itself throughout the right upper lung zone as an alveolar filling process with very poorly defined borders. The CT scan confirmed this finding. There was no cavitation at this time. This was confirmed invasive *Aspergillus* fungal disease.

(316). This opportunistic infection is associated with a high mortality.

CRYPTOCOCCUS NEOFORMANS INFECTION

The *Cryptococcus neoformans* organism is responsible for a variety of roentgenographic appearances—isolated or multiple nodules, areas of infiltrate, and diffuse nodular and interstitial infiltrates indistinguishable from tuberculosis. The more severe manifestations reflect increasing immune compromise, especially in AIDS (317), leukemia, and lymphoma. Cryptococcal meningitis can dominate the clinical picture in these patients (318, 319). The presence of multiple lung nodules can simulate or mask the concomitant presence of lung cancer (320).

PHYCOMYCETES AND MUCORMYCOSIS INFECTION

Infections by phycomycetes and mucormycosis occur rarely but have a high mortality. Mucor manifests with both pulmonary and sinus involvement, the latter with frequent vascular invasion and extension to involve the intracranial structures.

CYTOMEGALOVIRUS INFECTION

Involvement of the lungs by cytomegalovirus is most commonly seen in lymphoma patients, transplant patients, and patients with AIDS, and is related to a defect in cell-mediated T-lymphocyte immunity. Involvement of the lungs is manifested by interstitial shadows present mainly at the lung bases. This opportunistic infection may be present concomitantly with involvement of the lungs by *P. carinii* infection.

CONCLUSION

Carefully performed imaging studies have assumed a central role in the evaluation of neoplasms. In addition to the conventional chest radiograph, an entire gamut of imaging examinations exist that may be requested to characterize pathologic processes within

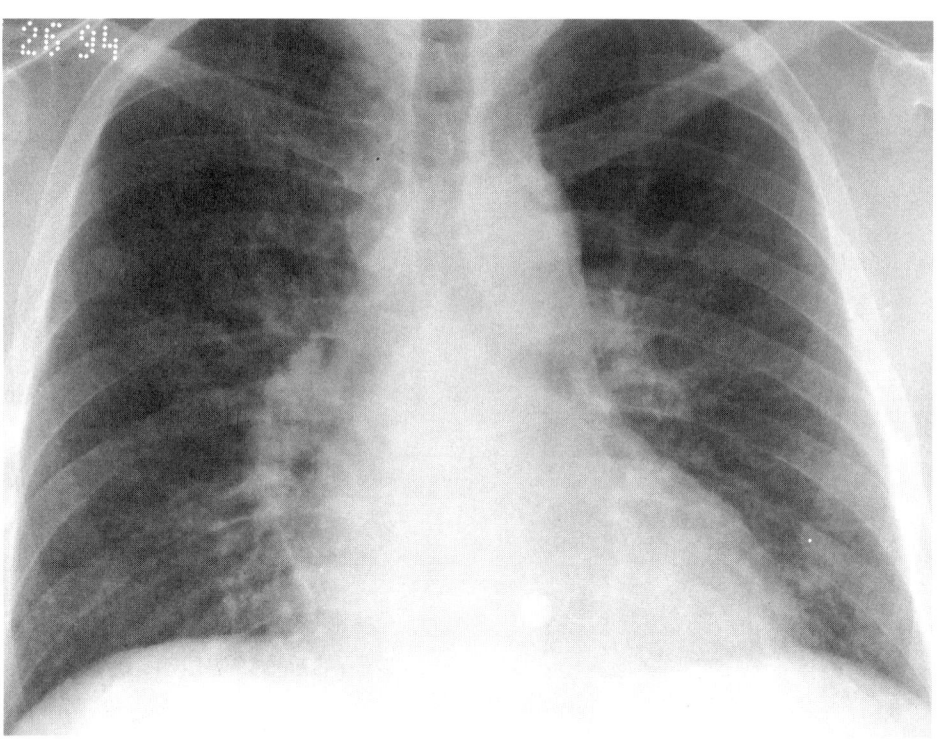

FIGURE 6.35. Opportunistic infection. PA chest radiograph in a patient treated for acute myelogenous leukemia with carboplatin. After the administration of carboplatin, the patient developed nadir sepsis with shortness of breath. PA chest radiograph revealed bilateral parahilar and lower lung zone infiltrates, most prominent at the left base and in the retrocardiac region. The radiographic appearance alone is nonspecific, but the clinical history and radiographic findings strongly suggested opportunistic infection. *Klebsiella* was diagnosed from sputum cytology.

the thorax. These imaging examinations are useful for the detection and characterization of neoplastic processes. The imaging appearance, however, frequently is nonspecific. More sophisticated examinations such as CT, MRI, and nuclear medicine procedures and endoscopic ultrasonography (for esophageal pathology) greatly enhance the accuracy of noninvasive staging and frequently affects the choice of therapy. Imaging examinations are also crucial to the follow-up of patients who have been treated by any modality. The evolution of the postoperative chest, as well as response to chemotherapy, may be followed closely with plain chest radiographs. Detection of recurrence or progression of disease, as well as the presence of complications of treatment, may be evaluated accurately by these modalities.

The issue of choice of examination is crucial in an era of cost containment. The basic initial chest radiograph retains an important role in detecting abnormalities, which then often are further characterized, most frequently by CT. The use of CT has become so common that it constitutes an early routine diagnostic evaluation. A variety of nuclear medicine procedures have also become routine, specifically, bone scanning and evaluation of pulmonary function.

The indication for more complex forms of imaging, some of them investigational, should be performed routinely only in consultation with the imaging physician. Possible benefits of these more complex (and more expensive) procedures should be clearly apparent, for example, the use of PET-FDG scanning in evaluation of solitary pulmonary nodules. In the future this modality may well be used for staging of lung cancer. These modalities, however, should not be requested without consultation with the imaging specialist.

Organisms causing pneumonia in the healthy population (*Streptococcus pneumoniae*, *Staphylococcus aureus*, *Pseudomonas aeruginosa*, *Klebsiella*) (Fig. 6.35) may also occur in immune-compromised patients, with a tendency to wider intraparenchymal dissemination. In addition, these patients respond more slowly to antibiotic therapy because of compromised white cell function. Tuberculosis may occur in immunocompromised patients, most notably AIDS patients, in whom it is relatively common. In other diseases involving compromise of immune function, it is uncommon, but its sporadic appearance makes it particularly important to diagnose. In addition, this pathogen represents a particular threat to the non-immunocompromised health care worker. *Nocardia asteroides* infection appears in patients on steroids and/or chemotherapy and results in a subacute pulmonary inflammatory process. *Legionella pneumophila* and *Legionella micdadei* infection occurs in patients on steroids and in renal transplant patients (321). Overwhelming acute pneumonias can be related to either varicella-zoster or Herpes simplex virus.

References

1. Coleman RE. Radiol Clin North Am 1993;31:721–959.
2. Armstrong P, Wilson AG, Dee P. Imaging of diseases of the chest. Chicago: Year Book Medical Publishers, 1990.
3. Fraser RG, Pare JAP, Pare PD, Fraser RS, Genereux GP. Diagnosis of diseases of the chest. Philadelphia: Saunders, 1991:IV.
4. Naidich DP, Zerhouni EA, Siegelman SS, Kuhn JP. Computed tomography and magnetic resonance of the thorax. New York: Raven Press, 1991.
5. Janerich DT, Thompson WD, Varela LR, Greenwald P, et al. Lung cancer and exposure to tobacco smoke in the household. N Engl J Med 1990;323:632–636.
6. Garfinkel L, Silverberg E. Lung cancer and smoking trends in the United States over the past 25 years. Cancer 1991;41:137–146.
7. Brower M, Ihde DC, Johnston-Early A. Treatment of extensive stage small cell bronchogenic carcinoma: effects of variation in intensity of induction chemotherapy. Am J Med 1983;75:993–1000.
8. Levenson RM Jr, Saurbrunn BJ, Ihde DC, et al. Small cell lung cancer: radionuclide bone scan for assessment of tumor extent and response. Am J Radiol 1981;137:31–35.
9. Perrin-Resche I, Bizais Y, Bube T, Fiche M. How does iliac crest bone marrow biopsy compare with imaging in the detection of bone metastasesin small cell cancer. Eur J Nucl Med 1993;20:420–425.
10. Balban EP, Walker BS, Cox DO, et al. Detection and staging of small cell lung carcinoma with a technetium-labelled monoclonal antibody in comparison with standard imaging methods. Clin Nucl Med 1992;17:439–445.
11. Fontana RS. Early diagnosis of lung cancer (editorial). Am Rev Respir Dis 1977;116:399–402.
12. Higgins GA, Shields TW, Keehn RJ. The solitary pulmonary nodule: ten-year follow up of Veterans Administration–Armed Forces Cooperative Study. Arch Surg 1975;110:570–575.
13. Jackman RJ, Good CA, Clagett OT, Bordlee RP, Salk D, Abrams PC, Sheehan RG, et al. Survival rates in peripheral bronchogenic carcinoma up to four centimeters in diameter presenting as solitary pulmonary nodules. J Thorac Cardiovasc Surg 1969;57:1–8.
14. Brogdon BG, Kelsey CA, Moseley RD. Factors affecting perception of pulmonary lesions. Radiol Clin North Am 1983;21:633–654.
15. Fontana RS, Sanderson DR, Taylor WF, et al. Early lung cancer detection: results of the initial (prevalence) radiologic cytologic screening in the Mayo Clinic study. Am Rev Respir Dis 1984;130:561–565.
16. Frost JK, Ball WC, Levin ML, et al. Early lung cancer detection: results of initial (prevalence) radiologic any cytologic screening in the Johns Hopkins study. Am Rev Respir Dis 1984;130:549–554.
17. Melamed MR, Flehinger BJ, Zaman MB, et al. Screening for early lung cancer: results of the Memorial Sloan–Kettering study in New York. Chest 1984;86:44–53.
18. Spencer H. Carcinoma of the lung. In: Pathology of the lung. 2nd ed. New York: Pergamon, 1969:849–869.
19. Theros EG. Varying manifestations of peripheral pulmonary neoplasms: a radiologic-pathologic correlative study. AJR Am J Roentgenol 1977;128:893–914.
20. Kuriyama K, Tateishi R, Doi O, et al. CT-pathologic correlation in small peripheral lung cancers. AJR Am J Roentgenol 1987;149:1139–1143.
21. Chaudhuri MR. Primary pulmonary cavitating carcinomas. Thorax 1973;28:354–366.
22. Stewart JG, MacMahon H, Viborny CJ, et al. Dystrophic calcification in carcinoma of the lung: demonstration by CT. AJR Am J Roentgenol 1987;149:29–30.
23. Muhm JR, Miller EW, Fontana RS, et al. Lung cancer detected during a screening program using four month chest radiographs. Radiology 1983;148:609–615.
24. Huhti E, Saloheimo M, Sutinen S. The value of roentgenologic screening in lung cancer. Am Rev Respir Dis 1983;128:395–398.
25. Heelan RT, Flehinger BJ, Melamed MR, Zaman MB, Perchick WB, Caravelli JF, Martini N. Non–small cell lung cancer: results of the New York Screening Program. Radiology 1984;151:289–293.
26. Ginsberg RJ, Rubinstein L. A randomized comparative trial of lobectomy vs. limited resection for patients with T1 N0 non-SCLC lung cancer. Journal of the International Association for the Study of Lung Cancer. 6th World Conference on Lung Cancer, Melbourne, Australia, Nov 1991.
27. Byrd RB, Carr DT, Miller WE. Radiographic abnormalities in carcinoma of the lung as related to histological cell type. Thorax 1969;24:573–575.
28. Byrd RB, Miller WE, Carr DT, et al. The roentgenographic appearance of squamous cell carcinoma of the bronchus. Mayo Clin Proc 1968;43:327–332.
29. Byrd RB, Miller WE, Carr DT, et al. The roentgenographic appearance of large cell carcinoma of the bronchus. Mayo Clin Proc 1968;43:333–336.
30. Byrd RB, Miller WE, Carr DT, et al. The roentgenographic appearance of small cell carcinoma of the bronchus. Mayo Clin Proc 1968;43:337–341.
31. Lehar TJ, Carr DT, Miller WE, et al. Roentgenographic appearance of bronchogenic adenocarcinoma. Am Rev Respir Dis 1967;96:245–248.
32. Fraser RG, Pare JAP. Diagnosis of diseases of the chest. 2nd ed. Philadelphia: Saunders, 1979.
33. Golden R. The effect of bronchostenosis upon the roentgen-ray shadows in carcinoma of the bronchus. AJR Am J Roentgenol 1925;13:21.
34. Johnson J. Discussions. J Thorac Surg 1957;34:308–309.
35. Crowe JK, Brown LR, Muhm JR. Computed tomography of the mediastinum. Radiology 1978;128:75.
36. Shevland JE, Chiu LC, Schapiro RL, Young JA, Rossi NP. The role of conventional tomography and computed tomography in assessing the resectability of primary lung cancer: a preliminary report. J Comput Assist Tomogr 1978;2:1.
37. Faling LJ, Pugatch RD, Jung-Legg Y, Daly BDT Jr, Hong WK. CT scanning of the mediastinum in the staging of bronchogenic carcinoma. Am Rev Respir Dis 1981;124–690.
38. Daly BDT, Faling LJ, Pugatch RD, et al. Computed tomography: an effective technique for mediastinal staging in lung cancer. J Thorac Cardiovasc Surg 1984;88:486–494.
39. Glazer GM, Orringer MB, Gross BH, Quint LE. The mediastinum in non–small cell lung cancer: CT-surgical correlation. AJR Am J Roentgenol 1984;142:1101–1105.
40. Goldstraw GM, Kurzer M, Edwards D. Preoperative staging of lung cancer: accuracy of computed tomography versus mediastinoscopy. Thorax 1983;38:10–15.
41. Khan A, Gersten KC, Garvey J, et al. Oblique hilar tomography, computed tomography, and mediastinoscopy for prethoracotomy staging of bronchogenic carcinoma. Radiology 1985;156:295–298.
42. Lewis JW Jr, Madrazo BL, Gross SC, et al. The value of radiographic and computed tomography in the staging of lung carcinoma. Ann Thorac Surg 1982;34:553–558.

43. Osborne DR, Korobkin M, Ravin CE, et al. Comparison of plain radiography, conventional tomography, and computed tomography in detecting intrathoracic lymph node metastases from lung carcinoma. Radiology 1982;142:157–161.
44. Richey HM, Matthews JI, Helsel RA, Calle H. Thoracic CT scanning in the staging of bronchogenic carcinoma. Chest 1984;85:218–221.
45. Ratto GB, Mereu C, Motta G. The prognostic significance of preoperative assessment of mediastinal lymph nodes in patients with lung cancer. Chest 1988;98:807–813.
46. Staples CA, Müller NL, Miller RR, et al. Mediastinal nodes in bronchogenic carcinoma: comparison between CT and mediastinoscopy. Radiology 1988;167:367–372.
47. McKenna RJ Jr, Libshitz HI, Mountain CE, McMurtrey MJ. Roentgenographic evaluation of mediastinal nodes for pre-operative assessment in lung cancer. Chest 1985;88:206–210.
48. Libshitz HI. CT of mediastinal lymph nodes in lung cancer: is there a "state of the art"? AJR Am J Roentgenol 1983;141:1081–1085.
49. Cohen AM, Creviston S, LiPuma JP, Evans KG, Nelems B. Nuclear magnetic resonance imaging of the mediastinum and hili: early impressions of its efficacy. AJR Am J Roentgenol 1983;141:1163–1169.
50. Levitt RG, Glazer HS, Roper CL, et al. Magnetic resonance imaging of mediastinal and hilar masses: comparison with CT. AJR Am J Roentgenol 1985;145:9–14.
51. Webb WR, Jensen BG, Sollitto R, et al. Bronchogenic carcinoma: staging with MR compared with staging with CT and surgery. Radiology 1985;156:117–124.
52. Heelan RT, Martini NR, Westcott JW, et al. Carcinomatous involvement of the hilum and mediastinum: computed tomographic and magnetic resonance evaluation. Radiology 1985;156:111–115.
53. Martini N, Heelan R, Westcott J, et al. Comparative merits of conventional, computed tomographic, and magnetic resonance imaging in assessing mediastinal involvement in surgically confirmed lung cancer. J Thorac Cardiovasc Surg 1985;90:639–648.
54. Musset D, Grenier P, Carette MF, et al. Primary lung cancer staging: prospective comparative study of MR imaging with CT. Radiology 1986;160:607–611.
55. Patterson GA, Ginsberg RJ, Poon PY, et al. A prospective evaluation of magnetic resonance imaging, computed tomography, and mediastinoscopy in the preoperative assessment of mediastinal node status in bronchogenic carcinoma. J Thorac Cardiovasc Surg 1987;94:679–684.
56. Poon PY, Bronskill MJ, Henkelman RM, et al. Mediastinal lymph node metastases from bronchogenic carcinoma: detection with MR imaging and CT. Radiology 1987;162:651–656.
57. Laurent F, Drouillard J, Dorcier F, et al. Bronchogenic carcinoma staging: CT vs MR imaging—assessment with surgery. Eur J Cardiothorac Surg 1988;2:31–36.
58. Grenier P, Dubray B, Carette MF, Frija G, Musset D, Chastang C. Preoperative thoracic staging of lung cancer: CT and MR evaluation. Diagn Intervent Radiol 1989;1:23–28.
59. Epstein DM, Stephenson LW, Gefter WB, van der Voorde F, Aronchik JM, Miller WT. Value of CT in the preoperative assessment of lung cancer: a survey of thoracic surgeons. Radiology 1986;161:423–427.
60. Webb RW, Gatsonis C, Zerhouni EA, et al. CT and MR imaging in staging non–small cell bronchogenic carcinoma: report of the radiologic diagnostic oncology group. Radiology 1991;178:705–713.
61. Heelan RT, Demas BE, Caravelli JF, et al. Superior sulcus tumors: CT and MR imaging. Radiology 1989;170:637–641.
62. Mitchell DG, Crovello M, Matteucci T, Petersen RO, Miettinen MM. Benign adrenocortical masses: diagnosis with chemical shift MR imaging. Radiology 1992;185:345–351.
63. Burt M, Heelan RT, Coit D, McCormack PM, Bains MS, Martini N, Rusch V, et al. Prospective evaluation of unilateral adrenal masses in patients with operable non–small cell lung cancer. J Thorac Cardiovasc Surg 1994;107:584–9.
64. Burt MG, Vitelli C, Fels A. Predicting post-lobectomy pulmonary function: a prospective evaluation of quantitative radionuclide perfusion scanning (PLS) in patients with non–small cell lung scanning. Abstr Biol Assoc Med P. Rico 1990;82(4):178.
65. Eagle KA, Corey CM, Newell JB, Darling RC. Combining clinical and thallium data optimizes pre-operative assessment. Ann Intern Med 1989;110:859–866.
66. de Lima R. Bronchial adenoma. Chest 1980;77:81.
67. Paladugu RR, Benfield JR, Pak HY, et al. Bronchopulmonary Kulchitzky cell carcinomas: a new classification scheme for typical and atypical carcinoids. Cancer 1985;55:1303.
68. Berge T, Linell F. Carcinoid tumours. Frequency in a defined population during a 12-year period (abstract). Acta Pathol Microbiol Scand 1976;84:322.
69. Arrigoni MG, Woolner LB, Bernatz PE. Atypical carcinoid tumors of the Lung. J Cardiovasc Thorac Surg 1972;64:413.
70. Salyer DC, Salyer WR, Eggleston JC. Bronchial carcinoid tumors. Cancer 1975;36:1522.
71. Felson B. Mucoid impaction (inspissated secretions) in segmental bronchial obstruction. Radiology 1976;133:9–16.
72. Pugatch RD, Gale ME. Obscure pulmonary masses: bronchial impaction revealed by CT. AJR Am J Roentgenol 1983;141:909–914.
73. Altman RL, Miller WE, Carr DT, et al. Radiographic appearance of bronchial carcinoid. Thorax 1973;28:433–434.
74. Giustra PE, Stassa G. The multiple presentations of bronchial adenoma. Radiology 1969;93:1013–1019.
75. Ranchod M, Levine GD. Spindle-cell carcinoid tumors of the lung. A clinicopathologic study of 35 cases. Am J Surg Pathol 1980;4:315.
76. Kremming EP, Kwekkeboom DJ, Bakker WH, et al. Somatostatin receptor scintigraphy with (In 111-DTPA-d-Phe1) and (I 123-Tyr3)-octreotide: the Rotterdam experience with more than 1000 patients. Eur J Nucl Med 1993;20:716–731.
77. Spizarny DL, Shepard J-AO, McLoud TC, et al. CT of adenoid cystic carcinoma of the trachea. AJR Am J Roentgenol 1986;146:1129.
78. Klaesmann PG, Olson JL, Eggleston JC. Mucoepidermoid carcinoma of the bronchus. An electron microscopic study of the low grade and the high grade variants. Cancer 1979;43:1720.
79. Yousem SA, Hochholzer L. Mucoepidermoid tumors of the lung. Cancer 1987;60:1346.
80. Davis SD, Henschke CI, Chamides BK, et al. Intrathoracic Kaposi sarcoma in AIDS patients: radiographic-pathologic correlation. Radiology 1987;163:495–500.
81. Sivit CJ, Schwartz AM, Rockoff SD. Kaposi's sarcoma of the lung in AIDS: radiologic-pathologic analysis. AJR Am J Roentgenol 1987;148:25–28.
82. Woolfenden JM, Carrasquillo JA, Larson SM, et al. Acquired immunodeficiency syndrome: Ga 67 citrate imaging. Radiology 1987;162:383–387.
83. Abdel-Dayem HM, Scott A, Macapinlac H, Larson SM. Tracer imaging in lung cancer. Eur J Nucl Med 1994;21:57–81.

84. Ohtomo K, Araki T, Yashiro N, et al. Pulmonary blastoma in children. Radiology 1983;147:101–104.
85. Siegelman SS, Khouri NF, Scott WW, et al. Pulmonary hamartoma: CT findings. Radiology 1986;160:313–317.
86. Poirier TJ, Van Ordstrand HS. Pulmonary chondromatous hamartoma: report of seventeen cases and review of the literature. Chest 1971;59:50–55.
87. Webb WR. Radiologic evaluation of the solitary pulmonary nodule. AJR Am J Roentgenol 1990;154:701–708.
88. Trunk G, Gracey DR, Byrd RB. The management and evaluation of the solitary pulmonary nodule. Chest 1974;66:236–239.
89. Cahan WG, Castro EB, Hajdu SI. The significance of a solitary lung shadow in patients with colon carcinoma. Cancer 1974;33:414–421.
90. O'Keefe ME Jr, Good CA, McDonald JR. Calcification in solitary nodules of the lung. AJR Am J Roentgenol 1957;77:1023–1033.
91. Mayo JR, Webb WR, Gould R, et al. High-resolution CT of the lungs: an optimal approach. Radiology 1987;163:507–510.
92. Kuriyama K, Tateishi R, Doi O, et al. CT-pathologic correlation in small peripheral lung cancers. AJR Am J Roentgenol 1987;149:1139–1143.
93. Stark P. Multiple independent bronchogenic carcinomas. Radiology 1982;145:599–601.
94. Bower SL, Choplin RH, Muss HB. Multiple primary bronchogenic carcinomas of the lung. AJR Am J Roentgenol 1983;140:253–258.
95. Siegelman SS, Zerhouni EA, Leo FP, et al. CT of the solitary pulmonary nodule. AJR Am J Roentgenol 1980;135:1–13.
96. Siegelman SS, Khouri NF, Leo FP, Fishman EK, Braverman RM, Zerhouni EA. Solitary pulmonary nodules: CT assessment. Radiology 1986;160:307–312.
97. Proto AV, Thomas SR. Pulmonary nodules studied by computed tomography. Radiology 1985;153:149–153.
98. Huston J, Muhm JR. Solitary pulmonary nodules: evaluation with a CT reference phantom. Radiology 1989;170:653–656.
99. Larson SM. Positron emission tomography in oncology and allied diseases. Principles and Practice of Oncology Updates 1989;3:1–12.
100. Patz EF, Lowe VJ, Hoffman JM, et al. Focal pulmonary abnormalities: evaluation with F-18 fluorodeoxyglucose PET scanning. Radiology 1993;188:487–490.
101. Wahl RL, Qumt LE, Greenough RL, Meyer CR, White RI, Orringer MB. Staging of mediastinal non–small cell lung Ca with FDG-PET, CT and fusion images: preliminary prospective evaluation. Radiology 1994;191:371–377.
102. Patz EF, Lowe VJ, Hoffman JM, Paine SS, Harris LK, Goodman PC. Persistent or recurrent bronchogenic carcinoma: detection with PET and 2-[F-18]-deoxy-D-glucose. Radiology 1994;191:379–372.
103. Herman PG, Hessel SJ. The diagnostic accuracy and complications of closed lung biopsies. Radiology 1977;125:11–14.
104. Khouri NF, Stitik FP, Erozan YS, et al. Transthoracic needle aspiration biopsy of benign and malignant lung lesions. AJR Am J Roentgenol 1985;144:281–288.
105. vanSonnenberg E, Casola G, Ho M, et al. Difficult thoracic lesions: CT-guided biopsy experience in 150 cases. Radiology 1988;167:457–461.
106. Naidich DP, Sussman R, Kutcher WL, Aranda CP, Garay SM, Ettenger NA. Solitary pulmonary nodules: CT-bronchoscopic correlation. Chest 1988;93:595–598.
107. Halvorsen RA Jr, Thompson WM. Computed tomographic staging of gastrointestinal tract malignancies. Part I. Esophagus and stomach. Invest Radiol 1987;22:2–16.
108. Halvorsen RA Jr, Thompson WM. CT of esophageal neoplasms. Radiol Clin North Am 1989;27:667–685.
109. Thompson WM, Halvorsen RA Jr., Fister WL, et al. Computed tomography for staging esophageal and gastroesophageal cancer: re-evaluation. AJR Am J Roentgenol 1983;141:951–958.
110. Picus D, Balfe DM, Koehler RE, et al. Computed tomography in the staging of esophageal carcinoma. Radiology 1983;146:433–438.
111. Gayet B, Frija J, Cahuzac J, Fekete F. The usefulness of computed tomography in esophageal carcinoma. A prospective and "blind" study. Gastroenterol Clin Biol 1988;12:23–28.
112. Grosser G, Wimmer B, Ruf G. Computed tomography for carcinoma of the esophagus. A prospective study. Fortschr Geb Roentgenstr Nuklearmed Ergänzungsbd 1985;143:288–293.
113. Muhling T, Kuklinski MR, Hubsch T, Witte J. Computed tomography of oesophageal carcinoma. A correlation of computer tomographic and postoperative findings. Fortschr Geb Roentgenstr Nuklearmed Ergänzungsbd 1985;143:189–193.
114. Takashima S, Takeuchi N, Shiozaki H, Kobayashi K, et al. Carcinoma of the esophagus: CT vs. MR imaging in determining resectability. AJR Am J Roentgenol 1991;156:297–302.
115. Quint LE, Glazer GM, Orringer MB. Esophageal imaging by MR and CT: study of normal anatomy and neoplasms. Radiology 1985;156:727–731.
116. Tio TL, Cohen P, Conne PP, et al. Endosonography and computed tomography of esophageal carcinoma: preoperative classification compared to the new (1987) TNM system. Gastroenterology 1989;96:1478–1486.
117. Ziegler K, Sanft C, Zeitz M, et al. Evaluation of endosonography in TN staging of esophageal cancer. Gut 1991;32:16–20.
118. Vilgrain V, Mompoint D, Palazzo L, et al. Staging of esophageal carcinoma: comparison of results with endoscopic sonography and CT. AJR Am J Roentgenol 1990;155:277–281.
119. Coppage L, Shaw C, Curtis AM. Metastatic disease to the chest in patients with extrathoracic malignancy. J Thorac Imag 1987;2(4):24–37.
120. Willis RA. The spread of tumours in the human body. 3rd ed. London: Butterworth, 1973.
121. Spencer H. Pathology of the lung. 4th ed. Philadelphia: Saunders, 1985.
122. Crow J, Slavin G, Kreel L. Pulmonary metastasis: a pathologic and radiologic study. Cancer 1981;47:2595–2602.
123. Gilbert HA, Kagan AR. Metastases: incidence, detection and evaluation without histologic confirmation. In: Weiss L, ed. Fundamental aspects of metastasis. Amsterdam: North-Holland, 1976.
124. Libshitz HI, Baber CE, Hammond CB. The pulmonary metastases of choriocarcinoma. Obstet Gynecol 1977;49:412–416.
125. Dodd GD, Boyle JS. Excavating pulmonary metastases. AJR Am J Roentgenol 1961;85:277–293.
126. Chaudhuri MR. Cavitary pulmonary metastases. Thorax 1970;25:375–381.
127. Deck FW, Sherman RS. Excavation of metastatic nodules in the lungs. Radiology 1959;72:30–34.
128. Wright FW. Spontaneous pneumothorax and pulmonary malignant disease: a syndrome sometimes associated with cavitating tumours. Clin Radiol 1976;27:211–222.
129. D'Angio GJ, Iannaccone G. Spontaneous pneumothorax as a complication of pulmonary metastases in malignant tumors of childhood. AJR Am J Roentgenol 1961;86:1092–1102.

130. Spittle MR, Heal J, Harmer C, et al. The association of spontaneous pneumothorax with pulmonary metastases in bone tumours of children. Clin Radiol 1968;19:400–403.
131. Dines DE, Cortese DA, Brennan MD, et al. Malignant pulmonary neoplasms predisposing to spontaneous pneumothorax. Mayo Clin Proc 1973;48:541–544.
132. Maile CW, Rodan BA, Godwin JD, et al. Calcification in pulmonary metastases. Br J Radiol 1982;55:108–113.
133. Chen JTT, Dahmash NS, Ravin CE, et al. Metastatic melanoma to the thorax: report of 130 patients. AJR Am J Roentgenol 1981;137:293–298.
134. Dwyer AJ, Reichart CM, Woltering EA, et al. Diffuse pulmonary metastasis in melanoma: radiographic pathologic correlation. AJR Am J Roentgenol 1984;143:983–984.
135. Webb WR, Gamsu G. Thoracic metastasis in malignant melanoma: a radiographic survey of 65 patients. Chest 1977;71:176–181.
136. Swett HA, Wescott JL. Residual nonmalignant pulmonary nodules in choriocarcinoma. Chest 1974;65:560–562.
137. Vogelzang NJ, Stenlund R. Residual pulmonary nodules after combination chemotherapy of testicular cancer. Radiology 1983;146:195–197.
138. Libshitz HI, Jing BS, Wallace S, et al. Sterilized metastases: a diagnostic and therapeutic dilemma. AJR Am J Roentgenol 1983;140:15–19.
139. Cahan WG. Lung cancer associated with cancer primary in other sites. Am J Surg 1955;89:494–499.
140. Cahan WG, Montemayor PB. Cancer of the larynx and lung in the same patient. J Thor Cardiovas Surg 1962;44:309–320.
141. Cahan WG, Castro El B, Hajdu SI. The significance of a solitary lung shadow in patients with colon carcinoma. Cancer 1974;33:414–420.
142. Ghaed N, Thrall JH, Pinsky SM. Detection of extraosseous metastases from osteosarcoma with Tc(99) polyphosphate bone scanning. Radiology 1974;112:373.
143. Schlumberger M, Tubiana M, De Vathaire F. Long term results of treatment of 283 patients with lung and bone metastases from differentiated thyroid cancer. J Clin Endo Metas 1986;63:960–967.
144. Bramman SS, Whitcomb ME. Endobronchial metastasis. Arch Intern Med 1975;135:543–547.
145. Albertini RE, Ekberg NL. Endobronchial metastasis in breast cancer. Thorax 1980;35:435–440.
146. Baumgartner WA, Mark JBD. Metastatic malignancies from distant sites to the tracheobronchial tree. J Thorac Cardiovasc Surg 1980;79:499–503.
147. Mountain CF, McMurtrey MJ, Hermes KE. Surgery for pulmonary metastasis: a 20-year experience. Ann Thorac Surg 1984;38:323–330.
148. Morrow CE, Vassilopoulos PP, Grage TB. Surgical resection for metastatic neoplasms of the lung: experience at the University of Minnesota Hospitals. Cancer 1980;45:2981–2985.
149. Marincola FM, Mark JBD. Selection factors resulting in improved survival after surgical resection of tumors metastatic to the lungs. Arch Surg 1990;125:1387–1393.
150. Shaner EG, Chang AE, Doppman JL, et al. Comparison of computed and conventional whole lung tomography in detecting pulmonary nodules: a prospective radiology-pathology study. AJR Am J Roentgenol 1978;131:51–54.
151. Muhm JR, Brown LR, Crowe JK, et al. Comparison of whole lung tomography and computed tomography for detecting pulmonary nodules. AJR Am J Roentgenol 1979;131:981–984.
152. Peuchot M, Libshitz HI. Pulmonary metastatic disease: radiologic-surgical correlation. Radiology 1987;164:719–722.
153. Heaston DK, Putman CE, Rodan BA, et al. Solitary pulmonary metastases in high risk melanoma patients: a prospective comparison of conventional and computed tomography. AJR Am J Roentgenol 1983;141:169–174.
154. Chiles C, Ravin CE. Intrathoracic metastases from an extrathoracic malignancy: radiographic approach to patient evaluation. Radiol Clin North Am 1985;23:427–438.
155. Feuerstein IM, Jicks DL, Pass HI, et al. Pulmonary metastases: MR imaging with surgical correlation—a prospective study. Radiology 1992;182:123–129.
156. Panicek DM. MR imaging for pulmonary metastases? Radiology 1992;182:10–11.
157. Reed CR. Chest radiology patterns and differential diagnoses. Chicago: Year Book Medical Publishers, 1981:58–106.
158. Lee JKT, Sagel SS, Stanley RJ. Computed body tomography with MRI correlation. 2nd ed. New York: Raven Press, 1989.
159. Kaplan HS. Hodgkin's disease. 2d ed. Cambridge, MA: Harvard University Press, 1980.
160. Castellino RA, Blank N, Hoppe RT, et al. Hodgkin disease: contributions of chest CT in the initial staging evaluation. Radiology 1986;160:603–605.
161. Filly R, Blank N, Castellino RA. Radiographic distribution of intrathoracic disease in previously untreated patients with Hodgkin's disease and non-Hodgkin's lymphoma. Radiology 1976;120:277–281.
162. Edwards CL, Hayes RL. Tumor scanning with gallium citrate. J Nucl Med 1969;10:103–105.
163. Front D, Ben Haim S, Israel O. Lymphoma: predictive of Ga-(67) scintigraphy after treatment. Radiology 1992;182:359–363.
164. Tumeh SS, Rosenthal DS, Kaplan WD, English RJ, Holman BL. Lymphoma: evaluation with Ga(67) SPECT. Radiology 1987;164:111–114.
165. Kostacoglu L, Yeh SDJ, Portlock C, Heelan R, Yao TJ, Niedzwiecki D, Larson SM. Validation of gallium-67 citrate single photon emission tomography in biopsy confirmed residual Hodgkin's disease. J Nucl Med 1992;33:345–350.
166. U.S. National Cancer Institute. National Cancer Institute–sponsored study of classification of non-Hodgkin's lymphoma: summary and description of a working formulation for clinical usage. Cancer 1982;49:2112–2135.
167. Shields AF, Porter BA, Churchley S, et al. The detection of bone marrow involvement by lymphoma using magnetic resonance imaging. J Clin Oncol 1987;5:225–230.
168. Kirn D, Maneh P, Shaffer K, Pinkus G, Shipp MA, Kaplan WD, Tung N, et al. Large cell and immunoblastic lymhphoma of the mediastinum: prognostic features and treatment outcome in 57 patients. J Clin Oncol 1993;11:1336–1343.
169. Kaplan WD. Residual mass and negative gallium scintigraphy in treatment of lymphoma: when is the gallium scan really negative (editorial)? J Nucl Med 1990;31:369–371.
170. Weinberg B, Rose JS, Efremidis SC, Kirshner PA, Gribetz D. Posterior mediastinal teratoma (cystic dermoid): diagnosis by computerized tomography. Chest 1980;77:694–695.
171. Dobranowski J, Martin LFW, Bennett WF. Case report. CT evaluation of posterior mediastinal teratoma. J Comput Assist Tomogr 1987;11:156–157.
172. Seltzer SE, Herman PG, Sagel SS. Differential diagnosis of mediastinal fluid levels visualized on computed tomography. J Comput Assist Tomogr 1984;8:244–246.
173. Fulcher AS, Proto AV, Jolles H. Case report. Cystic teratoma of the mediastinum: demonstration of fat-fluid level. AJR Am J Roentgenol 1990;154:259–260.

174. Shin MS, Ho KJ. Computed tomography of primary mediastinal seminomas. J Comput Assist Tomogr 1983;7:990–994.
175. Levitt RG, Husband JE, Glazer HS. CT of primary germ-cell tumors of the mediastinum. AJR Am J Roentgenol 1984;142:73–78.
176. Blomlie V, Lien HH, Fossa SD, Jawbsen AB, Stenwig AE. Computed tomography in primary non–seminomatous germ cell tumors of the mediastinum. Acta Radiol 1988;29:289–292.
177. Lee KS, Im JG, Han CH, Kim CW, Kim WS. Pictorial essay. Malignant primary germ sell tumors of the mediastinum: CT features. AJR Am J Roentgenol 1989;153:947–951.
178. Weibreb JC, Mootz A, Cohen JM. MRI evaluation of mediastinal and thoracic inlet venous obstruction. AJR Am J Roentgenol 1986;146:679–684.
179. Baron RL, Lee JKT, Sagel SS, Peterson RR. Computed tomography of the normal thymus. Radiology 1982;142:121–125.
180. Moore AV, Korobkin M, Olanow W, Heaston DK, Ram PC, Dunnick NR, Silverman PM. Age-related changes in the thymus gland: CT-pathologic correlation. AJR Am J Roentgenol 1983;141:241–246.
181. Francis IR, Glazer GM, Bookstein FL, Gross BH. The thymus: reexamination of age-related changes in size and shape. AJR Am J Roentgenol 1985;145:249–254.
182. Dixon AK, Hilton CJ, Williams GT. Computed tomography and histologic correlation of the thymic remnant. Clin Radiol 1981;32:255–257.
183. Goldstein G, Mackey IR. The human thymus. St. Louis: Warren H. Green, 1969.
184. Goldberg RE, Haaga JR, Yulish BS. Case report. Serial CT scans in thymic hyperplasia. J Comput Assist Tomogr 1987;11:539–540.
185. Chen J, Weisbrod GL, Herman SJ. Computed tomography and pathologic correlations of thymus lesions. J Thorac Imag 1988;3:61–65.
186. Cohen M, Hill CA, Cangir A, Sullivan MP. Thymic rebound after treatment of childhood tumors. AJR Am J Roentgenol 1980;135:151–156.
187. Choyke PL, Zeman RK, Gootenberg JE, Greenberg JN, Hoffer F, Frank JA. Thymic atrophy and regrowth in response to chemotherapy: CT evaluation. AJR Am J Roentgenol 1987;149:269–272.
188. Gelfand DW, Goldman AS, Law FJ, MacMillan BG, Larson D, Abston S, Schreiber JT. Thymic hyperplasia in children recovering from thermal burns. J Trauma 1972;12:813–817.
189. Doppman JL, Oldfield EH, Chrousos GP. Rebound thymic hyperplasia after treatment of Cushing's syndrome. AJR Am J Roentgenol 1986;147:1145–1147.
190. Rossleigh MA, Murray IP, Mackey DW, Bargwanna KA, Nayanar VV. Pediatric solid tumors: evaluation by gallium-67 SPECT studies. J Nucl Med 1990;31:168–172.
191. Mink JH, Bein ME, Sukov R, Herrmann C Jr, Winter J, Sample WF, Mulder D. Computed tomography of the anterior mediastinum in patients with myasthenia gravis and suspected thymoma. AJR Am J Roentgenol 1978;130:239–246.
192. Keesey J, Bein M, Mink J. Detection of thymoma in myasthenia gravis. Neurology 1980;30:233–239.
193. Baron RL, Lee JKT, Sagel SS, Levitt RG. Computed tomography of the abnormal thymus. Radiology 1982;142:127–134.
194. Fon GT, Bein ME, Mancuso AA, Keesey JC, Lupetin AR, Wong WS. Computed tomography of the anterior mediastinum in myasthenia gravis. A radiologic-pathologic correlative study. Radiology 1982;142:135–141.
195. Keen SJ, Libshitz HI. Thymic lesions. Experience with computed tomography in 24 patients. Cancer 1987;59:1520–1523.

196. Maggi G, Giaccone G, Donadio M, Ciuffreda L, Dalesio O, Leria G, Trifiletti G, et al. Thymomas. A review of 169 cases, with particular reference to results of surgical treatment. Cancer 1986;58:756–776.
197. Fujimura S, Kondo T, Handa M, Shiraishi Y, Tamahashi N, Nakada T. Results of surgical treatment for thymoma based on 66 patients. J Thorac Cardiovasc Surg 1987;93:708–714.
198. Krueger JB, Sagerman RH, King GA. Stage III thymoma: results of postoperative radiation therapy. Radiology 1988;168:855–858.
199. Zerhouni EA, Scott WW, Baker RR, Wharam MO, Siegelman SS. Invasive thymomas: diagnosis and evaluation by computed tomography. J Comput Assist Tomogr 1982;6:92–100.
200. Scatariage JC, Fishman EK, Zerhouni EA, Siegelman SS. Transdiaphragmatic extension of invasive thymomas. AJR Am J Roentgenol 1985;144:31–35.
201. Brown LR, Muhm JR, Sheedy PF, Unni KK, Bermatz PE, Hermann RC. The value of computed tomography in myasthenia gravis. AJR Am J Roentgenol 1983;140:31–35.
202. Baron RL, Sagel SS, Baglan RJ. Thymic cysts following radiation therapy for Hodgkin's disease. Radiology 1981;141:593–597.
203. Lewis CR, Manoharan A. Benign thymic cysts in Hodgkin's disease: report of a case and review of published cases. Thorax 1987;42:633–634.
204. Jaramillo D, Perez-Atayde A, Griscom NT. Apparent association between thymic cysts and prior thoracotomy. Radiology 1989;172:207–209.
205. Lagrange W, Dahm HM, Karstens J, Feichtinger J, Mittermayer C. Melanocystic neuroendocrine carcinoma of the thymus. Cancer 1987;59:484–488.
206. Herrera L, Oz M, Lally J, Davies A. Thymolipoma simulating pulmonary sequestration. J Pediatr Surg 1982;17:313–315.
207. Becker DV, Hurley JR. Treatment of thyroid carcinoma with Radioiodine. In: Gottschalk A, Hoffer PB, Potchen EJ, eds. Diagnostic nuclear medicine. 2nd ed. Baltimore: Williams & Wilkins, 1988:792–814.
208. Binder RE, Pugatch RD, Faling LJ, Kanter RA, Sawin CT. Case report. Diagnosis of posterior mediastinal goiter by computed tomography. J Comput Assist Tomogr 1980;4:550–552.
209. Glazer GM, Axel L, Moss AA. CT diagnosis of mediastinal thyroid. AJR Am J Roentgenol 1982;138:495–498.
210. Silverman PM, Newman GE, Korobkin M, Moore AV, Coleman RE. Computed tomography in the evaluation of thyroid disease. AJR Am J Roentgenol 1984;141:897–902.
211. Bashist B, Ellis K, Gold RP. Computed tomography of intrathoracic goiters. AJR Am J Roentgenol 1983;140:455–460.
212. Radecki PD, Arger PH, Arenson RL, Jennings AS, Coleman RG, Mintz MC, Kressel HY. Thyroid imaging: comparison of high-resolution real-time ultrasound and computed tomography. Radiology 1984;153:145–147.
213. Stark DD, Clark OH, Gooding GAW, Moss AA. High-resolution ultrasonography and computed tomography of thyroid lesions in patients with hyperparathyroidism. Surgery 1983;94:863–868.
214. Katz JF, Kane RA, Reyes J, Clarke MP, Hill TC. Thyroid nodules; sonographic-pathologic correlation. Radiology 1984;151:741–745.
215. Charkes ND, Maurer AH, Siegel JA, Radecki PD, Malmud LS. MR imaging in thyroid disorders: correlation of signal intensity with Graves disease activity. Radiology 1987;164:491–494.
216. Noma S, Nishimura K, Togashi K, Itoh K, Fujisawa I, Nakano Y, et al. Thyroid gland: MR imaging. Radiology 1987;164:495–499.

217. Norris EH. The parathyroid adenoma: a study of 322 cases. International Abstracts in Surgery 1947;84:1–41.
218. Satava RM, Beahrs OH, Scholz DA. Success rate of cervical exploration for hyperparathyroidism. Arch Surg 1975;110:625–627.
219. Cates JD, Thorsen K, Lawson TL, Middleton WD, Foley WD, Wilson SD, Krubsack AJ. CT evaluation of parathyroid adenomas: diagnostic criteria and pitfalls. J Comput Assist Tomogr 1988;12:626–629.
220. Spritzer CE, Gefter WB, Hamilton R, Greenberg BM, Axel L, Kressel HY. Abnormal parathyroid glands: high-resolution MR imaging. Radiology 1987;162:487491.
221. Auffermann W, Gooding GAW, Okerlund MD, Clark OH, Thrurnher S, Levin KE, Higgins CB. Diagnosis of recurrent hyperparathyroidism: comparison of MR imaging and other imaging techniques. AJR Am J Roentgenol 1988;150:1027–1033.
222. Kneeland JB, Krubsack AJ, Lawson TL, Wilson SD, Collier BD, Froncisz W, Jesmanowicz A, et al. Enlarged parathyroid glands: high-resolution local coil MR imaging. Radiology 1987;162:143–146.
223. Kim K, Koo BC, Davis JT, Franco-Saenz R. Primary myelolipoma of mediastinum. J Comput Assist Tomogr 1984; 8:119–123.
224. Kountz PD, Molina PL, Sagel SS. Case report. Fibrosing mediastinitis in the posterior thorax. AJR Am J Roentgenol 1989;153:489–490.
225. Black WC, Armstrong P, Daniel TM, Cooper PH. Case report. Computed tomography of aggressive fibromatosis in the posterior mediastinum. J Comput Assist Tomogr 1987;11:153–155.
226. Kumar AJ, Kuhajda FP, Martinez CR, Fishman EK, Jezic DV, Siegelman SS. CT of extracranial nerve sheath tumors. J Comput Assist Tomogr 1983;7:857–865.
227. Burk DL, Brunberg JA, Kanal E, Latchaw RE, Wolf GL. Spinal and paraspinal neurofibromatosis: surface coil MR imaging at l.5T. Radiology 1987;162:797–801.
228. Dietrich RB, Kangarloo H, Lenarsky C, Feig SA. Neuroblastoma: the role of MR imaging. AJR Am J Roentgenol 1987;148:927–942.
229. Siegel MJ, Jamroz GA, Glazer HS, Abramson CL. MR imaging of intraspinal extension of neuroblastoma. J Comput Assist Tomogr 1986;10:593–595.
230. Francis PA, Rigas JR, Kris MG, Pisters KMW, Orazem JP, Woolley KJ, Heelan RT. Phase II trial of docetaxel (Taxotere) in patients with stage III and IV non–small cell lung cancer. J Clin Oncol 1994;12:1232–1237.
231. Sahn SA: The pleura. Am Rev Respir Dis 1988;138:184–234.
232. Leff A, Hopewell PC, Costello J. Pleural effusion from malignancy. Ann Intern Med 1978;88:532–537.
233. Chernow B, Sahn SA. Carcinomatous involvement of the pleura: analysis of 96 patients. Am J Med 1977;63:695–702.
234. Meyer PC. Metastatic carcinoma of the pleura. Thorax 1966; 21:437–443.
235. Salyer WR, Eggleston JC, Erozan YS. The efficacy of pleural needle biopsy and of pleural fluid cytology in the diagnosis of malignant neoplasm involving the pleura. Chest 1975;67:5.
236. Scerbo J, Keltz H, Stone DJ. A prospective study of closed pleural biopsies. JAMA 1971;218:377–380.
237. Ryan CJ, Rodgers RF, Unni KK, Hepper NGG. The outcome of patients with pleural effusion of indeterminate cause at thoracotomy. Mayo Clin Proc 1981;56:145–149.
238. Zerhouni EA, Scott WW, Baker RR, Wharam MO, Siegelman SS. Invasive thymomas: diagnosis and evaluation by computed tomography. J Comput Assist Tomogr 1982;6:92–100.
239. Moran CA, Travis WD, Rosado-de-Christenson ML, Koss MN, Rosai J. Thymomas presenting as pleural tumors: report of eight cases. Am J Surg Pathol 1992;16:138–144.
240. Webb WR, Jeffrey RB, Godwin JD. Thoracic computed tomography in superior sulcus tumors. J Comput Assist Tomogr 1981;5:361–365.
241. Glazer HS, Duncan-Meyer J, Aronberg DJ, et al. Pleural and chest wall invasion in bronchogenic carcinoma: CT evaluation. Radiology 1985;157:191.
242. McLoud TC, Filion RB, Edelman RR, Shepard JO. MR imaging of superior sulcus carcinoma. J Comput Assist Tomogr 1989;13:233–239.
243. Webb WR, Jensen BJ, Sollitto R, et al. Bronchogenic carcinoma: staging with MR compared with staging with CT and surgery. Radiology 1985;156:117.
244. Hagger AM, Pearlberg JL, Froelich JW, et al. Chest wall invasion by carcinoma of the lung: detection by MR imaging. AJR Am J Roentgenol 1987;148:1075–1087.
245. England DM, Hochholzer L, McCarthy MJ. Localized benign and malignant fibrous tumors of the pleura. A clinicopathologic review of 223 cases. Am J Surg Pathol 1989;13:640.
246. Dervan PA, Tobin B, O'Connor M. Solitary (localized) fibrous mesothelioma: evidence against mesothelial cell origin. Histopathology 1986;10:867.
247. Hernandez FJ, Fernandez BB. Localized fibrous tumors of pleura: a light and electron microscopic study. Cancer 1974; 34:1667.
248. Said JW, Nash G, Banks-Schlegel S, et al. Localized fibrous mesothelioma: an immunohistochemical and electron microscopic study. Hum Pathol 1984;15:440.
249. El-Naggar AK, Ro JY, Ayala AG, et al. Localized fibrous tumor of the serosal cavities. Immunohistochemical, electron-microscopic, and flow-cytometric DNA study. Am J Clin Pathol 1989;92:561.
250. Berne AS, Heitzman ER. The roentgenologic signs of pedunculated pleural tumors. AJR Am J Roentgenol 1962;87:892.
251. Hayward RH. Migrating lung tumor. Chest 1974;66:77.
252. Dedrick CG, McLoud TC, Shepard JO, Shipley RT. Computed tomography of localized pleural mesothelioma. AJR Am J Roentgenol 1985;144:275–280.
253. Lee KS, Im JG, Choe KO, Kim CJ, Lee BH. CT findings in benign fibrous mesothelioma of the pleura: pathologic correlation in nine patients. AJR Am J Roentgenol 1992;158:983–986.
254. Mendelson DS, Meary E, Buy JN, Pigeau I, Kirschner PA. Localized fibrous pleural mesothelioma: CT findings. Clin Imag 1991;15:105–108.
255. Spizarny DL, Gross BH, Shepart JO. CT findings in localized fibrous mesothelioma of the pleural fissure. J Comput Assist Tomogr 1986;10:942–944.
256. Yousem SA, Flynn SD. Intrapulmonary localized fibrous tumor: intraparenchymal so-called localized fibrous mesothelioma. Am J Clin Pathol 1988;89:365–369.
257. Briselli M, Mark EJ, Dickerson GR. Solitary fibrous tumors of the pleura: eight new cases and review of 360 cases in the literature. Cancer 1981;47:2678.
258. Rabinowitz JG, Efremidis SG, Cohen B, et al. A comparative study of mesothelioma and asbestosis using computed tomography and conventional chest radiography. Radiology 1982; 144:453.
259. Rusch VW, Godwin JD, Shuman WP. The role of computed tomography scanning in the initial assessment and the follow-up of malignant pleural mesothelioma. J Thorac Cardiovasc Surg 1988;96:171–177.

260. Kawashima A, Libshitz HI. Malignant pleural mesothelioma: CT manifestations in 50 cases. AJR Am J Roentgenol 1990;155:965–969.
261. Rosenow EC. Chemotherapeutic drug-induced pulmonary disease. Semin Respir Med 1980;2:89–96.
262. Cooper JAD, White DA, Matthay RA. Drug-induced pulmonary disease. I. Cytotoxic drugs. Am Rev Respir Dis 1986;133:321–340.
263. Cooper JAD, White DA, Matthay RA. Drug-induced pulmonary disease. II. Noncytotoxic drugs. Am Rev Respir Dis 1986;133:488–505.
264. Gefter WB. Drug-induced disorders of the chest. In: Taveras JM, Ferrucci JT, eds. Radiology: diagnosis-imaging-intervention. Philadelphia: Lippincott, 1986.
265. Cooper JAD. Drug-induced pulmonary disease. Clin Chest Med 1990;11:1–194.
266. Israel-Biet D, Labrune S, Huchon GJ. Drug-induced lung disease: 1990 review. Eur Respir J 1991;4:465–478.
267. Lehne G, Lote K. Pulmonary toxicity of cytotoxic and immunosuppressive agents: a review. Acta Oncol 1990;29:113–124.
268. Rubin SA, ed. Lung and heart disease associated with drug therapy and abuse (review). J Thorac Imaging 1991;6:1–86.
269. Moinuddin M. Radionuclide scanning in the detection of drug-induced lung disorders. J Thorac Imaging 1991;6:62–67.
270. White DA, Stover DE. Severe bleomycin-induced pneumonitis: clinical features and response to corticosteroids. Chest 1984;86:723–728.
271. Bellamy EA, Husband JE, Blaquiere RM, et al. Bleomycin-related lung damage: CT evidence. Radiology 1985;156:155–158.
272. Jules-Elysee K, White DA. Bleomycin-induced pulmonary toxicity. Clin Chest Med 1990;11:1–20.
273. Kuhlman JE. The role of chest computed tomography in the diagnosis of drug-related reactions. J Thorac Imaging 1991;6:52–61.
274. Sostman HD, Matthay RA, Putman CE. Methotrexate-induced pneumonitis. Medicine 1976;55:371–388.
275. Twohig KJ, Matthay RA. Pulmonary effects of cytotoxic agents other than bleomycin. Clin Chest Med 1990;11:31–54.
276. Haupt HM, Hutchins GM, Moore GW. Ara-C lung: noncariogenic pulmonary edema complicating cytosine arabinoside therapy of leukemia. Am J Med 1981;70:256–261.
277. Anderson BS, Cogan BM, Keating MJ, et al. Subacute pulmonary failure complicating therapy with high dose Ara-C in acute leukemia. Cancer 1985;56:2181–2184.
278. Tjon A, Tham RTO, Peters WG, et al. Pulmonary complications of cytosine arabinoside therapy: radiographic findings. AJR Am J Roentgenol 1987;149:23–27.
279. Conant EF, Fox KR, Miller WT. Pulmonary edema as a complication of interleukin-2 therapy. AJR Am J Roentgenol 1989;152:749–752.
280. Mann H, Ward JH, Samlowski WE. Vascular leak syndrome associated with interleukin-2: chest radiographic manifestations. Radiology 1990;176:191–194.
281. Purtilo DT. Immune deficiency predisposing to Epstein-Barr virus induced lymphoproliferative diseases: the X-linked lymphoproliferative syndrome as a model. Adv Cancer Res 1981;34:279–312.
282. Starzl TE, Nalesnik MA, Porter KA, et al. Reversibility of lymphomas and lymphoproliferative lesions developing under cyclosporine-steroid therapy. Lancet 1984;1:583–587.
283. Harris KM, Schwartz ML, Slasky BS, Nalesnik M, Makowka L. Posttransplantation cyclosporine-induced lymphoproliferative disorders: clinical and radiological manifestations. Radiology 1987;162:697–700.
284. Boxt LM, Katz J. Effects of drugs on the radiographic appearance of the heart. J Thorac Imaging 1991;6:76–84.
285. Schwartz RG, Zaret BL. Diagnosis and treatment of drug induced myocardial disease. In: Maggia FM, ed. Cancer treatment and the heart. Baltimore: John Hopkins Press, 1982;173–197.
286. Libshitz HI. Thoracic radiotherapy changes. In: Herman PG, ed. Iatrogenic thoracic complications. New York: Springer-Verlag, 1983:141–160.
287. Moss WT, Brand WN, Battifora H. Radiation oncology: rationale, technique, results. 5th ed. St. Louis: Mosby, 1979:253–288.
288. Glazer HS, Lee JKT, Levitt RG, et al. Radiation fibrosis: Differentiation from recurrent tumor by MR imaging: work in progress. Radiology 1985;156:721–726.
289. Libshitz HI, Shuman LS. Radiation-induced pulmonary change: CT findings. J Comput Assist Tomogr 1984;8:15–19.
290. Bell J, McGiven D, Bullimore J, et al. Diagnostic imaging of the post-irradiation changes in the chest. Clin Radiol 1988;39:109–119.
291. Farmer W, Ravin C, Schachter EN. Hyperlucent lung after radiation therapy. Am Rev Respir Dis 1975;112:255–258.
292. Wyman SM, Weber AL. Calcifications in intrathoracic nodes in Hodgkin's disease in the chest. Radiology 1969;93:1021–1024.
293. Huvos AG, Woodward HQ, Cahan WB, et al. Post irradiation osteogenic sarcoma of bone and soft tissue. A clinico-pathologic study in 66 patients. Cancer 1985;55:1244–1255.
294. Rosenow EC, Wilson WR, Cockerill FR. Pulmonary disease in the immunocompromised host. Mayo Clin Proc 1985;60:473–478.
295. Suster B, Akerman M, Orenstein M, et al. Pulmonary manifestations of AIDS: review of 106 episodes. Radiology 1986;161:87–93.
296. Katzenstein ALA, Askin FB. Interpretation and significance of pathologic findings in transbronchial lung biopsy. Am J Surg Pathol 1980;4:223–234.
297. Leight GS, Michaelis LL. Open lung biopsy for the diagnosis of acute diffuse pulmonary infiltrates in the immunosuppressed patient. Chest 1978;73:477–482.
298. Rossiter SJ, Miller C, Churg AM, et al. Open lung biopsy in the immunosuppressed patient. Is it really beneficial? J Thorac Cardiovasc Surg 1979;77:338–345.
299. Simmons JT, Suffredini AF, Lack EE. Nonspecific interstitial pneumonitis in patients with AIDS: radiologic features. AJR Am J Roentgenol 1987;149:265–268.
300. Oldham SAA, Castello M, Jacobson FL, et al. HIV-associated lymphocytic interstitial pneumonia: radiologic manifestation and pathologic correlation. Radiology 1989;170:83–87.
301. Tenholder MF, Hooper RG. Pulmonary infiltrates in leukemia. Chest 1980;78:468–473.
302. Krowka MJ, Rosenow EC, Hoagland HC. Pulmonary complications of bone marrow transplantation. Chest 1985;87:237–246.
303. Pagani JJ, Kangarloo H, Gyepes MT, et al. Radiographic manifestations of bone marrow transplantation in children. AJR Am J Roentgenol 1979;132:883–890.
304. Gedroyc WMW, Reidy JF. The early chest radiographic changes of *Pneumocystis* pneumonia. Clin Radiol 1985;36:331–334.
305. Turbiner EH, Yeh HD, Rosen PP, et al. Abnormal gallium scintigraphy in *Pneumocystis carinii* pneumonia with a normal chest radiograph. Radiology 1978;127:437–438.

306. Coleman DL, Haltner RS, Luce JM, et al. Correlation between gallium lung scans and fiberoptic bronchoscopy in patients with suspected *Pneumocystis carinii* pneumonia and the acquired immune deficiency syndrome. Am Rev Respir Dis 1984;130:1166–1169.
307. Woolfenden JM, Carrasquilo JA, Larson SM, et al. Acquired immunodeficiency syndrome. Ga-67 citrate imaging. Radiology 1987;162:383–387.
308. Cohen BA, Pomeranz S, Rabinowitz JG, et al. Pulmonary complications of AIDS: radiologic features. AJR Am J Roentgenol 1984;143:115–122.
309. Bier S, Halton K, Krivisky B, et al. *Pneumocystis carinii* pneumonia presenting as a single pulmonary nodule. Pediatr Radiol 1986;16:59–60.
310. Cross AS, Steigbigel RT. *Pneumocystis carinii* pneumonia presenting as localized nodular densities. N Engl J Med 1974; 291:831–832.
311. Gefter WB, Weingrad TR, Epstein DM, et al. "Semi-invasive" pulmonary aspergillosis. A new look at the spectrum of *Aspergillus* infections of the lung. Radiology 1981;140:313–321.
312. Kuhlman JE, Fishman EK, Siegelman SS. Invasive pulmonary aspergillosis in acute leukemia: characteristic finding on CT, the CT halo sign and the role of CT in early diagnosis. Radiology 1985;157:611–614.
313. Libshitz HI, Pagani JJ. Aspergillos and mucormycosis: two types of opportunistic fungal pneumonia. Radiology 1981;140: 301–306.
314. Buff SJ, McLelland R, Gallis HA, et al. *Candida albicans* pneumonia: radiographic appearance. AJR Am J Roentgenol 1982; 138:645–648.
315. Degregorio MW, Lee WMF, Linker CA, et al. Fungal infections in patients with acute leukemia. Am J Med 1982;73:543–548.
316. Pagani JJ, Libshitz HI. Opportunistic fungal pneumonias in cancer patients. AJR Am J Roentgenol 1981;137:1033–1039.
317. Kovacs JA, Kovacs AA, Polis M, et al. Cryptococcosis in acquired immunodeficiency syndrome. Ann Intern Med 1985; 103:533–538.
318. Balmes JR, Hawkins JG. Pulmonary cryptococcosis. Semin Respir Med 1987;9:180–186.
319. Kerkering TM, Duma RJ, Shadomy S. The evolution of pulmonary cryptococcosis: clinical implications from a study of 41 patients with and without compromising host factors. Ann Intern Med 1981;94:611–616.
320. Duperval R, Hermans PE, Brewer NS, et al. Cryptococcosis, with emphasis on the significance of isolation of *Cryptococcus neoformans* from the respiratory tract. Chest 1977;72: 13–19.
321. Pope TL, Armstrong P, Thomas R, et al. Pittsburgh pneumonia agent: chest film manifestations. AJR Am J Roentgenol 1983; 138:237–241.

7

PULMONARY FUNCTION EVALUATION VIS À VIS TUMOR TREATMENT

Hani Shennib, Kevin Lachapelle, and Neil Colman

The only person that I had met who lived with only one lung was a woman who had spent the last 30 years playing Camille on a chaise lounge. True she seemed happy enough, but it certainly was not a role that I envied (1).

The American Cancer Society estimated that 172,000 cases of lung cancer would be detected in 1994 in the United States (2). It also is estimated that nearly 20% of the population with lung cancer will have resection with curative intent (3). However, surgical therapy is possible only in a minority of patients presenting with metastatic disease, locally advanced mediastinal involvement, or poor pulmonary function. Surgery traditionally has been the main curative treatment for lung cancer, but some success has been achieved in phase II trials of preoperative chemotherapy and radiotherapy followed by surgery in patients with locally advanced lung cancer involving mediastinal lymph nodes (4, 5). There is a suggestion that patients with stage IIIA non–small cell lung cancer have improved survival with preoperative chemotherapy compared with surgery alone (6). Patients who may have been refused operative therapy until recently because of poor pulmonary function are now being offered surgery because of improvements in preoperative assessment (7) and the advent of limited pulmonary resections (8). The number of patients offered potentially curative therapy thus will increase as a result of a multimodal approach to lung cancer treatment that includes surgery, radiotherapy, and chemotherapy.

Patients with lung cancer often have co-morbid conditions such as chronic obstructive lung disease (9) and cardiovascular disease caused by prolonged tobacco exposure. Before beginning any therapy, an assessment of the patient's pulmonary function should be determined accurately (10). The assessment of pulmonary function before surgical therapy for lung carcinoma has been described in the literature for more than 35 years and is a major part of the general preoperative evaluation. The effect and reduction of pulmonary function caused by radiotherapy and chemotherapy are not as well defined but may be important for several reasons: (*a*) patients often are excluded from surgery on the basis of poor pulmonary function and frequently are offered palliative radiotherapy; (*b*) patients may receive preoperative radiotherapy, e.g., superior sulcus tumors; and (*c*) patients may be part of clinical studies of combined preoperative chemotherapy and radiotherapy.

This chapter outlines the assessment of pulmonary function before surgery, radiotherapy, and chemotherapy. More specifically, a logical method using a step-wise approach to preoperative pulmonary function testing is stressed. A clear understanding of lung function and of the effects that surgery, radiotherapy, and chemotherapy have on the integrity of pulmonary function is essential to enable selection of the appropriate therapeutic modality for each patient.

BASIS OF PULMONARY FUNCTION TESTING

A number of preoperative tests are available that determine the adequacy of pulmonary function before lung resection; these range from simple spirometric tests to the more complicated exercise test. The basis of lung function assessment rests in the understanding of lung volumes, lung capacity, and flow rates.

The lung can be divided into four volumes and four capacities (Fig. 7.1). The tidal volume is the amount of gas exhaled and inhaled during each breath. The expiratory reserve volume is the additional amount of gas that can be expelled at the end of normal expiration. The residual volume (RV) is the amount of gas remaining after maximal expiration, and

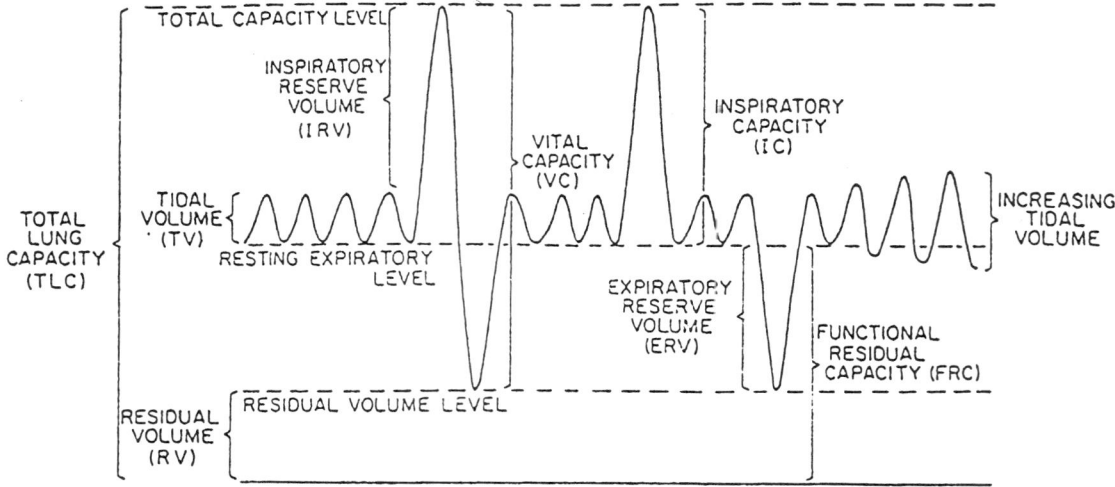

FIGURE 7.1. Spirometric volumes.

the inspiratory reserve volume is the amount of additional gas that can be inhaled after normal inspiration. The total lung capacity (TLC) is the amount of gas in the lung at the end of maximal inspiration whereas the vital capacity (VC) is the amount of gas that can be expelled after maximal inspiration. The inspiratory capacity is the amount of gas that can be inspired after a quiet inspiration, and the functional residual capacity (FRC) is the volume of gas that remains in the lung after normal expiration.

The determination of FRC, RV, and TLC requires either helium gas inhalation or body plethysmography, but the latter is more accurate and is used more commonly. The rest of the volumes and capacities can be determined using simple spirometry. Standards for normality are based on age, sex, height, weight, and race, with an abnormal value occurring if there is a difference of ±20% from the predicted mean value.

Forced expiratory and inspiratory flows generally are performed once the lung volumes and capacities are known. The VC usually is measured as a forced vital capacity (FVC) because the gas is expelled during forced expiration. When the measured FVC is coupled with the amount of gas exhaled during the first second of the FVC maneuver the ratio of the forced expiratory volume in 1 second (FEV_1) to the FVC is obtained (Fig. 7.2). Three to five measurements are made, and the highest sum of the FEV_1 and FVC is used. This ratio is very sensitive for assessing the degree of airway obstruction in patients with chronic obstructive pulmonary disease (COPD) and usually is reduced markedly from the normal value of 75% (Fig. 7.2). Another indicator of airflow obstruction is the forced expiratory flow between 25% and 75% of the FVC

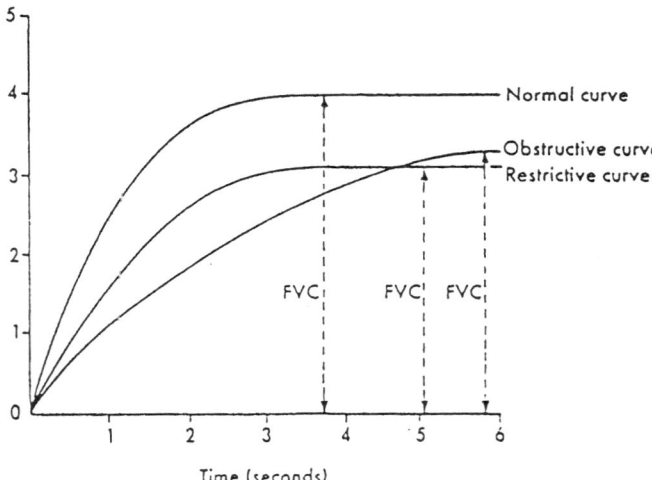

FIGURE 7.2. Timed vital capacity.

($FEF_{25\%-75\%}$). This test measures the rate of airflow occurring between 25% and 75% of the volume expired during the FVC. Patients also may have a pattern of lung dysfunction that is restrictive in nature: the lung volumes are reduced but the FEV_1 to FVC ratio is preserved. A measure that also correlates with FEV_1 is the maximal voluntary ventilation (MVV), which records the ventilation that can be achieved during 15 seconds of maximal inspiration and expiration. It not only tests for airway obstruction but also for lung compliance and muscle strength (11).

Rather than plot a graph of volume versus time as is done for FEV_1 and FVC, a flow versus volume loop can be constructed during maximal expiration and inspiration. The rate of flow in liters per second is plotted at various lung volumes, and a characteristic expi-

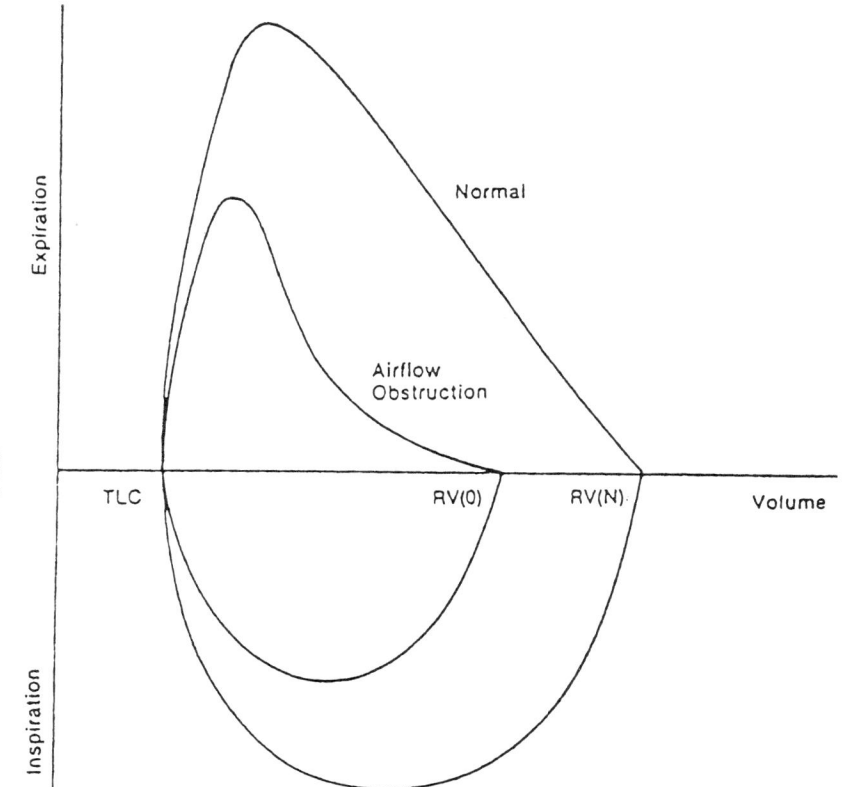

FIGURE 7.3. Flow-volume curves.

ratory and inspiratory graph is produced (Fig. 7.3). Patients with airway obstruction have a reduced peak flow rate at TLC, a scooped out portion of the graph during the latter part of the exercise, and an increase in RV. The contour of the terminal part of the curve may be abnormal in patients with early airways disease even when the FEV_1 to FVC ratio is normal. In addition, the contour of the expiratory and inspiratory flow-volume loop can localize lesions, thus causing upper airway obstruction (12). The obstruction can be classified as intrathoracic or extrathoracic and as fixed or variable (Figs. 7.4 and 7.5). A fixed lesion that is either intrathoracic or extrathoracic is not affected by pleural pressure changes during forced expiration and inspiration, and a plateau is seen on both the expiratory and inspiratory limbs of the curve. A variable lesion that is intrathoracic reduces flow during expiration because the upper airway is compressed by the increase in pleural pressure, and a plateau is seen on the expiratory curve. The inspiratory flow is not affected because the airway is distended by the decreased pleural pressure during inspiration. Conversely, a variable extrathoracic lesion causes a plateau to occur on forced inspiration because the surrounding atmospheric pressure is greater than the intratracheal pressure. Upon expiration the intratracheal pressure distends the airway and the expiratory curve is not affected. A reduced FEV_1 and FVC, therefore, may not be caused by COPD but rather may reflect an underlying anatomic lesion.

EFFECT OF SURGERY ON LUNG FUNCTION

The basis for the continued use of pulmonary function tests stems from the physiologic alterations that occur after pulmonary surgery and the early reports in the literature of increased mortality after thoracotomy in patients with COPD (13). The effects of thoracic surgery on lung function generally are caused by three interrelated processes: general anesthesia, the surgical incision and the body's response to the surgical stress, and the extent of lung resection.

GENERAL ANESTHESIA

Inhalation agents such as isoflurane and enflurane that are used in general anesthesia are significant respiratory depressants (14, 15), as are intravenous narcotics (15). Patients with COPD are more sensitive to inhalation agents and are at risk of developing hy-

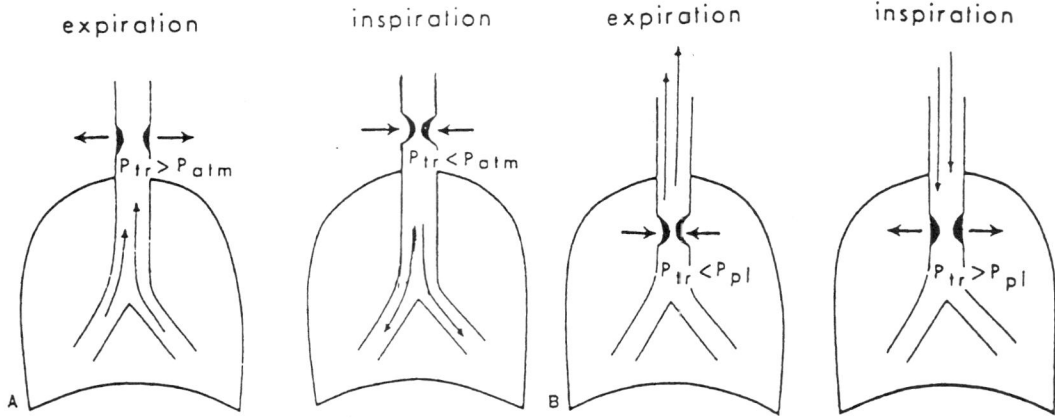

FIGURE 7.4. Intrathoracic and extrathoracic upper airway obstruction. Effects of resection.

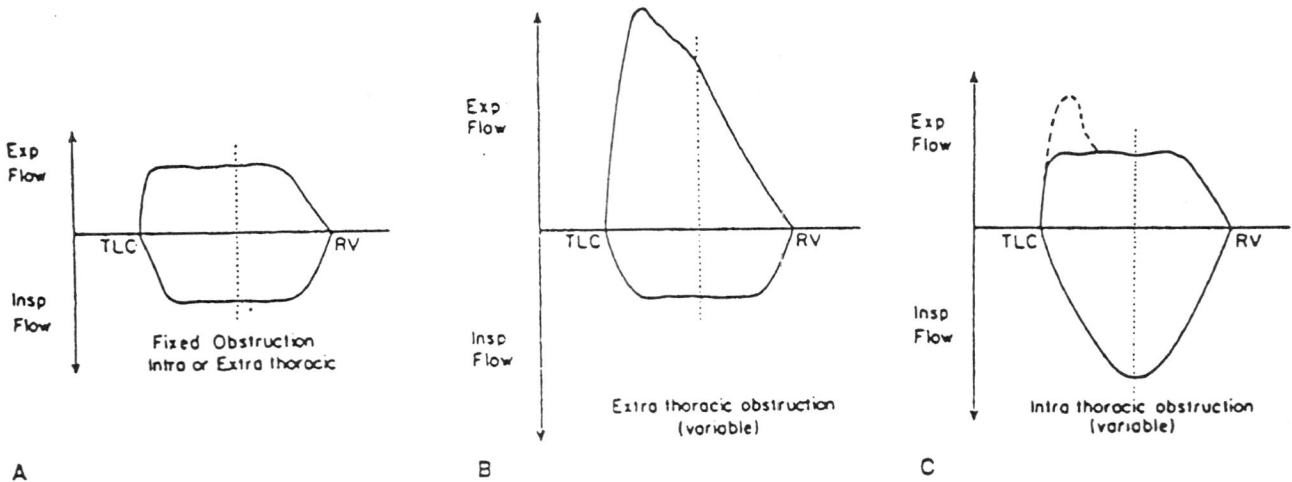

FIGURE 7.5. Flow-volume loops in upper airway obstruction.

percarbia and respiratory depression even in the postoperative period (16). General anesthesia also causes a reduction of approximately 0.5 L in the FRC (17), which is unaltered by the use of positive end-expiratory pressure (18). The reduction in FRC and the loss of diaphragm tone with induction of anesthesia promote the formation of atelectasis (19). Atelectasis contributes to postoperative arterial hypoxemia by producing areas of ventilatory-perfusion mismatch (shunt). Arterial hypoxemia also occurs because the normal vasoconstricting response to hypoxia is inhibited after general anesthesia (20). Furthermore, tracheobronchial secretions are poorly cleared in the postoperative period either because of poor mucociliary function (21) or increased viscosity (22). Coupled with increased secretions, a decreased ventilatory drive, and a reduction in lung volumes, it is clear that general anesthesia contributes to postoperative pulmonary morbidity and mortality.

SURGICAL INCISION

The alterations of pulmonary function directly related to the type of thoracic incision are difficult to separate from changes occurring because of general anesthesia. The major effects attributable to thoracic incisions are chest wall compliance and postoperative pain. After a standard posterolateral thoracotomy, chest wall compliance may be decreased by up to 75% (23), which results in a significant elevation in the work of breathing (24). A decreased compliance results in decreased total volumes as well as a reduction in the VC (25, 26). This reduction in lung volumes coupled with postoperative pain may lead to alveolar hypoventilation with respiratory acidosis and a decrease in oxygen saturation that may last up to 10 days postoperatively (27). A standard thoracotomy results in severe postoperative pain, which prevents adequate coughing, clearing of secretions, early mobilization, and patient cooperation.

Postoperative pain is a major driving force behind the body's response to surgical stress (28). The neuroendocrine response to pain promotes corticotropin release from the anterior pituitary with release of cortisol and epinephrine from the adrenal gland (29). These catabolic hormones promote insulin resistance, gluconeogenesis, and increased amino acid mobilization for wound healing (29). Aldosterone and antidiuretic hormone also are released in response to both pain and changes in serum osmolarity and tonicity. In conjunction with cortisol, these hormones promote sodium and water retention and increase the extracellular fluid compartment in the periphery of the lung and the lung itself. The increase in extracellular lung water can result in ventilation-perfusion abnormalities (29). Patients with limited cardiac reserve may be prone to heart failure because of the fluid retention as well as the increase in heart rate and myocardial contractility caused by catecholamines. The combination of increased lung water, heart failure, and postoperative pain may reduce the FRC by as much as 50% of preoperative values (30). However, there have been significant recent advances in postoperative pain management, and it now is accepted that continuous narcotic epidural analgesia is superior to intravenous narcotics both in terms of pain relief and of prevention of respiratory depression (31).

Epidural analgesia also is associated with improved postoperative pulmonary function (32), a reduction in the work of breathing (33), and a reduction in overall postoperative morbidity and mortality compared with the use of intravenous narcotics (34, 35). Modulation of the stress response may be responsible for these improved results with epidural anesthesia. Improvements in postoperative pain management also have helped to alleviate the anxiety, immobility, and sense of helplessness that often occur after a traditionally painful thoracotomy.

The changes in pulmonary function that occur after a thoracotomy not associated with a pulmonary resection usually resolve within 4 to 6 weeks (36). Some investigators have found that a muscle-sparing thoracotomy, compared with a standard thoracotomy, results in a significant reduction in postoperative pain as measured by a visual scale and by narcotic requirements in the first 24 hours postoperatively (37). However, there were no differences in postoperative spirometry values, muscle strength, and perioperative complications.

A median sternotomy has been suggested by some as an alternative to a standard thoracotomy for certain pulmonary resections because of decreased postoperative pain and improved chest wall mechanics (25). Cooper et al. (38) compared spirometric data among patients undergoing thoracotomy or sternotomy and found a significant improvement in VC and peak flows in sternotomy patients at 4 and 7 days postoperatively. Other authors have stressed that a median sternotomy results in decreased pain and shorter hospital stays, compared with thoracotomy (39, 40). Despite these advantages, the exposure from a median sternotomy makes resection of the left lower lobe, superior sulcus tumor, and posterior chest wall difficult and at times impossible. It may be a useful approach, however, in the patient with poor preoperative pulmonary function and an accessible tumor.

Thoracoscopy has been used traditionally as a diagnostic procedure, but it is rapidly becoming a frequently used therapeutic modality since the advent of video-assisted thoracic surgery (VATS). It is now possible to perform wedge resections as well as lobectomies in highly selected patients (41–44). Because it involves only two to three small (1-cm) incisions and a 6- to 8-cm access thoracotomy, it generally is thought that both postoperative pulmonary function and pain are improved after VATS, compared with thoracotomy. In a retrospective comparison of VATS and thoracotomy wedge resection, it was found that patients subjected to thoracoscopy required less postoperative analgesia (42). A nonrandomized prospective study (45) of selected patients compared thoracoscopic lung resection and standard thoracotomy; it also showed reduced postoperative pain in VATS patients in addition to significant early improvement in the FEV_1. The lung function was similar, however, at 3 weeks after surgery. Currently, there are no randomized prospective studies with large enough sample sizes that compare VATS and standard thoracotomy and, thus, the true benefit of this popular procedure in terms of postoperative pain, pulmonary function, morbidity, and mortality as well as tumor recurrence and overall long-term survival is unknown. Despite a variety of surgical approaches that can be used for pulmonary resection, a standard thoracotomy is the incision generally favored by most thoracic surgeons who treat lung cancer because of the excellent exposure it provides and the ability to sample bronchial and mediastinal lymph nodes more completely. The use of VATS in the treatment of high-risk surgical patients may be an alternative to thoracotomy and is discussed below.

EXTENT OF LUNG RESECTION

Whereas the adverse pulmonary effects of general anesthesia and the thoracic incision usually are short-lived and can be modulated to some degree, the effect of removing a portion of lung generally is permanent. The effect of lung resection on pulmonary function depends on the extent of the resection performed and the function of the area removed. For example, if a lobectomy is performed for a 4-cm lesion with obstructing pneumonitis, it can be expected that the postoperative pulmonary function will be similar to the preoperative value because the resected lobe probably did not contribute to preoperative function. Clearly, pneumonectomy causes greater changes in function than does lobectomy. In a review of 36 postpneumonectomy cases 1 year after surgery (46), it was found that the percentage of predicted value for TLC, VC, and MVV, based on two lungs, was 70%, 53%, and 47%, respectively. In a similar postpneumonectomy study (47), the TLC was 60% of predicted for two lungs, whereas the VC was 50% of predicted and the MVV was 35% to 40%. The preoperative values were not given in these studies, thus the true extent of the reduction is not known. Assuming normal preoperative predicted values, the TLC is noted to be elevated disproportionately for one lung, whereas the postoperative VC and MVV are intuitively correct. After a pneumonectomy the remaining lung hyperinflates and shifts the mediastinum in an attempt to obliterate the operated side. The TLC is relatively expanded for one lung, but this expansion occurs to the benefit of the residual volume and not of the VC. In studies in which the preoperative values are known, the TLC is reduced by 40% (48), whereas the FEV_1 is reduced by 25.8% (49). Similarly, the diffusing capacity also is reduced by approximately 40% after pneumonectomy (48). After a lobectomy the TLC is reduced by 13% (50) to 26% (48), and the VC is reduced by approximately 10% (50). Similarly, the MVV diminishes by nearly 20% (51). Segmental and wedge resections, however, are associated with minimal reduction in pulmonary function (52).

In conclusion, the effects of surgery on lung function can be profound and are multifactorial. The goal of the preoperative pulmonary assessment (see below) thus is the determination with some degree of certainty whether a patient can withstand the proposed lung resection safely without postoperative respiratory insufficiency while at the same time offering a curative procedure.

PREOPERATIVE PULMONARY ASSESSMENT

The ideal preoperative pulmonary assessment should be able to answer three questions before subjecting a patient to lung resection: (a) What is the tolerable extent of surgical resection? (b) What is the predicted perioperative morbidity and mortality? (c) What is the predicted quality of life with the remaining pulmonary function? A single preoperative pulmonary assessment cannot answer these questions, and there is a paucity of data concerning quality of life indices after pulmonary resection. Practically, the main objective of preoperative pulmonary function assessment has been to predict postoperative morbidity and mortality and to spare patients at a prohibitively high risk a needless thoracotomy. However, what constitutes prohibitively high risk is not well defined considering that lung cancer has a 100% mortality if untreated (53). Reported mortality rates after thoracotomy vary widely, ranging from 10.6% (54) to 29.6% (55) for pneumonectomy and from 1.9% (56) to 14.3% (56) for lobectomy. The largest single-institution study reported a 2% overall mortality among 961 patients undergoing lung resection (57). The Lung Cancer Study Group has reported their 30-day operative mortality in 2220 lung resections among 12 participating institutions. Overall mortality was 6.2% for pneumonectomies and 2.9% for lobectomies (58); nearly half of the deaths were caused by postoperative pulmonary complications and 17% were cardiac related. These figures may be viewed as the gold standard for perioperative mortality, considering the reputation of the institutions involved and the low death rate. However, the actual mortality after pneumonectomy in the general community may be 11.6% (59); this figure may be more reflective of the current standard of care.

A number of spirometric values have been suggested that place a patient into a high-risk group for pulmonary surgery. Most of these values are based on retrospective data, and the true mortality of these high-risk patients after surgery is not known because they often are excluded from prospective studies. A number of high-risk patients are able to undergo surgery without complications, and therefore the onus is on the physician, surgeon, and patient to decide if the risks of surgery outweigh the potential benefits. A step-wise approach to the pulmonary evaluation of the preoperative candidate places emphasis on using simple screening tests to identify high-risk patients followed by more elaborate investigations to select those patients who may benefit from surgery. This approach is supported by a number of investigators and has been reviewed previously (10, 60–64).

IDENTIFICATION OF THE HIGH-RISK PATIENT

The following tests form the cornerstone of preoperative pulmonary function assessment: spirometry and lung volumes, diffusing capacity, and arterial blood gas measurements. Specific abnormalities found in these tests can identify patients at high risk for complications after pulmonary surgery.

SPIROMETRY AND LUNG VOLUMES

Gaensler and coworkers (65) were among the first to report the use of routine spirometry in predicting mortality after thoracic surgery. They found that patients with an MVV of less than 50% of predicted, coupled with an FVC of less than 70% of predicted, had a combined early and late postoperative mortality of 50%, compared with a 5.3% mortality in patients with an MVV of more than 50% of predicted. Similarly, Mittman (66) correlated a number of spirometric and lung volume measurements with postoperative death. He supported previous data by demonstrating a 5% mortality in patients with an MVV of more than 50% and a 70% mortality in those with an MVV of less than 50% coupled with electrocardiogram (EKG) abnormalities. He also showed that an elevated RV to TLC ratio of more than 50% was associated with a mortality of 36%, versus a mortality of 12% if the ratio was less than 50%. Stein and associates (67) showed that a reduction in the FVC, FEV_1, or single-breath N2 meter test, or an increased RV to TLC ratio was associated with a postoperative respiratory complication rate of 70%, compared with a 3% complication rate if these values were normal.

Furthermore, Boushy and colleagues (68) recognized that patients over 60 years of age with an FEV_1 of less than 2 L and an FEV_1 to FVC ratio of less than 50% of predicted suffered a 40% mortality after thoracotomy and various degrees of lung resection. Lockwood (69) has tried to categorize patients, based on their lung function test results, into four risk groups. The very high risk group includes patients with the following limits: RV to TLC ratio of more than 47%; FEV_1 of less than 1.2 L or 35% of the FVC; or MVV of less than 28 L per minute. These patients would be expected to have a 1 in 1.04 risk of suffering a cardiopulmonary complication after thoracotomy.

The application of specific spirometric limits for patients undergoing pulmonary resection has been advocated by Miller and Hatcher (8). In a recent review involving 2340 patients, they demonstrated excellent clinical results by selecting patients for surgery based on the following preoperative criteria: (a) for pneumonectomy: FEV_1 of more than 2 L, $FEF_{25\%-75\%}$ of more than 1.6 L, and MVV of more than 55%; (b) for lobectomy: FEV_1 of more than 1 L, $FEF_{25\%-75\%}$ of more than 0.6 L, and MVV of more than 40%; and (c) for wedge resection: FEV_1 of more than 0.6 L, $FEF_{25\%-75\%}$ of more than 0.6 L, and MVV of more than 35%. Mortality rates for pneumonectomy were 8%; for lobectomy, 3%; and for wedge resection, 1%. This study also demonstrates that patients with relatively poor function and at high risk as defined by Lockwood (69) can tolerate minimal pulmonary resection.

There are several problems that have been noted with spirometric and lung volume data. Not all investigators have found simple spirometric pulmonary assessment predictive of postoperative morbidity and mortality after thoracic surgery (71–73). In a retrospective report of complications after pneumonectomy, Keagy et al. (73) classified patients as high risk based on an FVC of less than 70%, an FEV_1 of less than 1.5 L, and an FEV_1 to FVC ratio of less than 0.6 and found no difference in the complication rate between these patients and the low-risk group. This report has been criticized because of potential selection bias because the physicians referring the patients for surgery were not blinded (60), and those patients with the worst pulmonary function or other co-morbid disease may not have been referred for surgery. Similarly, Kearney et al. (74), in a recent prospective review of 331 patients, found that a preoperative FEV_1 of less than 1 L was not associated with increased postoperative complications, although the review of daily notes was the method used to detect complications.

These conflicting results of spirometric evaluation may be attributable to improved postoperative care over time, the retrospective nature of the studies, and the lack of uniformity in the definition of a pulmonary complication. Physicians should be cautious about refusing patients surgical therapy based solely on simple tests of pulmonary function because well-selected patients with poor pulmonary function may do well after surgery. A further complicating issue regarding spirometric data lies in the use of absolute numbers to correlate postoperative morbidity and mortality. Because the predicted spirometric values are based on sex, age, and height (75), a short elderly women and a tall young man with similar absolute spirometric values will have very different percentages of normal volumes. Some investigators therefore think that the use of "percentage of normal" would be more appropriate than absolute volumes (61, 76). Finally, prospective data exist in patients with these spirometric limits, such that the true risk of operating on these patients is unknown. Spirometric limits that suggest high risk have been obtained using retrospective studies and have not been substantiated with prospective studies, thus again the true risk of operating on these patients is unknown. However, most investigators (61–63) conclude that spirometric and lung volume data at least can identify a potentially high-risk surgical candidate who might need further evaluation.

DIFFUSION CAPACITY

The diffusing capacity (DLCO) is another simple test that can be done at the same time as the spirometric and lung volume assessment. A predicted value is calculated using alveolar ventilation, age, and sex (77). The volume of carbon monoxide that is taken up by the patient's lungs during a 10-second breath hold after a maximal inspiration of a mixture of air and carbon monoxide is recorded (64). The calculation value is a measure of the alveolar surface area, alveolar membrane integrity, and pulmonary capillary blood volume. Coleman et al. (78) demonstrated that a reduced DLCO correlated with the number of postoperative complications in patients undergoing noncancer pulmonary resection. Similarly, Markos and his associates (79) showed that a low DLCO preoperatively was a sensitive predictor of postoperative complications after lobectomy. In the most widely cited study (80), among 20 patients, a DLCO percentage predicted of not more than 60% was associated with a 25% mortality and a 45% complication rate, compared with a 4.8% mortality and a 20% morbidity in 145 patients with a DLCO of more than 60% predicted. In this study DLCO was the most sensitive indicator of mortality and the only predictor of morbidity; a significant reduction in DLCO was noted even when spirometric data were considered acceptable. Because DLCO measures both the alveolar membrane surface area and its integrity, it may be more sensitive to subtle emphysematous changes usually not detected by routine spirometry (81).

ARTERIAL BLOOD GAS

The measurement of arterial oxygen pressure (PaO_2) as well as arterial carbon dioxide pressure ($PaCO_2$) often is done before pulmonary resection, but neither PaO_2 nor $PaCO_2$ has been tested as predictors of postoperative complications. It generally is thought that preoperative hypercapnia, defined as a $PaCO_2$ of more than 45 mm Hg, is an absolute contraindication to surgery (62, 82, 83), based primarily on the observation that patients with severe COPD and hypercapnia have a shortened survival (84). However, there are no large retrospective studies and certainly no prospective data to substantiate a nonoperative approach in patients with hypercapnia. In fact, of 30 patients with a $PaCO_2$ of more than 45 mm Hg, Kearny and colleagues (74) demonstrated a respectable 13% complication rate and no mortality. Others have shown that patients with hypercapnia are likely to have severe COPD and are at risk for respiratory complications and prolonged postoperative mechanical ventilation (85).

Similarly, arterial hypoxemia, defined as a PaO_2 of less than 60 mm Hg on room air is considered by some to preclude surgery (62, 79). However, as noted previously (86), hypoxemia may develop because of right to left intrapulmonary shunting caused by an atelectatic lung in patients with cancerous lesions obstructing the airways, and this condition may be relieved once resected. No absolute blood gas value can be viewed as prohibiting surgery, thus patients with hypercapnia and hypoxemia should be considered for further evaluation.

In conclusion, these general screening tests help the clinician decide on the need for further evaluation. Guidelines based on available data, albeit imperfect, are listed in Table 7.1. These limits are not meant to replace clinical judgment in the decision-making process because it is known that some patients classified as high risk do very well postoperatively, and some patients without these risk factors die after surgery. Clearly, other factors such as advanced age (87), poor nutritional status (58, 88), borderline cardiac function

TABLE 7.1 Identification of the High-Risk Patient

Spirometry and lung volumes
 FEV_1, <2 L
 FEV_1/FVC, <50%
 $FEF_{25\%-75\%}$, <1.6 L
 MVV, <50%
 RV/TLC, >50%
Diffusion capacity
 DLCO, <60%
Arterial blood gas
 $PaCO_2$, >45 mm Hg
 PaO_2, <60 mm Hg

Abbreviations. FEV_1, forced expiratory volume in 1 second; FVC, forced vital capacity; FEF, forced expiratory flow between 25% and 75% of the FVC; MVV, maximal voluntary ventilation; RV, residual volume; TLC, total lung capacity; DLCO, diffusing capacity; $PaCO_2$, arterial carbon dioxide pressure; PaO_2, arterial oxygen pressure.

(89), and other co-morbid diseases (90) influence the postoperative course and must be included in the total preoperative evaluation of the surgical patient. These guidelines should be used to help select patients requiring more sophisticated testing. In general, patients who are not in this high-risk category should be able to tolerate a conventional thoracotomy and resection, including pneumonectomy, with acceptable mortality, i.e., less than 10%. Therefore, any lesser procedure may also proceed with an acceptable complication rate.

EVALUATION OF THE HIGH-RISK PATIENT

Once the patient has been categorized into the high-risk group, the goal of the subsequent evaluation is, first, to determine the extent of surgical resection that both cures the patient and avoids postoperative respiratory insufficiency; and, second, to determine the most appropriate surgical approach (Fig. 7.7). It is especially important that this group of high-risk patients be staged completely and accurately to minimize needless thoracotomy; this process should include mediastinal node sampling. To further define operability in this group of patients, more advanced methods of pulmonary function testing are used commonly to help the decision-making process. These include split-lung function using radionuclide lung scanning and cardiovascular exercise testing. Previously used techniques such as bronchospirometry (91), the lateral position test (92), and pulmonary artery hemodynamics (93)—tests that enabled differentiation of the function of each separate lung—are time consuming, require significant attention to detail, at times are uncomfortable, and are invasive (e.g., pulmonary artery hemodynamics). These tests have largely been replaced by the more accurate and simpler quantitative lung scan. The exercise test generally is reserved for patients who require more rigorous investigation after the quantitative lung scan has been performed.

QUANTITATIVE RADIONUCLIDE LUNG SCANNING

Quantitative radionuclide lung scanning has been developed over the last 25 years in an attempt to predict the postoperative pulmonary function of patients before surgical resection. Two scanning methods have generally been used and studied. One is a ventilation scan using ^{133}Xe radioactive gas (94), and the other is a perfusion study employing ^{99m}Tc-labeled macroaggregates (95). Both measure the percentage contribution of the nonoperated lung tissue to the total function; this value is multiplied by the preoperative spirometric measure to obtain the predicted postoperative value.

Postoperative FEV_1 = preoperative FEV_1 × the percentage of total function from the remaining lung

Kristersson and coworkers (94) first used ^{133}Xe ventilation for the quantification of differential lung function in patients prior to pneumonectomy. After ventilation with the radioactive substance, a gamma counter is used to determine the percentage of lung function contributed by the remaining lung tissue by counting the emanating radiation from the contralateral lung. The predicted postoperative FVC and FEV_1 and the true postoperative FVC and FEV_1 at 1 month and 1 year correlated well (coefficients of .73 and .63, respectively). Olsen and colleagues (95) demonstrated that ^{99m}Tc macroaggregate infusion also could be used to calculate postoperative pulmonary function, again by calculating the percentage of total radiation from the nonoperated lung. Good correlation coefficients of .705 for the FVC and .72 for the FEV_1 were found between the predicted values and those obtained at 6 weeks postoperatively (Fig. 7.6). The FVC and FEV_1 generally were predicted to be lower than the actual values, thus the authors concluded that a margin of safety existed with these predictions. A number of other investigators also have found good correlation between the predicted value and the true postoperative measure (79, 96–99); only one reported study has cast doubt on the use of quantitative lung scanning to predict postoperative function. Although some have extolled the merits of one scan over another, it appears that the accuracy of ventilation and perfusion is equivalent. Wernly and coworkers (100) analyzed both perfusion and ventilation scans in 85 patients and com-

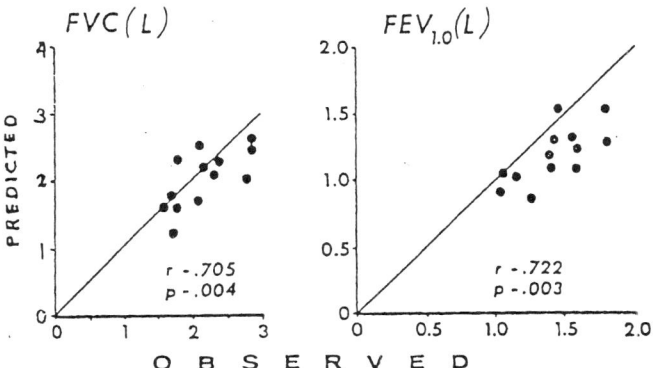

FIGURE 7.6. Quantitative perfusion scan's prediction of postoperative lung function.

FIGURE 7.7. Proposed flow sheet for preoperative assessment.

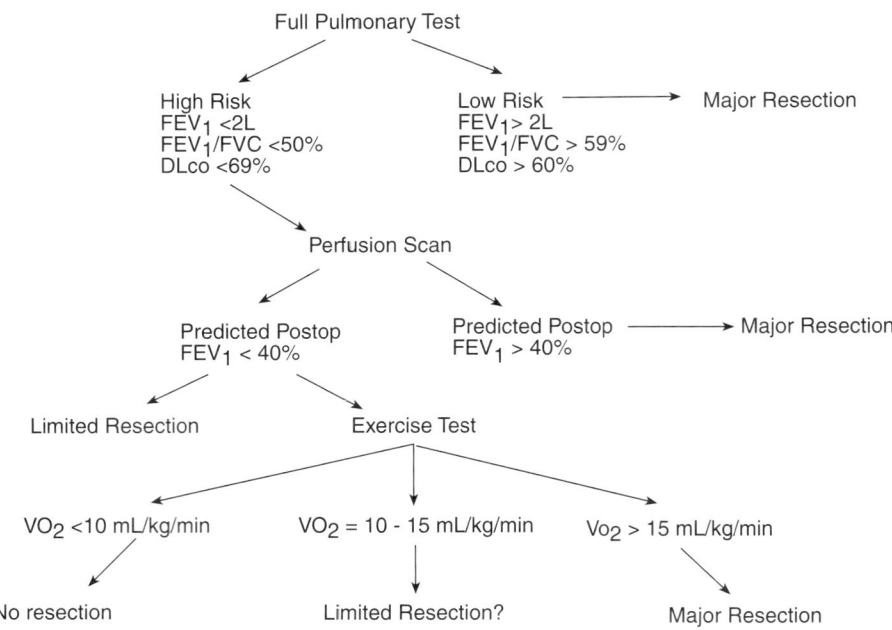

pared the predicted postoperative FEV_1 using each method to the measured postoperative FEV_1, concluding that there was no significant difference among the various techniques. Markos (79) reported similar findings and found a correlation coefficient of .91 between perfusion and ventilation scan estimates for patients subjected to pneumonectomy and a correlation of .89 for patients undergoing lobectomy.

The usefulness of quantitative radionuclide lung scanning hinges on its ability to predict the postoperative pulmonary function of a patient before the pulmonary resection. Theoretically, such information would allow the physician and surgeon to select patients considered to have adequate postoperative function, as determined by radionuclide lung scanning, for surgical resection. Alternatively, the predicted postoperative function may be considered inadequate and the proposed intervention may be altered so that, for example, a patient who may not tolerate a pneumonectomy may be offered a lobectomy or even a wedge resection if complete resection was anticipated with these lesser procedures.

The problem with these predictions is that the cutoff levels of acceptable postoperative pulmonary function are defined arbitrarily. The most frequently quoted value is that a patient must have a postoperative FEV_1 of at least 800 mL. This figure, as clearly stated by Gass and Olsen (61), is based on the personal experience of Olsen and colleagues (101) with the activity level of patients with COPD as well as on the increased finding of hypercapnia in patients with an FEV_1 of 800 mL (102). The second problem with this arbitrary value is that it does not take into account differences in sex, height, and age. Despite these shortcomings, several studies have shown the usefulness of quantitative lung scanning in selecting high-risk patients for surgery. Boysen and coworkers (103), in a prospective fashion, used the perfusion lung scan in a high-risk group of patients with an FEV_1 of less than 2 L before pneumonectomy. All patients with a predicted postoperative FEV_1 exceeding 800 mL were offered surgery. Thirty-three patients had surgery with five perioperative deaths (15%) reported, a mortality rate that was considered acceptable.

In a follow-up study, Boysen and associates (104) looked at overall long-term survival in 38 high-risk patients with an FEV_1 of less than 2 L or an MVV of less than 50% of predicted; these patients were selected for a pneumonectomy on the basis of a predicted postoperative FEV_1 of more than 800 mL as determined by perfusion scanning. The 1- and 2-year survival rates were 23 (60%) of 38 and 13 (34%) of 38, respectively. Importantly, there was only one death in the first year related to respiratory insufficiency, whereas eight patients were thought to have died of metastatic disease. Rather than use an arbitrary predicted FEV_1 limit, Markos and coworkers (79) in a prospective study using perfusion lung scanning, found that a postoperative predicted FEV_1 of 40% predicted was a good cutoff value in selecting patients for surgery. Half (3 of 6) of the patients with values below 40% died, whereas no mortality was recorded in 47 patients with a predicted postoperative FEV_1 of 40% predicted. In a recent study (74), predicted postoperative FEV_1 was the best indicator for complications after lung resection; the risk increased for each 0.2-L decrease in predicted postoperative function. The highest complication rate for both respiratory (15%) and cardiac events (19%) was in patients with a predicted postoperative FEV_1 of less than 1 L. These studies indicate that perfusion lung scanning is a reliable method for selecting high-risk patients for surgery and for predicting postoperative mortality. A predicted postoperative FEV_1 of more than 800 mL or a predicted postoperative FEV_1 of more than 40% predicted appear to be reasonable levels for recommending surgical therapy, including pneumonectomy. Patients with results below these cutoff limits should be evaluated further with an exercise test. Alternatively, the proposed extent of the surgical resection may be modified to limit the reduction in postoperative pulmonary function.

EXERCISE TEST

The exercise test has become a useful adjunct in the preoperative evaluation of the surgical patient. Whereas quantitative lung scanning provides information on regional pulmonary perfusion or ventilation, exercise testing has the potential of assessing the reserve of the oxygen transport system while under stress. Certainly, surgery is a major stress, and the appeal of exercise testing stems from the perception that adequate performance on one stress test equates with a successful outcome on another. The simplest form of exercise testing is the stair climb. In a retrospective study, it was found that patients who could climb two flights of stairs had an 11% mortality after pneumonectomy, whereas 2 of 4 patients who could not complete one flight of stairs preoperatively died (82). Other authors have tried to correlate the ability to climb steps to the results of routine pulmonary function tests (105) and postoperative complications (106). Although there was some correlation among the number of stairs climbed, parameters such as FVC and FEV_1, and complications such as prolonged intubation, both studies were inconclusive. Presently, there are no prospective studies on stair climbing, and recommendations concerning its use must await further clinical trials.

More formal exercise testing uses either a treadmill (107) or a cycle ergometer (78). A number of physiologic parameters are monitored including pulse, blood pressure, pulse oximetry, ECG, oxygen uptake (VO_2), carbon dioxide output (VCO_2), and minute ventilation (V_e). An important measure of cardiopulmonary-vascular fitness is VO_2. As the patient exercises, the increased muscle utilization of oxygen causes an increase in cardiac output, an increase in ventilation, and an increase in oxygen uptake in an effort to meet the oxygen requirements of the muscle. For example, an average-sized adult consumes 200 mL of oxygen per minute while resting but more than 1400 mL of oxygen minute during a tennis game (108). With the patient exercising on a cycle ergometer, the oxygen uptake is determined at increasing workloads. Eventually, a point is reached at which higher workloads do not result in higher oxygen consumption; this plateau is known as the VO_2max. This level is associated with maximal aerobic power, and further work induces anaerobic metabolism and an exaggerated V_e. In patients with COPD, the ventilatory reserve is not sufficient to obtain a leveling off of VO_2, thus the exercise test continues until the patient stops because of dyspnea or fatigue or the exercise is stopped because of ECG abnormalities. This oxygen uptake is more appropriately referred to as VO_2peak. The oxygen uptake is calculated and can be expressed as liters per minute or milliliters per kilogram per minute and can be correlated to the predicted value based on sex, age, and weight (109).

A number of studies have tried to correlate performance on the exercise test with postoperative outcome. In 1982, Eugene and associates (110) studied 19 patients with cycle ergometry and measured VO_2peak in all patients. They found that patients with a VO_2peak of less than 1 L/minute had a 75% mortality, whereas patients with a measured value of more than 1 L/minute survived. Smith and coworkers (111) compared routine pulmonary function tests to VO_2peak in 22 patients undergoing thoracotomy and pulmonary resection. He found that FEV_1, FVC, MVV, and DLCO were not predictive of postoperative complications; however, only 5 patients in the group would have been considered high risk according to present criteria (Table 7.1). They did find that patients with complications had significantly reduced VO_2peak levels compared with those who had no complications. Only 1 of 10 patients with a VO_2peak of more than 20 mL/kg/minute had a complication, whereas all 6 patients with a VO_2peak of less than 15 mL/kg/minute had a complication. Colman (28), however, in a prospective study of postthoracotomy complications among 59 patients, found that preoperative exercise performance as determined by VO_2peak did not predict morbidity.

Included in this study were complications such as excessive blood loss, prolonged air leak, and wound infection, which are more reflective of an error in surgical technique and thus would not be predicted by exercise testing. Bechard and Wetstein (70) used VO_2peak as an adjunct to regular spirometric testing. Fifty patients were selected for surgical resection based on strict criteria. A patient undergoing a pneumonectomy had an FEV_1 of more than 1.7 L; a lobectomy, more than 1.2 L; and a wedge resection, more than 0.9 L. Patients with a VO_2 of less than 10 mL/kg/minute had a 29% (2 of 7) mortality and a 43% (3 of 7) morbidity, whereas those with a VO_2 of more than 20 mL/kg/minute had no (0 of 15) mortality or morbidity. Patients between these values suffered no mortality (0 of 28) but had a 10.7% complication rate (3 of 28). This study suggests that adherence to strict guidelines for pulmonary resection yields acceptable overall morbidity and mortality but that exercise testing is a useful tool to further stratify patients into high-risk groups, especially those with VO_2 of less than 10 mL/kg/minute.

Morice and associates (7) extended the use of exercise testing specifically to the evaluation of the patient who is considered inoperable by routine pulmonary function testing. Patients were considered inoperable if they had an FEV_1 of less than 40% predicted, a predicted postoperative FEV_1 of less than 33% predicted, or an arterial PCO_2 of less than 45 mm Hg. Patients with an exercise test showing a VO_2peak of more than 15 mL/kg/minute were offered surgery. Among 8 patients, only 2 had complications after surgery, and there were no deaths. In a similar study involving a larger cohort of patients, Walsh and coworkers (13) found identical results. Using the same criteria for inoperability as described by Morice et al. (7), 69 high-risk patients with resectable lesions had exercise testing. Patients were offered surgery if their VO_2 level was more than 15 mL/kg/minute, and the rest were referred for radiation, chemotherapy, both treatments, or observation. Of 21 patients with resections, there were no deaths and only 5 minor complications. The median survival of the surgical group was 48 months, whereas the median survival of the nonoperative group was only 15 months. This study suggests that by using specific exercise testing criteria, even patients deemed inoperable by standard pulmonary function testing can have aggressive surgical therapy with a good outcome.

Whether exercise testing represents a cost-effective modality for assessing operative risk is unknown and depends on the indication for which it is being used. As previously noted, some investigators (71–74) have concluded that spirometry does not predict postoperative complications adequately and thus is not helpful in identifying the high-risk patient. There is controversy on this point, but it would be foolhardy to suggest that all patients regardless of pulmonary function be evaluated with an exercise test. This test is costly, requires a high level of technical expertise, and would not be reasonable to use indiscriminately because the vast majority of patients with adequate preoperative pulmonary function have a benign postoperative course. Exactly which patients will benefit from preoperative exercise testing and exactly what cutoff level of VO_2max should be applied is not known. These authors think that the previously presented data suggest that spirometry, blood gas, and diffusion capacity tests identify a high-risk patient. Further testing with a perfusion scan will predict postoperative function, and, if adequate, surgery should proceed. Exercise testing should be done in high-risk patients whose predicted postoperative function is deemed inadequate. Only further studies will substantiate this approach.

RADIATION THERAPY AND LUNG FUNCTION

Thoracic irradiation of the patient with lung cancer has been used in a wide variety of clinical settings. Most commonly, radiation therapy is given for the palliation of local symptoms such as chest wall pain, obstructive atelectasis, hemoptysis, or superior vena cava syndrome (112, 113). This form of therapy also has been used as a mode of primary therapy with curative intent for the elderly, those refusing surgery, or those too ill to undergo surgical resection (114–121). It has been used preoperatively (122–126), postoperatively in an attempt to improve cure rates and for local control in patients with regional and nodal metastases (127–139), and as an adjuvant to surgery and/or chemotherapy in several protocols (135, 140–147).

Lung parenchyma is quite sensitive to the effects of irradiation. An early pneumonic phase, occurring 1 to 3 months after the completion of radiation therapy, may be asymptomatic or clinically may mimic acute or subacute pneumonia (148). It may be followed by a progressive fibrotic process that can evolve over 1 or 2 years (149). Symptomatic and functional consequences of these effects can be anticipated. However, there are a number of determinants of the severity of these reactions.

The risk of developing lung injury from radiation is proportional to the total dose of irradiation (150).

Only 5% of patients developed radiation pneumonitis after 2650 cGy delivered to the entire lung volume (in 20 fractions over 4 weeks), whereas 50% developed radiation pneumonitis when 3050 cGy was delivered to the same volume of lung with the same fractionation schedule (148). Doses in excess of 6000 cGy invariably led to severe radiation pneumonitis (151).

The volume of lung irradiated also is very important in determining the extent of lung injury. A dose of irradiation given to only 25% of the total lung volume may not cause any symptoms, but the same dose delivered to the entire volume of both lungs would probably be fatal (152).

Fractionation of the delivered dose allows repair of sublethal damage to normal tissue; malignant tissue retains its sensitivity to the effects of irradiation. A higher dose of radiation can thus be delivered to the tumor with a lessening of effect on normal tissue (153). A variety of radiation schemes have been used to take advantage of this phenomenon (139, 154, 155). Regardless of the dosing schedule, the dose-response curve remains very steep (156); the position of the curve may be altered by changes in dose fractionation.

A number of other circumstances may augment the risk of developing radiation pneumonitis. Treatment of a previously irradiated area triples the risk of developing radiation pneumonitis (148). Atelectatic lung is said to be more prone to radiation effects, but this observation is disputed by some investigators (157). Rapid withdrawal of systemic corticosteroids begun before or during irradiation can precipitate symptomatic radiation pneumonitis (158). As discussed below, concomitant administration of a number of chemotherapeutic agents can augment the risk of radiation damage to the lung (159).

In patients with compromised lung function, the same caution taken when considering surgery must apply to the consideration of any radiation therapy strategy. At one extreme, irradiation of the entire lung can lead to the functional equivalent of a pneumonectomy. Rarely, lung tissue outside of the radiation field can be involved with radiation pneumonitis (160), perhaps because of the triggering of a hypersensitivity response (161). In general terms, the functional changes seen are restrictive. There is a loss of lung volume and a reduction in the diffusing capacity (162–164). The magnitude of these changes parallels the extent of damage to the lung. Under other circumstances, radiation therapy might improve lung function, e.g., when leading to establishment of bronchial patency, and thereby relieving atelectasis (163, 165). In a group of 19 patients with severe airflow obstruction (FEV_1, 37% predicted) reported by Choi (135), high-dose radiation therapy given directly to a parenchymal mass was well tolerated; only two patients had a decrease of lung function of more than 10%. Thus, with careful attention to dose, volume treated, fractionation, and the particular situation of the individual patient, radiation therapy can safely be given to patients, including those with severe compromise of lung function.

EFFECTS OF CHEMOTHERAPY ON LUNG FUNCTION

Many of the drugs used in the chemotherapy of lung cancer can affect the lungs adversely. Some of these agents also enhance the toxicity of radiation therapy. These reactions are important. In their own right, they can be a cause of substantial morbidity and even mortality (179). Toxicity of drugs in the lung also must be distinguished from progression of tumor, opportunistic infection, alveolar hemorrhage, pulmonary thromboembolism, congestive heart failure, and radiation-induced changes (202). With few exceptions, the pretreatment condition of the patient does not influence the risk of pulmonary drug toxicity (200). However, poor performance status influences survival independent of therapy (170) and appears to influence the probability of response to therapy (204). Therefore, patients with debilitating impairment of lung function because of underlying obstructive lung disease may not be good candidates for protocols that include chemotherapy in the setting of non–small cell carcinoma. In this setting, aggressive protocols for the treatment of small cell carcinoma probably should be avoided.

The most common lung injury response to chemotherapeutic agents is the development of interstitial pneumonitis and fibrosis. Table 7.2 lists agents that have been reported to affect this response; agents

TABLE 7.2 Chemotherapeutic Drugs Causing Interstitial Fibrosis

DRUG	REFERENCE NO.
Bleomycin	171
Mitomycin C	175, 194
Busulfan	182
Cyclophosphamide	169, 185, 195, 196
Chlorambucil	186
Melphalan	187
Nitrosoureas	175, 188
Methotrexate	190, 195, 196
Azathioprine	192
Vinblastine (in combination with mitomycin C)	193, 194

used in the treatment of non–small cell and small cell lung cancers have been highlighted in this and all other tables. Patients present with subacute to insidious onset of shortness of breath on exertion. Dry cough is common, and fever may be present (175, 177, 202). Tachypnea may be notable, and inspiratory crackles can be auscultated. Radiologically, diffuse reticulo-nodular interstitial lung disease is present (176, 202). Associated air-space disease is sometimes seen (180). On occasion, particularly when bleomycin is used, lung nodules imitating metastatic disease can be a manifestation of lung toxicity (202). Lung function testing reveals a restrictive process, with loss of lung volume, preservation of flow rates, and a low diffusing capacity. Hypoxemia accompanies these changes (178, 175).

Fever, breathlessness, and dry cough of subacute to acute onset characterize the clinical presentation of hypersensitivity pneumonitis. Eosinophilic infiltrates and granuloma formation are seen pathologically, and peripheral eosinophilia may be present (175). The radiologic and functional consequences of this type of drug reaction are similar to those of interstitial pneumonitis and fibrosis, but the clinical features of hypersensitivity pneumonitis make this more likely to be confused with opportunistic infection. Table 7.3 lists agents that have caused this type of lung reaction.

Rarely, some agents have caused the acute onset of noncardiogenic pulmonary edema. Table 7.4 lists these drugs. This disastrous response to lung injury has occurred in direct relation to administration of the drugs or even 3 to 4 weeks after drug administration (175). Fever is not seen, and patients have the abrupt onset of breathlessness. Diffuse air-space disease is noted radiologically, and hypoxemia is prominent

TABLE 7.3 Chemotherapeutic Drugs Causing Acute Pneumonitis

DRUG	REFERENCE NO.
Bleomycin	172, 173
Methotrexate	191, 195, 196
Procarbazine	189, 196

TABLE 7.4 Chemotherapeutic Drugs Causing Acute Pulmonary Edema

DRUG	REFERENCE NO.
Cyclophosphamide	169, 183, 195, 196
Cytosine arabinoside	199
Methotrexate	195, 196
Mitomycin C	180
Interleukin-2	203

TABLE 7.5 Chemotherapeutic Drugs Enhancing Radiation Toxicity in the Lung

DRUG	REFERENCE NO.
Adriamycin	167, 195, 196
Bleomycin	174, 175
Cisplatin	125, 140, 168, 194, 201
5-Fluorouracil	198
Methotrexate	195, 196
Cyclophosphamide	169, 184, 195, 196
Vincristine	197

(174). The diagnosis is one of exclusion; other causes of both cardiac (fluid overload, ischemia, cardiac drug toxicity) and noncardiogenic (adult respiratory distress syndrome with sepsis) pulmonary edema must be excluded.

The administration of vinca alkaloids with mitomycin C has been associated with the development of asthma (205). In this situation, lung function changes would be obstructive in nature with a reduction of the FEV_1 and a reduction in the FEV_1 to FVC ratio.

The enhanced toxicity of irradiation has been attributed to a number of chemotherapeutic agents. Table 7.5 lists such agents. Protocol design must take into account these important interactions, because radiation pneumonitis has been fatal in these circumstances (179).

References

1. Key M. What it is like to lose a lung? BMJ 1985;290:142–143.
2. Boring CC, Squires TS, Tong T, Montgomery S. Cancer statistics, 1994. CA Cancer J Clin 1994;44:7–26.
3. Graves EJ. 1989 Summary: National Hospital Discharge Survey. CDC Advance Data 1991;199(6):1–8.
4. Martini N, Kris MG, Flehinger BJ, et al. Preoperative chemotherapy for stage IIIa (N2) lung cancer: the Sloan-Kettering experience with 136 patients. Ann Thorac Surg 1993;55:1365–1374.
5. Rusch VW, Albain KS, Crowly JJ, et al. Surgical resection of stage IIIa and IIIb nonsmall cell lung cancer after concurrent induction chemoradiotherapy: a Southwest Oncology Group trial. J Thorac Cardiovasc Surg 1993;105:97–106.
6. Rosell R, Gomez-Codina J, Camps C, et al. A randomized trial comparing preoperative chemotherapy plus surgery with surgery alone in patients with non–small cell lung cancer. N Engl J Med 1994;330:153–158.
7. Morice RC, Peters EJ, Ryan BM, Putman JB, Ali MK, Roth JA. Exercise testing in the evaluation of patients at high risk for complications from lung resection. Chest 1992;101:356–361.
8. Miller JI, Hatcher CR. Limited resection of bronchogenic carcinoma in the patient with marked impairment of pulmonary function. Ann Thorac Surg 1987;44:340–343.
9. Lange P, Nyboe J, Appleyard M, et al. Ventilatory function and chronic mucus hypersecretion as predictors of death from lung cancer. Am Rev Respir Dis 1990;141:613–617.

10. Position Paper of the American College of Physicians. Preoperative pulmonary function testing. Ann Intern Med 1990;112:793–794.
11. Aldrich T, Arora N, Rocheseter D. The influence of airway obstruction and respiratory muscle strength on maximal voluntary ventilation in lung disease. Am Rev Respir Dis 1982;126:195.
12. Lavelle T, Rotman H, Weg J. Isoflow-volume curves in the diagnosis of upper airway obstruction. Am Rev Respir Dis 1978;117:845.
13. Walsh GL, Morice RC, Putman JB, Nesbitt JC, McMurtrey MJ, Ryan BM, et al. An aggressive surgical approach is justified in high-risk patients with lung cancer identified by exercise oxygen consumption testing. Ann Thorac Surg 1994; in press.
14. Knill RL, Kieraszewicz HT, Dodgson BG, et al. Chemical regulation of ventilation during isoflurane sedation and anesthesia in humans. Can Anesth Soc J 1983;30:607–614.
15. Knill RL. Control of breathing: effects of analgesic, anesthetic and neuromuscular blocking drugs. Can Anesth Soc J 1988;35:S4–S8.
16. Pietak S, Weenig CS, Hickey RF, et al. Anesthetic effects on ventilation in patients with chronic obstructive pulmonary disease. Anesthesia 1975;42:160–166.
17. Hedenstierna G, Strandberg A, Brismar B, et al. Functional residual capacity, thoracoabdominal dimensions, and central blood volume during general anesthesia with muscle paralysis and mechanical ventilation. Anesthesia 1985;62:247–254.
18. Froese AB, Bryan AC. Effects of anesthesia and paralysis on diaphragmatic mechanics in man. Anesthesia 1974;41:242–255.
19. Hedenstierna G. New aspects on atelectasis formation and gas exchange impairment during anesthesia. Clin Physiol 1989;9:407–417.
20. Marshall C, Lindgren L, Marshall BE. Effects of halothane, enflurane, and isoflurane on hypoxic pulmonary vasoconstriction in rat lungs in vitro. Anesthesia 1984;60:304–308.
21. Lichtiger M, Landa JF, Hirsch JA. Velocity of tracheal mucus in anesthetized women undergoing gynecologic surgery. Anesthesia 1975;42:753–756.
22. Pizov R, Takahashi M, et al. Halothane inhibition of ion transport of the tracheal epithelium. Anesthesia 1992;76:985–989.
23. Ellison RG, Hall DP, Talley RE, et al. Analysis of ventilatory and respiratory function after 82 thoracic and non-thoracic operations. Am Surg 1960;26:485–491.
24. Peters RM, Wellons HA, Htwe TM. Total compliance and work of breathing after thoracotomy. J Thorac Cardiovasc Surg 1969;57:348–355.
25. Steed WW. Physiologic studies following thoracic surgery I: Immediate effects of thoracoplasty. J Thorac Surg 1952;23:453–464.
26. Smith TC, Cook FD, Dekornfeld TJ, et al. Pulmonary function in the immediate postoperative period. J Thorac Cardiovasc Surg 1960;39:788.
27. Siebecker KL, Sadler PE, Mendenhall JT. Postoperative ear oximeter studies on patients who have undergone pulmonary resection. J Thorac Surg 1958;36:88–91.
28. Kehlet H. Modification of responses to surgery and anesthesia by neural blockade. In: Cousins MJ, Bridenbough PO, eds. Neural blockade in clinical anesthesia and management of pain. Philadelphia: JB Lippincott, 1987:145.
29. Wilmore DW. Homeostasis, bodily changes in trauma and surgery. In: Sabiston DC, ed. The biological basis of modern surgical practice. Philadelphia: WB Saunders, 1991:19.
30. Spence AA. Pulmonary changes after surgery. Reg Anesth 1982;7(Suppl):S119–S121.
31. Logas WG, El-Baz N, El-Ganzouri A, et al. Continuous thoracic epidural analgesia for postoperative pain relief following thoracotomy: a randomized prospective study. Anesthesia 1984;67:787–791.
32. Shulman MS, Sandler AN, Bradley JW, et al. Postthoracotomy pain and pulmonary function following epidural and systemic morphine. Anesthesia 1984;61:564–575.
33. Sabanathan S, Bickford Smith PJ, Pradhan GN, et al. Continuous intercostal nerve block for pain relief after thoracotomy. Ann Thorac Surg 1988;46:425–426.
34. Yeager MP, Glass DD, Neff RK, et al. Epidural anesthesia and analgesia in high-risk surgical patients. Anesth 1987;66:726–736.
35. Tuman KJ, McCarthy RJ, March R, et al. Effects of epidural anesthesia and analgesia on coagulation and outcome after major vascular surgery. Anesth Analg 1991;66:696–704.
36. Gorlin R, Knowles JH, Storey CF. Effects of thoracotomy on pulmonary function. Patients with localized pulmonary disease. J Thorac Surg 1957;34:242–249.
37. Hazelrigg SR, Landreneau RJ, Boley TM, et al. The effect of muscle-sparing versus standard posterolateral thoracotomy on pulmonary function, muscle strength, and postoperative pain. J Thorac Cardiovasc Surg 1991;101:394–401.
38. Cooper JD, Nelems JM, Pearson FG. Extended indications for median sternotomy in patients requiring pulmonary resection. Ann Thorac Surg 1978;26:413–420.
39. Asaph JW, Keppel JF. Midline sternotomy as a standard treatment of primary pulmonary neoplasms. Am J Surg 1984;147:589–592.
40. Meng RL, Jensik RJ, Kittle F, et al. Median sternotomy for synchronous bilateral pulmonary operations. J Thorac Cardiovasc Surg 1980;80:1–7.
41. Kirby TJ, Mack MJ, Landreneau RJ, Rice TW. Initial experience with video-assisted thoracoscopic lobectomy. Ann Thorac Surg 1993;56:1239–1247.
42. Allen MS, Deschamps C, Lee RE, Trastek VF, Daly RC, Pairolero PC. Video-assisted thoracoscopic stapled wedge excision for indeterminate pulmonary nodules. J Thorac Cardiovasc Surg 1993;106:1048–1052.
43. Walker WS, Carnochan FM, Pugh GC. Thoracoscopic pulmonary lobectomy: early operative experience and preliminary clinical results. J Thorac Cardiovasc Surg 1993;106:1111–1117.
44. Shennib HA, Landreneau R, Mulder DS, Mack M. Video-assisted thoracoscopic wedge resection of T1 lung cancer in high-risk patients. Ann Surg 1993;218:555–560.
45. Landreneau RJ, Hazelrigg SR, Mack MJ, et al. Postoperative pain-related morbidity: video-assisted thoracic surgery versus thoracotomy. Ann Thorac Surg 1993;56:1285–1289.
46. Burrows B, Harrison RW, Adams WE, Humphreys RW, Long ET, Reimann AF. The postpneumonectomy state. Clinical and physiologic observations in thirty-six cases. Am J Med 1960;28:281–297.
47. Jones JC, Robinson JL, Meyer BW, Motley HL. Primary carcinoma of the lung: a follow-up study including pulmonary function studies of long-term survivors. J Thorac Cardiovasc Surg 1960;39:144–158.
48. Dietker F, Lister W, Burrows B. The effects of thoracic surgery on the pulmonary diffusing capacity. Am Rev Respir Dis 1960;81:830–838.

49. Legge JS, Palmer KNV. Effect of lung resection for bronchial carcinoma on pulmonary function in patients with and without chronic obstructive bronchitis. Thorax 1975;30:563–565.
50. Berend N, Woolcock AJ, Marlin GA. Effects of lobectomy on lung function. Thorax 1980;35:145–150.
51. Nikly J, Villemin J. Capacite vitale et volume expiratoire maximal/second avant et apres exerese pour tuberculose pulmonaire. Bull Soc Med Passy 1960;26:31–51.
52. Miller RD, Bridge EV, Fowler WS, et al. Pulmonary function before and after pulmonary resection in tuberculous patients. J Thoracic Surg 1958;35:651–661.
53. Gass GD, Olsen GN. Preoperative pulmonary function testing to predict postoperative morbidity and mortality. Chest 1986;89:127–135.
54. Cook JW, Robicsek F, Daugherty HK, Selle JG, Sanger PW, Scott WP. The late results of surgical treatment of lung cancer. N C Med J 1978;39:541–544.
55. Hepper NG, Bernatz PE. Thoracic surgery in the aged. Chest 1960;37:298–303.
56. Vincent RG, Takita H, Lane WW, Gutierrez AC, Pickren JW. Surgical therapy of lung cancer. J Thorac Cardiovasc Surg 1976;71:581–591.
57. Nagasaki F, Flehinger BJ, Marini N. Complications of surgery in the treatment of carcinoma of the lung. Chest 1982;82:25–29.
58. Ginsberg RJ, Hill LD, Eagan RT, et al. Modern thirty-day operative mortality for surgical resections in lung cancer. J Thorac Cardiovasc Surg 1983;86:654–658.
59. Romano PS, Mark DH. Patient and hospital characteristics related to in-hospital mortality after lung cancer resection. Chest 1992;101:1332–1337.
60. Marshall CM, Olsen GN. The physiologic evaluation of the lung resection candidate. In: Olsen GN, ed. Clinics in chest medicine. Philadelphia: WB Saunders, 1993:305–320.
61. Gass DG, Olsen GN. Preoperative pulmonary function testing to predict postoperative morbidity and mortality. Chest 1986;89:127–135.
62. Tisi GM. Preoperative evaluation of pulmonary function. Am Rev Respir Dis 1979;119:293–310.
63. Reilly JJ, Mentzer SJ, Sugarbaker DJ. Preoperative assessment of patients undergoing pulmonary resection. Chest 1993;103:342S–345S.
64. Crapo RO, Morris AH. Standardized single breath normal values for carbon monoxide diffusing capacity. Am Rev Respir Dis 1981;123:185–189.
65. Gaensler EA, Cugell DW, Lindgren I, Verstraeten JM, Smith SS, Strieder JW. The role of pulmonary insufficiency in mortality and invalidism following surgery for pulmonary tuberculosis. J Thorac Surg 1955;29:163–187.
66. Mittman M. Assessment of operative risk in thoracic surgery. Am Rev Respir Dis 1961;84:197–207.
67. Stein M, Koota GM, Simon M, Frank HA. Pulmonary evaluation of surgical patients. JAMA 1962;181:765–770.
68. Boushy SF, Billig DM, North LB, et al. Clinical course related to preoperative and postoperative pulmonary function in patients with bronchogenic carcinoma. Chest 1971;59:383–391.
69. Lockwood P. Lung function test results and the risk of postthoracotomy complications. Respiration 1973;30:529–542.
70. Bechard D, Wetstein L. Assessment of exercise oxygen consumption as a preoperative criterion for lung resection. Ann Thorac Surg 1987;44:344–349.
71. Reichel J. Assessment of operative risk of pneumonectomy. Chest 1972;62:570–576.
72. Didolkar MS, Moore RH, Takita H. Evaluation of the risk of pulmonary resection for bronchogenic carcinoma. Am J Surg 1974;127:700–703.
73. Keagy BA, Schorlemmer GR, Murray GF, Starek PJK, Wilcox BR. Correlation of preoperative pulmonary function testing with clinical course in patients after pneumonectomy. Ann Thorac Surg 1983;36:253–257.
74. Kearney DJ, Lee TH, Reilly JJ, DeCamp M, Sugarbaker DJ. Assessment of operative risk in patients undergoing lung resection (importance of predicted pulmonary function). Chest 1994;105:753–759.
75. Morris JF, Koski A, Johnson LC. Spirometric standards for nonsmoking healthy adults. Am Rev Respir Dis 1971;103:57–67.
76. Deslauriers J. In: Miller JI. Physiologic evaluation of pulmonary function in the candidate for lung resection (discussion). J Thorac Cardiovasc Surg 1993;105:347–352.
77. Gaensler EA, Wright GW. Evaluation of respiratory impairment. Arch Environ Health 1966;12:146–189.
78. Coleman NC, Schraufnagel DE, Rivington RN, Pardy RL. Exercise testing in evaluation of patients for lung resection. Am Rev Respir Dis 1982;125:604–606.
79. Markos J, Mullan BP, Hilman DR, Musk AW, Antico VF, Lovegrove FT, Carter MJ, Finucane KE. Preoperative assessment as a predictor of mortality and morbidity after lung resection. Am Rev Respir Dis 1989;139:902–910.
80. Ferguson MK, Little L, Rizzo L, Popovich KJ, Glonek GF, Leff A, et al. Diffusing capacity predicts morbidity and mortality after pulmonary resection. J Thorac Cardiovasc Surg 1988;96:894–900.
81. Gleb AF, Gold WM, Bruch HR, Nadel JA. Physiologic diagnosis of subclinical emphysema. Am Rev Respir Dis 1973;107:50–63.
82. Van Nostrand D, Kjesberg MO, Humphry EW. Pre-resectional evaluation of risk from pneumonectomy. Surg Gynecol Obstet 1968;127:306.
83. Shields TW. Carcinoma of the lung. In: Shields TW, ed. General thoracic surgery. Philadelphia: Lea & Febiger, 1984:919–926.
84. Traver GA, Cline MG, Burrows B. Predictors of mortality in chronic obstructive pulmonary disease. Am Rev Respir Dis 1979;119:895–902.
85. Milledge I, Nunn JF. Criteria of fitness for anesthesia in patients with chronic obstructive lung disease. BMJ 1975;3:670–673.
86. Dunn WF, Scanlon PD. Preoperative pulmonary function testing for patients with lung cancer. Mayo Clin Proc 1993;68:371–377.
87. Cole WH. Medical differences between the young and the aged. J Am Geriatr Soc 1970;18:589–614.
88. Harvey KB, Ruggiero CS, Regan JA, et al. Hospital morbidity-mortality risk factors using nutritional assessment. Clin Res 1978;26:581A.
89. Goldman L, Caldera DL, Nussbaum SR, et al. Multifactorial index of cardiac risk in noncardiac surgical procedures. N Engl J Med 1977;297:845–850.
90. Owens WD, Felts JA, Spritnaqgel EL Jr. ASA physical status classification: a study of consistency of ratings. Anesthesiology 1978;49:239–243.
91. Neuhaus H, Cherniack NS. A bronchospirometric method of estimating the effect of pneumonectomy on the maximum breathing capacity. J Thorac Cardiovascular Surg 1968;55:144–148.

92. Bergan F. A simple method for determinations of the relative functions of the right and left lung. Acta Chir Scand 1960;253:58–63.
93. Carlens E, Hanson HE, Nordenstrom B. Temporary unilateral occlusion of the pulmonary artery. J Thorac Surg 1951;22:527–536.
94. Kristersson S, Lindell S, Strandberg L. Prediction of pulmonary function loss due to pneumonectomy using ^{133}Xe-radiospirometry. Chest 1972;62:696–698.
95. Olsen GN, Block AJ, Tobias JA. Prediction of post-pneumonectomy pulmonary function using quantitative macroaggregate lung scanning. Chest 1974;66:13–16.
96. Demeester TR, Van Heertum RL, Karas JR, et al. Preoperative evaluation with differential pulmonary function. Ann Thorac Surg 1974;18:61–71.
97. Ali MK, Mountain C, Miller JM, et al. Regional pulmonary function before and after pneumonectomy using xenon. Chest 1975;68:288–296.
98. Corris PA, Ellis DA, Hawking T. et al. Use of radionuclide scanning in the preoperative estimation of pulmonary function after pneumonectomy. Thorax 1987;42:285–291.
99. Gass GD, Olsen GN. Preoperative pulmonary function testing to predict postoperative morbidity and mortality. Chest 1986;89:127–135.
100. Wernly JA, Demeester TR, Kirchner PT, Myerowitz PD, Oxford DE, Golomb HM. Clinical value of quantitative ventilation-perfusion lung scans in the surgical management of bronchogenic carcinoma. J Thorac Cardiovasc Surg 1980;80:535–543.
101. Olsen GN, Block AJ, Swenson EW, Castle JR, Wynne JW. Pulmonary function evaluation of the lung resection candidate: a prospective study. Am Rev Respir Dis 1975;111:379–387.
102. Segall JJ, Butterworth BA. Ventilatory capacity in chronic bronchitis in relation to carbon dioxide reduction. Scand J Respir Dis 1966;47:215–224.
103. Boysen PG, Block JA, Olsen GN, Moulder PV, Harris JO, Rawitscher RE. Prospective evaluation for pneumonectomy using the ^{99m}Technetium quantitative perfusion scan. Chest 1977;72:422–425.
104. Boysen PG, Harris JO, Block AJ, Olsen GN. Prospective evaluation for pneumonectomy using perfusion scanning. Chest 1981;80:163–166.
105. Bolton JWR, Weiman DS, Haynes JL, et al. Stair climbing as an indicator of pulmonary function. Chest 1987;92:783–787.
106. Olsen GN, Bolton JWR, Weiman DS, et al. Stair climbing as an exercise test to predict the postoperative complications of lung resection. Chest 1991;99:587–590.
107. Reichel J. Assessment of operative risk of pneumonectomy. Chest 1972;62:570–576.
108. Gordon EE. Energy costs of activities in health and disease. Arch Intern Med 1958;101:702–713.
109. Jones NL, Makrides L, Hitchcock C, et al. Normal standards for an incremental progressive cycle ergometer test. Am Rev Respir Dis 1985;131:700–708.
110. Eugene J, Brown SE, Light RW, et al. Maxium oxygen consumption: a physiologic guide to pulmonary resection. Surg Forum 1982;33:260–262.
111. Smith TP, Kinasewitz GT, Tucker WY, Spillers WP, George R. Exercise capacity as a predictor of post-thoracotomy morbidity. Am Rev Respir Dis 1984;129:730–734.
112. Israel L, Bonnadonna G, Sylvester R, et al. Lung cancer: progress in therapeutic research. Controlled study with adjuvant radiotherapy in operable squamous cell carcinoma of the lung. In: Muggia, Rosensweig, eds. New York: Raven Press, 1979:443–452.
113. Cox JD, Komaki R, Byhardt RW. Is immediate chest radiotherapy obligatory for any or all patients with limited-stage non–small cell cancer of the lung? Cancer Treat Rep 1983;67:327–330.
114. Phillips TL, Miller TJ. Should asymptomatic patients with inoperable bronchogenic carcinoma receive immediate radiotherapy? Am Rev Respir Dis 1978;117:405–410.
115. Shields TM. Preoperative radiation therapy in the treatment of bronchial carcinoma. Cancer 1972;30:1388–1394.
116. Patterson R, Russell MH. Clinical trials in malignant disease: IV. Lung cancer. Value of postoperative radiotherapy. Clin Radiol 1962;13:141–144.
117. van Houtte P, Rocmans P, Smets P, et al. Postoperative radiation therapy in lung cancer: a controlled trial after resection of curative design. Int J Radiat Oncol Biol Phys 1980:983–986.
118. Perez CA, Stanley K, Grundy G, et al. Impact of irradiation technique and tumor extent in tumor control and survival of patients with unresectable non–oat cell carcinoma of the lung. Cancer 1982;50:1091–1099.
119. Komaki R, Cox JD, Hartz AJ, et al. Characteristics of long-term survivors after treatment for inoperable carcinoma of the lung. Am J Clin Oncol 1985;8:362–370.
120. Holsti LR, Mattson K. A randomized study of split-course radiotherapy of lung cancer: long term results. Int J Radiat Oncol Biol Phys 1980;6:977–981.
121. Lee RE, Carr DT, Childs DS. Comparison of split-course radiation therapy and continuous radiation therapy for unresectable bronchogenic carcinoma: 5 year results. AJR Am J Roentgenol 1976;126:116–122.
122. Cox JD, Azarnia N, Byhardt RW, et al. A randomized phase I/II trial of hyperfractionated radiation therapy in patients with stage III non–small cell lung carcinoma: report of Radiation Therapy Oncology Group 83-11. J Clin Oncol 1990;8:1543–1555.
123. Saunders MI, Dische S. Continuous hyperfractionated, accelerated radiotherapy (CHART) in non–small cell carcinoma of the bronchus. Int J Radiat Oncol Biol Phys 1990;19:1211–1215.
124. Armstrong BA, Perez CA, Simpson JR, et al. Role of irradiation in the management of superior vena cava syndrome. Int J Radiat Oncol Biol Phys 1987;13:531–539.
125. Murren JR, Buzaid AC. Chemotherapy and radiation for the treatment of non–small cell cancer: a critical review. Clin Chest Med 1993;14:161.
126. Noordijk EM, Poest Clement EVD, Hermans J, et al. Radiotherapy as an alternative to surgery in elderly patients with resectable lung cancer. Radiother Oncol 1988;13:83–89.
127. Plowman PN, EmElwain TJ, Meadows AT. Complications of cancer management. Butterworth Heinemann, 1991:232–249.
128. Gross NJ. Pulmonary Effects of Radiation Therapy. Ann Intern Med 1977;86:81–92.
129. Fanta CH. Respiratory complications. In: Holland JF, Frei E, Bast RC, Kufe DW, Morton DL, Weichselbaum RR, eds. Cancer medicine. 3rd ed. Philadelphia: Lea & Febiger, 1993:2349–2358.
130. Fraser RG, Pare JAP, Pare PD, Fraser RS, Genereux eds. Diagnosis of diseases of the chest. 3rd ed. Philadelphia: WB Saunders, 1991:2480–2571.
131. Komaki R. Preoperative and postoperative irradiation for cancer of the lung. J Belge Radiol 1985;68:195–198.
132. Warram J. Preoperative irradiation of cancer of the lung: final report of a therapeutic trial. Cancer 1975;36:914–925.

133. Paulson DL. Carcinoma in the superior pulmonary sulcus. Ann Thorac Surg 1979;28:3–4.
134. Turrisi AT III. The integration of platinum and radiotherapy in the treatment of lung cancer. Semin Oncol 1991;18:81–89.
135. Choi NC, Kanarek DJ, Kazemi H. Physiologic changes in pulmonary function after thoracic radiotherapy for patients with lung cancer and role of regional pulmonary function studies in predicting postradiotherapy pulmonary function before radiotherapy. Cancer Treat Sympos 1985;2:119–130.
136. Rusch VW, Albain KS, Crowley JJ, Rice TW, Lonchyna V, McKenna R Jr, Livingston RB, et al. Southwest Oncology Group trial: surgical resection of stage IIIA and stage IIIB non–small cell lung cancer after concurrent induction chemoradiotherapy. J Thorac Cardiovasc Surg 1993;105:97–104.
137. Johnson DH, Einhorn LH, Bartolucci A, et al. Thoracic radiotherapy does not prolong survival in patients with locally advanced, unresectable non–small cell lung cancer. Ann Intern Med 1990;113:33.
138. Vines E, Baeza MR, Pertuze J, Matura G. Radiotherapy in the treatment of non–small cell lung cancer. Rev Med Chil 1992;120(3):267–274.
139. Johnson DH, Bass D, Einhorn LH, et al. Combination chemotherapy with or without thoracic radiotherapy in limited-stage small-cell cancer: a randomized trial of the Southeastern Cancer Study Group. J Clin Oncol 1993;11(7):1223–1229.
140. Schaake-Koning C, van den Bogaert W, Dalesio O, et al. Effects of concomitant cisplatin and radiotherapy on inoperable non–small-cell lung cancer. N Engl J Med 1992;326(8):524–530.
141. Armstrong JG, Rosenstein MM, Shank BM, et al. Twice daily irradiation for limited small cell lung cancer. Int J Radiat Oncol Biol Phys 1991;21(5):1269–1274.
142. Carlson RW, Sikic BI, Gandara DR, et al. Late consolidative radiation therapy in the treatment of limited-stage small cell lung cancer. Cancer 1991;68(5):948–958.
143. Johnson DH, Strupp J, Greco FA, et al. Neoadjuvant cisplatin plus vinblastine chemotherapy in locally advanced non–small cell lung cancer. Cancer 1991;68(6):1216–1220.
144. Umeko S, Okimoto N, Soejima R. Atelectatic lung escaping radiation pneumonitis. Chest 1992;101(3):879–880.
145. Awan AM, Weichselbaum RR. Palliative radiotherapy. Hematol Oncol Clin North Am 1990;4(6):1169.
146. Vokes EE. Sequential combined modality therapy for stage III non–small cell lung cancer. Hematol Oncol Clin North Am 1990;4(6):1133–1142.
147. Seagren SL. Radical radiation therapy for lung cancer. Hematol Oncol Clin North Am 1990;4(6):1093–1099.
148. Wara WM, Phillipa TL, Margolis LW, et al. Radiation pneumonitis: a new approach to the derivation of time-dose factors. Cancer 1973;32:547–552.
149. Castellino RA, Glatstein E, Turbow MM, Rosenberg S, Kaplan HS. Latent radiation injury of the lungs or heart activated by steroid withdrawal. Ann Intern Med 1974;80:593–599.
150. Trask CWL, Joannides T, Harper PG, et al. Radiation-induced lung fibrosis after treatment of small cell carcinoma of the lung with very high-dose cyclophosphamide. Cancer 1985;55:57–60.
151. Rubin P, Dasarett GW. Clinical radiation pathology. Philadelphia: WB Saunders 1968;I.
152. Shahian DM, Neptune WB, Elis FH Jr. Pancoast tumors: improved survival with preoperative radiotherapy. Ann Thorac Surg 1987;43:32–38.
153. Rubin P. The Franz Buschke lecture: late effects of chemotherapy and radiation therapy: a new hypothesis. Int J Radiat Oncol Biol Phys 1984;10:5–34.
154. Lung Cancer Study Group. Effects of postoperative mediastinal radiation on completely resected stage II and stage III epidermoid cancer of the lung. N Engl J Med 1986;315:1377–1381.
155. Kaskowitz L, Graham MV, Emami B, et al. Radiation therapy alone for stage I non–small cell lung cancer. Int J Radiat Oncol Biol Phys 1993;27(3):517–523.
156. Roswit B, White DC. Severe radiation injuries of the lung. AJR Am J Roentgenol 1977;129:127–136.
157. Gibson PG, Bryant DH Morgan GW, et al. Radiation-induced lung injury: a hypersensitivity pneumonitis? Ann Intern Med 1988;109:288–291.
158. Cooper G Jr, Guerrant JL, Harden AG, et al. Some consequences of pulmonary irradiation. AJR Am J Roentgenol 1961;85:865–874.
159. Brindle JS, Shaw EG, Su JQ, et al. Pilot study of accelerated hyperfractionated thoracic radiation therapy in patients with unresectable stage III non–small cell lung carcinoma. Cancer 1993;72(2):405–409.
160. Deely TJ. The effects of radiation on the lungs in the treatment of carcinoma of the bronchus. Clin Radiol 1960;11:33–39.
161. Rodman T, Karr S, Close HP. Radiation reaction in the lung. Report of a fatal case in a patient with carcinoma of the lung, with studies of pulmonary function before and during prednisone therapy. N Engl J Med 1960;262:431–434.
162. Murray N, Coy P, Pater JL, et al. Importance of timing for thoracic irradiation in the combined modality treatment of limited-stage small-cell lung cancer. J Clin Oncol 1993;11(2):336–344.
163. Salazar OM, Rubin P, Brown JC, Feldstein ML, Keller BE. Predictors of radiation response in lung cancer. Cancer 1976;37:2636–2650.
164. Hoffbrand BI, Gillam PMS, Heaf PJD. Effect of chronic bronchitis on changes in pulmonary function caused by irradiation of the lungs. Thorax 1965;20:303–308.
165. Bangma PJ. Postoperative radiotherapy. In: Deely TJ, ed. Modern radiotherapy. Carcinoma of the bronchus. New York: Appleton-Century-Crofts, 1972:163.
166. Byhardt RW, Martin L, Pajak TF, et al. The influence of field size and other treatment factors on pulmonary toxicity following hyperfractionated irradiation for inoperable non–small cell cancer—analysis of a Radiation Therapy Oncology Group protocol. Int J Radiat Oncol Biol Phys 1993;27(3):537–544.
167. Selawry OS. Response of bronchogenic carcinoma to Adriamycin. Cancer Chemother Rep 1975;6:349–351.
168. Pannettiere FJ, Vance RB, Stuckey WJ, et al. Evaluation of single-agent cisplatin in the management of non–small cell carcinoma of the lung: a Southwest Oncology Group Study. Cancer Treat Rep 1983;67:399–400.
169. Ettinger DS, Karp JE, Abeloff ME, et al. Intermittent high-dose cyclophosphamide chemotherapy for small cell carcinoma of the lung. Cancer Treat Rep 1978;62:413–424.
170. Capewell S, Sudlow MF. Performance and prognosis in patients with lung cancer: the Edinburgh Lung Cancer Group. Thorax 1990;45:951–956.
171. Bennett JM, Reich SD. Bleomycin. Ann Intern Med 1979;90:945–948.
172. Yousem SA, Lifson JD, Colby TV. Chemotherapy-induced eosinophilic pneumonia: relation to bleomycin. Chest 1985;88:103–106.

173. Holoye PY, Luna MA, MacKay B, et al. Bleomycin hypersensitivity pneumonitis. Ann Intern Med 1978;88:47–49.
174. Samuels ML, Johnson DE, Holoye PY, et al. Large-dose bleomycin therapy and pulmonary toxicity: a possible role of prior radiotherapy. JAMA 1976;235:1117–1120.
175. Cooper JAD Jr, White DA, Matthay RA. Drug-induced pulmonary disease. Part 1: cytotoxic drugs. Am Rev Respir Dis 1986;133:321–340.
176. Balikian JP, Jochelson MS, Bauer KA, et al. Pulmonary complications of chemotherapy regimens containing bleomycin. AJR Am J Roentgenol 1982;139:455–461.
177. Batist G, Andrews JL Jr. Pulmonary toxicity of antineoplastic drugs. JAMA 1979;246:1449–1453.
178. Pascual RS, Mosher MB, Sikand RS, et al. Effects of bleomycin on pulmonary function in man. Am Rev Respir Dis 1973;108:211–217.
179. Iacovino JR, Leitner J, Abbas AK, et al. Fatal pulmonary reaction from low doses of bleomycin. An idiosyncratic tissue response. JAMA 1976;235:1253–1255.
180. Jolivet J, Giroux L, Laurin S, et al. Microangiopathic hemolytic anemia, renal failure, and noncardiogenic pulmonary edema: a chemotherapy-induced syndrome. Cancer Treat Rep 1983;67:429–434.
181. Budzar AU, Legha SS, Luna MA, et al. Pulmonary toxicity of mitomycin. Cancer 1980;45:236–244.
182. Oliner H, Schwartz R, Rubio F, et al. Interstitial pulmonary fibrosis following busulfan therapy. Am J Med 1961;31:134–139.
183. Maxwell I. Reversible pulmonary edema following cyclophosphamide treatment. JAMA 1974;229:137–138.
184. Trask CW, Joannides T, Harper PG, et al. Radiation-induced lung fibrosis after treatment of small cell carcinoma of the lung with very high-dose cyclophosphamide. Cancer 1985;55:57–60.
185. Mark GJ, Lehimgar-Zadeh A, Ragsdale BD. Cyclophosphamide pneumonitis. Thorax 1978;33:89–93.
186. Godard P, Marty JP, Michel FB. Interstitial pneumonia and chlorambucil. Chest 1979;76:471–473.
187. Goucher G, Rowland V, Hawkins J. Melphalan-induced pulmonary interstitial fibrosis. Chest 1980;77:805–806.
188. Mitsudo SM, Greenwald ES, Banerji B, et al. BCNU lung: drug-induced pulmonary changes. Cancer 1984;54:751–755.
189. Ecker MD, Jay B, Keohane MF. Procarbazine lung. AJR Am J Roentgenol 1978;131:527–628.
190. Schwartz, IR, Kajani MK. Methotrexate therapy and pulmonary disease. JAMA 1969;210:1924.
191. Ridley MG, Wolfe CS, Mathews JA. Life-threatening acute pneumonia during low-dose methotrexate treatment for rheumatoid arthritis: a case report and review of the literature. Ann Rheum Dis 1988;47:784–788.
192. Bedrossian CWM, Sussman J, Conklin RH, et al. Azathioprine-associated interstitial pneumonitis. Am J Clin Pathol 1984;82:148–154.
193. Rao SX, Ramaswamy G, Levin M, et al. Fatal acute respiratory failure after vinblastine-mitomycin therapy in lung carcinoma. Arch Intern Med 1985;145:1905–1907.
194. Burkes, RL, Ginsberg RJ, Shepherd FA, et al. Induction chemotherapy with mitomycin, vindesine and cisplatin for stage III unresectable non–small-cell cancer: results of the Toronto phase III trial. J Clin Oncol 1992;10:580–586.
195. Buccheri GF, Ferrigno D, Curcio A, et al. Continuation of chemotherapy versus supportive care alone in patients with inoperable non–small cell lung cancer and stable disease after two or three cycles of MACC. Cancer 1989;63:428–432.
196. Trovo MG, Tirelli U, De Paoli A, et al. Combined radiotherapy and chemotherapy with CAMP in 64 consecutive patients with epidermoid bronchogenic carcinoma, limited disease: a prospective study. Int J Radiat Oncol Biol Phys 1982;8:1051–1054.
197. Holoye PY, Samuels ML. Cyclophosphamide, vincristine, and sequential split-course radiotherapy in the treatment of small cell lung cancer. Chest 1975;76:675–679.
198. Mira JG, Miller TP, Crowley JJ. Chest irradiation vs chest RT and chemotherapy with or without prophylactic brain RT in localized non–small cell cancer: a Southwest Oncology Group study. Proc Am Soc Ther Radiat Oncol 1990;19:145.
199. Haupt HM, Hutchins GM, Moore GW. Ara-C lung: noncardiogenic pulmonary edema complicating cytosine arabinoside therapy of leukemia. Am J Med 1981;70:256–261.
200. Blum RH, Carter SK, Agre K. A clinical review of bleomycin—a new antineoplastic agent. Cancer 1973;31:903–914.
201. Turrisi AT. The integration of platinum and radiotherapy in the treatment of lung cancer. Semin Oncol 1991;18:81–87.
202. Fanta CH. Respiratory complications in cancer medicine. 3rd ed. In: Holland JF, Frei E, Bast RC, et al., eds. Philadelphia: Lea & Febiger, 1993:2349–2358.
203. Mann H, Ward JH, Samlowski WE. Vascular leakage syndrome associated with interleukin-2; chest radiographic manifestations. Radiology 1990;176:191–194.
204. Dewys WD, Begg C, Lavin PT, et al. Prognostic effect of weight loss prior to chemotherapy in cancer patients. Am J Med 1980;69:491–497.
205. Hoelzer KL, Harrison BR, Luedke SW, et al. Vinblastine-associated pulmonary toxicity in patients receiving combination therapy with mitomycin and cisplatin. Drug Intell Clin Pharmacol 1986;20:287–289.

8

Treatment Evaluation

Jean-Pierre Pignon and Rodrigo Arriagada

In the usual circumstance, advances in therapeutics come from a succession of small improvements. When such small differences are to be established, only carefully conducted trials will be able to provide definite information (1).

This chapter describes the principles of clinical trials with emphasis on the design and conduct of randomized trials. It also addresses the problems related to treatment evaluation in lung cancer.

RATIONALE OF CLINICAL TRIALS

To improve patient care, we need to know whether a new treatment will achieve better results than the standard treatment or than the absence of treatment when there is no well-established therapy. One possibility is the comparison of different treatment approaches (e.g., radical thoracic radiotherapy and no radiotherapy), using databases, e.g., computer-stored medical records for treatment description and a tumor registry for patient outcome. With the technological advances in data processing and the possibility of cross-linking databases, a large amount of information can now be collected on a large number of patients (2, 3). Such nonexperimental surveys are based on observations of patient groups receiving different kinds of treatments (4). Arguments in favor of databases are reduced cost; the rapid availability of results; the study of unselected populations, which facilitates the generalization of results; and avoidance of randomization (5). Even if databases are very useful for descriptive data on treatment morbidity in a general population and may prompt further research in cases of discrepancies with previous published data (6), they do not permit unbiased comparison of treatments.

The main problem is that treatments are selected according to patient prognostic factors and comorbidity, different pretreatment assessments, and physicians' skills (7, 8). However, databases are often developed for purposes other than treatment evaluation—e.g., reimbursement of health care by insurers—and covariate collection and data checking (e.g., missing data, coding) could be inappropriate. Another alternative is the performance of a historical comparison of two prospective series of patients included in a well-defined protocol. This approach is more reliable for treatment selection, administration, and evaluation (4). A traditional way of decreasing biases in such group comparisons is the use of adjustments on pertinent covariates. However, such covariates should be known and their assessment should be reliable (2). Furthermore, the statistical methods that rely heavily on modeling are difficult to check and understand. The choice of the model must be appropriate because results may vary with the model used (2, 9).

The clinical trial has been defined as "any form of planned experiment which involves patients and is designed to elucidate the most appropriate treatment of future patients with a given medical condition" (10). It is usual to distinguish four phases in the evaluation of a treatment

Phase I trial: study of the clinical pharmacology and the relationship between toxicity and the treatment dose schedule, in search of a maximum tolerated dose;

Phase II trial: identification of promising treatments in specific tumor sites;

Phase III trial: comparison of a new treatment to the standard treatment;

Phase IV trial: detection of rare or late-occurring side effects.

The first three phases are based on experimental methodology as described in the 19th century by scientists such as Claude Bernard (11). They imply the prospective use of a standard treatment in a group of persons selected according to predefined criteria. The aim is to answer one or a few specific questions by assessing prespecified endpoints(s)—a criterion for evaluating treatment effect. Schwartz et al. (1) pointed out that "the essential core of this methodology has been its statistical component." Other key components are: good ideas that rely on researchers with insight and imagination; safety that relies on animal experiments prior to clinical applications and on the first clinical phases of treatment development; good clinical monitoring; and respect for ethical principles.

Phase IV trials can rely on either randomized studies or surveys. Epidemiological surveys, based on observation, are the key tools used to determine disease etiology. In such studies, it is difficult to demonstrate cause and effect relationships. Hill (12) proposed guidelines for scientifically establishing causality in cancer. To fulfill the proposed criteria, several well-performed studies are needed (13). It is therefore much more difficult to conclude that a treatment effect exists with surveys than with randomized trials because of the inherent difference in methodology between methods (14–16).

In lung cancer, different kinds of treatments should be evaluated and may be grouped in three classes, as shown in Table 8.1: preventive treatment, treatment with a curative intent, and symptomatic and palliative treatment.

Trials on lung cancer prevention could concern either the general population, or focus on a high-risk population (heavy smokers, asbestos workers) or patients who have had lung cancer (secondary prevention). Interventions currently evaluated include prevention or cessation of tobacco use (17), and vitamin administration, e.g., vitamin A, synthetic retinoids, beta carotene (18, 19). The results of a Finnish trial (20) showed that beta carotene had a possible harmful effect on the incidence of lung cancer. This unexpected result supports the skeptics who contested a potentially beneficial effect of vitamins because it was suggested by epidemiologic or preclinical experimental data only. Prevention trials are singular with respect to the endpoint, the selected population, and the statistical methods. Several clinical and statistical reports have been published on this topic (18, 19, 21–24).

Clinical trials on symptomatic treatment and ancillary care should be encouraged because they can lead to an improvement in the quality of life and can foster active clinical research collaboration with paramedics and patients. The sample size needed is smaller than that required for trials aimed at improving treatment efficacy. Three reasons may explain the smaller sample size needed: the useful difference expected between treatments is larger than that expected for survival in adjuvant settings, quantitative endpoints are often used, and a short-term follow-up is sufficient to obtain valid results.

This chapter focuses on prospective trials evaluating treatments with a curative intent.

TRIAL PROTOCOL

Writing the protocol is a key step in the trial design. The quality of this document plays a role in the success of the trial and should be the result of multidisciplinary collaboration among clinicians, biologists, and statisticians. It should describe the scientific background and the trial design, and become the operation manual for running the trial (10). The protocol should clearly answer why and how the trial will be performed. Scientific and ethics committees, and funding agencies will use this document to judge whether the trial is worthwhile and feasible, and whether it will be well performed. Clinicians should estimate the workload implied by the trial. The trial coordinators should evaluate the additional staff needed, the overall cost, and the duration of the trial. Table 8.2 lists the parts required in a protocol. The scientific background should include a critical review, with references of all relevant preclinical and clinical studies, including ongoing trials. A synthesis of the results of previous trials may be necessary. How the proposed trial relates to those summarized should be stated.

The main trial objectives include a concise definition of the hypotheses under investigation. Because of the number of patients needed, most trials should be

TABLE 8.1. Types of Treatment in Lung Cancer

Preventive treatment (primary or secondary prevention)
  Tobacco use: prevention and cessation
  Retinoid and beta carotene
Treatment with a curative intent
  Surgery
  Chemotherapy
    Adjuvant to surgery or radiotherapy
    Neoadjuvant (preoperative)
  Radiotherapy
    Thoracic: external radiotherapy, brachytherapy
      Adjuvant (preoperative, intraoperative, postoperative)
      Radical
    Cranial: prophylactic
    Unconventional fractionation
    Radiosensitizers
  Immunotherapy
  Combined modalities
Symptomatic and palliative treatment
  Chemotherapy
  Thoracic radiotherapy, cranial radiotherapy
  Antibiotics, antiemetics, analgesics, hematopoetic growth factors
  Neodymium: YAG laser, photodynamic therapy for bronchial obstruction
  Combined modalities

TABLE 8.2. Main Chapters of a Clinical Trial Protocol

Scientific background
Specific objectives
Study design
Eligibility of patients
Pretreatment evaluation
Registration (randomization) of patients
Treatment plan, procedures in case of toxicity
Criteria for evaluating the treatment effect and methods to assess them
Procedures in case of treatment failure and protocol deviations
Statistical considerations: sample size, planned analyses
Informed consent and ethical considerations
Data forms and data handling
Names and addresses of the trial staff members and participants

restricted to one or two primary objectives. Secondary objectives, such as toxicity, are usually included. The study design should ensure that at least all primary objectives will be attained (25). The best studies are those in which "either positive or negative results are informative for patient management and for developing better treatments" (8). The protocol should clearly state the trial design and whether an early stopping rule will be used. Inclusion criteria, treatment schedules, and methodology used for treatment evaluation should be described accurately and in detail.

The protocol should answer all practical questions that may be raised by investigators during the accural period and follow-up of patients. These recommendations ensure good trial compliance and avoid recourse to a single individual for practical problems, e.g., the decision to interrupt treatment after the occurrence of a well-known toxicity. The following parameters should be described in the treatment schedule: drug and radiation doses, practical administration and technical details, treatment duration and schedule, and procedures in the event of toxicity (treatment interruption or decreased doses) or no response (minimum duration of treatment, second-line treatment). Some decisions should be stated in the protocol, such as the choice of a second-line treatment being at the discretion of the investigator.

The role of the statisticians is not limited to computing the sample size. Their collaboration at different steps during the preparation of the trial may be fruitful. A good description of the planned analysis and handling of protocol deviations avoids data dredging. The organization of the trial structure, as well as the administrative responsibilities, should be described clearly. The full address, including telephone and telefax numbers, of the trial staff should be included.

PATIENT SELECTION

Phase I trials are conducted in patients whose cancers make them unsuitable candidates for an established treatment. Usually, there is no selection by tumor type because the main goal of the study is the assessment of toxicity. This goal implies selection of patients with unimpaired organ function.

In phase II trials, the emphasis is on tumor response to treatment, which depends on the primary site and histologic type. Thus, phase II trials are performed on specific tumor sites in patients with measurable disease. In lung cancer, for instance, it is well-established that the chemosensitivity and radiosensitivity of small cell lung cancer is higher that of non–small cell lung cancer (NSCLC) (26, 27). However, the relative chemosensitivity of histologic NSCLC subtypes is unclear (28). Tumor responses may vary with the performance status and previous treatment (28 ,29). Sörensen and Hansen (28) propose that new drugs be tested in patients with a good performance status, "minimum extent of disease, and minimum amount of previous therapy" to increase the probability of detecting response to treatment because the likelihood of response is lower and of toxicity, higher in patients with a poor prognosis. Because there are other active treatments for lung cancer, inclusion of untreated patients may be ethically difficult. Moore and Korn (29) suggest a phase II design, termed the window-of-opportunity design, with a good likelihood of detecting tumor response. Such a trial would include previously treated patients with recurrent disease and previously untreated patients who, in the absence of early response to the new treatment, will receive salvage therapy.

For phase III trials, the choice of inclusion criteria is dictated by a trade-off between the extrapolation of results to as large a population as possible and the selection of patients with highly responsive tumors (8, 24). In any case, patients included should be suitable for any of the treatments being compared, e.g., chemotherapy and surgery. Two arguments favor highly selected patients (8, 30, 31): (a) the selection of a homogeneous high-risk population increases the statistical power; and (b) the selection of young patients with a good performance status and without concurrent disease increases the likelihood of detecting a treatment effect. Another argument is that if a valid cause and effect relationship has been established by a randomized study, the result is likely to hold, at least qualitatively, in another setting (31).

Several arguments favor unselected populations (30, 32): (a) the extrapolation of results to the real clinical world is straightforward; (b) precise estimates of the treatment effect in the general population are important; (c) costly selection procedures based on tests not routinely used in general hospitals are avoided and a rapid accrual is possible; (d) loss of power, if any, associated with the heterogeneous population is balanced by the increase in sample size; and (e) subset analyses based on a priori hypotheses could help to identify patients who may obtain a major treatment benefit.

Indeed, both approaches have been useful in treatment development. Schwartz and Lellouch (33) have drawn the distinction between explanatory and pragmatic trials. In the former, the aim is the establishment of whether a treatment is effective, whereas in the latter, the objective is the determination of its usefulness in general practice. Some phase III trials, such as those in advanced disease, are more explanatory, but most have a pragmatic goal. A trial including a highly selected population is useful, as a first step, to demonstrate treatment efficacy. Such a study should be confirmed by a further trial that includes a nonselected population when a new treatment may have important implications for public health.

Of course, between the two ends of the spectrum, there is ample room for compromise. Elderly persons are often excluded from trials, both because of their age and their associated diseases. Because the age of the population is increasing, with more than 55% of cancers in the European Community occurring in patients over 65 years old (34), more resources should be devoted to designing specific studies for older patients, who are at an increased risk of toxicity (34). Table 8.3 compares the incidence of three major cancer sites in Western countries with the number of patients included in adjuvant chemotherapy trials. Even if there is a smaller proportion of patients with lung cancer initially treated by surgery compared with patients having breast or colon cancer, the proportion of patients randomized in adjuvant chemotherapy trials is quite small; in fact, it is even smaller than that achieved with chemotherapy alone in childhood leukemia (39). This disease is one of the few for which steady and continuing improvement in survival has been observed (39, 40).

Deacon and Peto (39) estimated that less than 7.5% of eligible patients with head and neck cancer in either the United Kingdom or the United States were entered in published randomized trials on combined modality therapy. The proportion of patients from the target population actually included in trials during the 1980s is between 6% and 41% in the studies reviewed

TABLE 8.3. Comparison of Annual Incidence and Number of Patients Included in Adjuvant Chemotherapy Trials Performed for Lung, Breast, and Colorectal Cancers

TUMOR SITE	NO. OF NEW CASES PER YEAR		TOTAL NO.	
	USA[a]	EC[b]	PATIENTS	TRIALS
Lung	152,000	158,000	5,000	18[c]
Breast	136,000	135,000	23,000	58[d]
Colon/rectum	147,000	137,000	18,000	49[e]

Abbreviations: USA, United States; EC, European Community.
[a]Estimation for 1988. From Fraumeni. JF Jr, Hoover RN, Devasa SS, Kinlen LJ. Epidemiology of cancer: In: DeVita VT, Hellman S, Rosenberg SA, eds. Cancer: principles and practice of oncology. 3d ed. Philadelphia: JB Lippincott, 1989:396–420.
[b]Estimation for 1978–1982. Jensen OM, Esteve J, Moller H, Renard H. Cancer in the European Community and its member states. Eur J Cancer 1990;26:1167–1256.
[c]Trials between 1965 and 1991. From Non–Small Cell Lung Cancer Collaborators Group. Chemotherapy in non–small cell lung cancer: a meta-analysis using updated individual patient data from 52 randomised clinical trials. BMJ 1995: in press.
[d]Trials before 1985. From Early Breast Cancer Trialists' Collaborative Group. Systemic treatment of early breast cancer by hormonal, cytotoxic or immune therapy: 133 randomised trials involving 31,000 recurrences and 24,000 deaths among 75,000 women. Lancet 1992; 339:1–15, 71–85.
[e]Trials before 1987. M. Clarke, personal communication for the Colorectal Cancer Collaboration Secretariat.

by Begg (30). These proportions are related not only to restrictive inclusion criteria but also to reticence of patients or physicians (30, 41, 42). The description of eligible patients who were not included and of ineligible patients (42) is useful as a means of convincing clinicians of the possibility of generalizing the results; it also can be used to estimate the treatment impact on a general population. Because such additional studies encumber a trial and could slow down its accrual, they should be performed only when favorable conditions exist, such as when clinicians are enthusiastic about the trial and/or the data are limited or uncomplicated.

A physician's reticence (41) to include patients in randomized trials is secondary to ethical issues or difficulties in obtaining a written informed consent as well as to the rigidity of the protocol design, inconvenience for patients, and additional time commitments. The development of large-scale trials in oncology was only possible because these concerns were taken into account. Programs have been developed in North America and Europe to include community hospitals and to improve patient accrual. Some studies have demonstrated the good quality of participation of such centers (43, 44). Mobilization of public opinion with the help of lay people has been suggested to promote participation in randomized clinical trials (45). Such actions prepare people to sign informed consent forms by giving them—outside the context of a recent diagnosis of cancer—information about cancers, their treatments, and the need for research and clinical randomized trials. For example, in the United States and England, groups at high risk of AIDS infection are actively participating in treatment evaluation (46).

ENDPOINTS

The choice of criteria for evaluating treatment is a key issue in treatment evaluation. It determines the size and duration of the trial and its relevance. The endpoint should be meaningful clinically and should assess patient welfare. A well-defined endpoint is essential to perform an unbiased treatment evaluation. This evaluation includes the definition of follow-up procedures, tests to be performed, guidelines for test interpretation, and methods for summarizing results.

Duration of overall survival, the usual main endpoint for phase III trials is objective, clinically meaningful, and easy to update. To obtain the approval of the U.S. Food and Drug Administration, a new anticancer treatment when compared with no treatment (or a standard treatment), must either prolong survival or improve the quality of life (47).

Endpoints such as disease free survival, progression free survival, or the response rate are usually used as secondary endpoints in randomized trials. There are several justifications for using endpoints other than survival: (a) to obtain information on treatment effect after a shorter observation time; (b) to conclude with a smaller number of patients as the dilution of treatment difference by intercurrent deaths or by effective second-line therapy is avoided; and (c) to limit this "dilution effect" provides a more direct appreciation of the treatment effect and is more relevant for clinicians. The use of these endpoints as surrogates of survival assumes that they are good predictors of overall survival whatever the type of tumor and type of treatment (48). However, this is not a general fact because an adjuvant treatment inducing second cancers may improve disease free survival without a change in overall survival if these events are not taken into account. There are several examples of trials, including lung cancer trials, in which an improvement in response rate is not translated into an improvement of overall survival (49, 50).

Before using a time dependent endpoint, one should define the zero time and the event(s) considered. If the first day of treatment can be an adequate zero time for nonrandomized trials, the date of randomization should be used for randomized trials. When the interval between the date of randomization and the first day of treatment is different between the two arms, a slight bias occurs when they are compared if the first day of treatment is used. There are no international definitions of disease free survival, local relapse free survival, distant relapse free survival, or progression free survival. For example, some authors censor, for survival, those patients who die from causes other than cancer (specific cancer survival); others censor patients with second tumors for disease free survival. As such a choice could skew the results, the reason for censoring such patients should be discussed (51). For the estimation of disease free survival, it is better to include events such as relapses, second cancers, or death, whichever comes first, and to describe the pattern of events. The lack of agreement in defining these types of endpoints, and its consequences on the results, imply the necessity of always describing in detail the method chosen.

In trials with a combined therapy arm, the description of the number of relapses according to site (locoregional versus distant) and the use of actuarial analysis are important for the interpretation of the results (52). For relapse free survival, all patients beginning therapy (phase II) or all patients randomized should be included (phase III). Thus, when two treatments are compared, the difference in complete response rates can be taken into account. Figure 8.1 shows an example (53) of such a comparison where the beginning of the curves at less than 100% corresponds to the rates of complete remission.

Considerable variability in the response rates for the same treatment (28) could be explained not only by differences in patient characteristics but also by differences in the methods used for tumor assessment and by errors in measurement (54, 55). Because of these errors, reporting minor responses or stable disease should be abandoned unless of very long duration (55, 56). Frequent and elaborate investigations lead to the detection of fewer complete responses or recurrent disease earlier than the use of sporadic routine investigations. For example, the systematic use of bronchoscopic biopsy in locally advanced NSCLC assessment has changed the rate of complete responses (57). Thus, follow-up procedures should be standardized and identical in the different arms of a randomized trial. A blind review of tumor responses is the best way to obtain unbiased assessment of tumor response, and the use of a second-party review has been recommended (58). The adoption of standard criteria, such as those proposed by the World Health Organization, Eastern Coopera-

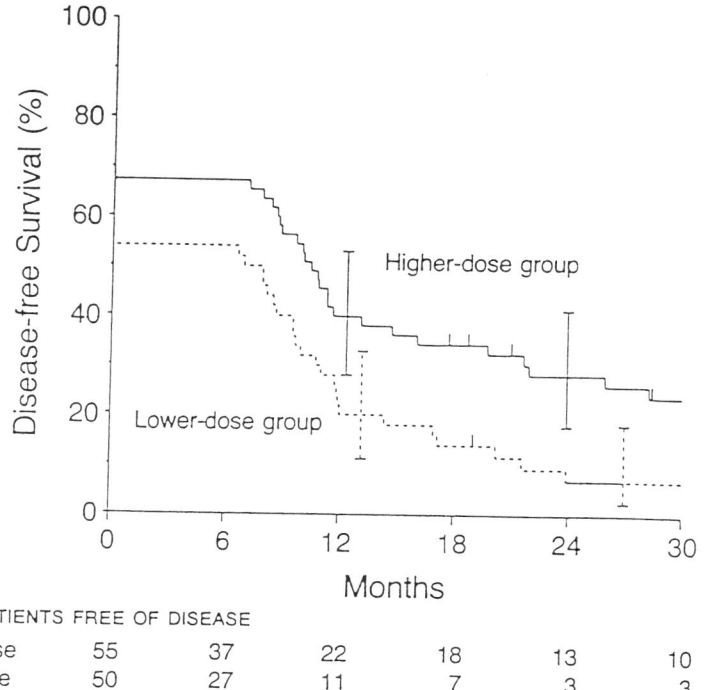

FIGURE 8.1. Example of disease free survival curves according to treatment group. Only patients in complete remission were considered free of disease. Disease free survival rates are given with 95% confidence intervals. (Reprinted with permission from Arriagada R, Le Chevalier T, Pignon JP, et al. Initial chemotherapeutic doses and survival in patients with limited small cell lung cancer. N Engl J Med 1993;329:1848–1852.)

tive Oncology Group (ECOG), and European Organization for Research and Treatment of Cancer (EORTC) (59, 60), is necessary for the evaluation of tumor response. These general criteria should be completed with site specific criteria.

In spite of several publications on the risks of comparing the survival of responders and nonresponders (56, 58, 61–66) and the refusal to publish such comparisons by *Cancer Treatment Reports*, 6 of 25 phase II trials and 4 of 10 randomized trials published during the first semester of 1990 in *Cancer* used such comparisons (J. P. Pignon, personal communication). The comparison of the survival of responders and nonresponders is biased in several ways. Patients who die early are by definition nonresponders. Even if this time bias is corrected (61), the comparison continues to be biased: responders may have a more favorable prognosis regardless of the treatment received. They may have a more favorable profile for known prognostic factors, e.g., tumor burden, previous treatment, performance status, as well as unknown prognostic factors. Conclusions about treatment efficacy should never be drawn with this method (Fig. 8.2). In a randomized trial evaluating two chemotherapy regimens, the comparison of survival that is limited to two groups of responders is not an appropriate method of evaluation. The two chemotherapy regimens could select patients with different prognostic factors, response could occur at a different time after the start of the treatment, and survival could be better with one of the treatments in nonresponders (67, 68).

Toxicity is an important endpoint. Short-term and long-term toxicity should be studied. Well-established criteria such as the World Health Organization scale for acute toxicity of chemotherapy (59) are used commonly. Cost is another endpoint that will be used increasingly in the future. The assistance of economists could be sought to take into account indirect costs such as sick leave. Direct costs (drugs, consultations, hospital admissions) should not always be considered the sole criteria of economic evaluation because, in some cases, indirect costs may be the main component.

Evaluation of the quality of life is increasingly being used, particularly for palliative treatments (69), and tremendous progress has been made in developing psychometrically robust indexes (70). Before it can be considered adequate for measuring the quality of life, an index should be feasible, reliable (reproducible), valid (measuring the appropriate parameters), and responsive to changes in the quality of life (71). A quality of life index is often a multidimensional construction composed minimally of four domains: the physical functional status; disease-related and treatment-related physical symptoms; psychologic functioning; and social functioning. The multidimensional nature of the quality of life should be respected, and self-rating by patients is preferred to observer rating because the

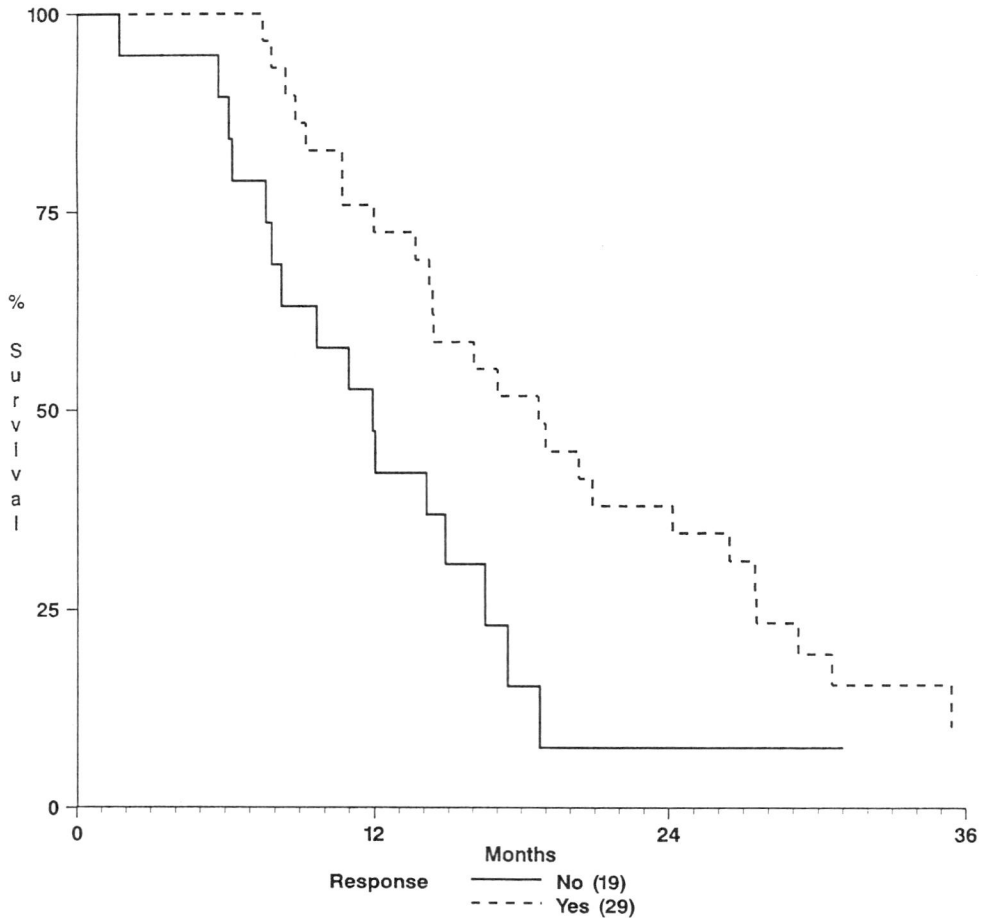

FIGURE 8.2. Comparison of survival between responders and nonresponders to intraarterial chemotherapy in patients with liver metastases. The survival difference was significant in favor of responders ($P = .02$). There was an imbalance in a well-established prognostic factor: 59% of responders versus 84% of nonresponders had more than four liver metastases ($P = .06$). After exclusion of early deaths ($n = 4$), the survival difference was not significant. (Reproduced with permission from Pignon JP, Ducreux M, Rougier PH, Lasser PH. Danger de la comparaison de la survie des répondeurs et des non-répondeurs à une chimiothérapie dans les essais de phase II en Cancérologie. Gastroenterol Clin Biol 1991;15:A140.)

correlation between both ratings is poor (69). Modular assessments with a core questionnaire and disease specific and/or treatment specific modules have been proposed as the best strategy to facilitate cross-study comparisons and permit a good specificity for addressing particular clinical issues (72). This strategy has been developed by the European Organization for Research and Treatment of Cancer (73). In the United States, Hollen et al. (74) are developing an instrument, the Lung Cancer Symptom Scale, that focuses on measuring the physical and functional dimensions of the quality of life in individuals with lung cancer. Other groups have used the association of different specific indexes for different dimensions of quality of life (75). Investigation on the quality of life should be mandatory to be useful in a clinical trial, and a high standard of data collection and processing should be ensured (70, 76). Several groups have managed successfully the practical problems of performing a trial with the evaluation of the quality of life (69, 76).

Analysis of quality of life data is associated with particular statistical issues such as the handling of repeated measurements (with missing data) and the analysis of multiple endpoints. Other methods have been proposed to evaluate some aspects of the quality of life such as survival without symptoms (77), survival without symptoms or toxicity (78), or a change in performance status or body weight (79, 80). Such methods study only a part of a multidimensional problem and rely mainly on observer evaluation; they are often used only on a subgroup of patients and have not been evaluated with the same degree of precision as quality of life indexes (69, 81).

STUDY DESIGN
PHASE II DESIGN

Phase II studies can be divided into two phases depending on the objectives addressed (82). During the first phase (phase II-A), the main goal is screening new drugs and obtaining more data on toxicity and pharmacology. When the first results of a new drug are encouraging, new phase II studies (phase II-B) are performed. The main goal of such studies is to search for new indications, such as usefulness in other tumor types, and to evaluate new combinations including a new drug. At this step, if promising results are observed, a phase III trial should be started as soon as possible. In the phase II-A studies, there is room for the two-stage design proposed by Gehan in 1961 (83). This method allows for early stopping if the drug is not effective. For example, if no response is observed with the first 14 patients, it is concluded that the response rate is below 15% with a risk of false-negative results (type II error) of 5%. Among the other multistage designs are those proposed by Simon (84) and Fleming (85). The Fleming design allows early stopping for both low and high efficacy. Group sequential methods such as the triangular test have also been proposed (86). In phase II-B trials, a randomized design is a appropriate, allowing rapid progression to a phase III trial and limiting the selection bias often observed in small one-arm trials (87–89).

PHASE III DESIGN

WHY RANDOMIZATION IS NEEDED

The major advantages of randomization (7, 10, 16, 90) are threefold: it eliminates biases in treatment assignment, avoids biases secondary to a conscious or unconscious selection of patients to receive one of the treatments; it achieves a balance in known and unknown prognostic factors between treatment groups; and it provides a basis for the standard methods of statistical analysis such as significance tests. Sacks et al. (91), in a review of trials with historical and randomized controls in six kinds of treatments, showed that 79% of the former found that therapy was better than control and that only 20% of the latter reached the same conclusion. This discrepancy between results of trials evaluating the same treatment is largely caused by the worse outcome of the historical control groups compared with the randomized control groups. The retrospective collection of the data for the historical control group, and the changes in the methods of staging, ancillary care, and patient referral patterns that occur with time, explain why trials with historical controls tend to overestimate the value of new treatments (8, 10, 90). The technologic advances in disease staging can produce the so-called Will Rogers or stage migration phenomena (39, 92, 93): because of a shift of patients from an early to an advanced stage, the results apparently are improved within each stage, but overall results remain unchanged. Table 8.4 shows a theoretical example of this temporal drift of stages. The aim of controlled trials is not only to learn which is the best treatment, but also to obtain the best estimation of the size of the treatment effect. Thus, an unbiased estimation of the treatment effect is needed.

Selection criteria (to obtain good historical controls) and adjustment by prognostic factors have been proposed so that unbiased comparisons can be performed (94). This method implies that such controls are available and that outcome can be predicted accurately with known prognostic factors. Control groups from randomized trials are expected to be good historical control groups. Pocock (95) compared 19 pairs of the same treatment arms in consecutive randomized trials and found a significant difference in outcome in four pairs, showing that the use of historical controls, even from randomized trials, could lead to biased comparisons. There are two cases in which historical comparisons can be used legitimately: (*a*) when the treatment effect is substantial and the prognosis of the disease is highly predictable before the use of the new treatment; and (*b*) when accrual of a sufficient number of patients is impossible through international collaboration, such as in rare diseases. In these cases, a well-performed historical comparison is better than no comparison, but this comparison should be interpreted cautiously (96).

RANDOMIZATION METHODS

Systematic assignment methods such as those based on odd/even numbers, for example date of birth, may result in a bias that is sufficient to invalidate the trial results. This is also true for any random method for which investigators are aware of treatment allocation before patient inclusion (10, 97, 98). To avoid any sizable imbalance during the accrual between the number of patients randomized in each arm, randomization usually is performed by random permuted blocks. For example, if the size of the block is four, for every four patients, two are randomized to arm A and two to arm B. Pocock (10) and Simon (8) have pro-

TABLE 8.4. Stage Migration Phenomena: Better Staging Produces a Spurious Improvement of Survival Within Stage Without an Improvement in Overall Survival

STAGE	PERIOD 1			PERIOD 2		
	NO. OF PATIENTS	NO. OF 2-YEAR SURVIVORS	2-YEAR SURVIVAL RATE (%)	NO. OF PATIENTS	NO. OF 2-YEAR SURVIVORS	2-YEAR SURVIVAL RATE (%)
Limited	250	25	10	100	18	18[a]
Extensive	250	0	0	400	7	2[a]
Total	500	25	5	500	25	5

[a] $P = .03$ (one-sided Fisher exact test) for the comparison between periods in each stage.

vided practical examples of such a method. If the clinician knows the size of the block, he or she could predict the treatment allocated to the last patient of each block. Use of envelopes could result in bias if the envelopes are opened before the decision to include a patient (98).

As unbiased assignment is essential, with randomization by telephone call being the most used method (99). A central registration office oversees the verification of eligibility criteria immediately before treatment assignment. It should also check that the agreement of patients and physicians has been obtained before randomization. Confirmation of the allocated treatment by mail or telefax is advisable. These different measures result in a lower number of ineligible patients after randomization (99). In trials in which patients receive more than one treatment, such as chemotherapy after surgery or maintenance chemotherapy after induction chemotherapy, randomization should be delayed until the patient is ready to receive the randomized treatments (10, 100, 101). This delay avoids including patients who may become ineligible after the first treatment. For instance, in a trial testing adjuvant chemotherapy versus no therapy, randomization is performed after recovery from surgery. Durrleman and Simon (101) have discussed several examples of such trials and have provided quantitative data to evaluate the impact of early randomization.

Several investigators have reviewed randomization methods (10, 99, 102, 103). An imbalance in prognostic factors may occur in small randomized trials. The probability of it occurring decreases as the size of the trial increases. Stratified randomization, which allows balanced randomization for each prognostic stratum, has been proposed to limit this problem. The simplest method is the preparation of a separate randomization list using random permuted blocks for each stratum. Stratification factors should have an established independent prognostic value and be easily and reliably obtainable before randomization. Stage, performance status, and weight loss have been proposed in NSCLC (104). Osterlind (105) recently reviewed the confounding factors in the evaluation of treatment effect in lung cancer. There are several advantages of stratified randomization: (a) trial results are more credible when prognostic factors are balanced according to treatment arms; (b) adjusted analyses are avoided when an imbalance occurs such as in a nonstratified scheme; and (c) the power of the analysis is optimized. In a large-scale trial, the likelihood of an imbalance between treatment arms is small, making stratification unnecessary (10, 100). When random permuted blocks are used within each stratum, the number of strata increases rapidly with the number of prognostic factors, e.g., 5 factors (age, weight loss, performance status, stage, histology) with 2 levels result in 32 strata. In multicenter trials, it is worthwhile to stratify according to center. Treatment effect could vary according to center because of differences in patient referral patterns and local skills. Stratification by center could result in a considerable increase in the number of strata. Because of the small number of patients in each stratum, major imbalances may occur. Thus, overstratification may be detrimental (10). The minimization method (106) can accommodate a large number of stratification factors, e.g., 10–20 (107). Its aim is the optimization of the balance between the numbers of patients in each treatment arm within each level of the prognostic factors throughout the accrual period. Based on the distribution of previously randomized patients, the next treatment allocation is the one offering the best balance between treatments for each level of the prognostic factors. This method is more useful in small trials or when interim analyses are planned (108).

The standard practice is to randomize in a 1:1 ratio. The statistical power is maximal in this case. However, in some cases unequal randomization is advisable, for instance when there is (a) unequal experience with the two drugs compared, (b) overenthusiasm for new drugs, and (c) ethical concern regarding an untreated arm. Peto (32) advocates the wide use of randomized phase II trials with unequal randomization. Pocock (10) considers that "there is a reasonable case for more widespread use of unequal randomization," but he shows that a randomization ratio higher than 3:1 is undesirable because of the considerable loss of statistical power. In oncology, only a few trials have been performed with the unequal randomization design (10, 109).

TRIAL SIZE

To plan a trial and determine its feasibility, it is essential to estimate how many patients should be included. The size of a clinical trial depends on the answers to four questions:

1. What is the main purpose of the trial and its foremost endpoint? Example: Does a new multidrug regimen B improve the percentage of complete responses in metastatic NSCLC?
2. What type of statistical analysis will be performed? Continuing the example used in 1, *above*: rates of complete response are compared by a χ^2 test. The test is two sided and has a 5% risk of erroneously concluding that there is a treatment effect (type I error).
3. What are the results expected with the standard treatment? For example, the standard regimen A leads to 30% complete responses.
4. What is the treatment difference considered worth detecting with a reasonable degree of certainty? To continue the example: one hopes to increase the complete response rate to 50% and would prefer a 90% chance of detecting this increase (type II error, 10%).

In the above example, 268 patients are needed (110). The usual methods for the determination of the sample size are based on the simplified assumption that only one statistical test concerning the main endpoint is performed at the end of the trial. The null hypothesis tested is the absence of a difference in the probability of response ($P_A - P_B = 0$). If the alternative hypothesis is that the new treatment is better than the standard treatment, the test is one sided. If the alternative hypothesis is that the new treatment is either better or worse than the standard treatment, then the test is two sided. The level of the significance test, or risk α (type I error or false-positive rate), is the probability of concluding that there is a difference, when in fact there is none. The probability of concluding that there is no significant difference, when there really is a difference, is called risk β (type II error or the false-negative rate). The statistical power or probability of detecting a difference that is equal to $P_A - P_B$ corresponds to $1 - \beta$.

An estimation of results for the standard treatment is based on previous studies. The treatment difference sought depends on the level of optimism of the investigators. Thus, the sample size is only an estimation based on clinical hypotheses and statistical assumptions and certainly is not a magic number.

Simon (8) and Pocock (10) have given further details on sample size determination. George (111) reviewed the methods available for phase III trials. For all analyses of time dependent events such as survival, it is the number of events and not the number of patients that is critical. Table 8.5 shows examples of sample size when a log rank test is used to compare two survival rates (112). It illustrates the variations in sample size when the results of standard treatments are changed (Table 8.5*b*) when a one-sided rather than two-sided test is used (Table 8.5*c*), and when the type II error is increased (Table 8.5*d*). Other methods have been proposed to account for the duration of accrual and the length of follow-up (111).

Ambiguous or erroneous interpretation of trial results is frequent (113) because of the limits of the trial size. Sample size determination should be associated with an estimation of the accrual rate, which is often too optimistic. Collaboration with other groups may be necessary to recruit patients within a reasonable period. When accrual exceeds 3 or 4 years, the accrual rate may decrease because of loss of interest and controversies over ethical issues after the results of other trials.

In oncology, a common design is the inclusion of between 100 and 300 patients in two equal-sized treatment groups. Such moderately sized developmental trials are needed to evaluate new treatments and new modes of treatment delivery. These trials are time consuming and potentially costly. Their cost results from one or several of the following factors: (*a*) a patient selection based on new or expensive tests; (*b*) systematic collection of prognostic factors, data on toxicity, compliance, and secondary endpoints; (*c*) careful monitoring of treatment quality and data collection. According to the type of treatment evaluated and its stage of development, some or all of these factors are essential to the trial design. In oncology, two designs need special mention, i.e., the factorial design and the large-scale trial (or mega-trial) design; the first is interesting because it is more efficient in terms of sample size, and the second because it allows for the detection of a more realistic treatment effect. Other trial designs have been discussed by Simon (114) and Pocock (10).

TABLE 8.5. Number of Patients (Deaths) by Treatment Arm for Comparison of Survival Rates (Logrank Test) by Survival Rate of the Control Arm (P_1), Survival Rate of the Investigational Arm (P_2), Type I Error (α), Type II Error β, and Type of Test (One-Sided Versus Two-Sided)

Two-sided test, $\alpha = 0.05$, $\beta = 0.05$

			P_2			
	20%	25%	30%	35%	40%	45%
$P_1 = 15\%$	1171	336	168	105	74	56
	(966)	(269)	(131)	(79)	(54)	(40)

Two-sided test, $\alpha = .05$, $\beta = .05$

			P_2			
	50%	55%	60%	65%	70%	75%
$P_1 = 45\%$	2481	630	284	162	105	74
	(1301)	(315)	(135)	(73)	(45)	(30)

One-sided test, $\alpha = 0.05$, $\beta = 0.05$

			P_2			
	20%	25%	30%	35%	40%	45%
$P_1 = 15\%$	975	280	140	88	62	47
	(804)	(224)	(109)	(66)	(45)	(33)

Two-sided test, $\alpha = 0.05$, $\beta = 0.20$

			P_2			
	20%	25%	30%	35%	40%	45%
$P_1 = 15\%$	707	203	102	64	45	34
	(584)	(163)	(79)	(48)	(33)	(24)

Adapted with permission from Machin D, Campbell MJ. Statistical tables for the design of clinical trials. Oxford: Blackwell Scientific Publications, 1987.

FACTORIAL DESIGN

Peto (32) and Byar (115) advocated a wider use of factorial designs, in particular the 2 × 2 design, which would answer two questions rather than one with little or no extra difficulties or cost. To compare two treatments, A and B, versus no treatment, patients can be randomized into four groups: neither treatment, A alone, B alone, or both together. Then, to study the effect of A, for example, the results of the comparison A + B versus B and A versus no treatment are combined. This design assumes that the effect of A is not conditional on the presence or absence of B. However, the test required to detect such an interaction has a low power (115, 116). As pointed out by Crowley (117), in oncology it is not always possible to give no treatment or both treatments. For example, when chemotherapy and radiotherapy are combined, it may be necessary to lower the treatment doses because of overlapping toxicity. When a significant interaction is present, the study should be analyzed as a four-arm trial; as a result there is a substantial loss in statistical power (8). In SCLC, factorial design has been used to study the role of chemotherapy and prophylactic cranial irradiation (118). Such a design could be used, for example, to compare two adjuvant chemotherapy regimens and to study their duration (3 versus 6 months).

LARGE-SCALE TRIAL AND PROSPECTIVE POOLED ANALYSIS

In adult solid tumors, treatments achieving an improvement of 10% or more in absolute survival are exceptional (39, 98, 119). To detect a survival benefit below 10% in the adjuvant setting implies performing trials in which more than 1000 patients are included, because the survival rates are often higher than 40% in the control group (120). Such an improvement could have major impact on public health for common diseases, e.g., lung cancer or myocardial infarction (121). For treatment with mild toxicity, e.g., tamoxifen in breast cancer (122) or intraportal 5-fluorouracil in colorectal cancer (123), a 5% to 10% improvement in survival is worthwhile. In the past, the trial size has been too small to detect a moderate and yet clinically relevant treatment effect (39, 120, 121). The problem worsens as we move from comparisons between treatment and no treatment to those between different treatments because the expected difference is even smaller. Among the 14 randomized trials included in the NSCLC overview on the role of chemotherapy in the adjuvant setting, 5 included fewer than 200 patients (37). The National Surgical Adjuvant Breast Project has performed several large-scale trials but at a high cost because their designs were similar to the moderately sized trials. Several large trials in cardiovascular diseases (24) have been performed at a relatively low cost because of the simple inclusion criteria and the small amount of data collected (few prognostic factors, main endpoints). Only trials asking important questions, such as whether adjuvant chemotherapy is worthwhile in lung cancer, are likely to succeed in including a large number of patients. In this type of trial, broad inclusion criteria can be used with some variation from one center to another and a broad definition of treatments (e.g., range of doses of chemotherapy or radiotherapy) to facilitate intergroup collaboration (119, 121). Such trials could include a large number of unselected patients in a short period. Their results are easy to extrapolate to a large population. One key principle for these trials is that if quantitative interaction is common, unexpected qualitative interaction is extremely rare (121). In this context, a qualitative interaction corresponds to a treatment effect pointing to opposite directions in different subgroups (e.g., stage of disease), and a quantitative interaction corresponds to a variation in the size of treatment effects without a change in direction. Participation in a large-scale trial could be an efficient way of diffusing a new treatment. Large-scale trials are currently ongoing in colorectal, breast, lung, ovarian, and head and neck cancer.

An alternative to large-scale trials and intergroup trials is the prospective pooling of several similar average-sized trials performed in parallel (104). With this design, collaboration between data centers and their correspondents is maintained and intergroup collaboration is improved. This kind of flexible organization could decrease trial costs. It is also useful when some information on toxicity, compliance, and secondary endpoints is needed.

Phase IV Design

Ray et al. (124) recently stressed the need for a better evaluation of drugs after their approval for clinical use. Because some treatments may induce clinically significant but rare or late-occurring side effects, e.g., benign lung disease secondary to lung fibrosis or a second malignancy, the best approach is to ensure that all patients included in randomized trials are followed up for an extended period. Even if some large trials have succeeded in identifying such side effects (125, 126), it may be necessary to combine the results of several trials for events with a low incidence (127, 128). The conclusions of this type of study may be limited if reports of toxicity are not standardized. Alternative methods are cohort studies or nested case control studies, but causality is certainly more difficult to establish with observational studies (13). Kaldor and Lasset (129) discussed the results and the methodologic problems related to clinical series, population-based series, and case control studies when evaluating the incidence of second malignancies after treatment of Hodgkin's disease. Surveys using population-based cancer registries are cost effective when studying the risk of a second malignancy compared with those performed in the general population. For treatments including combined radiotherapy and chemotherapy, an assessment of long-term morbidity is essential because it may limit the feasibility of such treatments (130).

Analysis

Significance Tests and Confidence Interval

In general, the P value of the statistical test is overemphasized. The P value is the probability of obtaining a difference as large as the one observed when in fact there is no difference. It provides information on the extent to which results are reliable but nothing about its clinical significance. A small treatment difference, although clinically negligible, can be statistically significant with a large sample size, whereas a 20% difference may be statistically nonsignificant because of the small sample size (65). Table 8.6 gives an example of the relation between the P value and sample size. It is misleading to use the significance of the statistical test (usually $P \leq .05$) to justify the main conclusion of a trial. The P value of a one-sided test is generally half that of the corresponding two-sided test. The results of a two-sided test with a borderline significance (e.g., $P = .06$) become significant if a one-sided test is used. The one-sided test is based on the hypothesis that the new treatment could only be superior to the control

TABLE 8.6. Changes in 95% Confidence Interval and P Value When the Sample Size Increases

Sample Size	Relative Risk	95% Confidence Interval	P Value (Two-Sided)
100	0.82	(0.38–1.79)	.62
500	0.82	(0.58–1.16)	.26
1,000	0.82	(0.64–1.05)	.11
2,500	0.82	(0.70–0.96)	.0125
5,000	0.82	(0.73–0.91)	<.001
10,000	0.82	(0.76–0.89)	<.0001

Note. The treatment effect corresponds to a relative risk of 0.82. Such a relative risk is observed when overall survival improves from 50% to 55%.

arm. Such was not the case in a trial on the suppression of arrhythmia after myocardial infarction. This trial was stopped prematurely because of increased mortality in the treated group. A one-sided test had been planned in the protocol (131). Estimating the treatment difference with a confidence interval, which has a high probability of containing the true difference, is clinically more relevant. The confidence interval narrows as the sample size increases, as shown in Table 8.6. The use of confidence intervals is now a requirement in many major medical journals. Simon (132), and Gardner and Altman (133) discuss the usefulness of the confidence interval and describe the methods used to compute it. If a significant difference has not been demonstrated, the confidence interval indicates whether a clinically relevant difference has been missed and whether another trial with a large sample size is warranted.

EXCLUSION OF PATIENTS FROM ANALYSIS

Exclusion of patients before randomization could limit the generalization of the trial results to other populations, but it does not have an impact on the validity of results. In contrast, any exclusion after randomization may lead to a biased treatment comparison because of an imbalance of prognostic factors in the remaining population or because the exclusions are dependent on treatment assignment and treatment effect (98, 100, 134). When a moderate difference between treatments is expected, an analysis based on all randomized patients by treatment allocation (intention-to-treat analysis) is the best method of distinguishing between no effect and a moderate effect. Discussions about exclusions generally focus on two main categories of patients: ineligible patients and noncompliant patients. Their inclusion in the trial may result in an underestimation of the treatment effect. Exclusion of ineligible patients is possible only when based on objective criteria (e.g., age) or a blind review of data collected before randomization (e.g., pathologic review). Good trials only have few ineligible patients. Some investigators prefer retaining such patients to obtain results more applicable to general practice. Exclusion of noncompliant patients should certainly be avoided because of the high risk of a biased comparison (115, 135). In the Coronary Drug Project (136), whatever the treatment received (clofibrate or placebo), patients with a poor compliance had a high mortality rate compared with patients with good compliance. In the first trials of a new treatment, data on compliance are important if feasibility is to be established. Poor compliance could explain the absence of a significant treatment effect. Good monitoring should detect such a problem during the conduct of the trial. Gail (31) in oncology and May et al. (135) in cardiovascular disease provide several examples of patient exclusion. When an analysis is performed on eligible patients, an intention-to-treat analysis should also be performed to test the consistency of results.

SUBGROUP ANALYSIS

Prognostic factors are collected in clinical trials to (a) adjust for an imbalance between treatment arms, (b) increase the power of the comparison by accounting for these factors, and (c) perform subgroup analyses (10, 137). From a clinical perspective, it is important to know whether a group of patients will benefit more from a new treatment than from another treatment. Subgroup analyses are a useful means of generating hypotheses. However, the risk of obtaining such findings purely by chance is high. For example, if treatments A and B are compared in 10 subgroups, the probability of observing at least one significant test is 40% by chance alone (100, 116). The following guidelines have been proposed to limit this risk: (a) plan, a priori, a limited number of subgroup analyses in the protocol, (b) perform such analyses only when the difference is significant in the overall population, (c) use conservative tests for interactions between the treatment and covariates instead of conventional tests comparing treatment arms in each subset, (d) present the results with their confidence interval, (e) interpret the results in the light of a biological rationale and of results based on other endpoints or other trials, and (f) validate the results in a future trial (10, 98, 115, 116, 138).

SURVIVAL ANALYSIS AND COMPETING RISKS

Because the duration of follow-up differs for patients included in a clinical trial, appropriate methods should be used to estimate survival rates (e.g., Kaplan-Meier estimate), to compare survival curves (e.g., log rank test) and to account for covariates (e.g., Cox model). Several publications have described these methods for nonstatisticians (8, 134, 139, 140). Differences in follow-up procedure could lead to a biased comparison of disease free survival curves because disease recurrence could be detected earlier in the group with a larger number of follow-up visits (141). Losses to follow-up could invalidate the results of a trial because the reason for missing follow-up visits could be related to the treatment itself (31, 141). The number of patients lost to follow-up is a good index of the quality of a trial. Use of national death registries may be an efficient way of obtaining information on the date of death for patients lost to follow-up.

Median survival, the time at which 50% of patients are alive, often is used to summarize survival curves. This method is appropriate when the death rate is high and there is no crossing once the median is reached. Figure 8.3 provides an example of survival curves with an identical median but a different long-term outcome. The comparison of medians cannot be recommended because they could be a misleading summary of survival curves (142). Repeated statistical tests comparing survival rates at different times is also inappropriate (134). When survival curves cross, interpretation of the log rank test is difficult. In this case, the comparison of the curves before and after crossing may be proposed, but strong a priori hypotheses are needed to justify crossing and its time of occurrence to obtain a definite conclusion. The interruption of the curve when there are fewer than 5 patients at risk has been proposed to avoid misinterpretation of a plateau at the end of the curve (139).

Competing risks between death and other events are a frequent problem in oncology. For instance, in a trial including patients with head and neck cancer, death related to a second primary disease or a benign disease related to alcohol or tobacco use could occur before a recurrence of a primary lesion. In patients treated with a local treatment, the analysis of the pattern of failure (local versus metastatic) is of interest to better understand the treatment effect. The actuarial method frequently used to estimate local recurrence and distant metastasis rates often is biased because the different failure types are not independent (143). Two methods have been proposed: analysis of the time to first failure and the distribution of sites of the first failure (143), and estimation of event specific cumulative functions assuming competing risks (144). With the latter method, unbiased event specific curves can be plotted.

INTERIM ANALYSES

Interim analyses are performed to detect a treatment difference clearly larger or smaller than that expected at the beginning of the trial. Table 8.7 shows the main advantages and disadvantages of interim analyses. When interim analyses lead to the early conclusion of a trial, related costs are decreased and it is possible to proceed more rapidly to another trial. This result not only is important from an ethical viewpoint, but also because research resources and the number of available patients are limited. Thus, if the trial concludes in favor of one of the treatments, patients would benefit earlier from the best treatment, and the number of patients treated with a less effective treatment would be decreased. The only way to control the overall significance level (type I error) and the power of the trial is through the use of formal statistical methods to perform interim analyses. Repeated interim analyses lead to an increase in the overall type I error and a decrease in the statistical power. For example, if 5 or 10 interim analyses are planned at regular intervals and each at a 5% significance level, then the type I error is 14.2% and 19.3%, respectively (145).

Group sequential methods have been developed to detect earlier whether one treatment is superior to

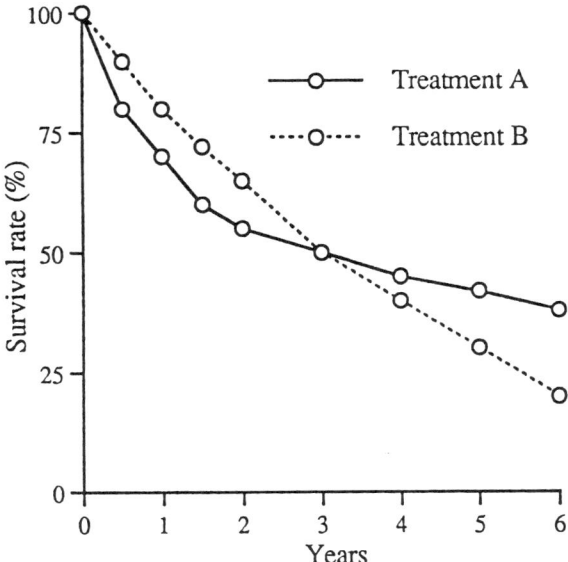

FIGURE 8.3. Example of discrepancy between median and survival rates: both treatments A and B have a 3-year median, but the survival rate differences are 12% at 5 years and 18% at 6 years, respectively.

TABLE 8.7. Advantages and Disadvantages of Trials with Early Stopping Rules Compared with the Fixed-Sample Size Trial

ADVANTAGES	DISADVANTAGES
Decreased number of patients to be included	Decreased precision in the estimation of the treatment effect
Decreased duration of trial	Overestimation or underestimation bias of treatment effect
Decreased cost	More work for the data center
Earlier report of results	Decreased power for estimation of late treatment effects
More ethical for individuals	Less ethical for community

TABLE 8.8. Trial Using a Four-Stage Group Sequential Method

	POCOCK[a]	FLEMING ET AL.[b]	O'BRIEN & FLEMING[c]	PETO & HAYBITTLE[d]
Analysis 1	.018	.0067	.0001	.001
Analysis 1	.018	.0083	.004	.001
Analysis 1	.018	.0098	.019	.001
Analysis 1	.018	.0402	.043	.049

Note. Significance level (type I error) at each stage to maintain an overall significance level of .05 (two-sided test).
[a]From Pocock SJ. Group sequential methods in clinical trials. Biometrika 1977;64:191–199.
[b]From Fleming TR, Harrington DP, O'Brien PC. Designs for group sequential tests. Controlled Clin Trials 1984;5:348–361.
[c]O'Brien PC, Fleming TR. A multiple testing procedure for clinical trials. Biometrics 1979;35:549–556.
[d]From Peto R, Pike MC, Armitage P, et al. Design and analysis of randomized clinical trials requiring prolonged observation of each patient. I. Introduction and design. Br J Cancer 1976;34:585–612; and Haybittle JL. Repeated assessment of results in clinical trials of cancer treatment. J Radiol 1971;44:793–797.

another (100, 146–149). With these methods, the number of interim analyses should be prespecified. Table 8.8 depicts a four-stage trial—three interim analyses and one final analysis—and the P values below which the observed difference is considered statistically significant. These methods and others, such as the triangular test and the α-spending function are discussed elsewhere (150–152). Methods are available for the conduct of interim analyses that were not planned in the protocol (151). Fleming et al. (153) and Pignon and Arriagada (108) discussed problems related to interim analysis in phase III trials with a long-term follow-up. In such trials, it is not unusual to observe a large difference between treatments a short time after beginning treatments, which decreases after a longer period. Nevertheless, the long-term results are often more clinically relevant, and appropriate methods should be used to study them (108, 153). Methods have also been developed for the early stopping of a trial when the difference is lower than that expected (8, 152), but the use of some of these methods has been criticized (154).

When the trial results advocate an early interruption, the lower the number of patients the higher the risk that chance alone will account for the results, even if there is no statistical difference in known prognostic factors between arms of the trial. Furthermore, adjustments for several covariates may be impossible when the number of patients is small. In any case, when there is a discrepancy between adjusted and unadjusted results, the trial conclusions are less convincing. To avoid any data dredging, the following information should be included in the protocol: (a) a list of factors to be checked for imbalance, (b) timing of adjusted interim analyses, and (c) methodology. Each interim analysis should be performed with accurate, comprehensive, updated data. Delays or errors in the processing of data forms could invalidate the analysis (155). Thus, the use of interim analyses implies more work than a fixed-sample design for investigators and for the data center.

One important consequence of early stopping is the decreased precision of results because of the reduced sample size achieved. A difference between treatments may be exaggerated because, when the observed difference is randomly greater than the actual difference, the chance of stopping is higher than when the observed difference is randomly smaller than the actual difference (154, 156).

There are several examples in the literature of an early significant difference that was not corroborated by a longer follow-up (157). If an early difference leads to the interruption of the trial, the resultant statistical power may not be sufficient to evaluate long-term survival. Furthermore, the ability to perform relevant subset analyses may be decreased or lost (155). Premature presentation or publication of interim analyses before the end of accrual or after a short follow-up is generally inappropriate (8, 154).

One randomized trial comparing radiotherapy plus chemotherapy to radiotherapy alone in locally advanced NSCLC and using the O'Brien-Fleming rule—a frequently used sequential group method—is a good example of interim analysis. The planned sample size was 240 patients. The data monitoring committee recommended that the trial be stopped in March 1987, after the fifth interim analysis, when 163 patients were included (158). The trial was closed for accrual 2 months later (158). Its results were presented at the 1988 American Society for Clinical Oncology meeting and published in 1990 (159), and results after 5 years of follow-up were presented at the 1993 meeting of the same group (160). Table 8.9 shows the increase in the

TABLE 8.9. Evolution of p Values with Increased Follow-Up in a Trial Using the O'Brien-Fleming Stopping Rule

"STAGE" (REFERENCE NO.)	NO. OF PATIENTS ANALYSED/ RANDOMIZED (NO. OF FAILURES)	p VALUES LOGRANK TEST/ COX MODEL	MEDIAN FOLLOW-UP
Decision to stop (158)	105/163 (56)	.0015/.0008	8 months
Publication (159)	155/180 (126)	.0066/.0075	34 months
Long-term results (160)	155/180 (?)	.01/?	>5 years

P value with time despite the increasing number of events. This trial has been criticized because (a) 14% of patients were ineligible, (b) the treatment effect was not estimated, and (c) the overestimation bias was not discussed (154, 161). Finally, investigators encouraged the conduct of confirmatory trials (158). Preliminary results of an intergroup trial (162) have corroborated their findings. There was no early stopping in the latter trial, and the difference in median survival was 2.4 months instead of 4 months in the initial study (159).

In case of early stopping, if the follow-up of a published trial is too short, editors should be notified of subsequent results after an additional period of follow-up and should publish a letter or a brief report from the main investigator if there is a significant change in the conclusions (51). Pocock (154) discussed other problems related to the publication of interim analysis.

ETHICS

INFORMED CONSENT AND RANDOMIZATION

Ethics and scientific committees have been organized worldwide to protect patients and ensure that the international declarations on research on human subjects such as the Declaration of Helsinki (163) are respected (Table 8.10). Clinical trials should address important questions and answer them reliably. Although fraud in the conduct of clinical trials is exceptional (164), inadequately conducted studies because of ignorance regarding methodology are more frequent (98). Commitment to a high scientific standard should be extended to the interpretation and publication of the trial (98, 165). Randomized trials have been criticized because they "generate a fundamental conflict of interest within the patient-physician relationship,"

TABLE 8.10. Extracts from the Declaration of Helsinki: Recommendations for Guiding Medical Doctors in Biomedical Research Involving Human Subjects

"research involving human subjects must conform to generally accepted scientific standard"
"concern for the interests of the subject must always prevail over the interest of science and society"
"in any research on human beings, each potential subject must be adequately informed of the aims, methods, anticipated benefits and potential hazards of the study"
"[the patient] should be informed that he/she is at liberty to abstain from participation in the study and that he/she is free to withdraw his/her consent to participate at any time"

From World Health Association. Declaration of Helsinki: recommendation for guiding medical doctors in biomedical research involving human subjects. Helsinki: World Medical Association, 1964.

particularly in life-threatening diseases (166, 167). Physicians should both act in the best interests of the patient and promote the progress of health care based on advances in scientific knowledge. Patients may be randomized only if the physician in charge is uncertain whether one treatment is better than another. This decision should account for possible toxicities and the opinion of the international clinical community (168). The history of the evaluation of medical treatment should be considered before endorsing the preliminary results of a new treatment. There are several examples of widely used and poorly evaluated treatments that were ineffective or toxic, as shown afterward (169, 170). The process of obtaining informed consent is difficult, both for the patient who has just been informed of his/her disease and for physicians, who must explain that they do not know which is the best treatment (171–174). Tattersall and Simes (175) reviewed the issues relating to informed consent. Surveys have shown public sympathy for clinical trials (176, 177). Patients participating in clinical trials may have a better survival than patients treated outside trials (178). Furthermore, there is no evidence of detrimental effect of such participation on survival (178). Because written informed consent is used increasingly worldwide, more time should be devoted to teaching medical students and informing the public about ethical and scientific issues surrounding clinical trials.

Because of the existence of a double standard when a treatment is given inside or outside of a clinical trial, Segelov et al. (179) suggested informed consent as a requirement for nonparticipation in a trial. Chalmers (180) questioned the ethics of not including aged patients. Zelen (181, 182) proposed randomization before obtaining informed consent to facilitate accrual in randomized trials. In this case, informed consent is requested either in the experimental treatment arm only (single randomized consent design) or in both arms (double randomized consent design). Patients are asked whether they accept the randomized treatment or not. If they refuse they receive the treatment used for the other arm or another treatment. Analysis is performed on all randomized patients. This method assumes that the increase in accrual would balance the dilution of the estimated treatment effect because patients did not receive the allocated treatment. However, such was not usually the case in the few trials using this design (183). Furthermore, the insufficiency of the information communicated to the patient has been a cause for ethical concern.

To facilitate accrual in large-scale trials, the Oxford group (184, 185) proposed basing randomization on the uncertainty principle. The physician in charge only considers for randomization patients for whom there is considerable uncertainty regarding the choice between the treatments compared. However, if the physician is reasonably certain that one of the treatments is not appropriate in a particular case, the patient should not be randomized. The uncertainty area changes from one physician to another; for example, in a trial comparing intraportal 5-fluorouracil in colorectal cancer, one surgeon will randomize only Duke's stages B and C, a second physician will randomize all stages, and a third, only young patients. Because of the planned large sample size, the entire spectrum of patients is included and the trial answers both general and specific questions. The main advantage of this method is the drastic reduction in the number of eligibility criteria. Such a method has been used in several trials on cardiovascular diseases and oncology (184, 185).

INTERIM ANALYSES AND DATA MONITORING COMMITTEE

The ultimate goal of randomized trials is not only to demonstrate which is the best treatment in a particular clinical setting, but also to change current therapeutic practice, because a maximal number of patients will benefit from the new treatment. In general, the results of a single trial are not sufficient to convince the medical community that results are valid and applicable to all patients with similar characteristics, and that therapeutic benefits clearly outweigh side effects. If the trial results are equivocal or misleading, patient participation in the trial would have been pointless and thousands of other patients could be treated inappropriately in the future. Thus, ethics concerning individual patients, i.e., the decision to stop the trial, should be balanced against ethics pertaining to the community as a whole, i.e., the ability to choose the best treatment for patients in the future (154, 156, 157).

Treatment effect statistics are not the only contributing factor in the decision to stop a trial. Others, such as treatment toxicity and new results from other trials, should also be considered. Because it is often difficult to reach such a decision, the assistance of experts not directly involved in the trial should be sought (155, 186). In major trials, independent data monitoring committees often are involved in the decision to stop a trial early (154). They review the results of each interim analysis and issue recommendations for the trial coordinators. Pignon et al. (187) recently described experiences with such a process. If results of an interim analysis are given to all trial participants, some investigators may stop entering patients before the final conclusion of the trial and accrual slows; this problem has been experienced by some cooperative groups (155). Thus, results of interim analyses should only circulate within the data monitoring committee. The monitoring of trials currently in practice in Europe and the United States has been reviewed recently (188). Indeed, accrual of the planned sample size in a short period is the best way to limit ethical problems. In this case, however, it may not be possible—except when a short-term effect is studied—to stop accrual before the end of the trial in the event of an unexpected detrimental effect.

REPORTING RESULTS OF CLINICAL TRIALS

Bailar and Mosteller (189) described and explained the guidelines adopted by the International Committee of Medical Journal Editors for statistical reporting in articles to be published. Following two meetings organized by the World Health Organization, recommendations on the standardization of the reporting of results of cancer treatments also were published (59). Simon and Wittes (58) proposed methodologic guidelines for the reporting of clinical trials, and they have been adopted by major cancer journals. Specific guidelines have also been proposed for trials in lung cancer (52, 104).

Criteria for patient selection, the randomization method used, treatment administration, the follow-up procedure, and the evaluation of endpoints should be discussed (51, 58, 63). The a priori hypotheses (treatment difference considered worthwhile, statistical power) and the sample size estimated in the protocol should be given. The use of interim analyses and the reasons for the early stopping of a trial should be reported. The reader should know whether a particular analysis has not been planned in the protocol for subgroup analysis and adjustment for prognostic factors. Whenever possible, the presentation of statistical methods and data should be done in a way such that the analysis could be reproduced or data used to perform other analyses. For instance, all denominators of proportions should be given. The total number of patients randomized per arm; the number, in the event of exclusion; and the reasons for exclusion from the analysis should be described for each arm. With this information, it is possible to compute results, e.g., response rate, in a different way (63). The use of different methods to study the same criterion should be reported, and any discrepancies in results should be discussed. If these methods lead to similar results, a detailed report of the simplest method will suffice, e.g., the log rank test or Cox's model. An exact P value is more informative than is an expression such as $P < 05$. The reader should be able to transform a one-sided result into a two-sided result or to combine data from several trials (189). Investigators also should report the estimation of treatment effects along with their confidence intervals and the statistical power of the trial.

Reporting a time dependent endpoint implies defining the zero point and the event considered, describing its assessment (tests performed, frequency of examination), and the duration of follow-up (59, 190). The number of events observed should be noted for a better appreciation of the amount of information available in a survival analysis. Dates defining the accrual period and the cutoff date for analysis should be reported. When survival curves are given with the number of patients at risk, the number of failures per time interval, and the standard error for survival rates, it is possible to appraise the maturity of the data and the stability of the curves. Median follow-up is often used as a measure of quality. Unfortunately, there is no standard definition for this term (191). Relative risks with their confidence interval are a good summary of a survival comparison. Because of its clinical value, an absolute difference in survival between treatments—or survival rates for each treatment—at some relevant time points is always useful. Relative risks or survival curves with logarithmic ordinates could give the illusion of a strong treatment effect (192). A comparison of survival based on all randomized patients and including death from any cause should be reported because it is the best method for comparing trial results.

Baar and Tannock (63) showed how high-quality and low-quality reporting of the same data could lead to opposite conclusions. Zelen (51) proposed a list of six potential biases to be addressed when comparing a nonrandomized trial with an external control group: (a) physician selection, (b) patient self-selection (informed consent leads to self-selected subgroups), (c) methods for diagnosis and staging, (d) supportive care and patient management, (e) patient evaluation and the quality of follow-up, and (f) prognostic factors. If information on statistical methodology is too long, some of that information could be given in an appendix or sent to readers on request.

META-ANALYSIS

Meta-analysis (or overview) of randomized clinical trials (193) is defined as the use of formal statistical methods to combine the results of separate but similar trials. Unlike a literature review, which is mainly a qualitative process, meta-analysis is a quantitative synthesis of all available data. The advantages of meta-analysis are numerous: (a) an increase in statistical power; (b) the ability to resolve apparently discordant trial results; (c) the improvement in the estimation of the size of the treatment effect; and (d) answers to new questions not previously addressed in individual trials. If most of trials addressing closely related questions are undersized, a review of them exclusively based on P values will conclude that only a few trials are significantly in favor of the new treatment; this result could lead to the erroneous conclusion that the new treatment is ineffective. With meta-analyses, an apparent discrepancy between trials disappears because of an increase in statistical power. Thus, the detection of a moderate, but worthwhile effect is possible. Furthermore, this methodology is an efficient means of expanding the scope of some trials. For instance, survival can be analyzed in a set of trials that included a limited number of patients and whose main endpoint was tumor response.

The most difficult and sensitive step in this kind of study is the choice of selection criteria for trials to be included in the meta-analysis. The authors of this type of investigation should therefore provide the list of included and excluded trials in their publication (194). The more specific the question under study, the more pertinent the results of the meta-analysis will be. However, it may be impossible to find enough patients in trials evaluating this specific question. In such cases, it would be preferable not to perform the meta-analysis and to state publicly that more relevant trials are warranted. Indeed, a large-scale trial is more apt to answer a specific question than a meta-analysis of several trials. Consequently, large trials should be encouraged as well as prospective pooled analysis. Close collaboration between clinicians and statisticians is needed to select inclusion criteria of similar trials, including large numbers of patients, to answer a relevant question with sufficient power and without biases.

The increased use of meta-analyses (195) has led to critical publications on the value of the method from clinical or statistical points of view (8, 196, 197). As shown in Table 8.11, the quality of a meta-analysis is largely dependent on the quality of individual trials. It is always possible to repeat a meta-analysis, but a badly designed or performed trial is definitively lost for the scientific community. Criteria aimed at identifying well-conducted meta-analyses have been proposed (194) as well as guidelines to improve their quality (194, 198).

Meta-analysis is based on the statistical principle (193) that all errors, be they random (play of chance)

TABLE 8.11. Main Factors that Influence the Quality of Meta-Analyses

Factors related to individual trials
    Randomization procedure
    Postrandomization exclusion
    Characteristics of follow-up in each treatment arm
    Evaluation of endpoints
Factors related to trial publication
    Publication bias
    Retrieval bias
Factors related to the meta-analysis itself
    Relevance of the question
    Adopted inclusion criteria and compliance with these criteria
    Choice of endpoints
    Available follow-up
    Statistical power of the meta-analysis
    Choice and interpretation of subgroup analyses
    Choice and interpretation of indirect comparisons

or systematic (biases), must be small if a moderate effect or the absence of an effect is evaluated. To comply with this principle, it is necessary: (*a*) to include only properly randomized trials, i.e., trials in which treatment assignment is totally unpredictable; (*b*) to use an unequivocal endpoint, such as survival, or another objective criterion of evaluation; and (*c*) to perform the analysis on all patients ever randomized (in all trials ever performed on that specific subject) according to the allocated treatment (intent-to-treat analysis). The same considerations on randomization and patient exclusion procedures discussed for trials are, of course, valid for meta-analysis because the most moderate bias could have an effect on the results of the study. The two other key features are the comparability of follow-up between treatment arms and the objectivity of endpoint evaluation. Overall survival is the most frequently used endpoint in cancer meta-analyses. The use of other criteria such as disease free survival could enhance the interest of results, but because this criterion may differ from trial to trial and be difficult to obtain from all trials, it should always be used in conjunction with overall survival.

Trials that obtain significant results are more likely to be published (199). Trials that indicate an apparent large effect may be published prematurely (200) or published more easily in well-known journals. Thus, meta-analysis is subject to publication bias, as is any type of literature-based review. The retrieval of trials through a computer search is insufficient and should be supplemented by other methods (201). The constitution of registries of randomized trials will improve the retrieval of such studies in the future and decrease publication bias.

The Mantel-Haenszel-Peto method is appropriate for the majority of meta-analyses in oncology, but its limitations should be known (122). This method is not specific to meta-analysis and is simply a χ^2 analysis, stratified by trial, using a particular estimator of the odds ratio proposed by Peto. This estimate corresponds to a weighted average of the estimations of the differences in treatment in each trial added. This method is easy to perform and understand. Results can be verified by readers because the data required are usually given in the publication (202) and they can perform additional analyses if they wish to explore related questions. Figure 8.4 gives an example of the results of a meta-analysis. This kind of figure is the best way to study heterogeneity between trials (193). Sometimes it is more useful to attempt to explain why treatment effects from a group of trials are heterogeneous compared with others rather than to estimate an average treatment effect. If the endpoint chosen is overall survival, the literature-based review allows only the study of the survival rate at a fixed time during the follow-up, e.g., 2-year survival rates, and not the whole survival curve, which is possible with individual data-based meta-analyses. However, under specific conditions, e.g., a death rate below 75% (203), both methods may give similar results. The point estimate method is less powerful than the comparison of whole survival curves, particularly if the death rate is high.

Meta-analyses permit subgroup analyses; for example, the results for young and old patients can be compared. Indirect comparisons of the results of trials using long-term tamoxifen versus those using short-term tamoxifen can also be performed (38). These analyses are very useful for the design of future trials aimed at directly testing the generated hypotheses. It is usually impossible to conduct these analyses based on published data, either because the subgroup analysis has not been published for all trials or because of insufficient data in the publications.

The use of individual data may improve the quality of meta-analyses in several ways. Unpublished data may be included, thus decreasing publication bias. The absence of a peer review is counter-balanced by the possibility of directly checking the trial quality with the investigators. For example, it is possible to determine whether the randomization was performed adequately by checking the balance between the two treatment arms (number of patients, distributions) and by analyzing the distribution of randomization dates.

Collaboration between coordinators of the meta-analysis and investigators may help to identify new studies, to improve the relevance of the question posed, and to interpret the results and design future trials. Under such circumstances, meta-analysis would not only be an improved quantitative review of all

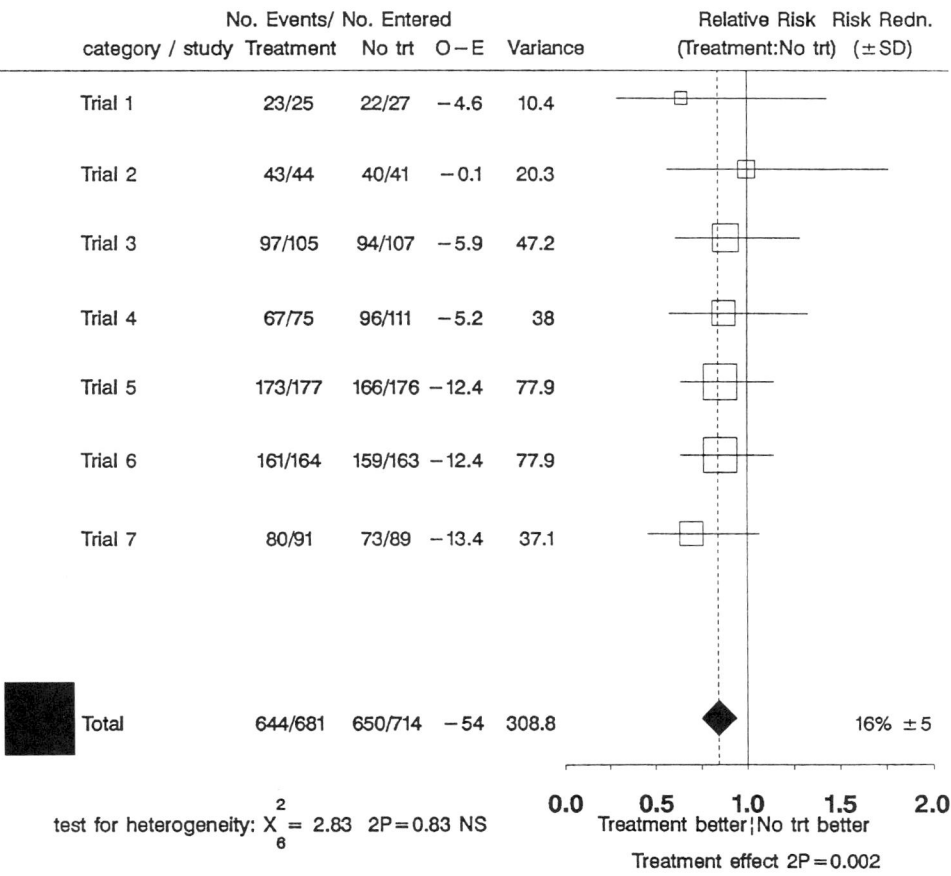

FIGURE 8.4. Example of meta-analysis graph: relative risk of deaths with treatment compared with no treatment (No trt). The open square represents the relative risk (RR) for individual trials and the horizontal line its 95% confidence interval. The area of each open square is proportional to the amount of information from the corresponding trial. The vertical line drawn through unity indicates equivalence or no difference between treatments, relative risk to the right of this line favors the no-treatment group, and those to the left favor the treatment group. The pooled relative risk and its 95% confidence interval are represented by the black diamond. The percentage of the reduction in the relative risk of death is given with its standard deviation. See the Early Breast Cancer Trialists' Collaborative Group (122) and Pignon et al. (204) for a detailed description of the method used.

available randomized data but also a prospective international collaborative endeavor.

Data on patients who were randomized but excluded from published analyses could be retrieved. For example, in a meta-analysis on the role of thoracic radiotherapy in limited small cell lung cancer (198, 204), the proportions of excluded patients were initially 5% in the control arm and 9% in the treatment arm. These proportions were decreased to less than 2% in both arms with the help of investigators.

A better evaluation of long-term survival is possible with an updated follow-up. The best example is the meta-analysis on early breast cancer: the initial median follow-up of the published trials was 5 years (205), and the results after 10 years of follow-up have now been published through a second meta-analysis (32).

A more powerful analysis can be performed using the log rank test, stratified by trials. This method is only applicable if individual data are available. An updated follow-up of each patient further increases the power of the analysis.

Subgroup analyses can be conducted if covariates are available for each patient. A major drawback of meta-analyses based on individual data is that a period of 2 to 3 years is needed before they can be completed. Of course, there is still room for reviews based only on the literature, either as a first step in a study (123) or when a relatively large difference is expected between two treatment arms (more than 10%) (206), but the limitations of this approach should be discussed carefully in the publications (198). Stewart and Parmar (207) analyzed in detail an example of a discrepancy between a meta-analysis based on literature that concluded in favor of the new treatment and a meta-analysis based on individual data that concluded that there was a nonsignificant difference, although the second study had a larger statistical power. They concluded that "unpublished trials, excluded patients, a short follow-up, and fixed timepoint analysis all tend to contribute to an overestimate of the treatment effect." In another example of the role of radiotherapy in SCLC (208), consistent results were found with both methods.

Nicolucci et al. (209), after reviewing randomized trials on lung cancer treatment, concluded that a meta-analysis of existing trials would not be constructive; however, their review was based only on trials published as full papers before 1987. Table 8.12 lists the

TABLE 8.12. Meta-Analyses of Randomized Trials, Performed or Ongoing, in Lung Cancer

	META-ANALYSIS BASED ON	
SUBJECT	INDIVIDUAL DATA (REFERENCE NO.)	LITERATURE (REFERENCE NO.)
Small cell lung cancer		
CT and TRT versus TRT[a]	SCLC meta-analysis (204)	Warde and Payne (210)
PCI versus none[b]	PCI overview[c]	
Non–small cell lung cancer		
CT versus none	NSCLC overview[d] (37)	Grilli et al.[f] (211) Souquet et al.[f] (212)
CDDP versus none	NSCLC collaboration[e]	

Abbreviations: CT, chemotherapy; TRT, thoracic radiotherapy; PCI, prophylactic cranial irradiation; CDPP, cisplatin.
[a]In patients with limited disease.
[b]In complete responders.
[c]R. Arriagada, personal communication on behalf of the PCI Overview Collaborative Group.
[d]In three different settings: surgery plus CT, radical radiotherapy with or without CT, and supportive care with or without CT.
[e]O. Dalesio, personal communication on behalf of the NSCLC Collaboration Group.
[f]In supportive care setting.

FIGURE 8.5. Relation between meta-analysis and randomized clinical trials, and interpretation of the results of meta-analyses according to the results of the significance tests.

meta-analyses of randomized trials performed or currently in progress in lung cancer. Meta-analyses are only one of the tools available for treatment evaluation, and their results should be updated regularly to facilitate decision making regarding treatment. A successful meta-analysis should lead to the design of new trials. As a result of the NSCLC overview (37), large-scale trials on the role of adjuvant cisplatin-based chemotherapy are currently ongoing. Figure 8.5 illustrates the relationship between randomized trials and meta-analysis.

IMPACT OF CLINICAL TRIALS ON CLINICAL PRACTICE

The impact of clinical trials on clinical practice is variable, from no influence at all to marked changes taking many years (213–219). For instance, despite the results of meta-analyses and large-scale trials, aspirin and fibrinolytic treatment have not been disseminated optimally (215, 218, 220). Physicians are more likely to adopt a treatment when trial results are summarized as the relative difference in event rates rather than if the absolute difference is used (216, 217, 219). Research studies on the reasons that guide therapeutic

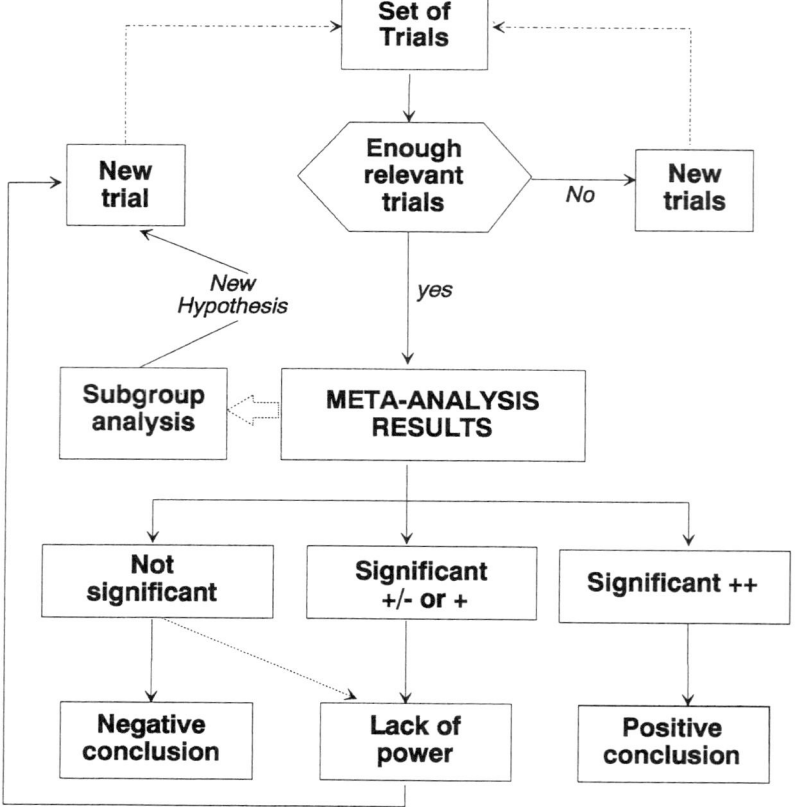

choice and on the mechanisms of dissemination of trial results are limited (214, 218, 221). Results of large, multicenter randomized trials are more likely to influence clinical practice than are other trials (221). Participants in trials are more likely to adopt their own trial results (218, 221). To obtain the rapid dissemination of new therapeutic results, the National Cancer Institute uses clinical announcements—brief communications sent to practicing physicians (222). Another process used to disseminate therapeutic results is the consensus conference. Both methods have been criticized and merit further evaluation (223, 224).

Acknowledgments

We are grateful to L. Saint Ange for editing the manuscript, to G. Feris for secretarial assistance, and to S. Iacobelli for preparing the figures.

References

1. Schwartz D, Flamant R, Lellouch J. Clinical trials. 1980. London: Academic Press, 1980.
2. McDonald CJ, Hui SL. The analysis of humongous databases: problems and promises. Stat Med 1991;10:511–518.
3. Ellwood PM. A technology of patients experience. N Engl J Med 1988;318:1549–1556.
4. Byar DP. Why data bases should not replace randomized clinical trials. Biometrics 1980;36:337–342.
5. Greenfield S. The state of outcome research: are we on target?. N Engl J Med 1989;320:1142–1143.
6. Anonymous. Databases for health care outcomes. Lancet 1989;i:195–196.
7. Green SB, Byar DP. Using observational data from registries to compare treatments: the fallacy of omnimetrics. Stat Med 1984;3:361–370.
8. Simon RM. Design and conduct of clinical trials. In: DeVita VT, Hellman S, Rosenberg SA, eds. Cancer: principles and practice of oncology. 3rd ed. Philadelphia: JB Lippincott, 1989:396–420.
9. Arriagada R, Auquier A. Difficulties in evaluating non-randomized studies. Radiat Oncol 1989;15:307–312.
10. Pocock SJ. Clinical trials. A practical approach. Chichester, England: John Wiley, 1983.
11. Bernard C. Introduction to experimental medicine. New York: Dover Reprint, 1956.
12. Hill AB. The environment and disease: association or causation?. Proc R Soc Med 1965;58:295–300.
13. Kleinbaum DG, Kupper LL, Morgenstern H. Epidemiologic research: principles and quantitative methods. New York: Van Nostrand Reinhold, 1982.
14. MacMahon B, Pugh TF. Epidemiology: principles and methods. Boston: Little, Brown, 1970.
15. Feinstein A. The role of observational studies in the evaluation of therapy. Stat Med 1984;3:341–351.
16. Moses LE. Statistical concepts fundamental to investigations. N Engl J Med 1985;312:890–897.
17. Silagy C, Mant D, Fowler G, Lodge M. Meta-analysis on efficacy of nicotine replacement therapies in smoking cessation. Lancet 1994;343:139–142.
18. Boone CW, Kellof GJ, Malone WE. Identification of candidate cancer chemopreventive agents in their evaluation in animals models and human clinical trials: a review. Cancer Res 1990;50:2–9.
19. Benner SE, Lippman SM, Hong WK. Chemoprevention strategies for lung cancer and upper aerodigestive tract cancer. Cancer Res 1992;52:2758S–2763S.
20. The Alpha-Tocopherol, Beta-Carotene Cancer Prevention Study Group. The effect of vitamin E and beta carotene on the incidence of lung cancers and other cancers in male smokers. N Engl J Med 1994;330:1029–1035.
21. Byar DP. Some statistical considerations for design of cancer prevention trials. Prev Med 1989;18:688–699.
22. Freedman LS, Green SB. Statistical designs for investigating several intervention in the same study: methods for cancer prevention trials. J Natl Cancer Inst 1990;82:910–914.
23. Prentice SJ. Opportunities for enhancing efficiency and reducing cost in large scale disease prevention trials: a statistical perspective. Stat Med 1990;9:161–172.
24. Wittes J, Duggan J, Held P, Yusuf S. Proceedings of "cost and efficiency in clinical trials." Stat Med 1990;9:1–199.
25. Armitage P, Flamant R, Gehan EA. Controlled therapeutic trials in cancer. Part I. The methodology. Geneva: Union Internationale Contre le Cancer (UICC), Technical Report 1974;14:1–24.
26. Carmichael J, Hickson UD. Mechanisms of cellular resistance to cytotoxic drugs and X-irradiation. Int J Radiat Oncol Biol Phys 1991;20:197–202.
27. Duchesne GM, Cassoni AM, Pera MF. Radiosensitivity related to neuroendocrine and endodermal differentiation in lung carcinoma lines. Radiother Oncol 1988;13:153–161.
28. Sörensen JB, Hansen HH. Review of methodological problems in the interpretation of phase II trials in non–small-cell lung cancer. In: Arriagada R, Le Chevalier T, eds. Treatment modalities in lung cancer. Antibiotics and chemotherapy. Basel: Karger, 1988;41:57–64.
29. Moore TD, Korn EL. Phase II trial design considerations for small cell lung cancer. J Natl Cancer Inst 1992;84:150–154.
30. Begg CB. Selection of patients for clinical trials. Semin Oncol 1988;15:434–440.
31. Gail MH. Eligibility exclusions, losses to follow-up, removal of randomized patients, and uncounted events in cancer clinical trials. Cancer Treat Rep 1985;69:1107–1113.
32. Peto R. Clinical trial methodology. Biomedicine 1978;28:24–36.
33. Schwartz D, Lellouch J. Explanatory and pragmatic attitudes in therapeutic trials. J Chronic Dis 1967;20:637–648.
34. Monfardini S, Aapro M, Ferruci L, Zagonel V, Scalliet P, Fentiman I. Commission of the European Communities: "Europe Against Cancer" Programme. European School of Oncology advisory report on cancer treatment in the elderly. Eur J Cancer 1993;29A:2325–2330.
35. Fraumeni JF Jr, Hoover RN, Devesa SS, Kinlen LJ. Epidemiology of cancer. In: DeVita VT, Hellman S, Rosenberg SA, eds. Cancer: principles and practice of oncology. 3rd ed. Philadelphia: JB Lippincott, 1989:396–420.
36. Jensen OM, Esteve J, Moller H, Renard H. Cancer in the European Community and its member states. Eur J Cancer 1990;26:1167–1256.
37. Non–Small Cell Lung Cancer Collaborative Group. Chemotherapy in non–small cell lung cancer: a meta-analysis using updated individual patient data from 52 randomised clinical trials. BMJ 1995: in press.
38. Early Breast Cancer Trialists' Collaborative Group. Systemic treatment of early breast cancer by hormonal, cytotoxic or immune therapy: 133 randomised trials involving 31,000 recur-

rences and 24,000 deaths among 75,000 women. Lancet 1992;339:1–15, 71–85.
39. Deacon J, Peto J. Clinical trial design and evaluation of combined chemotherapy and radiotherapy. In: Horwich A, ed. Combined radiotherapy and chemotherapy in clinical oncology. London: E Arnold, 1992:1–13.
40. Gehan EA. Progress of therapy in acute leukemia 1948–1981: randomized versus non-randomized clinical trials. Controlled Clin Trials 1982;3:199–207.
41. Benson AB, Prokop Pregler JP, Bean JA, Rademaker AW, Eshler B, Anderson K. Oncologists' reluctance to accrue patients onto clinical trials: an Illinois Cancer Center Study. J Clin Oncol 1991;9:2067–2075.
42. Charlson ME, Horwitz RI. Applying results of randomized trials to clinical practice: impact of losses before randomization. BMJ 1984;289:1281–1284.
43. Begg CB, Carbone PP, Elson PJ, Zelen M. Participation of community hospitals in clinical trials. Analysis of five years of experience in the Eastern Cooperative Oncology Group. N Engl J Med 1982;306:1076–1080.
44. Koretz MM, Jackson PM, Torti FM, Carter SK. A comparison of the quality of participation of community affiliates and that of universities in the Northern California Oncology Group. J Clin Oncol 1983;1:640–644.
45. Baum M. New approach for recruitment into randomised trials. Lancet 1993;341:812–813.
46. Institute of Medical Ethics Working Party on the Ethical Implications of AIDS. AIDS, ethics and clinical trials. BMJ 1992;305:699–701.
47. Johnson JR, Temple R. Food and Drug Administration requirements for approval of new anticancer drugs. Cancer Treat Rep 1985;69:1155–1157.
48. Ellenberg SS, Hamilton JM. Surrogate endpoints in clinical trials: cancer. Stat Med 1989;8:405–413.
49. Advanced Colorectal Cancer Meta-Analysis Project. Modulation of fluorouracil by leucovorin in patients with advanced colorectal cancer: evidence in terms of response rate. J Clin Oncol 1992;10:896–903.
50. Rosso R, Salvati F, Ardizzoni A, et al. Etoposide versus etoposide plus high dose cisplatin in the management of advanced non–small cell lung cancer. Cancer 1990;66:130–134.
51. Zelen M. Guidelines for publishing papers on cancer clinical trials: responsibilities of editors and authors. J Clin Oncol 1983;1:164–169.
52. Ihde DC. How should we report results of clinical trials of combined chemotherapy and chest irradiation in limited stage small cell lung cancer?. In: R Arriagada, T Le Chevalier, eds. Treatment modalities in lung cancer. Antibiotic and chemotherapy. Basel: Karger, 1988;41:65–69.
53. Arriagada R, Le Chevalier T, Pignon JP, et al. Initial chemotherapeutic doses and survival in patients with limited small cell lung cancer. N Engl J Med 1993;329:1848–1852.
54. Moertel CG, Hanley JA. The effect of measuring error on the results of therapeutic trials in advanced cancer. Cancer 1976;38:388–394.
55. Warr D, McKinney S, Tannock I. Influence of measurement error on assessment of response to anticancer chemotherapy: proposal for new criteria of tumor response. J Clin Oncol 1984;2:1040–1046.
56. Tannock I, Murphy K. Reflection on medical oncology: an appeal for better clinical trials and improved reporting of their results. J Clin Oncol 1983;1:66–70.
57. Arriagada R, Le Chevalier T, Quoix E, et al., for the GETCB, the FNCLCC, and the CEBI Trialists. Astro plenary: effect of chemotherapy on locally advanced non–small cell lung carcinoma: a randomized study of 353 patients. Int J Radiat Oncol Biol Phys 1991;20:1183–1190.
58. Simon R, Wittes RE. Methodologic guidelines for reports of clinical trials. Cancer Treat Rep 1985;69:1–3.
59. Miller AB, Hoogstraten B, Staquet M, Wrinler A. Reporting results of cancer treatment. Cancer 1981;47:207–214.
60. Oken MM, Creech RH, Tormey DC, et al. Toxicity and response criteria of the Eastern Cooperative Oncology Group. Am J Clin Oncol 1982;5:649–655.
61. Anderson JR, Cain KC, Gelber RD. Analysis of survival by tumor response. J Clin Oncol 1983;1:710–719.
62. Anderson JR, Cain KC, Gelber RD, Gelman RS. Analysis and interpretation of the comparison of survival by treatment outcome variables in cancer clinical trials. Cancer Treat Rep 1985;69:1139–1146.
63. Barr J, Tannock I. Analyzing the same data in two ways: a demonstration model to illustrate the reporting and misreporting of clinical trials. J Clin Oncol 1989;7:969–978.
64. Weiss GB, Bunce H III, Hokanson JA. Comparing survival of responders and non responders after treatment: a potential source of confusion in interpreting cancer clinical trials. Controlled Clin Trials 1983;4:43–52.
65. Parmar MKB. Pitfalls and biases in the reporting and interpretation of the results of clinical trials. Lung Cancer 1994;10 (Suppl):S135–S141.
66. Pignon JP, Ducreux M, Rougier Ph, Lasser Ph. Danger de la comparaison de la survie des répondeurs et des non-répondeurs à une chimiothérapie dans les essais de phase II en Cancérologie. Gastroenterol Clin Biol 1991;15:A140.
67. Gralla RJ, Casper ES, Kelsen DP, et al. Cisplatin and vindesine combination chemotherapy for advanced carcinoma of the lung: a randomized trial investigating two dosage schedules. Ann Intern Med 1981;95:414–420.
68. Sculier JP, Klastersky J, Giner V, et al., for the European Lung Cancer Working Party. Phase II: randomized trial comparing high-dose cisplatin with moderate-dose cisplatin and carboplatin in patients with advanced non–small cell lung cancer. J Clin Oncol 1994;12:353–359.
69. Osoba D. Lessons learned from measuring health-related quality of life in oncology. J Clin Oncol 1994;12:608–616.
70. Aaronson NK. Quality of life assessment in clinical trials: methodologic issues. Controlled Clin Trials 1989;10:195S–208S.
71. Donovan K, Sanson-Fisher RW, Redman S. Measuring quality of life in cancer patients. J Clin Oncol 1989;7:959–968.
72. Aaronson NK. Assessing the quality of life of patients in cancer clinical trials: common problems and common sense solutions. Eur J Cancer 1992;28A:1304–1307.
73. Bergman B, Aaronson NK, Ahmedzai S, Kaasa S, Sullivan M, for the European Organization for Research and Treatment of Cancer (EORTC) Study Group on Quality of Life. The EORTC QLQ-LC13: a modular supplement to the EORTC core quality of life questionnaire (QLQ-C30): for use in lung cancer clinical trials). Eur J Cancer 1994;30A:635–642.
74. Hollen PJ, Gralla RJ, Kris MG, Potanovich LM. Quality of life assessment in individuals with lung cancer: testing the lung cancer symptom scale (LCSS). Eur J Cancer 1993;29A(Suppl 1):S51–S58.
75. Abratt RP. IASLC workshop on improving quality of life and the supportive management of patients with lung cancer. Lung Cancer 1994;10:375–380.
76. Morris J, Goddard M. Economic evaluation and quality for life assessments in cancer clinical trials: the CHART trial. Eur J Cancer 1993;29A:766–770.

77. Nordic Gastrointestinal Tumor Adjuvant Therapy Group. Expectancy of primary chemotherapy in patients with advanced asymptomatic colorectal cancer: a randomized trial. J Clin Oncol 1992;10:904–911.
78. Goldhirsch A, Gelber RD, Simes RJ, Glasziou P, Coates AS, for the Ludwig Breast Cancer Study Group. Costs and benefits of adjuvant therapy in breast cancer: a quality-adjusted survival analysis. J Clin Oncol 1989;7:36–44.
79. Ganz PA, Figlin RA, Haskell CM, La Sotto N, Siau J, for the UCLA Solid Tumor Study Group. Supportive care versus supportive care and combination chemotherapy in metastatic non–small cell lung cancer. Does chemotherapy make a difference?. Cancer 1989;63:1271–1278.
80. Poon MA, O'Connell MJ, Moertel CG, et al. Biochemical modulation of fluorouracil: evidence of significant improvement of survival and quality of life in patients with advanced colorectal carcinoma. J Clin Oncol 1989;7:1407–1418.
81. Feldstein ML. Quality-of-life-adjusted survival for comparing cancer treatments. A commentary on TWIST and Q-TWIST. Cancer 1991;67:851–854.
82. Pignon JP. Essais de phase II en Cancérologie: quoi de neuf? Pour une plus grande coopération multicentrique et multidisciplinaire. Gastroenterol Clin Biol 1992;16:131–133.
83. Gehan EA. The determination of the number of patients required in a preliminary and a follow-up trial of a new chemotherapy agent. J Chronic Dis 1961;13:346–353.
84. Simon R. Optimal two-stage designs for phase II clinical trials. Controlled Clin Trials 1989;10:1–10.
85. Fleming TR. One-sample multiple testing procedure for phase II clinical trials. Biometrics 1982;38:143–151.
86. Bellisant E, Benichou J, Chastang Cl. A comparison of methods for phase II cancer clinical trials: advantages of the triangular test, a group sequential method. Lung Cancer 1994;10: S105–S115.
87. Simon R, Wittes RE, Ellenberg SS. Randomized phase II trials. Cancer Treat Rep 1985;69:1375–1381.
88. Carter SK. Clinical aspect in the design and conduct of phase II trials. In: ME Buyse, MJ Staquet, RJ Sylvester, eds. Cancer clinical trials. Methods and practice. Oxford: Oxford University Press, 1988:223–238.
89. Storer BA. A sequential phase II/III trial for binary outcomes. Stat Med 1990;9:229–235.
90. Byar DP, Simon RM, Friedewald WT, et al. Randomized clinical trials: perspectives on some recent ideas. N Engl J Med 1976;295:74–80.
91. Sacks H, Chalmers TC, Smith H Jr. Randomized versus historical controls for clinical trials. Am J Med 1982;72:233–240.
92. Feinstein AR, Sosin DM, Wells CK. The Will Rogers phenomenon. Stage migration and new diagnostic techniques as a source of misleading statistics for survival in cancer. N Engl J Med 1985;312:1604–1608.
93. Arriagada R, Le Chevalier T. Progrès thréapeutiques dans les cancers bronchiques à petites cellules. Press Med 1988;17: 1851–1856.
94. Gehan EA. The evaluation of therapies: historical control studies. Stat Med 1984;3:315–324.
95. Pocock SJ. Randomized clinical trials (letter). BMJ 1977;1: 1161.
96. Moses LE. The series of consecutive cases as a device for assessing outcomes of interventions. N Engl J Med 1984;311: 705–710.
97. Chalmers TC, Celano P, Sacks HS, Smith H Jr. Bias in treatment assignment in controlled clinical trials. N Engl J Med 1983;309:1358–1361.
98. Nowak R. Problems in clinical trials go far beyond misconduct. Science 1994;264:1538–1541.
99. Pocock SJ, Lagakos SW. Practical experience of randomization in cancer trials: an international survey. Br J Cancer 1982; 46:368–375.
100. Peto R, Pike MC, Armitage P, et al. Design and analysis of randomized clinical trials requiring prolonged observation of each patient. I. Introduction and design. Br J Cancer 1976;34: 585–612.
101. Durrleman S, Simon R. When to randomize? J Clin Oncol 1991;9:116–122.
102. Kalish LA, Begg CB. Treatment allocation methods in clinical trials: a review. Stat Med 1985;4:129–144.
103. Simon R. A decade of progress in statistical methodology for clinical trials. Stat Med 1991;10:1798–1817.
104. Hansen HH, Perry M, Arriagada R, et al. Treatment evaluation. Lung Cancer 1994;10(Suppl 1):S7–S9.
105. Osterlind K. Factors confounding evaluation of treatment effect. Lung Cancer 1994;10(Suppl 1):S97–S103.
106. Taves DR. Minimization: a new method of assigning patients to treatment and control groups. Clin Pharmacol Ther 1974; 15:443–453.
107. Therneau TM. How many stratification factors are "too many" to use in a randomization plan? Controlled Clin Trials 1993; 14:98–108.
108. Pignon JP, Arriagada R. Early stopping rules and long-term follow-up in phase III trials. Lung Cancer 1994;10(Suppl 1): S151–S159.
109. Scheithauer W, Rosen H, Kornek GV, Sebesta C, Depisch D. Randomised comparison of combination chemotherapy plus supportive care with supportive care alone in patients with metastatic colorectal cancer. BMJ 1993;306:752–755.
110. Casagrande JT, Pike MC, Smith PG. An improved formula for calculating sample size for comparing two binomial distributions. Biometrics 1978;34:483–486.
111. George SL. The required size and length of a phase III clinical trial. In: ME Buyse, MJ Staquet, RJ Sylvester, eds. Cancer Clinical trials. Methods and practice. Oxford: Oxford University Press, 1988:287–310.
112. Machin D, Campbell MJ. Statistical tables for the design of clinical trials. Oxford: Blackwell Scientific Publications, 1987.
113. Freiman JA, Chalmers TC, Smith H Jr, Kuebler RR. The importance of beta, the type II error and sample size in the design and interpretation of the randomized controlled trial. Survey of 71 "negative" trials. N Engl J Med 1978;299:690–694.
114. Simon R. A critical assessment of approaches to improving the efficiency of cancer clinical trials. In: Scheurlen H, Kay R, Baum M, eds. Recent results in cancer research. Heidelberg: Springer-Verlag, 1988;111:18–26.
115. Byar DP. Assessing apparent treatment-covariate interactions in randomized clinical trials. Stat Med 1985;4:255–263.
116. Simon R. Statistical tools for subset analysis in clinical trials. In: Scheurlen H, Kay R, Baum M, eds. Recent results in cancer research. Heidelberg: Springer-Verlag 1988;111:55–66.
117. Crowley J. Discussion. Cancer Treat Rep 1985;10:1079–1080.
118. Seydel HG, Creech R, Pagano M, et al. Combined modality treatment of regional small cell undifferentiated carcinoma of the lung: a cooperative study of the RTOG and ECOG. Int J Radiat Oncol Biol Phys 1983;9:1135–1141.
119. Souhami RL. Large-scale studies. In: Williams CJ, ed. Introducing new treatments for cancer. Practical, ethical and legal problem. Chichester, England: John Wiley, 1992:173–187.
120. Freedman LS. The size of clinical trials in cancer research: what are the current needs?. Br J Cancer 1989;59:396–400.

121. Yusuf S, Collins R, Peto R. Why do we need some large, simple randomized trials? Stat Med 1984;3:409–420.
122. Early Breast Cancer Trialists' Collaborative Group. Treatment of early breast cancer. Worldwide evidence 1985–1990. Oxford: Oxford University Press, 1990.
123. Gray R, James R, Mossman J, Stenning S. AXIS. A suitable case for treatment. Br J Cancer 1991;63:841–845.
124. Ray WA, Griffin MR, Avorn J. Evaluating drugs after their approval for clinical use. N Engl J Med 1993;329:2029–2032.
125. Stott H, Fox W, Girling DJ, Stephens RJ, Galton DAG. Acute leukemia after busulphan. BMJ 1977;2:1513–1517.
126. Arriagada R, Rutqvist LE. Adjuvant chemotherapy in early breast cancer and incidence of new primary malignancies. Lancet 1991;338:535–538.
127. Boice JD, Greene MH, Killen JY, et al. Leukemia and preleukemia after adjuvant treatment of gastrointestinal cancer with semustine (methyl-CCNU). N Engl J Med 1983;309:1079–1084.
128. Chalmers TC, Berrier J, Hewitt P, et al. Meta-analysis of randomized controlled trials as a method of estimating rare complications of non-steroidal anti-inflammatory drug therapy. Aliment Pharmacol Ther 1988;2S:9–26.
129. Kaldor JM, Lasset C. Second malignancies following Hodgkin's disease. In: Somers R, Henry-Amar M, Meerwaldt JH, Carde P, eds. Treatment strategies in Hodgkin's disease. Paris: Colloque INSERM/John Libbey Eurotext, 1990;196:139–150.
130. Vokes EE, Weichselbaum RR. Concomitant chemoradiotherapy: rationale and clinical experience in patients with solid tumors. J Clin Oncol 1990;8:911–934.
131. Cardiac Arrhythmia Suppression Trial Investigators. Preliminary report: effect of encainide and flecainide on mortality in a randomized trial of arrhythmia suppression after myocardial infarction. N Engl J Med 1989;321:406–412.
132. Simon R. Confidence intervals for reporting results of clinical trials. Ann Intern Med 1986;105:429–435.
133. Gardner MJ, Altman DG. Statistics with confidence. London: British Medical Journal, 1989.
134. Peto R, Pike MC, Armitage P, et al. Design and analysis of randomised trials requiring prolonged observation of each patient. II. Analysis and examples. Br J Cancer 1977;35:1–39.
135. May GS, Demets DL, Friedman LM, Furberg C, Passamani E. The randomized clinical trials. Bias in analysis. Circulation 1981;64:669–673.
136. The Coronary Drug Project Research Group. Influence of adherence to treatment and response of cholesterol on mortality in the Coronary Drug Project. New Engl J Med 1980;303:1038–1041.
137. Simon R. Importance of prognostic factors in cancer clinical trials. Cancer Treat Rep 1984;68:185–192.
138. Bulpitt CJ. Subgroup analysis. Lancet 1988;2:31–34.
139. Peto J. The calculation and interpretation of survival curves. In: Buyse ME, Staquet MJ, Sylvester RT, eds. Cancer Clinical trials. Methods and practice. Oxford: Oxford University Press, 1988;361–380.
140. Christensen E. Multivariate survival analysis using Cox's regression model. Hepatology 1987;7:1346–1358.
141. Buyse M. Potential and pitfalls of randomized clinical trials in cancer research. Cancer Surv 1989;8:91–105.
142. Breslow N. Comparison of survival curves. In: ME Buyse, MJ Staquet, RT Sylvester, eds. Cancer clinical trials. Methods and practice. Oxford: Oxford University Press, 1988:381–406.
143. Gelman R, Gelber R, Henderson IC, Coleman CN, Harris JR. Improved methodology for analyzing local and distant recurrence. J Clin Oncol 1990;8:548–555.
144. Arriagada R, Kramar A, Le Chevalier T, de Cremoux H, for the French Cancer Centers' Lung Group. Competing events determining relapse free survival in limited small-cell lung carcinoma. J Clin Oncol 1992;10:447–451.
145. McPherson K. Statistics: the problem of examining accumulating data more than once. N Engl J Med 1974;290:501–502.
146. Haybittle JL. Repeated assessment of results in clinical trials of cancer treatment. J Radiol 1971;44:793–797.
147. Pocock SJ. Group sequential methods in clinical trials. Biometrika 1977;64:191–199.
148. O'Brien PC, Fleming TR. A multiple testing procedure for clinical trials. Biometrics 1979;35:549–556.
149. Fleming TR, Harrington DP, O'Brien PC. Designs for group sequential tests. Controlled Clin Trials 1984;5:348–361.
150. Benichou J, Chastang C. Use of the triangular test in the analysis of randomized clinical trials when the response is censored: application to two trials in lung cancer. In: Arriagada R, Le Chevalier T, eds. Treatment modalities in lung cancer. Antibiotics and chemotherapy. Basel: Karger, 1988;41:83–91.
151. Geller NL. Planned interim analysis and its role in cancer clinical trials. J Clin Oncol 1987;5:1485–1490.
152. Souhami RL, Whitehead J. Workshop on early stopping rules in cancer clinical trials. Robinson College, Cambridge, U.K., 13–15 April 1993. Stat Med 1994;13:1289–1499.
153. Fleming TR, Green SJ, Harrington DP. Consideration for monitoring and evaluating treatment effects in clinical trials. Controlled Clin Trials 1984;5:55–66.
154. Pocock SJ. When to stop a clinical trial. BMJ 1992;305:235–240.
155. Green SJ, Fleming TR, O'Fallon JR. Policies for study monitoring and interim reporting of results. J Clin Oncol 1987;5:1477–1484.
156. Pocock SJ, Hughes MD. Practical problems in interim analyses, with particular regard to estimation. Controlled Clin Trials 1989;10:209S–221S.
157. Bartelink H, Jassem J. Early presentation of results in clinical trials: an ethical dilemma for medicine and science. Eur J Cancer 1990;26:419.
158. Propert KJ, Kim K. Group Sequential methods in multi-institutional cancer clinical trials. In: Peace KE, ed. Biopharmaceutical sequential statistical applications. New York: Marcel Dekker, 1992:133–153.
159. Dillman RO, Seagren SL, Propert KJ, et al. A randomized trial of induction chemotherapy plus high-dose radiation versus radiation alone in stage III non–small cell lung cancer. N Engl J Med 1990;323:940–945.
160. Dillman RO, Seagren SL, Herndon J, Green MR. Randomized trial of induction chemotherapy plus radiation therapy versus RT alone in stage III non–small cell lung cancer (NSCLC: five-year follow-up of CALGB 84-33). Proc Am Soc Clin Oncol 1993;12:329.
161. Souhami RL, Spiro SG, Cullen M. Chemotherapy and radiation therapy as compared with radiation therapy in stage III non–small cell lung cancer (letter). N Engl J Med 1991;324:1136.
162. Sause W, Scott C, Taylor S, et al. RTOG 8808 ECOG 4588, preliminary analysis of a phase III trial in regionally advanced unresectable non–small cell lung cancer. Proc Am Soc Clin Oncol 1994;13:325.
163. World Medical Association. Declaration of Helsinki: recommendation for guiding medical doctors in biomedical research involving human subjects. In: Mason JK, McCall Smith RA, eds. Laws and medical ethics. London: Butterworth, 1991:446–449.

164. Cohen J. Clinical trial monitoring: hit or miss?. Science 1994;264:1534–1537.
165. Altman DG. Statistics and ethics in medical research. BMJ 1980;281:1182–1184.
166. Truog RD. Randomized controlled trials of potentially life-saving therapies: are they ethical. Coron Artery Dis 1993;4:835–836.
167. Hellman S, Hellman DS. Of mice but not men. Problems of the randomized clinical trial. New Engl J Med 1991;324:1585–1589.
168. Freedman B. Equipoise and the ethics of clinical research. N Engl J Med 1987;317:141–145.
169. Passamani E. Clinical trials: are they ethical? N Engl J Med 1991;324:1589–1592.
170. Poland RL. Randomized clinical trials (letter). N Engl J Med 1991;325:1513.
171. Thornton HM. Breast cancer trials: a patient's viewpoint. Lancet 1992;339:44–45.
172. Cavalli R. Randomized trials: what's the problem? Ann Oncol 1992;3:96.
173. Williams CJ, Zwitter M. Informed consent in European multicentre randomised clinical trials: are patients really informed?. Eur J Cancer 1994;30A:907–910.
174. Tobias JS, Houghton J. Is informed consent essential for all chemotherapy studies? Eur J Cancer 1994;30A:897–899.
175. Tattersall MHN, Simes RJ. Issues of informed consent. In: Williams CJ, ed. Introducing new treatments for cancer. Practical, ethical and legal problem. Chichester, England: John Wiley 1992:79–90.
176. Kemp N, Skinner E, Toms J. Randomized clinical trials of cancer treatment: a public opinion survey. Clin Oncol 1984;10:155–161.
177. Cassileth BR, Lusk EJ, Miller DS, Hurwitz S. Attitudes toward clinical trials among patients and the public. JAMA 1982;248:968–970.
178. Stiller C. Survival of patients in clinical trials and at specialist centres. In: Williams CJ, ed. Introducing new treatments for cancer: practical, ethical and legal problems. Chichester, England: John Wiley, 1992:119–136.
179. Segelov E, Tattersall MHN, Coates AS. Redressing the balance: the ethics of not entering an eligible patient on a randomised clinical trial: point of view. Ann Oncol 1992;3:103–105.
180. Chalmers TC. Ethical implications of rejecting patients for clinical trials. JAMA 1990;263:865.
181. Zelen M. A new design for randomized clinical trials. N Engl J Med 1979;300:1242–1245.
182. Zelen M. Randomized consent designs for clinical trials: an update. Stat Med 1990;9:645–656.
183. Parmar MKB. Randomization before consent: practical and ethical considerations. In: Williams CJ, ed. Introducing new treatment for cancer. Practical, ethical and legal problem. Chichester, England: John Wiley 1992:189–201.
184. Stenning S. "The uncertainty principle": selection of patients for cancer clinical trials. In: Williams CJ, ed. Introducing new treatments for cancer. Practical, ethical and legal problem. Chichester, England: John Wiley, 1992:161–172.
185. Collins R, Doll R, Peto R. Ethics of clinical trials. In: Williams CJ, ed. Introducing new treatments for cancer. Practical, ethical and legal problem. Chichester, England: John Wiley, 1992:49–65.
186. Chalmers TC, Block JB, Lee S. Controlled studies in clinical cancer research. N Engl J Med 1972;287:75–78.
187. Pignon JP, Arriagada R, Le Chevalier T, et al. Triangular test and randomized trials: practical problems in a small cell lung cancer trial. Stat Med 1994;13:1415–1422.
188. Ellenberg SS, Geller G, Simon R, Yusuf S. Proceedings of the workshop on "practical issues in data monitoring of clinical trials." Stat Med 1993;12:415–615.
189. Bailar JC, Mosteller F. Guidelines for statistical reporting in articles for medical journals. Amplifications and explanations. Ann Intern Med 1988;108:266–273.
190. Rudnick SA, Feinstein AR. An analysis of the reporting of results in lung cancer drug trials. J Natl Cancer Inst 1980;64:1337–1343.
191. Shuster JJ. Median follow-up in clinical trials (letter). J Clin Oncol 1991;9:191–192.
192. Mueller CB. Breast cancer: reporting results with inflationary arithmetic. Am J Clin Oncol 1994;17:86–92.
193. Yusuf S, Simon R, Ellenberg S. Proceedings of the workshop on methodologic issues in overviews of randomized clinical trials. Stat Med 1987;6:217–409.
194. Sacks HS, Berrier J, Reitman J, Ancona-Berk VA, Chalmers TC. Meta-analysis of randomized controlled trials. N Engl J Med 1987;316:450–455.
195. Gelber RD, Goldhirsch A. Meta-analysis: the fashion of summing-up evidence. Part I. Rationale and conduct. Ann Oncol 1991;2:461–468.
196. Goldman L, Feinstein AR. Anticoagulants and myocardial infarction: the problem of pooling, drowning, and floating. Ann Intern Med 1979;90:92–94.
197. Thompson SG, Pocock SJ. Can meta-analyses be trusted?. Lancet 1991;338:1127–1130.
198. Pignon JP, Arriagada R. Meta-analyses of randomized clinical trials: how to improve their quality?. Lung Cancer 1994;10 (Suppl 1):S135–S141.
199. Dickersin K, Chan S, Chalmers TC, Sacks HS, Smith H. Publication bias and clinical trials. Controlled Clin Trials 1987;8:343–353.
200. Simes J. Publication bias: the case for an international registry of clinical trials. J Clin Oncol 1986;4:1529–1541.
201. Pignon JP, Ducreux M, Rougier P. Meta-analysis of adjuvant chemotherapy in gastric cancer: a critical reappraisal (letter). J Clin Oncol 1994;12:877–878.
202. Pignon JP, Arriagada R. Meta-analysis of thoracic radiotherapy for small cell lung cancer (letter). N Engl J Med 1992;328:1425–1426.
203. Buyse M, Ryan LM. Issues of efficiency in combining proportions of deaths from several clinical trials. Stat Med 1987;6:565–576.
204. Pignon JP, Arriagada R, Ihde DC, et al. A meta-analysis of thoracic radiotherapy for small-cell lung cancer. N Engl J Med 1992;327:1618–1624.
205. Early Breast Cancer Trialists Collaborative Group. Effects of adjuvant tamoxifen and of cytotoxic therapy on mortality in early breast cancer. An overview of 61 randomized trials among 28,896 women. N Engl J Med 1988;319:1681–1692.
206. Poynard T, Pignon JP. Duodenal ulcer. Analyses of 293 randomized clinical trials. Montrouge: John Libbey Eurotext, 1989.
207. Stewart LA, Parmar MKB. Meta-analysis of the literature or of individual patient data: is there a difference? Lancet 1993;341:418–422.
208. Pignon JP, Arriagada R. Meta-analysis (letter). Lancet 1993;341:964–965.
209. Nicolucci A, Grilli R, Alexanian AA, Apolone G, Torri V,

Liberati A. Quality, evolution, and clinical implications of randomized, controlled trials on the treatment of lung cancer. A lost opportunity for meta-analysis. JAMA 1989;262:2101–2107.
210. Warde P, Payne D. Does thoracic irradiation improve survival and local control in limited-stage small cell carcinoma of the lung? A meta-analysis. J Clin Oncol 1992;10:890–895.
211. Grilli R, Oxman AD, Julian JA. Chemotherapy for advanced non–small cell lung cancer: how much benefit is enough?. J Clin Oncol 1993;11:1866–1872.
212. Souquet PJ, Chauvin F, Boissel JP, et al. Polychemotherapy in advanced non–small cell lung cancer: a meta-analysis. Lancet 1993;342:19–21.
213. Garnier HS, Flamant R, Fohanno C. Assessment of the role of randomized clinical trials in establishing treatment policies. Controlled Clin Trials 1982;3:227–234.
214. Boissel JP. Impact of randomized clinical trials on medical practices. Controlled Clin Trials 1989;10:120S–134S.
215. Lamas GA, Pfeffer MA, Hamm P, Wertheimer J, Rouleau JL, Braunwald E, for the SAVE investigators. Do the results of randomized clinical trials of cardiovascular drugs influence medical practice? New Engl J Med 1992;327:241–247.
216. Forrow L, Taylor WC, Arnold RM. Absolutely relative: how research results are summarized can affect treatment decisions. Am J Med 1992;92:121–124.
217. Naylor CD, Chen E, Strauss B. Measured enthusiasm: does the method of reporting trial results alter perceptions of therapeutic effectiveness? Ann Intern Med 1992;117:916–921.
218. Ketley D, Woods KL. Impact of clinical trials on clinical practice: example of thrombolysis for acute myocardial infarction. Lancet 1993;342:891–894.
219. Bobbio M, Demichelis B, Giustetto G. Completeness of reporting trials results: effect on physicians' willingness to prescribe. Lancet 1994;343: 1209–1211.
220. Moher M, Johnson N. Use of aspirin by general practitioners in suspected acute myocardial infarction. BMJ 1994;308:760.
221. Stephens R, Gibson D. The impact of clinical trials on the treatment of lung cancer. Clin Oncol 1993;5:211–219.
222. Friedman MA. The clinical announcement policy of the National Cancer Institute. In: Williams CJ, ed. Introducing new treatments for cancer. Practical, ethical and legal problem. Chichester, England: John Wiley, 1992:413–419.
223. Smith T. Achieving a consensus on cancer treatment. In: Williams CJ, ed. Introducing new treatments for cancer. practical, ethical and legal problem. Chichester, England: John Wiley, 1992:437–445.
224. Omura GA. Cancer clinical alerts: less than wise. In: Williams CJ, ed. Introducing new treatments for cancer. practical, ethical and legal problem. Chichester, England: John Wiley, 1992:421–436.

9

Modern Principles of Radiation Therapy

Paul Van Houtte, Stéphane Simon, and René Regnier

The practice of radiotherapy requires a knowledge of the disease treated (oncology), the physics of the radiation (radiophysics), and the effect on normal tissue and tumors (radiobiology). The progress in radiation oncology made during recent decades resulted not only from major improvements in technical equipment but also from a better understanding of the interaction between radiation and tumors, thus leading to the development of new treatment modalities. In this brief review of radiophysics and radiobiology, only basic principles are discussed. Several textbooks are available for more details (1–7).

BASIC CONCEPTS OF RADIATION PHYSICS

Atomic and Nuclear Structures

The atom may be seen as a central core composed by protons with a positive electric charge and neutrons surrounded by small orbiting particles, the electrons, bearing a negative charge. A neutral atom must have the same number of positive and negative charges. The electrons revolve around the nucleus on specific orbits: a specific energy links the negatively charged particles, the electrons, with the positive charges of the protons located in the nucleus. This energy decreases as the electrons orbit farther from the nucleus. To move an electron from one orbit to another one farther from the nucleus, energy must be supplied to the particle; this process is called excitation. Ionization is the process of removing an electron completely from the atom, thus creating an ion, a charged particle that is unstable and interacts to reach a steady state.

Absorption of Radiation in Matter

X-rays and τ-rays may be considered a series of photons each representing a quantity of energy. When photons penetrate a tissue, they either pass through or interact with the atomic electrons or with the nucleus, thus, there is a probability of interaction leading to an attenuation and diffusion of the entering beam. This probability depends on the specific mass attenuation for the beam energy considered and on the thickness of the tissue.

The photon may interact with the matter in several ways, but only three are relevant for radiation oncology. In the photoelectric effect, the total energy of the photon is transferred to an orbital electron; this electron, usually located on an orbit close to the nucleus, is ejected with an energy equal to the photon minus the binding energy of the electron. This electron loses its energy through excitation and ionization processes with nearby atoms and molecules. The atom is left with a vacancy on one of its orbits that is filled by an electron located farther away with the emission of a characteristic x-ray. Photoelectric absorption varies with the cube of the atomic number. This variation explains the shielding efficacy of lead and the better absorption in bones of lower energy x-rays (orthovoltage) in which this effect is predominant. The Compton effect represents an interaction between an incident photon and a loosely bound electron; the incident photon is scattered in a different direction with less energy, and the electron gains the fraction of the energy lost by the photon. The expulsed electron thereafter loses its energy through Coulomb's interactions with other charged particles of the medium. This interaction is not dependent on the atomic number (Z). The third interaction is the pair production in which positive and negative electrons are created in the vicinity of a nucleus at the same time; however, this interaction requires a photon with a minimum energy of 1.022 MeV. This interaction is highly dependent on the Z number.

The relative importance of these three interaction processes depends on the photon energy and the Z number. With superficial x-ray machines, the photoelectric process dominates, whereas for linear accelerators or telecobalt units (photons having an energy in excess of 1 MeV), the absorption mainly results from a Compton interaction.

TYPES OF CLINICAL RADIATION

The radiation used in clinical practice is called ionizing radiation. During absorption in tissues, ionizing radiation produces the ejection of an orbital electron, creating an ion. Different types of radiation are available, e.g., electromagnetic or particulate (electrons, protons, neutrons, π-mesons, ions). Except for electrons, most of the other particulate radiations are used primarily in clinical research rather than in daily clinical practice.

Electromagnetic radiation can be represented by a varying electrical and magnetic field traveling at the speed of light in a vacuum. This group includes visible light; radio, infrared, and ultraviolet light; and x-rays and τ-rays. The sinusoidal wave is characterized by its wavelength and frequency. The energy of the radiation is directly proportional to the frequency and inversely proportional to the wavelength: when the latter decreases, the energy increases. This wave representation explains the propagation of the radiation. Although electromagnetic waves have no rest mass, the quantum theory considers them to be little packets of energy called photons, a representation that better explains their interaction with the matter. The photon energy is directly proportional to its frequency through a constant of proportionality, Planck's constant (numerical value, 6.625×10^{-34} joule-seconds).

EXTERNAL RADIATION THERAPY TREATMENT EQUIPMENT

Before 1951 most treatment units available were x-ray machines producing only photon beams with limited penetration. The degree of penetration is used to differentiate the different machines: contact units are used to treat superficial tumors such as skin cancers, and the orthovoltage units operate in the range of 200 to 300 kVp.

In the 1950s the development of supervoltage units (cobalt 60 [^{60}Co] and cesium 137 [^{137}Cs] teletherapy, betatron, linear accelerator, and, more recently, microtron units) radically changed radiotherapy practice by offering better performing machines, both in terms of beam energy available and accuracy. Telecobalt units were introduced after 1951 and are still used widely. They emit two high-energy τ-rays (1.17 and 1.33 MeV) and have a high specific activity (the physical size of the source can be kept very small, reducing the problem of beam focalization). The main advantage of this machine is the stability of the beam intensity and its reliability. The major concerns relate to radioprotection issues, e.g., the source needs to be replaced because of the decay of the isotope (half-life, 5.26 years).

Modern betatron units can produce photon beams with energies of more than 40 MV. They are obtained by an acceleration of electrons by magnetic induction in a circular structure. X-ray beams are obtained by making the electrons strike a target in heavy metal; otherwise, the electrons can be extracted, providing electron beams. The main limitations of the betatron are the large size of the machine, the low dose rate, and the small size of the field available for clinical use (less than 20 cm × 20 cm).

Linear accelerators are becoming the most common machines in radiation therapy departments. The linear accelerator uses high-frequency electromagnetic waves to accelerate electrons to high energy through a microwave accelerator structure; it can produce photon or electron beams of different energies. Linear accelerators or telecobalt units are now designed to work in an isocentric way: the source of the radiation rotates around a horizontal axis (the gantry axis). This design allows the patients to stay in the same position during the treatment while the machine turns around them in the different fields, increasing the treatment accuracy. Cyclotrons are used to produce proton or neutron beams. The microtron combines the principles of a linear accelerator and a cyclotron.

RADIATION BEAMS: ADVANTAGES AND DRAWBACKS

Each radiation beam has some advantages and drawbacks; depending on the goal of the treatment, the role of the radiophysicists and radiation oncologists is the selection of the most appropriate radiation beams for each individual clinical situation. Megavoltage radiation produced by telecobalt units and linear accelerators offers numerous advantages:

Skin-sparing effect: in contrast to earlier x-ray units, the maximum absorbed dose is no longer located at the level of the skin but rather a few millimeters or centimeters below, depending on the energy output of the unit (Fig. 9.1).
This high energy allows a better penetration into the tissues, enabling treatment of deeply located tumors.

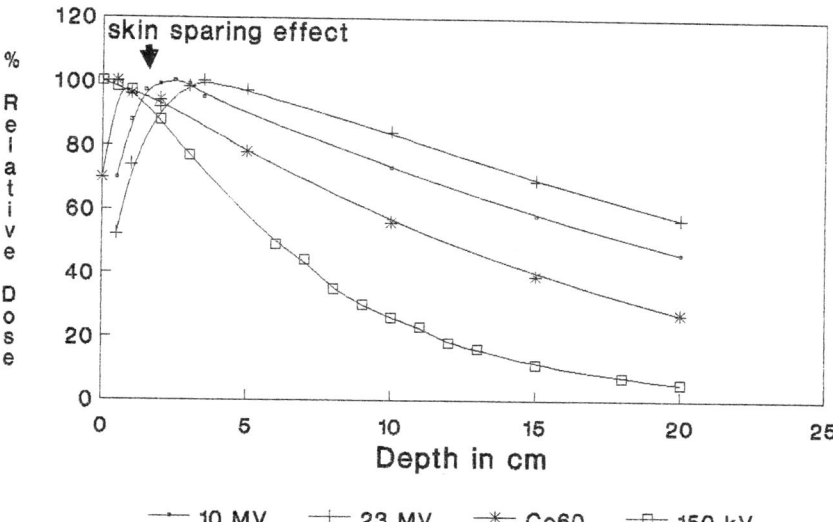

FIGURE 9.1. Examples of the central axis percentage depth dose for different photon beams.

A better collimation permits the reduction of side scatter and the beam's focalization, increasing the accuracy of the treatment.

Within this energy range, the interaction takes place through the Compton effect, independently from the atomic number: this feature avoids increasing dose absorption into the bone.

The available field sizes are larger, reducing the need to treat with several adjacent fields and eliminating the problems of gaps between adjacent fields.

Because the maximum range of an electron in a medium is proportional to its energy, electron beams offer the main advantage of a sharp fall-off in depth dose. The dose is then rather uniform from the surface to the depth at which the fall-off region begins (Fig. 9.2). Disadvantages include the fact that the dose approaches 90% of the maximum dose within the first few millimeters, reducing the skin-sparing effects. Another problem with electron beams is that their range is modified markedly by bones or air cavities.

Heavier charged particles such as protons, ions, and π-mesons show a better radiation dose distribution because of the Bragg peak, i.e., the maximum dose absorption situated within a narrow region with a relative sparing until that peak and a perfect sparing after it. Furthermore, some of those charged particulate beams (i.e., ions, but excluding accelerated protons and π-mesons) and neutron beams producing recoil protons show greater radiobiologic differences because of their high linear energy transfer (LET), defined as the density of absorbed energy along the trajectory of a charged particle by unit length. The LET is expressed in kiloelectron volts per micrometer. In some cases the radiobiologic differences of high LET radiations might offer several advantages, but these particle beams are still not part of the daily clinical armamentarium.

DOSE DISTRIBUTION AND UNITS

The plot of dose along the central axis into tissue from the point of beam entry is called the central axis depth dose curve. The data are expressed as a percentage of the absorbed dose to a fixed reference point on the central axis, the point of maximum absorbed dose. The depth dose curves vary with the distance between the source and the skin, the beam energy, and the field size. The data usually are presented as isodose curves: these curves refer to lines of equal absorbed dose within the matter or the patient. They usually are expressed as percentages and are normalized to specific reference points.

Several devices have been developed to modify the characteristics of the beams. Tissue compensators and wedges are used to compensate for some anatomic distortion leading either to overdosage or underdosage of some areas. The wedge-shaped filters are constructed of lead or brass, shift the isodose of different angles, and are interposed in the radiation beam to cause a planned asymmetry in the isodose curves. Currently, special beam modifier devices may be built with different thicknesses to improve the dose distribution in all directions.

In radiation practice, the inverse square law plays an important role, i.e., for the radiation spreading from a source, the intensity of the radiation varies inversely with the square of the distance between the source and

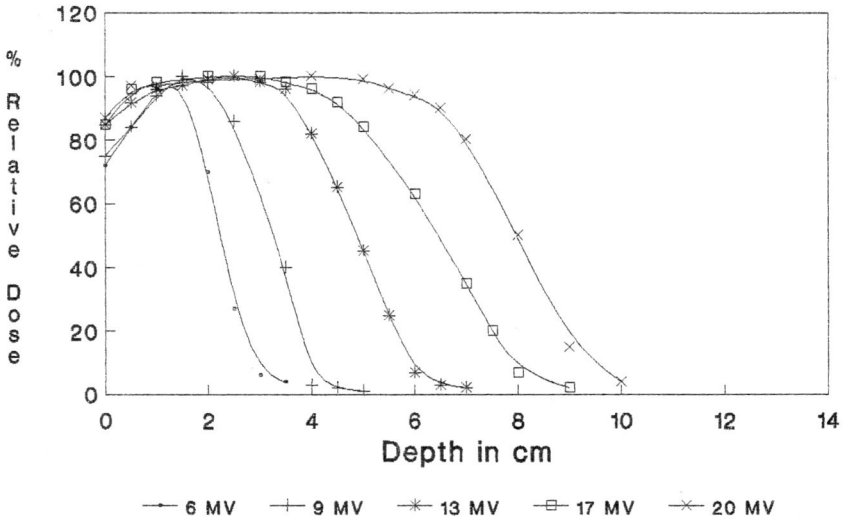

FIGURE 9.2. Examples of the central axis percentage depth dose for different electron beams.

the point considered. This law has more influence on short source skin distance, low energy machines, and brachytherapy techniques.

The fundamental quantity necessary to describe the interaction of radiation with the matter is the amount of energy absorbed per unit of mass. Currently, the recommended absorbed dose unit is the Gray (Gy), which represents the absorption of one joule per kilogram. This unit replaces the term rad, which is the absorption of 100 ergs per gram of tissue. One Gray is equivalent to 100 rad. Note that these are only physical units and do not necessarily translate into biologic effect.

BRACHYTHERAPY AND PHYSICS

In brachytherapy techniques radioactive isotopes are inserted into the patient to deliver the radiation dose. The different radioactive elements emit three main different types of radiation: α particles (two positive charges and two neutrons corresponding to a helium nucleus), β particles (particles similar to electrons but that can also carry an elementary positive charge), and τ-rays, which are electromagnetic radiation. α-Particles are not relevant for clinical practice because of their very short penetration and high toxicity.

Radioactive isotopes are characterized by their decay constant, half-life, and type of radiation. The activity describes the number of disintegrations per unit of time of a sample. In the past the activity was expressed in curies: one curie being equal to the number of disintegrations in 1 second of 1 g of radium 226; this measure is equivalent to 3.7×10^{10} disintegrations. The unit currently used is the Becquerel (Bq), which corresponds to one disintegration per second.

TABLE 9.1. Characteristics of Radioisotopes Used for Brachytherapy

		ENERGY		
ISOTOPE	HALF-LIFE	α	β	γ (MEV)
Radium 226	1600 hr	+	+	0.011–2.45
Cesium 137	30 yr	...	+	0.004–0.662
Cobalt 60	5 yr	...	+	1.17 + 1.33
Iridium 192	74 d	...	+	0.009–0.872
Iodine 125	60 d	...	...	0.004–0.035
Gold 198	2.7 d	...	+	0.01–1.09
Yttrium 90	64 hr	...	+	...
Phosphorus 32	14 d	...	+	...

Table 9.1 presents some of the most commonly used isotopes in brachytherapy. Most isotopes used in clinical practice have photon radiation energy below 1 MeV except for ^{60}Co and radium sources. During the last decade, radium sources, which originally were used at the many cancer centers, have been replaced increasingly for radioprotection reasons (radium decays to a harmful radioactive gaseous compound, and the radon and high-energy photon radiation pose shielding problems) and because of the higher flexibility of the new radioisotope sources, such as iridium wires or cesium sources. The inverse square law governs the dose distribution and has a major impact on results. The geometric distribution of the different sources is the keystone of the success of an implant. The radioisotopes may be kept in a special envelope designed to filter the undesirable radiation such as α particles or low-energy β radiation. Different applicators have been designed to hold the sources in position; often they are built to push the tissues away from the source, thus reducing the rapid fall-off of the dose,

or they have some special shielding design that decreases the dose to specific area.

PRINCIPLES OF RADIOBIOLOGY

The interaction of ionizing radiation with the matter proceeds through a cascade of events from the initial ionization and excitation process to the later biologic or genetic effects. If the former, events take only a fraction of seconds; the latter requires weeks, months, or years to develop. Several stages are considered:

The physical stage is characterized by ionization and excitation process.

In the physicochemical stage, ionizations produced by radiation are random events. Molecules not affected by the initial physical process may undergo radiation-related changes because of energy transfer from other ionized molecules. There are two types of chemical changes: the direct effect on important target molecules, mainly the DNA, and the indirect effect, produced by a series of intermediary radiation products. Because tissues and cells are composed primarily of water, the indirect reaction mostly involves water molecules creating oxidizing radicals (hydroxyl groups) and highly reducing radicals (H^+ and free electrons). These radicals may interact to form molecular hydrogen and hydrogen peroxide. The lifetime of free radicals, because of their high reactivity, is very short, thus the interactions take place within a short distance (less than 20 angstroms). The direct or indirect effects induce changes in the nucleic acids (change or loss of base, single- and double-strand breakage, hydrogen bond breakage between strands), in proteins (damage to chain groups and modifications in their structure), and in lipids (formation of peroxides, which is particularly important for the lipids included in the cell membranes).

The biologic stage represents the response of the tissues and organs to the chemical products induced by the radiation. Acute or late effects, including issues relating to genetics and carcinogenesis, are the possible clinical expression.

In clinical practice the radiation cell kill is caused by the loss of the capacity for clonogenic cells to proliferate or divide. In fact, cells that are sufficiently damaged die during one of the following mitosis stages and lose their capacity for sustained cell division. This phenomenon explains the delay between the administration of radiation and the clinical effects: often the tumor clearance is seen weeks or months after completion of the radiation therapy, especially for slowly dividing tumors such as prostatic or rectal cancers.

Programmed cell death or apoptosis also occurs after radiation. This form of cell death is more important in lymphomas and is almost absent in sarcomas (8). Because experimentally this process peaks in the first hours after irradiation of tumors, apoptosis may be the prominent factor for tumors responding quickly to a low radiation dose. Radiation exposure also produces a mitotic delay through a temporary block of cells in the G2 phase of the cell cycle. Rapid cell death of nondividing or dividing cells requires single doses in excess of 50 Gy, which are not used in clinical practice.

CELL SURVIVAL AND SURVIVAL CURVES

Radiation effects on dividing cells are random events. The proportion of surviving cells decreases as the radiation dose increases. For most mammalian cells, after an initial "shoulder," the radiation killing is exponential (Fig. 9.3); thus, for a given dose increment, the same proportion of cells is killed but not the same number. In the low-dose region, the shoulder represents a reduced efficiency of cell killing. These

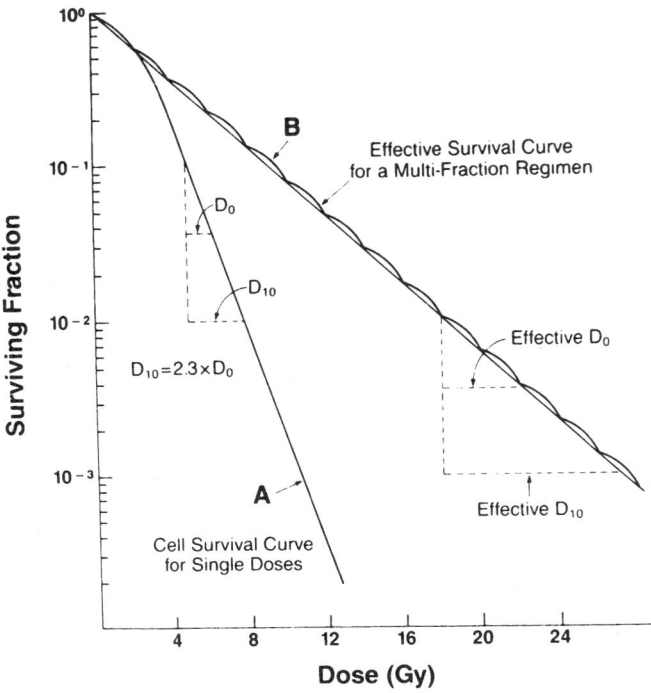

FIGURE 9.3. Survival curve for one or several fractions. If the time interval between fractions is long enough to allow full repair of sublethal damage, the shoulder of the survival curve is reproduced. (From Hall EJ. Radiobiology for the radiologist. 4th ed. Philadelphia: Lippincott, 1994.)

survival curves are described by their shoulder (the dose difference needed to achieve the same killing effect [Dq] or the extrapolation number [n]) and their slope (the dose required to reduce the survival to 37% in the exponential part of the curve [Do]) (Fig. 9.3). The survival curves differ for different species (bacteria, mammalian cells), types of tumor cells, and growth conditions.

After irradiation the cells may be damaged lethally, or the lesions induced may be subject to some repair process. Two types of repair damage are considered: potentially lethal damage and sublethal damage. Most of these repair processes take place in the first few hours after irradiation. Thus, if a second course of irradiation is given, this additional irradiation repeats the same survival curve shape with the initial shoulder. Therefore, the cell kill by two courses of half-fraction radiation separated by a few hours is less than that of a single fraction; thus a much larger radiation dose is required to achieve the same degree of cell killing with a fractionated radiation course. The dose difference needed to achieve the same killing effect is a measure of the sublethal damage repair. There must be a difference in dose needed to achieve the same killing effect between the tumor and normal tissues for fractionation to offer some clinical advantage.

Potential lethal damage repair represents another form of cell recovery. If cells are held under poor conditions (i.e., conditions that stop or slow the normal cell division), cells may even have time to repair potential lethal damage. Weichselbaum (9) correlated the tumor cell potential lethal damage repair measured in vitro with the tumor radioresistance. In brachytherapy technique the irradiation is given continuously over a period of time. If the dose rate is low enough, such as the low or medium dose rate used in clinical practice, the radiation may be considered a series of small fractions reproducing the survival curve with the shoulder. As a limit, for very low dose rates in brachytherapy or for many small fraction doses in external radiotherapy, the survival curve coincides with the tangent at the origin of the survival curve observed after high-dose-rate brachytherapy or a single fraction of external radiation. Varying the dose rate modifies the survival curve. This result is particularly true for dose rates between 10 to 200 cGy/hour. Experimental data confirmed an increase in radiation effect with small fraction doses in the range of 0.5 Gy (10).

OXYGEN AND RADIATION

Oxygen has been shown to be one of the most important modifiers of the radiation response. The earliest demonstration was done by Schwartz in 1910: the radiation effect on his skin was reduced if a compression was made during the treatment. The level of cell killing in cell culture is directly dependent on the degree of oxygenation at the time of irradiation. The dose required to produce the same effect under hypoxic conditions is approximately 3 times greater than the that required under fully oxygenated circumstances. The oxygen enhancement ratio (OER) is this ratio.

The radiosensitivity of cells increases rapidly for an oxygen concentration of 0.5% for cells in culture. This sensitivity corresponds to an oxygen partial pressure of about 5 mm Hg (11). Normal tissues, except cartilage or mouse skin, are considered to be well oxygenated because their oxygen tension is similar to that of the venous blood (20 to 40 mm Hg). The oxygen enhancement ratio varies according to the type of radiation. For radiation with a low LET, such as x- or τ-rays or electrons, the oxygenation enhancement ratio is between 2.5 and 3, whereas for high-speed neutrons, this ratio is approximately 1.6.

The presence of hypoxic cells and the role of reoxygenation during a course of radiation are two other important contributions. In a study of bronchial cancers, Thomlinson and Gray (12) showed the presence of necrotic areas within a tumor for diameters greater than 0.3 mm. The presence of well-oxygenated viable cells represents a small cord of less than 180 μm. Calculations of oxygen diffusion from capillaries predicted that the oxygen tension would decrease to zero at a distance between 150 to 200 μm. Because proliferation is taking place close to the capillaries, hypoxic cells are pushed to a more anoxic condition and ultimately die. An apparent paradox exists: because hypoxic cells are quite resistant to conventional radiation, no tumor could be cured by radiation. In a classic experience, van Putten and Kallman (13) followed the outcome of hypoxic cells during a course of fractionated radiation. Because hypoxic cells are considered radioresistant, their relative percentage should increase during the treatment, but this was not the case; rather, the percentage remained unchanged (13). One possible explanation was that during a course of radiation, some hypoxic cells were becoming oxygenated, i.e., reoxygenated. The kinetics of this reoxygenation process may vary among tumors. Carcinomas appear to exhibit more extensive reoxygenation than sarcomas because of different rates of tumor shrinkage and natural cell loss.

The clinical importance of this oxygen effect has led to a large number of studies, both experimental and clinical, addressing the problem of anemia, hyperbaric oxygen, and hypoxic radiosensitizers (14–17). Anemia has been shown in several articles dealing with cervical cancers and lung and head and neck tumors, to reduce the probability of local control by radiation (15–17). In a classic study, Bush et al. (15) showed that the local control for cervical cancer was reduced from 77% to 50% in the presence of a hemoglobin level of less than 12 g/dL. Furthermore, after transfusion, the local control rose to 84%. Dische et al. (16) showed a similar effect for lung cancer and hemoglobin levels (Fig. 9.4). Most patients treated for lung cancers have a long history of heavy tobacco smoking and may have altered lung functions and higher concentrations of carboxyhemoglobin, thus reducing the oxygen available.

Current larger studies are ongoing in the Accelerated Radiotherapy with Carbogen and Nicotinamide program, which is investigating two factors: time and oxygenation. In the laboratory carbogen has been used to sensitize hypoxic cells to radiation; this sensitization has led to better tumor control, especially with accelerated radiation regimes (18). Furthermore, Nicotinamide, a vitamin B complex, is used to overcome the acute hypoxia caused by closure and opening of small vessels. The preliminary results have shown the feasibility of such an approach with encouraging results: four of eight patients with bronchogenic cancer experienced a complete radiologic regression (19).

RECRUITMENT

The radiosensitivity of cells depends on their position in the growth cycle. Proliferating cells are in general more sensitive than nonproliferating cells. The cells are more sensitive at or near the mitosis: mitotic phase (M) and phase G2 are the most sensitive, whereas cells in the late G1 and S phases are reaching a maximum of resistance. Furthermore, the radiation may delay the cell progression through its cell cycle. The duration of this delay depends on the radiation dose and cell position within its growth cycle; the longest delay is observed for cells in the G2 phase.

This differential cell cycle effect of radiation both in terms of radiosensitivity and delay in cell progression may tend to synchronize the cell population in one phase preferentially. Furthermore, as proliferating cells are destroyed, cells may be recruited from the nonproliferating compartment. The clinical exploitation of this blockade in a more radiosensitive phase is quite difficult because of the wide range of cell cycles, the shortness of the blockade, and the low number of proliferating clonogenic cells.

REPOPULATION

During a course of fractionated radiation, the main concern is the risk of increased proliferation within the tumor, leading to an increased number of clonogenic cells. For acute-responding tissues, such as the skin, mucosa, or bone marrow, a cell depletion induces an increased proliferation of surviving cells; this repopulation starts after a few weeks and enables compensation for the tissue deficits. In contrast, proliferation for late-responding tissues does not begin until the completion of a conventional radiation course. The key question is knowing if repopulation also occurs for tumors during the radiation course. Experimental data suggest that for rapidly proliferating tumors, repopulation occurs during a fractionated radiation course (20).

In 1988 Withers et al. (21), from a review of literature data, suggested that for head and neck tumors there is no evidence of significant proliferation during the first 3 weeks; this proliferation occurs after 3 weeks, and an additional dose of 60 cGy/day is neces-

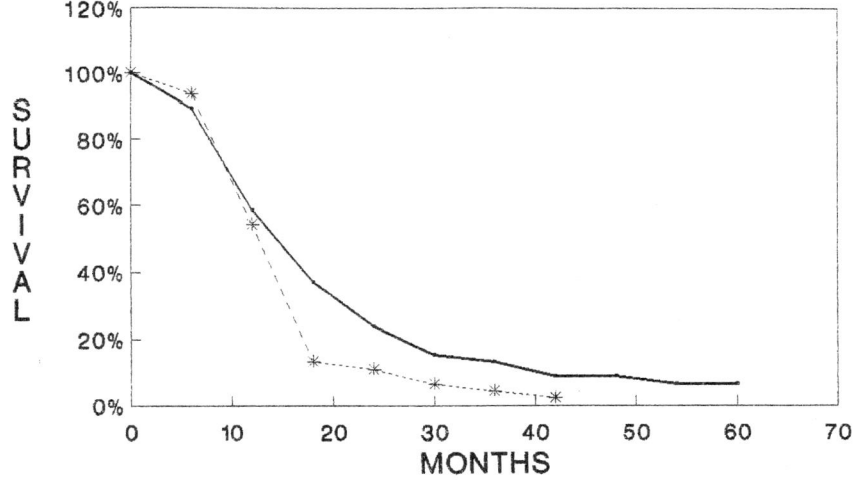

FIGURE 9.4. Hemoglobin level and survival of inoperable lung cancers. (Redrawn from Dische S, Saunders MI, Warburton MF. Hemoglobin, radiation morbidity and survival. Int J Radiat Oncol Biol Phys 1986;12:1335–1337.)

sary to overcome it. Several reports have shown a decrease in tumor control for split-course schedules or treatments interrupted or lasting longer than the planned schedule (6 or 7 weeks) (22–26).

TUMOR GROWTH

The growth of a tumor often is measured by its volume doubling time, which is affected by different factors: the cell cycle, the number of cells proliferating, and the cellular loss. Indeed, within a tumor there are proliferating and nonproliferating cells. The growth fractions describe the proportion of cells proliferating. The growth of a tumor also is affected by the loss of cells either because of migration, differentiation, or necrosis. Thus, the growth rate depends on the proliferation and the cell loss. The potential doubling time (Tpot) is the rate at which a cell population should grow in the absence of cellular loss; Tpot is proportional to the duration of the S phase and inversely proportional to the fraction of proliferating S phase cells (the labeling index). For most epithelial cancers, Tpot varies between 3 and 10 days, whereas the volume doubling time of the tumors ranges from 30 to 170 days. Thus, the percentage of cell loss is more than 80% (Table 9.2) (27–30).

MATHEMATICAL MODELS

Many mathematical models, based on hypotheses of cellular lethality, have been proposed for analyzing these survival curves. The multitarget model component was based on the assumption that each mammalian cell contains a fixed number of targets; these targets all must be inactivated to suppress the reproductive capacity of the cells. This effect was supposed to explain the shoulder part of the curve.

The linear-quadratic model has become increasingly more popular among clinicians, especially for new fractionation studies. Kellerer and Rossi (31, 32) based their hypothesis on fundamental microdosimetric concepts of energy deposition: that the damage induced by radiation results from the interaction of at least two sublesions. They proposed that:

$$S = e - \alpha D - \beta D2$$

where S is the surviving fraction. This equation has an initial shoulder but does not end in a straight line. Chadwick and Leenhouts (33, 34) in 1981 proposed that double-strand breaks in DNA arise either because of a single particle damaging both strands (with a probability proportional to the dose) or random ionizations producing lesions by chance on opposite strands close enough to produce a double-strand break (with a probability proportional to the square of the dose). The biologic effect (E) may be described by the equation

$$E = \alpha D + \beta D2$$

where D corresponds to the total dose delivered (30, 35, 36). Different ratios of α and β have been proposed for early-reacting tissues and late-reacting tissues and for tumors.

The main problems with this approach probably are an underestimation of the effects at a very low radiation dose and an overestimation at a very high dose; the curves continue to bend and are not the classic straight line. A time factor has been added to this equation. The term target does not correspond to a specific structure within the cells that leads to cell death but rather to a probability of events leading to cell death.

BASIC PRINCIPLES OF CLINICAL RADIOTHERAPY

THE THERAPEUTIC RATIO

The basic goal of treatment remains the cure of a patient's cancer while preserving his appearance and the functioning of the organs. This, of course, would be an ideal situation; generally in clinical practice, however, some residual damage is accepted as the price necessary for cure. This principle applies not only to the work of radiation oncologists but also to that of medical oncologists or surgeons, and it has led to the concept of the therapeutic ratio. The relationship between radiation dose and the probability of tumor con-

TABLE 9.2. Tumor Volume and Potential Doubling Times of Primary Tumors

	TUMOR VOLUME DOUBLING TIME	POTENTIAL DOUBLING TIME (TPOT)
Lung		
Epidermoid	84–100 d	15 d
Small Cell	35 d	4 d
Large Cell	90 d	5 d
Adenocarcinoma	144–185 d	17 d
Colorectal cancer	96–630 d	7.5 d
Breast cancer	90–166 d	10 d
Lymphoma	15–70 d	2–15 d
Burkitt's	3 d	1 d

From Schiffer LM, Cellular proliferation in tumor and normal tissues. In: Perez CA, Brady LW, eds. Principles and practice of radiation oncology. Philadelphia: JB Lippincott, 1987:56–66.

trol for a homogeneous population is a sigmoidal curve, i.e., as the dose increases more clonogenic cells are destroyed. The same principle applies to normal cells and tissues. Thus, the therapeutic ratio could be translated as the difference between the dose required for tumor control and that inducing permanent damage.

In most clinical circumstances, the best therapeutic ratio is a compromise based on clinical judgment. If radiation oncologists decide to avoid all possible late damage, they also will have fewer patients cured. Several parameters influence this therapeutic ratio, including the tumor characteristics, the radiobiologic responses, the factors associated with the radiation treatment (dose, fractionation, volume, techniques), and the normal tissue tolerance.

TUMOR CHARACTERISTICS

Tumor characteristics include clinical parameters such as pathology, presentation, and size. Tumors classified as radiosensitive include lymphomas, seminomas, and dysgerminomas; radioresistant tumors include sarcomas, melanomas, and glioblastomas. Squamous cell carcinomas and adenocarcinomas have an intermediate sensitivity. Radiosensitivity and radiocurability are two different concepts. For instance, a prostatic cancer shows a slow response to radiation but cure may be achieved, whereas a disseminated lymphoma may have a fast, complete, local remission without any hope of cure.

The tumor volume is a critical factor. When the tumor increases in size, the number of cells increases and the dose required to control the tumor must be higher. This dose-volume relationship has been shown for different head and neck tumors and cervical cancers (Fig. 9.5) (6). For lung cancers there is now a clear suggestion of dose effect—at least for doses between 40 and 70 Gy given conventionally (26, 37, 38) (Fig. 9.6). Furthermore, there is a suggestion of volume effect. In the well-known dose study of the Radiation Therapy Oncology Group (RTOG) (37), the data showed an effect of both dose and tumor size; however, the number of cases was too small to draw the same conclusions as for head and neck cancers.

The general appearance of the tumor also influences local control in that exophytic tumors are more easily controlled than infiltrative lesions. The presence of tumor necrosis was reported by Gelinas and Fletcher (39) to increase the risk of local recurrence for head and neck cancers. Low hemoglobin levels and poor Karnofsky performance status also are associated with poor outcome (16, 40).

PREDICTIVE ASSAYS

Nevertheless, the parameters mentioned certainly are neither specific and nor relevant for the treatment of an individual patient because of the wide variation in response and tumor heterogeneity. One current area of research is the development of tests predicting the radiation treatment outcome, independently of known clinical factors, so that the radiation schedule may be adapted to individual needs. These may be divided into tests evaluating tumor cell survival and parameters of the tumor's radiosensitivity, either cellular (e.g., tumor cell kinetics) or extracellular (e.g., tumor hypoxia, vascularity index) (41).

The cellular radiosensitivity of different human cell lines may be measured by in vitro clonogenic assays. Different parameters are used to describe the radiosensitivity of the cell line, including the extrapolation number, the dose required to reduce survival to

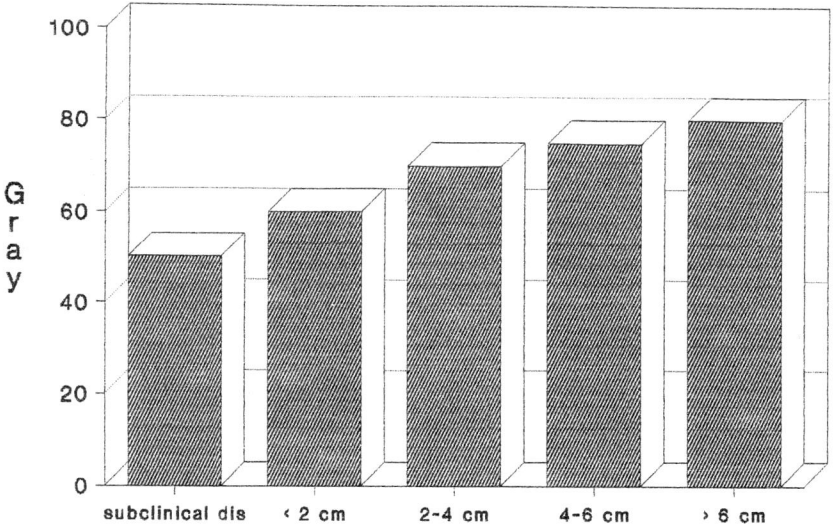

FIGURE 9.5. Ninety percent tumor control probability in squamous cell carcinoma of the upper aerodigestive tract as it relates to radiation dose delivered with a conventional radiation schedule (2 Gy per fraction). The influence of tumor volume is illustrated. (Adapted from Fletcher GH, ed. Textbook of radiotherapy. 3rd ed. London: Henry Kimpton Publishers, 1980.)

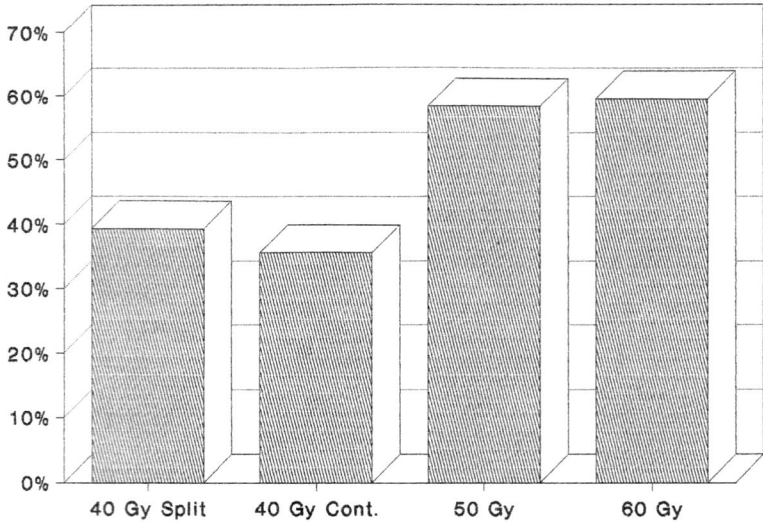

FIGURE 9.6. Influence of local radiation dose on the ultimate local control of epidermoid lung carcinoma. The results of RTOG trial 73-01 are shown. (Modified from Perez CA, Pajak TF, Rubin P, Simpson SR, et al. Long-term observations of the patterns of failure on patients with unresected non–oat cell carcinoma of the lung treated with definitive radiotherapy. Cancer 1987;58:1874–1881.)

37%, and the α and β values. More recently, the surviving fraction of cells at a dose of 2 Gy (SF2) was found to correlate well with the clinical sensitivity of different tumors (Table 9.3) (41–46). Deacon et al. (45) reported an SF2 of 18.7% for tumors considered highly radiosensitive (lymphoma, neuroblastoma, myeloma), between 43 and 46 for tumors with an intermediate sensitivity (breast, bladder, colon, lung), and 52% for tumors considered radioresistant (glioblastoma, melanoma, osteosarcoma). Girinsky et al. (46) observed that patients treated with radiation for cervical or head and neck cancers had a higher local control rate (93% versus 68%) when the SF2 was above or below 36%. The main problems with such an approach are related to the ability to obtain the cell line in culture.

Micronuclei, the formation of acentric chromosome fragments, is a common lesion induced by ionizing radiation. The number of micronuclei increases with the radiation dose and indicates the loss of reproductive capacity (47). In in vitro experiments, it predicts cell survival. Streffer et al. (48) observed, in a series of patients treated preoperatively with radiation for rectal cancer, an increased risk of local failure if there was a reduction in the number of micronuclei observed.

Tetrazolium dye is a marker of viable cells and mitochondrial activity. Carmichael et al. (49) used this assay to estimate the cell survival after chemotherapy and radiotherapy. The main advantage is the short time required to obtain a response, i.e., less than 1 week, but there are drawbacks related to the risk of culture contamination by nonmalignant cells and the loss of reproductive capacity allowing one or more cell division.

Hypoxia has been shown to render tumor cells more resistant to ionizing radiation. The clinical impact of hemoglobin levels, treatment with hyperbaric oxygen, or hypoxic radiosensitizers such as misonidazole suggests that hypoxia may be a limiting factor for treatment. Several attempts have been made to quantify tumor hypoxia, including direct measurement of oxygen partial pressure using microelectrodes, assessment of vascular supply (intercapillary distance), or detection of anaerobic metabolism. Höckel et al. (50) found a close correlation between the intratumoral level of pO_2 and survival of cancers of the cervix treated by radiotherapy (Fig. 9.7). A gross measurement of hypoxia may perhaps be misleading because hypoxic clonogenic cells may be only a small fraction of the total number.

Different methods have been developed to monitor tumor proliferation rates: thymidine labeling with 5-bromodeoxyuridine (BUdR) or iododeoxyuridine (IUDR) (two thymidine analogues) are recognized by a monoclonal antibody and measured by flow cytometry; and, more recently, with Ki^{67}, an antibody that specifically recognizes an antigen on proliferating cells. The iododeoxyuridine method is quite simple and requires an intravenous injection and a small biopsy a few hours later. Several investigators have reported a good correlation between Tpot value and treatment outcome. In a European Organization for the Research and Treatment of Cancer (EORTC) trial, use of a conventional radiation schedule with a dose of 2 Gy per fraction was associated with a poor outcome for tumors with a fast Tpot (less than 4 days); in contrast, an accelerated radiation program was beneficial only for patients with a fast Tpot (Fig. 9.8) (28, 29, 51). Additional prospective studies on a large number of pa-

TABLE 9.3. Survival Curve Parameters and Surviving Fraction at 2 Gy for Histologic Groups of Human Tumor Cell Lines

Histologic Group	α (Gy^{-1})	β (Gy^{-2})	N	Do (Gy)	S2 (%)
	(Mean Values/Coefficient of Variation [%])				
Glioblastomas	0.241/86	0.029/37	12/71	1.44/28	58/34
Melanomas	0.255/69	0.053/56	73/265	1.04/27	51/28
Squamous cell cancers	0.273/39	0.045/25	5/38	1.28/11	49/18
Adenocarcinomas	0.311/117	0.055/79	37/166	1.04/26	48/37
Lymphomas	0.451/42	0.051/126	1.8/79	1.48/34	34/27
Oat cell cancers	0.650/37	0.081/183	1.8/104	1.51/70	22/42

From Malaise EP, Fertil B, Chavaudra N, Guichard M. Distribution of radiation sensitivities for human tumor cells of specific histological types: comparison of in vitro and in vivo data. Int Radiat Oncol Biol Phys 1986;12:617–624.
Abbreviations. Do, dose required to reduce the survival to 37% in the exponential part of the curve; SF2, surviving fraction of cells at a dose of 2 Gy.

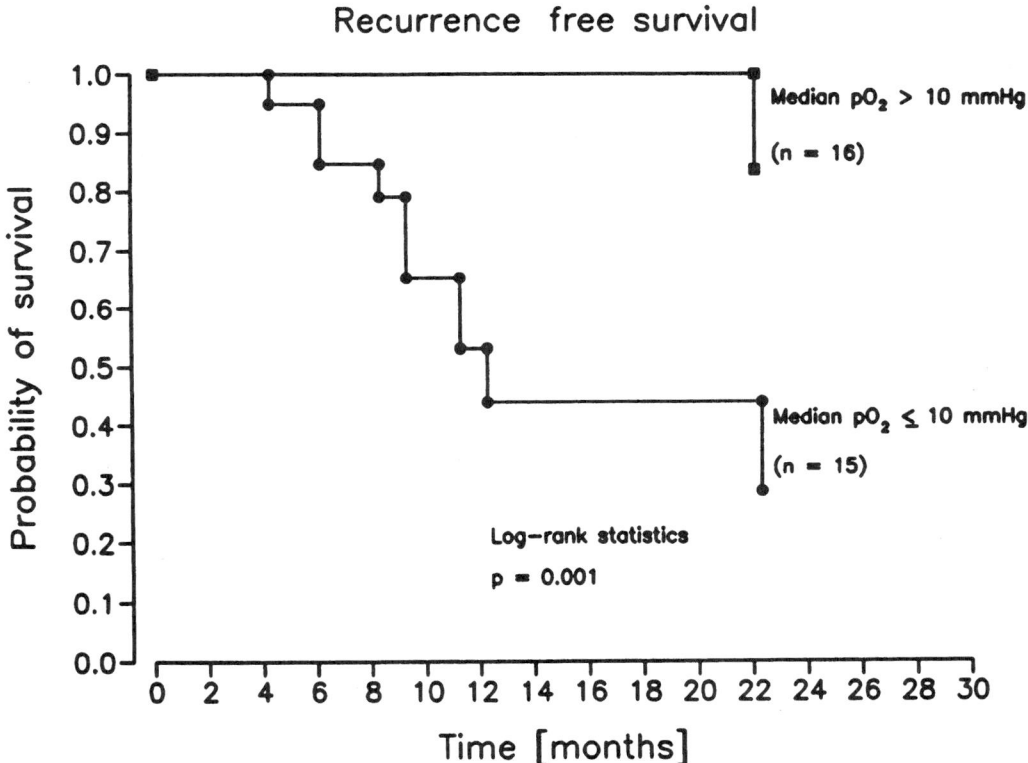

FIGURE 9.7. Influence of pO$_2$ level on the local control of advanced cervical cancer treated with radiation therapy. (From Höckel M, Knoop C, Schlenger K, et al. Intratumoral pO$_2$ predicts survival in advanced cancer of the uterine cervix. Radiother Oncol 1993;26: 45–50.)

tients may help to clarify the clinical usefulness of the Tpot value. There are several limitations and uncertainties with Tpot measurements, including the differentiation in a biopsy specimen between malignant and nonmalignant cells, especially in the case of diploid cells in the presence of tumor heterogeneity.

Some predictive assays of radiosensitivity appear to offer encouraging results, but additional data are required before they are integrated into daily clinical practice. Indeed, these assays must be compared and combined with other well-known prognostic factors such as tumor stage, volume, and histology. Furthermore, the response to treatment depends on several factors including the number of clonogenic cells, the microenvironment, the cell repair capacity, and the tumor cell heterogeneity (41, 44). Most reported series included only a limited number of cases, thus they cannot be used to draw a final conclusion.

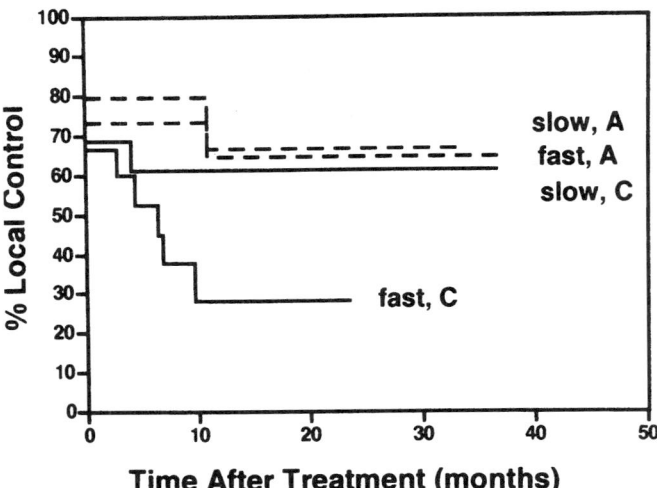

FIGURE 9.8. Impact of Tpot value on local control of different head and neck tumors relative to the radiation schedule. For a slow Tpot of more than 4 days, the radiation schedule did not influence the outcome. In contrast, for a fast Tpot of 4 days or less, the accelerated fractionated schedule (A) yielded better local control than conventional fractionation (C). (From Begg AC, Hofland I, Van Glabekke M, Bartelink H, Horiot JC. Predictive value of potential doubling time for radiotherapy of head and neck tumor patient: results from the EORTC Cooperative trial 22851. Semin Radiat Oncol 1992;2:22–25.)

NORMAL TISSUE TOLERANCE

The limiting factor of radiotherapy is the risk of inducing severe damage to normal tissues. With increasing radiation doses, more and more neoplastic cells are killed to achieve the complete destruction of all clonogenic cells, a prerequisite for cure. Unfortunately, the same principle also applies to normal tissues. Classically, the sequence of events is divided in acute reactions, usually within the first months of the treatment, and late events seen after several months or years. The latter often are characterized by a form of chronicity.

The normal tissues of the body have been classified by their proliferative and growth activities as rapidly proliferating tissues and slowly proliferating tissues. The former group, characterized by an active proliferation as well as by maintenance of a steady-state number, includes the bone marrow, intestinal epithelium, skin, and mucosa. Slowly proliferating tissues include the liver, lung, kidney, and connective tissues. Rapidly proliferating tissues also are characterized by a hierarchical structure: the mature functional cells are produced by the division of stem cells, and an intermediate group is composed of cells in the process of maturation with proliferating capacity remaining. A classic example of such a system is the mucosa of the small bowel. The progenitor cells are located in the base of the crypt; dividing cells migrate up and undergo maturation in the upper third of the crypt before migrating to the villus as differentiated functionals at which point they are lost. This system is normally in balance with a fast renewal and a short turnover time. After a radiation dose of a few Grays, the number of cells undergoing mitosis is progressively reduced within the proliferating zone of the crypt, leading to a sharp and progressive reduction of the villus. After 24 hours a regeneration is seen with a shortening of the cell cycle and an extension of the proliferative zone to compensate for the cellular loss. Thus, the ability of such tissue to regenerate depends on the survival of stem cells. Acute effects are related to the balance between the cellular loss of stem cells and the regeneration possibilities of the tissue. In a slow renewal or nonrenewal system, no change is observed during the radiation course. Late damage may occur several weeks, months, or years after treatment. Two different theories have been proposed. Late damage results (a) from lesions induced to the vasculoconnective cells of an organ, particularly the endothelial cells, leading to a decrease in the blood flow, or (b) from a depletion of stem cells within the different tissues (21, 52).

Another important concept is based on the organization and function of a tissue or organ. In the case of localized skin damage, active proliferation of adjacent areas provides a rapid repair process, whereas for the kidney, the nephron represents a subunit that cannot be repopulated from adjacent areas. Furthermore, localized lung damage (fibrosis) may be compensated for functionally by an hypertrophy of adjacent alveoli. For small bowel, however, severe late damage (stenosis) leads to major symptom damage because the function of the whole system is impaired. This also is true for the central nervous system in which a localized necrosis may have a disastrous outcome.

The concept of tolerance dose has been introduced as an aid to the radiotherapist, but it never should replace clinical judgment and analysis of the balance between benefit and risk. Rubin and Casarett (52) proposed the concept of tolerance dose 5/5 (TD 5/5) or tolerance dose 5/50 (TD 50/5)—doses that result in no more than 5% or 50% severe complications, respectively, within a period of 5 years Table 9.4 presents the tolerance doses for several thoracic organs by the volume treated, but those figures are only valid for conventional treatments (2 Gy per fraction, 5 fractions per week) (53). The recent progress in computed treatment planning probably will be quite helpful as a means of better refining the importance of the volume treated.

TABLE 9.4. Normal Thoracic Tissue Tolerance Doses to Radiotherapy

	TD 5/5[a]			TD 50/5[a]			
VOLUME TREATED	1/3 (Gy)	2/3 (Gy)	3/3 (Gy)	1/3 (Gy)	2/3 (Gy)	3/3 (Gy)	ENDPOINTS
Lung	45	30	17.5	65	40	24.5	Pneumonitis
Heart	60	45	40	70	55	50	Pericarditis
Esophagus	60	58	55	72	70	68	Stenosis
Rib cage	50			65			Fracture
Brachial plexus	62	61	60	77	76	75	Nerve damage
Spinal cord	5 cm	10 cm	20 cm	5 cm	10 cm	20 cm	Myelitis
	50	50	47	70	70	—	Necrosis

From Emami B, Lyman J, Brown A, et al. Tolerance of normal tissue to therapeutic irradiation. Int J Radiat Oncol Biol Phys 1991;21:109–122.
Abbreviation. TD, tolerance dose.
[a]The tolerance dose inducing a 5% (TD 5/5) or a 50% (TD 50/5) incidence of damage with a 5-year period of observation.

CARCINOGENIC RISK

Another concern is the risk that radiation therapy could later induce the development of second tumors. This risk was recognized shortly after the Roentgen discovery. Early practitioners working without any radioprotection developed skin cancers and leukemia. Current information about human tolerance is provided by patients exposed in the past to radiation for benign disease, survivors of the atomic bomb blasts at Hiroshima and Nagasaki, workers exposed accidentally to radiation, and patients treated for cancer with radiotherapy.

Generally, it can be said that nearly all tissues are susceptible to the development of a radiation-induced tumor.

There are no signs allowing for differentiation of a radiation-induced tumor from another tumor; only an increased incidence of such a pathology in a population may allow elucidation of the role of radiation. Compared with natural tumors, the so-called radiation-induced cancer has the same nature, prognosis, and sensitivity to radiation. A radiation-induced tumor is not radioresistant per se, but the doses already received by the tissues after therapeutic radiation may not allow retreatment of the tumor with ionizing radiation (a problem of radiotolerance). There is a latency period, varying from years to decades, between the time of exposure and the detection of the tumor. Leukemias are observed after a shorter period (3 to 5 years) than are solid tumors (more than 10 years) (54).

Moderate radiation doses, when applied to a large volume of bone marrow, may induce leukemias. This effect was observed in a series of 14,000 patients treated between 1933 and 1954 for spondylitis with radiation (doses between 2 and 6 Gy), the number of leukemia cases increased 5 times, whereas the number of solid tumor cases was 1.5 times higher than in a control group (55). This risk of second leukemias also was found to be increased by a factor of 2 in an epidemiologic study of women treated for cervical cancer (56). Higher radiation doses seem to be required to induce a significant number of secondary solid tumors. Although the same rate of cancers was observed among women treated with surgery or radiation for cervical cancers, the relative risk of developing a second cancer in specific organs receiving a relatively higher radiation doses was found to be as high as 2.7. This incidence was seen mainly for the bowel and bladder, but the doses received were lower than those used to cure a cancer (57).

The volume of tissue irradiated also influences the risk. The relative risk of occurrence of a second cancer is only increased significantly after the subtotal or total nodal irradiation used in Hodgkin's disease (58). Age also may modulate the risk, perhaps in some circumstances because of hormonal variations. After irradiation for Hodgkin's disease or breast cancer, the relative risk of development of a second cancer in the breast is 2 to 4 times higher for women younger than 30 to 35 years (59–61).

With these possible exceptions, the risk of developing a second cancer several years after the radiation treatment is not a reason to eliminate the use of this successful treatment. In almost all situations, this risk is quite low compared with risk factors such as tobacco smoking or other environmental risks. Indeed, in a study of 82,000 women treated for cervical cancer, an increase in development of a second cancer, mainly lung cancer, was observed among women treated with surgery or radiation because of the higher incidence of tobacco smoking in this group compared with the gen-

TABLE 9.5. Risk of Second Cancers After Treatment of 82,000 Women with Cancers of the Cervix

	RADIOTHERAPY		SURGERY	
	OBSERVED	EXPECTED	OBSERVED	EXPECTED
Number of second cancers with follow-up of more than	3324	3062	479	435
10 years	1401	1251	190	181
Smoking habit	71%	34%	...	...

From Boice JD, Day NE, Andersen A, et al. Second cancers following treatment for cervical cancer. An International collaboration among cancer registries. J Natl Cancer Inst 1985;74:955–975.

eral population (62) (Table 9.5). Excluding possible tobacco-induced cancers, only an excess of 125 cancers may be related to the radiation, a figure far below the expected number calculated from other experiences. In their conclusions, Boice et al. (62) noticed that despite the large number of patients included in the study, only a few second cancers (less than 5%) were linked convincingly to radiation.

FRACTIONATION

HISTORICAL BACKGROUND

The success of radiation therapy not only is based on the tumor radiosensitivity and normal tissue tolerance but also on the fractionation used. Indeed, when radiotherapy treatment was performed in a single fraction or a few fractions, leading to severe acute and late reactions, the benefit of dividing the treatment into a series of small fractions was noticed rapidly. In a classic experiment on ram testicles, Regaud showed that sterilization was possible without inducing skin necrosis when the dose was divided into four fractions instead of one. Fractionation is aimed at taking advantage of the four basic principles of radiobiology (reoxygenation, reparation, repopulation, and redistribution). During the last 20 years, radiotherapists have realized the importance of the fraction size and the differences between acute and late effects. In the 1960s and 1970s, fractionation was changed in some centers from five fractions per week to three or four fractions while keeping the same weekly doses. It was thought that 10 Gy per week was safe (63). Nevertheless, this increase in fraction size without any total dose reduction led to a significant increase in late effects (6, 64–66).

Formerly, many clinicians thought that there was a correlation between the severity of acute effects and the occurrence of late effects (63). If this is partially true for classic schedules, new fractionation programs, such as split-course or hyperfractionated schedules, may either decrease or increase the acute effects while keeping the risk of late effects unchanged. Until the end of the 1960s, the Strandqvist formula, which related time and dose, was used to compare different radiation schedules; this formula considers the amount of recovery because of treatment protraction but not the fraction number (67). In 1969 Ellis (68) introduced the nominal standard dose concept and the roentgen equivalent therapy (ret) unit. This formula was based on the skin reaction and also accounts for the dose, the total exposure time, and the number of fractions. Although this formula was a great step forward because of the recognition of the fractionation role, it did not recognize the different responses of tissues and tumors (the same exponents are applied for all tissues) and in repopulation. This was particularly true for large fractions and short treatments. The same comments applied to derived formulas such as the cumulative radiation effect (CRE) or the time-dose fractionation (TDF).

More recently, Fowler (30) and Barendsen et al. (20) introduced the linear quadratic models that distinguish between cell killing because of nonrepairable lesions and that caused by repairable damage (69). The different mathematical models aim to compare different radiation schedules. They are a help to the radiation oncologist, but they must never replace clinical judgment.

BIOLOGIC PRINCIPLES OF FRACTIONATED RADIOTHERAPY

Thames et al. (69) and Fowler (30) summarized the basic radiobiologic principles involved in a fractionated course of radiotherapy, outlining the differences in response of early- and late-reacting tissue and tumors. The physician should remember that cells are damaged at the time of the irradiation, but that most of the time, they die only when they try to divide. Effects on tissue and the proliferation process are seen only after clonogenic cell death; thus, for early-reacting tissue this effect is observed a few weeks after the start of radiation therapy, whereas for late-reacting tissue, it occurs several months later.

Late complications are observed in slowly proliferating or nonproliferating tissues. The time factor is not an important parameter (these tissues are not spared by increasing the length of the radiation treatment), but the fraction size has a major influence. Large fractions increase the risk of complication. Indeed, the dose-response curve shows a rapid increase

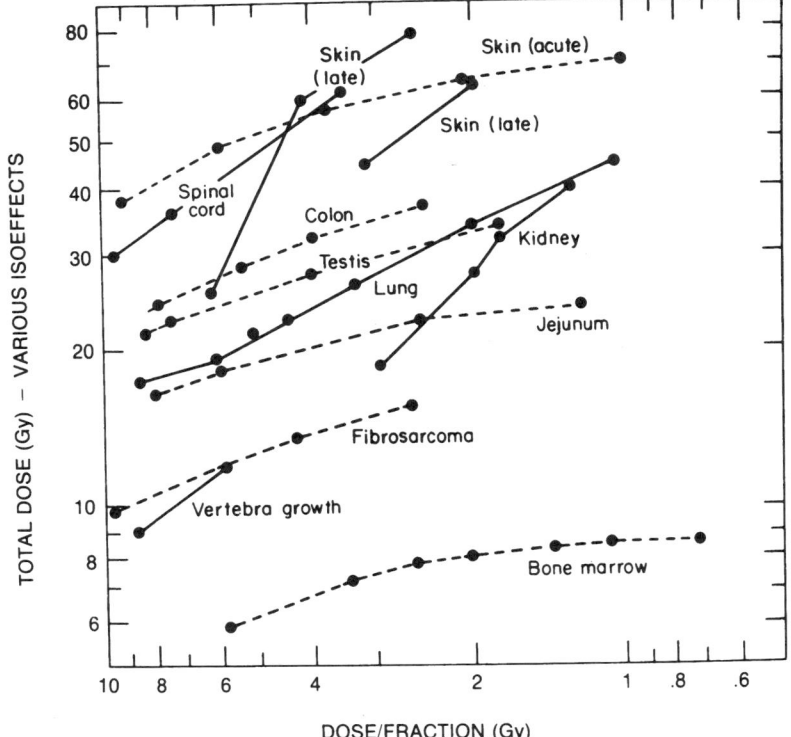

FIGURE 9.9. Isoeffect curves for acute reactions (*dashed line*) and late effects (*solid lines*). The total dose necessary to achieve a specific effect is plotted as a function of dose per fraction. The isodoses for late effects show a steeper increase with a larger dose per fraction than does the isodose for acute effects. (From Withers HR. Biologic basis for altered fractionation schemes. Cancer 1985;55:2086–2095.)

over the dose per fraction range used in classic clinical practice (Fig. 9.9) (69, 70).

Early complications are observed in rapidly proliferating tissues such as the skin, bowels, and mucosa. Increasing the treatment time has a sparing effect with the exception that below 2 weeks, shortening the treatment duration has an adverse effect. Thus, these acute effects are less dependent on the fraction size than are late effects, and they are related to the dose per day and the weekly dose (Table 9.6).

Tumors are very heterogeneous with wide variations in tumor types and individuals. As shown earlier, a dose of 2 Gy allows for sterilization of 50% of the viable cells of most tumors except sarcomas, glioblastomas, and melanomas. Most tumors have a fraction size dependence very close to that of the rapidly proliferating tissue, and their Tpot is close to 5 days for most epithelial tumors. The key question is knowing, in a specific tumor, when repopulation begins to compensate for cell loss. Several recent observations suggest that breaks in the treatment or longer overall exposure times have an adverse effect and require an additional radiation dose (50 to 70 cGy per day), probably to compensate for a short Tpot (21–25). Redistribution in the cell cycle and reoxygenation occurring during a fractionated radiation course are two mechanisms that increase its effectiveness.

TABLE 9.6. α–β Values of Different Tissues

EARLY-RESPONDING TISSUES	α–β (GY)
Skin	9–12
Jejunum	6–10
Colon	10–11
Spermatogenic cells	12–13
Bone marrow	9
LATE-RESPONDING TISSUES	α–β (GY)
Spinal cord	1.7–4.9
Kidney	0.5–5
Lung	2.5–4.5
Liver	1.4–3.5
Bladder	3.1–7
Skin	2.5–4.5

FRACTIONATION SCHEDULE

The type of radiation fractionation used until recently involved the delivery of a single treatment per day (usually 1.8 or 2 Gy), 5 to 6 times per week for 3 to 7 weeks depending on the type of tumor treated and the goal of the treatment. This method is referred to as conventional fractionation. Table 9.7 summarizes the different types of radiation schedules.

Split-course schedules use daily fractions for 1 to 2 weeks followed by a rest period of from 2 to 4 weeks and a second course of daily irradiation. The daily radiation dose is usually higher than 2 Gy. This technique was advocated by Scanlon in 1960 (71) and Sambrook in 1965 (72). Both investigators observed a better treatment tolerance. Theoretically, this rest period was thought to allow a better tumor reoxygenation of hypoxic cells. The main advantage of this approach is an improved convenience for patients and physicians by reducing the number of fractions, the rest period, and the possibility, in cases of progression, of not delivering the second radiation course. Nevertheless, a split-course schedule also has major drawbacks: the rest period allows for tumor repopulation, and the high fraction size increases the risk of late damage.

Several trials were conducted. Generally, split-course radiation schedules were found to be no more efficient than continuous irradiation, but, even worse, some proposed schedules were clearly inferior, such as the well-known program of Adamson and Cavanaugh: 20 Gy in five fractions over 1 week and repeated after 3 weeks of rest (73, 74).

A hypofractionated schedule delivers less than 4 fractions per week, usually with a large fraction size (4 to 6 Gy). In fact, such an approach often was used either for technical convenience (overloaded treatment units, patients living a long distance from the radiation facilities) or to adapt the treatment to take full advantage of some radiosensitizers, such as the trials with hyperbaric oxygen or misonidazole. Such high fraction size has led to an increase in late effects, especially in the absence of total dose or volume reduction, but also to a lower local control (65, 66).

The basic principle of hyperfractionation is the delivery of smaller than the classic fraction doses 2 to 3 times per day with a 4- to 6-hour interval between fractions, without reducing the total treatment time; the fraction size usually is between 100 and 130 cGy. This approach is designed to take advantage of the fraction size impact on acute and late effects and on tumor volume. The goal is maintenance of the same level of late complications while increasing the total dose and improving tumor control. Acute reactions are expected to be increased. The RTOG also investigated this approach in non–small cell lung cancer, defining the optimal schedule through a series of phase II trials.

Accelerated fractionated schedules imply the delivery of several fractions per day while reducing the total treatment time. The critical issue with this approach is the tolerance of rapidly proliferating normal tissues. Thus, it often is necessary to introduce a rest period. For example, the EORTC radiotherapy group introduced a break, because of mucosal reactions, of 3 to 4 weeks after delivery of 48 Gy of radiation with fractions of 1.6 Gy 3 times per day over 2 weeks (75). To avoid the problem of the rest period and the risk of repopulation, Dische and Saunders (76) developed a continuous hyperfractionated accelerated radiotherapy (CHART) schedule: three fractions of 1.5 Gy are delivered daily during 12 consecutive days (including weekends). The acute reactions were observed after treatment completion, but the late damage was not increased except at the level of the spinal cord; a reduction of dose below 40 Gy was required because of the problem of sublethal damage recovery (76, 77) (Fig. 9.10).

Thus, a new and very important issue with this kind of approach is the importance of the recovery kinetics from sublethal damage. In conventional treatment, the time interval between two fractions is as long as 24 hours. In contrast, when delivering several treatments per day, the physician is faced with the

TABLE 9.7. Fractionation Schedules in Radiotherapy Practice

Schedule	Fractions	Dose (Gy)	Fraction Day	Week
Conventional	||||| ||||| ||||| ||||| |||||	2	1	5
Split-course	||||| REST |||||	2–4	1	5
Hypofractionated	I I I I I I I I	>2	1	<5
Hyperfractionated	||||| ||||| ||||| ||||| |||||	1–1.3	2	10
Accelerated hyperfractionated	||||| ||||| REST ||| |||||	>1.2	2–3	10–15
Accelerated hyperfractionated	||||| ||||| ||||| |||||	>1.2	2–3	10–15
CHART	|||||||||||| ||||||||||||	1.5 (8-hour interval)	3	21

Abbreviation. CHART, continuous hyperfractionated accelerated therapy.

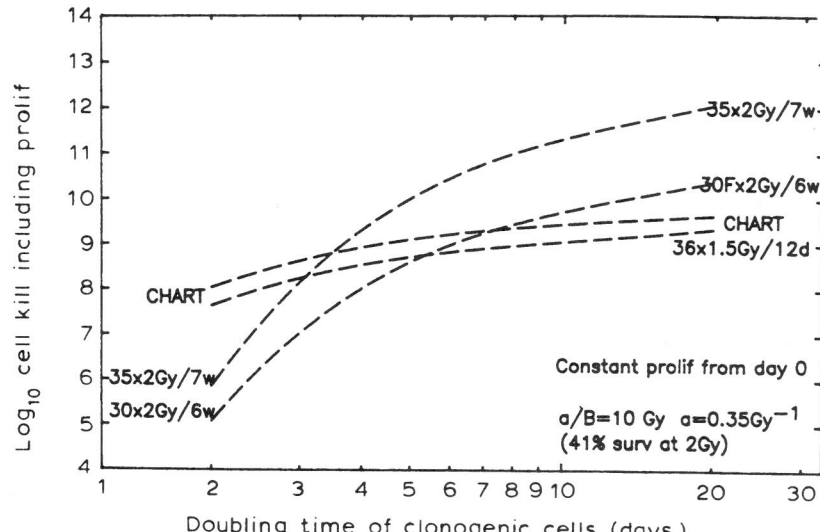

FIGURE 9.10. Influence of the doubling time of clonogenic cells on the calculated log cell kill for different radiation schedules. There is a clear loss of effectiveness for the conventional radiation schedule when the doubling time decreases. The different parameters are assumed to be 0.35 Gy for α and 10 Gy for α/β, and a constant proliferation throughout the treatment. (From Fowler JF. Fractionation and therapeutic gain. In: Steel GG, Adams GE, Horwich A, eds. The biological basis of radiotherapy. 2nd ed. Amsterdam: Elsevier, 1989:182–207.)

problem of performing the procedure within the normal working hours (8 to 10 hours) with an interval between fractions of from 4 to 6 hours. For example, the full recovery at the level of the spinal cord requires more than 6 hours; the total delivered dose thus needed to be reduced to avoid this severe late damage (76, 78).

The concomitant boost technique is a form of an accelerated schedule in which the classic cone-down boost is not delivered after the basic large radiation fields but rather as a second daily treatment during the delivery of those large fields. The aim of this approach is the reduction of the overall treatment time without increasing the fraction size. This approach is designed to overcome the problem of tumor repopulation without increasing the risk of late damage.

CLINICAL RADIATION PROCEDURE

The modern practice of radiation therapy is a complex multistep procedure requiring the cooperation and skills of several professionals (physicians involved in the imaging procedures, nurses, technologists, physicists, dosimetrists, nutritionists).

The initial step of any radiation treatment is a precise clinical evaluation of the patient and the extent and nature of the disease. The clinical evaluation is based on all sources of information available: clinical examination, imaging procedures such as computed tomography (CT), magnetic resonance imaging (MRI), radiography, radionuclide tests, laboratory tests, and surgical information. This evaluation must allow for a precise staging of the tumor and the decision to treat or not to treat the patient. The possible benefits as well as the side and late effects induced by the radiation, the possible alternative treatments, and their integration into a multidisciplinary approach must be taken into account.

After the decision to treat, the different target volumes must be defined; the palpable or visible extent of the tumor represents the gross tumor volume (79). A margin must be added to this volume to include direct local subclinical spread; the resulting figure is the clinical target volume. Additional volume may be added to cover, for example, the possible regional lymph nodes. These volumes are based purely on anatomic-topographic and biologic considerations without taking into account the technical factors of the treatment. For radiation treatment planning, margins must be added to the clinical target volume to account for the variation in size and position of tissues during treatment (e.g., patient movement, breathing during treatment) and for the possible variation in the daily set-up. This figure represents the planning target volume, which is more a geometrical concept used to ensure that the clinical target volume receives the prescribed dose. Furthermore, the radiation oncologist must define the different critical structures.

The next step is treatment planning. In the early 1970s, the advent of CT and the introduction of computed treatment planning revolutionized the radiation treatment approach. CT is now the basic treatment planning tool, but it must be performed with the patient in the position used for the radiation treatment, thus requiring use of a similar flat table. Furthermore, because CT contains electron density data, factors can be calculated to correct inhomogeneities in tissue density. Actual treatment plans are performed through a library of isodose distribution of the entire spectrum of

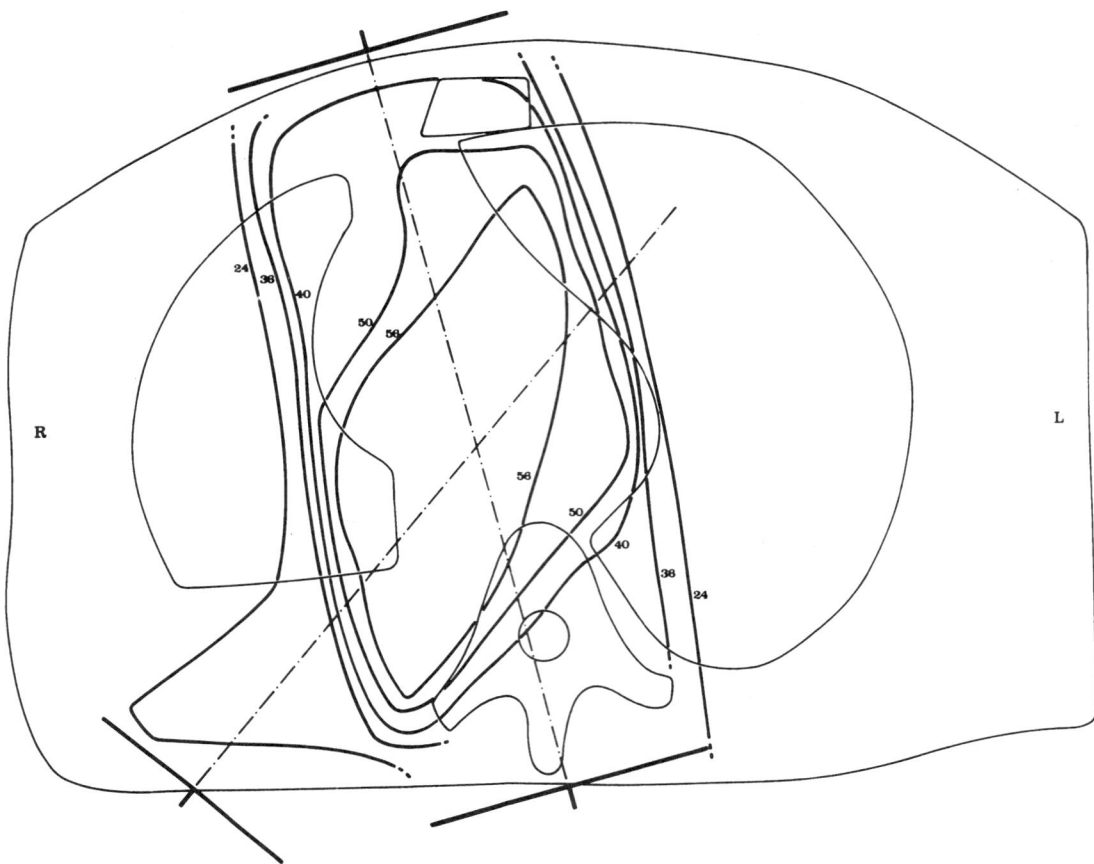

FIGURE 9.11. Example of dose distribution after a right pneumonectomy. A dose of 56 Gy is delivered to the mediastinum with a three-field technique, thus limiting the dose to the spinal cord and the remaining left lung.

beam energies and modalities available in the department (Fig. 9.11).

The goal is to individualize the treatment and ideally to obtain a complete description of the radiation dose distribution in the three dimensions throughout the volume of interest within the body. Thus, to plan individual treatment, it is necessary to have at least one cross-sectional contour of the patient and to report the position of the target volume and critical structures. In the past treatment planning was performed by making a manual contour of the patient using, for example, lead wires and then sets of isodose curves that were manually reported on the contour.

Dose calculations once were performed in one or a few planes. Currently, three-dimensional (3D) treatment planning is becoming available (80) (Fig. 9.12). This approach allows for refinement of the treatment and movement from simply shaped fixed beams to a mixed beam approach; it also allows for the use of increasingly more complicated set-ups that even approach the complexity of conformal therapy. Three-dimensional treatment planning allows for the development of dose-volume histograms; this information, in turn, helps to improve the understanding of the problems of normal tissue tolerance because most late effects appear to be dose as well as volume related. Furthermore, the 3D treatment planning system provides dose reconstructions that show the coverage of the target volume and critical structures. It also generates a beam's eye view digital image of how the simulation field should look.

A diagnostic x-ray unit, the simulator, is used to take radiographs of each treatment portal. The geometric parameters are identical to the different treatment units. Some centers now use CT-designed simulators. Another important step is the provision of proper immobilization, which can be done with foam, plastic, or plaster, and of a marking technique, either permanent (tattoos) or temporary, to ensure the daily reproducibility of the treatment.

The daily radiation treatment implies the delivery of the radiation in the conditions defined by the treatment plan and the reproducibility of these conditions several times. Included in this plan are the treatment

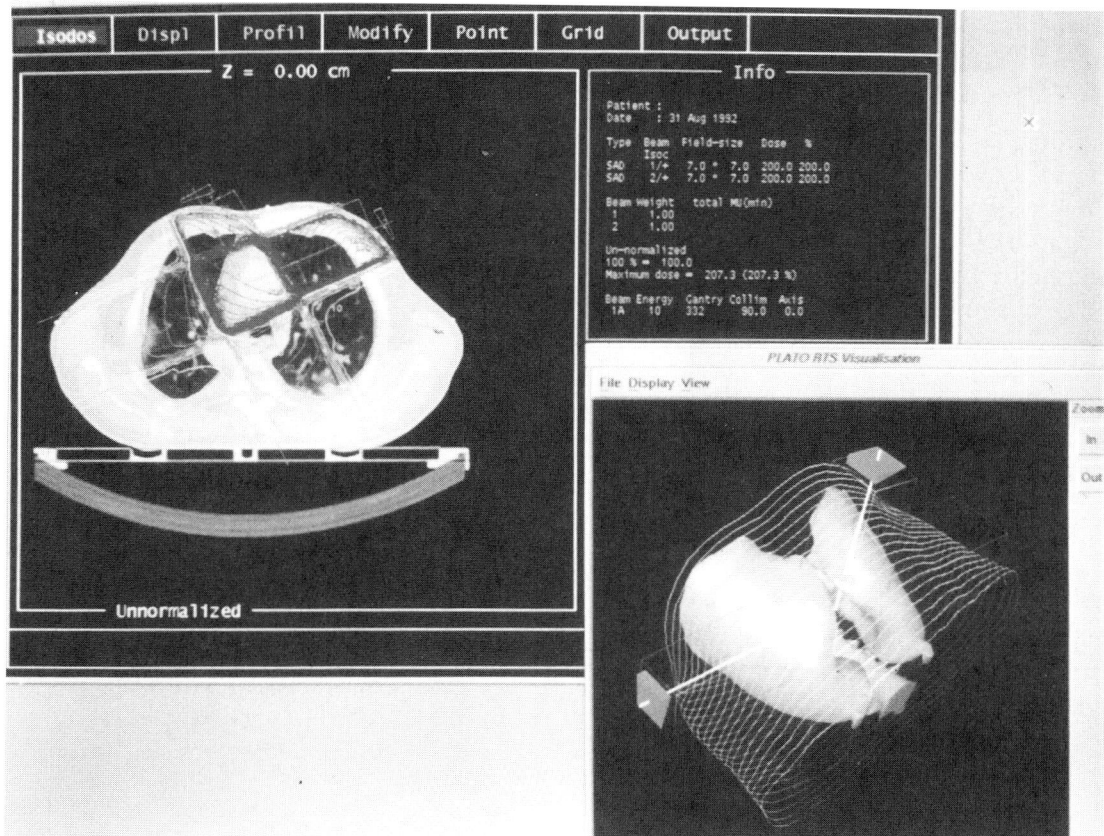

FIGURE 9.12. Example of 3D treatment planning for lung cancer. (Courtesy of Nucletron International, Veanandal, The Netherlands.) See color plates.

parameters (field sizes, beam angles, beam energy, wedge filters), the patient's position, and the quality of the radiotherapy unit. Indeed, the best treatment planning system is meaningless if physicians cannot ensure a proper and precise daily set-up. In 1986 Horiot and colleagues (81) noted that "in most instances, improvement in radiotherapy in visited centers is not dependent upon an increase in megavoltage equipment. It depends rather on improved integration of tumor localization, treatment planning, simulation and quality control during treatment". Quality assurance and reproducibility of daily treatments are the cornerstone of a successful treatment. Several tools are quite useful in reducing the risk of errors and improving the accuracy of the treatment. A routine machine calibration is necessary, including checks of the simulator and lasers, routine in vivo dosimetry, and computer programs that control the individual treatment parameters on the different units. Special devices and lasers are helpful in subsequently placing the patient in the same position. Conventional portal verification films and on-line portal imaging are two systems used to reduce the risk of set-up errors.

Portal films can be made with the supervoltage unit and then compared to the simulator films to control reproducibility; the former often are of poor quality because of the supervoltage radiation, which is absorbed primarily by a Compton process. The main drawbacks of conventional portal verification films are the time required for processing and reviewing and the high cost of materials and handling if repeated verifications are performed during a course of treatment. On-line portal imaging systems provide, within a few seconds, a view of the field treated, allowing either the modification of the field position or the cessation of treatment. Video-based systems can acquire an image in less than 1 second, and the scanning liquid ion chamber design requires 6 seconds to obtain an image. The low operating costs and simplicity of operation allow the repetition of the procedure for each field and at each session. The main problems are related to the initial investment cost and the limited resolution of images for some localizations or angles (82, 83).

During the radiation treatment, the physician must evaluate the patient regularly to determine the individual tolerance and tumor response to the radiation. Indeed, adequate supportive care may be helpful in reducing the possible side effects. This care must be carried out in close cooperation with the nursing staff, the referring physician, and primarily the general practitioner because most patients are treated as outpatients. After treatment the radiation oncologist must continue to follow the patient both to detect a possible relapse and to observe and treat the potential late effects induced by the radiation.

In a recent survey of radiation practice for non–small cell lung cancer, the responses were available from 114 radiotherapists from 38 countries (84). Concerning the radiation facilities available, 98% had access to a linear accelerator, 99% to CT scan for treatment planning, 87% to individualized blocks, and 76% to lung factors corrections. However, there is a wide variety of calculation methods that range from fixed value (21%) to pixel by pixel calculated values (29%). Three-dimensional treatment planning was used routinely only in 14% of the centers. The progress in radiobiology had a major impact on daily radiation practice: only 6% of the radiotherapists are using the split-course technique and 2.7% are using fewer than four fractions per week.

SPECIAL RADIATION TECHNIQUES
Brachytherapy

Soon after the radium was discovered by Marie Curie, it was used to treat cancers. In 1904 Danlos prepared surface applicators to treat skin lesions. During the two world wars, brachytherapy techniques using radium were developed for the treatment of gynecologic cancers—and the debate had begun about the importance of the dose rate. Heyman at the Radiumhemmet in Stockholm treated cervical cancers with three equal implants lasting for 24 hours, whereas Regaud in Paris found better results with a treatment extended over several days using low-intensity radium. During the last 20 years, brachytherapy techniques have experienced a renewal because of the new radioelements available, the introduction of precise dose distribution, the possibilities of afterloading techniques that increase the radioprotection of the medical staff, and a better understanding of the radiobiologic principles applying to brachytherapy techniques.

Implants are classified as permanent (with the sources remaining indefinitively in the patient) and temporary (the sources being placed in the patient for a fixed and limited period). Table 9.1 summarizes the main characteristics of the different radioelements currently available. Permanent implants, besides causing possible radioprotection problems, have several drawbacks because of the long duration of radiation exposure: (a) a slow and progressive decrease in the dose rate leading to dose calculation problems, (b) the risks of source displacement over time, and (c) the impossibility of modifying the source position in case of misplacement. This approach is used primarily for tumor locations unapproachable for a temporary implant. In the past radioactive sources were implanted directly into patients, leading to an exposure of the medical staff, the use of standardized forms of implantations, and limited dosimetry possibilities (the only variable parameter being the duration of implantation). Today, afterloading techniques are increasingly more popular and involve placing catheters, taking radiographs with dummy sources, performing a dose distribution study, and, finally, inserting the radiation source in the right configuration (Figs. 9.13 and 9.14). This approach allows for optimization of the dose distribution to the patient while reducing the radiation exposure of the medical staff. Furthermore, remote afterloading machines are now used more commonly and replace the manual placement of the radioactive sources.

Brachytherapy techniques also are classified by the dose rate: the low dose rate (LDR) delivers 0.4 to 2 Gy/hour, the medium dose rate delivers between 2 and 12 Gy/hour, and the high dose rate delivers more than 12 Gy/hour or more than 0.2 Gy/minute. High-dose-rate brachytherapy technique has become more popu-

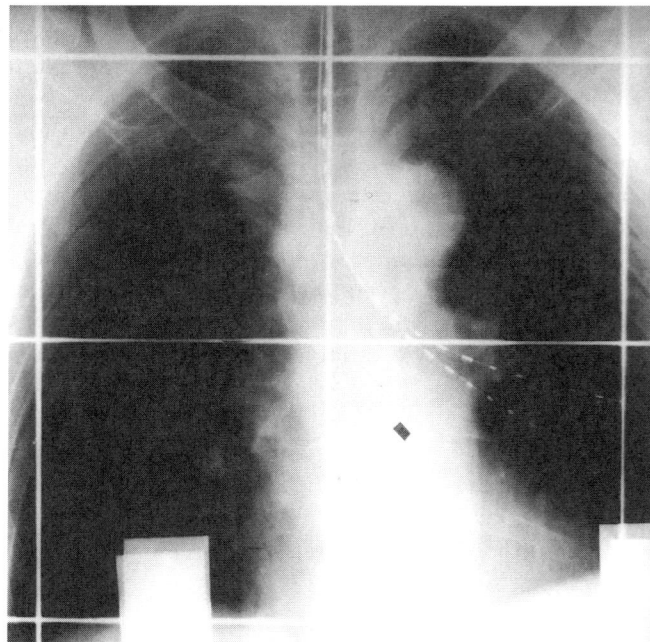

FIGURE 9.13. Radiographs with two dummy catheters used to check the position of the sources in this case of endobronchial brachytherapy.

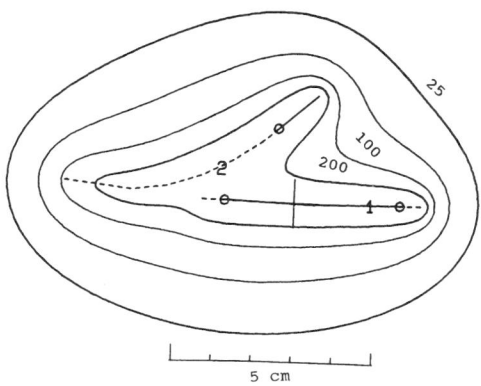

FIGURE 9.14. Dose distribution with two iridium wires. Notice the rapid fall off of the dose.

lar because it offers several advantages. (a) The treatment can be carried out on an outpatient basis, which decreases the total cost, in the same shielded room, thus eliminating the need for an operating room or general anesthesia. (b) There is no need for source preparation, thus reducing staff exposure. (c) Treatment times are shorter, allowing for treatment of more patients. (d) There is less risk of applicator and source displacements during the treatment because the time is shorter. The latter also increases patient comfort. On the negative side, this approach requires the physician to fractionate the treatment and to adjust the total dose. Pulse-dose-rate brachytherapy is a new method combining the principle of high dose rate and hyperfractionation; numerous small radiation doses are delivered over time with a small time interval. The aim is the simulation of continuous irradiation through use of a high number of fractions, allowing for the advantage of the repair process.

The impact of the dose rate variation should be considered relative to the possible radiobiologic effects and clinical data (85, 86). The classic survival curve for mammalian cells shows that the second part of the curve becomes increasingly more shallow when the dose rate is reduced. This reduction in cell killing is caused by repair of sublethal damage. The repair process for most tissues has a half-time of 1 to 2 hours. Redistribution within the cell cycle takes a few days for proliferating tissue. Repopulation takes a few weeks for active renewal tissue such as the human mucosa (2 to 3 weeks with a conventional fractionated schedule), but a longer period for late-reacting tissues. Reoxygenation may affect the tumors on a time scale, probably, of days. Thus, the repair process, lasting several minutes or days, is the most important process affecting treatment duration. For very low dose rates, cell cycle progression may be an important factor in that cells may accumulate in the G2 phase, a more radiosensitive part of the cycle. If the treatment is extended over a longer period, then repopulation may occur within the normal tissue and the tumor. Furthermore, for a high dose rate, the fraction size has a greater influence on late damage than on early reaction.

The impact of the dose rate in clinical brachytherapy is well known. Nevertheless, until recently, there was a major controversy between clinicians and radiobiologists. Relevant series did not show any difference in tumor control or late damage for treatments given in 3 to 10 days, whereas all radiobiologic data suggested a great difference, especially for slowly proliferating tissue. Within the dose range of 50 to 200 cGy per hour, Lambin et al. (87) observed an increased incidence in late damage when higher dose rates were used to treat cervical cancer. The percentage of complications, regardless of the grade, rose from 32% for a dose rate of 0.38 Gy/hour to 54% for a dose rate of 0.73 Gy/hour; severe late damage (grades 3 and 4) was observed, respectively, in 9 and 13 patients in each group, which each included 102 women. The reference isodose of 60 Gy was identical for both dose rates. In a series of two consecutive articles on breast and tongue cancers, Mazeron et al. (88, 89) observed a correlation between tumor control or late damage and dose rate (Fig. 9.15).

Interstitial implants of the lung are used mainly for gross residual disease in the lung parenchyma, chest wall, or mediastinum. The technique requires a surgical procedure. Permanent radioactive sources (gold Au 198 or iodine 125) may be implanted using a nomogram to determine the number of seeds required to cover the tumor volume. Another approach is the insertion of plastic catheters for an afterloading approach with iridium wires (90). Hilaris and Martini (91) reported their results with 340 patients treated only with a permanent implantation. The 5-year survival rate was 46% for 13 patients with stage I disease and 7% for those with stage III tumors. A 68% local control rate was reported.

Recently, endobronchial brachytherapy has been developed because of technical progress in the design of applicators, sources, and afterloading machines. In the past, radon 222 or iodine 125 seeds were placed during a rigid bronchoscopy with some success. However, at the time this was a very difficult procedure that included problems with radiation exposure of the medical staff, acute effects caused by edema or hemorrhage, and radiation source displacements and poor geometry. Currently, flexible catheters are introduced during a flexible fiberbronchoscopy. Radiographs are

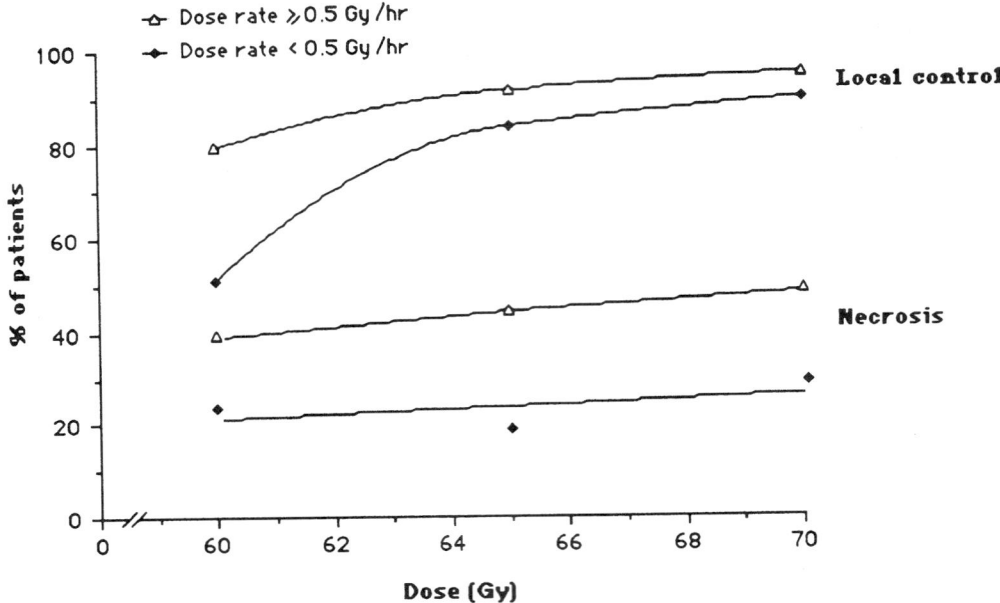

FIGURE 9.15. Influence of the dose rate on local control and necrosis for a pelvilingual tumor treated with iridium. Notice the steepness of the local control curve for low dose rate. (From Mazeron JJ, Simon JM, Le Pechoux C, et al. Effect of dose rate and local control on complications in definitive irradiation of T1-2 squamous cell carcinoma of the mobile tongue and floor of the mouth with interstitial iridium 192. Radiother Oncol 1991;21:39–47.)

taken to verify their position and afterwards as a dose distribution study, and the treatment may be performed using, for example, a high-dose-rate afterloading unit. This approach has been used to treat recurrent endobronchial tumors, as a boost to complete an external course of radiation, or as a palliative treatment to relieve a bronchial obstruction (92–94).

THREE-DIMENSIONAL CONFORMAL/DYNAMIC RADIATION THERAPY

The introduction of new computer technology, both for treatment planning and computer-driven treatment systems, has led to the development of conformal radiation therapy. Conformal therapy aims to match precisely the borders of the treated volume to the clinical target volume while reducing as much as possible the amount of normal tissue irradiated. The main goal of this new technology follows directly from the general philosophy of radiation research over the years: that volume reduction helps to increase the dose to the target area for the purpose of achieving better local control and thus improvement in survival. Of course, a prerequisite is that the local control of the tumor has a great impact on the possible metastatic spread and thus on patient survival. Several requirements must be fulfilled when using this technology:

The precise definition of tumor volume and organs at risk through the use of modern imaging systems with 3D reconstruction.

Optimization of radiation technique by use of multiple fields of irradiation, dynamically controlled rotation of the linear accelerator, and dynamic computer-controlled multileaf collimation, allowing modification of the beam collimation during the rotation of the linear accelerator.

Precise set-up of the patient (perfect immobilization and possibilities for an on-line imaging system for position verification) (95, 96).

For example, a photon beam is shaped dynamically by a multileaf collimator to conform to the tumor projection while the linear accelerator is rotating around the patient. The precision achieved by such a technique raises questions about our ability to define the clinical target volume with such precision, the limits of imaging procedures such as CT or MRI to define precisely the tumor extent within 1 or 2 mm, and, finally, the reproducibility of the daily treatments including patient movement, tumor displacement during the radiation course, and possible anatomic variation resulting, for example, from weight loss.

Conformal radiotherapy may be an alternative to increasing doses above 70 Gy while keeping the dose to the spinal cord or the contralateral lung within the accepted tolerated limits. Ha et al. (97) evaluated the gain from such an approach in six patients with a non–small cell lung cancer. A minimum target dose of 80 Gy could be given to three of the six patients if a technique other than conventional treatment was used, two could be treated adequately by either method, and one could not receive the prescribed dose regardless of the method used. In a similar study, Armstrong et al. (98) noticed that only two of nine patients received a minimal dose of more than 70 Gy with a conventional planning but that, with 3D conformal radiation therapy planning, nine patients could receive more than 70 Gy to the tumor while reducing significantly the dose to the esophagus and lung parenchyma. This approach allows for the initiation of studies on radiation dose escalation.

INTRAOPERATIVE RADIATION THERAPY

The main limitation of radiotherapy is the tolerance of normal tissues. Intraoperative radiation therapy (IORT) has been introduced to overcome this problem of normal tissue tolerance by delivering the radiation to the target area while keeping or protecting these normal tissues. In fact, IORT is a very old technique that was used in the early practice of radiotherapy to overcome the technical limitations of the available equipment (e.g., orthovoltage machines with low deep penetration). This approach was then developed by Abe and his colleagues in Japan, taking advantage of the dose distribution of electron beams. IORT implies delivery of a high single radiation dose during a surgical procedure. This approach offers several advantages. (*a*) The surgical procedure allows for visualization of the tumor directly and thus for limitation of the radiation precisely to the desired target volume. (*b*) Surgery allows removal of some sensitive organs or structures from the treatment field. (*c*) The use of electron beams whose penetration into tissue depends directly on their energy allows for limiting the radiation to the treated area. The main problems of this approach relate to the practical organization and delivery of a single high-dose fraction. The practical organization certainly is one of the greatest problems because in most centers the operating room and the radiation facilities are not in the same unit, thus requiring transportation of the patient (Fig. 9.16). (Few centers have a dedicated IORT machine placed in an operating room.)

This single high-dose fraction has raised many questions, especially regarding normal tissue tolerance. A series of studies has been carried out on dogs in an attempt to define the tolerance doses both on normal organs or after surgery. Large abdominal blood vessels tolerate doses in excess of 40 Gy, whereas

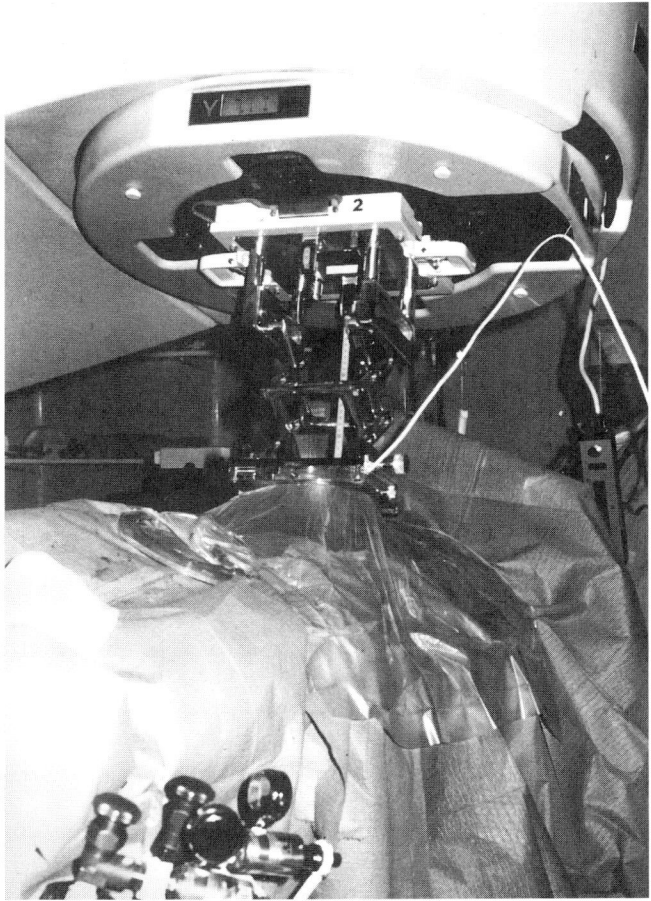

FIGURE 9.16. Intraoperative radiotherapy. The cone is fixed to the linear accelerator through a special device with a sterile drape covering the surgical bed. See color plates.

many functioning organs such as the kidney, duodenum, small bowel, and ureter exhibit some damage from doses in excess of 15 to 20 Gy (99). Tochner et al. (100) specifically evaluated the tolerance of thoracic organs. The trachea and large blood vessels can tolerate doses in excess of 20 Gy, whereas the tolerance of the esophagus, heart, and lung is limited, with severe damage seen with doses of 20 Gy; thus the latter requires either shielding or limiting, to the absolute minimum, the amount of lung volume treated. Dutreix and colleagues (101) tried to calculate the equivalent dose to conventional 2 Gy fractions. They reported that for early-reacting tissue a single IORT fraction of 20 Gy should be equivalent to 28 fractions of 2 Gy (56 Gy), and for late effects, to 30 fractions or 60 Gy. These figures are offered for illustrative purposes and should be used with caution.

The clinical experience with IORT primarily relates to the treatment of abdominal tumors. There is only very limited experience with IORT for lung cancer, although this technique may be interesting as a means of increasing the total dose delivered to the tumor. Calvo et al. (102) treated 34 patients with stage III lung cancer and showed the feasibility of this approach. IORT was used as a boost, delivering single doses of 10 to 15 Gy, and was followed by a course of external radiation (46 to 50 Gy over 5 weeks). They observed two cases of life-threatening complications related to the IORT: one massive hemoptysis and one bronchopleural fistula. With a short period of observation (median follow-up, 1 year), the estimated local control rate was 30%. Arian-Shad et al. (103) treated 24 patients and reported one fatal case of intrabronchial hemorrhage (the tumor initially invaded the pulmonary vein). Sixteen of the 18 patients completing the IORT treatment and external radiation remained free of local recurrence.

QUALITY OF TREATMENT

Radiotherapy is limited by factors related to the tumor (inherent radiosensitivity, unknown microscopic extension, or distant metastases), to biologic factors (hypoxia, repair of sublethal damage, tumor cell repopulation), normal tissue tolerance, and to physical and technical issues. The search for the means of reducing and optimizing the radiation treatment must remain one of our major commitments. This optimization implies improvement in the definition of tumor localization, avoidance of heterogeneous dose distribution in the treatment planning, and insurance of a good transmission of information and reproducibility of the daily treatments (81, 104).

Locoregional control of the disease is an absolute requirement for the cure of a patient's cancer, but it also reduces the risk of distant metastatic spread. This correlation has been reported for cancer of the prostate, head and neck, breast, cervix, and endometrium (105–107). During the last decade, local control also has been recognized as a critical factor in lung cancer. Perez et al. (108) reported a better survival for the first 3 years after radiation therapy in the case of intrathoracic tumor control evaluated at 6 months (Fig. 9.17). In a recent meta-analysis, Pignon et al. (109) reported an improvement in survival for limited small cell carcinoma when thoracic radiation therapy was added to chemotherapy.

During recent years, several studies have outlined clearly the importance and impact of treatment quality (dose, technique, fractionation) on the outcome of patients treated for lung cancer. Treatment interruptions delaying the completion of planned radiation therapy may have a negative impact on survival. In a recent re-

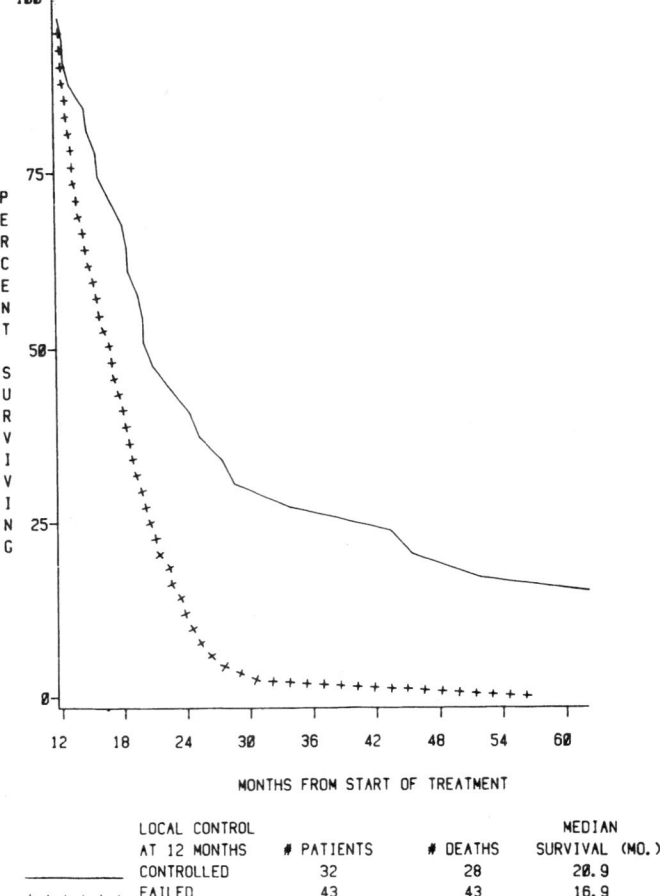

FIGURE 9.17. The importance of local control, evaluated at 12 months, on the survival of patients treated with radiation for inoperable lung cancer (RTOG protocol 73-01). (From Perez CA, Bauer M, Edelstein S, Gillespie BW, Birch R. Impact of tumor control on survival in carcinoma of the lung treated with irradiation. Int J Radiat Oncol Biol Phys 1986;12:539–548.)

view of the RTOG (25) experience with hyperfractionated schedules, the 2-year survival rates for patients with favorable prognosis (performance status, greater than 90%; weight loss, less than 15%; and no N3 disease) dropped from 33% to 14% if the radiation therapy had been delayed.

The radiation technique is another important factor not only for the control of the primary tumor but also for the avoidance of severe late effects. In the 1970s, a common practice of thoracic radiotherapy was the introduction of a so-called spinal cord block to avoid treating the spinal cord to doses exceeding its tolerance. The technique was simple and involved block shielding of the spinal cord; of course, the block also protected the central extension of the tumor and the involved mediastinal lymph nodes, an undesirable effect. With the progress in treatment planning and the emergence of CT, it is now easy to deliver the dose to

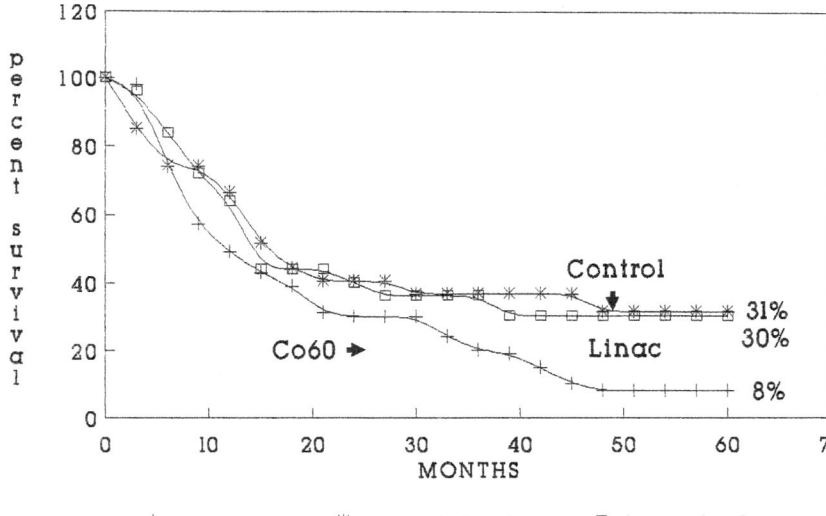

FIGURE 9.18. Influence of the radiation technique on survival after a pneumonectomy. (From Phlips P, Roemans P, Vanderhoeft P, Van Houtte P. Postoperative radiotherapy after pneumonectomy: impact of modern treatment facilities. Int J Radiat Oncol Biol Phys 1993;27:525–529.)

the primary tumor and the mediastinum while protecting the spinal cord (through the use of oblique or lateral fields). Several quality control studies reviewed the radiotherapy performed within trials, and they clearly demonstrated a negative impact of protocol deviation on local control and survival (37, 110).

In the experience of the authors (111), a poor survival after irradiation, especially in the case of a pneumonectomy, was observed in a randomized trial evaluating the role of postoperative radiotherapy for lung cancer. This effect was thought to be caused by the radiation technique used (three fields from a telecobalt unit), leading to an increased morbidity. In a recent review, the survival of patients treated with postoperative radiotherapy after a pneumonectomy for a T3, N1 or N2 tumor was similar to that of a group of patients operated for only an N0 tumor; those irradiated patients had an initial CT scan for treatment planning and were treated with a linear accelerator (Fig. 9.18) (112). This survival was achieved primarily by reducing complications while maintaining local control.

Radiation therapy is a complex procedure involving several steps: treatment prescription, treatment preparation, and treatment execution. Errors caused by an inadequate transfer of information can have a detrimental effect on the final results. Leunens et al. (113) reported their experience in verifying this treatment chain in a series of 464 patients. Each new treatment required the transfer of approximately 52 pieces of data, thus, 24,128 pieces of information had to be transferred. The total number of errors was 139 (0.6%), but 26% of the new treatments were affected. Errors involved the simulation (wrong field size, treatment unit), the data input for the calculation of the dose and the monitoring units, the preparation of the treatment chart, and the verification system on the machine. Interestingly, most of these errors could be detected by in vivo dosimetry and portal imaging. Furthermore, this report implies the need to institute a system to verify the whole treatment set-up at the beginning of the actual therapy to reduce the number of human errors as much as possible.

Within the complex treatment chain, the daily set-up is one of the most important tasks but also the weakest link because control procedures are more difficult to perform daily. Portal films are one way to check the accuracy of radiation fields and to offer a means of comparison with the intended simulated field. Byhardt et al. (114) reported as early as 1978 a localization error for lung irradiation of 13%. This error was caused by field malposition 68% of time. Rodrigus and colleagues (115) reported 46 field placement errors among 142 films taken during a radiation course; these problems included patient malposition (8), field malposition (8), and shielding block malposition (26).

These examples outline the complexity of modern radiation treatments and the necessity for using an adequate and proper technique in the management of lung cancer. Improving treatment accuracy will allow clinicians to increase the radiation dose, which may translate into better local tumor control and increased survival.

REFERENCES

1. Johns H, Cunningham J, eds. The physics of radiology. 4th ed. Springfield IL: CC Thomas, 1983.
2. Bleehen NM, ed. Radiobiology in radiotherapy. Berlin: Springer-Verlag, 1988.
3. Hall EJ, ed. Radiobiology for the radiologist. 4th ed. Philadelphia: Lippincott, 1994.

4. Steel GG, Adams GE, Horwich A, eds. The biological basis of radiotherapy. 2nd ed. Amsterdam: Elsevier, 1989.
5. Tubiana M, Dutreix J, Wambersie A, eds. Radiobiologie. Paris: Hermann, 1986.
6. Fletcher GH, ed. Textbook of radiotherapy. 3rd ed. London: Henry Kimpton Publishers, 1980.
7. Scherer E, Streffer C, Trott KR, eds. Radiopathology of organs and tissues. Berlin, Heidelberg: Springer-Verlag, 1991.
8. Stephens LC, Ang KK, Schultheiss TE, Milas L, Meyn R. Apoptosis in irradiated murine tumors. Radiat Res 1991;127:308–316.
9. Weichselbaum RR. Radioresistant and repair proficient cells may determine radiocurability in human tumors. Int J Radiat Oncol Biol Phys 1986;12: 637–639.
10. Joiner MC, Denekamp J, Maughan RL. The use of "top-up" experiments to investigate the effect of very small doses per fraction in mouse skin. Int J Radiat Biol 1986;49:565–580.
11. Gray LH, Conger AD, Ebert M, Hornsey S, Scott OC. The concentration of oxygen dissolved in tissues at the time of irradiation as a factor in radiotherapy. Br J Radiol 1953;26:638–648.
12. Thomlinson RH, Gray LH. The histological structure of some human lung cancers and the possible implications for radiotherapy Br J Cancer 1955;9:539–549.
13. van Putten LM, Kallman RF. Oxygenation status of a transplantable tumor during fractionated radiation therapy. J Natl Cancer Inst 1968;40:441–451.
14. Dische S. Hyperbaric oxygen: the Medical Research Council trials and their clinical significance. Br J Radiol 1979;51:888–894.
15. Bush RS, Jenkin RD, Allt WE, et al. Definitive evidence for hypoxic cells influencing cure in cancer therapy. Br J Cancer 1978;37:302–306.
16. Dische S, Saunders MI, Warburton MF. Hemoglobin, radiation morbidity and survival. Int J Radiat Oncol Biol Phys 1986;12:1335–1337.
17. Overgaard J, Sand Hansen H, Jorgensen K, Hjelm Hansen M. Primary radiotherapy of larynx and pharynx carcinoma: an analysis of some factors influencing local control and survival. Int J Radiat Oncol Biol Phys 1986;12:515–522.
18. Rojas A. Radiosensitisation with normobaric oxygen and carbogen. Radiother Oncol 1991;20:65–70.
19. Dische S, Rojas A, Rugg T, Hong A, Michael BD. Carbogen breathing: a system for use in man. Br J Radiol 1993;64:1081–1091.
20. Barendsen GW, Broerse JJ. Experimental radiotherapy of a rat rhabdomyosarcoma with 15 MeV neutrons and 300 kV x-rays. II. Effects of fractionated treatments applied five times a week for several weeks. Eur J Cancer 1970;6:89–109.
21. Withers HR, Taylor JMG, Maciejewski B. The hazard of accelerated tumor clonogen repopulation during radiotherapy. Acta Oncol 1988;27:131–146.
22. Parsons JT, Bova FJ, Million RR. A reevaluation of split course technique for squamous cell carcinoma of the head and neck. Int J Radiat Oncol Biol Phys 1980;6:1645–1652.
23. Girinsky T, Rey A, Roche B, et al. Overall treatment time in advanced cervical carcinomas: a critical parameter in treatment outcome. Int J Radiat Oncol Biol Phys 1993;27:1051–1056.
24. Keane TJ, Fyles A, O'Sullivan B, Barton M, Maki E, Simm J. The effect of treatment duration on local control of squamous carcinoma of the tonsil and of the cervix. Semin Radiat Oncol 1992;2:26–28.
25. Cox JD, Pajak TF, Asbell S, et al. Interruptions of high-dose radiation therapy decrease long-term survival of favorable patients with unresectable non–small cell carcinoma of the lung: analysis of 1244 cases from 3 Radiation Therapy Oncology Group (RTOG) trials. Int J Radiat Oncol Biol Phys 1993;27:493–498.
26. Perez CC, Pajak TF, Rubin P., et al. Long-term observations of the patterns of failure in patients with unresectable non–oat cell carcinoma of the lung treated with definitive radiotherapy: report by the Radiation Therapy Oncology Group. Cancer 1987;59:1874–1881.
27. Schiffer LM. Cellular proliferation in tumor and normal tissues. In: Perez CA, Brady LW, eds. Principles and practice of radiation oncology. Philadelphia: Lippincott, 1987:56–66.
28. Begg AC, Hofland I, Van Glabekke M, Bartelink H, Horiot JC. Predictive value of potential doubling time for radiotherapy of head and neck tumor patient: results from the EORTC Cooperative trial 22851. Semin Radiat Oncol 1992;2:22–25.
29. Corvo R, Giaretti W, Sanguineti G, et al. Potential doubling time in head and neck tumors treated by primary radiotherapy: preliminary evidence for a prognostic significance in local control. Int J Radiat Oncol Biol Phys 1993;27:1165–1172.
30. Fowler JF. Brief summary of radiobiological principles in fractionated radiotherapy. Semin Radiat Oncol 1992;2:16–21.
31. Kellerer AM, Rossi HH. The theory of dual radiation action. Curr Top Radiat Res 1972;8:85–158.
32. Kellerer AM, Rossi HH. A generalized formulation of dual radiation action. Radiat Res 1978;75:471–488.
33. Chadwick KH, Leenhouts HP. A molecular theory of cell survival. Phys Med Biol 1973;18:78–87.
34. Chadwick KH, Leenhouts HP, eds. The molecular theory of radiation biology. Berlin, Heidelberg, New York: Springer, 1981.
35. Withers HR, Thames HD, Peters LJ. A new isoeffect curve for change in dose per fraction. Radiat Oncol 1983;1:187–191.
36. Scalliet P, Cosset JM, Wambersie A. Application of the LQ model to the interpretation of absorbed dose distribution in the daily practice of radiotherapy. Radiother Oncol 1991;22:180–189.
37. Perez CA, Stanley K, Grundy G, et al. Impact of irradiation technique and tumor extent in tumor control and survival of patients with unresectable non–oat cell carcinoma of the lung. Report by the Radiation Therapy Oncology Group. Cancer 1982;50:1091–1099.
38. Hazuka M, Turrisi AT, Lutz ST, et al. Results of high-dose thoracic irradiation incorporating beam's eye view display in non–small cell lung cancer: a retrospective multivariate analysis. Int J Radiat Oncol Biol Phys 1993;27:273–284.
39. Gelinas M, Fletcher GH. Incidence and causes of local failure of irradiation in squamous cell carcinoma of the faucial arch, tonsillar fossa and base of tongue. Radiology 1973;108:383–387.
40. Cox JD, Komaki R, Eisert DR. Irradiation for inoperable carcinoma of the lung and high performance status. JAMA 1980;244:1931–1933.
41. Peters LJ, Brock WA, Johnson T, Meyn RE, Tofilon JP, Milas L. Potential methods for predicting tumor radiocurability. Int J Radiat Oncol Biol Phys 1986;12:459–468.
42. Fertil B, Malaise EP. Intrinsic radiosensitivity of human cell lines is correlated with radioresponsiveness of human tumours. Analysis of 101 published survival curves. Int J Radiat Oncol Biol Phys 1985;11:1699–1707.
43. Malaise EP, Fertil B, Chavaudra N, Guichard M. Distribution of radiation sensitivities for human tumor cells of specific histological types: comparison of in vitro to in vivo data. Int J Radiat Oncol Biol Phys 1986;12:617–624.

44. Raaphorst GP. Prediction of radiotherapy response using SF2: is it methodology or mythology? Radiother Oncol 1993;28:187–188.
45. Deacon J, Peckham MJ, Steel G. The radioresponsiveness of human tumours and the initial slope of the cell survival curve. Radiother Oncol 1984;2:317–324.
46. Girinsky T, Lubin R, Pignon JP, et al. Predictive value of in vitro radiosensitivity parameters in head and neck cancers and cervical carcinomas: preliminary correlations with local control and overall survival. Int J Radiat Oncol Biol Phys 1992;25:3–7.
47. Midander J, Révész L. The frequency of micronuclei as a measure of cell survival in irradiated cell population. Int J Radiat Oncol Biol Phys 1980;38:237–241.
48. Streffer C, van Beuningen D, Gross E, Schabronath J, Eigler FW, Rebmann A. Predictive assays for the therapy of rectum carcinoma. Radiother Oncol 1986;5:303–310.
49. Carmichael J, Degraff WG, Gazdar AF, Minna JD, Mitchell JB. Evaluation of tetrazolium based semi-automated colorimetric assay. 2. Assessment of radiosensitivity. Cancer Res 1987;47:943–946.
50. Höckel M, Knoop C, Schlenger K, et al. Intratumoral pO2 predicts survival in advanced cancer of the uterine cervix. Radiother Oncol 1993;26:45–50.
51. Awwad HK, Khafagy Y, Barsoum M, et al. Accelerated versus conventional fractionation in the postoperative irradiation of locally advanced head and neck cancer: influence of tumor proliferation. Radiother Oncol 1992;25:261–266.
52. Rubin P, Casarett G. A direction for clinical radiation pathology. The tolerance dose. Front Radiat Ther Oncol 1972;6:1–16.
53. Emami B, Lyman J, Brown A, et al. Tolerance of normal tissue to therapeutic irradiation. Int J Radiat Oncol Biol Phys 1991;21:109–122.
54. Jablon G. Epidemiologic perspectives in radiation carcinogenesis In: Boice JD, Fraumani JF, eds. Radiation carcinogenesis. New York: Raven Press, 1984:1–8.
55. Smith PG. Late effects of x-ray treatment of ankylating spondylitis. In: Boice JD, Fraumani JF, eds. Radiation carcinogenesis. New York: Raven Press, 1984:107–118.
56. Boice JD, Blettner M, Kleinerman RA, et al. Radiation dose and leukemia risk in patients treated for cancer of the cervix. J Natl Cancer Inst 1987;79:1295–1311.
57. Boice JD, Engholm G, Kleinerman RA, et al. Radiation dose and second cancer risk in patients treated for cancer of the cervix. Radiat Res 1988;116:3–55.
58. Somers R, Henry-Ammar M, Meerwaldt JK, Carde P, eds. Treatment strategy in Hodgkin's disease. London: Colloques Inserm John Libbey Eurotext, 1990;186.
59. Hancock SL, Trucker MA, Hoppe RT. Breast cancer after treatment of Hodgkin's disease. J Natl Cancer Inst 1993;85:25–31.
60. Donaldson SS. Lessons from our children. Int J Radiat Oncol Biol Phys 1993;26:739–749.
61. Storm HH, Anderson M, Boice JD, et al. Adjuvant radiotherapy and risk of contralateral breast cancer. J Natl Cancer Inst 1992;84:1245–1249.
62. Boice JD, Day NE, Andersen A, et al. Second cancers following radiation treatment for cervical cancer. An international collaboration among cancer registries. J Natl Cancer Inst 1985;74:955–975.
63. Buschke F, Parker RG, eds. Radiation therapy in cancer management. New York: Grune & Stratton, 1972.
64. Gallez-Marchal D, Fayolle M, Henry-Amar M, LeBourgeois JP, Rougier P, Cosset JM. Radiation injuries of the gastrointestinal tract in Hodgkin's disease: the role of exploratory laparotomy and fractionation. Radiother Oncol 1984;2:93–99.
65. Cox JD. Large-dose fractionation. Cancer 1985;55:2105–2111.
66. Dische S, Martin WMC, Anderson P. Radiation myelopathy in patients treated for carcinoma of the bronchus using a six fraction regime of radiotherapy Br J Radiol 1981;54:29–35.
67. Stranqvist M. Stubien uber die kumulative wirking der Roentgenstrahlen bei fraktioerrun. Acta Radiol 1944;55:1–300.
68. Ellis F. Dose, time and fractionation: a clinical hypothesis. Clin Radiol 1969;20:1–7.
69. Thames HD, Withers HR, Peters LJ, Fletcher GH. Changes in early and late radiation responses with altered fractionation: implications for dose-survival relationships Int J Radiat Oncol Biol Phys 1982;8:219–226.
70. Withers HR. Biologic basis for altered fractionation schemes. Cancer 1985;55:2086–2095.
71. Scanlon PW. Initial experience with split-dose periodic radiation therapy. AJR Am J Roentgenol 1960;84:632–644.
72. Sambrook DK. Split-course radiation therapy in malignant tumors. AJR Am J Roentgenol 1965;91:37–45.
73. Abramson N, Cavanaugh PJ. Short-course radiation therapy in carcinoma of the lung: a second look. Radiology 1973;108:686–687.
74. Perez CA, Pajak TF, Rubin P, et al. Long-term observations of the pattern of failure in patients with unresectable non–oat cell carcinoma of the lung treated with definitive radiotherapy. Cancer 1987;59:1874–1881.
75. van Den Bogaert W, van der Schueren E, Horiot JC, et al. Early results of the EORTC randomized clinical trial on multiple fractions per day (MFD) and misonidazole in advanced head and neck tumors. Int J Radiat Oncol Biol Phys 1986;12:587–591.
76. Dische S, Saunders M. Continuous, hyperfractionated, accelerated radiotherapy (CHART): an interim report upon late morbidity. Radiother Oncol 1989;16:65–72.
77. Fowler JF. Fractionation and therapeutic gain. In: Steel GG, Adams GE, Horwich A, eds. The biological basis of radiotherapy. 2nd ed. Amsterdam: Elsevier, 1989:182–207.
78. Wong CS, Van Dyk J, Simpson WJ. Myelopathy following hyperfractionated accelerated radiotherapy for anaplastic thyroid carcinoma. Radioth Oncol 1991;20:3–9.
79. Landberg T, Wambersie A, Chavaudra J, Dobbs J, Hanks G, Johansson K-A, Möller T, et al., eds. Prescribing, recording and reporting photon beam therapy. Bethesda, MD: International Commission on Radiation Units and Measurements (ICRU), Report 50, 1993.
80. Smith AR, Purdy JA. Three-dimensional photon treatment planning. Report of the collaborative working group on the evaluation of treatment planning for external photon beam radiotherapy. Int J Radiat Oncol Biol Phys 1991;21:1–265.
81. Horiot JC, Johansson KA, Gonzalez DG, van der Schueren E, van den Bogaert W. Quality assurance control in the EORTC cooperative group of radiotherapy. 1. Assessment of radiotherapy staff and equipment. Radiother Oncol 1986;6:275–284.
82. Boyer A, Antonuk L, Fenster A,, et al. A review of electronic portal imaging devices (EPIDs). Med Phys 1992;19:1–16.
83. Verellen D, de Neve W, Van Den Heuvel F, Coghe M, Louis O, Storme G. On-line portal imaging: image quality defining parameters for pelvic fields: a clinical evaluation. Int J Radiat Oncol Biol Phys 1993;27:945–952.
84. Van Houtte P, Gregor A, Phlips P. International survey of radiotherapy practice for radical treatment of non–small cell lung cancer. Lung Cancer 1994;11:S128–S138.

85. Steel GG, Down JD, Peacock JH, Stephens TC. Dose-rate effects and the repair of radiation damage. Radiother Oncol 1986;5:321–331.
86. Scalliet P, Landuyt W, van der Schueren E. Kinetics of repair: its influence in low dose rate irradiations. Radiother Oncol 1988;11:249–251.
87. Lambin P, Gerbaulet A, Kramer A, et al. Phase III trial comparing two low dose rates in brachytherapy of cervix carcinoma. Report at 2 years. Int J Radiat Oncol Biol Phys 1993;25:405–412.
88. Mazeron JJ, Simon JM, Crook J, et al. Influence of dose rate on local control of breast carcinoma treated by external beam irradiation plus iridium 192 implant. Int J Radiat Oncol Biol Phys 1991;21:1173–1177.
89. Mazeron JJ, Simon JM, Le Pechoux C, et al. Effect of dose rate and local control on complications in definitive irradiation of T1-2 squamous cell carcinoma of the mobile tongue and floor of the mouth with interstitial iridium 192. Radiother Oncol 1991;21:39–47.
90. Nag S. Brachytherapy for lung cancer: review. Cancer Treat Symp 1985;2:49–56.
91. Hilaris BS, Martini N. Interstitial brachytherapy in cancer of the lung: a 20 year experience. Int J Radiat Oncol Biol Phys 1979;5:1951–1956.
92. Raju PI, Roy T, McDonald RD, et al. Ir-192, low dose rate endobronchial brachytherapy in the treatment of malignant air way obstruction. Int J Radiat Oncol Biol Phys 1993;27:677–680.
93. Speiser BL, Spratling L. Remote afterloading brachytherapy for the local control of endobronchial carcinoma. Int J Radiat Oncol Biol Phys 1993;25:579–588.
94. Speiser BL, Spratling L. Radiation bronchitis and stenosis secondary to high dose rate endobronchial irradiation. Int J Radiat Oncol Biol Phys 1993;25:589–598.
95. Leibel SA, Ling CC, Kutcher GJ, Mohan R, Cordon-Cordo C, Fuks Z. The biological basis for conformal three-dimensional radiation therapy. Int J Radiat Oncol Biol Phys 1991;21:805–811.
96. Powlis WD, Smith AR, Cheng E, et al. Initiation of multileaf collimator conformal radiation therapy. Int J Radiat Oncol Biol Phys 1993;25:171–180.
97. Ha CS, Kijewski PK, Langer MP. Gain in target dose from using computer controlled radiation therapy (CCRT) in the treatment of non–small cell lung cancer. Int J Radiat Oncol Biol Phys 1993;26:335–339.
98. Armstrong JG, Burman C, Leibel S, et al. Three-dimensional conformal radiation therapy may improve the therapeutic ratio of high dose radiation therapy for lung cancer. Int J Radiat Oncol Biol Phys 1993;26:685–689.
99. Sindelar WF, Kinsella T, Tepper J, Travis EL, Rosenberg SA, Glatstein E. Experimental and clinical studies with intraoperative radiotherapy. Surg Gynecol Obstet 1983;157:205–220.
100. Tochner ZA, Pass HI, Sindelar WF, et al. Long term tolerance of thoracic organs to intraoperative radiotherapy. Int J Radiat Oncol Biol Phys 1991;22:65–69.
101. Dutreix J, Cosset JM, Girinsky T. Equivalent biologique des doses uniques utilisées en irradiation peropératoire. Bull Cancer Radiother 1990;77:125–134.
102. Calvo FA, Ortiz De Urbina D, Abuchaibe O, et al. Intraoperative radiotherapy during lung cancer surgery: technical description and early clinical results. Int J Radiat Oncol Biol Phys 1990;19:103–109.
103. Arian-Schad KS, Juettner FM, Ratzenhofer B, et al. Intraoperative plus external beam irradiation in nonresectable lung cancer: assessment of local response and therapy-related side effects. Radiother Oncol 1990;19:137–144.
104. Dutreix A. When and how can we improve precision in radiotherapy? Radiother Oncol 1984;2:275–292.
105. Suit HD, Westgate SJ Impact of improved local control on survival. Int J Radiat Oncol Biol Phys 1986;12:453–458.
106. DeVita VT, Lippman M, Hubbard SM, Ihde DC, Rosenberg SA. The effect of combined modality therapy on local control and survival. Int J Radiat Oncol Biol Phys 1986;12:487–502.
107. Leibel S, Fuks Z. Is local failure a cause of or a marker for metastatic dissemination in carcinoma of the cervix? Int J Radiat Oncol Biol Phys 1992;24:377–380.
108. Perez CA, Bauer M, Edelstein S, Gillespie BW, Birch R. Impact of tumor control on survival in carcinoma of the lung treated with irradiation. Int J Radiat Oncol Biol Phys 1986;12:539–548.
109. Pignon JP, Arriagada R, Ihde DC, et al. A meta-analysis of thoracic radiotherapy for small-cell lung cancer. N Engl J Med 1992;327:1618–1624.
110. White JE, Chen T, McCracken J, et al. The influence of radiation therapy control on survival, response and sites of relapse in oat cell carcinoma of the lung. Preliminary report of a Southwest Oncology Group Study. Cancer 1982;50:1084–1090.
111. Van Houtte P, Rocmans P, Smets P, et al. Postoperative radiation therapy in lung cancer: a controlled trial after resection of curative design. Int J Radiat Oncol Biol Phys 1980;6:983–986.
112. Phlips P, Rocmans P, Vanderhoeft P, Van Houtte P. Postoperative radiotherapy after pneumonectomy: impact of modern treatment facilities. Int J Radiat Oncol Biol Phys 1993;27:525–529.
113. Leunens G, Verstraete G, Van Den Bogaert W, Van Dam J, Dutreix A, van der Schueren E. Human errors in data transfer during the preparation and delivery of radiation treatment affecting the final result: "garbage in, garbage out." Radiother Oncol 1992;23:217–222.
114. Byhardt RW, Cox JD, Hornburg A, Liermann G. Weekly localisations films and detection of field placement errors. Int J Radiat Oncol Biol Phys 1978;4:881–887.
115. Rodrigus P, Van den Weyngaert D, Van den Bogaert W. The value of treatment portal films in radiotherapy for bronchial carcinoma. Radiother Oncol 1987;9:27–31.

Section II

Lung Cancer: General

10

PATHOLOGY OF LUNG CANCER

Armando E. Fraire

INTRODUCTION

Lung cancer remains a major cause of morbidity and mortality in Western countries and a growing problem in emerging nations. For 1995, the American Cancer Society predicted the occurrence of 169,000 new cases of lung cancer in the United States alone (1). An understanding of the various facets of lung cancer is thus a major concern for health care workers. In particular, an understanding of the pathology of lung cancer and the definition of its various forms and histologic cell types may lead to the development of specific treatment modalities. This chapter reviews the traditional approaches to diagnostic pulmonary cytology, surgical pathology, and the newly emerging immunodiagnostic techniques for each of the major cell types of epithelial lung cancer. In addition, this chapter examines some of the controversial issues that confront pathologists today, including the distinction between adenocarcinoma and mesothelioma, and it discusses the applications and potential impact of flow cytometry and molecular diagnostics as further refinements of lung cancer pathology.

Lung cancer is predominantly a disease of older individuals with a median age of approximately 60 years; most cases occur between the ages of 40 and 70 (2–4). A small percentage of cases, ranging from 0.2% to 2.5%, occur among younger individuals (3, 4). A major shift has occurred in the male to female ratios of lung cancer, and the male predominance has declined steadily over the past three decades, reflecting the growing popularity of smoking and the growing incidence of the disease among women (2, 5). In one recent study encompassing a large hospital population, the male to female ratio fell from 3.4:1 in 1972 to 1.5:1 in 1986 (5). More recently, in 1993, a national male to female ratio of 1.5:1.0 was cited by Yesner (6). Earlier reports, in contrast, had noted male to female ratios of 10:1 in 1962, decreasing to 5:1 in 1975 (7). Lung cancer has thus become the leading cause of cancer death among women as well as men (1).

CLASSIFICATION

In 1924, Marchesani proposed the classification of lung cancer into four major histopathologic types, based on 26 cases seen at the Pathological Anatomical Institute in Innsbruck (8, 9). The four types were: (*a*) basal cell carcinoma, (*b*) polymorphocellular carcinoma, (*c*) keratinizing squamous cell carcinoma, and (*d*) cylindrical cell adenocarcinoma. This simple yet functional classification remained the standard for many years. Therapeutic necessities, however, led to multiple revisions and expansions during ensuing years. The chronology and evolution of the various classifications culminated in 1981 with the Second World Health Organization (WHO) classification scheme (9). The WHO classification schema and its basis have been reviewed previously in detail (10). This WHO classification scheme of lung cancer, shown in an abbreviated form in Table 10.1, has become an international standard. Nonetheless, the clinical necessity to segregate small cell lung cancers (SCLCs) has led to the creation and general acceptance of a practical, but unofficial, classification that divides primary lung cancers into two main subgroups: SCLCs and non–small cell lung cancers (NSCLCs). In the histologic classification of SCLC, a more functional and prognostically oriented subclassification was proposed originally and was used by the Veterans Administration Lung Group (11, 12); it was then modified and updated by The International Association for the Study of Lung Cancer (see Small Cell Lung Cancer, below) (13–15). Future classifications of lung cancers probably will be derived from both the developing immunodiagnostic studies and the further understanding of lung cancer biology.

TABLE 10.1. Histologic Classification of Lung Tumors

Epithelial tumors
  Benign
    Papillomas
      Squamous cell papilloma
      "Transitional" papilloma
    Adenomas
      Pleomorphic adenoma ("mixed" tumor)
      Monomorphic adenoma
      Others
  Dysplasia
  Carcinoma in situ
  Malignant
    Squamous cell carcinoma (epidermoid carcinoma)
    Variant
      Spindle cell (squamous) carcinoma
    Small cell carcinoma
      Oat cell carcinoma
      Intermediate cell type
      Combined oat cell carcinoma
    Adenocarcinoma
      Acinar adenocarcinoma
      Papillary adenocarcinoma
      Bronchioalveolar carcinoma
      Solid carcinoma with mucus formation
    Large cell carcinoma
    Variants:
      Giant cell carcinoma
      Clear cell carcinoma
    Adenosquamous carcinoma
    Carcinoid tumor
    Bronchial gland carcinomas
      Adenoid cystic carcinoma
      Mucoepidermoid carcinoma
      Others
    Others

The World Health Organization histological typing of lung cancers: 2nd edition. Am J Clin Pathol 1982;77:123–136.

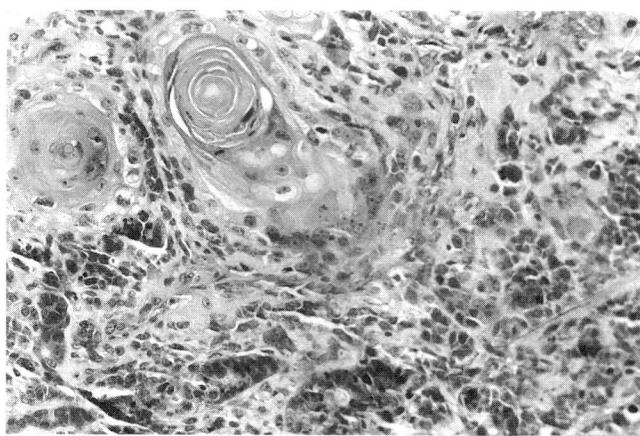

FIGURE 10.1. Small cell carcinoma. Combined (IASCL) subtype. Note the islands of squamous component nested among small carcinoma cells. (From Fraire AE, Johnson EH, Yesner R, et al. Prognostic significance of histopathologic subtype and stage in SCLC. Hum Pathol 1992;23:520–528.)

TUMOR HETEROGENEITY

One of the greatest problems in the classification and treatment of lung cancers is the tremendous heterogeneity seen in these tumors. Lung cancers often are composed of variable mixtures of cell types. This heterogeneity may pose a problem in the accurate histologic classification. A common mixture of cell types is the presence of glandular components in squamous cell carcinomas or squamous elements within an otherwise typical adenocarcinoma. Less commonly, small cell carcinoma may be seen admixed with either squamous cell carcinoma or adenocarcinoma (Fig. 10.1). This cellular heterogeneity of lung cancer has long been known, but only a few studies have attempted to quantify such heterogeneity. Roggli et al. (16) examined 1001 slides from 100 consecutive lung tumors in a blinded and randomized fashion to determine the extent of tumor heterogeneity. Of 66 heterogeneous cancers, 21 showed minor heterogeneity whereas 45 showed major heterogeneity (16). In contrast, Olcott (17) and Willis (18) previously reported a considerably greater proportion of homogeneity in lung cancers, with 77% of cases showing only one cell type. The Roggli et al. study (16), however, yielded findings remarkably similar to those reported by Reid and Carr (19), who identified only 37% of 138 lung cancers as homogeneous. To assess the clinical usefulness of recognizing heterogeneity of lung cancer, a further analysis (20) was undertaken of 91 of the 100 cancers reported previously by Roggli et al. (16). These 91 cases included 65 surgically resected patients with 5 years of follow-up. Survival was analyzed with regard to age, sex, stage, predominant histologic pattern, and presence or absence of major cell type heterogeneity. In this study stage was reported as the only significant predictor of survival ($P < .0001$). For the present, lung cancer heterogeneity appears to have little influence on perceptible clinical outcomes. However, it may be important for accurate histopathologic diagnosis, and considering the changing understanding of lung cancer biology, it may eventually prove useful despite the ever-diminishing size of biopsy specimens.

The heterogeneity of lung tumors also can be appreciated and refined at the level of electron microscopy. In one recent series, 26 of 44 lung carcinomas showed evidence of ultrastructural heterogeneity manifested as combined features of squamous, glandular, or neuroendocrine differentiation as illustrated in Figures 10.2 and 10.3 (21). Ultrastructural heterogeneity has been observed even within tumors showing uniform phenotypic features by light microscopy. In a prospective study of 24 lung scar adenocarcinomas, Herrera et al. (22) drew attention to the expression of

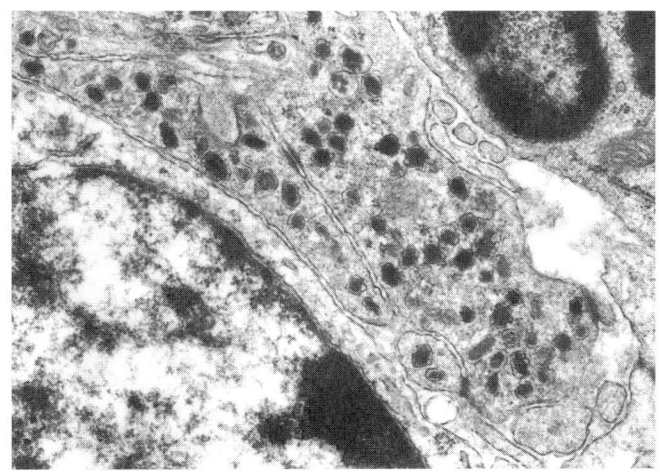

FIGURE 10.2. Cytoplasmic extension in which numerous dense core granules are seen denoting neuroendocrine differentiation. Electron micrograph magnification, ×19500. (From Mooi WJ, Dingemans KP, Wagenaar SS, et al. Ultrastructural heterogeneity of lung carcinomas: representativity of samples for electron microscopy in tumor classification. Hum Pathol 1990;21:1227–1234.)

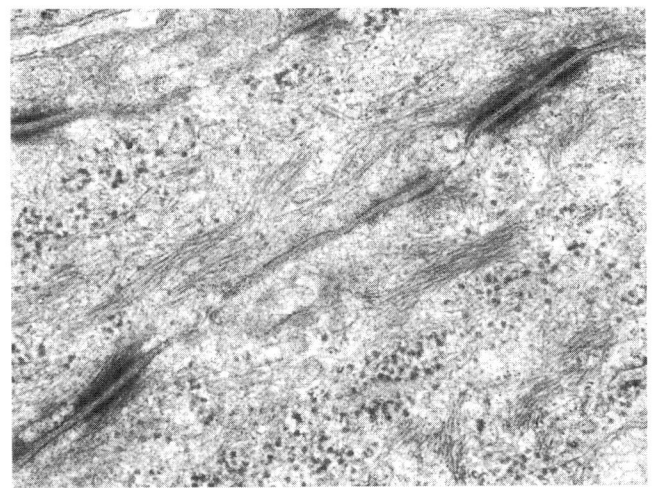

FIGURE 10.3. Large desmosomes with attached tonofibrils running into the cytoplasm of two adjacent tumor cells. This configuration denotes squamous differentiation. Electron micrograph magnification, ×67.300. (From Mooi WJ, Dingemans KP, Wagenaar SS, et al. Ultrastructural heterogeneity of lung carcinomas: representativity of samples for electron microscopy in tumor classification. Hum Pathol 1990;21:1227–1234.)

mucous, Clara, and alveolar cell ultrastructural morphology, suggesting that heterogeneity exists even within apparently uniform tumor morphotypes. Thus, the attempt to correlate heterogeneity by light microscopy with clinical outcome may have underestimated the magnitude of the heterogeneity, and attempts at such correlations using ultrastructural criteria may be more fruitful.

HISTOPATHOLOGY

The establishment of a tissue diagnosis holds a special place in clinical chest medicine (23). Usually, physicians will not embark on a treatment plan for lung cancer without a tissue diagnosis and will require, at a minimum, a tissue diagnosis of either small cell carcinoma or NSCLC. Biopsies, especially those from bronchoscopies or needle biopsies, may be too small, too distorted, or nonrepresentative for optimum interpretation. Furthermore, because lung cancers may express more than one cell type, a specific histologic diagnosis may be difficult. Additionally, there is considerable interobserver and even intraobserver variability in the classification of lung cancer. This variability of tissue diagnosis is illustrated by a carefully designed study of intraobserver and interobserver variability in which five experienced pathologists gave two independent readings of 50 different tissue slides from patients with lung cancers, encompassing a wide range of histologic types (24). Significant disagreements between the first and second readings of the same slide by the same pathologist occurred in a range between 2% and 20% for the least and the most consistent readers, respectively (24). These results underscore the subjectivity of tissue diagnoses.

Centralized pathology reviews have evolved from the necessity to have uniform and objective criteria in establishing a histologic diagnosis, and these centralized panels have provided some additional experience on interobserver correlation in histologic interpretation conducted in a multiple-institution setting (11). The central review in cooperative studies of the Radiation Therapy Oncology Group evaluated 807 biopsies from NSCLCs from 249 hospitals and clinics in 25 states, Canada, and Puerto Rico (11). This study concluded that pathologists in general have no difficulty in separating small cell from non–small cell carcinomas, and that central review is not required for such a distinction. However, overall agreement rates between referring pathologists and the (central) referee for adenocarcinoma was only 80%, with this agreement rate decreasing to 73% in cases of poorly differentiated adenocarcinoma (11). Interobserver variability in the subtyping of adenocarcinoma also was reviewed blindly by a panel of three pathologists (25). One hundred and eighty-nine cases of adenocarcinoma were suitable for examination. Overall agreement in the determination of the histopathologic subtype was obtained in only 41% of the 189 cases. However, the overall agreement for a subset of 53 cases in which tissue was obtained via thoracotomy was 88%, more than double the overall rate of agreement. The investigators concluded that the quality of the resultant diagnosis was superior with the larger quantity of material that was presumed to be better preserved in cases derived from thoracotomy. They based their conclusions on the higher rate of agreement obtained with the larger tissue samples.

PATHOLOGY REPORTS

Modern surgical pathology reports should achieve uniformity of data to facilitate retrieval of meaningful information that will help to establish a prognosis and assist in the formulation of treatment protocols. One approach to achieving such uniformity is to use a disease specific template. An example of the surgical pathology template for the reporting of surgically resected lung cancers, currently in use at the University of Massachusetts Medical Center, is shown in Table 10.2. Regarding the incorporation of immunostaining data into surgical pathology reports, a recent communication from the Council of the Association of Directors of Anatomic and Surgical Pathology (27) suggests that the following immunostaining data be included in the pathology report:

1. The nature of the material studied should be noted, e.g., paraffin section, frozen section, or other tissue preparation.
2. The immunoreagents used should be described specifically, e.g., AE1/AE3 rather than just cytokeratins.
3. The results of the staining for each antibody should be reported in sufficient detail to justify the interpretation, e.g., in some cases positive or negative results suffice, but in others, cellular patterns of staining or localization within cellular compartments must be stated.

Although many laboratories in the United States already use this practice, it is expected that many others still need to adopt these or similar guidelines.

TABLE 10.2. Template Used Currently at University of Massachusetts Medical Center for Lung Cancer Surgical Pathology Reports

Histopathologic cell type
Degree of tumor differentiation
Tumor size, tridimensional in centimeters
Bronchial margin of resection: Yes/No
Distance of tumor from bronchial margin in centimeters
Pleural involvement: Yes/No
Vascular invasion: Yes/No
Associated intrapulmonary changes/qualify
Pathologic stage (pTNM) (26)
Flow cytometry
Immunostaining report
Comments

CYTOLOGY

Cytologic assessment, such as endobronchial or fine-needle aspiration (FNA) material, has become the primary method for obtaining a diagnosis in suspected lung cancer (28). Cytologic assessment includes the analysis of induced sputum, bronchial brushings and washings, transbronchial FNA cytology, and radiologically guided percutaneous FNA cytology.

SPUTUM CYTOLOGY AND BRONCHOALVEOLAR LAVAGE

The accuracy of sputum cytology depends primarily on the adequacy of the expectorated material. Handling and processing of the specimen may also influence the overall yield of sputum cytology. Compton et al. (29) compared the conventional Saccomanno technique to the Cytic thin prep processor (Cytic Corporation, Mallborough, MA), a new automated processing instrument. Fifty specimens, both positive and negative for tumor, were processed by the Saccomanno method and by the thin prep processor. These workers found that the thin prep processor yielded smears with adequate cellular material, enhanced nuclear detail, and a decrease in the obscuring background material, compared with the conventional Saccomanno technique.

The adequacy of a sputum specimen is determined by the presence of carbon-bearing alveolar macrophages (28). A specimen without these macrophages is likely to contain little more than saliva, and it should be regarded as unsatisfactory (28). The overall diagnostic sensitivity of sputum cytology is low (less than 20%) and not considered efficacious, compared with other minimally invasive techniques such as bronchoscopy (30). Sputum cytology thus is not suitable for mass screening, and as a screening technique it has not as yet been found to alter the mortality even among selected high-risk populations. However, it can be useful as an initial diagnostic step in symptomatic patients (31) and offers a relatively inexpensive method for establishing a diagnosis. Sputum cytology may be particularly important for individuals living in remote areas with very limited access to hospital care. Methods that increase the sensitivity and diagnostic yield of sputum cytology are highly desirable.

The majority of lung cancers are diagnosed with advanced stages of disease when only palliative therapies can be offered to the patient (32). In this situation the least invasive diagnostic method is preferable. Bocking et al. (32) evaluated the diagnostic accuracy of sputum specimens using paraffin-embedded, hematoxylin and eosin–stained sections of 4297 sputum samples obtained from 1889 patients, 219 of whom were proven to have lung cancer. When patients provided three adequate specimens, the diagnostic sensitivity was 85.4%. These findings suggest that sputum cytology has the potential for high diagnostic accuracy and that paraffin-embedded sputum samples may represent a valuable addition for the detection of lung cancer from sputum specimens.

Most squamous cell carcinomas are located centrally, and their exfoliated cells usually are found in sputum or other cytologic preparations. In well-differentiated squamous cancers, tumor cells occur predominantly as single cells or can be seen in small groups. Cytoplasmic orangeophilia can be prominent. Nuclei are generally dense and may assume bizarre shapes. Nucleoli are usually inconspicuous or absent. Tumor necrosis is manifested as debris and degenerating cells in the background. Tadpole-shaped cells, fiber cells, and cellular cannibalism are excellent indicators of squamous differentiation.

Because of the usual peripheral location of most adenocarcinomas, exfoliated cells from an adenocarcinoma are found less commonly in respiratory secretions. When present, they can vary considerably in size, ranging from 15 to 60 μm in diameter (31). The tumor cells tend to arrange themselves in tissue fragments and clusters (Fig. 10.4). At times there are abortive microlumens, helpful features that allow recognition of their glandular nature. The nuclear membrane may show irregular contours and usually contains one or two prominent nucleoli. Cytoplasmic vacuolation may be present, and mucin production may be identified in approximately half of the cases with the aid of a mucicarmine stain. Glandular structures, cell balls or papillary structures, cylindrical cells, and nuclear grooving are major diagnostic criteria for the diagnosis of adenocarcinoma (33). van Hoeven et al. (34) compared 17 cytomorphologic features of bronchoalveolar carcinoma with florid nonneoplastic bronchiolar and alveolar cell proliferations. Useful features that were statistically significant in the recognition and diagnosis of bronchoalveolar carcinoma included two-dimensional or three-dimensional tissue aggregates, bridgelike connections between cells, intranuclear inclusions, and a paucity of multinucleated forms. Because of its potential clinical significance, Auger and associates (35) undertook a study searching for discriminating factors that may help to separate bronchoalveolar carcinoma from conventional adenocarcinoma of the lung. Good discriminating signs of bronchoalveolar carcinoma included prominence of monolayered sheets, nuclear grooves, fine chromatin pattern, extra cellular mucin and minimal cellular pleomorphism.

Cytologic evaluation of large cell carcinoma is fraught with considerable difficulties. These difficulties, in part, appear to be related to an overgrowth of undifferentiated cellular components, which can be related to advanced clinical stage, rather than to an inadequacy of cytologic preparation or suboptimal performance by a screener (36). Other difficulties in correctly diagnosing large cell carcinoma can be illustrated when early-stage large cell lung cancers are considered. Barbazza et al. (36) reviewed 100 consecutive cases of stage I-II lung cancers. In these cases the accuracy rates, as assessed by subsequent tissue samples, for adenocarcinoma, squamous cell carcinoma, and small cell carcinoma were 91.6%, 98%, and 100%, respectively. However, not a single case of large cell carcinoma was identified by cytology among the 100 cases. The lack of cytologic identification in this series illustrates the problem of correctly diagnosing large cell carcinoma by cytologic means alone.

Respiratory secretions from patients with small cell carcinoma may contain tumor cells in loose groupings or single tumor cells, with little recognizable cytoplasm. The cells of small cell carcinoma, although usually referred to as small, are in fact quite large and can measure up to 22 to 24 μm, about 3 times the size of small lymphocytes. Nuclear molding and tumor necrosis are common, and the nuclear chromatin often has both a stippled fine and coarse pattern, the so-called salt and pepper chromatin pattern. Nucleoli are most often inconspicuous. Presence of nucleoli, particularly prominent nucleoli, should cast doubt on the diagnosis or should suggest the possibility of a mixed small and large cell carcinoma.

Alveolar cell hyperplasia, seen in a variety of nonneoplastic lung diseases, is particularly prominent in diffuse alveolar damage and viral and chemical pneumonitis as well as in individuals who recently received chemotherapy or radiation therapy (37). Stanley et al. (38) reviewed the cytologic findings in bronchoalveolar

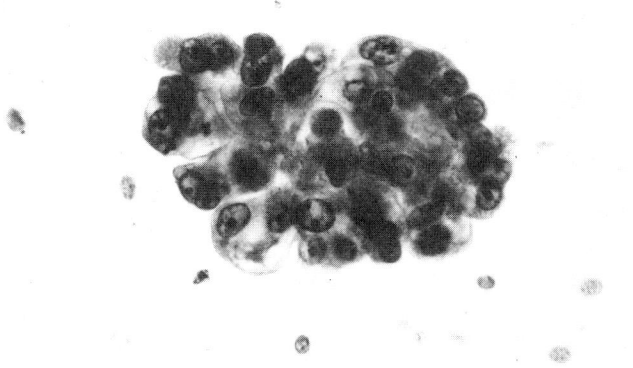

FIGURE 10.4. Cytologic appearance of adenocarcinoma. Note the clustering effect and large cells with prominent nucleoli.

lavage fluid from 38 patients with adult respiratory distress syndrome and found type II pneumocyte hyperplasia in 12 of the 38 patients. Most of these 12 patients had sepsis as the probable cause of their adult respiratory distress syndrome, although some had mycoplasma pneumonitis, cardiogenic shock, or a history of a recent coronary artery bypass. The hyperplastic type II pneumocytes occurred singly or in cohesive groups. In some cells the nuclei appeared angulated, and some showed macronucleoli features that are generally regarded as atypical and worrisome for malignancy. Stanley and associates (38) caution, however, that in patients with such cytologic findings, the clinical history and findings may be more helpful than the cytologic findings in ruling out a diagnosis of malignancy.

FINE-NEEDLE ASPIRATION CYTOLOGY

The role of FNA cytology in the diagnosis of lung cancer has grown at a rapid pace in the United States (39). This procedure is accurate, simple, and inexpensive compared with thoracotomy or thoracoscopic lung biopsies. Peripheral lesions are approached percutaneously, usually with CT guidance, whereas lesions located more centrally are often quite accessible using the Wang transbronchial aspiration needle. The nature of the malignancy can be established in the majority of cases when there is adequate cellularity of the specimen and the presence of characteristic nuclear features is exhibited by well-preserved neoplastic cells. The diagnostic yield of FNA can be further enhanced by use of ancillary studies. In a recent study of 345 percutaneous aspirations, immunocytochemistry and electron microscopy provided significant additional information in 40% and 67% of the cases, respectively (39). The use of immunocytochemical studies in cytologic material also is gaining widespread acceptance (39). Antibodies against prostatic specific antigen, prostatic acid phosphatase, HMB-45 (a melanoma specific antigen), and thyroglobulin appear particularly useful in separating primary lung neoplasms from metastatic cancers arising in the prostate, skin, and thyroid gland, respectively (40). Walts et al. (41) examined the usefulness of chromogranin as a marker of neuroendocrine cells in cytologic material and demonstrated positive immunoreactivity in all of 6 pulmonary carcinoid tumors and in 9 of 10 extrapulmonary neuroendocrine tumors, a finding that substantiates the efficacy of this immunostain in these clinical entities. In their study (41), 20 small cell carcinomas of pulmonary origin were all chromogranin negative, reflecting the paucity of neurosecretory granules in small cell carcinomas.

Using a computerized morphometry system, Burns and coworkers (42) evaluated criteria for the cytologic diagnosis of large cell carcinoma and adenocarcinoma of the lung. A logistic regression identified cell area, nucleolar to nuclear area ratio, and cell and nuclear form factors as significant contributors to the discrimination of large cell carcinoma from adenocarcinoma, with a positive predictive value of 92%. Thus, cell image analysis techniques represent yet another modality of cytopathology using complementary technology, in this instance, high-resolution optical scanners. Using this technology cells in cytologic preparations are divided into small squares, or pixels, of a resolution of usually 0.5 to 1 mm (28). Data derived from this technology have led to the determination of atypia status indices that can be used to quantify the degree of cytologic dysplasia and that may have the potential for use in diagnosis and patient follow-up (28).

Although histopathologic recognition of heterogeneity is well documented (16), the ability of cytopathologists to recognize cellular heterogeneity in cytopathologic specimens is less well documented. Khiyami et al. (43) studied 63 patients with lung cancers previously characterized by tissue sections as heterogeneous ($n = 22$) or homogeneous ($n = 41$). A panel of three cytopathologists independently reviewed the 63 cytologic samples without knowledge of their previous histopathologic characterization. The 63 samples included sputa, bronchial brushings, bronchial washings, fine-needle aspirates, and pleural fluids. A diagnosis of positive for malignancy was rendered by at least one cytopathologist in 25 (39%) of the 63 cases. Eight of these 25 cases had previously been characterized histopathologically as heterogeneous, but only 3 (37%) of the 8 cases were recognized as heterogeneous by cytopathology. These findings indicate that it is possible to diagnose heterogeneous lung cancer cell types correctly by cytopathologic methods, although the accuracy is not as great as by histopathology. The overall sensitivity in that study was low (37%), suggesting that for adequate determination of cellular heterogeneity in lung cancer, cytopathologic and histopathologic methods should be used together in a complementary fashion (43).

FLOW CYTOMETRY

The majority of malignant cells derived from human cancers are characterized by increased DNA content and aneuploidy (44). This feature suggests that flow cytometry could be used to measure DNA content in respiratory secretions either alone or as a supplement to conventional cytologic methods. Early flow cytometric studies suggested the value of aneuploidy in finding cancerous cells (45, 46). Fuhr et al. (47) evaluated 168 samples of respiratory secretions including 10 bronchial brushings, 49 effusions, and 109 lung fine-needle aspirates using flow cytometry and conventional cytology results as the standard. They found a sensitivity and specificity of 86% and 96%, respectively, suggesting that flow cytometry may be useful as a valuable adjunct in the diagnosis of lung cancer (47).

SQUAMOUS CELL CARCINOMA

Squamous cell carcinoma, once the most common cell type of lung cancer, has shown a declining trend in frequency over the past three decades. In a large hospital-based study of 1391 patients from Houston, the percentage of squamous cell carcinomas in men decreased from 51.8% in 1972 to 42.7% in 1986 (5). A similar decrease in the incidence of squamous cell carcinoma in women also was noted in that study. A decrease in the frequency of squamous cell carcinoma was further documented in another recent large study from Memphis involving 4928 patients (48). Previously, a series from Roswell Park had shown that squamous cell carcinomas represented 48% of all lung cancers. Thirteen years later, however, the percentage at that institution had fallen to 38% (7). These figures illustrate the changes in the frequency of histopathologic diagnoses that have taken place over the past three decades. The cause of these changes remains unknown; however, a decrease in smoking among men and the increasing popularity of smoking filtered cigarettes may be responsible for some of these changes.

Early in their development, squamous cell carcinomas do not form a discrete tumor mass. As the disease progresses, focal mucosal thickening may occur, eventually leading to the formation of an endobronchial tumor mass. It is generally agreed that approximately 90% of squamous cell carcinomas arise in subsegmental or larger bronchi. They usually appear as fungating endobronchial masses composed of gray, white, or yellow tissue, and they have a tendency to grow centrally toward the main stem bronchus and to infiltrate the underlying bronchial cartilage, lymph nodes, and adjacent lung parenchyma. In time, this progression may lead to the formation of large nodular masses (Fig. 10.5). Obstructive as well as organizing pneumonia may be seen around the main tumor mass. This finding is clinically important because it may blur the outlines of the tumor mass radiographically, thereby limiting the usefulness of radiographic studies in determining tumor size and preoperative staging. Squamous cell carcinomas also may arise from periph-

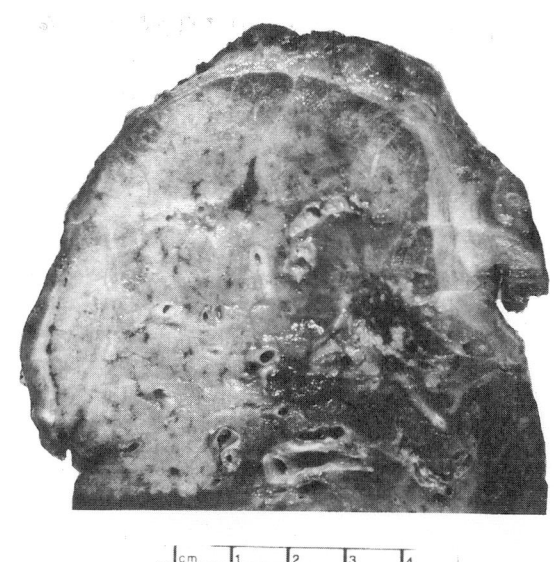

FIGURE 10.5. Squamous cell carcinoma (gross appearance). Note the large gray-tan tumor mass largely replacing and expanding the right upper lobe. Centimeter scale.

eral airways, sometimes presenting as solitary subpleural tumor masses that are similar to peripheral adenocarcinomas.

As defined by the WHO, well-differentiated squamous cell carcinomas show microscopic evidence of orderly stratification, intercellular bridges, and keratinization with pearl formation (9). In contrast, poorly differentiated squamous cell carcinomas show only minimal expression of these features, which often are discerned only with difficulty. Necrosis is observed commonly in squamous cell carcinoma (Fig. 10.6) and may lead to cavitation when extensive.

SQUAMOUS CELL CANCER MARKERS

Squamous cell carcinomas express immunoreactivity for antibodies directed against high molecular weight cytokeratins, epithelial membrane antigen and human milk fat globule antigen (49–51). In addition, squamous cell carcinomas may, on occasion, express immunoreactivity for B72.3 and Leu-M1 (Table 10.3) (10). Immunoreactivity for carcinoembryonic antigen (CEA) is equivocal, with conflicting reports being published (Table 10.3). Rarely, some squamous cell carcinomas express receptors for autocrine growth factors such as epidermal growth factor and transforming growth factor–α (51–53).

Human papilloma virus (HPV) has been implicated in the malignant transformation of squamous epithelium, leading to the development of squamous cell

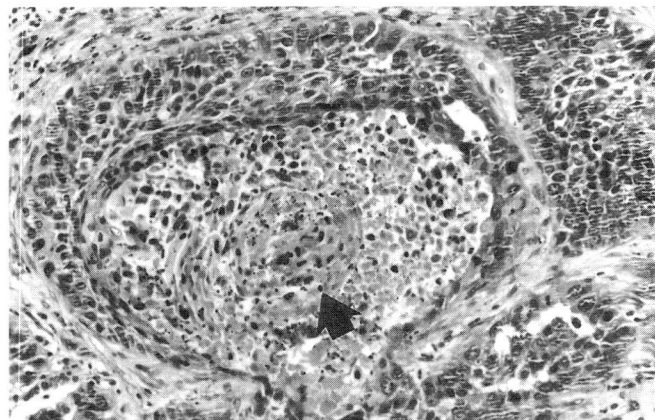

FIGURE 10.6. Histologic appearance of squamous cell carcinoma with moderate degree of differentiation. Large islands of tumor cells show central areas of keratinization and necrosis (arrow). Hematoxylin and eosin stain; magnification, ×200.

carcinoma. Although HPV DNA has been identified in a high proportion of cervical and anorectal carcinomas, few studies have tested for the presence of HPV DNA in pulmonary squamous cell carcinomas. Le and associates (54) used polymerase chain reaction techniques to identify HPV DNA in 4 of 7 patients, aged 45 or younger. However, none of 14 patients aged 65 or older had evidence of HPV DNA in their tumor cells. Using in situ hybridization and HPV DNA probes 6/11, 16/18, and 31/33/35, Yousem et al. (55) found HPV DNA in 6 of 20 squamous cell carcinomas and in 1 of 6 cases of large cell carcinomas. All three HPV serotypes were represented among the positive probes. None of 32 other tumors, including some adenocarcinomas and small cell carcinomas, was positive with the HPV DNA probes (55). The significance of these findings remains unclear. However, the authors suggested that HPV may act as a tumor promoter in concert with other viral or chemical carcinogens.

Involucrin, a soluble protein precursor of the cross-linked envelope of stratified squamous cells, has been shown to be a marker for squamous differentiation in a variety of lung tumors, particularly non–small cell carcinoma. Said et al. (56) stained 25 squamous cell carcinomas with involucrin and found immunoreactivity in all of the 25 tumors. In contrast, only 2 of 16 small cell carcinomas and 2 of 20 adenocarcinomas stained positively. Investigators at the University of Massachusetts studied 17 cases of non–small cell carcinomas, with 10 (58.8%) being focally positive for involucrin (unpublished observation). These findings further support the potential usefulness of this marker to identify squamous differentiation in some lung cancers, or possibly to correlate differentiation with clinical outcomes. For example, involucrin may prove helpful in identifying the combined SCLC and NSCLC components as defined by the pathology panel of the IASLC (14).

Tenascin, an extracellular matrix glycoprotein, can be found in healing wounds and myotendinous, cartilaginous, and smooth muscle tissues as well as in basement membranes of endothelial and epithelial tissues (57–59). Using a novel monoclonal antibody that detects tenascin in formalin-fixed, paraffin-embedded tissues, Soini and coworkers (60) found tenascin expressed in 10 of 27 pulmonary squamous cell carcinomas and 2 of 27 adenocarcinomas, suggesting that tumor cells, as well as normal lung tissue, are capable of tenascin expression. The variable expression of tenascin in lung tumors and walls of nonneoplastic alveoli may be of biologic relevance regarding tumor spread because tenascin, being deposited on the walls of the alveolar septa, may function as an adhesive protein for neoplastic cells (60, 61).

A considerable body of evidence has accumulated to document an inherent resistance to chemotherapeutic agents in non–small cell carcinomas. A novel study suggests that such chemotherapy resistance may be caused by the overexpression of heat shock protein HSP-27 in some carcinomas (62). Among 56 tumors, all of 14 squamous cell carcinomas overexpressed HSP-27, when tested by immunoperoxidase techniques. In contrast, only 3 (18.2%) of 11 small cell carcinomas overexpressed this marker, suggesting that HSP-27 may correlate with some of the chemoresistance observed in non–small cell carcinomas (62).

Squamous histology in lung cancers is reportedly an important prognostic factor. Gail et al. (63) analyzed 392 cases of non–small cell carcinoma and divided them into squamous (189 cases) and nonsquamous (203 cases) histology. The recurrence rates per person per year were 0.105 and 0.207, respectively, for the two types, suggesting a favorable impact of squamous cell histology on prognosis. In the study by Katlic and Carter (64), the overall 5-year survival rate for poorly differentiated squamous cell carcinoma was 7%, whereas it was 20% for moderately differentiated and 39% for well-differentiated squamous cell carcinomas. The difference between the poorly differentiated group and the combined moderately and well-differentiated groups reached statistical significance (64). However, studies that adjusted for stage of disease have suggested that the tumor, node, metastasis (TNM) stage remains the most important factor in prognosis, thus obscuring the effect of the degree of differentiation (65, 66).

TABLE 10.3. Immunohistochemical Features of Common Lung Neoplasms

TYPE OF NEOPLASM	ANTIGENS TESTED FOR								
	LMWCK	HMWCK	CEA	HMFGP	NSE	CG	LEU₂ M1	B72.3	BerEP4
Squamous CA	+	+	±	±	...	...	±[a]	±[a]	±[a]
Adenocarcinoma	+	±	+	+	±	...	±[b]	±[b]	±[b]
Large cell CA	+	±	±	±	±	...	±[c]	±[c]	±[c]
Small cell CA	+	±	±	±	±	±	...[d]	...[d]	...[d]
Mature carcinoid	+	±	±	±	+	+	...[d]	...[d]	...[d]
Atypical carcinoid	+	±	±	±	+	±	...[d]	...[d]	...[d]
Large cell neuro-endocrine CA	+	±	±	±	+	±	...[d]	...[d]	...[d]

Modified from Hammar SP. Common neoplasms. In: Dail DH, Hammar SP, eds. Pulmonary pathology, 2nd ed. New York, Berlin: Springer-Verlag, 1993;1123–1278.

Abbreviations: LMWCK, low molecular weight cytokeratin; HMWCK, high molecular weight cytokeratin; CEA, carcinoembryonic antigen; HMFGP, human milk fat globule protein; NSE, neuron specific enolase; CG, chromogranin; CA, carcinoma; +, positive reaction; −, negative reaction. Some reports were positive and others were negative.

[a]Most frequently negative. If positive, it is usually focal and often in cell membrane distribution.
[b]Positive in 30% to 50% of cases in Hammar's experience.
[c]Positive in 20% to 30% of cases in Hammar's experience.
[d]Information was inadequate to state results.

ADENOCARCINOMA

Because of the apparent shift in the histologic pattern of lung cancer, adenocarcinoma may now be the leading cell type (48, 67). Bronchoalveolar carcinoma (BAC), a subtype of adenocarcinoma, may also be increasing in frequency (52, 67, 68). The rising frequency of adenocarcinoma also has been reported in Japan (69), where it is the most common type of lung cancer. In Western and developed nations, adenocarcinomas are found primarily in the lung periphery, whereas in a series from India (70), nearly 50% of adenocarcinomas were located more centrally. Adenocarcinomas also appear to be the predominant form of lung cancer in human immunodeficiency virus (HIV)–infected individuals (71, 72), although it is not clear whether this finding is specific to HIV-infected patients or is a reflection of the overall increase in the incidence of adenocarcinoma.

With its peripheral presentation, adenocarcinoma can often be found in a subpleural location. The underlying pleura may be retracted, creating a puckering effect. Grossly, adenocarcinoma appears as gray tissue with focal black pigmentation. A relationship with segmental or subsegmental airways is seldom discerned. Adenocarcinomas may sometimes occur as a solitary nodule, but closer inspection also may reveal satellite nodules near the tumor mass. BAC, however, is more likely to present as a multicentric tumor (73). Rarely, adenocarcinoma encases the lung in a fashion similar to that in mesothelioma, as seen in Figure 10.7.

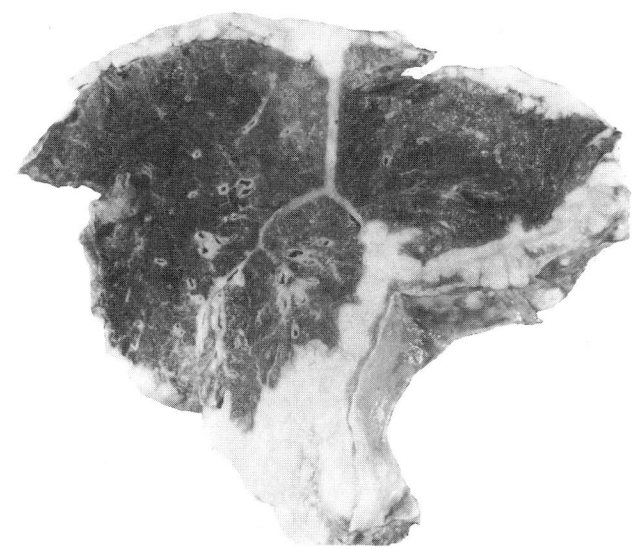

FIGURE 10.7. Mesotheliomalike adenocarcinoma, gross appearance. Note the tumor growth encasing lung with extension along the interlobar septum.

The WHO classification (9, 10) divides adenocarcinoma into four subtypes: acinar, papillary, bronchoalveolar, and solid with mucin production. A defining feature of adenocarcinoma of the lung is its ability to produce mucinous substances. This feature prompted the reclassification of solid tumors with mucin production out of the large cell carcinoma category in the WHO I system (1967) to the adenocarcinoma category in the WHO II system (1981). However, with the exception of the mucinous variant of BAC, mucin production is seldom a truly prominent characteristic of adenocarcinoma. The overall frequency of mucin production is not known, but approximately half of these tumors are mucin positive when tested histochemically with mucicarmine stains.

Scroggs and coworkers (74) pointed out the presence of intracytoplasmic globular eosinophilic bodies in six adenocarcinomas of the lung. These bodies stained brightly with periodic acid-Schiff (PAS) and were homogenous ultrastructurally. These authors suggested that such bodies may represent secretory glycoproteins that accumulate in areas of cell injury. Similar but larger bodies were reported in 27 of 105 surgically resected adenocarcinomas by Nakanishi et al. (75). Psammoma bodies can be seen in primary papillary adenocarcinomas (76), but they can also be seen in metastatic cancers from the thyroid, ovary, pancreas, and other sites that produce papillary neoplasms.

Adenocarcinoma of the lung may spread into the bronchial epithelium in a fashion similar to that occurring in Paget's tumor. Higashiyama et al. (77) reported a Paget's-like spread of adenocarcinoma cells with in situ involvement of bronchial glands and ducts by adenocarcinoma cells. This pattern of spread appears similar to that of extramammary Paget's disease in the perineum, vulvar, and anorectal areas.

Relatively discrete adenomas, single or multiple, that are composed of atypical alveolar cells with increased nuclear cytoplasmic ratio have been regarded by some as the early stage of adenocarcinoma (78). Less well-outlined hyperplastic changes of alveolar epithelial cells also have been implicated as a possible precursor lesion of adenocarcinomas and particularly of BACs. A nonnodular hyperplasia of the alveolar epithelial cells has been implicated similarly as a possible precursor lesion of adenocarcinoma (79). A recent study of 41 patients with surgically resected adenocarcinoma of the lung sought to determine the frequencies of association between alveolar cell hyperplasia and atypical alveolar cell hyperplasia (80). The criteria used to look for alveolar cell hyperplasia included a single-row arrangement of cuboidal or columnar cells along the alveolar walls and cellular morphology distinct from terminal bronchiolar epithelium (79). Atypical alveolar cell hyperplasia was considered whenever nuclear size was double the size of neighboring alveolar cell hyperplasia and/or in cases with nuclear irregularity or hyperchromatism. Alveolar cell hyperplasia was identified in 24 of the 41 cases of adenocarcinoma. Atypical alveolar cell hyperplasia was demonstrated further in 6 of the 24 cases of alveolar cell hyperplasia (80). These findings suggest that alveolar cell hyperplasia and atypical alveolar cell hyperplasia are common histopathologic features found in 24 and 6 of the 41 adenocarcinoma cases, respectively (80). Shimosato et al. (81) analyzed the nuclear DNA content of atypical adenomatous hyperplasia of the lung and found diploidy, polyploidy, or aneuploidy, suggesting an abnormal clonal expansion. Cases that stained positively for proliferating cell nuclear antigen (PCNA) were few in number in typical adenomatous hyperplasia, but they were increased in areas with greater cell atypia (81). Shimosato et al. (81) suggested that such lesions are neoplastic, representing either an early adenoma or an extremely well-differentiated adenocarcinoma with a bronchoalveolar growth pattern. Further recent data supporting the thought that atypical alveolar cell hyperplasia may represent a precancerous lesion were presented by Kawai and associates (82). These investigators assessed cases of alveolar cell hyperplasia and atypical alveolar cell hyperplasia for $p53$ immunoreactivity. Mutations of the $p53$ gene occurred in three of eight cases of atypical alveolar cell hyperplasia but not in any of the five cases of alveolar cell hyperplasia. Unique pulmonary nodules bearing a resemblance to bronchoalveolar carcinomas sometimes occur in adolescents receiving systemic chemotherapy for other tumors (83). These lesions also may represent precursor lesions (83). In two such cases reported by Travis et al. (83), CEA immunopositivity was identified in both cases and aneuploidy in one of the two.

Asbestos is a recognized risk for mesothelioma of the pleura and various types of epithelial lung cancers, including adenocarcinoma. However, the simultaneous occurrence of mesothelioma and adenocarcinoma in patients with known asbestos exposure is uncommon. Cagle et al. (84) reported the unique development of both mesothelioma and adenocarcinoma in a 62-year-old insulation worker who also had a significant smoking history. The two tumors were physically separate and had immunophenotypes consistent with mesothelioma and adenocarcinoma, respectively. Although asbestos exposure and lung cancer are probably related causally, the cell type distribution of asbestos-related lung cancers has not been defined clearly. In a case control study of 41 surgical and 106 autopsy tissue samples in men, Mollo et al. (85) identified a trend toward a greater association between asbestos and adenocarcinomas in autopsy series but not in their surgical series.

BRONCHOALVEOLAR CARCINOMA

BAC is a type of lung cancer that is widely recognized as a variant of adenocarcinoma. The true frequency of BAC is not known. However, the frequency, when expressed as a percentage of total lung cancers, appears to be on the rise. In the study of Auerbach and Garfinkel (67), the frequency of this tumor more than doubled over an 18-year period. Barsky and associates (86) investigated the frequency of BAC in successive 5-year periods from 1955 to 1990. Over these time periods, BAC rose from less than 5% to 24%, a difference that proved to be statistically significant ($P < .0001$) (85). First described in the 19th century, BAC has been the subject of considerable research and interest (87). As with most adenocarcinomas, BACs develop at the periphery of the lung. Grossly, these tumors may present as single or multiple nodules or, uniquely, as a diffuse "pneumonic" form in which the tumor infiltrates the alveoli and often is mistaken for a pneumonia. Hybrid forms of adenocarcinoma containing foci of bronchoalveolar morphology can also occur. At present, there appears to be no quantitative criteria that separate this hybrid form from the pure forms. To provide some degree of standardization in the nomenclature, it would be most helpful to note the principal pattern, e.g., acinar or papillary, and to provide an estimate of the percentage of the bronchoalveolar component. BAC and the papillary type of adenocarcinoma share similar morphologic features that may make it difficult to distinguish them. A diagnostic triad may help to separate true papillary carcinomas from BAC (76): (a) a papillary component with fibrovascular cores comprising more than 75% of the lesion, (b) secondary and tertiary papillary branching, and (c) tufting.

Up to 38% of the papillary tumors are likely to have psammoma bodies, and 20% are likely to show dirty necrosis (76). Twenty-nine tumors fulfilling these criteria had diminished disease free survival for stages I and II, suggesting that papillary tumors represent a distinct clinical entity with a considerably worse prognosis than BAC (76). BAC typically grows along unaltered preexisting alveolar walls. This form of growth is known as the lepidic type of growth pattern. Ultrastructurally, these cells have features of nonneoplastic type II pneumocytes and/or Clara cells. Manning and associates (88) distinguished two types of BAC based in part on their ability to produce mucin. Type I tumors with abundant mucin production had a poor prognosis with 26% of patients surviving 5 years; type II tumors with lesser mucin production had a much better outcome with 72% of the patients surviving 5 years.

The bronchiolar Clara cell has been proposed as the putative cell of the origin of nonmucinous variants of BACs. First described in 1937 by Max Clara (89), these cells are nonciliated bronchiolar epithelial cells, usually found in the peripheral airways at the level of the terminal bronchiole. Clara cells are metabolically active and are involved with the production and processing of various proteins with surfactant properties. The bronchiolar mucosa is lined by a single layer of cuboidal cells consisting of ciliated cells and nonciliated Clara cells. Ultrastructural characterization has been particularly helpful in the diagnosis of BAC. Clara cells have characteristic, large, electron dense granules that may secrete surfactantlike granules (90). Demonstration of such granules may help to differentiate a BAC from other adenocarcinomas (52). BAC bears some morphologic resemblance to pulmonary tumors of sheep, known as Jaagsiekte disease, and spontaneous and urethane-induced pulmonary tumors in mice (91–93). Rarely, BAC develops in the setting of generalized amyloidosis. One such case was described recently in a 51-year-old woman with a long-standing history of progressive systemic sclerosis with autopsy-proven amyloid deposits in the heart and adrenal glands (94). A case of papillary BAC with myoepithelial cells was reported recently by Dekmezian and coworkers (95). Ultrastructurally and microscopically, this unique tumor showed features of Clara cell and myoepithelial differentiation.

SCAR ADENOCARCINOMA

Although carcinoma arising in the setting of diffuse pulmonary fibrosis may be regarded as an example of a scar carcinoma, Shimosato et al. (81) suggest that in most scar adenocarcinomas the central fibrosis forms after the development of the carcinoma, not before. This concept is supported by the observation that in the earliest stage of adenocarcinoma a fibrotic focus is usually absent and that collagen is also absent in areas with dense aggregates of elastic fibers (81). Cagle et al. (96) followed 22 patients with resected pulmonary scar adenocarcinoma for 10 or more years. The degree of collagen in the scar was an important predictor of long-term survival in these patients. Four of eight patients whose scars contained abundant collagen died of their disease. Yoneda (97) drew attention to the possibility that scar adenocarcinomas may not represent a single clinicopathologic entity. This author reviewed 17 cases of scar carcinoma found among 112 surgically resected lung carcinomas in a geographic region endemic for histoplasmosis. Type I scar carcinomas, the mucinous type, appeared more desmoplastic. Type II, the nonmucinous type, appeared to have arisen around preexisting histoplasmic granulomas, which incorporated yeast organisms, suggesting that scar carcinomas can have a varied expression. A unique patient with a synchronous double scar carcinoma, reported by Jackson et al. (98), had a large cell carcinoma in the right upper lobe and an adenocarcinoma in the right lower lobe.

IMMUNOCYTOCHEMISTRY

Adenocarcinomas express low molecular weight cytokeratins, high molecular weight cytokeratins, CEA, and epithelial membrane antigen (51, 99). In addition, adenocarcinomas may express immunoreactivity to S-100, Leu-M1, B72.3, vimentin, and neuron specific enolase (Table 10.3) (80, 100, 101). The main clinical application of CEA is to distinguish adenocarcinomas, which generally are positive for CEA, from mesotheliomas, which are negative for it. (51, 102). Desmin, neurofilaments, tubulin, and fibrillary acidic proteins generally are not found in adenocarcinomas (51).

Vimentin, a cytoplasmic protein, is the most ubiquitous of the intermediate filament proteins (103, 104) and is expressed by the pulmonary counterparts of soft tissue sarcomas and by some large cell carcinomas of the lung (100). Its relevant clinical use lies in its application to distinguishing primary pulmonary adenocarcinomas from malignant pleural mesotheliomas, with most sarcomatoid (fibrous) mesotheliomas having the ability to express vimentin along with cytokeratin. Caution should be exercised, however, because occasionally some adenocarcinomas also have the ability to express vimentin.

Distinctive α-fetoprotein–producing pulmonary adenocarcinomas also have been reported (105). Studies that differentiate adenocarcinoma from mesothelioma have considerable clinical and medicolegal importance. Brown and associates (106) analyzed 32 cases of malignant mesothelioma and 103 pulmonary adenocarcinomas using a panel of seven immunohistochemical markers consisting of B72.3, CA 125, CEA, Leu-M1, PAS, secretory (mucin) component, and vimentin (Table 10.4). Using this panel approach to diagnosis, the best single marker phenotype was a negative CEA (97.1% specific and 96.9% sensitive for mesothelioma). The most discriminating two-marker phenotype was a negative B72.3 and negative CEA (99.0% specific and 96.9% sensitive for mesothelioma) (Table 10.4) (106). A positive result for either B72.3 or CEA nearly always ruled out mesothelioma. Noguchi et al. (107) reported the immunohistochemical properties of 9 cases of mesothelioma and 21 cases of pulmonary adenocarcinoma. They found that none of the 9 mesotheliomas was immunoreactive for CEA or surfactant apoprotein. In contrast, 13 (62%) of the 21 lung adenocarcinomas were positive for these markers ($P < .01$), suggesting their usefulness in the differential diagnosis of these two neoplasms. Currently, reliance on a battery of immunohistochemistry results appears to be a useful adjunct in distinguishing these two neoplasms.

The search for specific markers that may assist in the distinction of primary from metastatic lung tumors is another issue of considerable clinical relevance. Although significant efforts have been made to find specific markers to make such a distinction, commercially distributed immunomarkers remain unavailable. Two markers from the progenitor cells of peripheral airways and tumors derived from them are the 10 kilodalton Clara cell protein and the major surfactant-associated protein A. Using in situ hybridization techniques, Broers et al. (108) studied expression of genes encoding these two proteins in 19 pairs of nonneoplastic and neoplastic tissue from resected human lungs. One of 19 adenocarcinomas expressed the Clara cell protein and 5 of 17 adenocarcinomas expressed the surfactant protein A. A separate study by investigators from the same laboratory examined these two markers of peripheral airways differentiation using paraffin sections from 247 primary and metastatic non–small cell carcinomas (109). Among patients with primary lung adenocarcinomas, 14 (19%) of 73 and 21 (30%) of 70 adenocarcinomas stained positively for surfactant protein A and the Clara cell antigen, respectively. In contrast, only 2 of 75 and 4 of 75 nonpulmonary neoplasms stained positively for surfactant protein A and the Clara cell antigen, respectively (109). These results provide useful tools for studying the biology of lung cancers, and they underscore the importance of these two antibodies as potentially specific markers for tumors of lung origin (108, 109).

Simultaneous expression patterns of CEA and intercellular adhesion molecule 1 appear to be an inherent characteristic of tumor cells (110). Nonomura and associates (110) studied the expression of these two antigens in 24 pulmonary adenocarcinomas. They suggested that the abnormal expression of these two antigens appears to play a role in the physiologic behavior of tumor cells, and they may be involved in intercellular recognition and binding. This expression in turn may be related to tumor cell differentiation and

TABLE 10.4. Immunohistochemical Features of Malignant Mesothelioma and Adenocarcinoma of the Lung

TUMOR TYPE	B72.3	CA 125	CEA	LEU-M1	PAS	SC	VIM
Mesothelioma	0	3.1	3.1	6.3	9.4	0	65.6
Adenocarcinoma	90.3	14.6	97.1	76.7	66.0	62.1	19.4

From Brown RW, Clark GM, Allred DC. A panel approach of distinguishing malignant epithelial mesotheliomas from adenocarcinomas of the lung by immunohistochemistry. Mod Pathol 1991;4:113A.
Abbreviations. PAS, periodic acid-Schiff; SC, secretory component; VIM, vimentin.

metastatic potential. As pointed out by Furukawa et al. (111), Langerhans' cell granules have been identified in some adenocarcinomas including BAC. In a series of 40 stage I adenocarcinomas, these authors demonstrated Langerhans' granules in 31 (77.5%) of the 40 cases, using immunostaining for the S-100 protein. The possible clinical significance of this finding is not known, but the presence of Langerhans' histiocytes in adenocarcinomas does appear to have some prognostic significance. The CD1 (OKT6) antibody is currently accepted as a more specific marker for Langerhans' histiocytes, with greater specificity than the S-100 protein. Using the anti-CD1 monoclonal antibody, Fox and colleagues (112) quantified the occurrence of Langerhans' histiocytes in 41 tumors, 8 of which were adenocarcinomas. Patients whose tumors contained fewer than two Langerhans' cells per high-power field had a better prognosis than those that had more than two Langerhans' histiocytes per high-power field.

MORPHOMETRY

Morphometry may be useful in the differentiation of atypical adenomatous hyperplasia from adenocarcinoma of the lung by providing objective and reproducible criteria (113). Using this diagnostic tool, Mori et al. (113) assigned lesions previously diagnosed by light microscopy as atypical adenomatous hyperplasia to the category of adenocarcinoma. However, using this criteria lesions also were found that had overlapping features of atypical adenomatous hyperplasia and adenocarcinoma.

LARGE CELL CARCINOMA

Large cell carcinomas constitute fewer than 15% of all lung cancers and are tumors that fail to express either glandular or squamous differentiation at the level of light microscopy (5, 7, 113). Although termed large cell carcinomas, these tumors are made up of cells that have been shown morphometrically to have a smaller cell size than cells of its closely related kin, the adenocarcinoma (42).

Simultaneous usage of the terms large cell carcinoma and non–small cell carcinoma have led inevitably to some confusion. More differentiated tumors, such as squamous cell carcinoma and adenocarcinoma, are non–small cell carcinomas, but so are large cell undifferentiated carcinomas (87). Mackay et al. (87, 114) have thus proposed that the term large cell carcinoma be viewed as synonymous with large cell undifferentiated carcinoma. Although undifferentiated at the light microscopic level, large cell carcinomas may have features of either squamous cell carcinoma or adenocarcinoma ultrastructurally. (90). Using electron microscopy, some large cell carcinomas may show the presence of intracytoplasmic tonofilaments, mucin droplets, or even electron dense granules that are indicative of neuroendocrine differentiation. In some series squamous or adenocarcinomatous differentiation can be detected in nearly 50% of these cases using ultrastructural or immunohistochemical techniques (87), and an additional 20% of the cases can show neuroendocrine differentiation (115).

Large cell carcinoma occurs as a bulky gray-pink tumor mass, usually located at the periphery of the lung, grossly similar to adenocarcinoma (116). Large cell carcinomas are seldom multiple. About half of large cell carcinomas involve subsegmental bronchi or larger airways. Cavitation is not a common feature, but necrosis is seen often. Large cell carcinoma metastasizes in a pattern quite similar to that of adenocarcinoma with a predilection for mediastinal lymph nodes, pleura, adrenal glands, bone, and the central nervous system. As defined by the WHO (9), large cell carcinomas are made up of epithelial cells with large nuclei, well-outlined cell boundaries, and prominent nucleoli (8, 9). The nucleoli are usually large, and they represent features that help to distinguish these tumors from small cell carcinomas. These cells may occur as solid sheets or amorphous aggregates. Rarely, large cells are seen admixed with small darker cells, simulating the mixed or variant morphology small cell cancer

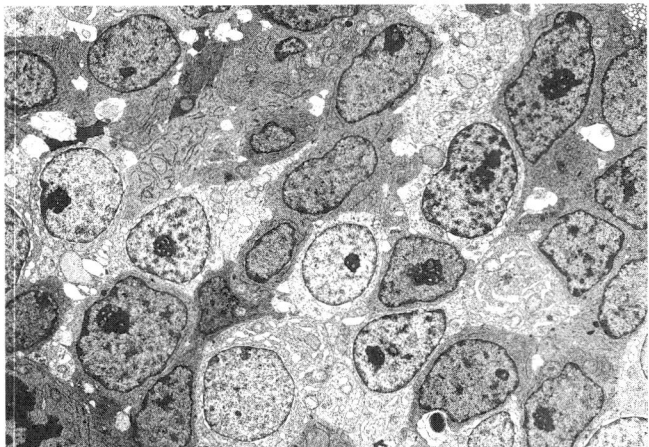

FIGURE 10.8. Undifferentiated large cell carcinoma with a component of smaller darker cells simulating the mixed (small cell and large cell) IASLC subtype of small cell carcinoma. Electron micrograph magnification, ×4700. (From Mackay B, Lukeman JM, Ordóñez NG. Tumors of the lung. In: Bennington JL, ed. Major problems in pathology. Philadelphia: Saunders, 1991;24:115.)

subtype (Fig. 10.8). Two variants of large cell carcinoma are recognized by the WHO: (*a*) giant cell, and (*b*) clear cell carcinoma.

Giant cell carcinoma was first described by Nash and Stout (117) as a distinct clinical entity generally associated with a rapid clinical course and poor prognosis with median survival of only 6 to 8 months. However, the concept of giant cell carcinoma of the lung as an entity with a greater aggressive biologic behavior has been challenged recently. In a study of 16 cases, Ginsberg et al. (118) found a median survival for the group of 14 months with 5 of the 16 patients alive and disease free after a median follow-up of 51 months (range, 20 to 116 months). In this study the 5 surviving patients had early-stage disease (stage I or II), and all patients with stage IIIA, IIIB, and IV disease died of the disease, thus verifying the influence of stage in the survival of patients with this type of lung cancer. Grossly, giant cell carcinomas have no distinguishing features, but they tend to be voluminous and focally necrotic (116). Microscopically, giant cell carcinomas are made up of very large, plump, often bizarre-looking cells showing trapping of leukocytic neutrophils within their cytoplasm, a phenomenon that has been regarded as a form of emperipolesis (119).

Leukocytosis in association with malignancy has been well described. Leukocytosis and neutrophilia are known to occur particularly in association with giant cell carcinoma. One possible explanation for the leukocytosis is the production of colony-stimulating factor by tumor cells (120). Using radioimmunoassay, enzyme-linked immunoabsorbent assay, and colony-forming unit granulocyte–macrophage assay, Sawyers et al. (120) demonstrated the presence of colony-stimulating factor in pleural fluid of two patients with peripheral blood leukocytosis and eosinophilia. One of the patients had squamous cell carcinoma and the other had adenocarcinoma. Ten of 11 patients with pleural effusions of various origins did not have evidence of colony-stimulating factor by these assays (120).

Clear cell carcinomas of lung are exceedingly rare tumors (116). They must be distinguished from benign ("sugar") clear cell tumors of the lung. Benign clear cell tumors of the lung are strongly PAS positive, a feature that is useful in the differential diagnosis of these two tumors. Metastatic clear cell carcinoma from other organs such as the kidney or adrenal gland may pose a diagnostic problem by mimicking clear cell carcinoma of lung.

IMMUNOHISTOCHEMISTRY

Immunophenotypic subsets of large cell carcinoma, including exocrine, endocrine, and mixed subtypes, were categorized by Gould and coworkers (121). The immunophenotypical profiles were carried out on the basis of immunoresponsiveness to chromogranin A, synaptophysin, and the mucinlike glycoprotein A-80. Significantly, in this series of 50 surgically resected large cell carcinomas, pure exocrine phenotypes ($n = 38$) appeared to have a survival advantage when compared with the other phenotypes. The ultrastructural and immunoperoxidase features of large cell carcinoma of the lung were assessed by Capelozzi-Delmonte et al. (122). These researchers studied large cell carcinoma with cytokeratin, CEA, and neuron specific enolase, and they subdivided 41 tumors into five groups: squamous, glandular, adenosquamous, neuroendocrine, and undifferentiated. With the possibility of further subclassification of lung cancers, these studies encourage efforts to diagnose large cell carcinoma more accurately (122).

Morphometry of large cell carcinoma appears to contribute little to its distinction from poorly differentiated adenocarcinoma. Burns and associates (42) examined the nucleolar to nuclear ratio, cell area, cell form factor, and nuclear form factor. Then, using logistic regression they attempted to separate large cell carcinoma from adenocarcinoma morphometrically. The classification efficiency was only 61%, compared with the histopathologic review.

SMALL CELL CARCINOMA

Small cell carcinoma represents 20% to 25% of all cases of lung cancer (5, 123). In the United States, small cell lung carcinoma is the seventh most frequent cause of cancer death (123). A strong relationship exists between SCLC and cigarette smoking. (124). Most SCLCs are located centrally, presenting in the main stem or lobar bronchi. SCLCs tend to disseminate early and widely into the hilar and mediastinal nodes, often forming very bulky masses. The current WHO classification (9) of lung tumors recognizes three types of SCLC:

1. Oat cell carcinoma: a malignant tumor composed of uniform small cells, generally larger than lymphocytes, having dense round or oval nuclei, diffuse chromatin, inconspicuous nucleoli, and very sparse cytoplasm.
2. Small cell carcinoma, intermediate cell type: a malignant tumor composed of small cells, with nuclear characteristics similar to those of oat cell but with more abundant cytoplasm. The cells may be polygonal or fusiform and are less regular in appearance than those of oat cell carcinoma.
3. Combined oat cell carcinoma: a tumor in which there is a definite component of oat cell carcinoma with squamous cell and/or adenocarcinoma.

Despite numerous studies, there is no convincing evidence that these subtypes have prognostic importance (14, 15, 125–127). A special panel convened by the IASLC at Gleneagles, Scotland, in 1984 reviewed the subclassification of small cell carcinoma (128). The IASLC pathology panel proposed that the terms oat cell and intermediate cell be deleted and that small cell carcinomas be subdivided into three subtypes: (a) (classic) small cell carcinoma, (b) mixed (small/large cell) type, and (c) combined squamous cell carcinoma. The latter was added to encompass tumors with a substantial amount of differentiated (squamous or glandular or both) components (Fig. 10.1). These subtypes were proposed on the basis of potential prognostic significance (128).

SCLCs often show areas of necrosis, grossly, although they are not as prone to cavitation as are squamous cell carcinomas. Microscopically, there may be a peculiar staining of the walls of vessels by an intensely basophilic material near areas of necrosis. As shown by Azzopardi (129), this nuclear cuffing appears to be nuclear DNA material from necrotic cells. Rarely, a small cell carcinoma is seen in a rosette formation, but sheets of haphazardly arranged tumor cells divided by thin fibrous or necrotic septa are seen more commonly. Trabecular, organoid, and ribbonlike morphologic patterns can also be seen. Foci of squamous differentiation may be found, but this change is more often seen in treated patients at surgery or in autopsy material. Metastases are seen early in at least two thirds of patients at presentation and may involve liver, adrenal gland, bone, central nervous system, and bone marrow. Twijnstra and coworkers (130) evaluated the significance of histologic subtypes, as defined by the Pathology Committee of the IASLC, in 100 cases of SCLC and found no significant differences among the various subtypes in their propensity to metastasize to the brain.

Small cell carcinomas express low molecular weight cytokeratin but are seldom reactive to high molecular weight cytokeratins. Immunoreactivity to CEA, human milk fat globule protein, and chromogranin can be variable (Table 10.3). SCLC cells are immunoreactive to synaptophysin, L-dopa decarboxylase, neuron specific enolase, creatine BB kinase, bombesin (gastric-releasing peptide), calcitonin, and various gut and brain peptide hormones (131, 132). This richness and variety of cellular constituents suggest that SCLC is a highly functional and differentiated rather than undifferentiated neoplasm (132). Loss of the biochemical and biologic properties of this neoplasm is associated morphologically with its morphologic conversion to an undifferentiated large cell tumor (133).

PROGNOSIS

Without treatment, the prognosis of SCLC is extremely poor (134, 135). Although some reports of long-term survival have appeared in the medical literature, most studies cite median durations of survival ranging from 6 to 24 months, depending on the clinical stage (136). The prognostic significance of the IASLC subclassification scheme for SCLC has remained uncertain. A recent study of 149 patients tested the reproducibility and prognostic impact of this subclassification system (15). The tissue slides from the 149 patients with initial diagnoses of SCLC (114 cases) and undifferentiated carcinoma (35 cases) were reclassified blindly as SCLC or non–small cell carcinoma by a panel of five pathologists with no knowledge of the initial diagnosis. The SCLCs were catalogued into the three subtypes outlined by the IASLC panel. Consensus diagnosis (defined as agreement by at least three of the five pathologists) was achieved in 144 (96.6%) of the 149 cases. Of these 144 cases, 124 were reclassified as SCLC; 115 (92.9%) were subclassified as small cell, 5 (4.0%) as mixed, and 4 (3.2%) as combined subtypes. Twenty cases were classified as non–small cell carcinoma. This study showed that the combined and mixed subtypes were very infrequent (15).

The clinical significance of variant morphology small cell lung carcinoma, using the 1984 IASLC classification system, was assessed by Aisner and associates (137). These investigators identified 22 cases with the combined small cell and large cell (variant) subtype from among 507 evaluable patients. On a second concordance review, only 10 cases remained classified as small cell and large cell. Four of these 10 patients achieved complete response to treatment, and the survival of either the initially identified or concordance identified combined subhistology groups was not distinguishable from the cases having the classic small cell subtype. Other studies looking at the prognostic significance of small cell carcinoma subtypes are shown in Table 10.5.

ADENOSQUAMOUS CARCINOMA

As defined by the WHO (9), adenosquamous carcinoma is a neoplasm composed of malignant squamous and glandular cellular elements (Figs. 10.9 and 10.10). The frequency of this tumor ranges from 0.4% to 4.0% (9, 10). In a series of 2160 primary lung tumors from Japan, adenosquamous carcinomas represented 2.6% of all tumors (138). Adenosquamous carcinomas are almost always located peripherally and are prone to disseminate early, with a concurrent poor prognosis. Relatively little has been written regarding this tumor. However, several large series have addressed the issue of survival in these tumors. Sridhar and associates

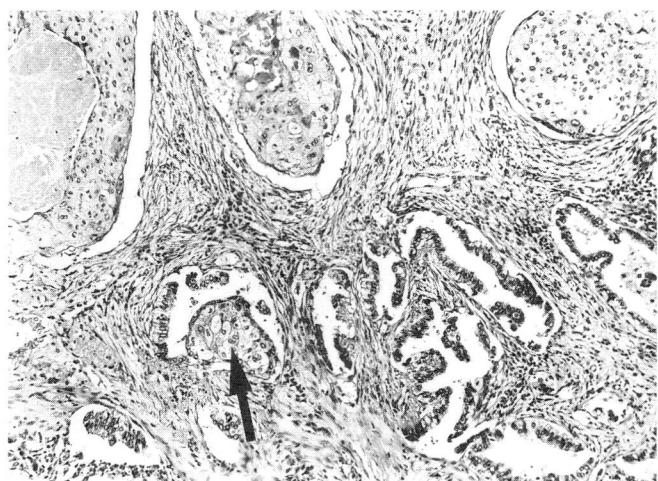

FIGURE 10.9. Adenosquamous carcinoma of lung showing coexisting well-differentiated adenocarcinoma (lower) and well-differentiated squamous cell carcinoma (upper). Note the nest of squamous cell carcinoma protruding into neoplastic glandular lumen (arrow). Hematoxylin and eosin stain; magnification, ×144. (From Ishida T, Kaneko S, Yokohama H, et al. Adenosquamous carcinomas of the lung. Clinical pathologic and immunohistochemical features. Am J Clin Pathol 1992;97:678–685.)

(139) evaluated a series of 127 patients with adenosquamous carcinoma and reported a 5-year survival of 62% for patients with localized disease. However, the median duration of survival for patients with regional and distant disease was only 8 and 4 months, respectively.

In adenosquamous carcinoma the squamous cell carcinoma components lie adjacent or side to side with the adenocarcinoma components (114). In contrast,

TABLE 10.5. Small Cell Lung Cancer Literature Review of Mixed Small Cell Lung Cancer Subtypes

SOURCE/YEAR	NO. OF CASES[a]	DIAGNOSIS[b]	VALIDATION OF SURVIVAL[c]	SIGNIFICANCE
Matthews, 1981	18,121 (14.8)	Not stated	Worse	Not stated
Radice et al., 1982	19,158 (12)	2 (2)[d]	Worse	$P < .005$
Hirsch et al., 1983	27,200 (14)	1 (1)	Worse	$P < .01$
Bepler et al., 1989	13,249 (5)	2 (3)[e]	Better[f]	Not significant
Aisner et al., 1990	24,550 (4.4)	2 (2)[g]	Better[h]	Not significant
Fraire et al., 1992	5,115 (4)	3 (5)	Better	$P = .009$

Modified from Fraire AE, Johnson EH, Yesner R, et al. Prognostic significance of histopathologic subtype and stage in small cell lung cancer. Hum Pathol 1992; 23:520–528.
[a]Number of mixed histology cases/total number of cases (percentage of mixed histology cases).
[b]Number under this heading refers to the number of pathologists validating the diagnosis.
[c]Survival of patients with mixed subtypes compared with pure or classic small cell subtypes.
[d]No comments on how discordant diagnoses were resolved.
[e]In case of discordance between the diagnoses of two pathologists, a third pathologist determined the final diagnosis.
[f]In this study the 2-year survival rates for the oat cell and mixed (small cell/large cell) subtypes were 7% and 15%, respectively.
[g]Concordance between the two pathologists was achieved in only 11 (45.8%) of 24 of the cases.
[h]Complete remission rates for the mixed and pure (classic) small cell subtypes were 33% and 19%, respectively.

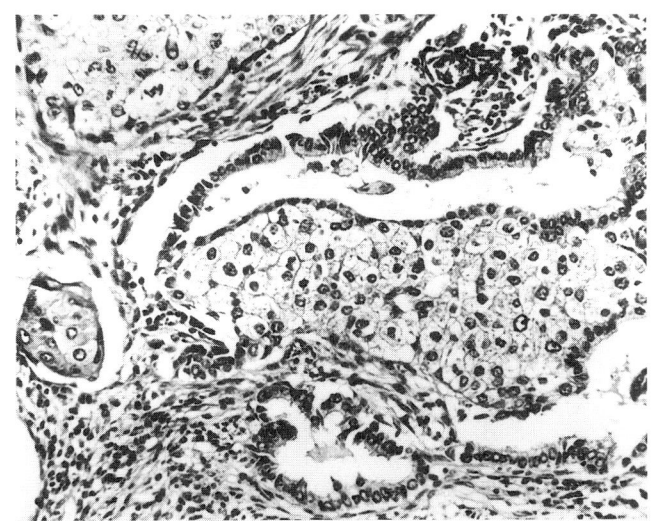

FIGURE 10.10. Adenosquamous carcinoma of lung showing the transition from glandular to squamous components. Hematoxylin and eosin stain; magnification, ×144. (From Ishida T, Kaneko S, Yokohama H, et al. Adenosquamous carcinomas of the lung. Clinical pathologic and immunohistochemical features. Am J Clin Pathol 1992;97:678–685.)

mucoepidermoid tumors show the same two cell components but mixed in a more intimate or mingled fashion (114). Ishida and colleagues (139a) proposed separation of adenosquamous carcinomas into three subgroups: (a) a predominant glandular type in which the squamous component may have originated within foci of preexisting squamous metaplasia, (b) a mixed type derived possibly from transition of undifferentiated carcinoma into two different cell types, and (c) a predominantly squamous type bearing resemblance to high-grade mucoepidermoid carcinoma. In the series of Ishida et al. (139a), the overall prognosis of eleven adenosquamous carcinomas (encompassing all three subgroups) did not differ from other non–small cell carcinoma. However, in the study by Takamori et al. (138), the results conflict with the series of Ishida's series (139a). In the experience of Takamori et al. (138), adenosquamous carcinomas showed a poorer prognosis than tumors that were pure adenocarcinomas or squamous cell carcinomas.

NEUROENDOCRINE TUMORS

Neuroendocrine tumors remain a subject of controversy. Uncertainty exists regarding their classification, criteria for diagnosis, and predictors of behavior and therapy (140). Hammar (10) has outlined a taxonomy for these tumors. In an ascending order of complexity, cellular atypia and clinical behavior, this taxonomy encompass tumorlets, typical and atypical carcinoids (the latter can also be referred to as well-differentiated neuroendocrine carcinoma), large cell neuroendocrine carcinoma, and lastly, small cell carcinoma.

TUMORLETS

Literally tiny tumors, tumorlets may be regarded as cellular proliferations rather than true neoplasms. Although first described in 1926 (141), they did not become known as tumorlets until 1955. The endocrine nature of tumorlets has been documented by immunostaining and electron microscopy (141). Although metastasis from tumorlets to lymph nodes has been reported, these events remain very infrequent (141).

CARCINOID (TYPICAL AND ATYPICAL) TUMORS

Once considered benign and classified as bronchial adenomas, bronchial carcinoid tumors are now regarded as malignant tumors. Since first described in the 19th century, carcinoid tumors have been the subject of considerable interest. The earliest accounts are credited to Heschl in 1877 and Mullen in 1882 (142). Modern knowledge, however, dates to Hamperl's (142) description of tumors currently classified as typical or well-differentiated carcinoid tumors. Hamperl further recognized the similarities between bronchial carcinoid tumors and their gastrointestinal counterparts. Formerly thought to be incapable of regional or distant dissemination, carcinoid tumors are known now to spread locally and to metastasize in about 10% of the cases (143). Therefore, the term bronchial adenoma, which implies a benign tumor, has been discarded. Bronchial carcinoids are rare neoplasms representing approximately 5% of all lung tumors (144). Although generally accepted as neuroendocrine in nature, the progenitor cell of a carcinoid tumor has not been established with certainty (143). Possible cells of origin include the Kulchitsky cell, located within the bronchial wall (145), or amine precursor uptake and deamination system cells that are thought to have migrated to the bronchial wall from the neural crest (146). However, recently introduced evidence suggests that an undifferentiated bronchial epithelial stem cell may represent the actual cell of origin (143, 147).

Most carcinoid tumors are located centrally, but some do arise from the peripheral airways (Table 10.6) (148). Although solitary carcinoid tumors are usually seen, multiple carcinoids do occur, and in this setting

TABLE 10.6. Primary Sites of Typical Bronchial Carcinoid Tumors[a]

Site	Central (84%)	Peripheral (16%)	Total
Right lung	104	22	126
Left lung	79	12	91

Modified from Okike N, Bernatz PE, Woolner LB. Carcinoid tumors of the lung. Ann Thorac Surg 1976;22:270–275.
[a]n = 203; some patients had more than one tumor.

they are likely to be peripheral rather than central (149). First described in 1953 by Felton, peripheral carcinoid tumors have a variety of morphologic patterns, including a spindle cell appearance (148–151). Microscopically, typical (mature) carcinoid tumors have an organoid pattern with cytologically bland cells arranged in nests, ribbons, or trabecular arrangements. These nests or ribbons are separated from each other by delicate strands of connective tissue stroma containing a rich capillary network (Fig. 10.11). This vascularization renders carcinoid tumors susceptible to bleeding, particularly when subjected to instrumentation during endoscopic procedures. The delicate fibrovascular stroma of carcinoid tumors may undergo extensive hyalinization and, occasionally, bony metaplasia. The overlying bronchial mucosa frequently is intact, and thus cytologic examination of sputum usually is negative. In 1972, Arrigoni and associates (152) laid the foundation for the histopathologic recognition of atypical carcinoids: tumors that appear to represent intermediate forms between the indolent typical carcinoid tumors and the highly malignant SCLC. Atypical carcinoid tumors are now referred to as well-differentiated to moderately differentiated neuroendocrine carcinomas, and they differ from their typical counterpart by the presence of focal necrosis, nuclear atypia, increased mitotic activity, and some loss of the organoid architectural pattern (151, 152).

Despite the frequent presence of hormonal products within neurosecretory granules, most bronchial carcinoid tumors manifest initially with only local symptoms related to bleeding or airway obstruction (143). Rarely, they present with systemic hormonal symptoms (143). Numerous hormonal and other neuroendocrine peptides, vasoactive amines, kinins, endorphins, and other similar products have been recognized in carcinoid tumors. A list of such products is tabulated in Table 10.7 (143). Some histopathologic features such as vascular invasion and ploidy status appear to be important prognostic factors for carcinoid tumors (153, 154). El Naggar and associates (151) found statistically significant associations between an-

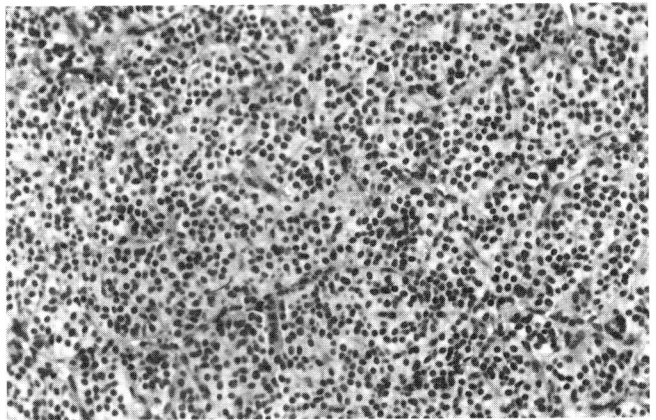

FIGURE 10.11. Histologic appearance of typical bronchial carcinoid. Note the small round uniform cells arranged in a nesting pattern. Hematoxylin and eosin stain; magnification, ×200.

TABLE 10.7. Bronchial Carcinoid Tumors Neuroendocrine Protein Products

Peptides
  Amylase
  Bombesin
  Calcitonin
  Corticotropin
  Corticotropin-releasing hormones
  Gastrin
  Glucagon
  Growth hormone–releasing factor
  Human chorionic gonadotropin
  Insulin
  Melanocyte-stimulating hormone
  Motilin
  Neurotensin
  Pancreatic polypeptide
  Secretin
  Somatostatin
  Substance K
  Substance P
  Vasoactive intestinal polypeptide
  Vasopressin
Vasoactive amines
  Catecholamines
  Histamine
Kinins
  Bradykinins
  Tachykinins (neurokinin A)
Endorphins and enkephalins
  β-Endorphin
  Leu-enkephalin
  Met-enkephalin
  Pan-opioid
Other
  Kallikrein
  Prostaglandins

From Davila DG, Dunn WG, Tazelar HD, Pairolero PC. Bronchial carcinoid tumors. Mayo Clin Proc 1993;68:795–803.

euploidy and tumor size, as well as vascular invasion and lymph node involvement in their study of 47 cases of bronchopulmonary carcinoid tumors. Histologically, atypical carcinoid tumors with diploid DNA content pursued a less aggressive course than their aneuploid counterparts (151).

LARGE CELL NEUROENDOCRINE CARCINOMAS

These lung carcinomas have been the focus of considerable interest (115, 121, 155–158). This interest stems, in part, from the awareness that squamous cell carcinomas, adenocarcinomas, and large cell carcinomas may show evidence of neuroendocrine differentiation, when scrutinized by the electron microscope or by modern immunostaining techniques (115). Features that identify neuroendocrine differentiation include dense core granules, high levels of L-dopa decarboxylase, and the manufacturing of a variety of hormonal substances and neuropeptides (147). These features are shared ostensibly by their putative progenitors, the pulmonary endocrine cells. Large cell neuroendocrine carcinomas cannot be distinguished from large cell carcinomas without neuroendocrine features by means of light microscopy; however, Hammar (10) intimates that large cells with large vesicular nuclei and prominent nucleoli betray their ultrastructural makeup. As noted in Table 10.3, large cell neuroendocrine carcinomas consistently express low molecular weight cytokeratins and neuron specific enolase but variably express high molecular weight cytokeratins, CEA, human milk fat globule protein, and chromogranin. In a study of 12 large cell carcinomas showing evidence of neuroendocrine differentiation, 5 (55%) died of their disease within 3 years (115). In contrast, most of the patients with large cell carcinomas lacking neuroendocrine differentiation were free of disease within a similar time frame. A separate study of 35 cases and those reported in the literature concluded that the prognosis of large cell carcinomas with neuroendocrine differentiation lies somewhere between that of atypical carcinoid tumors and of small cell carcinomas (159). However, larger series of patients are needed to document significant differences in survival (158, 159).

OTHER EPITHELIAL LUNG CANCERS

A diverse but rare group of primary nonmesenchymal lung tumors do not fit established categories of lung cancer and currently await further classification. A partial list of such tumors includes basaloid carcinoma, sarcomatoid carcinoma, lung carcinoma with spindle cell components, the so-called mucinous cystic tumors of lung, and primary mucinous adenocarcinoma of the lung with signet ring components.

On review of 115 poorly differentiated lung cancers obtained from a pool of 671 resected cases over a 7-year period, Brambilla and coworkers (160) identified 38 cases of basal cell (basaloid) carcinoma, an apparent new morphologic and phenotypic pulmonary entity with distinct prognostic significance. A lobular growth pattern, peripheral palisading, small hyperchromatic cells with nucleoli, scant cytoplasm, and high mitotic rate were cardinal histopathologic features that helped to distinguish this clinically aggressive neoplasm from other non–small cell cancers (Fig. 10.12). In the series of Brambilla and coworkers (160), patients with this histology had a poor prognosis, with a median survival of 22 months for stage I and II disease. Although relatively uncommon in the lung, basaloid carcinomas also are known to occur in the upper airway, oropharynx, esophagus, and uterine cervix. As pointed out by Saldana and Mones (161), the histopathologic diagnosis of these tumors is fraught with difficulties, especially when the tissue specimen is a small crushed transbronchial biopsy. A nesting arrangement of the tumor cells with peripheral palisading (Fig. 10.12) is a cardinal histopathologic feature for these tumors regardless of their anatomic location.

Lung tumors with coexisting mesenchymal and epithelial malignant components include pulmonary

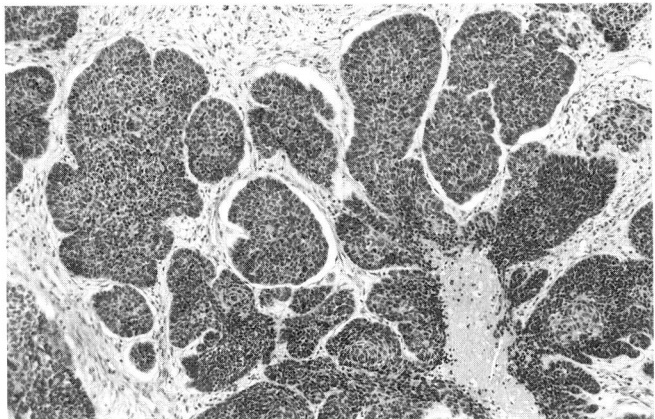

FIGURE 10.12. Basaloid carcinoma of lung. Note the solid lobular pattern with peripheral palisading of tumor cells. Magnification, ×100. (From Brambilla E, Moro D, Veale D, et al. Basal cell [basaloid] carcinoma of the lung; a new morphologic and phenotypic entity with separate prognostic significance. Hum Pathol 1992;23: 993–1003.)

blastomas, carcinosarcomas, and sarcomatoid carcinomas (162–164). The first two neoplasms have been well categorized, but sarcomatoid carcinomas, akin to those occurring in the esophagus, larynx, and other sites, are not well defined. Fourteen cases of sarcomatoid carcinoma of the lung studied by Chen and associates (165) showed clear male predominance (12 men, 2 women), history of smoking (13 of 14), and advanced stage (10 were stage III and one was stage IV disease) at presentation. These investigators suggested that appropriate epithelial markers or ultrastructural evaluation be used to establish an epithelial differentiation. Immunoreactivity for cytokeratin appeared to be helpful, with 9 of 12 tested carcinomas showing positive immunostaining for this marker. Four of the tumors that were cytokeratin positive also reacted positively with the epithelial membrane antigen.

Among 16 cases of lung carcinoma with spindle cell components studied by Matsui et al. (166), 6 had squamous cell carcinoma, 4 had adenocarcinoma, 5 had adenosquamous carcinoma, and 1 had large cell carcinoma as their epithelial components. Immunohistochemistry showed positive reactions for keratin, epithelial membrane antigen, or CEA to a varying degree according to the histologic types. The spindle cell elements revealed a positive immunoreaction for keratin in all but one case. Mesenchymal markers, such as desmin, actin, and myosin, were all negative. These investigators thought that the spindle cell components in these 16 cases represented mesenchymal features with partial or complete loss of epithelial features (166). These findings further suggest that sarcomatoid carcinomas and carcinomas with spindle cell carcinoma show significant histopathologic overlap. Whether they represent a single pathologic entity or parts of a spectrum of neoplasms awaits further clarification.

IMMUNOHISTOCHEMISTRY AND FLOW CYTOMETRY

During the past few years, many monoclonal antibodies have made the transition successfully from research to clinically useful tools. The immunophenotypic profiles of most of the primary lung neoplasms are delineated in Table 10.3. The use of these antibodies and flow cytometry have become important adjuncts in establishing the diagnosis and prognosis of lung cancers. However, although these antibodies are generally specific, cross-reactivity with other tissues can occur; thus, a useful guideline in immunopathology is the avoidance of reliance on the expression of single markers for a given diagnosis.

IMMUNOHISTOCHEMISTRY

Successful immunostaining techniques require the presence and preservation of the target antigen(s). The loss of such antigens may be caused by fixation delays or excessive heat during fixation, or during embedding. Rarely, antigen loss may be encountered in poorly differentiated tumors. Vimentin, a ubiquitous molecule that is uniformly distributed in most tissue samples, is uniquely suited as an internal control for monitoring antigenic loss in formalin-fixed tissue material (167). Battifora (167) aptly referred to vimentin as a reporter molecule, and he advocated its use to monitor alterations of other antigenic molecules. Thus, vimentin has a place not only in the study of sarcomatoid tumors and epithelial lung tumors but also in assessing antigen loss.

A fibrillary meshwork found within most eukaryotic cells, collectively known as the cytoskeleton, comprises three types of fibrils, microfilaments, intermediate filaments, and microtubules. Within the family of intermediate filaments, five proteins, including cytokeratins, are currently recognized. The intermediate filament proteins are presented in Table 10.8 together with tissue tumors in which they are often found (103). One of the five intermediate filaments, cytokeratins are especially important because they are found in epithelia, and high molecular weight cytokeratins are found in complex epithelia. Antibodies specific for high molecular weight cytokeratins react with squamous and ductal (i.e., complex) epithelia (103, 168). Commercial antibodies against intermediate filaments can sometimes be useful in distinguishing poorly differentiated primary and metastatic neoplasms of the lung because the normal pseudostratified epithelium of the airways expresses a combination of low and high molecular weight cytokeratins (169). Tumors that react to cytokeratin antibodies include squamous cell and adenocarcinomas of lung and breast, and adenocarcinomas of the pancreas, among many others. Usually non-

TABLE 10.8. Intermediate Filaments

PROTEINS	TISSUES	TUMORS
Keratins	Epithelium	Carcinomas
Desmin	Muscle	Muscle sarcomas
Glial fibrillary acidic proteins	Astroglia	Gliomas
Neurofilaments	Neurons	Neuroblastomas
Vimentin	Mesenchyme	Non–muscle sarcomas

From Elias JM. Immunohistopathology. A practical approach to diagnosis. Chicago: American Society of Clinical Pathologists Press, 1990.

reactive tumors include lymphomas, sarcomas, melanomas, gliomas, and adenocarcinomas arising from organs made up of simple epithelium such as hepatocellular carcinoma. Rarely, poorly differentiated nonepithelial tumors such as large cell lymphomas may also express cytokeratin (170). In these instances gene rearrangement studies, or more comprehensive evaluation with immunohistochemical panels for epithelial and lymphoid markers, usually resolve the diagnostic problem (170).

Cytokeratin immunostaining may sometimes be useful in the detection of nodal metastasis. Sedmak and coworkers (171) applied cytokeratin immunostaining to a variety of axillary nodes removed from patients with breast and other cancers, and they demonstrated that this technique is at least as effective as conventional staining with hematoxylin and eosin. The applicability of this technique to nodal diagnosis in lung cancer remains to be established. Cytokeratins, however, can be somewhat limited as a diagnostic aid because they can sometimes be expressed by some other tumors such as sarcomas (e.g., malignant fibrous histiocytomas, leiomyosarcomas, and Ewing's sarcomas) as well as some gliomas and astrocytomas (103, 172).

The epithelial membrane antigen, which occurs in milk fat globule membranes, was first assumed to be specific to epithelial cells (103, 173). However, this antigen was subsequently demonstrated in a variety of nonepithelial cells, including mesothelial cells, plasma cells, histiocytes, fibroblasts, and neoplastic T lymphocytes (103, 174, 175). Thus, although most carcinomas express the marker, its use as a diagnostic aid is limited by its expression in the wide variety of other tumors.

CEA is expressed in normal epithelium throughout the body including the epithelium of the respiratory tract (51). Immunostaining with antibodies against CEA reveals strong luminal staining of adenocarcinomas, and variable staining of squamous cell carcinomas and large cell carcinomas with only weak focal staining in SCLC (51). As a rule, most adenocarcinomas of the lung express CEA, but mesotheliomas generally do not.

S-100 protein is a highly soluble acidic protein (21 to 24 kilodaltons), which is found in glial and Schwann cells (103). S-100, however, can also be found in cells not of neural origin, including cells from poorly differentiated carcinomas (176). This wide distribution limits the usefulness of S-100 in pulmonary pathology, narrowing its role largely to the detection of suspected Langerhans' cells in some lung carcinomas and as an aid in the differential diagnosis of metastatic malignant melanoma.

Lectins are carbohydrate-binding proteins of nonimmune origin (177), and the binding sites for these lectins are found in the plasma membrane of various epithelial cells (178). The expression of lectin proteins appears to correlate with the maturity or differentiation of normal or neoplastic cells (177, 178). Various lectin antibodies stained tumor cells in 35% to 100% of the cases with a greater percentage of reactivity obtained in the better differentiated (acinar) adenocarcinomas and a lesser percentage of reactivity in the poorly differentiated (solid) adenocarcinomas in an autopsy series of 54 cases (178). Lectin immunostaining patterns for adenocarcinomas are shown in Table 10.9 (178).

Chromogranins are a family of secretory proteins that have a widespread occurrence in neuroendocrine granules (179, 180). Chromogranin A was the first member of this family of proteins, which was identified in the bovine adrenal medulla (181, 182). Chromogranin A, in contrast to the cytoplasmic marker neuron specific enolase, is regarded as a granular marker (51). SCLCs are poorly granulated, such that chromogranin antibodies have only limited value in their diagnosis (51). However, chromogranin A is frequently and strongly expressed in most bronchial carcinoids (143).

FLOW CYTOMETRY

Flow cytometry as a measure of cellular DNA content and nuclear ploidy has helped to increase understanding of the biology of lung cancer as well as many other cancers. The introduction of newer methodology by Hedley et al. (183) permitted the use of flow cytometry analysis to archival paraffin-embedded tissue. In general, the finding of aneuploidy on flow cytometry in lung cancer has generally shown the tumor of origin to have a more virulent behavior. In a 5-year follow-up study of 187 previously untreated cases of NSCLC, Volm et al. (184) identified shorter survival periods in patients with aneuploid lung cancers. This shorter survival was independent of stage. Similar results were obtained by Zimmerman et al. (185) in a group of 100 patients with NSCLC. Miyamoto et al. (186) evaluated the prognostic significance of nuclear DNA content of tumors from 112 patients with NSCLC. A higher rate of 5-year survival occurred in the diploid group (61%) than in the DNA aneuploid group (35%). Although this difference was statistically significant, the DNA content was not a major independent prognostic factor in tumors classified as adenocarcinomas. These studies sug-

TABLE 10.9. Reactions of Primary Adenocarcinoma of the Lung to Lectins and PE-10[a]

Histologic Type	WGA	Suc WGA	SBA	PNA	RCA-1	UEA-1	PE-10
Acinar (n = 17)	59	100	88	76	100	88	35
Papillary (n = 21)	69	81	85	77	88	69	42
Solid (n = 11)	64	91	91	64	64	45	18

From Sugiyama K, Kawai T, Nakanishi K, Susuki M. Histochemical reactivities of lectins and surfactant apoprotein in pulmonary adenocarcinomas and their metastasis. Mod Pathol 1992;5:273–276.
Abbreviations. WGA, wheat germ agglutin; Suc WGA, succynilated WGA; SBA, soybean agglutinin; PNA, peanut agglutinin; RCA-1, ricinus communis; UEA, ulex Europaeus agglutinin; PE-10, Anti–human pulmonary surfactant apoprotein.
[a] n = 54.

gest that ploidy may be a very important predictor of survival, but further study is needed to define its exact role. Flow cytometry, however, was not able to distinguish which tumors were likely to recur. In a study of 102 patients with T1, N0 disease, Schmidt et al. (186a) prospectively evaluated both recurrent and nonrecurrent tumors (51 patients each) to identify subsets with unfavorable tumors. Ploidy abnormalities and proliferative cell rates were not significantly different between the recurrent and control cases, suggesting that flow cytometry analysis has a limited role in guiding postoperative management.

Although potentially useful for prognosis, the usefulness of tumor cell DNA content determined by flow cytometry has been limited in most sites by sampling and by the heterogeneity of the tumor. Sara and El-Naggar (187) obtained three separate tissue samples from each of 28 surgically resected NSCLCs to determine the DNA variability of the lung tumor. An FNA for flow cytometry also was obtained from the center of the resected NSCLC. Twenty-three (82%) of the tumors were aneuploid, and 5 (18%) were diploid. Four (17%) of the 23 aneuploid tumors showed DNA heterogeneity expressed as additional stem lines in at least one of the three tissue samples. In general, these authors observed good correlation between the results obtained from the FNA and the three tissue samples, suggesting that, as opposed to tumors in other anatomic sites, the majority of NSCLCs display little intratumoral DNA heterogeneity. Confirmation of these findings is needed, however.

MOLECULAR DIAGNOSTICS

Another area of considerable progress in the understanding of lung cancer is derived from new evolutions in molecular biology that have considerable importance for diagnosis and prognosis of lung cancers.

ONCOGENES

Genes associated with lung cancer are usually normal cellular genes that, when activated (protooncogenes), result in enhanced cellular growth, or when altered or lost cease to inhibit growth (188, 189). Protooncogene activation may occur by point mutations, overexpression, or loss of normal cell cycle dependent regulation (188). Oncogenes associated with lung cancer include the *myc* and *ras* families, the *neu, myb, raf,* and *bcl*-1 and *bcl*-2 genes (Table 10.10).

myc Oncogenes are activated by overexpression through amplification. Overexpression of *myc* oncogenes in SCLC cell lines has been associated with shortened survival and limited or absent response to chemotherapy (190) (Fig. 10.13). *myc* Oncogene amplification also has been observed in metastatic tumors and after treatment (191, 192). This shortened survival

TABLE 10.10. Molecular Changes in Lung Cancer: Comparison of Small Cell Lung Cancer with Non–Small Cell Lung Cancer

Gene/Site	SCLC	NSCLC
Oncogenes		
myc	~10%	Rare[a]
ras	Rare	~20%
HER-2*neu*	Rare	~30%
Antioncogenes		
Ch 3p[b]	~100%	50%–80%
rb gene	~100%	15%
p53 gene	≈100%	47%
Ch 9p	≈35%	~35%
Ch 5q[b]	~40%	≈40%–50%

Modified from Gazdar AF. Molecular markers for the diagnosis and prognosis of lung cancer. Cancer 1992;69:1592–1599.
Abbreviations. SCLC, small cell lung cancer; NSCLC, non–small cell lung cancer.
[a] Amplification is rare, but overexpression may be relatively common.
[b] This antioncogene may represent the *MCC* and *APC* genes frequently involved in colon cancer.

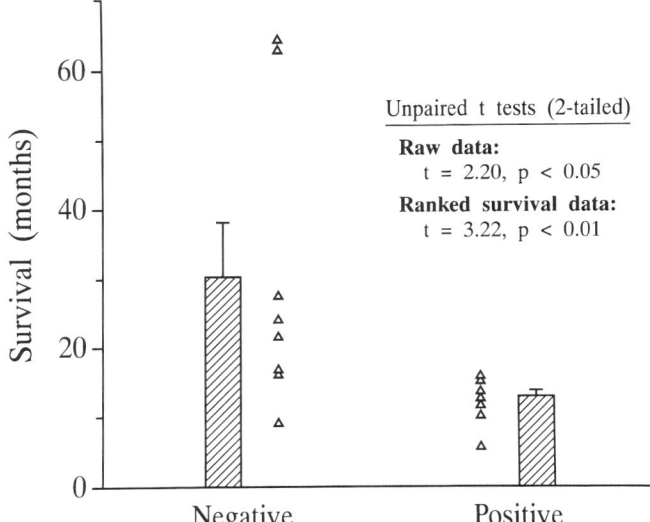

FIGURE 10.13. Difference in survival for patients who are negative and positive for N-*myc* expression. Bars show plus or minus standard error of mean (SEM). (From Funa K, Steinholz L, Nou E, Bergh J. Increased expression of N-*myc* in human small cell lung cancer biopsies predicts lack of response to chemotherapy and poor prognosis. Am J Clin Pathol 1987;88:216–220.)

in SCLC associated with an increased expression of the *myc* oncogene is in accord with prior reports drawing attention to the association of *myc* amplification and rapid tumor progression in children with neuroblastoma (193), cerebellar medulloblastoma (194), neuroesthesioneuroblastoma (195), and retinoblastoma (196). *myc* Amplification in human lung cancers other than SCLC is rare but does occur. Kashii and coworkers (197) studied 30 human lung cancer cell lines and found an adenocarcinoma amplifying the N-*myc* oncogene but not the c-*myc* or L-*myc* or k-*ras* oncogenes. Interestingly, this adenocarcinoma had histology typical of adenocarcinoma, and the CEA was strongly positive in the culture medium. N-*myc* oncogene amplification also was described in a patient with a primary lung adenocarcinoma with neuroendocrine differentiation (198).

In contrast to *myc* oncogenes, *ras* protooncogenes are activated by mutation. The three protooncogenes, H-*ras*, K-*ras*, and N-*ras*, constitute this family of oncogenes. In experimental models *ras* mutations have been associated with: specific mutagens such as alkylating agents, a metastatic phenotype, and an inherent resistance to cytotoxic therapy (188, 199, 200). Whereas *myc* oncogenes have been found amplified predominantly in metastatic tumors and in tumors after treatment, *ras* oncogenes typically have been found mutated in primary tumor specimens (201) and occur in approximately 20% of NSCLCs (Table 10.10). Such *ras* mutations appear to correlate with a decreased disease free survival among patients with adenocarcinoma, despite aggressive surgical resection (201, 202).

The *p53* gene appears to be a commonly mutated gene in human cancers. The p53 protein binds to specific DNA sequences, blocking progression through the cell cycle. The p53 protein, a nuclear phosphoprotein, was first identified in extracts of cells transformed by SV40 (203). In normal cells, p53 exhibits a very short half-life (5 to 20 minutes) and thus is undetectable by standard immunohistochemical methods (204). However, tumor cells with genetic alterations of *p53* frequently have been found to express readily detectable levels of p53 (205).

After Vogelstein et al. (206) reported *p53* gene alterations in colorectal carcinomas, other investigators found that *p53* mutations were relevant to the prognosis and clinical behavior of many human neoplasms (207, 208). For example, *p53* mutations are seen more frequently in young patients and in patients with squamous histology (188). In addition, detection of *p53* mutations may prove useful in the detection of precancerous lesions. Bennett et al. (208) studied human lung tissues containing preinvasive lesions using a polyclonal anti-p53 rabbit antiserum. Nuclear staining was noted in none of 15 patients with a normal mucosa and none of 3 patients with squamous metaplasias. However, this staining was positive in 2 of 5 mild dysplasias, 9 of 10 severe dysplasias, 12 of 12 in situ carcinomas, and both cases of microinvasive carcinomas. These findings suggest that p53 immunostaining may be useful in the early detection of lung cancer in individuals with increased risk factors.

The protooncogene *bcl-2* has been proposed as a regulator of programmed cell death, also known as apoptosis, in a variety of cells (209). Recently, Pezzella et al. (210) reported *bcl-2* protein expression in 25% of 80 squamous cell carcinomas and 12% of 42 adenocarcinomas. In the adjacent normal respiratory epithelium, *bcl-2* was expressed only in basal cells. Survival at 5 years was higher among patients with *bcl-2* positive tumors, both in the group as a whole ($P < .01$) and in the subgroup with squamous cell carcinoma ($P < .02$). Patients 60 years of age or older who had *bcl-2* positive tumors had the best survival statistics, both in the group as a whole ($P < .02$) and in the group with squamous cell carcinoma ($P < .01$). The authors concluded that *bcl-2* is abnormally expressed in some lung cancers and that its expression may have prognostic importance. In the author's laboratory at the University of Massachusetts Medical Center, *bcl-2* protein expression was studied recently in 47 surgically resected adenocarcinomas (210a). A control group of 7 patients with squamous carcinomas showed immunoreactivity in 4 of the 7 (Fig. 10.14). Twenty-five of the 47 adenocarcinomas were immunoreactive. Among *bcl-2* positive adenocarcinomas, there appeared to be a survival advantage compared with *bcl-2* negative adenocarcinomas. However, with this small number of patients, the survival difference did not reach a level of statistical significance (210a).

HISTOPATHOLOGIC PROGNOSTIC FACTORS

As defined by the TNM classification system, local tumor invasion can alter the prognosis. Invasion of the visceral pleura by carcinoma of the lung adversely impacts on tumor stage and hence on the patient's prognosis. Gallagher and Urbanzki (211) retrospectively analyzed 23 patients with peripheral T2, N0, M0 lung cancers with invasion of the visceral pleura (Fig. 10.15). Compared with a group of matched controls, patients with pleural invasion by squamous cell carcinoma had a significantly shorter survival ($P = .0236$), suggesting the need for histologic assessment for invasion of the visceral pleura by peripheral lung cancers. This report strongly supports the need for consistent inclusion of pleural assessment in all cases of surgically resected lung cancer, and possibly for the modification of the staging system to indicate this involvement.

Tumor necrosis (Fig. 10.16) appears to represent an adverse predictor of survival in patients with carcinoma of lung (212) as well as other malignancies such

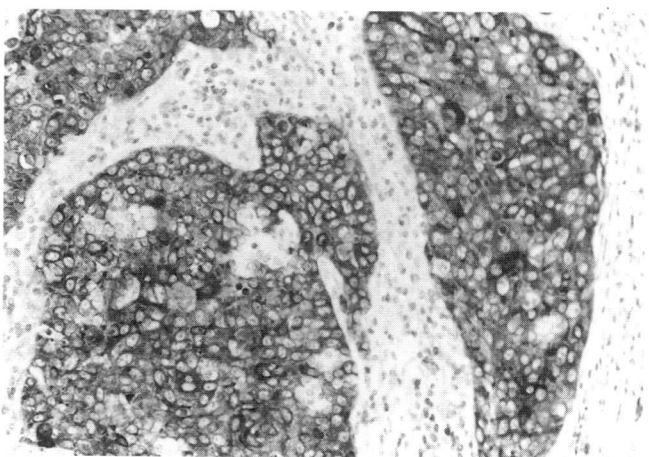

FIGURE 10.14. *bcl-2* Immunohistologic stain showing moderately strong reactivity in cells from a squamous cell carcinoma (2+ in a scale of 1 to 3+). Magnification, ×400.

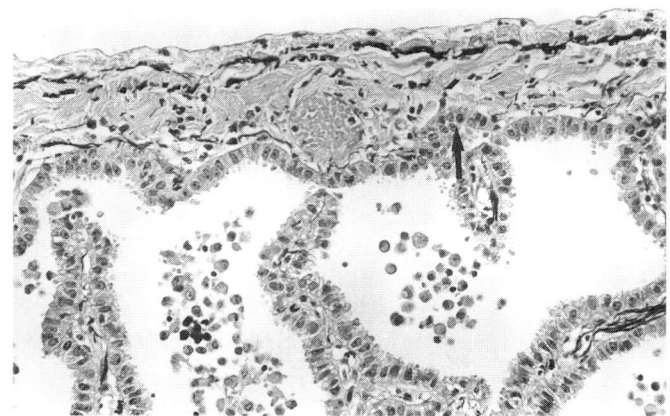

FIGURE 10.15. Adenocarcinoma invading through the pleural internal elastic lamina (*arrow*). Movat's stain; magnification, ×390. (From Gallagher B, Urbanski SJ. The significance of pleural elastic invasion by lung carcinoma. Hum Pathol 1990;21:512–517.)

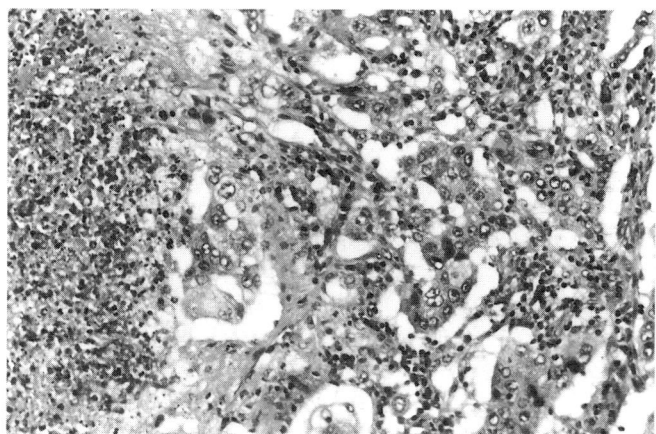

FIGURE 10.16. Tumor necrosis. Note the well-preserved adenocarcinoma on the middle and right thirds of the field shown and the extensive necrosis on the far left. Hematoxylin and eosin stain; magnification, ×400

as breast cancer (213). Elson et al. (212) showed a statistically significant association between the extent of tumor necrosis and survival in 47 surgically resected carcinoma of lung. However, in that study the necrosis was quantified subjectively by a group of histopathologists. In a subsequent study, Shahab et al. (214) objectively examined the extent of tumor necrosis by computer-assisted morphometry in 28 patients with surgically resected carcinoma of lung. Comparing the extent of tumor necrosis in two subsets of patients, these workers confirmed earlier observations that the extent of tumor necrosis is significantly adversely related to the probability of survival.

Some of the reported adverse differences in the prognosis of adenocarcinoma compared with squamous cell carcinomas may in part be related to a higher frequency of vascular invasion in adenocarcinomas. Haque et al. (215) compared 26 squamous cell carcinomas and 20 adenocarcinomas. Vascular invasion was seen in 19% of the squamous cell carcinomas and 55% of the adenocarcinomas. The mean survival for patients with squamous cell carcinoma and adenocarcinomas was 25 and 15.5 months, respectively.

Although histopathologic prognostic variables for large cell carcinoma have not yet been well documented, intercellular cohesion may be an important histopathologic predictor of survival. Ishida et al. (216) divided 54 large cell carcinomas into those with compact and those with loosely structured tumor patterns. The survival rates were 46% and 28% for the two subgroups, respectively. Neuroendocrine differentiation in large cell carcinoma also appears to have some prognostic implications. Wick et al. (115) compared 12 large cell carcinomas with neuroendocrine differentiation and 15 large cell carcinomas lacking such differentiation. A distinctly worse prognosis was seen for the latter group. In that study neuroendocrine differentiation was defined as the expression of neuron specific enolase, Leu-7, synaptophysin, and chromogranin, and by the content of dense granules on electron microscopy. Because most large cell carcinomas are not studied in this fashion, the frequency of this association is not well understood.

Brown et al. (217) tested the usefulness of PCNA as a prognostic marker in stage I NSCLC. PCNA was found in 73% of 84 stage I tumors. However, when patients were stratified into favorable and unfavorable groups, there were no significant differences in the mean percentage of PCNA positive tumor cells, suggesting that PCNA immunostaining has limited value in determining the outcome of stage I NSCLCs.

Morphologic abnormalities of the nucleolus have long been recognized as possible indicators of malignancy (218). In particular, macronucleoli, deeply eosinophilic nucleoli, and angulated nucleoli appear to be particularly significant. Correlations between nucleolar organizer regions as visualized by silver techniques (Agnor's) have been described in a variety of breast and other human tumors (219, 220) and are said to be related to the proliferative activity and rate of cell growth. Ogura et al. (221) studied 58 adenocarcinomas of the lung for the purpose of correlating Agnor's stain results with tumor growth rate, as estimated by tumor doubling times and chest radiographs. They found an inverse correlation between Agnor count and tumor doubling time (221). These data suggest that Agnor counts may be useful as an index of proliferative activity in lung cancer. Agnor score may also assist in determining proliferative activity of precancerous lesions of the bronchial epithelium. Abe et al. (220) performed Agnor counts in five normal bronchial epithelium, nine atypical metaplasia, five in situ carcinomas, and seven microinvasive squamous cell carcinomas. There was a highly significant difference between Agnor counts in atypical squamous metaplasia and carcinoma in situ. This difference is particularly relevant because the distinction between highly atypical squamous metaplasia and in situ carcinoma may, at times, be very difficult using light microscopy.

Increased deposition of basement membrane by tumor cells has been suggested to represent a sign of favorable prognosis independent of tumor stage. Ten Velde et al. (222) used polyclonal antibodies against type II human collagen in 68 patients with squamous cell lung carcinoma to assess basement membrane substances. Twenty seven of 62 patients had extensive basement membrane deposition, which had a significant effect on survival independent of tumor stage. Desmosomes and intercellular junctions function to maintain cohesiveness between epithelial cells. The notion that loss of cohesiveness among tumor cells may lead to metastatic spread of tumor cells has been entertained for years (223). McDonagh et al. (224) counted the number of intercellular junctions per area of tissue section in 76 cases of lung cancer by means of electron microscopy. These authors found that the number of intercellular bridges is inversely related to the ability of the tumor to spread and metastasize. Furthermore, the number of intercellular junctions in this study did appear to be related inversely to tumor stage, suggesting the potential usefulness of this diagnostic tool in the assessment of prognosis in patients with lung cancer.

ACKNOWLEDGMENTS

The author thanks Ms. Beryl Edney for the preparation of the manuscript, Drs. Bruce Woda and German Pihan for reviewing the introduction and molecular diagnostic sections, Dr. Frank Reale for reviewing the introduction and cytology sections, and Dr. Adi Gazdar for providing helpful data on the update and modification of Table 10.10, which compares molecular changes in small cell and non–small cell lung cancers.

REFERENCES

1. Wingo PA, Tong T, Boldens S. Cancer statistics, 1995. Ca: A Cancer Journal for Clinicians. American Cancer Society, Atlanta, GA, 1995;45:8–30.
2. Cotran RS, Kumar V, Robbins SL. In: Robbins SL, ed. Pathologic basis of disease. 4th ed. Philadelphia: Saunders, 1989: 797.

3. Roviaro GC, Varoli F, Zannini P, et al. Lung cancer in the young. Chest 1985;64:456–459.
4. Rocha MP, Fraire AE, Guntupalli KK, Greenberg SD. Lung cancer in the young. Cancer Detect Prev 1994;18:349–355.
5. Fraire AE, Cooper SP, Greenberg SD, Buffler PA. Carcinoma of the lung: changing cell distribution and histopathologic cell types. In: Fenoglio-Preisser CM, Wolff M, Rilke F, eds. Progress in surgical pathology. Blue Bell, PA: Field and Wood Medical Publishers, 1992;XII:129–149.
6. Yesner R. Lung cancer: pathogenesis and pathology. Clin Chest Med 1993;14:17–30.
7. Vincent RG, Pickren JW, Lane WW, et al. The changing histopathology of lung cancer: a review of 1682 cases. Cancer 1977;39:1617–1655.
8. Deiyberg L, Liebow AA, Vehlinger EA. Histological typing of lung tumors, International Histological Classification of Tumors. Geneva: World Health Organization, 1967; No. 1.
9. The World Health Organization histological typing of lung tumors. 2nd ed. Am J Clin Pathol 1982;77:123–136.
10. Hammar SD. Common neoplasms. In: Dail DH, Hammar SP, eds. Pulmonary pathology. 2nd ed. New York: Springer-Verlag, 1993:1123–1278.
11. Yesner R, Seydel GH, Asbell SO, et al. Biopsies of non–small cell lung cancer: central review in cooperative studies of the radiation therapy oncology group. Mod Pathol 1991;4:432–440.
12. Yesner R, Fraire AE, Zhang XB, et al. Traditional histology in the diagnosis of SCLC: is it useful? Cancer Ther Control 1991;2:31–38.
13. Yesner R. Classification of lung cancer histology. N Engl J Med 1985;312:652–653.
14. Hirsch FR, Matthews MJ, Aisner S, et al. Histopathologic classification of small cell lung cancer. Changing concepts and terminology. Cancer 1988;62:973–977.
15. Fraire AE, Johnson EH, Yesner R, et al. Prognostic significance of histopathologic subtype and stage in small cell lung cancer. Hum Pathol 1992;23:520–528.
16. Roggli VL, Vollmer RT, Greenberg SD, et al. Lung cancer heterogeneity: a blinded and randomized study of 100 consecutive cases. Hum Pathol 1985;16:569–579.
17. Olcott CT. Cell types and histologic patterns in carcinoma of lung: observations on the significance of tumors containing more than one type of cell. Am J Pathol 1955;31:975–995.
18. Willis RA. Pathology of tumors. 4th ed. London: Butterworth, 1967.
19. Reid JD, Carr AH. The validity and value of histological and cytological classification of lung cancer. Cancer 1961;14:673–698.
20. Fraire AE, Roggli VL, Vollmer RT, et al. Lung cancer heterogeneity: prognostic implications. Cancer 1987;60:370–379.
21. Mooi WJ, Dingemans KP, Wagenaar SS, et al. Ultrastructural heterogeneity of lung carcinomas: representativity of samples for electron microscopy in tumor classification. Hum Pathol 1990;21:1227–1234.
22. Herrera GA, Turbat-Herrera EA, Alexander B. Ultrastructural heterogeneity of pulmonary scar adenocarcinomas. Correlations with patients survival. Ultrastruct Pathol 1988;12:265–277.
23. Underwood JCE. Introduction to biopsy interpretation and surgical pathology. New York: Springer-Verlag, 1981:7.
24. Feinstein AR, Gelfman NA, Yesner R, et al. Observer variability in the histopathologic diagnosis of lung cancer. Am Rev Respir Dis 1970;101:671–684.
25. Sorensen JB, Hirsch FR, Gazdar A, Olsen JE. Interobserver variability in histopathologic subtyping and grading of pulmonary adenocarcinoma. Cancer 1993;71:2971–2976.
26. American Thoracic Society. Clinical staging of primary lung cancer. Am Rev Respir Dis 1983;127:1–6.
27. Council of the Association of Directors of Anatomic and Surgical Pathology. The incorporation of immunostaining data in anatomic pathology reports (editorial). Mod Pathol 1993;6:238.
28. Greenberg SD. Recent advances in pulmonary cytopathology. Hum Pathol 1983;14:901–912.
29. Compton J, Bogle E, Barch M, et al. Sputum cytology: a comparison of two methods, the conventional Saccomanno preparation and the Thin Prep processor. Acta Cytol 1993;37:55A.
30. Fraire AE, Underwood RD, McLarty JW, Greenberg SD. Conventional respiratory cytology versus fine needle aspiration cytology in the diagnosis of lung cancer. Acta Cytol 1991;35:385–388.
31. Saccomanno G. Diagnostic pulmonary cytology. 2nd ed. Chicago: American Society of Clinical Pathologists Press, 1986:102.
32. Böcking A, Biesterfeld S, Chatelain R, et al. Diagnosis of bronchial carcinoma on sections of paraffin-embedded sputum. Sensitivity and specificity of an alternative to routine cytology. Acta Cytol 1992;36:37–47.
33. Zusman-Harach SB, Harach HR, Gibbs AR. Cytologic features of non–small cell carcinoma of the lung in fine needle aspirates. J Clin Pathol 1991;44:997–1002.
34. van Hoeven KH, Zaman SS, Slott S, Gupta P. The distinction of bronchioalveolar carcinoma from hyperplastic pulmonary proliferations: cytologic clues for diagnosis. Acta Cytol 1993;37:131A.
35. Auger M, Katz RL, Johnston DA. The differentiating fine needle aspiration cytologic features of bronchioalveolar carcinomas from adenocarcinoma of lung: a statistical analysis (abstract 115A). Acta Cytol 1993;37:825.
36. Barbazza R, Toniolo L, Pinarello A, et al. Accuracy of bronchial aspiration cytology in typing operable (stage I-II) pulmonary carcinomas. Diagn Cytopathol 1992;8:3–7.
37. Katzenstein AA, Askin FB. Surgical pathology of non-neoplastic lung disease. 2nd ed. Philadelphia: Saunders, 1990.
38. Stanley MW, Henry-Stanley MJ, Gajl-Peczacska KJ, Bitterman PB. Hyperplasia of type II pneumocytes in acute lung injury. Cytologic findings of sequential bronchoalveolar lavage. Am J Clin Pathol 1992;97:669–677.
39. O'Reilly PE, Brueckner J, Silverman JF. Value of ancillary studies in fine needle aspiration cytology of the lung. Acta Cytol 1994;38:144–150.
40. Kline TS. Lung, handbook of fine needle aspiration cytology. 2nd ed. London: Churchill Livingstone, 1988:266–278.
41. Walts AE, Said JW, Shintaku P, Lloyd RV. Chromogranin as a marker of neuroendocrine cells in cytologic material: an immunocytochemical study. Am J Clin Pathol 1985;84:273–277.
42. Burns TR, Teasdale TA, Greenberg SD. Use of morphometry as an aid in the differential diagnosis of large cell carcinoma of the lung. Anal Quant Cytol Histol 1993;15:101–106.
43. Khiyami A, Fraire AE, Greenberg SD, et al. Recognition of lung cancer heterogeneity in cytopathologic specimens (abstract). Acta Cytol 1990;34:62A.
44. Barlogie B, Raber MN, Schumann J, et al. Flow cytometry in clinical cancer research. Cancer Res 1983;43:3982–3997.

45. Schneller J, Eppich E, Greenebaum E, et al. Flow cytometry and Feulgen cytophotometry in evaluation of effusions. Cancer 1987;59:1307–1313.
46. Chretien MF, Chassevent A, Malrani K, Rebel A. Flow cytometric DNA analysis in the diagnosis of lung tumors. Anal Quant Cytol Histol 1988;10:251–255.
47. Fuhr JE, Kattine AA, Sullivan TA, Nelson HS. Flow cytometric analysis of pulmonary fluids and cells for the detection of malignancies. Am J Pathol 1992;141:211–215.
48. El-Torky M, El-Zeky F, Hall C. Significant changes in the distribution of histologic types of lung cancer. Cancer 1990;65:2361–2367.
49. Gatter KC, Dunnill MS, Pulford KAF, et al. Human lung tumours. A correlation of antigenic profile with histological type. Histopathology 1985;9:805–823.
50. Sheppard MN, Morittu L, Moss F, et al. A study of epithelial, neuroendocrine and natural killer cell antibodies in adult lung and lung tumors. Lung Cancer 1988;4:70–72.
51. Sheppard MN. Immunohistochemistry and in situ hybridization in the diagnosis of lung cancer. Lung Cancer 1993;9:119–134.
52. Hirsch FR, Rygaard K. The role of the pathologist in the clinical management of lung cancer in the 90's. Lung Cancer 1993;9:111–118.
53. Battista P, Pizzicannella G, Vitullo P, et al. The epidermal growth factor in pulmonary carcinoids: immunohistochemical evidence of growth-promoting circuits. Mod Pathol 1993;6:162–166.
54. Le TN, Moser TG, Shroyer L, et al. Detection of human papillomavirus by polymerase chain reaction in squamous cell carcinomas of the lung of young versus old patients (abstract). Am J Clin Pathol 1994;101:375A.
55. Yousem SA, Ohori NP, Sonmez-Alpan E. Occurrence of human papillomavirus DNA in primary lung neoplasms. Cancer 1992;69:693–697.
56. Said JW, Nash G, Sassoon AF, et al. Involucrin in lung tumors. A specific marker for squamous differentiation. Lab Invest 1983;49:563–568.
57. Chiquet-Ehrismann R. What distinguishes tenascin from fibronectin? Federation of American Societies of Experimental Biology Journal 1990;4:2598–2604.
58. Erickson HP, Bourdon MA. Tenascin. An extracellular matrix protein prominent in specialized embryonic tissues and tumors. Annu Rev Cell Biol 1989;5:71–92.
59. Chuong C-M, Chen H-M. Enhanced expression of neural cell adhesion molecules and tenascin (Cytotactin) during wound healing. Am J Pathol 1991;138:427–440.
60. Soini Y, Paako P, Nuorva K, et al. Tenascin immunoreactivity in lung tumors. Am J Clin Pathol 1993;100:145–150.
61. Bourdon MA, Ruoslahti E. Tenascin mediates cell attachment through an RGD-dependent receptor. J Cell Biol 1989;108:1149–1155.
62. Jagirdar J, Sahu S, Ahuja S, et al. Heat shock protein 27 (HSP-27) in lung carcinomas. Clinical pathologic correlation. Mod Pathol 1994;7:151A.
63. Gail MH, Eagan RT, Feld R, et al. Prognostic factors in patients with resected stage I non–small cell lung cancer. A report from the lung study group. Cancer 1984;54:1802–1813.
64. Katlic M, Carter D. Prognostic implications of histology, size and location of primary tumors. In: Muggia FM, Rosencweig M, eds. Lung cancer: progress in therapeutic research. New York: Raven Press, 1979:143–150.
65. Greenberg SD, Fraire AE, Kinner BM, Johnson EH. Prognosis in carcinoma of the lung: tumor cell type versus staging. In: Rosen PP, Fechner RE, eds. The prognosis of carcinoma of the lung: pathology annual. Norwalk, CT: Appleton-Lange, 1987;2:387–405.
66. Mountain CF, Greenberg SD, Fraire AE. Tumor stage in non–small cell carcinoma of lung. Chest 1991;99:1258–1260.
67. Auerbach O, Garfinkel L. The changing pattern of lung carcinoma. Cancer 1991;68:1973–1977.
68. Falk RT, Pickle LW, Fontham ETH, et al. Epidemiology of bronchioloalveolar carcinoma. Cancer Epidemiology, Biomarkers and Prevention 1992;1:339–344.
69. Asamura H, Nakajima T, Mukai K, et al. DNA cytofluorometric and nuclear morphometric analyses of lung adenocarcinoma. Cancer 1989;64:1657–1664.
70. DaCosta N, Sivaraman A, Kinare SG. Carcinoma of lung with special reference to adenocarcinoma (an autopsy study of 122 cases). Ind J Cancer 1993;30:42–47.
71. Fraire AE, Awe R. Lung cancer in association with human immunodeficiency virus infection. Cancer 1992;70:432–436.
72. Crawley J, Klukowicz A, Safirstein BH, Khan A. HIV seropositivity as a poor prognostic indicator in primary carcinoma of lung. Chest 1993;104:45S.
73. Miller RR. Bronchioloalveolar cell adenomas. Am J Surg Pathol 1990;14:904–912.
74. Scroggs MW, Roggli VL, Fraire AE, Sanfilippo F. Eosinophilic intracytoplasmic globules in pulmonary adenocarcinomas: a histochemical, immunohistochemical and ultrastructural study of six cases. Hum Pathol 1989;20:845–849.
75. Nakanishi K, Kawai T, Susuki M. Large intracytoplasmic body in lung cancer compared with Clara cell granule. Am J Clin Pathol 1987;88:472–477.
76. Silver SA, Askin FB. True papillary carcinoma of the lung: A distinct clinico pathologic entity. Mod Pathol 1994;7:194A.
77. Higashiyama M, Doi O, Kodama K, et al. Extra-mammary Paget's disease of the bronchial epithelium. Arch Pathol Lab Med 1991;115:185–188.
78. Miller RR, Nelems B, Evans KG, et al. Glandular neoplasia of the lung. A proposed analogy to colonic tumors. Cancer 1988;61:1009–1014.
79. Nakanishi K. Alveolar epithelial hyperplasia and adenocarcinoma of the lung. Arch Pathol Lab Med 1990;114:363–368.
80. Rao SK, Fraire AE. Alveolar cell hyperplasia in association with surgically resected adenocarcinoma of lung. An immunohistochemical profile. Mod Pathol 1995;8:165–169.
81. Shimosato Y, Noguchi M, Matsuno Y. Adenocarcinoma of the lung: its development and malignant progression. Lung Cancer 1993;9:99–108.
82. Kawai T, Hiroi S, Nakanishi K, et al. P-53 gene mutations in alveolar epithelial hyperplasia (AEH) of the lung. Mod Pathol 1994;7:151A.
83. Travis WD, Linnoila RI, Horowitz M. et al. Pulmonary nodules resembling bronchioloalveolar carcinoma in adolescent cancer patients. Mod Pathol 1988;1:372–377.
84. Cagle PT, Wessels R, Greenberg SD. Concurrent mesothelioma and adenocarcinoma of the lung in a patient with asbestosis. Mod Pathol 1993;6:438–441.
85. Mollo F, Piolatto G, Bellis D, et al. Asbestos exposure and histologic cell types of lung cancer in surgical and autopsy reviews. Int J Cancer 1990;46:576–580.
86. Barsky SH, Cameron R, Osann KE, et al. Rising incidence of bronchoalveolar lung carcinoma and its unique clinico-pathologic features. Cancer 1994;73:1163–1170.

87. Mackay B, Lukeman JM, Ordóñez NG. Tumors of the lung. In: Bennington JL, ed. Major problems in pathology. Philadelphia: Saunders, 1991;24:115.
88. Manning JT, Spjut HJ, Tschen JA. Bronchioloalveolar adenocarcinoma. The significance of two histopathologic types. Cancer 1984;54:525–534.
89. Smith MS, Greenberg SD, Spjut HJ. The Clara cell: a comparative ultrastructural study in mammals. Am J Anat 1979;155:15–30.
90. Gazdar AF, Linnoila RI. The pathology of lung cancer: changing concepts and newer diagnostic techniques. Semin Oncol 1988;15:215–225.
91. Greenberg SD, Smith MN, Spjut HJ. Bronchiolo-alveolar carcinoma—cell of origin. Am J Clin Pathol 1975;63:153–167.
92. Brooks RE. Pulmonary adenoma of strain A mice: an electron microscopic study. J Natl Cancer Inst 1968;411:719–742.
93. Nisbet DJ, Mackay JMK, Smith W, et al. Ultrastructure of sheep pulmonary adenomatosis (Jaagsiekte). J Pathol 1971;103:157–162.
94. Benharroch D, Sukenik S, Sacks M. Bronchioloalveolar carcinoma and generalized amyloidosis complicating progressive systemic sclerosis. Hum Pathol 1992;23:839–841.
95. Dekmezian R, Ordonez NG, Mackay B. Bronchioloalveolar adenocarcinoma with myoepithelial cells. Cancer 1991;67:2356–2360.
96. Cagle PT, Cohle SD, Greenberg SD. Natural history of pulmonary scar cancers. Clinical and pathologic implications. Cancer 1985;56:2031–2035.
97. Yoneda K. Scar carcinomas of the lung in a histoplasmosis area. Cancer 1990;65:164–168.
98. Jackson D, Greenberg SD, Howell JF. Pulmonary scar carcinoma: a case with two primaries. Cancer 1984;54:361–366.
99. Marchevsky AM. Malignant epithelial tumors of the lung. In: Marchevsky AM, ed. Surgical pathology of lung neoplasms. New York, Basel: Marcel Dekker, 1990;44:105.
100. Upton MP, Horohashi S, Tome Y, et al. Expression of vimentin in surgically resected adenocarcinomas and large cell carcinomas of lung. Am J Surg Pathol 1986;10:560–567.
101. Cherwitz D, Swanson P, Drier J, Wick M. S-100 protein reactivity in poorly differentiated carcinomas: an immunohistochemical comparison with malignant melanoma. Lab Invest 1987;56:13A.
102. Said JW. Immunohistochemistry of lung tumors. In: Marchevsky AM, ed. Surgical pathology of lung neoplasms. New York, Basel: Marcel Dekker, 1990;44:635–651.
103. Elias JM. Immunohistopathology. A practical approach to diagnosis. Chicago: American Society of Clinical Pathologists Press, 1990.
104. Cote RJ, Thomson TM, Cordon-Cardo C. Intermediate filaments. In: Russo J, ed. Immunocytochemistry in tumor diagnosis. Boston: Martinus Nijhoff Publishers, 1985;72.
105. Ishikura H, Kanda M, Ito M, et al. Hepatoid adenocarcinoma: a distinctive histological subtype of alpha fetoprotein producing lung carcinoma. Virchows-A Pathol Anat Histopathol 1990;417:73–80.
106. Brown RW, Clark GM, Allred DC. A panel approach of distinguishing malignant epithelial mesotheliomas from adenocarcinomas of the lung by immunohistochemistry. Mod Pathol 1991;4:113A.
107. Noguchi M, Nakajima T, Hirohashi S, et al. Immunohistochemical distinction of malignant mesothelioma from pulmonary adenocarcinoma with anti-surfactant apoprotein, anti-Lewis[a] and anti-Tn[53] antibodies. Hum Pathol 1989;20:53–57.
108. Broers JL, Jensen SM, Travis WD, et al. Expression of surfactant associated protein-A and Clara cell 10 kilodalton mRNA in neoplastic and non-neoplastic human lung tissue as detected by in situ hybridization. Lab Invest 1992;66:337–346.
109. Linnoila RI, Jensen SM, Steinberg SM, et al. Peripheral airway cell marker expression in non–small cell lung carcinoma. Association with distinct clinicopathologic features. Am J Clin Pathol 1992;97:233–243.
110. Nonomura A, Mizukami Y, Shimizu J, et al. Simultaneous detection of intercellular adhesion molecule-1 (CD54) and carcinoembryonic antigen in lung adenocarcinoma. Mod Pathol 1994;7:155–159.
111. Furukawa T, Watanabe S, Sato Y, et al. Heterogeneity of histiocytes in primary lung cancer stained with anti S-100 protein, lysozyme and OKT6 antibodies. Jpn J Clin Oncol 1984;14:647–657.
112. Fox SB, Jones M, Dunnill MS, et al. Langerhans cells in human lung tumours: an immunohistological study. Histopathology 1989;14:269–275.
113. Mori M, Chiba R, Takahashi T. Atypical adenomatous hyperplasia of the lung and its differentiation from adenocarcinoma. Characterization of atypical cells by morphometry and multivariate cluster analysis. Cancer 1993;72:2331–2340.
114. Mackay B. Large cell carcinomas. In: Saldaña MJ, ed. Pathology of pulmonary disease. Philadelphia: JB Lippincott, 1994:571.
115. Wick MR, Berg LC, Hertz M. Large cell carcinoma of the lung with neuroendocrine differentiation. A comparison with large cell "undifferentiated" pulmonary tumors. Am J Clin Pathol 1992;97:796–805.
116. Carter D, Eggleston JC. Tumors of the lower respiratory tract. Atlas of tumor pathology, second series. Fascicle, 17. Washington, DC: Armed Forces Institute of Pathology, 1980.
117. Nash G, Stout AP. Giant cell carcinoma of the lung: report of 5 cases. Cancer 1958;11:369–376.
118. Ginsberg SS, Buzaid AC, Stern H, Carter D. Giant cell carcinoma of the lung. Cancer 1992;70:606–610.
119. Yanuck MD, Greenberg SD, Fraire AE. Large cell carcinoma of lung: assessment of clinical stage and histopathologic variables as prognostic factors. Houston Med 1991;7:42–46.
120. Sawyers CL, Golde DW, Quan S, Nimer SD. Production of granulocyte-macrophage colony stimulating factor in two patients with lung cancer, leukocytosis and eosinophilia. Cancer 1992;69:1342–1346.
121. Gould VE, Tomanova R, Monson R, et al. Immunophenotypic subsets of large cell pulmonary carcinomas. Mod Pathol 1994;7:150A.
122. Capelozzi-Delmonte V, Alberti O, HN Saldiva P. Large cell carcinoma of the lung: ultrastructural and immunohistochemical features. Chest 1986;90:524–527.
123. Einhorn LH. Introduction: small cell lung cancer. In: Gralla RJ, Einhorn LH, eds. Treatment and prevention of small cell lung cancer and non–small lung cancer. London: The Royal Society of Medicine Services, 1989:1–2.
124. Morabia A, Wynder EL. Cigarette smoking and lung cancer cell types. Cancer 1991;68:2074–2078.
125. Brereton HD, Matthews MM, Costa J, et al. Mixed anaplastic small-cell and squamous-cell carcinoma of the lung. Ann Intern Med 1978;88:805–806.
126. Radice PA, Matthews MJ, Ihde DC, et al. The clinical behavior of "mixed" small cell/large cell bronchogenic carcinoma compared to "pure" small cell subtypes. Cancer 1982;50:2894–2902.

127. Bepler G, Neumann K, Holle R. et al. Clinical relevance of histopathologic subtyping in small cell lung cancer. Cancer 1989;64:74–79.
128. Yesner R. Classification of lung cancer histology. N Engl J Med 1985;312:652–653.
129. Azzopardi JG. Oat-cell carcinoma of the bronchus. J Pathol Bacteriol 1959;78:513–519.
130. Twijnstra A, Thunnissen FB, Lassouw G, et al. The role of the histologic sub-classification of tumor cells in patients with small-cell carcinoma of the lung and central nervous system metastases. Cancer 1990;65:1812–1815.
131. Shimosato Y, Nakatima T, Hirohashi S, et al. Biological, pathologic and clinical features of small cell lung cancer. Cancer Lett 1986;33:241–258.
132. Abe K, Kameya T, Yamaguchi K, et al. Hormone-producing lung cancers. In: Becker KL, Gazda F, eds. Endocrine lung in health and disease. Philadelphia: Saunders, 1984:549–595.
133. Abeloff MD, Eggleston JC, Mendelsohn G, et al. Changes in morphologic and biochemical characteristics of small cell carcinoma of the lung. Am J Med 1979;66:757–764.
134. Osterlind K, Ihde DC, Ettinger DS, et al. Staging and prognostic factors in small cell carcinoma of the lung. Cancer Treat Rep 1983;67:3–9.
135. Hansen HH, Dombernowsky P, Hirsch FR. Staging procedures and prognostic features in small cell anaplastic bronchogenic carcinoma. Semin Oncol 1978;5:280–287.
136. Aisner J. Treatment of limited-disease small cell lung cancer. Semin Oncol 1992;19:51–58.
137. Aisner SC, Finkelstein DM, Ettinger DS, et al. The clinical significance of variant cell morphology small-cell carcinoma of the lung. J Clin Oncol 1990;8:402–408.
138. Takamori S, Noguchi M, Morinaga S, et al. Clinical pathologic characteristics of adenosquamous carcinoma of the lung. Cancer 1991;67:649–654.
139. Sridhar KS, Bounassi MJ, Raub W, Richman SP. Clinical features of adenosquamous lung carcinoma in 127 patients. Am Rev Respir Dis 1990;142:19–23.
139a. Ishida T, Kaneko S, Yokohama H, et al. Adenosquamous carcinomas of the lung. Clinical pathologic and immunohistochemical features. Am J Clin Pathol 1992;97:678–685.
140. Yousem SA. Pulmonary carcinoid tumors and well differentiated neuroendocrine carcinomas. Is there room for atypical carcinoid (editorial)? Am J Clin Pathol 1991;95:763–764.
141. Whitwell F. Tumorlets of the lung. J Pathol Bacteriol 1955;70:529–541.
142. Hamperl H. Uber Gutartige Bronchialtumoren (Cylindrome und Carcinoide). Virchows Arch (A) 1937;300:46–88.
143. Davila DG, Dunn WG, Tazelar HD, Pairolero PC. Bronchial carcinoid tumors. Mayo Clin Proc 1993;68:795–803.
144. Sdyer DC, Sdyer WR, Eggleston JF. Bronchial carcinoids. Cancer 1975;36:1522–1537.
145. Bensch KG, Corrin B, Pariente R, Spencer H. Oat cell carcinoma of the lung: its origin and relationship to bronchial carcinoid. Cancer 1968;22:1163–1172.
146. Pearse AGE. The diffuse neuroendocrine system and the APUD concept: related "endocrine" peptides in brain, intestine, pituitary, placenta, and aneurin cutaneous glands. Med Biol 1977;55:115–125.
147. Gould VE, Linnoila VE, Faber LP, et al. Neuroendocrine neoplasms of the bronchopulmonary tract: a classification of the spectrum of carcinoid to small cell carcinoma and intervening variants. Lab Invest 1983;49:519–537.

148. Bonikos DS, Bensch KG, Jamplis RW. Peripheral pulmonary carcinoid tumors. Cancer 1976;37:1469–1477.
149. Felton WL, Liebow AA, Lindskog G. Peripheral and multiple bronchial adenomas. Cancer 1953;6:555–567.
150. Ranchod M, Levine GD. Spindle cell carcinoid tumors of the lung. A clinico pathologic study of 35 cases. Am J Surg Pathol 1980;4:315–331.
151. El-Naggar AK, Ballance W, Abdul-Karim FW, et al. Typical and atypical bronchopulmonary carcinoids. Am J Clin Pathol 1991;95:828–834.
152. Arrigoni MG, Woolner LB, Bernatz PE. Typical carcinoid tumors of the lung. J Thorac Cardiovasc Surg 1972;64:413–421.
153. Mills SE, Cooper PH, Walver AN, Kron IL. Atypical carcinoid tumors of the lung. Am J Surg Pathol 1982;6:643–654.
154. Paladugu RR, Benfield JR, Pak HY, et al. Bronchopulmonary Kulchitsky cell carcinomas: a new classification scheme for typical and atypical carcinoids. Cancer 1985;55:1303–1311.
155. MacDowell EM, Wilson TS, Trump BF. Atypical endocrine tumors of the lung. Arch Pathol Lab Med 1981;105:20–28.
156. Hammond ME, Sause WT. Large cell neuroendocrine tumors of the lung. Cancer 1985;56:1624–1629.
157. Piehl MR, Gould VE, Warren WH, et al. Immunohistochemical identification of exocrine and neuroendocrine subsets of large cell lung carcinomas. Pathol Res Pract 1988;183:675–682.
158. Warren WH, Faber LP, Gould VE. Neuroendocrine neoplasms of the lung: a clinicopathologic update. J Thorac Cardiovasc Surg 1989;98:321–332.
159. Travis WD, Linnoila I, Tsokos MG, et al. Neuroendocrine tumors of the lung with proposed criteria for large-cell neuroendocrine carcinoma: an ultrastructural, immunohistochemical, and flow cytometric study of 35 cases. Am J Surg Pathol 1991;15:529–543.
160. Brambilla E, Moro D, Veale D, et al. Basal cell (basaloid) carcinoma of the lung; a new morphologic and phenotypic entity with separate prognostic significance. Hum Pathol 1992;23:993–1003.
161. Saldana MJ, Mones JM. Squamous cell carcinoma. In: Saldana MJ, ed. Pathology of pulmonary disease. Philadelphia: Lippincott, 1994:545–554.
162. Humphrey PA, Scroggs MW, Roggli VL, Shelbourne JD. Pulmonary carcinomas with a sarcomatoid element. An immunocytochemical and ultrastructural analysis. Hum Pathol 1988;19:155–165.
163. Battifora H. Spindle cell carcinoma: ultrastructural evidence of squamous origin and collagen production by the tumor cells. Cancer 1976;37:2275–2282.
164. Addis BJ, Corrin B. Pulmonary blastoma, carcinosarcoma and spindle cell carcinoma. An immunohistochemical study of keratin intermediate filaments. J Pathol 1985;147:291–301.
165. Chen JL, Lee JS, Sahin AA, et al. Sarcomatoid carcinoma of the lung. Immunohistochemical and ultrastructural studies of 14 cases. Cancer 1992;69:376–386.
166. Matsui K, Kitagawa M, Miwa A. Lung carcinoma with spindle cell components: sixteen cases examined by immunohistochemistry. Hum Pathol 1992;23:1289–1297.
167. Battifora H. Assessment of antigen damage in immunohistochemistry. The Vimentin Internal Control. Am J Clin Pathol 1991;96:669–671.
168. Franke WW, Schiller DL, Moll R. et al. Diversity of cytokeratins: differentiation-specific expression of cytokeratin polypeptides in epithelial cells and tissues. J Mol Biol 1981;153:933–959.

169. Cooper D, Schermer A, Sun TT. Classification of human epithelia and their neoplasms using monoclonal antibodies to keratins. Strategies, applications and limitations. Lab Invest 1986;52:243–256.
170. Frierson HF, Bellafiore FJ, Gaffey MJ, et al. Cytokeratin in anaplastic large cell lymphoma. Mod Pathol 1994;7:317–321.
171. Sedmak DD, Meineke TA, Knetchtges L. Detection of metastatic breast carcinoma with monoclonal antibodies to cytokeratins. Arch Pathol Lab Med 1989;113:786–789.
172. Norton AJ, Thomas JA, Isaacson PG. Cytokeratin-specific monoclonal antibodies are reactive with tumors of smooth muscle derivation: an immunocytochemical and biologic study using antibodies to intermediate filament cytoskeletal proteins. Histopathology 1987;11:487–499.
173. Heyderman E, Steele K, Ormerod MG. A new antigen on the epithelial membrane in immunoperoxidase localization in normal and neoplastic tissue. J Clin Pathol 1979;32:35–39.
174. Rabkin M, Kjeldsberg C. Epithelial membrane antigen staining of lesions derived from dendritic cells and other histiocytes (abstract). Lab Invest 1987;56:62A.
175. Pinkus GS, Kurtin PJ. Epithelial membrane antigen: a diagnostic discriminant in diagnostic pathology. Immunohistochemical profile in epithelial, mesenchymal and hematopoietic neoplasms using paraffin sections and monoclonal antibodies. Hum Pathol 1985;16:929–942.
176. Drier JK, Swanson PE, Cherwitz DL, Wick MR. S-100 protein immunoreactivity in poorly differentiated carcinomas: Immunohistochemical comparison with malignant melanoma. Arch Pathol Lab Med 1987;111:447–452.
177. Alvarez-Fernandez E, Carretero-Albinana L. Lectin histochemistry of normal bronchopulmonary tissues and common forms of bronchogenic carcinoma. Arch Pathol Lab Med 1990;114:475–481.
178. Sugiyama K, Kawai T, Nakanishi K, Susuki M. Histochemical reactivities of lectins and surfactant apoprotein in pulmonary adenocarcinomas and their metastasis. Mod Pathol 1992;5:273–276.
179. Wiedenmann B, Huttner WB. Synaptophysin and chromogranins/secretogranins—widespread constituents of distinct types of neuroendocrine vesicles and new tools in tumor diagnosis. Virchows Arch B Cell Pathol 1989;58:95–121.
180. Fisher Colbrie R, Hagn C, Schober M. Chromogranins A, B and C: widespread constituents of secretory vesicles. Ann N Y Acad Sci 1987;493:120–134.
181. Helle KB. Some chemical and physical properties of the soluble protein fraction of bovine adrenal chromaffin granules. Mol Pharmacol 1966;2:298–310.
182. Lloyd RV, Wilson BS. Specific endocrine tissue marker defined by monoclonal antibody. Science 1983;222:628–630.
183. Hedley DW, Friedlander ML, Taylor LW, et al. Method for analysis of cellular DNA content of paraffin-embedded pathological material using flow cytometry. J Histochem Cytochem 1983;31:1333–1335.
184. Volm M, Hahn EW, Mattern J, et al. Five year follow up study of independent clinical and flow cytometric prognostic factors for the survival of patients with non–small cell carcinoma. Cancer Res 1988;48:2923–2928.
185. Zimmerman PV, Hawson GAT, Bint MH, Parsons PG. Ploidy as a prognostic determinant in surgically treated lung cancer. Lancet 1987;2:530–533.
186. Miyamoto H, Harada M, Isobe A, et al. Prognostic value of nuclear DNA content and expression of the ras oncogene product in lung cancer. Cancer Res 1991;51:6346–6350.
186a. Schmidt RA, Rusch SW, Piantadosi S. A flow cytometric study of non–small cell lung cancer classified as T1N0. Cancer 1992;69:78–85.
187. Sara A, El-Naggar AK. Intratumoral DNA content variability. A study of non–small cell lung cancer. Am J Clin Pathol 1991;96:311–317.
188. Gazdar AF. Molecular markers for the diagnosis and prognosis of lung cancer. Cancer 1992;69:1592–1599.
189. Viallet J, Minna JD. Dominant oncogenes and tumor suppressor genes in the pathogenesis of lung cancer. Am J Respir Cell Mol Biol 1990;2:225–232.
190. Funa K, Steinholz L, Nou E, Bergh J. Increased expression of N-myc in human small cell lung cancer biopsies predicts lack of response to chemotherapy and poor prognosis. Am J Clin Pathol 1987;88:216–220.
191. Johnson BE, Ihde DC, Makuch RW, et al. myc Family oncogene amplification in tumor cell lines established from small lung cancer patients and its relationship to clinical status and course. J Clin Invest 1987;79:1629–1634.
192. Noguchi M, Hirohashi S, Hara F, et al. Heterogeneous amplification of myc family oncogenes in small cell lung carcinomas. Cancer 1990;66:2053–2058.
193. Seager RC, Brodeur GM, Sather H, et al. Association of multiple copies of the N-myc oncogene with rapid progression of neuroblastomas. N Engl J Med 1985;313:1111–1116.
194. Tomlinson FH, Jenkins RB, Scheithauer BW, et al. Aggressive medulloblastoma with high-level N-myc amplification. Mayo Clin Proc 1994;69:359–365.
195. Castaneda VL, Cheah MSC, Saldivar VA, et al. Cytogenetic and molecular evaluation of clinically aggressive esthesioneuroblastoma. Am J Pediatr Hematol Oncol 1991;13:62–70.
196. Lee W-H, Murphree AL, Benedict WF. Expression and amplification of the N-myc gene in primary retinoblastoma. Nature 1984;309:458–460.
197. Kashii T, Mizushima Y, Nakagawa K, et al. Amplification of the N-myc oncogene in an adenocarcinoma cell line of the lung. Anticancer Res 1992;12:621–624.
198. Saksela K, Bergh J, Nilsson K. Amplification of the N-myc oncogene in an adenocarcinoma of the lung. J Cell Biochem 1986;31:292–304.
199. Barbacid M. ras Genes. Annu Rev Biochem 1987;56:779–827.
200. Greenberg AH, Egan SE, Wright JA. Oncogenes and metastatic progression. Invasion Metastasis 1989;9:360–378.
201. Davila DG, Williams DE. The etiology of lung cancer. Mayo Clin Proc 1993;68:170–182.
202. Slebos RJC, Kibbelaar RE, Dalesio O, et al. K-ras oncogene activation as a prognostic marker in adenocarcinoma of the lung. N Engl J Med 1990;323:561–565.
203. Lane DP, Crawford LV. T-antigen is bound to a host protein in SV-40 transformed cells. Nature 1979;278:261–263.
204. Ulrich SJ, Anderson CW, Mercer WE, et al. The p53 tumor suppressor protein, a modulator of cell proliferation. J Biol Chem 1992;267:15259–15262.
205. Jensen RA, Page DL. p53: The promising story continues to unfold (editorial). Hum Pathol 1993;24:455–456.
206. Vogelstein B, Kinzler KW. p53 Function and dysfunction. Cell 1992;70:523–526.
207. Baker SJ, Fearon ER, Nigro JM, et al. Chromosome 17p deletions and p53 gene mutations in colorectal carcinomas. Science 1989;244:217–221.
208. Bennett WP, Borkowsky A, Colby TV, et al. p53 Mutation and immunopositivity in the pathogenesis of human bronchogenic carcinoma. Mod Pathol 1993;6:129A.

209. Korsmeyer SJ. bcl-2 Initiates a new category of oncogene regulators of cell death. Blood 1992;80:879–886.
210. Pezzella F, Turley H, Kuzu I, et al. bcl-2 Protein in non–small cell lung carcinoma. N Engl J Med 1993;369:690–694.
210a. Rao SK, Woda BA, Savas L, Fraire AE. Immunohistochemical detection of bcl-2 protein in adenocarcinoma of lung. Presented at the XX International Congress of the International Academy of Pathology, Hong Kong, October 1994.
211. Gallagher B, Urbanski SJ. The significance of pleural elastic invasion by lung carcinoma. Hum Pathol 1990;21:512–517.
212. Elson CE, Roggli VL, Vollmer RT, et al. Prognostic indicators for survival in stage I carcinoma of lung. A histologic study of 47 cases. Mod Pathol 1988;1:288–291.
213. Carter D, Elkins RC, Pipkin RD, et al. Relationship of necrosis and tumor border to lymph node metastases and 10 year survival in carcinoma of breast. Am J Surg Pathol 1978;2:39–46.
214. Shahab I, Fraire AE, Greenberg SD, et al. Morphometric quantitation of tumor necrosis in stage I non–small cell carcinoma of lung: prognostic implications. Mod Pathol 1992;5:521–524.
215. Haque AK, Adegboyega P, Sanchez RL. Vascular invasion in carcinoma of lung. Mod Pathol 1993;6:131A.
216. Ishida T, Kaneko S, Tateishi M, et al. Large cell carcinoma of the lung. Prognostic implications of histopathologic and immunohistochemical subtyping. Am J Clin Pathol 1990;93:176–182.
217. Brown RW, Fraire AE, Roggli V, Cagle PT. Assessment of proliferative fraction by PCNA in stage I non–small cell lung cancer. Mod Pathol 1993;6:129A.
218. Busch H, Smetana K. Nucleoli of tumor cells. In: Busch H, Smetana K, eds. The nucleus. New York: Academic Press, 1970:448–471.
219. Smith R, Croker J. Evaluation of nucleolar organizer region–associated proteins in breast malignancy. Histopathology 1988; 13:95–99.
220. Abe S, Ogura S, Kunikane H, et al. Nucleolar organizer regions in precancerous and cancerous lesions of the bronchus. Cancer 1991;67:472–475.
221. Ogura S, Abe S, Sukoh N, et al. Correlation between nucleolar organizer regions visualized by silver staining and the growth rate in lung adenocarcinoma. Cancer 1992;70:63–68.
222. Ten Velde GP, Havenith MG, Volovics A, Bosman FT. Prognostic significance of basement membrane deposition in operable squamous cell carcinomas of the lung. Cancer 1991;67:3001–3005.
223. Coman DR. Decreased mutual adhesiveness, a property of cells from squamous cell carcinoma. Cancer Res 1944;4:625–629.
224. McDonagh D, Vollmer RJ, Shelbourne JD. Intercellular junctions and tumor behavior in lung cancer. Mod Pathol 1991;4:436–440.

11

Molecular Biology in the Diagnosis, Prognosis, and Therapy of Lung Cancer

David P. Carbone

MOLECULAR ORIGINS OF GENETIC LESIONS CONTRIBUTING TO LUNG CANCER

Lung cancer is unique among the common cancers in that an estimated 85% of cases are caused by a single (although complex) environmental factor, i.e., tobacco smoke (1, 2). The lungs are exposed to the environment with every breath, and they are a very efficient route for the access of addictive and/or carcinogenic compounds directly into the bloodstream. One such compound, nicotine, is both addictive and susceptible to conversion into potent nitrosamine carcinogens. Two of the best studied nitrosamines, nicotine-derived nitrosamine ketone (NNK) and N'-nitrosonornicotine (NNN), are both potent and specific lung carcinogens. Minute doses of NNK administered subcutaneously, orally, or topically produce tumors, predominantly lung, in laboratory animals (3). Another class of carcinogens in tobacco smoke is the polycyclic hydrocarbons, such as benzo(a)pyrene. Other inhaled pollutants such as radon or asbestos, as well as inherited genetic factors, can compound the risk associated with smoking.

GENETIC DAMAGE TO ONCOGENES LEADS TO LUNG CANCER

What molecular events lie between chronic exposure to tobacco smoke and lung cancer? Covalent carcinogen adducts form with many molecules within the cell, including proteins, lipids, and DNA. Because dysregulated growth is passed from a cancer cell to its daughters in the absence of further carcinogen exposure, the essential target in cancer development is thought to be the genetic material itself, and many of the known carcinogens in cigarette smoke can act to damage directly DNA. It currently is thought that multiple genetic lesions, perhaps 10 to 20 or more, are required to cause a normal cell to lose all of the normal growth regulatory pathways and become a cancer.

This DNA damage can result in the activation of a growth stimulatory gene (a dominant oncogene) or the inactivation of a growth suppressing gene (a tumor suppressor gene). In the simplest case, activation of a dominant oncogene involves a single nucleotide substitution, resulting in the alteration of an amino acid in the gene product. This activation would have to occur only in one of the two copies of the gene, a fact that has allowed the isolation of dominant oncogenes in human cells by transfection studies in which tumor DNA is introduced into nontumorigenic cells. DNA fragments with the capability of transforming these cells into tumorigenic ones are then identified by molecular techniques. Sequence analysis of these genes in a variety of tumors has revealed activating point mutations or regulatory alterations.

Recessive oncogenes are characterized by somatic abnormalities that result in loss of function. A prototypical tumor suppressor gene could be inactivated by point mutation, but both copies would have to be damaged to result in complete loss of function. One way for a cell to uncover a defective tumor suppressor gene would thus be by deletion of the normal allele. This deletion can be large and span hundreds of other genes, and the detection of such hemizygous loss is an important indication that a tumor suppressor gene may lie somewhere within the limits of the deletion.

Their recessive nature allows their silent transmission to progeny, and inherited lesions in tumor suppressor genes have been described. Inherited abnormalities in dominant oncogenes have thus far been found only in transgenic laboratory model systems. Knudson et al. (4) first postulated that, although these genes act in a recessive manner at the cellular level, the mode of inheritance of tumor suppressor genes appears to be dominant when cancer predisposition is analyzed in cancer pedigrees. This dominance results from the fact that two inactivating events in a single cell at the genetic level are required for tumor development. In sporadic cancer, both inactivating lesions are acquired somatically in the same cell, a rare occurrence, resulting in only a fraction of the individuals in a population getting cancer. In hereditary cancer caused by germline transmission of a mutant tumor suppressor gene, however, one lesion is transmitted in the germline and the second inactivating event occurs during the lifetime of the individual as a somatic mutation. A normal rate of random somatic events would cause nearly every individual inheriting one defective copy of the gene to develop cancer. Familial retinoblastoma, Wilms' tumor, renal cancer associated with the von Hippel-Lindau syndrome, and colon cancer with familial adenomatous polyposis syndrome are examples of tumors arising because of the inactivation of tumor suppressor genes.

METHODS OF GENETIC ANALYSIS

Early evidence of genetic abnormalities in lung cancer came from studies of chromosomal abnormalities in cancer cells. As opposed to leukemias and lymphomas, solid tumors often have unstable numbers of chromosomes and a plethora of chromosomal abnormalities, including interstitial and terminal deletions, duplications, balanced and unbalanced translocations, ring chromosomes, and centromereless chromosome fragments called "double minutes." Although these chromosomal abnormalities appeared initially to show no consistent pattern, suggesting the involvement of specific chromosome regions, certain common regions of loss in lung cancers ultimately were identified. The first was a very common loss of chromosomal material on chromosome 3p (5–7). Cytogenetics has implicated several other chromosomal regions in lung cancer as well, including 1p, 3q, 5q, 9p, 11p, 13q, and 17p (7, 8); identification of these regions has led to the discovery of several new tumor suppressor genes. Because the chromosome rearrangements often are complex, small fragments of chromosomes involved in translocations can be difficult to identify by unaided light microscopy. A new technique called fluorescence in situ hybridization (FISH) and the related technique, comparative genomic hybridization, allow not only identification of translocated chromosomal fragments but also rapid screening of the entire tumor genome for both regional losses and gains of material. In this technique tumor and normal DNA are fluorescently labeled in different colors and simultaneously hybridized onto normal chromosomes. If the tumor DNA has lost or gained genetic material in a given chromosomal region, that region has an imbalance of the two different colors. This technique has been applied successfully to small cell lung cancer (SCLC) and has indicated loss of 3p, 5q, 10q, 13q, and 17p, and amplification of sequences on 3q, 5p, 8q, and 17q (9). These findings agree with the cytogenetic data.

DNA damage visible at a light microscopic level involves at least tens of millions of bases of DNA. Locating responsible genes within the region of a 30-megabase deletion requires molecular techniques. As mentioned above, a hallmark of a tumor suppressor gene involved in a tumor is the loss of a defined region of a chromosome containing the gene. Detecting such loss depends on the ability to distinguish between the two copies of a given region of DNA in tumor cells. There are a variety of subtle ways in which individuals are different at the genetic level (approximately one difference every few hundred bases of DNA in unrelated individuals); because everyone inherits one copy of every somatic chromosome from each parent, there are many such polymorphisms throughout the genome. Most of these involve noncoding regions of the DNA and are without discernible phenotype. Such polymorphisms can, however, allow one to distinguish the two otherwise identical copies of a region of DNA, thus allowing the detection of the loss of one of the two alleles in the tumor tissue compared to normal cells. Polymorphic differences can result in the loss or acquisition of a restriction enzyme site, and this effect is the basis of restriction fragment length polymorphism (RFLP) analysis. Sequences repeated in tandem often vary in the number of repeats between individuals, and this effect can be detected as differences in the size of polymerase chain reaction (PCR) fragments. Techniques, such as genomic mismatch scanning, are being developed that are capable of detecting any single base difference in thousands of bases. Multiple polymorphic probes corresponding to many different regions of the genome may be used to screen for regions of frequent DNA loss in a particular tumor. This technique is referred to as allelotyping.

Once candidate genes or regions are identified, analysis of the molecular details of the lesions occurring in tumors becomes possible. Such detailed analysis can be performed by direct DNA sequencing, or it may consist of such screening techniques as mutant selective oligohybridization, RNase protection, chemical mismatch cleavage, single-strand conformation polymorphism analysis, or denaturing gradient gel electrophoresis. These techniques can detect the presence of even a single base alteration in several hundred base pairs of DNA, and thus can be used as screening tools to survey large numbers of tumors.

DOMINANT ONCOGENE LESIONS IN LUNG CANCER

Genes capable of converting normal cells to cancer cells were first identified in oncogenic retroviruses. The oncogenes carried by the oncogenic retroviruses (prefixed by v-) have been found to have normal cellular homologues called protooncogenes (prefixed by c-) that often are found to be key cellular regulatory proteins. Perhaps the best studied example is the retroviral gene from the Harvey and Kirsten rat sarcoma viruses, whose genes v-H-*ras* and v-K-*ras* have the cellular homologues c-H-*ras*, c-K-*ras*, and N-*ras*. Other examples of oncogenes include *myc*, *raf*, *myb*, *fos*, and *jun*.

THE *RAS* FAMILY

These genes code for 21 kDa proteins attached to the inner surface of the cytoplasmic membrane via a posttranslationally added farnesyl group, which is essential for its function. They are homologous to G proteins and are thought to mediate signal transduction by a similar mechanism. G proteins exist in two states, guanosine diphosphate (GDP)–bound and guanosine triphosphate (GTP)–bound. Only the (GTP)-bound form is effective at transmitting a growth response, and there is a dynamic interconversion between the two forms. Growth stimuli (mitogens or growth factors) cause the substitution of GTP for GDP, activating *ras*, whereas the intrinsic GTPase activity (along with GTPase activating protein [GAP]) catalyzes the conversion of *ras* back to the inactive GDP-bound form. *ras* Mutations are frequent in human tumors (10, 11), and usually occur by missense substitutions at codons 12, 13, or 61, all of which directly affect the GTP catalytic site and consequently block GTPase activity. These GTPase-deficient *ras* mutants thus are locked into the growth stimulatory GTP-bound form (Fig. 11.1).

In a series of 77 non–small cell lung cancer (NSCLC) and 42 SCLC cell lines, Mitsudomi et al. (12) found *ras* mutations exclusively in NSCLC, and predominantly in K-*ras* codon 12 (Table 11.1). Introduction of a mutant *ras* into an SCLC cell line caused it to acquire characteristics more like NSCLC (13, 14). The lack of *ras* mutations in SCLC suggests a molecular specificity to this genetic abnormality and may reflect different pathogenetic mechanisms.

In studies of resected lung cancer specimens, mutations are found nearly exclusively in adenocarcinomas (Table 11.1) (16). The increased incidence of mutations

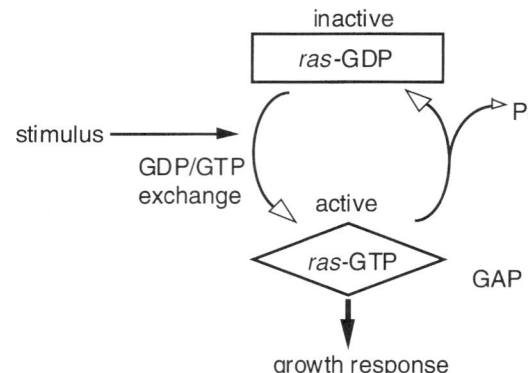

FIGURE 11.1. A model for *ras* function as an intermediate in the growth response.

TABLE 11.1. Incidence and Location of *ras* Mutations in Lung Cancer Cell Lines

CANCER TYPE	K-RAS 12	K-RAS 13	K-RAS 61	H-RAS 61	N-RAS 61	TOTAL (%)
NSCLC	42	6	4	2	2	55/233 (24)
Adenocarcinoma						
Cell lines	6	4	0	0	1	11/44 (25)
Tumors	28	1	1	1	0	30/88 (34)
Other						
Cell lines	8	1	3	1	1	14/33 (42)
Tumors	0	0	0	0	0	0/68 (0)
Small cell cancer						
Cell lines	0	0	0	0	0	0/42 (0)
Tumors	0	0	0	0	0	0/2 (0)

Data from Mitsudomi T, Viallet J, Mulshine JL, Linnoila RI, Minna JD, Gazdar, AF. Mutations of *ras* genes distinguish a subset of non–small-cell lung cancer cell lines from small-cell lung cancer cell lines. Oncogene 1991;6:1353–1362; Cabone DP, Mitsudomi T, Chiba I, et al. p53 Immunostaining positivity is associated with reduced survival and is imperfectly correlated with gene mutations in resected non–small cell lung cancer. Chest 1994: in press; and Rodenhuis S, Slebos RJC, Boot AJM, et al. Incidence and possible clinical significance of K-ras oncogene activation in adenocarcinoma of the human lung. Cancer Res 1988;48:5738–5741.

in x-ray adenocarcinoma cell lines may reflect either de novo *ras* mutation during cell line establishment or selection for that small subset of x-ray adenocarcinomas that exhibit the occasional naturally occurring mutation. In the resected tumor specimens, these mutations were almost exclusively in K-*ras* codon 12. Gene amplification is uncommon for *ras* in lung cancer (17, 18), and these mutations are stable and are present in both primaries and subsequent metastases (19).

THE *MYC* GENE FAMILY

The v-*myc* oncogene was isolated from the avian myelocytomatosis retrovirus, and the cellular homologues c-*myc*, N-*myc*, and L-*myc* were identified by homology. L-*myc* was discovered to be amplified in SCLC (20). Functionally, *myc* is a short-lived nuclear phosphoprotein that participates in transcriptional regulation.

In contrast to *ras* genes, which are activated by point mutations, *myc* genes are rarely found to be mutant, but rather appear to be activated by overexpression, either by up-regulation or gene amplification. N-*myc* and L-*myc* gene amplification is seen in 10% to 20% of SCLC tumor samples taken before chemotherapy (21). In cell lines established after chemotherapy and clinical relapse, 11 of 25 had amplified *myc* genes (five c-*myc*, three N-*myc*, and three L-*myc*) (44%) (22). c-*myc* Amplification is associated with the variant phenotype of SCLC (23) and with shortened patient survival (22). When RNA expression is evaluated rather than DNA amplification, 80% to 90% of SCLC tumors show overexpression relative to normal or fetal lung tissues (24). NSCLC only very infrequently shows amplification of c-*myc* (2 of 47 tumors), and these two were adenocarcinomas with normal *ras* genes (25). Thus, *myc* amplification not only is associated with a class of lung tumor (SCLC), but also with exposure to chemotherapy, a particular subtype (variant SCLC), and poor survival.

Growth Factor Receptors

Another class of oncogenes bears homology to membrane tyrosine kinase growth factor receptors. c-*erb*B-1 encodes the epidermal growth factor receptor (EGFR), and c-*erb*B-2 (also called HER2*neu*) encodes a gene, originally isolated from rat neuroblastomas, with structural similarity to EGFR. Schneider et al. (26) studied 60 NSCLC tumor samples for abnormalities in the c-*erb*B-2 gene. Eleven human lung cancer cell lines, including four derived from SCLC and seven from NSCLC, also were examined for altered c-*erb*B-2 gene expression. Amplification of the c-*erb*B-2 gene was rare in NSCLC (2 of 60). Four of four SCLC cell lines demonstrated minimal or nondetectable expression of c-*erb*B-2 mRNA compared with high levels of expression by seven of seven NSCLC lines. The highest expression levels were seen in four of four adenocarcinomas. Immunohistochemical HER2*neu* overexpression was correlated with decreased survival in NSCLC (27), and overexpression may enhance metastatic potential (28). Antibodies to HER2*neu* may be useful either directly or by sensitizing tumors to chemotherapy (29).

EGFRs are found predominantly in NSCLC as well (41 of 48 tumors) (30), and the production of EGF-like activity by lung cancer cells raises the possibility of an autocrine loop. Some NSCLCs have been shown to express a mutant form of the EGFR, detectable by antibodies to a novel extracellular domain protein sequence (31).

A variety of other oncogenes have been evaluated in lung cancer. c-*myb* Is a nuclear oncogene whose level has been inversely associated with differentiation. It is expressed in SCLC but not NSCLC (32). c-*raf* Is an oncogene located at 3p25 that frequently is deleted in lung cancer, as well as in every case of SCLC examined (33).

There is evidence that c-*kit*, a tyrosine kinase receptor thought to be involved in hematopoiesis, and its ligand, stem cell factor, are expressed simultaneously in SCLC but not in NSCLC (34, 35). Similarly, platelet-derived growth factor (PDGF), a potent mitogen, and its receptor are found to be expressed in primary lung cancers and cell lines (36, 37). Both of these form potential autocrine growth self-stimulatory loops. *myc* Overexpression also has been correlated with expression of c-*kit* (38).

Somatostatin receptors are expressed in SCLC and NSCLC tumors and are being targeted both for imaging and therapy with somatostatin analogs (39, 40).

Tumor Suppressor Genes in Lung Cancer

Retinoblastoma

The *retinoblastoma* (Rb) gene is located on chromosome 13q and encodes a nuclear phosphoprotein that appears to regulate the cell cycle by binding to G1 cyclins and the transcription factor E2F (41–43). This binding itself seems to be regulated by Rb phosphorylation, and lack of cell-cycle dependent phosphorylation often is a clue that the Rb protein is defective. Children who inherit a defective rb allele are at great risk of multiple, often bilateral, retinoblastomas, and these tumors result from somatic inactivation (by mutation or deletion) of the remaining allele. Rb also can be bound and inactivated by a variety of DNA tumor virus gene products including SV40 large T antigen, adenovirus E1A, and human papillomavirus E7; this event may allow the virus to force quiescent cells into the cell cycle to facilitate viral replication.

Most SCLCs (more 95%) have absent or abnormal Rb protein, whereas only a fraction of NSCLC is affected (44). Most of these mutations involve the "pocket region" of Rb that is involved in its binding to other proteins. Further evidence of the involvement of Rb in lung cancer comes from studies of individuals who are carriers of abnormal genes and either statistically escape or survive retinoblastoma. These patients develop nonocular tumors at 10 times the expected rate, and prominent among these tumors is SCLC, which has a 15-fold excess risk (45). The presence of the inherited Rb mutation has been demonstrated in a patient who survived retinoblastoma, but who developed SCLC at age 28 (46). The level of Rb protein expression in NSCLC has been evaluated for clinical impact, but none was found (47, 48).

When the normal Rb gene is reintroduced into RB negative human lung cancer cells via retroviral transduction, they lose tumorigenicity in nude mice (49), even though the tumors clearly have multiple genetic lesions.

p53

p53 Is a nuclear phosphoprotein whose gene is located on chromosome 17p. It has been shown to have specific DNA binding and transcriptional activation capabilities. It is the most frequent somatic genetic alteration in human cancer. p53 Has complex physiologic effects, acting as a dominant oncogene when mutant (becoming tumorigenic when introduced into primary, x-ray malignant rodent cells along with activated *ras*) and as a tumor suppressor gene (suppressing transformation and cell proliferation) when normal. When homozygously deleted in the germline of mice, the mice are phenotypically normal at birth, but they have a high incidence of tumors (50). This finding indicates that development and differentiation can occur normally but that there is an increased susceptibility to subsequent genetic events leading to cancer.

p53 Is very frequently abnormal in lung cancer, with somatically acquired mutations being found in less than 50% of NSCLC and less than 90% of SCLC (51, 52). The mutations found in p53 in human lung cancer are of all types: missense, nonsense, splicing, and large deletions, and they occur throughout the open reading frame, in contrast to the limited substitutions found in activated *ras*. Missense mutations are most frequent in exons 5 through 8 (53) (Fig. 11.2) and also are associated with prolonged protein half-life and thus with an increased steady-state protein level. All normal cells express low levels of p53, usually below the level of detection of immunohistochemistry, but mutant proteins with a prolonged half-life become readily detectable. This fact forms the basis for a simple screening test of clinical material for the presence of p53 mutations, even though it misses about one third of the lesions, mostly splicing and nonsense mutations (54).

The locations of missense mutations in *p53* are similar among different tumor types, but there may be a preference for mutations between codons 150 and 160 in NSCLC. Codon 175 mutations are very common in colon cancer, but they are uncommon in lung cancer. The significance of these differences is unclear. When lung cancer tumors are evaluated for somatic mutations in the *p53* and *ras* oncogenes, a different pattern of base alterations is seen compared with that in other tumors. There is a preference for G to T transversions in lung cancer and for G to A transitions in colon cancer (51, 53). There also is a strand asymmetry, with unequal numbers of G to T changes compared with changes of C to A (the complementary change). The explanation for these findings, if confirmed, may lie in the types and specificities of carcinogens involved in lung cancer pathogenesis.

p53 Also can be inactivated by binding to viral or cellular proteins in the absence of mutation. SV40 T antigen, as well as adenovirus and papillomavirus proteins, can bind and effectively inactivate p53. A cellular protein called MDM2 also binds and inactivates p53, and it is found to be overexpressed in some tumors; however, its role in lung cancer is unclear. Human papilloma virus (HPV) or adenovirus proteins also are probably not present in established tumors (48), although they may still play a role in the transient loss of growth control in preneoplastic cells that are infected naturally.

Transfection of wild-type p53 into lung cancer cells with mutant or deleted p53 suppresses growth in vitro and tumorigenicity in mice with severe combined immunodeficiency disease (SCID) (55). Missense mutations in p53 often have been shown to lack the ability to activate transcription, or they become temperature sensitive in this property: active at 32° and inactive at 37° (56). The x-ray crystal structure shows that the DNA binding domain of p53 is a β-sandwich structure, and many of the common sites of mutation affect DNA-p53 contact sites (57).

If p53 is primarily a transcriptional regulator, elucidation of the function of genes or pathways regulated by p53 could shed light on its role as a tumor suppressor. One crucial pathway probably involves the induction of apoptosis. Apoptosis is a form of planned cell death that occurs normally in the process of development of an organism. It also is known as programmed cell death or active cell death. It refers to the activation of an energy dependent internal program in a cell that actively causes the death of the cell. A variety of reports link wild-type p53 with the ability of a cell to undergo apoptosis (58). A myeloid leukemia cell line expressing a temperature sensitive mutant p53 was observed to undergo apoptosis upon a temperature-induced shift to the wild-type conformation (59). When p53 expression was induced in colon cancer cells, they were induced to undergo apoptosis (60). The role of p53 in apoptosis is supported further by the observa-

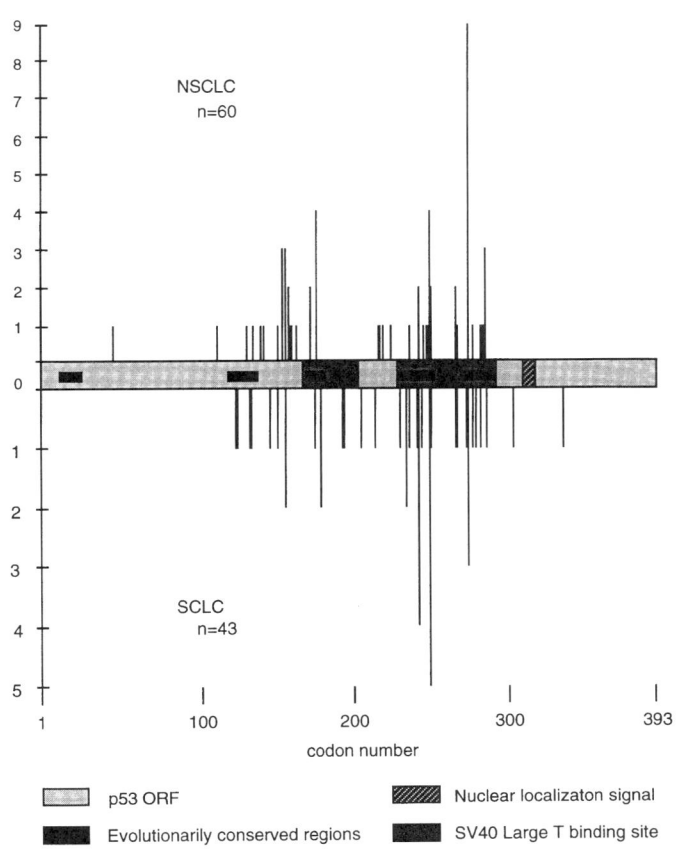

FIGURE 11.2. A histogram depicting the locations of p53 missense mutations in SCLC and NSCLC tumors and cell lines, compiled from various published and unpublished sources. The regions that are highly conserved through evolution, and those that are postulated to be involved in nuclear localization and binding to the SV40 large T binding site, are indicated. (Published data from Caron de Fromental C, Soussi T. *TP53* tumor suppressor gene: a model for investigating human mutagenesis. Genes Chromosom Cancer 1992;4:1–15.)

tion that thymocytes, although very sensitive to radiation-induced apoptosis in normal mice, are resistant in p53 knockout mice (61). These data all suggest that wild-type p53 function somehow facilitates the cell's ability to undergo apoptosis.

A possible link between p53-mediated transcriptional activation and apoptosis has come from the study of cell cycle control after radiation-induced DNA damage. If cells with normal p53 are subjected to DNA-damaging doses of x-irradiation, they normally arrest at the G1-S phase in the cell cycle. Cells with mutant p53, however, fail to arrest and proceed through the S phase (62). It is thought that this G1-S arrest allows cells to repair the DNA damage before undergoing DNA replication, or if the cells are under continued growth stimulation from other pathways (the "clash" hypothesis), it induces apoptosis. Cells with mutant p53 are incapable of using this checkpoint and proceed through the S phase, at which point any damaged DNA becomes fixed in the genome and is passed to the cell's progeny. This process—shown diagrammatically in Figure 11.3—potentially initiates a cascade of genetic alterations that leads to cancer.

One gene that is highly induced by p53 is WAF-1 (63), or Cip-1 (64). This protein binds to cyclins A, D1, E, and cdk2 and is a potent inhibitor of the phosphorylation of cdk and RB. Thus, expression of this gene directly inhibits cell cycling, and loss of expression via inactivation of the transcriptional activity of p53 would directly cause loss of this aspect of cell cycle control, making WAF-1/Cip-1 a tumor suppressor gene. Consistent with this hypothesis is the fact that transfection of this gene into tumor cells directly inhibits growth. It also provides a link between the functional roles of p53 and RB and appears to be a direct mediator of the growth suppressive properties of p53. The relevance of the findings linking apoptosis and cell cycle control to p53 in lung cancer therapeutics remains undetermined.

CHROMOSOMES 3P AND 9P

The short arm of chromosome 3 was one of the first chromosomal regions identified as a frequent site of somatic deletion (6), but to date no convincing target gene has been identified. There appear to be three regions on 3p that are lost (65, 66): around 3p25, 3p21, and 3p14. The gene for von Hippel-Lindau disease, a cancer predisposition syndrome characterized by pheochromocytomas and multiple renal cell carci-

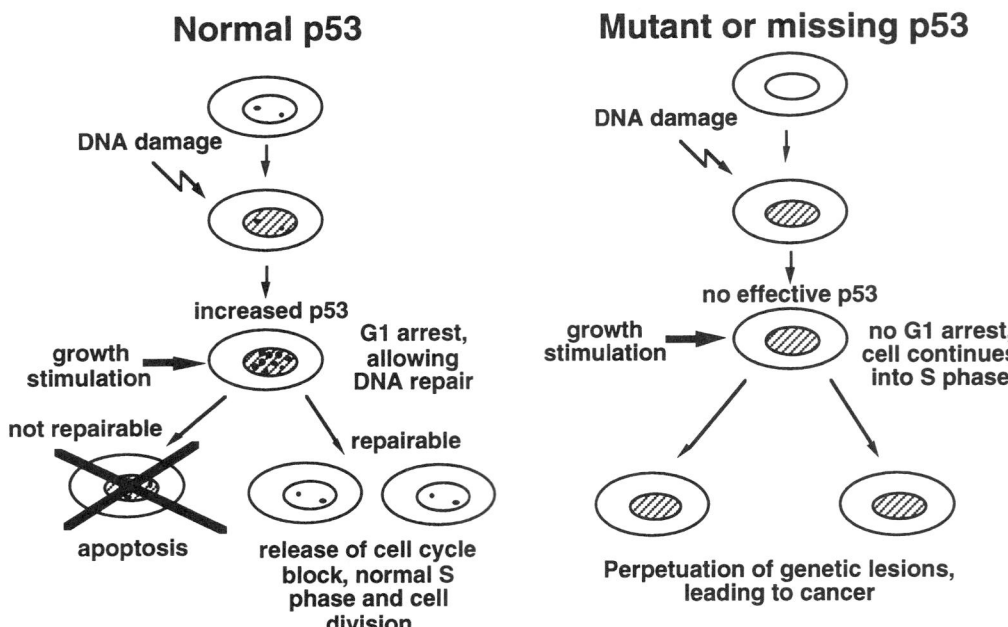

FIGURE 11.3. A model depicting p53-mediated cell cycle arrest as a means of preventing perpetuation of genetic lesions.

nomas, has been cloned and mapped to 3p25 (67). This gene only infrequently is involved in lung cancer, however, and some other gene in the region may play a more prominent role (68). Several groups have found somatic deletions in the 3p21 region, and several candidate genes have been cloned (69–74); however, none thus far has demonstrated convincing frequent somatic alterations. The human DNA mismatch repair gene hMLH1, which is involved in hereditary x-ray polyposis colon cancer, has been cloned and localized to 3p21, but it has not been identified convincingly as being important in the development of lung cancer. Deletions in the 3p14 region are being characterized as well, with no convincing gene candidates as yet identified (75–77).

Hemizygous and homozygous deletion of genetic material within the interferon gene cluster on chromosome 9p has been observed in lung cancer (8, 78). This deletion may indicate the presence of a tumor suppressor gene in that region. Recently, a candidate tumor suppressor gene named *p16* or *MTS1* was identified as homozygously deleted in tumor cell lines (79). This gene is an inhibitor of cyclin dependent kinase, and its role in lung cancer genesis is being studied, although it appears that mutation frequencies in fresh tumors are considerably lower than in cell lines (80).

MCC/APC REGION ON CHROMOSOME 5Q IN LUNG CANCER

Chromosome 5q frequently shows loss of heterozygosity in colon cancer, and the mutated in colon cancer (*MCC*) gene on 5q21 was found to be mutated somatically in many cases (81, 82). The familial adenomatous polyposis syndrome, which is associated with a high frequency of colon cancer, also mapped to 5q21, and germline mutations were found in a nearby gene, the adenomatous polyposis coli (*APC*) gene. While screening for mutations in these genes in lung cancer, D'Amico et al. (83) found no somatic mutations, but they did find an extremely high frequency of loss of heterozygosity (80%) in SCLC and a lower frequency of loss (20%) in NSCLC. These findings indicate yet another chromosome region in which a tumor suppressor gene may reside (84, 85).

TELOMERASE

The telomeres of eukaryotic chromosomes are made up of short, tandem, repeat sequences thought to be involved in protecting chromosomal material from end-to-end fusion or exonucleolytic degradation (86–88). The level of telomerase, the enzyme responsible for elongation of these repeats, and the length of the repeats are higher in germ cells than in senescent cells. This characteristic is thought to be related to replicative capacity, i.e., young cells have long repeats, whereas senescent cells have short ones. Inappropriately high levels of telomerase may cause long repeats and contribute to the lack of growth control exhibited by cancer cells. There is some evidence that this phenomenon is observed in lung cancer and that long repeats are associated with a worse prognosis (89). Further studies are needed to characterize this effect and develop treatments that block telomerase in cancer cells.

GENETIC INSTABILITY AND LUNG CANCER

Instability and loss of genetic material have long been known as a frequent (and perhaps universal) characteristic of cancer. Recently, two genes, mutl (*hMLH1*) and muts (*hMSH2*), involved in the detection and repair of DNA mismatch mutations, have been shown to cause hereditary nonpolyposis colon cancer (90–93) when defective alleles are inherited. Individuals inheriting a defective allele and one normal allele have normal mismatch repair capabilities in their somatic cells; however, cancers arising in these individuals lose the second copy and become deficient in mismatch repair. These tumors have an interesting propensity toward difficulty in accurately replicating DNA, particularly in stretches of dinucleotide repeats. These are regions in the DNA that occur approximately every 20 to 30 kilobases; these kilobases are composed of alternating repeats of two nucleotides, e.g., CACA-CACA. Typically, the number of these repeats is variable among individuals and is the basis for PCR-based fingerprinting assays. Within an individual, however, they are thought to be stable. In hereditary nonpolyposis colon cancer (HNPCC) patients, tumor cells are found to have different numbers of these repeats compared with the normal somatic cells in the same patient (94, 95). This same phenomenon has been observed in lung cancer (96). The functional connection between this instability and the cancer phenotype, particularly point mutations and deletions of oncogenes, is still unclear, but they do represent a new class of acquired and inherited genetic abnormalities. Interestingly, *hMLH1* maps to 3p21.3, a deletional hotspot in SCLC. Whether *hMLH1* is the gene thought to be involved in lung cancer in this region remains to be shown. The frequency and relevance of lesions in either of these genes also is unclear in lung cancer, although a preliminary report has found evidence of genomic instability in SCLC (96).

ORDER OF EVENTS IN LUNG CANCER PATHOGENESIS

Once the cancer is clinically evident, many of the oncogene lesions described above are relatively stable. When variously staged SCLC tumors and resulting metastases are evaluated, there is some evidence that the earliest stage tumors may have a somewhat lower incidence of p53 abnormalities, but that metastases always have the same mutation as each other and the primary (19, 97). Also, SCLC cell lines almost always have mutations identical to those found in the tumors from which they were derived. *ras* Mutations also are stable with disease progression (19). c-*myc* Amplification, however, seems to be associated with relapsed SCLC tumors after cytotoxic therapy, and thus it is a progression event.

Most epithelial tumors, including lung cancer, however, do not arise de novo from normal epithelia but rather are associated with a series of morphologic changes that may last for from 5 to 15 years or longer (98, 99). Almost certainly, some of the molecular events must precede the onset of invasive cancer. Because of the problems associated with sequential sampling of the bronchial tree, the precise order of molecular events that leads to invasive cancer is difficult to establish. Instead, spatially separated preoplastic lesions in resection specimens from patients with known cancer often are evaluated in an attempt to recapitulate temporally separated genetic changes. Modern PCR-based techniques, coupled with microdissection of paraffin-imbedded tissues, make this analysis possible. These techniques also allow detection of molecular abnormalities in small, crushed, bronchial biopsies and in exfoliated cells (100, 101). Loss of DNA material from the short arm of chromosome 3 and p53 mutations has been detected in carcinoma in situ lesions (102). In addition, cytogenetic changes and overexpression of growth factors have been described in morphologically normal epithelium (103). Similarly, *ras* mutations are present in very early stage lung tumors, but the time of their appearance has not been well characterized. Some clues to the impact of specific changes also may come from the study of bronchial epithelial cells in culture and their response to introduction of oncogenes (104) or selective inhibition of oncogene expression using antisense technologies. Knowledge of the timing and role of individual genetic lesions will both extend our understanding of oncogenesis and provide possibilities for early detection and intervention.

INHERITED PREDISPOSITION TO LUNG CANCER

Although lung cancer has an unequivocal statistical linkage to smoking, there is marked individual variation in the susceptibility to developing the disease. The high incidence of lung cancer and the presence of known potent and prevalent environmental factors make identification of other factors contributing to these differences a complex problem. It is increasingly evident from case studies, however, that hereditary and genetic influences play important roles in determining this host susceptibility (105). Multivariate analyses of clinical data on lung cancer incidences have demonstrated a significant excess of deaths related to lung and other cancers among relatives of patients compared with population controls (106). In a model of recessive inheritance, it has been predicted that a gene with a population frequency of 0.3 to 0.5 that carried a relative risk for lung cancer of 50 to 100 would cause a twofold to fourfold increased risk of cancer among siblings of affected patients (107); population studies have shown approximately the same results (108). There also is a significantly increased chance of a parent having had lung cancer and of an increased predisposition to lung cancer in persons who have chronic airways obstruction (109, 110).

There are some families in which members are afflicted with two or more primary cancers occurring in metachronous fashion (111, 112). The Li-Fraumeni familial cancer syndrome is one such example of familial cancer, with neoplasms ranging from osteosarcomas to brain tumors, leukemia, and breast cancers arising at a relatively young age (113, 114). In addition, segregation analysis of families identified an autosomal dominant pattern of transmission. Survivors of hereditary retinoblastoma are at higher risk of developing lung cancer as adults, and they develop them at an earlier age than the general population (115). The relatives of index cases, if they are carriers of the Rb gene, also have a 15-fold increased risk of lung cancer compared with controls (45). Inactivation of both alleles at the Rb locus has been confirmed following characterization of the gene (116, 117). The presence of the inherited Rb mutation has been demonstrated in a patient who survived retinoblastoma, but who developed SCLC at age 28 (46). Thus, the Rb gene is the stereotypic tumor susceptibility gene that can be inherited and somatically mutated in some cases of lung cancer. Germline mutations in another tumor suppressor gene, *p53*, have been identified in families with Li-Fraumeni syndrome (118, 119). Although this tumor suppressor gene frequently is found to be mutated somatically in lung cancer, there have been only rare cases of lung cancer in individuals inheriting mutant alleles. This finding would suggest that *p53* is not the preferred "first hit" in the development of lung cancer and that some as yet unknown gene, perhaps located in chromosome 3p, may be the primary susceptibility gene.

Increased activity of CYP1A1, a p450 gene, also has been seen in lung cancer cells themselves, compared with normal lung tissue in the same patient, suggesting that direct dysregulation of the gene may occur in the process of carcinogenesis (120).

The finding of variability among individuals in their metabolic handling of xenobiotics, including carcinogens, has lead to the speculation that the metabolic profile of smokers plays a significant role in lung cancer susceptibility. The cytochrome P450s are a family of highly polymorphic microsomal monooxygenase enzymes that are implicated because of their ability to bioactivate procarcinogens to reactive electrophilic compounds, which can form adducts with DNA and generate genetic mutations (121, 122). Such speculations have been supported by observations, including the association of lung cancer risk to debrisoquine metabolism and inducibility of P450 enzymes by smoking. Debrisoquine is an antihypertensive agent that is hydroxylated by a P450 enzyme, P450 2D6. Accordingly, individuals can be identified as extensive or poor metabolizers of debrisoquine, with the former group of smokers having about a 10-fold relative risk of developing lung cancer, independent of smoking or asbestos exposure (123).

Elevated expression of one such p450 gene, called CYP1A1 or aryl hydrocarbon hydroxylase (AHH), is strongly associated with increased susceptibility to aryl hydrocarbon–induced carcinogenesis (124). Because AHH can metabolize known promutagenic and procarcinogenic polycyclic aromatic hydrocarbons present in cigarette smoke, it also has been implicated in lung carcinogenesis. This gene is located on human chromosome 15q22-qter (125) and is inducible readily by exposure to its substrates, including cigarette smoke (126). This induction is mediated by the aromatic hydrocarbon receptor and varies widely among individuals. Strains of animals with higher expression are more susceptible to the chemical carcinogen 3-methylcholanthrene (127), but proving an association with human lung cancer has been complicated by the fact that changes in smoking habits brought about by the diagnosis of cancer can affect expression levels. Carefully controlled studies have shown a strong association for human lung cancer (124, 128), however, as well as for altered gene regulation in lung cancer patients (120, 129).

Other enzymes involved in the detoxification of carcinogens in cigarette smoke are the glutathione S-transferases (GSTs). These enzymes can inactivate polycyclic aromatic hydrocarbons by conjugating them with intracellular glutathione to form inactive, water soluble metabolites (130). Genetic polymorphisms of the *GST1* gene result in interindividual variation of several thousandfold in the activity of the encoded enzyme GST-μ (131). One of the most common alleles actually is a deletion, or null allele. About 50% of the white population is homozygous for this allele, 42% are heterozygous, and 9% are homozygous for the active allele. Smokers with a high activity of this enzyme have a lower risk for lung carcinoma than smokers with no or low activity (relative risk, 0.30; 95% confidence interval, 0.11–0.79) (132). The same correlation was found when expression was detected immunohistochemically in lung tissue rather than enzymatically (132).

Other enzymes induced or reduced by cigarette smoke include microsomal epoxide hydroxylase, UDP-glucuronosyltransferase, and dimethylnitrosamine demethylase (133). It thus is likely that an individual's net risk of lung cancer upon exposure to a complex mixture of carcinogens such as tobacco smoke is a summation of the contribution of multiple genes. Several enzymes may interact along parallel or sequential metabolic pathways to determine the ultimate concentration of reactive chemical species to which the genetic material is exposed.

MOLECULARLY BASED APPROACHES TO DIAGNOSIS AND PROGNOSIS OF LUNG CANCER

Specific knowledge about molecular genetic lesions detected in an individual's cells may alter clinical management in a variety of ways. These include genetic counseling, early detection, prognostication, detection of residual disease, and molecularly based therapies.

Inheritance of particular genes may sufficiently predispose an individual to cancer to warrant more intensive screening or more vigilant risk avoidance. As discussed above, the inherited risk factors for lung cancer, in particular, are not well defined enough to warrant genetic counseling. The contribution of cigarette smoking to multiple adverse health effects is so large that smoking cessation should be recommended to everyone, regardless of genetic background. It is striking, however, that certain individuals develop lung disease and/or cancer after only moderate or no tobacco use and others with heavy abuse histories fail to develop any symptoms at all. It remains to be shown how much of this variation is stochastic and how much is genetic, but there may be identifiable subpopulations who are at particularly high risk because of genetic factors.

In addition, the genetic signatures of cancer may be detectable before the disease becomes apparent clinically, potentially allowing early detection or chemoprevention. Several studies of smokers using standard cytologic and radiographic screening techniques have shown that it is possible to identify tumors earlier, and that these patients tend to be diagnosed at an earlier stage and are more likely to be resected for cure than are their unscreened counterparts (134–137). However, none of these studies has demonstrated a clear survival advantage. It is now possible to detect genetic lesions associated with cancer in individual exfoliated cells or in tiny biopsy specimens in other tumors (100, 138). Detection of mutant oncogenes may ultimately be standard screening practice for lung cancer in otherwise nondiagnostic sputa or biopsies. Genetic signatures also could be used to help identify subtypes; the finding of a *ras* mutation would argue strongly for adenocarcinoma or large cell carcinoma and against small cell subtypes.

Once an individual is known to have cancer, molecular features of the tumor cells may help guide the selection of standard therapies. These features could be used to select subsets for more intensive staging, adjuvant therapy, or more aggressive or alternative therapies.

In one study of *ras* mutations in resected NSCLC (16), it was found that K-*ras* mutations tended to occur in tumors that were smaller and less differentiated than those without mutations. The presence of a K-*ras* codon 12 mutation, however, was a strong adverse prognostic factor for survival (139). These two findings appear to be contradictory, but actually the finding of K-*ras* mutations seems to be identifying a subset of patients who do badly even though their tumors appear to be resectable. Because these series included only resectable tumors, this finding says that *ras* mutant tumors appear to be resectable clinically only when they are detected earlier than their *ras* normal counterparts. Positive immunohistochemical staining for *ras* has been correlated with adverse outcome as well. In a retrospective study of 116 resected NSCLCs, immunostaining was a strong independent prognostic determinant of survival (140); the same result was seen in 112 resected NSCLC patients when analyzed by flow cytometry (141). No *ras* mutational analyses were done, however, and *ras* expression level may be correlated with the presence of a mutation and not an independent risk factor. Clinical studies are being designed that use the presence of mutant *ras* genes to select a subset of patients for adjuvant chemotherapy.

As mentioned above, mutation of p53 often results in a prolonged protein half-life and overexpression of the protein. This overexpression is detectable by immunostaining on paraffin sections and has been used as a screening test for the presence of p53 mutations. There is some disagreement in the literature about the prognostic significance of p53 mutations or overexpression. One study showed that overexpression of p53 is associated with a poor prognosis in lung cancer (142), but another found no such association (143). No genetic mutation analysis was done in either of these studies. Another study showed that mutations were correlated with poor prognosis but immunostaining was not done (144). Yet another study, which evaluated both staining and mutations in NSCLC, found an imperfect correlation between the two, as well as reduced survival, but not mutations, with positive immunostaining (15).

Molecular markers may allow guidance regarding when to switch, stop, or restart therapies, assuming that effective regimens were available. It is possible that bone marrows, nodes, or surgical margins that are negative by light microscopy could be found to be positive by PCR molecular genetic techniques. This finding could be used to upstage patients and either alter therapy or prevent toxicity from futile local therapy in the presence of metastatic disease.

MOLECULARLY BASED APPROACHES TO THERAPY OF LUNG CANCER

The genetic lesions responsible for the development of cancer may prove to be ideal targets for future rationally designed therapy. These lesions are not only specific for tumors and not found in normal cells, but they are thought to be fundamental to the maintenance of the malignant phenotype. Following is a brief review of some of the therapeutic approaches that are under development in the United States and elsewhere.

Activated *ras* requires posttranslational lipid modification for activity (145), and inhibition with mevalonate inhibits its ability to support transformation (146). More active and more specific compounds are being developed for potential use as anticancer agents. One such agent was developed recently at the University of Texas Southwestern by Drs. Michael Brown and Joseph Goldstein (147). This compound specifically inhibited the growth of cells transformed by *ras*, and experiments designed to test its effectiveness against human lung cancer cells growing in culture are in progress.

Another promising therapeutic approach is gene therapy, i.e., the use of genetic material as an anticancer agent. There are two basic approaches. The first involves removing a portion of the tumor, introducing the therapeutic gene ex vivo, rendering this tumor replication incompetent with radiation or drugs, and reintroducing it into the patient in the form of a tumor vaccine with the hope of stimulating a tumor specific immunity that eradicates the residual viable tumor in the patient. The second approach involves introducing the therapeutic gene into the tumor cells in vivo, which results in a direct cytotoxic effect and/or systemic protective immunity. The vaccine approach is based on the hypothesis that (*a*) a significant component of escape from immune surveillance is a poor induction of a primary response in vivo, and (*b*) if a strong response could be induced artificially, this response would effectively kill the cells that were unable to induce this response. The latter effect has been thought of as an inadequate helper response, involving an inadequate local concentration of immune regulatory cytokines in the vicinity of the tumor. Recently, it has been shown that the introduction of various cytokine genes can induce antitumor responses against the gene-modified tumor as well as systemic responses against a non–gene-modified tumor at distant sites. The expression of cytokine genes in tumor cells is thought to flag the otherwise tolerated tumor cells as foreign to the immune system, thus allowing the generation of an effective immune response that reacts against metastatic malignant tumors. The development of gene therapy has made it possible to produce cytokines locally in tumor deposits continuously with minimal release into the systemic circulation. The current list of cytokines that can arrest tumor growth after gene transfer into tumor cells includes: IL-2 (148–152), IL-4 (151, 153, 154), IL-6 (155, 156), IL-7 (157, 158), IL-12 (159–161), TNF (162), IFN-g (152, 163), and GM-CSF (164). The *MHC* genes (165–168) and B7, a costimulatory molecule as the ligand for CD28 (169, 170), are also potential immunomodulatory therapeutic genes.

There are many genes that appear to be involved directly in the induction or maintenance of the malignant phenotype. These include mutant *ras* and p53, overexpressed HER2*neu*, *myc*, and others. Wild-type tumor suppressor genes can be reintroduced in vivo and produce an antitumor effect (171, 172). Alternatively, dominant oncogenes can be inactivated in cancer cells by the introduction of a plasmid that causes the expression of an antisense RNA, which anneals to the sense message and renders it translationally inactive. Antisense *ras*, p53, and HER2*neu* trials in lung cancer are currently being initiated (173, 174). This approach again relies on the introduction of these genes into every tumor cell. It thus is unlikely to have an effect on metastatic disease, unless it also aids in the induction of an immune response, although control of local disease in itself is a worthwhile goal. The major challenges in the practical application of gene therapy of lung cancer lie in the discovery of more powerful therapeutic genes, the unraveling of their modes of action, and the development of efficient technologies capable of targeting them into lung cancer cells. It is possible, but unlikely, that there will be a single genetic remedy for all cancer types because of the wide variability in their genetic etiologies.

Additional therapeutic strategies include the interruption of autocrine growth loops. Antibodies against gastrin-releasing peptide have been shown to block human lung cancer cell growth, both in vitro and in nude mouse models (175). A trial in humans is being conducted. Both radiolabeled and toxin-conjugated antibodies that bind to tumor targets have been developed, and they have stable linkages and high affinity for their targets (176). These targets could be lung cancer surface antigens themselves or unique antigens present on the endothelium of tumor microvasculature (177).

The numerous molecularly characterized genetic lesions involved in the development of lung cancer could result in the production of proteins that would be very attractive targets for immunotherapy, assuming that the mutant form could be recognized as distinct from the normal form. This recognition then would be absolutely specific for tumor, not normal tissue, and the tumor would not lose the epitope easily, because the continued presence of the oncogene is required to maintain the malignant phenotype. The recent finding that intracellular proteins are processed normally and presented on the surface of the cell in the context of class I MHC molecules makes this approach feasible (178). Lung cancers often have downregulated antigen processing/presentation capability (179), but this effect can be overcome in experimental situations with low doses of γ-interferon, which up-regulates all aspects of antigen processing and presentation. It has been shown recently in a murine model that tumor cells expressing a particular mutant p53 can be killed by vaccinating animals with a peptide corresponding to the mutation in the tumor cells (180). Whether this translates into an effective therapy in humans remains to be determined.

CONCLUSION

Lung cancer has long been recognized as a heterogeneous collection of diseases with different histologies, growth properties, and endocrine and clinical properties. Molecular biology has revealed a multitude of genetic lesions that have given rise to new levels of complexity, but there are certain patterns emerging from these data. Histologic types of lung cancers and even clinically relevant subsets within a histologic type can now be related to certain patterns of molecular lesions. Hopefully, molecular early detection, chemoprevention, and rationally derived therapies based on these findings will begin to decrease mortality from this disease in the near future.

REFERENCES

1. Doll R, Hill A. Lung cancer and other causes of death in relation to smoking. A second report on the mortality of British doctors. Br Med J 1956;2:1071–1081.
2. Doll R, Gray R, Hafner B, Peto, R. Mortality in relation to smoking: 22 years' observations on female British doctors. Br Med J 1980;280:967–971.
3. Hecht S, Hoffmann D. Tobacco-specific nitrosamines, an important group of carcinogens in tobacco and tobacco smoke. Carcinogenesis 1988;9:875–884.
4. Knudson AJ, Hethcote HW, Brown BW. Mutation and childhood cancer: a probabilistic model for the incidence of retinoblastoma. Proc Natl Acad Sci U S A 1975;72:5116–5120.
5. Whang-Peng J, Kao-Shan C, Lee E, et al. A specific chromosome defect associated with human small-cell lung cancer: deletion 3p(14-23). Science 1982;215:181–182.
6. Whang-Peng J, Bunn P Jr, Kao-Shan C, et al. A non-random chromosomal abnormality, del 3p(14-23) in human small cell lung cancer. Cancer Genet Cytogenet 1982;6:119–134.
7. Whang-Peng J, Knutsen T, Gazdar A, et al. Nonrandom structural and numerical chromosome changes in non–small-cell lung cancer. Genes Chromosom Cancer 1991;3:168–188.
8. Lukeis R, Irving L, Garson M, Hasthorpe, S. Cytogenetics of non–small cell lung cancer: analysis of consistent non-random abnormalities. Genes Chromosom Cancer 1990;2:116–124.
9. Ried T, Petersen I, Holtgreve-Grez H, et al. Mapping of multiple DNA gains and losses in primary small cell lung carcinomas by comparative genomic hybridization. Cancer Res 1994;54:1801–1806.
10. Bos J. *ras* Oncogenes in human cancer: a review. Cancer Res 1989;49:4682–4689.
11. Grand RJA, Owen D. The biochemistry of *ras* p21. Biochem J 1991;279:609–631.
12. Mitsudomi T, Viallet J, Mulshine JL, Linnoila RI, Minna JD, Gazdar, AF. Mutations of *ras* genes distinguish a subset of non–small-cell lung cancer cell lines from small-cell lung cancer cell lines. Oncogene 1991;6:1353–1362.
13. Mabry M, Nakagawa T, Nelkin B, et al. v-Ha-*ras* oncogene insertion: a model for tumor progression of human small cell lung cancer. Proc Natl Acad Sci U S A 1988;85:6523–6527.
14. Doyle LA, Mabry M, Stahel RA, Waibel R, Goldstein LH. Modulation of neuroendocrine surface antigens in oncogene-activated small cell lung cancer lines. Br J Cancer Suppl 1991;14:39–42.
15. Carbone DP, Mitsudomi T, Chiba I, et al. p53 Immunostaining positivity is associated with reduced survival and is imperfectly correlated with gene mutations in resected non–small cell lung cancer. Chest 1994: in press.
16. Rodenhuis S, Slebos RJC, Boot AJM, et al. Incidence and possible clinical significance of K-*ras* oncogene activation in adenocarcinoma of the human lung. Cancer Res 1988;48:5738–5741.

17. Heighway J, Hasleton PS. c-Ki-*ras* amplification in human lung cancer. Br J Cancer 1986;53:285–287.
18. Mitsudomi T, Steinberg SM, Oie HK, et al. *ras* Gene mutations in non–small cell lung cancers are associated with shortened survival irrespective of treatment intent. Cancer Res 1991; 51:4999–5002.
19. Li S, Rosell R, Urban A, et al. K-*ras* point mutation: a stable tumor marker in non–small cell lung carcinoma. Lung Cancer 1994;11:19–27.
20. Nau MM, Brooks BJ, Battey J, et al. L-*myc*, a new *myc*-related gene amplified and expressed in human small cell lung cancer. Nature 1985;318:69–73.
21. Johnson B, Makuch R, Simmons A, Gazdar A, Burch D, Cashell A. *myc* Family DNA amplification in small cell lung cancer patients' tumors and corresponding cell lines. Cancer Res 1988;48:5163–5166.
22. Johnson BE, Ihde DC, Makuch RW, et al. *myc* Family oncogene amplification in tumor cell lines established from small cell lung cancer patients and its relationship to clinical status and course. J Clin Invest 1987;79:1629–1634.
23. Brennan J, O'Connor T, Makuch RW, et al. *myc* Family DNA amplification in 107 tumors and tumor cell lines from patients with small cell lung cancer treated with different combination chemotherapy regimens. Cancer Res 1991;51:1708–1712.
24. Takahashi T, Obata Y, Sekido Y, et al. Expression and amplification of *myc* gene family in small cell lung cancer and its relation to biological characteristics. Cancer Res 1989;49: 2683–2688.
25. Slebos R, Evers S, Wagenaar S, Rodenhuis S. Cellular protooncogenes are infrequently amplified in untreated non–small cell lung cancer. Br J Cancer 1989;59:76–80.
26. Schneider PM, Hung MC, Chiocca SM, et al. Differential expression of the c-erbB-2 gene in human small cell and non–small cell lung cancer. Cancer Res 1989;49:4968–4971.
27. Kern JA, Schwartz DA, Nordberg JE, et al. p185*neu* Expression in human lung adenocarcinomas predicts shortened survival. Cancer Res 1990;50:5184–5187.
28. Yu D, Wang SS, Dulski KM, Tsai CM, Nicolson GL, Hung MC. c-erbB-2/*neu* overexpression enhances metastatic potential of human lung cancer cells by induction of metastasis-associated properties. Cancer Res 1994;54:3260–3266.
29. Shepard HM, Lewis GD, Sarup JC, et al. Monoclonal antibody therapy of human cancer: taking the HER2 protooncogene to the clinic. J Clin Immunol 1991;11:117–127.
30. Cerny T, Barnes D, Hasleton P, et al. Expression of epidermal growth factor receptor (EGF-R) in human lung tumours. Br J Cancer 1986;54:265–269.
31. Garcia de Palazzo IE, Adams GP, Sundareshan P, et al. Expression of mutated epidermal growth factor receptor by non–small cell lung carcinomas. Cancer Res 1993;53:3217–3220.
32. Griffin C, Baylin S. Expression of the c-*myb* oncogene in human small cell lung carcinoma. Cancer Res 1985;45: 272–275.
33. Graziano SL, Pfeifer AM, Testa JR, et al. Involvement of the RAF1 locus, at band 3p25, in the 3p deletion of small-cell lung cancer. Genes Chromosom Cancer 1991;3:283–293.
34. Hibi K, Takahashi T, Sekido Y, et al. Coexpression of the stem cell factor and the c-*kit* genes in small-cell lung cancer. Oncogene 1991;6:2291–2296.
35. Sekido Y, Obata Y, Ueda R, et al. Preferential expression of c-kit protooncogene transcripts in small cell lung cancer. Cancer Res 1991;51:2416–2419.
36. Antoniades HN, Galanopoulos T, Neville GJ, O'Hara CJ. Malignant epithelial cells in primary human lung carcinomas coexpress in vivo platelet-derived growth factor (PDGF) and PDGF receptor mRNAs and their protein products. Proc Natl Acad Sci U S A 1992;89:3942–3946.
37. Bravo M, Vásquez R, Rubio H, Salazar M, Pardo A, Selman M. Production of platelet-derived growth factor by human lung cancer. Respir Med 1991;85:479–485.
38. Plummer HD, Catlett J, Leftwich J, et al. c-*myc* Expression correlates with suppression of c-*kit* protooncogene expression in small cell lung cancer cell lines. Cancer Res 1993;53: 4337–4342.
39. O'Byrne K, Carney D. Somatostatin and the lung. Lung Cancer 1993;10:151–172.
40. Thomas F, Brambrilla E, Friedmann A. Transcription of somatostatin receptor subtype 1 and 2 genes in lung cancer. Lung Cancer 1994;11:111–114.
41. Dowdy SF, Hinds PW, Louie K, Reed SI, Arnold A, Weinberg RA. Physical interaction of the retinoblastoma protein with human D cyclins. Cell 1993;73:499–511.
42. Ewen ME, Sluss HK, Whitehouse LL, Livingston DM. TGF beta inhibition of Cdk4 synthesis is linked to cell cycle arrest. Cell 1993;74:1009–1020.
43. Kato J, Matsushime H, Hiebert SW, Ewen ME, Sherr CJ. Direct binding of cyclin D to the retinoblastoma gene product (pRb) and pRb phosphorylation by the cyclin D–dependent kinase CDK4. Genes Dev 1993;7:331–342.
44. Harbour JW, Lai S-L, Whang-Peng J, Gazdar AF, Minna JD, Kaye FJ. Abnormalities in structure and expression of the human retinoblastoma gene in SCLC. Science 1988;241: 353–357.
45. Sanders B, Jay M, Draper G, Roberts, E. Non-ocular cancer in relatives of retinoblastoma patients. Br J Cancer 1989;60: 358–365.
46. Weir TE, Condie A, Leonard RC, Prosser J. A familial *RB1* mutation detected by the HOT technique is homozygous in a second primary neoplasm. Oncogene 1991;6:2353–2356.
47. Reissmann PT, Koga H, Takahashi R, et al. Inactivation of the retinoblastoma susceptibility gene in non–small-cell lung cancer. The Lung Cancer Study Group. Oncogene 1993;8: 1913–1919.
48. Shimizu E, Coxon A, Otterson GA, et al. RB protein status and clinical correlation from 171 cell lines representing lung cancer, extrapulmonary small cell carcinoma, and mesothelioma. Oncogene 1994;9:2441–2448.
49. Huang H-J, Yee J-K, Shew J-Y, et al. Suppression of the neoplastic phenotype by replacement of the *RB* gene in human cancer cells. Science 1988;242:1563–1566.
50. Donehower LA, Harvey M, Slagle BL, et al. Mice deficient for p53 are developmentally normal but susceptible to spontaneous tumours. Nature 1992;356:215–221.
51. Chiba I, Takahashi T, Nau MM, et al. Mutations in the *p53* gene are frequent in primary, resected non–small cell lung cancer. Oncogene 1990;5:1603–1610.
52. D'Amico D, Carbone D, Mitsudomi T, et al. High frequency of somatically acquired *p53* mutations in small cell lung cancer cell lines and tumors. Oncogene 1992;7:339–346.
53. Caron de Fromental C, Soussi T. *TP53* tumor suppressor gene: a model for investigating human mutagenesis. Genes Chromosom Cancer 1992;4:1–15.
54. Bodner SM, Minna J, Jensen SM, et al. Expression of mutant p53 proteins in lung cancer correlates with the class of *p53* gene mutation. Oncogene 1992;7:743–749.

55. Takahashi T, Carbone D, Takahashi T, et al. Wild-type but not mutant p53 suppresses the growth of human lung cancer cells bearing multiple genetic lesions. Cancer Res 1992;52: 2340–2343.
56. Unger T, Nau MM, Segal S, Takahashi T, Minna JD. p53: A transdominant regulator of transcription whose function is ablated by mutations occurring in human cancer. European Molecular Biology Organization Journal 1992;11:1383–1390.
57. Cho Y, Gorina S, Jeffrey PD, Pavletich NP. Crystal structure of a p53 tumor suppressor-DNA complex: understanding tumorigenic mutations (comments). Science 1994;265:346–355.
58. Symonds H, Krall L, Remington L, et al. p53-Dependent apoptosis suppresses tumor growth and progression in vivo. Cell 1994;78:703–711.
59. Yonish-Rouach E, Resnitzky D, Lotem J, Sachs L, Kimchi A, Oren M. Wild-type p53 induces apoptosis of myeloid leukaemic cells that is inhibited by interleukin-6. Nature 1991; 352:345–347.
60. Shaw P, Bovey R, Tardy S, Sahli R, Sordat B, Costa J. Induction of apoptosis by wild-type p53 in a human colon tumor-derived cell line. Proc Natl Acad Sci U S A 1992;89.
61. Clarke AR, Purdie CA, Harrison DJ, et al. Thymocyte apoptosis induced by p53-dependent and independent pathways. Nature 1993;362:849–852.
62. Kastan MB, Plunkett BS, Kuerbitz SJ. p53 Protein is a cell cycle checkpoint following DNA damage. Proceedings of the American Association for Cancer Research 1992;33:169.
63. el-Deiry WS, Tokino T, Velculescu VE, et al. WAF1, a potential mediator of p53 tumor suppression. Cell 1993;75:817–825.
64. Harper JW, Adami GR, Wei N, Keyomarsi K, Eledge SJ. The p21 Cdk-interacting protein Cip1 is a potent inhibitor of G1 cyclin kinases. Cell 1993;75:805–816.
65. Maestro R, Gasparotto D, Vukosavljevic T, Barzan L, Sulfaro S, Boiocchi M. Three discrete regions of deletion at 3p in head and neck cancers. Cancer Res 1993;53:5775–5779.
66. Hibi K, Takahashi T, Yamakawa K, et al. Three distinct regions involved in 3p deletion in human lung cancer. Oncogene 1992;7:445–449.
67. Latif F, Duh FM, Gnarra J, et al. von Hippel-Lindau syndrome: cloning and identification of the plasma membrane Ca(++)-transporting ATPase isoform 2 gene that resides in the von Hippel-Lindau gene region. Cancer Res 1993;53: 861–867.
68. Sekido Y, Bader S, Latif F, et al. Molecular analysis of the von Hippel-Lindau disease tumor suppressor gene in human lung cancer cell lines. Oncogene 1994;9:1599–1604.
69. Miller Y, Minna J, Gazdar A. Lack of expression of aminoacylase-1 in small cell lung cancer. Evidence for inactivation of genes encoded by chromosome 3p. J Clin Invest 1989;83: 2120–2124.
70. Daly MC, Xiang RH, Buchhagen D, et al. A homozygous deletion on chromosome 3 in a small cell lung cancer cell line correlates with a region of tumor suppressor activity. Oncogene 1993;8:1721–1729.
71. Yamakawa K, Takahashi T, Horio Y, et al. Frequent homozygous deletions in lung cancer cell lines detected by a DNA marker located at 3p21.3-p22. Oncogene 1993;8:327–330.
72. Gemmill RM, Varella-Garcia M, Smith DI, et al. A 2.5-Mb physical map within 3p21.1 spans the breakpoint associated with Greig cephalopolysyndactyly syndrome. Genomics 1991;11: 93–102.
73. Lukeis R, Ball D, Irving L, Garson OM, Hasthorpe S. Chromosome abnormalities in non–small cell lung cancer pleural effusions: cytogenetic indicators of disease subgroups. Genes Chromosom Cancer 1993;8:262–269.
74. Kok K, van den Berg A, Veldhuis PM, et al. A homozygous deletion in a small cell lung cancer cell line involving a 3p21 region with a marked instability in yeast artificial chromosomes. Cancer Res 1994;54:4183–4187.
75. Daly MC, Douglas JB, Bleehen NM, et al. An unusually proximal deletion on the short arm of chromosome 3 in a patient with small cell lung cancer. Genomics 1991;9:113–119.
76. Bardenheuer W, Szymanski S, Lux A, et al. Characterization of a microdissection library from human chromosome region 3p14. Genomics 1994;19:291–297.
77. Boldog FL, Gemmill RM, Wilke CM, et al. Positional cloning of the hereditary renal carcinoma 3;8 chromosome translocation breakpoint. Proc Natl Acad Sci U S A 1993;90:8509–8513.
78. Olopade OI, Buchhagen DL, Minna JD, et al. Deletions of the short arm of chromosome 9 that include the alpha and beta interferon genes are associated with lung cancers (abstract 1814). Proceedings of the American Association for Cancer Research, 1991;32:305.
79. Kamb A, Gruis NA, Weaver-Feldhaus J, et al. A cell cycle regulator potentially involved in genesis of many tumor types. Science 1994;264:436–440.
80. Cairns P, Mao L, Merlo A, et al. Rates of p16 (MTS1) mutations in primary tumors with 9p loss (letter). Science 1994;265: 415–417.
81. Kinzler KW, Nilbert MC, Vogelstein B, et al. Identification of a gene located at chromosome 5q21 that is mutated in colorectal cancers (comments). Science 1991;251:1366–1370.
82. Ashton-Rickardt PG, Wyllie AH, Bird CC, et al. MCC, a candidate familial polyposis gene in 5q.21, shows frequent allele loss in colorectal and lung cancer. Oncogene 1991;6:1881–1886.
83. D'Amico D, Carbone DP, Johnson BE, Meltzer SJ, Minna JD. Polymorphic sites within the MCC and APC loci reveal very frequent loss of heterozygosity in human small cell lung cancer. Cancer Res 1992;52:1996–1999.
84. Nishisho I, Nakamura Y, Miyoshi Y, et al. Mutations of chromosome 5q21 genes in FAP and colorectal cancer patients. Science 1991;253:665–669.
85. Kinzler KW, Nilbert MC, Su LK, et al. Identification of FAP locus genes from chromosome 5q21. Science 1991;253:661–665.
86. Counter CM, Avilion AA, LeFeuvre CE, et al. Telomere shortening associated with chromosome instability is arrested in immortal cells which express telomerase activity. European Molecular Biology Organization Journal 1992;11:1921–1929.
87. Hastie ND, Dempster M, Dunlop MG, Thompson AM, Green DK, Allshire RC. Telomere reduction in human colorectal carcinoma and with ageing (comments). Nature 1990;346: 866–868.
88. Hiyama E, Hiyama K, Yokoyama T, Ichikawa T, Matsuura Y. Length of telomeric repeats in neuroblastoma: correlation with prognosis and other biological characteristics. Jpn J Cancer Res 1992;83:159–164.
89. Shirotani Y, Hiyama K, Ishioka S, et al. Alteration in length of telomeric repeats in lung cancer. Lung Cancer 1994;11:29–41.
90. Bronner CE, Baker SM, Morrison PT, et al. Mutation in the DNA mismatch repair gene homologue hMLH1 is associated with hereditary non-polyposis colon cancer. Nature 1994; 368:258–261.
91. Papadopoulos N, Nicolaides NC, Wei YF, et al. Mutation of a mutL homolog in hereditary colon cancer. Science 1994; 263:1625–1629.

92. Leach FS, Nicolaides NC, Papadopoulos N, et al. Mutations of a mutS homolog in hereditary nonpolyposis colorectal cancer. Cell 1993;75:1215–1225.
93. Fishel R, Lescoe MK, Rao MR, et al. The human mutator gene homolog MSH2 and its association with hereditary nonpolyposis colon cancer. Cell 1993;75:1027–1038.
94. Ionov Y, Peinado MA, Malkhosyan S, Shibata D, Perucho M. Ubiquitous somatic mutations in simple repeated sequences reveal a new mechanism for colonic carcinogenesis. Nature 1993;363:558–561.
95. Thibodeau SN, Bren G, Schaid D. Microsatellite instability in cancer of the proximal colon. Science 1993;260:816–819.
96. Merlo A, Mabry M, Gabrielson E, Vollmer R, Baylin SB, Sidransky D. Frequent microsatellite instability in primary small cell lung cancer. Cancer Res 1994;54:2098–2101.
97. Sameshima Y, Matsuno Y, Hirohashi S, et al. Alterations of the p53 gene are common and critical events for the maintenance of malignant phenotypes in small-cell lung carcinoma. Oncogene 1992;7:451–457.
98. Saccomanno G, Archer VE, Auerbach O, Saunders RP, Brennan LM. Development of carcinoma of the lung as reflected in exfoliated cells. Cancer 1974;33:256–270.
99. Carter D. Pathology of the early squamous cell carcinoma of the lung. Pathol Ann 1978;13:131–147.
100. Sidransky D, Von Eschenbach A, Tsai YC, et al. Identification of p53 gene mutations in bladder cancers and urine samples. Science 1991;252:706–709.
101. Mitsudomi T, Lam S, Shirakusa T, Gazdar AF. Detection and sequencing of p53 gene mutations in bronchial biopsy samples in patients with lung cancer (comments). Chest 1993;104:362–365.
102. Sundaresan V, Ganly P, Hasleton P, et al. p53 And chromosome 3 abnormalities, characteristic of malignant lung tumours, are detectable in pre-invasive lesions of the bronchus. Oncogene 1992;7:1989–1997.
103. Sozzi G, Miozzo M, Tagliabue E, et al. Cytogenetic abnormalities and overexpression of receptors for growth factors in normal bronchial epithelium and tumor samples of lung cancer patients. Cancer Res 1991;51:400–404.
104. Bonfil R, Reddel R, Ura H, et al. Invasive and metastatic potential of a v-Ha-ras transformed human bronchial epithelial cell line. J Natl Cancer Inst 1989;81:587–594.
105. Tokuhata G. Familial factors in human lung cancer and smoking. Am J Public Health 1964;54:25–32.
106. Sellers T, Ooi W, Elston R. Increased familial risk for non–lung cancer among relatives of lung cancer patients. Am J Epidemiol 1987;126:237–246.
107. Peto J. Genetic predisposition to cancer. In: Cairns J, Lyon JL, Skolneck M, eds. Cancer incidence in defined populations. New York: Cold Spring Harbor Laboratory Press. 19??;4:203–213.
108. Ooi WL, Elston RC, Chen VW, Bailey WJ, Rothschild H. Increased familial risk for lung cancer. J Natl Cancer Inst 1986;76:217–222.
109. Samet J, Humble C, Pathak D. Personal and family history of respiratory disease and lung cancer risk. Am Rev Respir Dis 1986;134:466–470.
110. Skillrud D, Offord K, Miller R. Higher risk of lung cancer in chronic obstructive pulmonary disease. Ann Intern Med 1986;105:503–507.
111. Lynch HT, Guirgis HA, Lynch PM, Lynch JF, Harris RE. Familial cancer syndromes: a survey. Cancer 1977;39:1867–1881.
112. Li FP, Fraumeni JPJ, Mulvihill JJ, et al. A cancer family syndrome in twenty-four kindreds. Cancer Res 1988;48:5358–5362.
113. Li FP, Fraumrni JFJ. Soft-tissue sarcomas, breast cancer, and other neoplasms. A familial syndrome? Ann Intern Med 1969;71:747–752.
114. Li FP, Fraumeni JFJ. Prospective study of a family cancer syndrome. JAMA 1982;247:2692–2694.
115. Leonard R, MacKay T, Brown A, Gregor A, Crompton G, Smyth J. Small-cell lung cancer after retinoblastoma. Lancet 1988;2:1503.
116. Lee WH, Bookstein R, Hong F, Young LJ, Shew JY, Lee EY. Human retinoblastoma susceptibility gene: cloning, identification, and sequence. Science 1987;235:1394–1399.
117. Dunn JM, Phillips RA, Becker AJ, Gallie BL. Identification of germline and somatic mutations affecting the retinoblastoma gene. Science 1988;241:1797–1800.
118. Srivastava S, Zou Z, Pirollo K, Blattner W, Chang EH. Germline transmission of a mutated p53 gene in a cancer-prone family with Li-Fraumeni syndrome. Nature 1990;348:747–749.
119. Malkin D, Li FP, Strong LC, et al. Germ line p53 mutations in a familial syndrome of breast cancer, sarcomas, and other neoplasms. Science 1990;250:1233–1238.
120. McLemore T, Adelberg S, Czerwinski M, et al. Altered regulation of the cytochrome P4501A1 gene expression in pulmonary carcinoma cell lines. J Natl Cancer Inst 1989;81:1787–1794.
121. Gelboin H. Carcinogens, drugs, and cytochromes P-450. New Engl J Med 1983;309:105–107.
122. Guengerich, FP. Roles of cytochrome P-450 enzymes in chemical carcinogenesis and cancer therapy. Cancer Res 1988;48:2946–2954.
123. Caporaso N, Hayes RB, Dosemeci M, et al. Lung cancer risk, occupational exposure, and the debrisoquine metabolic phenotype. Cancer Res 1989;49:3675–3679.
124. Kouri RE, McKinney CE, Slomiany DJ, Snodgrass DR, Wray NP, McLemore TL. Positive correlation between high aryl hydrocarbon hydroxylase activity and primary lung cancer as analyzed in cryopreserved lymphocytes. Cancer Res 1982;42:5030–5037.
125. Jaiswal AK, Gonzalez FJ, Nebert DW. Human P1-450 gene sequence and correlation of mRNA with genetic differences in benzo(a)pyrene metabolism. Nucleic Acids Res 1985;13:4503–4520.
126. Reducing the health consequences of smoking: 25 years of progress. A Report of the Surgeon General. ed. Rockville, MD: U.S. Department of Health and Human Services, 1989.
127. Kouri RE, Ratrie H, Whitmire CE. Evidence of a genetic relationship between susceptibility to 3-methyl-cholanthrene-induced subcutaneous tumors and inducibility of aryl hydrocarbon hydroxylase. J Natl Cancer Inst 1973;51:197–200.
128. Yoshikawa M, Arashidani K, Kawamoto T, Kodama Y. Aryl hydrocarbon hydroxylase activity in human lung tissue: in relation to cigarette smoking and lung cancer. Environ Res 1994;65:1–11.
129. McLemore TL, Adelberg S, Liu MC, et al. Expression of CYP1A1 gene in patients with lung cancer: Evidence for cigarette smoke-induced gene expression in normal lung tissue and for altered gene regulation in primary pulmonary carcinomas. J Natl Cancer Inst 1990;82:1333–1339.
130. Tsuchida S, Sato K. Glutathione transferases and cancer. Crit Rev Biochem Mol Biol 1992;27:337–384.

131. Seidegård J, Pero RW. The hereditary transmission of high glutathione transferase activity towards trans-stilbene oxide in human mononuclear leukocytes. Hum Genet 1985;69:66–68.
132. Nazar-Stewart V, Motulsky AG, Eaton DL, et al. The glutathione S-transferase mu polymorphism as a marker for susceptibility to lung carcinoma. Cancer Res 1993;53(Suppl 10):2313S–2318S.
133. Petruzzelli S, Camus A-M, Carrozzi L, et al. Long-lasting effects of tobacco smoking on pulmonary drug-metabolizing enzymes: a case-control study on lung cancer patients. Cancer Res 1988;48:4695–4700.
134. Edell ES, Cortese DA. Bronchoscopic localization and treatment of occult lung cancer. Chest 1989;96:919–921.
135. Flehinger BJ, Melamed MR, Zaman MB, Heelan RT, Perchick WB, Martini N. Early lung cancer detection: results of the initial (prevalence) radiologic and cytologic screening in the Memorial Sloan–Kettering study. Am Rev Respir Dis 1984;130:555–560.
136. Frost JK, Ball W Jr, Levin ML, et al. Early lung cancer detection: results of the initial (prevalence) radiologic and cytologic screening in the Johns Hopkins study. Am Rev Respir Dis 1984;130:549–554.
137. Fontana RS, Sanderson DR, Taylor WF, et al. Early lung cancer detection: results of the initial (prevalence) radiologic and cytologic screening in the Mayo Clinic study. Am Rev Respir Dis 1984;130:561–565.
138. Sidransky D, Tokino T, Hamilton SR, et al. Identification of *ras* oncogene mutations in the stool of patients with curable colorectal tumors. Science 1992;256:102–105.
139. Slebos RJ, Kibbelaar RE, Dalesio O, et al. K-*ras* oncogene activation as a prognostic marker in adenocarcinoma of the lung. N Engl J Med 1990;323:561–565.
140. Nishio H, Nakamura S, Horai T, Ikegami H, Matsuda M. Clinical and histopathologic evaluation of the expression of Ha-*ras* and *fes* oncogene products in lung cancer. Cancer 1992;69:1130–1136.
141. Miyamoto H, Harada M, Isobe H, et al. Prognostic value of nuclear DNA content and expression of the *ras* oncogene product in lung cancer. Cancer Res 1991.
142. Quinlan DC, Davidson AG, Summers CL, Warden HE, Doshi HM. Accumulation of p53 protein correlates with a poor prognosis in human lung cancer. Cancer Res 1992;52:4828–4831.
143. McLaren R, Kuzu I, Dunnill M, Harris A, Lane D, Gatter KC. The relationship of p53 immunostaining to survival in carcinoma of the lung. Br J Cancer 1992;66:735–738.
144. Horio Y, Takahashi T, Kuroishi T, et al. Prognostic significance of *p53* mutations and 3p deletions in primary resected non–small cell lung cancer. Cancer Res 1993;53:1–4.
145. Jackson JH, Cochrane CG, Bourne JR, Solski PA, Buss JE, Der CJ. Farnesol modification of Kirsten-*ras* exon 4B protein is essential for transformation. Proc Natl Acad Sci U S A 1990;87:3042–3046.
146. Schafer W, Kim R, Sterne R, Thorner J, Kim S, Rine J. Genetic and pharmacological suppression of oncogenic mutations in *ras* genes of yeasts and humans. Science 1989;245:379–385.
147. James GL, Goldstein JL, Brown MS, et al. Benzodiazepine peptidomimetics: potent inhibitors of *ras* farnesylation in animal cells (comments). Science 1993;260:1937–1942.
148. Ley V, Langlade DP, Kourilsky P, Larsson SE. Interleukin 2-dependent activation of tumor-specific cytotoxic T lymphocytes in vivo. Eur J Immunol 1991;21:851–854.
149. Fearon ER, Pardoll DM, Itaya T, et al. Interleukin-2 production by tumor cells bypasses T helper function in the generation of an antitumor response. Cell 1990;60:397–403.
150. Gansbacher B, Zier K, Daniels B, Cronin K, Bannerji R, Gilboa E. Interleukin 2 gene transfer into tumor cells abrogates tumorigenicity and induces protective immunity. J Exp Med 1990;172:1217–1224.
151. Ohe Y, Podack ER, Olsen KJ, et al. Combination effect of vaccination with IL2 and IL4 cDNA transfected cells on the induction of a therapeutic immune response against Lewis lung carcinoma cells. Int J Cancer 1993;53:432–437.
152. Gastl G, Finstad CL, Guarini A, et al. Retroviral vector-mediated lymphokine gene transfer into human renal cancer cells. Cancer Res 1992;52:6229–6236.
153. Golumbeck PT, Lazenby AJ, Levitsky HI, et al. Treatment of established renal cancer by tumor cells engineered to secrete interleukin-4. Science 1991;254:713–716.
154. Tepper RI, Pattengale PK, Leder P. Murine interleukin-4 displays potent anti-tumor activity in vivo. Cell 1989;57:503–512.
155. Mullen CA, Coale MM, Levy AT, et al. Fibrosarcoma cells transduced with the *IL-6* gene exhibited reduced tumorigenicity, increased immunogenicity, and decreased metastatic potential. Cancer Res 1992;52:6020–6024.
156. Porgador A, Tzehoval E, Katz A, et al. Interleukin 6 gene transfection into Lewis lung carcinoma tumor cells suppresses the malignant phenotype and confers immunotherapeutic competence against parental metastatic cells. Cancer Res 1992;52:3679–3686.
157. Aoki T, Tashiro K, Miyatake S, et al. Expression of murine interleukin 7 in a murine glioma cell line results in reduced tumorigenicity in vivo. Proc Natl Acad Sci U S A 1992;89:3850–3854.
158. McBride WH, Thacker JD, Comora S, et al. Genetic modification of a murine fibrosarcoma to produce interleukin 7 stimulates host cell infiltration and tumor immunity. Cancer Res 1992;52:3931–3937.
159. Zeh HJD, Hurd S, Storkus WJ, Lotze MT. Interleukin-12 promotes the proliferation and cytolytic maturation of immune effectors: implications for the immunotherapy of cancer. J Immunother 1993;14:155–161.
160. Soiffer RJ, Robertson MJ, Murray C, Cochran K, Ritz J. Interleukin-12 augments cytolytic activity of peripheral blood lymphocytes from patients with hematologic and solid malignancies. Blood 1993;82:2790–2796.
161. Lotze MT, Zeh HJD, Elder EM, et al. Use of T-cell growth factors (interleukins 2, 4, 7, 10, and 12) in the evaluation of T-cell reactivity to melanoma. J Immunother 1992;12:212–217.
162. Blankenstein T, Qin ZH, Uberla K, et al. Tumor suppression after tumor cell-targeted tumor necrosis factor alpha gene transfer. J Exp Med 1991;173:1047–1052.
163. Gansbacher B, Bannerji R, Daniels B, Zier K, Cronin K, Gilboa E. Retroviral vector-mediated γ-interferon gene transfer into tumor cells generates potent and long lasting antitumor immunity. Cancer Res 1990;50:7820–7825.
164. Dranoff G, Jaffee E, Lazenby A, et al. Vaccination with irradiated tumor cells engineered to secrete murine granulocyte-macrophage colony-stimulating factor stimulates potent, specific, and long-lasting anti-tumor immunity. Proc Natl Acad Sci U S A 1993;90:3539–3543.
165. Wallich R, Bulbuc N, Hämmerling GJ, Katzav S, Segal S, Feldman M. Abrogation of metastatic properties of tumour cells by

165. de novo expression of H-2K antigens following *H-2* gene transfection. Nature 1985;315:301–305.
166. Hui K, Grosveld F, Festenstein H. Rejection of transplantable AKR leukaemia cells following MHC DNA-mediated cell transformation. Nature 1984;311:750–752.
167. Tanaka K, Isselbacher KJ, Khoury G, Jay G. Reversal of oncogenesis by the expression of a major histocompatibility complex class I gene. Science 1985;228:26–30.
168. James RF, Edwards S, Hui KM, Bassett PD, Grosveld F. The effect of class II gene transfection on the tumourigenicity of the H-2K-negative mouse leukaemia cell line K36.16. Immunology 1991;72:213–218.
169. Townsend SE, Alison JP. Tumor rejection after direct costimulation of CD8+ T cells by B7-transfected melanoma cells. Science 1993;259:368–370.
170. Chen L, Ashe S, Brady WA, et al. Costimulation of antitumor immunity by the B7 counterreceptor for the T lymphocyte molecules CD28 and CTLA-4. Cell 1992;71:1093–1102.
171. Fujiwara T, Mukhopadhyay T, Cai DW, Morris DK, Roth JA, Grimm EA. Retroviral-mediated transduction of *p53* gene increases TGF-beta expression in a human glioblastoma cell line. Int J Cancer 1994;56:834–839.
172. Fujiwara T, Cai DW, Georges RN, Mukhopadhyay T, Grimm EA, Roth JA. Therapeutic effect of a retroviral wild-type p53 expression vector in an orthotopic lung cancer model (comments). J Natl Cancer Inst 1994;86:1458–1462.
173. Roth JA. Oncogenes: what role in cancer therapy? Contemp Oncol 1993;May:40–52.
174. Georges RN, Mukhopadhyay T, Zhang Y, Yen N, Roth JA. Prevention of orthotopic human lung cancer growth by intratracheal instillation of a retroviral antisense K-*ras* construct. Cancer Res 1993;53:1743–1746.
175. Avis IL, Kovacs TO, Kaspryzk PG, et al. Preclinical evaluation of an anti-autocrine growth factor monoclonal antibody for treatment of patients with small-cell lung cancer. J Natl Cancer Inst 1991;83:1470–1476.
176. Vitetta ES, Thorpe PE. Immunotoxins containing ricin or its A chain. Semin Cell Biol 1991;2:47–58.
177. Burrows FJ, Watanabe Y, Thorpe PE. A murine model for antibody-directed targeting of vascular endothelial cells in solid tumors. Cancer Res 1992;52:5954–5962.
178. Hunt DF, Henderson RA, Shabanowitz J, et al. Characterization of peptides bound to the class I MHC molecule HLA-A2.1 by mass spectrometry. Science 1992;255:1261–1263.
179. Doyle A, Martin WJ, Funa K, et al. Markedly decreased expression of class I histocompatibility antigens, protein, and mRNA in human small-cell lung cancer. J Exp Med 1985;161:1135–1151.
180. Yanuck M, Carbone DP, Pendleton CD, et al. A mutant p53 tumor suppressor protein is a target for peptide-induced CD8+ cytotoxic T cells. Cancer Res 1993;53:3257-3261.

12

CLINICAL PRESENTATION AND STAGING OF LUNG CANCER

Ashokakumar M. Patel and James R. Jett

CLINICAL PRESENTATION OF LUNG CANCER

INTRODUCTION

The clinical manifestations and diverse presentations of primary bronchogenic carcinoma continue to be common diagnostic and therapeutic challenges of clinical practice. Lung cancer is the most common cause of cancer death in the United States and many other countries. Estimates from the American Cancer Society for 1995 are 169,000 new diagnoses of lung cancer and 157,400 deaths from lung cancer (1). Most distressing is that the 5-year survival rates are still less than 15% for all stages of lung cancer combined (1).

The early detection of lung cancer, preferably before the onset of symptoms, is very important prognostically and deserves further discussion. Identification of asymptomatic patients with lung cancer is difficult because mass screening appears impractical and plain chest roentgenograms rarely detect carcinomas less than 1 cm in diameter (2, 3). Shimizu and associates (4) reported 5-year survival rates of 25% among lung cancer patients presenting with symptoms compared with 56% for an asymptomatic group detected by screening. Similar results were observed in the Mayo Lung Screening Project (5). The influence of tumor stage on prognosis is reviewed below.

A variety of risk factors have been reported (Table 12.1), but the strongest association with lung cancer is cigarette smoking (6, 7). An awareness of these risk factors may aid the physician in suspecting lung cancer in the asymptomatic patient.

The estimated doubling time or rate of growth of different lung tumors is variable (approximately 30 to 200 days) and also influences the chance of early detection (13). Despite the recognition of risk factors and characteristics of tumor growth, many patients with lung cancer present with symptoms and advanced disease.

The symptomatic presentations of lung cancer may result from one of three major processes: (*a*) local tumor growth, (*b*) intrathoracic or extrathoracic metastasis, and/or (*c*) a paraneoplastic syndrome (Table 12.2). The spectrum of presenting pulmonary complaints in patients with lung cancer is broad, ranging from no symptoms to cough (45% to 75%), weight loss (45% to 70%), dyspnea (40% to 60%), chest pain (30% to 45%), hemoptysis (25% to 35%), and hoarseness (10% to 15%) (14–18). Table 12.3 summarizes the relative frequency of symptoms and signs commonly associated with lung cancer. Unusual manifestations associated with bronchogenic carcinoma may occur from paraneoplastic phenomena or metastasis to unusual sites (16, 19–27). It is important to be aware of the potential complications that may result from the local growth, as well as from the metastatic and paraneoplastic effects of pulmonary malignancy. Because successful treatment of lung cancer depends on early detection, recognizing the risk factors (Table 12.1) and clinical manifestations (Table 12.2) becomes even more imperative.

LOCAL TUMOR GROWTH

Symptoms from local growth of a malignancy depend on the initial location and size of the tumor, as well as on the involvement of surrounding structures. The location of the tumor is classified typically as either central (major bronchi, hilum, or mediastinum) or peripheral (distal to major bronchi, pleura, or chest wall). The squamous cell and small cell types of lung cancer are often central, whereas adenocarcinomas and large cell carcinomas are often peripheral lesions. Local growth of centrally occurring lesions may produce symptoms such as cough, hemoptysis, or wheezing; ob-

TABLE 12.1. Risk Factors Associated with Lung Cancer

Cigarette smoking (6,7)
Obstructive lung disease (8)
Age (uncommon <45 years) (9)
Occupation (10)
    Asbestos
    Radon (uranium)
    Arsenic
    Nickel
    Chromium
    Vinyl Chloride
    Bis(chloromethyl) ether
    Chloromethyl methyl ether
    Acrylonitrile
    Beryllium
    Cadmium
Human immunodeficiency virus (11)
Familial (12)

Note. Reference numbers appear in parentheses.

TABLE 12.2. Patterns of Initial Clinical Manifestations of Lung Cancer

ASYMPTOMATIC
SYMPTOMATIC
Local growth
  Central
    Endobronchial
    Compression or invasion of adjacent structures
      Esophagus
      Trachea
      Nerve involvement (phrenic, recurrent laryngeal, brachial plexus, sympathetic chain, vagus)
      Superior vena cava
      Thoracic duct
      Pericardium/heart
  Peripheral
    Lung parenchyma
    Pleura
    Chest wall
Metastatic Disease
  Hematogenous, especially liver, central nervous system, adrenals, bone
  Lymphangitic
  Interalveolar
Paraneoplastic (nonmetastatic) syndromes

From Patel AM, Peters SG. Clinical manifestations of lung cancer. Mayo Clin Proc 1993;68:273–277.

TABLE 12.3. Approximate Frequency of Presenting Symptoms and Signs of Lung Cancer

SYMPTOMS/SIGNS	APPROXIMATE FREQUENCY (%)
Cough	45–75
Weight loss	45–70
Dyspnea	40–60
Chest pain	30–45
Hemoptysis	25–35
Other pain (bone, shoulder)	25
Clubbing, hypertrophic osteoarthropathy	21, 5
Hoarseness	5–18
Dysphagia	2
Wheezing	2

Data from Anderson HA, Prakash UBS. Diagnosis of symptomatic lung cancer. Semin Respir Med 1982;3(3):165–175; Grippi MA. Clinical aspects of lung cancer. Semin Roentgenol 1990;25(1):12–24; Chute CG, Greenberg ER, Baron J, et al. Presenting conditions of 1539 population-based lung cancer patients by cell type and stage in New Hampshire and Vermont. Cancer 1985;56:2107–2111; and Hyde L, Hyde CI. Clinical manifestations of lung cancer. Chest 1974;65:299–306.

struction with postobstructive pneumonitis; dysphagia or recurrent aspiration (esophageal compression); hoarseness (recurrent laryngeal nerve involvement); superior vena cava syndrome (see below); chylothorax (thoracic duct compression); or palpitations and syncope (pericardial irritation/cardiac involvement) (28–31). Cavitation of the tumor or postobstructive pneumonitis may produce fever, chills, pleuritic chest pain, and/or a productive cough mimicking an infectious process or abscess (32).

Cough is the most common presenting symptom in patients with lung cancer (17). Although a history of cigarette smoking is often a confounding factor in patients presenting with persistent cough (17), abnormalities in the cough pattern, hemoptysis, or radiographic changes should raise the index of suspicion for bronchogenic carcinoma. Bronchorrhea—a cough productive of voluminous amounts of thin, mucoid secretions—occurs in less than 15% of patients with advanced bronchoalveolar carcinoma and rarely with other cell types (14, 33, 34). Hemoptysis may be a presenting symptom in 20% to 35% of patients with lung cancer (14, 15, 35). The incidence of lung cancer in patients presenting with hemoptysis and a nonlocalizing chest radiograph has been reported to be between 2.5% and 9% in some bronchoscopic series (35–37). The role of fiberoptic bronchoscopy in patients with hemoptysis and a normal or nonlocalizing chest radiograph is controversial. The study by Poe and colleagues (35) indicates that bronchoscopy performed in patients who are 50 years old or older, males, and those having a smoking history of more than 40 pack-years may have the highest diagnostic yield for lung cancer. Despite the low yield, some experts advocate bronchoscopy in any patient with repeated hemoptysis even if the chest radiograph remains normal during the interval.

Peripheral lesions may be associated with pleural and/or chest wall extension resulting in chest pain, dyspnea, or cough. Pleural involvement occurs in approximately 8% to 25% of patients with lung cancer and is asymptomatic in approximately 25% of these cases (38, 39). When symptomatic, the major complaints are dyspnea, cough, and chest pain (38). Malignant pleural effusions are most commonly caused by lung cancer and are most frequently associated with adenocarcinoma. They denote a T4 lesion and, hence, such patients are considered unresectable (40). However, in patients with a malignant effusion, it is essential to perform a cytologic examination to determine the presence or absence of malignant cells in the pleural fluid, as well as to determine the cell type. In two series of 73 and 78 patients with lung cancer and pleural effusions with negative cytologic evaluation, four and eight patients, respectively, were deemed resectable and disease free 2 to 14 years after surgery (41, 42). Thoracoscopy is useful in the evaluation of an exudative pleural effusion with a negative cytologic evaluation (40–44). However, it is our practice to have at least two negative pleural fluid cytology results before performing a diagnostic thoracoscopy. Other presentations of malignant pleural involvement include pleural-based masses and spontaneous pneumothorax (45, 46).

Persistent chest wall pain may occur from tumor extension into the mediastinum, pleura, or chest wall. Although rarely symptomatic, chest wall involvement may occur by seeding of a needle tract and present as a palpable nodule over a prior thoracentesis or needle biopsy site (47–49). In addition, local extension of lung cancer may produce symptoms caused by neurologic impingement on the brachial plexus (Pancoast or apical tumors), the cervical sympathetic chain (Horner's syndrome), the recurrent laryngeal nerve (almost always the left recurrent nerve because of the intrathoracic anatomy) (30), and/or the phrenic nerve (hemidiaphragm paralysis) (50).

PANCOAST TUMOR

Pancoast tumors, initially described more than 60 years ago, typically present with: (*a*) pain over the shoulder and medial scapula, (*b*) radicular pain with or without muscle wasting along the ulnar nerve distribution, and (*c*) Horner's syndrome with ptosis, miosis, and hemifacial anhydrosis (51, 52). Although most superior sulcus tumors are squamous cell carcinomas, any histologic type of lung cancer may be found. Small cell carcinoma has been described in 1% to 2% of superior sulcus tumors (53, 54). Magnetic resonance imaging (MRI) may more accurately delineate chest wall or brachial plexus invasion when compared with conventional computed tomography (CT), although the clinical practice in this area is evolving (55). These noninvasive imaging modalities may be useful in evaluating difficult diagnostic cases, e.g., a smoker presenting with shoulder pain who has a normal plain chest roentgenogram. Transthoracic needle aspiration is coming into common use for tissue diagnosis, but bronchoscopy may yield a tissue diagnosis and simultaneously allows assessment of the bronchial anatomy (56).

SUPERIOR VENA CAVA SYNDROME

Since its initial description by Hunter in 1757, major changes in the prevalence of etiologic factors and therapeutic approaches to superior vena cava (SVC) syndrome have been reported (57, 58). Bronchogenic carcinoma is the etiology in 65% to 80% of more recent cases of SVC syndrome (58–61). SVC syndrome results most commonly from extrinsic compression of the superior vena cava with secondary intraluminal thrombosis. Major complaints consist of facial fullness or flushing, headache, dyspnea, cough, and occasionally upper extremity edema (58, 62). Less commonly, pain, dysphagia, and syncope may occur. Accompanying physical findings include prominent venous patterns over the upper trunk and face, papilledema, facial cyanosis, and occasionally pleural effusion (Fig. 12.1). Although bronchogenic carcinoma is now the most common etiology of SVC syndrome, previously common causes such as tuberculosis and fibrosing mediastinitis should be considered (58). The SVC syndrome was previously considered a radiotherapeutic emergency. Although this is no longer considered true, an expeditious diagnosis should be obtained so that appropriate therapy can be initiated (63). Radiation therapy and/or chemotherapy may be effective in ameliorating the signs and symptoms of SVC obstruction if small cell carcinoma or lymphoma is discovered (61, 63, 64).

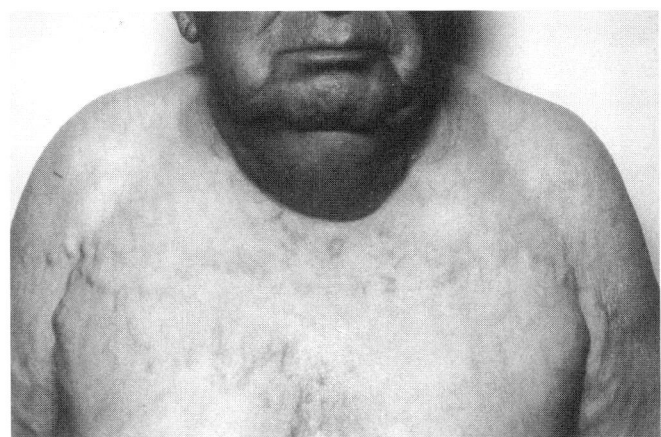

FIGURE 12.1. Superior vena cava obstruction in a patient with bronchogenic carcinoma.

METASTATIC DISEASE

The clinical manifestations of metastatic lung cancer may result from hematogenous, lymphangitic, or interalveolar dissemination (14, 65). Hematogenous spread to virtually all sites has been reported but occurs most frequently to the liver, adrenal glands, central nervous system, and bones (Table 12.4). Metastases occur earlier and most frequently in small cell carcinoma. Hepatic and adrenal metastases are often asymptomatic, and laboratory and radiologic evaluation is usually needed to detect spread to these structures (66–71). Elevations in lactate dehydrogenase, alkaline phosphatase (liver isoenzyme), and serum glutamic–oxaloacetic transaminase (SGOT) were seen in 79%, 71%, and 56%, respectively, of 34 patients with small cell lung cancer and verified liver metastases (67). Imaging modalities such as abdominal CT, nuclear medicine scintigraphy, and abdominal ultrasonography have all been useful for detection of hepatic and adrenal metastases, although reported sensitivities vary between 25% and 55% (66–71). In two series of otherwise operable non–small cell lung cancer patients, 4% and 8% of patients had a unilateral adrenal mass and less than half of these were proven malignant (68, 69). The accuracy of CT-assisted needle biopsy of adrenal masses has been reported to be 96%; however, the sensitivity of CT detection of adrenal metastasis may be only 40% (70, 71).

Metastatic involvement of bone frequently occurs with lung cancer, especially small cell lung cancer, producing osteolytic lesions in the vertebra, pelvis, and femur (14, 15). Radioisotope bone scanning may show increased uptake in 30% to 50% of patients with bronchogenic carcinoma (Fig. 12.2B), often in the absence of bone pain, elevated serum calcium, or alkaline phosphatase levels (72–74).

Autopsy series in patients with lung cancer indicate frequencies of brain metastasis of 30% and 45% (39, 75, 76). Seventy percent of patients presenting with symptomatic brain metastasis as the initial manifestation of malignancy will have a primary lung cancer (77, 78). Other neurologic presentations relate to extradural spinal cord compression, diffuse meningeal carcinomatosis, and paraneoplastic complications (79). Brain metastases with bronchogenic carcinoma are so frequent that it is advisable to obtain a CT scan evaluation of the brain in a patient with known lung cancer and any neurologic complaint.

In addition to hematogenous metastases from primary lung cancer to the liver, adrenal glands, bone, and brain, tumor embolism may occur. Tumor embolism (endovascular metastasis) from primary lung cancers as well as pulmonary emboli from tumors originating in distant sites has been reported recently by several authors (80–85). Goldhaber and associates (85) reviewed autopsies on 73 patients with solid tumors and pulmonary embolism. Seventeen patients (23%) had major tumor embolism to the lungs. Lung cancer and breast cancer were the most common malignancies in these patients. Only 1 of 17 patients had the tumor embolism correctly diagnosed antemortem. When the diagnosis is suspected, microvascular cytology can be obtained at the time of pulmonary angiography (82, 83). Negative cytologic results would not exclude the diagnosis. Tumor emboli may also involve cerebral vessels, in addition to the pulmonary circulation. In the Cornell series (84), cerebral infarction was caused by tumor emboli in 12 patients.

The detection of lymphatic spread is important in the staging of lung cancer. Lymphangitic carcinomatosis involving the lung parenchyma has characteristic features on high-resolution CT (86, 87). The high-resolution CT findings of uneven nodular thickening of interlobular septa and bronchovascular bundles in a patient with a suspected or previous known malignancy are almost pathognomonic of lymphangitic spread. Associated symptoms of cough, dyspnea, or fever depend on the extent of parenchymal involvement, the presence of a pleural effusion or atelectasis, and the type of tumor.

Interalveolar spread of lung cancer, as one mechanism of multicentric involvement, may occur predom-

TABLE 12.4. Approximate Frequency of Metastatic Involvement of Organ System by Lung Cancer

LOCATION	APPROXIMATE FREQUENCY (%)
Extrathoracic	
Liver	15–45
Brain	20–45
Bone	25–30
Lymph nodes	15–60
Kidney	20
Other	5–15
Intrathoracic	
Pleura	10–25
Cardiac	20–30
Pancoast syndrome	4–8
Superior vena cava syndrome	4

Data from Anderson HA, Prakash UBS. Diagnosis of symptomatic lung cancer. Semin Respir Med 1982;3(3):165–175; Grippi MA. Clinical aspects of lung cancer. Semin Roentgenol 1990;25(1):12–24; and Auerbach O, Garfinkel L, Parks JR. Histologic types of lung cancer in relation to smoking habits, year of diagnosis, and site of metastases. Chest 1975;64:382–387.

inantly with bronchoalveolar carcinoma (33). Bronchorrhea is rarely the presenting feature of bronchoalveolar carcinoma and usually indicates extensive pulmonary involvement (14). The nodular variant of bronchoalveolar carcinoma may be less prone to such interalveolar dissemination (88) and, hence, more amenable to surgical resection.

Metastatic disease associated with primary bronchogenic carcinoma most commonly occurs by lymphohematogenous spread, but occasionally interalveolar dissemination may occur. Common sites of metastasis include intrathoracic lymph nodes, pleura, and mediastinum, and extrathoracic sites including the liver, adrenal glands, brain, and bones. The clinical presentation depends on the site of metastatic involvement, in addition to local characteristics and the histologic type of bronchogenic carcinoma.

PARANEOPLASTIC SYNDROMES

The paraneoplastic syndromes are a group of clinical disorders associated with malignancy; they are not directly related to the physical effects of primary or metastatic tumor. Certain disorders such as digital clubbing and hypertrophic pulmonary osteoarthropathy may also occur in nonmalignant conditions and have been present for more than 2400 years (89). Such syndromes occur in 10% to 20% of patients with bronchogenic carcinoma and illustrate the systemic nature of malignancy (Table 12.5) (14, 15, 90). Differentiating true paraneoplasia from other processes related to malignancy can be difficult. Occult metastasis or obstruction by tumor, adverse effects of therapy, vascular abnormalities, primary fluid and electrolyte disturbances, and infection can mimic paraneoplasia. In addition, the degree of expression of paraneoplastic symptoms may be unrelated to the total bulk of the primary tumor, and may either precede the diagnosis of malignancy, occur later in the clinical course, or be the first sign of recurrence. Hence, a high index of suspicion and exclusion of other diagnostic possibilities are essential when evaluating patients with lung cancer who may have a paraneoplastic process.

Although recent advances in immunobiology and cytogenetics have provided insight into the potential mechanisms of paraneoplasia, many of the phenomena remain poorly understood. In the 1970s, Nathanson and Hall (91) discussed potential mechanisms of paraneoplasia that included: (*a*) embryogenic derepression in tumor cells resulting in the production of various hormones and either stimulatory or inhibitory polypeptides; (*b*) antigen-antibody interactions with antigenic products released by tumor cells or during cellular breakdown; and (*c*) neurovascular reflexes. The hormonal and autoimmune mechanisms for paraneoplastic disorders have been characterized further (92–96). The recognition of a paraneoplastic syndrome may result in earlier diagnosis and treatment of the underlying lung cancer, and in some cases, alleviation of the remote effects (93, 95).

SYSTEMIC DISORDERS

Constitutional symptoms such as weight loss resulting from anorexia and cachexia, fever, and generalized malaise occur in at least 20% of patients with bronchogenic carcinoma (14). The etiologic factors remain elusive, but cytokines such as tumor necrosis factor, interleukin-1, and prostaglandins may be involved in addition to local tumor effects (97). Anemia, infection (most commonly postobstructive pneumonitis), malnutrition, fluid and electrolyte disturbances, and adverse drug effects should also be excluded before attributing the symptoms to a primary paraneoplastic process. Placebo-controlled trials confirm the beneficial effect of megestrol acetate in some patients with cancer anorexia and cachexia (98).

Orthostatic hypotension sometimes occurs on the basis of paraneoplastic autoimmunity (99). Rheumatologic disorders, such as hypertrophic pulmonary osteoarthropathy (HPO), dermatomyositis, polymyositis, and rarely systemic lupus erythematosus, have also been associated with pulmonary neoplasia (100, 101). Other uncommon systemic paraneoplastic disorders associated with lung cancer are marantic endocarditis, lactic acidosis, hypouricemia, and several cutaneous conditions listed in Table 12.5 (101–104).

CUTANEOUS PARANEOPLASIA

Table 12.5 lists several cutaneous syndromes reported with intrathoracic malignancy. The pathophysiologic mechanisms of these disorders are currently unknown. Digital clubbing is a favorite sign for bedside teaching in pulmonary medicine. It may occur in hereditary, nonpulmonary and pulmonary disorders, including bronchogenic carcinoma (105). Neurogenic (vagally mediated), hormonal (high estrogen or growth hormone), and vascular (arteriovenous shunting with local tissue hypoxia) mechanisms have been proposed for clubbing and HPO (106).

Clubbing refers to the soft-tissue subungual thickening that most commonly involves the fingernails and is usually asymptomatic. HPO is an uncommon entity characterized by a painful symmetric arthropathy

TABLE 12.5. Paraneoplastic Syndromes Associated with Lung Cancer

Systemic	Endocrine or metabolic	Hematologic
Anorexia, cachexia, weight loss[a]	Cushing's syndrome[a]	Anemia[a]/polycythemia
Fever	Hypercalcemia[a]	Hypercoagulability
Orthostatic hypotension	Hyponatremia[a]	Thrombocytopenic purpura
Nonbacterial thrombotic endocarditis	Hyperglycemia	Dysproteinemia (including amyloidosis)
Dermatomyositis/polymyositis	Hypertension	Leukocytosis/leukoerythroblastic reaction
Systemic lupus erythematosus	Acromegaly	Eosinophilia
Cutaneous	Hyperthyroidism	**Neurologic**
Acquired hypertrichosis lanuginosa	Hypercalcitoninemia	Peripheral neuropathy[a]
Bazex's syndrome (acrokeratosis)	Gynecomastia	Lambert-Eaton myasthenic syndrome[a]
Clubbing[a]	Galactorrhea	Necrotizing myelopathy
Dermatomyositis[a]	Carcinoid syndrome	Cerebral encephalopathy
Erythema gyratum repens	Hypoglycemia	Visual loss
Exfoliative dermatitis (erythroderma)	Hypophosphatemia	Necrotizing myelopathy
Hypertrophic pulmonary osteoarthropathy	Lactic acidosis	Visceral neuropathy
Superficial thrombophlebitis	Hypouricemia	**Renal**
Tripe palms	Hyperamylasemia	Glomerulopathies
Acanthosis nigricans		Tubulointerstitial disorders
Acquired ichthyosis		
Acquired palmoplantar keratoderma		
Dermatitis herpetiformis		
Erythema annulare centrifugum		
Extramammary Paget's disease		
Florid cutaneous papillomatosis		
Pemphigus vulgaris		
Pityriasis rotunda		
Pruritus		
Sign of Leser-Trelat		
Sweet's syndrome		
Vasculitis		

Modified from Patel AM, Davila DG, Peters SG. Paraneoplastic syndromes associated with lung cancer. Mayo Clin Proc 1993;68:278–287.
[a]Indicates the more common paraneoplastic syndromes associated with bronchogenic carcinoma.

(usually of the ankles, wrists, and knees), proliferative periostitis (usually of the long bones), and possibly neurovascular changes of the hands and feet. HPO is often, but not always, accompanied by clubbing. Nail changes and joint symptoms of HPO may precede pulmonary symptoms resulting in consultations with a chiropractor, orthopedist, or rheumatologist before the diagnosis of lung cancer is suspected or made. Radiographic changes involve characteristic periosteal thickening of the long bones with soft tissue swelling. A technetium-99m (^{99m}Tc) phosphonate bone scan typically demonstrates marked uptake of radioactive material in the areas of periostitis (Fig. 12.2A). Bronchogenic carcinoma, most commonly large cell or adenocarcinoma, accounts for more than 80% of HPO in adults (107). In a review of 1879 patients undergoing thoracotomy for lung lesions, 5% of the patients with primary lung cancer and HPO had small cell histology (107).

ENDOCRINE PARANEOPLASIA

Excess "ectopic" cortisol production, hypercalcemia, and syndromes of inappropriate antidiuretic hormone release are the most common paraneoplastic endocrine manifestations associated with lung cancer. Other endocrine disorders associated with bronchogenic carcinoma have been reported but are much less common (Table 12.5). Several mechanisms have been proposed to explain the paraneoplastic release of peptide hormones from lung tumors and other malignancies. Gene derepression and hypomethylation, cellular dedifferentiation, migration of hormone-secreting amine precursor uptake, and decarboxylating (APUD) cells to the lung, and dys-differentiation of transformed cells are theories that only partly account for these phenomena (96, 108–112). In addition, recent data suggest that normal lung is capable of synthesizing proopiomelanocortin (POM) (3), a precursor for adrenocorticotropin (ACTH), albeit in minimal amounts (112, 113). Thus, enhanced expression of baseline production is another mechanism for "ectopic or inappropriate" hormonal syndromes (113). Many other potential mediators released from lung tumors that contribute to paraneoplastic endocrine phenomena have been reported and warrant further study (114–122).

Criteria for attributing an elevated hormone level

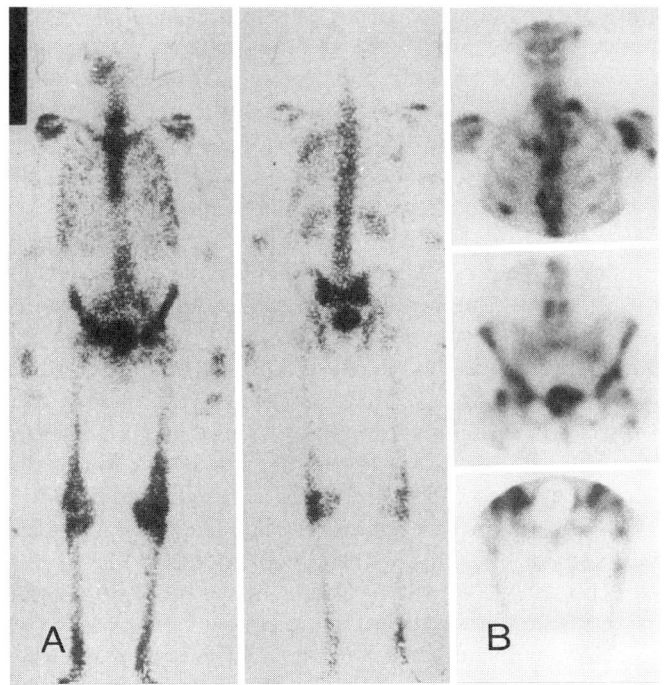

FIGURE 12.2. A. Radioisotope bone scan demonstrating increased uptake in regions of periostitis in a patient with hypertrophic pulmonary osteoarthropathy. B. Contrast Figure 12.2A with the radioisotope uptake pattern in a patient with bony metastases from lung cancer.

to paraneoplasia include: (a) temporal correlation of the serum concentration of the hormone with a change in tumor size, i.e., increased concentration associated with increased tumor burden or decreased serum concentrations with tumor excision or regression; (b) an elevated pulmonary venous to arterial concentration gradient of the hormone and increased hormone concentrations in the tumor by comparison with adjacent uninvolved lung tissue; and (c) ability of the tumor cells to synthesize and secrete a relevant protein product (112). The extent of evaluation for the source of the excess hormone level is, in practice, usually dictated by the severity of symptoms, degree of metabolic derangement, tumor type, stage of disease, and treatment plans.

CUSHING'S SYNDROME

Cushing's syndrome is caused by the chronic effects of an excess of glucocorticoid hormone. It was originally described in patients with pituitary adenomas (Cushing's disease) that were secreting ACTH. The classic signs and symptoms include truncal obesity, cutaneous striae, moon facies, buffalo hump, proximal myopathy and weakness, osteoporosis, diabetes mellitus, hypertension, and personality changes (123).

Many lung carcinomas contain proopiomelanocortin (POMC) polypeptide, and increased serum levels of ACTH may be detectable in up to 50% of patients with lung cancer (124). Other neoplastic sources of ACTH include thymic, neural crest, and carcinoid tumors (114, 125). Small cell lung cancer (SCLC) may have the greatest enzymatic ability to process the POMC polypeptide into its bioactive components, yet only about 1% to 5% of patients with SCLC develop signs and symptoms of Cushing's syndrome (126–128). This limited clinical expression is due partly to the rapid evolution of SCLC, and the release of a biologically inactive form of the hormone. In contrast, bronchial carcinoid tumors are the most common ectopic cause of Cushing's syndrome, comprising 28% to 38% of cases in two recent series (129, 130). In addition to ACTH and POMC, corticotropin-releasing hormone production by lung tumors may also result in excess cortisol secretion (115).

Approximately 15% to 20% of cases of Cushing's syndrome result from ectopic ACTH/corticotropin-releasing hormone production, most commonly by small cell cancer or bronchial carcinoid (123, 125, 129, 130). Patients with ectopic Cushing's syndrome typically have a rapid onset of symptoms and progressive course, although some have a more gradual onset resembling pituitary dependent Cushing's syndrome (123). With the more rapid growing small cell lung cancer, patients often do not have the classic signs and symptoms. In these cases weight loss, edema, proximal myopathy, and hypertension are the prominent features. Hypokalemic alkalosis and glucose intolerance are usually present. This difference in presentation may be the result of the rapid growth of the malignancy, relatively high levels of ACTH, and the fact that patients may not live long enough to develop the more classic features of the syndrome.

Screening for ectopic hypercortisolism may be done by assessing 24-hour urine free cortisol levels or response to overnight dexamethasone (1 mg) suppression. If these are elevated, further testing for suppressibility using high-dose dexamethasone (2 mg every 6 hours for eight doses) and plasma ACTH levels are necessary (130–132). Although the majority of lung cancer patients with ectopic Cushing's syndrome do not suppress cortisol and ACTH production with the high-dose dexamethasone test, pulmonary carcinoid tumors suppress approximately half the time (125, 131, 133). Because approximately 15% to 30% of patients with pituitary dependent Cushing's syndrome also fail to suppress with the high-dose dexamethasone test, caution must be taken when assigning the tissue source of the hormones (114, 131). Recently, assays for differentially processed hormone fragments by tumor tissue have been advocated in determining the source of the POMC (134).

If tumor removal is not possible, treatment of the excess cortisol production is dictated by the clinical condition and prognosis of the patient. Adrenal inhibitors such as aminoglutethimide, metyrapone, or more recently ketoconazole have been advocated for symptomatic relief (135–137). Ketoconazole blocks corticosteroid production by inhibition of cholesterol side-chain cleavage, 17-hydroxylase and 11-hydroxylase (138). The usual dose is 300 to 400 mg twice a day (137–139). Treatment may be associated with a rapid decrease in cortisol production, and acute hypoadrenalism has been reported to occur within 1 to 2 weeks on occasion. Therefore, after the initial treatment with higher dose (800 mg/day), the dose should be lowered to maintain normal cortisol levels (123, 137, 139). Patients on ketoconazole should be monitored for liver enzyme abnormalities. The use of RU486, octreotide (a somatostatin analogue) (140), selective adrenal arterial embolization (141), and bilateral adrenalectomy, alone or in combination, have also been suggested. The latter option may be the best treatment for the incurable patient who has a 1- to 2-year prognosis. A reduced hormone level following treatment of the tumor by surgery, chemotherapy, and/or radiation serves both diagnostic and therapeutic purposes. However, Shepherd et al. (142) reported that patients with SCLC and associated Cushing's syndrome have a reduced survival (median survival, 3.6 months) despite chemotherapy. This was thought to result from their higher frequency of infections secondary to the excessive corticosteroid secretion.

Hypercalcemia

The most common malignancies associated with hypercalcemia are tumors of lung, kidney, breast, head and neck, and hematologic malignancies such as myeloma and lymphoma (143–146). Hypercalcemia associated with lung cancer was thought to result from direct invasion of bone by tumor cells, or from tumor-secreted hormones, if bone involvement was absent. However, clinical and molecular findings challenge these assumptions (143, 147–150). First, bone involvement is found more often with SCLC, yet the incidence of hypercalcemia is less common than in the non–small cell subtypes. Squamous cell carcinoma is the cell type most frequently associated with hypercalcemia (144). Second, although humoral mechanisms of hypercalcemia are likely in cases without metastases to bone, similar mechanisms may also be operative in cases with bone involvement. Recent identification and cloning of a parathyroid hormone–related peptide (PTHrP) in hypercalcemic patients with lung cancer, including those with bony metastases, has been accomplished (151–155). The PTHrP molecule has many properties that are similar to PTH, including increasing bone resorption, renal tubular calcium reabsorption, renal phosphorous excretion, and urinary cyclic adenosine monophosphate excretion, but other functions differ (156). PTHrP messenger ribonucleic acid (mRNA) is also found in many nonneoplastic tissues, but normal circulating levels are lower than those observed in humoral hypercalcemia of malignancy (157). In addition, other mediators, such as prostaglandins and various cytokines, have been implicated in hypercalcemia associated with lung cancer (148, 158). Some of these factors may not be synthesized directly and released from lung tumor cells, but rather may originate from stimulated immune cells of the host (159).

Hypercalcemia normally results in suppression of parathyroid hormone secretion; however, PTHrP and similar cytokines are secreted autonomously by the tumor. These parathyroid hormone-related proteins cause renal calcium reabsorption and impair the normal renal defense mechanism (calciuria against hypercalcemia). Additionally, hypercalcemia interferes with the renal mechanisms for reabsorption of sodium and water, thus resulting in polyuria. The polyuria may not be matched by adequate fluid intake because of nausea, vomiting, and other gastrointestinal symptoms and may lead to dehydration. Dehydration decreases glomerular filtration and further aggravates the hypercalcemia.

Hypercalcemia in lung cancer patients should be suspected if symptoms of anorexia, nausea, vomiting, abdominal pain, weakness, lethargy, and constipation are present. Confusion and coma, renal failure, and nephrocalcinosis are late manifestations associated with marked hypercalcemia. Cardiovascular effects include shortened QT interval, broadened T wave, heart block, ventricular arrhythmias, and asystole. The diagnostic approach to hypercalcemia in lung cancer involves confirming an elevated serum ionized calcium concentration (or disproportionate increase in serum calcium relative to the serum albumin), normal or reduced serum phosphate level, and exclusion of other causes of hypercalcemia such as primary hyperparathyroidism (elevated immunoreactive PTH level) and drug-related hypercalcemia (e.g., thiazide diuretics). Metastases to bone may produce an elevated bone fraction of the serum alkaline phosphatase concentration and abnormal bone radiographs or bone scan results. A PTHrP level may be increased in blood and/or tumor tissue in patients with hypercalcemia associated with lung cancer (with or without bone invasion), but the sensitivity of current radioimmunoassays are only about 50% (154).

Mild elevation of the serum calcium may not require treatment, and the decision to treat should be based on the patient's symptoms. For patients with widely metastatic and incurable malignancy, it may be most appropriate to give supportive care only without specific therapy for the hypercalcemia. Otherwise, most individuals with serum calcium values of at least 12 to 13 mg/dL should be treated. The four basic goals of treatment of hypercalcemia are: (*a*) correct dehydration; (*b*) increase renal excretion of calcium; (*c*) inhibit bone resorption; and (*d*) treat the underlying malignancy (143). Initial treatment should be with intravenous normal saline using 3 to 6 L per 24 hours while monitoring carefully for volume overload. The next step after the patient has been rehydrated is to add a diuretic, which increases calcium excretion. Loop diuretics, such as furosemide and ethacrynic acid, are best (145, 160, 161). Thiazides should not be used because they increase calcium resorption in the distal tubule.

Second-line therapy has until recently involved such agents as calcitonin and/or mithramycin with varying degrees of success and toxicity (161–163). However, because the primary mechanism of hypercalcemia in lung cancer is now considered to be increased bone resorption, agents that specifically inhibit this process are probably most important. The bisphosphonates, etidronate and pamidronate, have shown efficacy in studies of lung cancer patients with and without evidence of bony metastases (143, 164–167). The bisphosphonates bind to bone and inhibit resorption. These compounds have poor gastrointestinal absorption and are best used intravenously. Etidronate is generally given as a 2- to 4-hour infusion over 3 to 5 days. Pamidronate is most commonly given as a single 24-hour infusion and normalizes the serum calcium in at least 70% of patients. In a randomized trial comparing pamidronate and etidronate, Gucalp and associates (167) achieved normal serum calcium levels within the first week in 70% and 40% of patients, respectively. The duration of normocalcemia was greater for pamidronate with a median of 7 days (range, 1 to 31 days). There was no difference in response in those with or without bony metastasis. Adverse effects are generally mild and transient, but bone pain and fever may occur. Asymptomatic hypocalcemia occurred in 5% to 10% or patients treated by Gucalp and coworkers (167).

A newer agent, gallium nitrate, also inhibits bone resorption and has the ability to lower serum calcium regardless of whether bony involvement is present, and in both epithelial and nonepithelial-derived tumors (168–170). This latter experience has not always been the case with conventional therapy nor with bisphosphate administration (169, 171). In a randomized control trial of gallium nitrate versus etidronate for hypercalcemia patients, gallium therapy was superior for normalization of serum calcium (82% versus 43%) (170). Normocalcemia was maintained for a median of 8 days (range, 0–54+) in the patients treated with gallium versus zero days (range, 0–23+) following etidronate therapy. The main drawbacks of gallium use are the need to treat patients for 5 days with a continuous infusion of the drug and potential nephrotoxicity.

Calcitonin inhibits bone resorption, increases renal calcium excretion, and has a rapid onset of action. However, it is a relatively weak agent, and when used alone does not usually normalize the serum calcium of patients with marked hypercalcemia (143). The duration of action is short lived. The most common indication for calcitonin may be when there is an urgent need for lowering the calcium (12 to 24 hours) while waiting for the greater effects of the slower acting agents. An additional benefit may be the relief of pain in some patients with skeletal metastasis.

In general, patients with lung cancer and hypercalcemia, resulting either from metastasis or secretion of a parathyroid hormone-related protein or other hypercalcemic factor, do not respond satisfactorily to corticosteroids. Our initial approach is to rehydrate the patient adequately and induce calcium diuresis with loop diuretics. If additional treatment is needed, they are then treated with a 24-hour infusion of pamidronate. Plicamycin is a less common alternative to pamidronate if there are no contraindications to its use. When rapidity of onset of action is important (severe hypercalcemia), then calcitonin is the first drug of choice while waiting for the onset of action of more potent hypocalcemic agents. The development of specific parathyroid hormone receptor antagonists may also provide better long-term control of hypercalcemia in these patients, but further studies are necessary.

The prognosis in patients with hypercalcemia associated with lung cancer is poor. The hypercalcemia usually indicates a large tumor burden (often squamous cell histology) and is seldom associated with resectable disease (145, 160, 172). The median survival in patients with hypercalcemia and no further treatment of the underlying malignancy was 30 to 45 days in two recent series (145, 160).

SYNDROME OF INAPPROPRIATE ANTIDIURETIC HORMONE RELEASE

Ectopic production of antidiuretic hormone (ADH) or arginine vasopressin is most commonly associated with SCLC. The syndrome of inappropriate antidiuretic hormone release (SIADH) has also been documented in nonmalignant pulmonary conditions (173–177). Although 50% to 75% of patients with SCLC have elevated ADH levels, only 1% to 5% of patients develop symptoms attributed to SIADH (120, 121, 175, 178–180). In addition, some patients with SCLC and normal arginine vasopressin levels have elevated levels of atrial natriuretic factor, suggesting alternate mechanisms for deranged sodium homeostasis (121, 181, 182). Other malignancies associated with SIADH include bronchial carcinoid, esophagus, duodenum, pancreas, bladder, head and neck, lymphoma, and thymoma. Additionally, nonmalignant conditions including pulmonary disease (usually infections); central nervous system disorders such as head trauma, space-occupying lesions, and cerebrovascular accidents; and drugs have been associated with SIADH. Drugs most commonly associated with SIADH include chlorpropamide, carbamazepine, tricyclic antidepressants, thiazide diuretics, morphine, cyclophosphamide, and vincristine.

Patients, especially those with known lung cancer, exhibiting symptoms of confusion, unexplained seizures, or a decreased level of consciousness or coma should be evaluated for hyponatremia. Symptoms appear to relate to the rapidity of change in the serum sodium rather than the absolute serum sodium value (183). The usual diagnostic criteria for SIADH include: (*a*) hyponatremia associated with serum hypo-osmolality (less than 275 mOsm/kg); (*b*) inappropriately elevated urine osmolality (more than 200 mOsm/kg) relative to serum osmolality; (*c*) elevated urine sodium (more than 20 mEq/L); (*d*) clinical euvolemia without edema; and (*e*) normal renal (serum creatinine, less than 1.5 mg/dL), and adrenal and thyroid function. The serum uric acid is usually but not always low, and the urine osmolality to serum osmolality ratio is frequently more than 2. Other etiologies of hyponatremia to be excluded are decreased solute intake; renal, adrenal, or thyroid disease; congestive heart failure; cirrhosis; and drug effects. Hyponatremia is not always found in patients with elevated ADH levels and impaired urine concentrating capacities (176, 179). Inappropriate thirst, in addition to high ADH levels, can also contribute to hyponatremia.

Treatment of this disorder depends on the severity of symptoms and includes fluid restriction, enhancing free water excretion, and, when possible, treatment of the underlying malignancy (180, 184). Other recommended treatment strategies include demeclocycline and possibly, lithium carbonate in refractory cases (185–188). List et al. (180) reviewed 350 cases of SCLC seen over 5 years and noted that 40 (11%) met a strict definition of SIADH similar to that outlined above. There was no difference in frequency of SIADH in patients with limited or extensive stage disease. Of the 40 patients with SIADH, 33 had the syndrome at initial presentation. The serum sodium normalized within 3 weeks of initiation of chemotherapy in 80% of patients and in 88% by 6 weeks. The presence of SIADH did not affect the response to chemotherapy or overall survival when compared with a group matched for stage of disease. Eventually, SIADH recurred in 22 of 31 patients who experienced disease relapse after an initial response to chemotherapy. In general, the serum levels of arginine vasopressin correlated with the clinical syndrome, response to therapy, and relapse of disease. In patients with mild or no symptoms, fluid restriction of 500 to 1000 mL per 24 hours is the initial treatment of choice (184). Demeclocycline (900 to 1200 mg/day) induces a dose dependent nephrogenic diabetes insipidus and blocks the action of antidiuretic hormone on the renal tubule. The onset of action varies from a few hours to a few weeks, thus it is not recommended in the acute treatment of severe hyponatremia. Adverse effects include skin photosensitivity, nephrotoxicity, and gastrointestinal upset. Relative contraindications include chronic renal failure, liver disease, and congestive heart failure because demeclocycline is excreted in the urine and the bile. Lithium has also been used for treatment of SIADH, but its effects on the kidney are inconsistent, and it is associated with frequent side effects related to the digestive, cardiac, thyroid, and central nervous systems. Accordingly, demeclocycline is the preferred treatment (187).

In patients with more severe or life-threatening symptoms related to hyponatremia (serum sodium, less than 115 mEq/L) treatment consists of intravenous fluids with 0.9% saline with supplemental potassium and diuresis with a loop diuretic such as intravenous furosemide (183). Rarely, 300 mL of 3% saline given over 3 to 4 hours may be necessary in combination with furosemide (189, 190). Saline without diuretic is not ultimately effective in raising the sodium concentration. Patients with minimal or no symptoms should not have rapid correction of the sodium concentration. The rate of correction of the sodium is best limited to 2 mEq/L/hour or a maximum of 20 mEq/L/day to a serum concentration of 120 to 130 mEq/L (189–193). More rapid correction has been associated with development of central pontine myelinolysis, which results in flaccid quadriplegia, cranial nerve abnormalities manifesting as pseudobulbar palsy, alteration in mental status, and subsequent death (191, 192).

HEMATOLOGIC SYNDROMES

Anemia occurs in approximately 20% of patients with bronchogenic carcinoma (14). Anemia may be caused by chronic disease, iron deficiency, cytoreductive effects of chemotherapy, hemolysis, bone marrow infiltration, or red cell aplasia (194). Disturbances in other bone marrow elements attributed to a possible paraneoplastic syndrome from lung cancer include eosinophilia or leukocytosis with either leukemoid or leukoerythroblastic reaction on peripheral blood smear examination (195).

Lung cancer has been implicated in altered coagulation, resulting in thrombotic and hemorrhagic diatheses. Trousseau (196) alluded to the potential association of venous thrombosis and malignancy in 1865. Potential mechanisms involved in hypercoagulability are incompletely understood and include platelet activation, thrombocytosis, release of procoagulant substances by the tumor cell or from monocyte-macrophage stimulation, and dysfibrinogenemia (197–199).

There may be an increased incidence of malignancy associated with thrombotic episodes such as deep venous thrombosis (DVT) and pulmonary embolism (200–203). A recent prospective report by Prandoni and associates (200) demonstrated that patients with idiopathic DVT have an increased risk of subsequent overt malignant disease. During a 2-year observation period, the incidence of newly diagnosed cancer was 1.9% in patients with secondary DVT (predisposing factor such as recent surgery, trauma, or immobilization), 7.6% in patients with idiopathic DVT, and 17.1% in patients with recurrent idiopathic DVT (200). The extent of investigations performed to search for an occult malignancy in patients with idiopathic deep venous thromboembolism is debatable (201, 202). Further evaluation appears most useful for patients with unusual types of thromboses, e.g., migratory thrombophlebitis, Budd-Chiari syndrome, upper extremity DVT, major cerebral vessel thrombosis, nonbacterial thrombotic endocarditis (NBTE), or disseminated intravascular coagulation (198).

Recurrent DVT or pulmonary emboli may occur despite therapeutic doses of coumarin. In these circumstances, alternative therapeutic options include subcutaneous heparin with or without the placement of an inferior vena cava filter, or occasionally, thrombolytic agents (only in severe, acute cases) (198). In contrast to thrombotic events, bleeding episodes unrelated to direct tumor involvement may result from thrombocytopenia, DIC, dysproteinemias, or amyloidosis.

The association of NBTE and malignancy is well documented (102, 204, 205). NBTE is generally defined as vegetations on the heart valves or wall that contain fibrin and platelets, but without evidence of infection. Whereas NBTE was previously considered an incidental finding at autopsy, it is now clearly recognized as a significant cause of morbidity and mortality. In an autopsy series from Memorial Hospital (102), NBTE was identified in 75 patients from 7840 postmortem examinations. The incidence of NBTE was highest in patients with lung cancer and occurred in 7.7% of bronchiolar and 7.1% of adenocarcinomas of the lung. In a review of cerebrovascular complications in patients with cancer, Graus and colleagues (205) observed cerebral embolic infarction in 42 of 86 patients with pathologically documented NBTE and careful autopsy examination of the brain. Non–small cell lung cancer (NSCLC) was the most common malignancy in this group. Cerebral infarction was symptomatic in 32 (76%) of these individuals antemortem and was associated with clinical evidence of other systemic emboli in 19 patients (205).

NEUROLOGIC SYNDROMES

A variety of neurologic syndromes have been associated with lung cancer and are thought to occur through autoimmune mechanisms (Table 12.5) (92, 94, 206, 207). Small cell carcinoma is the most common type of lung cancer associated with paraneoplastic autoimmune neurologic syndromes. Symptoms may precede the diagnosis of the lung cancer by many months or may be the first sign of tumor recurrence. Direct metastatic effects, or metabolic or infectious processes contributing to the neurologic findings, must be excluded. The severity of the neurologic symptoms is unrelated to tumor bulk; in fact, a primary malignancy may be undetected antemortem despite disabling symptoms (208).

SUBACUTE PERIPHERAL NEUROPATHY

Subacute sensory neuropathy is the most characteristic peripheral neuropathy associated with small cell carcinoma of the lung. Symptoms may precede the diagnosis of SCLC by several months (209). Type I antineuronal nuclear antibody (ANNA-1) and anti-Hu antibodies have been described recently (99, 206, 209–211). These two antibodies are thought to be the same in that they both are directed against nuclei. The Hu antigen and the antigen for ANNA-I are expressed in both SCLC and neuronal tissue. The ANNA-I is distinguished from the antinuclear antibodies found in immune disorders such as systemic lupus erythematosus by the selective binding to neuronal elements (99). The anti-Hu antibody is defined more specifically in that it has also been shown to identify a protein of 35 to 40 kDa molecular mass on Western blot tests of cerebral cortex neurons (211). The ANNA-I binds to the nucleus and cytoplasm, but not to the nucleolus of virtually all neurons in the central and peripheral nervous system, including sensory and autonomic ganglia, myenteric plexus, and cells of the adrenal medulla (99). ANNA-I or anti-Hu antibodies should not be confused with the anti-Purkinje cell cytoplasmic antibody or anti-Yo antibodies that are more characteristically found in patients with subacute cerebellar degeneration as a manifestation of gynecologic or breast carcinoma (99, 208, 212, 213). The ANNA-I and anti-Hu antibody are present both in the serum and spinal fluid of patients with sensory neuropathy and/or encephalomyelitis and SCLC. It is thought to be very uncommon for a patient with SCLC and the previously described neurologic findings to have no autoantibody. Approximately 15% of patients with SCLC and no paraneoplastic manifestations may have an ANNA-I or anti-Hu antibody, but it is usually at a lower titer than that observed in individuals with paraneoplastic syndromes (211).

It is uncertain how frequently the ANNA-I antibody occurs in patients with NSCLC with or without neurologic paraneoplastic syndromes. Curiously, the ANNA-I antibody may present months or years before the diagnosis of lung cancer. In a patient with the appropriate neurologic findings, positive ANNA-I and significant smoking history, a diligent diagnostic evaluation should be undertaken. The most helpful diagnostic test is probably the CT or MRI of the chest with careful attention to mediastinal or hilar nodes. The abnormality may occasionally be very subtle. Random bone marrow evaluation is not indicated, because most of these patients have limited stage disease (214). The immunocytochemical pattern of nuclear staining differentiates ANNA-1 from the anti-Purkinje cell antibodies found in patients with paraneoplastic cerebellar degeneration associated with ovarian and breast carcinomas (99, 208). Kimmel and colleagues (209) recommend serologic testing for ANNA-1 in any middle-aged or elderly patient with a peripheral sensory neuropathy of indeterminate cause (particularly in smokers) and, if detected, careful investigation for an occult cancer.

It has been suggested that patients with neurologic paraneoplastic syndromes and SCLC may have a better prognosis than those without paraneoplastic syndromes (214, 215). In one recent series, 95% of patients with paraneoplastic syndromes, anti-Hu antibodies, and SCLC were found to have limited stage disease (214). Whether the better prognosis is related to the autoimmune phenomenon or just to the early stage disease is a moot point. In a report of three patients with long-term survival, it was suggested that that the antitumor immune response may be responsible for the unusually long survival of these patients (215). Regression of the neurologic syndromes may occur after the treatment of SCLC but is not the rule. Ideally, the SCLC should be diagnosed and treated expeditiously in an effort to prevent further neurologic deterioration.

Lambert-Eaton Myasthenic Syndrome

The association between a myasthenic disorder and lung cancer was first described in 1953 (216). Definitive electrophysiologic distinction between Lambert-Eaton myasthenic syndrome (LEMS) and myasthenia gravis was made by Lambert and colleagues (217, 218). The syndrome is characterized by proximal muscle weakness with a postexertional facilitation in strength, hyporeflexia, and autonomic dysfunction. Symptoms are most pronounced in the pelvic girdle and thigh muscles, although dysarthria, dysphagia, diplopia, or ptosis may occur. Electromyography characteristically shows a reduced amplitude of the compound muscle action potential that enhances immediately after 10 to 15 seconds of maximal voluntary contraction, or during high-frequency nerve stimulation (e.g., 30 Hz). Approximately 50% of patients with LEMS have a malignancy, with small cell carcinoma of the lung being the most common (219, 220). The manifestations of LEMS may occur as long as 2 to 4 years before the diagnosis of SCLC. Other malignancies that have been found with LEMS include systemic mastocytosis, endometrial cancer, colon cancer, mixed parotid tumor, and renal cell carcinoma (219, 220).

The pathophysiology of LEMS has been delineated in part. The defect in neuromuscular transmission is caused by antibody-mediated impairment of the presynaptic neuronal calcium channel activity, which impairs the nerve–stimulus-induced release of acetylcholine (220). The production of anticalcium channel antibodies reflects an autoimmune response to voltage-gated calcium channels expressed by the cancer cells. These tumor ionic channels appear to be related antigenically to calcium channels at the motor nerve terminals (219). The stimulus is unknown for the 40% to 50% of cases without evidence of cancer.

Lennon and Lambert (220, 221) have described a radioimmunoassay for detecting antibodies that react with calcium channel components extracted from small cell lung carcinoma. This assay is most useful as a diagnostic tool for LEMS in symptomatic patients with characteristic weakness; 75% of patients with a proven primary lung cancer are seropositive, and 43% of patients without evidence of lung cancer are seropositive (220). Approximately 10% of patients with SCLC without evidence of LEMS are seropositive in this test (V. A. Lennon, unpublished observation). Current therapeutic options, in addition to treatment of any associated malignancy, include use of 3,4-diaminopyridine, an agent that enhances acetylcholine release from the nerve terminal; plasmapheresis; anticholinesterases (adjuvant therapy); and immunosuppressive agents such as corticosteroids and azathioprine (223, 224). Guanidine hydrochloride and 4-aminopyridine are no longer recommended because of toxicity.

INTESTINAL DYSMOTILITIES

Chronic intestinal pseudo-obstruction usually presents with nausea, vomiting, early satiety, abdominal discomfort, weight loss, and altered bowel habits caused by abnormal gastrointestinal motility. The association of chronic intestinal pseudo-obstruction and malignancy was first reported by Ogilvie in 1948 (225). Subsequently, several investigators reported cases associated with small cell carcinoma of the lung (226–228). In a retrospective study of five patients with intestinal pseudo-obstruction associated with SCLC, Lennon and colleagues (228) found that four patients had serum antibodies to myenteric and submucosal neural plexuses of the jejunum and stomach. These are in fact antibodies of ANNA-1 specificity (99, 229). The majority of these patients continued to deteriorate symptomatically despite treatment of the underlying malignancy. Lennon and colleagues (229) recently reported finding ANNA-1 prospectively as a marker of SCLC in patients presenting with a broader spectrum of intestinal dysmotility disorders.

LIMBIC ENCEPHALITIS

The presentation of this rare entity is often dramatic with prominent mental status changes or acute psychosis (230, 231). The associated malignancy is usually SCLC, although primary malignancies of the ovary, breast, stomach, uterus, kidney, and colon have been reported also. ANNA-1 antibodies usually are detectable in patients who have limbic encephalitis with SCLC (V. A. Lennon, unpublished observation) (92, 208). There is no known effective therapy at this time.

NECROTIZING MYELOPATHY

Necrotizing myelopathy is an unusual neurologic paraneoplastic syndrome characterized by a relatively acute, rapidly ascending paraplegia that culminates in rapid deterioration and death (232). This rare entity should be considered after exclusion of other known causes of spinal cord necrosis, such as ischemic injury, complications of radiation or chemotherapy, opportunistic infections, and nutritional deficiency. ANNA-1 has also been reported with myelopathy.

VISUAL PARANEOPLASTIC SYNDROME

Rapid, binocular loss of vision is a rare paraneoplastic syndrome reported with SCLC. Antibodies to small cell carcinoma antigens in the serum and cerebrospinal fluid were immunologically cross-reactive with identical retinal antigens (233). The possible relationship or identity of this antibody to ANNA-1 has not been investigated. The prognosis for recovery of vision is poor, and no beneficial therapy is known.

RENAL PARANEOPLASIA

Carcinoma of the lung is also associated with (paraneoplastic) glomerulopathies, especially nephrotic syndrome caused by membranous nephropathy in adults (234–236).

Renal involvement may be caused by metastasis in 20% of patients with lung cancer, is usually clinically silent, and often portends a poor prognosis (95, 101, 237, 238). Approximately 10% of adults with nephrotic syndrome may have an underlying malignancy, most commonly carcinoma of the lung or gastrointestinal tract, or lymphoma (234, 239–241). Renal biopsy specimens often reveal the typical granular subepithelial deposits of immunoglobulin and complement seen in membranous nephropathy not associated with cancer (234). Several studies support an immunopathologic mechanism for lung cancer–associated nephropathy (242, 243). Antineoplastic treatment may improve renal function, and return of proteinuria may signify tumor recurrence (241, 244, 245).

Hence, the paraneoplastic syndromes associated with lung cancer are diverse and epitomize the systemic nature of human malignancy. The underlying mechanisms of paraneoplasia are multifactorial and include the excessive release of hormones or products from target organs in response to cytokines released by the tumor, the "ectopic" production of hormonelike peptides, and autoimmune phenomena. Increased understanding of these mechanisms should lead to earlier detection, i.e., initial or recurrent lung cancer diagnosis and better insight into the process of lung carcinogenesis. Until further data are available to define more markers for many of the proposed paraneoplastic disorders, physicians are left with phenomena that require exclusion of metastatic processes and other nonparaneoplastic etiologies, as well as a high index of clinical suspicion before diagnosis. Therapeutic options are aimed primarily at treating the underlying malignancy, but this action does not always improve the paraneoplastic symptoms. Pamidronate, demeclocycline, ketoconazole, and 3,4-diaminopyridine may be useful for specific paraneoplastic phenomena such as hypercalcemia, SIADH, hypercortisolemia, and LEMS, respectively. Other diagnostic and therapeutic alternatives should become available, furthering our understanding of the paraneoplastic processes.

Summary

The clinical manifestations of lung cancer are diverse. The goal of effective early detection must be the identification of asymptomatic high-risk patients. Unfortunately, most patients are symptomatic at the time of diagnosis. These presenting symptoms may result from local tumor extension, metastatic disease, or paraneoplastic phenomena, and depend partly on the specific cell type involved. The location of the tumor, rapidity of tumor growth, mode of dissemination, and the symptoms or signs produced also influence the clinical presentation. Finally, a high index of suspicion is prudent in improving the early detection of clinical manifestations associated with this common malignancy.

Staging of Lung Cancer
Non–small Cell Lung Cancer

Tumor stage, performance score, weight loss, and cell type are the most significant prognostic variables in lung cancer (246–248).Therefore, once the diagnosis of lung cancer is suspected and confirmed histologically, the extent or stage of the malignancy must be determined. A system of classifying anatomic extent of lung cancer by the status of the primary tumor (T), regional lymph nodes (N), and metastases (M) (TNM) was proposed originally in 1946 by Pierre Denoix (249). Such a systematic definition of neoplastic burden has proven successful in allowing meaningful analysis and communication concerning the assessment of diagnostic and therapeutic results. NSCLC accounts for approximately 70% to 80% of all pulmonary neoplasms. The TNM staging system has since become internationally accepted in this regard for the clinical and pathologic staging not only of NSCLC cancers, but of many other malignancies as well (250, 251).

In the 1970s, to refine the classification of lung cancer extent, the American Joint Committee on Cancer (AJCC) and other organizations proposed a staging scheme based on the TNM system (252–254). According to this classification, tumor extent was defined as stage I, II, or III disease. Stage I (operable) included patients with T1 N0 M0; T1, N1, M0; or T2, N0, M0 disease. Stage II (also operable) consisted of only T2, N1, M0 disease. All other tumors (i.e., all T3, N2, and M1 disease) constituted stage III disease, which was, by 1973 standards, inoperable. A report of 2000 cases of bronchogenic carcinoma studied by the American Task Force for Lung Cancer clearly showed that the stage of disease at presentation influenced prognosis in squamous, adenocarcinoma, and large cell lung tumors (252). In contrast, for small cell carcinoma the anatomic extent of disease as judged by this staging system was unsuccessful in predicting outcome because of the propensity for early, widespread dissemination with this cell type (252).

With further application of the 1973 AJCC staging categories, it was apparent that changes were required to improve prognostication and to determine resectability more precisely (250, 251, 255). Reclassification of patients with nodal involvement or extensive local disease, as well as the creation of a T4 category, was undertaken. The final results from several international consensus conferences involving the AJCC, Union Internationale Contre Cancer (UICC), and German and Japanese TNM committees were published by Mountain in 1986 (256). This revised system (Table 12.6; Fig. 12.3) has since been implemented widely and its clinical value reported by several investigators (257–264). Analysis of large patient series have shown the revised AJCC staging system to be a more descriptive prognostic index than the prior system for NSCLC (257, 262, 264). These studies illustrate the usefulness of this system as a consistent, accurate, clinical and surgical-pathologic staging method. Such a tool is also of paramount importance in establishing and comparing future treatment regimens in NSCLC.

The main TNM revisions were in the T3 and T4 categories for the primary tumor descriptions and the N2 and N3 categories for regional nodal spread, and a new definition for the M1 category delineating the site(s) of distant metastasis. The T3 category now refers to those patients with tumors with limited, circumscribed, extrapulmonary extension that invades either the chest wall (including superior sulcus tumors

TABLE 12.6 *TNM Staging of Non–Small Cell Lung Cancer*

PRIMARY TUMOR (T)
TX Tumor proven by presence of malignant cells in bronchopulmonary secretions but not visualized roentgenographically or bronchoscopically, or any tumor that cannot be assessed, such as in retreatment staging
T0 No evidence of primary tumor
TIS Carcinoma in situ
T1 A tumor that is not more than 3 cm in greatest dimension, surrounded by lung or visceral pleura, and without evidence of invasion proximal to a lobar bronchus at bronchoscopy[a]
T2 A tumor larger than 3 cm in greatest dimension, or a tumor of any size that either invades the visceral pleura or has associated atelectasis or obstructive pneumonitis that extends to a hilar region. At bronchoscopy, proximal extent of demonstrable tumor must be within a lobar bronchus or at least 2 cm distal to carina. Any associated atelectasis or obstructive pneumonitis must involve less than an entire lung.
T3 A tumor of any size with direct extension into the chest wall (including superior sulcus tumors), diaphragm, or mediastinal pleura or pericardium without involving the heart, great vessels, trachea, esophagus, or vertebral bodies; or a tumor in the main bronchus within 2 cm of carina without involving it
T4 A tumor of any size with invasion of the mediastinum or involvement of the heart, great vessels, trachea, esophagus, vertebral bodies, or carina; or with the presence of malignant pleural effusion[b]

NODAL INVOLVEMENT (N)
N0 No demonstrable metastatic involvement of regional lymph nodes
N1 Metastatic involvement of lymph nodes in peribronchial or ipsilateral hilar region, or both, including direct extension
N2 Metastatic involvement of ipsilateral mediastinal lymph nodes and subcarinal lymph nodes
N3 Metastatic involvement of contralateral mediastinal lymph nodes, contralateral hilar lymph nodes, or ipsilateral or contralateral scalene or supraclavicular lymph nodes

DISTANT METASTATIC INVOLVEMENT (M)
M0 No (known) distant metastatic lesion
M1 Distant metastatic involvement present; specify site(s)

TNM categories and stage grouping from Mountain CF. A new international staging system for lung cancer. Chest 1986;89:225S–233S.
[a]An uncommon superficial tumor of any size with its invasive component limited to the bronchial wall, which may extend proximal to the main bronchus, is classified as T1.
[b]Most pleural effusions associated with lung cancer are caused by tumor. In a few patients, however, cytopathologic examination of pleural fluid (on more than 1 specimen) is negative for tumor, and the fluid is not bloody and is not an exudate. In such cases in which these elements and clinical judgment dictate that the effusion is unrelated to tumor, the disease should be staged T1, T2, or T3, and the effusion should be excluded as a staging element.

TNM STAGE GROUPING

Occult carcinoma	TX	N0	M0
Stage 0	TIS	N0	M0
Stage I	T1	N0	M0
	T2	N0	M0
Stage II	T1	N1	M0
	T2	N1	M0
Stage IIIa	T3	N0	M0
	T3	N1	M0
	T1-3	N2	M0
Stage IIIb	Any T	N3	M0
	T4	Any N	M0
Stage IV	Any T	Any N	M1

without vertebral body invasion), pericardium, diaphragm, or mediastinal pleura; these tumors are generally considered resectable by current surgical techniques. In addition, the T3 category includes tumors in the main bronchus within 2 cm of the carina without involvement of the carina. Invasion of the heart, great vessels, trachea, esophagus, spine, or carina designates a T4 lesion and is currently considered unresectable. A small number of patients with tumor involvement limited to the main carina have undergone successful resection of the tumor with tracheobronchial reconstruction, suggesting a potentially salvageable subgroup in carefully selected cases (265–268). Malignant pleural effusions associated with lung cancer are also designated T4 lesion disease. However, in a few patients in whom the effusion is not judged to be related to malignancy, i.e., when pleural fluid analyses are negative for tumor and indicate nonbloody, transudative characteristics, the new staging system permits designation of such tumors as either T1, T2, or T3 without regard for the effusion. According to the current (1986) TNM classification the N1 category is restricted to involvement of intrapulmonary or ipsilateral hilar nodes, and the N2 category to ipsilateral mediastinal involvement, including subcarinal lymph nodes. The N3 descriptor to contralateral involvement of mediastinal and/or hilar nodes as well as supraclavicular and scalene nodal metastases (ipsilateral or contralateral).

As is evident from Table 12.5, combination of the TNM elements results in 19 possible subsets that can be grouped further to depict five stages of disease extent. In addition, there is a stage 0 category for in situ lung carcinoma (designated TIS) and for occult lung cancer (TX). Furthermore, the extent of hilar and mediastinal nodal involvement, intraoperatively, has been further classified in an effort to standardize the surgical-pathologic staging of primary bronchogenic carcinoma (Fig. 12.4) (269). This nomenclature, recommended by the AJCC, aims to describe the location of the lymph nodes relative to fixed structures such as the trachea, bronchi, aortic arch, and other vascular structures (269). Finally, the M1 category delineates unresectable disease due to distant metastases.

USE OF TNM SUBSETS/STAGE GROUPINGS

OCCULT CARCINOMA

Patients having malignant cells in sputum or bronchoscopic secretions without other evidence of tumor, either bronchoscopically or radiographically, are considered to have occult carcinoma (designated as TX, N0, M0), for which a stage classification is not

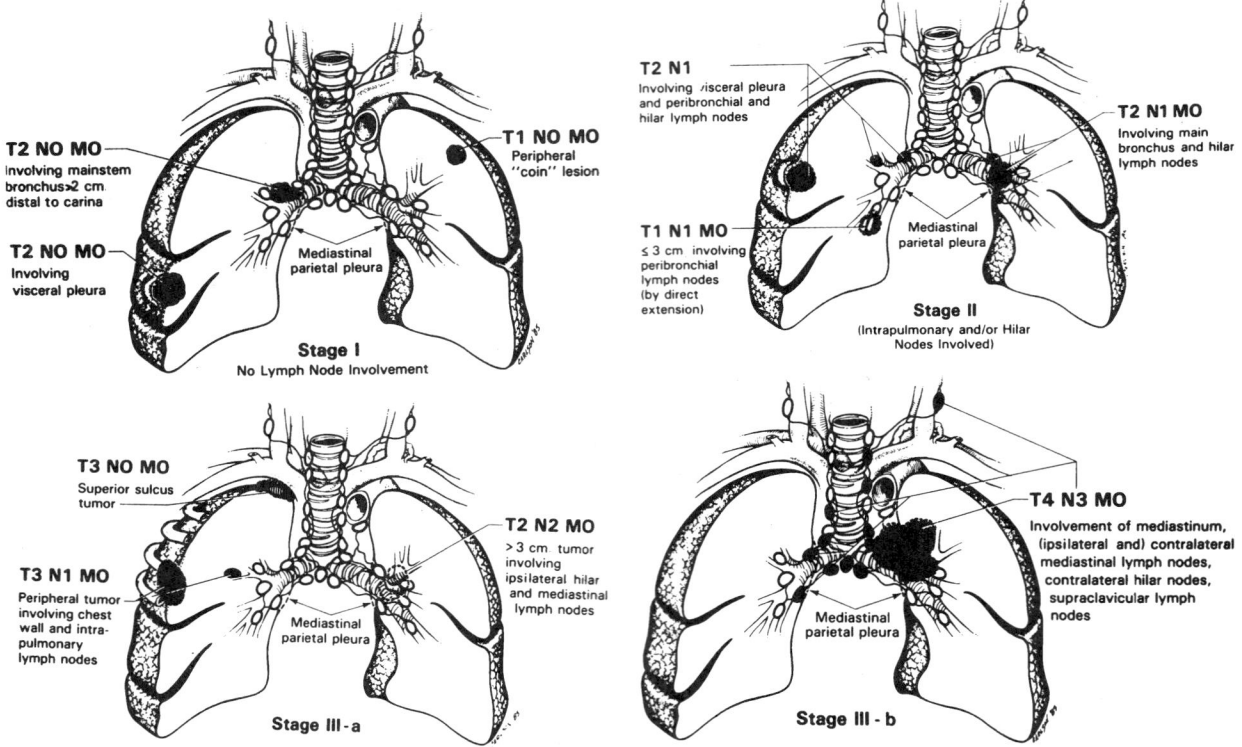

FIGURE 12.3. Stage I, II, IIIa, and IIIb disease. (From Mountain CF, Greenberg SD, Fraire AE. Tumor stage in non–small cell carcinoma of the lung. Chest 1991;99:1258–1260.)

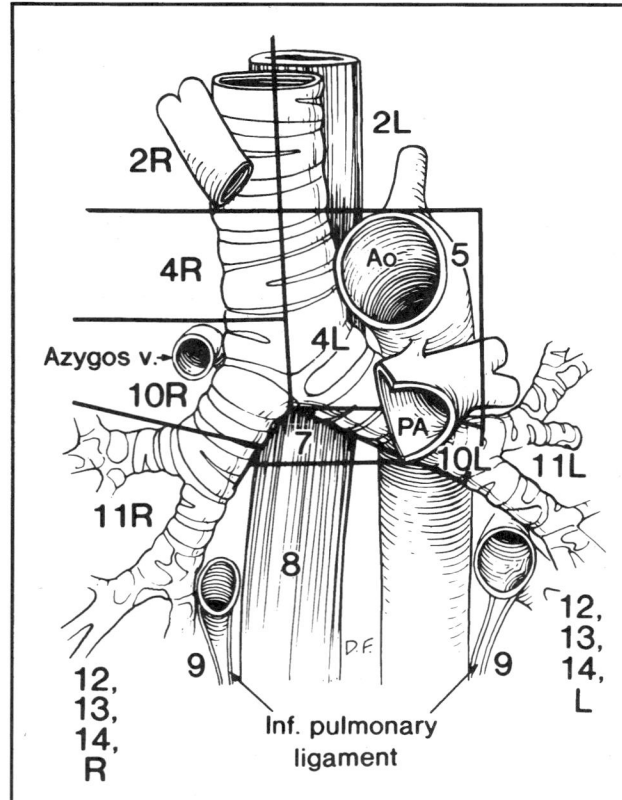

Superior Mediastinal Nodes

2R = Right upper paratracheal nodes
Between intersection of caudal margin of innominate artery with trachea and the apex of the lung (suprainnominate nodes)

2L = Left upper paratracheal nodes
Between top of aortic arch and apex of lung (supra-aortic nodes)

4R = Right lower paratracheal nodes
Between intersection of caudal margin of innominate artery with trachea and cephalic border of azygos vein

4L = Left lower paratracheal nodes
Between top of aortic arch and carina

10R = Right tracheobronchial nodes
From cephalic border of azygos vein to origin of right upper lobe bronchus

10L = Left tracheobronchial nodes
Between carina and left upper lobe bronchus (medial to ligamentum arteriosum)

Aortic Nodes

5 = Aortopulmonary nodes
Subaortic and para-aortic nodes. Lateral to the ligamentum arteriosum (proximal to first branch of left pulmonary artery)

6 = Anterior mediastinal nodes
Anterior to ascending aorta or innominate artery (not shown)

Inferior Mediastinal Nodes

7 = Subcarinal nodes
Caudal to the carina of the trachea

8 = Paraesophageal nodes
Dorsal to the posterior wall of the trachea and to the right or left of the midline of the esophagus

9 = Inferior pulmonary ligament nodes
Nodes within the pulmonary ligament

N1 Nodes

11 = Interlobar nodes
12 = Lobar nodes
13 = Segmental nodes
14 = Subsegmental nodes

FIGURE 12.4. Intraoperative staging scheme for lymph node involvement in lung cancer. (From Tisi GM, Friedman PJ, Peters RM, et al. Clinical staging of primary lung cancer. Official statement of the American Thoracic Society. Am Rev Respir Dis 1983;127:659–664.)

assigned. For patients with a positive sputum cytology and no evidence of lung cancer, an upper respiratory tract (otolaryngologic) neoplasm must be excluded.

STAGE 0

Stage 0 refers to carcinoma in situ similar to other cancers defined at this stage (TIS or carcinoma in situ).

STAGE I

In stage I, the lesion is completely contained within the lung without evidence of lymph node or other metastases (i.e., T1, N0, M0 or T2, N0, M0). Patients with stage I disease are candidates for definitive surgical treatment, and a favorable prognosis is anticipated. Naruke and coworkers (262) recently reported that patients with clinically staged (preoperative) T1, N0, M0 and T2, N0, M0 disease had 5-year postoperative survival rates of 65% and 42%, respectively. In the same study, patients with pathologically staged (postoperative) T1, N0, M0 and T2, N0, M0 disease had 5-year survival rates of 76% and 57%, respectively. Other series have also shown a survival advantage for T1, N0, M0 versus T2, N0, M0 disease (255, 270). Although not all studies concur, T1, N1, M0 disease appears to have a worse prognosis than either T1, N0, M0 or T2, N0, M0 disease, supporting the reassignment of T1, N1, M0 disease to stage II (255, 270).

STAGE II

Stage II malignancy is completely within the lung and ipsilateral intrapulmonary node(s) by either direct extension or metastasis (i.e., T1, N1, M0 or T2, N1, M0). Patients in this stage are also candidates for surgical resection. After clinical staging, Mountain (256) reported postoperative 5-year survival rates of approximately 30% for patients with stage II disease. For pathologic stage II disease, Naruke and associates (262) reported 5-year survival rates of 40%, with Williams and colleagues (255) noting a survival of 50% for pathologically staged T1, N1, M0 disease.

STAGE III

Stage III disease continues to be refined in an effort to identify those patients with extrapulmonary extension of tumor who may benefit from surgical intervention. The category has been divided further into stage IIIa (potentially resectable in some cases) and IIIb (generally regarded as unresectable) (271). Stage IIIa refers to disease with extrapulmonary tumor extension that may be associated with limited nodal involvement, specifically to the ipsilateral mediastinal and subcarinal lymph nodes (i.e., T3, N0, M0; T3, N1, M0; or T1-3, N2, M0). The anticipated overall postoperative 5-year survival rate for resected stage IIIa disease is approximately 22% (262) to 28% (272), but it may be as high as 50% for the T3, N0, M0 subset (273). Trials evaluating multimodality therapies and neoadjuvant strategies for stage IIIa disease are in progress (274). In contrast to stage IIIa, stage IIIb disease refers to extrapulmonary extension of tumor to (*a*) contralateral lymph nodes involving the hilum and/or mediastinum, (*b*) ipsilateral or contralateral supraclavicular/scalene nodes, (*c*) extensive mediastinal invasion without distant metastases (i.e., T1-3, N3, M0; T4, N1-3, M0), or (*d*) malignant pleural effusion without distant metastases (T4, N1-3, M0).

STAGE IV

Stage IV refers to metastases to distant organs or remote lymph nodes (i.e., any T or N with M1 disease). These patients are not generally considered surgical candidates.

SMALL CELL LUNG CANCER

Recent statistics suggest that SCLC accounts for approximately 20% to 30% of all pulmonary neoplasms (275, 276). The staging of small cell carcinoma of the lung is challenging because of early, widespread dissemination of this neoplasm as well as its frequent association with various paraneoplastic syndromes (90, 95, 277, 278). The alternative staging system (to the TNM scheme) of limited and extensive disease for SCLC was initially proposed by the Veterans Administration Lung Cancer Study Group (VALG) (279). Several studies indicate that the VALG staging system is an independent prognostic indicator for patients with SCLC and that it is used more commonly than the TNM system for SCLC (280, 281). Currently, limited disease is defined as tumor confined to one hemithorax and its regional lymph nodes (hilar or mediastinal) with or without ipsilateral supraclavicular node involvement. Extensive disease refers to spread beyond these limits. Contralateral hilar mediastinal and/or supraclavicular node involvement usually is included in the limited disease category if all of the disease can be safely encompassed in one radiation portal. The presence of an ipsilateral malignant pleural effusion has variably been included or excluded from the limited stage definition, but it is generally considered extensive stage disease (277, 279, 282–284). The extent of disease and performance score are the two most important prognostic factors for SCLC (280, 281).

Several limitations to the current definitions of limited and extensive disease in SCLC have been recognized. For example, Livingston et al. (282) suggested that the prognosis in patients with SCLC and unilateral pleural effusions treated with combination chemotherapy is similar to that in patients treated for limited disease. However, more recent studies have shown poorer survival in these individuals; currently, patients with malignant pleural effusions are classified as extensive stage disease in most trials conducted by the cooperative oncology groups (284). Involvement of contralateral cervical or supraclavicular lymph nodes may respond to treatment better than do intraabdominal metastases (66). Furthermore, SVC syndrome caused by SCLC can result from a small tumor and thus does not necessarily confer a poor prognosis (285). Further revision of the existing criteria for limited and extensive stage disease in SCLC may be necessary to improve prognostication in such subgroups.

CLINICAL APPROACH TO STAGING OF LUNG CANCER

The clinical evaluation of patients with lung cancer includes an accurate estimate or determination of the anatomic extent of tumor involvement as well as a careful preoperative assessment to identify those at high risk for perioperative morbidity and mortality (286). To prognosticate accurately, preoperative (clinical) staging should reflect postoperative (pathologic) staging as closely as possible. Feinstein and colleagues (287) showed that technological improvements altering preoperative stage clearly influenced predictive accuracy. The importance of knowing the staging method used when comparing survival results among various studies cannot be overemphasized. For example, patients preoperatively staged without imaging modalities of higher resolution, such as computed chest tomography, would be expected to be judged erroneously as having more limited tumor extent than the same patient staged with CT. Therapeutic options and prognosis in patients with lung cancer may also be influenced by co-morbid disorders, patient compliance, and consent to therapy. Support for the use of physiologic staging using a clinical-severity classification scheme in improving prognostic precision was proposed by Feinstein and Wells (288). Hence, the sensitivity, specificity, and accuracy of diagnostic modalities, physiologic considerations, comorbidity, and the histologic features of lung cancer influence staging and prognosis.

The clinical staging of NSCLC requires a detailed history and physical examination for co-morbid illnesses, functional status, and evidence of metastatic spread and/or paraneoplastic complications as well as baseline complete blood cell count and serum chemistry profile (289). Pulmonary function tests are recommended for patients undergoing thoracotomy or radiotherapy. Imaging with plain chest roentgenogram and CT of the chest (CT), extended to include the upper abdomen (liver, adrenals, spleen), and/or abdominal ultrasonography are considered part of the basic evaluation by many investigators; we would agree with this approach. Cytologic evaluation of any pleural effusion is also recommended for purposes of staging. Bronchoscopy is very useful for assessing vocal cord function, endobronchial anatomy and involvement, and specimen retrieval, as well as the uncommon detection of synchronous primary lesions. Transcarinal needle aspiration is useful for assessing subcarinal metastases, but mediastinoscopy and/or thoracotomy are still required when mediastinal involvement cannot be proven (290–291). Histologic proof of metastatic involvement is needed in some cases, especially for solitary metastasis such as adrenal enlargement. Further imaging using radioisotope bone scans, CT or MRI of the head, abdominal ultrasonography, and/or assisted biopsy procedures such as percutaneous fine-needle aspiration of an adrenal mass are reserved for patients with focal complaints or suspected metastases to these sites (71, 75–81).

CT of the chest, extended to include the upper abdomen through the liver and adrenal glands, is recommended prior to mediastinoscopy and/or thoracotomy for all patients with presumably operable NSCLC (292). At present, CT is the most effective noninvasive technique for the evaluation of mediastinal adenopathy. Using a nodal size of 1 cm or larger, the reported sensitivity of CT is 64% to 79% and the specificity is between 62% and 66% (293–297). Accuracy of CT detection of mediastinal spread may be increased further by the adjunct use of radiolabeled monoclonal antibodies such as NR-LU-10 (298), but this technique is still under investigation.

The clinical approach to staging patients with SCLC requires knowledge of the status of certain frequent metastatic sites such as the lymph nodes, central nervous system, liver, adrenal glands, bone, and bone marrow. Hence, in addition to the basic evaluation discussed above for NSCLC, the staging evaluation for SCLC often involves exclusion of extrathoracic metastases by CT of the chest (extended to include the liver and adrenal glands), and CT or MRI of the head (283). Bone scans should be obtained on patients with bony symptoms or elevation of serum calcium and/or alkaline phosphatase. Bone marrow aspiration and biopsies are necessary only in the setting of staging for clinical trials. Biopsies of any other symptomatic or suspicious lesion(s) may be required to assess the extent of metastatic disease. Staging tests that are experimental at present include MRI, cytogenetic markers (*myc*, *ras*), DNA histograms (for ploidy analysis), and the other tumor markers (ACTH, ADH, and calcitonin; creatinine kinase–BB; gastrin-releasing peptide [bombesin]; chromogranin-A; and neuron specific enolase).

CONCLUSION

There is an increasing demand for accurate preoperative and intraoperative staging of bronchial carcinoma with respect to neoadjuvant therapy protocols and lung-sparing operations. The adherence to similar staging schemes by all physicians facilitates precise and unambiguous communication. By providing a systematic means for valid comparisons of therapeutic results among different centers, staging systems such as those discussed assist interinstitutional coordination of care and prognostication. The current TNM staging system for NSCLC has provided more meaningful analysis and communication of information concerning the anatomic extent of disease with better delineation of extensive local disease than previous systems. These revisions allow for better refinement of treatment options based on current therapeutic alternatives and also improve prognostication. For SCLC, an alternative system to TNM staging involves "limited" or "extensive" categories with differing therapeutic and prognostic implications. These clinical and surgical-pathologic staging systems, in addition to other physiologic considerations, should continue to be modified as our understanding of lung cancer and various diagnostic and therapeutic modalities advances.

SUMMARY

The diverse presentations of lung cancer are common, challenging, diagnostic and therapeutic problems in clinical practice. The manifestations of lung cancer may result from either local tumor growth, metastatic disease, and/or paraneoplastic phenomena.

Because lung cancer is the most common cause of cancer death and most patients present with symptomatic, advanced disease, it is important to recognize predisposing factors and the varying presentations to enhance earlier detection and therapeutic intervention. In addition to obtaining histologic confirmation of suspected primary lung cancer, accurate staging of the lung cancer is essential for providing precise, unambiguous communication of disease extent to facilitate meaningful analysis of therapeutic interventions and prognostication. The current diagnostic and staging strategies for patients with lung cancer will be refined further as understanding of the pathophysiology of lung cancer evolves and technologic advances complement our clinical acumen.

ACKNOWLEDGMENT

We are deeply indebted to Sheila Roth for her secretarial assistance in the preparation of this manuscript.

REFERENCES

1. Wingo PA, Tong T, Bolden S. Cancer statistics, 1995. CA Cancer J Clin 1995;45:8–30.
2. Goldmeier E. Limits of visibility of bronchogenic carcinoma. Am Rev Respir Dis 1965;91:232–239.
3. Statement on early lung cancer detection. Am Rev Respir Dis 1984;130:565–570.
4. Shimizu N, Ando A, Teramoto S, et al. Outcome of patients with lung cancer detected via mass screening as compared to those presenting with symptoms. J Surg Oncol 1992;50:7–11.
5. Fontana RS, Sanderson DR, Taylor WF, et al. Early lung cancer detection: results of the initial (prevalence) radiologic and cytologic screening in the Mayo Clinic Study. Am Rev Respir Dis 1984;130:561–565.
6. Capewell S, Sankaran R, Lamb D, et al. Lung cancer in lifelong non-smokers. Thorax 1991;46:565–568.
7. Loeb LA, Ernster VL, Warner KE, et al. Smoking and lung cancer: an overview. Cancer Res 1984;44:5940–5958.
8. Tockman MS, Antonisen NR, Wright EC, et al. Airways obstruction and the risk for lung cancer. Ann Intern Med 1987;106:512–518.
9. Bourke W, Milstein D, Giura R, et al. Lung cancer in young adults. Chest 1992;102:1723–1729.
10. Whitesell PL, Drage CW. Occupational lung cancer. Mayo Clin Proc 1993;68:183–188.
11. Fraire AE, Awe RJ. Lung cancer is associated with human immunodeficiency virus infection. Cancer 1992;70:432–436.
12. Ambrosone CB, Rao U, Michalek AM, et al. Lung cancer histologic types and family history of cancer: analysis of histologic subtypes of 872 patients with primary lung cancer. Cancer 1993;72:1192–1198.
13. Geddes DM. The natural history of lung cancer: a review based on rates of tumour growth. Br J Dis Chest 1979;73:1–17.
14. Andersen HA, Prakash UBS. Diagnosis of symptomatic lung cancer. Semin Respir Med 1982;3(3):165–175.
15. Grippi MA. Clinical aspects of lung cancer. Semin Roentgenol 1990;25(1):12–24.
16. Chute CG, Greenberg ER, Baron J, et al. Presenting conditions of 1539 population-based lung cancer patients by cell type and stage in New Hampshire and Vermont. Cancer 1985;56:2107–2111.
17. Hyde L, Hyde CI. Clinical manifestations of lung cancer. Chest 1974;65:299–306.
18. Patel AM, Peters SG. Clinical manifestations of lung cancer. Mayo Clin Proc 1993;68:273–277.
19. Greenberg E, Divertie MB, Woolner LB. A review of unusual systemic manifestations associated with carcinoma. Am J Med 1964;36:106–120.
20. Saito H, Shimokata K, Yamada Y, et al. Umbilical metastasis from small cell carcinoma of the lung. Chest 1992;101(1):288–289.

21. Olsson CA, Moyer JD, Lafeite RO. Pulmonary cancer metastatic to the kidney. J Urol 1971;105:492–496.
22. Cantera JM, Hernandez AV. Bilateral parotid gland metastasis as the initial presentation of a small cell lung carcinoma. J Oral Maxillofac Surg 1989;47(11):1199–1201.
23. Monforte R, Ferrer A, Montserrat JM, et al. Bronchial adenocarcinoma presenting as a lingual tonsillar metastasis. Chest 1987;92(6):1122–1123.
24. Wegener M, Borsch G, Reitemeyer E, Schafer K. Metastasis to the colon from primary bronchogenic carcinoma presenting as occult gastrointestinal bleeding—report of a case. Z Gastroenterol 1988;26(7):358–362.
25. Morgan LW, Linberg JV, Anderson RL. Metastatic disease first presenting as eyelid tumors: a report of two cases and review of the literature. Ann Ophthalmol 1987;9(1):13–18.
26. McKenzie CR, Rengachary SS, McGregor DH, et al. Subdural hematoma associated with metastatic neoplasms. Neurosurgery 1990;27(4):619–625.
27. McEvoy M, Ryan E, Neale G, et al. Unilateral hyperhydrosis: an unusual presentation of bronchial carcinoma. Ir J Med Sci 1982;151(2):51–52.
28. Strauss BL, Matthews MJ, Cohen MH, et al. Cardiac metastases in lung cancer. Chest 1977;71:607–611.
29. Adenle AD, Edwards JE. Clinical and pathologic features of metastatic neoplasms of the pericardium. Chest 1982;81(2):166–169.
30. Terris DJ, Arnstein DP, Nguyen HH. Contemporary evaluation of unilateral vocal cord paralysis. Otolaryngol Head Neck Surg 1992;107:84–90.
31. Martini N, Goodner J, D'Angio GJ, et al. Tracheoesophageal fistula due to cancer. J Thorac Cardiovasc Surg 1970;59:319–324.
32. Wallace RJ, Cohen A, Awe RJ, et al. Carcinomatous lung abscess. Diagnosis by bronchoscopy and cytopathology. JAMA 1979;242:521–522.
33. Daly RC, Trastek VF, Pairolero PC, et al. Bronchoalveolar carcinoma: factors affecting survival. Ann Thorac Surg 1991;51:368–377.
34. Shimura S, Takishima R. Bronchorrhea from diffuse lymphangitic metastasis of colon carcinoma to the lung. Chest 105(1):308–310, 1994.
35. Poe RH, Israel RH, Marin MG, et al. Utility of fiberoptic bronchoscopy in patients with hemoptysis and a nonlocalizing chest roentgenogram. Chest 1988;93:70–75.
36. Oneil KM, Lazarus AA. Hemoptysis: indication for bronchoscopy. Arch Intern Med 1991;151:171–174.
37. Schraufnagel D, Margolis B. Bronchoscopy for hemoptysis. Chest 1990;97:1502.
38. Chernow B, Sahn SA. Carcinomatous involvement of the pleura. An analysis of 96 patients. Am J Med 1977;63:695–702.
39. Auerbach O, Garfinkel L, Parks JR. Histologic types of lung cancer in relation to smoking habits, year of diagnosis, and site of metastases. Chest 1975;64:382–387.
40. Johnston WW. The malignant pleural effusion: a review of cytopathologic diagnoses of 584 specimens from 472 consecutive patients. Cancer 1985;56:905–909.
41. Decker DA, Dines DE, Payne WS, et al. The significance of a cytologically negative pleural effusion in bronchogenic carcinoma. Chest 1978;74:640–642.
42. Canto A, Ferrer G, Romagosa V, et al. Lung cancer and pleural effusion: clinical significant and study of pleural metastatic locations. Chest 1985;87:649–652.
43. Menziers R, Charbonneau M. Thoracoscopy for the diagnosis of pleural disease. Ann Intern Med 1991;114:271–276.
44. Lynch TJ Jr. Management of malignant pleural effusions. Chest 1993;103(Suppl 4):385S–389S.
45. Dines DE, Cortese DA, Brennan MD, et al. Malignant pulmonary neoplasms predisposing to spontaneous pneumothorax. Mayo Clin Proc 1973;48:541–544.
46. Sahn SA. Pleural effusion in lung cancer. Clin Chest Med 1993;14:189–200.
47. Seyfer AE, Walsh DS, Graeber GM, et al. Chest wall implantation of lung cancer after thin-needle aspiration biopsy. Ann Thorac Surg 1989;48(2):284–286.
48. Muller N, Bergun C, Miller R, et al. Seeding of malignant cells into the needle tract after lung and pleural biopsy. J Can Assoc Radiol 1986;37:192–194.
49. Ryd W, Hagmar B, Ericksson O. Local tumour cell seeding by fine-needle aspiration biopsy. Acta Pathol Microbiol Immunol Scand 1983;91(1):17–21.
50. Piehler JM, Pairolero PC, Gracey DR, et al. Unexplained diaphragmatic paralysis: a harbinger of malignant disease? J Thorac Cardiovasc Surg 1982;84:861–864.
51. Pancoast HK. Importance of careful roentgen-ray investigations of apical chest tumors. JAMA 1924;83(18)1407–1411.
52. Pancoast HK. Superior pulmonary sulcus tumor. Tumor characterized by pain, Horner's syndrome, destruction of bone and atrophy of hand muscles. JAMA 1932;99(17):1391–1396.
53. Paulson DL. Carcinomas in the superior pulmonary sulcus. J Thorac Cardiovasc Surg 1975;70:1095–1104.
54. Johnson DH, Haimsworth JD, Greco FA. Pancoast's syndrome and small cell lung cancer. Chest 1982;82(5):602–606.
55. Heelan RT, Bemas BE, Caravelli JF, et al. Superior sulcus tumors: CT and MR imaging. Radiology 1989;170:637–641.
56. O'Connell RS, McLoud TC, Wilkins EW. Superior sulcus tumor: radiographic diagnosis and workup. AJR Am J Roentgenol 1983;140:25–30.
57. Hunter W. The history of an aneurysm of the aorta with some remarks on aneurysms in general. Med Obs Inq (Lond) 1757;1:323–357.
58. Parish JM, Marschke RF, Dines DE, et al. Etiologic considerations in superior vena cava syndrome. Mayo Clin Proc 1981;56:407–413.
59. Bell DR, Woods RL, Levi JA. Superior vena caval obstruction: a ten-year experience. Med J Aust 1986;145:566–568.
60. Abner A. Approach to the patient who presents with superior vena cava obstruction. Chest 1993;103(Suppl 4):394S–397S.
61. Urban T, Lebeau B, Chastang C, et al. Superior vena cava syndrome in small cell lung cancer. Arch Intern Med 1993;153:384–387.
62. Rodrigues N, Straus MJ. Superior vena caval syndrome. In: Straus MJ, ed. Lung cancer: clinical diagnosis and treatment. 2nd ed. Philadelphia: Grune & Stratton, 1983:323–333.
63. Schraufnagel DE, Hill R, Leech JA, et al. Superior vena caval syndrome. Is it a medical emergency? Am J Med 1981;70:1169–1174.
64. Sculier JP, Evans WK, Feld R, et al. Superior vena caval obstruction syndrome in small cell lung cancer. Cancer 1986;57:847–851.
65. Hansen HH. Diagnosis in metastatic sites. In: Straus MJ, ed. Lung cancer: clinical diagnosis and treatment. 2nd ed. Philadelphia: Grune & Stratton, 1983:185–200.
66. Mirvis SE, Whitley NO, Aisner J, et al. Abdominal CT in the staging of small cell carcinoma of the lung: incidence of metas-

tases and effect on prognosis. AJR Am J Roentgenol 1987;148: 845–847.
67. Dombernowsky P, Hirsch FR, Hansen HH, et al. Peritoneoscopy in the staging of 190 patients with small cell anaplastic carcinoma of the lung with special reference to subtyping. Cancer 1978;41:2008–2012.
68. Oliver TW, Bernardino ME, Miller JI, et al. Isolated adrenal masses in non–small cell bronchogenic carcinoma. Radiology 1984;153:217–218.
69. Ettinghausen SE, Burt ME. Prospective evaluation of unilateral adrenal masses in patients with operable non–small cell lung cancer. J Clin Oncol 1991;9:1462–1466.
70. Silverman SG, Mueller PR, Pinkney LP, et al. Predictive value of image-guided adrenal biopsy: analysis of results of 101 biopsies. Radiology 1993;187:715–718.
71. Allard P, Yankaskas BC, Fletcher RH, et al. Sensitivity and specificity of computed tomography for the detection of adrenal metastatic lesions among 91 autopsied lung cancer patients. Cancer 1990;66:457–462.
72. Michel F, Soler M, Imhof E, et al. Initial staging of non–small cell lung cancer: value of routine radioisotope bone scanning. Thorax 1991;46:469–473.
73. Tritz DB, Doll DC, Ringenberg QS, et al. Bone marrow involvement in small cell lung cancer. Clinical significance and correlation with routine laboratory variables. Cancer 1989;63:763–766.
74. Levitan N, Byrne RE, Bromer RH, et al. The value of the bone scan and bone marrow biopsy in staging small cell lung cancer. Cancer 1985;56(3):652–654.
75. Tarver RD, Richmond BD, Klatte EC. Cerebral metastases from lung carcinomas: neurological and CT correlation. Radiology 1984;153:689–692.
76. Halpert B, Erickson EE, Fields WS. Intracranial involvement from carcinoma of the lung. Arch Pathol 1960;69:93–103.
77. Merchut MP. Brain metastases from undiagnosed systemic neoplasms. Arch Intern Med 1989;149:1076–1080.
78. Newman SJ, Hansen HH. Frequency, diagnosis, and treatment of brain metastases in 247 consecutive patients with bronchogenic carcinoma. Cancer 1974;33:492–496.
79. Kim RY, Spencer SA, Meredith RF, et al. Extradural spinal cord compression: analysis of factors determining functional prognosis—prospective study. Radiology 1990;176:279–282.
80. Schriner RW, Ryu JH, Edwards WD. Microscopic pulmonary tumor embolism causing subacute cor pulmonale: a difficult antemortem diagnosis. Mayo Clin Proc 1991;66(2):143–148.
81. Kvale PA. The cancer patient with dyspnea: unusual cause? Mayo Clin Proc 1991;66(2):215–218.
82. Masson RG, Ruggieri J. Pulmonary microvascular cytology: A new diagnostic application of the pulmonary artery catheter. Chest 1985;88:908–914.
83. Masson RG, Krikorian J, Lukl P, et al. Pulmonary microvascular cytology in the diagnosis of lymphangitic carcinomatosis. N Engl J Med 1989;321:71–76.
84. Graus F, Rogers LR, Posner JB. Cerebrovascular complications in patients with cancer. Medicine 1985;64:16–35.
85. Goldhaber SZ, Dricker E, Buring JE, et al. Clinical suspicion of autopsy-proven thrombotic and tumor pulmonary embolism in cancer patients. Am Heart J 1987;114:1432–1435.
86. Munk PL, Muller NL, Miller RR, Ostrow DN. Pulmonary lymphangitic carcinomatosis: CT and pathologic findings. Radiology 1988;166:705–709.
87. Muller NL, Miller RR. Computed tomography of chronic diffuse infiltrative lung disease. Am Rev Respir Dis 1990;142(5):1206–1215.
88. Tao LC, Delarue NC, Sanders D, Weisbrod G. Bronchioloalveolar carcinoma: a correlative clinical and cytologic study. Cancer 1978;42:2759–2767.
89. Martinez-Lavin M, Mansilla J, Pineda C, et al. Evidence for hypertrophic pulmonary osteoarthropathy in human skeletal remains from pre-Hispanic Mesoamerica. Ann Intern Med 1994;120:238–241.
90. Patel AM, Davila DG, Peters SG. Paraneoplastic syndromes associated with lung cancer. Mayo Clin Proc 1993;68:278–287.
91. Nathanson L, Hall TC. A spectrum of tumors that produce paraneoplastic syndromes. Lung tumors: how they produce their syndromes. Ann N Y Acad Sci 1974;230:367–377.
92. Andersen NE. Anti-neuronal autoantibodies and neurologic paraneoplastic syndromes. Aust NZ J Med 1989;19:379–387.
93. Markman M. Response of paraneoplastic syndromes to antineoplastic therapy. West J Med 1986;144:580–585.
94. Grunwald GB. Autoimmune paraneoplastic syndromes: manifestations and mechanisms. In: Fishman AP, ed. Update: pulmonary diseases and disorders. New York: McGraw-Hill, 1992:137–146.
95. Bunn PA Jr, Ridgway EC. Paraneoplastic syndromes. In: DeVita VT, Hellman S, Rosenberg SA, eds. The principles and practice of oncology. 4th ed. Philadelphia: JB Lippincott, 1993:2026–2071.
96. Daughaday WH. Endocrine manifestations of systemic disease (symposium). Endocrinol Metab Clin North Am 1991;20(3):453–564.
97. Nelson KA, Walsh D, Sheehan FA. The cancer anorexia-cachexia syndrome. J Clin Oncol 1994;12:213–225.
98. Loprinzi CL, Ellison N, Schaid DJ, et al. Controlled trial of megestrol acetate for the treatment of cancer anorexia and cachexia. J Natl Cancer Inst 1990;8:287–297.
99. Altermatt HJ, Rodriguez M, Scheithauer BW, et al. Paraneoplastic anti-Purkinje and type I anti-neuronal nuclear autoantibodies bind selectively to central, peripheral, and autonomic nervous system cells. Lab Invest 1991;65:412–420.
100. Sigurgeirsson B, Lindelof B, Edhag O, et al. Risk of cancer in patients with dermatomyositis or polymyositis. N Engl J Med 1992;326(6):363–367.
101. Bunn PA Jr. Paraneoplastic syndromes. In: Wyngaarden JB, Smith LH Jr, Bennett JC, eds. Cecil textbook of medicine. 19th ed. Toronto: WB Saunders, 1992;159:1032–1034.
102. Rosen P, Armstrong D. Nonbacterial thrombotic endocarditis in patients with malignant neoplastic diseases. Am J Med 1973;54:23–29.
103. Doolittle GC, Wurster MW, Rosenfeld CS, Bodensteiner DC. Malignancy-induced lactic acidosis. South Med J 1988;81(4):533–536.
104. Cooper DJ. Oat cell carcinoma and severe hypouricemia. N Engl J Med 1973;288:321–322.
105. Hansen-Flaschen J, Nordberg J. Clubbing and hypertrophic osteoarthropathy. Clin Chest Med 1987;8(2):287–298.
106. Shneerson JM. Digital clubbing and hypertrophic osteoarthropathy: the underlying mechanisms. Br J Dis Chest 1981;75:113–129.
107. Stenseth JH, Clagett OT, Woolner LB. Hypertrophic pulmonary osteoarthropathy. Dis Chest 1967;52:62–68.
108. Gellhorn A. Ectopic hormone production in cancer and its implication for basic research on abnormal growth. Adv Intern Med 1969;15:299–316.

109. Feinberg AP, Vogelstein B. Hypomethylation distinguishes genes of some human cancers from their normal counterparts. Nature 1983;301:89–92.
110. Abelev GI. α-Fetoprotein as a marker of embryonic specific differentiation in normal and tumor tissues. Transplant Rev 1974;20:3–37.
111. Russo IH, Russo J. Hormone production by tumors: ectopia or gene derepression? Cancer Growth Prog 1989;4:123–132.
112. Baylin SB, Mendelsohn G. Ectopic (inappropriate) hormone production by tumors: mechanisms involved and the biological and clinical implications. Endocr Rev 1980;1:45–77.
113. DeBold CR, Menefee JK, Nicholson WE, et al. Proopiomelanocortin gene is expressed in many normal tissues and in tumors not associated with ectopic adrenocorticotropin syndrome. Mol Endocrinol 1988;2:862–870.
114. Schteingart DE. Ectopic secretion of peptides of the proopiomelanocortin family. In: Daughaday WH, ed. Endocrine manifestations of disease. Endocrinol Metab Clin North Am 1991 (Sept):453–471.
115. Schteingart DE, Lloyd RV, Akil H, et al. Cushing's syndrome secondary to ectopic corticotropin-releasing hormone-adrenocorticotropin secretion. J Clin Endocrinol Metab 1986;62(2):770–775.
116. Zarati A, Kovacs K, Flores M, et al. ACTH and CRF-producing bronchial carcinoid associated with Cushing's syndrome. Clin Endocrinol (Oxf) 1986;24(5):523–529.
117. Seyberth HW, Segre GV, Morgan JL, et al. Prostaglandin as mediators of hypercalcemia associated with certain types of cancer. N Engl J Med 1975;293:1278–1283.
118. Freed RM, Voelkel EF, Rice RH, et al. Two squamous cell carcinomas not associated with humoral hypercalcemia produce a potent bone resorption stimulating 1a, 1b factor which is interleukin-1 alpha. Endocrinology 1989;125:742–751.
119. Yoneda T, Alsim MM, Chaney JB, et al. Hypercalcemia in a human tumor is due to tumor necrosis factor production by host immune cells. J Bone Miner Res 1989;4:826.
120. Moses AM, Scheinman SJ. Ectopic secretion of neurohypophyseal peptides in patients with malignancy. Endocrinol Metab Clin North Am 1991;20(3):489–506.
121. Bliss DP Jr, Battey JF, Linnoila RI, et al. Expression of the atrial naturetic factor gene in small cell lung cancer tumors and tumor cell lines. J Natl Cancer Inst 1990;82:305–310.
122. Boizel R, Halimi S, Labat F, et al. Acromegaly due to a growth hormone-releasing hormone-secreting bronchial carcinoid tumor: further information on the abnormal responsiveness of the somatotroph cells and their recovery after successful treatment. J Clin Endocrinol Metab 1987;64(2):304–308.
123. Schteingart DE. Cushing's syndrome. Endocrinol Metab Clin North Am 1989;18:311–338.
124. Mendelsohn G, Baylin SB. Ectopic hormone production: biological and clinical implications in hormones and cancer. Prog Clin Biol Res 1984;142:291–316.
125. Limper AH, Carpenter PC, Scheithauer BW, et al. The Cushing syndrome induced by bronchial carcinoid tumors. Ann Intern Med 1992;117:209–214.
126. Odell WD, Wolfsen AR, Bachelot I, et al. Ectopic production of lipocortin by cancer. Am J Med 1979;66:631–638.
127. Hansen M, Bork E. Peptide hormones in patients with lung cancer. Recent Results Cancer Res 1985;99:180–186.
128. Hansen M, Pedersen AG. Tumor markers in patients with lung cancer. Incidence of SIADH and ectopic ACTH. Chest 1986;89(Suppl):219S–224S.
129. Jex RK, van Heerden JA, Carpenter PC, et al. Ectopic ACTH syndrome: diagnostic and therapeutic aspects. Am J Surg 1985;149:276–282.
130. Howlett TA, Drury PL, Perry L, et al. Diagnosis and management of ACTH dependent Cushing's syndrome: comparison of the features in ectopic and pituitary ACTH production. Clin Endocrinol (Oxf) 1986;24:699–713.
131. Kaye TB, Crapo L. The Cushing syndrome: an update on diagnostic tests. Ann Intern Med 1990;112:434–444.
132. Oldfield EH, Doppman JL, Nieman KL, et al. Petrosal sinus sampling with and without corticotropin-releasing hormone for the differential diagnosis of Cushing's syndrome. N Engl J Med 1991;325:897–905.
133. Malchoff CD, Orth DN, Abboud C, et al. Ectopic ACTH syndrome caused by a bronchial carcinoid tumor responsive to dexamethasone, metyrapone and corticotropin releasing factor. Am J Med 1988;84:760–764.
134. Vieau D, Massias JF, Girard F, et al. Corticotropin-like intermediate lobe peptide as a marker of alternate proopiomelanocortin processing in ACTH producing nonpituitary tumors. Clin Endocrinol 1989;31: 691–700.
135. Jeffcoate WJ, Rees LH, Tomlin S, et al. Metyrapone in long-term management of Cushing's disease. BMJ 1977;2:215–217.
136. Schteingart DE, Conn JW. Effects of aminoglutethimide upon adrenal function and cortisol metabolism in Cushing's syndrome. J Clin Endocrinol Metab 1967;27:1657–1666.
137. Sonio W, Boscaro M, Paoletta A, et al. Ketoconazole treatment in Cushing's syndrome: experience in 34 patients. Clin Endocrinol 1991;35:347–352.
138. Sonio N. The use of ketoconazole as an inhibitor of steroid production. N Engl J Med 1987;317:812–818.
139. McCance DR, Hadden DR, Kennedy L, et al. Clinical experience with ketoconazole as a therapy for patients with Cushing's syndrome. Clin Endocrinol 1987;27:593–599.
140. Bertagna X, Favrod-Coune C, Escourolle H, et al. Suppression of ectopic adrenocorticotropin secretion by the long-acting somatostatin analog octreotide. J Clin Endocrinol Metab 1989; 68:988–991.
141. Blunt SB, Pirmohamed M, Chaterjee VKK, et al. Use of adrenal artery embolization in severe ACTH-dependent Cushing's syndrome. Postgrad Med J 1989;65:575–579.
142. Shepherd FA, Laskey J, Evans UK, et al. Cushing's syndrome associated with ectopic corticotropin production and small cell lung cancer. J Clin Oncol 1992;10:21–27.
143. Bilezikian JP. Management of acute hypercalcemia. N Engl J Med 1992;326:1196–1203.
144. Bender RA, Hansen H. Hypercalcemia in bronchogenic carcinoma: a prospective study of 200 patients. Ann Intern Med 1974;80:205–208.
145. Ralston SH, Gallacher SJ, Patel U, et al. Cancer-associated hypercalcemia: morbidity and mortality. Ann Intern Med 1990; 112:499–504.
146. Vasilopoulou-Sellin R, Newman BM, Taylor SH, et al. Incidence of hypercalcemia in patients with malignancy referred to a comprehensive cancer center. Cancer 1993;71:1309–1312.
147. Ralston S, Gardner MD, Fogelman I, et al. Hypercalcemia and metastatic bone disease: is there a causal link? Lancet 1982; 2:903–905.
148. Ralston SH. The pathogenesis of humoral hypercalcemia of malignancy. Lancet 1987;2:1443–1446.
149. Mundy GR, Ibbotson KJ, D'Souza SM, et al. The hypercalcemia of cancer. Clinical implications and pathogenic mechanisms. N Engl J Med 1984;310(26):1718–1727.

150. Yoshimoto K, Yamasaki R, Sakai H, et al. Ectopic production of parathyroid hormone by small cell lung cancer in a patient with hypercalcemia. J Clin Endocrinol Metab 1989;68:976–981.
151. Budayr AA, Nissenson RA, Klein RF, et al. Increased serum levels of a parathyroid hormone-like protein in malignancy-associated hypercalcemia. Ann Intern Med 1989;111:807–812.
152. Burtis WJ, Wu TL, Insogna KL, Stewart AF. Humoral hypercalcemia of malignancy. Ann Intern Med 1988;108(3):454–457.
153. Broadus AE, Mangin M, Ikeda K, et al. Humoral hypercalcemia of cancer: identification of a novel parathyroid hormone-like peptide. N Engl J Med 1988;319:556–563.
154. Kao PC, Klee GG, Taylor RL, Heath H III. Parathyroid hormone-related peptide in plasma of patients with hypercalcemia and malignant lesions. Mayo Clin Proc 1990;65(11):1399–1407.
155. Mosley JM, Kubota M, Diefenbach-Jagger H, et al. Parathyroid hormone-related protein purified from a human lung cancer cell line. Proc Natl Acad Sci U S A 1987;84:5048–5052.
156. Yates AJP, Gutierrez GE, Smolens P, et al. Effects of a synthetic peptide of a parathyroid hormone-related protein on calcium homeostasis, renal tubular calcium absorption and bone metabolism. J Clin Invest 1988;81:932–938.
157. Ikeda K, Weir EC, Mangin M, et al. Expression of messenger ribonucleic acids encoding a parathyroid hormone-like peptide in normal human and animal tissues with abnormal expression in human parathyroid adenomas. Mol Endocrinol 1988;2:1230–1236.
158. Mundy GR, Ibbotson KJ, D'Souza SM. Tumor products and the hypercalcemia of malignancy. J Clin Invest 1985;76:391–394.
159. Dominguez J, Mundy G. Monocytes mediate osteoclastic bone resorption by prostaglandin production. Calcif Tissue Int 1986;31:29–34.
160. Campbell JH, Ralston SH, Boyle IT, et al. Symptomatic hypercalcemia in lung cancer. Respir Med 1991;85:223–227.
161. Stevenson JC. Current management of malignant hypercalcemia. Drugs 1988;36:229–238.
162. Wisneski LA, Croom WP, Silva OL, et al. Salmon calcitonin in hypercalcemia. Clin Pharmacol Ther 1978;24:219–222.
163. Perlia CP, Gubisch NJ, Wolter J, et al. Mithramycin treatment of hypercalcemia. Cancer 1970;25:389–394.
164. Singer FR, Ritch PS, Lad TE, et al., and the Hypercalcemia Study Group. Treatment of hypercalcemia of malignancy with intravenous etidronate. Arch Intern Med 1991;151:471–476.
165. Pamidronate. Med Lett Drugs Ther 1992;34(861):1–2.
166. Fulmer DH, Dimich AB, Rothschild EO, et al. Treatment of hypercalcemia: comparison of intravenously administered phosphate, sulfate and hydrocortisone. Arch Intern Med 1972;129:923–930.
167. Gucalp R, Ritch P, Wiernik PH, et al. Comparative study of pamidronate disodium and etidronate disodium in the treatment of cancer-related hypercalcemia. J Clin Oncol 1992;10:134–142.
168. Gallium for hypercalcemia of malignancy. Med Lett Drugs Ther 1991;33(843):41–42.
169. Warrell RP, Israel R, Frisone M, et al. Gallium nitrate for acute treatment of cancer-related hypercalcemia. Ann Intern Med 1988;108:669–674.
170. Warrell RP, Murphy WK, Schulman P, et al. A randomized, double-blind study of gallium nitrate compared with etidronate for acute control of cancer-related hypercalcemia. J Clin Oncol 1991;9:1467–1475.
171. Thiebaud D, Jaeger P, Burckhardt P. Response to retreatment of malignant hypercalcemia with the bisphosphate AHPrBP (APD): respective role of kidney and bone. J Bone Miner Res 1990;5:221–226.
172. Coggeshall J, Merrill W, Hande K, et al. Implications of hypercalcemia with respect to diagnosis and treatment of lung cancer. Am J Med 1986;80:325–328.
173. Hou S. Syndrome of inappropriate antidiuretic hormone secretion. In: Reichlin S, ed. The neurohypophysis. Physiological and clinical aspects. New York: Plenum Press, 1984:165.
174. DeFronzo RA, Goldberg M, Agus ZS. Normal diluting capacity in hyponatremic patients: reset osmostat or a variant of the syndrome of inappropriate antidiuretic hormone secretion. Ann Intern Med 1976;84:538–542.
175. Maurer LH, O'Donnell JF, Kennedy S, et al. Human neurophysins in carcinoma of the lung: relation of histology, disease stage, response rate, survival and syndrome of inappropriate antidiuretic hormone secretion. Cancer Treat Rep 1983;67:971–976.
176. Padfield PL, Morton JJ, Brown JJ, et al. Plasma arginine vasopressin in the syndrome of inappropriate antidiuretic hormone excess associated with bronchogenic carcinoma. Am J Med 1976;61:825–831.
177. Vorherr H. Para-endocrine tumor activity with emphasis on ectopic ADH secretion. Oncology 1974;29:382–416.
178. North WG. Biosynthesis of vasopressin and neurophysins. In: Gash DM, Doer GJ, eds. Vasopressin, principles and properties. New York: Plenum Press, 1987:175.
179. Comis RL, Miller M, Ginsberg SJ. Abnormalities in water homeostasis in small cell anaplastic lung cancer. Cancer 1980;45:2414–2421.
180. List AF, Hainsworth JD, Davis BW, et al. The syndrome of inappropriate secretion of antidiuretic hormone in small cell lung cancer. J Clin Oncol 1986;4:1191–1198.
181. Kamoi K, Ebe T, Hasegawa A, et al. Hyponatremia in small cell lung cancer: mechanisms not involving inappropriate ADH secretion. Cancer 1987;60:1089–1093.
182. Gross AJ, Steinberg SM, Reilly JG, et al. Atrial natriuretic factor and arginine vasopressin production in tumor cell lines from patients with lung cancer and their relationship to serum sodium. Cancer Res 1993;53:67–74.
183. Decaux G, Waterlot Y, Genette F, et al. Treatment of the syndrome of inappropriate secretion of antidiuretic hormone with furosemide. N Engl J Med 1981;304:329–330.
184. Miyagawa CI. The pharmacologic management of the syndrome of inappropriate secretion of antidiuretic hormone. Drug Intell Clin Pharmacy 1987;20:527–531.
185. Cherrill DA, Stote RM, Birge JR, et al. Demeclocycline treatment in the syndrome of inappropriate antidiuretic hormone secretion. Ann Intern Med 1975;83:654–656.
186. DeTroyer A. Demeclocycline: treatment for syndrome of inappropriate antidiuretic hormone secretion. J Am Med Assoc 1977;237:2723–2726.
187. Forrest JN, Cox M, Hong C, et al. Superiority of demeclocycline over lithium in the treatment of chronic syndrome of inappropriate secretion of antidiuretic hormone. N Engl J Med 1978;298:173–177.
188. White MG, Fetner CD. Treatment of the syndrome of inappropriate secretion of antidiuretic hormone with lithium carbonate. N Engl J Med 1975;292:390–392.
189. Hantman D, Rossier B, Zohlman R, et al. Rapid correction of hyponatremia in the syndrome of inappropriate secretion of antidiuretic hormone. Ann Intern Med 1973;78:870–875.

190. Berl T. Treating hyponatremia: what is all the controversy about? Ann Intern Med 1990;113:417–419.
191. Arieff AI. Hyponatremia, convulsions, respiratory arrest and permanent brain damage after elective surgery in healthy women. N Engl J Med 1986;314:1529–1535.
192. Ayus CJ, Krothapalli RK, Arieff AI. Treatment of symptomatic hyponatremia and its relation to brain damage: a prospective study. N Engl J Med 1987;317:1190–1195.
193. Narins RG. Therapy of hyponatremia: does haste make waste? N Engl J Med 1986;314:1573–1575.
194. Steinberg D. Anemia and cancer. CA Cancer J Clin 1989;39(5):296–304.
195. Ramaiah RS, Biagi RW. Eosinophilia: an unusual presentation of carcinoma of the lung. Practitioner 1982;226:1805–1806.
196. Trousseau A. Lectures on clinical medicine delivered at the Hotel-Dieu, Paris. London: New Sydenham Society, 1865:292–332.
197. Nachman RL, Silverstein R. Hypercoagulable states. Ann Intern Med 1993;119:819–827.
198. Patterson WP, ed. Symposium on coagulation and cancer. Semin Oncol 1990;17(2):137–237.
199. Schafer AI. The hypercoagulable states. Ann Intern Med 1985;102:814–828.
200. Prandoni P, Lensing AWA, Buller HR, et al. Deep-vein thrombosis and the incidence of subsequent symptomatic cancer. N Engl J Med 1992;327(16):1128–1133.
201. Griffin MR, Stanson AW, Brown ML, et al. Deep venous thrombosis and pulmonary embolism. Risk of subsequent malignant neoplasms. Arch Intern Med 1987;147:1907–1911.
202. Gore JM, Applebaum JS, Green HL, et al. Occult cancer in patients with acute pulmonary embolism. Ann Intern Med 1982;96:556–560.
203. Goldberg RJ, Seneff M, Gore JM. Occult malignant neoplasm in patients with deep venous thrombosis. Arch Intern Med 1987;147:251–253.
204. Henson RA. Unusual manifestations of bronchial carcinoma. Proc R Soc Lond [Biol] 1953;46:859–861.
205. Graus F, Rogers LR, Posner JB. Cerebrovascular complications in patients with cancer. Medicine 1985;64:16–35.
206. Andersen NE, Rosenblum MK, Graus F, et al. Autoantibodies in paraneoplastic syndromes associated with small-cell lung cancer. Neurology 1988;38:1391–1398.
207. Posner JB, Furneaux HM. Paraneoplastic syndromes. In: Waksman BH, ed. Immunologic mechanisms in neurologic and psychiatric disease. New York: Raven Press, 1990.
208. Lennon VA. Anti-Purkinje cell cytoplasmic and neuronal nuclear antibodies aid diagnosis of paraneoplastic autoimmune neurological disorders (letter). J Neurol Neurosurg Psychol 1989;52:1438–1439.
209. Kimmel DW, O'Neill BP, Lennon VA. Subacute sensory neuronopathy associated with small cell lung carcinoma: diagnosis aided by autoimmune serology. Mayo Clin Proc 1988;63:29–32.
210. Graus F, Cordon-Cordo C, Posner JB. Neuronal anti-nuclear antibody in sensory neuronopathy from lung cancer. Neurology 1985;35:538–543.
211. Dalmau J, Furneaux HM, Grolla RJ, et al. Detection of the anti-Hu antibody in the serum of patients with small cell lung cancer: a quantitative Western blot analysis. Ann Neurol 1990;27:544–552.
212. Furneaux HM, Rosenblum MK, Dalmau J, et al. Selective expression of Purkinje cell antigens in tumor tissue from patients with paraneoplastic cerebellar degeneration. N Engl J Med 1990;322:1844–1851.
213. Hetzel DJ, Stanhope CR, O'Neill BP, et al. Gynecologic cancer in patients with subacute cerebellar degeneration predicted by anti-Purkinje cell antibodies and limited in metastatic volume. Mayo Clin Proc 1990;65:1558–1563.
214. Dalmau J, Graus F, Rosenblum MK, et al. Anti-Hu associated paraneoplastic encephalomyelitis/sensory neuropathy: a clinical study of 71 patients. Medicine 1992;71:59–72.
215. Darnell RB, DeAngelis LM. Regression of small cell lung cancer in patients with paraneoplastic neuronal antibodies. Lancet 1993;341:21–22.
216. Anderson HJ, Churchill-Davidson HC, Richardson AT. Bronchial neoplasm with myasthenia: prolonged apnea after administration of succinylcholine. Lancet 1953;2:1291–1293.
217. Lambert EH, Eaton LM, Rooke ED. Defect of neuromuscular conduction associated with malignant neoplasms. Am J Physiol 1956;187:612–613.
218. Eaton LM, Lambert EH. Electromyography and electrical stimulation of nerves in diseases of the motor unit: observations on a myasthenic syndrome associated with malignant tumours. JAMA 1957;161:1117–1124.
219. O'Neill JH, Murray NMF, Newsom-Davis J. The Lambert-Eaton myasthenic syndrome: a review of 50 cases. Brain 1988;3(3):577–596.
220. Lennon VA, Lambert EH. Autoantibodies bind solubilized calcium channel—conotoxin complexes from small cell lung carcinoma: a diagnostic aid for Lambert-Eaton myasthenic syndrome. Mayo Clin Proc 1989;64(12):1498–1520.
221. Lambert EH, Lennon VA. Selected IgG rapidly induces Lambert-Eaton myasthenic syndrome in mice: complement independence and EMG abnormalities. Muscle Nerve 1988;11:1133–1145.
222. Oguro-Okano M, Griesmann GE, Wilben ED, et al. Molecular diversity of neuronal type calcium channels identified in small cell lung carcinoma. Mayo Clin Proc 1992;67(12):1150–1159.
223. Lundh H, Nilsson O, Rosen I. Current therapy of the Lambert-Eaton myasthenic syndrome. Prog Brain Res 1990;84:163–170.
224. McEvoy KM, Windebank AJ, Daube JR, et al. 3,4-Diaminopyridine in the treatment of Lambert-Eaton myasthenic syndrome. N Engl J Med 1989;321(23):1567–1571.
225. Ogilvie H. Large intestine colic due to sympathetic deprivation: a new clinical syndrome. BMJ 1948;2:671–673.
226. Schuffler MD, Baird HW, Fleming CR, et al. Intestinal pseudoobstruction as the presenting manifestation of SMA neuropathy of the gastrointestinal tract. Ann Intern Med 1983;98(2):129–134.
227. Sodhi N, Camilleri M, Camoriano JK, et al. Autonomic function and motility in intestinal pseudoobstruction caused by paraneoplastic syndrome. Dig Dis Sci 1989;34(12):1937–1942.
228. Lennon VA, Sas DF, Busk MF, et al. Enteric neuronal autoantibodies in pseudoobstruction with small-cell lung carcinoma. Gastroenterology 1991;100:137–142.
229. Lennon VA. Enteric neuronal autoantibodies in pseudoobstruction with small cell lung cancer (reply to letter). Gastroenterology 1991;101:1143–1144.
230. Newman NJ, Bell IR, McKee AC. Paraneoplastic limbic encephalitis: neuropsychiatric presentation. Biol Psychiat 1990;27(5):529–542.
231. Ralston SH, Fogelman I, Lowe GD. Oat cell carcinoma of bronchus presenting as an acute psychiatric illness in young women. Postgrad Med 1982;58(683):562–563.
232. Ojeda VJ. Necrotizing myelopathy associated with malignancy. A clinicopathologic study of two cases and literature review. Cancer 1984;53(5):1115–1123.

233. Grunwald GB, Kornguth SE, Towfighi J, et al. Autoimmune basis for visual paraneoplastic syndrome in patients with small cell lung carcinoma. Cancer 1987;60:780–786.
234. Martinez-Maldonado, M, Benabe JE. Nonrenal neoplasms and the kidney (chapter XII, 82). In: Schrier RW, Gottschalk CW, eds. Diseases of the kidney. 5th ed. Toronto: Little, Brown, 1993:III:2265–2273.
235. Davison M, Thomson D. Malignancy-associated glomerular disease. In: Cameron S, et al., eds. Oxford textbook of clinical nephrology. New York: Oxford University Press, 1992;1:475–486.
236. Striker L, Striker GE. A. renal parenchymal disease. In: Massry SG, Glassock RJ, eds. Textbook of nephrology. Baltimore: Williams & Wilkins, 1989;56:977–981.
237. Olsson CA, Moyer JD, Laferte RO. Pulmonary cancer metastatic to the kidneys: a common renal neoplasm. J Urol 1971;105:492–496.
238. Wagle DG, Moore RH, Murphy GP. Secondary carcinomas of the kidney. J Urol 1975;114:30–32.
239. Lee JC, Yamauchi H, Hopper J Jr. The association of cancer and the nephrotic syndrome. Ann Intern Med 1966;64:41–51.
240. Row PG, Cameron JS, Turner DS, et al. Membranous nephropathy: long term follow up and association with neoplasm. Q J Med 1975;44:207–239.
241. Froom DW, Franklin WA, Hano JE, et al. Immune deposits in Hodgkin's disease with nephrotic syndrome. Arch Pathol 1972;94:547–553.
242. Eagen JW, Lewis EJ. Glomerulopathies of neoplasia. Kidney Int 1977;11:297–306.
243. Lewis MG, Laughridge LM, Phillips TM. Immunological studies in nephrotic syndrome associated with extrarenal malignant disease. Lancet 1971;2:134–135.
244. Barton CH, Vaziri ND, Speak GS. Nephrotic syndrome associated with adenocarcinoma of the breast. Am J Med 1980;68:308–312.
245. Plager J, Stutzman L. Acute nephrotic syndrome as a manifestation of active Hodgkin's disease. Am J Med 1971;50:56–66.
246. Kemeny M, Block LR, Braun DW Jr, Martini N. Results of surgical treatment of carcinoma of the lung by stage and cell type. Surg Gynecol Obstet 1978;147:865–871.
247. Stanley KE. Prognostic factors for survival in patients with inoperable lung cancer. J Natl Cancer Inst 1980;65:25–32.
248. Lipford EH III, Eggleston JC, Lillemoe KD, et al. Prognostic factors in surgically resected limited stage, non–small cell carcinoma of the lung. Am J Surg Pathol 1984;8:357–365.
249. Denoix PF. Enquete permanent dans les centres anticancereux. Bull Inst Natl Hyg 1946;1:70–75.
250. Sobin LH, Hermanek P, Hutter RVP. TNM classification of malignant tumors: a comparison between the new (1987) and old editions. Cancer 1988;61:2310–2314.
251. Patel AM, Dunn WF, Trastek VF. Staging systems of lung cancer. Mayo Clin Proc 1993;68:475–482.
252. Mountain CF, Carr DT, Anderson WA. A system for the clinical staging of lung cancer. Am J Roentgenol Radium Ther Nucl Med 1974;120(1):130–138.
253. Ishikawa S. Staging system on TNM classification for lung cancer. Jpn J Clin Oncol 1973;3(1):19–30.
254. Harmer EM, ed. TNM classification of malignant tumours. 3rd ed. Geneva: International Union Against Cancer, 1978:41–45.
255. Williams DE, Pairolero PC, Davis CS, et al. Survival of patients surgically treated for stage I lung cancer. J Thorac Cardiovasc Surg 1981;82(1):70–76.
256. Mountain CF. A new international staging system for lung cancer. Chest 1986;89:225S–233S.
257. Mountain CF. The new international staging system for lung cancer. Surg Clin North Am 1987;67(5):925–935.
258. Mountain CF. Value of the new TNM staging system for lung cancer. Chest 1989;96(1):47S–50S.
259. Mountain CF, Greenberg SD, Fraire AE. Tumor stage in non–small cell carcinoma of the lung. Chest 1991;99:1258–1260.
260. Mountain CF, Lukeman JM, Hammar SP, et al. Lung cancer classification: the relationship of disease extent and cell type to survival in a clinical trials population. J Surg Oncol 1987;35:147–156.
261. Friedman PJ. Lung cancer: update on staging classifications. AJR Am J Roentgenol 1988;150:261–264.
262. Naruke T, Goya T, Tsuchiya R, et al. Prognosis and survival in resected lung carcinoma based on the new international staging system. J Thorac Cardiovasc Surg 1988;96:440–447.
263. Little AG, Stitik FP. Clinical staging of patients with non–small cell lung cancer. Chest 1990;97(6):1431–1438.
264. Plaja S, Puccia V, Russo A, et al. Carcinoma of the lung, stage III: experience with the new TNM-AJCC classification. Scand J Thorac Cardiovasc Surg 1988;22:139–141.
265. Mathisen DJ, Grillo HC. Carinal resection for bronchogenic carcinoma. J Thorac Cardiovasc Surg 1991;102(1):16–23.
266. Deslauriers J, Gaulin P, Beaulieu M, et al. Long-term clinical and functional results of sleeve lobectomy for primary lung cancer. J Thorac Cardiovasc Surg 1986;92(5):871–879.
267. Delarue NC, Eschapasse H, eds. International trends in general thoracic surgery. Philadelphia: WB Saunders, 1985:1.
268. Faber LP, Jensik R, Kittle CF. Results of sleeve lobectomy for bronchogenic carcinoma in 101 patients. Ann Thorac Surg 1984;37:279–285.
269. Tisi GM, Friedman PJ, Peters RM, et al. Clinical staging of primary lung cancer. Official statement of the American Thoracic Society. Am Rev Respir Dis 1983;127:659–664.
270. Roeslin N, Chalkiadakis G, Dumont P, Witz JP. A better prognostic value from a modification of lung cancer staging. J Thorac Cardiovasc Surg 1987;94:504–509.
271. Van Raemdonck DE, Schneider A, Ginsberg RJ. Surgical treatment for higher stage non–small cell lung cancer. Ann Thorac Surg 1992;54:999–1013.
272. Mountain CF. Expanded possibilities for surgical treatment of lung cancer: survival in stage IIIa disease. Chest 1990;97(5):1045–1051.
273. Piehler JM, Pairolero PC, Weiland LH, et al. Bronchogenic carcinoma with chest wall invasion: factors affecting survival following en bloc resection. Ann Thorac Surg 1982;34:684–691.
274. Ginsberg RJ. Multimodality therapy for stage IIIa (N2) lung cancer; an overview. Chest 1993;103(Suppl 4):356S–359S.
275. Iannuzzi MC, Scoggin CH. Small cell lung cancer. Am Rev Respir Dis 1986;134:593–608.
276. Mountain CF. Clinical biology of small cell carcinoma. Relationship to surgical therapy. Semin Oncol 1978;5:272–279.
277. Abrams J, Doyle LA, Aisner J. Staging, prognostic factors, and special considerations in small cell lung cancer. Semin Oncol 1988;15(3):261–277.
278. Østerlind K, Ihde DC, Ettinger DS, et al. Staging and prognostic factors in small cell carcinoma of the lung. Cancer Treat Rep 1983;67(1):3–9.
279. Zelen M. Keynote address on biostatistics and data retrieval. Cancer Chemother Rep 1973;4(2):31–42.
280. Sagman U, Maki E, Evans WK, et al. Small cell carcinoma of the lung: derivation of a prognostic staging system. J Clin Oncol 1991;9:1639–1649.
281. Maksymiuk A, Jett JR, Earle JD, et al. Sequencing and sched-

ule effects of cisplatin plus etoposide in small cell lung cancer: results of a north central cancer treatment group randomized clinical trial. J Clin Oncol 1994;12:70–76.
282. Livingston RB, McCraken JD, Trauft CJ, et al. Isolated pleural effusion in small cell lung carcinoma: favorable prognosis. Chest 1982;81:208–215.
283. Ihde DC, Pass HI, Eli JG. Small cell lung cancer. In: DeVita VT, Hellman S, Rosenberg SA, eds. The principles and practice of oncology. 4th ed. Philadelphia: JB Lippincott, 1993:723–758.
284. Albain KS, Crowlye JJ, Leblanc M, Livingston RB. Determinants of improved outcome in small cell lung cancer: an analysis of the 2,580 patients: Southwest Oncology Group database. J Clin Oncol 1990;8:1563–1574.
285. Nogeire C, Muncer F, Botstein C. Long survival in patients with bronchogenic carcinoma complicated by superior vena cava obstruction. Chest 1979;75:325–329.
286. Reilly JJ Jr, Mentzer SJ, Sugarbaker DJ. Preoperative assessment of patients undergoing pulmonary resection. Chest 1993;103(4):342S–345S.
287. Feinstein AR, Sosin DM, Wells CK. The Will Rogers phenomenon: stage migration and new diagnostic techniques as a source of misleading statistics for survival in cancer. N Engl J Med 1985;312(25):1604–1608.
288. Feinstein AR, Wells CK. A clinical-severity staging system for patients with lung cancer. Medicine 1990;69(1):1–33.
289. Ginsberg RJ, Kris MG, Armstrong JG. Non–Small cell lung cancer. In: DeVita VT, Hellman S, Rosenberg SA, eds. The principles and practice of oncology. 4th ed. Philadelphia: JB Lippincott, 1993:673–723.
290. Schenk DA, Chambers SL, Derdak S, et al. Comparison of the Wang 19-gauge and 22-gauge needles in the mediastinal staging of lung cancer. Am Rev Respir Dis 1993;147:1251–1258.
291. Utz JP, Patel AM, Edell ES. The role of transcarinal needle aspiration in the staging of bronchogenic carcinoma. Chest 1993;104(4):1012–1016.
292. Pearson FG. Staging of the mediastinum: role of mediastinoscopy and computed tomography. Chest 1993;103(4):346S–348S.
293. Patterson GA, Ginsberg RJ, Poon PY, et al. A prospective evaluation of magnetic resonance imaging, computed tomography, and mediastinoscopy in the preoperative assessment of mediastinal node status in bronchogenic carcinoma. J Thorac Cardiovasc Surg 1987;94:679–684.
294. Libshitz HI, McKenna RJ Jr, Haynie TP, et al. Mediastinal evaluation in lung cancer. Radiology 1984;151:295–299.
295. Staples CA, Muller NL, Miller RR, et al. Mediastinal nodes in bronchogenic carcinoma: comparison between CT and mediastinoscopy. Radiology 1988;167:367–372.
296. McCloud TC, Bourgouin PM, Greenberg RW, et al. Bronchogenic carcinoma: analysis of staging in the mediastinum with CT by correlative lymph node mapping and sampling. Radiology 1992;182:319–322.
297. Gross BH, Glazer GM, Orringer MD, et al. Bronchogenic carcinoma metastatic to normal sized lymph nodes: frequency and significance. Radiology 1988;166:74–77.
298. Rusch V, Macapinlac H. Heelan R, et al. NR-LU-10 monoclonal antibody scanning. J Thorac Cardiovasc Surg 1993;106:200–204.

13

PROGNOSTIC FACTORS

Kell Østerlind and Jens Benn Sørensen

INTRODUCTION

Lung cancer is the leading cause of cancer death in males and the second or third cause in females in most of the world. Antitobacco campaigns have recently resulted in slightly decreasing incidence rates in males in North America and other Western countries, whereas rates in females are still increasing. Epidemiologic data show a close relationship between incidence and mortality rates without a significant effect of clinical endeavors to improve treatment, even after the introduction of chemotherapy in the early 1970s (1, 2). The overall 5-year survival rate is still about only 5%. Minimal disease at the time of diagnosis is the most important prognostic determinant in small cell as well as non–small cell lung cancer (NSCLC). Early diagnosis through screening of high-risk groups has not proved to be effective; the strategy is expensive, and overall treatment results are not significantly improved (3, 4).

Why, then, do we care so much about prognostic factors in lung cancer when the outlook for most patients in general terms could be characterized as "bad" or "very bad"? Historically, the interest in prognostic factors can be traced to progress in cancer surgery and radiotherapy in the middle of the century with a renaissance after introduction of combination chemotherapy of small cell lung cancer (SCLC) some 20 years ago. Inspired by progress in treatment of Hodgkin's disease and childhood lymphoblastic leukemia, the 1970s and 1980s became an era of randomized trials. Chemotherapy of lung cancer was not another success story, however, especially regarding long-term results; the survival difference among treatment arms in many trials often was small, thus treatment efficacy evaluation was at risk of being confounded by incidental differences in prognostic characteristics (5). Pretreatment prognostic stratification is now routine in randomized trials, and prognostic factors are increasingly important in the selection of patients for phase II trials and for individual planning of therapy outside of trials. Selection may be necessary because of limitations in health care resources and ethical concerns about balancing side effects and the chances of a beneficial effect of chemotherapy treatment—especially in patients with NSCLC. This balance is crucial in the evaluation of new agents, and inclusion criteria in phase II trials are therefore much more restrictive today than they were 10 years ago. Inclusion requires favorable prognostic attributes such as good performance status, no brain or liver metastases, and no major abnormalities in biochemical tests. Prognostic factor data are mandatory to enable comparison of results of a trial with those of similar trials; they also support estimates of the expected outcome when a trial plans to introduce an investigative regimen as a general treatment policy.

Prognostic factors for general clinical use include such variables as age, sex, performance status, stage of disease, and routine biochemical test results. Histopathologic features, flow cytometry, identification and quantitation of tumor specific compounds in tissue, and cytogenetic examinations require surgically sampled specimens, i.e., a thoracotomy in patients without distant metastases. Clinical use of these types of prognostic variables is thus restricted to patients with operable tumors, i.e., less than 5% of patients with SCLC and only about 25% of patients with non–small cell carcinomas. Investigations on the prognostic impact of tumor characteristics are warranted, nevertheless, to associate new laboratory research with clinical behavior of the tumor. Of special interest for the clinician are tumor markers in blood. Ideally, they should be tumor specific and the concentration should be correlated to tumor volume or other biologic characteristics that influence the prognosis. To be useful as a prognostic factor, a tumor marker should occur in abnormal concentrations in a majority of patients at the time of diagnosis, and the spectrum of values should be broad, with a simple negative relationship to survival.

STATISTICAL METHODS

A prognostic factor is a variable with a statistically significant relationship to survival. Survival does not have a definitive value before the patient is dead, but with simple statistical models, such as the Kaplan-Meier estimation, it is possible to estimate the probability of being alive at a certain time after initiation of observation (6). A 95% confidence interval on the estimate is calculated as $\pm 1.96 \times SE$ (standard error of the estimate). The confidence limits may be useful when a certain benchmark value is mentioned, e.g., the estimated 2-year survival; however, graphically confidence ranges disturb the visual impression of the figure (Fig. 13.1). A difference between survival estimates for two series of patients can be tested with specific tests, such as the log rank test (Mantel-Cox) or the generalized Wilcoxon test (Gehan). As a zero hypothesis it is postulated that there are identical death hazards in the two groups. Supposing proportionality between death hazards in two groups, the proportionality factor must be close to 1 if the zero hypothesis is correct. The test statistic is χ^2 distributed, and the zero hypothesis is usually rejected if $P > .05$. The proportionality assumption can be tested with a plot of the cumulative hazard functions. If the survival curves cross, as in the example, it is normally not reasonable to assume proportionality between death hazards. The log rank test can also be used for characteristics for which it would be more natural to split the series into more than two groups. If there is a hierarchical order among groups, a test for trend should be used (7). Statistical software packages such as BMDP (BMDP Statistical Software, Inc., University of California, Los Angeles, CA) (8) for personal computers are of great practical help, and the program documentation, including examples with simple data files, may often improve the understanding of the statistical methods.

A multivariate model is necessary if the influence of several concurrent factors is to be investigated. The most common method is Cox' proportional hazards regression model (9):

$$H(t) = H_0(t) \times \exp(z_1\beta_1 + z_2\beta_2 + z_3\beta_3 + ... + z_n\beta_n)$$

This model postulates that the death hazard $H(t)$ for any patient is proportional to an empirical baseline hazard $H_0(t)$, which is the death hazard function for patients in whom all the regression variables (z) are zero. In a stepwise computer analysis, a set of best fitting coefficients (β), with significant contribution in the equation, are obtained. The stepwise process is called forward if the variables are included one by one (and discarded again if their influence is insignificant); the reverse process is called the backward procedure.

Interactions among variables may result in minor differences between final models obtained with the two procedures, thus both procedures are often carried out, combined with tests for interactions, for proportionality, and for variation with time. For interpretation of the model, it is important that all $z = 0$ codes are related to clinically meaningful attributes, e.g., normal laboratory tests and normal findings at imaging procedures.

The proportionality assumption is tested with log-log plots (Fig. 13.1), which must be made for all variables in the final model. If the principle is violated for one of the pivotal factors, it may be necessary to stratify the model for this factor or to establish two separate models (8–10).

The Cox model assumes the same influence of each variable (i.e., a fixed β-value) throughout the data and constant interaction between two variables, if interaction occurs. Focal problems related to fit, in one or the other end of the "prognostic spectrum," are supposed to reflect stochastic variation and therefore are suppressed in the fitting process. Unanticipated biologic peculiarities may thus be overlooked. The advantage is that the risk of overfitting is reduced. If peculiarities are suspected, such as a hypothesis based on laboratory research, other statistical models are optional, e.g., the recursive partition and amalgamation method (RECPAM) (11). RECPAM is based on statistical clustering theories. For example, the patient material is split, step by step, like a branching tree, to a minimum of 30 patients in a branch; every branch ends in a terminal node (Fig. 13.2). Survival data from different terminal nodes are compared, and if differences are small, relative to predefined criteria, nodes are merged (or amalgamated) to form final prognostic classes. The resulting tree thus has similarities to the stepwise order of a clinical examination program. Specific variables may be influential in some, but not in other, parts of the tree, which may inspire new biologic hypotheses; the risk of overfitting should always be kept in mind, however.

PROGNOSTIC FACTORS IN SMALL CELL LUNG CANCER

Prognostic factor studies in SCLC can be subdivided into those on classical clinical characteristics, tumor markers combined with general clinical variables, and new biologic tumor characteristics. The aims of the first type are simple predictive models for use in treatment trials or clinical practice. Tumor markers may improve clinical practice two ways: improvements in the separation of prognostic subgroups

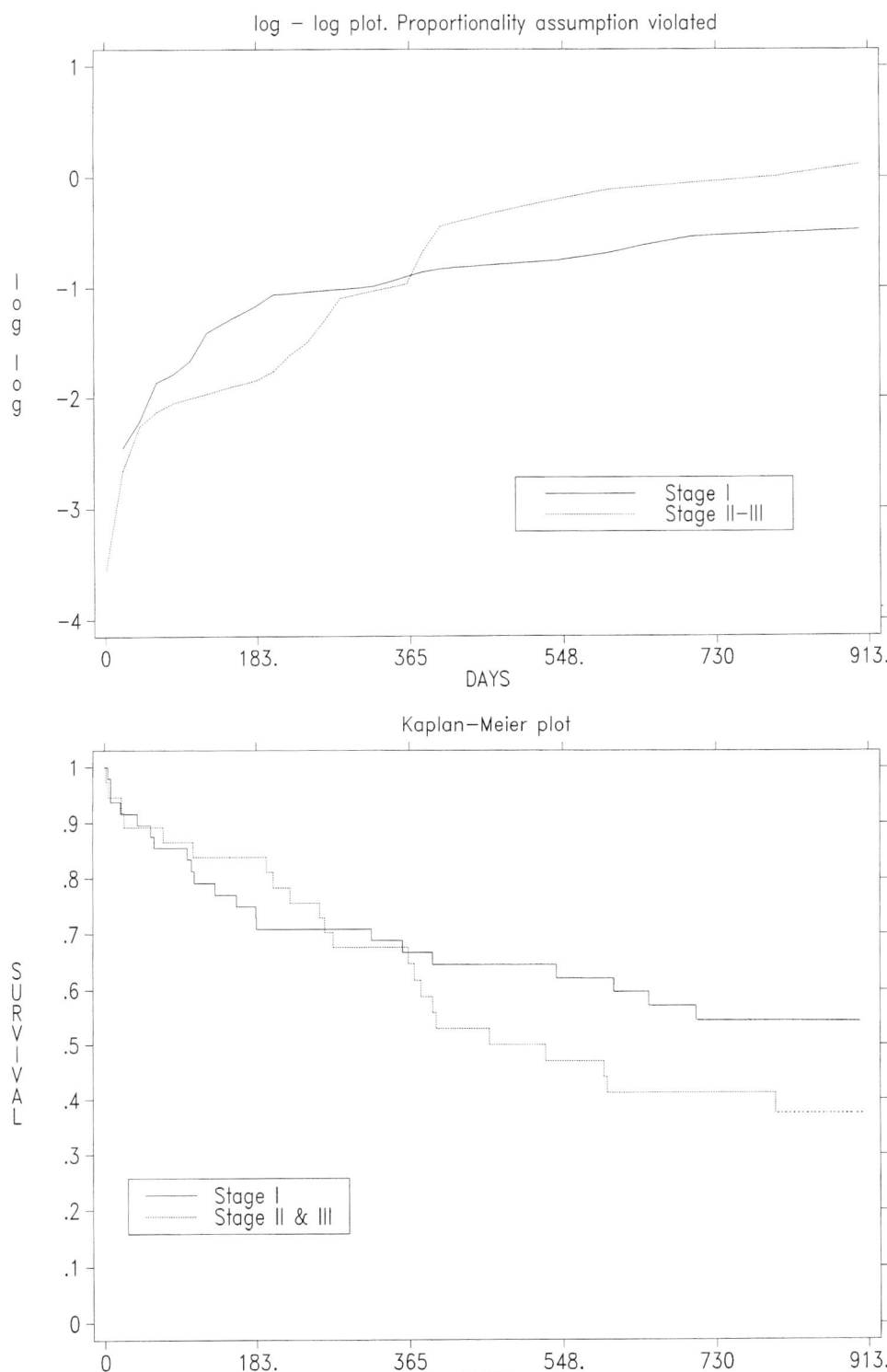

FIGURE 13.1. Upper panel. Kaplan-Meier plots of survival in a series of 108 patients with adenocarcinoma of the lung. Curves cross, thus the log rank test is an inappropriate statistical test. Lower panel. Cox proportional hazards model on the same series, stratified by stage of disease. The curves are not parallel, and the stage thus is dubious as a variable in the Cox model.

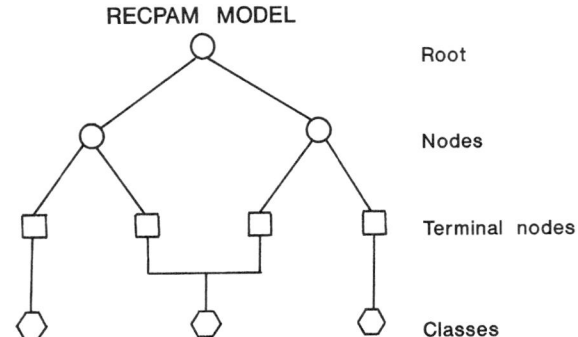

FIGURE 13.2. Recursive partioning and amalgamation model (RECPAM) is a treelike prognostic classification method. By convention, bad risk patients go left at a split. An insignificant difference in survival between two patients in two (or more) terminal nodes leads to amalgamation into one common class.

and reduction or elimination of staging. Investigations on new molecular features are important for clarification of tumor biology, even if there is no immediate desire to add them to clinical prognostic models.

CLINICAL PROGNOSTIC FACTOR MODELS

Some of the larger prognostic factor studies published since 1985 are summarized in Table 13.1 (12–20). The stage of disease and pretreatment performance status are dominating factors in all studies. The typical outcome of staging is summarized in Table 13.2. Most adverse for the prognosis are metastases to the bone marrow, liver, or brain, whereas the prognostic impact of spread to pleura, skin, or peripheral lymph nodes, or the presence of an abnormal bone scan have less impact on the death hazard in univariate as well as multivariate analyses (13, 17, 20, 21). Disease stage thus is a compound factor dependent on the number and type of staging procedures. It is clear that the demarcation between limited-stage and extensive-stage disease has changed with the introduction, during the past two decades, of better imaging techniques. Abdominal computed tomography (CT) scans or ultrasonography have replaced isotope scans and peritoneoscopy. Generally, this stage migration results in a reduced proportion of patients in the good prognosis group and improved survival data in both groups (22). For example, replacement of abdominal ultrasonography with CT scans resulted in migration and better prognosis for the remaining group of patients with limited disease (23). It even seems possible to make further substaging of limited disease dependent on whether mediastinal lymph node metastases are apparent at mediastinoscopy and/or on the chest roentgenograms (24). Patients with brain metastases rarely become long-term disease free survivors, but the influence of this variable is often insignificant in multivariate models probably because the brain is more accessible to chemotherapy than originally supposed. Another reason is that the brain, in contrast to the liver and bone marrow, tolerates combined treatment with chemotherapy and radiotherapy. Selection may also play a role, however; symptomatic brain metastases may quickly deteriorate the performance status of the patient, hindering inclusion in trials on which prognostic factor analyses have been based. Abnormal values of lactate dehydrogenase (LDH) and alkaline phosphatase are other important prognostic determinants. The two features are partly correlated, but LDH is elevated in 55% to 60% of newly diagnosed patients compared with elevated alkaline phosphatase in 40% of patients. This finding may explain why LDH tends to overrule alkaline phosphatase when both are included in the same Cox model (13). Abnormal values of LDH seem to reflect tumor burden (25), ruling out a variable such as "number of metastatic sites" in extensive-stage disease.

Hyponatremia (of less than 136 mmol/L) is observed in approximately 20% of patients. In about half of these patients, the condition is part of an inappropriate antidiuretic hormone secretion, although this syndrome is not invariably associated with a poor prognosis (26). Age and gender have prognostic impact in some series. The influence of age is especially characterized by an inferior outlook in patients older than 65 or 70 years. Poor tolerance of intensive chemotherapy tends to augment this influence (27), whereas exclusion from trials of patients in poor shape because of concurrent diseases, such as chronic bronchitis or early dementia, tends to attenuate the apparent impact of age. Part of this selection process may take place in offices referring patients to the oncology center.

The proportion of female patients varies among centers in different countries, from 15% to 35%, reflecting differences in smoking habits among women. The proportion seems to be steady in North America (17, 18), whereas we have noticed an increase from 25% to 35% in the Copenhagen Lung Cancer Group patient series from the period 1973 through 1987. Generally, the prognosis in females is better than that in males, especially long-term survival (28, 29), but the trend is not significant in all series (Table 13.1). Better prognosis in females compared with males is not restricted to lung cancer. The reason presumably is multifactorial and has not yet been clarified.

Other laboratory tests, such as hemoglobin and white blood cell (WBC) counts and plasma urate and bicarbonate concentrations, have been proved to influ-

TABLE 13.1. Clinical Prognostic Factors in Small Cell Lung Cancer: Results from Multivariate Analyses

Variable	A[a] (371)	B[b] (874)	C[c] (407)	D[d] (333)	E[e] (1521)	F[f] (411)	G[g] (2580)	H[h] (411)	I[i]
Poor performance status	+	+	+	+	+	+	+	+	+
Extensive disease	+	+	+	+[j]	+	+[j]	+	+	+[k]
LDH	...	+	+	ns	...	+	+	+	+
Alkaline phosphatase	+	ns	+	ns	...	+	...	ns	ns
Alanine transaminase	ns	ns	ns	+	...	ns	...	ns	ns
Hyponatremia	+	+	+	ns	...	ns	...	ns	ns
Hypoalbuminemia	+	...	ns	+	...	ns	...	ns	ns
Age	ns	+	ns	ns	ns	ns	+	+	ns
Male sex	ns	+	ns	ns	+	+	+	ns	ns

Abbreviations. +, statistically significant; ns, not significant.
[a]Souhami et al., 1985 (12).
[b]Østerlind et al., 1986 (13).
[c]Cerny et al., 1987 (14).
[d]Vincent et al., 1987 (15).
[e]Spiegelman et al., 1989 (16).
[f]Dearing et al., 1990 (17).
[g]Albain et al., 1990 (18).
[h]Allan et al., 1990 (19).
[i]Sagman et al., 1991 (20).
[j]Liver metastases.
[k]Separate influence of brain and liver metastases.

TABLE 13.2. Metastatic Spread of Disease at Pretreatment Staging in Small Cell Lung Cancer: Examples From Three Large Series

Site of Metastases	NCI[a] (411) (%)	Toronto[b] (614) (%)	Copenhagen[c] (1651) (%)
Brain	11	6	7
Bone	25	26	...
Bone marrow	23[d]	16	20[d]
Liver[e]	25	28	27
Nodes/soft tissue	8	12	14
Extensive disease	66	53	51

[a]Data from Dearing et al., 1973 through 1987 (17).
[b]Data from Sagman et al., 1974 through 1986 (20).
[c]Data from Østerlind et al., 1973 through 1987 (13).
[d]Bilateral iliac crest examinations.
[e]Isotope scintigraphy, peritoneoscopy, ultrasonography (with or without biopsies), and CT scans-procedures changing over time.

ence the prognosis in a few studies (Table 13.1). Clinically, it seems reasonable that anemia or a increased WBC, because of airway infections, may be associated with an inferior prognosis, but varying "penetrance" in multivariate analyses of these "weaker" prognostic factors can result from stochastic biologic variation. The influence of these features may also be correlated to, and thus overshadowed by, strong factors such as performance status and disease stage. It is therefore reasonable to exclude them from a general prognostic factor system.

A GENERAL PROGNOSTIC FACTOR SYSTEM

No general prognostic factor system exists. The International Organization for the Study of Lung Cancer (IASLC) has published recommendations for staging procedures and prognostic factors in treatment trials (30), but no unique system has been established. There may be several reasons: many investigators do not feel a need for one common system; some think we do not have enough data to establish a system; no exact recommendations have been established regarding how to handle prognostic factors in treatment trials; exact requirements for staging (including options on staging procedures) have not been formulated; and it has not been decided whether "stage" could be excluded or should be included—either as a "normal" prognostic factor or as a global stratification factor. A specific statistical method must also be chosen; should it be the proportional hazards model or the RECPAM method? Exclusion of stage would simplify the system and spare clinical resources, but stage is the strongest determinant of long-term survival. Omission of stage as a variable results in a system that underestimates and overestimates the prognosis in limited- and extensive-stage disease, respectively (19). An initiative to simplify and standardize a prognostic factor system in SCLC has been taken by Rawson and Peto (31). Among their primary aims were the reduction of factors to the most influential minimum, division of patients into three equally sized groups based on prognostic score, and establishment of separate models for early (less than 6-month) and subsequent (6- to 24-month) periods of follow up. The last issue was prompted by observed changes in influence over time for some factors. Disease stage was an important prognostic factor in both periods and was integrated as a conventional variable in the suggested models (Table 13.3).

TUMOR MARKERS

A steadily increasing number of tumor markers are detected in SCLC, and some of them are known to be related to prognosis. Table 13.4 (32–39) includes a summary of six of the most extensively studied markers plus LDH. LDH is included because it is an important factor in the clinical prognostic factor models, and because both serum concentrations and influence on the prognosis are correlated to that of the tumor markers, despite the fact that LDH is less tumor specific in its origin (25). Thus, serum LDH is correlated linearly to serum concentrations of neuron specific enolase (NSE) (34, 37), thymidine kinase (TK), and tissue polypeptide antigen (TPA) (37). Similarly, serum concentrations of NSE, TK, TPA, and creatine kinase BB (CK-BB) are all correlated (33, 37), whereas serum carcinoembryonic antigen (CEA) is not well correlated to either NSE or CK-BB (33). Serum levels of all markers are generally higher in extensive-stage compared with limited-stage disease, but the difference between stages is not equally pronounced for the various compounds (Table 13.5). With the exception of CK-BB and CEA, pretreatment marker levels are abnormal in more than 50% of the total series of patients. Considering these similarities and correlations, it is reasonable that only one or two factors will remain in a multivariate analysis that includes a larger set of markers; there is no contradiction in the fact that the four multivariate analyses mentioned in Table 12.4 do not lead to identical results. According to van der Gaast et al. (37), combined determination of TK, TPA, and LDH—or the combination of disease extent and a marker—does not result in more prognostic information than is offered by one of these variables alone.

Based on current data it can be concluded that CEA has no role as a pretreatment prognostic factor in SCLC because it is less reliable than the other six markers, including LDH, NSE, TK, TPA, chromogranin A (ChrA), and probably also CK-BB. These markers are each candidates for a future prognostic factor system, but more prospective investigations in larger series are necessary to conclude definitively which is best. This decision will also be influenced by cost and other useful characteristics of the marker, such as impact on long-term survival and early prediction of relapse, for which one study proves ChrA to be more sensitive than NSE (38). In the same study LDH was as good as NSE in predicting relapse, thus it may still be too early to delete LDH from the pretreatment laboratory program in SCLC.

GROWTH FACTORS

Tumor secretion of peptides with endocrine activity may result in the well-known and clinically interesting Cushing's syndrome and syndrome of inappropriate antidiuretic hormone secretion. These conditions may negatively influence prognosis in univariate analyses (26), but the complex set of criteria required for the diagnosis of these syndromes makes them impractical as prognostic factors. Other peptides have local activity as autocrine growth factors and thus have a direct biologic impact on the prognosis. The most extensively investigated of these peptides is the bombesinlike peptide, gastrin-releasing peptide (GRP). The half-life of this compound in blood is supposed to be very short, and plasma GRP escapes detection with general radioimmunoassays (40). It seems possible, however, to detect GRP with a highly sensitive radioimmunoassay method (41), as well as with the prehormone pro-GRP, which seems to be

TABLE 13.3. Prognostic Factors Related to Survival after Diagnosis in Small Cell Lung Cancer: Cox Analyses

VARIABLE	FIRST 6 Mo (1960 PATIENTS)	6–24 Mo (1310 PATIENTS)
Poor performance status	++	++
Alkaline phosphatase	++	+
Extensive disease	++	++
Age	+	ns
Hyponatremia	+	++
Male sex	+	ns

Data from Rawson NSB, Peto J. An overview of prognostic factors in small cell lung cancer. A report from the Subcommittee for the Management of Lung Cancer of the United Kingdom Coordinating Committee on Cancer Research. Br. J Cancer 1990;61:597–604.

Abbreviations. +, statistically significant; ++, statistically significant and mandatory for optimal separation of the patients into three equally sized prognostic strata; ns, not significant.

TABLE 13.4. Tumor Markers with Prognostic Influence in Small Cell Lung Cancer.

VARIABLE	STUDY (NO. OF PATIENTS)							
	A[a] (43)	B[b] (195)	C[c] (85)	D[d] (125)	E[e] (37)	F[f] (69)	G[g] (159)	H[h] (92)
NSE	+	+	+	ns	+	ns	+	+
CK-BB	...	+	...	...	...	...	...	...
TK	...	...	...	ns	...	+	...	...
TPA	...	...	...	+	...	ns	...	...
ChrA	...	...	...	...	...	...	ns	...
CEA	...	+	ns	ns	...	...	ns	...
LDH	...	...	ns	ns	...	+	ns	...

Abbreviations. +, statistically significant; ns, not significant; NSE, neuron specific enolase; CK-BB, creatinine kinase BB; TK, thymidine kinase; TPA, tissue polypeptide antigen; ChrA, chromogranin A; CEA, carcinoembryonic antigen; LDH, lactate dehydrogenase.
[a]Data from Akoun et al., 1987 (32).
[b]Data from Jaques et al., 1988 (33).
[c]Multivariate analysis, Cox model. Data from Jørgensen et al., 1988 (34).
[d]Multivariate analysis, Cox model. Data from Gronowitz et al., 1990 (35).
[e]Data from Harding et al., 1990 (36).
[f]Multivariate analysis, Cox model. Data from van der Gaast et al., 1991 (37).
[g]Multivariate analysis, Cox model. Data from Johnson et al., 1993 (38).
[h]Data from Szturmowicz et al., 1993 (39).

TABLE 13.5. Incidence of Abnormal Blood Levels of Six Tumor Markers in Limited and Extensive Stage Small Cell Lung Cancer

STUDY/VARIABLE (REFERENCE NO.)	LIMITED STAGE (%)	EXTENSIVE STAGE (%)
Jaques et al. (33)		
NSE	60	70
CEA	44	44
CK-BB	14	39
van der Gaast et al. (37)		
NSE	90	95
TK	38	68
TPA	36	79
Johnson et al. (38)		
NSE	77	85
CEA	20	47
ChrA	50	71

Abbreviations. ChrA, chromogranin A; NSE, neuron specific enolase; CEA, carcinoembryonic antigen; CK-BB, creatine kinase BB; TK, thymidine kinase; TPA, tissue polypeptide antigen.
Cutoff levels. NSE, >12.5 ng/mL; CEA >3 ng/mL in Jaques et al.; CK-BB, >10 ng/mL; TK, >5 U/mL; TPA, >100 U/mL; ChrA, >50 ng/mL.

much more stable in plasma compared with GRP (42); however, the possible prognostic value of these tests has not yet been clarified. Another aspect of GRP as a growth factor is its local regulation, such as degradation, a process catalyzed by cell surface endopeptidase CD10/neutral endopeptidase 24.11 (43). It is interesting that cigarette smoke inactivates this enzyme.

If autocrine growth factors can be detected in blood, and if plasma concentrations are well correlated to processes occurring in the microenvironment in the tumor, these compounds may be both specific and sensitive as clinical prognostic predictors. Furthermore, they may provide qualitative information about the neoplasm that, in the future, may open possibilities for more individualized treatment strategies.

Investigations on relationships between defective oncogenes and characteristics of the malignant cell have led to a new category of prognostic factors. Detection of defective oncogenes requires tissue specimens of "surgical" quality, which cannot be obtained routinely in SCLC. No relationship between oncogene abnormalities and the prognosis has yet been proved in SCLC. Amplification of the *myc* family oncogenes has been proved in 15% to 31% of treated tumors but only in 8% of untreated tumors (44). Studies on cell lines suggest an association between *myc* amplification and variant subtype morphology (45). This subtype has analogies to the histopathologic "combined" subtype, which is associated with a significantly inferior prognosis in clinical series (46, 47). Histopathologic subtyping has never found a place among other clinical prognostic factors, however, because approximately 50% of the diagnostic biopsies are technically insufficient to enable classification—and probably often too small to be representative (46).

PROGNOSTIC FACTORS IN NON–SMALL CELL LUNG CANCER

The study populations in NSCLC are usually divided into patients with resectable and those with nonresectable tumors, respectively. This separation occurs because of the very different treatment and outlook with respect to survival in these two groups.

When using the current prognostic factors describing clinical, histologic, and clinical chemistry features, however, the prognosis is not predicted completely because a large fraction of the variability in survival remains unexplained. This is most likely the case because the prognostic variables noted above are, in reality, epiphenomena of the true cellular and molecular characteristics of NSCLC. Little is known about the biologic model of the disease itself, but the literature on this topic is increasing rapidly, thereby promising a better understanding of the disease and a more accurate prediction of outcome, which ultimately may be used for selection of treatment. An update on the current knowledge of prognostic variables in NSCLC that have been established through multivariate analyses follows. The studies reviewed describe prognostic factors for survival solely in NSCLC patients and provide clear descriptions of the variables included in the multivariate analyses. These studies are divided by whether resectable tumors, nonresectable tumors, or all stages of disease, respectively, were included. Results presented in abstracts are not included. Finally, some of the biologic factors that have shown promising results in preliminary analyses are considered.

MULTIVARIATE ANALYSES OF PROGNOSTIC FACTORS FOR SURVIVAL IN RESECTABLE NSCLC

Twenty studies (48–67), including a total of 3500 patients with resected NSCLC, are summarized in Table 13.6. It is apparent that none of the variables has been evaluated in all 20 studies. Definite prognostic factors for long-term survival include good performance status, low stage, and low lymph node category (N in the TNM classification system). Low tumor category (T) also was a major predictor of survival in many trials, but the variables describing T and N were not independent and significant predictors of survival in all studies evaluating these factors. This observation might be explained by the phenomenon that T and N categories may be less important in Cox multivariate regression analysis when the stage of disease is included in the analyses as well. In most studies including these variables, there was a significant prediction by either T and N or by stage.

Possible prognostic factors listed in Table 13.6 include variables that have not been evaluated extensively but that have been attributed as having an inde-

TABLE 13.6. Multivariate Analyses of Prognostic Factors in 20 Studies Including 3500 Resected NSCLC Tumors

PROGNOSTIC FACTOR	POSITIVE STUDIES/ TOTAL EVALUATED (NO.)
Definite	
Performance status	3/3
Stage	9/9
T stage	5/13
N stage	5/8
Possible	
Postoperative infection	2/2
Perioperative blood transfusion	2/2
DNA ploidy	3/5
Minor importance	
Age	1/8
Gender	1/9
Histology	3/12
Differentiation	1/4
Extent of resection	3/9
Preliminary	
Tumor giant cells	1/1
Plasma cell infiltration	1/1
Solid ACL/other ACL subtypes	1/1
Satellite pulmonary nodules	1/1
FEV_1	1/1
WBC	1/3
Hemoglobin level preoperatively	1/1
Intratumoral blood vessel invasion	1/2
ras Mutation	1/1
p53 Mutation	1/1
p53 Protein expression	1/1
Tumor-associated antigen 43-9F	1/1
Proliferative activity	1/2
Cell line establishment	1/1

Abbreviations. ACL, adenocarcinoma of the lung; FEV_1, forced expiratory volume in 1 second.

pendent impact on survival in more than half of the studies. Such is the case for postoperative infections, perioperative blood transfusions, and DNA ploidy.

The impact of infections, including empyema, pneumonia, or wound infection in the postoperative period, was evaluated by Gail et al. (48), whereas Deslaurier et al. (52) included in one group patients with major postoperative complications, such as pleuropneumonia, bronchopleural fistulas, and respiratory failure. Both trials reported a significant deterioration of survival outlook, a finding, however, that probably is associated less with the biologic characteristics of the malignant disease than with the treatment.

The effect of perioperative blood transfusion has been a significant prognostic variable in two studies (53, 63). Both studies included exclusively stage I patients and observed 5-year survival rates of 53% and 62% for patients with blood transfusions and 81% and 76% for patients without, respectively. Thus, any perioperative transfusions significantly worsen the patient's prognosis. This association may be due to an adverse effect of the transfusion itself, or may serve as a marker for another yet undetermined risk factor.

The ploidy status of the DNA has been investigated in five studies (58, 62, 64, 66, 67) and was an independent predictor of survival in three of them (62, 64, 67). Survival was poorest in patients with DNA aneuploid tumors, and the same pattern, although not significant, was observed in one of the two negative studies (66) but not in the other (58).

Other less evaluated prognostic factors are outlined in Table 13.6. Because these factors have been evaluated or were positive in only one trial, none can be claimed to be established prognostic factors. They should be evaluated further for confirmation or rejection as predictors of survival in this patient group.

A number of variables have been evaluated relatively intensively and have been shown to be important in only a few studies (Table 13.6). These variables may thus be of minor importance as predictors of survival in resected NSCLC patients. This was the case for variables describing age, gender, histology, histologic degree of differentiation, and extent of operation (usually evaluated as lobectomy compared with a larger resection).

With respect to histology, both Gail et al. (48) and Deslaurier et al. (52) observed an independent and significant prediction for long-term survival among patients with squamous cell carcinoma compared with patients with nonsquamous histology, although these observations were not confirmed in the study by Lipford et al. (49). However, the latter study revealed a significantly worse prognosis for patients having large cell carcinoma. In contrast, nine studies (54, 58–60, 62–65, 67) did not find any independent prognostic impact of histology. Overall, these 12 studies suggest that the influence of different histologic types of resected NSCLC is minor when other variables are also taken into consideration.

MULTIVARIATE ANALYSES OF PROGNOSTIC FACTORS FOR SURVIVAL IN NONRESECTABLE NSCLC

Fourteen studies (68–81), including a total of 5875 patients with inoperable NSCLC included in chemotherapy trials with or without radiotherapy, have reported data on multivariate analyses of variables predicting survival. The prognostic variables carrying significant and independent information are outlined in Table 13.7. Also included in this table is a

TABLE 13.7. Multivariate Analyses of Prognostic Factors in Nonresectable NSCLC

	POSITIVE STUDIES/TOTAL EVALUATED (NO.)	
PROGNOSTIC FACTOR	CHEMOTHERAPY ± RADIOTHERAPY (N = 5875)	RADIOTHERAPY ALONE (N = 1565)
Definite		
Performance status	13/14	1/1
New international staging	4/5	1/1
Possible		
LDH	4/8	...
Gender	7/11	1/1
Albumin	2/4	...
Minor importance		
Weight loss	3/11	1/1
Histology	2/7	...
Age	1/9	1/1
Preliminary		
T stage	1/1	1/1
N stage	...	1/1
Metastases to		
Liver	3/7	...
Bone	2/6	...
Subcutaneous	1/1	...
0/1 Extrathoracic metastasis	1/1	...
WBC	1/2	...
Aspartic aminotransferase	1/2	...
Hemoglobin	1/2	...
Calcium	1/1	...
Chemotherapy/BSC	1/1	...
Cisplatin/no cisplatin	1/1	...

Data from 14 studies including 5875 patients treated with chemotherapy or chemotherapy plus radiotherapy and one study including 1565 patients treated with radiotherapy alone.
Abbreviations. BSC, best supportive care.

recent large study evaluating independent prognostic factors in 1565 patients treated with radiotherapy in four clinical trials (82). Performance status has been evaluated individually in all 15 studies listed in Table 13.7 and was significant in 14 of them, indicating that performance status is still the best-documented prognostic variable in NSCLC patients.

The new international staging system, as described by Mountain in 1986 (83), has been evaluated in six multivariate analyses; of those, this analysis offered independent and significant additional information on survival outlook in five of the studies (75, 79–82). Thus, the importance of the new staging system has now been firmly documented as an independent prognostic factor for survival both among resected patients and nonresectable patients receiving other treatments.

Other variables that may be possible predictors of good prognosis, although less intensively evaluated, are low LDH, female gender, and normal plasma albumin level (Table 13.7). Variables of minor importance, as indicated by lack of significant influence in the majority of studies in which they were evaluated, include weight loss, histology, and age (Table 13.7.)

The relative importance of other potential variables should be explored further in patients with nonresectable tumors. This also holds true for a number of biochemical variables, such as WBC count, and aspartic aminotransferase, hemoglobin, and calcium levels. However, these variables may be less logical theoretically as prognostic indicators than the anatomic stage of the disease possesses.

The impact of chemotherapy versus best supportive care and of cisplatin-based chemotherapy versus cytostatic treatment without cisplatin has been evaluated by Rapp et al. (73) and Albain et al. (76), respectively. The Canadian multicenter study by Rapp and colleagues (73) showed both an enhanced survival for patients receiving chemotherapy and also that chemotherapy—as opposed to best supportive care only—was an independent predictor of survival in the 137 patients evaluated in the study.

Albain et al. (76) analyzed data from 2531 patients with inoperable NSCLC from the Southwest Oncology Group treated between 1974 and 1988. The use of cisplatin was an additional independent predictor of improved outcome in multivariate analyses after adjustments for year of accrual and all other prognostic variables. Although the effect of cisplatin was modest, the data allow the conclusion that it is real and not due to concurrent occurrence of other favorable prognostic variables. These data allow a cautious optimism regarding the development of more effective chemotherapy against this disease, but the issue should also be studied further.

MULTIVARIATE ANALYSES INCLUDING PATIENTS WITH ALL STAGES OF NSCLC

Six studies (84–89), including a total of 1701 patients with NSCLC of all stages and treated with either surgery, irradiation, or chemotherapy, have reported data on multivariate analyses of variables predicting survival. The prognostic variables carrying significant and independent information are outlined in Table 13.8. Again, not all variables have been included in all analyses, which somewhat limits conclusions. However, as in studies evaluating solely resectable or solely nonresectable tumors, both performance status and stage of disease carried significant and independent in-

TABLE 13.8. Multivariate Analyses of Prognostic Factors Including 1821 NSCLC Patients

Prognostic Factor[a]	Positive Studies Total Evaluated (No.)
Definite	
Performance status	2/2
Stage	5/6
Possible/minor importance	
Weight loss	1/1
Gender	3/6
T stage	1/2
N stage	1/2
LDH	1/2
Preliminary	
DNA ploidy	1/1
Tissue polypeptide antigen	1/1
Smoking habit (pack years)	1/1
Cell line establishment	1/1
Erythrocyte sedimentation rate	1/1
p53 Mutation	1/1
Probably not	
Age	0/5
Histology	0/3

Data from 6 studies including patients with all stages and treated with either surgery, irradiation, or chemotherapy.
[a]Variables relating to treatment have not been reviewed in this table.

formation on prognosis in nearly all studies evaluating these parameters, being positive in two of two and in five of six studies, respectively (Table 13.8). Stage was not a significant variable in a multivariate analysis by Stevenson et al. (86), which instead observed as significant a variable dividing patients into palliative or curative treatment status. Probably, this summarizing variable overrules the information regarding stages.

With respect to information on tumor (T) and lymph node (N) status, these variables were significant in one (84) of two (84, 88) multivariate analyses. In the study by Buccheri et al. (88), the significant impact of stage probably reduced the influence of T and N.

Among the preliminary variables, Stevenson et al. (86) reported that the ability to establish cell lines from tumor specimens was a detrimental survival factor compared with patients from whom cell lines could not be established. A similar observation was reported by Ichinose et al. (67). It has been speculated that the worse prognoses of patients who were cell line positive may reflect an enhanced metastatic potential and enhanced chemoresistance of the tumor cells in these patients (86).

BIOLOGIC FACTORS

In addition to stage of disease and performance status of the patient, many other factors are important for predicting the prognosis in NSCLC. These factors include the biologic properties inherent in the tumor cells themselves. The majority of these factors are currently considered preliminary because they have not usually been evaluated against other variables in multivariate testing. However, the literature is rapidly expanding in this field, as recently outlined by Szabo and Mulshine (90). Some of the biologic factors that have shown promising results in preliminary analyses are discussed below and are outlined in Table 13.8.

Neuroendocrine Markers

A subgroup of NSCLC, morphologically indistinguishable from other NSCLCs by conventional microscopy, exhibits some of the neuroendocrine features of SCLC (91, 92) and may be more responsive to chemotherapy than NSCLC tumors without these features (93–96). In these studies a variety of techniques were used to detect the expression of neuroendocrine markers, including immunohistochemical staining, electron microscopy, biochemical or immunologic assays, and molecular probes.

Four studies have reported the prognostic significance of neuroendocrine differentiation in clinical trials. In one by Graziano et al. (95), 52 NSCLC tumors were analysed immunohistochemically. Multiple neuroendocrine markers were significantly more frequent among chemotherapy responders than among nonresponders (38% versus 0%). Linnoila et al. (93) also observed a significantly higher response rate among neuroendocrine positive patients compared with patients whose tumors lacked these markers. There was, however, no significant impact on survival observed. Berendsen et al. (94) found neuroendocrine markers in 31% of 141 biopsy specimens from NSCLC patients, more frequently in adenocarcinoma. A multivariate analysis of the importance of neuroendocrine differentiation in NSCLC suggested that the observance of more than 50% positively stained tumor cells with a MOC-1 antibody was a negative prognostic factor.

Another study was reported by Skov et al. (96), who examined the prognostic impact of histologic demonstration of ChrA and NSE in 114 patients with nonresectable NSCLC treated with chemotherapy. Forty-four percent of the patients with more than 10% positive NSE cells responded to chemotherapy compared with 17% of the patients with fewer than 10% positive cells ($P < .025$). There was no similar impact of ChrA positivity, and no impact on survival was noted.

The prognostic value of pretreatment serum NSE level was evaluated in NSCLC patients of all stages by Diez et al. (97). Serum NSE was not related to stage or to histologic type. Patients with low NSE levels (less than 15 ng/mL) experienced significantly longer 2-year survival rates than patients whose initial levels were more than 15 ng/mL (70% versus 47%; $P < .05$).

From these studies it appears that the presence of neuroendocrine differentiation in NSCLC is an important biologic factor that should be evaluated further in multivariate analyses in clinical trials to show its relevance in the clinical behavior of these tumors. The current data suggest that the presence of neuroendocrine differentiation in NSCLC predicts a higher responsiveness to chemotherapy, which has not yet, however, translated into significant prolongation of survival.

Oncogenes and Oncogene Products

Oncogenes have been the basis for much research, and the prognostic importance of the presence of activating mutations in the *ras* oncogene in pulmonary adenocarcinoma has been demonstrated by Slebos et al. (98). A subsequent study by Rodenhuis and Slebos (99) confirmed the presence of *ras* mutations in approximately one third of the 69 cases. Despite apparently radical resection, the prognosis for patients with *ras* mutations was worse than for patients without this defect (death in 12 of 19 compared with 22 of 50; median observation time, 47 months). Studies by Sugio et al. (100) and Harada et al. (101) also disclosed a significant difference in survival in favor of *ras* negative patients. Similar results were presented by a group from the National Cancer Institute (NCI) who used the Cox proportional hazards model to show a shortened survival for patients with any type of *ras* mutation (102). The finding agrees with the observation by Harada et al. (101), who also found the presence of *ras* oncogene mutation to be an independent adverse prediction of survival in 116 surgically treated NSCLC patients. These studies suggest that the *ras* oncogene mutation identifies a poor-prognosis subgroup and that it should be explored further.

Amplification of the *myc* family of oncogenes has been found in 10% to 15% of lung cancers. An analysis of L-*myc* in 252 patients, of whom 237 had NSCLC, showed three possible patterns of restriction fragment length polymorphism with long, short, or both long and short fragments upon digestion of DNA by the enzyme *Eco*R1. Patients with long-only patterns live significantly longer than did those with the other two patterns in a univariate analysis (103).

Mutation in the gene coding for the p53 tumor suppressor protein is common in a variety of tumors. It also has been reported frequently in NSCLC, with structural abnormalities of the *p53* gene occurring in 60 (52%) of 115 surgical specimens (104). The finding is important because mutation of the *p53* gene coding for a tumor suppression protein leads to overexpression of the protein and loss of its tumor-suppression properties. Using an immunoperoxidase detection system, Quinlan et al. (105) examined 114 cases of stage I and II NSCLC and observed that accumulation of p53 protein had a significant, negative prognostic value. This finding, however, was not supported in two other studies (106, 107), which found no correlation with patient survival. Two studies (59, 89) have reported the presence of p53 mutation to be a significant prognostic variable in multivariate analyses (Tables 13.6 and 13.8).

Other oncogene products have also been considered important, such as the c-*erb*B-2 protein, which was studied in 203 NSCLC patients by Tateishi et al. (108). Immunohistochemical staining was positive in 28% of the adenocarcinomas and 2% of the squamous cell carcinomas; survival was significantly shorter for patients with c-*erb*B-2 positive tumors (Table 13.9).

Kern et al. (109) evaluated the p185*neu* protein product of the HER2*neu* protooncogene. This protein has characteristics of a tyrosine kinase growth factor receptor and may be important in human carcinogenesis. The expression of p185*neu* protein was a significant determinant of poor survival in patients with NSCLC with adenocarcinoma histology but not with squamous cell histology (109).

DNA PLOIDY

Aneuploidy (abnormal chromosomal number) has been evaluated for prognostic impact in several studies (109–111). Two recent studies (109, 110) observed that patients with diploid tumors had longer survival times than patients with aneuploid tumors, but the studies included both NSCLC and SCLC tumors. Another study by Isobe et al. (112) included 130 patients with NSCLC and similarly observed a more favorable survival for patients with a diploid DNA pattern compared with patients with aneuploid patterns ($P < .001$). In addition, a recent study by Volm et al. (84) showed an independent and significant impact of DNA ploidy on survival (Table 13.8).

CARBOHYDRATE ANTIGENS

Oncofetal antigens are alterations of the normal classic blood group antigens and are frequently expressed by tumor cells. The tumors often lose the mature blood group A and B determinants, whereas the precursor antigen H and H-related antigens often increase reciprocally. The presence of blood group antigens A, B, and H was assessed immunohistochemically in tumor samples from 164 resected NSCLC patients by Lee et al. (113). Survival of 28 patients with blood type A or AB who had primary tumors negative for blood group antigen A was significantly shorter than that of the 43 patients with antigen A-positive tumors ($P < .001$) and of the 93 patients with blood type B or O ($P = .002$). Expression of blood group antigen B or H in tumor cells did not correlate with survival. A Cox regression analysis showed that the expression of blood group antigen A in tumor cells added significantly to the prediction of overall survival provided by other potential prognostic variables in the patients with blood types A and AB. Thus, the expression of blood group antigen A in tumor cells seems to be an important favorable prognostic factor in NSCLC.

Miyake et al. (114) evaluated the binding of the monoclonal antibody MIA-15-5, which defines H, Le^y, and Le^b antigens in a study of 149 lung cancer patients, 141 of whom had NSCLC. Survival was significantly worse for MIA-15-5 positive patients compared with MIA-15-5 negative patients when analyzing the whole patient population as well as patients with only adenocarcinoma; it was most pronounced in the 67 patients with squamous cell carcinoma. The 5-year sur-

TABLE 13.9. Biologic Characteristics Attributed to Prognostic Impact in NSCLC Patients

VARIABLES
Neuroendocrine differentiation
Oncogenes
K-*ras* mutation
p-53 mutation
L-*myc* mutation
Oncogene products
p53 protein
c-*erb*B-2 protein
p185*neu* protein
DNA ploidy
Carbohydrate antigens
ABH blood group
Le^y and Le^b antigens
Le^x antigen (4C9) antigen
DBA binding site
Growth factors
Epidermal growth factor receptor
Proliferative activity
Ki67-related antigen

vival rate was 20.9% in the antigen positive group and 58.6% in the antigen negative group. Multivariate analysis with the Cox regression model indicated that among the variables tested, MIA-15-5 positivity had the best correlation with 5-year mortality, followed by lymph node status (N stage) and tumor size (T stage).

Two other carbohydrate markers, the 4C9 antigen, which is an Lex antigen, and the Dolichos biflorus agglutinin (DBA) binding site, which is an N-acetylgalactosamine marker, was examined histochemically in tumors and in normal tissue of 100 patients with NSCLC and two patients with SCLC (115). Survival rates varied significantly, especially among the 16 patients with tumors that expressed DBA binding sites but not 4C9 antigen (4C9−, DBA+); these patients had fewer metastases and significantly better prognosis than patients with tumors of other carbohydrate profiles.

Evidence has now accumulated showing that cell-surface carbohydrate structures are important in the interactions between cells and between the cell and the extracellular matrix, which in turn is closely linked to growth and differentiation, malignant transformation and progression, and metastases. Changes in major blood group antigens (ABH) and related antigens are among the most common alterations, and their prognostic value has now been substantiated in several studies. This seems to be a rather unique clinical situation, in which simple modifications of cell surface carbohydrates are responsible for tumor progression and metastases and for differences in clinical outcome. These results open prospects for future scientifically well-founded forms of therapy for patients with an otherwise poor prognosis.

GROWTH FACTORS

Increased expression of epidermal growth factor receptor (EGFr) has been reported in NSCLC when compared with normal lung (116). Veale et al. (117) examined survival in 19 surgically treated patients who were characterized for EGFr resection specimens. A high level of EGFr was a significant negative predictor of survival. If these results are confirmed, an EGFr assay may be clinically useful in selecting resected patients with a poor prognosis for adjuvant therapy.

The proliferative activity of NSCLC was evaluated for the presence of Ki67-related antigen using an immunohistochemical technique by Scagliotti et al. (118). Ki67 is a monoclonal antibody that detects a nonhistone protein expressed in all phases of the cell cycle except G0 and probably early G1, thereby serving as a marker of proliferative activity. Disease free survival was significantly lower in completely resected patients with a high Ki67 score at diagnosis than in patients with a low score ($P < .03$). Thus, growth fraction may serve as a prognostic parameter in resected NSCLC.

CONCLUSION

The stage of disease, performance status, serum LDH, and hyponatremia are the most important clinical prognostic factors in SCLC. Prognostic classification based on these variables requires an algorithm, but no internationally accepted algorithm has yet been established. A first step toward developing a common system would be agreement about the choice of statistical method.

Serum tumor markers, such as NSE, TPA, and TK, do not identify qualitatively different subgroups with outlooks distinct from that of other patients. Typically, there is a positive relationship between the serum concentration and the death hazard. There is a linear correlation between LDH and most of the new markers, as there is among the markers. Currently, none of the new markers, compared with the others, seems to have significant advantages as a prognostic factor.

Definite prognostic factors in completely resected NSCLC are performance status and stage. T and N status also are important, although less so when stage, serving as a summarizing variable, is included in the analysis. The two former variables are also the most important in patients with nonresectable disease. Variables describing age, histology, gender, and weight all have been confirmed as having a prognostic impact in fewer studies than did performance status and age.

In preliminary analyses, a large number of variables describing biologic features of the tumors have been confirmed as having a prognostic impact in NSCLC patients. This is the case for variables such as neuroendocrine differentiation, oncogenes, and oncogene products, DNA ploidy status, and presence of carbohydrate antigens, growth factors, and proliferative activity of the tumors.

Future studies are warranted to document further the value of these variables as accurate predictors of the prognosis of patients with NSCLC. Doing so will enable oncologists to make treatment decisions on a firmer basis than is currently possible.

REFERENCES

1. Ferlay J. Cancer in five continents. Unit of descriptive epidemiology. Lyon, France: International Association for Research on Cancer, 1992;VI.

2. Hansen J, Olsen JH. Respiratory system. In: Carstensen B, Storm HH, eds. Survival of Danish cancer patients 1943–1987. Acta Pathol Microbiol Immunol Scand 1993;101(Suppl 33):77–98.
3. Frost JK, Ball WC, Levin ML, et al. Early lung cancer detection: results of the initial (prevalence) radiologic and cytologic screening in the Johns Hopkins Study. Am Rev Respir Dis 1984;130:549–554.
4. Flehinger BJ, Kimmel M, Polyak T, Melamed MR. Screening for lung cancer. The Mayo lung project revisited. Cancer 1993; 72:1573–1580.
5. Rothman KJ. Epidemiologic methods in clinical trials. Cancer 1977;39:1771–1775.
6. Peto R, Pike MC, Armitage P, et al. Design and analysis of randomized clinical trials requiring prolonged observation of each patient. II. Analysis and examples. Br J Cancer 1977;35:1–39.
7. Tarone RE. Test for trend in life table analysis. Biometrika 1975;62:679–682.
8. Dixon WJ, Brown MB, Engelman L, Jennrich RI, eds. BMDP statistical software. Los Angeles, Oxford: University of California Press, 1990.
9. Cox DR. Regression models and life-tables. J R Stat Soc 1972;34:187–220.
10. Concato J, Feinstein AR, Holford TR. The risk of determining risk with multivariable models. Ann Intern Med 1993;118: 201–210.
11. Ciampi A, Lawless JF, McKinney SM, Singhal K. Regression and recursive partition strategies in the analysis of medical survival data. J Clin Epidemiol 1988;41:737–748.
12. Souhami RL, Bradbury I, Geddes DM, Spiro SG, Harper PG, Tobias JS. Prognostic significance of laboratory parameters measured at diagnosis in small cell carcinoma of the lung. Cancer Res 1985;45:2878–2882.
13. Østerlind K, Andersen PK. Prognostic factors in small cell lung cancer: multivariate model based on 778 patients treated with chemotherapy with or without irradiation. Cancer Res 1986;46:4189–4194.
14. Cerny T, Blair V, Anderson H, Bramwell V, Thatcher N. Pretreatment prognostic factors and scoring system in 407 small-cell lung cancer patients. Int J Cancer 1987;39:146–149.
15. Vincent MD, Ashley SE, Smith IE. Prognostic factors in small cell lung cancer: a simple prognostic index is better than conventional staging. Eur J Cancer Clin Oncol 1987;23:1589–1599.
16. Spiegelman D, Maurer LH, Ware JH, Perry MC, Chahinian AP. Prognostic factors in small-cell carcinoma of the lung: an analysis of 1521 patients. J Clin Oncol 1989;7:344–354.
17. Dearing MP, Steinberg SM, Phelps R, Anderson MJ, Mulshine JL, Ihde DC. Outcome of patients with small-cell lung cancer: effect of changes in staging procedures and imaging technology on prognostic factors over 14 years. J Clin Oncol 1990;6:1042–1049.
18. Albain KS, Crowley JJ, LeBlanc M, Livingston RB. Determinants of improved outcome in small-cell lung cancer: an analysis of the 2580-patient Southwest Oncology Group data base. J Clin Oncol 1990;8:1563–1574.
19. Allan SG, Stewart ME, Love S, Cornbleet MA, Smyth JF, Leonard CF. Prognosis at presentation of small cell carcinoma of the lung. Eur J Cancer 1990;26:703–705.
20. Sagman U, Maki E, Evans WK, et al. Small-cell carcinoma of the lung: derivation of a prognostic staging system. J Clin Oncol 1991;9:1639–1649.
21. Ihde DC, Makuch RW, Carney DN, et al. Prognostic implications of stage of disease and sites of metastases in patients with small cell carcinoma of the lung treated with intensive combination chemotherapy. Am Rev Respir Dis 1981;123:500–507.
22. Feinstein AR, Sosin DM, Wells CK. The Will Rogers phenomenon. Stage migration and new diagnostic techniques as a source of misleading statistics for survival in cancer. N Engl J Med 1985;312:1604–1608.
23. Hirsch FR, Østerlind K, Ingeman Jensen L, et al. The impact of abdominal computerized tomography on the pretreatment staging and prognosis of small cell lung cancer. Ann Oncol 1992;3:469–474.
24. Shepherd FA, Ginsberg RJ, Haddad R, et al. Importance of clinical staging in limited small-cell lung cancer: a valuable system to separate prognostic subgroups. J Clin Oncol 1993;11:1592–1597.
25. Sagman U, Feld R, Evans WK, et al. The prognostic significance of pretreatment serum lactate dehydrogenase in patients with small-cell lung cancer. J Clin Oncol 1991;9:954–961.
26. Hansen M, Hammer M, Hummer L. Diagnostic and therapeutic implications of ectopic hormone production in small cell carcinoma of the lung. Thorax 1980;35:101–106.
27. Østerlind K, Lassen U, Herrstedt J, JØrgensen M, Hansen HH. Is intensive combination chemotherapy feasible in old patients with small cell lung cancer (SCLC)? The Copenhagen group experience 1973–1987. Ann Oncol 1992;3(Suppl 5):37.
28. Østerlind K, Hansen HH, Hansen M, Dombernowsky P, Andersen PK. Long-term disease-free survival in small-cell carcinoma of the lung: a study of clinical determinants. J Clin Oncol 1986;4:1307–1313.
29. Johnson B, Steinberg SM, Phelps R, Edison M, Veach SR, Ihde D. Female patients with small cell lung cancer live longer than male patients. Am J Med 1988;85:194–196.
30. Stahel R, Aisner J, Ginsberg R, et al. Staging and prognostic factors in small cell lung cancer. Lung Cancer 1989;5:119–126.
31. Rawson NSB, Peto J. An overview of prognostic factors in small cell lung cancer. A report from the subcommittee for the management of lung cancer of the United Kingdom coordinating committee on cancer research. Br J Cancer 1990;61: 597–604.
32. Akoun GM, Scarna HM, Milleron BJ, Bénichou MP, Herman DP. Serum neuron-specific enolase. A marker for disease extent and response to therapy for small-cell lung cancer. Chest 1985;87:39–43.
33. Jaques GJ, Bepler G, Holle R, Wolf M. Prognostic value of pretreatment carcinoembryonic antigen, neuron-specific enolase, and creatine kinase-BB levels in sera of patients with small cell lung cancer. Cancer 1988;62:125–134.
34. JØrgensen LGM, Østerlind K, Hansen HH, Cooper EH. The prognostic influence of serum neuron specific enolase in small cell lung cancer. Br J Cancer 1988;58:805–807.
35. Gronowitz JS, Bergström R, Nôu E, et al. Clinical and serologic markers of stage and prognosis in small cell lung cancer. A multivariate analysis. Cancer 1990;66:722–732.
36. Harding M, McAllister J, Hulks G, et al. Neurone specific enolase (NSE) in small cell lung cancer: a tumour marker of prognostic significance? Br J Cancer 1990;61:605–607.
37. van der Gaast A, van Putten WLJ, Oosterom R, Cozijnsen M, Heekstra R, Splintor TAW. Prognostic value of serum thymidine kinase, tissue polypeptide antigen and neuron specific enolase in patients with small cell lung cancer. Br J Cancer 1991;64:369–372.
38. Johnson PWM, Joel SP, Love S, et al. Tumour markers for prediction of survival and monitoring of remission in small cell lung cancer. Br J Cancer 1993;67:760–766.

39. Szturmowicz M, Roginska E, Roszkowski K, Kwick S, Filipecki S, Rowinska-Zakrzewska E. Prognostic value of neuron-specific enolase in small cell lung cancer patients. Lung Cancer 1993;8:259–264.
40. Bork E, Hansen M, Urdal P, et al. Early detection of response in small cell bronchogenic carcinoma by changes in serum concentrations of creatine kinase, neuron specific enolase, calcitonin, ACTH, serotonin and gastrin releasing peptide. Eur J Cancer Clin Oncol 1988;24:1033–1038.
41. Maruno K, Yamaguchi K, Abe K, et al. Immunoreactive gastrin-releasing peptide as a specific tumor marker in patients with small cell lung carcinoma. Cancer Res 1989;49:629–632.
42. Holst JJ, Hansen M, Bork E, Schwartz TW. Elevated plasma concentrations of C-flanking gastrin-releasing peptide in small-cell lung cancer. J Clin Oncol 1989;7:1831–1838.
43. Shipp MA, Tarr GE, Chen C-Y, et al. CD10/neutral endopeptidase 24.11 hydrolyzes bombesin-like peptides and regulates the growth of small cell carcinomas of the lung. Proc Natl Acad Sci U S A 1991;88:10662–10666.
44. Brennan J, O'Connor T, Makuch RW, et al. *myc* Family DNA amplification in 107 tumors and tumor cell lines from patients with small cell lung cancer treated with different combination chemotherapy regimens. Cancer Res 1991;51:1708–1712.
45. Gazdar AF. Molecular markers for the diagnosis and prognosis of lung cancer. Cancer 1992;69(Suppl):1592–1599.
46. Hirsch FR, Østerlind K, Hansen HH. The prognostic significance of histopathologic subtyping of small cell carcinoma of the lung according to the classification of the World Health Organization. A study of 375 consecutive patients. Cancer 1983;52:2144–2150.
47. Aisner SC, Finkelstein DM, Ettinger DS, Abeloff MD, Ruckdeschel JC, Eggleston JC. The clinical significance of variant-morphology small-cell carcinoma of the lung. J Clin Oncol 1990;8:402–408.
48. Gail MH, Eagan RT, Feld R, et al. Prognostic factors in patients with resected stage I non–small cell lung cancer. A report from the Lung Cancer Study Group. Cancer 1984;54:1802–1813.
49. Lipford HH, Sears DL, Eggleston JC, More CW, Littlemore KD, Baker RR. Prognostic factors in surgically resected limited-stage, non–small cell carcinoma of the lung. Am J Surg Pathol 1984;8:357–365.
50. Chastang C, Lebeau B, Charpak Y, Decroix G. Prognostic factors from a randomized clinical trial in resected lung cancer. Stat Med 1985;4:279–285.
51. Søorensen JB, Badsberg JH. Prognostic factors in resected stage I and II adenocarcinomas of the lung. A multivariate regression analysis of 137 consecutive patients. J Thorac Cardiovasc Surg 1990;99:218–226.
52. Deslaurier J, Brisson J, Cartier R, et al. Carcinoma of the lung. Evaluation of satellite nodules as a factor influencing prognosis after resection. J Thorac Cardiovasc Surg 1989;97:504–512.
53. Little AG, Wu H-S, Ferguson MK, et al. Perioperative blood transfusion adversely affects prognosis of patients with stage I non–small-cell lung cancer. Am J Surg 1990;160:630–632.
54. Harada M, Dosaka-Akita H, Miyamoto H, Kuzumaki N, Kawakami Y. Prognostic significance of the expression of *ras* oncogene product in non–small cell lung cancer. Cancer 1992;69:72–77.
55. Fontanini G, Macchiarini P, Pepe S, et al. The expression of proliferating cell nuclear antigen in paraffin sections of peripheral, node-negative non–small cell lung cancer. Cancer 1992;70:1520–1527.
56. Macchiarini P, Fontanini G, Hardin JM, Pingitore R, Angeletti CA. Most peripheral, node-negative, non–small-cell lung cancers have low proliferative rates and no intratumoral and peritumoral blood and lymphatic vessel invasion. J Thorac Cardiovasc Surg 1992;104:892–899.
57. Stipa S, Danesi DT, Modini C, et al. The importance of heterogeneity and of multiple site sampling in the prospective determination of deoxyribonucleic acid flow cytometry. Surg Gynecol Obst 1993;176:427–434.
58. Møorkve O, Halvorsen OJ, Skjaerven R, Stangeland L, Culsvik A, Lacrum OD. Prognostic significance of p53 protein expression and DNA ploidy in surgically treated non–small cell lung carcinomas. Anticancer Res 1993;13:571–578.
59. Horio Y, Takahashi T, Kuroishi T, et al. Prognostic significance of p53 mutations and 3p deletions in primary resected non–small cell lung cancer. Cancer Res 1993;53:1–4.
60. Pena CM, Rice TW, Ahmad M, Medendorp S. Significance of perioperative blood transfusions in patients undergoing resection of stage I and II non–small-cell lung cancers. Chest 1992;102:84–88.
61. Battifora H, Sorensen HR, Mehta P, et al. Tumor-associated antigen 43-9F is of prognostic value in squamous cell carcinoma of the lung. Cancer 1992;70:1867–1872.
62. Liewald F, Hatz R, Storck M, et al. Prognostic value of deoxyribonucleic acid aneuploidy in primary non–small-cell lung carcinomas and their metastases. J Thorac Cardiovasc Surg 1992;104:1476–1482.
63. Tartter PI, Burrows L, Kirschner P. Perioperative blood transfusion adversely affects prognosis after resection of stage I (subset N0) non–oat cell lung cancer. J Thorac Cardiovasc Surg 1984;88:659–662.
64. Zimmerman PV, Hawson GAT, Bint MH, Parsons PG. Ploidy as a prognostic determinant in surgically treated lung cancer. Lancet 1987;230:530–533.
65. Alama A, Costantini M, Repetto L, et al. Thymidine labelling index as prognostic factor in resected non–small cell lung cancer. Eur J Cancer 1990;26:622–625.
66. van Bodegom PC, Baak JPA, Stroet-van Galen C, et al. The percentage of aneuploid cells is significantly correlated with survival in accurately staged patients with stage 1 resected squamous cell lung cancer and long-term follow up. Cancer 1989;63:143–147.
67. Ichinose Y, Hara N, Ohta M, et al. Is T factor of the TNM staging system a predominant prognostic factor in pathologic stage I non–small-cell lung cancer? J Thorac Cardiovasc Surg 1993;106:90–94.
68. Miller TP, Chen TT, Coltman CA, et al. Effect of alternating combination chemotherapy on survival of ambulatory patients with metastatic large-cell and adenocarcinoma of the lung. A Southwest Oncology Group study. J Clin Oncol 1986;4:502–508.
69. Finkelstein DM, Ettinger DS, Ruckdeschel JC. Long-term survivors in metastatic non–small cell lung cancer: an Eastern Cooperative Oncology Group study. J Clin Oncol 1986;4:702–709.
70. Einhorn LE, Loehrer PJ, Williams SD, et al. Random prospective study of vindesine versus vindesine plus high-dose cisplatin versus vindesine plus cisplatin plus mitomycin C in advanced non–small-cell lung cancer. J Clin Oncol 1986;4:1037–1043.
71. Evans WK, Nixon DW, Daly JM, et al. A randomized study of oral nutritional support versus ad lib nutritional intake during chemotherapy for advanced colorectal and non–small cell lung cancer. J Clin Oncol 1987;5:113–124.
72. O'Connell JP, Kris MG, Gralla RJ, et al. Frequency and prognostic importance of pretreatment clinical characteristics in

patients with advanced non–small cell lung cancer treated with combination chemotherapy. J Clin Oncol 1986;4:1604–1614.
73. Rapp E, Pater JL, Willan A, et al. Chemotherapy can prolong survival in patients with advanced non–small-cell lung cancer: report of a Canadian multicenter randomized trial. J Clin Oncol 1988;6:633–641.
74. Sukurai M, Shinkai T, Eguchi K, et al. Prognostic factors in non–small cell lung cancer: multiregression analysis in the National Cancer Center Hospital (Japan). J Cancer Res Clin Oncol 1987;115:563–566.
75. Søorensen JB, Badsberg JH, Olsen J. Prognostic factors in inoperable adenocarcinoma of the lung: a multivariate regression analysis of 259 patients. Cancer Res 1989;49:5748–5754.
76. Albain KS, Crowley JJ, LeBlanc M, Livingston RB. Survival determinants in extensive-stage non–small-cell lung cancer: the Southwest Oncology Group experience. J Clin Oncol 1991;9:1618–1626.
77. Shinkai T, Eguchi K, Sasaki Y, et al. A prognostic-factor risk index in advanced non–small-cell lung cancer treated with cisplatin-containing combination chemotherapy. Cancer Chemother Pharmacol 1992;30:1–6.
78. Kojima A, Shinkai T, Eguchi K, et al. Analysis of three-year survivors among patients with advanced inoperable non–small cell lung cancer. Jpn J Clin Oncol 1991;21:276–281.
79. Kawahara M, Furuse K, Kodama N, et al. A randomized study of cisplatin versus cisplatin plus vindesine for non–small cell lung carcinoma. Cancer 1991;68:714–719.
80. Bonomi P, Gale M, Rowland K, et al. Pre-treatment prognostic factors in stage III non–small cell lung cancer patients receiving combined modality treatment. Int J Radiat Oncol Biol Phys 1991;20:247–252.
81. Pujol JL, Cooper EH, Lehmann M, et al. Clinical evaluation of serum tumour marker CA 242 in non–small cell lung cancer. Br J Cancer 1993;67:1423–1429.
82. Graham MV, Geitz LM, Byhardt R, et al. Comparison of prognostic factors and survival among black patients and white patients treated with irradiation for non–small-cell lung cancer. J Natl Cancer Inst 1992;84:1731–1735.
83. Mountain CF. A new international staging system for lung cancer. Chest 1986;89:225–233.
84. Volm M, Mattern J, Müller T, Drings P. Flow cytometry of epidermoid lung carcinomas: relationship of ploidy and cell cycle phases to survival. A five-year follow up study. Anticancer Res 1988;8:105–112.
85. Hilsenbeck SG, Raub WA Jr, Sridhar KS. Prognostic factors in lung cancer based on multivariate analysis. Am J Clin Oncol 1993;16:301–309.
86. Stevenson H, Gazdar AF, Phelps R, et al. Tumor cell lines established in vitro: an independent prognostic factor for survival in non–small-cell lung cancer. Ann Intern Med 1990;113:764–770.
87. Hannisdal E, Engan T. Blood analyses and survival in symptom- and survey-detected lung cancer patients. J Intern Med 1991;229:337–341.
88. Buccheri G, Ferrigno D, Vola F. Carcinoembryonic antigen (CEA), tissue polypeptide antigen (TPA) and other prognostic indicators in squamous cell lung cancer. Lung Cancer 1993;10:21–33.
89. Mitsudomi T, Oyama T, Kusano T, Osaki T, Nakanishi R, Shirakusa T. Mutations of the p53 gene as a predictor of poor prognosis in patients with non–small-cell lung cancer. J Natl Cancer Inst 1993;85:2018–2023.
90. Szabo E, Mulshine J. Epidemiology, prognostic factors and prevention of lung cancer. Curr Opin Oncol 1993;5:302–309.
91. Carney DN. Lung cancer biology. Curr Opin Oncol 1991;3:288–296.
92. Linnoila I. Pathology of non–small cell lung cancer. New diagnostic approaches. Hematol Oncol Clin North Am 1990;4:1027–1051.
93. Linnoila RI, Jensen S, Steinberg S, et al. Neuroendocrine differentiation in non–small cell lung cancer correlates with favorable response to chemotherapy (abstract). Proc Am Soc Clin Oncol 1989;8:248.
94. Berendsen HH, de Leij L, Poppema S, et al. Clinical characterization of non–small-cell lung cancer tumors showing neuroendocrine differentiation features. J Clin Oncol 1989;7:1614–1620.
95. Graziano SL, Mazid R, Newman N, et al. The use of neuroendocrine immunoperoxidase markers to predict chemotherapy response in patients with non–small-cell lung cancer. J Clin Oncol 1989;7:1398–1406.
96. Skov BG, Sørensen JB, Hirsch FR, Larsson LI, Hansen HH. Prognostic impact of histologic demonstration of chromogranin A and neuron-specific enolase in pulmonary adenocarcinoma. Ann Oncol 1991;2:355–360.
97. Diez M, Torres A, Ortega L, et al. Value of serum neuron-specific enolase in non–small cell lung cancer. Oncology 1993;50:127–131.
98. Slebos RJC, Kibbaelaar RE, Dalesio O, et al. K-ras oncogene activation as a prognostic marker in adenocarcinoma of the lung. N Engl J Med 1990;32:561–565.
99. Rodenhuis S, Slebos RJC. Clinical significance of ras oncogene activation in human lung cancer. Cancer Res 1992;52(Suppl 6):2665S–2669S.
100. Sugio K, Ishida T, Yokoyama H, Inoue T, Sugimachi K, Sasazuki T. ras Gene mutations as a prognostic marker in adenocarcinoma of the human lung without lymph node metastases. Cancer Res 1992;52:2903–2906.
101. Harada M, Dosaka-Akita H, Miyamoto H, Kuzumaki N, Kawakami Y. Prognostic significance of the expression of ras oncogene product in non–small cell lung cancer. Cancer 1992;69:72–77.
102. Mitsudomi T, Steinberg SM, Oie HK, et al. ras Gene mutations in non–small cell lung cancers are associated with shortened survival irrespective of treatment intent. Cancer Res 1991;51:4999–5002.
103. Kawashimi K, Nomura S, Hirai H, et al. Correlation of L-myc RFLP with metastasis, prognosis, and multiple cancer in lung cancer patients. Int J Cancer 1992;50:557–561.
104. Kishimoto Y, Murakami Y, Shiraishi M, Hayakhi K, Sekia T. Aberrations of the p53 tumor suppressor gene in human non–small cell carcinomas of the lung. Cancer Res 1992;52:4799–4804.
105. Quinlan DC, Davidson AG, Summers CL, Wender HE, Doshi HM. Accumulation of p53 protein correlation with a poor prognosis in human lung cancer. Cancer Res 1992;52:4828–4831.
106. Mitsudomi T, Steinberg SM, Nau MM, et al. p53 Gene mutations in non–small cell lung cancer cell lines and their correlation with the presence of ras mutations and clinical features. Oncogene 1992;7:171–180.
107. McLaren R, Kuzu I, Dunnill M, Harris A, Lane D, Catter KC. The relationship of p53 immunostaining to survival in carcinoma of the lung. Br J Cancer 1992;66:735–738.
108. Tateishi M, Ishidu T, Mitsudomi T, Kanedo S, Sugimachi K. Prognostic value of c-erb B-2 protein expression in human

lung adenocarcinoma and squamous cell carcinoma. Eur J Cancer 1991;27:1372–1375.
109. Kern JA, Schwartz DA, Nordberg JE, et al. p185neu Expression in human lung adenocarcinomas predicts shortened survival. Cancer Res 1990;50:5184–5191.
110. Ogawa J, Tsurumi T, Inoue H, Shohtsu A. Relationship between tumor DNA ploidy and regional lymph node changes in lung cancer. Cancer 1992;69:1688–1695.
111. Miyamoto H, Karado M, Isobe H, et al. Prognostic value of nuclear DNA content and expression of the ras oncogene product in lung cancer. Cancer Res 1991;51:6346–6350.
112. Isobe H, Miyamoto H, Shimizi T, et al. Prognostic and therapeutic significance of the flow cytometric nuclear DNA content in non–small cell lung cancer. Cancer 1990;65:1391–1395.
113. Lee JS, Ro JY, Sahin AA, et al. Expression of blood-group antigen A—a favorable prognostic factor in non-small-cell lung cancer. New Engl J Med 1991;324:1084–1090.
114. Miyake M, Taki T, Hitomi S, Hakomori S-I. Correlation of expression of H/Ley/Leb antigens with survival in patients with carcinoma of the lung. N Engl J Med 1992;327:14–18.
115. Matsumoto H, Muramatsu H, Muramatsu T, Shimazu H. Carbohydrate profiles shown by a lectin and a monoclonal antibody correlate with metastatic potential and prognosis of human lung carcinomas. Cancer 1992;6~9:2084–2090.
116. Veale D, Kerr N, Gibson GJ, Harris AL. Characterisation of epidermal growth factor receptor in primary human non–small cell lung cancer. Cancer Res 1989;49:1313–1317.
117. Veale D, Kerr N, Gibson GJ, Kelly PJ, Harris AL. The relationship of quantitative epidermal growth factor receptor expression in non–small cell lung cancer to long term survival. Br J Cancer 1993;68:162–165.
118. Scagliotti GV, Micela M, Gubetta L, et al. Prognostic significance of Ki67 labelling in resected non small cell lung cancer. Eur J Cancer 1993;29A:363–365.

Section III

Therapeutic Approaches to Non–Small Cell Lung Cancer

14

Treatment of Stage I and II Disease

Nael Martini and Robert J. Ginsberg

Surgical treatment of lung cancer is still regarded as the most effective method of controlling the primary tumor, provided a complete resection is possible and the risks of the procedure are low. It is the therapy of choice for early-stage non–small cell lung cancer (NSCLC) and generally is offered to all patients with stage I or II disease.

The 5-year survival rate after complete resection of a lung cancer is stage dependent. Incomplete resections invariably do not cure. Many recent series show that approximately 70% of patients with stage I resected NSCLC survive 5 years, and 80% never have a recurrence (1–6). At the other extreme, only a handful of patients with stage IIIB disease are ever resected or cured completely.

The number of patients that present with early lung cancer depends on the referral pattern of a given center or hospital. At Memorial Sloan–Kettering Cancer Center, nearly one third of all patients seen with lung cancer have stage I or II disease (Fig. 14.1). Nearly all have an excellent performance status at presentation. They also have a favorable prognosis if treated surgically. Many are asymptomatic. They include patients who participate in lung cancer screening programs, individuals who receive a routine chest roentgenogram as part of a preemployment medical clearnace, and patients undergoing cardiorespiratory assessment as part of preadmission screening for elective surgery. Patients with symptomatic disease found at this early stage usually present with symptoms related to an intrabronchial tumor (e.g., cough, hemoptysis, dyspnea).

The three categories of early localized lung cancer include occult carcinomas of the lung as well as stage I and stage II cancers.

OCCULT LUNG CARCINOMAS

Few patients with lung cancer are diagnosed before it becomes apparent on chest roentgenograms, and this group accounts for less than 1% of the lung cancer population (7–9). In this group, diagnosis usually is established on sputum cytology (e.g., participants in a lung cancer detection program) or by bronchoscopy in patients presenting with an unexplained cough or hemoptysis and a normal chest roentgenogram.

LOCALIZATION

For cancers detected on sputum cytology, the fact that the patient has a positive sputum cytology does not necessarily mean that the patient has lung cancer. For instance, cancer cells may originate from a head and neck primary. After a negative head and neck evaluation, localization of occult lung tumors is accomplished by fiberoptic bronchoscopy. If a lesion is seen, a biopsy is obtained for confirmation. If it is not seen, repeated positive brushings from an isolated segment are acceptable for localization. Otherwise, diagnosis is deferred and bronchoscopy repeated in 2 to 3 months. Recently, fluorescent staining of bronchial mucosa with hematoporphyrin derivatives or laser-induced autofluorescence have improved bronchoscopic localization (10, 11).

TREATMENT

After localization, the treatment of choice for these early squamous cell tumors is surgical removal of the primary tumor by lobectomy, pneumonectomy, or segmentectomy. Frequently, sleeve resections combined with these procedures can be used to preserve lung function. Because most occult lung cancers are located in the major airways, wedge resections usually are not possible. Histologically, 90% of occult lung cancers are squamous carcinomas, and 10% are either adenocarcinomas or large cell carcinomas. Surgical treatment is curative in this small group of patients. Memorial Sloan–Kettering Cancer Center has not ob-

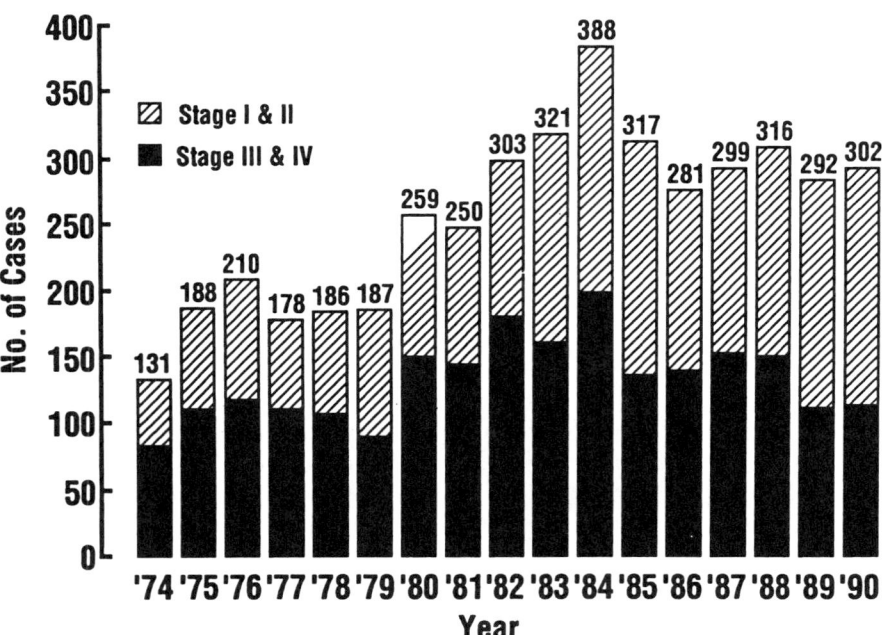

FIGURE 14.1. Yearly accrual of NSCLC patients by clinical stage: the Memorial experience, 1974–1990.

served a single case of recurrent tumor after resection despite follow-up periods of 20 or more years. Unfortunately, the risk of a patient developing a *new* cancer is as high as 45%. In an unpublished series from Toronto, all patients treated by radiotherapy died of recurrent cancer.

Photodynamic therapy, using transbronchoscopic laser-induced photoexcitation of a hematoporphyrin derivative has been shown to be effective in eradicating occult in situ endobronchial lung cancers and can be considered as an alternative therapy, especially in patients who cannot tolerate a surgical resection (12). Once invasive carcinoma has been identified, treatment with hematoporphyrins is not curative, and primary resection is necessary.

STAGE I DISEASE

Stage I disease is the most common form of early lung cancer seen by most physicians. Many such cases are detected on routine chest roentgenograms in patients who present for unrelated medical conditions or as part of a routine annual examination. Many are discreet peripheral tumors, presenting as "coin lesions."

PREOPERATIVE STAGING

Computed tomographic (CT) scans are done routinely on these patients to assess nodal involvement in the mediastinum and to detect metastases in the liver and the adrenal glands. Routine mediastinoscopy remains controversial and probably is unnecessary if the CT scan is negative. Moreover, if the alkaline phosphatase level is normal, routine multiorgan screening for metastases in the absence of signs and symptoms of metastatic disease is unrewarding because it has an overall true-positive rate of less than 1% (13).

TREATMENT

For patients with clinical stage I disease, surgical resection is the treatment of choice whenever possible. However, at the time of final pathologic staging, despite all preoperative efforts, a significant number of patients are found to be understaged. In a prospective validation of the International Union Against Cancer TNM Classification, the data of 3823 patients were analyzed in terms of concordance between clinically and pathologically confirmed TNM stages (14). The agreement in stage I disease was 61%.

For many stage I patients, lobectomy is the surgical treatment of choice because it encompasses all disease and preserves lung function. Infrequently, with more proximal tumors, pneumonectomy is required, although, with proximally placed tumors, a sleeve lobectomy often is sufficient for cure and allows preservation of functioning pulmonary tissue.

It has been the practice at Memorial Sloan–Kettering Cancer Center to use mediastinal lymph node dissection as part of the standard surgical resection for lung cancer, believing that this approach provides the best possible final pathologic staging of disease. Whether this technique provides a greater opportunity of cure (allowing occult mediastinal lymph node disease to be resected completely) has never been demonstrated in a randomized trial. However, with the experience that incompletely resected disease rarely is cured, one must believe without scientific proof that a complete mediastinal lymph node dissection will allow a more complete resection, allowing occult N1 and N2 disease to be detected and removed.

Although resections less extensive than a lobectomy (e.g., segmentectomy or wedge resection) can be used in patients with compromised pulmonary function and despite earlier reports of their efficacy in managing stage I patients, recent analyses have demonstrated a much higher local recurrence rate and, in one report, a poorer 5-year survival (15, 16). For these reasons, limited resection cannot be recommended as standard therapy in the management of stage I lung cancer. It must be reserved for patients who cannot tolerate a lobectomy but who can be resected completely by this lesser operation.

RESULTS OF SURGICAL THERAPY: THE MEMORIAL EXPERIENCE

Results were reported recently with surgical treatment of 598 patients with stage I tumors (2). The male to female ratio was 1.9 to 1, and the median age was 62 years. The primary tumor was located in the upper lobe in 67% of the patients, in the middle or lower lobes in 30%, and in the main bronchus in 3%.

The histology was squamous carcinoma in 233 patients and nonsquamous carcinoma in 365 (adenocarcinoma, 253; bronchoalveolar carcinoma, 98; large cell carcinoma, 14).

There were 291 T1 tumors (49%), and 307 T2 tumors (51%). Lobectomy was performed in 85% of the patients, pneumonectomy in 4%, and wedge resection or segmentectomy in 11%. Of the latter group, nearly 90% had T1 tumors. A mediastinal lymph node dissection was carried out in 560 patients (94%) and lymph node sampling and no formal dissection in 38 (6%).

Ninety-nine percent of the patients were followed for a minimum of 5 years or until death (median follow-up, 91 months). There was a 2.3% mortality rate. The overall 5- and 10-year survival rates (Kaplan-Meier) were 75% and 67%, respectively (Fig. 14.2). Patients with T1 tumors fared better than those with T2 tumors. Survival in patients with T1 tumors was 82% at 5 years and 74% at 10 years, compared with 68% at 5 years and 60% at 10 years for those with T2 tumors. ($P < .0004$) (Fig. 14.3).

Tumor size also influenced survival with significant P values among the four groups: tumors less than 1 cm, 1 to 3 cm, greater than 3 to 5 cm, and greater than 5 cm (Fig. 14.4). Patients with T2 tumors, by virtue of visceral pleural involvement but with tumors not more than 3 cm in diameter, had survival rates comparable to patients without visceral pleural involvement (Fig. 14.5). The validity of classifying these patients as T2 (versus T1) by virtue of visceral pleural involvement alone is questionable.

As with other recent reports (15–17), the Memorial experience confirms that patients undergoing a pulmonary resection less extensive than a lobectomy had a poorer survival and higher local recurrence rate, with the 5- and 10-year survival for pneumonectomy or lobectomy being 77% and 70% respectively, compared with 59% and 35% in patients with lesser resections ($P = .026$).

RECURRENCE AND NEW CANCERS

During the course of follow-up, 159 patients (27%) developed recurrence, most within 5 years of treatment, although 9% developed a recurrence later than 5 years (18). The first sites of recurrence in the overall group of patients were mostly distant and were not influenced by histology (local, 20%; regional, 8%; and distant, 72%). The most common site of distant metastases was the brain.

Resections less extensive than lobectomy and no lymph node dissection had adverse effects on recurrence. Fifty percent of patients who had wedge resection or segmentectomy had a recurrence ($P = .00002$), half of which were local or regional recurrences. Of patients who had no formal lymph node dissection, 55% had recurrence ($P = .00008$), 71% of which were local or regional recurrences. Only 5% of all recurrences were local or regional in patients who had mediastinal lymph node dissection.

The incidence of recurrence was influenced also by the T factor and by tumor size in centimeters. This experience was statistically significant between T1 and T2 tumors ($P = .0004$) and between tumors not more than 3 cm and those greater than 3 cm ($P = .03$).

An interesting observation was the number of second primary cancers occurring in the surviving patients. There were 206 patients who had second cancers, an overall incidence of 34%. This was similar among histologies. One third of the multiple cancers were lung cancers. (Table 14.1).

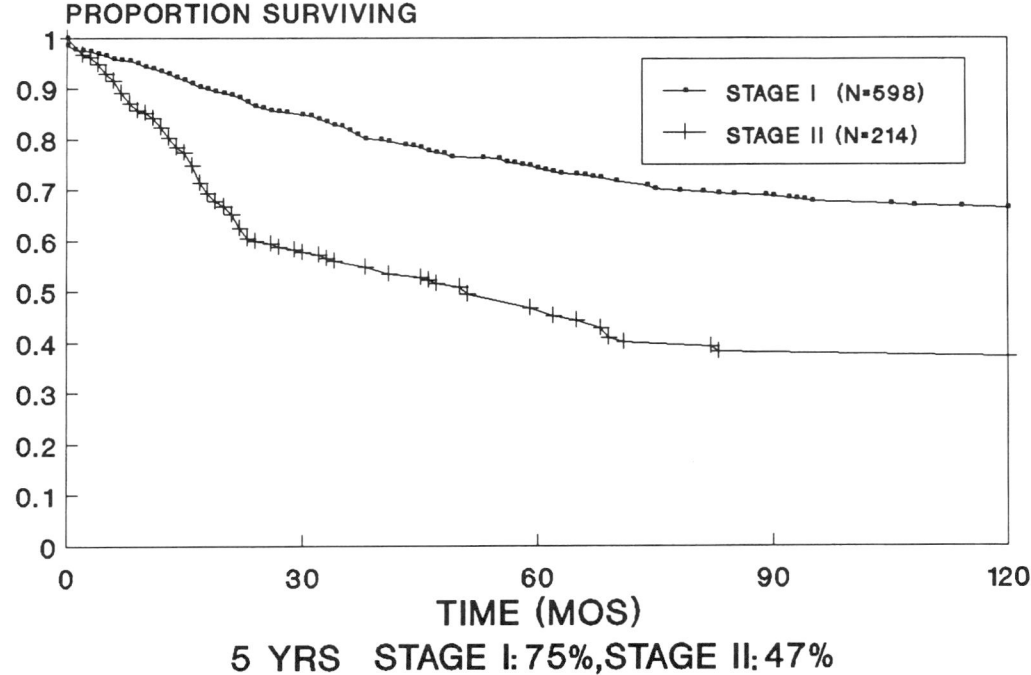

FIGURE 14.2. Survival post complete resection in stage I and II lung cancer.

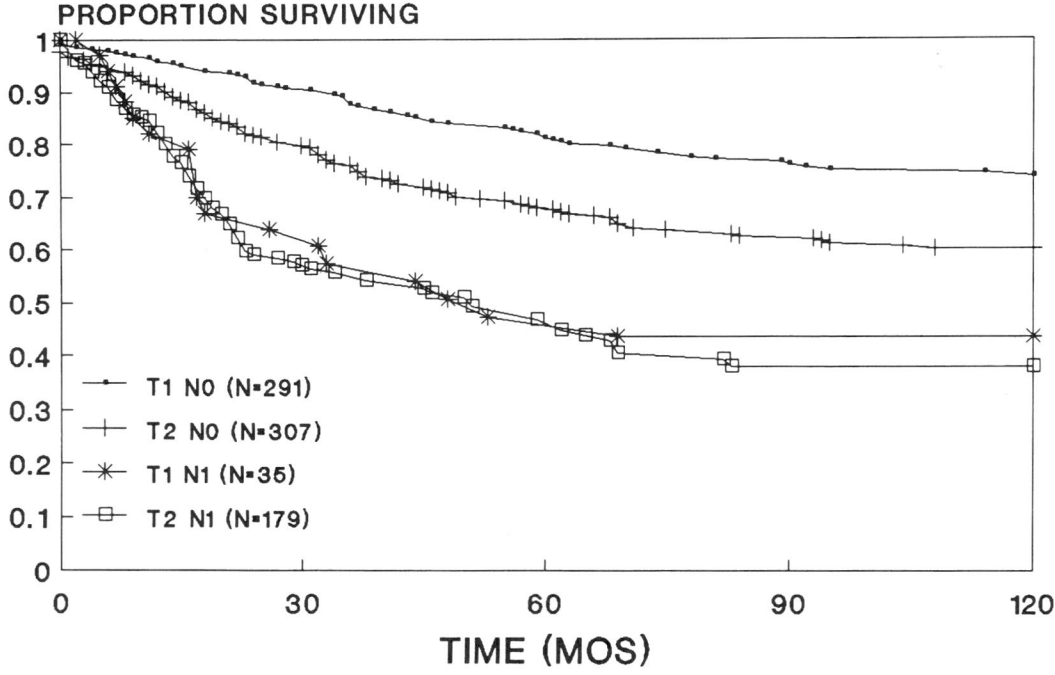

FIGURE 14.3. Survival post resection by T factor in stage I and II lung cancer.

PREDICTORS OF SURVIVAL

Other than tumor stage, there have been no confirmed predictors of survival. In the past, vascular or lymphatic invasion and tumor differentiation were implicated without substantiation (19). Recently, blood vessel invasion was reported to be a main predictor of recurrence in T1, N0, M0 NSCLCs (20). Recent interest in genetic markers has suggested that K-*ras* oncogene expression in tumors (especially adenocarcinoma) may be a predictor of poor survival (21). Other

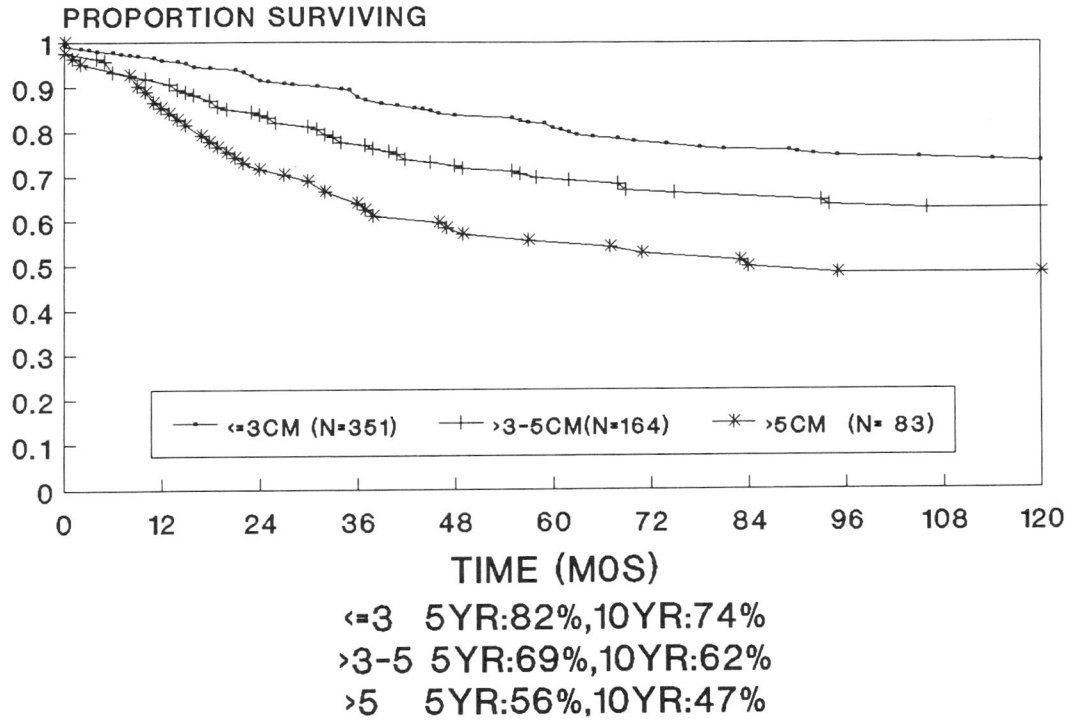

FIGURE 14.4. Survival post resection by tumor size in centimeters in stage I lung cancer.

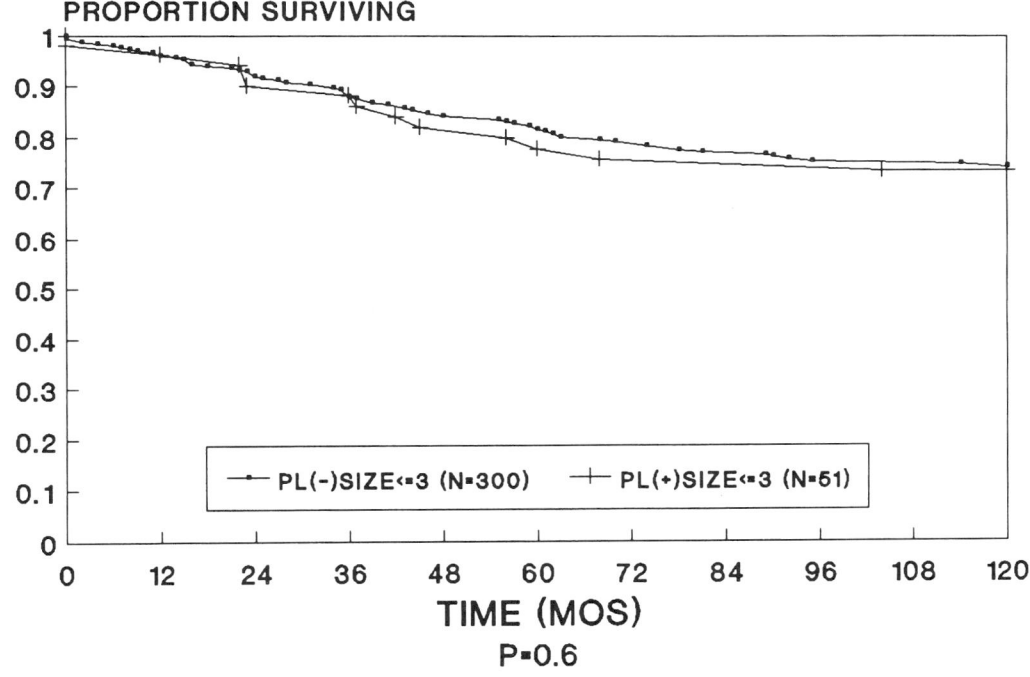

FIGURE 14.5. Survival post resection by visceral pleural involvement in small stage I lung cancer.

TABLE 14.1 *Criteria for Diagnosis of Multiple Lung Cancers*

Metachronous tumors
  Histology different
  Histology the same, if:
    Free interval between cancers is at least 2 years or:
    Origin from carcinoma in situ or:
    Second cancer in different lobe or lung, but:
      No carcinoma in lymphatics common to both
      No extrapulmonary metastases at time of diagnosis
Synchronous tumors
  Tumors physically distinct and separate
  Histology:
    Different
    Same, but in different segment, lobe, or lung, if:
      Origin from carcinoma in situ
      No carcinoma in lymphatics common to both
      No extrapulmonary metastases at time of diagnosis

predictors that have yet to be substantiated include the presence of blood group antigen A, deletion of the *p53* gene, and the presence of aneuploidy. Although there are reports that note that DNA assessment is valuable (22, 23), it was not prognostic in the Memorial experience (24–26), nor in that of the Lung Cancer Study Group (LCSG) (1).

ALTERNATIVE TREATMENTS

The effects of primary chemotherapy in stage I disease are unknown. Radiation therapy is considered an alternative treatment to surgery in patients who cannot undergo or refuse treatment by surgery. Only a limited number of reports in the literature refer to the results of radiation therapy with curative intent in early lung cancer. Smart and Hilton (27) reported the results of external radiation therapy in 33 patients with good performance status, technically resectable lesions, and no evidence of mediastinal node involvement. The 5-year survival rate was 33%. Schumacher in 1976 (28) reported his experience with external radiation therapy in stage I and II patients. His 5-year survival rate was 31% (13 of 42 patients). Cooper et al. (29) reported a 5-year survival rate of 6% for patients with operable lung cancer treated by radiation alone (4 of 67 patients).

Intraoperative brachytherapy also is an effective alternative to resection for patients with small lesions and no mediastinal lymph node metastases who are considered unresectable at thoracotomy mainly because of the presence of severe obstructive pulmonary disease that precludes adequate resection. Fifty-five such patients with stage I or II tumors received an interstitial implant and nearly half also received external radiation therapy postoperatively (30). Local control was attained in 62% of patients. The overall 5-year survival (Kaplan-Meier) was 32%, and the median survival was 23 months. This rate is similar to that of prior reports of the use of external radiation therapy.

ADJUVANT THERAPY

The role of adjuvant radiotherapy, chemotherapy, or a combination of both after surgical resection for stage I lung cancer is still unclear. Several randomized trials in the past two decades have failed to show a survival benefit when adjuvant therapy is added to surgical resection. A host of immunopotentiators and chemotherapeutic agents has been tested as adjuvants in resected stage I disease. A survival advantage was noted initially in patients treated with intrapleural bacille Calmette–Guérin (BCG) (32). However, this rate was not confirmed in a large multicenter study by the LCSG (33, 34). Other immunotherapeutic agents used were cutaneous BCG, levamisole, and *Corynebacterium parvum*. They also have not been shown to be effective. In a recent study by the LCSG (35), patients with completely resected T2, N0 tumors were randomized to receive either CAP (cyclophosphamide, Adriamycin [doxorubicin], cisplatin) chemotherapy or no further treatment. There was no benefit demonstrated for the CAP chemotherapy.

At this time, no adjuvant treatment is recommended for patients with stage I disease after resection.

CHEMOPREVENTION

There has been recent interest in the prevention of second primary tumors after curative therapy in early lung cancer (36, 37). Because Vitamin A and the retinoids were found to be strong inhibitors of epithelial cancer progression in experimental carcinogenesis, several randomized studies are currently in progress to assess the merits of retinoids in improving the disease free interval by preventing secondary aerodigestive cancers or recurrences. Pastorino et al. (37) have demonstrated a beneficial effect of postoperative vitamin A treatment in the prevention of second primary tumors. The data are still viewed as preliminary and will require several years of follow-up before definitive conclusions can be drawn. A nationwide study in the United States is now accruing patients to answer this question in a large randomized controlled study. At this time, it is recommended that retinoids and vitamin A be offered only in protocol settings.

STAGE II DISEASE

Tumors confined to the lung or bronchus with involvement of hilar or bronchopulmonary nodes as the sole site of tumor spread are classified as stage II tumors. They make up fewer than 5% of all NSCLCs and, in the Memorial experience, account for less than 10% of all resected tumors.

Once lymph node metastases are present, even when confined to the ipsilateral hemithorax without mediastinal involvement, the results of curative therapy are much worse than those for stage I disease. Although surgery is still the prime method of curative treatment, fewer than 50% of patients survive tumor free beyond 5 years. Efforts have been made to supplement the surgical treatment in these patients by radiation therapy, chemotherapy, or both. To date, there has been no concrete evidence that any adjuvant therapy is beneficial.

RESULTS OF SURGICAL THERAPY: THE MEMORIAL EXPERIENCE

The experience at Memorial Sloan–Kettering Cancer Center on the surgical treatment of stage II lung cancer was reviewed recently. From 1973 to 1989, 214 patients had undergone a complete resection of their stage II lung cancer with a mediastinal lymph node dissection (38).

Thirty-five patients had T1, N1 lesions, and 179 had T2, N1 tumors. The male to female ratio was 2 to 1, and the median age was 62 years. Ten percent of the tumors were in the main bronchus beyond 2 cm of the carina, 51% in the upper lobes, 36% in the lower lobes, and 4% in the right middle lobe. There were 116 adenocarcinomas and 98 squamous cancers. Included under adenocarcinomas were 18 bronchoalveolar cancers and 9 large cell carcinomas. Eighty-three percent of the patients with T1 lesions had adenocarcinomas. In T2 lesions, adenocarcinomas and squamous cancers were of equal frequency.

Lobectomy was the procedure of choice in most patients. Sixty-eight percent had a lobectomy, 31% a pneumonectomy, and 1% a wedge resection or segmentectomy. Of interest was the fact that half of the patients had a single N1 node involved and 85% of the patients had nodal involvement at a single N1 level.

The overall survival rate after resection (Kaplan-Meier) was 47% at 5 years. Deaths from unrelated causes were considered withdrawals. There was no difference in survival between patients with T1 and T2 tumors (Fig. 14.2). Favorable prognostic factors included the number of involved nodes and the size of the lesion. There was a significant difference in survival between patients with tumors 3 cm or smaller in diameter and those 5 cm or greater (Fig. 14.6). Also, patients with single sites of N1 disease fared better than those with multiple sites. The best survival was obtained in patients with small tumors (no more than 3 cm) and a single N1 node, and the worst survival was seen in those with large tumors (at least 5 cm) and multiple N1 nodes (52% versus 37%, respectively) (Fig. 14.7). The location of the primary tumor, the location of the N1 nodes, the histology, the extent of the surgical resection, and the presence or absence of visceral pleural involvement had no appreciable impact on survival.

There were more local or regional recurrences in patients with squamous cancers and more distant metastases in patients with adenocarcinoma.

ADJUVANT THERAPY

The incidence of local or regional recurrence was reduced in the Memorial series by the administration of postoperative radiation therapy. However, there was no impact on survival by the addition of postoperative radiation therapy. Recurrence rates were high despite resection. Most patients who did not respond to the initial therapy developed distant metastases, suggesting the need for an effective systemic treatment, but the specific regimens that might benefit this group of patients are still undetermined.

Two large cooperative studies have attempted to address this group of patients. The LCSG (39) randomized 189 resected stage II patients by histology to receive adjuvant treatments. Those with resected squamous cancers were treated by postoperative external radiation or received no further treatment. This study concluded that in squamous carcinoma, postoperative radiation therapy reduced local and regional recurrence but had no impact on survival.

The LCSG, in another trial comparing postoperative irradiation with chemoirradiation, reported some advantages in the time to recurrence of combined adjuvant radiation and chemotherapy in adenocarcinoma (40). However, this latter study did not compare or assess adjuvant treatment with chemotherapy alone and with no adjuvant treatment.

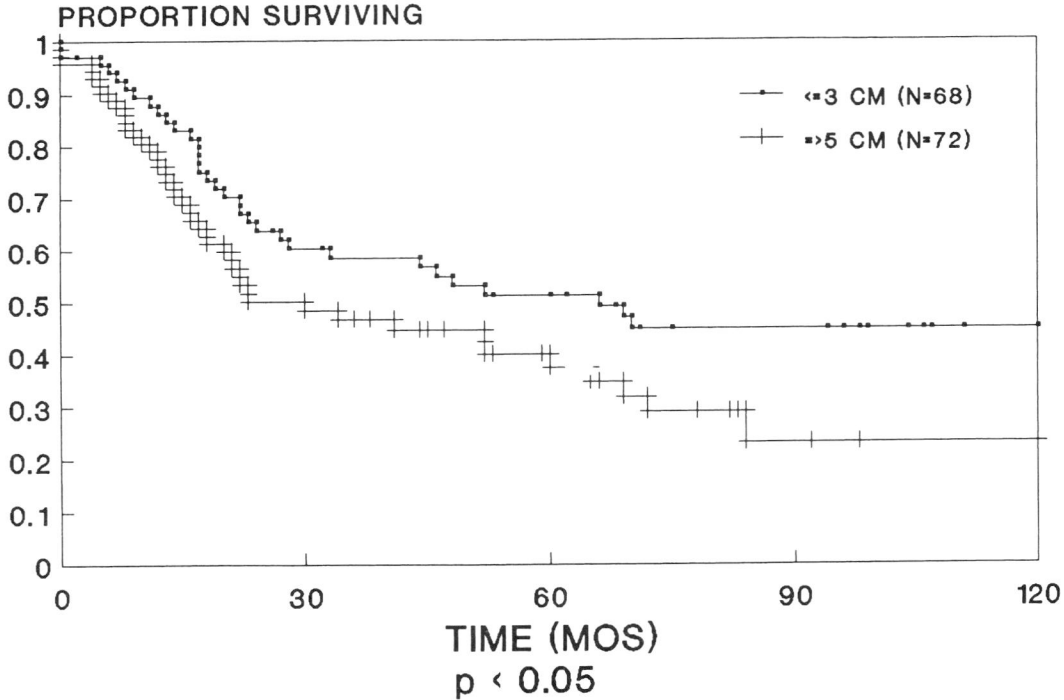

FIGURE 14.6. Survival post resection by tumor size in centimeters in stage II lung cancer.

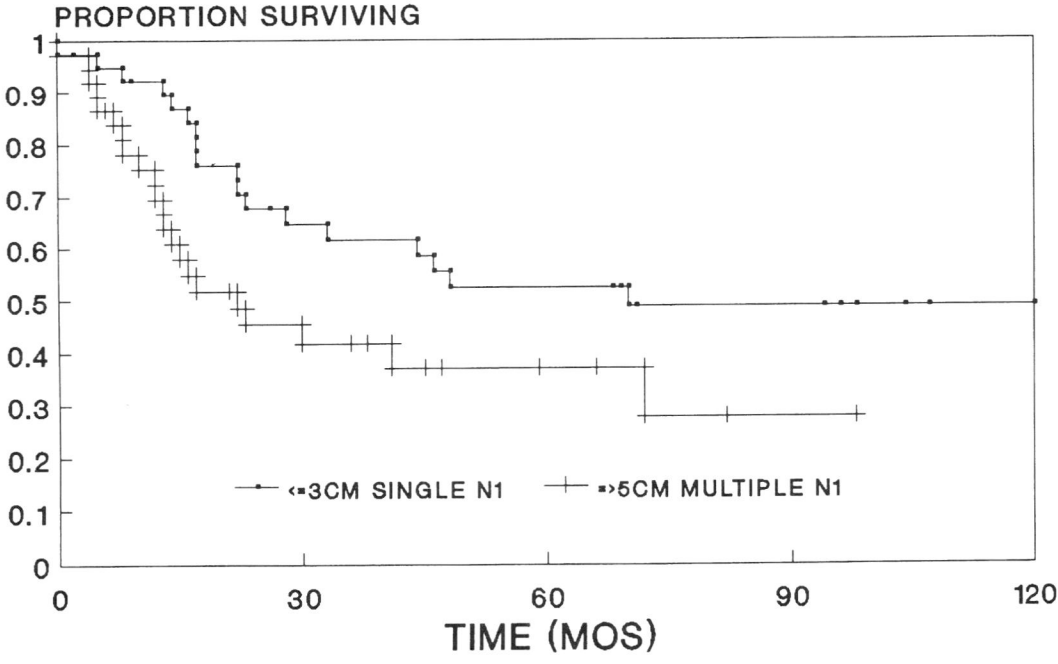

FIGURE 14.7 Survival post resection by tumor size and number of involved N1 nodes in stage II lung cancer.

In resected stage II adenocarcinomas, postoperative adjuvant trials of chemotherapy, immunotherapy, or combinations of the two have had little effect on the survival rate in randomized studies (41–44). The LCSG also reported a survival difference between patients with squamous carcinoma and adenocarcinoma, and between those with T1 and T2 lesions, that was not observed in the Memorial series.

Another large cooperative trial conducted by the Ludwig Lung Cancer Study Group from Europe (45) evaluated resected stage II carcinomas for survival and recurrence. There were 253 patients with stage II disease entered into the study (81 staged T1, N1 and 172 staged T2, N1). Only median survival rates were reported; these indicated that patients with T1 lesions lived twice as long as patients with T2 disease (median T1 survival, 4.8 years; T2 survival, 2.3 years).

Naruke from the National Cancer Center Hospital of Japan (4) reported 221 patients with completely resected stage II lung cancer and showed an overall 5-year survival of 43%, similar to the Memorial experience, but a 5-year survival of 52% for patients with T1 lesions and 38% for those with T2 lesions ($P = .05$). There was no difference in survival by histology in his series.

In an earlier study by the Veterans Administration Surgical Oncology Cooperative Group (46, 47), 152 patients with resected stage II lung cancer had shown no significant difference in survival at 3 years between T1 and T2 lesions (T1, 37%; T2, 40%). A more recent report of the M. D. Anderson experience combined with that of the LCSG (48) reported 317 patients with resected stage II lung cancer. The 5-year survival was 54% for those with T1 lesions ($n = 67$) and 40% for patients with T2 lesions ($n = 250$). These differences in observation among the various series may reflect differences in case material and in the method of lymph node assessment among the various institutions.

A recent Finnish study using CAP chemotherapy as adjuvant treatment, but for a longer period than any of the LCSG trials, has demonstrated an improved survival in the treated group (49). Presently, an American cooperative trial comparing postoperative radiotherapy and postoperative chemoradiotherapy includes patients with completely resected stage II and stage III disease. Physicians must await the results of this trial to see if the original LCSG report suggesting improved survival with chemoradiotherapy is confirmed.

Because most patients fail in distant sites and more than 50% of patients with stage II disease are not cured by surgery alone, the role of induction chemotherapy before surgery is being investigated, even in this earlier stage of disease.

At Memorial Sloan–Kettering Cancer Center, induction therapy is being tested in this subset of patients. Because patients with large tumors (5 cm or greater in diameter) with N0 or N1 disease have a poorer survival rate than those with smaller tumors within the same stage, physicians at this center have embarked on induction chemotherapy with MVP (mitomycin, vinblastine, high-dose cisplatin) in patients with T2, N0 or T2, N1 tumors greater than 5 cm in diameter.

ROLE OF MINIRESECTION AND THORACOSCOPY IN STAGE I OR II DISEASE

Pulmonary resection has been the accepted treatment for early-stage lung cancer. Initially, pneumonectomy was the treatment of choice, regardless of the stage or location of the disease. With the development of techniques for hilar dissection, lobectomy became a feasible alternative, and, for the past 30 years, this procedure has been accepted as the minimal resection of choice in lung cancer when the site and stage allowed a complete resection by this lesser operation. Lobectomy continues to be the procedure of choice for early-stage lung cancer limited to a single lobe, even if a lesser resection could encompass all disease (2, 50). However, in the past two decades, limited resections have been used for selected indications; with the enthusiasm now generated for video-assisted thoracoscopic procedures, such resections have been promulgated for early-stage lung cancer treatment.

Lesser pulmonary resections (segmental resection, wedge resection, precision cautery dissection) were used initially as compromise operations in patients with lung cancer who suffered from poor pulmonary reserve and who could withstand a thoracotomy but not a lobectomy (51–59). Both segmental and wedge resections have been used for this compromise operation.

Despite being a compromise procedure and despite some locally advanced tumors being treated in this fashion, retrospective reports suggested a reasonable 5-year survival rate when a lesser resection is used as a compromise procedure. In many cases, incomplete resections were performed necessarily, and the local recurrence rate of lesser resections in this group of patients was significant. Most authors, including those from the Memorial Sloan–Kettering Cancer Center, thought that because of the high local recurrence rate, the use of lesser resection should not be advised in patients who could tolerate a lobectomy (16, 54, 57, 60, 61).

More recently, patients presenting with bilateral synchronous or metachronous primry tumors have been managed, on a selective basis, with standard pulmonary resections if required, but with lesser resections whenever possible to preserve as much pulmonary function tissue as possible (61–63). The use of lesser resections for this indication does not appear to have compromised the ability to cure.

In 1973, Jensik et al. (64) reported the first experience with elective segmental resection as the treatment of choice in early-stage lung cancer. Since that first report, many other centers have adopted this approach and have published their updated results. In the larger series the survival rate appears comparable to that expected from standard lobectomy in the treatment of stage I carcinoma (1, 17, 26, 34, 54, 60). There has been a persistent fear that local recurrence could prove to be a major problem. Until recently, none of the historical series has demonstrated local recurrence to be the case. However, there is general agreement that patients suitable for this type of resection should have T1, N0 tumors, peripherally located, and preferably not transgressing a segmental plane. The postoperative mortality and morbidity from this lesser resection has been acceptable and is comparable to that seen with lobectomy for stage I lung cancer.

In 1982, the LCSG (60) initiated a prospective trial of limited resection (segmentectomy or wedge resection) compared with lobectomy for the management of patients staged at operation to have peripheral T1, N0 lung cancers. In instituting this trial, the LCSG imposed rigid criteria for entry into the protocol including a peripheral tumor without nodal involvement, tumor not visible on bronchoscopy, and tumor measuring 3 cm or less on plain chest radiographs. All patients were able to tolerate a lobectomy. Follow-up included analysis of postoperative morbidity and mortality; pulmonary function evaluations at 6, 12, and 18 months; and an analysis of local recurrence rates and ultimate survival.

The late results have now been reported in abstract form and show no significant difference in perioperative mortality or pulmonary function in the two arms (15, 60). The trial has been closed for 4 years. At a minimum 3-year follow-up, there was a significant increase in the local recurrence rate and decreased survival after the limited resection (16).

A recent retrospective analysis from Rush-Presbyterian–St. Luke's Medical Center (65) confirms this result. From 1980 to 1988, 173 patients had undergone either a standard lobectomy or a segmental resection for stage I (T1, N0 or T2, N0) carcinoma. Sixty-eight patients had undergone segmentectomy, and 105 had a lobectomy. There was no significant difference in the 5-year survival when the tumor was no more than 3 cm in diameter. There was, however, more than a fourfold increase in the incidence of local or regional recurrence.

The local or regional recurrence rate was 22.7% after segmental resection versus 4.9% after lobectomy. This finding was true even among tumors less than 2 cm in diameter. Most of the local or regional recurrences were detected 18 to 36 months after resection, and most arose within the lung. In several cases, the recurrence was detected early enough that the patients were able to undergo an additional resection successfully, often with long-term survival. For all of these reasons, resections less extensive than a lobectomy should be performed only in compromise situations. Thoracoscopic approaches for the treatment of lung cancer should continue to follow the oncologic principles outlined above, i.e., lobectomy plus, at a minimum, adequate lymph node sampling.

SUMMARY

In early-stage NSCLC, a complete resection is the treatment of choice. In most patients, a lobectomy suffices, although a pneumonectomy may be required in certain cases. Lesser resections (wedge or segment) should be reserved for patients who cannot tolerate a lobectomy. To preserve lung function, lesser resections also have been advocated when synchronous or metachronous tumors occur.

With the advent of video-assisted surgical techniques, wedge resections have become popular and have been advocated in low-risk patients, but without additional supportive data. Early results have shown a disturbingly high incidence of local recurrence within the lung (i.e., along the staple line), and in 20 cases implantation of tumor at the chest wall port site has been reported (66).

Although postoperative radiotherapy has been used in stage II patients and has decreased the incidence of locoregional recurrence, the ultimate survival has not been altered. Except for one recent study, adjuvant chemotherapy has never been demonstrated to be of value in treating early-stage disease. Although chemoradiotherapy has demonstrated a minimal improved survival, the role of this treatment is still being investigated. Induction therapy before resection in patients thought to have clinical stage II disease also is being investigated.

Patients who cannot tolerate a surgical resection should be offered radiotherapy as the primary local control treatment. Recent studies suggest that the addition of chemotherapy to primary radiotherapy improves the likelihood of long-term success in more locally advanced disease and may well prove to be the treatment of choice when radiotherapy is the primary method of local control.

REFERENCES

1. Gail MH, Eagan R, Feld R, et al. Prognostic factors in patients with resected stage I non–small cell lung cancer. A report from the Lung Cancer Study Group. Cancer 1984;54:1802–1813.
2. Martini N, Bains MS, Burt ME, et al. Incidence of local recurrence and second primary tumors in resected stage I lung cancer. J Thorac Cardiovasc Surg 1995;109:1–10.
3. Martini N, Beattie EJ. Results of surgical treatment in stage I lung cancer. J Thorac Cardiovasc Surg 1977;74:499–505.
4. Naruke T, Goya T, Tsuchiya R, Suemasu K. Prognosis and survival in resected lung carcinoma based on the new international staging system. J Thorac Cardiovasc Surg 1988;96:440–447.
5. Pairolero P, Williams DE, Bergstralh EJ, Piehler JM, Bernatz PE, Payne WS. Postsurgical stage I bronchogenic carcinoma: morbid implications of recurrent disease. Ann Thorac Surg 1984;38:331–338.
6. Williams DE, Pairolero PC, Davis CS, et al. Survival of patients surgically treated for stage I lung cancer. J Thorac Cardiovasc Surg 1981;82:70–76.
7. Cortese DA, Pairolero PC, Bergstralh EJ, et al. Roentgenographically occult lung cancer: a ten-year experience. J Thorac Cardiovasc Surg 1983;86:373–380.
8. Flehinger BJ, Kimmel M, Melamed MR. The effect of surgical treatment on survival from early lung cancer. Implications for screening. Chest 1992;101:1013–1018.
9. Martini N, Zaman MB, Melamed MR. Early diagnosis in carcinoma of the lung. In: Roth JA, Ruckdeschel JC, Weisenburg TH, eds. Thoracic oncology. Philadelphia: WB Saunders, 1989:133–141.
10. Hayata Y, Kato H, Konaka C, et al. Hematoporphyrin derivative and laser photoradiation in the treatment of lung cancer. Chest 1982;81:269–277.
11. Lam S, MacAulay C, Hung J, et al. Detection of dysplasia and carcinoma in situ with a lung imaging fluorescence endoscopic device. J Thorac Cardiovasc Surg 1993;105:1035–1040.
12. Hayata Y, Kato H, Konaka C, et al. Photoradiation therapy with hematoporphyrin derivative in early and stage I lung cancer. Chest 1984;86:169–177.
13. Ramsdell JW, Peters RM, Taylor AT Jr, et al. Multiorgan scans for staging lung cancer. J Thorac Cardiovasc Surg 1977;73:653–659.
14. Bulzebruck H, Bopp R, Drings P, et al. New aspects in the staging of lung cancer. Prospective validation of the International Union Against Cancer TNM classification. Cancer 1992;70:1102–1110.
15. Ginsberg RJ, for the Lung Cancer Study Group. Limited resection for peripheral T1N0 tumors. Lung Cancer 1988;4:A80.
16. Ginsberg RJ, Rubinstein L, for the Lung Cancer Study Group. A randomized comparative trial of lobectomy vs limited resection for patients with T1 N0 non–small cell lung cancer (abstract 304). Lung Cancer 1991;7 (Suppl): 83.
17. Read RC, Yoder G, Schaeffer RC. Survival after conservative resection for T1 N0 M0 non–small cell lung cancer. Ann Thorac Sug 1990;49:391–400.
18. The Lung Cancer Study Group, prepared by Thomas PA Jr, Rubinstein L. Malignant disease appearing late after operation for T1 N0 non–small lung cancer. J Thorac Cardiovasc Surg 1993;106:1053–1058.
19. Shields TW. Prognostic significance of parenchymal lymphatic vessel and blood vessel invasion in carcinoma of the lung. Surg Gynecol Obstet 1983;157:185–190.
20. Macchiarini P, Fontanini G, Hardin MF, et al. Blood vessel invasion by tumor cells predicts recurrence in completely resected T1 N0 M0 non–small-cell lung cancer. J Thorac Cardiovasc Surg 1993;106:80–89.
21. Slebos RJC, Kibbelaar RE, Dalesio O, et al. K-*ras* oncogene activation as a prognostic marker in adenocarcinoma of the lung. N Engl J Med 1990;323:561–565.
22. Cibas ES, Melamed MR, Zaman MB, Kimmel M. The effect of tumor cell DNA content on the survival of patients with stage I adenocarcinoma of the lung. Cancer 1989;63:1552–1556.
23. Rice TW, Bauer TW, Gephardt GN, Medendorp SV, McLain DA, Kirby TJ. Prognostic significance of flow cytometry in non–small-cell lung cancer. J Thorac Cardiovasc Surg 1993;106:210–217.
24. Schmidt RA, Rusch VW, Piantadosi S. A flow cytometric study of non–small cell lung cancer classified as T1N0. Cancer 1992;69:78–85.
25. Thomas P, Rubinstein L, Lung Cancer Study Group. Cancer recurrence after resection: T1 N0 non–small cell lung cancer. Ann Thorac Surg 1990;49:242–247.
26. Volm M, Hahn EW, Mattern J, Muller T, Vogt-Moykopf I, Weber E. Five-year follow-up study of independent clinical and flow cytometric factors for the survival of patients with non–small cell lung carcinoma. Cancer Res 1988;48:2923–2928.
27. Smart J, Hilton G. Radiotherapy of cancer of the lung. Results in a selected group of cases. Lancet 1956;270:880–881.
28. Schumacher W. The use of high-energy electrons in the treatment of inoperable lung and bronchogenic carcinoma. In: Kramer S, Suntharalingam N, and Zinninger GF, eds. High-energy photons and electrons: clinical applications in cancer management. New York: John Wiley & Sons, 1976:255–284.
29. Cooper JD, Pearson FG, Todd TRJ, et al. Radiotherapy alone for patients with operable carcinoma of the lung. Chest 1985;87:289–292.
30. Hilaris BS, Nori D, Martini N. Results of radiation therapy in stage I and II unresectable non–small-cell lung cancer. Endocurietherapy/Hyperthermia Oncology 1986;2:15–21.
31. Kaplan EL, Meier P. Nonparametric estimation from incomplete observations. J Am Stat Assoc 1958;53:457–481.
32. McKneally MF, Maver C, Kausel HW. Regional immunotherapy of lung cancer with BCG. Lancet 1976;21:377–379.
33. Mountain CF, Gail MH. Surgical adjuvant intrapleural BCG treatment for stage I non–small cell lung cancer. Preliminary report of the National Cancer Institute Lung Cancer Study Group. J Thorac Cardiovasc Surg 1981;82:649–657.
34. Moores DWO, McKneally M. Treatment of stage I lung cancer (T1N0M0, T2N0M0). Surg Clin North Am 1987;57:5:937–943.
35. Feld R, Rubinstein L, Thomas PA, Lung Cancer Study Group. Adjuvant chemotherapy with cyclophosphamide, doxorubicin and cisplatin in patients with completely resected stage I non–small cell lung cancer. J Natl Cancer Inst 1993;85:299–306.

36. Lippman SC, Hong WK. Not yet standard: retinoids versus second primary tumors (editorial). J Clin Oncol 1993;11:1204–1207.
37. Pastorino U, Infante M, Maioli M, et al. Adjuvant treatment of stage I lung cancer with high-dose vitamin A. J Clin Oncol 1993;11:1216–1222.
38. Martini N, Burt ME, Bains MS, McCormack PM, Rusch VW, Ginsberg RJ. Survival after resection of stage II non–small cell lung cancer. Ann Thorac Surg 1992;54:460–466.
39. Lung Cancer Study Group, prepared by Weisenburger TH, Gail M. Effects of postoperative mediastinal radiation in complete resected stage II and stage III epidermoid cancer of the lung. N Engl J Med 1986;315:1377–1381.
40. Holmes EC, Gail M, for the Lung Cancer Study Group. Surgical adjuvant therapy for stage II and III adenocarcinoma and large-cell undifferentiated carcinoma. J Clin Oncol 1986;4:710–715.
41. Holmes EC. Treatment of stage II cancer (T1N1 and T2N1). Surg Clin North Am 1987;67:5:945–949.
42. Holmes EC, Hill LD, Gail M, for the Lung Cancer Study Group. A randomized comparison of the effects of adjuvant therapy on resected stages II and III non–small cell carcinoma of the lung. Ann Surg 1985;202:335–340.
43. Newman SB, DeMeester TR, Golomb HM, Hoffman PC, Little AG, Raghavan V. Treatment of modified stage II (T1N1M0, T2N1M0) non–small cell bronchogenic carcinoma. A combined modality approach. J Thorac Cardiovasc Surg 1983;86:180–185.
44. Shields TW, Yee J, Conn JH, Robinette CD. Relationship of cell type and lymph node metastasis to survival after resection of bronchial carcinoma. Ann Thorac Surg 1975;20:501–510.
45. Ludwig Lung Cancer Study Group. Patterns of failure in patients with resected stage I and II non–small cell carcinoma of lung. Ann Surg 1987;205:67–71.
46. Shields TW, Humphrey EW, Matthews M, Eastridge CE, Keehn BS. Pathologic stage grouping of patients with resected carcinoma of the lung. J Thorac Cardiovasc Surg 1980;80:400–405.
47. Immerman SC, Vanecko RM, Fry WA, Head LR, Shields TW. Site of recurrence in patients with stage I and II carcinoma of the lung resected for cure. Ann Thorac Surg 1981;32:23–27.
48. Mountain CF. A new international staging system for lung cancer. Chest 1986;89(Suppl):225–233.
49. Niiranen A, Niitamo-Korhonen S, Kouri M, Assendelft A, Mattson, Pyrhonen S. Adjuvant chemotherapy after radical surgery for non–small cell lung cancer: a randomized study. J Clin Oncol 1992;10:1927–1932.
50. Martini N, McCaughan BC, McCormack PM, Bains MS. The extent of resection for localized lung cancer. Lobectomy. In: Kittle CF, ed. Current controversies in thoracic surgery. Philadelphia: WB Saunders, 1986:171–174.
51. Bennett WF, Smith RA. Segmental resection for bronchogenic carcinoma. A surgical alternative for the compromised patient. Ann Thorac Sug 1979;27:170–172.
52. Errett LE, Wilson J, Chiu RC-J, Munro DD. Wedge resection as an alternative procedure for peripheral bronchogenic carcinoma in poor-risk patients. J Thorac Cardiovasc Surg 1985;90:656–661.
53. Hoffmann TH, Ransdell HT. Comparison of a lobectomy and wedge resection for carcinoma of the lung. J Thorac Cardiovasc Surg 1980;79:211–217.
54. Jensik RJ. The extent of resection for localized lung cancer: Segmental resection. In: Kittle CF, ed. Current controversies in thoracic surgery. Philadelphia: WB Saunders, 1986:175–182.
55. Kulka F, Forai I. The segmental and apical resection of primary lung cancer. Proceedings of the IVth World Conference on Lung Cancer, 1985:81.
56. Kutschera W. Segment resection for lung cancer. Thorac Cardiovasc Surg 1984;32:102–104.
57. McCormack PM, Martini N. Primary lung carcinoma: results with conservative resection in treatment. N Y State J Med 1980;80:612–616.
58. Miller JI, Hatcher CR Jr. Limited resection of bronchogenic carcinoma in the patient with marked impairment of pulmonary function. Ann Thorac Surg 1987;44:240–343.
59. Stair JM, Womble J, Schaefer RF, Read RC, et al. Segmental pulmonary resection for cancer. Am J Surg 1985;150:659–664.
60. Ginsberg RJ, for the Lung Cancer Study Group. Limited resection for peripheral T1N0 tumors. Lung Cancer 1988;4(Suppl):A80.
61. Jensik RJ, Faber LP, Kittle CF, Meng RL. Survival following resection for a second primary bronchogenic carcinoma. J Thorac Cardiovasc Surg 1981;92:658–668.
62. Martini N, Ghosn P, Melamed MR. Local recurrence and new primary carcinoma after resection. In: Delarue NC, Eschapasse H, eds. International trends in general thoracic surgery. Philadelphia: WB Saunders, 1985;1:164–169.
63. Martini N, Melamed MR. Multiple primary lung cancers. J Thorac Cardiovasc Surg 1975;70:606–612.
64. Jensik RJ, Faber LB, Milloy FJ, Monson DO. Segmental resection for lung cancer. A fifteen year experience. J Thorac Cardiovasc Surg 1973;66:563–572.
65. Warren WH, Faber LP. Segmentectomy versus lobectomy in patients with stage I pulmonary carcinoma. Five-year survival and patterns of intrathoracic recurrence. J Thorac Cardiovasc Surg 1994;107:1087–1094.
66. Downey RJ, McCormack P, Locicero J, for the VTSSG. Dissemination of tumor following video-assisted thoracoscopy: a report of twenty-one cases. Ann Thorac Surg: in press.

15

Surgical Management of Stage IIIA Non–Small Cell Lung Cancer

Valerie W. Rusch and Yevgeniy Gincherman

INTRODUCTION

Stage III non–small cell lung cancer (NSCLC) includes a group of locally advanced tumors that do not have evidence of distant metastatic disease. Stage III is subdivided into stage IIIA, which designates tumors that are potentially resectable, and stage IIIB, which includes tumors usually considered unresectable (Table 15.1). Of the 140,000 patients diagnosed each year in the United States with NSCLC, approximately 30,000 have stage III disease (1). The overall 5-year survival rates in this group of patients range from 0% to 30%, but the majority of patients have a 10% or less chance of cure. Because of the number of patients affected and the poor prognosis of stage III disease, even small improvements in the treatment of these tumors can significantly impact the high overall mortality rate of lung cancer.

Despite the attempt to refine the staging system by subdividing stage III into IIIA and IIIB, both of these categories encompass heterogeneous groups of patients. Stage IIIA includes patients who have tumors that are designated T3 by virtue of involvement of the chest wall, pericardium, diaphragm, or proximal airway, and tumors that are N2 by virtue of involvement of the ipsilateral mediastinal lymph nodes (Table 15.1). In general, advanced T status disease is more amenable to surgical resection as the primary form of treatment than are patients with N2 disease, because T status is associated with a better long-term survival and a lower risk of distant metastatic disease. However, even within the categories of T3, N0-1 tumors and of N2 nodal disease, there are tumor subsets that differ in behavior and prognosis (2, 3). Treatment of these tumor subsets is effective only if it is based on an understanding of their diverse biologic behavior.

During the past decade, the management of stage III disease has been the most controversial and rapidly evolving area of lung cancer treatment. A standard of care for stage III NSCLC has not yet been established fully, but much has been learned about staging, proper patient selection for surgical resection, and the feasibility and validity of combined modality treatment. This chapter focuses on stage IIIA NSCLC and provides a perspective of both the tenets and controversies surrounding treatment for these patients.

CLINICAL PRESENTATION

Patients with stage IIIA NSCLC often present with symptoms because of the locally advanced nature of their tumors. T3 tumors involving the pericardium or diaphragm may be asymptomatic, but those involving the chest wall usually cause pain. Although ill-defined in many cases, this pain becomes localized and intense when tumors extend deeply into the chest wall to involve the intercostal nerves or ribs. T3 tumors involving the main stem bronchi produce hemoptysis, shortness of breath, wheezing, atelectasis, and postobstructive pneumonia (Figs. 15.1A, B, and C). N2 disease is often asymptomatic but may lead to symptoms if extensive nodal involvement compresses the proximal airways or superior vena cava (Fig. 15.2).

The presence of stage IIIA disease is usually evident on both plain chest radiographs and on chest computed tomography (CT) scan. A mass is often visible adjacent to the chest wall, diaphragm, or pericardium; however, even a CT scan cannot always distinguish whether the mass is adherent, invasive, or merely adjacent to these structures (Figs. 15.3A, B, and C), unless there are obvious findings such as associated rib destruction or elevation of the hemidiaphragm

TABLE 15.1. International TNM Staging System for Non–Small Cell Lung Cancer

T: Primary Tumor and Extent
- TX   Primary tumor cannot be assessed
- T0   No evidence of primary tumor
- TIS Carcinoma in situ
- T1   Primary tumor limited to ipsilateral parietal and/or visceral pleura
- T2   Tumor invades any of the following: ipsilateral lung, endothoracic fascia, diaphragm, pericardium
- T3   Tumor invades any of the following: ipsilateral chest wall muscle, ribs, mediastinal organs, or tissues
- T4   Tumor extends to any of the following: contralateral pleura or lung by direct extension; peritoneum or intraabdominal organs by direct extension; cervical tissues

N: Lymph Nodes
- NX   Regional lymph nodes cannot be assessed
- N0   No regional lymph node metastases
- N1   Metastases in ipsilateral bronchopulmonary or hilar lymph nodes
- N2   Metastases in ipsilateral mediastinal lymph nodes
- N3   Metastases in contralateral mediastinal, internal mammary, supraclavicular, or scalene lymph nodes

M: Metastases
- MX   Presence of distant metastases cannot be assessed
- M0   No (known) distant metastasis
- M1   Distant metastasis present

STAGE GROUPING

Occult carcinoma	TX	N0	M0
Stage 0	TIS	N0	M0
Stage I	T1	N0	M0
	T2	N0	M0
Stage II	T1	N1	M0
	T2	N1	M0
Stage IIIA	T1	N2	M0
	T2	N2	M0
	T3	N0, N1, N2	M0
Stage IIIB	Any T	N3	M0
	T4	Any N	M0
Stage IV	Any T	Any N	M1

caused by phrenic nerve involvement. The addition of magnetic resonance (MR) imaging to CT rarely aids in making this distinction (4–8). T3 disease involving the proximal main stem bronchus can be a subtle radiographic finding, particularly if there is no peribronchial disease. The tumor within an airway may not be visible on a chest radiograph and may only be suspected by virtue of associated postobstructive atelectasis or pneumonia (Figs. 15.4A and B). Endobronchial tumors are more likely to be visible on an amber chest radiograph or on CT scan (Fig. 15.4C).

Bulky extranodal N2 disease, also termed "clinical N2 disease," may be evident on plain chest radiographs. These findings are seen most frequently in patients who have right upper lobe tumors with metastasis to the right paratracheal lymph nodes (Fig. 15.2). Extensive subcarinal lymph node involvement can cause elevation and splaying of the main carina (Fig. 15.5A and B), and extensive involvement of the subaortic lymph nodes obliterates the space normally visible between the aorta and the left main pulmonary artery. CT scans can confirm the suspicion of mediastinal adenopathy (Figs. 15.6A, B, C, and D) and provide better definition of the location of enlarged lymph nodes than do plain radiographs. In general, any lymph node larger than 1 cm in diameter on CT scan is considered abnormal and potentially suspicious for metastatic disease (9, 10).

DIAGNOSIS AND STAGING

A tissue diagnosis usually is obtained easily in patients with stage IIIA NSCLC via percutaneous needle biopsy if the tumor is peripheral, or by bronchoscopy if it is located centrally. Bronchoscopy may not be diagnostic if a centrally located tumor does not have an endobronchial component. In this situation, transbronchial biopsy or transthoracic fine-needle aspiration may be required.

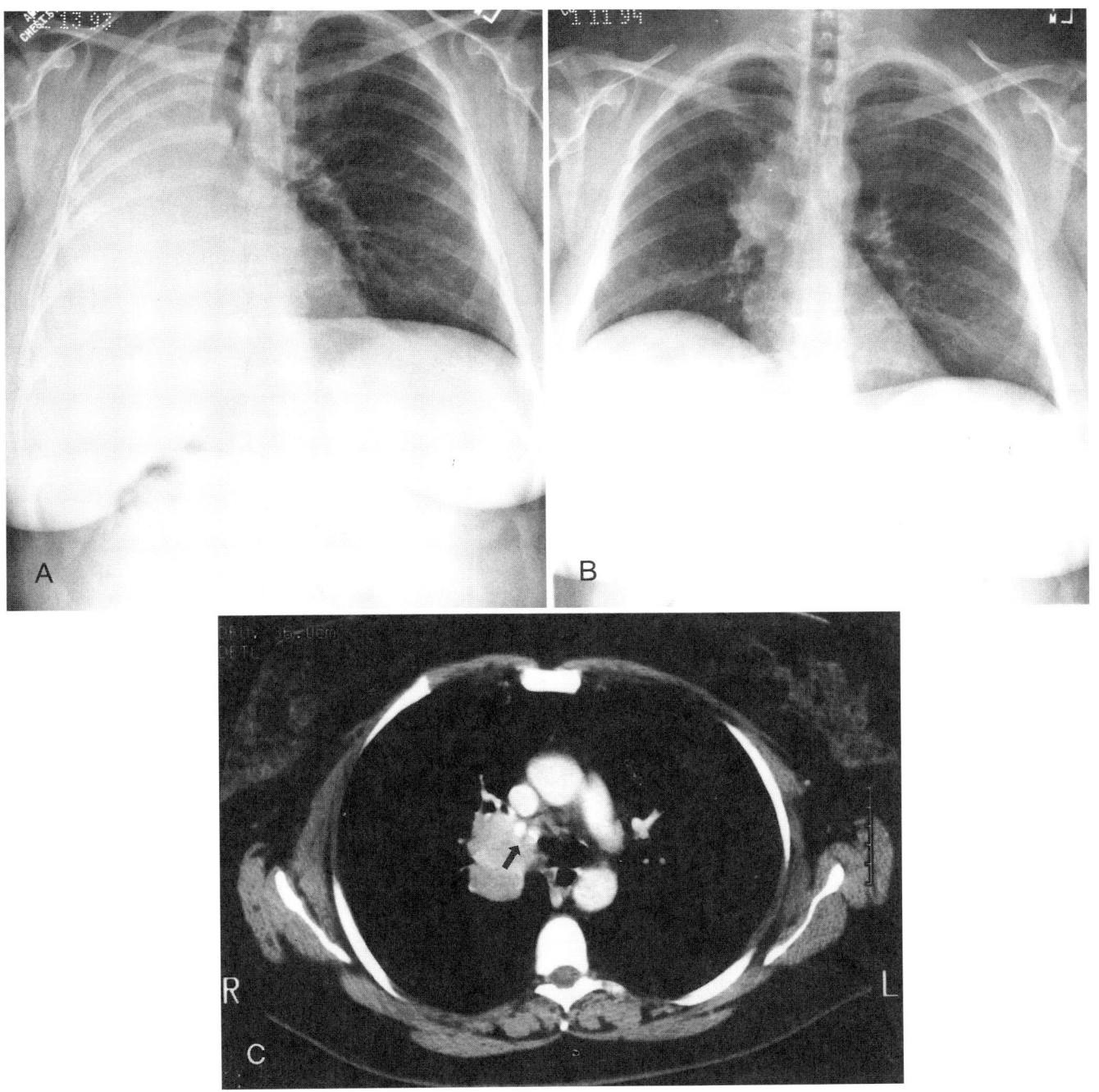

FIGURE 15.1. **A.** Primary squamous cell cancer of the right upper lobe extending into the right main stem bronchus and distal trachea. The patient presented with cough, hemoptysis, and shortness of breath. **B.** After laser resection of the tracheal and main stem bronchial component of the tumor, the lung has reexpanded and the extent of the primary tumor is visible on plain chest radiograph. **C.** The CT scan suggests that the tumor may extend into the mediastinum (*arrow*) and that the mediastinal lymph nodes may be involved. However, the patient proved to have a T3, N0 tumor that was completely resected by pneumonectomy.

Accurate staging is the most important and complex aspect of the evaluation of stage IIIA tumors. The first step is to exclude the presence of distant metastases by a thorough physical examination that includes a search for suspicious supraclavicular lymph nodes, abnormal pulmonary findings suggestive of airway obstruction or pleural effusion, abdominal or flank tenderness caused by liver or adrenal metastases, hepatomegaly, neurologic deficits indicative of spine or central nervous system metastases, and subcutaneous metastases.

A good quality chest radiograph delineates the primary tumor, and may also suggest mediastinal nodal involvement, direct extension of the tumor into the

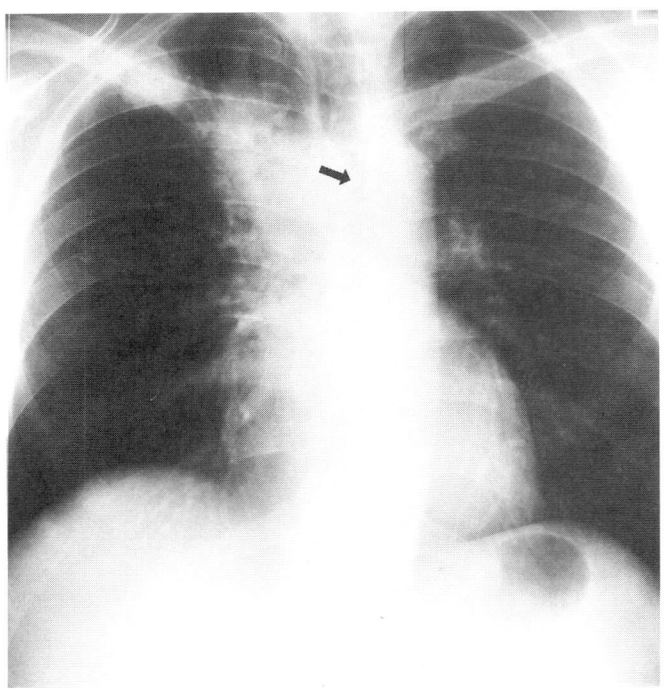

FIGURE 15.2. Chest radiograph of a patient who had a stage IIIA N2 adenocarcinoma of the right upper lobe. The N2 disease produced extrinsic compression of the trachea (*small arrow*). The patient failed to respond to initial treatment with radiation and chemotherapy. The N2 disease progressed into T4 disease, eroding through the wall of the distal trachea and right main stem bronchus and producing high-grade airway obstruction.

chest wall or mediastinum, and rib or pulmonary metastases distinct from the primary tumor. In contrast to earlier stage lung cancers, the high risk of micrometastatic disease in stage III tumors routinely warrants a complete metastatic workup including a chest and abdominal CT scan, a CT or MR scan of the brain, and a bone scan.

The assessment of the patient's overall medical condition is particularly important in determining the treatment of a stage III NSCLC. Many of these patients are now considered for multimodality treatment with some combination of chemotherapy, radiation therapy, and surgical resection. Cardiopulmonary disease caused by age, smoking, and exposure to synergistic carcinogens (e.g., asbestos), and occupational diseases (e.g., industry-related hearing loss), can limit the use of some treatment options. A careful history and physical examination should be performed to screen for these potential problems. In-depth evaluation of pulmonary reserve by pulmonary function testing, including diffusion capacity and rest and exercise arterial blood gases, and by ventilation perfusion lung scanning is almost always necessary. Any clinical suspicion of coronary artery disease should be investigated further by a stress thallium scan, stress radionuclide angiogram, or stress echocardiogram. Abnormal findings on these noninvasive cardiac tests, or prior known significant coronary artery disease, may require cardiac catheterization, with or without angioplasty, before initiating treatment for the patient's lung cancer. The history and physical examination should include a search for an abdominal aortic aneurysm or underlying carotid artery and peripheral vascular disease. If suspected, these should be evaluated further by Doppler examination and abdominal ultrasound. Renal insufficiency and hearing loss may preclude the use of cisplatin-based chemotherapy. A creatinine clearance calculated from the serum creatinine level and a clinical assessment of hearing on physical examination are adequate screening tests, but a 12- or 24-hour measured creatinine clearance and a formal audiogram may be necessary for definitive evaluation.

If extrathoracic spread has been excluded and the patient's general condition permits consideration of a pulmonary resection, the extent of direct mediastinal invasion and airway involvement, as well as the status of the mediastinal lymph nodes, should be assessed. Although CT can determine tumor size and proximity to other structures, it cannot distinguish tumor proximity to the mediastinum or chest wall from actual invasion; it also is relatively inaccurate in evaluating mediastinal lymph nodes (11, 12). The distinction between parietal pleural invasion (T3) versus simple tumor proximity to the chest wall and inflammatory adhesions (T2) is not clinically important because both are amenable to complete surgical resection. MR scanning adds to the information provided by CT only when invasion of the vertebral body or neural foramina are suspected or when there is involvement of the superior sulcus.

Bronchoscopy is important in evaluating the endobronchial extent of tumor. Biopsies of the main stem bronchus and main carina should be obtained to determine whether the primary tumor is T2, T3, or T4 (Table 15.1).

An accurate determination of the degree of mediastinal lymph node involvement in these patients is essential. Mediastinoscopy with systematic sampling of paratracheal, subcarinal, and tracheobronchial nodes remains the most accurate means of assessment (9, 10). CT scanning alone is much less accurate. Numerous studies have shown that using a 1-cm cutoff for defining positive lymph nodes on CT scan gives a sensitivity of only 64% to 79% and a specificity of 62% to 66% (5–14). These inaccuracies occur because of the finding of carcinoma in small unsuspected lymph nodes, yielding a significant false-negative rate. Similarly, carcinoma may not be present in large lymph nodes that are merely hyperplastic because of local in-

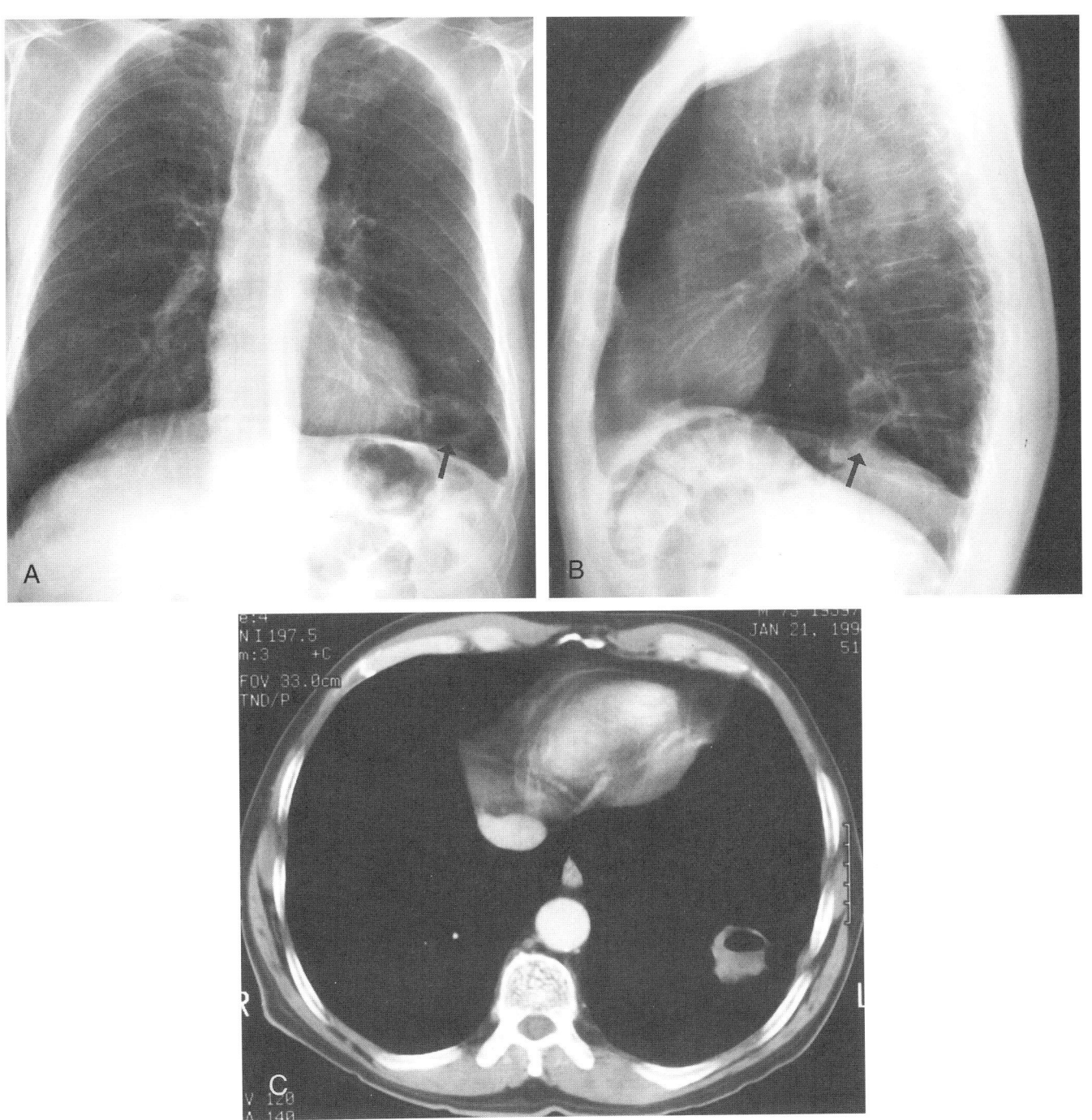

FIGURE 15.3. A. Left lower lobe cavitary squamous cell cancer (*arrow*). B. The lateral chest radiograph demonstrates the mass more clearly and suggests involvement of the diaphragm (*arrow*). C. The diaphragmatic involvement of this T3, N0 tumor was not shown by the preoperative CT scan.

fection surrounding the primary tumor. MRI imaging has a similar diagnostic ability.

A false-negative or false-positive CT scan has serious implications. For example, a false-negative scan may subject a patient to an extensive operation in the presence of N2 or N3 disease in which cure after surgical resection alone is unlikely. A false-positive scan may lead to unnecessary exposure to a neoadjuvant treatment with its attendant morbidities when a straightforward surgical resection was indicated. Because the morbidity of mediastinoscopy is minimal and the consequences of false-negative or false-positive CT scan are serious, mediastinoscopy should be used more frequently. In a retrospective review of 1000 medi-

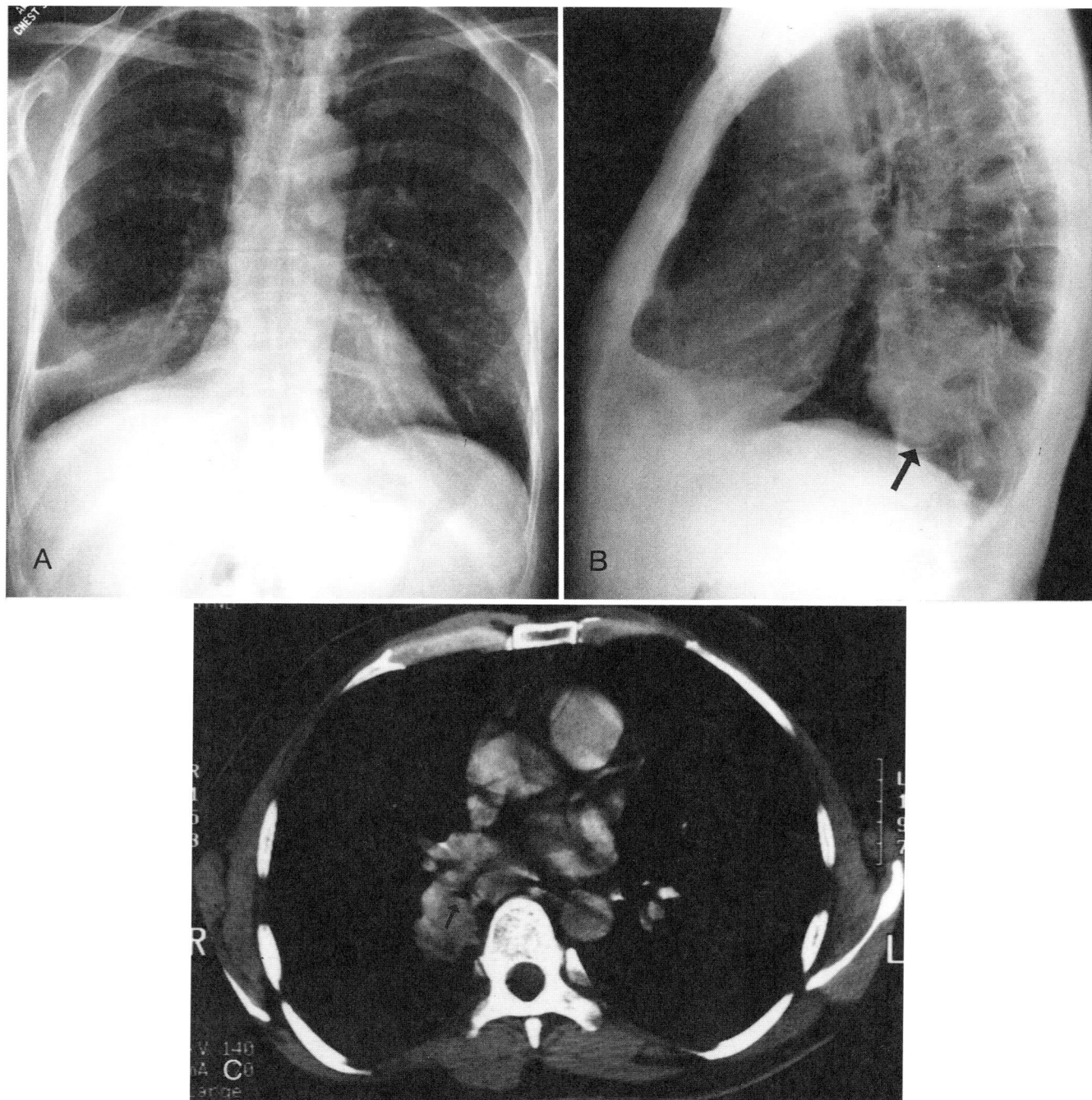

FIGURE 15.4. NSCLC originating in the right lower lobe bronchus and extending into the bronchus intermedius. A. On the posteroanterior (AP) chest radiograph, the most notable finding is the postobstructive collapse of the right lower lobe. B. The mass and associated collapse and consolidation are more easily appreciated on the lateral chest radiograph (*arrow*). C. The CT scan on this same patient shows the endobronchial tumor in the bronchus intermedius (*small arrow*) and suggests extension of the tumor into the mediastinum. However, the patient proved to have a T2, N0 tumor at thoracotomy.

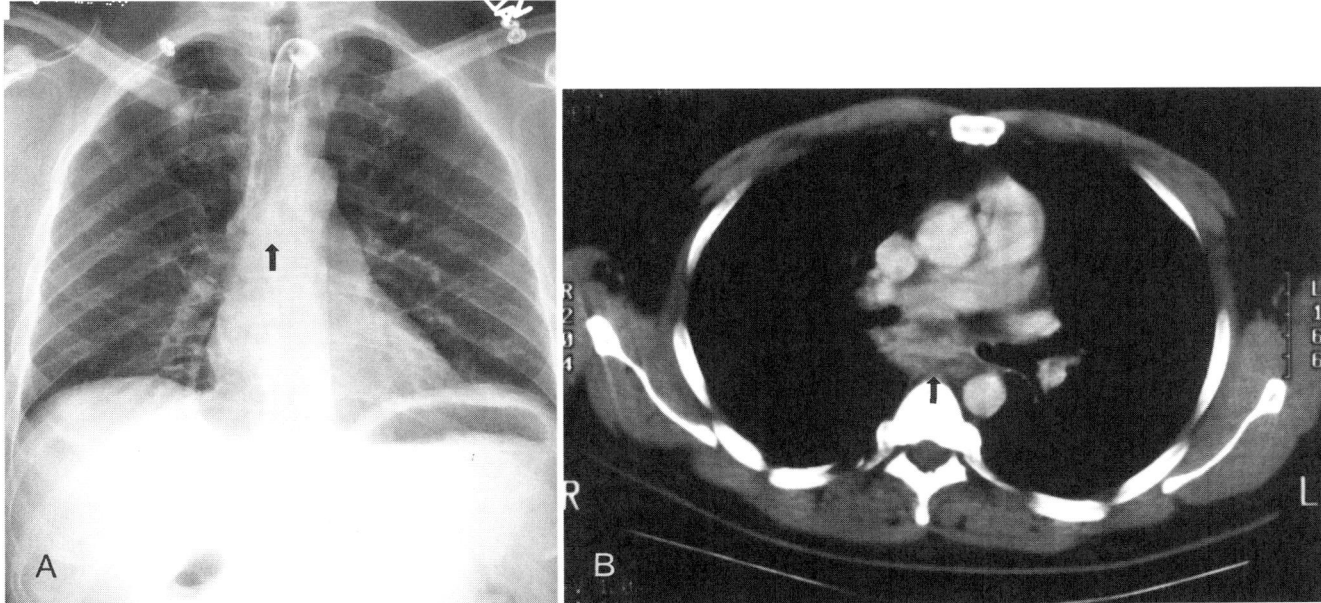

FIGURE 15.5. A. Subcarinal adenopathy in a patient who developed a new primary lung cancer after previously undergoing a hemilaryngectomy for an early laryngeal cancer. Despite the tracheal stent inserted to palliate the proximal airway obstruction, widening of the main carina is still visible on the chest radiograph (*arrow*). B. The massive subcarinal nodal involvement is clearly visible on the CT scan (*arrow*).

astinoscopies, no operative death occurred and a 2.3% morbidity rate was observed. Morbidity consisted of hemorrhage, pneumothorax, wound infection, and recurrent nerve palsy (15). In patients with left upper lobe lesions or suspicious aortopulmonary window nodes, extended mediastinoscopy (16, 17), a Chamberlain procedure, or thoracoscopy can be performed if the CT scan suggests that the extent of nodal involvement may preclude a complete resection (18, 19).

MANAGEMENT OF T3 TUMORS INVOLVING THE CHEST WALL

Direct extension of primary lung cancers into the chest wall was originally thought to be an indication of incurability. However, since the 1960s, several retrospective series have shown that surgical resection leads to long-term survival in carefully selected patients (Table 15.2). Operative mortality ranges from 3% to 16% in these series and reflects the frequency of postoperative respiratory failure, which in turn is related to the extent of pulmonary resection, the size and location of the chest wall defect, and the methods of chest wall reconstruction. Long-term survival is related to the completeness of surgical resection and to the presence of nodal disease. A few patients with N1 disease, but virtually no patients with N2 disease, survive 5 years. Local recurrence occurs rarely after complete resection of the primary tumor, with distant metastases being the predominant form of relapse in most patients. Survival does not appear to be influenced by whether the chest wall is resected in continuity or separately from the primary tumor, but a resection that is microscopically incomplete because of tumor remaining in the chest wall is associated with higher local recurrence and a poorer overall survival rate (20–28). Therefore, the proper management of patients with T3 chest wall tumors includes a mediastinoscopy to exclude the presence of N2 disease and wide resection of the involved area of chest wall in conjunction with a pulmonary resection. If the location of chest wall involvement makes it technically difficult to resect this area en bloc with the primary tumor (e.g., paravertebral chest wall extension), a discontinuous resection is acceptable, but the completeness of resection should be documented carefully by frozen sections intraoperatively.

Because the numbers of patients who have T3 chest wall tumors is small, there has been no prospective study of treatment for these patients. Based on the reported retrospective experience, surgical resection has become the standard of care for patients with T3, N0-1 NSCLCs. The role of adjuvant or neoadjuvant therapy remains unclear. Both preoperative and postoperative radiation have been used in a highly individualized manner with perhaps some improvement in local control, but with no clear impact on overall survival (29). It would seem logical to incorporate

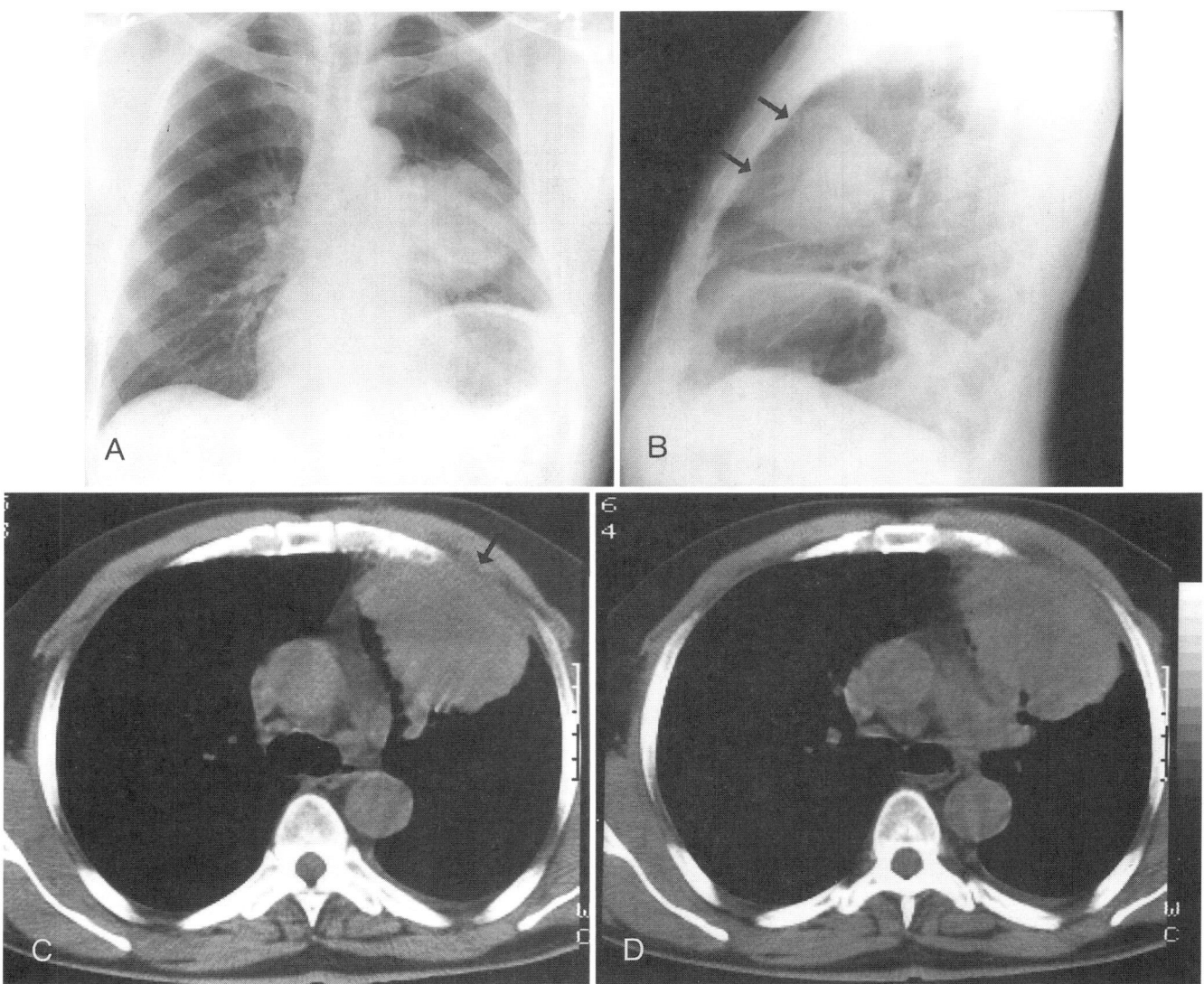

FIGURE 15.6. Left upper lobe mass involving the chest wall, pericardium, and phrenic nerve. **A.** The elevation of the hemidiaphragm caused by involvement of the phrenic nerve is obvious on the PA chest radiograph. **B.** The chest wall involvement is suggested by the lateral chest radiograph (*arrows*). **C.** The CT scan on the same patient clearly shows extension of the tumor into the chest wall (*arrow*), and **D.** suggests involvement of the pretracheal lymph nodes. The patient proved to have a T3, N0 squamous cell cancer with chest wall and pericardial involvement and is alive and disease free 4 years after surgical resection and postoperative radiation.

TABLE 15.2. Results of Surgical Resection in Selected Series of Patients with T3 Non–Small Cell Lung Cancers

Author, Year (Reference)	No. Patients	Operative Mortality	5-Year Survival, All Patients	5-Year Survival, All Patients	5-Year Survival, All Patients
Grillo, 1966 (28)	33	9%	10%	0%	NS
Geha, 1967 (25)	74	4%	32%	0%	0%
Jamieson, 1979 (26)	43	16%	7%	0%	NS
Paone, 1982 (21)	32	3.1%	35%	0%	0%
Patterson, 1982 (29)	35	8.5%	38%	0%	0%
Piehler, 1982 (20)	66	15%	33%	N/A	7.4%
McCaughan, 1984 (23)	125	4%	40%	0%	16%
Allen, 1991 (24)	52	3.8%	26%	0%	N/A
Albertucci, 1992 (22)	30	13%	30%	NS	0%

Note. The cancers are T3 by virtue of direct extension into the chest wall. Note the adverse prognostic impact of incomplete resection and N2 disease.
Abbreviations. N/A, not applicable; NS, not stated.

chemotherapy in the management of these patients because of the high risk of distant relapse. Patients with T3, N0 tumors have been included sporadically in some trials of neoadjuvant therapy for stage III NSCLC, but the number of patients treated in this manner is too small to draw any conclusions about the validity of this approach.

Some of the original concerns about surgical resection for T3, N0 tumors stemmed from the technical problems of performing a chest wall reconstruction. Early efforts at chest wall reconstruction were hampered by the inadequacies of available prosthetic materials, which made it difficult to tailor the reconstruction to the size and contour of the chest wall defect, and to prevent late complications of infection or erosion into adjacent structures. The use of a Marlex mesh–methylmethacrylate sandwich (Figs. 7A, B, and C) was a major technical advance in reconstruction of the bony chest wall. This simple technique, originally developed at Memorial Sloan-Kettering Cancer Center (30), provides complete stability with proper size and contour even for very extensive reconstructions (Fig. 15.5). Defects underlying the scapula from the first through the fourth ribs, or those located very posteriorly under the paraspinous muscles, do not require chest wall reconstruction. A minimal defect underlying the tip of the scapula at the level of the fifth or sixth rib can be reconstructed with a double layer of Marlex mesh without methylmethacrylate, simply to prevent the tip of the scapula from moving in and out of the chest wall defect with shoulder motion. Small lateral or anterior defects of less than 10 cm in diameter can also be reconstructed with a double layer of Marlex mesh or with a Gortex patch, but larger defects are best reconstructed with a Marlex mesh–methylmethacrylate sandwich. This technique prevents the potential respiratory morbidity caused by paradoxical chest motion and provides an optimal cosmetic result.

MANAGEMENT OF T3 TUMORS INVOLVING THE MEDIASTINUM AND DIAPHRAGM

In contrast to T3 tumors extending into the chest wall, less information is available about the results of surgical resection for T3 tumors involving the diaphragm or mediastinal soft tissues. These patients have sometimes been included in larger series evaluating the treatment of all types of T3 tumors (31). The largest series addressing this issue reported 225 patients having operations at Memorial Sloan-Kettering Cancer Center from 1974 to 1984 (32). This series classified as T3 some tumors that would now be designated T4 because of involvement of mediastinal organs such as major vessels and the esophagus. Thus, the 5-year survival of 7% reported for the entire group of patients reflects the advanced T status and inability to resect many of these tumors completely. A more recent evaluation, from the same institution, of T3 tumors involving the mediastinum or diaphragm has shown that complete surgical resection is associated with a 5-year survival of 30%—if there is no evidence of mediastinal nodal involvement (33). These results suggest that the incidental finding of mediastinal soft-tissue or diaphragmatic involvement at thoracotomy should not preclude proceeding with resection as long as a complete resection can be performed. If the preoperative CT scan suggests involvement of the diaphragm or mediastinum, it is important to perform mediastinoscopy to avoid operating on patients who also have N2 disease and therefore would have a very poor prognosis with surgical resection alone.

MANAGEMENT OF T3 TUMORS INVOLVING THE MAIN STEM BRONCHI

Patients with T3 tumors involving the main stem bronchi are selected for surgical resection using the same guidelines as for patients with other types of T3 tumors. The presence of N2 disease is associated with virtually no chance of survival at 5 years unless the nodal involvement represents direct extension of the primary tumor (e.g., into the subcarinal lymph nodes) (34). Therefore, it is particularly important to perform a thorough mediastinoscopy to ensure that the potentially higher risk operation required to resect these tumors is warranted. To plan the resection, a detailed bronchoscopy should also be performed with biopsies of the main carina, lateral distal tracheal wall, and main stem and relevant lobar bronchi. Patients who present with high-grade airway obstruction often benefit from laser resection of the tumor in the main stem bronchus before pulmonary resection. Reexpansion of the lung and resolution of associated postobstructive pneumonitis decreases the risk of the subsequent bronchopulmonary resection.

The extent of resection required for T3 tumors involving the main stem bronchi depends on the length of airway involvement and the presence or absence of peribronchial tumor. Very early tumors that do not extend outside the bronchial wall can be removed completely by bronchial resection alone (35, 36). On the left side, this may simply require a resection and end-to-end anastomosis of the main stem bronchus. On the

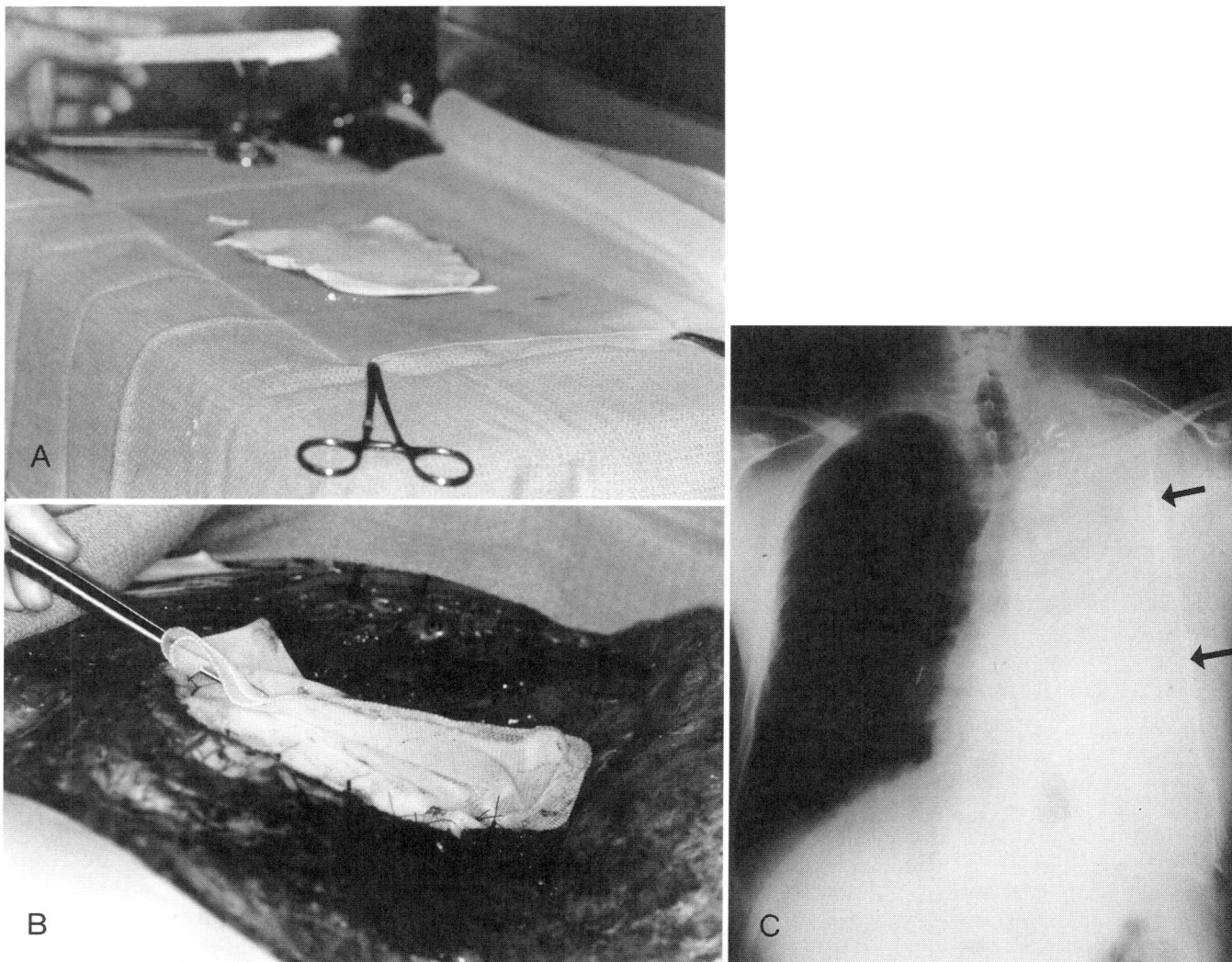

FIGURE 15.7. A. Creation of a Marlex mesh–methylmethacrylate prosthesis for chest wall reconstruction. The size of the chest wall defect is outlined on the Marlex mesh, and a 1- to 2-cm rim of mesh is left around this. Methylmethacrylate is spread over the area of the defect between the two layers of Marlex. The prosthesis is allowed to harden before being sutured in place to avoid placing the intrathoracic structures in contact with the exothermic reaction caused by hardening of the methylmethacrylate. B. The prosthesis is sutured in place. C. An extreme example of how an entire lateral chest wall can be reconstructed using a Marlex-methylmethacrylate sandwich (*arrows*). The patient had a pneumonectomy and chest wall resection and reconstruction for a locally advanced primary pulmonary sarcoma.

right side, the short length of the main stem bronchus usually dictates performing a right upper lobe sleeve resection with reanastomosis of the bronchus intermedius to the main carina.

By contrast, the presence of peribronchial tumor mandates a pulmonary resection in addition to the bronchial resection because of involvement of hilar vessels or adjacent pulmonary parenchyma. An adequate bronchial margin can usually be obtained by dividing the main stem bronchus flush with the carina and hand sewing the bronchial stump. This technique allows more bronchus to be resected than if a stapler is used for bronchial closure. Rarely, a sleeve lobectomy or pneumonectomy is required to obtain sufficient bronchial length for a complete resection (37). The techniques for sleeve pneumonectomy and intraoperative management of the airway have been well described, primarily in the context of resection of T4 tumors involving the distal trachea or main carina (38, 39). The end-to-end bronchial anastomosis is performed with a completely open technique using interrupted absorbable suture (Fig. 15.8). Fine running suture can be used to close the membranous portion of the bronchus. The airway can be managed in a variety of ways, including intermittent apnea or jet ventilation (Figs. 15.9*A*, *B*, and *C*), or by use of a specially de-

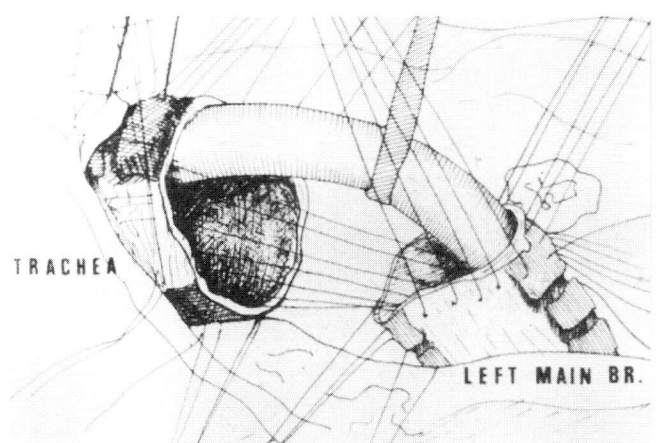

FIGURE 15.8. Technique for performing the bronchial anastomosis after sleeve pneumonectomy. A small-caliber long endotracheal tube has been passed across the anastomosis, which is performed with interrupted absorbable sutures.

signed, small-caliber, long endotracheal tube extending across the anastomosis. Reported perioperative mortality rates for sleeve pneumonectomy range from 10% to 29% in the hands of surgeons experienced in this operation. Complications include pneumonia in the remaining lung, and infection and respiratory failure related to anastomotic dehiscence. Meticulous attention to surgical technique and anesthetic management are crucial to achieving an acceptably low operative morbidity and mortality.

It is somewhat difficult to judge the results of surgical resection of T3 tumors involving the main stem bronchi because these patients are often included in series reporting sleeve lobectomy for more distally located tumors or in series reporting sleeve pneumonectomy for T4 tumors (40, 41). Nakahashi and colleagues (31) reported that four of five patients whose T3 tumors were confined to the main bronchus survived 5 years. However, peribronchial tumor or nodal involvement decrease the survival rate at 5 years to within the range of 15% to 30%. Five-year survival is rare when N2 nodes distant from the primary tumor are involved by metastatic disease. Careful patient selection based on bronchoscopy and mediastinoscopy is key to achieving long-term survival.

SURGICAL RESECTION FOR N2 DISEASE

The most controversial and complex part of the treatment of stage IIIA NSCLC is the management of patients with N2 disease. Reported 5-year survival rates after resection for N2 disease are usually 20% to 30%, but they range from a low of zero to a high of 40%

(42–44). This variation reflects the extent of mediastinal nodal involvement, the T status of the primary tumor, and the ability to perform a complete resection. With respect to mediastinal nodal involvement, adverse prognostic factors include the presence of extracapsular nodal disease, multiple levels of involved lymph nodes, or presence of superior mediastinal nodal metastases (45–57).

Many reported series present an inappropriately optimistic view of the benefit of surgical resection for N2 disease because they focus on highly selected groups of patients. The experience reported by Martini (56) places surgical resection for N2 disease in proper perspective because it examines the outcome of treatment of all patients with N2 disease, not just a small subset. From 1974 to 1981, the group at Memorial Sloan–Kettering Cancer Center saw 1598 patients with NSCLC, of whom 706 had mediastinal nodal metastases. Ultimately, only 151 patients, or 21% of all patients with N2 disease, had complete potentially curative resections of their primary tumors and all accessible mediastinal lymph nodes. The survival for these 151 patients was 29% at 5 years. However, the 33 patients who had "clinical N2" disease, i.e., mediastinal nodal involvement extensive enough to be visible on a chest radiograph or at bronchoscopy, had only an 8% survival at 3 years. Thus, only 16.7% of all patients benefited long term from surgical resection.

Outcome in this group of patients was influenced further by the T status of the primary tumor, with T2 or T3 tumors faring significantly worse than T1 tumors. These results have been corroborated by the experience of several other groups (Table 15.3). The Toronto group (45) reported that patients who had mediastinal nodal metastases identified at mediastinoscopy had a 5-year survival rate of 15%, whereas patients who had a negative mediastinoscopy and microscopic lower mediastinal nodal disease detected at thoracotomy had a 5-year survival rate of 41%. In a separate series (48), the Toronto group found that patients who had left upper lobe tumors with mediastinal nodal metastases confined to the aortopulmonary window nodes had a 5-year survival rate of 42%.

In a retrospective analysis of 163 patients with N2 disease, the Lung Cancer Study Group found that involvement of multiple levels of mediastinal nodes, i.e., subcarinal plus paratracheal nodes was associated with a significantly worse survival than nodal disease at a single level (49).

In more recent series, Watanabe and colleagues (52) reported that 53 patients with N2 disease who had a complete resection and involvement of the mediastinal nodes suspected on the preoperative CT scan experienced a 5-year survival rate of 20%. Thirty-one

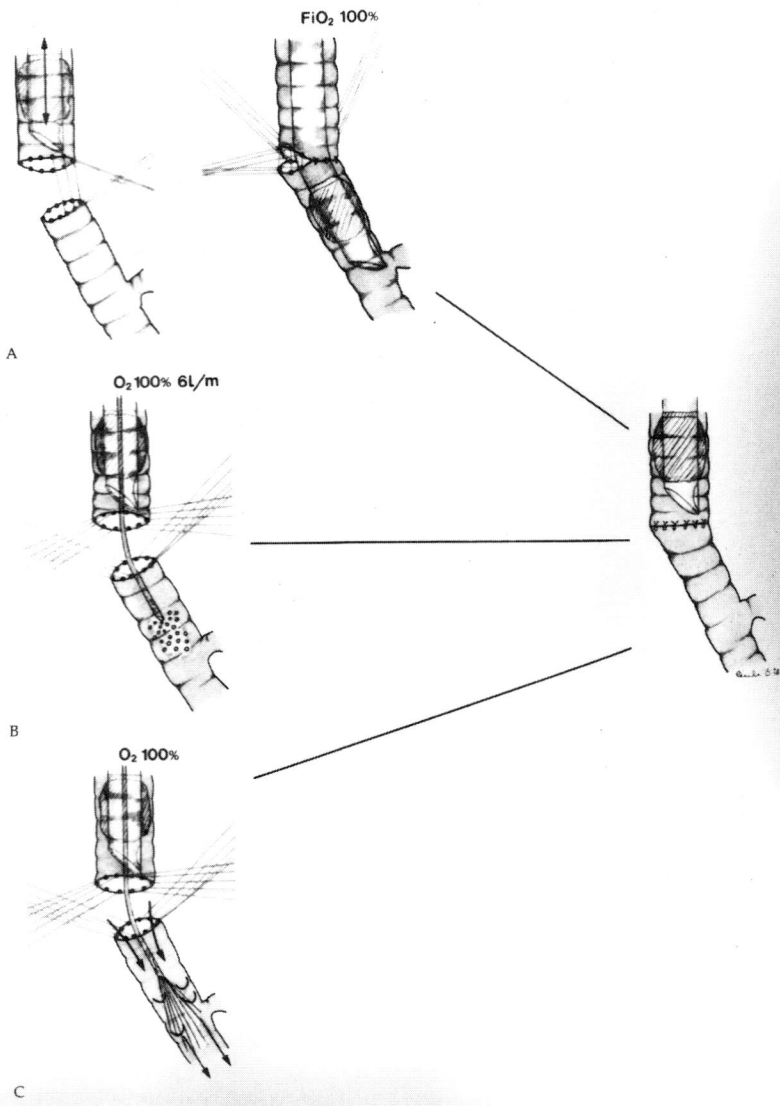

FIGURE 15.9. Anesthetic techniques for sleeve pneumonectomy. **A.** Small-caliber single-lumen tube ventilation across an anastomosis. **B.** Apneic oxygenation. **C.** Jet ventilation (FiO_2, inspired fraction of oxygen).

patients who had N2 disease and complete resection, but no mediastinal adenopathy on preoperative CT scan, had a 5-year survival rate of 33% (52). Goldstraw and colleagues (54) reported a 5-year survival of 20% in 127 patients with N2 disease who had a complete resection and who did not have mediastinal nodal involvement detected by preoperative CT scan or mediastinoscopy.

In a recent review, Shields (55) emphasized that the subset of patients with N2 disease who might benefit from surgical resection as their primary form of treatment represents only about 10% of all patients with NSCLC and 15% to 20% of all patients with N2 disease. Because of the inaccuracy of CT scanning in diagnosing involved mediastinal lymph nodes correctly, mediastinoscopy with systematic biopsies of the subcarinal and both paratracheal regions remains the most accurate way of staging patients with possible N2 disease. Most surgeons now consider performing resections only on those patients who have a T1 or T2 primary tumor and who also have single level, intranodal, N2 disease.

Moreover, two small randomized clinical trials have now challenged the concept of offering surgical resection as the primary treatment to any patient with N2 disease. Rosell and colleagues (58) randomized 60 patients with stage IIIA NSCLC (16 of whom did not have N2 disease) to surgical resection or to three cycles of cisplatin-based chemotherapy followed by surgical resection. Median survival was significantly longer (26 versus 8 months) in the patients receiving preoperative chemotherapy compared with patients going directly to surgical resection. A similar study from the

TABLE 15.3. Overall Survival in Selected Retrospective Series

AUTHOR, YEAR (REFERENCE)	NO. OF PATIENTS	5-YEAR SURVIVAL (%)
Abbey Smith, 1978 (43)	56	28.5
Naruke, 1978 (44)	64	18.8
Kirschner, 1979 (42)	35	11.4
Pearson, 1982 (45)	141	0–41
Kirsh, 1982 (46)	136	21.3
Martini, 1983 (56)	151	29
Rubinstein, 1985 (47)	18	0
Patterson, 1987 (48)	35	28–42
Thomas, 1988 (49)	335	20–50
Naruke, 1988 (50)	242	19.2
Mountain, 1990 (51)	118	21
Watanabe, 1991 (52)	153	17–24
Daly, 1993 (53)	37	28
van Klaveren, 1993 (57)	48	10
Goldstraw, 1994 (54)	130	20.1

Note. Surgical resection was the primary treatment for patients with stage IIIA N2 disease.

M. D. Anderson Cancer Center confirms these results (59). Both trials were stopped early because of the highly significant differences between the two study arms. These two studies suggest that it may be appropriate to consider all patients with N2 disease diagnosed at mediastinoscopy for induction chemotherapy. Unfortunately, because pretreatment mediastinoscopy was not mandated in either trial, some patients who did not have N2 disease were included. The small numbers of patients enrolled in each of these studies, lack of systematic pretreatment staging, and unusually poor survival of patients in the control arm cast doubt on the results of both trials.

RATIONALE FOR NEOADJUVANT THERAPY

Although a few patients with minimal N2 disease may benefit from surgical resection as their primary form of treatment, most patients have more extensive nodal involvement and are not candidates for this approach. Until 10 years ago, the standard treatment for such patients was radiation. The survival rates after radiation are harder to interpret than after surgical resection because most series included a mixture of stage IIIA and IIIB patients, and they did not define the precise extent of nodal involvement (60–62). Sequential trials by the Radiation Therapy Oncology Group showed that high-dose, continuous radiation yields the best chance of local control (63). A recent trial of high-dose hyperfractionated radiation (to a maximum dose of 79.2 Gy) suggested that it might confer a small improvement in overall survival (64); however, in previous experience the 5-year survival after radiation alone has been 10% or less.

Distant metastatic disease is the dominant form of relapse after either surgical resection or radiotherapy. This is somewhat influenced by the effectiveness of local treatment. Twenty-nine percent of patients who received only 4000 cGy of split-course radiation relapsed in distant sites, whereas 47% of patients given 6000 cGy of continuous radiation developed distant disease (63). Eighty percent of patients with N2 disease who undergo complete surgical resection and postoperative mediastinal radiation relapse in distant sites, particularly in the brain. It is possible that patients whose local disease remains uncontrolled do not survive long enough to manifest distant metastases. The fact that half of patients relapse within 1 year, and 80% within 2 years of surgical resection, suggests that micrometastases are present at the time of operation. The poor long-term survival after radiation or surgical resection, and the risk of distant metastatic disease, have prompted the development of multimodality therapy for stage III NSCLC, with chemotherapy being the primary form of treatment.

EARLY TRIALS OF NEOADJUVANT THERAPY

The concept of neoadjuvant therapy dates to 1955 when Bromley (65) used a dose of approximately 45 Gy before surgical resection to treat 66 patients. At operation, no viable tumor was found in 29 (47%) of 62 patients, but 10 patients died of complications in the first month, and only 2 patients were alive 5 years postoperatively. At the time, the natural history of NSCLC was not as well understood, the methods of staging not as accurate, and the importance of distant metastases not fully recognized. Effective chemotherapy did not exist, and it was hoped that an approach that increased resectability might lead to better long-term survival. Thus, early neoadjuvant trials focused on using preoperative radiation.

Several subsequent studies explored this approach further (66–72). In 1964, Bloedorn (69) used 60 Gy of radiation to treat 109 patients with inoperable lung cancer preoperatively. Fifty-two patients (48%) underwent resection, but the postoperative mortality rate was 35% and the 1-year survival rate was only 20%. The Veterans Administration carried out two trials that randomized patients to immediate surgery versus surgery preceded by 40 to 50 Gy of radiation (70–72). Twenty-seven percent (23 of 86) of patients in the irradiated group had no viable tumor in the resected specimen, but radiation did not improve the resectability or survival rates, which were about 8% at 5 years. Operative mortality was 12% in both groups, but the incidence of bronchopleural fistula was 10% in the irradiated patients and only 3% in the nonirradiated patients (71–72).

The design of these trials was flawed by a lack of pretreatment staging, and by use of widely varying amounts of radiation and excessively long intervals between radiation and surgical resection. Nevertheless, it was apparent that aggressive local treatment did not improve long-term survival, even though radiation could sterilize tumor in a significant number of patients. From 50% to 80% of patients developed distant metastases during or shortly after treatment, emphasizing the need for systemic therapy in stage III NSCLC.

RECENT NEOADJUVANT THERAPY TRIALS

Recognition of the risk of metastatic disease and the advent of effective chemotherapy radically altered the approach to stage III NSCLC. Chemotherapy has become the primary treatment, with surgical resection and/or radiation added to optimize control of loco-regional disease. Although the long-term survival advantage of neoadjuvant therapy over more conventional forms of treatment, such as radiation therapy alone, remains incompletely proven, the concept of neoadjuvant therapy has become very popular and is now often used outside of the setting of clinical trials.

A large number of neoadjuvant therapy trials have now been performed. Most of these have been phase II studies that were designed to test the feasibility of this treatment. It is difficult to assess whether one neoadjuvant regimen is superior to others because of wide variations in the type of induction therapy and the eligibility criteria among trials. The initial neoadjuvant trials using induction chemotherapy were developed in the early 1980s when less information about the natural history of stage III lung cancer was available. Therefore, they included a very heterogeneous patient population. A better understanding of the natural history of early stage lung cancer, and the advent of the new International Staging System in 1986 that separated stage III into IIIA and IIIB, has allowed recent trials to focus on more uniform patient populations. Consequently, it has become easier to design clinical trials for stage III patients and to interpret response and survival rates.

Although many different treatment regimens have been used in neoadjuvant trials, they can be grouped into two major categories: chemotherapy and radiation without surgical resection, and chemotherapy or chemoradiotherapy followed by surgical resection.

TRIALS OF CHEMOTHERAPY AND RADIATION WITHOUT SURGICAL RESECTION

The feasibility of combined chemotherapy and radiation, without surgical resection, for stage III NSCLC has been demonstrated in several phase II trials. More importantly, there have now been several phase III randomized trials comparing radiation alone and combined treatment with radiation and chemotherapy (73). The results of these trials cannot be equated with trials of neoadjuvant therapy that include surgical resection, because the patients entered on nonsurgical trials are staged clinically without the benefit of mediastinoscopy. Therefore, nonsurgical trials may include patients with mixtures of stage IIIA and IIIB cancers or some patients who have earlier stage disease but are thought erroneously to be stage III by virtue of mediastinal adenopathy on CT scan.

Three different strategies have been investigated for combining chemotherapy and radiation. The concept of alternating chemotherapy and radiation has been explored in phase II trials but has not been tested in randomized trials. Phase III trials comparing radiation with chemotherapy and radiation have been conducted; these trials have used either sequential treatment with induction chemotherapy followed by radiation, or concurrent chemotherapy and radiation (73, 74). Both of these approaches have theoretical advantages. Sequential treatment potentially allows more intensive chemotherapy and higher radiation doses, whereas concurrent chemotherapy and radiation potentially allows both radiosensitization and effective systemic therapy, provided the combined toxicity is tolerable.

The results of six major phase III trials comparing radiation alone with sequential chemotherapy and radiation are outlined in Table 15.4. All of these trials have confirmed the feasibility of combined modality treatment, and some have demonstrated modest treatment advantages (e.g., better control of systemic disease) (75–80). However, only the trial conducted by the Cancer and Leukemia Group B (CALGB) has shown a significant improvement in overall survival for the chemoradiotherapy arm (73). An intergroup trial by the Radiation Therapy Oncology Group and the Eastern Cooperative Oncology Group was performed to

TABLE 15.4. Results of Phase III Trials Comparing Radiotherapy Alone to Sequential Chemoradiotherapy for Stage III Non–Small Cell Lung Cancer

Author, Year (Reference)	No. of Patients	Chemotherapy	Radiotherapy (Gy)	Group	Survival Median (Mo.)	2-Year (%)
van Houtte et al., 1984 (79)	59	CDDP/VP-16	55 (C)	CT-RT	11	...
				RT	11	...
Dillman et al., 1990 (75)	180	CDDP/Vbl	60 (C)	CT-RT	13.8	26
				RT	9.7	13
Mattson et al., 1988 (78)	228	CAP	55 (S)	CT-RT	11.0	19
				RT	10.4	17
Morton et al., 1988 (80)	121	MACC	60 (C)	CT-RT	10.5	23
				RT	9.7	12
Trovo et al., 1990 (77)	111	CAMP	4500 (C)	CT-RT	11.7	15
				RT	10	15
Le Chevalier et al., 1991 (76)	353	VCPC	65 (C)	CT-RT	12	21
				RT	10	14

Abbreviations. CDDP, cisplatin; VP-16, etoposide; CAP, cyclophosphamide, doxorubicin, cisplatin; MACC, methotrexate, doxorubicin, cyclophosphamide, lomustine; CAMP, cyclophosphamide, doxorubicin, methotrexate, procarbazine; (C), continuous course; RT, radiotherapy; CT-RT, chemoradiotherapy.

TABLE 15.5. Results of Phase III Trials Comparing Radiotherapy with Concurrent Chemoradiotherapy for Stage III Non–Small Cell Lung Cancer

Author, Year (Reference)	Total No. of Patients	Chemotherapy	Radiotherapy (Gy)	Group	Survival Median (Mo.)	2-Year (%)
Ansari et al., 1991 (84)	200	CDDP, days 1, 22, 43	60	Concurrent	9	5
			60	Radiation	10	9
Trovo et al., 1991 (83)	180	Daily CDDP	60 (C)	Radiation	No diff	...
			45 (C)	Concurrent	No diff	...
Schaake-Koning et al., 1992 (81)	334	Weekly CDDP	55 (S)	Concurrent	...	19
		Daily CDDP		Concurrent	...	26
				Concurrent	...	13
Sadeghi et al., 1991 (82)	154	CAP	40 (S)	Concurrent	~20	~40
			40 (S)	Radiation	~14	~35

Abbreviations. CDDP, cisplatin; CAP, cyclophosphamide, doxorubicin, cisplatin; (C), continuous course; (S), split course; No diff, no difference.

confirm the results of the CALCB trial. This three-arm randomized trial compared standard fractionation radiotherapy, hyperfractionated radiotherapy, and sequential chemotherapy and radiation as structured in the CALGB trial. Preliminary results indicate that patients in the chemoradiotherapy arm experienced a better survival than those receiving either form of radiotherapy alone.

At least four randomized trials (81–84) comparing radiation with concurrent radiation and chemotherapy have been reported (Table 15.5). Two of these, the trial by the European Organization for Research and Treatment of Cancer (EORTC) and that by the Lung Cancer Study Group (LCSG), have shown a benefit for the combined modality arm (81, 82). The EORTC trial showed improved overall survival for patients who received daily cisplatin and concurrent radiation. The LCSG trial, performed in patients who had earlier stage disease (positive surgical margins or the highest mediastinal node positive after surgical resection), found an improved recurrence free survival in the chemoradiotherapy arm. The benefit in overall survival was lost after the third year of follow-up.

The variable results among phase III trials comparing radiation with chemotherapy and radiation may be related to several factors, including differences in total radiation dose and method of administration (split versus continuous course); differences in chemotherapy dose, especially with respect to cisplatin; and differences in patient selection based on staging criteria. Recent phase II studies have demonstrated the feasibility of using concurrent high-dose continuous radiation with high total dose cisplatin (85–89). Taken as a whole, the results of multiple phase II and III trials show that combined treatment with chemotherapy and radiation can be administered safely to patients with stage III NSCLC and that it leads to a modest but real survival benefit compared with radiotherapy alone.

Neoadjuvant Trials That Include Surgical Resection

These trials also have used two different treatment strategies: induction chemotherapy alone, or concurrent chemotherapy and radiation before surgical resection. The rationale for chemotherapy alone as induction treatment is that it potentially allows greater dose intensity, as well as the use of some drugs such as mitomycin, which cannot be administered with radiation. Proponents of this approach think that chemotherapy provides induction treatment that is as effective as combined chemotherapy and radiation. They also think that separating the two modalities allows the use of radiation postoperatively when a higher total dose can be given. Proponents of concurrent preoperative chemotherapy and radiation believe that this approach provides adequate systemic treatment of micrometastatic disease, and more effective control of bulky primary and mediastinal tumor.

Neoadjuvant Trials Using Chemotherapy Alone Before Surgical Resection

Several small phase II trials have shown the feasibility of combining induction chemotherapy with subsequent pulmonary resection in patients with initially unresectable stage III NSCLCs (90–93). The best-known regimen of this type is the one developed at Memorial Sloan–Kettering Cancer Center. As noted previously, Martini and colleagues (56) identified a large group of patients with N2 disease who did not benefit from surgical resection as their primary form of treatment. Patients who had mediastinal nodal involvement so bulky that it was visible on a chest radiograph (clinical N2 disease) had only an 8% 3-year survival. Therefore, in 1984 they initiated a trial of high-dose cisplatin-based chemotherapy for patients with clinical N2 disease, followed by surgical resection in patients who showed a response to induction therapy. Vindesine or vinblastine and, subsequently, mitomycin were added to the cisplatin to form the so-called MVP regimen. Postoperative radiation was given to patients who had persistent mediastinal nodal tumor at thoracotomy, and all patients received two additional cycles of chemotherapy postoperatively. The initial results of this trial have been confirmed in a recent report of all 136 patients treated with this regimen from 1984 to 1991 (94). The major response rate to induction chemotherapy was 77% (105 of 136), and the complete resection rate was 65% (89 of 136). There was no histologic evidence of tumor in the resected specimens of 19 patients, for a complete pathologic response rate of 21% (19 of 89). The overall survival of all 136 patients at 5 years was 17%, with a median survival of 19 months, a distinct improvement over the historical survival rate for this group of patients. There were seven treatment-related deaths in the entire series (5% treatment-related mortality), five of which occurred postoperatively (95).

After the initial report of this trial, two other groups—the Toronto group and the LCSG—undertook confirmatory trials. Neither of these trials included postoperative radiation, but both used an induction MVP chemotherapy regimen identical to the one developed at the Memorial Sloan–Kettering Cancer Center (95). All of the patients in these two trials had N2 disease proven by mediastinoscopy, but the LCSG study also included a few patients who were designated stage IIIB by virtue of T4 disease. In the Toronto trial, the overall response rate was 65% (25 of 39), and the complete resection rate was 46% (18 of 39). The overall survival at 3 years was 26%, and the median survival was 18.6 months. There was a 15% treatment-related mortality (6 of 39), due mainly to four patients who died of sepsis during induction treatment because of postobstructive pneumonia (96). In a preliminary report of the LCSG trial, the overall response rate was 46%, the complete resection rate was 36%, and the treatment-related mortality was 12.5%. Follow-up was too short to provide accurate information about survival (97).

The cumulative data from these three studies demonstrate that neoadjuvant therapy with MVP is both a feasible and effective treatment. The low mortality rate of the Memorial trial (95) may reflect careful patient selection and management by physicians experienced in the use of this regimen. As usual, it is difficult to reproduce the results of a single-institution trial in a multiinstitutional setting. Enthusiasm for the MVP regimen in the oncology community at large has been tempered by the perceived risk of mitomycin-induced pulmonary toxicity, especially postoperative adult respiratory distress syndrome (ARDS), and the side effects of high-dose cisplatin. Many oncologists think that similar results can be achieved with less toxic regimens. Retrospective analysis of the Memorial experience identified 12 patients (8.8%) thought to have mitomycin-related pulmonary toxicity. This toxicity appeared to be dose related, occurred only in patients who had received a total dose of 24 mg/m^2, and responded to treatment with corticosteroids (95).

NEOADJUVANT TRIALS USING COMBINED CHEMOTHERAPY AND RADIATION BEFORE SURGICAL RESECTION

Most of the reported neoadjuvant trials have used combined chemotherapy and radiation as induction treatment (Table 15.6). One of the first trials of this type was performed by the LCSG (98). Thirty-nine patients with clinical stage III disease received three cycles of chemotherapy with cyclophosphamide, doxorubicin, and low-dose (60 mg/m^2) cisplatin (CAP), and 1500 cGy of concurrent radiation in 300 cGy fractions with chemotherapy cycles two and three. The overall response rate to induction therapy was 51% (20 of 39 patients), and 33% (13 of 39 patients) subsequently had a complete resection at thoracotomy. There were no treatment-related deaths, but the overall survival at 2 years was only 8%, with a median survival of 11 months.

Subsequently, the LCSG performed a neoadjuvant trial of cisplatin (75 mg/m^2), 5-fluorouracil (5-FU), and partially concurrent low-dose radiation (3000 cGy in 15 fractions) in 85 patients with stage IIIA (N2) or stage IIIB disease (99). The overall response rate was 56% (48 of 85), and the complete resection rate was 34% (29 of 85). Four (7%) of 54 patients died postoperatively, and the median survival for all 85 patients was 13 months.

The Rush-Presbyterian group has performed two sequential neoadjuvant trials of low-dose cisplatin (60 mg/m^2) chemotherapy and concurrent radiation in patients with clinical stage III disease (100). In the first 56 patients, 5-FU was added to the cisplatin, whereas subsequent patients also received etoposide (VP-16). All patients received 4000 cGy of split-course radiation administered concurrently with the four cycles of induction chemotherapy. The toxicity of this induction regimen was significant, but there was only one treatment-related death. Of the 130 patients entered in the study, 85 were considered potential candidates for surgical resection, and 62 (73%) ultimately underwent thoracotomy. The complete resection rate was 68% (58 of 85), and the operative mortality rate was 5% (3 of 62). The overall survival rate for all 85 patients was 40% at 3 years, with a median survival of 22 months. The addition of VP-16 to the induction regimen did not appear to increase the response or resectability rates significantly.

The CALGB performed a similar neoadjuvant study that used high-dose cisplatin (100 mg/m^2), vinblastine, and 5-FU with 3000 cGy of radiation in 15 fractions as induction therapy in patients with stage IIIA disease (101). The overall response rate was 51% (21 of 41), and the complete resection rate was 61% (25 of 41). Toxicity was substantial with a 15% (6 of 41) treatment-related mortality, but the median survival was 15.5 months.

TABLE 15.6. Results of Representative Neoadjuvant Trials for Stage III Non–Small Cell Lung Cancer Using Induction Chemotherapy Followed by Surgical Resection

				SURVIVAL	
INSTITUTION/GROUP, YEAR (REFERENCE)	ELIGIBLE STAGE (NO. OF PATIENTS)	CHEMOTHERAPY	RADIOTHERAPY	MEDIAN (MO.)	2-YEAR (%)
LCSG, 1987 (98)	IIIA, III (39)	CAP × 3	3000 cGy (S) 10 fractions	11	8
Rush-Presbyterian, 1989 (100)	IIIA (including 19 N0 patients) (85)	CDDP (60 mg/m^2) − 5-FU ± VP-16 × 4	4000 cGy (S) 20 fractions	21 8	40 (3y)
LCSG, 1991 (99)	IIIA, III (85)	CDDP (75 mg/m^2) + 5-FU × 2	3000cGy (C) 15 fractions	13	~20
CALGB, 1992 (101)	IIIA (including 8 N0-1 patients) (41)	CDDP (100 mg/m^2) + Vbl + 5-FU × 2	3000cGy (C) 15 fractions	15.5	~30
SWOG, 1993 (102)	IIIA, IIIB (146)	CDDP (50 mg/m^2) days 1, 8 + VP-16 × 2	4500cGy (C) 30 fractions	17	40

Abbreviations. CDDP, cisplatin; Vbl, vinblastine; 5-FU, 5 fluorouracil; CAP, cyclophosphamide, doxorubicin, cisplatin; VP-16, etoposide; (C), continuous course; (S), split course

The most recent and largest phase II neoadjuvant trial using concurrent chemotherapy and radiation was performed by the Southwest Oncology Group (102). This study intentionally enrolled both stage IIIA and IIIB patients, including patients with N3 disease, but mandated pathologic documentation of initial tumor stage, usually by mediastinoscopy. The induction therapy was cisplatin (50 mg/m^2 on days 1, 8, 28, and 36), VP-16 (50 mg/m^2 on days 1 through 5 and 29–33) with 4500 cGy of concurrent radiation in 25 fractions. All patients underwent subsequent thoracotomy unless they had evidence of progressive disease. Interim analysis of the first 75 patients showed that 91% (68 of 75) were eligible for thoracotomy and that 73% (55 of 75) had a complete resection. The operative mortality rate was 6% (4 of 63), and the overall treatment-related mortality was 14% (9 of 63). The 2-year survival rate was 40%, and the median survival was 17 months, with as yet no apparent difference in survival between the stage IIIA and IIIB patients.

Two notable differences between the SWOG trial and earlier neoadjuvant trials were the use of higher dose continuous radiation (i.e., 4500 cGy rather than 3000 cGy continuous or 4000 cGy split course) and the fully concurrent manner in which the chemotherapy and radiation was administered. Two small single-institution trials have investigated the use of fully concurrent high-dose cisplatin and high-dose continuous radiation. Yashar and colleagues (103) treated 36 stage IIIA (N2) patients with two cycles of cisplatin (25 mg/m^2/day for 4 days) and VP-16 (100 mg/m^2 on days 2 and 4) and 55 Gy of radiation. All 36 patients underwent thoracotomy, and 31 (86%) has a pulmonary resection, of whom 27 had a pneumonectomy. There were two operative deaths (5.6%), and six patients required prolonged intubation because of ARDS. Three patients developed a bronchial stump leak. The overall survival at 3 years was 34%.

In another similar study, Fowler and colleagues (104) treated 13 patients with stage IIIA (N2) disease with two cycles of cisplatin (20 mg/m^2 on days 1 through 5), 5-FU (640 to 800 mg/m^2 on days 1 through 5), VP-16 (days 1, 3, and 5), and 60 Gy of concurrent radiation in 30 fractions. All 13 patients underwent pulmonary resection, 6 by lobectomy and 7 by pneumonectomy. However, ARDS developed in 1 lobectomy patient and 5 of the 7 pneumonectomy patients, and it led to death in 2 patients. Three pneumonectomy patients developed bronchial stump leaks, and 1 ultimately died of related complications. The trial was closed to patient accrual because of the high morbidity and mortality in these 13 patients. An additional 27 patients who received the same induction therapy, but who did not go to thoracotomy, apparently tolerated treatment without major toxicity.

IS THERE AN OPTIMAL NEOADJUVANT REGIMEN?

Concurrent chemotherapy and radiation has been the most common induction treatment for unresectable stage III NSCLCs, but caution should be exercised in drawing conclusions from the numerous reported neoadjuvant trials. There are considerable differences among these trials with respect to eligibility criteria, accuracy of pretreatment staging, and induction regimens. Some trials (e.g., the LCSG and SWOG trials) included both stage IIIA (N2) and IIIB (T4 and N3), whereas other trials (e.g., the Rush-Presbyterian trial) intentionally included some tumors that were stage IIIA but not N2 (T3, N0-1), and a few patients who had stage IIIB (T4) tumors. Other trials (e.g., the Memorial trial) included patients with stage IIIA (N2) tumors but no stage IIIB tumors. The inclusion of these different tumor stages accounts in part for the differences in response, resectability, and survival rates. In addition, the staging of patients before induction therapy was primarily clinical in early neoadjuvant trials. Greater experience with this form of treatment, the advent of the new International Staging System, and a growing appreciation of the heterogeneity of stage III disease has led to the use of more stringent staging in recent studies, such as the SWOG trial.

The criteria for taking patients to thoracotomy after induction treatment also vary among these trials. Some trials, particularly the early ones, offered patients surgical resection only if they had a radiographic response to induction therapy. Other trials mandated thoracotomy in all patients unless they show evidence of progressive disease. Therefore, the resectability rates are not comparable among various trials. Both the Rush-Presbyterian and the SWOG trials (100, 102) have shown that there can be a discrepancy between radiographic and pathologic response, and that resectability is not necessarily linked to radiographic response (Figs. 15.10 and 15.11). The response, resectability, and survival rates are also not reported uniformly. In some cases, the resectability rates are reported as a percentage of the patients who had a radiographic response, and only the survival rate of patients who had a resection are emphasized. In reality, these rates should be reported as percentages of the total number of patients entered into the study. The use of a smaller denominator falsely suggests better results.

Taken as a whole, trials of neoadjuvant therapy

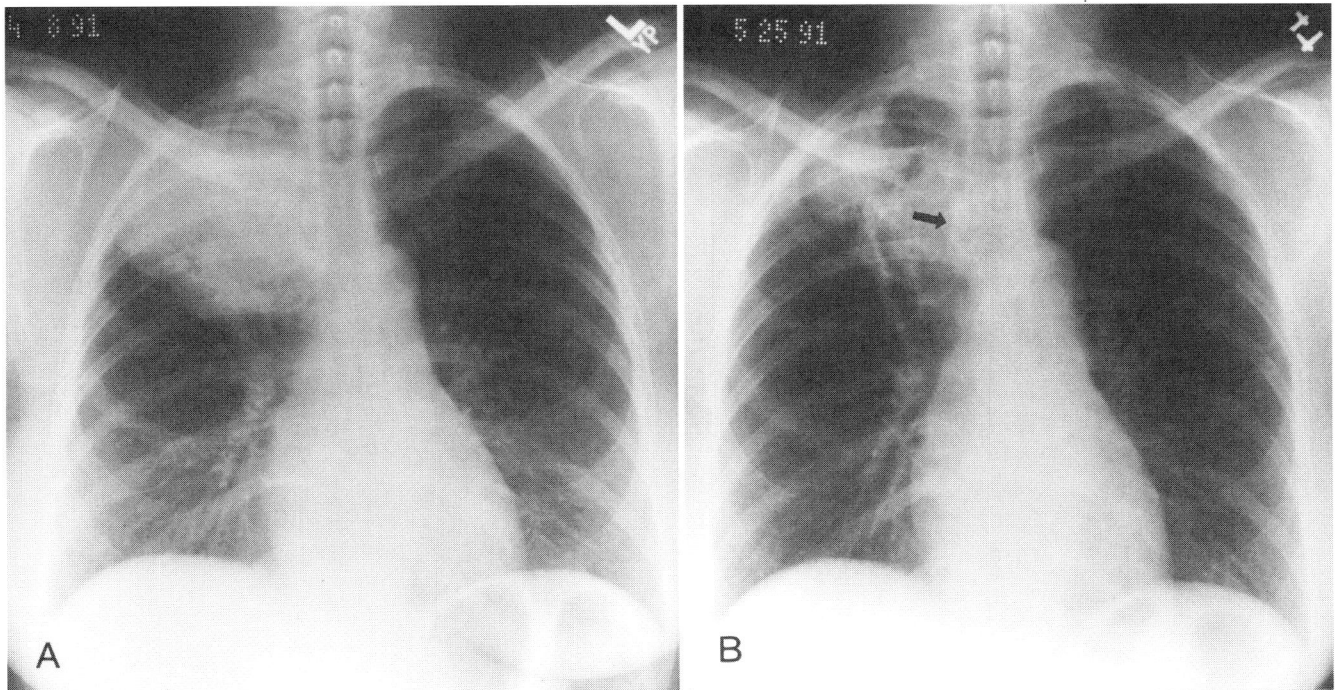

FIGURE 15.10. A. Example of the difference between radiographic and pathologic response in a patient who received neoadjuvant therapy for stage IIIA (N2) right upper lobe NSCLC. B. The chest radiograph after induction treatment shows a partial response, but the primary tumor and right paratracheal adenopathy (*arrow*) are still visible. At thoracotomy, there were only scattered microscopic foci of active tumor.

have demonstrated the feasibility of combined modality treatment in stage III NSCLC. The resectability and survival rates of these locally advanced tumors appear to be at least 50% greater than they were historically with surgical treatment alone. Induction regimens that use high-dose cisplatin (100 mg/m^2 or greater), or high-dose radiation (4000 cGy or greater), seem to produce higher response rates. However, radiation doses of 5500 cGy or higher have been associated with a prohibitive risk of postoperative ARDS and bronchial stump leaks in patients undergoing pneumonectomy. In the Memorial experience (95), induction therapy with chemotherapy alone has been as effective as concurrent chemotherapy and radiation, but unfortunately the MVP regimen has been associated with greater toxicity and lower response rates in the multi-institutional setting. Thus, regimens that use standard dose cisplatin (100 mg/m^2 in single or divided dose) with a synergistic agent such as VP-16 and moderate doses of concurrent radiation (40 or 45 Gy), are effective and may be administered more easily to the general population of lung cancer patients. In all trials to date, the major form of relapse has been distant metastatic disease, underscoring the need for more effective systemic treatment.

IMPORTANT PRINCIPLES OF NEOADJUVANT THERAPY

Successful neoadjuvant treatment of patients with stage III disease requires a truly multidisciplinary effort with close collaboration among medical oncologists, radiation oncologists, surgeons, and anesthesiologists. Repeat staging and pulmonary resection must be integrated in a timely manner so that no more than 4 to 5 weeks elapse after the completion of induction treatment. The same is true for the resumption of postoperative chemotherapy, if planned.

The surgeon must bring to the management of these patients greater technical expertise, and a broader knowledge of oncology and cardiopulmonary physiology, than is necessary in the care of patients with early stage lung cancers. The technical difficulty of resection after induction therapy is difficult to quantify, but all surgeons experienced in this area acknowledge that pulmonary resection in patients who have received neoadjuvant therapy is technically challenging. The hilum and mediastinum are often surrounded by dense fibrosis that makes it hard to identify normal anatomic planes and to distinguish the boundaries of the tumor. Complex resections such as intrapericardial

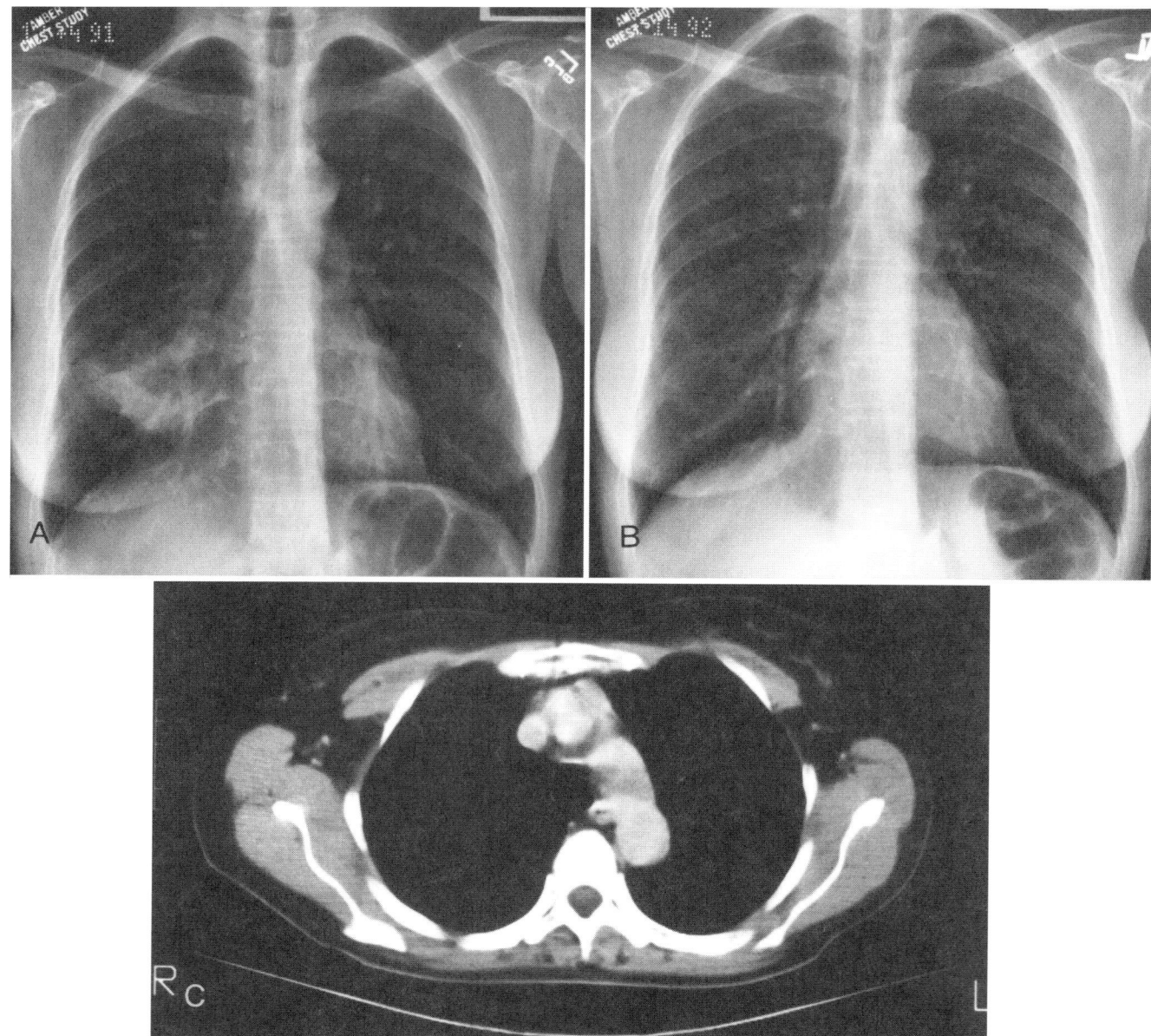

FIGURE 15.11. A. Another example of the difference between radiographic and pathologic response in a patient who had a large right middle lobe primary tumor with N2 disease in the right paratracheal nodes. B. After induction chemotherapy, the patient appeared to have had a complete response by chest radiograph, and C. by CT scan, which no longer showed paratracheal adenopathy. However, at thoracotomy the patient had residual active tumor in the right paratracheal nodes.

pneumonectomy or en bloc chest wall resection are frequently necessary.

The risk of perioperative complications is increased because of the extent of the primary tumor and the toxicity of induction therapy. Surgeons must be aware of the potential perioperative toxicities associated with various chemotherapeutic agents, chronic steroid treatment, and radiation therapy. Perioperative fluid management is always critical. It is important to avoid exacerbating cisplatin-induced nephrotoxicity by volume depletion, but equally important to avoid fluid overload in patients whose pulmonary vascular bed may be compromised by preoperative therapy (e.g., mitomycin, radiation), antecedent pulmonary disease, and extent of pulmonary resection. The surgeon must discuss the potential risks with the anesthesiologist preoperatively, so that anesthetic technique, intraoperative fluid management, inspired oxygen level, and perioperative pain management can be optimized. Failure on the surgeon's part to understand or foresee potential problems related to the patient's multimodality treatment can have disastrous consequences. The very low morbidity and mortality reported in some of the single-institution studies of neoadjuvant therapy, such as the Memorial trial, in part reflect the expertise and close collaboration of all involved physicians in the management of these challenging cases.

The decision about whether to continue chemotherapy and/or radiation postoperatively has usually been based on the findings at operation, the completeness of resection, and the presence or absence of mediastinal nodal involvement. It is often impossible to determine whether residual active tumor remains within an area of dense fibrosis, and the surgeon can be faced with making difficult intraoperative decisions about the extent of pulmonary resection. Frozen section results may be misleading under these circumstances because extensive fibrosis can mask a small number of viable malignant cells. Because the completeness of resection may affect long-term survival, it is generally best in this situation to err on the side of extensive resection, provided the patient's overall condition permits. No matter what the extent of pulmonary resection, meticulous staging, particularly nodal staging, should be performed, and the specimens again individually labeled for the pathologist according to the American Thoracic Society map. Reinforcement of the bronchial stump with muscle or omental flaps is sometimes indicated, depending on the type of induction treatment the patient has received and the extent of pulmonary resection.

Continued vigilance by the surgeon is necessary throughout the postoperative period to avoid complications. As illustrated by some of the previously mentioned neoadjuvant trials, the potential risk of serious postoperative complications is greater after neoadjuvant therapy than after standard pulmonary resection, but that risk can be kept to an acceptable level by meticulous perioperative care.

CONCLUSION

The management of stage IIIA NSCLC remains complex and is evolving rapidly. Surgical resection is the appropriate primary treatment of T3, N0-1 tumors involving the chest wall, mediastinum, diaphragm, or main stem bronchi. The presence of distant metastases, and of N2 disease, should be excluded by CT scans and by mediastinoscopy before offering such patients a thoracotomy and resection. No clear benefit has been shown for adjuvant therapy in this group of patients.

A small minority of patients with N2 disease may benefit from surgical resection. These include patients with single-level, microscopic, completely resectable nodal disease, particularly if confined to the lower mediastinum. However, three recent trials suggest that even this small subset of patients may benefit from induction chemotherapy before surgical resection (58, 59, 105).

Most patients with stage IIIA N2 NSCLC are not candidates for surgical resection as their initial form of treatment. Experience during the past 10 years has clearly demonstrated the feasibility of neoadjuvant therapy in patients with stage III NSCLCs, particularly stage IIIA. A variety of induction regimens have produced resectability and survival rates that appear superior to the historical experience with either surgical resection or radiation alone. There is no single "standard" neoadjuvant therapy, but regimens incorporating high-dose cisplatin, with or without moderate-dose radiation, have achieved the best results with acceptable toxicity. Careful surgical management of these patients can lead to complete resection of residual disease with an operative risk comparable to that of standard pulmonary resection. The next important question is whether neoadjuvant therapy including surgical resection is superior to nonsurgical treatment with intensive chemotherapy and high-dose radiation. Large, prospective randomized phase III trials are currently in progress within the clinical cooperative groups to answer this question and to determine the optimal treatment of the large number of patients diagnosed each year with stage III NSCLC.

REFERENCES

1. Boring CC, Squires TS, Tong T. Cancer statistics, 1993. Cancer 1993;43:7–26.
2. Naruke T, Goya T, Tsuchiya R, Suemasu K. Prognosis and survival in resected lung carcinoma based on the new international staging system. J Thorac Cardiovasc Surg 1988;96:440–447.
3. Van Raemdonck DE, Schneider A, Ginsberg RJ. Surgical treatment for higher stage non–small cell lung cancer. Ann Thorac Surg 1992;54:999–1013.
4. Patterson GA, Ginsberg RJ, Poon PY, et al. A prospective evaluation of magnetic resonance imaging, computed tomography, and mediastinoscopy in the preoperative assessment of mediastinal node status in bronchogenic carcinoma. J Thorac Cardiovasc Surg 1987;94:679–684.
5. Martini N, Heelan R, Westcott J, et al. Comparative merits of conventional, computed tomographic, and magnetic resonance imaging in assessing mediastinal involvement in surgically confirmed lung carcinoma. J Thorac Cardiovasc Surg 1985;90:639–648.
6. Webb WR, Gatsonis C, Zerhouni EA, et al. CT and MR imaging in staging non–small cell bronchogenic carcinoma: report of the Radiologic Diagnostic Oncology Group. Radiology 1991;178:705–713.

7. Webb WR, Jensen BG, Sollitto R, et al. Bronchogenic carcinoma: staging with MR compared with staging with CT and surgery. Radiology 1985;156:117–124.
8. Heelan RT, Martini N, Westcott JW, et al. Carcinomatous involvement of the hilum and mediastinum: computed tomographic and magnetic resonance evaluation. Radiology 1985; 156:111–115.
9. Pearson FG. Staging of the mediastinum: role of mediastinoscopy and computed tomography. Chest 1993;103: 346S–348S.
10. Libshitz HI, McKenna RJ, Haynie TP, et al. Mediastinal evaluation in lung cancer. Radiology 1984;151:295–299.
11. Pennes DR, Glazer GM, Wimbish KJ, Cross BH, Long RW, Orringer MB. Chest wall invasion by lung cancer: limitations of CT evaluation. AJR Am J Roentgenol 1984;144:507–511.
12. Glazer HS, Duncan-Meyer J, Aronberg DJ, Moran JF, Levitt RG, Sagel SS. Pleural and chest wall invasion in bronchogenic carcinoma: CT evaluation. Radiology 1985;157:191–194.
13. Staples CA, Muller NL, Miller RR, et al. Mediastinal nodes in bronchogenic carcinoma: comparison between CT and mediastinoscopy. Radiology 1988;167:367–372.
14. McCloud TC, Bourgouin PM, Greenberg RW, et al. Bronchogenic carcinoma: analysis of staging in the mediastinum with CT by correlative lymph node mapping and sampling. Radiology 1992;182:319–322.
15. Luke WP, Todd TRJ, Cooper JD. Prospective evaluation of mediastinoscopy for assessment of carcinoma of the lung. J Thorac Cardiovasc Surg 1986;91:53–56.
16. Ginsberg RJ, Rice TR, Goldberg M, et al. Extended cervical mediastinoscopy: a single staging procedure for bronchogenic carcinoma of the left upper lobe. J Thorac Cardiovasc Surg 1987;94:673–678.
17. Lopez L, Varela A, Fleixinet J, et al. Extended cervical mediastinoscopy: prospective study of 50 patients. Ann Thorac Surg 1994;57:555–558.
18. McNeill TM, Chamberlain JM. Diagnostic anterior mediastinotomy. Ann Thorac Surg 1966;2:532–539.
19. Schreinemakers HHJ, Joosten HJM, Mravunac M, Lacquet LK. Parasternal mediastinoscopy. Assessment of operability in left upper lobe lung cancer: a prospective analysis. J Thorac Cardiovasc Surg 1988;95:298–302.
20. Piehler JM, Pairolero PC, Weiland LH, at el. Bronchogenic carcinoma with chest wall invasion: factors affecting survival following en bloc resection. Ann Thorac Surg 1982;34:684–691.
21. Paone JF, Spees EK, Newton CG, et al. An appraisal of en bloc resection of peripheral bronchogenic carcinoma involving the thoracic wall. Chest 1982;81:203–207.
22. Albertucci M, DeMeester TR, Rothberg M, et al. Surgery and management of peripheral lung tumors adherent to the parietal pleura. J Thorac Cardiovasc Surg 1992;103:8–13.
23. McCaughan BC, Martini N, Bains MS, McCormack PM. Chest wall invasion in carcinoma of the lung. Therapeutic and prognostic implications. J Thorac Cardiovasc Surg 1985;89: 836–841.
24. Allen MS, Mathisen DJ, Grillo HC, et al. Bronchogenic carcinoma with chest wall invasion. Ann Thorac Surg 1991;51: 948–951.
25. Geha AS, Bernatz PE, Woolner LB. Bronchogenic carcinoma involving the thoracic wall. Surgical treatment and prognostic significance. J Thorac Cardiovasc Surg 1967;54:394–402.
26. Jamieson MPG, Walbaum PR, McCormack RJM. Surgical management of bronchial carcinoma invading the chest wall. Thorax 1979;34:612–615.
27. Trastek VF, Paorolero PC, Piehler JM, et al. En bloc non–chest wall resection for bronchogenic carcinoma with parietal fixation. J Thorac Cardiovasc Surg 1984;87:352–358.
28. Grillo HC, Greenberg JJ, Wilkins EW Jr. Resection of bronchogenic carcinoma involving thoracic wall. J Thorac Cardiovasc Surg 1966;51:417–421.
29. Patterson, GA, Ilves R, Ginsberg RJ, et al. The value of adjuvant radiotherapy in pulmonary and chest wall resection for bronchogenic carcinoma. Ann Thorac Surg 1982;34:692–697.
30. McCormack PM, Bains MS, Martini N, et al. Methods of skeletal reconstruction following resection of lung carcinoma invading the chest wall. Surg Clin North Am 1987;67:979–986.
31. Nakahashi H, Yasumoto K, Ishida T, et al. Results of surgical treatment of patients with T3 non–small cell lung cancer. Ann Thorac Surg 1988;46:178–181.
32. Burt ME, Pomerantz AH, Bains MS, et al. Results of surgical treatment of stage III lung cancer invading the mediastinum. Surg Clin North Am 1987;67:987–1000.
33. Martini N, Yellin A, Ginsberg RJ, et al. Management of non–small cell lung cancer with direct mediastinal involvement. Ann Thorac Surg 1994;58:1447–1451.
34. Mehran R, Deslauriers J, Guojin L, et al. Survival related to nodal status after sleeve resection for primary lung cancer. J Thorac Cardiovasc Surg 1994;107:576–583.
35. Newton JR Jr., Grillo HC, Mathisen DJ. Main bronchial sleeve resection with pulmonary conservation. Ann Thorac Surg 1991;52:1272–1280.
36. Belli L, Meroni A, Rondinara G, Beati CA. Bronchoplastic procedures and pulmonary artery reconstruction in the treatment of bronchogenic cancer. J Thorac Cardiovasc Surg 1985;90: 167–171.
37. Dartevelle PG, Khalife J, Chapelier A, et al. Tracheal sleeve pneumonectomy for bronchogenic carcinoma: report of 55 cases. Ann Thorac Surg 1988;46:68–72.
38. Deslauriers J, Beaulieu M, Bénazéra A, McClish A. Sleeve pneumonectomy for bronchogenic carcinoma. Ann Thorac Surg 1979;28:466–474.
39. Roviaro GC, Varoli F, Rebuffat C, et al. Tracheal sleeve pneumonectomy for bronchogenic carcinoma. J Thorac Cardiovasc Surg 1994;107:13–18.
40. Tedder M, Anstadt MP, Tedder SD, Lowe JE. Current morbidity, mortality and survival after bronchoplastic procedures of malignancy. Ann Thorac Surg 1992;54:387–391.
41. Faber LP. Results of surgical treatment of stage III lung carcinoma with carinal proximity. The role of sleeve lobectomy versus pneumonectomy and the role of sleeve pneumonectomy. Surg Clin North Am 1987;67:1001–1014.
42. Kirschner PA. Lung cancer. Surgical significance of mediastinal lymph-node metastases. N Y State J Med 1979;12: 2036–2039.
43. Smith RA. The importance of mediastinal lymph node invasion of pulmonary carcinoma in selection of patients for resection. Ann Thorac Surg 1978;25:5–11.
44. Naruke T, Suemasu K, Ishikawa S. Lymph node mapping and curability at various levels of metastasis in resected lung cancer. J Thorac Cardiovasc Surg 1978;76:833–839.
45. Pearson FG, DeLarue NC, Ilves R, et al. Significance of positive superior mediastinal nodes identified at mediastinoscopy in patients with resectable cancer of the lung. J Thorac Cardiovasc Surg 1992;83:1–11.
46. Kirsh MM, Sloan H. Mediastinal metastases in bronchogenic carcinoma: influence of postoperative irradiation, cell type, and location. Ann Thorac Surg 1982;33:459–463.

47. Rubinstein I, Baum GL, Bubis JJ, Kalter Y, Lieberman Y. Prognosis of patients with adenocarcinoma of the lung and mediastinal lymph node metastases undergoing pulmonary resection. Respiration 1985;47:70–72.
48. Patterson GA, Piazza D, Pearson FG, et al. Significance of metastatic disease in subaortic lymph nodes. Ann Thorac Surg 1987;43:155–159.
49. Thomas PA, Piantadosi S, Mountain CF. Should subcarinal lymph nodes be routinely examined in patients with non–small cell lung cancer? J Thorac Cardiovasc Surg 1988; 95(5):883–887.
50. Naruke T, Goya T, Tsuchiya R, Suemasu K. The importance of surgery to non–small cell carcinoma of lung with mediastinal lymph node metastasis. Ann Thorac Surg 1988;46:603–610.
51. Mountain CF. Expanded possibilities for surgical treatment of lung cancer. Survival in stage IIIa disease. Chest 1990; 97:1045–1051.
52. Watanabe Y, Shimizu J, Oda M, et al. Aggressive surgical intervention in N2 non–small cell cancer of the lung. Ann Thorac Surg 1991;51:253–261.
53. Daly BDT, Mueller JD, Faling LJ, et al. N2 lung cancer: Outcome in patients with false-negative computed tomographic scans of the chest. J Thorac Cardiovasc Surg 1993;105: 904–911.
54. Goldstraw P, Mannam GC, Kaplan DK, Michail P, Shields TW. Surgical management of non–small cell lung cancer with ipsilateral mediastinal node metastasis (N2 disease). J Thorac Cardiovasc Surg 1994;107:19–28.
55. Shields TW. The significance of ipsilateral mediastinal lymph node metastasis (N2 disease) in non–small cell carcinoma of the lung. A commentary. J Thoracic Cardiovasc Surg 1990; 99:48–53.
56. Martini N, Flehinger BJ, Zaman MB, Beattie EJ Jr. Results of resection in non–oat cell carcinoma with mediastinal lymph node metastases. Ann Surg 1983;198:386–397.
57. van Klaveren RJ, Festen J, Otten HJAM, Cox AL, de Graff R, Lacquet LK. Prognosis of unsuspected but completely resectable N2 non–small cell lung cancer. Ann Thorac Surg 1993;56:300–304.
58. Rosell R, Gómez-Codina J, Camps C, et al. A randomized trial comparing preoperative chemotherapy plus surgery with surgery alone in patients with non-small-cell lung cancer. N Engl J Med 1994;330:153–158.
59. Roth JA, Fossella F, Komaki R, et al. A randomized trial comparing perioperative chemotherapy and surgery with surgery alone in resectable stage IIIA non–small cell lung cancer. J Natl Cancer Inst 1994;86:673–680.
60. Roswit B, Patno ME, Rapp R, et al. The survival of patients with inoperable lung cancer: a large-scale randomized study of radiation therapy versus placebo. Radiology 1968;90:688–697.
61. Curran WJ, Stafford PM. Lack of apparent difference in outcome between clinically staged IIIA and IIIB non–small cell lung cancer treated with radiation therapy. J Clin Oncol 1990;8(3):409–415.
62. Johnson DH, Einhorn LH, Bartolucci A, et al. Thoracic radiotherapy does not prolong survival in patients with locally advanced, unresectable non–small cell lung cancer. Ann Intern Med 1990;113:33–38.
63. Perez CA, Pajak TF, Rubin P, et al. Long-term observations of the patterns of failure in patients with unresectable non–oat cell carcinoma of the lung treated with definitive radiotherapy: Report by the Radiation Therapy Oncology Group. Cancer 1987;59:1874–1881.
64. Cox JD, Azarnia N, Byhardt RW, et al. A randomized phase I/II trial of hyperfractionated radiation therapy with total doses of 60.0 Gy to 79.2 Gy: possible survival benefit with 69.6 Gy in favorable patients with Radiation Therapy Oncology Group stage III non–small cell lung carcinoma: Report of Radiation Therapy Oncology Group 83-11. J Clin Oncol 1990;8:1543–1555.
65. Bromley LL, Szur L. Combined radiotherapy and resection for carcinoma of the bronchus, experience with 66 patients. Lancet 1955;2:937–941.
66. Payne DG. Pre-operative radiation therapy in non–small cell cancer of the lung. Lung Cancer 1991;7:47–56.
67. Sherman DM, Neptune W, Weichselpaum R, et al. An aggressive approach to marginally resectable lung cancer. Cancer 1978;41:2040–2045.
68. Kirschner PA. Lung cancer: preoperative radiation therapy and surgery. N Y State J Med 1981;3:339–342.
69. Bloedorn FG, Cowley RA, Cuccia CA, et al. Preoperative irradiation in bronchogenic carcinoma. AJR Am J Roentgenol 1964;92(1):77–87.
70. Shields TW, Higgins GA Jr, Lawton R, et al. Preoperative x-ray therapy as an adjuvant in the treatment of bronchogenic carcinoma. J Thorac Cardiovasc Surg 1970;59(1):49–61.
71. Shields TW. Preoperative radiation therapy in the treatment of bronchial carcinoma. Cancer 1972;30(5):1388–1394.
72. Warram J, et al. Preoperative irradiation of cancer of the lung: final report of a therapeutic trial. Cancer 1975;36:914–925.
73. Bleehen NM. Combined radiotherapy with chemotherapy for inoperable non–small cell lung cancer. Lung Cancer 1991; 7:85–89.
74. Green MR. Sequential chemotherapy and radiotherapy for initial management of stage IIIA and stage IIIB non–small cell lung cancer—induction chemotherapy. Lung Cancer 1991; 7:77–84.
75. Dillman RO, Seagren SL, Propert KJ, et al. A randomized trial of induction chemotherapy plus high-dose radiation versus radiation alone in stage III non–small cell lung cancer. N Engl J Med 1990;323:940–945.
76. Le Chevalier T, Arriagada R, Quoix E, et al. Radiotherapy alone versus combined chemotherapy and radiotherapy in nonresectable non–small cell lung cancer: first analysis of a randomized trial in 353 patients. J Natl Cancer Inst 1991;83:417–423.
77. Trovo MG, Minatel E, Veronesi A, et al. Combined radiotherapy and chemotherapy versus radiotherapy alone in locally advanced epidermoid bronchogenic carcinoma: a randomized study. Cancer 1990;65:400–404.
78. Mattson K, Holsti LR, Holsti P, et al. Inoperable non–small cell lung cancer: radiation with or without chemotherapy. Eur J Cancer Clin Oncol 1988;24(3):477–482.
79. van Houtte P, Klastersky J, Nguyen H, et al. Comparative randomized study of chest radiotherapy preceded or not by chemotherapy with cisplatin, etoposide, and vindesine for the treatment of NSCLC (abstract). Proc Am Assoc Cancer Res 194;25:785.
80. Morton RF, Jett JR, McGinnis WL, et al. Thoracic radiation therapy alone compared with combined chemoradiotherapy for locally unresectable non–small cell lung cancer: a randomized, phase III trial. Ann Intern Med 1991;115:681–686.
81. Schaake-Konig C, van den Bogaert W, Kalesio O, et al. Effects of concomitant cisplatin and radiotherapy on inoperable non–small cell lung cancer. N Engl J Med 1992;326:524–530.
82. Sadeghi A, Payne D, Rubenstein L, et al, and the Lung Cancer Study Group. Combined modality treatment for resected ad-

vanced non–small-cell lung cancer: local control and local recurrence. Int J Radiat Oncol Biol Phys 1991;15:89–97.
83. Trovo MG, Minatel E, Franchin G, et al. Radiotherapy (RT) versus RT enhanced by cisplatin (DDP) in stage III non–small cell lung cancer (NSCLC): randomized cooperative study (abstract). Lung Cancer 1991;7(Suppl):590.
84. Ansari R, Tokars R, Fisher W, et al. A phase III study of thoracic irradiation with or without concomitant cisplatin in locoregional unresectable non–small cell lung cancer (NSCLC): a Hoosier Oncology Group (HOG) protocol (abstract). Proc Am Soc Clin Oncol 1991;10:A823.
85. Langer C, Curran W, Catalano R, et al. Encouraging 2-year survival in phase II trial of simultaneous thoracic radiation therapy (RT) and multi-agent chemotherapy for locally advanced non–small cell lung cancer (NSCLC) (abstract). Proc Am Soc Clin Oncol 1992:298.
86. Friess GG, Baikadi M, Harvey WH. Concurrent cisplatin and etoposide with radiotherapy in locally advanced non–small cell lung cancer. Cancer Treat Rep 1987;71:681–684.
87. Vokes EE, Vijayakumar S, Hoffman PC, et al. 5-Fluorouracil with oral leucovorin and hydroxyurea and concomitant radiotherapy for stage III non–small cell lung cancer. Cancer 1990;66:437–442.
88. Shaw E, Jett J, McGinnis W, et al. Pilot study of accelerated hyperfractionated thoracic radiation therapy (AHTRT) concomitant with VP-16/CDDP (EP) chemotherapy for inoperable stage III M0 non–small cell lung cancer (abstract). Proc Am Soc Clin Oncol 1992:393.
89. Hazuka M, Crowley J, Bunn P, et al. Concurrent daily low-dose cisplatin (LDCP) combined with chest irradiation (RT) in locally advanced non–small cell ung cancer: Preliminary results of a Southwest Oncology Group (SWOG) study (abstract). Proc Am Soc Clin Oncol 1992:295.
90. Kirn DH, Lynch TJ, Mentzer SJ, et al. Multimodality therapy of stage IIIA N2 non–small cell lung cancer: impact of preoperative chemotherapy on resectability and downstaging. J Thorac Cardiovasc Surg 1993;106:669–702.
91. Takita H, Regal A-M, Antkowiak JG, et al. Chemotherapy followed by lung resection in inoperable non–small cell lung carcinomas due to locally far-advanced disease. Cancer 1986; 57:630–635.
92. Bitran JC, Golomb HM, Hoffman PC, et al. Protochemotherapy in non–small cell lung carcinoma. An attempt to increase surgical resectability and survival: a preliminary report. Cancer 1986;57:44–53.
93. Katsuki H, Shimada K, Koyama A, et al. Long-term intermittent adjuvant chemotherapy for primary, resected lung cancer. J Thorac Cardiovasc Surg 1975;70(4):590–605.
94. Martini N, Kris MG, Gralla RJ, et al. The effects of preoperative chemotherapy on the resectability of non–small cell lung carcinoma with mediastinal lymph node metastases (N2 M0). Ann Thorac Surg 1988;45:370–379.
95. Martini N, Kris MM, Flehinger BJ, et al. Preoperative chemotherapy of stage IIIa (N2) non–small cell lung cancer: The Memorial Sloan-Kettering experience with 136 patients. Ann Thorac Surg 1993;55:1365–1374.
96. Burkes RL, Ginsberg RJ, Shepherd FA, et al. Induction chemotherapy with mitomycin, vindesine, and cisplatin for stage III unresectable non–small cell lung cancer: results of the Toronto phase II trial. J Clin Oncol 1992;10(4):580–586.
97. Wagner H Jr, Lad T, Piantadosi S. Randomized phase II evaluation of preoperative radiation therapy and preoperative chemotherapy with mitomycin-c, vinblastine, and cisplatin in patients with technically unresectable stage IIIA and IIIB non–small cell lung cancer of the lung (abstract). Lung Cancer 1991;157(Suppl 7).
98. Eagan RT, Ruud C, Lee RE, et al. Pilot study of induction therapy with cyclophosphamide, doxorubicin, and cisplatin (CAP) and chest irradiation prior to thoracotomy in initially inoperable stage III M0 non–small cell lung cancer. Cancer Treat Rep 1987;71:895–900.
99. Weiden PL, Piantadosi S. Preoperative chemotherapy (cisplatin and fluorouracil) and radiation therapy in stage III non–small cell lung cancer: a phase II study of the Lung Cancer Study Group. J Natl Cancer Inst 1991;83:266–272.
100. Faber LP, Kittle CF, Warren WH, et al. Preoperative chemotherapy and irradiation for stage III non–small cell lung cancer. Ann Thorac Surg 1989;47:669–677.
101. Strauss GM, Herndon JE, Sherman DD, et al. Neoadjuvant chemotherapy and radiotherapy followed by surgery in stage IIIA non–small cell carcinoma of the lung: report of a cancer and leukemia group B phase II study. J Clin Oncol 1992; 10:1237–1244.
102. Rusch VW, Albain KS, Crowley JJ, et al. Surgical resection of stage IIIA and stage IIIB non–small-cell lung cancer after concurrent induction chemoradiotherapy: a Southwest Oncology Group trial. J Thorac Cardiovasc Surg 1993;105:97–106.
103. Yashar J, Weitberg AB, Glicksman AS, et al. Preoperative chemotherapy and radiation therapy for stage IIIa carcinoma of the lung. Ann Thorac Surg 1992;53:445–8.
104. Fowler WC, Langer CJ, Curran WJ, et al. Postoperative complications following combined neoadjuvant treatment of lung cancer. Ann Thorac Surg 1993;55:986–989.
105. Pass HI, Pogrebniak HW, Steinberg SM, et al. Randomized trial of neoadjuvant therapy for lung cancer: interim analysis. Ann Thorac Surg 1992;53:992–998.

16

SUPERIOR SULCUS TUMORS

Robert J. Ginsberg, David G. Payne, and Farid Shamji

The syndrome of pain in the shoulder and arm, sensorimotor symptoms in the involved upper limb, ipsilateral Horner's syndrome, and a lesion situated at the extreme apex of the lung was described by Henry Pancoast in 1932 (1). He labeled this entity a superior pulmonary sulcus tumor, emphasizing that it always occurred "at a definite location at the thoracic inlet," the word sulcus presumably referring to the groove made by the subclavian artery on the anterosuperior surface of the lung apex and its overlying cupola of the pleura.

The superior sulcus tumor is now considered a primary lung cancer that early in the disease progression extends beyond the lung to invade important local anatomic structures present in the thoracic inlet. It is estimated that between 2% and 4% of all primary lung cancers give rise to the distinct clinical picture known as Pancoast's syndrome.

These tumors have been singled out for special consideration because of their location in the thoracic inlet, which makes them difficult to detect on routine radiographs. They are also important because they cause symptoms that mimic cervical spine osteoarthritis or shoulder joint bursitis, thus resulting frequently in a delay in making the correct diagnosis.

HISTORICAL DESCRIPTION

In 1838 Edwin Hare, a house-surgeon to the Stafford County General Infirmary, wrote "Tumor Involving Certain Nerves" in the London Medical Gazette (2). This report was the first meticulous clinical and pathologic description of a tumor that resembles the superior sulcus tumor. Hare pointed out an important feature of this tumor is its propensity to extend along the nerve sheaths into the adjacent intervertebral foramina and cause epidural spinal cord compression.

In 1924 Henry Pancoast, a radiologist in Philadelphia, called attention to the "Importance of Careful Roentgen-Ray Investigations of Apical Chest Tumors" by reporting three patients (3). Eight years later, in 1932, Pancoast published his classic article on the superior pulmonary sulcus tumor in which he reported four more patients who had a similar clinical picture and findings including pain in the axilla and arm, weakness and wasting of the muscles of the hand, an ipsilateral Horner's syndrome, and an apical shadow with bone destruction on radiographs (1). Pancoast incorrectly regarded this picture as arising from an embryonal epithelial rest of the fifth branchial pouch. He rejected primary lung cancer as a cause because of the lack of metastatic disease, infrequent or absent pulmonary symptoms, and extreme peripheral location.

The true site of origin of this tumor, the lung, was recognized first by Tobias in 1932 when he described the same clinical syndrome in five patients (4). He called it the "apico-costo-vertebral syndrome," and the cause in four cases was carcinoma of the lung.

The first reported cure after treatment of a superior sulcus tumor was by Chardack and MacCallum in 1956 (5). The patient had a complete resection of the tumor followed by external irradiation to a dose of 6528 Gy in 54 days to the tumor bed. He died disease free of unrelated causes nearly 6 years later.

In 1961, Shaw et al. (6) advocated the use of a combined treatment, preoperatively irradiating the tumor to a dose of 30 Gy in 12 days, followed by a radical en bloc resection 3 weeks later. This regimen continues to be the most common treatment program for this tumor. When resection is complete, a cure is possible.

PATHOLOGIC CONSIDERATIONS

Peripheral tumors arising in the extreme apex of the lung at the thoracic inlet although still quite small, may involve the lower trunk of the brachial plexus, the roots of the eighth cervical and first and second thoracic nerves, the sympathetic chain, and the stellate

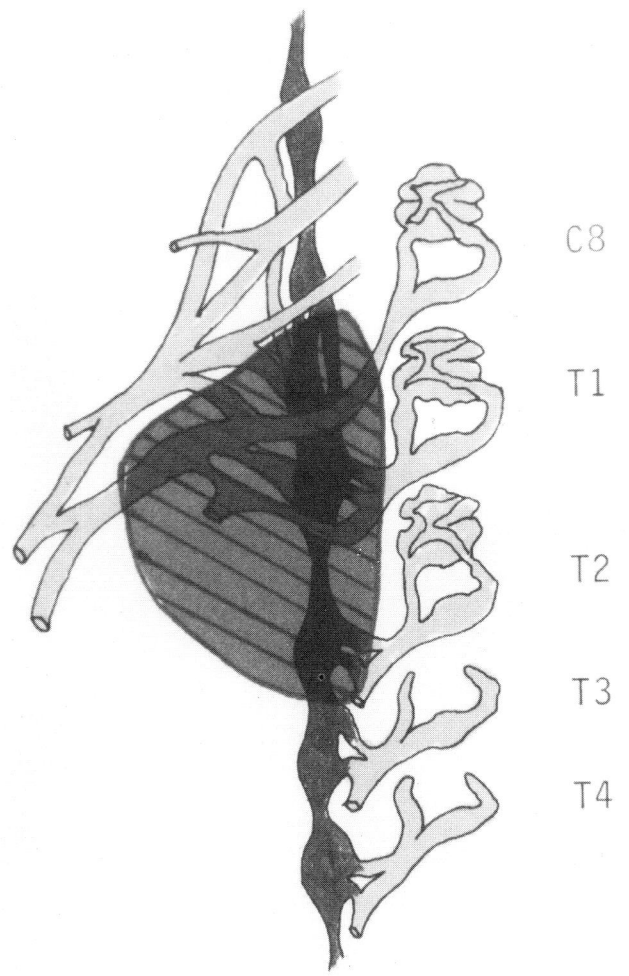

FIGURE 16.1. A diagrammatic representation of the superior sulcus tumor involving the lower and brachial plexus, stellate ganglion, and sympathetic chain.

ganglion (Fig. 16.1). Ultimately, there may be local destruction of adjacent upper ribs and thoracic vertebrae. Spread of the tumor though the intervertebral foramina may cause epidural spinal cord compression.

The characteristic clinical syndrome described by Pancoast can be produced by any lesion arising in the thoracic inlet because of the local anatomic relationships. Both benign and malignant processes have been described as causing some or all of the Pancoast's syndrome characteristics.

Of the primary lung cancers in this location, between 50% and 60% are squamous cell in histology, 30% are large cell, and 15% are adenocarcinoma. Small cell carcinomas are uncommon. The tumor grows slowly and early in its progression extends outside of the lung to involve the important anatomic structures present in the crowded thoracic inlet rather than the underlying lung tissue. By definition, the superior sulcus tumor is a T3 lesion by virtue of its local invasion until vertebral bony invasion, epidural extension, or major vascular involvement occur (T4). Spread of the tumor to the mediastinal lymph nodes and/or distant sites occurs late in its course. Of 151 cases reviewed by Herbut and Watson (7) in 1946, 67% were primary carcinomas of the lung; a further 14% were designated with uncertainty as primary carcinoma of the neck but probably represented lung cancers. The rest were secondary tumor deposits to the thoracic inlet from widespread primary lesions.

CLINICAL FEATURES

Initially confined to the lung tissue, the tumor may produce no definite local symptoms, the diagnosis being suggested by a routine chest radiograph with apical density in the form of a pleural thickening or mass.

Local spread of cancer involves the overlying visceral pleura and produces local parietal pleural irritation. This irritation is manifested by vague diffuse pain over the shoulder and upper chest without local tenderness. An incorrect diagnosis of a shoulder joint problem or cervical disk disease is made often, and the tumor may continue to grow undetected for some time. A delay in diagnosis of up to 18 months from the onset of symptoms is common.

In time, the tumor grows through the strong fascial layer—the suprapleural membrane (Sibson's fascia) overlying the lung apex and the cervical dome of the pleura. Thus begins the gradual invasion of the adjacent upper ribs, intervening intercostal muscles, adjoining vertebral bodies of the upper thoracic spine, the lower brachial plexus and its branches, upper thoracic sympathetic chain, and subclavian vessels. The character of the pain changes because of this local invasion. In addition to the nonspecific shoulder pain already present, the patient now may experience several other symptoms.

1. Severe local pain with marked tenderness because of involvement of the ribs—usually the first, second, and/or third rib—or adjacent vertebral body. The radiographic examination may not show bone involvement if only the periosteum is involved, because bone destruction occurs later as the tumor progresses.
2. Referred pain anteriorly along the segmental distribution of the intercostal nerves as the tumor invades the intercostal muscles and nerves, especially the intercostobranchial nerve (T2).

3. Pain in the lower part of the shoulder and inner aspect of the arm along the ulnar nerve distribution (C8, and T1 segments). This pain is caused by the tumor invading the lower trunk of the brachial plexus and occurs at a later stage in the course of the disease.

The arm pain, which may be severe and unremitting, may ultimately be accompanied by sensory loss in the same distribution and ultimately by wasting and weakness of the small muscles of the hand and of the medial forearm, wrist, and finger flexors.

Further neurologic manifestations result when the tumor progresses medially to involve the stellate ganglion, resulting in the classic Horner's syndrome. The Horner's syndrome is characterized by ipsilateral partial ptosis, the appearance of enophthalmos, a small pupil, and hypohidrosis of the face. Being a late manifestation of local cancer invasion, it is associated with a worse survival. Epidural spinal cord compression occurs if the tumor extends into an adjacent intervertebral foramen, along a nerve root. The presence of epidural spinal cord compression is suggested by increasing neuralgic pain (because of nerve root compression by direct invasion and edema); worsening brachial plexus involvement; symptoms of weakness, numbness, and tingling in the legs; and urinary retention. The outcome is devastating.

The lung cancer growing in the thoracic inlet can invade the lymphatics of the posterior chest wall gradually before entering the pulmonary lymphatic channels. This invasion may explain the occasional presence of tumor deposits in the supraclavicular or axillary lymph nodes without prior involvement of the regional hilar and mediastinal nodes. The incidence of cancer spread to the supraclavicular lymph nodes from superior pulmonary sulcus tumor is not known precisely. Spread to the hilar or mediastinal lymph nodes occurs in approximately 20% of the patients at the time of diagnosis.

DIAGNOSIS

CLINICAL DIAGNOSIS

The most common presenting symptom is the characteristic pain, which is often severe and sometimes is worsened by active or passive movements of the affected arm. More than 80% of patients complain of pain, often developing months before any other symptoms or signs. The diagnosis should be considered in all patients with symptoms suggestive of cervical osteoarthritis or shoulder bursitis, particularly because incomplete forms of the Pancoast's syndrome are found. The only hope of curing a superior pulmonary sulcus tumor is early diagnosis. Unfortunately, the correct diagnosis frequently is made too late, when the disease has progressed to a state that precludes effective relief of pain, let alone a cure.

RADIOGRAPHIC DIAGNOSIS

Pancoast in his original article in 1924 emphasized two important points: (a) the difficulty in seeing a lesion at the extreme apex of the lung on chest film, and (b) the sign that an apical primary lung cancer could produce extreme pain even when it is scarcely detectable radiographically. In the presence of suggestive symptoms, a normal chest radiograph does not rule out the diagnosis, and further early investigation, by apical lordotic chest radiographs or computed tomography (CT) scan should be considered.

These tumors, in their early stages, may produce a dense, irregular, somewhat crescentic shadow at the extreme lung apex, which is indistinguishable from apical pleural thickening resulting from other causes (Fig. 16.2). As they enlarge, they become clearly distinguishable as an apical mass, sometimes with invasion or destruction of the posterior parts of one or

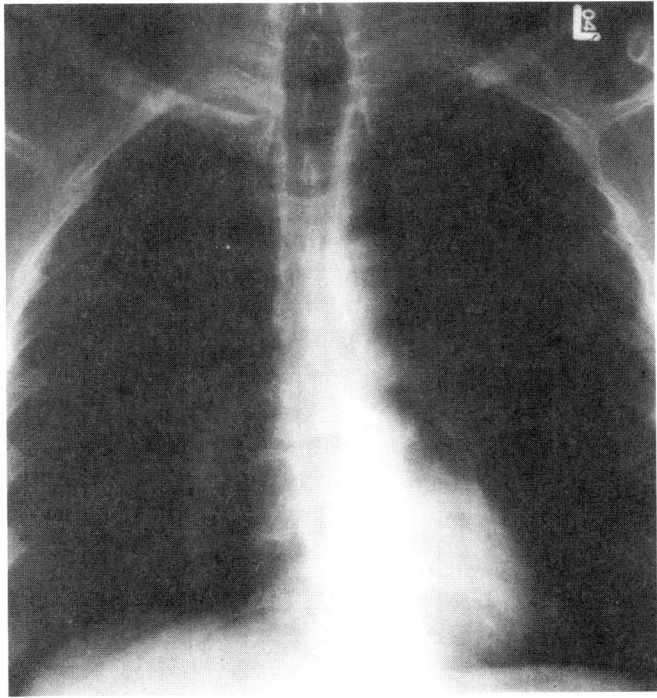

FIGURE 16.2. An early radiologic manifestation of a superior sulcus tumor with haziness in the right apex.

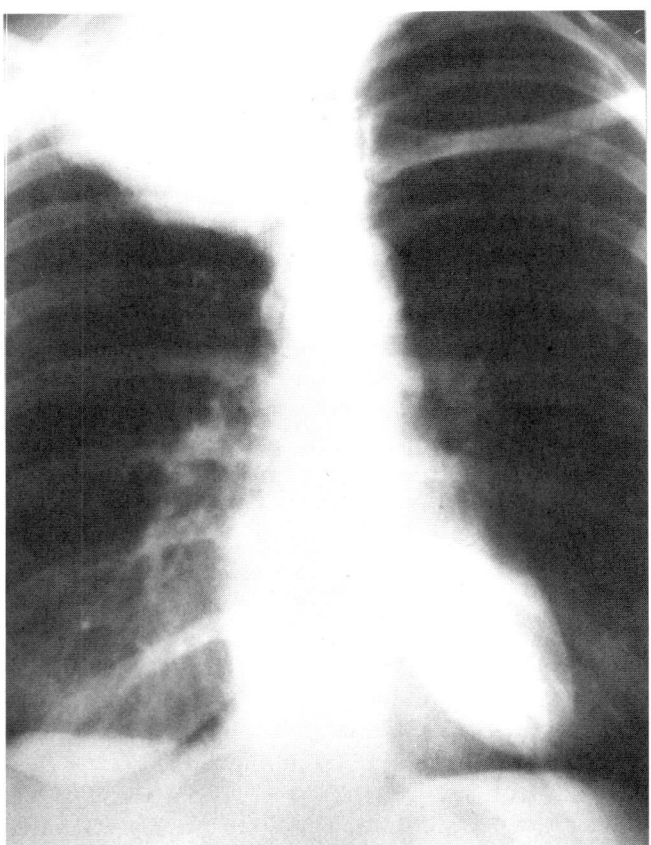

FIGURE 16.3. A large superior sulcus tumor presenting with the full-blown Pancoast syndrome.

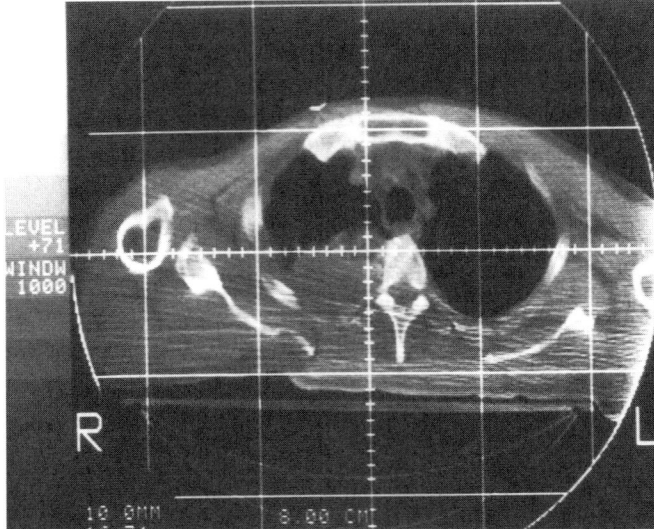

FIGURE 16.4. A CT scan demonstrating erosion of the posterior ribs and vertebral body.

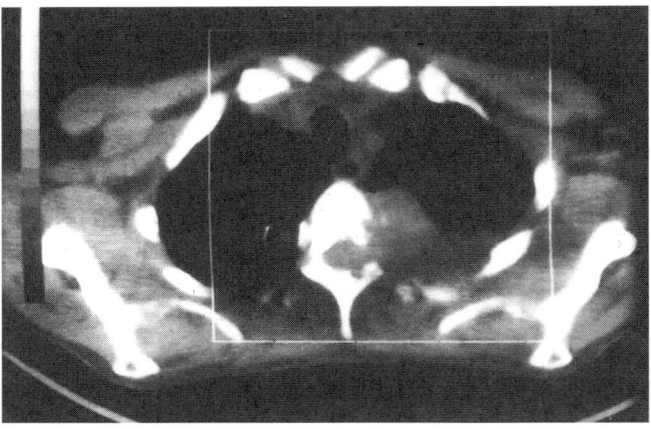

FIGURE 16.5. A CT scan demonstrating erosion of the posterior ribs and vertebral body.

more of the first three ribs. The transverse processes and vertebrae tend to be involved much later as the tumor progresses (Fig. 16.3).

The CT scan may demonstrate local invasion, suggesting inoperability, including direct invasion of the mediastinum, tumor encasing the subclavian artery, and destruction of the contiguous vertebral body (Fig. 16.4).

A myelogram combined with CT, or preferably a magnetic resonance imaging (MRI) study may be necessary to demonstrate tumor extension into an intervertebral foramen (Fig. 16.5). Such cancer spread can lead to gradual epidural spinal cord compression and may occur with little or no abnormality seen on radiographs or bone scans. MRI is valuable in assessment of local tumor invasion, particulary chest wall invasion, extension into the base of the neck to involve the brachial plexus and subclavian vessels, direct mediastinal extension, vertebral body invasion, and foramina spread; whenever possible, it should be included in the preoperative assessment (Fig. 16.6).

HISTOLOGIC CONFIRMATION

The diagnosis of superior sulcus carcinoma is often obvious, with more than 95% certainty, when all components of the Pancoast's syndrome, including bony destruction, are present. Establishment of a histologic diagnosis, however, is valuable in determining the exact histologic type of tumor and ruling out other etiologies before initiating treatment for superior sulcus tumors. (Table 16.1).

Fiberoptic bronchoscopy with bronchial washings from the affected upper lobe or transbronchial needle aspiration surgery may reveal the diagnosis. However, percutaneous fine-needle aspiration biopsy is simple and safe, and it is the most direct technique of estab-

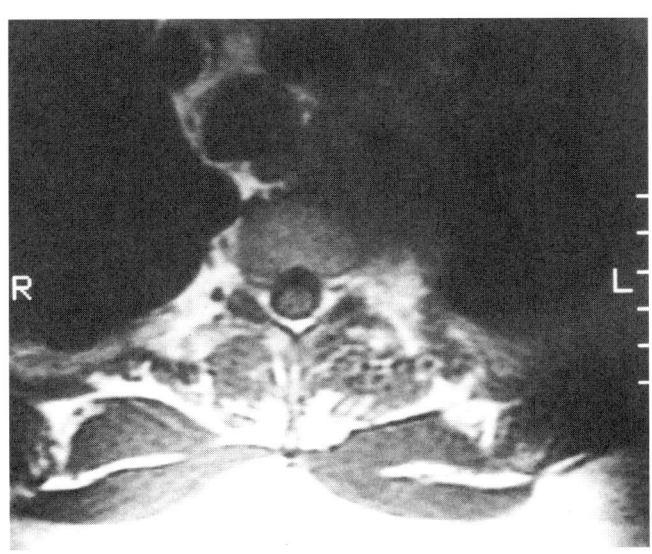

FIGURE 16.6. An MRI scan demonstrating invasion of the vertebral body, tracheal wall, and aorta.

TABLE 16.1. Differential Diagnosis of Superior Sulcus Lesions

SITE	DISEASE
Apical lung tissue	Metastatic tumor, tuberculosis, other inflammatory lesions
Apical pleura	Mesothelioma, benign pleural thickening
Brachial plexus, stellate ganglion, intercostal nerves	Neurogenic tumor
Superior mediastinum	Mediastinal tumors or cysts

lishing a cytologic diagnosis in superior sulcus carcinoma, with an overall accuracy of 92% (8). It can rule out other causes of the apical shadowing (e.g., tuberculosis, neurogenic tumor).

Needle-aspiration biopsy of a palpable scalene lymph node may provide quick confirmation of the diagnosis. A supraclavicular scalenotomy is now seldom used to obtain tissue for histologic diagnosis. Cervical mediastinoscopy can also be used to establish a diagnosis by both lymph node sampling and, when necessary, transpleural fine-needle aspiration biopsy of the apical lung lesion through the mediastinoscope. However, its more important role is in the proper staging of the cancer.

Exploratory thoracotomy for diagnosis is not recommended without first attempting a less invasive approach. This caution is particularly important because the treatment regimen for these patients often includes a preoperative course of radiation therapy.

METASTATIC WORKUP

Superior pulmonary sulcus tumors are locally invasive, and they tend to metastasize late; distant metastases occur in a small group of patients, approximately 8% to 14%. Despite this fact, because of the extensive surgery required for curative treatment, metastases should be sought by CT scan of the head and abdomen and by radionuclide bone scan.

MANAGEMENT

In recent years it has become evident that for superior pulmonary sulcus tumors, complete surgical excision, when possible, offers the most appreciable pain relief and survival, both in terms of quality and duration, and that it is the preferable primary treatment for local control when a complete resection is possible. Poor local control has a devastating outcome, ultimately increasing pain and suffering.

Selection of patients for curative treatment, whether by surgery, radiotherapy, or a combination of the two, is based on three factors:

1. Detailed noninvasive assessment of the local extent of disease in the thoracic inlet using CT and MR imaging. The findings, which indicate potentially unresectable disease, include direct tumor invasion of the mediastinum; tumor extending into the root of the neck and extensively invading the brachial plexus and encasing the subclavian vessels; destruction of the continguous vertebral body; extension of the tumor through an intervertebral foramen; and the presence of significant mediastinal lymph node enlargement.
2. Accurate staging of the cancer by mediastinal lymph node sampling (mediastinoscopy) and scanning for distant metastases in the bone, liver, adrenal glands, and brain. For this tumor, by definition a T3 lesion, long-term survival depends on the status of the mediastinal lymph nodes. Histologic confirmation of mediastinal nodal involvement indicates virtual incurability and a very poor outcome in most series (8). Patients with T3, N2 lesions rarely survive more than 2 years. Also, the presence of distant metastases rules out surgical resection for treatment. The role of routine scalene node biopsy to rule out supraclavicular disease has never been assessed.
3. Proper evaluation of the patients' general medical condition, cardiopulmonary function, and respiratory reserve.

The majority of patients presenting with superior sulcus tumors are inoperable at presentation. In a retrospective review of 174 patients at the Ontario Center Institute presenting between 1966 and 1982 (9), 121 had advanced disease at presentation that precluded surgery because of mediastinal or supraclavicular nodal metastasis, T4 tumors deemed inoperable, or distant metastases. Of the 53 patients with T3, N0 or N1 tumors, 36 were treated surgically, and 17 were treated by primary radiotherapy. In this series garnered from a regional referral center, less than one third of the patients presenting with superior sulcus tumors could be deemed operable at the time of presentation.

SURGICAL TREATMENT

CURATIVE TREATMENTS

Superior sulcus tumors originally were considered to be inoperable and incurable because of their relative inaccessibility and their invasion of important local structures in the thoracic inlet. Until 1961, even when radical resections were done, survival was poor because the local resection was usually incomplete; until then, surgical resection usually was employed mainly for palliation of pain (5). The addition of postoperative radiotherapy to incomplete palliative resections helped little, with minimal survival advantage compared to no treatment at all. Selectivity, based on careful cancer staging, has been the most important factor in deciding the best therapeutic approach. With improved selection of patients, after a curative resection 30% of patients can be expected to survive 5 years. In an attempt to increase the number of tumors that may be resected completely for cure, Shaw and colleagues (6) advocated preoperative radiotherapy, given a dose of 30 Gy in 10 fractions over 12 days, thereby increasing resectability, theoretically blocking lymphatics, and reducing seeding at the time of the operation. More recently, a dose of 45 Gy preoperatively has been used frequently to provide a more complete tumoricidal dosage and to increase resectability by further shrinkage of the tumor (Fig. 16.7).

Recent reports of improved survival after induction chemotherapy or chemoradiotherapy in stage IIIA disease makes these induction modalities worth assessing in the treatment of superior sulcus tumors. As yet, these multimodality approaches have not been evaluated completely.

Preoperative radiotherapy followed by extended

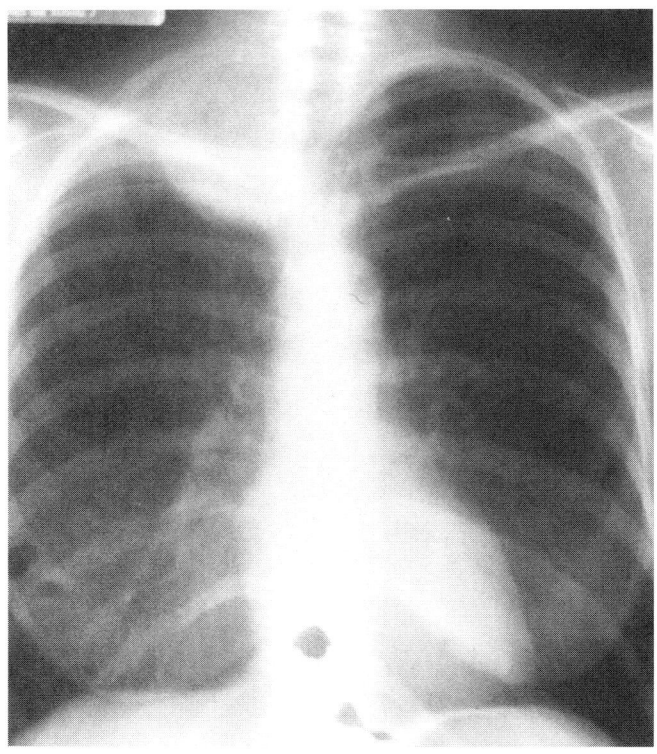

FIGURE 16.7. Tumor originally seen in Fig. 16.3 after preoperative radiotherapy to 30 Gy in 3 weeks.

en bloc resection has been accepted as the standard treatment for resectable tumors; resection is carried out 4 to 6 weeks after completion of radiotherapy (Fig. 16.8). An extended en bloc resection should include:

1. The chest wall and entire first rib and posterior parts of other involved ribs and, when necessary, lateral portions of upper thoracic vertebrae (up to one quarter of the body can be removed without undue instability), including their transverse processes as well.
2. Corresponding thoracic nerve roots divided at the intervertebral foramina.
3. A portion of the lower trunk of the brachial plexus, usually sacrificing the first thoracic nerve and preserving the eighth cervical nerve root.
4. A portion of the stellate ganglion and the thoracic sympathetic chain.
5. A pulmonary resection, preferably by lobectomy or occasionally by anatomic segmental or wedge resection (Fig. 16.9).
6. A complete mediastinal lymph node dissection.

The standard approach used to extract a superior sulcus tumor is a posterolateral thoracotomy incision

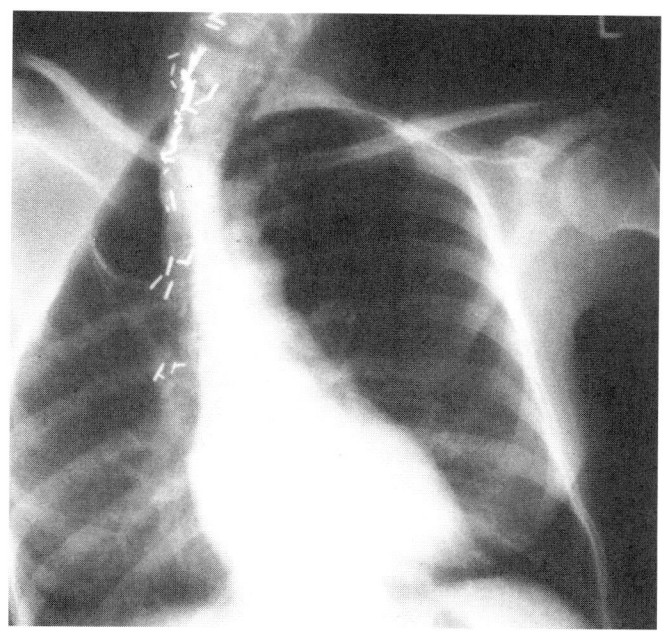

FIGURE 16.8. Tumor in Fig. 16.7 after complete resection en bloc with five ribs and partial vertebral bodies. Note the significant scoliosis. This patient is alive and well 20 years after resection.

that extends to the nape of the neck superiorly. In most instances, this approach provides the best surgical exposure. More recently, Dartevelle et al. (8) have advocated using an anterior transclavicular approach to deal with tumors situated more anteriorly in the thoracic inlet (Fig. 16.10).

Once the tumor has invaded the vertebral body or subclavian vessels (T4 disease) it is less likely that a complete resection can be achieved regardless of the approach. It is rare that long-term survival occurs after such a radical en bloc excision of vertebrae or vessels. However, recently Dartevelle et al. (8) using the anterior approach, has noted an improved long-term outcome by enabling a more complete resection.

The rationale for the radical en block resection is that when local resection is complete, then a cure is possible. If resection is incomplete, further radiotherapy may be added using either postoperative external-beam irradiation or intraoperative brachytherapy using interstitial implants or afterloading catheters.

Paulson (10), who pioneered this aggressive combined treatment, reported that in 75 patients there was a 31% actuarial 5-year survival rate for all patients, with a 44% 5-year survival rate if there were no nodal metastases; the resection rate was 99% in patients undergoing operations.

According to Hilaris et al. (11) preoperative radiotherapy increased the resectability rate without ad-

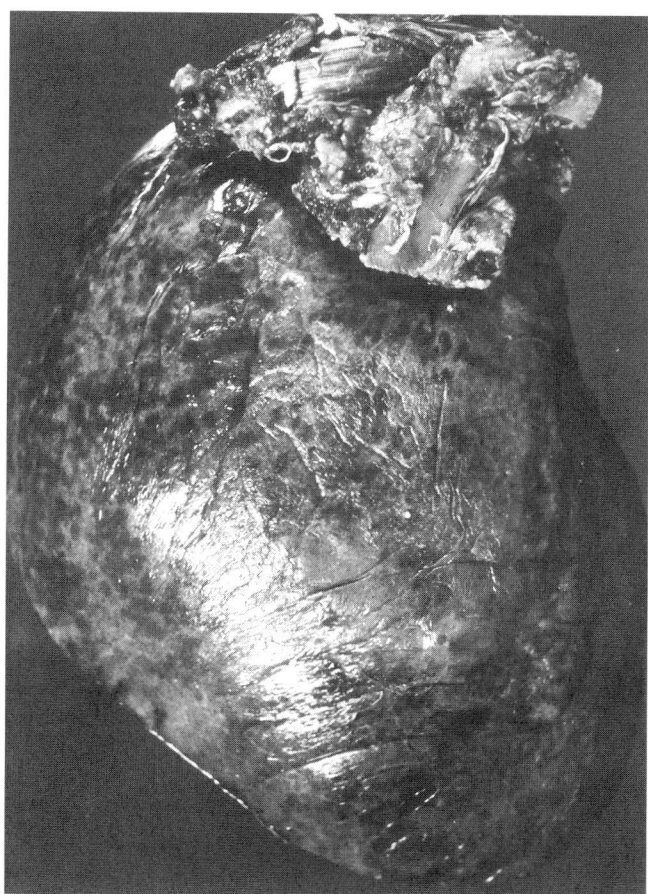

FIGURE 16.9. A right upper lobectomy specimen removed en bloc with the first three ribs.

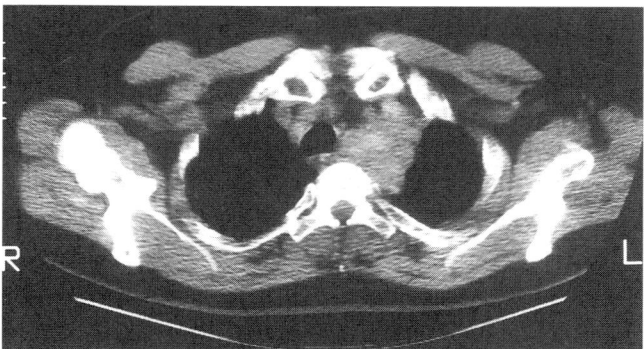

FIGURE 16.10. CT scan showing an anterior tumor abutting the subclavian vessels but not involving the posterior ribs. This tumor is suitable for an anterior approach.

versely affecting surgical morbidity and mortality and it improved actuarial 5-year survival rates. The real role of preoperative therapy has never been tested in a controlled fashion, however.

The importance of careful patient selection and cancer staging was confirmed by Stanford et al. (12) They reported a 5-year acturarial survival rate of approximately 50% with combined treatment when there was no evidence of cancer spread. In 1979, when Attar et al. (13) reported less-promising results of preoperative radiotherapy, not all of the 73 patients had resectable tumors; palpable, supraclavicular nodes were found in 18 patients, superior vena cava obstruction in 4, recurrent laryngeal nerve paralysis in 7, and phrenic nerve paralysis in 3 patients.

Recently at Memorial Sloan–Kettering Cancer Center, the results of surgical treatment in 124 patients who had undergone thoracotomy for superior sulcus tumors were analyzed. (14) (Table 16.2). Most received preoperative radiotherapy, but some had radiotherapy deferred to the postoperative period. One hundred patients were resected. The significant prognostic factors included the ability to resect completely, en bloc chest wall resection (versus extrapleural resection), and lobectomy (versus wedge resection) for the pulmonary component of the disease. The overall 5-year survival for resected patients was 30%, and for completely resected patients it was 41%. Fig. 16.11). In the group of patients with the best survival, i.e., those undergoing en bloc resection with lobectomy, a 60% 5-year survival was achieved. In this series, locoregional failure was significant in both completely resected and incompletely resected patients (72% of all failures); preoperative adverse factors included Horner's syndrome and clinically evident T4, N2 or N3 disease (Fig. 16.7).

In summary, surgical treatment for true superior pulmonary sulcus tumors must obtain complete local control of the cancer for cure. This control depends on proper selection of the patients, which in turn depends on accurate staging of the cancer. Operability and resectability should be defined carefully.

TABLE 16.2. Results of Thoracotomy for Superior Sulcus Tumors

	No. of Patients	Mo.	Survival 3 Yr (%)	5 Yr (%)
All thoracotomies	124	17	31	26
Incomplete resections	55	11	14	9
No resection	24	8	18	9
Wedge resection	22	11	10	10
Lobectomy	9	17	13	...
Complete resections	69	26	46	41
Wedge resection	47	21	39	33
Lobectomy	22	Not reached	60	60

PALLIATIVE SURGICAL TREATMENT

Poor local control of this tumor causes considerable suffering for the patient from intractable pain. These patients die in less than 2 years after enduring emotional, physiologic, and physical suffering. It is the pain caused by tumor invasion of the brachial plexus and nerve root compression in the intervertebral foramina that is the most difficult to control. Unfortunately, it has never been shown that a palliative surgical excision really palliates these symptoms for any significant time. However, when epidural compression is imminent, surgical maneuvers that alleviate this compression may be of value.

Interruption of the affected pain pathways to provide pain relief becomes necessary when antitumor treatment fails. The techniques currently used are percutaneous cervical cordotomy, selective posterior rhizotomy, stereotactic thalamotomy, commissural myelotomy, and rarely cingulotomy. When radical combined treatment for cure is not possible, other means of obtaining satisfactory pain relief must be considered, with radiotherapy being the most common but with surgery occasionally being required.

RADIOTHERAPY

Irradiation of superior sulcus tumors, as with other forms of lung cancer, may be considered as an exclusive treatment or as adjuvant to surgery (preoperatively or postoperatively). In addition, there is current interest in combined treatment with chemotherapy.

CURATIVE (PRIMARY) RADIOTHERAPY

The general question of whether superior sulcus tumors are biologically different from locally invasive NSCLCs has been discussed in several reports (15–17). A detailed comparison of clinically staged unresected superior sulcus tumors and other stage III cancers (all treated by radiotherapy alone) was performed by the Fox Chase group (15). In a review of 30 patients with superior sulcus tumors and 626 other stage III patients with disease, they found no significant differences in overall survival, local failure rates, or pattern of failure. Indeed, it is unlikely that the patterns of local and distant spread differ from those of other T3 tumors. This point is important because if true, it suggests that other clinical experience in treating lung cancer may be applied to this tumor. The reported experience of superior sulcus tumors has to some extent unduly emphasized surgical populations, who tend to have a better prognosis and who frequently have had other treat-

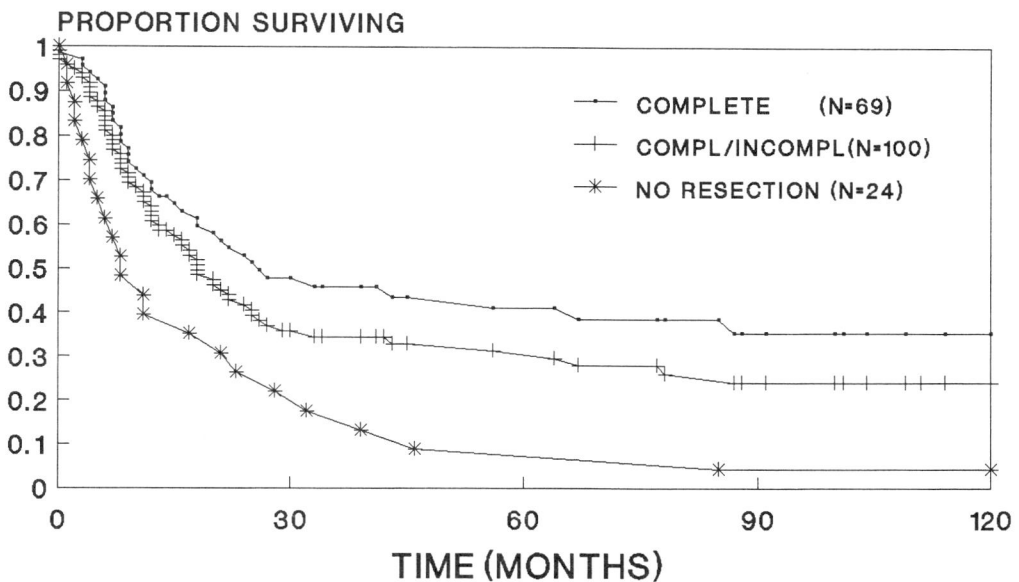

FIGURE 16.11. The 5- and 10-year survival of patients undergoing a complete resection, all patients undergoing resection, and patients not receiving resection at Memorial Sloan–Kettering Cancer Center.

ments (such as preoperative and/or postoperative radiotherapy) as well.

High-dose megavoltage radiotherapy for superior sulcus tumors demonstrated palliative benefit in the 1950s (18). Morris and Abadir (19) reported 22 patients treated with radiotherapy alone. They suggested that improved palliation was achieved using doses in excess of 60 Gy in 20 fractions, or equivalent. Since then various reports have sought evidence for a dose–local control relationship.

Komaki et al (20) reported a single-institution experience of 36 patients at the University of Wisconsin. One third of the patients had mediastinal involvement. The radiation dose varied from 40 to 64 Gy (1.8- to 2.4-Gy fractions), and fields encompassed mediastinal as well as primary tumor. They noted excellent symptom relief (86%; median duration, 12 months), local control in 17 of 36, with distant metastases in 9 of 17, and a 5-year overall survival of 23%. They emphasized the importance of using target volumes sufficient to treat mediastinal nodes as well as the tumor itself. Selection factors in this small series were not defined, but no factors prognostic for survival were identified in the analysis, except for the achievement of local control.

In a later report from the M.D. Anderson Cancer Center, Komaki and co-workers (21) reviewed 85 patients treated with a wide variety of combinations of surgery, radiation, and chemotherapy. The use of radiotherapy alone produced 2-year survivals in 7 (23%) of 31 and local control in 52% of unresectable tumors. Improved local control was associated with doses in excess of 65 Gy. A series from Rochester (22) found a 5-year survival of 18% in 31 patients treated with radiation alone (22 to 70 Gy). Local control again tended to be more likely with high radiation doses (more than 50 Gy) and more limited tumor extent.

There are no prospective studies of the dose–local control relationship. A 1992 series from the Veterans Administration (23) found a median survival of 14 months in 13 patients treated exclusively with radiotherapy. They emphasized the poor prognosis of patients considered unsuitable for resection at any time. Many of these series have noted distant failure in 40% to 50%, with the brain being at particular risk (20).

Although these and other reports emphasize local control as a prognostic factor predicting a favorable survival, this observation is not helpful in treatment decision making. Achievement of local control is a treatment effect, not a pretreatment prognostic factor. Thus, to associate local control with survival is simply a refinement of the old observation that responders to a given treatment live longer than nonresponders. This is not to deny the importance of achieving local control, which is of great palliative benefit as well as being a sine qua non for cure.

In appropriately selected patients, either surgery and/or radiotherapy may play a decisive role. Several studies have attempted a comparison between the combined regimen (radiation followed by surgery) and radiation alone (24, 25). The Memorial experience reported by Hilaris in 1974 (26) compared resectability in those receiving, or not receiving, preoperative irradiation. Complete resection was accomplished in 26% of those treated versus 9% in the untreated group. Other conclusions were that the survival of those treated with radiation alone was very poor, and that ultimate local control was not influenced by the use of preoperative radiation. However, these comparisons were uncontrolled.

Two reports from the University of California, Los Angeles, involving 28 (27) and 55 (28) patients, respectively, noted the grim prognosis associated with mediastinal adenopathy, and the superior survival associated with preoperative radiation (30 to 45 Gy) and surgery. Both reports emphasize the less favorable characteristics of the nonsurgical population. A 1991 study from Florida (16) compared these two approaches in a retrospective review of 32 patients receiving radiotherapy alone and 41 receiving preoperative radiotherapy followed by an attempted resection. They were careful to analyze by intention to treat and to comment extensively on the selection bias in the literature of this tumor. Despite the use of high doses of irradiation (65 Gy), local recurrence developed in 74%, the 5-year survival was 14%, and the treatment groups did not differ significantly in outcome. There was a substantial difference in the morbidity associated with the two treatments when the effects of the operation were taken into account.

ADJUVANT RADIOTHERAPY

Early descriptions of the tumor emphasized that the features of bone and nerve invasion were so characteristic that an extrapulmonary origin was considered for many years. Early reports of symptomatic responses to megavoltage radiotherapy (18) inspired combined modality approaches using radiotherapy and surgery. Treatment of this condition since has been influenced strongly by the reports of preoperative radiotherapy that first appeared in 1961 (6). There have been many subsequent series published, all characterized by uncertain selection criteria and a variety of treatment techniques. None is randomized, which reflects the relative rarity of the condition.

PREOPERATIVE RADIOTHERAPY

Shaw et al. (6) proposed that preoperative irradiation (30 to 35 Gy in approximately 2 weeks) would limit growth, block lymphatics, and destroy nests of malignant cells in perineural sheaths. They claimed evidence for this effect in histopathologic specimens, although control samples of tissue were not obtained before irradiation. Of the 18 patients in the initial report, 2 were disease free more than 3 years; the others had a follow-up of only up to 16 months. There were 5 patients with distant metastases and 1 had a local recurrence. This experience has been updated several times. A 1970 series (29) reported 57 patients selected and treated with preoperative irradiation. Twelve patients did not proceed to resection because of progression or refusal; 2 others died postoperatively and were excluded. The remaining 43 were then analyzed in terms of survival. Similarly, in the series of 131 patients reported in 1985, the analysis was actually based on the 78 patients completing the irradiation and surgery (not counting surgical mortality). The 5-year survival of these responding patients was 31%.

On the basis of an intent to treat analysis, in which the survival experience of all patients initially selected for treatment is analyzed, the 5-year survival would be substantially lower. The intention to treat analysis provides a much more realistic estimate of the effectiveness of therapy, including as it does all patients entering the selection process, not simply those who survive it. The value of this approach is now widely recognized (30). Any interpretation of the earlier literature must account for the fact that the analysis may be based on only the responders to the treatment. This factor has led to a somewhat uncritical enthusiasm in the literature for Paulson's method.

Nonetheless, this therapeutic approach has been practiced widely. All subsequent published series are retrospective, and most cover a long period during which surgical selection and technique may have changed, and the patient population may not have been stable because of changes in diagnostic methods. Control groups for comparison, if present, usually are based on the treatment selected rather than on host or tumor factors present at the time of treatment decision making; they are thus independent of treatment.

Certain general statements can be made, however. Tumors in this uncommon site may produce severe and troublesome symptoms, as noted by Pancoast. Without a satisfactory response to the initial treatment, the patient may develop severe and intractable problems before death. This progression has been the clinical justification for the aggressive approaches undertaken. Another important observation from the later series of Paulson (29) and others is the adverse prognosis associated with nodal involvement. This involvement, of course, is consistent with the behavior of bronchogenic carcinomas arising in other sites within the lung.

POSTOPERATIVE RADIOTHERAPY

The adjuvant role of postoperative radiotherapy in superior sulcus tumors is unknown and has not been explored properly. Many reports have included patients who were treated with postoperative radiotherapy (external and/or interstitial brachytherapy). This was often in response to an incomplete resection with known residual disease. In such cases the radiotherapy has, in effect, been interrupted, a practice that is thought to be disadvantageous radiobiologically and clinically. Because of case selection bias, it is impossible to draw definite conclusions about the efficacy of this approach. When the resection is complete, it is possible that local failure rates are improved somewhat but that overall survival rates are not altered, which is analogous to the experience of postoperative radiotherapy for completely resected cancer (31).

COMBINED MODALITY RADIOTHERAPY

Although many of the earlier reports have included administration of chemotherapy, there are no reports of its systematic use in this setting. Its contribution remains impossible to assess from existing data.

There is, however, increasing interest in the principle of induction chemotherapy (preoperative, neoadjuvant) for superior sulcus tumors. This concept has been proposed for several reasons. First, experience suggests the value of a preoperative therapy (although not established on a firm scientific basis). Second, overall results notwithstanding, many surgeons feel that any prior therapy that produced tumor shrinkage might lead to easier access at thoracotomy, and hence to increased resectability and reduced morbidity. Third, chemotherapy might have an effect on distant micrometastases, which are known to be important in the final outcome. Fourth, and most importantly, two recent large randomized trials in NSCLC have shown a modest but statistically significant benefit to the use of induction chemotherapy before high-dose radiation therapy in patients with stage III disease and generally favorable prognostic factors.

In locally advanced lung cancer, the Cancer and Leukemia Group B (CALGB) study (32, 33) found an increase in survival of 11% to 23% at 3 years when two cycles of vinblastine and cisplatin were administered before a course of radiotherapy to the primary tumor and mediastinum (60 Gy in 30 fractions). This study design was repeated in an intergroup study, and preliminary reports indicate a similar result (34). The response rates to chemotherapy alone were 4% complete and 22% partial in the CALGB study, whereas the combination of chemotherapy and radiation produced 19% complete and 27% partial responses. Another provocative result in locally advanced disease involving concurrent (not induction) chemotherapy was reported from the European Organization for the Research and Treatment of Cancer (35). In this study the addition of daily cisplatin to a regimen of high-dose radiotherapy resulted in improved rates of both local control and survival in a randomized trial. As noted, the cisplatin was given concurrently with (not before) the irradiation. This result may be relevant to the superior sulcus tumor, in which local control is such an important issue. Finally, there also has been a pilot program undertaken by the Southwest Oncology Group (36) that combined cisplatin with etoposide and concurrent radiotherapy (45 Gy in 25 fractions) for patients with bulky stage IIIA and selected IIIB disease. Three quarters of the patients were able to undergo resection, and one fifth of these patients had no tumor in the specimen.

These results cannot be considered directly applicable to the superior sulcus situation except by analogy. Nevertheless, an American intergroup trial has been proposed that would pilot an aggressive multimodality induction approach in patients with superior sulcus tumors, N0 or N1 disease as assessed by CT and mediastonoscopy, and medically fit for the whole program. This therapy would consist of etoposide, cisplatin, and concurrent irradiation (45 Gy in 25 fractions in 5 weeks) with nonprogressing patients proceeding to resection.

BRACHYTHERAPY

Intraoperative brachytherapy as an adjunct or definitive therapy was popularized at Memorial Sloan–Kettering

Cancer Center by Hilaris and colleagues (11). In incompletely resected patients or those who underwent thoracotomy without resection, it appeared that brachytherapy was useful in obtaining a 15% 5-year survival rate. However, this result never was compared with that for external beam radiation alone. In a recent analysis, use of brachytherapy as an adjunct after complete resection demonstrated no additional benefit when compared to the usual therapy for superior sulcus tumors, i.e., preoperative radiotherapy plus surgery or surgery followed by postoperative external-beam radiotherapy.

CONCLUSION

Apical chest tumors at one time were thought to be of a specific type and called superior pulmonary sulcus tumors or Pancoast tumors after the author who first drew attention to them and regarded them, incorrectly as it happened, as a specific type of extrapulmonary growth. In fact, their only peculiarity is their position, and most are primary lung cancers with no particular histologic predilection. These tumors tend to become locally invasive early in their progression, very often well before systemic spread occurs. The most common presenting symptom is the characteristic pain, present in more than 80% of patients.

Although it is likely that the natural history of tumors arising in the superior sulcus does not differ from that of other NSCLCs, a vigorous effort to achieve local control is important. Invasion of the chest wall, brachial plexus, mediastinum, or vertebral body carries grave consequences for the patient if unchecked. Initial evaluation to identify metastatic advanced nodal or local (T4) disease and the patient's general condition identify some patients whose prognosis or other considerations indicate treatment with palliative intent. Although this treatment usually means radiotherapy alone to doses in the range of 30 Gy in 10 fractions, the nature of the tumor and its location frequently suggest the need for high-dose radiotherapy to control symptoms or impending symptoms. Such patients would include those with vertebral body invasion, supraclavicular lymphadenopathy, or superior vena cava or other mediastinal invasion. Doses may reach 60 to 75 Gy, even though a dose control relationship for these tumors must be considered generally supported but not proven. Careful treatment planning is required to spare critical normal tissues, such as the spinal cord, from these high doses.

Potentially resectable patients should be evaluated with sophisticated imaging techniques, including MRI to determine the probability of residual disease remaining after surgery. If a complete resection with a margin of uninvolved tissue can be anticipated, surgery should be carried out.

At present, there is no scientific evidence to support preoperative radiotherapy in this subset of patients. On the contrary, to achieve the best possible local control, full-dose postoperative radiotherapy has at least a scientific basis.

If an incomplete resection is anticipated, three options present themselves. These are the traditional approach of preoperative radiation therapy, high-dose radiotherapy alone (or possibly with chemotherapy), or an experimental induction regimen of radiochemotherapy followed by resection, if possible. If the latter course is adopted, it is preferable that a collaborative protocol be followed. Only through participation of these patients in large-scale clinical trials can we expect to advance our knowledge of therapy for this challenging disease.

REFERENCES

1. Pancoast HK. Superior pulmonary sulcus tumors. Tumor characterized by pain, Horner's syndrome, destruction of bone and atrophy of hand muscles. JAMA 1932;99:1391–1396.
2. Hare ES. Tumor involving certain nerves. Lond Med Gaz 1838;1:16–18.
3. Pancoast HK. Importance of careful roentgen-ray investigations of apical chest tumors. JAMA 1924;83:1407–1411.
4. Hilaris BS, Martini N. Multimodality therapy of superior sulcus tumors. In: Bonica J, ed. Advances in pain research and therapy. New York: Raven Press, 1982;4:113–122.
5. Chardack WM, MacCallum JD. Pancoast tumor: five year survival without recurrence or metastases following radical resection and postoperative irradiation. J Thorac Surg 1956;31:535–542.
6. Shaw RR, Paulson DL, Lee JL. Treatment of the superior sulcus tumor by irradiation followed by resection. Ann Surg 1961;54:29–40.
7. Herbut PA, Watson JS. Tumor of thoracic inlet producing Pancoast syndrome: report of 17 cases and reviews of literature. Arch Pathol 1946;43:88–103.
8. Dartevelle PG, Chapelier AR, Macchiarini P, et al. Anterior transcervical thoracic approach for radical resection of lung tumors invading the thoracic inlet. J Thorac Cardiovasc Surg 1993;105:1025–1034.
9. Rice TW, Pringle JF, Sinclair JE, Cavanaugh KT, Ginsberg RJ. Superior sulcus tumors—results of treatment (abstract). IV World Conference on Lung Cancer. Lung Cancer 1985;2:44.
10. Paulson DL. Carcinomas in the superior pulmonary sulcus. J Thorac Cardiovasc Surg 1975;70:1095–1104.
11. Hilaris BS, Martini N, Wong GY, Dattatreyudu N. Treatment of superior sulcus tumor (Pancoast tumor). Surg Clin North Am 1987;67:965–977.
12. Stanford W, Barnes RP, Tucker AR. Influence of staging in superior sulcus (Pancoast) tumors of the lung. Ann Thorac Surg 1980;29:406–409.
13. Attar S, Miller JE, Satterfield J, et al. Pancoast's tumor: irradiation of surgery? Ann Thorac Surg 1979;28:578–586.
14. Ginsberg RJ, Martini N, Zaman M, Armstrong JG, Bains MS, Burt

ME, McCormack PM, et al. The influence of surgical resection and intraoperative brachytherapy in the management of superior sulcus tumor. Ann Thorac Surg 1994;57:1440–1445.
15. Herbert SH, Curran WJJ, Stafford PM, et al. Comparison of outcome between clinically staged, unresected superior sulcus tumors and other stage III non–small cell lung carcinomas treated with radiation therapy alone. Cancer 1992;69(2):363–369.
16. Neal CR, Amdur RJ, Mendenhall WM, et al. Pancoast tumor: radiation therapy alone versus preoperative radiation therapy and surgery. Int J Radiat Oncol Biol Phys 1991;21:651–660.
17. Van Houtte P, Rocmans P. Do superior sulcus tumors have a better prognosis than other lung cancer sites? Int J Radiat Oncol Biol Phys 1990;19(3):823–824.
18. Haas LL, Harvey RA, Langer SS. Radiation management of otherwise hopeless thoracic neoplasms. JAMA 1954;154:323–326.
19. Morris RW, Abadir R. Pancoast tumor: the value of high dose radiation therapy. Radiology 1979;132:717–719.
20. Komaki R, Roh J, Cox J, et al. Superior sulcus tumors: results of irradiation in 36 patients. Cancer 1981;48:1563–1568.
21. Komaki R, Mountain C, Holbert J, et al. Superior sulcus tumors: treatment selection and results for 85 patients without metastasis (M0) at presentation. Int J Radiat Oncol Biol Phys 1990;19(1):31–36.
22. VanHoutte P, MacLennan I, Poulter C, Rubin P. External Radiation in the management of superior sulcus tumor. Cancer 1984;54:223–227.
23. Taylor LQ, Williams AJ, Santiago SM. Survival in patients with superior pulmonary sulcus tumors. Respiration 1992;59:27–29.
24. Paulson DL. Technical considerations in stage III disease: the superior sulcus lesion. In: Delaru NC, Eschapasse H, eds: International trends in thoracic surgery. Philadelphia: WB Saunders 1985;I:121–133.
25. Miller JI, Mansour KA, Hatcher CR. Carcinoma of the superior pulmonary sulcus. Ann Thorac Surg 1979;28:44–47.
26. Hilaris BS, Martini N, Luomanen RKJ, et al. The value of preoperative radiation therapy in apical cancer of the lung. Surg Clin North Am 1974;54(4):831–840.
27. Beyer DC, Wiesenburger T. Superior sulcus tumors. Am J Clin Oncol 1986;9(2):156–161.
28. Anderson TM, May PM, Holmes EC. Factors affecting survival in superior sulcus tumors. J Clin Oncol 1986;4(11):1598–1603.
29. Paulson DL. The role of preoperative radiation therapy in the surgical management of carcinoma in the superior pulmonary sulcus. Front Radiat Ther Oncol 1970;5:177–187.
30. Simon R, Wittes RE. Methodologic guidelines for reports of clinical trials. Cancer Treat Rep 1985;69:1–3.
31. Payne DG. Is preoperative or postoperative radiation therapy indicated in non–small cell cancer of the lung? Lung Cancer 1994;10(Suppl 1):S205–S212.
32. Dillman RO, Seagren SL, Herndon J, et al. Randomized trial of induction chemotherapy plus radiation therapy vs RT alone in stage III non–small cell lung cancer (NSCLC): five year followup of CALGB 84-33 (abstract 1092). Proc Am Soc Clin Oncol 1993;12:329.
33. Dillman RO, Seagren SL, Propert KJ, et al. A randomized trial of induction chemotherapy plus high-dose radiation versus radiation alone in stage III non–small-cell lung cancer. N Engl J Med 1990;323(14):940–945.
34. Sause WT, Scott C, Taylor S, et al. Radiation Therapy Oncology Group (RTOG) 88-08 and Eastern Cooperative Oncology Group (ECOG) 4588: preliminary results of a phase III trial in regionally advanced unresectable non–small cell lung cancer. J Natl Cancer Insti 1995;87(3):198–204.
35. Schaake-Koning C, Van Den Bogaert W, Dalesio O, et al. Effects of concomitant cisplatin and radiotherapy on inoperable non–small-cell lung cancer. N Engl J Med 1992;326(8):524–530.
36. Rusch V, Albain KS, Crowley JJ, et al. Surgical resection of stage IIIA and stage IIIB non–small cell lung cancer after concurrent induction chemoradiotherapy. J Thorac Cardiovasc Surg 1994;105:97–106.

17

THERAPEUTIC OPTIONS IN LOCALLY ADVANCED NON–SMALL CELL LUNG CANCER (STAGE IIIB)

Thierry Le Chevalier and Rodrigo Arriagada

INTRODUCTION

Despite increased public awareness of the dangers of smoking and recent measures enacted in many countries to curtail smoking in the workplace and in other public places, cigarette smoking continues to be the leading cause of preventable morbidity and mortality in the industrialized world (1). Non–small cell lung carcinoma (NSCLC), which accounts for 80% of lung cancers, is tobacco related in more than 80% of cases (2). It is the leading cause of mortality from cancer in males in Western countries (3). Locally advanced NSCLC without distant metastases (stage III disease) involves a subset of patients considered inoperable at time of presentation because of a lack of benefit from initial surgical resection. Patients are classified conventionally as having stage IIIA disease when the tumor is marginally resectable or stage IIIB when it is definitively unresectable. For a long time thoracic radiotherapy has been the standard treatment of stage III patients. Considering the activity of new chemotherapeutic agents or regimens, a revision of the therapeutic strategies in such patients is needed. Additionally, the limits of thoracic radiotherapy call for a reevaluation of the role of surgery in local control after preoperative chemotherapy or combined chemotherapy and radiotherapy. Furthermore, the use of radio-sensitizers or new fractionated schedules of irradiation must be evaluated also. This chapter reports data and trends in staging procedures and discusses therapeutic approaches in patients with stage III NSCLC.

ANATOMY

The anatomy of the lungs is discussed elsewhere in this book. A succinct review of the main structures concerned by locoregional involvement of lung tumors is relevant here for a better understanding of the pathways of extension, limitations of surgical management, and complications related to radiotherapy on crucial organ structures.

Briefly, the right lung consists of three lobes: upper, middle, and lower. The lobes are separated from each other by two fissures: the oblique or major fissure, and the horizontal or minor fissure. The left lung consists of two lobes that are separated by a single fissure. The lingular portion of the left upper lobe corresponds to the middle lobe of the right. The trachea enters the superior mediastinum and bifurcates approximately at the level of the fifth thoracic vertebra. The hila of the lungs contain the bronchi, pulmonary arteries and veins, various branches from the pulmonary plexus, bronchial arteries and veins, and lymphatics.

The lung has a highly developed network of lymphatic vessels throughout its loose interstitial connective tissue, draining into the various regional lymph nodes (Fig. 17.1). The intrapulmonary lymph nodes may be connected to segmental bronchi or be located at the bifurcation of branches of the pulmonary artery. Most of the lymphatic drainage of both lungs ultimately reaches the right superior mediastinal and right supraclavicular areas.

From the radiologist's viewpoint (Fig. 17.2), the bronchopulmonary lymph nodes, located either along the lower portions of the main bronchi (hilar lymph nodes) or at the bifurcations of the main bronchi into lobar bronchi (interlobar nodes), form the hilar nodes. The mediastinal lymph nodes are divided into two groups: the superior, located above the bifurcation of the trachea (carina), including the upper paratracheal, pretracheal, retrotracheal, lower paratracheal nodes (azygos nodes), and a group of nodes located in the aortic window; and the inferior, located in the subcarinal region and inferior mediastinum, including the sub-

17 Therapeutic Options in Locally Advanced Non–Small Cell Lung Cancer (Stage IIIB)

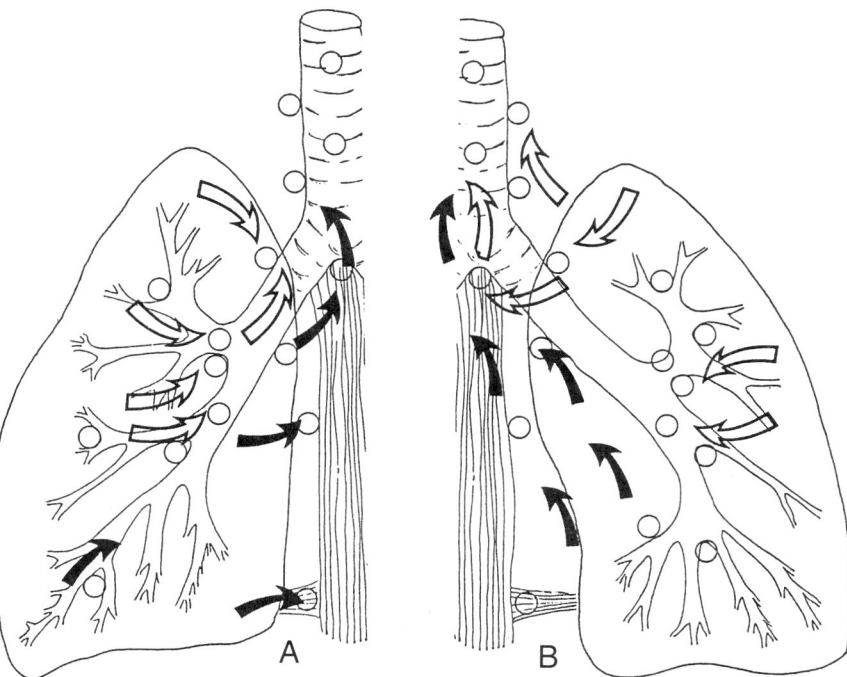

FIGURE 17.1. Regional lymphatic drainage. **A.** Right lung. **B.** Left lung. Note the drainage *(arrows)* from the lower lobes.

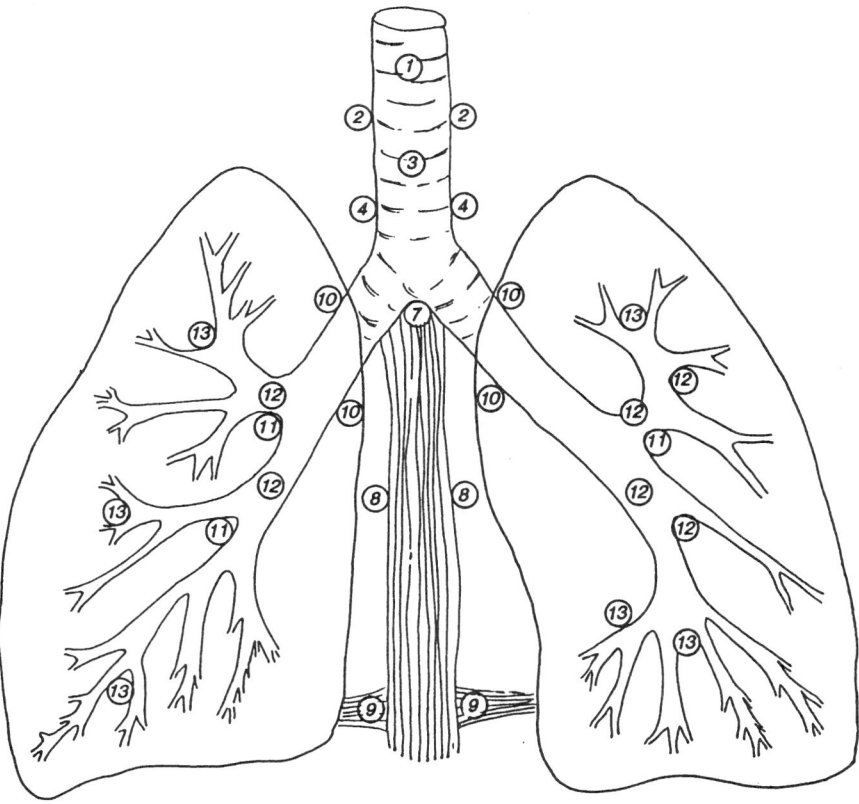

FIGURE 17.2. Lymph node distribution in N2-N3 disease showing mediastinal lymph nodes. Superior mediastinal nodes: 1, highest mediastinal; 2, upper paratracheal; 3, pretracheal or retrotracheal; 4, lower paratracheal (including azygos nodes). Aortic nodes: 5, subaortic (aortic window) (not shown); and 6, paraaortic (ascending aorta or phrenic) (not shown). Inferior mediastinal nodes: 7, subcarinal; 8, paraesophageal (below carina); 9, pulmonary ligament. Lymph node distribution in N1 disease: 10, hilar nodes; 11, interlobar nodes; 12, lobar nodes; 13, segmental nodes.

carinal, paraesophageal, and pulmonary ligament nodes. As a primary tumor grows in the lung parenchyma or the bronchial wall, it invades lymphatics and blood vessels, resulting in an extension to regional lymph nodes and distant metastases. In most cases lymphatic spread occurs before other metastatic sites develop.

Metastatic lymphatic spread of lung cancer follows these channels with tumors involving bronchopulmonary, mediastinal, and supraclavicular lymph nodes. The primary tumor can spread to adjacent structures, including the mediastinum (e.g., heart, esophagus), pleura, chest wall, vertebra, and diaphragm. The larger the locoregional involvement, the greater the risk of distant metastases, i.e., most commonly to bone, liver, adrenals, and brain.

PATHOLOGY

The World Health Organization established a histologic classification system for lung neoplasms (4). Four major cell types account for 95% of all primary lung tumors: squamous or epidermoid carcinoma, adenocarcinoma, large cell carcinoma, and small cell carcinoma. The other 5% consist of combined types. It is widely accepted that small cell lung carcinomas, which have clinical, biologic, and therapeutic specificities, are distinct, and that the other three histologic types, for which there are no major clinical or therapeutic differences, are pooled. These are the non–small cell lung carcinomas and represent approximately 80% of all lung tumors. Distant metastases develop more commonly in patients with adenocarcinoma or large cell carcinoma, whereas squamous cell carcinomas are more likely to metastasize locally (5). Nevertheless, there is no clear difference among the various types with regard to outcome of patients with locally advanced NSCLC or with identical staging. Furthermore, the biopsy specimen obtained in locally advanced disease is generally small and represents only a very limited part of the whole tumor. Thus, management of locally advanced NSCLC generally does not take the histology of the tumor into account.

STAGING

Staging of lung cancer is important because tumor, node, and metastasis (T, N, and M) findings influence the prospects for therapeutic management. According to the International Stage Classification system, locally advanced NSCLC refers to stage IIIA and stage IIIB. Stage III disease concerns patients for whom, despite the lack of macroscopic distant metastases, T or N extension obscures the prognosis. Two subsets of patients are considered: those for whom surgical resection, even if technically possible, is not clearly beneficial (stage IIIA), and those considered definitively unresectable or for whom it is futile to attempt the resection of all malignant tissue (stage IIIB).

The staging of patients with lung cancer consists of two parts: first, identification of the tumor location and extension (anatomic staging), and second, assessment of the patient's ability to withstand various antitumor treatments (physiologic staging). Although a complete clinical workup is part of good clinical practice, the comprehensiveness of the workup is much more debatable. The staging procedure may vary from one center to another, and there is no general consensus on its extent.

The current TNM classification of lung cancer is shown in Table 17.1 (6, 7). The T (tumor size), N (locoregional node involvement), and M (presence or absence of distant metastases) characteristics determine different stage groupings. The primary tumor is subdivided into four categories, depending on size, site, and local involvement (T1–4). Lymph node spread is subdivided into bronchopulmonary or hilar (N1), ipsilateral mediastinal (N2), and contralateral or supraclavicular involvement (N3), and metastases are either absent (M0) or present (M1). Staging was revised and updated in 1986 when Mountain (7) proposed a new international staging system based on the most recent diagnostic modalities and prognosis. Table 17.2 shows the staging system currently in use.

Stage IIIB disease includes patients with extensive pulmonary tumors (T4 and/or N3 disease). T4 tumors may invade the mediastinal structures (carina, trachea, heart and great vessels, esophagus, and vertebral bodies) and/or cause malignant pleural effusions. N3 disease includes patients with metastases to contralateral mediastinal or hilar nodes or ipsilateral or contralateral supraclavicular nodes (Table 17.1). In fact, staging is troublesome, particularly in patients with large N2 disease involving the mediastinal fat and those who should be considered T4 for the purpose of planning therapy. New attempts to clarify the international classification system have been proposed recently and will be valuable for improved assessment of reported clinical trials (8).

CLINICAL PRESENTATION

Malignancies produce clinical symptoms in three general ways: by direct effects resulting from invasion or compression of normal tissues; by release of cy-

TABLE 17.1. Tumor, Node, Metastasis (TNM Classification)

PRIMARY TUMOR (T)

TX, tumor proven by the presence of malignant cells in bronchopulmonary secretions but not visualized roentgenographically or bronchoscopically; or any tumor that cannot be assessed, as in a retreatment staging

T0, no evidence of primary tumor

TIS, carcinoma in situ

T1, a tumor that is ≤3 cm in greatest dimension, surrounded by lung or visceral pleura, and without evidence of invasion proximal to a lobar bronchus at bronchoscopy

T2, a tumor more than 3 cm in greatest dimension, or a tumor of any size that either invades the visceral pleura or has associated atelectasis or obstructive pneumonitis extending to the hilar region. At bronchoscopy, the proximal extent of demonstrable tumors must be within a lobar bronchus or at least 2 cm distal to the carina. Any associated atelectasis or obstructive pneumonitis must involve less than an entire lung.

T3, a tumor of any size with direct extension into the chest wall (including superior sulcus tumors), diaphragm, or the mediastinal pleura or pericardium without involving the heart, great vessels, trachea, esophagus, or vertebral body; or a tumor in the main bronchus within 2 cm of the carina without involving the carina

T4, a tumor of any size with invasion of the mediastinum; or one involving the heart, great vessels, trachea, esophagus, vertebral body, or carina, or the presence of malignant pleural effusion

NODAL INVOLVEMENT (N)

N0, no demonstrable metastasis to regional lymph nodes

N1, metastasis to lymph nodes in the peribronchial or ipsilateral hilar region or both, including direct extension

N2, metastasis to ipsilateral, mediastinal lymph nodes and subcarinal lymph nodes

N3, metastasis to contralateral mediastinal lymph nodes, contralateral hilar lymph nodes, ipsilateral or contralateral scalene, or supraclavicular lymph nodes

DISTANT METASTASES (M)

M0, no (known) distant metastasis

M1, distant metastasis present at specific site(s)

From Mountain CF. A new international staging system for lung cancer. Chest 1986;89:225–233.

TABLE 17.2. Stage Grouping

STAGE	TUMOR	NODES	METASTASIS
I	T1	N0	M0
I	T2	N0	M0
II	T1	N1	M0
II	T2	N1	M0
IIIA	T3	N0	M0
IIIA	T3	N1	M0
IIIA	T1	N2	M0
IIIA	T2	N2	M0
IIIA	T3	N2	M0
IIIB	Any T	N3	M0
IIIB	T4	Any N	M0
IV	Any T	Any N	M1

tokines, hormones, or other biologically active agents into the local and systemic environment; and by psychologic effects on the patient. Each of these factors may contribute to the extent of illness experienced by the patient.

All lung cancer patients should have a complete history and physical examination with determination of performance status (based on the Karnofsky index [9] or other performance status scale such those proposed by the Eastern Cooperative Oncology Group [ECOG] or the World Health Organization) and weight loss.

In the case of locally advanced disease, the main local symptoms are dyspnea, which is related to obstruction of a main bronchus or to a pleural effusion; pain, which results from chest wall involvement; hemoptysis; cough; hoarseness; infection; and superior vena cava syndrome (SVCS). Pericardial involvement can result in cardiac tamponade.

A malignant lesion may not cause symptoms in a patient with early-stage lung cancer. Lung tumors develop insidiously in many cases for a period of time, which explains why initial nonspecific complaints, e.g., weakness and weight loss, may be the sole clinical manifestations of this disease in a population of cigarette smokers who frequently develop cough and chronic bronchitis. In most cases tumors cause clinical problems as a result of local extension (with obliteration of normal tissues), i.e., as malignant cells proliferate in the confines of the involved organ, they may compromise oxygen exchange in involved alveoli. Another effect of localized tumor expansion is the compression of normal structures, with partial or complete obstruction of tubular organs, blood vessels, and lymphatics, thus producing blocked airflow through bronchi and obstruction of pulmonary venous return. Among patients with locally advanced disease, hemoptysis occurs in about half of cases (10). Dyspnea may result from large tumors, especially in the upper pulmonary lobes, with massive mediastinal involvement and bronchus obstruction; from pleural effusion; or from phrenic nerve involvement leading to paralysis of a hemidiaphragm. Chest pain can be related to chest wall or pleural involvement. Hoarseness reveals paralysis of the vocal cord related to left recurrent nerve involvement or entrapment in its thoracic pathway. Extension to the pericardium may result in cardiac tamponade. A tumor in the right lung or right mediastinal lymph node involvement can cause SVCS or Horner's syndrome. Infection is a frequent complication and can be the revealing symptom of the disease.

Most patients with inoperable NSCLC have symptoms related to their disease at the time of examination. The high incidence of such symptoms and their severity may require rapid specific treatment with careful management of each symptom. Although lung carcinoma can metastasize to almost any organ, the most common sites of involvement are the pleura (distant from the primary tumor), lung, lymph nodes, brain, adrenals, and liver (10).

DIAGNOSTIC WORKUP

The main biologic and histopathologic characteristics of NSCLC are discussed elsewhere in this book. Clinical and radiologic assessment are crucial for accurate staging of these patients, particularly in the case of bulky tumors and/or lymphatic involvement. Staging usually widens the screening for metastases in the most common sites at risk, i.e., bone, brain, adrenals, and liver.

Chest radiography and computed axial tomography (CT) scan are the best noninvasive imaging techniques and can clearly depict tumor extension and mediastinal involvement (11). Figures 17.3 and 17.4 show typical radiologic aspects of patients with T4 tumor or N3 contralateral lymph node extension.

More sophisticated imaging techniques include nuclear magnetic resonance imaging (MRI) (12) and gallium scanning (13). The use of transesophageal ul-

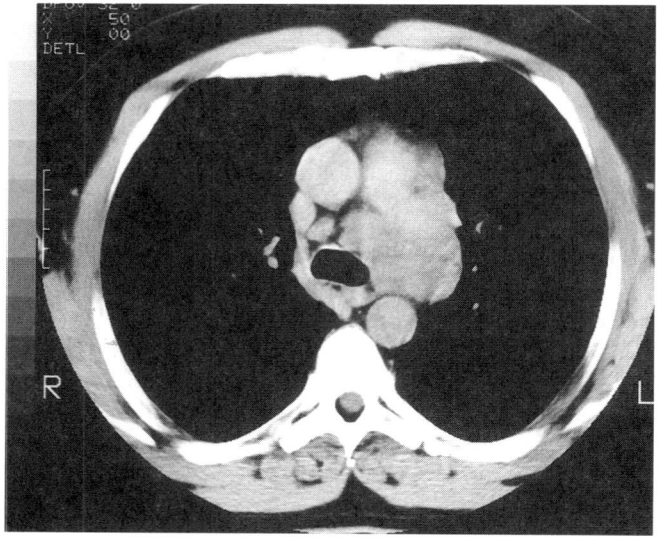

FIGURE 17.3. CT scan of a patient presenting with left lobar superior NSCLC (T4) involving the mediastinum.

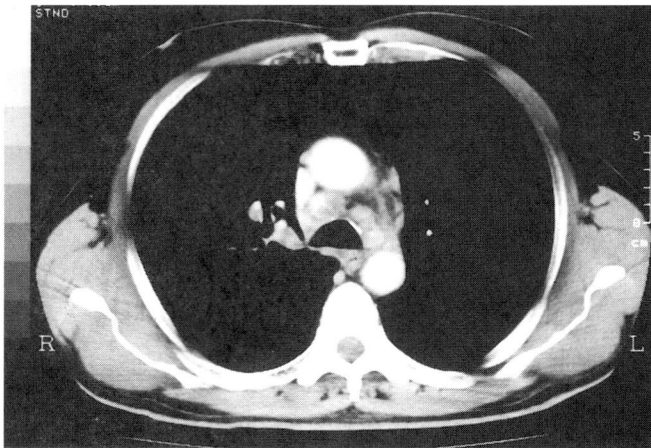

FIGURE 17.4. CT scan of a patient presenting with bilateral mediastinal lymph node involvement (N3).

trasound and an esophageal probe has been proposed recently to assess better the presence of lymph nodes (14). However, this technique has not offered a significantly better definition of stage III disease and has no clear impact on therapeutic strategies.

FIBEROPTIC BRONCHOSCOPY

Fiberoptic bronchoscopy is the main procedure used to stage the tumor and to determine whether a surgical procedure can be proposed. It provides meaningful information about the relationship among the tumor, carina, trachea, and contralateral main bronchus. It also may suggest subcarinal or laterotracheal lymph node involvement or eliminate other macroscopic or microscopic bronchial lesions. Furthermore, it establishes a pathologic diagnosis of the lesion.

MEDIASTINOSCOPY

Mediastinoscopy is an endoscopic examination of the mediastinum through a midline incision just above the thoracic inlet. It confirms mediastinal lymph node staging in addition to the information offered by the CT scan, and it facilitates treatment planning. This procedure is effective and safe (15). It is a valuable tool for staging of NSCLC before induction chemotherapy or chemoradiotherapy to determine whether a tumor is potentially resectable. It enables the physician to establish the definitive unresectability of the tumor, i.e., stage IIIB disease.

SUPERIOR VENA CAVA SYNDROME

SVCS is caused by stenosis or occlusion of the superior vena cava. It occurs frequently as a complication of NSCLC or a mediastinal tumor (16). Resulting symptoms include dyspnea, headache, and cough, whereas dysphagia, orthopnea, syncope, stridor, and mental confusion are less common. Clinical examination reveals distension of the jugular veins, and edema in the upper limbs, neck and face, and upper body collateral circulation. The nature of this obstruction is apparent in only the approximately 40% of patients in whom symptoms develop, whereas SVCS reveals the presence of a mediastinal tumor in almost one of two cases. With regard to the emergence of presentation, it can be difficult to obtain histologic proof of the malignancy before starting treatment.

Chest radiography is of limited value: widening of the mediastinum, the most frequent abnormality, is observed in approximately 80% of cases. A right hilar mass, bilateral pleural effusion, cardiomegaly, collapsed right upper lobe, or anterior mediastinal mass also can be seen.

CT scanning currently is the first-line diagnostic procedure to evaluate SVCS (17). The most common direct signs are SVC obstruction, displacement, compression, or invasion of the SVC by the mass lesion; indirect signs include the development of collateral circulation. CT scanning provides an evaluation of all abnormalities associated with the mediastinum before radiotherapy or chemotherapy and also can guide fiberoptic bronchoscopy or fine-needle biopsy to determine the etiology.

Venography provides a more precise location of the tumor mass and its effects on the SVC, including development of a collateral circulation, and it evaluates possible treatment with balloon angioplasty and installation of an expandable endovascular prosthesis (metallic stent) (18). MRI provides superior technical information but requires the availability of this imaging device. Patients also must remain supine during the procedure, which can be difficult because of their respiratory status.

EXTRATHORACIC ASSESSMENT

In locally advanced NSCLC, because of the high risk of distant disease, a routine workup assessing the most frequent metastatic sites is recommended, as shown in Table 17.3. In case of doubt more precise techniques can be proposed, and a cytologic or histologic procedure may be useful, as shown in Table 17.4.

TABLE 17.3. Diagnostic Workup Recommended in Locally Advanced NSCLC

Treatment	Routine Treatment	Research Protocol
Complete blood count + chemistries	+	+
Chest x-ray	+	+
Fiberoptic bronchoscopy	+	+
Chest CT scan	+	+
Liver/adrenal ultrasound or CT scan	+	+
Brain CT scan	+	+
Bone scan	...	+
NSE	...	+
CEA	...	+
LDH	...	+

Abbreviations. NSE, neuron specific enolase; CEA, carcinoembryonic antigen; LDH, lactic dehygrogenase.

TABLE 17.4. Diagnostic Workup for Metastases

Site	Standard Workup	In Case of Doubt
Bone	Bone scan	Radiography, CT scan, MRI
Liver	Ultrasound	CT scan, laparoscopy, MRI
Adrenals	Ultrasound or CT scan	Fine-needle biopsy
Lung	CT scan	Fine-needle biopsy
Brain	CT scan	MRI

Abbreviation. MRI, magnetic resonance imaging.

In investigational protocols, some additional tests may be ordered to decrease the risk of undetected distant metastases.

PROGNOSTIC FACTORS

Prognostic factors are patient or disease characteristics determined before the start of treatment that are significantly and independently correlated with disease progression or outcome. They are used primarily in selecting case management strategy, designing clinical trials, and improving the sensitivity of evaluations of therapy.

CLINICAL FACTORS

Many clinical prognostic factors have been analyzed. Their value is open to debate and is the subject of another chapter of this book. Briefly, the notion of local extension and metastatic dissemination (19–22) are the decisive features in the overall outcome.

Recent weight loss, generally qualified as a percentage of total weight, also is of prognostic importance (19–22). Prognosis is related closely to the patient's overall condition at the initial evaluation and involves the decision regarding whether to continue the workup and initiate aggressive therapy. In summary, clinical findings inform the physician mainly on the approach to be taken regarding additional laboratory investigations and curative treatment.

BIOLOGIC FACTORS

In addition to clinical findings, laboratory tests are done routinely in patients with bronchial tumors, and the prognostic value of some of them has been studied carefully. Among common criteria of prognostic value, leukocytosis and, particularly, increased neutrophilia (often related to the presence of physical signs suggesting metastases) as well as the proportion of lymphocytes should be noted. Similarly, hypoalbuminemia and an increased sedimentation rate carry a poor prognosis (19, 21, 23, 24).

The presence of two of these abnormalities carries a significantly poorer prognosis compared with their absence or the presence of only one sign (23). Also, elevated levels of lactate dehydrogenase (LDH) and alkaline phosphatase are observed most often in patients with metastases (20). More recently, a certain number of other biologic factors of prognostic value, such as ploidy, have been studied, as well as the thymidine labeling index and flow cytometric analysis (25–29). The above-mentioned biologic parameters are not specific and are not used currently in the management of NSCLC.

CONCEPT OF LOCAL CONTROL IN LOCALLY ADVANCED NSCLC

Absence of local control is a major problem in obtaining a long-term cure in locally advanced NSCLC because the 2-year rate of local failure is 90% after "curative" radiotherapy (30–33). The definition of local control varies widely from one medical team to another. There are several reasons for these variations. For instance, the definition of complete remission can include the use of chest radiography, thoracic CT scanning, fiberoptic bronchoscopy, and systematic biopsies. To determine the rate of local control reported in the literature, investigators may use different numerators in ratios: all patients (assumed to be controlled locally by treatment), all responders (partial or minor), or all patients with stable disease. In the denominator they can restrict their definition to complete responders, or all patients or only evaluable patients. Events considered in the actuarial determination of local control curves may include death and local recurrence, death and evidence of local progression (after stable disease), local recurrence only after complete or partial regression, or evidence of local progression only after any type of symptomatic control, i.e., including stabilization. The methodology used to calculate estimators of the local recurrence rate includes total events, censored events, or competing events (34, 35). If all of these possibilities are combined, there are more than 250 different ways to express local control, without taking into account the quality of follow-up and the different possibilities of plotting data graphically.

From these considerations it is clear that the definition of local control, as used today, has all the characteristics of a "soft" endpoint. This situation is far from ideal in the evaluation of treatments attempting to improve local control, because treatment response is the major endpoint in phase II studies.

Several recommendations are offered to clarify the treatment effect on local control by obtaining a "harder" endpoint: (*a*) to define the complete remission by a chest CT scan, fiberoptic bronchoscopy, and routine biopsies; (*b*) to include only complete remission patients in the numerator; (*c*) to include all patients in the denominator; (*d*) to include local recurrence after complete remission as the only event in the determination of local control curves; and finally, (*e*) to use a competing risk approach that provides the advantage of considering other events, such as distant metastatic recurrence, simultaneously (34, 35). At the least, reports and publications should state unambiguously which options are used in the definition of local control.

TREATMENT

Surgery is the only established curative treatment of NSCLC. When tumors cannot be resected because of significant thoracic extension or distant metastases, the potential for cure decreases drastically.

Although radiotherapy can play an important role in the control of such tumors, the main reason for therapeutic failure in partially or nonresected tumors is the development of resistance to radiation, thus leading to local or distant progression. In fact, in stage IIIB disease, which is considered unresectable, radiation is unfortunately merely palliative, and the long-term survival rate does not exceed 5% with the use of this single-treatment modality (30–33).

NSCLC usually has been considered poorly sensitive to chemotherapy (36, 37). It is therefore important to establish the precise value of chemotherapy in the treatment of this disease in earlier stages and not focus solely on the modest rates of survival observed in metastatic forms. Drugs are combined to prevent chemoresistance. If the drugs used are not cross-resistant and are comparable in overall safety, the risk of cell proliferation is reduced greatly. Although the advantage of combining drugs has been demonstrated in clinical practice, such as with the use of mechlorethamine, vincristine, procarbazine, and prednisone (MOPP) in the treatment of Hodgkin's disease (38), these combinations often are difficult to administer in lung cancer patients because of increased and unacceptable overall toxicity (39). A number of theoretical and experimental models have been developed to optimize treatment and prevent the proliferation of resistant cell clones. These models have highlighted the importance of dose intensity, a concept that is considered more typically in cases of chemosensitive malignancies, but that is evaluated rarely and perhaps underestimated in NSCLC (40).

Because combination chemotherapy could produce objective tumor regressions in advanced NSCLC, using chemotherapy for earlier stages of disease, such as regionally advanced disease, seemed reasonable. Thus, combined modality studies in patients with NSCLC have become a major area of clinical research.

The theoretical advantages of combining radiotherapy and chemotherapy are the spatial cooperation (between local irradiation and local and systemic chemotherapy effects) and the ability to prevent development of resistance to treatment. Even though examples of cross-resistance between radiotherapy and chemotherapy have been cited by some investigators, they are relatively rare, and the radiosensitivity of most chemoresistant tumor populations remains unchanged.

Moreover, because the toxic effects differ according to normal tissue type, it is possible to avoid any need for a reduction in either chemotherapy or radiotherapy doses; however, the timing of use of these two modalities remains debatable. Combinations used, timing, drug selection and doses, and radiation parameters are some of the major aspects of this multimodality treatment approach that are discussed in this chapter.

RADIOTHERAPY

For many years radiotherapy alone has been the treatment of choice for patients with stage IIIB NSCLC. The results obtained, however, have generally been disappointing. Many uncontrolled studies have been published showing a 1-year survival rate ranging from 29% to 58% and a 5-year survival rate ranging from 4% to 10% (41).

Only two randomized studies have been conducted in which an irradiated group was compared with an untreated group. The earliest of these studies was reported by Durrant et al. (42). In this study 249 patients were randomized to no treatment ($n = 63$) or radiotherapy, 40 Gy given by cobalt 60 (^{60}Co) or orthovoltage photon beams, to the primary tumor as well as the mediastinal nodes ($n = 62$). Another group of patients was given chemotherapy (nitrogen mustard) ($n = 63$), or a combination of radiotherapy and nitrogen mustard ($n = 61$). No advantage was found in any of the groups, and the mean survival time ranged from 8.3 to 8.8 months.

Moderate benefit in terms of median survival (although not statistically significant) was achieved in a large randomized trial conducted by Roswit et al. (43) comparing radiotherapy alone to no treatment. Most patients in the radiotherapy arm of the study were treated with 200 to 300 kV (orthovoltage). This old-fashioned technique has since the 1960s been replaced by megavoltage radiation (^{60}Co or high-energy photon beams produced by linear accelerators). This method led to a decrease in radiation-related side effects and enabled higher total doses to be delivered to the tumor. Some randomized trials also have sought to make such a comparison; all have encountered problems in recruiting patients because allowing half of the patients to receive no treatment, even when they are symptomatic, has not been accepted easily by either physicians or patients.

For many years there has been a considerable interest in the dose-time relationship in radiotherapy (44), and many studies assessing time-dose factors for NSCLC radiotherapy have been conducted.

RADIOTHERAPY PARAMETERS

Multiple parameters, such as the total dose of radiation, fraction size, volume and type of irradiated normal tissues, definition of the target volume, and quality control of radiotherapy techniques, should be considered in the management of stage IIIB NSCLC. These factors, which are reviewed in the chapter on radiotherapy elsewhere in this book, are of paramount importance in the planning and effects of combined approaches. Unfortunately, radiation parameters are poorly described in most study reports, and often it is difficult to determine the real reasons for the discrepant results found in the literature. For example, if the irradiated volume is exiguous, then there is a feasible explanation for a high rate of local recurrence at the border of the radiation fields; in contrast, the high incidence of related complications reported in some trials could be explained by an irradiated volume that is too large. Low doses can account for a high incidence of in-field recurrences, and doses that are too high may explain an increased rate of radiation complications.

The importance of the quality of radiotherapy has been stressed by many reports, and some of them have shown a significant impact on long-term local control and a potential survival benefit with adequate radiation technique (45–47). Indeed, all previous considerations are valid only if the quality of the radiotherapy delivered is good, whereas poor quality radiotherapy may obscure benefits and increase toxicity. Modern megavoltage radiotherapy standards include an unequivocal definition of the volumes to be treated, an unequivocal definition of the tumor dose (including considerations on fractionation), an optimal beam arrangement to cover the previously defined volume and to protect critical organs, computer dosimetry to describe dose distribution, film checking in the treatment machine to ensure reproducibility, and CT scanning–based planning. An example of treatment planning for a patient with stage IIIB NSCLC is shown in Figure 17.5. These standards should be used in randomized trials aimed at defining optimal treatment.

Total Dose

Prospective trials were conducted by the Radiation Therapy Oncology Group (RTOG) to investigate the question of dose intensity for control of locoregional tumor. An initial randomized study suggested that patients treated with a continuous course of 50 to 60 Gy over 5 to 6 weeks had better tumor control than those treated with lower doses (33, 46).

Since the 1980s, different regimens of hyperfractionated radiotherapy that could enable the total dose of radiation to be raised with no increase in morbidity were studied. Cox et al. (47) carried out studies in which patients were given a dose of 1.2 Gy per fraction twice a day with a 4- to 8-hour interfraction interval to total doses of 60, 64.8, 69.6, 74.4, and 79.2 Gy. A total of 848 patients were entered into the five nonrandomized groups of the study. Morbidity was similar among the different groups, even with a 20% to 30% increase in total dose. No overall difference in survival was observed among patients in the different fractionation regimen groups. However, a trend toward better survival was observed in favor of the higher dose groups.

Split-Course Radiotherapy

Split-course radiotherapy, whereby radiation therapy is followed by a resting interval, is another possible treatment schedule. It has been criticized by some because of the rebound effect of tumor cell proliferation during the period when therapy is discontinued. Nevertheless, it allows a rest period after 3 to 4 weeks of treatment and is probably more comfortable for patients. Two randomized studies, comparing continuous and split-course therapy, failed to show any survival difference (48, 49). Although Perez et al. (33) suggested a slightly better survival rate in patients treated with high-dose continuous treatment versus split-course radiotherapy in their preliminary report, this difference was no longer present after 3 years. The question of whether certain histologic subtypes of NSCLC benefit from split-course or continuous treatment remains unanswered.

Standard radiotherapy consists of giving 10 Gy per week, i.e., 60 Gy in 6 weeks. Radiation can be hypofractionated (i.e., using a high dose fraction) and given once or twice per week with the goal of causing as little discomfort as possible for the patient treated palliatively. Slawson et al. (50) reported a prospective, randomized, controlled trial on patients with NSCLC limited to the thorax and treated either with conventional radiotherapy (2 Gy per fraction 5 days each week to a total of 60 Gy) or with 5 Gy per fraction once each week up to a total of 60 Gy over 12 weeks. This study enrolled 120 patients, with a follow-up of between 12 and 66 months. One-year survival rates were 49% and 59%, respectively. Acute and late morbidity were comparable. The investigators concluded that there was an advantage of hypofractionated over standard radiotherapy on short-term survival.

Fractionation

Several trials have been conducted regarding the effect of fractionation in the the radiation treatment of locally advanced NSCLC (46–56). Two approaches are under evaluation to increase the radiation dose intensity: hyperfractionation, in which many small doses of radiation are delivered to increase the total dose; and accelerated fractionation, in which the overall duration of treatment is shortened. Hyperfractionation aims to provide the best ratio of efficacy to tolerance for the few patients who are potentially curable (44–47). One RTOG study was conducted to determine the upper limits of total dose possible with hyperfractionation using 1.2 Gy twice daily, 5 days per week (47). Total doses ranged from 60 Gy in 5 weeks to 79.2 Gy in 6.5 weeks, i.e., 32% higher than the dose considered tolerable with standard radiation. Results showed a similar survival at 5 years because of distant metastases. The investigators concluded that the greatest benefit in terms of response was achieved with a total dose 10% higher than that considered tolerable with standard fractionation, i.e., 69.6 Gy in 5.5 weeks.

Preliminary results have been reported recently from the RTOG-ECOG study, in which two of the three arms compared conventional radiotherapy (60 Gy total dose [2 Gy per fraction]) and a hyperfractionated

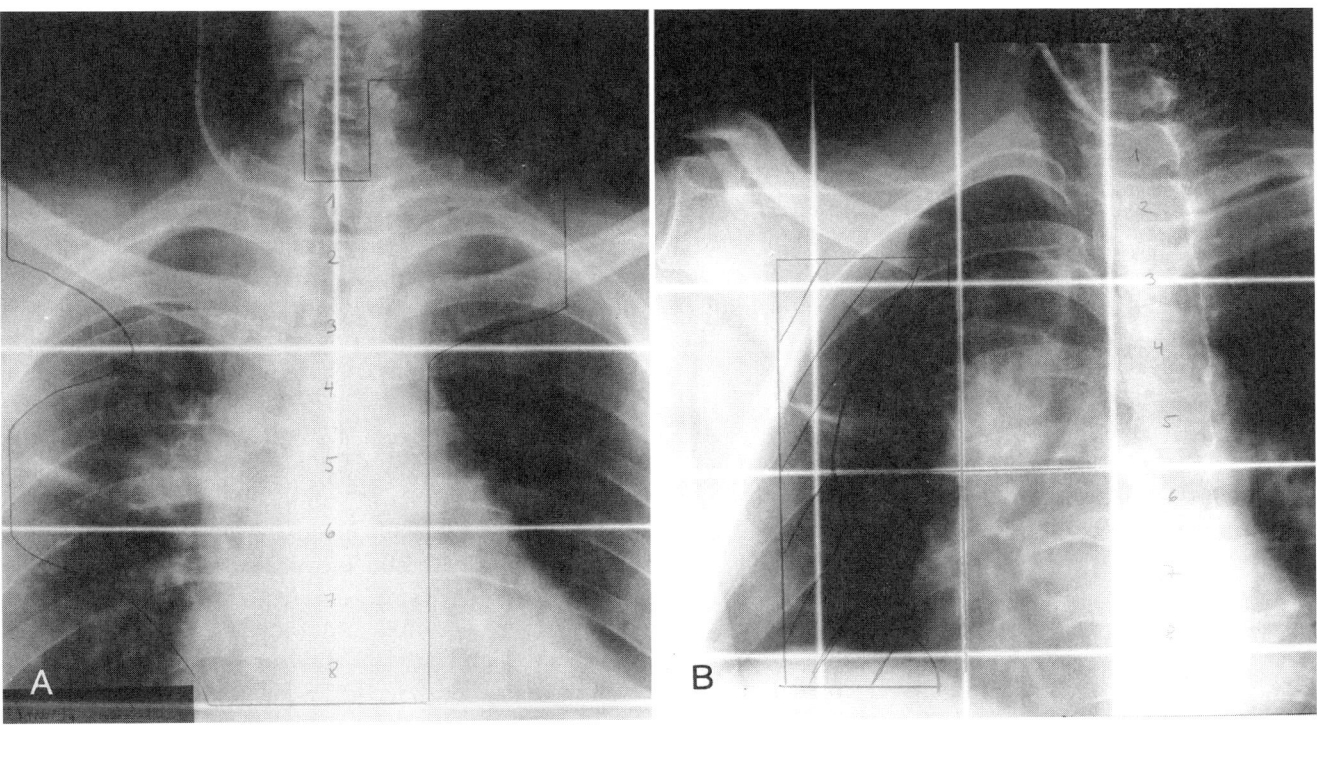
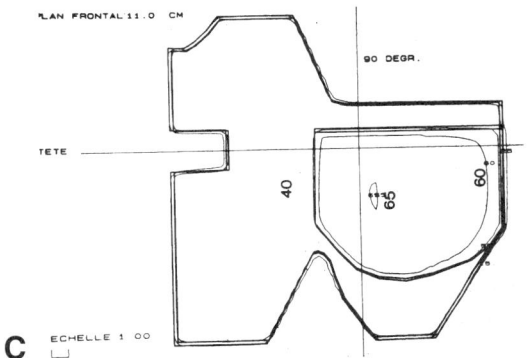
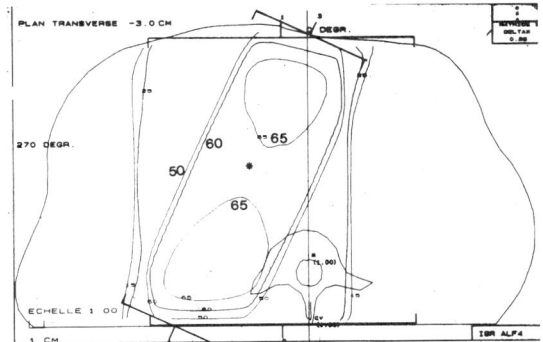

FIGURE 17.5. Radiation technique in the treatment of locally advanced NSCLC. **A.** Anteroposterior beam shaped by Cerrobend shielding, drawn in the simulator film. In this case, the field covers a limited atelectatic area of the right upper lobe considered to contain subclinical tumor. The total dose delivered by these fields is 40 Gy in conventional fraction. **B.** Oblique opposed fields to treat the macroscopic tumor and homolateral mediastinal nodes. These fields add 25 Gy in conventional fractionation without irradiation of the spinal cord. **C.** Computerized dosimetry in frontal plane showing the superposition of anteroposterior and oblique fields (photon beams of 18 MV). Bold numbers give the total dose in Gy. **D.** Computerized dosimetry in transverse plane. Doses are in Gy. The spinal cord receives a total dose of 42 Gy.

schedule in regionally advanced unresectable NSCLC (54). The preliminary results did not show any significant difference between these two radiation schedules (median survival and 1-year survival of 11.4 months and 46% versus 12.3 months and 51%, respectively).

In 1988 Emami et al. (55) reported a pilot study of rapid fractionation in T3-T4 NSCLC. A total of 56 patients received 75 Gy in 28 fractions over 5.5 weeks to the known tumor, whereas noninvolved lymph nodes received 50.4 Gy over the same period. Considering the total dose achieved and the poor prognosis of patients, it appeared that the incidence of complications was acceptable. This study concluded that further investigation of this regimen was justified.

The CHART regimen (continuous, hyperfractionated, accelerated radiotherapy), reported by Saunders et al. (53) at Mt. Vernon Hospital, in which 36 fractions are given over 12 consecutive days, combines both approaches and appears to be promising. Results of a pilot study of 76 evaluable patients with NSCLC showed that 40% achieved complete radiologic regression of disease. There was an improvement in survival in CHART patients compared with historical controls, with 60% alive at 1 year and 29% at 2 years. A randomized, controlled trial has begun in the United Kingdom comparing CHART with conventional radiotherapy. It is hoped that some 500 patients will be recruited over a 4-year period.

Another study, from Brindle et al. (56), showed similar promising results. Twenty-one patients with stage IIIA or IIIB disease were given 60 Gy in 40 fractions, at the rate of two fractions per day. The 1-, 2-, and 3-year survival rates were 48%, 29%, and 14%, respectively. The treatment produced an acceptable toxicity. Based on these results, a randomized trial comparing the new schedule to conventional radiotherapy in NSCLC (60 Gy, 30 fractions over 42 days) is now in progress.

CHART studies, although preliminary, seem to suggest that this treatment modality could be advantageous to some patients with stage III NSCLC, but definitive conclusions require further well-controlled studies.

CHEMOTHERAPY

The role of chemotherapy in locally advanced NSCLC is still debated, and no definitive consensus has been reached in this subset of patients. Approximately half of all patients treated with radiotherapy alone develop distant or both distant and local recurrences (30, 33). The low rate of cure and the high rate of metastases in stage IIIB NSCLC treated by radiotherapy alone have favored the inclusion of chemotherapy in treatment protocols and have even questioned the role of radiotherapy. In spite of low sensitivity to single agents based on reports in the literature, some multiple-drug regimens can induce partial or complete responses in NSCLC, especially when a vinca-alkaloid or etoposide is combined with cisplatin. Objective response rates ranging from 25% to 40% in inoperable NSCLC have been obtained with combined regimens, which nonetheless are unable to control the primary tumor adequately in the vast majority of cases (36, 37, 57). A number of phase II studies have evaluated preoperative chemotherapy in stage III NSCLC (58–67). These phase II studies indicate that patients with stage IIIA/B disease have higher objective response rates than those usually observed with the same chemotherapy in patients with more advanced disease. Table 17.5 shows reports of different regimens used in stage III disease. A brief clinical review of these studies indicates that 15% to 85% of patients can be resected subsequently, but the precise staging of these patients at the time of inclusion is not always established clearly, thus it is difficult to confirm that chemotherapy has made the tumor resectable. Other important information has been obtained. Studies using chemotherapy as the sole preoperative treatment modality have reported significant pathologically complete response rates, varying from 9% to 15% (61, 64, 65). Furthermore, in one of these studies, pathologically complete response predicted excellent survival with a median survival of 68 months and a 5-year survival of 54% (68).

Generally speaking, studies of preoperative chemotherapy have demonstrated definite clinical and pathologic activity in advanced NSCLC. However, there currently is no standard, universally accepted, combined chemotherapy regimen, and despite promising response rates reported with chemotherapy in stage III NSCLC, median survival often remains disappointing.

Few randomized studies comparing chemotherapy and radiotherapy in inoperable NSCLC have been performed. In one study Johnson et al. (69) sought to compare the survival of locally advanced NSCLC patients treated with single-drug chemotherapy, thoracic radiotherapy, or both modalities. In this trial 319 patients were assigned randomly to treatment either with vindesine only (3 mg/m^2/week), standard chest radiotherapy only (60 Gy over 6 weeks), or both modalities. Vindesine was administered for 6 weeks and then every other week to patients without disease progression. Patients with disease progression, while on vindesine or radiotherapy alone, were crossed over to radiotherapy or vindesine, respectively. Response to therapy was assessed at week 6. Results showed that the response rate was better in the radiotherapy arms of the study: radiotherapy alone, 30%; radiotherapy and vindesine, 34%; and vindesine alone 10% ($P = .001$). However, after a minimum follow-up of 42 weeks, no differences in survival were observed among the three groups. None of these treatments improved long-term survival; 5-year survival rates were 3%, 3%, and 1%, respectively ($P = .56$).

In another study reported by Kaasa et al. (70), 118 patients received 42 Gy in 15 fractions, and 115 patients received chemotherapy (cisplatin, 70 mg/m^2 on day 1, and etoposide, 100 mg/m^2 on day 1 with a double dose on days 2 and 3, repeated every 3 to 4 weeks). The response rate (complete plus partial response) was 42% after radiotherapy and 21% after chemotherapy ($P = .009$); however, median survival times, i.e., 10.6 and 10.5 months, respectively ($P = .81$), were similar.

COMBINED RADIOTHERAPY AND CHEMOTHERAPY

Traditionally, thoracic radiotherapy has been considered the standard treatment of locally advanced, medically inoperable NSCLC. When used alone, appropriately indicated, and correctly administered, radio-

TABLE 17.5. Induction Chemotherapy, as the Sole Preoperative Treatment, in Stage III NSCLC

Authors (Reference No.)	No. of Patients	Stages	Regimen	Response (%)	Resection (%)	Pathologically Complete Response (%)	Median Survival (Mo.)
Chapman et al. (58)	24	IIIA	CDDP/VLB	67	77	NA	NA
Bitran et al. (59)	20	III	CDDP/VDS/VP16	70	15	NA	9
Spain et al. (60)	22	III, IV	MVP	79	63	NA	19
Martini et al. (61)	136	IIIA (N2)	MVP	77	65	14	19
Vokes et al. (62)	27	IIIA, IIIB	CDDP/VP16/VDS	48	15	NA	8
Raut et al. (63)	32	I–III	CDDP/Bleo/MTX	74	86	NA	NA
Darwish et al. (64)	45	IIIA (N2)	CDDP/VP16	82	73	9	24.5
Pujol et al. (65)	33	IIIA, IIIB	CDDP/VP16/IFX	70	61	15	10
Fossella et al. (66)	13	IIIA	C/VP16	33	46	NA	NA
Burkes et al. (67)	35	IIIA	MVP	69	59	NA	19

Abbreviations. MTX, methotrexate; C, cyclophosphamide; CDDP, cisplatin; MVP, mitomycin/vinblastine/cisplatin; Bleo, bleomycin; IFX, ifosfamide; VDS, vindesine; NA, not available; VLB, vinblastine; VP16, etoposide.

therapy should produce approximately 20% to 25% complete remission rate and a 1- and 2-year survival rate of 45% and 25%, respectively. Long-term results, however, are poor: only 15% of patients survive beyond 2 years, and long-term survival does not exceed 5% in most studies including a large number of patients. Control of disseminated micrometastases requires effective systemic therapy. In addition, studies have indicated that some drugs such as 5-fluorouracil (5-FU) or cisplatin may serve as effective radiosensitizing agents (71).

The rationale for combining radiotherapy and chemotherapy in nonresectable NSCLC involves the following objectives (72, 73): (a) to improve the local control rate by delivering adequate total radiation doses, i.e., at least 55 Gy with conventional fractionation; (b) to avoid doses that are too high to prevent toxic effects on normal thoracic tissues; and (c) to decrease the distant metastasis rate by acting on micrometastases that exist at the time of presentation in more than 50% of cases.

The combined chemoradiotherapy can be administered either sequentially (i.e., one modality begins when the previous modality has concluded), concurrently (i.e., both treatment modalities are given simultaneously), or in an alternating mode (i.e., the modalities alternate). The technical aspects of these treatment schedules are developed in another chapter of this book.

Although randomized studies directly comparing chemotherapy and radiotherapy in inoperable NSCLC have not revealed any difference in survival between these two treatment modalities (69, 70), the value of adding radiotherapy to chemotherapy in stage III NSCLC has been assessed recently in a randomized study by Kubota et al. (74). In this study, after two cycles of chemotherapy, patients with locally advanced disease were randomized to receive thoracic radiation or no radiation. There were three chemotherapy regimens: (a) cisplatin, 100 mg/m^2 on day 1, and vindesine, 3 mg/m^2 on days 1, 8, and 15; (b) cisplatin, 80 mg/m^2 on day 1; vindesine, 3 mg/m^2 on days 1 and 8; and mitomycin, 8 mg/m^2 on day 1; (c) cisplatin, 80 mg/m^2 on day 1; etoposide, 100 mg/m^2 on days 2, 4, and 6; vindesine, 3 mg/m^2 on days 22 and 29; and mitomycin, 8 mg/m^2 on day 22. Radiotherapy consisted of 50- to 60-Gy total doses in 25 to 30 fractions. Sixty-three patients were enrolled, and all were evaluable. The median survival was similar for the two groups (461 days in the chemotherapy/radiotherapy group and 447 days in the chemotherapy alone group). The survival rate in the chemotherapy/radiotherapy group was 58% at 1 year, 36% at 2 years, and 29% at 3 years, compared with 66%, 9%, and 3% at 1, 2, and 3 years, respectively, in the chemotherapy alone group. It was concluded that in locally advanced NSCLC cisplatin-based chemotherapy followed by chest irradiation significantly increases the number of long-term survivors, compared with chemotherapy alone. This study evaluating the role of thoracic irradiation combined with chemotherapy, even considering the small number of patients, strongly suggested the efficacy of radiotherapy as part of a combined schedule.

SEQUENTIAL CHEMOTHERAPY-RADIOTHERAPY

The sequential use of chemotherapy and radiotherapy is the most conventional way to combine these modalities in NSCLC to avoid additive simultaneous toxicities.

PHASE II NONRANDOMIZED STUDIES

Many phase II studies have been reported in the last 20 years, often with encouraging results. In 1971–1972, Samuels et al. (75) treated 27 patients with locally advanced NSCLC using a combined chemoradiotherapy regimen consisting of bleomycin, vincristine, and methotrexate followed by split-course radiation therapy on an outpatient basis. Bleomycin was given in a fixed dose of 15 mg intramuscularly twice weekly for 3 weeks; vincristine, 2 mg intravenously once weekly for 3 weeks; and methotrexate, orally, 25 to 30 mg twice weekly for 3 weeks. After a 2-week rest period, split-course radiotherapy was started. One or two courses of radiotherapy, at a dose of 30 Gy in 10 fractions, were given. Chemotherapy, identical to the initial course of therapy, was resumed after recovery from radiotherapy. The 15 objective responders had a median survival time of 70 weeks. These results suggested that chemotherapy may be of contributive value.

In 1980 (76), 33 patients with locally advanced squamous cell carcinoma of the lung were entered in a phase II study that combined vindesine (1.5 mg/m^2 on day 1), lomustine (50 mg/m^2 on day 2 and 25 mg/m^2 on day 3), cisplatin (100 mg/m^2 on day 3), and cyclophosphamide (200 mg/m^2 on days 2 through 4) with thoracic radiotherapy at a total dose of 65 Gy. All patients were males, median age was 56.3 years, and median Karnofsky performance status was 80%. Two patients were considered unresectable because of major respiratory deficiency (one was staged T2, N2, and one was T2, NX). The remaining 31 patients were unresectable because of local extension, including six with supraclavicular node involvement. The treatment schedule consisted of two monthly cycles of the vindesine, lomustine, cisplatin, and cyclophosphamide (VCPC) regimen. All patients then received split-course irradiation of the tumor, mediastinum, and bilateral supraclavicular nodes at a total dose of 65 Gy; responders to chemotherapy received four additional cycles of chemotherapy. Fourteen patients (42%) had an objective response rate after the first two cycles of chemotherapy (2 complete and 12 partial responses). On final evaluation, 18 patients (54.5%) had a complete response and 6 (18%) achieved a partial response. Median survival of the whole population was 16 months, and treatment-related toxicity was acceptable. These results indicated that a randomized study comparing this combined modality treatment with radiotherapy alone was warranted.

Randomized Phase III Studies

Several phase III randomized studies have evaluated the role of chemotherapy added to radiotherapy by comparing radiotherapy alone to the combination of radiotherapy and chemotherapy. Major studies questioning this issue are presented and their main findings synthetically analyzed by the type of chemotherapy and the worldwide meta-analysis performed on individual data of most of these trials (77).

Trials with cyclophosphamide alone. In 1972 Bergsagel et al. (78) reported a trial on patients with nonresectable lung cancer limited to the thorax. Fifty-six patients with NSCLC were assigned randomly to treatment either with radiotherapy alone (40 Gy in 20 to 24 fractions) to the primary lesion and mediastinum, or the same radiotherapy with four or eight courses of high-dose intermittent cyclophosphamide (1 g/m^2 at 21-day intervals). It was observed that cyclophosphamide delayed the progression of metastatic lesions outside the irradiated field (median interval to progression, 192 days versus 114 days for radiotherapy alone), and prolonged survival (median, 306 days versus 216 days). Patients treated with combined chemoradiotherapy had a lower mortality rate during the first year of the study than did those treated with radiotherapy alone; long-term survival was similar in all three groups, however. It was concluded that even if cyclophosphamide was only minimally effective in the treatment of lung cancer, it was an active drug that should be considered in later trials of drug combinations.

Höst (79) conducted a study on 74 patients with unresectable non–small cell bronchogenic carcinoma who were allocated randomly to treatment either with radiotherapy alone or radiotherapy with adjuvant cyclophosphamide; the latter was given concurrently with radiation at a daily dose of 400 mg intravenously up to 40 mg/kg and then orally at a dose of 100 mg daily. Survival of patients treated with the combined modality was not increased, compared with that of patients treated with radiation alone.

Another trial was conducted by the Veterans Administration Lung Cancer Study Groups (80) on patients with nonresectable bronchogenic carcinoma. Upon entry, patients were divided into limited disease and extensive disease groups. Limited disease was defined as a tumor confined to one hemithorax. Of 1546 patients, 239 presented with limited disease. They were treated with megavoltage radiotherapy at a dose of 40 to 50 Gy in 4 to 6 weeks or the same irradiation plus cyclophosphamide, 300 mg/m^2/day intravenously for 5 days and then 200 mg/day orally until disease progression. Results did not show any significant difference between radiotherapy alone and the combination of radiotherapy and cyclophosphamide.

Simpson et al. (81) conducted a multicenter trial on 409 patients with inoperable NSCLC. Patients were randomized to receive cyclophosphamide at a dose of 1 g/m^2 every 3 weeks until progression or no chemotherapy after thoracic radiotherapy. Radiation consisted of three possible schedules: 40 Gy split course, 30 Gy continuous course, and 40 Gy continuous course. There were 316 evaluable patients. Palliation of symptoms was achieved in 60% of patients, and one fourth of patients became symptom free. Complete remission of local and regional tumor was achieved in 15% and a partial response in 26%. There were no significant differences between treatment arms in terms of objective response rates or median survival time (approximately 6 months).

In summary, cyclophosphamide was minimally effective in prolonging survival in patients treated with this agent in combination with radiotherapy.

OTHER SINGLE-DRUG TRIALS

Schallier et al. (82) performed a randomized study in patients with limited NSCLC to compare vinblastine as adjuvant treatment with radiotherapy. Forty-nine patients were randomized to receive radiotherapy to the tumor and mediastinum (55 Gy over 6 weeks) and vinblastine (6 mg/m^2 in weekly bolus injection) (group A, $n = 25$ patients), or radiotherapy alone at the same dose as for group A (group B, $n = 24$ patients). Response to therapy was observed in 12 of 18 patients in group A and in 8 of 20 in group B. A trend of benefit in terms of metastasis free survival ($P = .14$) and overall survival was observed in group A ($P = .14$). However, because of the small number of patients in each group, the statistical power of the analysis is very low.

White et al. (83) reported the results of a Southwest Oncology Group trial designed as a four-arm study of radiation with or without doxorubicin chemotherapy, with or without levamisole immunotherapy, in the treatment of limited squamous cell lung carcinoma. The aim of this study was to determine whether doxorubicin and/or levamisole added to radiation therapy could improve the local control rate or overall survival. Of 107 eligible patients, 14% had complete responses and 19% had partial responses. Complete plus partial response rates of the four individual treatment arms varied from 18% to 39%. Comparison based on chemotherapy, immunotherapy, previous surgery, and performance status showed no statistically significant difference in response rates or survival among the different groups. Survival of patients in the combined levamisole arms was found to be shorter ($P = .097$) than that of patients in the combined arms not receiving levamisole. Patients who received radiotherapy alone had the best survival. The main site of failure was the lung. Chemotherapy and/or immunotherapy were of no benefit.

In the randomized study conducted by Johnson et al. (69), which compared single-agent vindesine, thoracic radiotherapy, or both modalities in locally advanced NSCLC, median survival was 10, 9.4, and 8.6 months, respectively ($P = .58$). The investigators concluded that there was no established standard treatment in this population of patients.

In summary, the addition of doxorubicin, vindesine, or vinblastine used as single agents did not improve results obtained with radiotherapy alone in terms of survival. Table 17.6 summarizes the results of these studies.

Trials with non–cisplatin-containing multidrug regimens. In 1981 Anderson et al. (84) reported the results of a prospective randomized trial designed to evaluate the additive effect of doxorubicin and 5-FU following radiotherapy in inoperable NSCLC. Eighty-two patients were allocated to receive either radiotherapy alone (24 to 32 Gy), or the same dose of radiotherapy followed by four cycles of doxorubicin and 5-FU. Randomization of patients was done according to cell type. Radiotherapy was administered twice weekly with a total of eight fractions over 23 days. Chemotherapy was given as four cycles at 1-month intervals. Each cycle consisted of doxorubicin, 80 mg/m^2, and 5-FU, 1200 mg, both given intravenously. The first cycle of chemotherapy was given 51 days after day 1 of radiotherapy. Survival was better in the group receiving adjuvant chemotherapy for the 41 patients with squamous cell carcinoma; the median survival benefit was 2 months. The difference did not reach a significant level ($P = .25$).

Israel et al. (85) conducted a trial to evaluate the effects of chemotherapy and/or immunotherapy following radiation therapy in the treatment of unresectable NSCLC. Radiation consisted of 55 Gy to the tumor and 45 Gy to the mediastinum. Half of the patients achieved an objective response after radiotherapy and were randomized. A total of 238 patients, of whom 208 were included in the analysis, were randomized into four groups: (*a*) a control group; (*b*) 0.2 mL of intradermal bacille Calmette–Guérin every 4 months; (*c*) monthly chemotherapy with lomustine (100 mg/m^2), methotrexate (40 mg/m^2), and cyclophosphamide (1 g/m^2) every 4 weeks for 1 year; and (*d*) combination bacille Calmette Guerin and chemotherapy at the same dose and time schedule as above. The only significant finding was that chemotherapy was significantly superior in delaying both local recurrences and distant metastases, compared with the control group ($P = .02$). However, no significant difference was observed in terms of overall survival.

The North Central Cancer Treatment Group (86) designed a randomized trial comparing survival of patients with inoperable or unresectable stage III NSCLC treated with thoracic radiotherapy alone or in combination with chemotherapy. A total of 121 patients were

TABLE 17.6. Randomized Trials of Sequential Single-Agent Chemotherapy Combined with Radiotherapy

Author (Reference No.)	Chemotherapy	Radiotherapy Total Dose (Gy)	Radiotherapy Schedule	No. of Evaluable Patients	Median Survival	Survival at 2 Years (%)	Survival at 3 Years (%)	P Value
Bergsagel et al. (78)	Cyclophosphamide	40	Continuous	84	306 d	NA	NA	NA
		40	Continuous	39	216 d	NA	NA	NA
Höst (79)	Cyclophosphamide	40–50	Continuous	32	NA	NA	NA	NS
		40–50	Continuous	42	NA	NA	NA	
VALCSG (80)	Cyclophosphamide	40–50	Continuous	25	21.8 w	NA	NA	NS
		40–50	Continuous	22	20.5 w	NA	NA	
Simpson et al. (81)	Cyclophosphamide	40	Continuous	55	NA	NA	NA	NS
		40	Continuous	50	NA	NA	NA	
Schallier et al. (82)	Vinblastine	55	Continuous	25	79 w	NA	NA	$P = .14$
		55	Continuous	24	56 w	NA	NA	
White et al. (83)	Doxorubicin	30	Split	26	45 w	5	NA	$P = .530$
		30	Split	28	50 w	5	NA	
Johnson et al. (69)	Vindesine	60	Continuous	102	10 m	14	3	$P = .58$
		60	Continuous	104	9.4 m	12.5	3	

Abbreviations. NA, not available; d, day; w, week; m, month; NS, not statistically significant; VALCSG, Veterans Administration Lung Cancer Study Group.

enrolled and were stratified according to ECOG performance score, histologic cell type, tumor size, and institution. Thoracic radiotherapy consisted of a 50-Gy total dose over 5 weeks with a 10-Gy boost in five fractions to a small tumor field. Combined chemotherapy included methotrexate (40 mg/m^2), doxorubicin (40 mg/m^2), cyclophosphamide (400 mg/m^2), and oral lomustine (30 mg/m^2) (MACC) on day 1, repeated every 28 days. Two courses of chemotherapy were administered before and after thoracic radiotherapy in the combined modality arm. Patients with disease progression after radiotherapy alone were offered treatment with MACC. Major clinical responses were observed in 31 of 56 patients treated with combination therapy and in 37 of 58 treated with radiotherapy alone. Median survival time was the same in both groups (313 versus 317 days, respectively). The 1-, 2-, and 5-year survival rates after thoracic radiotherapy were 45%, 16%, and 7%, compared with 46%, 21%, and 5%, respectively, after combined treatment ($P = .69$). The investigators concluded that chemotherapy with MACC did not prolong survival of patients with stage III NSCLC treated with radiotherapy.

Petrovich et al. (87) reported the results of a randomized trial conducted by the Veterans Administration Lung Cancer Study Group that evaluated the addition of chemotherapy to radiotherapy in locally advanced lung tumors. A total of 346 patients, of whom 259 had histologically proven NSCLC, were included in this study. Radiotherapy consisted of 50 to 60 Gy given in from 28 to 42 days. The chemotherapy regimen included lomustine, 100 mg/m^2 orally every 6 weeks, and hydroxyurea, 1 g/m^2 orally twice weekly. Median survival ranged from 23 to 33 weeks depending on histologic subtype. No statistically significant difference was observed between the radiotherapy and chemoradiotherapy schedules.

Sidorowicz et al. (88) reported the results of a comparative study of radiotherapy and chemoradiotherapy in the treatment of limited NSCLC. Thoracic radiotherapy was delivered at a total dose of 50 to 60 Gy. Patients who were allocated to the combined modality arm received adjuvant MACC (methotrexate, 30 mg/m^2; doxorubicin, 40 mg/m^2; lomustine, 30 mg/m^2; and cyclophosphamide, 400 mg/m^2, given every 21 days) after completion of radiotherapy. Twenty-seven patients were randomized to radiotherapy alone and 25 to radiotherapy-MACC. In fact, only 16 of the latter 25 received chemotherapy. The average number of courses of MACC was five. No statistically significant difference was observed in the time to relapse (6 versus 8 months) or median survival (radiotherapy, 11 months; radiotherapy-MACC, 14 months), and the investigators concluded that there was no difference between radiotherapy alone and combined radiotherapy-MACC.

Trovo et al. (89) conducted a randomized trial on patients with inoperable NSCLC comparing radiotherapy alone with radiotherapy and combined cyclophosphamide, doxorubicin, methotrexate, and procarbazine (CAMP) chemotherapy consisting of cyclophosphamide, 300 mg/m^2 on days 1 and 8; doxorubicin, 20 mg/m^2 on days 1 and 8; methotrexate, 15 mg/m^2 on days 1 and 8; and procarbazine, 100 mg/m^2 orally on days 1 through 10, given every 4 weeks for 12 cycles. Radiotherapy consisted of 45 Gy in 15 fractions over 3 weeks. Nineteen of 49 patients treated with the combined modality therapy had an objective response, compared with 35 of 62 after radiotherapy alone. Median survival was 10 months in the combined treatment group compared with 11.7 months in the radiotherapy alone group.

In summary, results from these six trials show that a multidrug, non–cisplatin-based regimen can enhance the therapeutic effects of radiotherapy, but they are inconclusive in terms of median and long-term survival. These results are shown in Table 17.7.

Trials with cisplatin-based multidrug regimens. Alberti et al. (90) performed a randomized trial comparing immediate thoracic radiotherapy, chemoradiotherapy, or delayed radiotherapy in patients with inoperable NSCLC. Sixty-three patients were treated according to one of the following regimens: (*a*) immediate radiotherapy 2 times weekly at a dose of 4 Gy up to 52 to 56 Gy; (*b*) immediate chemotherapy (vindesine, 3 mg/m^2 on days 1 and 3; cisplatin, 80 mg/m^2 on day 2) for two to three courses, one every 4 weeks, followed by radiotherapy as in the first group; and (*c*) delayed radiotherapy at onset of symptoms. Fifty-two patients were evaluable. Response rates ranged from 76% to 78%, and median survival was 15, 19, and 11 months, respectively. These results suggested an advantage for immediate radiotherapy, but probably because of the small number of patients, no statistical difference was observed.

Brodin et al. (91) conducted a study for the Swedish Multicenter Group to evaluate the effects of chemotherapy in nonresectable squamous cell lung cancer. Patients were randomized to either three courses of chemotherapy before radiotherapy or radiotherapy only. The dose of radiation delivered was 56 Gy in 2 Gy fractions in both groups. Chemotherapy consisted of cisplatin, 120 mg/m^2 on day 1, and etoposide, 100 mg/m^2 intravenously on days 1, 2, and 3. A total of 330 patients were included. Median survival was approximately 9 months for both arms, and a nonsignificant difference was observed in favor of the combined modality arm.

Cardiello et al. (92) performed a trial on 51 patients with inoperable NSCLC who were randomized to treatment either with radiotherapy alone (55 Gy, split-course, to the primary tumor, mediastinum, and supraclavicular nodes), or radiotherapy (same schedule) combined with chemotherapy (cyclophosphamide, 400 mg/m^2; doxorubicin, 40 mg/m^2; and cisplatin, 40 mg/m^2) every 4 weeks for a total of six cycles. Median survival was 41 weeks after radiotherapy alone and 60 weeks in the combined modality, but this difference was not significant.

Crino et al. (93) conducted a trial on 66 patients with inoperable stage III NSCLC who were randomized to one of two treatment arms. Patients received either cisplatin, 100 mg/m^2 on day 1, and etoposide, 120 mg/m^2 on days 1, 2, and 3, every 3 weeks for three cycles, followed by radiotherapy of 56 Gy to the primary tumor lesion and 40 Gy to the mediastinum and bilateral supraclavicular nodes; or radiotherapy only at the same dose. Sixty-one patients were evaluable for survival and 58 for response and toxicity. The response rates were 53% and 32%, respectively. Median survival was 52 weeks for the combined treatment arm and 36 weeks for the radiation therapy arm. Toxicity was mild, and no treatment-related deaths occurred. No patients survived after 6 years of follow-up. No significant advantage was observed, possibly because of the small sample size.

TABLE 17.7. Randomized Trials of Sequential Non–Cisplatin-Based Regimens Combined with Radiotherapy

Author (Reference No.)	Chemotherapy	Radiotherapy Total Dose (Gy)	Schedule	No. of Evaluable Patients	Median Survival	Survival at 2 Years (%)	Survival at 5 Years (%)	P Value
Anderson et al. (84)	5-FU/DOX	24–32	Split	38	NA	14	NA	P = .25
		24–32	Split	43	NA	12	NA	
Israel et al. (85)	MTX/C/L	55	Continuous	49	62.4 w	NA	NA	NS
		55	Continuous	54	69.1 w	NA	NA	
Morton et al. (86)	MTX/DOX/C/L	60	Continuous	62	317 d	21	7	P = .69
		60	Continuous	63	313 d	16	5	
Petrovitz et al. (87)	Lomustine/Hydrea	50–60	Continuous	175	7.2 m	7	NA	P = .002
		50–60	Continuous	171	6.3 m	15	NA	
Sidorowicz et al. (88)	MTX/DOX/C/L	50–60	Continuous	25	14 m	NA	NA	NS
		50–60	Continuous	27	11 m	NA	NA	
Trovo et al. (89)	MTX/DOX/C/P	45	Continuous	49	10 m	NA	NA	NS
		45	Continuous	62	11.7 m	NA	NA	

Abbreviations. NA, not available; d, day; w, week; m, month; NS, not statistically significant; 5-FU, 5-fluorouracil; DOX, doxorubicin; MTX, methotrexate; C, cyclophosphamide; L, lomustine; P, prednisone.

The Cancer and Leukemia Group B (CALGB) (94) conducted a randomized trial of induction chemotherapy plus high-dose radiation compared with radiation alone for treatment of patients with stage III NSCLC. Eligibility criteria included absence of supraclavicular and/or scalene node involvement, presence of an excellent performance status, and loss of no more than 5% of body weight in the preceding 3 months. Patients were assigned randomly either to treatment with cisplatin (100 mg/m^2 given intravenously on days 1 and 29) and vinblastine (5 mg/m^2 intravenously on days 1, 8, 15, 22, and 29), followed by on radiotherapy on day 50 (60 Gy over 6 weeks); or to the same radiotherapy regimen started immediately and without chemotherapy. Both groups were comparable in terms of age, sex, performance status, histologic features, stage of disease, and completion of radiotherapy. Median survival was greater in the combined modality group (13.8 months versus 9.7 months, $P = .0066$). In the combined modality arm, 55% of patients were alive after 1 year, 26% after 2 years, and 23% after 3 years versus 40%, 13%, and 11%, respectively, in the radiotherapy alone arm. It was concluded that induction chemotherapy with cisplatin and vinblastine before radiotherapy significantly improved median survival and increased twofold the number of long-term survivors.

Long-term follow-up recently confirmed these initial results with a 5-year survival rate of 19% for the chemotherapy-radiotherapy group, compared with 7% for the radiotherapy alone group. This survival advantage was seen in both stage IIIA and IIIB subsets and for adenocarcinoma and squamous cell histologies (95). This trial was criticized because of early stopping. However, the preliminary analysis of an RTOG-ECOG trial (54) has confirmed the benefit of the combined approach. In this study the investigators compared standard radiotherapy at a dose of 60 Gy (2 Gy per fraction) with a hyperfractionated regimen and with induction chemotherapy combining vinblastine and cisplatin followed by the same standard radiation. Among the 452 patients entered and eligible, there was a significant short-term advantage in favor of the combined modality treatment (median survival, 13.8 months) compared with both radiation alone arms (median survival, 11.4 and 12.3 months, respectively; $P = .03$). This trial, in which the chemotherapy regimen was identical to that used in the CALGB study (94), confirmed the results.

Gregor et al. (96) conducted a trial to test the question of the choice of standard treatment for patients with inoperable NSCLC with minimal symptoms. They compared treatments for response, toxicity, and survival in this randomized trial with three arms: (a) radical radiotherapy at a dose of 50 Gy in 20 daily fractions over 4 weeks to the tumor; (b) the same irradiation regimen plus chemotherapy consisting of cisplatin, 100 mg/m^2 on day 1, and vindesine, 3 mg/m^2 on days 1 and 8, in two cycles given at 3-week intervals before radiotherapy; and (c) abstention from treatment with regular follow-up and palliative radiotherapy (30 Gy in 10 daily fractions) when symptoms occurred. There were 118 patients randomized. This trial was closed in 1989 and considered a failure because of difficulties in patient recruitment. Nevertheless, no differences were observed between the first two arms (median survival of 53 and 52 weeks, respectively).

In Seoul, Kim et al. (97) conducted a randomized comparison of chemotherapy with cisplatin, etoposide, and vinblastine plus radiation versus radiation alone in the treatment of stage III NSCLC. A total of 118 patients were entered and stratifed according to stage of disease (IIIA versus IIIB), performance status, weight loss, and histology. There were 28 responders in the combined treatment group (6 complete and 22 partial), and 32 in the radiotherapy only group (5 complete and 27 partial). Median survival was 15 months versus 9.7 months. There was no statistically significant difference in overall survival between the two treatment groups.

A large, multicenter, French randomized phase III trial (98, 99) was conducted on 353 patients with inoperable squamous cell and large cell lung carcinoma comparing the effects of radiotherapy alone—the standard therapy—versus a combination of radiotherapy with VCPC, a chemotherapy regimen previously evaluated in a phase II study (76). All patients entered in this trial were judged to have nonresectable disease after physical examination and bronchoscopic, radiologic, and nuclear diagnostic study. Eligibility criteria were as follows: age not more than 70 years, Karnofsky performance status greater than 50%, measurable or evaluable disease, no prior treatment, and no pleural effusion except for that in patients with biopsy-proven negative histology. Of interest, and in contrast to the CALGB 8433 study (94), 193 patients (55%) with a Karnofsky performance status between 60% and 80% and 18 patients (5%) with supraclavicular node involvement also were included. Patients were allocated randomly to one of two regimens: group A received radiotherapy alone, and group B received chemotherapy plus radiotherapy. Each group was planned to receive a total radiation dose of 65 Gy in conventional fractionation. Chemotherapy consisted of vindesine, 1.5 mg/m^2 on days 1 and 2; lomustine, 50 mg/m^2 on day 2 and 25 mg/m^2 on day 3; cisplatin, 100 mg/m^2 on day 2; and cyclophosphamide, 200 mg/m^2 on days 2 through 4.

Patients in the combined modality treatment group received three monthly cycles of VCPC as indicated above. Three additional courses of VCPC were administered after completion of radiotherapy in patients without disease progression. A total of 177 patients were given radiotherapy alone, and 176 were given the combined treatment. In the final assessment (5.6 and 7.7 months after randomization in groups A and B, respectively), 33 patients in group A had a complete response, 26 had a partial response, 33 were stabilized, and 75 had a progression versus 26, 25, 27, and 87, respectively, in group B. Median survival was 10 months in group A and 12 months in group B. Group A patients had a 41% 1-year overall survival, 14% at 2 years, and 4% at 3 years versus 51%, 21%, and 12%, respectively, for group B ($P < .02$) (Fig. 17.6). The distant metastasis rate was significantly lower in group B ($P < .001$), but there was poor local control in both groups with 20% and 18% complete responses at the end of induction treatment, respectively, and 1-year local control rate of only 17% and 15%, respectively. The conclusion was that there was a significant advantage in combining chemotherapy and radiotherapy in stage IIIB NSCLC, and that this benefit was provided by the systemic effect of chemotherapy.

Mattson et al. (100) performed a randomized multicenter trial evaluating split-course radiotherapy with or without combined chemotherapy in 238 patients with NSCLC confined to one hemithorax. Radiotherapy in both treatment groups consisted of 55 Gy in 20 fractions given over 7 weeks with a 3-week rest interval. Chemotherapy consisted of cyclophosphamide, 400 mg/m^2; doxorubicin, 40 mg/m^2; and cisplatin, 40 mg/m^2 (CAP). Two cycles of CAP were given before radiotherapy, one during the resting interval and six more after radiotherapy in the combined modality group. There was no significant difference between radiotherapy and the radiotherapy-chemotherapy arms with respect to objective response rates (44% versus 49%, respectively), median duration of response, local failure, distant progression of disease, or median survival (311 versus 322 days, respectively). It was concluded that chemotherapy did not contribute significantly to either local control or survival compared with radiotherapy alone.

Minet et al. (101) included 81 patients with unresectable NSCLC in a randomized trial comparing split-course irradiation alone with combined radiotherapy and chemotherapy (CAP plus vindesine). Radiotherapy consisted of 24 Gy in six fractions over 2 weeks with a 2-week rest period, followed by another 24 Gy over 2 weeks. Chemotherapy was as follows: cyclophosphamide, 400 mg/m^2; vindesine, 3 mg/m^2; doxorubicin, 40 mg/m^2; and cisplatin, 40 mg/m^2, all administered on day 1 and repeated at monthly intervals for 8 months. Survival and quality of life were evaluated. Survival was similar in both treatment groups. The investigators concluded that the efficacy of chemotherapy in combination with split-course radiation is similar to that of radiotherapy alone.

In a trial conducted by Van Houtte et al. (102), 59 patients were randomized to treatment with chest irradiation alone or chemotherapy followed by chest radiotherapy. Four cycles of chemotherapy were administered, each including cisplatin, 60 mg/m^2 on day 1; etoposide, 120 mg/m^2 on days 2, 4, and 8; and vindesine, 1.5 mg/m^2 on days 1 and 8. Cycles were repeated every 4 weeks unless the patient's disease progressed. Chest irradiation was the same in both arms of the study, i.e., 55 Gy over 5.5 weeks to the primary lung tumor with five fractions per week. Patients were reevaluated 4 weeks after completion of chest irradiation. Of 18 patients treated with chemotherapy, only 5 achieved an objective response, including 1 complete remission. Ten patients had disease progression during chemotherapy. At the end of radiotherapy, response rates were approximately similar in both groups: 8 responses in 19 patients treated with the combined approach and 17 of 31 treated with radiotherapy only. Survival was similar in both groups with a median survival of 11 months.

In summary, as shown in Table 17.8, only three of these trials reported a positive impact of the addition of chemotherapy to radiotherapy in locally advanced NSCLC. The benefit was approximately 2 months in terms of median survival. This benefit also was observed in terms of 2- and 3-year survival, and the recent report of the 5-year follow-up of the CALGB

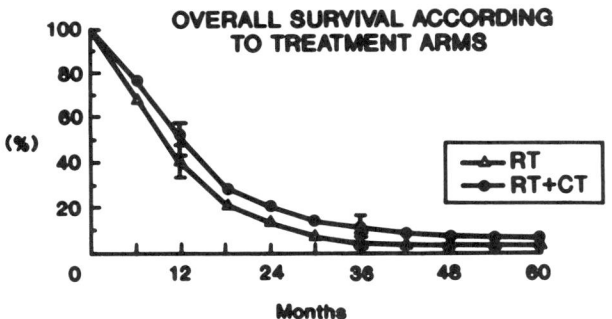

FIGURE 17.6. Survival curve of patients included in the French trial comparing radiotherapy alone to combined radiotherapy-chemotherapy in locally advanced NSCLC. (From Le Chevalier T, Arriagada R, Quoix E, et al. Radiotherapy alone versus combined chemotherapy and radiotherapy in non-resectable NSCLC: first analysis of a randomized trial in 353 patients. J Natl Cancer Inst 1991;83:417–423.)

TABLE 17.8. Randomized Trials of Sequential Cisplatin-Based Regimens Combined with Radiotherapy

Author (Reference No.)	Chemotherapy	Radiotherapy Total Dose (Gy)	Schedule	No. of Evaluable Patients	Median Survival	Survival at 2 Years (%)	Survival at 3 Years (%)	P Value
Alberti et al. (90)	CDDP/VDS	52–56	Continuous	14	19 m	NA	NA	$P = .06$
		52–56	Continuous	18	15 m	NA	NA	
Brodin and Nou (91)	CDDP/VP16	56	Continuous	330	9 m	NA	NA	NS
		56	Continuous	(total)	9 m	NA	NA	
Cardiello et al. (92)	CDDP/DOX/C	55	Split	51	60 w	NA	NA	NS
		55	Split	(total)	41 w	NA	NA	
Crino et al. (93)	CDDP/VP16	56	Continuous	33	52 w	30	NA	$P = .0559$
		56	Continuous	33	36 w	14	NA	
Dillman et al. (94, 95)	CDDP/VLB	60	Continuous	78	13.8 m	26	24	$P = .0066$
		60	Continuous	77	9.7 m	13	10	
Gregor et al. (96)	CDDP/VDS	50	Continuous	32	53 w	20	NA	NS
		50	Continuous	29	52 w	20	NA	
Kim et al. (97)	CDDP/VLB/VP16	NA	NA	43	15 m	NA	NA	NS
		NA	NA	46	9.7 m	NA	NA	
Le Chevalier et al. (98, 99)	CDDP/VDS/C/L	65	Continuous	176	12 m	21	11	$P < .02$
		65	Continuous	177	10 m	14	5	
Mattson et al. (100)	CDDP/DOX/C	55	Split	119	322 d	19	6	NS
		55	Split	119	311 d	17	8	
Minet et al. (101)	CDDP/DOX/VDS/C	48	Split	41	8 m	10	NA	NS
		48	Split	40	6.8 m	6	NA	
Sause et al. (54)	CDDP/VLB	60	Continuous	230	13.8 m	NA	NA	$P = .03$
		60	Continuous	222	11.4 m	NA	NA	
Van Houtte et al. (102)	CDDP/VDS/VP16	55	Continuous	18	11 m	7	7	NS
		55	Continuous	31	11 m	18	13	

Abbreviations. NA, not available; d, day; w, week; m, month; NS, not statistically significant; 5-FU, 5-fluorouracil; DOX, doxorubicin; MTX, methotrexate; C, cyclophosphamide; L, lomustine; P, prednisone; CDDP, cisplatin; VDS, vindesine; VLB, vinblastine.

84-33 study confirms a long-term advantage (95). Nevertheless, even though the P value reached a level of significance, the overall profile of the survival curves was not modified substantially by the addition of chemotherapy. The latter seemed only to produce a significant decrease in the rate of distant metastases but had no impact on local control, the main cause of failure in this subset of patients.

Results of the Meta-Analysis Using Individual Patient Data from Available Randomized Clinical Trials. This worldwide meta-analysis (77) was performed jointly by the Institut Gustave Roussy and the British Medical Research Council Cancer Trials Office, using updated individual patient data from 54 trials performed between 1961 and 1991, to clarify the role of chemotherapy in NSCLC. Among these, 22 involved studies comparing radiotherapy alone with the combination of chemotherapy and radiotherapy in patients with inoperable NSCLC. Two major categories of trials were considered based on whether cisplatin was included in the chemotherapy regimen. Trials of drugs given as a radiosensitizer were not included in this meta-analysis. A total of 3033 patients were evaluable, and 2814 deaths occurred. In two trials chemotherapy regimens involved the long-term use of cyclophosphamide. Vinca-alkaloids or etoposide were administered in five trials, and noncisplatin multidrug chemotherapy was used in five studies. Finally, there were 11 trials in which the chemotherapy regimen included cisplatin.

A total of 1780 patients were entered in studies in which cisplatin was part of the chemotherapy regimen, and among these 1696 deaths occurred. Two studies used the CAP regimen, three used cisplatin plus vindesine, and two others used cisplatin plus etoposide. Dosage of cisplatin ranged from 40 to 120 mg/m^2 per cycle, and total doses of cisplatin ranged from 120 to 800 mg/m^2. In these cisplatin-based trials, chemotherapy was started before radiotherapy in 10 studies. In other studies chemotherapy was given before radiotherapy in one, before and after in one, during radiotherapy in four, during and after radiotherapy in four, and after radiotherapy in six. Total radiation dose ranged from 32 to 65 Gy. It ranged from 50 to 65 Gy in the most recent cisplatin-based studies. Among 17 trials containing information on staging, 13 trials involved more than 70% stage III patients, whereas the other four had a more uniform distribution of stages I, II, and III inoperable tumors. Results show a statistically significant overall benefit of chemotherapy. The overall hazard ratio (HR) was 0.91 (P = .001), and the absolute survival benefit was 3% at 2 years and 2% at 5 years.

There was no statistical difference between trials (nonsignificant test for heterogeneity χ^2 = 22.34; degrees of freedom (df) = 24; P = .560), and no major difference in results was observed among the various chemotherapy regimens. This result was shown by the nonsignificant test for interaction ($\chi2$ = 1.91; df = 3; P = .592). Trials using long-term alkylating agents yielded a HR of 0.98 (P = .81), but the 95% confidence index (CI) is wide (0.83–1.16), and the result is not conclusive. Similarly, results with non–cisplatin-containing regimens had a HR of 0.98 (P = .88), with a 95% CI of 0.74 to 1.29. Trials in the vinca-alkaloid/etoposide category, with an HR of 0.87 (P = .23), did not significantly favor chemotherapy. The studies of cisplatin-based chemotherapy provided the most data (more than 50%) and the strongest evidence of an effect in favor of chemotherapy. The HR of 0.87 (P = .005) was equivalent to absolute survival benefits of 4% at 2 years and 2% at 5 years, with a 95% CI of 1% to 7% and 1% to 4%, respectively. Nevertheless, there is no evidence that results for the vinca-alkaloid/etoposide or other modern drug regimen categories are any different from those obtained in the cisplatin-based chemotherapy category.

CONCOMITANT RADIOTHERAPY AND CHEMOTHERAPY

Another way to combine chemotherapy and radiotherapy is to give them simultaneously. This modality is supposed to provide a better effect on local control. In contast, it also increases toxicity, and thus both modalities often need to be underdosed. If the radiosensitization obtained by chemotherapy can compensate for the decreased dose of radiotherapy, this type of combination a priori poses the problem of insufficient systemic treatment to control micrometastases.

Concomitant Trials

Several phase II trials have been conducted that attempt to define the best way to give concomitant chemotherapy and radiotherapy and to select the most active drugs for use for this type of combination.

In Italy, Bedini et al. (103) studied the effects of a continuous infusion of cisplatin (given at daily dose of 6 mg/m^2) and concomitant radiotherapy (50 Gy in a 25-fraction split course) in unresectable stage IIIA NSCLC. Treatment was administered on an outpatient basis. Toxicity was negligible, and the 2-year overall and progression free survival rates observed were 35% and 23%, respectively.

In another trial of concurrent carboplatin and radiotherapy for inoperable stage III NSCLC led by Belani (104), 37 patients with previously untreated unresectable stage III disease were treated with concurrent radiotherapy and weekly carboplatin in a single intravenous bolus of 75 mg/m^2/week (for the first six patients) and 100 mg/m^2/week in subsequent patients. Radiotherapy (1.8 to 2.0 Gy/day in five weekly fractions for a total of 60 Gy) was given concomitantly. Among the first 35 evaluable patients, there was 1 complete response and 11 partial responses, and 15 patients had stable disease. Median survival was 13 months. Overall, therapy was well tolerated.

Another phase II trial (105) was performed to evaluate the feasibility of a combined concurrent approach in an attempt to improve local control in advanced NSCLC. Thirty-four patients with a mean age of 56 years were entered. Treatment consisted of bifractionated radiotherapy (60 Gy total dose in 48 fractions in 24 days, 1.25 Gy per fraction) and cisplatin, 6 mg/m^2 administered each day of radiotherapy, plus vindesine, 2.5 mg/m^2 weekly during radiotherapy. Two complete cycles of cisplatin (120 mg/m^2, once in weeks 10 and 14) and vindesine (2.5 mg/m^2, once in weeks 11 through 13) were given after a 3-week rest period. Results showed that 18 patients (53%) had a complete response. Local control rates were 50% and 46% at 1 and 3 years, respectively. The 1-, 2- and 3-year overall survival rates were 52%, 33%, and 13%, respectively. Based on this phase II study, the investigators concluded that the combined concurrent approach may improve local control, compared with conventional approaches.

A phase II trial reported by Bardet et al. (106) was undertaken to evaluate the benefit of induction chemotherapy followed by concomitant chemoradiotherapy to improve local control in NSCLC. Forty-three patients, with a mean age of 59.8 years, who had stage IIIB NSCLC were entered and treated with etoposide (100 mg/m^2, days 1, 2, and 3) and carboplatin (350 mg/m^2, day 1); two cycles of therapy were administered on days 1 and 28. Chest irradiation was started on day 56 (2 Gy per fraction once daily, 5 days each week for a total dose of 66 Gy) together with carboplatin, 15 mg/m^2 daily. Patients who responded to induction chemotherapy received two additional cycles of etoposide-carboplatin. Results in 21 evaluable patients showed a partial response rate of 15%, stabilization of disease in 57%, and progression in 28%; the investigators concluded that a better drug combination should be used as induction treatment.

Reboul et al. (107) entered 92 patients with inoperable NSCLC into a trial evaluating the safety and efficacy of concurrent continuous infusion of cisplatin and thoracic radiotherapy. A total radiation dose of 70 Gy was delivered in 2-Gy daily fractions over 9 weeks with a 2-week rest period after 40 Gy. During the second week of each course of radiotherapy, patients were treated with cisplatin, 20 mg/m² for 5 days as a continuous infusion. Eighty-five patients were evaluable. There was an 82% overall response rate. Eleven patients who were then candidates for surgery underwent resection after a 40-Gy dose of radiation and one cycle of chemotherapy. Median survival of all patients was 11.4 months. Overall survival was 48%, 28%, and 25% at 12, 24, and 36 months, respectively. Patients who underwent surgical resection had a 2-year survival of 76% versus 21% for the other 74 patients. The authors concluded that concomitant chemoradiotherapy was well tolerated and that it produced good local control and survival benefit for patients who showed a complete response to therapy and underwent surgical resection.

Phase III Concomitant Trials

Recently, several phase III trials were developed that compared radiotherapy alone with concomitant chemoradiotherapy schedules. The results of some of these studies are already available.

The European Organization for Research and Treatment of Cancer (EORTC) conducted a three-arm randomized phase II followed by a phase III trial on 331 patients. The results were reported by Schaake-Koning et al. (108, 109). Group I received thoracic radiotherapy alone for 2 weeks (3 Gy given 10 times in five fractions per week), followed by a 3-week rest period, and then radiotherapy for 2 more weeks (2.5 Gy given 10 times in five fractions per week). Group II received the same radiotherapy schedule used in group I combined with 30 mg/m² of cisplatin given on the same first day of each treatment week. Group III was given the same radiotherapy used in group I, preceded daily by intravenous cisplatin, 6 mg/m². Results showed that survival was significantly improved in the daily cisplatin group, i.e., 54% at 1 year, 26% at 2 years, and 16% at 3 years, compared with 46%, 13%, and 2%, respectively, in the radiotherapy alone group ($P = .009$). Survival in the weekly cisplatin group was intermediate (44%, 19%, and 13%) and not significantly different from survival in either of the other two groups. The survival benefit of daily combined treatment resulted from improved control of local disease ($P = .003$). Survival without local progression was 59% at 1 year and 31% at 2 years in the daily cisplatin group; 42% and 30%, respectively, in the weekly cisplatin group; and 41% and 19% in the radiotherapy alone group. Toxicity of the concurrent schedules consisted mainly of nausea and vomiting.

Ball et al. (110) conducted a phase III randomized trial in Australia of concomitant radical accelerated radiotherapy and carboplatin chemotherapy in inoperable NSCLC. Sixty-nine patients were assigned randomly to one of four arms: arm I received conventional radiotherapy of 60 Gy in 30 fractions for 6 weeks; arm II had accelerated radiotherapy of 60 Gy in 30 fractions for 3 weeks; arm III had conventional radiotherapy (as in arm I) plus carboplatin, 70 mg/m²/day on days 1 through 5, weeks 1 and 5; or arm IV had intravenous accelerated radiotherapy (as in arm II) plus carboplatin during 1 week only. Toxicity consisted of nausea, vomiting, neutropenia, thrombocytopenia, and esophagitis. Patients in arm II had significantly more severe esophagitis than those in arm I ($P = .01$), and those in arm III had significantly more severe esophagitis than in arm I ($P = .01$). The investigators concluded that accelerated radiotherapy is associated with significantly more severe esophagitis. Results in terms of survival are awaited.

Kiseleva et al. (111) analyzed results obtained after radiotherapy or combined radiochemotherapy in 174 patients with inoperable lung cancer. This joint investigation was conducted in Hungary, Russia, and Czechoslovakia. Radiotherapy consisted of a total dose of 60 Gy administered to 98 patients, and combination radiochemotherapy (radiotherapy plus methotrexate, 2.5 mg/day for 1 to 5 days; and 5-FU, 250 mg twice weekly given simultaneously) was given to 76 patients. Mean survival after combined treatment was slightly superior (13.2 months versus 11.2 months after radiotherapy alone).

A phase III study of thoracic irradiation with or without concomitant cisplatin in locoregional unresectable NSCLC was conducted by the Hoosier Oncology Group (112). A total of 209 patients with locally advanced unresectable NSCLC were entered into a two-arm study comparing thoracic radiotherapy alone (1.8 to 2 Gy/day to a total of 60 Gy) and the identical radiotherapy plus cisplatin, 70 mg/m² on days 1, 22, and 43. There were 183 evaluable patients. Median follow-up was 28 months. There were 9% complete and 29% partial responses in the radiotherapy arm, and 38% of patients remained stable. In the combined arm, there were 12% complete and 37% partial responses, and 35% remained stable. In terms of tumor response or survival, this study failed to demonstrate a significant therapeutic advantage for radiotherapy plus concomitant weekly cisplatin compared with radiotherapy alone.

A randomized phase III clinical trial was conducted by Soresi et al. (113) to investigate whether radiotherapy together with concomitant weekly low-dose cisplatin could improve the overall response rate and locoregional disease control compared with radiotherapy alone. Ninety-five patients with unresectable NSCLC were enrolled: 50 were assigned to radiotherapy alone (50 Gy), and 45 were given the same radiotherapy plus 15 mg/m^2 of cisplatin intravenously weekly. Overall response rates of 50% and 64% were observed in the radiotherapy and radiotherapy plus cisplatin groups, respectively. No statistically significant difference was detected regarding median survival time ($P = .18$). A lower number of intrathoracic relapses was observed in the radiotherapy plus chemotherapy arm of the study (12 in the radiotherapy plus cisplatin arm versus 23 in the radiotherapy alone group, $P = .05$). Toxicity was mild.

In another study from Trovo et al. (114), 173 patients were randomized to daily-dose cisplatin with 45 Gy of continuous radiotherapy versus the same radiotherapy without cisplatin. Overall 2-year survival rates were, respectively, 15% and 20%, and this difference was not significant.

In summary, seven randomized trials questioning the benefit of concomitant radiotherapy and chemotherapy compared with radiotherapy alone have been published as shown in Table 17.9. Most trials do not show a significant difference in terms of survival. As performed for phase III trials comparing sequential combinations of radiotherapy and chemotherapy to radiotherapy alone, a meta-analysis based on individual data would probably clarify results of such an approach.

IS THERE A PLACE FOR ADJUVANT SURGERY?

Patients with stage IIIB disease usually are considered "definitely inoperable." In fact, a small number of these patients technically are completely resectable, i.e., some patients with T4 tumors and others with N3 disease. For example, a patient may have one supraclavicular homolateral lymph node involved or one right mediastinal lymph node when the primary tumor is in the left lower lobe. The classic approach to therapy in such patients is the combination of chemotherapy and radiotherapy, but this treatment modality offers poor local control as observed in several trials (98, 115). In most instances of mediastinal organ invasion by the primary tumor (T4) and/or contralateral mediastinal lymph node involvement or supraclavicular node involvement, surgical resection does not result in a complete resection. Palliative resections have not demonstrated any benefit. However, there have been scattered reports of long-term survival with aggressive surgical approaches. In fact, few studies have examined the role of preoperative radiation, chemoradiation, and chemotherapy prospectively in stage IIIB NSCLC patients.

Bedini et al. (103) performed a phase II study on 38 patients, of whom 27 had stage IIIB nonresectable NSCLC. They were treated with radiotherapy (50 Gy in a 25-fraction split course) and a concurrent continuous infusion of cisplatin (6 mg/m^2 daily). Eighteen patients underwent surgical resection; however, the exact number of patients initially staged IIIB who could un-

TABLE 17.9. Randomized Trials of Concomitant Chemoradiotherapy

Author (Reference No.)	Chemotherapy	Radiotherapy Total Dose (Gy)	Schedule	No. of Evaluable Patients	Median Survival	Survival at 2 Years (%)	Survival at 3 Years (%)	P Value
Schaake-Koning et al. (109)	CDDP, daily	55	Split	107	NA	26	16	
	CDDP, weekly	55	Split	110	NA	19	13	$P = .009$
		55	Split	114	NA	13	2	
Ball et al. (110)	CBDCA	60	Continuous					
	CBDCA	60	Accelerated	Ongoing	...	...	...	...
		60	Continuous					
		60	Accelerated					
Kiseleva et al. (111)	5-FU/MTX	60	Continuous	76	13.2 m	NA	NA	NS
		60	Continuous	98	11.2	NA	NA	
Ansari et al. (112)	CDDP	60	Continuous	93	35 w	15	NA	NS
		60	Continuous	90	41 w	9	NA	
Soresi et al. (113)	CDDP, weekly	50	Continuous	45	16 m	NA	NA	$P = 0.18$
		50	Continuous	50	11 m	NA	NA	
Trovo et al. (114)	CDDP, daily	45	Continuous	83	NA	20	NA	NS
		45	Continuous	90	NA	15	NA	

Abbreviations. NA, not available; w, week; m, month; NS, not statistically significant; MTX, methotrexate; CDDP, cisplatin; CBDCA, carboplatin; 5-FU, 5-fluorouracil.

dergo surgery was not available. Survival rates at 1, 2, and 3 years were 63%, 37%, and 24%, respectively. The investigators concluded that the good response and survival rates deserve further investigation.

In a trial started in early 1991 by Adelstein et al. (116), 32 patients with stage III NSCLC (including 12 with stage IIIB) were entered in a multimodality treatment protocol. Preoperative therapy consisted of cisplatin, 20 mg/m^2/day; 5-FU, 1000 mg/m^2/day; and etoposide, 75 mg/m^2/day, in continuous infusions over 4 days. Concurrent hyperfractionated radiation therapy was delivered at a dose of 1.5 Gy twice daily for a total dose of 27 Gy. Postoperatively, the same chemotherapy with a hyperfractionated radiation therapy dose of 13 to 36 Gy (total of 40 to 63 Gy) also was given to patients. A partial response was observed in 59% of patients after preoperative treatment, and 79% of patients could have a complete resection; 16% were not resectable; and one patient developed metastases. Nineteen patients were alive at the end of the study and disease free, despite a high treatment-related toxicity.

In the study reported by Pujol et al. (65), 3 of the 33 patients with bulky NSCLC had stage IIIB disease. Patients received a combination of cisplatin (25 mg/m^2), ifosfamide (1.5 g/m^2), and etoposide (100 mg/m^2) on days 1 through 4 of a 21-day cycle and repeated for three cycles. Patients who responded to chemotherapy underwent surgery 15 to 20 days after hematologic recovery. Five complete responses (15%) and 18 partial responses (55%) were obtained with chemotherapy. Twenty-one patients underwent thoracotomy, and tumor resection was possible in 20. A total resection was performed in 18 patients. Surgery induced no morbidity, and this induction regimen appeared to be highly effective in patients with stage III NSCLC.

A phase I-II study has been undertaken recently (117) in patients with stage IIIB disease to evaluate the feasibility of preoperative chemoradiotherapy. Chemotherapy combined 5-FU (1 g/m^2 on days 1, 2, and 3), cisplatin (100 mg/m^2 on day 1), and vinblastine (4 mg/m^2 on day 1) with concomitant accelerated thoracic radiotherapy (a total dose of 42 Gy given in two fractions of 1.5 Gy per day, 5 days per week). Of 13 patients entered in this trial, 8 became candidates for surgery, and resection was possible in 7 of them. There was no surgery-related morbidity. A phase III trial is planned to evaluate the role of surgical resection in stage IIIB NSCLC.

As shown in Table 17.10, most studies addressing the role of surgery in locally advanced NSCLC included both stages IIIA and IIIB. Response rates vary from 51% to 84% and resectability rates from 33% to 85%. Moreover, these trials are difficult to compare because of differing doses and scheduling of both radiotherapy and chemotherapy. Nevertheless, these results warrant further evaluation.

In any case a consensus exists among medical oncologists that surgery is not indicated as initial therapy in patients with stage IIIB NSCLC. Nevertheless, the very poor local control obtained suggests that more aggressive local treatment is required. To date, no study has demonstrated that survival can be prolonged by adjuvant surgery.

TREATMENT OF SUPERIOR VENA CAVA SYNDROME

Anticoagulant therapy should be initiated as soon as the diagnosis of SVCS is confirmed (16, 17). It can sometimes be sufficient by itself in paucisymptomatic cases. Radiotherapy is the main treatment for SVCS caused by malignancy (14, 16). It has been used at a dose of 4 Gy/day for the first 3 days, with subsequent decreasing doses up to a total of 30 to 40 Gy. Chemotherapy generally is used solely in NSCLC as adjuvant therapy after radiotherapy because this type of tumor is poorly chemosensitive and the use of cisplatin requires hydration. Venous bypass surgery with synthetic prostheses (128), usually used in cases of SVCS resulting from benign causes, is proposed rarely for SVCS related to malignancy. Vascular prostheses (expandable metallic stents) (18) have been developed recently for treatment of SVCS caused by extrinsic compression. With use of a suitable balloon catheter, dilation of the stenotic lumen is achieved carefully with installation of an expandable metallic stent. This treatment also requires anticoagulant therapy up to reepithelialization of the endoprosthesis. It generally produces complete relief of symptoms and recently has modified therapeutic strategies because chemotherapy can be started without problems of hydration.

PERSPECTIVES

Patients presenting with stage IIIB NSCLC represent a major challenge for the coming years. Despite recent advances in combined treatment modalities, these patients have a very poor prognosis, and their treatment is mainly palliative. The usefulness of chemotherapy in the treatment of patients with inoperable stage III NSCLC has been confirmed in a recent meta-analysis including 3000 patients, but the modest benefit observed deserves further investigation to improve long-term control substantially.

Bearing these considerations in mind, some major goals can be envisaged in the near future:

TABLE 17.10. Preoperative Chemoradiotherapy Trials in Stage III NSCLC

Author (Reference No.)	No. of Patients	Stages	Chemotherapy	Radiotherapy		Response (%)	Resection (%)	Median Survival (Mo.)
				Dose (Gy)	Schedule			
Eagan et al. (118)	39	III	CDDP/DOX/C	30	Sequential	51	33	11
Taylor et al. (119)	64	III	CDDP/5-FU	40	Concomitant	56	61	16
Recine et al. (120)	64	IIIA, IIIB	CCDDP/5-FU/VP16	40–67	Concomitant	84	36	13
Lokich et al. (121)	30	III	5-FU	30–60	Concomitant	91	NA	>12
Faber et al. (122)	64	III	CDDP/5-FU	40	Concomitant	NA	68	20
Faber et al. (122)	29	III	CDDP/5-FU/VP16	40	Concomitant	NA	76	34
Weiden and Piantadosi (123)	76	III	CDDP/5-FU	30	Concomitant	57	42	11
Strauss et al. (124)	32	IIIA	CDDP/5-FU/VLB	30	Concomitant	62	62	NA
Albain et al. (125)	65	IIIA, IIIB	CDDP/VP16	NA	Concomitant	65	65	NA
Skarin et al. (126)	41	IIIA	CDDP/DOX/C	30	Sequential	53	85	32
Sherman et al. (127)	21	III	CDDP/VDS	30	Sequential	56	62	27
Bedini et al. (103)	38	IIIA, IIIB	CDDP	50	Concomitant	83	47	14
Adelstein et al. (116)	32	IIIA, IIIB	CDDP/5-FU/VP16	27	Sequential	59	78	NA
Grunenwald et al. (117)	13	IIIB	CDDP/5-FU/VLB	42	Concomitant	NA	54	NA

Abbreviations. C, cyclophosphamide; CDDP, cisplatin; VDS, vindesine; 5-FU, 5-fluorouracil; DOX, doxorubicin; VLB, vinblastine; NA, not available.

1. Randomized trials need to be conducted with a large number of patients to evaluate promising new drugs. New combination regimens probably will increase the complete response rate and therefore improve the control of micrometastases.
2. New combined modality strategies should be employed, such as the use of multifractionated or accelerated fractionation radiation therapy. Major improvements can be expected using fractionation adjusted for particular tumor kinetics. It is now established that delayed complications are more strongly related to fractionation than to overall treatment time. Timing also must be evaluated better in chemotherapy-radiotherapy combination protocols.
3. Adjuvant surgery could be another modality that improves local control. Even though preliminary results are encouraging in some series of selected patients, its role remains to be defined. Together with other comparable studies, this aggressive approach to some stage IIIB NSCLC disease could improve long-term results because of better local control.
4. Symptomatic treatments such as laser therapy or cryotherapy (discussed elsewhere in this book) can be of great assistance for patients with obstructive tumors.
5. Another investigational approach, local gene therapy, is currently being studied and may be a new avenue of research for these patients (129).

CONCLUSION

Locally advanced NSCLC stage III disease involves a subset of patients without distant metastases considered inoperable at the time of presentation. For a long time radiotherapy has been widely accepted as the standard treatment of stage III NSCLC. A revision of the therapeutic strategies in such patients is warranted in light of recent progress in the treatment of metastatic disease with new chemotherapeutic regimens. Both poor local control and the short median survival of patients with stage IIIB disease have led to recent evaluations of combined chemotherapy and radiotherapy strategies, the use of new schedules of irradiation, and the impact of chemotherapy on survival. Other questions, such as the usefulness of possible adjuvant surgery or new biologic treatments, are still under investigation.

References

1. Bartecchi CE, Mackenzie TD, Schrier RW. The human costs of tobacco use (first of two parts). N Engl J Med 1994; 330:907–912.
2. Stanley KE. Lung cancer and tobacco: a global problem. Cancer Detect Prevent 1986;9:83–89.
3. Silverberg E, Lubera JA. Cancer statistics, 1988. CA Cancer J Clin 1988;38:5–22.
4. Kreyberg L. Histologic typing of lung tumors. In: Kreyberg L, ed. International Histologic Classification of Tumors. Geneva: World Health Organization, 1967:19–26.
5. Matthews MJ, Kanhouwa S, Pickner J, et al. Frequency of residual and metastatic tumors in patients undergoing curative surgical resection of lung cancer. Cancer Chemother Rep 1973;3:63–67.
6. Task Force on Lung Cancer. Staging of Lung Cancer, 1979. In: American Joint Committee for Cancer Staging and End Results Reporting: Manual for Staging of Cancer. Chicago: American Joint Committee, 1979.
7. Mountain CF. A new international staging system for lung cancer. Chest 1986;89:225–233.

8. Green MR. Unresectable stage III non–small cell lung cancer: lessons and directions from clinical trial research. J Natl Cancer Inst 1991;83:382–383.
9. Karnofsky D, Burchenal J. The clinical evaluation of chemotherapeutic agents in cancer. In: Macleod C, ed. Evaluation of chemotherapeutic agents. New York: Columbia University Press, 1949:191–205.
10. Minna JD. Neoplasms of the lung. In: Wilson JD, Braunwald E, Isselbacher KJ, Petersdorf RG, Martin JB, Fauci AS, eds. Harrison's principles of internal medicine. 12th ed. 1991.
11. Ginsberg RJ, Kris HG, Armstrong JG. Cancer of the lung. In: De Vita V, Hellman S, Rosenberg SA, eds. Cancer: principles and practice of oncology. 4th ed. Philadelphia: Lippincott, 1993;673–723.
12. Heelan R, Martini N, Wescott JW, et al. Carcinomas involving the hilum and mediastinum: computed tomographic and magnetic resonance evaluation. Radiology 1985;156:111–115.
13. Little AG, De Meester TR, Ryan JW. The use of radionuclide scans in lung cancer and thoracic surgery. Philadelphia: Saunders, 1986:122–128.
14. Little AG, Stitik FP. Clinical staging of patients with non small cell lung cancer. Chest 1990;97:1431–1438.
15. Luke WP, Pearson FG, Todd TRJ, et al. Prospective evaluation of the mediastinum for assessment of carcinoma of the lung. J Thorac Cardiovasc Surgery 1986;91:53–56.
16. Salsali M, Cliffton EE. Superior vena cava obstruction with lung cancer. Ann Thorac Surg 1968;6:437–442.
17. Painter TD, Karpf M. Superior vena cava syndrome: diagnostic procedures. Am J Med Sci 1983;285:2–6.
18. Putnam JS, Uchidia BT, Antonivic R, Rosch J. Superior vena cava syndrome associated with massive thrombosis: treatment with expandable wire stents. Radiology 1988;167:727–728.
19. Stanley KE. Prognostic factors for survival in patients with inoperable lung cancer. J Natl Cancer Inst 1980;65:25–32.
20. Albain KS, Crowley JJ, Leblanc M, Livingston RB. Survival determinants in extensive-stage non–small cell lung cancer: the Southwest Oncology Group experience. J Clin Oncol 1991;9:1618–1626.
21. Ihde DC, Minna JD. Non small cell lung cancer. Part I: biology, diagnosis and staging. Curr Probl Cancer 1991;15:61–104.
22. Feld R, Arriagada R, Ball DL, et al. Prognostic factors in non–small cell lung cancer. Lung Cancer 1991;7:3–5.
23. Nakahara D, Monden Y, Ohno K, Fujii Y, Hashimoto J, Kitagawa Y, Kawashima Y. Importance of biologic status to the post-operative prognosis of patients with stage III non small cell lung cancer. J Surg Oncol 1987;36:155–160.
24. Fatzinger P, de Meester TR, Derakjian H, Iascone C, Golomb HM, Little AG. The use of serum albumin for further classification of stage III non–oat cell lung cancer and its therapeutic implications. Ann Thorac Surg 1984;37:115–122.
25. Alama A, Costantini M, Repetto L, Conte PF, Serrano J, Nicolin A, Barbieri F, et al. Thymidine labelling index as prognostic factor in resected non–small cell lung cancer. Eur J Cancer 1990;26:622–625.
26. Ichinose Y, Hara N, Ohta M, Motohiro A, Kuda T, Aso H. Postoperative adjuvant chemotherapy in non–small cell lung cancer: prognostic value of DNA ploidy and post recurrent survival. J Surg Oncol 1991;46:15–20.
27. Isobe H, Miyamoto H, Shimizu T, et al. Prognostic and therapeutic significance of the flow cytometric nuclear DNA content in non–small cell lung cancer. Cancer 1990;65:1391–1395.
28. Sahin AA, Ro JY, El Naggar AK, et al. Flow cytometric analysis of the DNA content of non small cell lung cancer. Ploidy as a significant prognostic indicator in squamous cell carcinoma of the lung. Cancer 1990;65:530–537.
29. Volm M, Hahn EW, Mattern J, et al. Five-year follow-up of independent clinical and flow cytometric prognostic factors for survival of patients with non–small cell lung carcinoma. Cancer Res 1988;48:2923–2928.
30. Stanley K, Cox JD, Petrovich Z, Paig C. Patterns of failure in patients with inoperable carcinoma of the lung. Cancer 1981;47:2725–2729.
31. Saunders MI, Bennett MH, Dische S, Anderson PJ. Primary tumor control after radiotherapy for carcinoma of the bronchus. Int J Radiat Oncol Biol Phys 1984;10:499–501.
32. Perez CA, Bauer M, Edelstein S. Impact of tumor control on survival in carcinoma of the lung treated with irradiation. Int J Radiat Oncol Biol Phys 1986;12:539–547.
33. Perez CA, Pajak TF, Rubin P, et al. Long term observations of the patterns of failure in patients with unresectable non–oat cell carcinoma of the lung treated with definitive radiotherapy. Cancer 1987;59:1874–1881.
34. Gelman R, Gelber R, Henderson IC, et al. Improved methodology for analysing local and distant recurrence. J Clin Oncol 1990;8:548–555.
35. Kramar A, Arriagada R. Analysing local and distant recurrences. J Clin Oncol 1990;8:2086–2087.
36. Johnson M. Chemotherapy for unresectable non small cell lung cancer. Semin Oncol 1988;17:20–29.
37. Ihde DC. Chemotherapy of lung cancer. N Engl J Med 1992;327:1434–1441.
38. De Vita VT Jr, Simon RM, Hubbard SM, et al. Curability of advanced Hodgkin's disease with chemotherapy. Long-term follow up of MOPP-treated patients at the NCI. Ann Intern Med 1980;92:587–595.
39. Bonomi P, Finkelstein D, Ruckdeschel J, et al. Combination chemotherapy versus single agents followed by combination chemotherapy in stage IV non–small cell lung cancer. A study by the Eastern Cooperative Oncology Group. J Clin Oncol 1989;7:1602–1613.
40. Lazarus HM. Autologous bone marrow transplantation for the treatment of lung cancer. Semin Oncol 1993;20:72–79.
41. Damstrup L, Skovgaard, Poulsen H. Review of the curative role of radiotherapy in the treatment of non small cell lung cancer. Lung Cancer 1994;11:153–178.
42. Durrant KR, Ellis F, Black JM, et al. Comparison of treatment policies in inoperable bronchial carcinoma. Lancet 1971;1:715–719.
43. Roswit B, Patno ME, Rapp R, et al. The survival of patients with inoperable lung cancer. A large-scale randomized study of radiation therapy versus placebo. Radiology 1968;90:688–697.
44. Thames HD, Bentzen SM, Turesson I, et al. Time-dose factors in radiotherapy: a review of the human data. Radiother Oncol 1990;19:219–235.
45. Perez CA. Non–small cell carcinoma of the lung: dose-time parameters. Cancer Treat Symp 1985;2:131–142.
46. Perez CA, Stanley K, Rubin P, et al. A prospective randomized study of various irradiation doses and fractionation schedules in the treatment of inoperable non–oat cell carcinoma of the lung. Cancer 1980;45:2744–2753.
47. Cox JD, Azarnia N, Byhardt RW, et al. A randomized phase I/II trial of hyperfractionated radiation therapy with total doses of 60.0 Gy to 79.2 Gy: possible survival benefit with > 69.6 Gy in favorable patients with radiation therapy oncology group stage III non–small cell lung carcinoma. Report of radiation therapy oncology group 83-11. J Clin Oncol 1990;8:1543–1555.

48. Holsti LR, Mattson K. A randomized study of split course radiotherapy of lung cancer: long term results. Int J Radiat Oncol Biol Phys 1980;6:977–981.
49. Lee RE, Carr DT, Childs DS. Comparison of split-course radiotherapy and continuous radiation therapy for unresectable bronchogenic carcinoma: 5 years results. Am J Roentgenol Radium Ther Nucl Med 1976;126:116–121.
50. Slawson RG, Salazar OM, Poussin-Rosillo H, et al. Once a week versus conventional daily radiation treatment for lung cancer: final report. Int J Radiat Oncol Biol Phys 1988;15:61–68.
51. Petrovich Z, Stanley K, Cox JD, Paig C. Radiotherapy in the management of locally advanced lung cancer of all cell types. Cancer 1981;48:1335–1340.
52. Levitt SH, Bogardus CR, Ladd G. Split dose intensive radiation therapy in the treatment of advanced lung cancer: a randomized study. Radiology 1967;88:1159–1161.
53. Saunders MI, Dische S, Grosch EJ, et al. Experience with CHART. Int J Radiat Oncol Biol Phys 1991;21:871–878.
54. Sause W, Scott C, Taylor S, et al. RTOG 8808-ECOG 4588, preliminary analysis of a phase III trial in regionally advanced unresectable non–small cell lung cancer. Proc Am Soc Clin Oncol 1994;325:1072. Abstract.
55. Emami B, Perez CA, Herkovic A, Hederman MA. Phase I/II study of treatment of locally advanced (T3, T4) non–oat cell lung cancer with high dose radiotherapy (rapid fractionation): Radiation Therapy Oncology Study Group. Int J Oncol Biol Phys 1988;15:1021–1025.
56. Brindle J, Shaw EG, Su JQ, et al. Pilot study of accelerated hyperfractionated thoracic radiation therapy in patients with unresectable stage III non small cell lung carcinoma. Cancer 1993;72:405–409.
57. Splinter TAW. Chemotherapy in advanced non small cell lung cancer. Eur J Cancer 1990;10:1093–1099.
58. Chapman R, Lewis J, Kvale D, et al. A neoadjuvant trial in stage II and IIIA non small cell lung cancer with cisplatin and vinblastin chemotherapy (abstract 954). Proc Am Soc Clin Oncol 1990;9:246.
59. Bitran JD, Golomb HH, Hoffman PC, et al. Protochemotherapy in non–small cell lung cancer. An attempt to increase surgical resectability and survival. A preliminary results. Cancer 1986;57:44–53.
60. Spain RC. Neoadjuvant mitomycin C, cisplatin and infusion vinblastin in locally and regionally advanced non–small cell lung cancer: problems and progress from the perspective of long-term follow-up. Semin Oncol 1988;15:6–15.
61. Martini N, Kris MG, Flehinger BJ, et al. Preoperative chemotherapy for stage IIIa (N2) lung cancer: the Sloan-Kettering experience with 136 patients. Ann Thorac Surg 1993;55:1365–1374.
62. Vokes EE, Bitran JD, Hoffman PC, et al. Neoadjuvant vindesine, etoposide, and cisplatin for locally advanced non–small cell lung cancer. Chest 1989;96:110–113.
63. Raut Y, Huu N, Clavier J, et al. Surgery and chemotherapy. A new method of treatment for squamous cell bronchial carcinoma. J Thorac Cardiovasc Surg 1984;88:754–757.
64. Darwish S, Minoth V, Crino L, et al. Neoadjuvant cisplatin and etoposide for stage IIIA (clinical N2) non small cell lung cancer. Am J Clin Oncol 1994;17:64–67.
65. Pujol JL, Rossi JF, Le Chevalier T, et al. Pilot study of neoadjuvant ifosfamide, cisplatin and etoposide in locally advanced non–small cell lung cancer. Eur J Cancer 1990;26:798–801.
66. Fossella L, Ryan B, Dhingra H, et al. Interim report of a prospective randomized trial of neoadjuvant chemotherapy plus surgery versus surgery alone for stage IIIA non–small-cell lung cancer (NSCLC). Proc Am Soc Clin Oncol 1991;10:240.
67. Burkes RL, Ginsberg RJ, Shepherd FA, et al. Induction chemotherapy with mitomycin, vindesine and cisplatin for stage III unresectable non–small cell lung cancer. Results of the Toronto phase II trial. J Clin Oncol 1992;10:580–586.
68. Pisters KMW, Kris MG, Gralla JR, et al. Pathologic complete response in advanced non small cell lung cancer following preoperative chemotherapy: implications for the design of future non small cell lung cancer combined modality trials. J Clin Oncol 1993;11:1757–1762.
69. Johnson D, Einhorn L, Bartolucci A, et al. Thoracic radiotherapy does not prolong survival in patients with locally advanced unresectable non–small cell lung cancer. Ann Intern Med 1990;113:33–38.
70. Kaasa S, Thorud E, Höst H, et al. A randomized study evaluating radiotherapy versus chemotherapy in patients with inoperable non small cell lung cancer. Radiat Oncol 1988;11:7–13.
71. Dewit L. Combined treatment of radiation and cis-dichlorodiammine-platinum: a review of experimental and clinical data. Int J Radiat Oncol Biol Phys 1987;13:403–406.
72. Vokes EE, Weichselbaum RR. Concomitant chemoradiotherapy: rationale and clinical experience in patients with solid tumors. J Clin Oncol 1990;8:911–934.
73. Vokes EE. Investigation chemotherapy in multimodality therapy of non–small cell lung cancer. In: Meyer JL, Vaeth JM, eds. Radiotherapy/chemotherapy interactions in cancer therapy. Basel: Karger, 1991;26:64–71.
74. Kubota K, Furuse K, Kawahara M, et al. Role of radiotherapy in combined modality treatment of locally advanced non–small cell lung cancer. J Clin Oncol 1994;12:1547–1552.
75. Samuels ML, Barkley HT, Holoye PY, Rosenberg PJ, Smith TL. Combination chemotherapy with bleomycin, vincristine, and methotrexate plus split-course radiotherapy in the treatment of non–oat cell bronchogenic carcinoma. Cancer Chemother Rep 1975;59(Part 1):377–383.
76. LeChevalier T, Arriagada R, Baldeyrou P, et al. Combined chemotherapy (vindesine, lomustine, cisplatin, and cyclophosphamide), and radical radiotherapy in inoperable non-metastatic squamous cell carcinoma of the lung. Cancer Treat Rep 1985;69:469–472.
77. Pignon JP, Stewart LA, Souhami RL, Arriagada R. A meta-analysis using individual patient data from randomised clinical trials (RCTS) of chemotherapy (CT) in non small cell lung cancer (NSCLC). 2. Survival in the locally advanced (LA) setting (abstract 1109). Proc Am Soc Clin Oncol 1994;13:334.
78. Bergsagel DE, Jenkin RD, Pringle JF, et al. Lung cancer: clinical trial of radiotherapy alone versus radiotherapy plus cyclophosphamide. Cancer 1972;30:621–627.
79. Höst H. Cyclophosphamide as adjuvant to radiotherapy in the treatment of unresectable bronchogenic carcinoma. Cancer Chemother Rep 1973;4:161–164.
80. Veterans Administration Lung Cancer Study Groups. Preliminary report on nonresectable cancer of the lung. Cancer Chemother Rep 1974;58:359–364.
81. Simpson JR, Francis ME, Perez-Tamayo R, Marks RD, Rao DV. Palliative radiotherapy for inoperable carcinoma of the lung: final report on a RTOG multi-institutional trial. Int J Radiat Oncol Biol Phys 1985;11:751–758.
82. Schallier DC, De Neve WJ, De Greve L, et al. Is adjuvant treatment with vinblastine effective in reducing the occurrence of distant metastasis in limited squamous cell lung cancer? A randomized study. Clin Exp Metastasis 1988;6:39–48.

83. White J, Chen T, Reed R, et al. Limited squamous cell carcinoma of the lung: a Southwest Oncology Group randomized study of radiation with or without doxorubicin chemotherapy and with or without levamisole immunotherapy. Cancer Treat Rep 1982;66:1113–1120.
84. Anderson G, Deeley TJ, Smith C, Jani J. Comparison of radiotherapy alone and radiotherapy with chemotherapy using adriamycin and 5-fluorouracil in bronchogenic carcinoma. Thorax 1981;36:190–193.
85. Israel L, Depierre A, Dalesio O. Interim results of EORTC protocol 08742. Comparison after irradiation of locally advanced squamous cell bronchial carcinoma, of abstention, immunotherapy, combination chemotherapy or chemoimmunotherapy. In: Mathe G, Bonnadonna G, Salmon S. Recent results in cancer research. Berlin, Heidelberg: Springer-Verlag, 1982;80:214–218.
86. Morton R, Jett JR, McGinnis W, et al. Thoracic radiation therapy alone compared with combined chemoradiotherapy for locally unresectable non–small cell lung cancer: a randomized phase III trial. Ann Intern Med 1991;115:681–686.
87. Petrovich Z, Ohanian M, Cox J. Clinical research on the treatment of locally advanced lung cancer. Final report of VALG protocol 13 limited. Cancer 1978;42:1129–1134.
88. Sidorowicz E, Hirsch V, Hand R, et al. Comparison of radiotherapy and radiotherapy-MACC chemotherapy in limited non–small cell lung cancer (NSCLC) (abstract 277). IVth World Conference on Lung Cancer, Toronto, Canada, August 25–30, 1985:86.
89. Trovo MG, Minatel E, Veronesi A, et al. Combined radiotherapy and chemotherapy versus radiotherapy alone in locally advanced epidermoid bronchogenic carcinoma. Cancer 1990;65:400–404.
90. Alberti W, Nierderle N, Budach V, et al. Prospective randomised study comparing immediate radiotherapy (RT) chemo-plus radiotherapy (CT+RT) or delayed radiotherapy in non–small cell lung cancer (abstract B4, 149.22). Cancer Res Clin Oncol 1990;116(Suppl):503.
91. Brodin O, Nou E. Swedish Multicenter Group for the study of squamous cell carcinoma of the lung. Patients with non-resectable squamous cell carcinoma of the lung: a prospective, randomized study (abstract 615). Lung Cancer 1991;7(Suppl):165.
92. Cardiello C, Blanco VJ, Anac S, et al. Combined radiochemotherapy (RTCHT) versus radiotherapy (RT) in limited inoperable non small cell carcinoma of the lung (NSCLC). Proc Am Soc Clin Oncol 1985;4:692.
93. Crino L, Maranzano E, Meacci L, et al. Induction chemotherapy plus high dose radiotherapy versus radiotherapy alone in locally advanced unresectable non small cell lung cancer. Ann Oncol 1993;4:847–851.
94. Dillman RO, Seagren SL, Propert KJ, et al. A randomized trial of induction chemotherapy plus high-dose radiation versus radiation alone in stage III non–small cell lung cancer. N Engl J Med 1990;323:940–948.
95. Dillman RO, Seagren SL, Herndon J, et al. Randomized trial of induction chemotherapy plus radiation therapy versus RT alone in stage III non small cell lung cancer (NSCLC): five year follow-up of CALGB 84-33 (abstract 1092). Proc Am Soc Clin Oncol 1993;12:329.
96. Gregor A, Mac Beth F, Paul J, et al. Radical radiotherapy and chemotherapy in localized inoperable non small cell lung cancer: a randomised trial. J Natl Cancer Inst 1993;85:997–999.
97. Kim NK, Yang SH, Im YH, et al. A Phase III randomized comparison of neo-adjuvant chemotherapy with cisplatin, etoposide, and vinblastine (PEV) plus radiation versus radiation alone in stage III NSCLC (abstract 1098). Proc Am Soc Clin Oncol 1993;12:330.
98. Le Chevalier T, Arriagada R, Quoix E, et al. Radiotherapy alone versus combined chemotherapy and radiotherapy in non-resectable NSCLC: first analysis of a randomized trial in 353 patients. J Natl Cancer Inst 1991;83:417–423.
99. Le Chevalier T, Arriagada R, Tarayre M, et al. Significant effect of adjuvant chemotherapy on survival in locally advanced non small cell lung carcinoma (letter). J Natl Cancer Inst 1992;84:58.
100. Mattson K, Holsti L, Holsti P, et al. Inoperable non–small cell lung cancer: radiation with or without chemotherapy. Eur J Cancer Clin Oncol 1988;24:477–482.
101. Minet P, Bartsch P, Chevalier Ph, et al. Quality of life of inoperable non–small cell lung carcinoma. A randomized phase II clinical study comparing radiotherapy alone and combined radiotherapy. Radiother Oncol 1987;8:217–230.
102. Van Houtte P, Klastersky J, Renaud A, et al. Induction chemotherapy with cisplatin, etoposide, and vindesine before radiation therapy for NSCLC. In: Arriagada R, Le Chevalier T, eds. Treatment modalities in lung cancer. Antibiotics and chemotherapy. Basel: Karger, 1988;41:131–137.
103. Bedini AV, Tavecchio L, Milani F, et al. Non resectable stage III A-B lung carcinoma: a phase II study on continuous infusion of cisplatin and concurrent radiotherapy (plus adjuvant surgery). Lung Cancer 1993;10:73–84.
104. Belani CP. Multimodality therapy for regionally advanced non–small cell lung cancer. Semin Oncol 1993;20:302–314.
105. Arriagada R, Le Chevalier T, Bretel JJ, et al. Concurrent cisplatin-vindesine and bifractionated thoracic radiotherapy (RT) in locally advanced non small cell lung cancer (abstract 709). Lung Cancer 1994;11(Suppl 1):183.
106. Bardet E, Quoix E, Riviere A, et al. A phase II trial of induction chemotherapy followed by concomitant chemo-radiotherapy in stage IIIB non small cell lung cancer (NSCLC) (abstract 702). Lung Cancer 1994;11(Suppl 1):183.
107. Reboul F, Vincent P, Chauvet B, et al. Radiation therapy with concomitant continuous infusion cisplatin for unresectable nonsmall cell lung carcinoma. Int J Radiat Biol Phys 1994;28:1251–1256.
108. Schaake-Koning C, Maat B, Van Houtte P, et al. Radiotherapy combined with low-dose cis-diammine dichloroplatinum (II) (CDDP) in inoperable non–small cell lung cancer (NSCLC): a randomized three arm phase II study of the EORTC Lung Cancer and Radiotherapy Cooperative Groups. Int J Radiat Oncol Biol Phys 1990;19:967–972.
109. Schaake-Koning C, Van Den Bogaert W, Dalesio O, et al. Effects of concomitant cisplatin and radiotherapy on inoperable non–small cell lung cancer. N Engl J Med 1992;326:524–530.
110. Ball D, Bishop J, Smith J, Crennan E, O'Brien P, Davis S, Ryan G, et al. A phase III study of accelerated radiotherapy with and without carboplatin in non–small cell lung cancer (NSCLC): interim toxicity analysis. Lung Cancer 1994;11(Suppl 1):54–55.
111. Kiseleva ES, Pitskholaur A, Trakhtenberg KH, et al. Results of radiotherapy and combined chemotherapy and radiotherapy of inoperable lung cancer. Neoplasia 1983;30:573–580.
112. Ansari R, Tokar SR, Fisher W, et al. A phase III study of thoracic irradiation with or without concomitant cisplatin in locoregional unresectable non–small cell lung cancer (NSCLC): a Hoosier Oncology Group (HOG) protocol (abstract 823). Proc Am Soc Clin Oncol 1991;10:241.

113. Soresi E, Clerici M, Grilli R, et al. A randomized clinical trial comparing radiation therapy versus radiation therapy plus *cis*-dichlorodiammine platinum (II) in the treatment of locally advanced non–small cell lung cancer. Semin Oncol 1988;15(Suppl 7):20–25.
114. Trovo MG, Minatel E, Franchin G, et al. Radiotherapy versus radiotherapy enhanced by cisplatin in stage III non small cell lung cancer. Int J Radiat Oncol Biol Phys 1992;24:11–15.
115. Bardet E, Quoix E, Riviere A, et al. A phase II trial of induction chemotherapy followed by concomitant chemo-radiotherapy in stage IIIB non small cell lung cancer (NSCLC) (abstract 702). Lung Cancer 1994;11(Suppl 1):181.
116. Adelstein DJ, Rice TW, Tefft M, et al. Concurrent chemotherapy (CT) and hyperfractionated radiation therapy (HRT) followed by surgery for stage III non–small cell lung cancer (abstract 677). Lung Cancer 1994;11(Suppl 1):175.
117. Grunenwald D, Le Chevalier T, Arriagada R, et al. Surgical resection of stage IIIB non–small-cell lung cancer (NSLC) after concomitant induction chemo-radiotherapy. Preliminary results (abstract 703). Lung Cancer 1994;11(Suppl 1):181.
118. Eagan RT, Ruud C, Lee KE, et al. Pilot study of induction therapy with cyclophosphamide, doxorubicin, and cisplatin (CAP) and chest irradiation prior to thoracotomy in initially inoperable stage III M0 non–small cell lung cancer. Cancer Treat Rep 1987;71:895–900.
119. Taylor SG IV, Trybula M, Bonomi PD, et al. Simultaneous cisplatin fluorouracil infusion and radiation followed by surgical resection in regionally localized stage III, non–small cell lung cancer. Ann Thorac Surg 1987;43:87–91.
120. Recine D, Rowland K, Reddy S, et al. Combined modality therapy for locally advanced non–small cell lung carcinoma. Cancer 1990;66:2270–2278.
121. Lokich J, Chaffey J, Neptune W. Concomitant 5-Fluorouracil infusion and high-dose radiation for stage III non small cell lung cancer. Cancer 1989;64:1021–1025.
122. Faber LP, Kittle CF, Warren NH, et al. Preoperative chemotherapy and irradiation for stage III non–small-cell lung cancer. Ann Thorac Surg 1989;47:669–675.
123. Weiden P, Piantadosi S. Preoperative chemoradiotherapy in stage III non–small-cell lung cancer (NSCLC): a phase II study of the Lung Cancer Study Group (LCSG). Proc Am Soc Clin Oncol 1988;7:197.
124. Strauss G, Sherman L, Mathisen D, et al. Concurrent chemotherapy (CT) and radiotherapy (RT) followed by surgery (S) in marginally resectable stage IIIA non–small-cell lung carcinoma (NSCLC): a cancer and leukemia group B study. Proc Am Soc Clin Oncol 1988;7:203.
125. Albain K, Rusch V, Crowley J, et al. Concurrent cisplatin (DDP), VP16 and chest irradiation (RT) followed by surgery for stages IIIA and IIIB non–small-cell lung cancer (NSCLC): a Southwest Oncology Group (SWOG) study (#8805). Proc Am Soc Clin Oncol 1991;10:244.
126. Skarin A, Jochelson M, Sheldon T, et al. Neoadjuvant chemoradiotherapy in marginally resectable stage III M0 non–small-cell lung cancer: long term follow-up in 41 patients. J Surg Oncol 1989;40:266–274.
127. Sherman D, Strauss G, Schwartz J, et al. Combined modality therapy for regionally advanced stage III non–small-cell lung cancer (NSCLC) employing neoadjuvant chemotherapy (CT), radiotherapy (RT) and surgery (S). Proc Soc Clin Oncol 1987;6:167.
128. Doty DB. Bypass of superior vena cava: six years experience with spiral vein graft for obstruction of vena cava due to benign and malignant disease. J Thorac Cardiovasc Surg 1982;83:326–328.
129. Fujiwara T, Cai DW, Georges RN, et al. Therapeutic effect of a retroviral wildtype *p53* expression vector in an orthotopic lung cancer model. J Natl Cancer Inst 1994;86:1458.

18

ROLE OF SURGERY IN THE TREATMENT OF PATIENTS WITH SOLITARY METASTASIS FROM NON–SMALL CELL LUNG CANCER

Michael E. Burt

INTRODUCTION

The accepted standard of care for patients with metastatic non–small cell lung cancer (NSCLC) has traditionally been supportive care or chemotherapy. However, there appears to be a small group of patients with metastatic NSCLC who may benefit from resection of their metastasis. This group is defined as patients with a solitary metastatic focus of NSCLC and locoregional disease that has been controlled or is controllable.

It is estimated that in 1995 there will be 170,000 new cases of lung cancer diagnosed in the United States and that 158,000 patients will die of lung cancer (1). Of the new cases of lung cancer, 80% (136,000 patients) will have NSCLC. Because approximately 50% of all patients with a newly diagnosed NSCLC will have metastatic disease, 68,000 will have distant metastases at the time of initial presentation. Most of these patients will present with metastases at multiple sites; however, approximately 7%, or 4,800, will present with a solitary metastasis to the brain, lung, liver, bone, adrenal gland, or another less common site (2). This is a unique group of patients for whom an exploration has begun of an operative approach for control of both the metastatic and locoregional disease. To date, there are relatively few data to support an operative approach. Traditionally, these patients would be offered chemotherapy with the goal of prolonging life and palliating symptoms seen at presentation.

Although chemotherapy for patients with metastatic NSCLC has become an accepted standard, the data from randomized trials comparing supportive care with chemotherapy are conflicting. Table 18.1 summarizes the data of four randomized trials in patients with either locally advanced or stage IV NSCLC who have been treated with cisplatin-based chemo-therapy (3–6). The percentage of patients with stage IV disease who were randomized in these protocols ranged from 57% to 100%, and the dose of cisplatin ranged from 80 to 120 mg/M^2. In these trials of supportive care versus chemotherapy, the median survival in patients treated by supportive care alone ranged from 3.2 to 4.9 months, and from 4.7 to 8 months in patients randomized to cisplatin-based chemotherapy. Although these studies tended to show better survival for chemotherapy compared with supportive care, only the trial from the National Cancer Institute of Canada (5) demonstrated a statistically significant survival advantage (median survival, 7.4 months versus 3.9 months, respectively).

Regardless of the potential benefit from these forms of chemotherapy, the impact on survival for state IV disease remains modest at best. Alternative therapeutic strategies thus seem warranted, especially among subgroups with potentially better outcomes.

The bias in the literature (1–5) is that patients with a solitary site of metastasis receiving chemotherapy have a better prognosis than those with multiple sites of metastases, but the data supporting this perception are sparse. In a prospective study of solitary adrenal metastasis in otherwise operable patients with NSCLC performed at Memorial Sloan–Kettering Cancer Center, the median survival of patients with a solitary metastasis to the adrenal gland treated with cisplatin-based chemotherapy was 9 months, which is similar to the outcome of patients with multiple sites of metastases treated with the same regimen (7). Because patients with a solitary focus of metastatic disease from

TABLE 18.1. Results of Randomized Trials Comparing Supportive Care with Chemotherapy in Patients with Inoperable Non–Small Cell Lung Cancer

Study, Year (Reference No.)	No. of Patients	Stage IV (%)	CDDP (mg/m^2)	Median Survival (Mo)	P Value
NCI (Canada), 1988 (3)					
No chemo	50	90	0	3.9	...
Chemo (CAP)	43	86	40	5.7	.051
Chemo (VP)	44	82	120	7.4	.01
UCLA, 1989 (4)					
No chemo	26	100	0	3.2	...
Chemo (VP)	22	100	120	4.7	.09
Australia, 1990 (5)					
No chemo	91	59	0	3.9	...
Chemo (VP)	97	73	120	6.3	.33
Italy, 1991 (6)					
No chemo	61	57	0	4.9	...
Chemo (CECy)	62	60	80	8.0	.15

Abbreviations. Chemo, chemotherapy; CAP, cyclophosphamide, adriamycin, cisplatin; VP, vindesine, cisplatin; CDDP, cisplatin; CECy, cisplatin, etoposide, cyclophosphamide.
^{a}Compared with supportive care (no chemotherapy).

NSCLC treated with chemotherapy do not appear to have a better prognosis, the role of surgery in this group warrants exploration.

The data supporting resection of a solitary metastasis in NSCLC have been confined primarily to two groups: (a) patients with a solitary brain metastasis, and (b) those with a solitary adrenal metastasis. Data supporting resection of other solitary sites of metastasis, such as bone, liver, and contralateral lung, are less well supported.

SOLITARY BRAIN METASTASIS

The development of a brain metastasis in patients with NSCLC is both a common and a devastating event (8–11). Because brain metastasis develops before death in approximately 30% of patients with NSCLC, a brain metastasis thus will develop in approximately 40,000 patients with NSCLC in the United States during 1995. One realizes the size of this problem by comparing the estimated incidence of new primary cancers of other sites: in 1995 there will be 38,200 new cases of rectal cancer, 24,000 cases of pancreatic cancer, 22,800 cases of gastric carcinoma, and 12,100 cases of esophageal carcinoma. In addition, NSCLC is the most common tumor metastatic to the brain, accounting for 40% to 60% of all brain metastases (12). The natural history after development of a brain metastasis from NSCLC is one of progressive neurologic deterioration, with a median survival of approximately 1 month without therapy (13, 14). In this group, corticosteroids are usually administered and can produce a dramatic and rapid improvement in neurologic symptoms (15–18). Corticosteroids alone do little to prolong survival, however, and treated patients have a median survival of approximately 2 months (18–20). Because of this dismal prognosis, radiation therapy has been used in these patients. Early studies with full brain irradiation were encouraging, with approximately 80% of the patients demonstrating a benefit (21, 22). Subsequent work corroborated a palliative benefit, with little morbidity; unfortunately, the survival benefit was small, with most investigators reporting a median survival of only 3 to 6 months (23–27).

Given the dismal outlook for patients with NSCLC and a solitary brain metastasis using radiation therapy alone, early attempts were made to resect the brain metastasis, often with poor results (28, 29). Before the advent of steroids and modern neuroanesthesia and perioperative care, resection of brain metastasis was considered futile (29). With the modern era of neurosurgical techniques and perioperative care, resection of brain metastasis is possible with low mortality and an apparent increased survival benefit (30–32). Further refinement of indications and techniques for resection of brain metastasis allowed for routine consideration of surgical resection as a safe and viable option generally for patients with brain metastasis, and particularly for patients with NSCLC.

An example of a large solitary metastasis to the left frontal region discovered in a patient 6 months after a left pneumonectomy for a T2, N0, M0 squamous cell carcinoma is illustrated in Figure 18.1. This patient underwent craniotomy and resection of the large metastasis and was alive and well 2 years afterward, with only a residual scar seen on a recent brain MRI (Fig. 18.2). This example illustrates that even large metastatic lesions can be resected safely.

During the 1970s and early 1980s, there was continual debate among investigators regarding how best to treat patients with a solitary brain metastasis from NSCLC (27, 33). Without controlled trials comparing whole brain irradiation and surgery, patients were treated with various modalities depending on the bias of the physician.

In 1986 two retrospective studies (Mandell et al. [34] and Patchell et al. [35]) compared whole brain irradiation with surgical therapy plus whole brain irradiation in patients with a solitary NSCLC brain metastasis. Although both studies were retrospective, the results of the studies were similar, demonstrating a significant survival advantage for surgery plus whole brain irradiation compared with whole brain irradiation alone. The

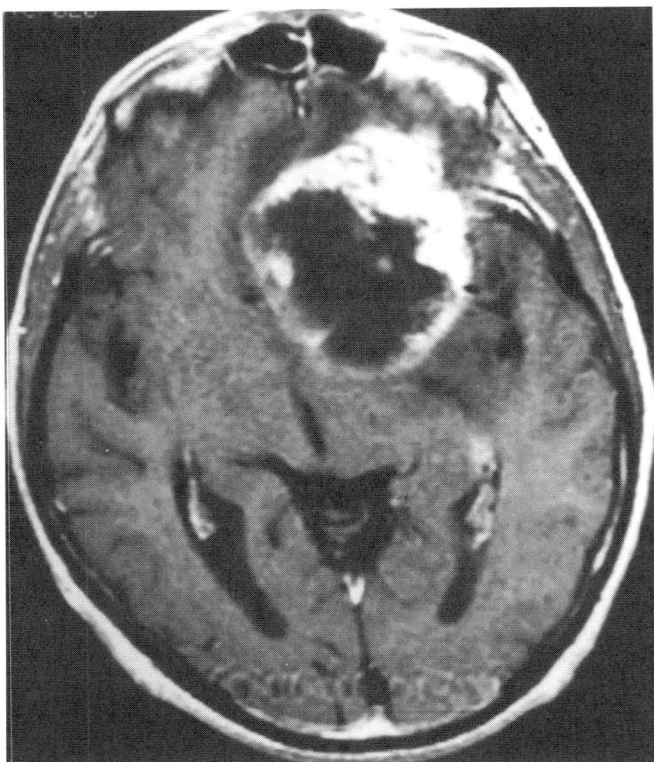

FIGURE 18.1. Brain MRI demonstrating a large left frontal mass in a patient with NSCLC.

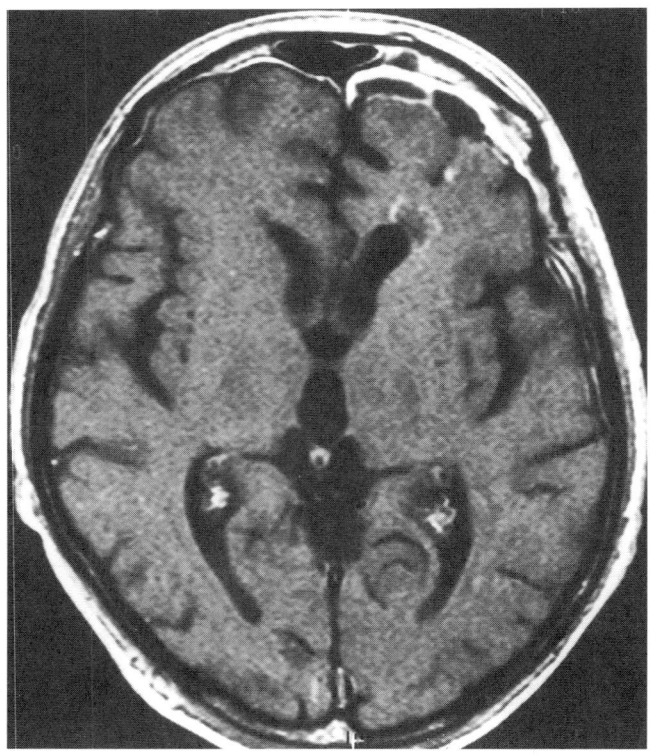

FIGURE 18.2. Brain MRI of the same patient shown in Figure 18.1 two years after resection of a metastasis from NSCLC.

group undergoing resection of the solitary brain metastasis had a median survival ranging from 16 to 19 months, compared with a median survival of from 4 to 6 months in the group receiving whole brain irradiation alone.

The randomized trial by Patchell et al. (36) compared resection followed by whole brain irradiation to whole brain irradiation alone in patients with a solitary brain metastasis from any site. Table 18.2 summarizes the data from this study: 72% to 83% of the patients entered in this trial had a solitary brain metastasis from NSCLC. The remaining patients had a metastasis from breast, gastrointestinal, or genitourinary carcinomas or melanoma. In addition, 36% to 39% of the patients also had metastases to other sites, in addition to metastasis to the brain. This randomized trial confirmed the survival advantage of surgery plus irradiation (median survival, 9.2 months) over whole brain irradiation alone (median survival, 3.4 months, $P < .01$) in patients with a solitary brain metastasis. In addition, this study showed that recurrence at the original site of the brain metastasis was significantly less, and that patients remained functionally independent significantly longer in the surgical group compared with the radiation therapy alone group. Although this study was not confined to patients with solitary brain metastasis from NSCLC, a large percentage of the patients did have NSCLC, and the overall advantage of surgery is highly suggestive that resection of a solitary brain metastasis from NSCLC translates into long-term survival.

A second prospective trial by Noordijk et al. (37) randomized 63 patients to resection plus whole brain irradiation versus radiation therapy alone in patients with a solitary brain metastasis from all sites. Approximately 50% of the patients had NSCLC, and the other patients had breast carcinoma, kidney carcinoma, mel-

TABLE 18.2. Randomized Trial of Resection plus Whole Brain Irradiation Versus Whole Brain Irradiation Alone in Patients with a Solitary Brain Metastasis

	WBRT	RESECTION + WBRT
Number of patients	23	25
Radiotherapy dose	3600 cGy	3600 cGy
Non–small cell lung cancer	83%	72%
Metastases to other sites	39%	36%
Recurrence in brain	52%	20% ($P < .02$)
Median survival	3.4 mo	9.3 mo ($P < .01$)
Median time with KS >70	1.9 mo	8.8 mo ($P < .005$)

Adapted from Patchell RA, Tibbs PA, Walsh JW, et al. A randomized trial of surgery in the treatment of single metastases to the brain. N Engl J Med 1990;322:494–500.
Abbreviations. WBFT, whole brain irradiation; KS, Karnofsky status.

anoma, and miscellaneous other primary malignant tumors. The median survival was significantly greater in the patients receiving resection plus full brain irradiation (median survival, 10 months) versus those receiving full brain irradiation alone (median survival, 6 months) ($P = .04$). In this study the majority of patients who died did so because of systemic disease. The investigators also noted that patients whose locoregional disease was stable had significantly prolonged survival compared with those whose locoregional disease had progressed.

At the Department of Surgery at Memorial Sloan–Kettering Cancer Center, results of a surgical approach to patients with brain metastasis from NSCLC were evaluated using a prospective database (created in 1972 by Joseph Galicich, M.D.) of all patients undergoing craniotomy for metastatic neoplasm. In this series there were 185 patients (89 men and 96 women) undergoing resection of a brain metastasis from NSCLC. The ages ranged from 34 to 75 years (median, 54 years) (38). Ninety percent of these patients smoked cigarettes for a median of 56 pack-years. Among these patients, the histology was adenocarcinoma in 70%, squamous cell carcinoma in 21%, and large cell carcinoma in 9%. All patients, by definition, had stage IV disease; however, excluding the M1 component of the brain metastasis, the locoregional disease was stage I in 38%, stage II in 7%, stage IIIA in 33%, stage IIIB in 16%, and stage IV (other metastatic sites) in 7%. A total of 120 patients (65%) presented with a metachronous lesion and 65 patients (35%) with a synchronous metastasis. Resection of the brain metastasis was considered complete in 94% and incomplete in 6% of the patients. There was a 3% 30-day and a 7% 60-day operative mortality. Of the 185 patients, 89% had resection of a single metastasis and 11%, multiple brain metastases. Of the patients with multiple brain metastases, 85% had a complete resection. Tumors were located infratentorially in 14% and supratentorially in 86%. Of note, 83% of the patients received either preoperative or postoperative whole brain irradiation, with 17% receiving no irradiation (Table 18.3).

The overall survival for these 185 patients undergoing craniotomy and resection of metastases from NSCLC was 58%, 17%, 13%, and 7% at 1, 3, 5, and 10 years, respectively (Fig. 18.3). The overall median survival for this group of patients was 14 months. To analyze prognostic variables that might predict survival in this group, a univariate analysis was performed; the results are compiled in Table 18.4. As can be seen from this analysis, resection of the primary locoregional chest disease had a significant impact on survival.

TABLE 18.3. Whole Brain Radiation in Patients Who Had Resection of a Brain Metastasis from Non–Small Cell Lung Cancer and Whole Brain Radiation Therapy

	Radiation Dose	
	Median (cGy)	Range (cGy)
Preoperative ($n = 32$)	3000	1000–6200
Postoperative ($n = 110$)	3000	600–6000
Preoperative and postoperative ($n = 11$)	4500	2100–8000
Total ($n = 153$)	3000	600–8000

There was a trend showing that the extent of the brain resection also impacted survival. Other variables—supratentorial versus infratentorial, synchronous versus metachronous, single versus multiple lesions, locoregional chest stage, early versus late metastasis, and whole brain irradiation versus no radiation therapy—did not significantly impact survival.

For patients presenting with an NSCLC and a solitary metastasis to the brain as their only evidence of systemic disease, the question arises regarding the best treatment of both the metastasis and the locoregional disease. From the retrospective reports showing a survival advantage for resection of an NSCLC brain metastasis and the two randomized trials showing a significant increase in survival for surgery plus whole brain irradiation, the treatment of choice of a solitary brain metastasis in patients with good performance status is resection. Whether whole brain irradiation impacts on the survival is uncertain. In one study (38) whole brain irradiation did not impact survival in a univariate or a multivariate analysis. In addition, when a case-controlled comparison of the 32 patients who did not receive whole brain irradiation after resection was matched to patients who did receive whole brain irradiation after resection, there was no significant impact on survival for the addition of whole brain irradiation to resection (39). These data suggest that if a complete resection of the brain metastasis were performed, whole brain irradiation would not impact survival or local recurrence in the brain. However, further study is needed to verify this concept.

The question then becomes how best to treat the locoregional disease in patients who present with a synchronous solitary brain metastasis from NSCLC and otherwise operable locoregional disease. From the literature it is not clear if the locoregional (i.e., T and N) stage or the treatment of the locoregional disease (i.e., resection, radiation therapy, or chemotherapy) affects survival. When the analysis was restricted to 65 patients undergoing resection of a synchronous NSCLC brain metastasis (38), it was found that the locore-

FIGURE 18.3. Actuarial overall survival of 185 patients undergoing resection of brain metastases from NSCLC (median survival, 14 months).

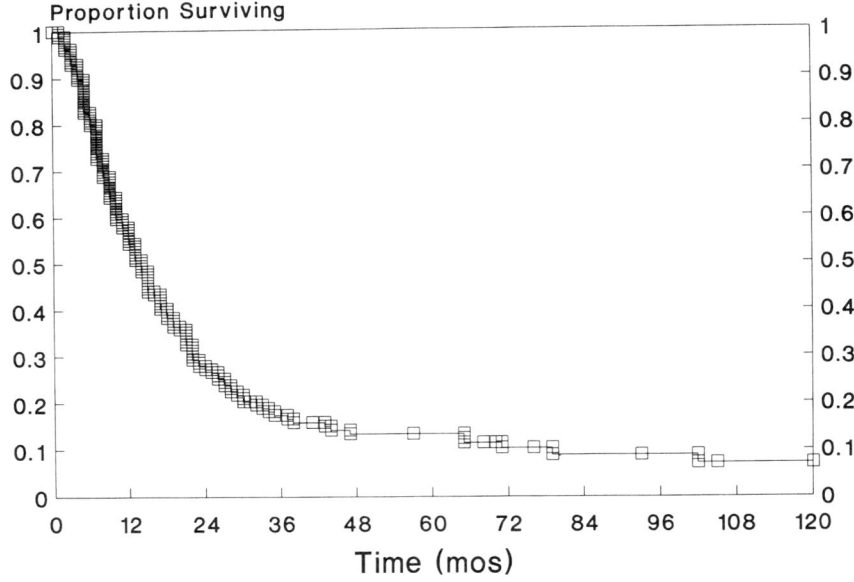

TABLE 18.4. Univariate Analysis of Prognostic Variables Affecting Survival in 185 Patients Undergoing Resection of Brain Metastases from Non–Small Cell Lung Cancer

VARIABLE	P VALUE
Resection of lung primary	.0006
Extent of brain resection	.09
Supra-tentorial versus infratentorial	.12
Synchronous versus metachronous	.24
Single versus multiple	.25
Locoregional chest stage	.3
Metachronous: early versus late	.69
Whole brain radiation versus none	.72

gional TN stage of patients undergoing resection of brain metastasis did not influence survival. There was no significant difference in survival between patients with early (stages I and II) or advanced (stages IIIA and IIIB) locoregional disease ($P = .30$). Approximately half of the patients underwent complete resection of the locoregional disease, and the remaining half either did not have an exploratory operation, or they had exploration and either did not have resection or had an incomplete resection. Sixty-one percent of these patients received radiation therapy, chemotherapy, or both. When analyzed by treatment, patients undergoing complete resection of the locoregional primary lung disease survived significantly longer (median, 21 months) than those with residual locoregional disease (median, 10 months) ($P = .0006$) (Fig. 18.4).

To clarify the effect of locoregional stage and resection of the locoregional chest disease, a multivariate analysis (Cox proportional hazards model) was performed, concluding that the locoregional stage did not significantly influence survival ($P = .97$), but that the resectability of the locoregional disease significantly prolonged survival ($P = .002$). Although it is highly possible that these differences are an artifact of patient selection, these data do suggest that resection of a solitary brain metastasis from NSCLC can translate into improved survival. The authors thus conclude that for patients with a solitary synchronous brain metastasis, both the primary and metastatic lesions should be excised surgically if they are potentially resectable.

SOLITARY ADRENAL METASTASIS

Adrenal metastases from NSCLC are common and have been reported in 18% to 42% of patients in autopsy series (40–44). Combining the autopsy series of Abrams et al. (40), Engleman et al. (41), and Matthews (42), there were 642 patients who died of NSCLC, of whom 39% had metastases to the adrenal gland. Although most of these patients also had metastases to other organs, there are patients who present with a solitary metastasis to the adrenal gland (7).

Because most investigators obtain a computed tomography (CT) scan of the chest and upper abdomen (that includes the liver and adrenal glands) during the evaluation of a patient with NSCLC (45–48), the number of adrenal masses discovered is increasing. A clinical problem arises when a patient with a potentially operable NSCLC also has a unilaterally enlarged adrenal gland. Data concerning the prevalence of adrenal metastasis from NSCLC in patients with otherwise operable disease are sparse. In a prospective

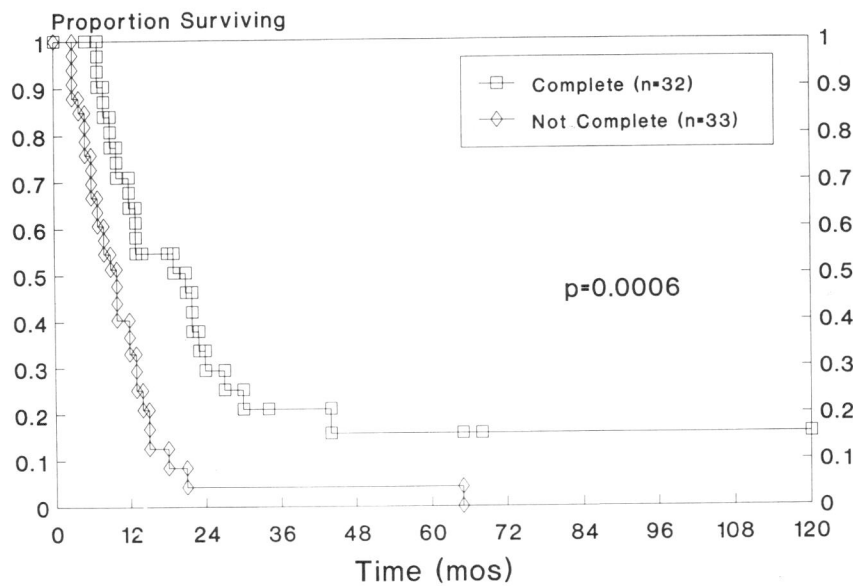

FIGURE 18.4. Actuarial survival of 65 patients undergoing resection of brain metastases from NSCLC stratified by treatment of the lung tumor. Thirty-two patients underwent complete resection of the locoregional lung disease, and 33 were either not explored or incompletely resected.

study, Oliver et al. (49) reported that 8% of 296 patients with operable NSCLC had a unilaterally enlarged adrenal gland found by CT scanning. Among the 23 patients with a unilaterally enlarged adrenal, 6 (26%) had metastatic deposits based on biopsy or follow-up CT scan. At Memorial Sloan–Kettering Cancer Center, of 246 patients with otherwise operable NSCLC, 10 patients (4%) had a unilaterally enlarged adrenal gland identified by a CT scan (7). All patients underwent biopsy, and 4 (40%) of the 10 were found to have metastasis to adrenals. From these two studies, it appears that approximately 4% to 8% of patients with otherwise operable NSCLC will have a unilaterally enlarged adrenal gland, and approximately 25% to 40% of these will be metastatic disease. One potentially could assume the opposite point of view, i.e., when a patient with operable NSCLC has a unilateral adrenal mass on CT scan, it could be benign because 60% to 74% ultimately prove to be benign. Most authors recommend that the CT scan performed as part of the evaluation of the patient with NSCLC include the upper abdomen to the level of the adrenal glands. The CT scan should not be used to distinguish between a metastatic and a benign adrenal mass, however. Even if a patient had a clinical stage I NSCLC, a unilateral adrenal mass should not be assumed to be benign because 25% to 40% of patients found to have a metastatic focus in the unilateral adrenal mass had clinical stage I as their locoregional disease (7, 50). Figure 18.5 depicts an abdominal CT scan in a 48-year-old man with a clinical stage I adenocarcinoma of the left upper lobe. Also depicted is a 2-cm left adrenal mass. Needle biopsy was nondiagnostic. A left adrenalectomy revealed complete

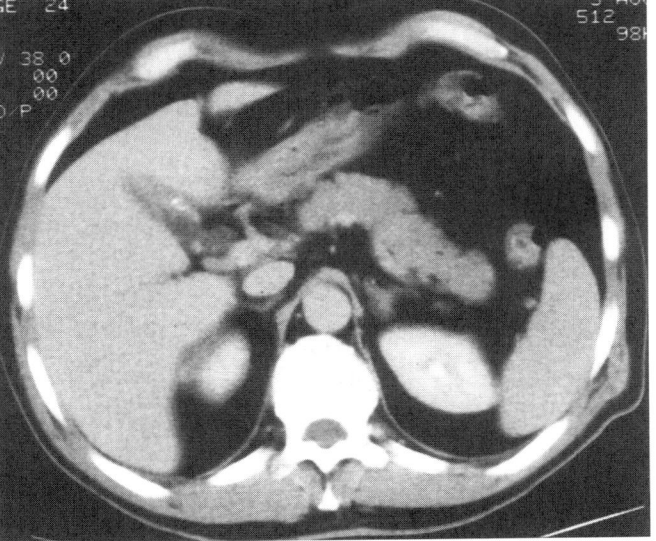

FIGURE 18.5. Abdominal CT scan of a patient with a clinical stage I NSCLC and a 2-cm left adrenal mass.

replacement with metastatic adenocarcinoma (Fig. 18.6).

Recent advances in magnetic resonance imaging (MRI) have led some investigators to suggest that MRI can accurately predict whether an adrenal mass in a patient with NSCLC is metastatic or benign. Early studies with 0.35 to 0.5 T superconducting magnets suggested that MRI could distinguish metastatic from benign lesions (51–54). As more data accumulated with this lower strength magnet, investigators cautioned against relying solely on MRI (55) and recommended biopsy when accurate histologic diagnosis was

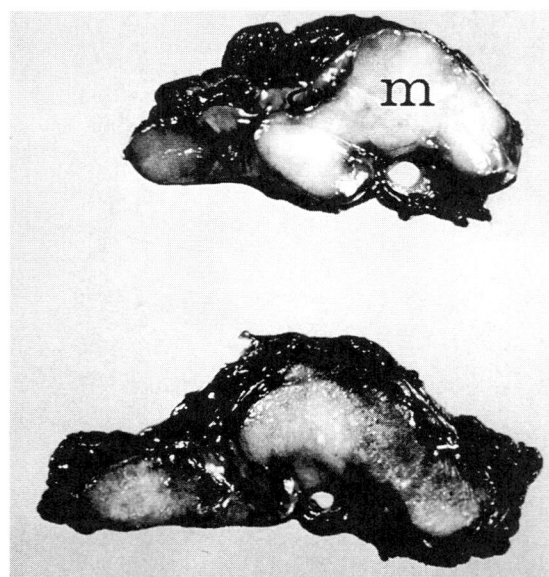

FIGURE 18.6. Resected left adrenal mass from the same patient shown in Figure 18.5 demonstrating complete replacement with metastatic adenocarcinoma of lung.

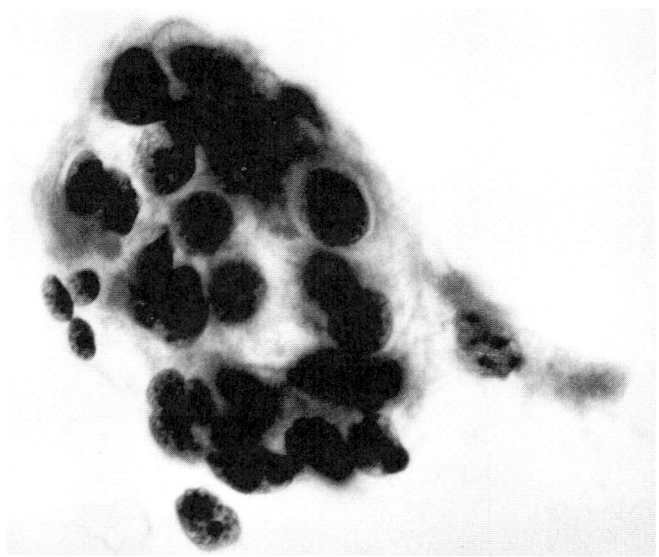

FIGURE 18.7. CT-guided aspiration needle biopsy of patient with a 2.5-cm right adrenal mass and a clinical stage II adenocarcinoma of lung, demonstrating metastatic adenocarcinoma.

crucial (56). With the development of a more powerful magnet (1.5 T), investigators have tried again to develop MRI criteria to predict whether an adrenal mass is benign or malignant (57, 58).

In a recent prospective study at Memorial Sloan–Kettering Cancer Center, 25 patients with otherwise operable NSCLC and a unilateral adrenal mass underwent MRI (1.5 T) by standard technique. Diagnosis of a benign or metastatic adrenal mass was based on the relative signal strengths of the enlarged adrenal on the T1- and T2-weighted pulsing sequences, compared with normal adrenal and liver. Four patients had metastatic NSCLC, and 21 had benign adrenal masses. The sensitivity of MRI for differentiating a benign from a malignant mass was 100%, the specificity was 24%, the false-positive rate was 67%, and the false-negative rate was 0%. These results preclude accepting MRI as a routine method for determining whether an adrenal mass is benign or malignant. Perhaps newer methods, such as in vivo chemical shift (59) or echoplanar MRI (60), may increase the specificity and decrease the false-positive rate. Therefore, until better imaging techniques become available, needle biopsy should remain the standard for distinguishing an adrenal adenoma from a NSCLC metastasis (Fig. 18.7).

Size alone also cannot be used to characterize adrenal masses as benign or malignant. Figures 18.8 and 18.9 show the CT scan and MRI of a 6.5-cm adrenal mass in a patient with an otherwise operable NSCLC. Needle biopsy was nondiagnostic, and a left adrenalectomy revealed a benign adenoma.

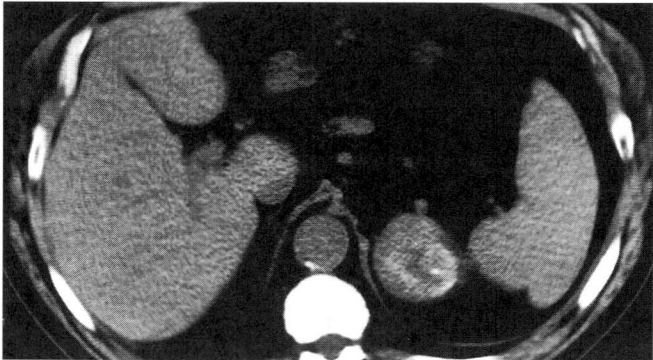

FIGURE 18.8. CT scan demonstrating a 6.5-cm left adrenal mass in an otherwise operable patient with a NSCLC.

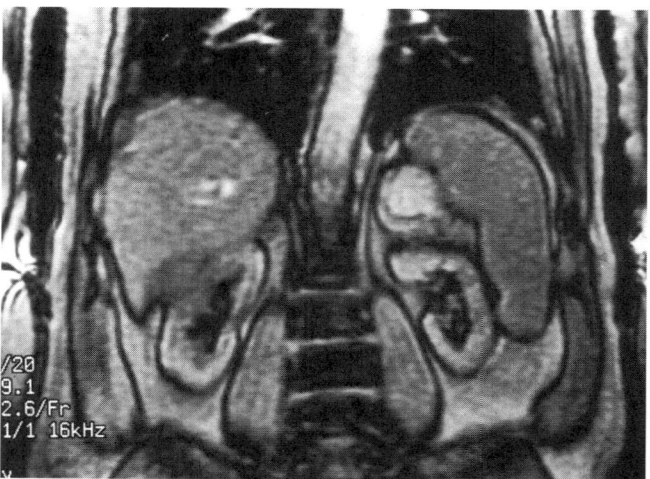

FIGURE 18.9. MRI (coronal view) of the same 6.5-cm left adrenal mass shown in Figure 18.8.

The importance of the etiology of an unilateral adrenal mass in determining prognosis cannot be overemphasized. A group of 37 patients with otherwise operable NSCLC and a unilateral adrenal mass was studied prospectively at Memorial Sloan–Kettering Cancer Center. In this data set, 9 patients had metastatic, and 28 patients had benign adrenal masses. Of the 28 patients with benign adrenal masses, 25 underwent pulmonary resection (5 after cisplatin-based chemotherapy for IIIA disease), 2 received radiation therapy for unresectable tumor, and 1 received preoperative chemotherapy but died of sepsis before surgery. Of the 9 patients with adrenal metastasis, 6 were treated with cisplatin-based chemotherapy alone, and 3 were treated with preoperative cisplatin-based chemotherapy and then pulmonary and adrenal resection. All 6 patients treated with chemotherapy alone died. Of the 3 patients treated with preoperative chemotherapy followed by resection of the adrenal metastases and the locoregional chest disease, all currently are alive, but the follow-up period at this time is short. The overall survival of patients with metastatic adrenal masses was significantly shorter than that of patients with benign masses (Fig. 18.10). As depicted, no patient with a solitary adrenal metastasis survived more than 2 years (median, 19 months).

A review of the literature yielded three series describing 11 patients with solitary adrenal metastases from NSCLC (61–63). Of these, 6 were synchronous and 5 metachronous; 6 were adenocarcinoma, 4 were large cell carcinoma, and 1 was squamous cell carcinoma. Nine patients underwent resection of the adrenal metastasis (1 received preoperative chemotherapy, 4 received postoperative chemotherapy, and 2 received postoperative radiation therapy); 2 patients received radiation therapy to the adrenal metastasis. The overall survival of these 11 patients was 34% at 5 years, with a median survival of 35 months. Obviously, these patients are a highly selective group. However, these data demonstrate a potential survival benefit for the resection of a solitary adrenal metastasis.

OTHER SOLITARY SITES OF METASTASIS

Data supporting the role of surgery in other solitary sites of metastatic NSCLC are particularly sparse. A recent review of the management of cancer metastatic to bone supports resection of bone metastases as a means of palliation in certain circumstances. At Memorial Sloan–Kettering Cancer Center, the outcome of 14 patients presenting metachronously with solitary metastases from NSCLC was reviewed recently. This analysis found metastasis to extrathoracic lymph nodes ($n = 5$), skeletal muscle ($n = 4$), bone ($n = 3$), small bowel ($n = 1$), and spleen ($n = 1$). All patients had previously undergone complete resection of the locoregional lung cancer at a mean of 19 months before the development of the metastasis. Histology of the metastasis included adenocarcinoma ($n = 8$), large cell carcinoma ($n = 1$), and squamous cell carcinoma ($n = 5$). The stage of these patients before development of a metastasis was: stage I ($n = 3$), stage II ($n = 6$), or stage IIIA ($n = 5$).

Thirteen patients had a complete resection of the metastasis (4 also received chemotherapy or radiation therapy), and 1 patient showed a complete response to curative radiation therapy for a metastasis to the

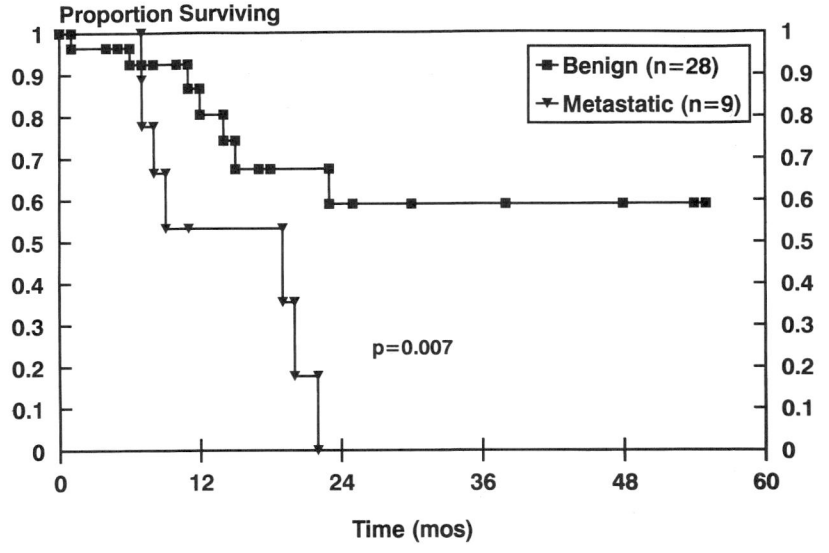

FIGURE 18.10. Actuarial survival of 37 patients with solitary adrenal masses and otherwise operable NSCLC stratified by whether the adrenal mass was benign or metastatic NSCLC.

humerus. The overall actuarial survival at 12 years was 91%, and 11 patients are currently alive with no evidence of disease at this point in time. Obviously, this is a retrospective analysis of a highly select group, but it does suggest that in a small but select number of patients, resection of a solitary metastasis may translate into long-term benefit.

CONCLUSIONS

In the United States in 1995, approximately 136,000 patients will present with NSCLC, of which approximately 50% will have metastatic disease. Although most patients will present with diffuse metastases, approximately 7% will present with a solitary focus of metastatic disease. In this unique group of patients, the data presented in this chapter suggest that a surgical approach to both locoregional chest disease and the metastasis warrants investigation. Thus far, chemotherapy alone has not made a large impact on survival in these patients.

With the initial encouraging results for resection of brain metastasis patients with NSCLC and the limited experience with solitary adrenal metastasis at Memorial Sloan–Kettering Cancer Center, a phase II trial has been developed to evaluate combination chemotherapy and surgery in these patients. Eligible patients are those with a solitary metastasis to the brain, adrenal gland, liver, bone, or lung. Histologic diagnosis must be obtained for both the metastasis and the locoregional disease. Brain metastasis are resected at presentation for diagnosis and therapy. Patients receive three cycles of high-dose cisplatin, mitomycin, and velban followed by resection of the locoregional chest disease and the metastasis (if not resected previously). They then receive two further cycles of cisplatin and velban post resection. To date, 18 patients have been entered on this trial, but the data are too preliminary to analyze. Hopefully, the use of combined modalities, including surgical resection, will permit greater local and systemic control among this select group of patients.

REFERENCES

1. Wingo PA, Tong T, Bolden S. Cancer statistics, 1995. CA Cancer J Clin 1995;45:8–30.
2. Albain KS, Crowley JJ, Le Blanc ML, Livingston RB. Survival determinants in extensive stage non–small cell lung cancer: the Southwestern Oncology Group experience. J Clin Oncol 1991;9:1618–1626.
3. Rapp E, Pater JL, Wilan A, et al. Chemotherapy can prolong survival in patients with advanced small-cell lung cancer: report of Canadian multicenter randomized trial. J Clin Oncol 1988;6:633–641.
4. Ganz PA, Figlin RA, Haskell CM, et al. Supportive care versus supportive care and combination chemotherapy in metastatic non–small cell lung cancer. Cancer 1989;63:1271–1278.
5. Woods RL, William CJ, Levi J, et al. A randomized trial of cisplatin and vindesine versus supportive care in advanced non–small cell lung cancer. Br J Cancer 1990;61:608–611.
6. Cellerino R, Tummarello D, Guidi F, et al. A randomized trial of alternating chemotherapy versus best supportive care in advanced non–small-cell lung cancer. J Clin Oncol 1991;9:1453–1461.
7. Ettinghausen SE, Burt ME. Prospective evaluation of unilateral adrenal masses in patients with operable non–small cell lung cancer. J Clin Oncol 1991;9:1462–1466.
8. Newman SJ, Hansen HH. Frequency diagnosis, and treatment of brain metastases in 247 consecutive patients with bronchogenic carcinoma. Cancer 1974;33:492–496.
9. Halpert B, Fields WS, De Bakey ME. Intracranial metastasis from carcinoma in the lung. Surgery 1954;35:346–349.
10. Figlin RA, Piantadosi S, Feld R. The Lung Cancer Study Group. Intracranial recurrence of carcinoma after complete surgical resection of stage I, II, and III non– small cell lung cancer. N Engl J Med 1988;318:1300–1305.
11. Komaki R, Cox JD, Start R. Frequency of brain metastases in adenocarcinoma and large cell carcinoma of the lung: Correlation with survival. Int J Radiat Oncol Biol Phys 1983;9:1467–1470.
12. Wright DC. Surgical treatment of brain metastases. In: Rosenberg SA, ed. Surgical treatment of metastatic cancer. New York: JB Lippincott, 1987:165–222.
13. Richards P, McKissock W. Intracranial metastases. BMJ 1963;1:15–18.
14. Stoier M. Metastatic tumors of the brain. Acta Neurol Scand 1965;41:262–268.
15. Galicich JH, French LA, Melby J. Use of dexamethasone in treatment of cerebral edema associated with brain tumors. Lancet 1961;81:46–53.
16. Kofman S, Garvin JS, Nagamani D, Taylor SS. Treatment of cerebral metastases from breast carcinoma with prednisolone. JAMA 1957;163:1473–1476.
17. Weinstein JD, Toy FJ, Jaffe ME, Goldberg HJ. The effect of dexamethasone on brain edema in patients with metastatic brain tumors. Neurology 1973;23:121–129.
18. Ruderman NB, Hall TC. Use of glucocorticoids in the palliative treatment of metastatic brain tumors. Cancer 1965;18:298–306.
19. Horton J, Baxter DH, Olson KB. The management of metastases to the brain by irradiation and corticosteroids. Am J Roentgenol Radium Ther Nucl Med 1971;3:334–335.
20. Posner JB. Brain tumor: current status of treatment and its complications. Arch Neurol 1975;32:781–784.
21. Chao J, Phillips R, Nickson JJ. Roentgen-ray therapy of cerebral metastases. Cancer 1954;7:682–689.
22. Chu FCH, Hilaris BS. Value of radiation therapy in the management of intracranial metastases. Cancer 1961;14:577–581.
23. Order SE, Hellman S, Von Essen CF, Kligerman MM. Improvement in quality of survival following whole brain irradiation for brain metastases. Radiology 1968;91:149–153.
24. Nisce LZ, Hilaris BS, Chu FCH. A review of experience with irradiation of brain metastases. Am J Roentgenol Radium Ther Nucl Med 1971;111:329–333.
25. Deutsch M, Parsons J, Mercado R. Radiotherapy for intracranial metastases. Cancer 1974;34:1607–1611.

26. Deeley TJ, Edwards JMR. Radiotherapy in the management of cerebral secondaries from bronchial carcinoma. Lancet 1968;1:1209–1213.
27. Cairncross JG, Kim JH, Posner JB. Radiation therapy for brain metastases. Ann Neurol 1980;7:529–541.
28. Grant FC. Concerning intracranial malignant metastases: their frequency and the value of surgery in their treatment. Ann Surg 1926;84:635–646.
29. Cushing H. Intracranial tumors: notes upon a series of two thousand verified cases with surgical mortality percentages pertaining thereto. Springfield, IL: Charles C. Thomas, 1932.
30. Flavell G. Solitary cerebral metastasis from primary bronchial carcinoma. Their incidental and case of successful removal. BMJ 1949;2:736–737.
31. Bakey L. Results of surgical treatment of intracranial metastasis from pulmonary cancer. J Neurosurg 1958;15:338–341.
32. Stortebecker TP. Metastatic tumors of the brain from a neurosurgical point of view: a follow-up study of 158 cases. J Neurosurg 1954;11:84–111.
33. Sundaresan N, Galicich JH. Surgical treatment of single brain metastasis from non–small cell lung cancer. Cancer Invest 1985;3:107–113.
34. Mandell L, Hilaris B, Sullivan M, et al. The treatment of single brain metastasis from non–oat cell lung carcinoma. Surgery and radiation versus radiation therapy alone. Cancer 1986;58:641–649.
35. Patchell RA, Cirrincione C, Thaler HT, Galicich JH, Kim JH, Posner JB. Single brain metastases: surgery plus radiation or radiation alone. Neurology 1986;36:447–453.
36. Patchell RA, Tibbs PA, Walsh JW, et al. A randomized trial of surgery in the treatment of single metastases to the brain. N Engl J Med 1990;322:494–500.
37. Noordijk EM, Vecht CJ, Haaxma-Reiche H, et al. The choice of treatment of single brain metastasis should be based on extracranial tumor activity and age. Int J Radiat Oncol Biol Phys 1994;29:711–717.
38. Burt ME, Wronski M, Arbit E, et al. Resection of brain metastasis from non–small cell lung carcinoma. Results of therapy. J Thorac Cardiovasc Surg 1992;103:399–411.
39. Armstrong JG, Wronski M, Galicich J, Arbit E, Leibel SA, Burt M. Postoperative radiation for lung cancer metastatic to the brain. J Clin Oncol 1994;12:2340–2344.
40. Abrams HL, Spiro R, Goldstein N. Metastases in carcinoma: analysis of 1000 autopsied cases. Cancer 1950;3:74–85.
41. Engleman RM, McNamara WL. Bronchogenic carcinoma: a statistical review of two hundred twenty-four autopsies. J Thorac Surg 1954;27:227–237.
42. Matthews MJ. Problems in morphology and behavior of bronchopulmonary malignant disease. In: Israel L, Chahinian AL (eds). Lung cancer: natural history, prognosis, and therapy. San Diego: Academic Press, 1976:23–62.
43. Ochsner A, De Bakey M. Carcinoma of the lung. Arch Surg 1941;42:209–258.
44. Glomset DA. The incidence of malignant tumors to the adrenals. Am J Cancer 1938;32:57–61.
45. Chapman GS, Kumar D, Redmond J III, Munderloh SH, Gandara DR. Upper abdominal computerized tomography scanning in staging non–small cell lung cancer. Thorax 1988;43:883–886.
46. Grant D, Edwards D, Goldstraw P. Computed tomography of the brain, chest, and abdomen in the preoperative assessment of non–small cell lung cancer. Thorax 1988;43:883–886.
47. Salvatierra A, Baamonde C, Llamas JM, Cruz F, Lopez-Pujol J. Extrathoracic staging of bronchogenic carcinoma. Chest 1990;97:1052–1058.
48. Whittlesey D. Prospective computed tomographic scanning in the staging of bronchogenic cancer. J Thorac Cardiovasc Surg 1988;95:876–982.
49. Oliver TW Jr, Bernardino ME, Miller JI, Mansour K, Greene D, David WA. Isolated adrenal masses in non–small cell bronchogenic carcinoma. Radiology 1984;153:217–218.
50. Burt M, Heelan RT, Coit D, et al. Prospective evaluation of unilateral adrenal masses in patients with operable non–small cell lung cancer. J Thorac Cardiovasc Surg 1994;107:584–589.
51. Reinig JW, Doppman JL, Dwyer AJ, Frank J. MRI of indeterminate adrenal masses. AJR Am J Roentgenol 1986;147:493–496.
52. Reinig JW, Doppman JL, Dwyer AJ, Johnson AR, Knop RH. Adrenal masses differentiated by MR. Radiology 1986;158:81–84.
53. Glazer GM, Woolsey EJ, Borrello J, et al. Adrenal tissue characterization using MR imaging. Radiology 1986;158:73–79.
54. Chang A, Glaser HS, Lee JKT, Ling D, Heiken JP. Adrenal gland: MR imaging. Radiology 1987;163:123–128.
55. Glazer GM. MR imaging of the liver, kidneys, and adrenal glands. Radiology 1988;166:303–312.
56. Chezma JL, Robbins SM, Nelson RC, Steinberg HV, Torres WE, Bernardino ME. Adrenal masses: Characterization with T-1 weighted MR imaging. Radiology 1988;166:357–359.
57. Kier R, McCarthy S. MR characterization of adrenal masses: field strength and pulse sequence considerations. Radiology 1989;171:671–674.
58. Baker ME, Blinder R, Spritzer C, Leight GS, Herfken RJ. Dunnick NR. MR evaluation of adrenal masses at 1.5 T. AJR Am J Roentgenol 1989;153:307–312.
59. Mitchell DG, Crovello M, Matteucci T, Petersen RO, Miettinen MM. Benign adrenocortical masses: diagnosis with chemical shift MR imaging. Radiology 1992;185:345–351.
60. Schwartz LH, Panicek DM, Koutcher JA, Heelan RT, Bains MS, Burt M. Echoplanar MR imaging for characterization of adrenal masses in patients with malignant neoplasms. AJR Am J Roentgenol 1995: in press.
61. Twomey P, Montgomery C, Clark O. Successful treatment of adrenal metastases from large cell carcinoma of the lung. JAMA 1982;248:581–583.
62. Raviv G, Klein E, Yellin A, Schneebaum S, Ben-Ari G. Surgical treatment of solitary adrenal metastases from lung carcinoma. J Surg Oncol 1990;43:123–124.
63. Reyes L, Parvez Z, Nemoto T, Regal AM, Takita H. Adrenalectomy for adrenal metastasis from lung carcinoma. J Surg Oncol 1990;44:32–34.

19

Management of Disseminated Non–Small Cell Lung Cancer

Rogerio C. Lilenbaum and Mark R. Green

INTRODUCTION

Approximately 130,000 patients are diagnosed with non–small cell lung cancer (NSCLC) each year in the United States (1). NSCLC is the second most common malignancy and the leading cause of cancer-related death in men and women in the United States. It has been estimated that only 10% to 15% of all patients diagnosed with NSCLC survive 5 years, a rather dismal figure that has not changed appreciably over the past several decades (2).

The International Staging System published in 1986 divided NSCLC into four stages (3). Approximately 25% to 30% of all patients diagnosed with NSCLC present with localized disease (stages I and II), partially amenable to curative surgical resection (4). However, a substantial proportion of these patients subsequently develop recurrent disease and require systemic treatment with chemotherapy. Another 30% to 35% of patients present with locally advanced disease (stage III), largely beyond the scope of primary surgical resection. Multimodality strategies, including chemotherapy, are being used more frequently in this group of patients (5). The remaining 40% of NSCLC patients have metastatic disease at the time of diagnosis (stage IV) and are also potential candidates for chemotherapy. Therefore, the vast majority of patients with NSCLC are candidates for systemic chemotherapy at some time during the course of their disease.

SINGLE-AGENT CHEMOTHERAPY

Until recently, only a few chemotherapeutic agents—cisplatin, ifosfamide, vinblastine, vindesine, mitomycin C, and possibly etoposide (6)—had demonstrated reproducible activity in advanced NSCLC patients. Combination regimens employing these agents have been shown to yield responses in up to 40% of selected patients with advanced NSCLC. The impact on survival, however, has been modest. Within the past few years, several new chemotherapeutic agents have shown promising activity in NSCLC (7) (Table 19.1). Whether these new agents, alone or in combination, will have a more substantial impact on survival of patients with advanced NSCLC remains to be determined.

CONVENTIONAL AGENTS

Cisplatin is one of the most widely used agents in the treatment of NSCLC. It produced an aggregate response rate of 21% in 10 single-agent trials involving more than 500 patients with advanced NSCLC disease (8). The importance of cisplatin dose intensity in the treatment of advanced NSCLC remains controversial. An early randomized study by Gralla et al. (9) compared cisplatin at a dose of 60 mg/m^2 versus 120 mg/m^2, each given in combination with a fixed dose of vindesine in 85 patients with advanced NSCLC. Although the response rates were equivalent, responding patients in the high-dose arm had a significantly prolonged survival duration. An initial phase II trial in NSCLC by Gandara et al. (10) suggested an increased response rate for cisplatin given at 100 mg/m^2 on days 1 and 8 every 4 weeks. In a subsequent randomized trial conducted by the Southwest Oncology Group (SWOG), this dose intensive regimen was compared with single-agent cisplatin given in standard doses (50 mg/m^2 on days 1 and 8) in patients with metastatic NSCLC (11). Response rates were similar: 12% in the standard arm and 14% in the high-dose arm. The European Organization for Research and Treatment of Cancer (EORTC) compared low-dose versus high-dose cisplatin in combination with a fixed dose of etoposide (12). There was no significant difference in response rates or survival. Toxicity was significantly increased

TABLE 19.1. Single Agents in Non–Small Cell Lung Cancer

CONVENTIONAL AGENTS	RESPONSE RATE (%)
Cisplatin	21
Ifosfamide	20
Vinblastine	27
Vindesine	16
Mitomycin	25
Etoposide	5–15
Carboplatin	9–16

NEW AGENTS	RESPONSE RATE
Irinotecan	32
Taxol	21–24
Taxotere	21–38
Navelbine	14–32
Chronic oral etoposide	4–23
Edatrexate	10–30
Gemcitabine	20–23

in all high-dose arms. These studies do not support a steep dose-response relationship for cisplatin in advanced NSCLC.

Single-agent carboplatin has an aggregate response rate of 10% in advanced NSCLC, lower than that reported for cisplatin (13). When evaluated in large cooperative groups, the Cancer and Leukemia Group B (CALGB) reported a 16% activity (14), whereas the Eastern Cooperative Oncology Group (ECOG) demonstrated a 9% response rate (15). The EORTC conducted the only randomized study comparing cisplatin (120 mg/m^2) versus carboplatin (325 mg/m^2), both given in combination with etoposide, in patients with advanced NSCLC (16). Response rates were higher in the cisplatin arm (27% versus 16%), but the difference did not reach statistical significance (P = .07). Median survival time was nearly identical (30 versus 27 weeks, respectively). Toxicity, mainly myelosuppression and renal function impairment, was significantly increased in patients receiving cisplatin.

Among the vinca alkaloids, vinblastine and vindesine are considered active drugs in NSCLC. Their response rates range from 11% to 28% in single-agent trials (17), and both agents have been used extensively in combination regimens. Recently, vinorelbine has emerged as a new semisynthetic vinca alkaloid with significant activity in NSCLC. Initial trials using a weekly dose of 25 to 30 mg/m^2 showed a response rate in the range of 30% in advanced NSCLC (18–19). Neutropenia was the principal toxicity. Neurotoxicity was mild, corroborating the preclinical data that vinorelbine spares the axonal microtubules compared with the traditional vinca alkaloids (20). A recent randomized study compared the single-agent activities of vinorelbine and vindesine in 150 patients with advanced NSCLC (21). Response rates, respectively, were 29.3% and 9.3% (P = .004), and median survival rates were 11.8 and 10.2 months, respectively (P = .72). Hematologic toxicity was similar in both arms.

Ifosfamide has shown consistent single-agent activity in advanced NSCLC. Response rates using doses in the range of 4 g/m^2 to 10 g/m^2 given in 1 day or over 5 days varied from 10% to 38%, respectively, with an aggregate of 20% (22). Ettinger (23) confirmed a pooled 21% overall response rate and a median survival of approximately 9 months in a review of 326 evaluable patients with advanced NSCLC treated with ifosfamide alone. The discordant experience reported by the SWOG (9% response in 113 patients) has not been published in article form (24). Hemorrhagic cystitis is the dose-limiting toxicity of ifosfamide without uroprotection with mesna. Neurotoxicity can also occur and is thought to relate to chloracetaldehyde, a metabolite of ifosfamide that structurally resembles chloral hydrate. The optimal dose and schedule of ifosfamide in the treatment of NSCLC are not clear. There is no clear dose-response relationship, and survival rates do not vary substantially with different doses or schedules of ifosfamide administration (23). Fractionated doses with mesna appear to be less toxic than single larger doses of ifosfamide.

Etoposide is a semisynthetic derivative of podophyllotoxin whose cytotoxic effects result from the inhibition of the nuclear enzyme topoisomerase II with subsequent formation of DNA strand breaks (25). The single-agent activity of etoposide in NSCLC using a standard multiple-day bolus administration schedule is in the range of 5% to 15% (26). Based on its schedule dependency documented in clinical trials (27), prolonged maintenance of threshold etoposide concentrations was envisioned to maximize the exposure of malignant cells during their sensitive phase of the cell cycle (28). This rationale prompted the use of chronic oral etoposide in NSCLC. In one study, a response rate of 23% was noted in 25 patients treated with oral etoposide 50 mg/m^2/day for 21 days (29). However, in a second study, the same schedule yielded only a 4% response rate in 43 patients (30). The reasons for this discrepancy are unclear and may reflect differences in the patient population.

The activity of mitomycin in NSCLC was recognized in the late 1970s. Single-agent studies using 10 to 20 mg/m^2 given every 3 to 6 weeks demonstrate a median response rate of 25% in a total of 207 evaluable patients (31). In a more recent trial, single-agent mitomycin produced a 30% response rate and a median survival of 4 months in 64 patients with metastatic squamous cell lung cancer (32). The toxicity associated with mitomycin can be severe. Cumulative myelotoxicity is well recognized. A thrombotic microangiopathy resembling the hemolytic-uremic syndrome and drug-induced interstitial lung disease are infrequent but well-known complications associated with mitomycin. Although dexamethasone reduces the frequency and severity of mitomycin-related lung injury, it may also reduce the response rates when given before mitomycin in combination with cisplatin and vinblastine (31).

NEW AGENTS

The taxanes, Taxol and Taxotere, are among the most exciting new agents for the treatment of NSCLC. Their unique mechanism of action is mediated through the promotion of microtubule assembly and subsequent inhibition of microtubule depolymerization (33). Single-agent Taxol has been tested in advanced NSCLC in two trials. The first, conducted at the M. D. Anderson Cancer Center, showed a 24% response rate with Taxol given at 200 mg/m^2 over 24 hours to 25 eligible patients (34). In the second trial, conducted by ECOG (35), Taxol at a dose of 250 mg/m^2 over 24 hours was given to 24 patients and yielded a response rate of 21%. Toxicities of Taxol include neutropenia, peripheral neuropathy, and arthralgias and myalgias. Hypersensitivity reactions were diminished significantly after the introduction of routine premedication with dexamethasone and H1 and H2 blockers. The optimal dose and schedule of Taxol in NSCLC are under active investigation. The 3-hour administration schedule significantly diminishes the myelosuppression observed with the 24-hour administration schedule (36).

Taxotere is a semisynthetic taxane analogue that has been evaluated in two recent single-agent trials at a dose of 100 mg/m^2 every 3 weeks. Response rates were 33% and 38%, respectively (37–38). Responses with lower doses seem to be inferior (39–40). Furthermore, a 21% response rate was observed in 44 platinum-refractory NSCLC patients, a provocative observation in previously treated patients with advanced NSCLC (41). Toxicities of Taxotere include neutropenia, skin rashes, and hypersensitivity reactions. A peculiar toxicity is a syndrome of fluid retention, including pleural effusions and ascites, associated with weight gain. Although release of cytokines has been postulated as a possible mechanism, the exact etiology of the syndrome remains unclear.

The camptothecin compounds are derived from the oriental plant Campthoteca acuminata. The sodium salt was first evaluated as an antineoplastic agent in the early 1970s, but response rates were disappointing and toxicity was severe (42). Two recently developed analogues have entered phase II clinical investigation. Irinotecan was initially tested in NSCLC by Japanese investigators (43). At 100 mg/m^2 weekly, a 31.9% response rate was reported in 72 chemotherapy naive patients. The most important toxicities were neutropenia and diarrhea. A low rate of largely reversible pulmonary toxicity also was observed. Topotecan is another semisynthetic camptothecin analogue that has demonstrated preliminary activity against a variety of solid tumors in phase I trials (44). When tested in advanced NSCLC, topotecan, 2 mg/m^2/day × 5 produced no responses in 20 patients in one trial (45). In a second trial, topotecan produced a response rate of 13.5% in 37 evaluable patients (46). Among the five responding patients, four had the squamous cell subtype and only one had adenocarcinoma. These disappointing results may reflect a schedule dependency of topotecan, and trials evaluating a prolonged administration of topotecan are ongoing (47). Further studies are necessary to define better the role of this agent in the treatment of NSCLC.

Traditional antimetabolites, such as methotrexate, 5-fluorouracil, or cytarabine, have shown little activity in NSCLC. More recently, the antifolate edatrexate and a new deoxycytidine analogue, gemcitabine, have demonstrated promising single-agent activity. Edatrexate is a water soluble methotrexate analogue that has been evaluated in three phase II trials in NSCLC (48–50). Using a weekly dose of 80 mg/m^2, response rates ranged from 10% to 30% in a total of 94 evaluable patients. Overall, edatrexate was well tolerated, producing minimal myelosuppression and moderate mucositis. Concomitant administration of leucovorin was found to ameliorate mucositis without affecting efficacy (51).

Gemcitabine also has undergone extensive testing as a single agent in NSCLC. Using doses that varied from 800 mg/m^2/week to 1750 mg/m^2/week × 3 every 4 weeks, a total of 211 patients in four different phase II trials have been evaluated (52–55). A consistent response rate in the range of 20% to 24% has been demonstrated. Gemcitabine is well tolerated with minimal hematologic toxicity. Nonhematologic toxicity is also mild and consists of flulike symptoms, skin rashes, mild elevations of liver enzyme levels, and peripheral edema.

COMBINATION CHEMOTHERAPY

The systemic treatment of NSCLC was initiated in the 1970s with nonplatinum-containing regimens such as CAMP (cyclophosphamide, doxorubicin, methotrexate, and procarbazine). Although evidence of efficacy could be shown in a small subset of patients (56), responses were brief in duration with no readily demonstrable impact on survival. Several combination regimens, with and without cisplatin, were tested subsequently in NSCLC. Over the years, many of these regimens were published as representing breakthroughs in the treatment of advanced NSCLC. Later randomized data, however, have invariably failed to confirm the claimed superiority. Despite several years of intensive clinical investigation, no particular chemotherapy regimen can be accepted as standard treatment for advanced NSCLC. The main principles of chemotherapy in advanced NSCLC have been summarized recently (57).

SINGLE-AGENT VERSUS COMBINATION CHEMOTHERAPY

Several trials compared cisplatin-containing combinations with single-agent treatment in advanced NSCLC (58–61) (Table 19.2). The results, in general, indicate a higher response rate for the combination regimens. However, despite a positive trend in some trials, median-term or long-term survival is usually not prolonged in patients treated with combination chemotherapy. This dissociation between response rate and survival can probably be explained by the relatively low activity level seen with most combinations (less than 50% objective response), and the absence of a substantial number of complete responders (fewer than 5%). Furthermore, some combination regimens may be associated with shorter survivals secondary to toxic effects.

COMBINATION REGIMENS

Table 19.3 shows response rates and median survival times for several combination regimens. The cisplatin and vindesine combination (PVd) was initially tested by Gralla et al. (9), who reported a 40% response rate in advanced NSCLC patients. Subsequent trials have confirmed an aggregate response of 26% among 691 evaluable patients (2). Equivalent response rates are observed with the combination of cisplatin and vinblastine (PVe), which is more readily available in the United States. A direct comparison between vindesine and vinblastine, both given in combination with cisplatin, showed no significant differences in response rates (33% versus 41%) or median survival times (18 versus 16 months), respectively (62). Toxicities were similar with the two regimens, but myelosuppression was more common with cisplatin and vinblastine.

The combination of cisplatin and vinorelbine (NVB-P) was studied in a recent, large three-arm randomized trial in comparison with cisplatin and vindesine (PVd) and single-agent vinorelbine (NVB) (63). An objective response was observed in 30% of patients in the NVB-P arm versus 19% in the PVd arm ($P = .02$) and 14% in the NVB arm ($P < .001$). Median survival times were 40, 32, and 31 weeks, respectively, and also

TABLE 19.2. Single-Agent Versus Combination Chemotherapy Randomized Trials

AUTHOR (REFERENCE)	DESIGN	NO. OF PATIENTS	RESPONSE RATE (%)	MEDIAN SURVIVAL (WK)
Rosso (58)	VP-16	103	7	24
	vs.			
	PE	113	26	32
Einhorn (59)	VDS	42	14	18
	vs.			
	PVd	41	20	26
	vs.			
	MVP	41	27	17
Klastersky (60)	CDDP	74	19	26
	vs.			
	PE	72	26	22
Luedke (61)	VDS	128	1	15
	vs.			
	PVd	125	19	20
	vs.			
	VDS/MITO	122	27	25
LeChevalier (63)	NVB	206	14	31
	vs.			
	NVB-CDDP	206	30	40[a]
	vs.			
	VDS-CDDP	200	19[b]	32

Abbreviations. PE, cisplatin + etoposide; VDS, vindesine; PVd, cisplatin + vindesine; MVP, mitomycin + vinblastine + cisplatin; CDDP, cisplatin; NVB, vinorelbine; MITO, mitomycin; VP-16, etoposide.
[a]$P = .04$ compared with VDS-CDDP; $p = .01$ compared with NVB. All other results are not statistically significant.
[b]Percent changed.

TABLE 19.3. Combination Chemotherapy

COMBINATIONS	RESPONSE RATE (%)	MEDIAN SURVIVAL (MO)
PVd	25–35	6.5–11
PVe	15–36	5.3–7.5
PE	12–38	5.3–8.3
MVP	20–46	5.5–6.0
NVB-P	30	10
PEI	26–44	6.0–7.7

Abbreviations. PVd, cisplatin + vindesine; PVe, cisplatin + vinblastine; PE, cisplatin + etoposide; MVP, mitomycin + vinblastine + cisplatin; NVB-P, vinorelbine + cisplatin; PEI, cisplatin + etoposide + ifosfamide.

were significantly superior in the NVB-P arm. Neutropenia was more pronounced in the NVB-P combination, whereas neurotoxicity was more frequent in the PVd arm. In this trial, the NVB-P combination compared favorably with the standard PVd regimen. Despite a lower response rate than that reported in phase II trials, vinorelbine alone represents an alternative for patients who are not candidates for cisplatin-containing regimens.

The combination of cisplatin and etoposide (PE) has been used widely in the treatment of NSCLC. Longeval and Klastersky (64) initially reported a 38% response rate and a median survival of 7.5 months using cisplatin at a dose of 60 mg/m^2 in 94 advanced NSCLC patients. Several other trials have studied the PE regimen with a pooled response rate of 28% in 647 patients (2). An early randomized trial compared PE versus PVd and a third regimen combining the three drugs (65). Response rates (30%, 35%, 22%, respectively) and survival times (29, 29, 28 weeks, respectively) were not significantly different, but toxicity was less in the PE arm.

The combination of mitomycin, vindesine, and cisplatin (MVP) yielded a 60% response rate and a median survival of 11 months in the initial study by Kris et al. (66). A more recent study using lower doses of cisplatin in the same regimen reported a 41% response rate (67). The substitution of vinblastine for vindesine in the MVP program was studied by Gralla et al. (68). The vinblastine-MVP regimen was associated with less hematologic toxicity and equivalent response rates compared with the vindesine-MVP combination. Furthermore, in an attempt to define the role of mitomycin in this combination, Gralla et al. (69) randomized 111 patients to receive cisplatin and vindesine, with or without mitomycin. Response to the MVP arm was twice as high (54% versus 27%), but median survival was not significantly improved (52 versus 46 weeks, respectively).

Several combinations involving ifosfamide have been reported. When used in combination with cisplatin, Drings et al. (70) reported a 35% response rate and a median survival of 8.3 months in 71 evaluable patients. Ifosfamide has been added to the cisplatin-vinca alkaloid combination (VIP) with response rates in the range of 14% to 62% (71–73). Another active combination is cisplatin with etoposide and ifosfamide (PEI), which produced response rates in the range of 26% to 44% (74–76).

LARGE RANDOMIZED TRIALS

A few large randomized studies have been reported in advanced NSCLC (Table 19.4). The first was

TABLE 19.4. Large Cooperative Group Randomized Trials

Study, Year (Reference)	No. of Patients	Treatment	Response (%)	Median Survival (wks)
ECOG, 1986 (77)	115	CAMP	17	25.1
	121	MVP	31	22.0
	124	PE	20	26.6
	126	PVd	25	26.0
ECOG, 1989 (15)	176	MVP	20	22.7
	175	PVe	13	25.01
	172	MVP/CAMP	13	25.0
	88	Carboplatin	9	31.7
	88	Iproplatin	6	26.1
SWOG, 1991 (79)	150	PE	16	21.2
	157	PE + MGBG	33	19.6
	156	PVe	24	23.6
	139	PVeMi	17	20
	138	FOMi/CAP	10	20

Abbreviations. CAMP, cyclophosphamide + doxorubicin + methotrexate + procarbazine; MVP, mitomycin + vinblastine + cisplatin; PE, cisplatin + etoposide; PVd, cisplatin + vindesine; PVe, cisplatin + vinblastine; MGBG, methylguazone; PVeMi, cisplatin + vindesine alternating with vinblastine + mitomycin; FOMi/CAP, fluorouracil + vincristine + mitomycin alternating with cyclophosphamide + doxorubicin + cisplatin.

published by ECOG in 1986 (77). The investigators randomly allocated 486 patients with metastatic NSCLC to CAMP, MVP, PE, or PVd. Response rates for each of the regimens were 17%, 31%, 20%, and 25%, respectively. The overall median survival time was 23.5 weeks and was not significantly different among treatments. Severe toxicity and fatality rates were significantly increased in patients with a performance status of 2 or less. A subsequent analysis of long-term survival indicated that 19% of all patients survived more than 1 year, and only 4% survived more than 2 years (78). The PE combination had the highest proportion of 1-year survivors (25%). Conversely, the MVP program, which had the best response rate, had significantly fewer 1-year survivors (12%) (P = .003).

A second large trial conducted by ECOG and published in 1989 compared MVP, PVe, MVP alternating with CAMP, and two single agents, carboplatin and iproplatin, followed by MVP, at the time of progression (15). The trial included 699 eligible patients with metastatic NSCLC. Although the MVP regimen used initially produced a significantly higher response rate, carboplatin followed by MVP was associated with significantly longer survival (31.7 weeks) (P = .008).

A more recent trial conducted by SWOG (79) randomized 680 evaluable patients to one of five cisplatin-containing regimens: PE, PE with methylguazone (PEM), PVe alone, PVe alternating with vinblastine and mitomycin, or FOMi/CAP (fluorouracil, vincristine, mitomycin/cyclophosphamide, doxorubicin, cisplatin). The overall response rate was 20%, ranging from 10% for FOMi/CAP to 33% for PEM. Duration of response ranged from 2.7 to 5 months, and overall survival ranged from 4.9 to 5.9 months; these rates were not significantly different among the five arms. Despite a higher response rate associated with PEM, toxicity was also more severe in this arm.

NEW STRATEGIES AND COMBINATIONS

A few innovative approaches and new combination regimens for the treatment of advanced NSCLC have been reported preliminarily. Murray et al. (80) designed a weekly, intensive chemotherapy regimen that combined cisplatin, vincristine, doxorubicin, and etoposide (CODE), administered over a total of 9 to 12 weeks. Fifty-three patients with advanced NSCLC were entered, and 33 (62%) responded, including 9% who achieved a complete response. The median survival was 42 weeks, and more than 40% of the patients were alive at 1 year. There were no treatment-related deaths, and only three episodes of febrile neutropenia were reported. Randomized studies evaluating this regimen are currently ongoing.

Among the new active drugs, the combination of cisplatin and irinotecan produced objective responses in 54% of patients with advanced NSCLC in a phase I-II trial (81). The addition of vindesine to the combination of cisplatin and irinotecan produced a 41% response rate in another phase I-II study in advanced NSCLC (82). A phase I study by Rowinsky et al. (83) showed 3 responses among 12 NSCLC patients treated with Taxol and cisplatin. This combination is currently being evaluated in phase II-III trials. Phase I studies testing cisplatin and gemcitabine in NSCLC have also reported encouraging results (84–85), and phase II studies are currently ongoing.

CHEMOTHERAPY VERSUS SUPPORTIVE CARE

PROGNOSTIC FACTORS

Numerous studies have analyzed the importance of several prognostic factors associated with survival in advanced NSCLC. A landmark report by Stanley (86) evaluated 77 prognostic factors in more than 5000 patients with advanced NSCLC. The most important factor affecting survival was the initial Karnofsky performance status (KPS), followed by the extent of disease and weight loss. More recently, O'Connell et al. (87) collected data on 378 advanced NSCLC patients receiving a cisplatin–vinca alkaloid combination chemotherapy. A KPS of 70 or less, presence of bone metastases, an elevated serum lactate dehydrogenase (LDH) level, male sex, and two or more extrathoracic metastatic sites were identified as important adverse prognostic factors. The first large randomized ECOG study (77) confirmed the relevance of KPS, bone metastases, and male sex; it also included prior weight loss and liver metastases as predictors of unfavorable survival.

A recent consensus report recognized KPS, extent or stage of disease, and weight loss as important prognostic factors for survival in advanced NSCLC (88). The identification of these factors are essential to interpret the results of clinical trials. Moreover, they may assist in the selection of patients with advanced NSCLC for treatment with systemic chemotherapy. Excessive toxicity can be avoided by excluding patients with less than optimal KPS from chemotherapy programs. Conversely, the possible beneficial effects of chemotherapy on survival can be evaluated more clearly in patients with favorable pretreatment characteristics.

RANDOMIZED TRIALS

Several randomized studies have compared combination chemotherapy with best supportive care (BSC) strategies in patients with advanced NSCLC (Table 19.5). Eight such studies, published from 1982 to 1993, involved a total of 808 patients (89–96). Differences in design among the trials included patient selection criteria, chemotherapy regimens, number of treatment cycles, and inclusion of other treatment modalities such as radiotherapy. Four studies showed a statistically significant survival benefit in favor of combination chemotherapy (90, 93 94, 96). In the study by Rapp et al. from the National Cancer Institute of Canada (94), 150 patients were entered in a three-arm trial of PVd versus CAP versus BSC. An additional 101 patients were entered in a two-arm schema comparing CAP with PVd. The overall response rates to CAP and PVd were 15.3% and 25.3%, respectively. Patients on the three-arm portion of the trial had a median survival of 32.6 in the PVd arm, 24.7 weeks in the CAP arm, and 17 weeks in the BSC arm. The differences were statistically significant for PVd and BSC ($P = .01$), and for CAP and BSC ($P = .05$). Toxicity in the chemotherapy arms was substantial, consisting of leukopenia, severe vomiting, and neurotoxicity, in a large proportion of patients.

The favorable results reported by Rapp et al. (94) were not confirmed in a subsequent larger trial reported by Wood et al. (95) containing twice as many patients and using the same chemotherapy employed in the Canadian study. Although the median

TABLE 19.5. Combination Chemotherapy Versus Best Supportive Care Randomized Trials

First Author (Reference)	No. of Patients	Chemotherapy	Median Survival CT	Median Survival BSC	P Value
Cellerino (89)	123	CDDP + CPA/MTX + CCNU + VP-16	8.5	5.0	.15
Cormier (90)	49	MACC	30.5	8.5	.005
Ganz (91)	63	PVe	19.9	14.4	.09
Kaasa (92)	87	PE	21.6	16.0	.5
Quoix (93)	43	PVd	27.5	9.7	.03
Rapp (94)	150	CAP	24.7	17.0	.05
		PVd	32.6		.01
Woods (95)	201	PVd	17.0	17.0	.075
Cartei (96)	102	CDDP + CPA + MITO	16.0	16.0	.0001

Abbreviations. CT, chemotherapy; BSC, best supportive care; CDDP + CPA/MTX + CCNU + VP-16, cisplatin + cyclophosphamide alternating with methotrexate + lomustine + etoposide; MACC, methotrexate + cyclophosphamide + lomustine; PVe, cisplatin + vinblastine; PE, cisplatin + etoposide; PVd, cisplatin + vindesine; CAP, cyclophosphamide + doxorubicin + cisplatin; MITO, mitomycin.

survival in the supportive care group in both trials was identical (17 weeks), the median survival for the chemotherapy patients in the Wood's trial was 27 weeks, a difference that did not reach statistical significance ($P = .07$).

Two recent meta-analyses compared the results of chemotherapy and BSC generated by the above trials. Souquet et al. (97) evaluated seven trials involving 706 patients and used the number of deaths at 3, 6, 9, 12, and 18 months as the endpoints. There was a significant reduction in the odds ratio for mortality at 3 and 6 months, but the difference became nonsignificant at 9, 12, and 18 months ($P = .01$ was chosen for statistical significance). In the second meta-analysis, Grilli et al. (98) evaluated six trials involving a total of 635 patients. Their analysis showed that chemotherapy was associated with a 24% reduction in the likelihood of death within 1 year. The effect of chemotherapy, however, varied with time. After starting treatment, there was a statistically significant risk reduction during the first 6 months, followed by a nonstatistically significant increased risk of death in the chemotherapy group between 7 and 9 months, and a nonsignificant risk reduction in favor of chemotherapy between 10 and 12 months. The mean potential gain in survival compared with supportive care was 6 weeks.

A third meta-analysis, using updated individual data, compared BSC with chemotherapy in 1190 patients (99). For cisplatin-based chemotherapy, an absolute improvement in survival of 10% at 1 year was noted (16% to 26%). Median survival increased from 6 to 8 months. The differences were highly statistically significant ($P = .00007$). Interestingly, alkylating agent chemotherapy resulted in a detrimental effect in median survival and survival at 1 year.

QUALITY OF LIFE

Although a definitive study addressing quality of life of NSCLC patients undergoing chemotherapy has not yet been published, preliminary reports indicate that chemotherapy can provide effective palliation of symptoms. Kris et al. (100) used visual analogue scores and showed a significant improvement in disease-related symptoms in the majority of patients with advanced NSCLC treated with combination chemotherapy. Specifically, the severity of cough, dyspnea, pain, and hemoptysis improved considerably after treatment with chemotherapy. Furthermore, the KPS improved in 44% and was maintained in 40% of patients receiving chemotherapy. Hardy et al. (101) treated 24 symptomatic patients with cisplatin-based chemotherapy. Although only five patients achieved an objective response (21%), tumor-related symptoms improved in 75% of patients. The overall benefit, however, was short lived, with a median duration of 7 weeks. Similarly, Fernandez et al. (102) reported an improvement in quality of life in 75% of 31 advanced NSCLC patients treated with cisplatin-based chemotherapy. Symptomatic improvement once again was observed in patients who did not achieve an objective response.

CONCLUSION

The outcome of patients with disseminated NSCLC remains poor. Although treatment options need to be tailored to individual patients, the data summarized in this chapter provide a rationale for offering systemic chemotherapy to a subset of advanced NSCLC patients. Cisplatin-based combinations have produced a significant survival advantage compared to BSC. The absolute survival gain, however, is modest and may be offset by adverse reactions associated with the treatment. Appropriate selection of patients for systemic chemotherapy is essential to avoid prohibitive toxicity. Chemotherapy can be offered to symptomatic patients with a good KPS who wish to undergo such treatment and fully acknowledge the risks and benefits of this approach. Furthermore, patients preferably should have measurable or evaluable disease so that response can be assessed objectively. Responses usually occur after the initial two courses. For responding patients, or for those with stable disease and clear improvement in disease-related symptoms, chemotherapy can be continued up to a total of four to six courses. Treatment should be discontinued in the remaining patients. Further testing of new chemotherapeutic agents and their incorporation into aggressive combination regimens hopefully will improve the outcome for patients with advanced NSCLC.

References

1. Boring CC, Squires TS, Tong T, et al. Cancer statistics, 1994. CA Cancer J Clin 1994;44:7–26.
2. Ginsberg RJ, Kris MG, Armstrong JG. Cancer of the lung. In: De Vita VT, Hellman S, Rosenberg SA, eds. Cancer: principles & practice of oncology. Philadelphia: JB Lippincott, 1993:673–758.
3. Mountain CF. A new international staging system for lung cancer. Chest 1986;89(Suppl):225S–233S.
4. Shields TW. Surgical therapy for carcinoma of the lung. Clin Chest Med 1993;14:121–147.
5. Lilenbaum RC, Green MR. Multimodality treatment of non–small cell lung cancer. Oncology 1994;8:25–31.
6. Johnson DH. Chemotherapy for unresectable non–small cell lung cancer. Semin Oncol 1990;17(Suppl 7):20–29.
7. Lilenbaum RC, Green MR. Novel chemotherapeutic agents in the treatment of non–small cell lung cancer. J Clin Oncol 1993;11:1391–1402.
8. Bunn PA Jr. The expanding role of cisplatin in the treatment of non–small cell lung cancer. Semin Oncol 1986;16(Suppl 6):1–12.
9. Gralla R, Casper E, Kelsen D. Cisplatin plus vindesine combination chemotherapy for advanced carcinoma of the lung: a randomized trial investigating two dosage schedules. Ann Intern Med 1981;95:414–420.
10. Gandara DR, Wold H, Perez EA, et al. Cisplatin dose intensity in non–small cell lung cancer: phase II results of a day 1 and day 8 high-dose regimen. J Natl Cancer Inst 1989;81:790–794.
11. Gandara DR, Crowley J, Livingston RB, et al. Evaluation of cisplatin intensity in metastatic non–small cell lung cancer: a phase III study of the Southwest Oncology Group. J Clin Oncol 1993;11:873–878.
12. Klastersky J, Sculier JP, Ravez P, et al. A randomized study comparing a high and a standard dose of cisplatin in combination with etoposide in the treatment of advanced non–small cell lung carcinoma. J Clin Oncol 1986;4:1780–1786.
13. Bunn PA. Clinical experiences with carboplatin (Paraplatin) in lung cancer. Semin Oncol 1992;19(Suppl 2):1–11.
14. Green MR, Kreisman H, Doll DC, et al. Carboplatin in non–small cell lung cancer: an update on the Cancer and Leukemia Group B experience. Semin Oncol 1992;19(Suppl 2):44–49.
15. Bonomi PD, Finkelstein DM, Ruckdeshel JC, et al. Combination chemotherapy versus single agents followed by combination chemotherapy in stage IV non–small cell lung cancer: a study of the Eastern Cooperative Oncology Group. J Clin Oncol 1989;7:1602–1613.
16. Klastersky J, Sculier JP, Lacroix H, et al. A randomized study comparing cisplatin or carboplatin plus etoposide in patients with advanced non–small cell lung cancer: European Organization for Research and Treatment of Cancer Protocol 17861. J Clin Oncol 1990;8:1556–1562.
17. Sorensen JB, Osterlind K, Hansen HH. Vinca alkaloids in the treatment of non–small cell lung cancer. Cancer Treat Rev 1987;14:29–41.
18. Depierre A, Lemarie E, Dabouis G, et al. A phase II study of Navelbine (vinorelbine) in non–small cell lung cancer. Am J Clin Oncol 1991;14:115–119.
19. Yokoyama A, Furuse K, Niitani H, et al. Multi-institutional phase II study of Navelbine (vinorelbine) in non–small cell lung cancer (abstract 957). Proc Am Soc Clin Oncol 1992;11:287.
20. Binet S, Chaineau E, Fellous A, et al. Immunofluorescence study of the action of navelbine, vincristine and vinblastine on mitotic and axonal microtubules. Int J Cancer 1990;46:262–266.
21. Furuse K, Niitani H, Sakuma A, et al. Randomized comparative phase II study of vinorelbine versus vindesine in previously untreated non–small cell lung cancer—interim result (abstract 286). 8th National Cancer Institute and European Organization for Research and Treatment of Cancer symposium on new cancer therapy, Program and Abstracts, 1994:143.
22. Johnson DH. Overview of ifosfamide in small cell and non–small cell lung cancer. Semin Oncol 1990;17(Suppl 4):24–30.
23. Ettinger DS. Ifosfamide in the treatment of non–small cell lung cancer. Semin Oncol 1989;16(Suppl 3):31–38.
24. Livinston RB. Perugia International Cancer Conference. Discussion. Semin Oncol 1988;15(Suppl 7):62–70.
25. Rowinsky E, Donehauer RC. Vinca alkaloids and epipodophyllotoxins. In: Perry MC, ed. The chemotherapy source book. Baltimore: Williams & Wilkins, 1992:359–383.
26. Ruckdeschel JC. Etoposide in the management of non–small cell lung cancer. Cancer 1991;67(Suppl):250–253.
27. Slevin ML, Clark PJ, Joel SP, et al. A randomized trial to evaluate the effect of schedule on the activity of etoposide in small cell lung cancer. J Clin Oncol 1989;7:1333–1340.
28. DeVore R, Hainsworth J, Greco FA, et al. Chronic oral etoposide in the treatment of lung cancer. Semin Oncol 1992;19(Suppl 14):28–35.
29. Waits TM, Johnson DH, Hainsworth JD, et al. Prolonged administration of oral etoposide in non–small cell lung cancer: a phase II trial. J Clin Oncol 1992; 292–296.
30. Saxman S, Loehrer PJ Sr, Logie K, et al. Phase II trial of daily oral etoposide in patients with advanced non–small cell lung cancer. Invest New Drugs 19911;9:253–256.
31. Spain RC. The case for mitomycin in non–small cell lung cancer. Oncology 1993;50(Suppl 1):35–52.
32. Veeder MH, Jett JR, Su JQ, et al. A phase III trial of mitomycin C alone versus mitomycin C, vinblastine, and cisplatin for metastatic squamous cell lung carcinoma. Cancer 1992;70:2281–2287.
33. Horwitz SB. Mechanism of action of Taxol. Trends Pharmacol Sci 1992;13:134–136.

34. Murphy WK, Fossela FV, Winn RJ, et al. Phase II study of Taxol in patients with untreated advanced non–small cell lung cancer. J Natl Cancer Inst 1993;85:384–387.
35. Chang A, Kim K, Glick J, et al. Phase II study of Taxol, merbarone, and piroxantrone in stage IV non–small cell lung cancer. J Natl Cancer Inst 1993;85:388–393.
36. Swenerton K, Eisenhauer E, Huiniuk WB, et al. Taxol in relapsed ovarian cancer: high versus low-dose and short versus long-infusion: a European-Canadian study coordinated by the NCI Canada clinical trials group (abstract 810). Proc Am Soc Clin Oncol 1993;12:256.
37. Francis PA, Rigas JR, Kris MG, et al. Phase II trial of docetaxel in patients with stage III and IV non–small cell lung cancer. J Clin Oncol 1994;12:1232–1237.
38. Fossella FV, Lee JS, Murphy WK, et al. Phase II study of docetaxel for recurrent or metastatic non–small cell lung cancer. J Clin Oncol 1994;12:1238–1244.
39. Miller VA, Rigas JR, Kris MG, et al. Phase II trial of docetaxel given at a dose of 75 mg/m^2 with prednisone premedication in non–small cell lung cancer (abstract 1226). Proc Am Soc Clin Oncol 1994;13:364.
40. Watanabe K, Yokoyama A, Furuse K, et al. Phase II trial of docetaxel in previously untreated non–small cell lung cancer (abstract 1095). Proc Am Soc Clin Oncol 1994;13:331.
41. Fossela FV, Lee JS, Shin DM, et al. Taxotere, an active agent for platinum-refractory non–small cell lung cancer: preliminary results of a phase II study (abstract 1115). Proc Am Soc Clin Oncol 1994;13.
42. Slichenmyer WJ, Rowinsky EK, Donehower RC, et al. The current status of camptothecin analogues as antitumor agents. J Natl Cancer Inst 1993;85:271–291.
43. Fukuoka M, Nitani H, Susuki A, et al. A phase II study of CPT-11, a new derivative of campthotecin, for previously untreated non–small cell lung cancer. J Clin Oncol 1992;10:16–20.
44. Rowinsky EK, Grochow LB, Hendricks CB, et al. Phase I and pharmacologic study of topotecan: a novel topoisomerase inhibitor. J Clin Oncol 1992;10:647–656.
45. Lynch TJ Jr, Kalish L, Strauss G, et al. Phase II study of topotecan in metastatic non–small cell lung cancer. J Clin Oncol 1994;12:347–352.
46. Perez-Soler R, Glisson BS, Kane J, et al. Phase II study of topotecan in patients with non–small cell lung cancer previously untreated (abstract 1114). Proc Am Soc Clin Oncol 1994;13:336.
47. Hochster H, Liebes L, Speyer J, et al. Phase I trial of low-dose continuous topotecan infusion in patients with cancer: an active and well tolerated regimen. J Clin Oncol 1994;12:553–559.
48. Kris MG, Gralla RJ, Potanovich LM, et al. Long term survival analysis of stage III and IV non–small cell lung cancer patients treated with edatrexate (abstract 408). Lung Cancer 1991;7:111.
49. Souhami RL, Rudd RM, Spiro SG, et al. Phase II study of edatrexate in stage III and IV non–small cell lung cancer. Cancer Chemother Pharmacol 1992;30:465–468.
50. Lee JS, Libshitz HI, Murphy WK, et al. Phase II study of 10-ethyl-10-deaza-aminopterin for stage IIIB or IV non–small cell lung cancer. Invest New Drugs 1990;8:299–304.
51. Lee JS, Libshitz HI, Fossella FV, et al. Improved therapeutic index by leucovorin of edatrexate, cyclophosphamide and cisplatin against non–small cell lung cancer. J Natl Cancer Inst 1992;84:1039–1040.
52. Anderson H, Lund B, Bach F, et al. Single-agent activity of weekly gemcitabine in advanced non–small cell lung cancer: a phase II study. J Clin Oncol 1994;12:1821–1826.
53. Abratt R, Bezwoda WK, Falkson G, et al. Efficacy and safety profile of gemcitabine in non–small cell lung cancer: a phase II study. J Clin Oncol 1994;12:1535–1540.
54. Fossella FV, Lippman S, Pang A, et al. Phase I/II study of gemcitabine by 30 minute weekly intravenous infusion 3 wks every 4 wks for non–small cell lung cancer (abstract 1082). Proc Am Soc Clin Oncol 1993;12:326.
55. Sheperd FA, Gatzemeier U, Gotfried M, et al. An extended phase II study of gemcitabine in non–small cell lung cancer (abstract 1096). Proc Am Soc Clin Oncol 1993;12:330.
56. Shepard KV, Golomb HM, Bitran JD, et al. CAMP chemotherapy for metastatic non–oat cell bronchogenic carcinoma. Cancer 1985;56:2385–2390.
57. Ihde DC. Chemotherapy of lung cancer. N Engl J Med 1992;327:1434–1441.
58. Rosso R, Salvati F, Ardizzoni A, et al. Etoposide versus etoposide plus high-dose cisplatin in the management of advanced non–small cell lung cancer: results of a prospective randomized FONICAP trial. Cancer 1990;65:130–134.
59. Einhorn LH, Loehrer PJ, Williams SD, et al. Random prospective study of vindesine versus vindesine plus high-dose cisplatin versus vindesine plus cisplatin plus mitomycin C in advanced non–small cell lung cancer. J Clin Oncol 1986;4:1037–1043.
60. Klastersky J, Sculier JP, Bureau G, et al. Cisplatin versus cisplatin plus etoposide in the treatment of advanced non–small cell lung cancer. J Clin Oncol 1989;7:1087–1092.
61. Luedke DW, Einhorn L, Omura G, et al. Randomized comparison of two combination regimens versus minimal chemotherapy in non–small cell lung cancer: a Southeastern Cancer Study Group trial. J Clin Oncol 1990;8:886–891.
62. Kris MG, Gralla RJ, Kalman LA, et al. Randomized trial comparing vindesine plus cisplatin with vinblastine plus cisplatin in patients with non–small cell lung cancer, with an analysis of methods of response assessment. Cancer Treat Rep 1985;69:387–395.
63. LeChevalier T, Brisgand D, Douillard JY, et al. Randomized study of vinorelbine and cisplatin versus vindesine and cisplatin versus vinorelbine alone in advanced non–small cell lung cancer: results of a European multicenter trial including 612 patients. J Clin Oncol 1994;12:360–367.
64. Longeval E, Klastersky J. Combination chemotherapy with cisplatin and etoposide in bronchogenic squamous cell carcinoma and adenocarcinoma. Cancer 1982;50:2751–2756.
65. Dhringra HM, Valdivieso M, Carr DT, et al. Randomized trial of three combinations of cisplatin with vindesine and/or VP-16 213 in the treatment of advanced non–small cell lung cancer. J Clin Oncol 1985;3:176–183.
66. Kris M, Gralla R, Wertheim M. Trial of the combination of mitomycin, vindesine and cisplatin in patients with advanced non–small. Cancer Treat Rep 1986;70:1091–1096.
67. Joss R, Burki K, Dalquen P, et al. Combination chemotherapy with mitomycin, vindesine, and cisplatin for non–small cell lung cancer. Cancer 1990;11:2426–2434.
68. Gralla RJ, Kris MG, Potanovich LM, et al. Enhancing the safety and efficacy of the MVP regimen (mitomycin + vinblastine + cisplatin) in 100 patients with inoperable non–small cell lung cancer (abstract 885). Proc Am Soc Clin Oncol 1989;8:227.
69. Gralla RJ, Kris MG, Burke, et al. The influence of the addition of mitomycin to vindesine plus cisplatin in a random assign-

ment trial in 120 patients with non–small cell lung cancer. Proc Am Soc Clin Oncol 1986;5:182.
70. Drings P, Abel N, Bulzebruck H, et al. Experience with ifosfamide combinations in non–small cell lung cancer. Cancer Chemother Pharmacol 1986;18(Suppl 2):34–39.
71. Rosell R, Abad-Esteve A, Moreno I, et al. A randomized comparison of two vindesine plus cisplatin containing regimens with the addition of mitomycin or ifosfamide in patients with non–small cell lung cancer. Lung Cancer 1988;4:120.
72. Schroeder M, Wellens W, Westerhausen M. Treatment of unresectable non–small cell lung cancer with cisplatin, ifosfamide, vindesine. Contrib Oncol 1987;26:369–371.
73. Ohnoshi T, Hiraki S, Ueoka H, et al. Phase II study of a three-drug combination of ifosfamide, cisplatin and vindesine in non–small cell lung cancer. Jpn J Cancer Chemother 1988;15:115–119.
74. Ardizzoni A, Fusco V, Gusilano M, et al. Etoposide, ifosfamide, and cisplatin in the treatment of advanced non–small cell lung cancer. Cancer Treat Rep 1987;71:1311–1312.
75. Shirinian M, Lee JS, Dhingra HH, et al. Phase II study of cisplatin, ifosfamide, and etoposide combination for advanced non–small cell lung cancer: final report. Semin Oncol 1992;19(Suppl 12):58–64.
76. Paccagnella A, Favaretto A, Brandes A, et al. Cisplatin, etoposide, and ifosfamide in non–small cell lung carcinoma. Cancer 1990;65:2631–2634.
77. Ruckdeschel JC, Finkelstein DM, Ettinger DS, et al. A randomized trial of the four most active regimens for metastatic non–small cell lung cancer. J Clin Oncol 1986;4:14–22.
78. Finkelstein DM, Ettinger DS, Ruckdeschel JC. Long-term survivors in metastatic non–small cell lung cancer: an Eastern Cooperative Oncology Group study. J Clin Oncol 1986;4:702–709.
79. Weick JK, Crowley J, Natale RB, et al. A randomized trial of five cisplatin-containing treatments in patients with metastatic non–small cell lung cancer: a Southwest Oncology Group study. J Clin Oncol 1991;9:1157–1162.
80. Murray N, Osoba D, Shah A, et al. Brief intensive chemotherapy for metastatic non–small cell lung cancer: a phase II study of the weekly CODE regimen. J Natl Cancer Inst 1991;83:190–194.
81. Masuda N, Fukuoka M, Takada M, et al. CPT-11 in combination with cisplatin for advanced non–small cell lung cancer. J Clin Oncol 1992;10:1775–1780.
82. Shinkai T, Arioka H, Kunikane H, et al. A phase I study of CPT-11 and cisplatin in combination with a fixed dose of vindesine in metastatic non–small cell lung cancer (abstract 1089). Proc Am Soc Clin Oncol 1993;12:328.
83. Rowinsky EK, Gilbert MR, McGuire WP, et al. Sequences of Taxol and cisplatin: a phase I and pharmacologic study. J Clin Oncol 1991;9:1692–1703.
84. Dunlop DJ, Cameron C, Dabouis G, et al. Phase I dose—escalation study of cisplatin in combination with gemcitabine in non–small cell lung cancer (abstract 1139). Proc Am Soc Clin Oncol 1994;13:342.
85. Cormier Y, Sheperd F, Burkes R, et al. Phase I study of gemcitabine and cisplatin for advanced non–small cell lung cancer (abstract 1140). Proc Am Soc Clin Oncol 1994;13:342.
86. Stanley KE. Prognostic factors for survival in patients with inoperable lung cancer. J Natl Cancer Inst 1980;65:25–32.
87. O'Connell JP, Kris MG, Gralla RJ, et al. Frequency and prognostic importance of pretreatment clinical characteristics in patients with advanced non–small lung cancer treated with combination chemotherapy. J Clin Oncol 1986;4:1604–1614.
88. Feld R, Arriagada R, Ball DL, et al. Prognostic factors in non–small cell lung cancer: a consensus report. Lung Cancer 1991;7:3–5.
89. Cellerino R, Tummarello D, Guidi F, et al. A randomized trial of alternating chemotherapy versus best supportive care in advanced non–small cell lung cancer. J Clin Oncol 1991;9:1453–1461.
90. Cormier Y, Bergeron D, LaForge J, et al. Benefit of polychemotherapy in advanced non–small cell bronchogenic carcinoma. Cancer 1982;50:845–849.
91. Ganz PA, Figlin RA, Haskel CM, et al. Supportive care versus supportive care and combination chemotherapy in metastatic non–small cell lung cancer. Does chemotherapy make a difference? Cancer 1989;63:1271–1278.
92. Kaasa A, Lund E, Thorod E, et al. Symptomatic treatment versus combination chemotherapy in patients with non–small cell lung cancer, extensive disease. Cancer 1991;67:2443–2447.
93. Quoix E, Dieterman A, Charbonneau J, et al. Disseminated non–small cell lung cancer: a randomized trial of chemotherapy versus palliative care. Lung Cancer 1988;4:A181.
94. Rapp E, Pater JL, Willan A, et al. Chemotherapy can prolong survival in patients with advanced non–small cell lung cancer. Report of a Canadian multicenter randomized trial. J Clin Oncol 1988;6:633–641.
95. Woods RL, Williams CJ, Levi J, et al. A randomized trial of cisplatin and vindesine versus supportive care only in advanced non–small cell lung cancer. Br J Cancer 1990;61:608–611.
96. Cartei G, Cartei F, Cantone A, et al. Cisplatin cyclophosphamide-mitomycin combination chemotherapy with supportive care versus supportive care alone for treatment of metastatic non–small cell lung cancer. J Natl Cancer Inst 1993;85:794–800.
97. Souquet PJ, Chauvin F, Boissel JP, et al. Polychemotherapy in advanced non–small cell lung cancer: a meta-analysis. Lancet 1993;342:19–21.
98. Grilli R, Oxman AD, Julian JA. Chemotherapy for advanced non–small cell lung cancer: how much benefit is enough? J Clin Oncol 1993;11:1866–1872.
99. Stewart LA, Pignon JP, Parmar MKB, et al. A meta-analysis using individual patient data from randomized clinical trials of chemotherapy in non–small cell lung cancer: survival in the supportive care setting (abstract 1118). Proc Am Soc Clin Oncol 1994;13:337.
100. Kris M, Gralla RJ, Potanovich L, et al. Assessment of pretreatment symptoms and improvement after edam + mitomycin + vinblastine in patients with inoperable non–small cell lung cancer (abstract 883). Proc Am Soc Clin Oncol 1990;9:229.
101. Hardy JR, Noble T, Smith IE. Symptom relief with moderate dose chemotherapy (mitomycin-C, vinblastine and cisplatin) in advanced non–small cell lung cancer. Br J Cancer 1989;60:764–766.
102. Fernandez C, Rosell R, Abad-Esteve A, et al. Quality of life during chemotherapy in non–small cell lung cancer patients. Acta Oncol 1989;28:29–33.

SECTION IV

THERAPEUTIC APPROACHES TO SMALL CELL LUNG CANCER

20

ROLE OF SURGERY IN THE MANAGEMENT OF SMALL CELL LUNG CANCER

Frances A. Shepherd

HISTORICAL BACKGROUND

The biologic nature of small cell lung cancer causes dissemination to regional lymph nodes and/or distant metastatic sites in more than 90% of patients at the time of initial presentation (1). Furthermore, most patients with tumors that clinically appear localized to the thorax probably have micrometastatic deposits at distant sites. These metastases have the potential to proliferate if only locoregional therapeutic modalities, such as surgery and/or radiotherapy, are employed. For these reasons, small cell lung cancer, which accounts for 20% to 25% of all primary bronchogenic carcinomas, represents less than 5% of cases in most surgical series. This fact also explains why most surgical series from the pre–chemotherapy era reported 5-year survival rates approaching zero for patients with small cell carcinoma. In 1975 Martini et al. (2) evaluated the Memorial Sloan–Kettering Cancer Center experience with small cell lung cancer over the 40-year period, 1931 to 1971. They found that only 7% of patients had surgically resectable tumors and only two patients survived longer than 5 years. These results were typical of those reported from virtually all centers before the 1970s.

Mountain's (3) review of the experience of the M. D. Anderson Hospital and Tumor Institute in the surgical management of 368 patients with pathologically proven small cell carcinoma of the lung revealed only one patient who survived longer than 5 years compared with 15% to 25% of patients with non–small cell disease (Fig. 20.1). Surprisingly, in this series the survival of patients with small cell carcinomas without lymph node involvement was inferior to that of patients with bronchopulmonary and/or hilar nodes, or even to those with mediastinal nodal involvement. Neither the location (central versus peripheral) nor the size of the primary tumor seemed to be prognostic, nor was the presence of atelectasis and/or pneumonitis associated with a significantly poorer outcome.

Because of the poor results obtained after operation, surgeons began questioning the appropriateness of surgery for patients with small cell lung cancer. This doubt gave rise to the important prospective randomized trail of the Medical Research Council of Great Britain (4, 5), in which 71 patients were randomized prospectively to undergo surgical resection and 73 to receive a course of radical radiotherapy. The radiotherapy dose and fractionation schemes, which were not standardized, consisted of a total dose of 30 Gy or more given during a period of from 20 to 40 days. The results of this trial were published in 1966, (4) and the 10-year follow-up results were published in 1973 (5). The median survival of patients in the surgical and radiotherapy arms was 199 and 300 days, respectively (Fig. 20.2), and at 5 years, one and three patients were alive in the surgery and radiotherapy arms, respectively ($P = .04$). At 10 years, only the three patients in the radiotherapy arm remained alive. It was concluded from this study that radical radiotherapy was preferable to surgery but that neither of the treatment policies was really effective. The investigators suggested that other therapeutic approaches (e.g., immunologic, chemotherapeutic, or various combination therapies) might be more successful and that it would be improbable that any advance in therapy could reduce significantly the overall death rate from this disease in the absence of successful smoking prevention programs. Is it not chastening to realize that 20 years later the same conclusions could be drawn from many of our lung cancer clinical research trials?

The results of the British Medical Research Council trial led some investigators to recommend a policy of preoperative radiotherapy followed by surgery for patients with small cell lung cancer. In a prospective phase II trial from the North Middlesex Hospital in

London, patients received low-dose preoperative radiotherapy (17.5 to 25 Gy) (6, 7). Based on early favorable results reported by Bates (6) and the lack of toxicity seen in the first 29 patients, the dose of radiotherapy was increased from 17.5 to 25 Gy; however, because researchers observed that the results deteriorated, they thus administered the original dose of 17.5 Gy preoperatively for the final 2 years of the study. Of the 90 patients who entered the study, only 73 underwent resection. Non–small cell lung cancer was identified in nine patients. Eight patients survived 5 years, but only two patients remained alive and disease free for more than 10 years postoperatively.

In a similar North American trial that included patients with both small cell and non–small cell lung cancer, patients received higher dose preoperative radiotherapy, 30 to 40 Gy in 2 weeks, followed by thoracotomy (8). No long-term survivors were seen for the small population of patients with oat cell carcinoma in this trial.

An analysis of relapse patterns in the early surgical and radiotherapy trials showed that patients were dying of systemic metastases, which suggested that no manipulation of local treatment modalities would result in significant long-term survival in the absence of effective systemic treatment. Bergsagel et al. (9) from the Princess Margaret Hospital were among the first to test the hypothesis that systemic chemotherapy might add to the effects of local radiotherapy. Their trial showed that a modest prolongation of survival could be achieved by treatment with single-agent low-dose cyclophosphamide. The British Medical Research Council Lung Cancer Working Party undertook a similar trial in which 125 patients were randomized prospectively to receive only 30 Gy of radiotherapy delivered in 15 fractions, or the same radiotherapy with systemic chemotherapy consisting of cyclophosphamide, 500 mg/m^2, given every 3 weeks, and chloroethylcyclohexylnitrosourea (CCNU) (lomustine), 50 mg/m^2 orally every 6 weeks. Prolongation of progression free survival was seen for patients in the chemotherapy arm, although overall survival was not improved and a long-term survival benefit was not seen (10).

At the same time, the principles of adjuvant chemotherapy were being applied to surgical patients. In the United States, large adjuvant chemotherapy trials were conducted by the Veterans Administration Surgical Oncology Group (VASOG), and most of their lung cancer trials contained a small proportion of patients with small cell tumors. In a trial of 417 patients with all cell types of lung cancer, no survival benefit was identified for patients who received postoperative adjuvant cyclophosphamide alone or cyclophosphamide and methotrexate combination therapy, compared with a no-treatment control group (11). Eighteen patients with small cell lung cancer were in-

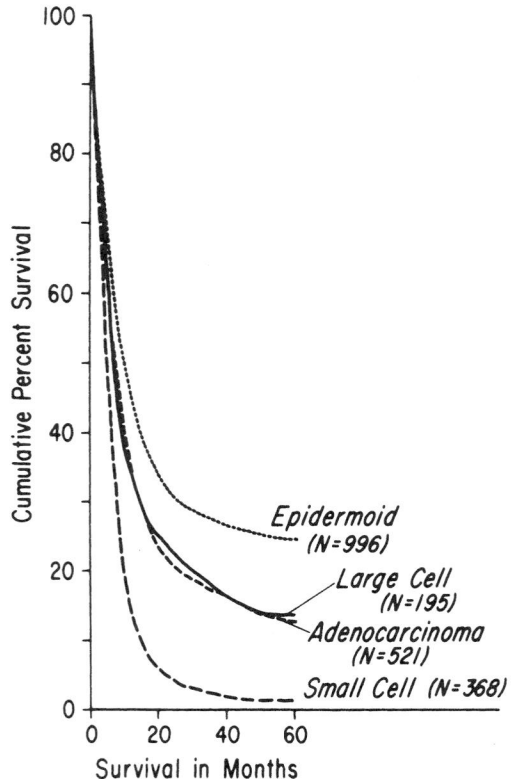

FIGURE 20.1. Bronchogenic carcinoma. Cumulative percentage of patients surviving based on morphology. (From Mountain C. Clinical biology of small cell carcinoma: relationship to surgical therapy. Semin Oncol 1978;5:272–279.)

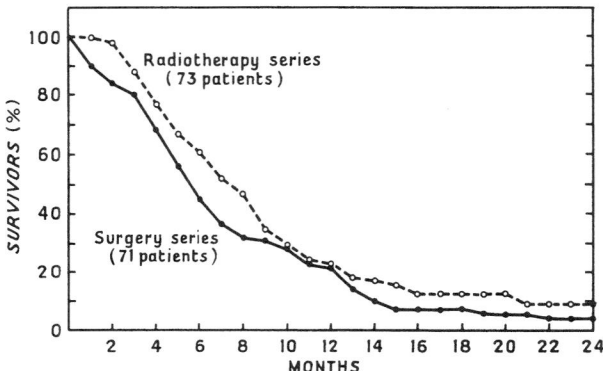

FIGURE 20.2. Survival in the radiotherapy and surgery treatment series (all patients). (From the Medical Research Council of Great Britain. Working-party on the evaluation of different methods of therapy in carcinoma of the bronchus comparative trial of surgery and radiotherapy for the primary treatment of small-celled, or oat-celled carcinoma of the bronchus. Lancet 1966;2:979–986.)

cluded in that trial. Of these, one of six patients in the cyclophosphamide-alone arm and three of nine patients in the cyclophosphamide and methotrexate arm were alive at 3 years, compared with none in the control group. The report of Shields et al. (11) was the first to suggest that adjuvant chemotherapy might prolong survival for patients with small cell lung cancer who had undergone complete surgical resection.

In 1982 Shields and colleagues (12) reviewed the results of four VASOG studies of adjuvant chemotherapy for lung cancer and undertook a separate analysis of the patients in these trials who had small cell pathology (Fig. 20.3). Of a total of 3133 men who underwent a curative resection for lung cancer, 148 (4.7%) had small cell tumors. In the first trial, 28 patients were randomized to receive nitrogen mustard and 27 to the control, and in the second trial, 26 received cyclophosphamide, and 20 no treatment. No survival advantage was seen for the treated patients in either of the single-agent chemotherapy trials. However, as discussed above, a small survival advantage was seen for patients in the combination chemotherapy arm of their third trial. In their fourth trial, in which patients were randomized to receive prolonged intermittent courses of lomustine and hydroxyurea or no further therapy, there was a survival benefit observed for the 11 treated patients compared with the 18 control patients. The survival differences did not reach statistical significance because of the small number of patients in these studies (Fig. 20.3).

Shields' analysis of patients with small cell carcinomas in the VASOG trials also demonstrated the importance of TNM (tumor, node, metastasis) staging for tumors of this cell type. Sixty percent of patients with T1, N0, M0 tumors were alive at 5 years, whereas there were almost no 5-year survivors among the patients who presented either with T2-3 tumors or with mediastinal lymph node involvement (Fig. 20.4]. Patients with T1 tumors with only hilar or bronchopulmonary nodes involved had an intermediate survival of approximately 30%. In fact, these survival results are similar to those of patients who have undergone complete surgical resection for non–small cell lung cancer of equivalent stage.

Although there was general acceptance by the 1970s that surgical resection was inappropriate for the majority of patients with small cell lung cancer, the observations of Shields and his colleagues suggested that there might be a subpopulation of patients with small cell cancers for whom a surgical approach could be considered. In a retrospective review of 40 patients with small cell lung cancer who underwent potentially curative resection between 1959 and 1972, Shore and Paneth (13) reported an overall 5-year survival rate of 25%. Four of 10 stage I patients (40%) achieved long-term survival compared with 9 of 26 patients (25%) who had hilar or mediastinal nodal involvement. Lennox et al. (14) observed that patients who had large proximal tumors or who required a pneumonectomy were less likely to achieve long-term survival. Their 2- and 5-year survival rates for patients who required only a lobectomy were 32% and 18%, respectively, compared with 14.4% and 7.2% for pneumonectomy patients. Only rarely does small cell lung cancer present as a solitary pulmonary nodule. Between 1958 and 1963, a total of 1134 patients with asymptomatic solitary pulmonary nodules were assessed by VASOG members (15); only 15 patients (4%) were found to have small cell pathology. Of these, 11 were able to undergo a curative surgical procedure; 1-, 5-, and 10-year survival rates for these were 63.6%, 36.4%, and 18.2%, respectively. Because most of these patients underwent surgery before the wide availability of chemotherapy, it may be assumed that approximately one third of them were cured by surgery alone as measured by survival at the 5-year mark.

It may be concluded from this historical review that local treatment alone, whether surgery or radiation, is inadequate therapy for most patients with small cell lung cancer. If surgery is to play any role, it must be in the context of a combined modality treatment program with systemic combination chemotherapy and perhaps radiotherapy as well.

RATIONALE FOR SURGERY

IMPROVED CONTROL AT THE PRIMARY SITE

The rationale for surgery in the management of small cell lung cancer has been summarized in Table 20.1. Small cell lung cancer is the most chemoresponsive of all the primary lung tumors. Response rates of 80% to 90% are achieved with current chemotherapy combinations, and a complete clinical response is seen in approximately 50% of patients with limited stage disease (16, 17). Unfortunately, however, most patients experience relapse shortly after discontinuing treatment, and the 2-year survival rate is 20% or less, even for patients with limited disease. The most frequent site of failure is the area of the primary tumor and its hilar and/or mediastinal draining lymph nodes. Clinically, 50% of patients fail initially at the primary site, and for half of those patients, the primary site may be

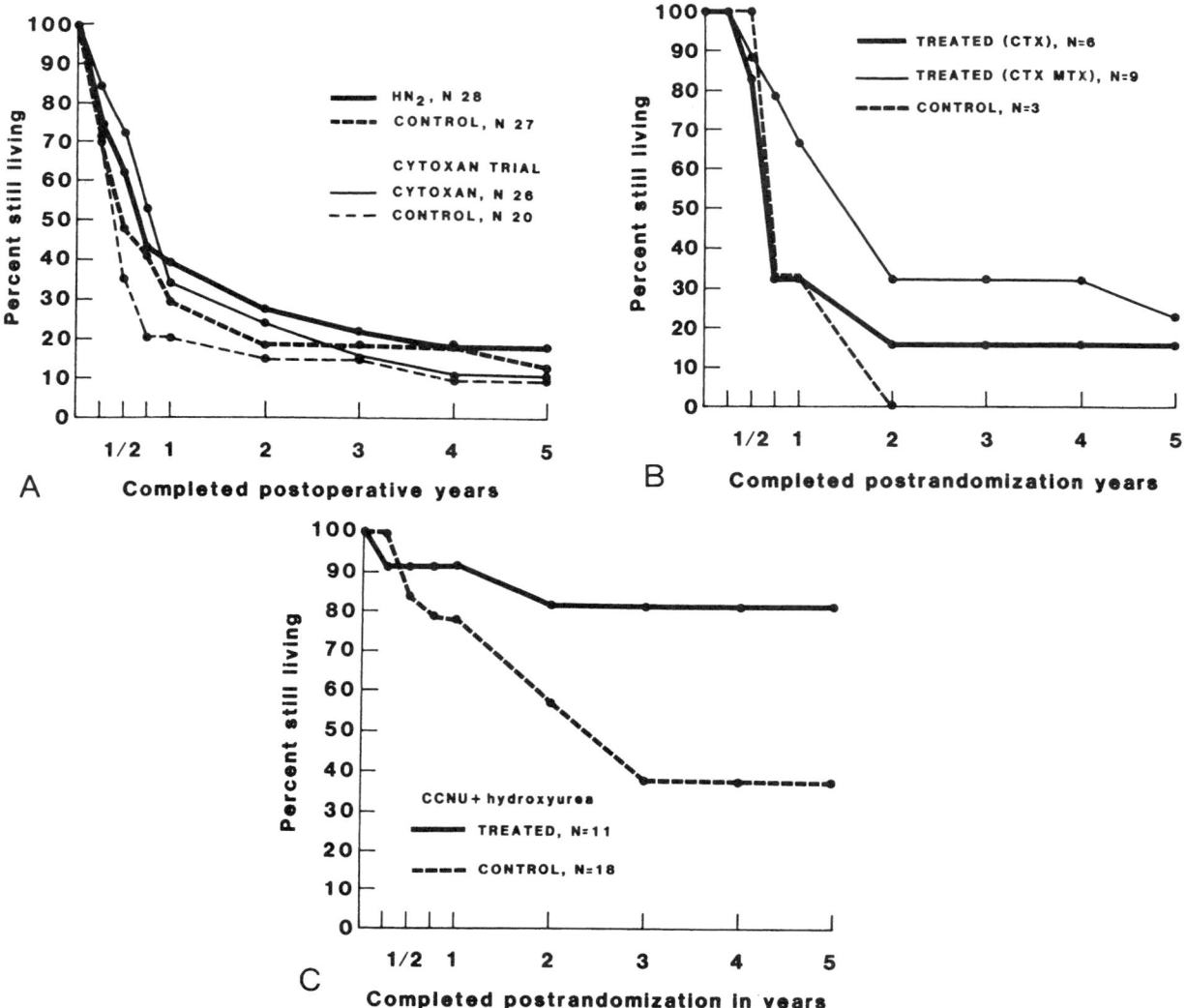

FIGURE 20.3. A. Survival of treated and control patients with undifferentiated small cell carcinoma in the nitrogen mustard (HN2) and cyclophosphamide (cytoxan) adjuvant chemotherapy. From VASOG lung trials. B. Survival of treated and control patients with undifferentiated small cell carcinoma in the prolonged intermittent cyclophosphamide (cytoxan) and methotrexate (MTX) adjuvant chemotherapy VASOG lung trial. C. Survival of treated and control patients with undifferentiated small cell carcinoma in the lomustine and hydroxyurea adjuvant chemotherapy VASOG lung trial. (From Shields TW, Higgins GA, Matthews MG, Keehn RJ. Surgical resection in the management of small cell carcinoma of the lung. J Thorac Cardiovasc Surg 1982;84:481–488.)

the *only* area of failure. These clinical observations have been confirmed in autopsy reviews, which have shown residual tumor at the primary site in 64%, and in the hilar and mediastinal lymph nodes in 53% of patients with limited disease who had achieved complete clinical response (18).

Modest improvement in control at the primary site may be achieved by the addition of thoracic irradiation. Most randomized trials have demonstrated that it is possible to reduce the local recurrence rate by approximately half, but a significant survival advantage has not been seen for patients in the radiotherapy arms of most studies. Because most of the prospective trials of thoracic irradiation were quite small, they did not have adequate statistical power to detect a 5% to 10% difference in survival at 5 years. For that reason two meta-analyses of thoracic radiotherapy were undertaken recently to determine whether the addition of thoracic irradiation contributed significantly to long-term survival for patients with limited small cell lung cancer (19, 20). The survival data for nearly 2000 patients in 16 trials were included in these analyses. Unfortunately, data on local control rates were available for only nine studies, but the meta-analysis showed

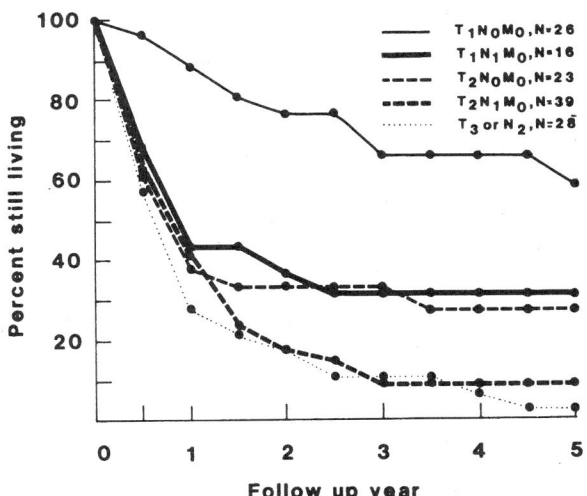

FIGURE 20.4. Survival computed by the life table method from postoperative day 30 (early trials) or from randomization (recent trials) by TNM classification for patients with undifferentiated small cell carcinoma who had undergone a curative resection in the VASOG lung trials. (From Shields TW, Higgins GA, Matthews MG, Keehn RJ. Surgical resection in the management of small cell carcinoma of the lung. J Thorac Cardiovasc Surg 1982;84:481–488.)

TABLE 20.1 Rationale for Surgery for Limited Small Cell Lung Cancer

---

Because small cell lung cancer is very chemosensitive, chemotherapy has the potential to eradicate micrometastic disease.

The most frequent site of relapse is the primary tumor and/or its regional lymph nodes, even in patients treated with thoracic irradiation.
- Surgery may improve control at the local site.

Mixed histology tumors respond poorly and incompletely to chemotherapy.
- Surgery may be helpful in the treatment of the non–small cell component.
- Late recurrences may be of the non–small cell type (a second primary) and should be resected if they meet standard criteria for operability.

Retrospective reviews suggest that with surgery and chemotherapy, the survival of patients with small cell lung cancer is similar to that of patients with non–small cell tumors of similar TNM stage.

---

that thoracic irradiation resulted in a reduction in local relapse rate from 47.9% to 23.3% ($P < .0001$) (19). Both analyses confirmed that a small but significant survival benefit was seen in patients who received radiotherapy (19, 20). The studies did not have the statistical power to show significant differences in the comparisons of early and late radiotherapy or of sequential and nonsequential radiotherapy (20).

The standard therapy for patients with limited small cell lung cancer now consists of combination chemotherapy and thoracic irradiation with or without prophylactic cranial irradiation. Recent trials suggest that the best results are achieved with the concurrent administration of radiation and chemotherapy early in the treatment course (with chemotherapy cycle one or two). Median survival of longer than 20 months and 5-year survival rates of approximately 20% have been reported (21). Even in the most successful combined modality treatment programs, isolated relapse at the primary site occurs in 20% to 25% of patients, and the cumulative risk of local recurrence approaches 50%.

The high local failure rate, despite the addition of radiation therapy, led several investigators to question whether surgical resection could improve local control. They postulated that control of bulk disease in the chest by surgery and eradication of the low-volume micrometastatic disease by systemic chemotherapy could result in an increased cure rate. Small retrospective reviews from several centers suggested that this might be the case. The University of Toronto Lung Oncology Group (22) reported only two local recurrences in 35 patients treated with combined modality therapy that included surgical resection. Similar results were reported by Comis et al. (23), who observed no local recurrences in 16 patients who underwent adjuvant surgical resection after induction chemotherapy.

MIXED HISTOLOGY TUMORS

Mixed histology tumors, in which small cell lung cancer is found in combination with other lung cancer histologies such as adenocarcinoma or squamous cell carcinoma, are seen in approximately 5% to 10% of cases (24). A review of patients with mixed histology tumors seen by Eastern Cooperative Oncology Group (25) oncologists revealed that these tumors were more likely to present as peripheral lesions on chest radiography, although other clinical characteristics were similar to those of the pure small cell lung cancer patients. On the whole, most of the patients in this review were treated on chemotherapy protocols, although it is interesting to note that four of the nine patients underwent surgery as part of their combined modality treatment. The percentage of patients with mixed small cell and non–small cell tumors appears to be higher in surgical series. The University of Toronto Lung Oncology Group (26) reported mixed histology in 14 (17.7%) of 79 patients who underwent initial surgery followed by adjuvant chemotherapy, and in 3 (7.5%) of 40 patients who had surgical resections after induction chemotherapy.

A combined modality treatment program may be appropriate for patients with limited stage tumors of mixed histology if standard surgical criteria are met. Because non–small cell lung cancers are less sensitive to chemotherapy, they are not likely to be controlled by systemic treatment. After initial treatment with chemotherapy for the small cell component, surgical resection of the non–small cell component might contribute significantly to the potential for cure in this small subgroup of patients.

LATE RECURRENCE AFTER PRIMARY TREATMENT

Several reviews have shown that long-term survivors of small cell lung cancer are at high risk of developing second primary tumors, in particular second primary lung cancers (27–30). A review of 47 patients who survived longer than 2 years after treatment at the M. D. Anderson Cancer Center identified 14 patients who had second malignancies; of these, seven had second primary lung cancers (27). In fact, their review suggested that a long-term survivor is more likely to have a second primary tumor than a relapse of small cell lung cancer. Although the patient population at risk for these second tumors is low because of the low cure rate for small cell lung cancer, clinicians seeing patients in follow-up must be aware that a new lesion on chest radiography may be a new primary tumor rather than a relapse. Such patients should be approached as though presenting with a lung mass for the first time. Histologic or cytologic confirmation of malignancy should be obtained; if non–small cell lung cancer pathology is found, the subsequent workup should be directed toward determining operability, because surgical resection has the potential to be curative for some of these patients.

ADJUVANT CHEMOTHERAPY AFTER SURGICAL RESECTION

The first suggestion that adjuvant chemotherapy after surgery might prolong survival arose from the review of Shields and colleagues (12) of the small cell lung cancer patients in four VASOG trials. Eighty patients in these trials received postoperative adjuvant chemotherapy, and a slight survival advantage was noted for patients in the later trials who received combination chemotherapy. Although there were too few patients for the results to be statistically significant and the chemotherapy administered would be considered inadequate by today's standards, the data suggested that after complete resection of bulk disease at the site of the primary tumor, additional systemic chemotherapy had the potential to eradicate micrometastatic tumor deposits. Some patients thus could achieve long-term survival, and even cure.

The favorable results seen in the VASOG trials led many groups to administer combination chemotherapy to all patients after complete resection of small cell lung cancer. The survival results from 10 of these trials are shown in Table 20.2 (12, 31–41). All of these studies were retrospective reviews, and thus they suffer from the inherent weaknesses of any retrospective assessment of a treatment policy. Nonetheless, important observations may be made from the studies.

For many of the patients in these series, surgery was undertaken because a preoperative diagnosis of small cell lung cancer had not been made. For some, it had not been possible to obtain adequate diagnostic tissue preoperatively, and for others, a diagnosis of non–small cell lung cancer had been made. Some of the latter patients were found subsequently to have mixed histology tumors with both small cell and non–small cell components; however, others had pure small cell tumors that had been diagnosed incorrectly preoperatively. Maassen and Greschuchna (35) reported that 18 of 24 patients had a correct histologic diagnosis of small cell lung cancer preoperatively. In a series of 63 patients reported by the University of Toronto Lung Oncology Group (36), only 18 had a correct preoperative diagnosis of small cell cancer. For 22 patients in the Toronto study, a diagnosis of malignancy had not been obtained preoperatively; biopsies from 18 patients had shown non–small cell lung cancer, and mixed histology tumors had been reported in five patients. Postoperatively, small cell lung cancer was seen in 54 patients and mixed histology tumors in nine. In contrast, the studies of Macchiarini et al. (39) and Davis et al. (41) were designed as prospective trials in which patients with small cell lung cancer were subjected initially to surgical resection followed by adjuvant systemic chemotherapy. In the Macchiarini trial, only patients with T1-3, N0 tumors were eligible, and in the Davis trial, participation was limited to patients with clinical stage I-II tumors.

In many of the reviews, chemotherapy was variable because most included patients seen over a period of 10 years or more. With the exception of the early trials reported by Shields et al. (12) and Hayata et al. (31), all patients were treated with combinations of drugs that would be considered adequate even today. A similar variation in the duration of chemotherapy also

TABLE 20.2. Survival According to Pathologic Stage for Patients Treated with Initial Surgery Followed by Adjuvant Chemotherapy for Small Cell Lung Cancer

Author, Year (Reference No.)	Number	Stage I	Stage II	Stage III	Total
Hayata, et al., 1978 (31)	Patients survival (5 yr)	27 / 26%	6 / 17%	39 / 0%	72 / 11%
Shields, et al., 1982 (12)	Patients survival (5 yr)	49 / 51%	55 / 20%	28 / 3%	132 / 28%
Meyer, et al., 1983 (32), 1984 (33)	Patients survival (5 yr)	6 / >50%	4 / 50%	10 / 0	30 / ?
Osterlind, et al., 1986 (34)	Patients survival (3½ yr)	18 / 22%	8 / ?	10 / ?	36 / 25%
Massen, et al., 1986 (35)	Patients survival (3 yr)	41 / 34%	19 / 21%	64 / 11%	124 / 20%
Shepherd, et al., 1986 (36)	Patients survival (5 yr)	19 / 48%	24 / 24%	20 / 24%	63 / 31
Karrer, et al., 1990 (37), Ulsperger, et al., 1991 (38)	Patients survival (4 yr)	63 / 61%	54 / 35%	40 / 35%	157 / ?
Macchiarini, et al., 1991 (39)	Patients survival (5 yr)	26 / 52%	... / ...	15 (T3, N0) / 13%	42 / 36%
Hara, et al., 1991 (40)	Patients survival (5 yr)	13 / 64%	10 / 42%	14 / 10.7%	37 / ?
Davis, et al., 1993 (41)	Patients survival (5 yr)	11 / 50%	16 / 35%	5 / 21%	32 / 36%

was seen and ranged from a single course of postoperative therapy to multiple courses for 18 months. Most groups administered approximately four to six cycles of treatment, and the long-term survival results do not suggest that this relatively brief course of treatment is inferior to more prolonged therapy.

Some patients also received local radiotherapy administered to the primary tumor bed and mediastinum as well as prophylactic cranial irradiation. In view of the variability in radiation treatment and the incomplete reporting in several series, no conclusions can be drawn concerning the advisability of trimodality therapy.

Because most patients with small cell lung cancer generally are not surgical candidates, the TNM staging system usually is not applied to this subtype of lung cancer. Instead, patients are classified simply as having limited disease (disease confined to the thorax and ipsilateral supraclavicular lymph nodes) or extensive disease (systemic metastatic involvement). The patients in the reviews summarized in Table 20.2 differ from patients with limited stage small cell lung cancer overall in that they all underwent pretreatment surgical resection, and therefore detailed pathologic staging is available. The survival results show clearly that the TNM staging system, which provides such important prognostic and therapeutic information for patients with non–small cell lung cancer, may also be prognostic for patients with limited small cell lung cancer.

Every study showed that the best survival was achieved by patients with pathologic stage I tumors, and the poorest survival was seen for patients with pathologic stage III tumors. For stage I patients, survival ranged from 22% at 3½ years in the Danish series (34) to 61% at 4 years in the International Society of Chemotherapy Lung Cancer Study Group (Fig. 20.5) (37, 38). Approximately 50% of the patients with stage I tumors were cured with combined modality treatment, which included surgical resection and adjuvant combination chemotherapy. In the early trials, few patients with stage III tumors achieved long-term sur-

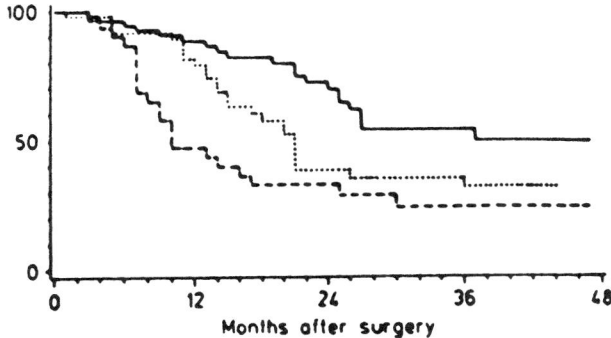

FIGURE 20.5. Life table survival curves for patients with small cell lung cancer according to lymph node involvement: patients classified N0, M0, n = 63 (solid line); N1, M0, n = 51 (dotted line); N2, M0, n = 32 (dashed line). (From Ulsperger E, Karrer K, Denck H, ISC–Lung Cancer Study Group. Multimodality treatment for small cell bronchial carcinoma. Eur J Cardiothorac Surg 1991;5:306–310.)

vival, but in the later studies, in which more aggressive combination chemotherapy regimens were employed, long-term survival ranged from 11% (35, 40) to 35% (37, 38). In all series the survival of stage II patients was intermediate between that of patients with stages I and III (Fig. 20.6). It is notable that these survival rates are similar to those seen after surgical resection for similarly staged patients with non–small cell lung cancer.

What should be concluded from this review? There is general agreement that local therapy alone, either surgery or radiotherapy, is inadequate treatment for most patients with limited small cell lung cancer. The survival rates reported in these series appear to be superior to the survival seen in patients who undergo surgery without adjuvant chemotherapy. Although these comparisons are retrospective, it is likely that the improved survival may be attributed to the postoperative chemotherapy and not to improvement in surgical techniques or supportive care. It seems appropriate, therefore, to recommend that combination chemotherapy be administered to patients who have undergone resection for limited small cell lung cancer, because the long-term survival benefits seem to more than justify the short-term toxicity of such treatment. The University of Toronto Lung Oncology Group (34, 42) recommend the use of no more than six treatment cycles, because survival does not seem to be superior for patients treated for more prolonged periods. Whether fewer than four to six cycles may also be adequate is unknown. In one study reported by Hara et al. (40), 11 patients received only one postoperative course of combination chemotherapy, and 26 patients received only two courses of chemotherapy followed by consolidation radiotherapy. Although the 5-year survival rates for stage I and II patients were excellent, only 10.7% of patients with stage III tumors were alive at 5 years. These results for stage III patients appear to be somewhat poorer than those achieved by other groups who administered a more prolonged course of adjuvant chemotherapy, although firm conclusions cannot be drawn from these retrospective analyses. Littlewood et al. (43) treated two young patients by pneumonectomy followed by a single course of very high dose chemotherapy and autologous bone marrow transplantation. Both patients relapsed, 118 and 80 weeks after treatment, respectively. It would appear, therefore, that a brief course (four to six treatment cycles) of standard dose combination chemotherapy should be the treatment of choice for patients at this time.

Although these retrospective trials support the recommendation for adjuvant chemotherapy after surgical resection, it is not possible to state with certainty which patients have the potential to derive the most benefit from adjuvant chemotherapy, and whether it is necessary to administer such treatment to all patients. Shah et al. (44) reported a 43.3% actual 5-year survival for 28 patients who underwent complete surgical resection without postoperative chemotherapy. The actual 5-year survival for patients with stage I disease was 51.1%, and surprisingly, it was 55.5% for stage III patients. No patient with stage II disease survived 5 years. More than half of the patients in this study had peripheral tumors, and their survival was better than that of patients who had central tumors. Peripheral stage I small cell lung cancer is uncommon, as shown by the VASOG study of solitary pulmonary nodules in which only 11 of 309 patients who underwent curative resection were found to have small cell tumors (15). The 5-year survival of the patients with small cell carcinomas was 36.4%, and their 10-year survival was 18.2%. The details of postoperative therapy, if any, for these patients were not provided, but it is likely that they did not receive aggressive combination chemotherapy. The 5-year survival rate for stage I patients appears to be less than that achieved in the trials of adjuvant chemotherapy, but one can only speculate whether superior survival might have been achieved with the addition of such treatment.

Conversely, it is not possible to draw firm conclusions concerning the contribution of the surgery to the overall survival of these patients. The survival of patients who undergo surgery cannot be compared directly with the survival seen in trials of standard chemotherapy and radiotherapy for limited disease small cell lung cancer. It must be remembered that

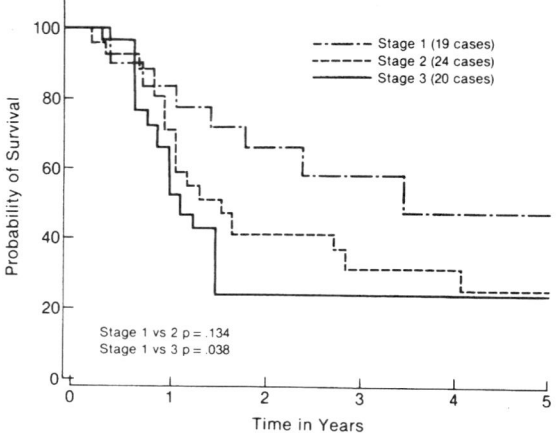

FIGURE 20.6. A comparison of survival by stage for patients treated with adjuvant chemotherapy after surgical resection for small cell lung cancer. (From Shepherd FA, Evans WK, Feld R, Young V, Patterson GA, Ginsberg R, Johansen E. Adjuvant chemotherapy following surgical resection for small cell carcinoma of the lung. J Clin Oncol 1988;6:832–838.)

surgical series include only a select subgroup of patients with limited disease from which patients with adverse prognostic factors, such as supraclavicular adenopathy, bulky primary tumors with superior vena cava obstruction, and/or pleural effusions, have been excluded specifically.

If surgery is to play a role in the treatment of small cell lung cancer, it probably will do so by improving control at the primary site. Relapse patterns were reported in only eight of the trials reviewed (32, 36, 39–43), but the results from those studies suggest that surgery did, indeed, improve local control, because isolated local relapse was seen in only 8 of the 201 patients in these studies (Table 20.3). It must be emphasized again, however, that these patients represent only a select subgroup of those with limited small cell cancer in that they were considered operable at the time of diagnosis. It is quite possible, therefore, that this high rate of local control was seen only because patients in these series had fewer locally advanced tumors and that the local control rate might have been equivalent with a combination of systemic chemotherapy and thoracic irradiation.

PROSPECTIVE TRIALS OF INDUCTION CHEMOTHERAPY FOLLOWED BY SURGICAL RESECTION

PHASE II TRIALS

It was clear to most investigators that the patient population in the series of initial resection followed by adjuvant chemotherapy represented only a subset of the entire limited stage small cell lung cancer group. Although the results achieved with this form of combined modality therapy were promising, such treatment might not be applicable to all patients. In an attempt to define further the role of surgery for this tumor, several groups initiated prospective studies of combined modality therapy that included systemic chemotherapy followed by surgery for certain patients with limited small cell lung cancer. In contrast to the studies reviewed in the previous section, the patients in these trials received initial induction chemotherapy, and surgery was undertaken as the adjuvant treatment for patients who had responded adequately to their induction therapy. A summary of nine such prospective phase II trials is presented in Table 20.4 (45–53).

In all of the trials, multiple courses of combination chemotherapy were administered preoperatively, and all studies employed regimens that contained several of the agents that are most active against small cell lung cancer (cyclophosphamide, doxorubicin, vincristine, etoposide, and cisplatin). There was considerable variability in the number of preoperative chemotherapy courses, ranging from two to six. The overall response to chemotherapy was greater than 88% in all studies except that of Baker et al. (46). In that trial patients received only two preoperative courses of chemotherapy, which may explain the low complete response rate of 3% and an overall response rate of only 54%. This result perhaps suggests that a longer course of induction chemotherapy would be advisable.

Not all responding patients proceeded to thoracotomy. Overall, approximately 60% of patients were considered to have responded adequately and to be medically fit for surgical exploration; of these patients, more than 80% could be completely resected. Therefore, approximately 50% of the patients who entered the studies were able to undergo complete surgical resection. Postsurgical morbidity and mortality were not reported for all studies, but it does not appear that the postoperative death rate or complication rates were significantly increased by the preoperative chemotherapy administered to these patients. Only three postoperative deaths were reported (48, 51, 53), all in patients who had required a complete pneumonectomy. Other postoperative complications included bronchopleural fistula formation, infection, and reversible supraventricular tachycardias, but it did not seem that the surgical complication rate was greater than that observed after similar procedures in patients who had not received chemotherapy.

Although the clinical response rate was high, the complete pathologic response rate was considerably lower, and almost all patients had residual tumor identified at the time of thoracotomy. With the exception of Benfield et al. (49), all investigators reported complete pathologic response in a small number of patients. The rate ranged from 4% (50) to 37% (47) and on average

TABLE 20.3. Sites of Relapse for Patients with Small Cell Lung Cancer Treated with Initial Surgery Followed by Adjuvant Chemotherapy

AUTHOR, YEAR (REFERENCE NO.)	NO. OF PATIENTS	NO. OF PATIENTS WITH RELAPSE		
		LOCAL ONLY	DISTANT ONLY	BOTH
Meyer, et al., 1983 (32)	10	...	1	...
Friess, et al., 1985 (42)	15	1	5	1
Shepherd, et al., 1986 (36)	63	2	26	5
Littlewood, et al., 1987 (43)	2	1	1	...
Macchiarini, et al., 1991 (39)	42	2	24	...
Hara, et al., 1991 (40)	37	2	?	...
Davis, et al., 1993 (41)	32	...	15	2
Total	201	8	72	8

TABLE 20.4. Prospective Phase II Trials of Induction Chemotherapy Followed by Surgery for Limited Small Cell Lung Cancer.

Author, Year (Reference No.)	No. of Patients	Clinical Stage			Chemotherapy	Response CR/PR (ORR%)	Surgery Thoracotomy/ CSR (%)	Complete Pathologic Response (%)
		I	II	III				
Prager, et al., 1984 (45)	39	2	12	25	CAVE × 2 × 4	13/21 (88)	11/8 (21)	2 (5)
Baker, et al., 1987 (46)	37	...	...	...	CAE × 2	1/19 (54)	20/20 (54)	2 (5)
Johnson, et al., 1987 (47)	24	3	7	14	CAV × 6 ± EP	? (100)	23/15 (62)	9 (37)
Williams, et al., 1987 (48)	38	...	...	...	CAE × 3	5/26 (82)	25/21 (55)	4 (11)
Benfield, et al., 1989 (49)	8	...	5	3	CAEV × 2	5/2 (88)	8/8 (100)	0
Shepherd, et al., 1989 (50)	72	21	16	35	CAV × 6 ± EP	27/30 (80)	38/33 (36)	3 (4)
Hara, et al., 1991 (51)	17	4	6	7	Various	4/10 (82)	17/17 (100)	?
Zatopek, et al., 1991 (52)	25	10	1	24	COPE × 3	10/14 (96)	14/10 (40)	5 (20)

Abbreviations. CR, complete response; PR, partial response; ORR, overall response rate; CSR, complete surgical resection; V, vincristine; E, etoposide; O, vincristine (Oncovin); P, cisplatin; C, cyclophosphamide; A, doxorubicin.

was approximately 10%. It is interesting that this complete pathologic response rate is similar to reported in studies of induction chemotherapy followed by surgery for patients with locally advanced (stage IIIA or IIIB) non–small cell lung cancer (54), a tumor that usually considered less sensitive to chemotherapy.

All investigators reported a strong correlation between survival and TNM stage (Fig. 20.7). Patients with pathologic stage I (T1-2, N0) tumors had the best prognosis, with 5-year survival rates that approached 70% for completely resected patients. Stage II and III patients fared less well, but all series reported a small number of patients with stage IIIA tumors (N2) who achieved long-term survival and appeared to be cured by their combined modality treatment program. The median survival for the entire group of patients who entered the trials (including those who did not proceed to thoracotomy) was reported for only six studies and ranged from 13 months to 33 months (46, 47, 49, 50, 51, 55). Several investigators reported the highest cure rate for patients who required only a lobectomy (46, 53), although this finding was not confirmed by all researchers (45, 47). Virtually no long-term survival was seen in patients who had unresectable tumors at the time of thoracotomy. Patients who achieved a complete pathologic response and who had no viable tumor identified at thoracotomy had the best survival. Williams et al. (46) reported that all five patients with a pathologically complete response were cured of their tumors, compared with only 20% of patients who were operable but who had viable small cell lung cancer present on pathologic review. None of their patients who had unresectable tumors was cured.

In general, most of these trials were feasibility studies of combined modality chemotherapy–surgery programs that were designed to determine whether surgery might contribute to long-term survival and cure by reducing the local recurrence rate. Although there was considerable variability in the local relapse rates, ranging from 0% (45) to 40% of completely resected patients (48), most series reported local failure rates of approximately 10% to 20% for patients who could undergo successful resection (Table 20.5) (45–47, 49–53, 55). Local control correlated with both the degree of response to chemotherapy and the completeness of the surgical resection. Of the patients who responded to chemotherapy and were eligible for surgical resection, approximately 15% had unresectable tumors. When these patients are added to those who relapsed locally, the local failure rate increases to more than 25% of the surgical patients. If this 25% were then added to the group who had local response inadequate to justify proceeding to thoracotomy, it perhaps becomes questionable whether surgery really contributed substantially to overall local control in the entire patient cohort identified, before treatment, as potential surgical candidates.

These phase II trials led to important observations that were useful in the design of subsequent randomized trials of surgery for limited small cell lung cancer. They demonstrated that combined modality treatment was feasible and that the preoperative administration of chemotherapy did not result in excessive or unacceptable postoperative morbidity or mortality. It was recognized by all investigators that the favorable survival observed in most of the studies might be the result of patient selection. The Toronto group emphasized the importance of selection bias after their review of limited stage small cell lung cancer treated at their institutions over a 10-year period (56). They reported a significant survival advantage for patients who had no clinical evidence of mediastinal node involvement. This group, which would include the type of patients who might be considered for surgery protocols, had a 20% cure rate with standard chemotherapy and radiation alone, compared with no

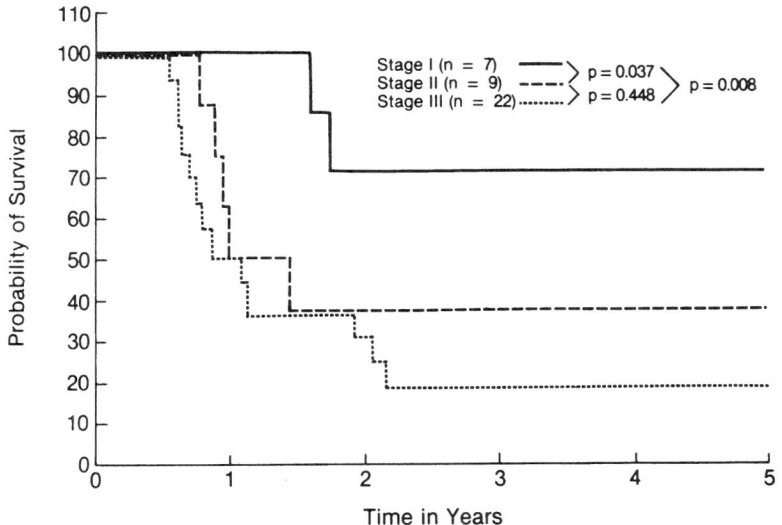

FIGURE 20.7. Comparison of survival by pathologic stage for 38 patients with small cell lung cancer treated with adjuvant surgical therapy after chemotherapy. (From Shepherd FA, Ginsberg RJ, Patterson GA, Evans WK, Feld R. Adjuvant chemotherapy following surgical resection for small cell carcinoma of the lung. J Thorac Cardiovasc Surg 1989;97:177–186.)

TABLE 20.5. Sites of Relapse for Patients with Small Cell Lung Cancer Treated with Induction Chemotherapy Followed by Surgery

Author, Year (Reference No.)	No. of Patients[a]	No. of Patients with Relapse[b]		
		Local Only	Distant Only	Both
Prager et al., 1984 (45)	11	...	4	...
Johnson et al., 1987 (47)	23	3	7	3
Williams et al., 1987 (48)	25	3	6	...
Benfield et al., 1989 (49)	8	...	6	1
Shepherd et al., 1989 (50)	38	3	20	2
Hara et al., 1991 (51)	17	3	7	...
Zatopec et al., 1991 (52)	14	...	5	...
Yamada et al., 1991 (55)	20	3	7	...
Muller et al., 1992 (53)	45	4	15	...
Total	201	19	70	6

[a]Number of patients who underwent thoracotomy.
[b]Excluding patients who were not resectable at time of thoracotomy.

long-term survival for patients with more advanced tumors. Prospective randomized trials were clearly needed to determine the true role of surgery for patients with limited small cell lung cancer.

RANDOMIZED TRIALS

In an attempt to determine whether the addition of surgery to combination chemotherapy and radiotherapy could prolong survival and improve the cure rate for patients with limited small cell lung cancer, the Lung Cancer Study Group initiated a prospective randomized trial of adjuvant surgical resection in 1983. Most patients with limited stage tumors were eligible for this trial, including those who had clinically evident mediastinal lymphadenopathy. Induction chemotherapy consisted of cyclophosphamide, doxorubicin, vincristine, and etoposide in the initial phase of the trial, but etoposide was dropped subsequently when a high degree of neutropenia was seen in the first cohort of patients. In the absence of toxicity or progressive disease, patients received five preoperative cycles of chemotherapy. They were then completely restaged and underwent medical assessment to determine their suitability for thoracotomy and pulmonary resection. Only after it was confirmed that patients were eligible to proceed to surgery were they randomized to receive either surgical resection followed by radiotherapy to the chest, 50 Gy over 5 weeks, and prophylactic cranial irradiation, 30 Gy over 3 weeks, or to the same radiotherapy regimen alone. The results of this trial were presented by Lad on behalf of the Lung Cancer Study Group (57). A total of 340 patients were registered on this trial. Their clinical response rate to chemotherapy was rather low at only 68%, and only 28% of patients achieved complete clinical response. Even though two thirds of the patients had responded at the completion of induction chemotherapy, only 144 (42%) of patients were randomized, 68 to receive surgery and radiotherapy, and 76 to receive radiotherapy alone. Of the 68 patients who were randomized to surgery, six did not undergo thoracotomy, but eight patients had off-study surgery and thus a total of 70 thoracotomies were performed. Fifty-eight patients were able to undergo resection of tumor (83%), and after pathologic review, 54 were thought to have had a complete resection (77%). A complete pathologic response was documented for 18% of patients who underwent surgery. Non–small cell pathology was identified in 11% of patients.

The median survival from enrollment for all patients was 14 months, and for the randomized patients it was 18 months. It was disappointing that when the survival of the patients who underwent surgical resection was compared with that of patients randomized to radiation alone, no difference could be seen in either median survival or long-term survival (Fig. 20.8). Because only half of the patients randomized in this study underwent surgical resection, and therefore pathologic staging, it is not possible to compare survival based on stage or TNM subgroup. The Toronto Group oncologists (50) were the first to draw attention to the discrepancy between clinical staging and pathologic staging for patients with small cell lung cancer, and they showed that clinical staging could not identify subgroups of patients with different prognoses (Fig. 20.9) (26). Similar results were found in the Lung Cancer Study Group study in which patients were very carefully staged at the time of surgery. For all patients it was a protocol requirement to submit lymph node samples from the intrapulmonary, hilar, paratracheal, and subcarinal lymph node stations. In fact, on average, 10 lymph nodes were submitted for each of the 70 patients who underwent thoracotomy. Clinical and surgical TNM stages after chemotherapy were the same in only 20 patients (29%), and, most frequently, patients moved into a more advanced stage (58). For the surgical group, no difference in resectability was identified for patients in any T or N subgroup, although there was a trend toward unresectability for patients with T3 tumors ($P = .08$). All pathologic T and N subsets in the surgical patients had similar survival.

How should the results of this Lung Cancer Study Group trial be interpreted, and are there any possible explanations for the lack of survival benefit seen in the surgical group? Survival was analyzed on an "intent-to-treat" basis, which, of course, is proper for any prospective randomized trial. It must be remembered, however, that 10% of the patients randomized to each of the arms did not receive their protocol-specified therapy. Six patients randomized to surgery declined operation, and of perhaps even greater significance, eight patients in the nonsurgical arm underwent thoracotomy and surgical resection. In a study of this size, a 10% protocol violation of this nature may have masked a small, but significant, survival advantage in one of the treatment arms.

The next question to be asked is why complete surgical resection was possible for only three quarters of the patients subjected to thoracotomy. Although the combination of cyclophosphamide, doxorubicin, and vincristine was considered standard therapy at the time, a disappointingly low response rate of only 65% was seen in this study. With newer regimens that incorporate etoposide and cisplatin and concurrent radiotherapy administered early in the treatment course, response rates of 90% are standard (23). It is possible, therefore, that a more complete response to chemotherapy could have resulted in a higher complete surgical resection rate. This, of course, is only speculation.

Seventeen percent of patients underwent "open and close" procedures with no attempt made to resect residual tumor. For some patients the residual tumor was unquestionably unresectable at the time of thoracotomy. For other patients, however, resection was abandoned when extensive scar tissue was identified at the location of the primary tumor and in the mediastinum. Response to chemotherapy often is accompanied by an intense local scirrhous reaction that makes surgical resection more difficult. Tumors that may appear initially to be unresectable because of fibrosis may, in fact, be resected safely with careful dissection of the tumor bed and mediastinum. Because of the large number of institutions participating in this study, any individual surgeon operated on only a handful of patients. It is possible that had this study continued longer, the overall resectability rate might have been higher. This conclusion is suggested by the observation that the resectability rate was somewhat higher for Lung Cancer Study Group surgeons than it was for surgeons in other centers who joined the trial later. This may have been because of the greater experience of

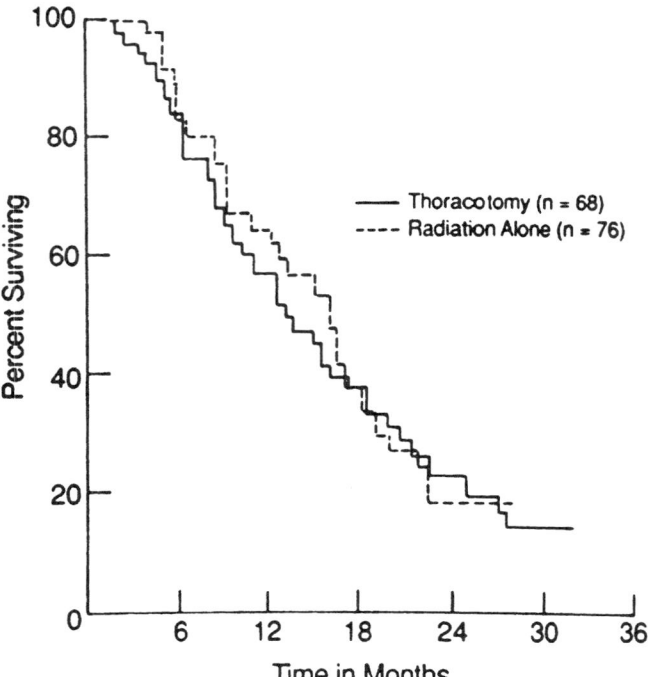

FIGURE 20.8. Comparison of survival for patients randomized to thoracotomy and radiation or radiation alone. (From Feld R, Shepherd FA. In Shields TW, ed. General thoracic surgery. 4th ed. Baltimore: Williams & Wilkins, 1994;95.)

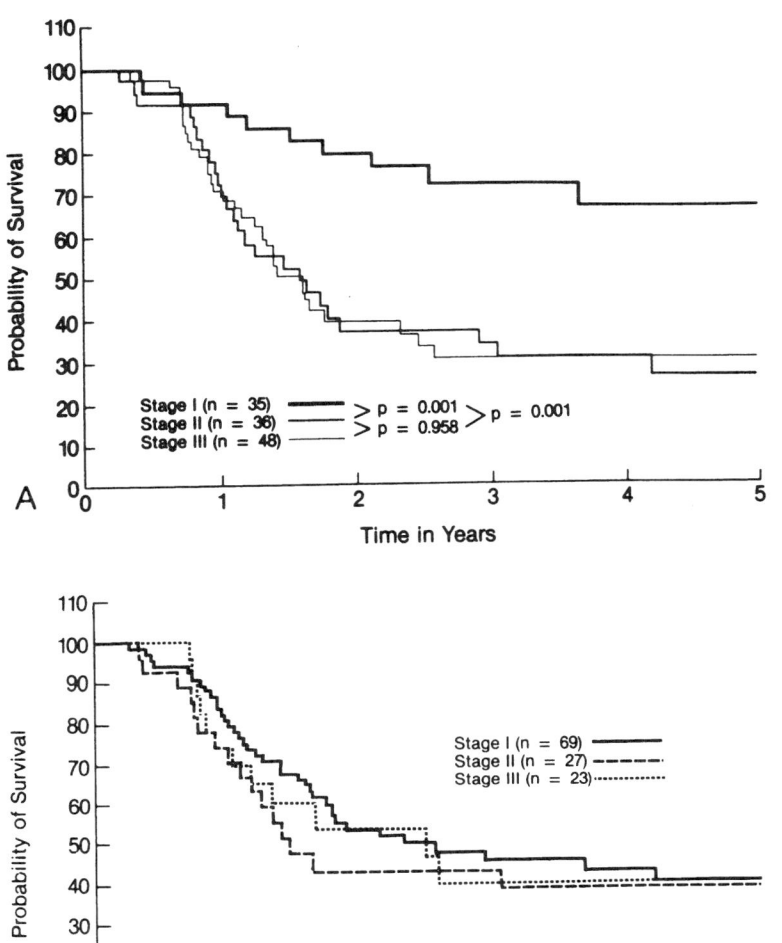

FIGURE 20.9. A. A comparison of survival by pathologic stage for 119 patients who underwent surgery for limited small cell lung cancer. B. A comparison of survival by pretreatment clinical stage for 119 patients who underwent surgery for limited small cell lung cancer.

the former group in operating on patients with both small cell and non–small cell cancers after induction chemotherapy.

Finally, patient selection undoubtedly played a large role in the results of this trial. All patients with limited disease, with the exception of those who had supraclavicular lymph node involvement or pleural or pericardial effusions, were eligible to enter this study. This policy meant that the majority of patients had stage III (N2 and/or T3) tumors. It has long been recognized that surgery plays a very limited role in the management of stage III patients with non–small cell lung cancer, and this trial suggests that the same is true for patients with small cell lung cancer. Because many, if not most, patients with limited small cell lung cancer have mediastinal node involvement (often bulky) at the time of initial presentation, it is clear that surgical resection will be potentially applicable only to the mi-

nority of patients with this disease. Nonetheless, it remains possible that patients with early stage disease (T1-2, N0 and perhaps nonbulky stage II) may benefit from a combined modality approach that includes surgery. Because so few patients are in this subgroup (probably less than 10%), it will probably never be possible to undertake a prospective randomized trial to prove or disprove that surgery is appropriate in this setting.

SALVAGE OPERATIONS FOR PATIENTS WITH SMALL CELL LUNG CANCER

At this time the combination of chemotherapy and thoracic irradiation administered either sequentially or concurrently remains the standard best treatment for limited small cell lung cancer; it results in overall response rates of greater then 90% and long-term survival for approximately 20% of patients. There are few satisfactory treatment options for patients who fail to respond to initial therapy or who relapse after a primary response, and only brief periods of palliation and prolongation of survival are achieved with second-line chemotherapy and/or radiotherapy. Several groups have evaluated whether surgery might be useful as salvage therapy for certain patients with limited small cell lung cancer. Yamada et al. (55) performed operations as salvage procedures on nine patients with limited small cell lung cancer 1½ to 2½ years after their initial diagnosis. Two patients had failed to respond to chemotherapy, six had achieved partial response, and one had experienced a complete response. No details were provided to explain why these patients had been selected for surgery. Four of the nine patients achieved long-term disease free survival that ranged from 3 to 11 or more years. Three of the long-term survivors had stage I tumors. These results were very similar to another cohort of 11 patients reported in the same article for whom surgery was offered as early consolidation treatment after completion of the primary chemotherapy. Once again, long-term survival was limited almost exclusively to patients with stage I tumors.

The Toronto Group (59) also reported their experience with salvage operations for 28 patients with limited small cell lung cancer. Eighteen of the 28 patients in their series had pure small cell tumors. Their overall median survival was 100 weeks, but only two patients survived 5 or more years (Fig. 20.10). In view of these small numbers, surgery cannot be recommended for patients with pure small cell tumors who fail to respond or who relapse after initial standard therapy. The only possible exception might be the rare patient with a true stage I tumor. If surgery is contemplated for any patient, mediastinoscopy should be undertaken preoperatively, because it is unlikely that any benefit will be derived if there is spread of the tumor to the mediastinal lymph nodes.

In a small percentage of patients, non–small cell carcinoma may be found in combination with small cell lung cancer. Investigators at Vanderbilt University found mixed histology tumors in only 9 (2%) of 429 cases (25). They may be seen somewhat more frequently in patients who have undergone surgery, and some reviews have reported rates of more than 10% (26). Non–small cell lung cancer is relatively resistant to chemotherapy, and even for chemoresponsive tumors, complete response is rare. Therefore, one would expect to find residual disease in a significant proportion of patients with mixed tumors at the completion of chemotherapy. In the series of salvage operations reported by Shepherd et al. (59) for the University of Toronto Group, eight patients had mixed histology tumors. The median survival for that group was 108 weeks, and four of the eight patients achieved long-term survival after operation. Three of those four patients had pathologic stage I tumors. Because a small number of patients with tumors of mixed histologic type may be cured by surgical treatment, consideration should be given to a second biopsy for patients who have localized, resistant, small cell lung cancer. Although very few patients fall into this favorable subgroup, it is important to take the steps necessary to identify them because curative therapy may be available.

Several investigators have reported that patients cured of small cell lung cancer have a higher risk of de-

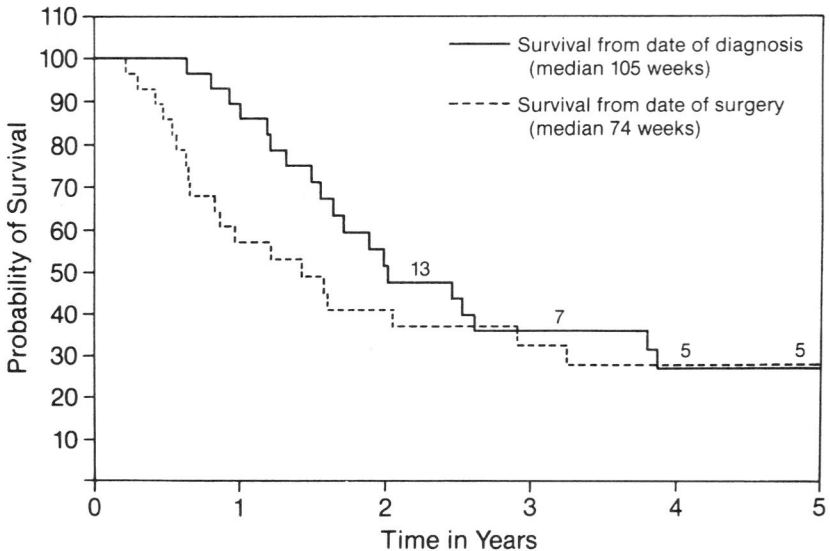

FIGURE 20.10. Survival of 28 patients who underwent salvage operations for SCLC. (From Shepherd FA, Ginsberg R, Patterson GA, Feld R, Goss PE, Pearson FG, Todd TJR, et al. Is there ever a role for salvage operations in limited small-cell lung cancer? J Thorac Cardiovasc Surg 1991;101(2):196–200.)

veloping second primary malignancies (27–30). In fact, a long-term survivor is more likely to have a second primary malignancy than a relapse of small cell lung cancer; many of these tumors arise in the upper aerodigestive tract, particularly in the lung. In the University of Toronto series (59), eight patients underwent surgical resection at the time of "relapse" following a long disease free interval after initial treatment for small cell lung cancer. Two of these eight patients were found to have non–small cell tumors, and both achieved long-term survival after surgery. It is recommended, therefore, that cytologic or histologic identification should be undertaken for long-term survivors of small cell lung cancer who develop a new lung lesion. If non–small cell pathology is documented, the patient should be staged completely, and surgery should be considered if the standard medical and surgical criteria for resection applied to all patients with non–small cell tumors are met. Once again, it must be recognized that any individual oncologist will see very few of these patients. Nonetheless, it is the responsibility of the medical oncologist to undertake the appropriate diagnostic tests and arrange for a surgical consultation because potentially curative therapy may be available.

SUMMARY

Even though most of the studies of surgery for small cell lung cancer were retrospective reviews or prospective phase II trials, many lessons can be learned from them. It is obvious that patient selection is the most important determinant in the results obtained. Most investigators have emphasized the importance of stage and have shown that, as with non–small cell lung cancer, the chance of long-term survival and cure is correlated strongly with pathologic TNM subgroup. In fact, any consideration of surgery for patients with small cell lung cancer should probably be limited to those with stage I and perhaps a small subgroup of stage II patients. Therefore, before surgery is contemplated, patients should undergo careful staging of the mediastinum with computed tomographic scanning and mediastinoscopy. Even with the most careful pretreatment staging, however, the clinical results may underestimate the extent of disease, as shown by both Shepherd et al. from the Toronto Group studies (50) and Lad et al. (58) in the prospective randomized trial of the Lung Cancer Study Group. Many groups have now shown that combined modality therapy with surgery, either before or after chemotherapy, is feasible. The toxicity is manageable, and the postoperative morbidity and mortality rates are not increased by chemotherapy even though surgery after chemotherapy may be more difficult because of the intense fibrous reaction to treatment that occurs in responding patients.

The results of the Lung Cancer Study Group trial (57) indicate that surgical resection will not benefit the majority of patients with limited small cell lung cancer. Unfortunately, the trial did not have the statistical power to demonstrate small but meaningful prolongations of survival for certain subgroups of patients. In general, the phase II studies suggest that the criteria of operability applied to non–small cell lung cancer are equally applicable to patients with small cell disease. Surgery could be considered, therefore, for patients with T1-2, N0 small cell tumors. Whether surgery is offered as the initial treatment or after induction chemotherapy does not seem to be important, as shown in Figure 20.11, a review of all surgical patients treated by

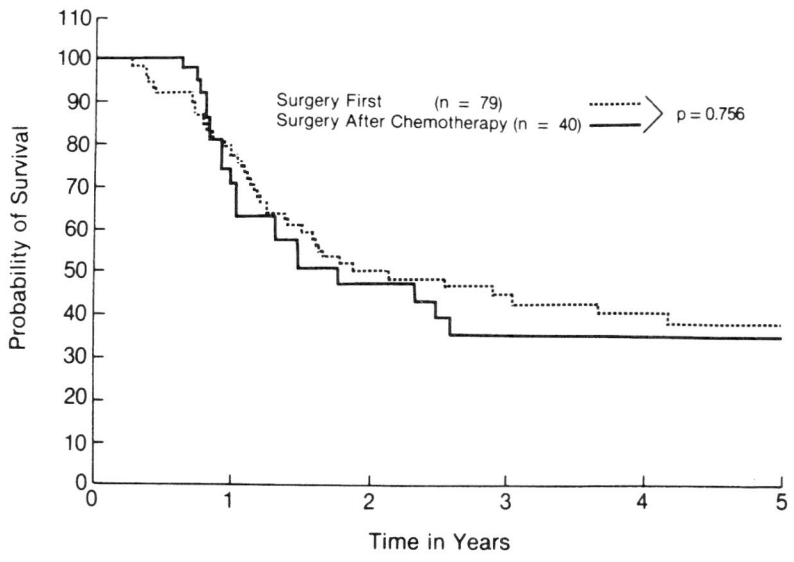

FIGURE 20.11. A comparison of the survival of patients with small cell lung cancer who had surgery first or surgery after chemotherapy. (From Shepherd FA, Ginsberg RJ, Feld R, Evans WK, Johansen E. Surgical treatment for limited small cell lung cancer. J Thorac Cardiovasc Surg 1991;101:385–393.)

the University of Toronto Thoracic Oncology Group (26). If a stage I small cell tumor is identified unexpectedly at the time of thoracotomy, complete resection and mediastinal lymph node dissection should be undertaken whenever possible. Chemotherapy should be administered postoperatively to all patients, even those with pathologic stage I tumors.

With respect to stage II disease, it is not possible to make generalized recommendations regarding surgery, and treatment decisions must be individualized. If surgery is to be part of the treatment approach, it probably should be offered as adjuvant treatment only to patients who have a demonstrated response to initial systemic chemotherapy. As was recommended for patients with stage I tumors, complete resection should be undertaken if small cell cancer is identified unexpectedly at thoracotomy, even if hilar or intrapulmonary lymph nodes are found to be positive. These patients should then receive a full course of adjuvant chemotherapy when they have recovered sufficiently from surgery.

Surgery is not recommended for patients with stage III tumors, even though most investigators have reported long-term survival for a small number of stage III patients. Most of these survivors had either T3 tumors or low-bulk microscopic involvement of mediastinal lymph glands that was identified only at surgery. Even though chemotherapy can result in dramatic shrinkage of bulky mediastinal tumors, the addition of surgical resection does not contribute significantly to long-term survival for the majority of patients, as shown conclusively by the Lung Cancer Study Group trial (59).

The final group of patients who may benefit from surgical resection are those with combined small cell and non–small cell tumors. If a mixed histology cancer is identified at diagnosis, the initial treatment should be chemotherapy to control the small cell component of the disease, and surgery should be considered for the non–small cell component. For limited stage patients who demonstrate an unexpectedly poor response to chemotherapy, as well as for patients who experience localized late relapse after treatment for pure small cell tumors, a repeat biopsy should be performed to rule out non–small cell pathology. Complete staging should be undertaken and surgery considered for stage I and II patients who are medically fit.

References

1. Hansen HH, Dombernowsky P, Hirsch FR. Staging procedures and prognostic features in small cell anaplastic bronchogenic carcinoma. Semin Oncol 1978;5:280–287.
2. Martini N, Wittes RE, Hilaris BS, et al. Oat cell carcinoma of the lung. Clin Bull 1975;5:144–148.
3. Mountain C. Clinical biology of small cell carcinoma: relationship to surgical therapy. Semin Oncol 1978;5:272–279.
4. Medical Research Council of Great Britain. Working party on the evaluation of different methods of therapy in carcinoma of the bronchus comparative trial of surgery and radiotherapy for the primary treatment of small-celled, or oat-celled carcinoma of the bronchus. Lancet 1966;2:979–986.
5. Fox W, Scadding JG. Medical Research Council comparative trial of surgery and radiotherapy for primary treatment of small-celled or oat-celled carcinoma of the bronchus. Ten-year follow-up. Lancet 1973;2:63–65.
6. Bates M, Levison V, Hurt R, Sutton M. Treatment of oat-cell carcinoma of bronchus by pre-operative radiotherapy and surgery. Lancet 1975;1:1134–1135.
7. Levison V. Pre-operative radiotherapy and surgery in the treatment of oat-cell carcinoma of the bronchus. Clin Radiol 1980;31:345–348.
8. Sherman DM, Neptune W, Weichselbaum R, Order SE, Piro AJ. An aggressive approach to marginally resectable lung cancer. Cancer 1978;41:2040–2045.
9. Bergsagel DE, Jenkin RDT, Pringle JF. Lung cancer: clinical trial of radiotherapy alone versus radiotherapy plus cyclophosphamide. Cancer 1972;30:621–627.
10. Medical Research Council Lung Working Party. Radiotherapy alone or with chemotherapy in the treatment of small-cell carcinoma of the lung. Br J Cancer 1979;40:1–10.
11. Shields TW, Humphrey EW, Eastridge CE, Keehn RJ. Adjuvant cancer chemotherapy after resection of carcinoma of the lung. Cancer 1977;40:2057–2062.
12. Shields TW, Higgins GA, Matthews MG, Keehn RJ. Surgical resection in the management of small cell carcinoma of the lung. J Thorac Cardiovasc Surg 1982;84:481–488.
13. Shore DF, Paneth M. Survival after resection of small cell carcinoma of the bronchus. Thorax 1987;35:819–822.
14. Lennox SC, Flavell G, Pollock DJ, Thompson VC, Wilkins JL. Results of resection for oat-cell carcinoma of the lung. Lancet 1968;2:925–927.
15. Higgins GS, Shields TW, Keehn RJ. The solitary pulmonary nodule. Ten-year follow-up of Veteran's Administration–Armed Forces Co-operative study. Arch Surg 1975;110:570–575.
16. Aisner J, Alberto P, Bitran J, et al. Role of chemotherapy in small cell lung cancer: a consensus report of the International Association for the Study of Lung Cancer Workshop. Cancer Treat Rep 1983;67:37–43.
17. Livingstone RB. Current chemotherapy of small cell lung cancer. Chest 1986;89:258S–263S.
18. Elliott JA, Østerlind K, Hirsch FR, Hansen HH. Metastatic patterns in small-cell lung cancer: correlation of autopsy findings with clinical parameters in 537 patients. J Clin Oncol 1987;5:246–254.
19. Warde P, Payne D. Does thoracic irradiation improve survival and local control in limited-stage small-cell carcinoma of the lung? A meta-analysis. J Clin Oncol 1992;10:890–895.
20. Pignon J-P, Arriagada R, Ihde D, Johnson DH, Perry MC, et al. A meta-analysis of thoracic radiotherapy for small-cell lung cancer. N Engl J Med 1992;327:1618–1624.
21. Murray N, Coy P, Pater J, Hodson I, Arnold A, et al. Importance of timing for thoracic irradiation in the combined modality treatment of limited-stage small-cell lung cancer. J Clin Oncol 1993;11:336–344.
22. Shepherd FA, Ginsberg RJ, Evans WK, Feld R, Cooper JD, et al. Reduction in local recurrence and improved survival in surgically treated patients with small cell lung cancer. J Thorac Cardiovasc Surg 1983;86:498–504.

23. Comis R, Meyer J, Ginsberg S, et al. The impact of TNM stage on results with chemotherapy and adjuvant surgery in small cell lung cancer (abstract C-884). Proc Am Soc Clin Oncol 1984;3:226.
24. Hirsch FR, Østerlind K, Hansen H. The prognostic significance of histopathologic subtyping of small-cell carcinoma of the lung according to the classification of the World Health Organization. Cancer 1983;52:2144–2150.
25. Magnum MD, Greco FA, Hainsworth JD, Hande KR, Johnson DH. Combined small-cell and non–small cell lung cancer. J Clin Oncol 1989;7:607–612.
26. Shepherd FA, Ginsberg RJ, Feld R, Evans WK, Johansen E. Surgical treatment for limited small-cell lung cancer. J Thorac Cardiovasc Surg 1991;101:385–393.
27. Heyne KH, Lippman SM, Lee JJ, Lee JS, Hong WK. The incidence of second primary tumors in long-term survivors of small-cell lung cancer. J Clinic Oncol 1992;10:1519–1524.
28. Sagman U, Lishner M. Maki E. Shepherd F, Haddad R, et al. Second primary malignancies following diagnosis of small-cell lung cancer. J Clin Oncol 1992;10:1525–1533.
29. Ihde DC, Tucker MA. Second primary malignancies in small-cell lung cancer: a major consequence of modest success. J Clin Oncol 1992;10:1511–1513.
30. Østerlind K, Hansen HH, Hansen M, et al. Mortality and morbidity in long-term surviving patients treated with chemotherapy with or without irradiation for small-cell lung cancer. J Clin Oncol 1986;4:1044–1052.
31. Hayata Y, Funatsu H, Suemasu K, Yoneyama T, Hashimoto K, Doi O, Ohota M. Surgical indications for small cell carcinoma of the lung. Jpn J Clin Oncol 1978;8:93–100
32. Meyer J, Comis RL, Ginsberg SJ, Burke WA, Ikins PM, DiFino S, et al. The prospect of disease control by surgery combined with chemotherapy in stage I and stage II small-cell carcinoma of the lung. Ann Thorac Surg 1983;36:37–43.
33. Meyer JA, Gullo JJ, Ikins PM, Comis RL, Burke WA, DiFino SM, Parker FB. Adverse prognostic effect of N2 disease in treated small-cell carcinoma of the lung. J Thorac Cardiovasc Surg 1984;88:495–501.
34. Østerlind K, Hansen M, Hansen HH, Dombernowsky P. Influence of surgical resection prior to chemotherapy on the long-term results in small-cell lung cancer. A study of 150 operable patients. Eur J Cancer Clin Oncol 1986;22:589–593.
35. Maassen W, Greschuchna D. Small-cell carcinoma of the lung—to operate or not? Surgical experience and results. Thorac Cardiovasc Surg 1986;34:71–76.
36. Shepherd FA, Evans WK, Feld R, Young V, Patterson GA, Ginsberg R, Johansen E. Adjuvant chemotherapy following surgical resection for small-cell carcinoma of the lung. J Clin Oncol 1988;6:832–838.
37. Karrer K, Denck H, Karnicka-Mlodkowska H, Drings P, Salzer GM, et al. The importance of surgery as the first step in multimodality treatment of small-cell bronchial carcinoma. Int J Clin Pharmacol Res 1990;X:257–263.
38. Ulsperger E, Karrer K, Denck H, ISC–Lung Cancer Study Group. Multi-modality treatment for small-cell bronchial carcinoma. Eur J Cardiothorac Surg 1991;5:306–310.
39. Macchiarini p, Hardin M, Basolo F, Bruno J, Chella A, Angeletti CA. Surgery plus adjuvant chemotherapy for T1-3N0M0 small-cell lung cancer. Am J Clin Oncol 1991;14:218–224.
40. Hara N, Ichinose Y, Kuda T, Asoh H, Yano T, Kawasaki M, Ohta M. Long-term survivors in resected and non-resected small-cell lung cancer. Oncology 1991;48:441–447.
41. Davis S, Crino L, Tonato M, Darwish S, Pelicci PG, Grignani F. A prospective analysis of chemotherapy following surgical resection of clinical stage I-II small-cell lung cancer. Am J Clin Oncol 1993;16:93–95.
42. Friess GG, McCracken JD, Troxell ML, Pazdur R, Coltman CA, Eyre HG. Effects of initial resection of small-cell carcinoma of the lung: a review of Southwest Oncology Group study 7628. J Clin Oncol 1985;3:964–968.
43. Littlewood TH, Smith AP, Bentley DP. Treatment of small-cell lung cancer by pneumonectomy and single course high dose chemotherapy. Thorax 1987;42:315–316.
44. Shah SS, Thompson J, Goldstraw P. Results of operation without adjuvant therapy in the treatment of small-cell lung cancer. Ann Thorac Surg 1992;54:498–501.
45. Prager RL, Foster JM, Hainsworth JD, Hande KR, Johnson DH, Wolff SN, Greco FA, et al. The feasibility of adjuvant surgery in limited-stage small cell carcinoma: a prospective evaluation. Ann Thorac Surg 1984;38:622–627.
46. Baker RR, Ettinger DS, Ruckdeschel JD, Eggleston JC, McKneally MF, Abeloff MD, Woll J, et al. The role of surgery in the management of selected patients with small-cell carcinoma of the lung. J Clin Oncol 1987;5:697–702.
47. Johnson DH, Einhorn LH, Mandelbaum I, Williams SD, Greco FA. Post chemotherapy resection of residual tumor in limited stage small cell lung cancer. Chest 1987;92:241–246.
48. Williams CJ, McMillan I, Lea R, Mead DJ, Thompson J, Sweetenham J, Herbert A, et al. Surgery after initial chemotherapy for localized small cell carcinoma of the lung. J Clin Oncol 1987;5:1579–1588.
49. Benfield GFA, Matthews HR, Watson DCT, Colling FJ, Cullen MH. Chemotherapy plus adjuvant surgery for local small cell lung cancer. Eur J Surg Oncol 1989;15:341–344.
50. Shepherd FA, Ginsberg RJ, Patterson GA, Evans WK, Feld R. A prosepctive study of adjuvant surgical resection after chemotherapy for limited small cell lung cancer. J Thorac Cardiovasc Surg 1989;97:177 – 186.
51. Hara N, Ohta M, Ichinose Y, Motohiro A, Kuda T, Asoh H, Kawasaki M. Influence of surgical resection before and after chemotherapy on survival in small cell lung cancer. J Surg Oncol 1991;47:53–61.
52. Zatopek N, Holoye P, Ellerbroek NA, Hong WK, Roth JA, Ryan B, Komaki R, et al. Resectability of small-cell lung cancer following induction chemotherapy in patients with limited disease (stage II-IIIb). Am J Clin Oncol 1991;14:427–432.
53. Muller LC, Salzer GM, Huber H, Prior C, Ebner I, Frommhold H, Prauer H-W. Multi modal therapy of small cell lung cancer in TNM stages I-IIIa. Ann Thorac Surg 1992;54:493–497.
54. Shepherd FA. Induction chemotherapy for locally advanced non–small cell lung cancer. Ann Thorac Surg 1993;55:1585–1592.
55. Yamada K, Saijo N, Kojima A, Ohe Y, Tamura T, Sasaki Y, Euguchi K, et al. A retrospective analysis of patients receiving surgery after chemotherapy for small cell lung cancer. Jpn J Clin Oncol 1991;21:39–45.
56. Shepherd FA, Ginsberg RJ, Haddad R, et al. Importance of clinical staging in limited small-cell lung cancer: a valuable system to separate prognostic subgroups. J Clin Oncol 1993;8:1592–1597.
57. Lad T, Thomas P, Piantadosi S. Surgical resection of small cell lung cancer—a prospective randomized evaluation (abstract 835). Proc Am Soc Clin Oncol 1991;10:224.
58. Lad T, Thomas P, Piantadosi S. Thoracotomy staging of small cell lung cancer (abstract 205). Lung Cancer 1991;7(Suppl):56.
59. Shepherd FA, Ginsberg RJ, Patterson GA, Feld R, Goss PE, Pearson FG, Todd TJR, et al. Is there ever a role for salvage operations in limited small-cell lung cancer? J Thorac Cardiovasc Surg 1991;101:196–200.

21

REGIONAL DISEASE

Rodrigo Arriagada and Thierry Le Chevalier

INTRODUCTION

Over the past decade, lung cancer has become the major cause of death from cancer in adults. The number of new cases of lung cancer in the European Community and the United States is estimated at 300,000 per year (1,2). For more than 20 years, small cell lung carcinoma (SCLC) has been recognized as a distinct clinical entity. Approximately 20% of lung cancer patients have tumors histologically classified as SCLC. About one third of these patients do not have evidence of macroscopic distant dissemination at the time of diagnosis, i.e., they have limited disease. Some improvement in survival has been seen in patients with limited disease. Results in patients with extensive disease have been less encouraging, but both improved quality of life and median survival time have been reported. This chapter focuses on the subgroup with limited disease; there are likely to be more than 20,000 European and American patients in this category each year.

The sensitivity of SCLC to radiotherapy (3–6) and combination chemotherapy has been well documented (7,8), and current management may include both.

The therapeutic approach to SCLC depends mainly on disease extent at the time of diagnosis. Different approaches have been used to improve results obtained with standard therapeutic regimens. Chemotherapy, radiotherapy, and even surgery may be an integral part of the treatment for patients with limited disease. Although new drug combinations have been introduced and some improvement in survival has been obtained, the best regimen and ways of using and scheduling thoracic radiation therapy have not been defined (9). Various regimens of intensive chemotherapy have been tested, but these are associated with increased toxicity. In this chapter, combined treatment modalities, timing, drug selection and doses, and radiation parameters are among the subjects discussed.

PATHOLOGY AND BIOLOGY

The main biologic and histopathologic characteristics of SCLC are discussed elsewhere in this book (see Chapters 10 and 12). Histologic studies define three types of small cell carcinomas (10): oat-cell tumors, intermediate (fusiform, polygonal) and combined (SCLC with squamous carcinoma or adenocarcinoma) types. Electron microscopy may show the neuroendocrine differentiation of these tumors and may help to establish the diagnosis.

Cytologic or enzymatic markers, such as bombesin, levodopa (L-Dopa) decarboxylase activity, or neuron specific enolase (NSE), by their presence or absence, can differentiate SCLC from non–small cell lung cancer (NSCLC) and confirm the neuroendocrine origin of the tumor cells. NSE enables evaluation of the amount of secreting neoplastic tissue. Increases in the blood concentrations, especially during the initial phase of therapy, reflect destruction of tumor tissue with release of this enzyme into the circulation. Other tumor markers include carcinoembryonic antigen, chromogranin A, creatine kinase BB, gastrin-releasing peptide, and other neuroendocrine peptides.

Cytogenetic analysis has shown that a large number of rearrangements, chromosomal deletions, and duplications occur. Loss of a fragment of chromosome 3p is especially common, although it is not specific for SCLC. The role of oncogenes, tumor suppressor genes, chromosomal deletions, and tumor growth factors is under investigation.

In SCLC, the high cell proliferation fraction and short cell cycle time are two biologic features that probably cause rapid tumor growth, predispose to early dissemination, and may account for the sensitivity of SCLC to chemotherapy and radiotherapy. Thus, the histologic cell type and its biologic characteristics may help to determine a different pattern of chemosensitivity and radiosensitivity (11). SCLC and typical carcinoid tumors are two well-defined entities, but a number of endocrine tumors are intermediate in pathologic appearance and clinical evolution. They are referred to as atypical neuroendocrine carcinomas (12). Another current problem is that of mixed bronchial tumors in which NSCLC elements are found in SCLC tumors. Electron microscopy studies have demonstrated that individual cells of combined tumors may exhibit multiple forms of differentiation (13). The definition of particular tumor-associated biologic factors that would predict sensitivity to treatment would be of major importance in optimizing different treatment schedules. In practice to date, the different subtypes of SCLC are treated identically.

DEFINITION

The treatment of patients with lung cancer is based on the crucial distinction between the histologic classification of the tumor as NSCLC or SCLC. At present, patients with limited SCLC treated by combined chemotherapy-radiotherapy have a better prognosis than those with locally advanced NSCLC. Generally speaking, SCLC differs in its clinical presentation (early development of metastases and responsiveness to both chemotherapy and radiotherapy) and biologic characteristics (short doubling time [14, 15] and tumor markers) from NSCLC. Table 21.1 summarizes some of the differences between small cell and non–small cell tumors. SCLC is characterized clinically by the fact that very often the disease has spread beyond the limits of surgical resectability when the diagnosis is made and management consists mainly of chemotherapy, with or without radiotherapy.

Staging procedures serve to divide SCLC into limited and extensive disease. The Veterans Administration Lung Cancer Study group (16) defined limited stage disease as a tumor confined to one hemithorax and any regional lymph nodes (mediastinal, contralateral hilar, and ipsilateral supraclavicular nodes). Extensive disease refers to more advanced or disseminated disease. The current definition of limited stage also tends to define whether the tumor is amenable to therapy with a tolerable extent of irradiation. Thus, many groups, among them the Institut Gustave-Roussy (IGR), include contralateral supraclavicular nodes in the definition of limited disease but exclude cytologically or histologically proven diffuse pleural involvement. Approximately one third of patients have limited disease and the remainder have extensive disease at the time of diagnosis (17). Staging procedures are based on clinical and laboratory workups, which are described below.

NATURAL HISTORY AND PATTERNS OF FAILURE

SCLC tumors have a shorter doubling time than do NSCLCs; the mean doubling time is approximately 50 days, but the range is wide—from 15 to 250 days—reflecting a significant cell heterogeneity (14, 15, 18). In general, the doubling time of the primary tumor is less than that of distant metastases (19), reflecting a biologic difference between tumor cells that metastasize and those that do not. This difference also is illustrated by patients with small peripheral primary tumors and large mediastinal masses. SCLC bronchial tumors spread early and very frequently to the hilar and mediastinal lymph nodes but also by hematogenous distant dissemination.

The natural history of SCLC is reflected partially in autopsy studies of metastatic patterns (20, 21) showing involvement of the liver in 62%, abdominal lymph nodes in 57%, adrenal glands in 39%, bone in 38%, and brain in 31%. In an autopsy study of 19 SCLC patients dying within 1 month of surgical resection, Matthews et al. (22) showed that 70% of patients had persistent thoracic disease and 63% had distant metastases. The rapid growth of the tumor causes major symptoms, which generally lead to some form of palliative treatment (low-dose radiotherapy or single-drug administration). In the Toronto study (23), the mean survival of 14 patients treated by 40 Gy of thoracic ra-

TABLE 21.1. Comparison Between Locally Advanced Small Cell and Non–Small Cell Lung Cancers

CRITERIA	LIMITED SCLC	NSCLC (STAGE IIIB)
Response to radiotherapy		
Objective tumor shrinkage	80%–90%	30%–50%
Complete response	Common (>50%)	Uncommon (<25%)
Response to combined chemotherapy		
Overall response rate	90%	30%–40%
Complete response rate	25%–50%	5%
2-Year local failure rate	40%	90%
2-Year distant metastasis rate	40%	50%
2-Year event free survival rate	25%	10%
Overall 5-year survival rate	15%	5%

diotherapy was 5 months compared with 10 months for the 27 patients also treated with cyclophosphamide.

Another early trial (3) compared surgery with radiotherapy. Patients treated by surgery alone had a very poor prognosis with an overall 5-year survival close to zero. Those treated by thoracic radiotherapy alone had a slightly better 5-year survival of 4%. The use of chemotherapy alone as given in randomized trials (24, 25) produces a 3-year survival of 9% and combined chemotherapy-radiotherapy a survival of 14%. The survival curves of these different treatment groups are shown in Figure 21.1 to illustrate both the natural history of the disease and the impact of different treatments. For comparison, a survival curve of patients with extensive disease also is plotted.

The poor prognosis of the disease is explained mainly by its high potential for early dissemination. It is evident from Figure 21.1 that patients with extensive disease are seldom cured. Current drug combinations thus are unable to sterilize overt metastases. However, they can control micrometastases and, most importantly, bulky thoracic disease, as suggested by the 7% of patients treated by chemotherapy alone who were alive at 5 years. This leads to the hypothesis that distant metastases are biologically different from the primary tumor and/or are constituted by tumor cells that have developed biologic characteristics that make them resistant to treatment (26, 27). It is possible that the need for rapid initiation of treatment is mainly to prevent the early emergence of resistant tumor cells. This effect, if any, would be more important than the avoidance of early dissemination per se, but it is possible that both factors may be highly correlated. In any case, the major cause of failure in SCLC is the development of treatment resistance, as shown by the 85% of patients dying even after current intensive radiotherapy-chemotherapy treatment. In these cases, tumor cells have become resistant to second-line drug therapy and radiation.

Patients treated with chemotherapy alone develop a high incidence of local recurrence, and such re-

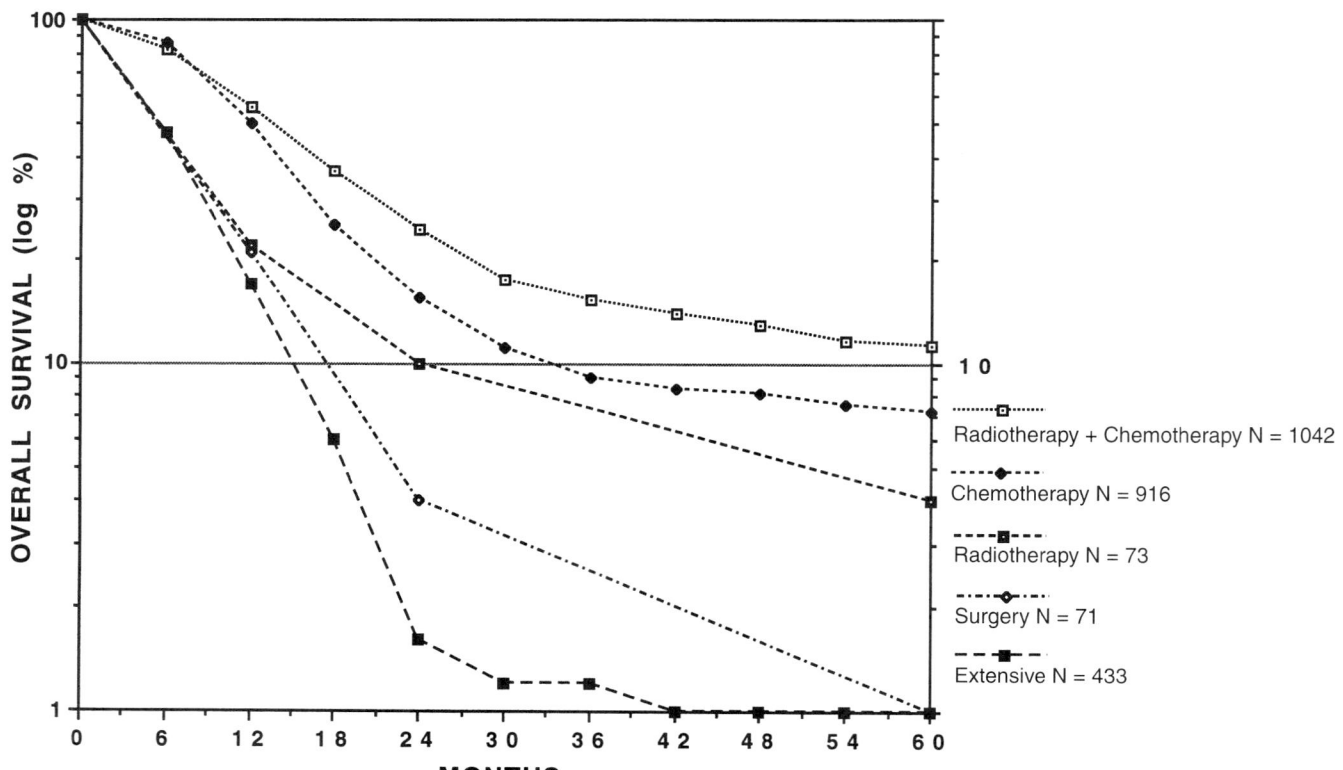

FIGURE 21.1. Overall survival of limited SCLC series. The definition of limited disease is not consistent because of the use of different staging procedures used since the late 1960s. (Surgery and radiotherapy series from Fox W, Scadding JG. Medical Research Council comparative trial of surgery and radiotherapy for primary treatment of small-cell or oat-celled carcinoma of the bronchus. Lancet 1973;2:63–65; Others from Pignon JP, Arriagada R, Ihde DC, et al. Effect of thoracic radiotherapy on mortality in limited small cell lung cancer. A meta-analysis of 13 randomized trials among 2,140 patients. N Engl J Med 1992;327:1618–1624.)

currences are more difficult to manage than primary tumors because of the emergence of chemoresistant cells (28, 29). Even if a complete remission is achieved, the tumor may still contain a very large number of viable cells that are the cause of disease recurrence. The problem of local recurrence in limited SCLC has been underestimated in recent years, mainly because of the emphasis on distant dissemination as the most important phenomenon in the natural history of SCLC. The analysis of the pattern of failure may give a good description of the natural history of patients being treated on current chemotherapy-radiotherapy regimens. Relapse free survival (RFS) is used widely to report results with local recurrence, distant metastasis, and death as endpoints; details on competing events usually are not included. The actuarial method of estimating the local recurrence or distant metastasis rate has been used frequently to assess patterns of failure. This latter procedure has been criticized for possible biases in the evaluation of event rates (30, 31). The main criticism is that this method assumes that the different failure rates are independent. However, it is highly likely that local and distant recurrences are interdependent phenomena. It may be more appropriate to assume competing risks among analyzed events.

In a previous study (32), results were reported in terms of the RFS obtained in 202 patients with limited SCLC treated at the Institut Gustave-Roussy and other participating centers since 1980 with four different consecutive protocols of alternating thoracic radiotherapy and chemotherapy. These protocols are described in detail below. At the end of induction therapy, 76% of patients were in complete remission. RFS variables were determined according to a model that assumed competing risks to define the first cause of failure (local disease, distant metastasis, or intercurrent death). Overall results showed a 2-year cumulative rate of failure of 75%. The causes of failure as the first event were local recurrence only in 33%, distant metastasis only in 25%, distant and local metastasis simultaneously in 9%, and intercurrent death in 8% of cases. These results are shown in Figure 21.2. From this study, it was concluded that: (*a*) the methodology of competing risks enables an unambiguous description of the first events in limited SCLC; and (*b*) local failure is the principal cause of failure in limited SCLC, even in a population treated with a high dose of thoracic radiotherapy. Therefore, local treatment is still suboptimal, and its improvement may lead to better treatment results.

The natural history of the disease may be modified by prognostic factors. Their careful analysis may allow for a better understanding of the disease biology and treatment effects. The study of prognostic factors is discussed further in Chapter 13. Briefly, the main prognostic factors, as determined by multivariate analysis, are common to other lung cancers, i.e., stage, performance status, and weight loss (33–36). In addition, sex, age, hyponatremia, levels of alkaline phosphatase, and initial lactate dehydrogenase and carcinoembryonic antigen levels have been shown to effect the prognosis in SCLC independently (33, 35, 37). However, as noted previously, it is important to compare new prognostic factors with well-established factors in series containing many hundreds of patients and using multivariate analysis adjustments.

DIAGNOSIS AND STAGING

Diagnosis

The main symptoms of SCLC are similar to those of other lung cancers and include cough, hemoptysis, chest pain, obstructive dyspnea, or signs secondary to pneumonitis. Less common are symptoms of esophageal compression, recurrent nerve paralysis, superior vena cava obstruction, or pleural effusion. Uncommon but more specific to SCLC are the manifestations of paraneoplastic syndromes such as Cushing's or Eaton-Lambert (myasthenialike) or inappropriate secretion of antidiuretic hormone.

Most SCLC tumors are detected on a chest radiograph as an abnormal lung opacity with hilar and/or mediastinal lymph nodes, atelectasis, or pneumonitis. Less often the tumor may be located peripherally with or without a pleural effusion. Cavitation is exceptional. Once the diagnosis of lung cancer is suspected, tissue diagnosis of the tumor and staging must be done to decide appropriate treatment.

Although radiologic studies can suggest a diagnosis and serve to guide other diagnostic procedures, they cannot replace histologic or cytologic examination of biopsy material. Fiberoptic bronchoscopy enables direct visualization of almost the entire tracheobronchial tree. In comparison, the older, rigid bronchoscope visualizes only lobar bronchi and some segmental bronchi. In addition to visualization, the aim of bronchoscopy is to provide biopsy specimens, brushings, or lung tissue of suspect bronchial lesions for culture and cytologic examination.

Baldeyrou et al. (38) assessed the value of fiberoptic bronchoscopy in 180 patients with SCLC between 1980 and 1986. This diagnostic procedure pro-

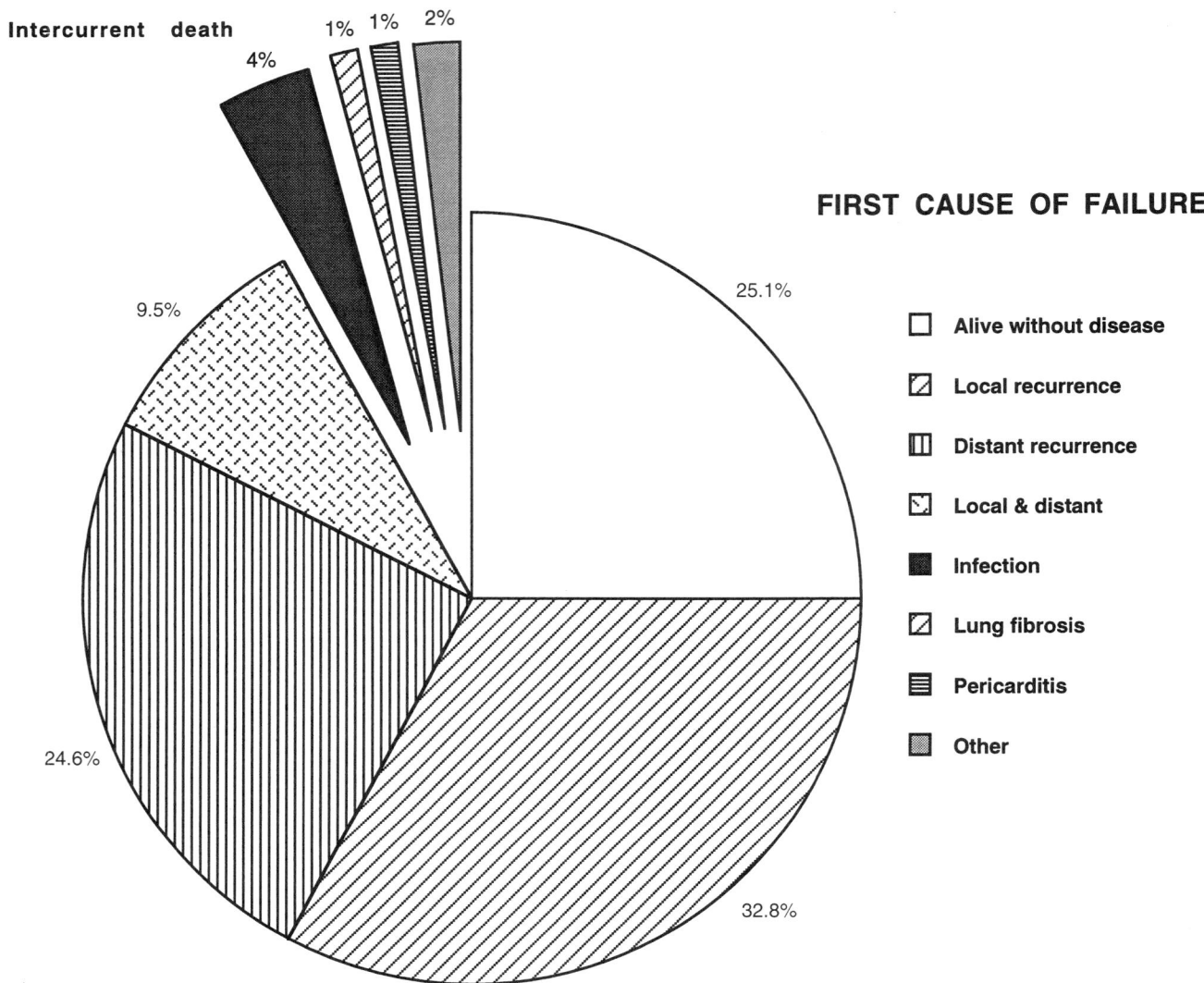

FIGURE 21.2. Pattern of treatment failure in a series of 202 patients with limited SCLC treated by alternating chemotherapy and radiotherapy.

vided the correct diagnosis in 93% of cases. In the remainder, mediastinoscopy or fine-needle biopsy were used. Indeed, if a suspect lesion is small and not accessible to fiberoptic bronchoscopy, direct-aspiration needle biopsy often is used. Fine-needle aspiration is safe and can provide diagnostic results in up to 80% of patients with pulmonary malignancy (39). If the diagnosis is still in doubt, a large-bore (22-gauge) cutting biopsy needle can provide an adequate amount of tissue for histologic examination and immunohistochemical techniques. Yang et al. (40) reported the results of a prospective study that compared cytologic examination of fine-needle aspiration specimens with histologic examination of core biopsies from 149 patients with thoracic tumors. Diagnostic accuracy was significantly higher in malignant tumors with the use of large-bore biopsy (97% versus 59% with fine-needle aspiration).

A proportion of SCLC patients present with major mediastinal involvement but without a visible primary tumor. In these cases, mediastinoscopy should be used to obtain biopsy specimens of mediastinal lymph nodes.

Baldeyrou et al. (38) recommended repeating the fiberoptic bronchoscopy to confirm complete remission and also following treatment to detect local recurrence and treatment sequelae. These findings could then be compared with chest radiograph and thoracic computed tomography (CT) scans. In conclusion, fiberoptic bronchoscopy is a valuable diagnostic method, both to establish the diagnosis and also to monitor the effects of treatment and possible disease recurrence.

Staging Procedures

Clinical and radiologic workups are crucial for accurate staging. Staging procedures vary from one center to another, and no general consensus has been reached regarding its extent. Pretreatment staging of patients with histologically confirmed SCLC includes a complete clinical examination, full blood cell count and biochemical profile, chest radiograph, fiberoptic bronchoscopy, chest CT scan, liver and adrenal ultrasound or CT scan, brain CT scan, and bone marrow biopsy. Other examinations can be added for research purposes, such as magnetic resonance imaging, bone scan, and determination of tumor markers such as neuron specific enolase and carcinoembryonic antigen, depending on the patient's symptoms and other findings. Chest films and CT scanning are used to evaluate tumor size and nodal involvement. CT scans are useful in planning chest radiation treatment, assessing the response to chemotherapy and radiotherapy, and, at follow-up, detecting tumor recurrence.

An analysis of the staging methods used is essential in the evaluation of clinical trials, because variations in staging procedures invalidate comparisons of different studies. Sophisticated staging techniques can identify subgroups of patients with a better prognosis, and as new therapeutic modalities are evaluated, the effectiveness of such new therapies will have to be evaluated in randomized studies, not through historical comparisons. A Danish group (41) recently published a prospective comparison of the use of abdominal CT scanning and ultrasound in the staging of SCLC. Seventy-seven patients underwent abdominal CT and ultrasound scanning, and 60 of these patients also underwent peritoneoscopy and biopsy. It was found that for hepatic metastases, the diagnostic sensitivity, specificity, and negative predictive value were similar for CT and ultrasound. However, an abdominal CT scan was a more sensitive method for diagnosing extrahepatic metastases.

Another group (42) showed that patients with brain metastases diagnosed by CT scanning have a significantly better overall prognosis than those detected with radionuclide studies. Conversely, patients who had hepatic metastases detected by liver biopsy had a longer survival than those identified by CT scanning.

In summary, the staging of SCLC is an essential part of the management of the disease because of the difference in prognosis between limited and extensive disease and hence the different treatment strategies.

Treatment Modalities

In limited SCLC, two problems arise: local tumor control and the treatment of micrometastases. Even if chemotherapy were a solution for both, the *complete* remission rate is below 50% and clearly is insufficient to ensure prolonged local control. For this reason, the addition of a local treatment—surgery or radiotherapy—should be considered.

The development and use of cytotoxic drugs and local treatments have proceeded in different directions. These differences arise from the strictly local effects of radiation and surgery rather than from the systemic effects of chemotherapy. The scheduling of local and systemic modalities poses both theoretical and practical problems that need to be resolved to obtain the best sequencing of treatment. This chapter reviews each treatment modality separately with their specific aspects before discussing the problem of treatment scheduling.

Surgery

Limited SCLC may present with local or regional lymph node involvement. Although current interest has focused on surgery as part of the multimodal management of SCLC (43), prospective studies have shown that few patients with limited SCLC are candidates for thoracotomy before or after chemotherapy. Only 10% of such patients may be treated with surgery (44). For example, in cases in which the primary tumor is T1 (no more than 3 cm in its largest dimension, with no evidence of proximal invasion of a lobar bronchus) or T2 (more than 3 cm in its largest dimension with invasion of the visceral pleura) and N0, surgical resection may be possible. The role of primary surgery in SCLC is discussed further in Chapter 20.

Radiotherapy

Treatment with radiation plays an important role in the management of lung cancer patients. It is widely recognized that chest irradiation decreases the local failure rate in regional SCLC. However, the main limiting factor is the tolerance of surrounding normal tissue to the administered radiation dose. General aspects of radiation biology have already been discussed. It is now clearly established (4, 6) that the response of lung cancer cells depends on the cell type. These studies have shown that SCLC is more radioresponsive than other histologic types. SCLC cell lines have nearly exponential radiation dose-response curves as opposed to NSCLC cells, which have shouldered radiation dose-response curves (6). The relatively high intracellular concentration of glutathione found in NSCLC tumor cells (45) may account for the radioresistance of this cell type by reducing the initial DNA damage. Induction of glutathione depletion may be used to increase radiosensitivity (46). However, Carmichael et al. (47) did not find any correlation between intracellular glutathione levels and inherent radiosensitivity. Preliminary studies (48) have shown that SCLC has a significant number of hypoxic tumor cells, thus hypoxic cell sensitizers such as nitroimidazoles or nitric oxide–releasing agents could be tested as agents to improve local control (49). The use of cytotoxic drugs such as cisplatin or paclitaxel is another approach to sensitizing tumor cells to radiation. The postulated mechanism of sensitization of such chemotherapeutic agents involves inhibition of cell repair and redistribution of cells into radiosensitive phases of the cell cycle.

In clinical practice, randomized trials performed in the 1980s showed that chest irradiation decreased the risk of thoracic recurrence and suggested a gain in long-term survival of approximately 5% to 10% in limited disease (50). These effects as well as radiation parameters, such as target volume, total dose, fractionation, and some technical aspects, are analyzed below.

CHEST IRRADIATION AND LOCAL FAILURE

Chemotherapy alone may produce a complete response rate of 30% to 40% in patients with limited disease (51), but approximately half of these patients will develop local recurrence within the first 2 years of follow-up. Combinations of radiotherapy and chemotherapy may produce a complete response in up to 80% of patients, and in approximately one third, thoracic disease will recur within 2 years. The theoretical curves of local control based on mean values of the literature are shown in Figure 21.3. It was possible to evaluate the local effect of radiotherapy in eight published randomized trials comparing chemotherapy alone with the combination of chest irradiation and chemotherapy. A review of the literature-based data comprising 1473 patients (52) is shown in Table 21.2. The overall odds ratio for the 2-year local failure is .32 (.26–.40), indicating that the risk of local failure may be decreased threefold with the addition of chest irradiation; this effect is highly significant ($P < .00005$). Such results should be interpreted cautiously because both the method used and publication bias may lead to an overestimation of the treatment effect, as discussed in Chapter 8.

CHEST IRRADIATION AND OVERALL SURVIVAL

The effect of chest irradiation on survival remained controversial until the early 1990s when a comprehensive meta-analysis based on individual patient data was performed on a series of 2140 patients with limited SCLC (25). This study is discussed below.

RADIOTHERAPY PARAMETERS

Several parameters, such as total radiation dose, fraction size, volume and type of irradiated normal tissues, definition of the target volume, and quality control of radiotherapy techniques, need to be considered. These factors are of paramount importance in the planning and effects of combined chemotherapy-radiotherapy. Unfortunately, they generally are described poorly in trial reports, and it is often difficult to determine the real reasons for the discrepant results found in the literature. For example, if the irradiated volume were too small, this would explain a high rate of local recurrence at the border of the radiation fields; in contrast, the high incidence of radiation-related complications reported in some trials could be explained by an irradiated volume that is too large. Low doses can account for a high incidence of in-field recurrences, and total doses or doses per fraction that are too high may explain an increased rate of radiation-related complications.

VOLUME TREATED

The standard recommendation (60, 61) is the treatment of the original tumor volume as defined before chemotherapy, with a 1.5- to 2-cm free margin. However, this recommendation is supported only by retrospective studies. Only one randomized trial, involving 191 patients, has been conducted on this subject (56). The overall intrathoracic recurrence rate was 32% in the "wide volume radiotherapy" arm compared with 28% in the "reduced volume radiotherapy" arm; this difference was not significant. In contrast, three retrospective studies (62–64) with a total of 159 patients showed that the use of inadequate portals was associated with a twofold to threefold increase in intrathoracic recurrences. This significant adverse effect could be related to major protocol violations because the recurrence rates were more than 50%. Institut Gustav-Roussy data (65) showed no increase in the local relapse rate in the event of inadequate coverage—strictly defined—of the initial tumor: 36% versus 33% in the case of adequate coverage. This finding agrees with the results of the randomized trial of Kies and colleagues (56), and it would suggest that tumor shrinkage after chemotherapy is sufficient to allow the tumor to be encompassed completely by limited fields. One

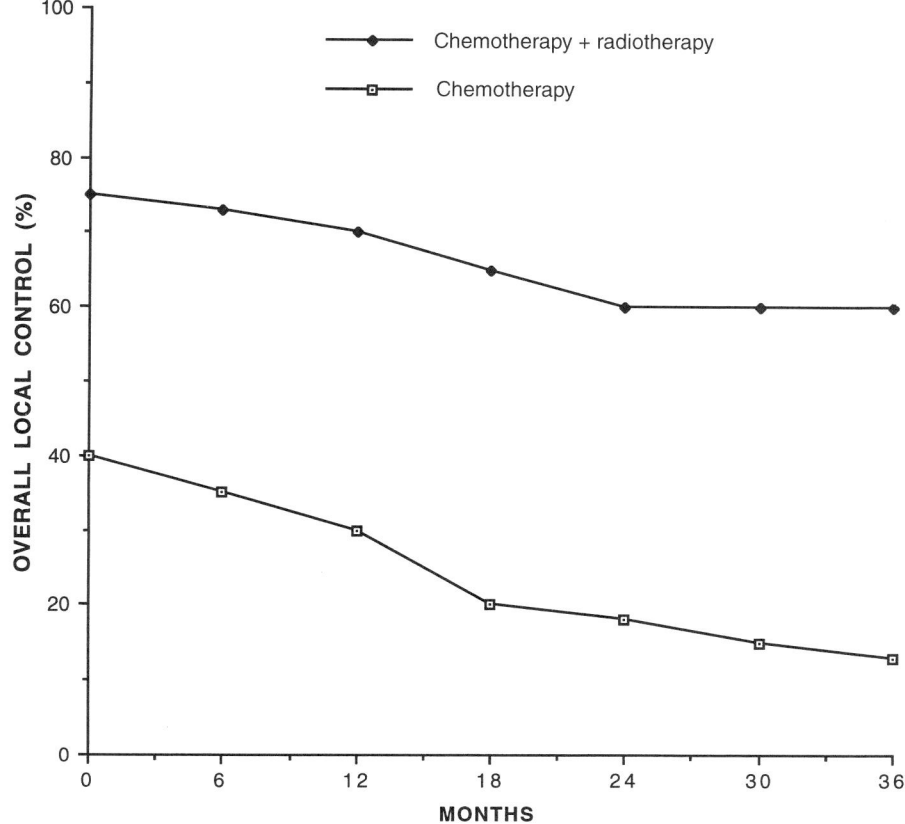

FIGURE 21.3. Theoretical curves of local control in limited SCLC. Only patients with complete remission have been considered locally controlled. Values for chemotherapy alone are the mean derived from the literature and assume a 40% complete remission rate with 50% of local recurrences occurring in the first 2 years of follow-up. Values for the combined approach correspond to those obtained with alternating chemotherapy and radiotherapy. (From Arriagada R, Le Chevalier T, Pignon JP, et al. Initial chemotherapeutic doses and survival in patients with limited small cell lung cancer. N Engl J Med 1993;329:1848–1852.)

TABLE 21.2. Literature-Based Review Evaluating the Effect of Thoracic Radiotherapy on the Thoracic Recurrence Rate

Trial (Reference No.)	No. of Events/Evaluated Patients		Local Failure (%)		Odds Ratio	P Value
	CT + RT	CT	CT + RT (%)	CT (%)		
Copenhagen (53)	35/57	51/60	61	85	.30	.004
NCI (54)	17/47	36/49	36	74	.22	<.0001
SECSG I (55)	84/149	104/142	56	73	.48	.003
SWOG (56)	20/40	38/53	50	72	.40	.033
Uppsala (57)	15/25	26/31	60	84	.30	.047
CALGB (58)	124/270	112/129	46	87	.18	<.0001
Okayama (59)	18/25	21/27	72	78	.74	.63
SECSG II (55)	88/147	163/222	60	73	.54	.006
Total	401/760	551/713	53	77	.34[a]	<.00001[b]

Adapted from Arriagada R, Pignon J, Le Chevalier T. The role of chest irradiation in small cell lung cancer. In: Hansen HH, ed. Lung Cancer V. Boston: Kluwer Academic Publishing, 1995:255–272.
[a]Range, .28–.43.
[b]Heterogeneity test, .02.

should not conclude immediately, however, that small fields should be recommended for treatment of these patients. These retrospective series clearly indicate that very limited fields fail to improve local control compared with treatments using chemotherapy alone. Three further arguments should be taken into account: (a) the difficulties encountered when attempting to define the meaning of adequate coverage, (b) the relatively small number of patients included in these studies, and (c) the fact that the most frequent site of relapse was inside the fields even when irradiation encompassed the original tumor volume (65). The latter finding probably indicates an inadequate dose level (66).

One solution might be the use of progressively shrinking fields, but this technique has not been evaluated prospectively. The amount of the surrounding lung that should be irradiated after chemotherapy is important inasmuch as it is linked closely to treatment toxicity and treatment failure. Turrisi et al. (67) include in the target volume only obvious abnormalities observed on CT scans, but they do not extend the fields to cover adjacent regional lymphatics such as supraclavicular or contralateral hilar regions. Wagner and Moffett (68) pointed out that recent results of the Eastern Cooperative Oncology Group (ECOG)/Radiation Therapy Oncology Group trial (69), in which such sites were not irradiated prophylactically, suggest that this omission did not lead to excessive local relapse rates.

In summary, further randomized and well-defined studies, using strict definitions of original and reduced tumor volumes and quality control of the radiation technique, are necessary to resolve this issue.

TOTAL RADIATION DOSE

Full doses of radiotherapy can be critical in obtaining a therapeutic gain. Some trials have concluded that radiation is ineffective; however, this conclusion may simply be the result of doses that were too low. Effective chemotherapy may possibly allow a decrease in the radiation dose necessary to produce consistent local control (70). However, the radiation dose level should not be decreased by more than 20% of the radiation dose necessary to obtain long-term control in the absence of chemotherapy. This implies that when combined with effective chemotherapy, i.e., that capable of inducing complete remissions, a radical dose of 70 Gy can be reduced to approximately 55 Gy. Unfortunately, many trials have reduced the radiation dose even further, to below 40 Gy (a dose in the lower range of that recommended for the treatment of subclinical disease). In general, these trials have reported little or no effect of adjuvant radiotherapy on many solid tumors in adult patients.

The optimal radiation dose level to be used in SCLC is still unknown. There has been only one randomized trial conducted on this subject (66). The comparison involved low-versus moderate-dose levels: 25 Gy in 10 fractions over 2 weeks versus 37.5 Gy in 15 fractions over 3 weeks. These doses are approximately equivalent to 28 Gy and 42 Gy in conventional (2 Gy per day) fractionation, respectively. The authors concluded that the use of a higher dose seemed to delay rather than prevent thoracic recurrence. All other data are derived solely from retrospective studies (71).

Local control at 2 years, based on the total radiation dose as reported in these series, is shown in Figure 21.4. Clearly, doses below 40 Gy are unable to control local disease, but nothing can be firmly stated about the effect of moderate (40 to 50 Gy) versus high radiation dose (more than 60 Gy). The wide variations observed in the local failure rate at each dose level as reported in the literature are probably related to different definitions of local failure in each center: (a) recurrence after complete remission versus overall local failure, (b) different protocols for assessing local failure, for example, elective bronchoscopy at fixed time intervals versus bronchoscopy only when the patient has symptoms, (c) overall failure versus first site of failure, (d) methodology used to report the results: total, censored, or competing event approaches (32). The French Cancer Centers' Lung Group analysis (32) did not show a significant difference in long-term local control in four consecutive alternating chemotherapy-radiotherapy protocols that delivered total radiation doses from 45 Gy to 65 Gy. However, the numbers of patients were small and the analyses were retrospective. There certainly is a need for a randomized trial testing of a moderate versus high total radiation dose, for example, 45 Gy versus 65 Gy or their biologic equivalent with nonconventional fractionation.

FRACTIONATION

Conventional fractionation, defined as five fractions of 2 Gy per week, allows a total radiation dose of as high as 70 Gy to be delivered to a limited mediastinal volume. The fraction size used in the 13 randomized trials included in the meta-analysis (25) varied between 2 and 4 Gy; a large fraction size could possibly account for the increased toxicity reported in some of these trials. The fraction size can be reduced and repeated a few hours later on the same day; this technique is termed hyperfractionated irradiation. With such a schedule the overall treatment time remains the same, but the total dose is slightly higher. The RTOG (74) has conducted consecutive studies in NSCLC using fractions of 1.2 Gy twice daily and increasing the total dose up to 79 Gy in a limited volume. Preliminary results were encouraging, but no significant differences in terms of overall survival were found in the intergroup randomized trial (75). However, as previously noted, NSCLC is less radiosensitive than SCLC, and probably SCLC is a better model for these kinds of studies.

The rationale for the use of unconventional fractionation has been discussed extensively in the literature (76, 77). It is based on the premise that normal

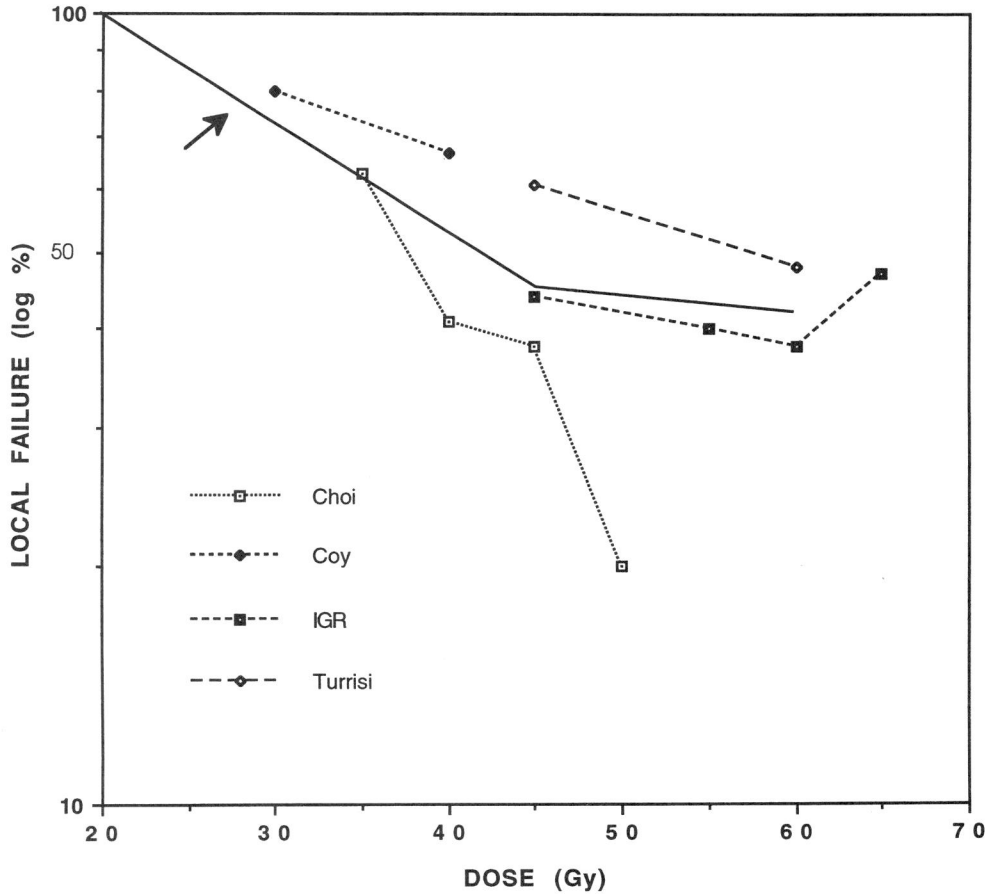

FIGURE 21.4. Local failure rate at 2 years based on the total radiation dose. A large heterogeneity exists in the results. This heterogeneity may be partially explained by the use of different radiation fractionation schedules, which are estimated conservatively in this figure. However, the major cause of heterogeneity is probably the different ways of assessing local control. A tentative line (*arrow*) of summary of results has been drawn. This line could suggest a plateau effect after a total dose of 50 Gy, but the numbers are too scanty to use to draw this conclusion. (Data from Arriadada R, Kramar A, Le Chevalier T, De Cremous H, for the French Cancer Centers' Lung Group. Competing events determining relapse-free survival in limited small-cell lung carcinoma. J Clin Oncol 1992;10:447–451; Coy P, Hodson BM, Payne D, et al. The effect of dose of thoracic irradiation on recurrence in patients with limited stage small cell cancer. Initial results of a Canadian multicenter randomized trial. Int J Radiat Oncol Biol Phys 1987;14:219–226; Choi NC, Carey RW. Reassessment of loco-regional failure rate in relation with radiation dose in combined modality approach of multidrug chemotherapy and radiotherapy for limited-stage small-cell lung carcinoma. In: Arriagada R, Le Chevalier T, eds. Treatment modalities in lung cancer. Antibiotics and chemotherapy. Basel: Karger, 1988;41:70–76; and Turrisi AT, Kim K, Johnson DH, et al., for the Eastern Cooperative Oncology Group. Daily (QD) v twice daily (BID) thoracic irradiation (TI) with concurrent cisplatin-etoposide (PE) for limited small cell lung cancer (LSCLC). Preliminary results on 352 randomized eligible patients. Lung Cancer 1994;11:172.)

tissues recover more rapidly than do tumor cells. Withers (78) pointed out that conventional fractionation may be a reasonable treatment for an average tumor but that greater individualization should be sought. Multiple daily fractionation schedules spare slowly responding tissues more than normal tissues as well as tumors that show an early response, suggesting that therapeutic gain may be obtained by reducing fractions to below 2 Gy. Thames et al. (79) concluded that the use of several fractions per day, either to reduce the overall time (accelerated treatment) or to increase the total dose (hyperfractionation), might improve therapeutic results. This approach might be particularly interesting in pure or oat cell SCLC, as demonstrated by Mitchell et al. (11) with exponential survival curves obtained from cell cultures. Looney and Hopkins (80) investigated the possibility of integrating multifractioned radiotherapy in an alternating chemotherapy-radiotherapy schedule. Small fraction sizes may allow higher total doses to be delivered with tolerable toxicity, improved local tumor control, and acceptable effects on normal tissue. The extreme radiosensitivity and high proliferation rate make SCLC a very promising model in which to test unconventional radiotherapy, especially accelerated hyperfractionation.

In practice, the optimal fractionation is unknown. Many pilot studies using concurrent chemotherapy and accelerated thoracic radiotherapy (81, 82) have obtained very promising results. However, more recently, Johnson et al. (69) reported a phase III randomized trial comparing cisplatin and etoposide plus concurrent thoracic radiotherapy; group A received single daily fractionation (45 Gy in 25 fractions over 33 days), and group B was given multiple daily fractions (45 Gy in 30 fractions over 19 days). Results in 358 evaluable patients showed that complete and overall response rates were similar. There was no difference in median survival (19 months) or in 2-year survival (43%). The authors claim a better local control rate for the unconventional radiotherapy arm (52% versus 39%), but there also was a significant increase in the incidence of esophagitis (31% versus 16%). A longer follow-up is needed to establish whether there is a therapeutic gain.

In the IGR series (32), 28 patients were treated with an alternating radiotherapy-chemotherapy schedule in which the first course of radiotherapy was given with accelerated hyperfractionation using reduced fields, thus avoiding the spinal cord. This first course consisted of a dose of 21 Gy (25 Gy for the first 4 patients) given in fractions of 1.4 Gy 3 times daily. Three of four patients receiving a higher dose developed a severe acute esophagitis; this complication was not observed in the subsequent patients for whom the radiation dose was decreased by 15%. The long-term results were no different from those observed with previous protocols used, including conventional fractionation, but a higher, albeit nonsignificant, incidence of deaths unrelated to cancer was recorded and probably was related to treatment toxicity. There are two possible explanations for toxicity in this specific protocol: (a) a higher initial dose of cisplatin (150 mg/m^2 given over 5 days), or (b) a 4-hour time gap between the three daily fractions. Currently, a time interval of at least 6 hours is recommended to allow repair of sublethal lesions in normal tissues (77).

Accelerated multifractionated radiotherapy is an interesting approach in the management of SCLC. However, its integration into combined schedules should be planned carefully and evaluated in prospective studies measuring efficacy and morbidity, because small changes in treatment parameters may have an unexpected impact on early and late toxicity.

QUALITY OF CHEST IRRADIATION

The importance of the quality of radiotherapy has been stressed by many reports. Some of these reports have shown a significant impact on long-term local control and a potential survival benefit with adequate radiation techniques (64, 83–85).

All previous considerations are valid only if the quality of radiotherapy delivery is good. Poor quality radiotherapy may overshadow benefits and increase toxicity. Modern megavoltage radiotherapy standards include: (a) a better definition of the volumes to be treated, (b) an unequivocal definition of the tumor dose, (c) prechemotherapy simulator film and CT scan–based planning, (d) optimal beam arrangement to cover the previously defined volume and protect critical organs, (e) computer dosimetry to calculate dose distribution, and (f) check films on the treatment machine to ensure treatment reproducibility. These standards need to be applied to randomized trials aimed at defining optimal treatment schedules.

RADIATION TECHNIQUE

Radiotherapy principles are discussed in Chapter 9. Renewed interest in combined chemotherapy-radiotherapy has led to technical improvements in the protocols used since 1979 at the Institut Gustave-Roussy, thus enabling the safe delivery of high-dose radiation to the chest while avoiding excessive irradiation of critical organs (86). This radiotherapy technique uses four to six high-energy photon beams (more than 15 megaelectron volts [MeV]). This method has several advantages: (a) dose distribution is fairly homogeneous within the target volume with two opposing beams and is less influenced by variations in patient thickness than that obtained with cobalt 60 (^{60}Co) photon beams; (b) the dose delivered to critical organs is usually lower than that with ^{60}Co photon beams because the contribution of photons scattered from the volume irradiated is smaller; and (c) corrections for inhomogeneities (air correction) are lower. This lower number of corrections is especially important when accurate data concerning the thickness and density of the entire irradiated lung are not available for all patients.

The reference point for the dose calculations is the isocenter of the oblique or lateral beams and is approximately at the center of the tumor. The dose delivered to the mediastinal lymph nodes is stated systematically as well as the dose delivered to the peripheral volume of the tumor.

A three-step procedure is used for each patient: (a) the limits of the initial tumor and mediastinal nodes involved are outlined by the radiotherapist or the pneumologist on frontal and lateral chest films, taking into account clinical, bronchoscopic, and radiologic data; (b) a target volume is drawn on simulator films; and (c) the safety margin of the antero posterior and lateral or oblique fields (distance between the target volume and the border of the fields) is measured. When the safety margin is at least 1 cm, the portals are considered adquate. However, in some cases, the radiation oncologist is obliged to arrive at a delicate balance between adequate coverage and an irradiated volume so large that there might be unacceptable toxicity. An example of treatment planning is shown in Figure 21.5.

CHEMOTHERAPY

Chemotherapy began to be used widely for the treatment of SCLC in the 1970s. Evidence of the efficacy of chemotherapy was provided by three randomized trials. The first evaluated the role of cyclophosphamide in locally advanced lung cancer (23); the only significant effect was found in patients with SCLC. The second trial (87) directly compared chemotherapy with cyclophosphamide and thoracic radiotherapy for patients with SCLC. The survival benefit for chemotherapy patients was moderate (13% at 18 months for the chemotherapy group versus 7% for the thoracic radiotherapy group), but it was judged sufficient to recommend the generalized use of chemotherapy. A third small trial involving 70 patients (88) compared thoracic radiotherapy with combined chemotherapy-radiotherapy. There was an advantage for the combined arm in terms of disease free survival.

The real benefit of chemotherapy was not clearly established in a larger population, becaue at the same time new staging procedures—bone scan, liver scan or ultrasound or CT scan, brain scan or CT scan, and bone marrow biopsy—were introduced to distinguish between limited and extensive disease. This change in assessment methods may have introduced a stage migration phenomenon leading to an overestimation of the treatment effect in nonrandomized trials (89, 90). This phenomenon is described in Chapter 8. If patients treated in randomized trials by chemotherapy alone are considered, the average 3-year survival rate is 9% (25), thus the maximum survival benefit caused by chemotherapy is approximately 5%, as shown in Figure 21.1. This moderate benefit fails to reflect the high response rates (more than 80%) yielded with chemotherapy, but it is consistent with the low complete remission rate, which is a firmer endpoint. The optimism induced by the high overall response rate explains why many teams discarded the use of thoracic radiotherapy in their therapeutic schedules.

In 1978, the Southwest Oncology Group (SWOG) (91) reported their experience with combination chemotherapy against SCLC using cyclophosphamide, doxorubicin, and vincristine (CAV). They reported a complete response (CR) rate of 41% and an overall response rate of 75% in patients with limited disease. Subsequently, CAV has been used by many others as standard therapy for SCLC. More recently, other combined regimens also have been shown to be similarly effective (9). The choice of active drugs is discussed in Chapter 22, but the most common combination regimens are listed in Table 21.3.

Attempts to avoid the emergence of chemoresistance have led to the use of a variety of combination chemotherapeutic regimens. All such protocols seek to expose the tumor to the maximum possible range of active antitumor agents, modified by the associated toxicities (98). The strategy behind such an approach is (a) the maximization of the cell kill per unit of time, and (b) the maximization of the potential number of cells against which the combination is active by minimizing the number of cells that are potentially resistant. Resistance to chemotherapy has been reviewed extensively (47, 99, 100). Only specific aspects of chemoresistance observed in SCLC are detailed below.

Twentyman (101) summarized some of the cellular mechanisms associated with resistance to anticancer drugs. These include overexpression of P glycoprotein (*MDR1* gene), changes in the activity of topoisomerase II, increased activity of glutathione, and altered intracellular drug distribution. A correlation between levels of P glycoprotein and response to chemotherapy in SCLC was observed. Multidrug resistance–associated protein also has been associated with alternative drug transport and has been shown to be overexpressed in some multidrug resistant lung cancer cell lines. The role of P-glyprotein overexpression in lung cancer remains uncertain (102). Saijo et al. (103) reported that resistance of lung cancer cells to vinca alkaloids and paclitaxel involved P-glycoprotein–mediated multidrug resistance. They also developed a paclitaxel resistant human SCLC cell line (H69/Tx1) with a different mechanism of drug resistance. This cell line was more sensitive to vinca alkaloids.

Ozols and O'Dwyer (104) administered buthionine sulfoximine, an inhibitor of γ-glutamyl cysteine synthesis, and melphalan in 34 drug resistant lung cancer patients. This regimen was intended to reduce lev-

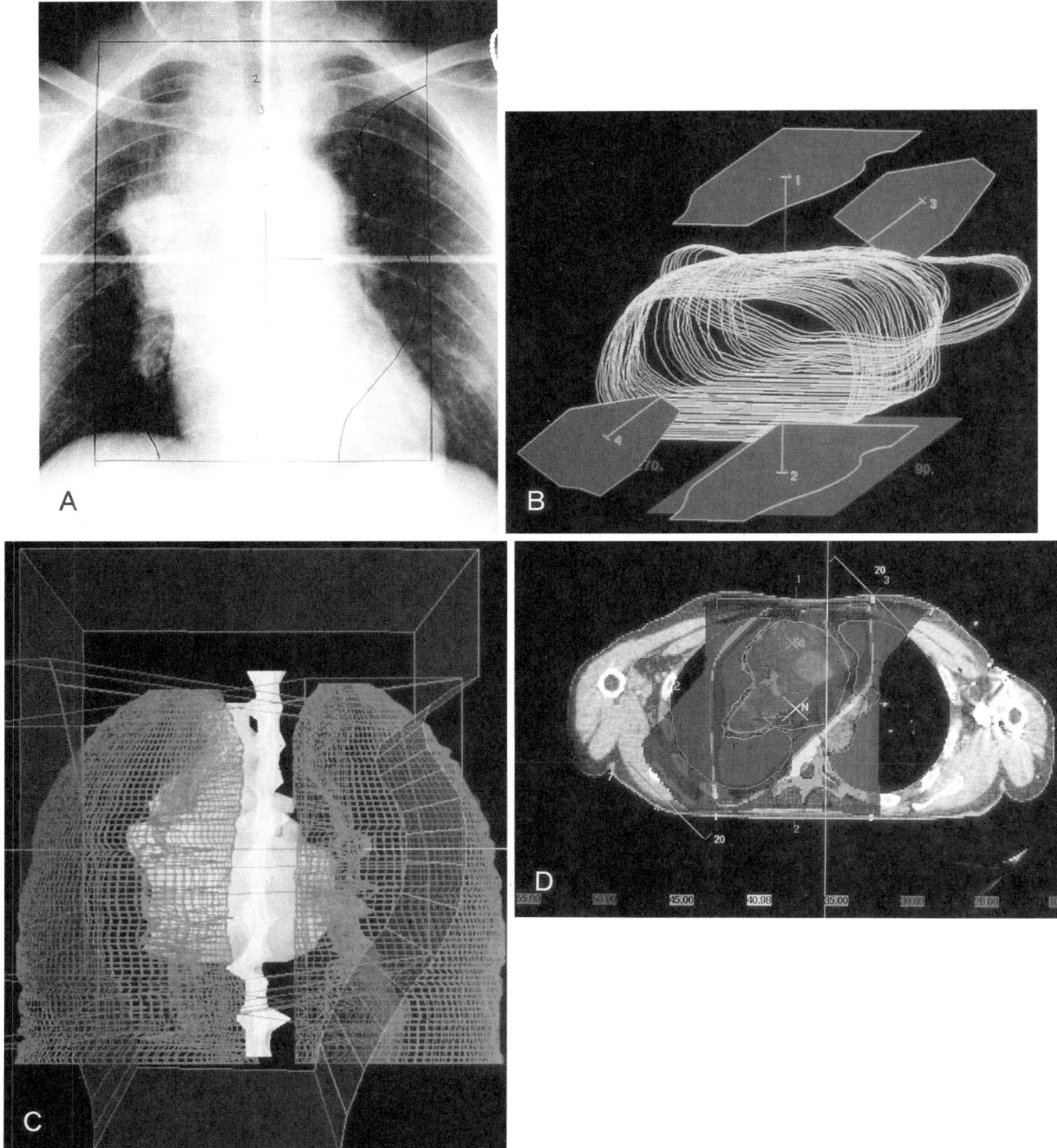

FIGURE 21.5. Radiation technique in the treatment of limited SCLC. **A.** Anteroposterior beam shaped by the shielding of a fusible alloy at low temperature (MCP70; Mining and Chemical Products, Ltd., Wembley, England), drawn in the prechemotherapy simulator film. B. through G. Tridimensional treatment planning done in a prechemotherapy CT scan for a patient with limited SCLC. **B.** The patient is treated by anteroposterior fields delivering a total dose of 40 Gy and by oblique fields delivering an additional 15 Gy. **C.** Lateral fields avoiding the spinal cord. Superimposed tumor and anatomic structures with geometric projects of radiation beams. Lungs, *(green)*, tumor volume *(yellow)*, spinal cord *(beige)*. **D.** Computed dosimetry in the transverse plane. The tumor volume receives between 50 and 55 Gy. The spinal cord receives 41 Gy. See color plates.

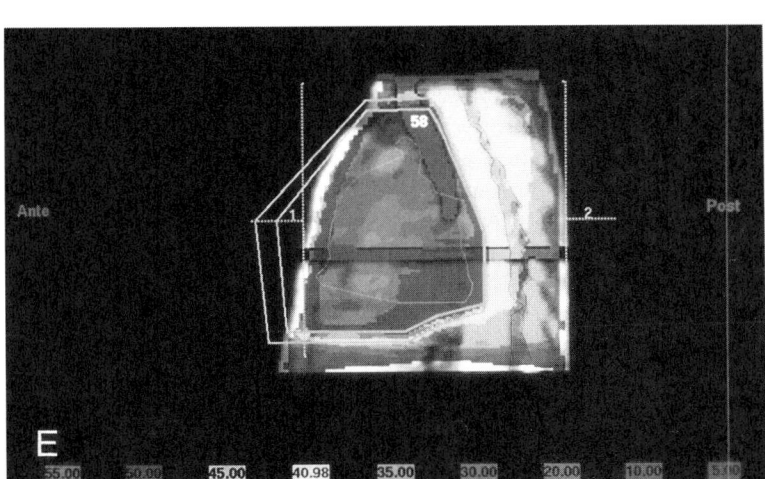
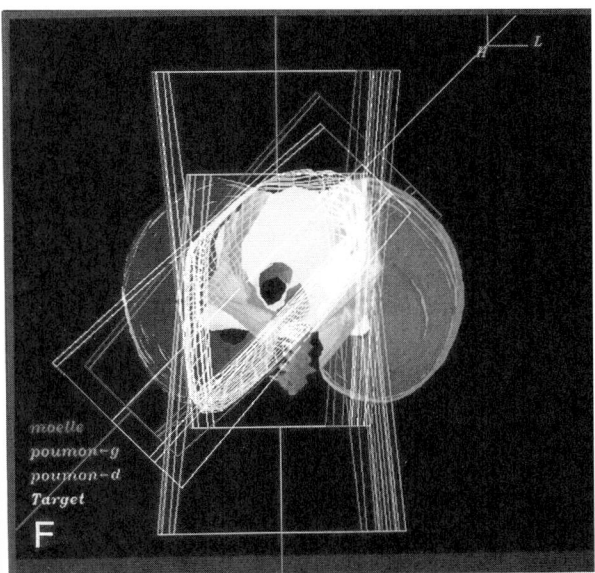
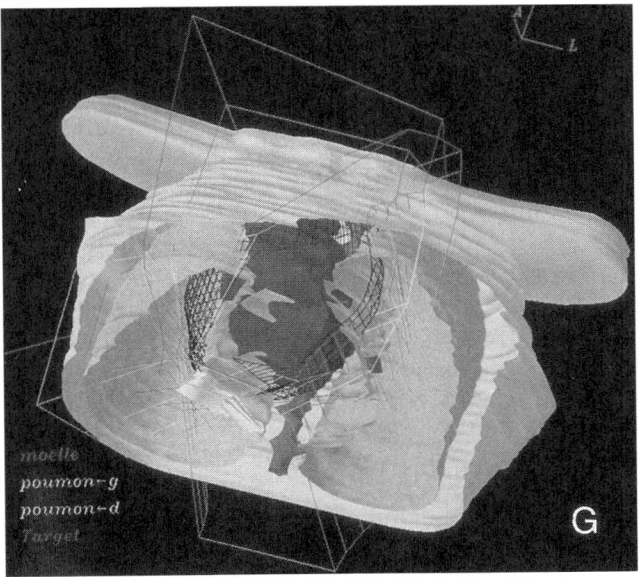

FIGURE 21.5—CONTINUED. E. Computed dosimetry in the sagittal plane. The spinal cord receives a homogenous dose of 41 Gy along the treated volume. F. Tridimensional view of anatomic structures and tumor volume with geometric projection of radiation beams. Target volume (*yellow*), left lung (*green*), right lung (*mauve*), spinal cord (*blue*). G. Tridimensional view of the treated volume. Lung (*yellow*), spinal cord (*blue*), target volume (*green*), 50% isodose area surrounding target volume (*red grid*). See color plates.

els of glutathione associated with drug resistance. At a dose of 10.5 g/m², the tested drug induced a depletion of glutathione in tumor cells of all patients. This study suggests that it is feasible to modulate factors associated with drug resistance.

Like radiotherapy, the use of chemotherapy involves many parameters such as alternating versus sequential therapy, drug doses (including intensification), dose scheduling, and maintenance chemotherapy.

ALTERNATING VERSUS SEQUENTIAL CHEMOTHERAPY

Evidence for early emergence of chemoresistance is based on both clinical trials and laboratory studies on tumor tissue and cell lines. Goldie and Coldman (105) proposed a mathematical model based on the probabilistic nature of spontaneously emerging resistant clones. A computer simulation was used to study the outcome of alternating therapy compared to that of sequential therapy using the same drug regimen. As-

TABLE 21.3. Most Common Chemotherapy Regimens Used in Small Cell Lung Cancer

ACRONYM (REFERENCE NO.)	DRUGS	DOSE (MG/M² IV)[a]	DAY(S)
MACC (92)	Methotrexate	30	1
	Doxorubicin	40	1
	Cyclophosphamide	400	1
	Lomustine	30 (PO)	1
CAV (91, 93–95)	Cyclophosphamide	750–1000	1
	Doxorubicin	45–50	1
	Vincristine	1.4	1
CDE (96)	Cyclophosphamide	1000	1
	Doxorubicin	45	1
	Etoposide	50	1–5
PACE (32)	Cisplatin	100	1
	Doxorubicin	40	1
	Cyclophosphamide	300–400	1–3
	Etoposide	75	1–3
PE (97)	Cisplatin	25	1–3
	Etoposide	100	1–3

[a] Administration is intravenous unless otherwise indicated.

suming the same log kill and similar mutation rates of resistance against each regimen, it was concluded that alternating chemotherapy should result in a greater cure rate.

The clinical experience of alternating chemotherapy schedules was reviewed by Elliot et al. in 1984 (106). They concluded that the five controlled studies done at the time had not demonstrated any advantage for alternating therapy. The results are summarized in Table 21.4. They suggested that the time at which alternate cycles are given may be very important as well as the role of possible confounding factors such as thoracic radiotherapy.

Since 1984, results from five large controlled trials have been published. One trial was limited to patients with extensive stage disease (115), whereas the others involved both patients with limited and extensive SCLC. Summarized results are included in Table 21.4.

An alternating regimen in the Stanford trial (111) was initiated with three cycles of the same combination (etoposide, doxorubicin, and methotrexate) followed by chest irradiation before an alternating combination was administered (procarbazine, vincristine, cyclophosphamide, and lomustine). The same alternating regimen, without radiation, resulted in significant prolongation of survival in patients with extensive disease; no significant difference was observed between alternating and sequential therapy in those with limited disease. The authors concluded that in the latter group thoracic radiotherapy could be a confounding factor.

In the Danish trial conducted in 1983 (110), radiation was not present as a confounding factor. Chest radiation was postponed until chemotherapy was completed in both the Canadian (112) and the German studies (113). Radiation was limited to responding patients in the Canadian study. In the latter trial, survival was significantly better in patients having extensive disease treated with the alternating regimen compared with those treated with a sequential schedule; however, there was no difference in the survival of patients with limited disease. Indeed, the Canadian trial (112) is the only one to test properly the alternating versus sequential schedules rather than more drugs versus fewer drugs.

The German trial (113) resulted in longer survival and higher response rates with an alternating regimen, regardless of disease stage. A phase III American intergroup trial (115) with 26 cooperating centers studied the combination of cisplatin and etoposide (PE) versus CAV versus the alternation of the two therapies for patients with extensive SCLC. Preliminary results based on 312 evaluable cases indicated that there were no significant differences in survival among the treatment arms. It also was observed that PE was no more effective than CAV.

Another study analyzed more specifically the drug sequencing of cisplatin and etoposide in SCLC (116). Five hundred and fifty-two patients with limited and extensive disease were randomized. There was a similar overall response rate in the four treatment arms. However, better results in terms of complete remission and survival were achieved in the treatment arm given a bolus administration of PE with the etoposide given after the cisplatin for the first two cycles of chemotherapy.

Although clinical experience does not undermine the Goldie-Coldman model, alternating chemotherapy has not produced any dramatic gain in the treatment of SCLC. However, experience acquired shows that close cooperation between biologists and clinicians is of major importance in designing clinical trials to investigate laboratory models of SCLC. It is probable that the Goldie-Coldman hypothesis has not been tested correctly because there is no assurance that the regimens evaluated include drugs without cross-resistance. A better understanding of the mechanisms of resistance to each drug will certainly improve the evaluation of the hypothesis.

DOSE EFFECT WITHIN THE STANDARD RANGE OF DOSES

It has been hypothesized that there is a dose-response relationship in the treatment of lung tumors

TABLE 21.4. Randomized Trials Comparing Alternating (A) and Sequential (S) Chemotherapy in Small Cell Lung Cancer

FIRST AUTHOR, YEAR (REFERENCE NO.)	REGIMEN	EVALUABLE (NO. OF PATIENTS)	MEDIAN SURVIVAL (MO)	COMMENTS
Alberto, 1981 (107)	S1: MTX, VCR, CPM, PCZ	30	8	$P = .10$
	S2: DOX, CCNU, CPM, PCZ, MTX, VCR, HU	30	8.5	...
	A: DOX, CCNU, CPM, PCZ, alt. MTX, VCR, HU	65	6	...
Krauss, 1981 (108)	S1: CPM, DOX, VCR, DTIC	29	10	NS
	S2: BCNU, PCZ, MTX, VBL	16	10	...
	A: S1 alt. S2	23	11	...
Aisner, 1982 (96)	S: CDE	53	LD: 16	NS
	A: CDE alt. CCNU, MTX, VCR, PCZ	56	LD: 12	...
Ettinger, 1982 (109)	S: CPM, CCNU	62	7.3	$P = .05$
	A: CPM, CCNU alt; DOX, VCR	76	9.5	...
Østerlind, 1983 (110)	C: CPM, CCNU, MTX, VCR	66	9	NS
	A: DOX, VP-16 alt. CPM, CCNU, MTX, VCR	64	9.5	...
Daniels, 1984 (111)	S: CPM, VCR, CCNU, PCZ	84	LD: 10	
	A: VP-16, DOX, MTX alt. CPM, VCR, CCNU, PCZ	78	LD: 16	NS. Significant difference for ED in favor of A
Feld, 1987 (112)	S: CAV and PE	290	LD: 15.5	NS. Significant difference for ED in favor of A ($P = .03$)
	A: CAV alt. PE	299	LD: 15	
Havemann, 1987 (113)	S: CAV	152	LD: 11.1	...
	A: VP-16, VCR, IFO alt. CDDP, DOX, VCR alt. CPM, MTX, CCNU	150	LD: 13.4	$P < .05$
Østerlind, 1989 (114)	S: CPM, CCNU, VCR, VP-16 + CDDP, DOX, VDN, MTX, HMM	225	LD: 9.5	$P < .05$ No difference for ED (31% of patients)
	A1: CPM, CCNU, VCR, MTX alt. VP-16 DOX, VCR	217	LD: 11.5	...
	A2: A1 + alt. CDDP, VDN, HMM	218	LD: 12	...
Roth, 1989 (115)	S1: PE	312	9.5	NS. All ED
	S2: CAV	...	9.8	...
	A: PE alt. CAV	...	9.5	...

Abbreviations. MTX, methotrexate; VCR, vincristine; CPM, cyclophosphamide; PCZ, procarbazine; DOX, doxorubicin; CCNU, lomustine; HU, hydroxyurea; VP-16, etoposide; DTIC, dacarbazine; BCNU, carmustine; VBL, vinblastine; VDN, vindesine; HMM, hexamethylmelamine; CDDP, cisplatin; IFO, ifosfamide; LD, limited disease; ED, extensive disease; NS, not significant; alt., alternating.

sensitive to chemotherapy. Toxicity associated with the different drugs used has been the major drawback in this approach. Different doses of chemotherapeutic agents have been tested, and an improved response rate (96% versus 45%) and better long-term survival were observed with high-dose versus standard-dose therapy with cyclophosphamide, methotrexate, and lomustine (117). A multivariate analysis of prognostic factors in 52 consecutive patients (118) identified two factors with an independent effect: the T classification (T1-2 versus T3) and the initial doses of cyclophosphamide and cisplatin actually given. These results were confirmed by a larger analysis of 131 patients with a longer follow-up (119). These analyses prompted investigators at the Institut Gustave-Roussy to conduct a randomized trial to test the hypothesis that moderate changes in initial chemotherapy doses may have an impact on overall survival. The hypothesis was supported by the results of the trial. A moderate increase of 20% and 25% in the initial dose of cisplatin and cyclophosphamide, respectively, increased the 2-year survival rate by 17% (120). The disease free survival was higher in the higher dose group; at 2 years, it was 28% in that group, compared with 8% in the lower dose group ($P = .02$) (see Figure 8.1). Early development of chemoresistance is a plausible explanation for the worse results obtained in the lower dose group. The results of this trial suggest that in clinical practice low initial doses should be avoided.

The effect of different doses of cyclophosphamide or ciplatin in patients with SCLC has been evaluated in six trials (120–125), summarized in Table 21.5. Most of these patients had extensive disease, and only one trial, other than the French study, included more than

TABLE 21.5. Randomized Trials Evaluating Dose Effect of Cyclophosphamide and Cisplatin in Small Cell Lung Cancer

First Author (Reference No.)	No. of Patients	Limited Disease (%)	Drug Tested	Intended Drug Dose (mg/m^2)	Median Survival	P Value	Comment
Arriagada (120)	105	100	CPM CDDP	900 vs. 1200 80 vs. 100	26% vs. 43%	.006	2-yr survival (log rank test)
Dinwoodie (121)	45	?	DOX CPM	50 vs. 70 750 vs. 1200	210 vs. 215 d	NS	Improved disease control but increased toxicity
Figueredo (122)	103	33	DOX CPM	50 vs. 60 1000 vs. 1500–2250	...	.36	Increased toxicity
Johnson (123)	298	0	DOX CPM	40 vs. 70 1000 vs. 1200	29 vs. 35 w	>.05	Increased toxicity
Ihde (124)	83	0	VP-16 CDDP	240 vs. 400 80 vs. 135	11 vs. 12 mo	.93	...
Mehta (125)	349	38	CPM	700 vs. 1500	36 vs. 41 w	.04	Increased effect in limited disease ($P = .02$)

Abbreviations. NS, not significant; DOX, doxorubicin; CPM, cyclophosphamide; VP-16, etoposide; CDDP, cisplatin.

100 patients with limited disease (125). In that study, survival was prolonged because of a 50% increase in the dose of cyclophosphamide. The results of the trial by Mehta and Vogl (125) and the French trial (120) do not support intensification of chemotherapy but rather suggest the need for a continued search for optimal doses within the range of standard treatments.

DOSE INTENSIFICATION

The dose effect shown previously may lead to the assumption that dose intensification, i.e., an increase of at least twofold the standard doses, could provide a further survival benefit. However, fatal treatment toxicity can be a major problem in this approach.

High-dose chemotherapy assumes that the increment in tumor cell kill is large enough to increase the cure rate (126). It also supposes that this increase in tumor cell kill is obtained in tumor cells that have escaped previous conventional drug doses. A third assumption is that the increase in tumor cell kill can be achieved with one or two cycles of chemotherapy if bone marrow aplasia is controlled adequately.

Cyclophosphamide and etoposide are the drugs most commonly used in this approach. Few studies (117, 121–124, 127) have been randomized; these trials were reviewed recently by Antman et al. (126). Despite the relatively small number of patients, it seems that high-dose chemotherapy gives a higher rate of tumor response, but any effect on survival is doubtful.

Humblet et al. (128) conducted a randomized trial with intensive high-dose treatment (cyclophosphamide, carmustine, and etoposide) and autologous bone marrow transplantation given to 23 patients in objective remisson after induction chemotherapy (methotrexate, vincristine, cyclophosphamide, and doxorubicin given for three cycles followed by two cycles of PE). These patients were compared with 22 patients receiving conventional doses of cyclophosphamide, carmustine, and etoposide. The complete remission rate increased in the late intensification group, from 39% to 79% after high-dose chemotherapy, compared with no changes in the conventional dose group; the result was a statistically significant increase in median RFS. There was, however, no improvement in overall survival because of high treatment-related toxicity and recurrence at the primary site.

Dose reductions and postponement of cycles of chemotherapy are made often because of potentially life-threatening bone marrow toxicity caused by chemotherapy. Currently available cytokines are able to reduce treatment-induced myelosuppression and febrile neutropenia. In conventional 3-week regimens, granulocyte–colony-stimulating factor allows a higher proportion of treatment cycles to be administered at full dose and on time, and it reduces the number of infections and complications associated with cytotoxic chemotherapy (129, 130). However, until now, dose and dose intensity could be increased by only up to twofold with cytokine use. Larger increases need stem cell or peripheral blood progenitor cell support. It still is necessary to include chest irradiation in the treatment schedule because despite the high response rate, relapses at the primary site are frequent (131). Another problem with dose intensification and the use of stem cell support is the high rate of bone marrow involvement when immunologic screening is used (132). Another approach would be the use of growth factors with a wider effect on blood cells, such as interleukin-3 (133) or the introduction of recently isolated specific compounds such as thrombopoietin or its derivatives (134). In any case, more randomized trials are needed in this area, but the recruitment of large numbers of patients remains a problem because of the restrictive inclusion criteria.

Results of these trials support the contention that there is a dose-response relationship in lung tumors sensitive to chemotherapy. However, dose intensification is limited by the treatment-related toxicity in this population. Currently, high-dose chemotherapy should be considered as experimental and cannot be regarded as a standard approach in the treatment of SCLC (9, 135, 136).

DOSE INTENSIFICATION USING WEEKLY CHEMOTHERAPY

The administration of weekly chemotherapy has been advocated to enhance treatment effect and decrease chemoresistance through the inhibition of accelerated repopulation and an increase in dose intensity. To obtain this effect, weekly chemotherapy should follow the basic rules of combined chemotherapy: (*a*) the use of only active drugs; (*b*) the use of drugs from different classes; (*c*) the use of drugs with nonoverlapping toxicity; (*d*) the use of drugs in their optimal dose range and schedule; and (*e*) the resting period between cycles of chemotherapy being as short as possible to enable the most sensitive target tissue, usually the bone marrow, to recover.

Mainly because of overlapping toxicity the use of weekly chemotherapy includes a wider range of drugs compared with standard treatments. Thus, the comparison also includes the evaluation of more versus fewer drugs. Weekly chemotherapy has been studied mainly in phase II trials. In 1993, Sculier et al. (137) published a randomized trial comparing weekly chemotherapy (doxorubicin, etoposide, and cyclophosphamide on day 1, cisplatin and vindesine on day 8, and methotrexate on day 15) with standard chemotherapy (cyclophosphamide and doxorubicin on day 1 and etoposide on days 1 through 3). Each cycle was repeated every 3 weeks for six courses. Ninety-two percent of patients were evaluable, 44% with limited disease. Objective responses were recorded in 69% and 62%, respectively, and 2-year survival was 8.5% and 7.9%, respectively. The authors noted that increased treatment delays in the investigational arm caused a decreased relative dose intensity.

Miles et al. (138) reported a phase II study with weekly chemotherapy using cisplatin on day 1 and etoposide on days 1 and 2, alternating with ifosfamide and doxorubicin on day 8, for a total of 12 weeks. The response rate was 92% with a CR rate of 48%, and median survival was 54 weeks. The same group recently published a randomized trial (139) that included 40 patients: it did not test the weekly schedule but rather the addition of granulocyte–colony-stimulating factor to the same protocol. Granulocyte–colony-stimulating factor significantly decreased dose reductions caused by neutropenia but not to a level that would allow an increase in dose intensity because of nonhematologic toxicity.

According to Murray (140), weekly treatment would not be advantageous because of the failure to increase dose intensity. The major advantage of this approach would be to provide a greater drug diversity with a given drug intensity, but weekly delivery does not allow granulocyte recovery. These concepts would support the use of rapid alternating regimens without cross-toxicity, such as cisplatin, vincristine, doxorubicin, and etoposide (141), a chemotherapy regimen that has obtained a 9% 5-year survival in patients with extensive disease included in a pilot study (140).

MAINTENANCE CHEMOTHERAPY

Maintenance chemotherapy was commonly administered in the late 1970s for patients with SCLC. At that time, high tumor response rates encouraged oncologists to prolong treatment to ensure long-term remission. Doubts about the benefits of maintenance chemotherapy arose when it was evident that long-term results were poor and that it probably was not to the patients' advantage to remain on therapy during their relatively short life span. Some noncomparative studies (94) suggested that prolonged treatment was unnecessary. Ten randomized trials, comprising a total of more than 1900 patients, have been conducted on this subject. The trials are summarized in Table 21.6. The largest studies have not shown any survival benefit for maintenance chemotherapy. Advantages for this treatment were found only in two small trials (142, 144) or in subgroup analyses of other trials. Ettinger et al. (148) concluded that when enough aggressive induction chemotherapy is given, maintenance treatment is unnecessary. From the overall results of the randomized trials, maintenance chemotherapy should not currently be considered as standard treatment.

IMMUNOTHERAPY

Therapies to restore immune function after aggressive treatment such as chemotherapy-radiotherapy have been investigated for many years. The development and clinical application of agents that modulate or stimulate the immune response attempted to increase the immune responsiveness of patients. Most studies on the role of immunotherapy in lung cancer have been conducted in NSCLC patients (152). However, some studies also have been done in SCLC using

TABLE 21.6. Randomized Trials Evaluating the Role of Maintenance Chemotherapy in Small Cell Lung Cancer

Trial, Year (Reference No.)	Induction CT	Thoracic RT[a]	Inclusion Criteria	Group	No. of Cycles	Evaluable (No. of Patients)	2-yr Overall Survival	Comments
CALGB 1980 (142)	CPM ± VCR, MTX	Yes	CR	CPM, VCR	UR	57[b]	33%	$P = .01$
				Control	0		9%	
Woods, 1984 (143)	CDDP, VP-16	Yes	CR + PR	CAV	10	49	50 w	Median survival
				Control	0	47		NS
Midlands SCLCG, 1986 (144)	CAV	Yes	CP + PR	CAV	8	45	Same	Only subgroup analyses, maintenance better in extensive but worse in limited disease
				Control	0	48	?	
MRC, 1989 (145)	VP-16, CPM, MTX, VCR	Yes	CR + PR	Same CT	6	131	<10%	$P = .27$
				Control	0	134	<10%	Advantage for CR?[c]
CRC, 1989 (146)	CPM, VCR, VP-16	No	All[d]	Same CT	4	305	<10%	$P = .085$
				Control	0	305	<10%	Maintenance worse if no chemotherapy at relapse[e]
Byrne, 1989 (147)	CDDP, VP-16 alt. CVM	Yes	CR	CVM	6	34	23%	$P = .05$
				Control	0	32	41%	
ECOG, 1990 (148)	CAV or CAV alt. HEM	No	CR	CAV	UR	18	17%	1-yr survival rates
				Control	0	18	5%	$P = .15$
				CAV alt. HEM	UR	25	23%	$P = .96$
				Control	0	25	20%	
PCG, 1992 (149)	CPM, CCNU, DOX VP-16	No	CR	Same CT	6	35	28%	$P = .041$
				Control	0	32	22%	
EORTC, 1993 (150)	CDE	No	All, except tumor progression	CDE	7	219	11%	$P = .70$
				Control	0	215	10%	
Mattson, 1992 (151)	CPM, VCR, VP-16	Yes	CR + PR	CPM, DOX, CDDP	6	59	<10%	NS
				Control[a]	0	87	<10%	

Abbreviations. CT, chemotherapy; RT, radiotherapy; CPM, cyclophosphamide; VCR, vincristine; MTX, methotrexate; CR, complete response; UR, until relapse; CDDP, cisplatin; VP-16, etoposide; PR, partial response; CAV, cyclophosphamide + doxorubicin + vincristine; alt., alternating; CVM, cyclophosphamide + vincristine + methotrexate; HEM, hexamethylmelamine + etoposide + methotrexate; PCG, Petites Cellules Group; CCNU, lomustine; DOX, doxorubicin; CDE, cyclophosphamide + doxorubicin + etoposide; NS, not significant.
[a]Mainly for limited disease.
[b]Total number as well as number evaluable.
[c]Subgroup analysis.
[d]Randomization before response evaluation.
[e]Second randomization.

agents such as bacille Calmette–Guérin (BCG) thymosin, interferons, and cytokines.

BCG is a strain of *Mycobacterium bovis* used for immunization against tuberculosis. BCG has been tested as a nonspecific adjuvant or immunostimulant in cancer therapy. It appears to act via activation of macrophages in combination with lymphoid cells.

A trial was conducted by the SWOG (153) on 254 patients to study the effect of BCG immunotherapy after combined chemotherapy-radiotherapy in extensive SCLC. Patients who received BCG had a response rate of 50% versus 46% in patients who did not receive BCG. Response duration was 20 weeks versus 23 weeks, respectively. There was no significant difference in overall survival.

Aisner and Wiernik (154) conducted a prospective randomized study on 38 patients treated with cyclophosphamide, doxorubicin, and etoposide and randomized to receive BCG immunotherapy. Twenty-four patients had extensive SCLC, and 15 had limited disease. BCG immunotherapy did not influence the response rate, drug toxicity, or survival, but it was associated with increased morbidity such as fever and/or serious infection.

Thymosin (thymosin fraction 5), a soluble product obtained from the calf thymus, also has been used in the immunotherapy of SCLC. Previous studies suggest that its mechanism of action consists of the reconstitution of immune defects rather than the enhancement of normal levels of cellular immunity. To investigate this hypothesis, Lipson et al. (155) conducted a study on 55 patients with SCLC who were randomized to receive subcutaneous doses of either (a) thymosin (60 mg/m^2) twice weekly during the first 6 weeks of intensive chemotherapy, or (b) no thymosin. No difference in overall response was observed in the three treatment groups ($P > .12$), but survival in the first group was significantly improved, compared with the chemotherapy alone group. It was concluded that patients with comparatively low levels of immunity may benefit from the administration of thymosin. However, these results were not confirmed by a second randomized trial (156) evaluating the role of thymosin (60 mg/m^2) in 67 patients. The addition of thymosin to a chemotherapy schedule that includes cyclophosphamide, vincristine, and doxorubicin alternating with PE did not alter the remission rate nor the length of survival.

Interferons are glycoproteins produced by cells in response to viral infections, immune stimulation, or chemical inducers. Biologic effects include inhibition of cell proliferation, differentiation of malignant cells, and stimulation of a variety of cells of the immune system (157). The wide variety of immunopotentiating effects may be used to restore depressed immune functions in treated SCLC patients. In the clinical setting, interferons have been evaluated mainly as maintenance therapy after clinical remission.

Mattson et al. (151) randomized 237 SCLC patients who were in complete or partial remission after a chemotherapy-radiotherapy schedule that included cyclophosphamide, vincristine, and etoposide to one of three arms of a trial that compared: (a) low-dose natural interferon-γ (3 million units per day, 5 days per week for 1 month, then 6 million units 3 times per week for 5 months; (b) maintenance chemotherapy (cyclophospamide, doxorubicin and cisplatin for six cycles and (c) observation only. Overall survival was significantly better for the interferon arm ($P = .05$). In a subgroup analysis, the difference was greater in 113 patients with limited disease. However, in a multivariate analysis adjusting for disease extension and other prognostic factors, the interferon effect was not significant (standard error [SE] = .1743; $P = .08$). The authors proposed including interferon as part of the induction treatment and administering it over a longer period.

More recently, Clamon et al. (158) studied the role of interleukin-2 in 24 patients who did not obtain complete remission after four cycles of cisplatin, doxorubicin, cyclophosphamide, and etoposide (PACE) chemotherapy. The CR rate was 17%, suggesting a non–cross-resistance with PACE therapy. However, a 45% incidence of life-threatening toxicity means that careful evaluation of the clinical use of this treatment is needed.

In summary, few large studies have evaluated the role of immunotherapy in SCLC patients. Previous studies on BCG or thymosin have not demonstrated any clinically significant antieoplastic activity. Recent promising results on the possible beneficial effect of γ-interferon raise hopes and emphasize the need for larger studies in this field.

ANTICOAGULANT THERAPY

Anticoagulants such as heparin or warfarin were advocated by Standford (159) and Zacharski (160), respectively, as adjuvant therapy in SCLC. The effect of treatment may be related to the anticoagulant mechanism itself (i.e., the decrease of microthrombosis or local fibrin so that tumor cells are more easily reached by cytotoxic agents), or to an antitumor effect by acting as antigrowth factors or by inhibition of angiogenesis. The possible effect of aspirin on the hematogenous spread of malignant disease has been investigated. Gasic et al. (161) showed that aspirin reduces the metastatic potential of tumor cells in animals; they attributed this effect to the inhibition of platelet aggregation.

Randomized trials evaluating the role of anticoagulant therapy in SCLC are summarized in Table 21.7. Zacharski et al. (162), in a Veterans Administration pioneering trial, studied 50 patients with limited or extensive SCLC who were randomized to receive either standard therapy (cyclophosphamide, vincristine, and methotrexate with thoracic radiotherapy) or the same therapy plus a dose of warfarin sufficient to prolong the prothrombin time to twice the control value. Median survival in the warfarin group was 50 versus 24 weeks in the control group ($P = .026$).

Chahinian et al. (92) conducted a randomized trial to evaluate warfarin in addition to methotrexate, doxorubicin, cyclophosphamide, and lomustine (MACC) chemotherapy in a Cancer and Leukemia Group B (CALGB) study. Despite improved response rates and failure free survival among the 153 patients with extensive SCLC treated with warfarin, overall survival was not significantly different. The authors support the role of warfarin in the treatment of SCLC, but because the difference in subgroup analyses was at the limit of clinical significance, warfarin should be considered an investigational agent in SCLC.

TABLE 21.7. Randomized Trials Evaluating the Role of Anticoagulant Therapy in Small Cell Lung Cancer

TRIAL, YEAR (REFERENCE NO.)	INDUCTION CT	THORACIC RT	INCLUSION CRITERIA	GROUP	TIME TREATMENT	EVALUABLE (NO. OF PATIENTS)	2-YR OVERALL SURVIVAL	COMMENTS
VACS, 1981 (162)	CPM, VCR, MTX	Yes	LD + ED	CT Id. + warfarin	...	50	24 w 50 w	Median survival, $P = .026$
CALGB, 1989 (92)	MACC	No	ED	MACC Id. + warfarin	UR UR	86 103	<10% <10%	$P = .17$
PCG, 1993 (163)	CPM, CCNU, DOX, VP-16	Optional	ED + LD	CCDE Id. + aspirin	6–12 cycles 18 months	150 153	10% 9%	$P = .90$
PCG, 1994 (164)	CCDE or CPM, CCNU, DOX, alt. VP-16, CDDP, VDN	Randomized for CR	ED + LD	Same CT Id. + heparin	8 cycles 5 w	139 138	9% 11%	$P = .01$

Abbreviations. PCG, Petites Cellules Group; CT, chemotherapy; RT, radiotherapy; CPM, cyclophosphamide; VCR, vincristine; MTX, methotrexate; LD, limited disease; ED, extensive disease; Id., same; MACC, methotrexate + doxorubicin + cyclophosphamide + lomustine; UR, until relapse; CCNU, lomustine; DOX, doxorubicin; VP-16, etoposide; CCDE, lomustine + cyclophosphamide + doxorubicin + etoposide; CDDP, ciplatin; VDN, vindesine; alt., alternating.

A multicenter, randomized trial was conducted by Lebeau et al. (163) on 303 patients with SCLC; 150 were treated with combined chemotherapy only and 153 with the addition of aspirin (1 g per day for 18 months). The response rate and survival were not increased in the aspirin-treated group ($P = .90$). An analysis based on disease extent did not modify that conclusion.

More recently, a group led by Lebeau (164) published a randomized trial evaluating the role of subcutaneous heparin given for 5 weeks starting at the first cycle of chemotherapy. Results showed a survival benefit from the use of heparin ($P = .01$). However, differences were more marked at 1 year (40% versus 30%) than at 2 or 3 years (11% versus 9% and 9% versus 6%, respectively). This trial illustrates that what is statistically significant may not be clinically significant or useful. The authors now wish to compare a short versus a long heparin dose schedule.

In summary, although anticoagulant therapy is interesting conceptually, the results obtained to date do not support its use as standard therapy.

COMBINED APPROACHES

The use of combined approaches has been investigated extensively over the past 20 years. Despite numerous trials, optimal schedules cannot yet be defined clearly. The role of thoracic surgery is discussed briefly before focusing on combined chemotherapy-radiotherapy.

ROLE OF ADJUVANT SURGERY

The role of surgery in the treatment of SCLC is controversial (165) (see Chapter 20). Although approximately 30% of patients may have limited disease at the time of diagnosis, only one third of them have SCLC that is potentially resectable surgically. Surgery is one approach used to improve local control as is thoracic radiotherapy. The main problem is that, despite the use of conventional radiotherapy and chemotherapy, locoregional disease recurrence is seen in approximately 50% of cases, and initial lack of local control affects 25%.

Surgery has been advocated in locally advanced SCLC (43, 166), but a recent randomized trial evaluating its role (167) failed to show any benefit when used as an adjunct to chemotherapy and radiotherapy. Surgical treatment thus should be restricted to patients with very limited disease, mainly stage I SCLC. There are some patients who present with peripheral lesions, undergo surgery first, and have the histologic diagnosis established only at that time. In these cases, further treatment with etoposide and cisplatin–based chemotherapy is recommended for a maximum of 6 monthly courses as well as postoperative thoracic radiotherapy delivering a total dose of 50 to 55 Gy in conventional fractionation or its radiobiologic equivalent. This choice of total radiation dose is empirical, as discussed previously. The good result observed in these patients, i.e., a 3-year survival of more than 30% (166), certainly is related to the early stage of the disease at diagnosis (T1-T2, N0-N1 disease). Unfortunately, only a small number of patients present with this very early stage disease. The benefits of surgery in patients with more advanced but limited forms of SCLC remain to be determined. A few patients who do not respond to induction chemotherapy or who experience disease recurrence may be considered for salvage surgical treatment.

COMBINED RADIOTHERAPY: RATIONALE AND SEQUENCING IN LIMITED SMALL CELL LUNG CANCER

Adjunctive thoracic radiotherapy significantly decreases the risk of local recurrence in limited SCLC (Table 21.2). The problem of drug resistance has led to use of the alternation of different drug regimens without cross-resistance (105). However, most of the tested chemotherapy schedules have a variable degree of cross-resistance. Local radiotherapy thus should be considered because of its effectiveness in controlling bulky tumor masses and because there is little cross-resistance between chemotherapy and radiotherapy (168–170). There are three theoretical reasons why combined chemotherapy-radiotherapy should be advantageous in chemosensitive tumors such as SCLC: (a) spatial cooperation, i.e., radiotherapy is used to control limited areas of bulky disease, whereas chemotherapy may eradicate smaller deposits of tumor that are outside the radiation field; (b) the impact of the tumor burden in the definitive long-term local control (Fig. 21.3); and (c) the early emergence of chemoresistant cells during chemotherapy.

Several comprehensive articles have reviewed various aspects of combined approaches (171–176). Two mechanisms may explain the effect of radiotherapy on survival: (a) local progression may be a direct cause of death in lung cancer patients; and (b) improved local control may result in a decrease in the incidence of distant metastases by avoiding redissemination, e.g., as is seen in some subsets of breast cancer patients (177). A high incidence of local recurrence has been observed among patients with very chemosensitive tumors treated with chemotherapy alone. These recurrences are more difficult to manage than primary tumors because of the emergence of chemoresistant cells (29, 178). The probability of developing drug resistant cells is much greater for bulky tumors (178), which often occur in lung cancer. The use of radiation and drugs may overcome resistance to treatment if their mechanisms of action are independent. In epithelial tumors, local radiotherapy can then be used because it can control bulky masses effectively. Radiation cell kill is related almost entirely to DNA damage, and it is the double strand break that is the critical lesion for cell death, unlike that of chemotherapy, for which there are many points of interaction within the cell, i.e., cell membrane, cytoplasm, and nucleus. However, cross-resistance may occur between both modalities, particularly after sequential combinations (174, 179, 180). Consequently, in theory the best method to prevent the development of resistance is the early administration of both modalities.

Chemotherapy achieves a high rate of clinical CR in SCLC. However, the high proportion of thoracic recurrences observed is ample evidence that a complete remission, as currently defined, has a limited meaning. If a tumor mass of 100 g is assumed, then the number of tumor cells can be estimated as 10^{11}. If this tumor decreases to less than 500 mg, it would disappear clinically and radiologically, and physicans would conclude that a clinical complete remission has been obtained. There would, however, still be 5×10^8 surviving cells. A 3 log cell kill may be sufficient to obtain a clinical and radiologically complete remission, but long-term tumor control would necessitate at least a 9 log cell kill, if the proportion of clonogenic tumor cells is assumed to be approximately 1% (174).

In a recent article (175), Tannock reviews the mechanisms that might lead to a therapeutic benefit. These mechanisms include the inhibition, using drugs, of repopulation during fractionated radiotherapy, the use of drugs with selective toxicity under hypoxic conditions, and the use of drugs that selectively sensitize cells to radiation. Repopulation of tumor cells during radiotherapy may be an important phenomenon, especially in tumors with rapid growth such as SCLC. Cancer cells may proliferate between dose fractions, thus decreasing the probability of local control. Withers et al. (77) reported the need for an increase in radiation dose when treatment was protracted beyond 3 to 4 weeks. Tumor repopulation may be stimulated by the initial cell killing. Beause most cytotoxic drugs have a high lethal toxicity for rapidly proliferating cells, concurrent chemotherapy-radiotherapy administration may produce a selective toxicity for the repopulating cells through their increased proliferation. Of course, this effect is beneficial only if the repopulation is more rapid in the tumor than in the normal tissues. Most normal mediastinal tissues, except those in the esophagus, contain slowly proliferating cells, thus thoracic tumors could be controlled better by concurrent administration. These considerations also would explain why esophageal reactions may be a limiting factor in the clinical application of concurrent schedules.

In the last two decades, many phase II and phase III studies have focused on chemotherapy and radiotherapy combinations. The combined approach has been shown to improve both the local control of bulky tumors and, in some randomized studies, the overall survival. Such goals can be achieved with acceptable toxicity if current radiotherapy techniques and doses are applied within a clinically tolerable combined schedule.

These hypotheses have been corroborated in clinical practice by the meta-analysis of 13 unconfounded randomized trials including 2573 patients with SCLC (25). These trials compared chemotherapy alone with the combination of chest irradiation and chemotherapy. Table 21.8 shows a summary of these randomized trials. The overall results showed a reduction of 14% in mortality ($P = .001$) in favor of the combined approach, as shown in Figure 21.6, for limited (2140 patients) and extensive disease (433 patients). There was no difference in treatment effect based on disease extent. The effect on mortality was translated into a 5.4% increase in the 3-year survival rate (14.3% versus 8.9%) for limited disease. The test for heterogeneity of results was not significant ($P = .15$).

The Copenhagen trial (53) showed borderline significance in favor of chemotherapy alone, as shown in Figure 21.6. A second analysis was performed without this trial. The pooled relative risk of death was then .82 (CI 95%, .75–.91) instead of .86 for the overall analysis; the test of heterogeneity produced a P value of .76 instead of .15. Treatment effect based on prognostic factors such as age, sex, and performance status also was analyzed. These analyses did not show significant differences except for age, which was a predictive factor of treatment effect. Radiotherapy afforded a greater benefit in younger patients, the test of trend for the treatment effect based on age being significant ($P = .01$). The relative risk of death ranged from .72 among patients less than 55 years old to 1.07 among patients more than 70 years old. Among younger patients the 3-year survival benefit was approximately 8%. The lack of effect of treatment in the older patients could be explained by increased toxicity.

The overall treatment effect observed represents a mean effect for the trials conducted from 1976 to 1988. It is interesting to note that 15 years elapsed between the initiation of the first trial (53) and the acquisition of a definite answer. This long interval clearly illustrates the need to analyze large numbers of patients when a moderate effect on survival, i.e., 5% to 10%, is expected. Small and even moderately large trials do not have enough statistical power to detect such a difference.

The demonstrated benefit of thoracic radiotherapy in terms of overall survival supports the general use of combined treatment in the management of limited SCLC (9). It is likely that a major benefit could be obtained if treatment variables were optimal. To date, the optimal combination still is unknown. As described previously, chest irradiation and combined chemotherapy-radiotherapy are composite parameters, and analysis of their effects can be equivocal. However, in numerous trials combined approaches have produced

TABLE 21.8. Randomized Trials Evaluating the Role of Chest Irradiation in Small Cell Lung Cancer

Trial (Reference No.)	Enrollment Period	Stage	Evaluable (No. of Patients)	Scheduling of CT/RT	First Day of RT	Dose (Gy)/ No. of Fraction
Copenhagen (53)	1976–79	LD	145	Concurrent	43	40/10[a]
Sydney (181)	1977–79	LD	94	Sequential	63	40/20
		ED	49			
NCI (54)	1977–86	LD	97	Concurrent	1–3	40/15
SECSG I (55)	1978–82	LD	295	Alternating	29	40/14[a]
London (182)	1979–82	LD	138	Sequential	85	40/20
		ED	247			
SWOG (56)	1980–83	LD	103	Sequential	85	48/22[a]
SAKK (183)	1980–84	LD	70	Sequential	127	42/25[a]
		ED				
Uppsala (57)	1980–84	LD	57	Sequential	77	40/20
		ED	65			
CALGB (58)	1981–84	LD	426	Concurrent	1 or 64	50/24
ECOG (184)	1981–85	LD	264	Sequential	43	50/25
Okayama (59)	1981–86	LD	56	Sequential	30	40/20
SECSG II (55)	1982–85	LD	322	Concurrent	1	45/15[a]
GETCB (185)	1986–88	LD	36	Sequential	224	32/8
		ED	18			

Abbreviations. LD, limited disease; ED, extensive disease.
[a]Split-course therapy.

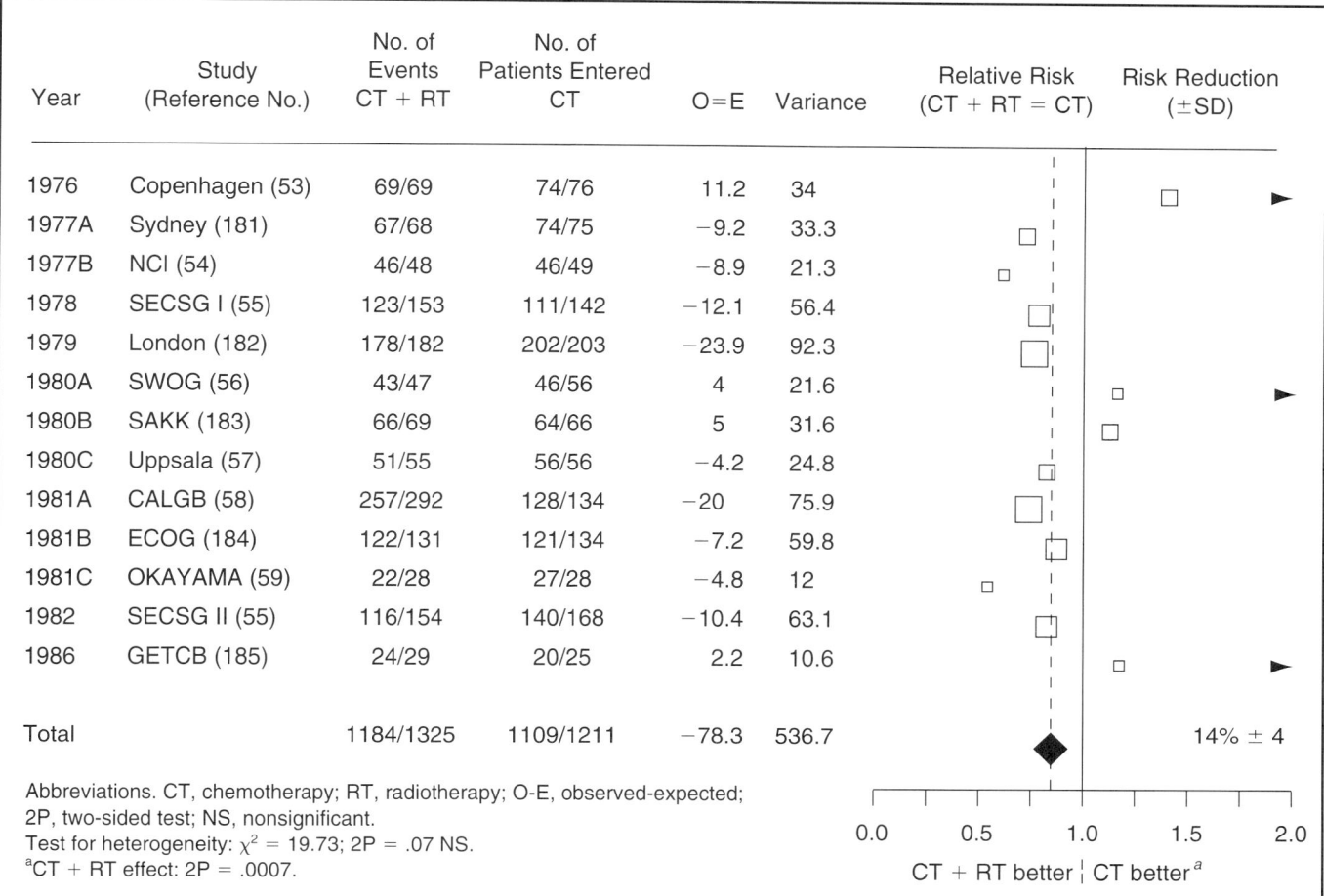

FIGURE 21.6. Meta-analysis of 13 randomized trials evaluating the role of thoracic radiotherapy and including 2536 patients, 2103 with limited and 433 with extensive disease. Results are shown in terms of relative risk of death among patients receiving both chemotherapy and radiotherapy (*CT + RT*), compared with patients receiving chemotherapy alone (*CT*). Each trial is summarized in a line. The first two digits before the trial name correspond to the year in which the trial was started. Each open square represents the relative risk for the trial, and each horizontal line is its 99% confidence interval; the area of each square is proportional to the amount of information from the corresponding trial. The broken line and the solid diamond represent the pooled relative risk of death and its 95% confidence interval. The percentage reduction in the pooled relative risk (±SD) was 14% ± 4%. The patients in the two combined treatment groups of the CALGB trial (early chemotherapy plus radiotherapy, and late chemotherapy plus radiotherapy) were added together for this analysis.

significantly increased toxicity (186–189). Indeed, acute and late toxicities can be increased and may overshadow any potential therapeutic gain. The critical aspects concerning the effect on the tumor and on toxicity include the type of cytotoxic agents, radiotherapy parameters, radiation and drug doses, and timing of chemotherapy-radiotherapy. Two fundamental aspects of the timing are discussed: early versus late radiotherapy and scheduling of combined chemotherapy-radiotherapy.

EARLY VERSUS LATE THORACIC RADIOTHERAPY

There are at least two theoretical reasons why thoracic radiotherapy should be given early. The first is the possible emergence of chemoresistant cells, and the second is tumor repopulation during treatment. If chemotherapy and radiation are given sequentially and in full doses, the consequence of this protracted administration may be a high level of tumor repopulation (76, 77). Occult distant metastases continue to proliferate if drug therapy is delayed. For example, if the tumor doubling time is 30 days, a delay of 2 months would permit a fourfold increase in the volume of metastases (174). Radiotherapy cannot be delayed for too long because chemotherapy often has only a limited effect on bulky tumors and can even induce the development of radioresistance. In view of the uncertainty regarding the extent of repopulation, the shortest possible interval between each treatment modality is advisable.

The indirect comparisons made in the SCLC meta-analysis (25) did not answer definitively whether preference should be given to early or late radiotherapy because the relative risk of death was similar in both groups of trials. The analysis limited to the trials with early radiotherapy, defined as radiation given within 60 days of the beginning of treatment gave a pooled relative risk of death of .88 (CI 95%, .78–.98) and .83 (CI 95%, .73–.93) when the Copenhagen trial (53) was excluded from this analysis. The study limited to the trials with late radiotherapy gave a pooled relative risk of .81 (CI 95%, .69–.94). No significant differences existed between these generated relative risks.

However, three randkmized studies have investigated this question directly, and their results are summarized in Table 21.9. The National Cancer Institute of Canada (NCIC) trial (190) showed a significant difference ($P = .016$) in favor of early radiotherapy given at day 22, compared with late radiotherapy given at day 106. However, in the CALGB trial (58) there was only a slight difference in favor of late radiotherapy (day 64), which may be explained by the nondelivery of full chemotherapy doses in the early radiotherapy arm (day 1) because of increased acute toxicity. In contrast, in the early radiotherapy arm of the NCIC trial, the initial drug dose delivery was not altered by thoracic radiotherapy because radiation was given only at the time of the second course of chemotherapy. These combined findings suggest that full initial doses of chemotherapy may have an influence on survival, as has been corroborated in the French trial described earlier (120). The Danish trial (191) did not show a significant difference. For the time being, most authors agree that the use of early radiotherapy is preferable, even if "early" may be not at the time of the first course of chemotherapy; however, further clinical research is needed to justify this view.

METHODS OF SCHEDULING COMBINED CHEMOTHERAPY-RADIOTHERAPY

For the scheduling of chemotherapy-radiotherapy, the following definitions (50) are used:

1. Concurrent chemotherapy-radiotherapy: combined modality therapy in which chemotherapy and radiotherapy are given simultaneously;
2. Alternating chemotherapy-radiotherapy: combined modality therapy in which radiotherapy is given on days of the chemotherapy cycle in which no chemotherapy is administered with no delay in chemotherapy beyond that occurring if chemotherapy were given alone.
3. Sequential chemotherapy-radiotherapy: administration of chemotherapy and radiotherapy separately, with chemotherapy followed by radiotherapy, radiotherapy followed by chemotherapy, or a delay in chemotherapy administration for delivery of radiotherapy.

No consensus exists regarding the optimal schedule, although a majority of investigators favor alternating or concurrent schedules. In the meta-analysis evaluating the role of thoracic radiotherapy (25), an indirect comparison was made between trials with or without sequential radiotherapy. An analysis limited to trials with sequential radiotherapy gave a pooled relative risk of death of .86 (CI 95%, .75–1). An analysis limited to trials with alternating or concurrent radiotherapy gave a pooled relative risk of .85 (CI 95%, .75–.96) and .79 (CI 95%, .69–.90) when the Copenhagen trial (53) was excluded; in the latter case, the heterogeneity test produced a P value of .78 instead of .03. In any case, no significant differences existed between the relative risks generated by sequential and nonsequential radiotherapy schedules. Some randomized trials are being conducted on this subject. European Organization for Research and Treatment of Cancer (EORTC) is comparing alternating and sequential regimens, and the Japanese Clinical Oncology Group is comparing concurrent and sequential schedules. It is hoped that these and other randomized trials will lead to a better understanding of the optimal schedules.

TABLE 21.9. Randomized Trials Evaluating the Timing of Thoracic Radiotherapy in Limited Small Cell Lung Cancer

TRIAL (REFERENCE NO.)	INDUCTION CT	PCI	THORACIC DOSE (GY/ NO. OF FRACTIONS)	NO. OF PATIENTS	FIRST DAY OF RT	2-YR SURVIVAL (%)	P VALUE
CALGB (58)	CPM, VCR, VP-16, alt. CPM, DOX, VCR	Yes	50/24	125	1	24	.08
				145	64	30	
NCIC (190)	CAV alt. CDDP, VP-16	Yes	40/15	155	22	40	.008
				153	106	33	
Aarhus (191)	CAV alt. CDDP, VP-16	Yes	40–45/22	97	1	20	NS
				98	126	18	

Abbreviations. CT, chemotherapy; PCI, prophylactic cranial irradiation; RT, radiotherapy; CPM, cyclophosphamide; VCR, vincristine; VP-16, etoposide; DOX, doxorubicin; CAV, cyclophosphamide + doxorubicin + vincristine; alt., alternating; CDDP, cisplatin; NS, not significant.

CONCURRENT APPROACHES

The theoretical and clinical reasons why preference should be given to concurrent or alternating radiotherapy-chemotherapy, as opposed to sequential radiotherapy-chemotherapy, have been analyzed previously (171, 173). The main advantage of concurrent combinations is that radiotherapy can be delivered early and without intervals between both modalities.

A U.S. National Cancer Institute (NCI) trial (54) reported a very high incidence of complications and lethal toxicity, although a survival benefit was obtained with the combined treatment. Severe toxicity included bone marrow aplasia, infections, and pulmonary and esophageal toxicity. For a time, these results were cited as the reason why concurrent administration should be avoided. However, the high rate of complications may have been caused by the use of a moderately concentrated radiation schedule (fractions of 2.66 Gy 5 times per week) and concurrent administration of methotrexate, high-dose cyclophosphamide and lomustine. These two factors were avoided in the CALGB and the NCIC trials (58, 190), and the toxicity seemed acceptable.

Turrisi (192) and other American groups (82) have conducted trials on concurrent PE chemotherapy and accelerated twice-daily radiotherapy for treatment of limited SCLC. Chemotherapy consisted of cisplatin and etoposide. Thoracic radiotherapy consisted of 30 fractions of 1.5 Gy given twice daily, 5 days per week (total dose, 45 Gy), with a 4- to 6-hour interval between each daily fraction. Tumor response to therapy was assessed at week 6 with restaging and subsequent cycles of therapy through week 25. In the first study, comprising 32 patients, the overall response rate was 91%. All pure small cell tumors responded completely. Two-year survival was 45%. This and other similar studies are summarized in Table 21.10.

Results of these trials showed that twice-daily, 1.5-Gy-per-fraction radiotherapy plus concurrent PE chemotherapy administered to selected patients had a substantial toxicity (esophagitis and bone marrow aplasia) but was very effective. However, it is not clear if the very good results reported are because of (a) the highly selected group of patients, e.g., histologic and biologic features of pure SCLC; (b) the use of a concurrent approach; or (c) the use of accelerated bifractionation. The latter hypothesis was tested recently in a randomized trial (69, 73) showing that bifractionation is probably not a major factor. At the same time, it is clear (Table 21.10) that a selection factor exists because overall results were not as good as reported in the previous pilot studies. Special attention should be paid to the development of late toxicity, such as esophageal stenosis, for which dilation is sometimes required; this effect has been recorded in more than 10% of patients in some of these series.

ALTERNATING APPROACHES

Alternating schedules that interdigitate a 1-week gap between the delivery of each modality make it possible to deliver both the radiotherapy and drugs early and regularly. They also permit the administration of drugs with specific toxicity, such as doxorubicin, when thoracic radiotherapy is to be given. Furthermore, these schedules capitalize on the tumor repopulation induced by the administration of each modality while avoiding the drawbacks of repopulation observed with sequential regimens or when the administration of the two modalities is separated by an excessively protracted interval. They are consistent with experimental data reported by Looney (194) using the rat hepatoma 3924A model. Many experiments combining radiotherapy and cyclophosphamide administration have enabled the definition of an optimal schedule: chemotherapy courses should be alternated with three courses of radiotherapy with an interval of 7 days between each treatment modality. This treatment achieved a cure rate of 60% compared with 0% when the animals were treated with a single modality. The use of three split courses of radiotherapy is open to criticism because of a decreased tumor effect resulting

TABLE 21.10. Clinical Studies Using Concurrent Bifractionated Radiotherapy-Chemotherapy in Limited Small Cell Lung Cancer

First Author (Reference No.)	No. of Patients	Concurrent Chemotherapy	Alternating Chemotherapy	Dose of Radiotherapy (Gy/Fraction/D)	2-Yr Survival (%)	Local Control (%)
Johnson (82)	41	PE	CAV	45/30/19	65	...
Turrisi (81)	32	PE	CAV	45/30/19	48	84
Turrisi (193)	40	PE	CAV	45/30/19	36	...
ECOG (69)[a]	182	PE	...	45/30/19	44	52

Abbreviations. PE, cisplatin + etoposide; CAV, cyclophosphamide + doxorubicin + vincristine.
[a]Randomized trial.

from tumor repopulation between the rest periods. This is true for tumors responding poorly to chemotherapy; however, in sensitive tumors the interdigitated chemotherapy probably precludes tumor repopulation between radiotherapy courses.

A clinical investigation was started at the Institut Gustave-Roussy in 1980, and these studies were later extended to four other cooperating centers. Detailed reports have been published previously (171, 195, 196). Thoracic radiotherapy was started 1 week after completion of the second course of chemotherapy and was given for 12 days with 1 week of no therapy between both modalities. Three courses of thoracic radiotherapy were alternated with chemotherapy, which continued for up to a total of six courses in the induction phase, as shown in Figure 21.7. Staging investigations included fiberoptic bronchoscopy, thoracic CT scan, bone marrow biopsy, bone scan, liver ultrasound or CT scan, and brain CT scan. All patients were restaged at 6 months, i.e., at the end of induction treatment, and at the completion of maintenance chemotherapy. Restaging was identical to that of the initial assessment, which included fiberoptic broncoscopy with systematic bronchial biopsies. A description of these trials is summarized in Table 21.11. Six consecutive studies were conducted from 1980 to 1991 and included a total of 346 patients with limited SCLC. Four trends can be noted in the treatment: (*a*) an increase in total radiation doses; (*b*) an increase in initial doses of cisplatin and etoposide; (*c*) prophylactic cranial irradiation was given systematically in the first two protocols and was randomized for complete responders in the later protocols; and (*d*) a decreasing number of maintenance chemotherapy cycles and absence of maintenance since 1987.

The population was 85% male. The mean age was 55 years, and the mean initial Karnofsky score was 85%. Ninety percent of patients had stage III disease at the time of inclusion. The complete remission rate at the end of the induction treatment was 75%. Overall survival is shown in Figure 21.8. The survival rate at 5 years is 16%. No significant differences were observed between the first four protocols. The use of a competing risk approach in the description of the causes of failure in the first 202 patients has been discussed in detail previously (32), and the results are shown in Figure 21.2. Local recurrence was a major cause of failure, although a high response rate was obtained with this combined chemotherapy-radiotherapy approach. Total radiation dose increments were added from the first to the third protocol to determine the maximum dose tolerated. The maximum total dose delivered was 65 Gy. There was no significant increase in radiation-related complications, but because there was no improvement in local control, participating investigators decided to use the total dose of 55 Gy as a standard treatment. The choice of this dose level remains empirical. Conventional fractionation was used in all but the fourth protocol, which included accelerated fractionation in the first course of thoracic radiotherapy (three fractions of 1.4 Gy per day). Because there was no clear improvement in local control, conventional fractionation was selected as the reference radiotherapy schedule for the next trial.

These protocols have proved to be feasible despite a high frequency of acute hematologic toxicity requiring stringent monitoring. The long-term survival rate is approximately 15% and remains among the highest actual survival rates reported in the literature. Despite these encouraging results, the superiority of alternating approaches over other chemotherapy-radiotherapy schedules has yet to be demonstrated in a randomized trial. The ECOG conducted a pilot study of alternating chemotherapy and twice-daily thoracic radiotherapy in 32 patients (197); overall results are similar to those obtained by the Institut Gustave-Roussy group. In the United Kingdom, the Medical Research Council (MRC) conducted a phase II trial in 24 patients according to the IGR-004 schedule of alternating chemotherapy and radiotherapy (198). Tumor remission and short-term survival rates were consistent with reported results of the Institut Gustave-Roussy (32). However, the authors concluded that because of early toxicity this kind of schedule was only feasible in a small proportion of centers in the United Kingdom. They decided not to embark on a randomized trial comparing an alternating to a sequential schedule. However, more recently, Bleehen et al. (199) published long-term results showing that patients with World Health Organization performance status grade 1 or 2 have a 2-year survival of approximately 15%, similar to comparable patients treated previously with a concurrent schedule. However, in patients with a performance status of grade 0, the 2-year survival is approximately 60% for the alternating schedule compared with 20% for the concurrent treatment. They concluded that the alternation of chemotherapy and radiotherapy

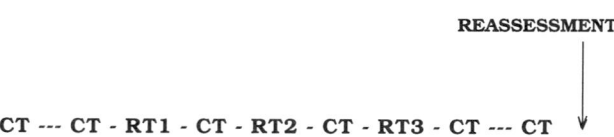

FIGURE 21.7. Schedule of the alternating chemotherapy and radiotherapy treatment used in the protocols of the Institute Gustave-Roussy and cooperating centers. CT, induction chemotherapy; RT1 and RT2, thoracic radiotherapy (anteroposterior fields); RT3, boost radiotherapy on tumor and mediastinum with spinal cord shielding; -, 1 week of rest.

TABLE 21.11. Summary of Alternating Radiotherapy-Chemotherapy Institut Gustave-Roussy and Cooperating Centers Studies

	INSTITUT GUSTAVE-ROUSSY STUDY NO. (YEARS)					
CHARACTERISTICS	002 (1980–81)	004 (1982–84)	006 (1985–86)	010 (1987–88)	012 (1989–91)	012B (1991–92)
Number of patients	28	81	64	29	105	39
Cyclophosphamide	300 × 4	300 × 4	300 × 3	300 × 4	R^a	300 × 4
Doxorubicin (mg/m^2)	40	40	40	40	40	40
Etoposide (mg/m^2)	75 × 3	75 × 3	100 × 3	75 × 5	75 × 3	75 × 3
Methotrexate (mg/m^2)	400	...	...	...	...	...
Cisplatin (mg/m^2)	...	100	120	30 × 5	R^a	100
Thoracic RT (Gy)	15-15-15	20-20-15	20-20-25	21^b-20-20	20-20-15	20-20-15
PCI (Gy)^c	30	30	24^d	24^d	24^d	24^d
Maintenance CT (number of cycles)	12	8	6	0	0	0

Abbreviations. RT, radiotherapy; PCI, prophylactic cranial irradiation; CT, chemotherapy.
^{a}Initial dose was randomized.
^{b}Multifractionated radiotherapy given by reduced radiation fields.
^{c}Fractions of 3 Gy.
^{d}Randomized for complete responders.

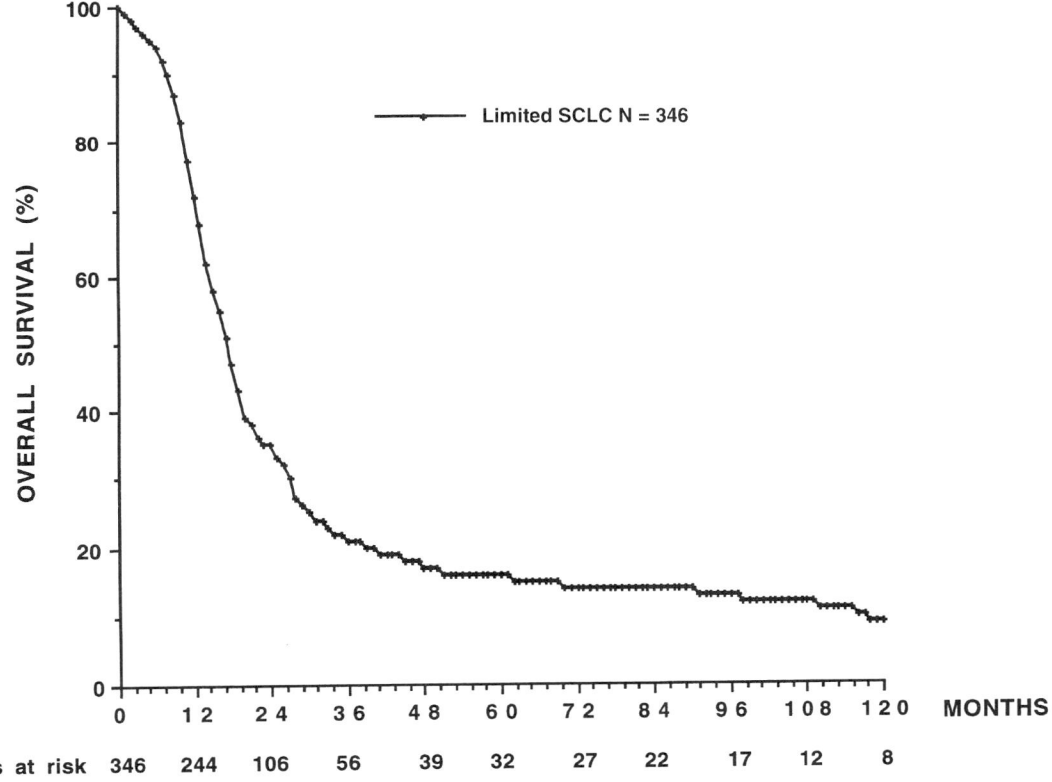

FIGURE 21.8. Overall survival rate in a series of 346 patients with limited SCLC treated by alternating chemotherapy and radiotherapy.

can offer to a subgroup of patients a better chance of cure with a higher risk of toxicity. Overall results of published alternating schedules are summarized in Table 21.12.

The EORTC Lung Cancer Study Group (200) initiated a randomized trial comparing a modified alternating schedule to a sequential combination of chemotherapy and radiation. Five cycles of cyclophosphamide, doxorubicin, and etoposide (CDE) chemotherapy were administered at 3-week intervals. Radiotherapy (50 Gy in 20 daily fractions) was given either after the fifth chemotherapy cycle or in four weekly courses of 12.5 Gy in five fractions. This shorter schedule was not considered feasible, and the group decided to use a 4-week interval as proposed in the IGR protocols (195, 201). Through the end of 1993, 293 of the 360 patients ini-

TABLE 21.12. Clinical Studies Using Alternating Chemo Radiotherapy in Limited Small Cell Lung Cancer

Study (Reference No.)	No. of Patients	Drugs Used	RT Dose (Gy) Per Series	2-Yr Overall Survival	4-Yr Overall Survival (%)	Local Control (%)
IGR (current study)	346	CPM, DOX, VP-16, CDDP (or MTX)[a]	15-15-15 20-20-15 20-20-25 21-20-20[b]	35%	17	58
ECOG (197)	34	PE ± CPM, VP-16	15-15-15[b]	47%	<30	59[c]
MRC (198)	22	CPM, DOX, VP-16, CDDP	20-20-15	32%	22	?
PCG (202)	67[d]	CDE	20-20-15	407 d[e]	...	?

Abbreviations. RT, radiation therapy; IGR, Institut Gustave-Roussy; CPM, cyclophosphamide; DOX, doxorubicin; VP-16, etoposide; CDDP, cisplatin; MTX, methotrexate; PE, cisplatin + etoposide; CDE, cyclophosphamide + doxorubicin + etoposide.
[a]Only first protocol.
[b]Accelerated radiotherapy.
[c]Complete remission rate.
[d]Randomized trial (alternating arm).
[e]Median survival.

tially planned had been randomized to either the alternating or the sequential arm. The results are awaited.

Finally, a Groupe Etude Treatment Cancers Bronchiques French trial (202) compared an alternating schedule with CDE chemotherapy (Table 21.12) and a concurrent approach in limited SCLC. One hundred and thirty-seven patients have been analyzed in a preliminary report (202). Differences were not significant, even though a trend favored the alternating arm in terms of overall survival ($P = .19$) and lethal toxicity (4% versus 11%). A very large number of patients probably will be needed to detect a significant difference between the schedules tested in these trials.

In summary, alternating approaches may be included and tested in phase III trials. The use of higher initial doses of chemotherapy and of unconventional fractionation in the delivery of thoracic radiotherapy are methods that are likely to improve long-term results.

TREATMENT OF ELDERLY PATIENTS AND TUMOR RELAPSES

Treatment of Elderly Patients

The treatment of elderly patients depends on the particular case and especially on the other medical problems that might make intensive combination chemotherapy difficult to administer. Less toxic treatments have been developed, the most popular being the use of oral etoposide as single agent at doses of 900 mg/m² per cycle (203). This treatment gives a response rate of 71% and a median survival of 16 months for limited disease.

Carney and Bryhe (204) studied the effect of oral etoposide alone or in combination with carboplatin. In a population of 63 elderly patients (median age, 72 years) treated with oral etoposide (200 mg/day for 5 days), an overall response rate of 76% was observed with a CR rate of 33% in limited disease. Ten percent of patients survived more than 2 years. The authors tested a consecutive combination of oral etoposide and carboplatin (300 mg/m² intravenously on day 1) in 83 elderly patients. Objective responses were observed in 81% and complete remission in 36% (53% in limited disease). The main value of such therapy is that the results are similar to those of more intensive treatment regimens but with less toxicity in an age group that generally has poor prognostic features. In addition, administration is easy, i.e., on an outpatient basis.

Recently, Murray et al. (205) reported a series of 55 elderly and infirm patients with limited SCLC treated with two cycles of chemotherapy: the first with CAV in and the second with PE, followed by chest irradiation (30 Gy in 10 fractions of 20 Gy in 5 fractions). The complete remission rate was 51%, and the 2- and 5-year survival rates were 29% and 18%, respectively. These encouraging results need confirmation, because, if confirmed, a major question about the duration of treatment in limited SCLC would be raised.

Treatment of Tumor Relapses

As seen in the natural history of the disease, approximately 90% of patients with SCLC have recurrences within the first 3 years of follow-up. The outlook after local or distant recurrence is poor, because second-line treatments are clearly less effective. In the case of isolated chest recurrence, local treatment should be considered, i.e., thoracic radiotherapy, if it was not given at the time of the primary treatment, or surgery in selected cases. In all cases, a histologic proof of recurrence should be obtained because in some cases a NSCLC component or a new primary tumor can be found (especially in long-term survivors). Even if the treatment of recurrences is unrewarding generally, this group of patients is suitable for the evaluation of new treatments or strategies to find mechanisms or drugs that reverse treatment resistance. Johnson (206) recently pointed out that the success of second-line treatment depends on the interval between cessation of the first treatment and the detection of recurrence as well as on the response to the primary therapy. When more than 1 year has elapsed, even retreatment with the original drugs may produce a second remission. In patients with a relapse, objective response rates are usually less than 30%. However, this response rate increases to 50% when a cyclophosphamide-based chemotherapy was given as primary treatment and PE was administered as a second-line chemotherapy. For 21 patients who previously were treated heavily, Faylona et al. (207) showed a response rate of 59% using a combination of etoposide, ifosfamide, and cisplatin. The median survival was 26 weeks. New agents with a different mechanism of action, such as taxanes or camptothecin derivatives, should certainly be tested in prospective trials.

TOXICITY AND LONG-TERM SURVIVAL

TREATMENT TOXICITY

One should remember that there is no therapeutic gain if lethal toxicity increases. Toxic effects on normal tissues have been the limiting factor in any therapeutic strategy whose aim is the eradication of malignant disease. Unfortunately, reports on toxicity are very heterogeneous, and it is difficult to determine clearly the intensity and extent of toxicity. Investigators at the Institut Gustave-Roussy have chosen to report results in SCLC under the heading of causes of death unrelated to cancer, including deaths not directly related to treatment toxicity (208). This simple procedure eliminates bias caused by medical interpretation of causes of death that may artificially reduce the rate of so-called lethal toxicity. For example, Figure 21.2 shows the overall rate of death unrelated to cancer (8%) in 202 patients with limited SCLC treated at the Institut Gustav-Roussy and participating centers.

Combined chemotherapy-radiotherapy schedules can produce severe and even life-threatening complications. Travis and Liao (209) conducted the studies in mice to determine the tolerance to the volume of lung tissue irradiated and the probability of radiation injury in the lung. They observed a volume dependent shift in the dose-response curves for breathing rate and mortality at 28 weeks, at the end of the pneumonitis phase. Reducing the volume of lung irradiated from 100% to 85% significantly increased the lethal dose 50% for death from pneumonitis by 3.5 Gy. These data suggested that only 15% of the lung was necessary to maintain lung function. Furthermore, the relation of morbidity to dose and volume irradiated depended on the part of the lung irradiated. Lastly, lung damage, as evidenced by histologic examination of pneumonitis, was observed in the irradiated area only. The authors hypothesize that clinical morbidity shows a marked volume effect but only after a threshold volume is damaged. After this volume is exceeded, the shape of the volume response curve is very steep.

Ward et al. (210) reported a search for clinically useful modifiers of radiation pneumonitis. Glucocorticoids have been shown to be effective against radiation pneumonitis but fail to improve lung fibrosis (211). Ward and colleagues (212) tested captopril (a converting enzyme inhibitor) to determine its antifibrosis action in rats. They found that this compound administered at doses 10 to 20 times that used to treat hypertension in humans reduced the severity of radiation pneumotoxicity and also the incidence of late malignancies within the radiation portals.

EARLY TOXICITY OF COMBINED TREATMENT MODALITIES

Because active drugs are used most commonly in combination, they can give a broad spectrum of toxicities. Among common side effects, those seen most frequently include nausea and vomiting; mucositis; alopecia; myelosuppression with possible infection, bleeding, or anemia; cardiotoxicity; nephrotoxicity; neurotoxicity; and homorrhage cystitis. Adverse events associated with thoracic radiotherapy include acute esophagitis and pneumonitis. Severe complications are observed in the tissues located within the irradiated thoracic volume. The symptomatic pneumonitis rate varies from 3% to 15% (213). This complication is related to the lung volume irradiated, the total radiation dose, and the number of fractions (211). Acute esophagitis is very common but usually is of mild to moderate intensity when radiation treatment is given in a dose that exceeds 30 Gy in conventional fractions; however, these transitory reactions rarely lead to treatment interruption. To decrease acute reactions it would be safer to avoid the administration, at least concurrently, of drugs such as bleomycin, mitomycin, and doxorubicin, which are associated with specific toxic effects on thoracic tissues.

In alternating protocols used by the Institut Gustave-Roussy and cooperating centers, acute toxicity was mainly hematologic. Most patients developed grade 3 or 4 granulocytopenia, thrombocytopenia, and anemia during the radiotherapy courses. Close monitoring was necessary, but radiation treatment was not interrupted except in cases of fever that exceeded 38.5°C or bleeding (mainly petechiae) requiring hospitalization. Interruptions generally were limited to 1 to 3 days. During induction treatment, mean drug doses were decreased by approximately 20%, based on the hematologic tolerance (201). Acute esophagitis generally was not a problem, except in the first four patients included in the protocol using accelerated radiotherapy. In these cases, it was sufficient to decrease the total dose of the first radiation course from 25 Gy to 21 Gy to reduce the acute mucosal reactions (214).

LATE TOXICITIES

The most common late complications after treatment with chemotherapy include cardiomyopathy, lung fibrosis, central and peripheral nervous system toxicity, and second malignancies. The percentage reduction in pulmonary function of lung cancer patients treated by radiotherapy is estimated at between 12% and 28% (213). However, asymptomatic radiographic changes occur in more than 90% (215, 216). High-dose cyclophosphamide may increase the risk of radiation-induced lung fibrosis (217). Late cardiotoxicity related to the use of doxorubicin is observed in fewer than 2% of patients (218), although new anthacyclines such as epirubicin are also potentially cardiotoxic.

Some cytotoxic drugs, such as cyclophosphamide, the nitrosoureas, bleomycin, and mytomycin C (219), may be implicated in the development of lung toxicity. However, lung fibrosis is related primarily to the lung volume irradiated. In concurrent chemotherapy-radiotherapy combinations, it may be observed in up to 30% of patients (186). In this trial (186), lung fibrosis was fatal in 6 of 11 patients who developed this complication. Histologic examination of the lung showed an interstitial pneumonitis, without any associated infection. The incidence of esophageal stricture also may be increased in concurrent chemotherapy-radiotherapy regimens.

Radiation myelitis is a catastrophic complication that can present more than 1 year after treatment. The threshold dose is more than 45 Gy at conventional fractionation (220), but the threshold decreases with increased fraction size or accelerated radiotherapy. This complication is unusual after treatment for lung cancer if good quality radiotherapy is performed.

Central nervous system toxicity possibly related to the use of chemotherapy and prophylactic cranial irradiation is discussed further in Chapter 23.

In the ICR series, neither esophageal stricture nor radiation myelopathy was observed. Severe pericarditis was observed in nine patients. However, limited pericardial effusion is seen in nearly all long-term survivors as detected by echocardiogram or thoracic CT scan. Systematic study by fibertoptic bronchoscopy allowed Baldeyrou et al. (38) to evaluate 70 patients in apparently complete remission at 1-year of follow-up. Ten percent had a tumor recurrence; all others except two had developed bronchial changes such as stenosis, hypervascularization, retraction, inflammatory signs, or infection. A high radiologic grade of lung fibrosis is often present, as reported previously (216). However, lung fibrosis generally was asymptomatic, and radiologic grading did not correlate with clinical symptoms. Three examples of lung fibrosis are shown in Figure 21.9. As shown in Figure 21.2, 8% of patients died free of neoplastic disease (32): in eight patients because of infectious disease, in two because of progressive lung fibrosis, in two because of pericarditis, in two because of neurologic symptoms without evidence of neurologic metastases, in one because of unexplained cachexia, and in one because of myocardial infarction.

LONG-TERM SURVIVAL

Previously, treatment with surgery or thoracic radiotherapy offered limited survival to patients with SCLC. With the modest improvement in cure rates and accrual of long-term survivors, the complications associated with chemotherapy, radiotherapy, and surgery have become apparent (218). Reporting of late toxicities has brought a new dimension to the management of patients with SCLC. The contribution of a specific treatment modality to a particular complication often is difficult to assess. Also, changing treatment approaches alter the range of treatment-related complications. Lastly, the extent to which early toxicity can predict later events remains to be determined.

Many series have reported a high incidence of new primary malignancies in long-term survivors (221–225). For instance, in a large series of 800 patients with SCLC treated in Toronto (223), the estimated relative risk for the development of secondary NSCLC tumors was 6.8 (CI 95%, 1.4–20). In the series of Johnson et al. (221) the estimated cumulative hazard function for the development of NSCLC was more than 25% at 9 years. In Copenhagen, Pedersen-Bjergaard et al, (226) reported a frequency of leukemia

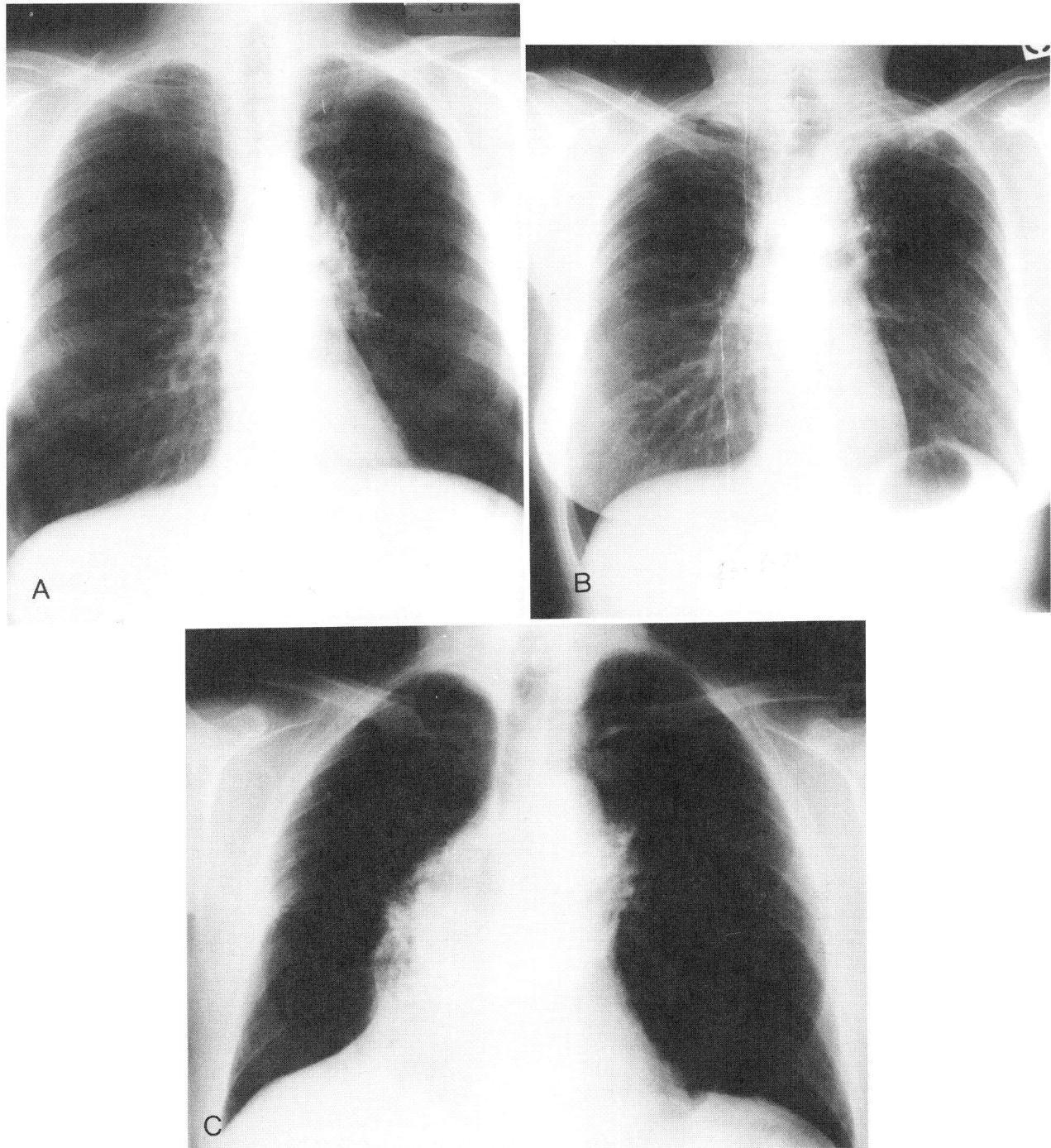

FIGURE 21.9. Examples of **A.** slight, **B.** moderate, and **C.** severe radiologic lung fibrosis observed at 2 years of follow-up in patients treated in the alternating chemotherapy-radiotherapy protocols. The three patients received a total radiation dose of 55 Gy in the mediastinum. (From Arriagada R, Cueto Ladron De Guevara J, Mouriesse H, et al. Limited small cell lung cancer treated by combined radiotherapy and chemotherapy: evaluation of a grading system of lung fibrosis. Radiother Oncol 1989;14:1–18.)

of 14% at 4 years, but it has been seen less frequently in other series (223, 227). Indeed, the estimation of second cancer rates is complicated by, for example, confusion over tumor recurrences, other competing risks, and underreporting (228). In the Institut Gustave-Roussy series of 346 patients (225), three late SCLC recurrences (at 5, 7, and 9 years) and 10 new primary malignancies (3 NSCLC, 2 gynecologic, 2 bladder, 1 larynx, 1 rectum, and 1 melanoma have been registered). An interesting observation is that cessation of smoking may be associated with a lower incidence of tobacco-related new primary malignancies, i.e., the relative risk of second primary NSCLC, decreases from 32 (CI 95%, 12–69) to 11 (CI 95%, 4–23) (225).

PERSPECTIVES

Combined treatments in solid tumors may provide a moderate survival benefit compared with treatment using a single modality. A large number of patients need to be evaluated in randomized trials to demonstrate a beneficial effect with combined treatment. If a survival benefit of 7% (intermediate between 5% and 10% is assumed), e.g., a change in the 2-year survival rate from 10% to 17%, a single trial would need more than 1000 patients to evaluate the question with α- and β-risks equal to .05. The assumed benefit of 7% is by no means negligible in limited SCLC because survival expectancy would be increased almost twofold.

Progress in improving survival in limited SCLC has been slow during the last two decades. The change in standard treatment from chest irradiation alone to chemotherapy alone in the 1970s increased the 5-year survival rate from roughly 5% to 10%. The combination of radiotherapy and chemotherapy in the 1980s yielded an additional benefit of 5%. Prophylactic cranial irradiation in complete responders might add a similar benefit (229). These moderate effects on survival should be tested in randomized trials with a large number of patients. Small- or medium-sized trials can result in equivocal answers or provide a mixture of positive and negative results; most of these contradictions may be caused by statistical variation.

Comprehensive meta-analyses using individual data may provide a solution to this problem. A case in point is the study that evaluated the role of chest irradiation in limited SCLC (25). One of the primary merits of this study was that it refuted the contention that meta-analysis was not a feasible means of evaluating the treatment effect in lung cancer (230). It also showed the advantages of meta-analyses based on individual data rather than on a review of the literature. The Pignon et al. study (25), summarized in Figure 21.5, concluded that chest irradiation afforded a survival benefit of 5% to 6% at 3 years; this conclusion is the mean effect of 13 randomized trials comprising more than 2000 patients. The next step will be to determine the optimal combined radiotherapy-chemotherapy schedule. One question has been answered, but many others are now emerging because combined approaches are multiparametric. It is inherent to scientific knowledge that each step forward generates new problems that are ever increasing in depth (231).

For the time being, physicians are unable to define the optimal combination required to treat limited SCLC. However, the most appropriate treatment for this disease is combination chemotherapy containing etoposide, cisplatin, and possibly cyclophosphamide, with chest irradiation to a minimum total dose of 50 Gy with a conventional fractionation schedule or its radiobiologic equivalent. Chest irradiation should be delivered without introducing a delay in the chemotherapy administration through the use of concurrent or alternating combined schedules.

The problems of defining optimal chest irradiation and optimal timing of chemotherapy and radiotherapy have been discussed. Because hundreds of patients are needed to test differences between two treatment approaches, it would be useless to compare very similar treatments. Years of research would be lost with this type of strategy. Treatments with rather extreme differences should be investigated (e.g., moderate versus high radiation doses, conventional versus unconventional fractionation, sequential versus nonsequential schedules) to test the validity of hypotheses. To optimize the management of SCLC with combined modalities, it is in the interest of patients that physicians investigate the questions raised, by conducting large randomized trials during the next few years.

Cytotoxic drugs with novel mechanisms of action also must be evaluated: the taxane derivatives (paclitaxel, docetaxel), which interfere with depolymerization of the tubulin molecules; camptothecin derivatives (topotecan, ironotecan), which target topoisomerase I; or difluorodeoxycytidine, a nucleoside analogue antimetabolite that disrupts DNA synthesis.

The increasing knowledge of SCLC biology allows investgators to test agents that could interfere with growth factors such as monoclonal antibodies or somatostatin analogues, or the manipulation of retinoic acid receptors or the correction of gene defects.

Another area is the evaluation of agents, such as verapamil or the triazine derivatives, that could reverse chemoresistance (232, 233).

Biologic response modifiers also should be evaluated, either to increase the treatment effect on tumor cells or to decrease toxicity to normal tissues (e.g., captopril to reduce radiation lung toxicity).

In conclusion, during the last 15 years, clinical research on limited SCLC has focused on combined chemotherapy-radiotherapy approaches. Overall, randomized trials on limited SCLC have shown that the combined approach is better than chemotherapy alone. A major trend in future clinical research on limited SCLC will be the exploration of optimizing combined approaches in randomized trials and other strategies that avoid or decrease the development of tumor cell resistance.

ACKNOWLEDGMENTS

The authors wish to thank all trialists who collaborated in the meta-analysis on the role of chest irradiation in limited SCLC (25). They also thank the Centre Hospitalier Intercommunal de Créteil, Hôpital A. Béclère, and Fondation Bergonié) participants in the IGR SCLC protocols, Mrs. M. Tarayre for data collection, Mrs. G. Feris for secretarial assistance, and Dr. J. A. Dewar for editing the manuscript. The IGR SCLC 010 protocol was partially supported by research grants ECC No. ST-A-000309; the IGR SCLC 010 and IGR SCLC 012 protocols were supported by research grant INSERM/CNAMTS No. 883063.

REFERENCES

1. Boring CC, Squires TS, Tong T. Cancer statistics. CA Cancer J Clin 1992;42:19–38.
2. Jensen OM, Esteve J, Moller H, Renard H. Cancer in the European Community and its member states. Eur J Cancer 1990; 26:1167–1256.
3. Fox W, Scadding JG. Medical Research Council comparative trial of surgery and radiotherapy for primary treatment of small-celled or oat-celled carcinoma of the bronchus. Lancet 1973;2:63–65.
4. Duchesne GM, Cassoni AM, Pera MF. Radiosensitivity related to neuroendocrine and endodermal differentiation in lung carcinoma lines. Radiother Oncol 1988;13:153–161.
5. Duchesne GM. Fundamental bases of combined therapy in lung cancer: cell resistance to chemotherapy and radiotherapy. Lung Cancer 1994;10(Suppl 1):S67–S72.
6. Carmichael J, Degraff W, Gamson J, et al. Radiation sensitivity of human cancer cell lines. Eur J Cancer Clin Oncol 1989; 25:527–534.
7. Einhorn LH, Fee WH, Farber MO, et al. Improved chemotherapy for small-cell undifferentiated lung cancer. JAMA 1976; 235:1225–1229.
8. Livingston RB, Einhorn LH, Bodey GP, et al. COMB (cyclophosphamide, oncovin, methyl-CCNU and bleomycin): a four-drug combination in solid tumors. Cancer 1975;36: 327–332.
9. Bunn PA, Van Zandwijk N, Pastorino U, et al. European School of Oncology. First Euro-American Forum on lung cancer treatment. Eur J Cancer 1994;30A:710–713.
10. World Health Organization. WHO Handbook for reporting the results of cancer treatment, Geneva: World Health Organization Offset Publication, 1979;48:319.
11. Mitchell JB, Morstyn G, Russo A, Carney DN. In vitro radiobiology of human lung cancer. Cancer Treat Symp 1985;2:3–10.
12. Gazdar AF, McDowell EM. Pathobiology of lung cancers. In: Biology of lung cancer: diagnosis and treatment. Rosen ST, Mulshine JL, Cuttita F, Abrams, PG, eds. New York: Marcel Dekker, 1988;1–42.
13. Chejfec G, Capella C, Solcia E, Jao W, Gould VE. Amphicrine cells, dysplasias and neoplasias. Cancer 1985;56:2683–2690.
14. Brigham BA, Bunn PA, Minna JD, Cohen MH, Ihde DC, Shackney SE. Growth rates of small cell bronchogenic carcinomas. Cancer 1978;42:2880–2886.
15. Charbit A, Malaise EP, Tubiana M. Relation between the pathological nature and the growth rate of human tumors. Eur J Cancer 1977;7:307–315.
16. Roswit B, Patno ME, Rapp R, Veinbergs A, Feder B, Stulbarg Cyprian BR. The survival of patients with inoperable lung cancer: a large-scale randomized study of radiation therapy versus placebo. Radiology 1968;90:688–697.
17. Minna JD, Pass H, Glatstein E, Ihde DC. Cancer of the lung. In: DeVita V, Hellman S, Rosenberg SA, eds. Principles and practice of oncology. 3rd ed. Philadelphia: JB Lippincott, 1989: 591–705.
18. Straus MJ. Characteristics of lung cancer. In: Straus MJ, ed. Lung cancer: clinical diagnosis and treatment. New York: Grune & Stratton, 1977;19–32.
19. Weiss W, Boucot KR, Cooper DA. Survival of men with peripheral lung cancer in relation to histologic characteristics and growth rate. Am Rev Respir Dis 1968;98:75–86.
20. Hansen HH. Diagnosis in metastatic sites. In: Straus MJ, ed. Lung cancer clinical diagnosis and treatment. New York: Grune & Stratton, 1983;185–200.
21. Newman SJ, Hansen HH. Frequency, diagnosis, and treatment of brain metastases in 247 consecutive patients with bronchogenic carcinoma. Cancer 1974;33:492–496.
22. Matthews MJ, Kanhouwa S, Pickren J, Robinette D. Frequency of residual and metastatic tumors in patients undergoing curative surgical resection for lung cancer. Cancer Chemother Rep 1973;4:63–67.
23. Bergsagel DE, Phil D, Jenkin RDT, et al. Lung cancer: clinical trial of radiotherapy alone versus radiotherapy plus cyclophosphamide. Cancer 1972;30:621–627.
24. Pignon JP, Arriagada R. Meta-analysis of radiotherapy for small cell lung cancer (reply). N Engl J. Med 1993;328:1425–1426.
25. Pignon JP, Arriagada R, Ihde DC, et al. Effect of thoracic radiotherapy on mortality in limited small cell lung cancer. A meta-analysis of 13 randomized trials among 2,140 patients. N Engl J Med 1992;327:1618–1624.
26. Fidler IJ, Hart IR. Biology diversity in metastatic neoplasms: origins and implications. Science 1982;217:998–1003.
27. Ura H, Bonfil RD, Reich R, et al. Expression of type IV collagen genes and its correlation with the tumorigenic, invasive, and metastatic abilities of oncogene-transformed human bronchial epithelial cells. Cancer Res 1987;47:1523–1528.
28. DeVita VT. Dose-response is alive and well. J Clin Oncol 1986;4:1157–1159.
29. Skipper HE, Schabel FM. Tumor stem cell heterogeneity: implications with respect to classification of cancers by chemotherapeutic effect. Cancer Treat Rep 1984;60:43–61.
30. Gelman R, Gelber R, Henderson IC, Coleman CN, Harris JR. Improved methodology for analyzing local and distant recurrence. J Clin Oncol 1990;8:548–555.
31. Kramar A, Arriagada R. Analyzing local and distant recurrence (letter). J Clin Oncol 1990;8:2086–2087.
32. Arriagada R, Kramar A, Le Chevalier T, De Cremoux H, for the French Cancer Centers' Lung Group. Competing events determining relapse-free survival in limited small-cell lung carcinoma. J Clin Oncol 1992;10:447–451.
33. Feld R, Arriagada R, Ball DL, Mattson K, Sorensen JB. Prognos-

tic factors in non–small cell lung cancer: a consensus report. Lung Cancer 1991;7:3–5.
34. Hansen HH, Perry M, Arriagada R, et al. Treatment evaluation in lung cancer. Lung Cancer 1994;10:S7–S9.
35. Rawson NSB, Peto J. An overview of prognostic factors in small cell lung cancer. Br J Cancer 1990;61:597–604.
36. Stahel R, Aisner J, Ginsberg R, et al. Staging and prognostic factors in small cell lung cancer. Lung Cancer 1989;5:1–8.
37. Sagman U, Feld R, Evans WK, et al. The prognostic significance of pretreatment serum lactate dehydrogenase in patients with small-cell lung cancer. J Clin Oncol 1991;9:954–961.
38. Baldeyrou P, Marrash R, LeChevalier T, Arriagada R. L'endoscopie bronchique dans le bilan diagnostique et évolutif des cancers broncho-pulmonaires à petites cellules. Bull Cancer 1987;74:511–515.
39. Shepherd FA. Screening, diagnosis, and staging of lung cancer. Curr Opin Oncol 1993;5:310–322.
40. Yang PC, Lee YC, Yu CJ, et al. Untrasonographically guided biopsy of thoracic tumors. Cancer 1992;69:2553–2560.
41. Hirsch FR, Osterlind K, Jensen LI, et al. The impact of abdominal computerized tomography on the pretreatment staging and prognosis of small cell lung cancer. Ann Oncol 1992;3:469–474.
42. Dearing MP, Steinberg SM, Phelps R, et al. Outcome of patients with small-cell lung cancer: effect of changes in staging procedures and imaging technology on prognostic factors over 14 years. J Clin Oncol 1990;8:1042–1049.
43. Ulsperger E, Shields T, Karrer K. The role of surgery in small cell lung cancer. Lung Cancer 1990;6:73–83.
44. Osterlind K. Surgery in small cell lung cancer: some quantitative aspects. A commentary. Lung Cancer 1990;6:84–86.
45. Hida T, Ariyoshi Y, Kuwabara M, et al. Glutathione S-transferase π levels in a panel of lung cancer cell lines and its relation to chemo-radiosensitivity. Jpn J Clin Oncol 1993;23:14–19.
46. Phillips TL, Mitchell JB, Degraff W, Russo A, Glatstein E. Variation in sensitising efficiency for SR 2508 in human cells dependent on glutathione content. Int J Radiat Oncol Biol Phys 1986;12:1627–1635.
47. Carmichael J, Hickson UD. Mechanisms of cellular resistance to cytotoxic drugs and X-irradiation. Int J Radiat Oncol Biol Phys 1991;20:197–202.
48. Groshar D, McEwan AJB, Parliament MB, et al. Imaging tumor hypoxia and tumor perfusion. J Nucl Med 1993;34:885–888.
49. Mitchell JB, Wink DA, Degraff W, Gamson J, Keefer LK, Krishna MC. Hypoxic mammalian cell radiosensitization by nitric oxide. Cancer Res 1993;53:5845–5848.
50. Arriagada R, Bertino Jr, Bleehen NM, et al. and the workshop participants. Consensus report on combined radiotherapy and chemotherapy modalities in lung cancer. In: Arriagada R, Le Chevalier T, eds. Treatment modalities in lung cancer. Antibiotics and chemotherapy. Basel: Karger, 1988;41:232–241.
51. Hansen HH. Management of small-cell cancer of the lung. Lancet 1992;339:846–849.
52. Arriagada R, Pignon JP, Le Chevalier T. The role of chest irradiation in small cell lung cancer. In: Hansen HH, ed. Lung cancer V. Boston: Kluwer Academic Publishing 1995:255–272.
53. Osterlind K, Hansen HH, Hansen HS, Dombernowsky P, Hansen M, Rorth M. Chemotherapy versus chemotherapy plus irradiation in limited small cell lung cancer. Results of a controlled trial with 5 years' follow-up. Br J Cancer 1986;54:7–17.
54. Bunn PA Jr, Lichter AS, Makuch RW, et al. Chemotherapy alone or chemotherapy with chest radiation therapy in limited stage small cell lung cancer: a prospective randomized trial. Ann Intern Med 1987;106:655–662.
55. Birch R, Omura GA, Greco FA, Perez CA. Patterns of failure in combined chemotherapy and radiotherapy for limited small cell lung cancer. Southeastern Cancer Group study experience. In: Wittes RD, Coleman CN, eds. Conference on the interaction of radiation therapy and chemotherapy. NCI 1986;6:265–270.
56. Kies MS, Mira JC, Crowley JJ, et al. Multimodal therapy for limited small cell lung cancer. A randomized study of induction combination chemotherapy with or without thoracic radiation in complete responders; and with widefield versus reduced volume radiation in partial responders: a Southwest Oncology Group study. J Clin Oncol 1987;5:592–600.
57. Nou E, Brodin O, Bergh J. A randomized study of radiation treatment in small cell bronchial carcinoma treated with two types of four-drug chemotherapy regimens. Cancer 1988;62:1079–1090.
58. Perry MC, Eaton WL, Propert KJ, et al. Chemotherapy with or without radiation therapy in limited small cell carcinoma of the lung. N Engl J Med 1987;316:912–918.
59. Ohnoshi T, Hiraki S, Kawahara S, et al. Randomized trial comparing chemotherapy alone and chemotherapy plus chest irradiation in limited stage small cell lung cancer: a preliminary report. Jpn J Clin Oncol 1986;16:271–277.
60. Bleehen NM, Radiotherapy for small cell lung cancer. Chest 1986;89:268S–276S.
61. Choi NC. Reassessment of the role of radiation therapy relative to other treatments in small-cell carcinoma of the lung. In: Choi NC, Grillo HC, eds. Thoracic oncology. New York: Raven Press, 1983:233–256.
62. Mantyla M, Nuranen A. The treatment volume in radiation therapy of small cell lung cancer (abstract 473). IV World Conference of lung cancer, Toronto, 1985:34.
63. Perez CA, Krauss S, Bartolucci AA, et al., and the Southeastern Cancer study Group. Thoracic and elective brain irradiation with concomitant or delayed multiagent chemotherapy in the treatment of localized small cell carcinoma of the lung: A randomized prospective study by the Southeastern Cancer Study Group. Cancer 1981;47:2407–2413.
64. White JE, Chen T, McCracken J, et al. The influence of radiation therapy quality control on survival, response and sites of relapse in oat cell carcinoma of the lung. Preliminary report of a Southwest Oncology Group Study. Cancer 1982;50:1084–1090.
65. Arriagada R, Pellae-Cosset B, Cueto Ladron De Guevara J et al. Alternating radiotherapy and chemotherapy schedules in limited small cell lung cancer: analysis of local chest recurrences. Radiother Oncol 1991;20:91–98.
66. Coy P, Hodson BM, payne D, et al. The effect of dose of thoracic irradiation on recurrence in patients with limited stage small cell lung cancer. Initial results of a Canadian multicenter randomized trial. Int J Radiat Oncol Biol Phys 1987;14:219–226.
67. Turrisi AT. Current radiotherapy perspectives for the treatment of limited small cell lung cancer. Lung Cancer 1994;11(Suppl 2):171–172.
68. Wagner H, Moffitt HL. Dose, volume, and fractionation issues in thoracic irradiation of small cell lung cancer. Lung Cancer 1994;11(Suppl 2):173–174.
69. Johnson DH, Kim K, Turrisi AT, et al, for the Eastern Cooperative Oncology Group. Cisplatin & etoposide + concurrent thoracic radiotherapy administered once versus twice daily for limited-stage small cell lung cancer: preliminary results of an intergroup trial. Proc Am Soc clin Oncol 1994;13:333.
70. Jenkin D, Chan H, Freedman M, et al. Hodgkin's disease

in children: treatment results with MOPP and low-dose, extended-field irradiation. Cancer Treat Rep 1982;66:949–959.
71. Turrisi A, Glover DJ. Thoracic radiotherapy variables: influence on local control in small cell lung cancer limited disease. Int J Radiat Oncol Biol Phys 1990;19:1473–1479.
72. Choi NC, Carey RW. Reassessment of loco-regional failure rate in relation with radiation dose in combined modality approach of multidrug chemotherapy and radiotherapy for limited-stage small-cell lung carcinoma. In: Arriagada R, Le Chevalier T, eds. Treatment modalities in lung cancer. Antibiotics and chemotherapy. Basel: Karger, 1988;41:70–76.
73. Turrisi AT, Kim K, Johnson DH, et al, for the Eastern Cooperative Oncology Group. Daily (QD) v twice (BID) thoracid irradiation (TI) with concurrent cisplatin-etoposide (PE) for limited small cell lung cancer (LSCLC). Preliminary results on 352 randomized eligible patients. Lung Cancer 1994;11:172.
74. Cox JD, Azarnia N, Byhart RW, Shin KH, Emami B, Pajak TF. A randomized phase I/II trial of hyperfractionated radiation therapy with total doses of 60.0 Gy to 79.2 Gy: possible survival benefit with ≥69.6 Gy in favorable patients with radiation therapy oncology group stage III non–small cell lung carcinoma: report of Radiation Therapy Oncology Group 83–11. J Clin Oncol 1990;8:1543–1555.
75. Sause WT, Scott C, Taylor S, et al. RTOG 8808 ECOG 4588, preliminary analysis of a phase III trial in regionally advanced unresectable non–small cell lung cancer. Proc Am Soc Clin Oncol 1994;13:325.
76. Tubiana M. Repopulation in human tumors. A biological background for fractionation in radiotherapy. Acta Oncol 1988;27:83–88.
77. Withers HR, Taylor JMG, Maciejewski B. The hazard of accelerated tumor clonogen repopulation during radiotherapy. Acta Oncol 1988;27:131–146.
78. Withers HR. Biologic basis for altered fractionation schemes. Cancer 1985;55:2086–2095.
79. Thames HD, Peters LJ, Withers HR, et al. Accelerated fractionation versus hyperfractionation: rationales for several treatments per day. Int J Radiat Oncol Biol Phys 1983;9:127–138.
80. Looney WB, Hopkins HA. The integration of multifractionated radiotherapy into combined chemotherapeutic-radiotherapeutic approaches to lung cancer treatment. In: Treatment modalities in lung cancer. Antibiotics and chemotherapy. Arriagada R, Le Chevalier T, eds. Basel: Karger, 1988;41:176–183.
81. Turrisi AT, Glover DJ, Mason BA. A preliminary report: concurrent twice-daily radiotherapy plus platinum-etoposide chemotherapy for limited small cell lung cancer. Int J Radiat Oncol Biol Phys 1988;15:183–187.
82. Johnson B. Concurrent approaches to combined chemotherapy and chest radiotherapy for the treatment of patients with limited stage small cell lung cancer. Lung Cancer 1994;10 (Suppl 1):S281–S287.
83. Kinzie JJ, Hanks GE, Maclean CJ, Kramer S. PCS outcome studies: Hodgkin's disease relapse rates and adquacy of portals. Cancer 1983;52:2223–2226.
84. Kramer S, Hanks GE, Maclean CJ. Paterns of failure: results of the Patterns of Care study in cancer of larynx, prostate, cervix and Hodgkins's disease. Cancer Treat Symp 1983;2:157–168.
85. Perez CA, Bauer M, Edelstein S, Gillespie BW, Birch R. Impact of tumor control on survival in carcinoma of the lung treated with irradiation. Int J Radiat Oncol Biol Phys 1986;12:539–547.
86. Chavaudra J, Arriagada R. Radiotherapy planning in lung cancer. Approach of the Institut Gustav-Roussy. Cancer Treat Symp 1985;2:87–91.
87. Medical Research Council Lung Cancer Working Party. Radiotherapy alone or with chemotherapy in the treatment of small-cell carcinoma of the lung: the results at 36 months. Br J Cancer 1981;44:611–617.
88. Krauss S, Perez C, Lowenbraun S, et al. Combined modality treatment of localized small cell lung carcinoma. A randomized study of the Southeastern Cancer Study Group. Cancer Clin Trials 1990;3:297–306.
89. Arriagada R, Le Chevalier T. Therapeutic advances in small cell bronchial cancers. Presse Med 1988;17:1851–1856.
90. Feinstein AR, Sosin DM, Wells CK. The Will Rogers phenomenon. Stage migration and new diagnostic techniques as a source of misleading statistics for survival in cancer. N Engl J Med 1985;312:1604–1608.
91. Einhorn LH Bond WH, Hornback N, Beng-Tek J. Long-term results in combined modality treatment of small cell carcinoma of the lung. Semin Oncol 1978;5:309–313.
92. Chahinian AP, Propert KJ, Ware JH, et al. A randomized trial of anticoagulation with warfarin and of alternating chemotherapy in extensive small-cell lung cancer by the Cancer and Leukemia Group B. J Clin Oncol 1989;7:993–1002.
93. Greco FA, Richardson RL, Snall JD, Stroup SL, Oldham RK. Small cell lung cancer: complete remission and improved survival. Am J Med 1979;66:625–630.
94. Feld R, Evans WK, DeBoer G, et al. Combined modality induction therapy without maintenance chemotherapy for small cell carcinoma of the lung. J Clin Oncol 1984;2:294–303.
95. Livingston RB, Mira JG, Ghen TT, McGavran M, Costanzi JJ, Samson M. Combined modality treatment of extensive small cell lung cancer: a Southwest Oncology Group study. J Clin Oncol 1984;2:585–590.
96. Aisner J, Whitacre M, Van Echo DA, Wesley M, Wiernik PH. Doxorubicin, cyclophosphamide and VP16-213 (ACE) in the treatment of small cell lung cancer. Cancer Chemother Pharmacol 1982;7:187–193.
97. Evans WK, Feld R, Murray N, et al. The use of VP-16 plus cisplatin during induction chemotherapy for small cell lung cancer. Semi Oncol 1986;13:10–16.
98. Goldie JH, Coldman AJ, Ng V, Hopkins HA, Looney WB. A mathematical and computer-based model of alternating chemotherapy and radiation therapy in experimental neoplasms. In; Antibiotics and chemotherapy. Treatment modalities in lung cnacer. Arriagada R, Le Chevalier T, eds. Karger, Basel. Antibiot Chemother. 1988;41:11–20.
99. Goldie AG. Drug resistance. In: Perry MC, ed. The chemotherapy source book. Baltimore: Williams & Wilkins, 1992:54–66.
100. Tannock If. Experimental chemotherapy. In: Tannock IF, Hill RP, eds. The basic science of oncology. 2nd ed. New York: McGraw-Hill, 1992:338–359.
101. Twentyman PR. Multidrug resistance in lung cancer. Lung Cancer 1994;11:203–204.
102. Doyle LA. Mechanisms of drug resistance in human lung cancer cells. Semin Oncol 1993;20:326–337.
103. Saijo N. Molecular mechanisms of drug resistance of lung cancer. Lung Cancer 1994;11:205–206.
104. Ozols RF, O'Dwyer P. Clinical reversal of drug resistance. Lung Cancer 1994;11:207–208.
105. Goldie GH, Coldman AG. The genetic origin of drug resistance in neoplasm: implications for systemic therapy. Cancer Res 1984;44:3643–3663.
106. Elliot JA, Osterlind K, Hansen H. Cyclic alternating "non cross resistant" chemotherapy in the management of small cell anaplastic carcinoma of the lung. Cancer Treat Rev 1984;11:103–113.

107. Alberto P, Berchtold W, Sonntag R, Barrelet L, Jungi F, Martz G, Obrecht P. Chemotherapy of small cell carcinoma of the lung: comparison of cyclic alternative combination with simultaneous combinations of four and seven agents. Eur J Cancer Clin Oncol 1981;17:1027–1033.

108. Krauss S, Lowenbraun S, Bartolucci A, Buchanan R, Birch R. Alternating non–cross resistant drug combinations in the treatment of small cell carcinoma of the lung. Cancer Clin Trials 1981;4:147–153.

109. Ettinger DS, Lagakos S. Phase III study of CCNU, cyclophosphamide, Adriamycin, vincristine and VP-16 in small cell carcinoma of the lung. Cancer 1982;49:1544–1554.

110. Østerlind K, Sorenson S, Hansen HH, et al. Treatment of advanced small cell carcinoma of the lung: continuous versus alternating combination chemotherapy. Cancer Res 1983;43:6085–6089.

111. Daniels JR, Chak LY, Sikic BI, et al. Chemotherapy of small cell carcinoma of lung: a randomized comparison of alternating and sequential combination chemotherapy programs. J Clin Ondcol 1984;2:1192–1199.

112. Feld R, Evans WK, Coy P, et al. Canadian multicenter randomized trial comparing sequential and alternating administration of two non–cross-resistant chemotherapy combinations in patients with limited small-cell carcinoma of the lung. J Clin Oncol 1987;5:1401–1409.

113. Havemann K, Wolf M, Holle R, et al. Alternating versus sequential chemotherapy in small-cell lung cancer. A randomized German multicenter trial. Cancer 1987;59:1072–1082.

114. Østerlind K. Alternating or sequential chemotherapy in small cell lung cancer? Lung Cancer 1989;5:55–59.

115. Roth JA, Johnson DH, Greco FA, et al. A phase III trial of etoposide and cisplatin versus cyclophosphamide, doxorubicin and vincristine versus alternation of the two therapies for patients with extensive small cell lung cancer: preliminary results. Proc Am Soc Clin Oncol 1989;8:225.

116. Maksymiuk AW, Jett JR, Earle JD, et al. Sequencing and schedule effects of cisplatin plus etoposide in small cell lung cancer—results of a North Central Cancer Treatment Group randomized clinical trial. J Clin Oncol 1994;12:70–76.

117. Cohen MH, Creaven PJ, Fossieck BE, et al. Intensive chemotherapy of small cell bronchogenic carcinoma. Cancer Treat Rep 1977;61:349–354.

118. Arriagada R, De The H, Le Chevalier T, et al. Limited small cell lung cancer: possible prognostic impact of initial chemotherapy doses. Bull Cancer 1989;76:605–615.

119. De Vathaire F, Arriagada R, De The H, et al. Dose intensity of initial chemotherapy may have an impact on survival in limited small cell lung carcinoma. Lung Cancer 1993;8:301–308.

120. Arriagada R, Le Chevalier T, Pignon JP, et al. Initial chemotherapeutic doses and survival in patients with limited small cell lung cancer. N Engl J Med 1993;329:1848–1852.

121. Dinwoodie WR, Lyman GH, Williams CC. Intensive combination chemotherapy and radiotherapy for small cell bronchogenic carcinoma (abstract C-675). Proc Am Assoc Cancer Res 1981;22:505.

122. Figueredo A, Hryniuk WM, Strautmanis I, Frank G, Rendell S. Co-trimoxazole prophylaxis during high-dose chemotherapy of small-cell lung cancer. J Clin Oncol 1985;3:54–64.

123. Johsnon DH, Einhorn LH, Birch R, et al., and the Southeastern Cancer Study Group. A randomized comparison of high-dose versus conventional-dose cyclophosphamide, doxorubicin, and vincristine for extensive-stage small-cell lung cancer: a phase III trial of the Southeastern Cancer Study Group. J Clin Oncol 1987;5:1731–1738.

124. Ihde D, Mulshine J, Kramer B, et al. Randomized trial of high versus standard dose VP16/cisplatin in extensive small cell lung cancer. Lung Cancer 1991;7(Suppl):135.

125. Mehta C, Vogl SE. High-dose cyclophosphamide in the induction chemotherapy of small cell lung cancer–minor improvements in the rate of remission and survival. Proc Am Assoc Cancer Res 1982;23:155.

126. Antman KH. Souhami RL. High dose chemotherapy in solid tumours. Ann Oncol 1993;4:S29–S44.

127. Hande Kr, Oldham RK, Fer MF, et al. Randomized study of high-dose versus low-dose methotrexate in the treatment of extensive small cell lung cancer. Am J Med 1982;73:413–419.

128. Humblet Y, Symann M, Bosly A, et al. Late intensification chemotherapy with autologous bone marrow transplantation in selected small-cell carcinoma of the lung: a randomized study. J Clin Oncol 1987;5:1864–1873.

129. Crawford J, Ozer H, Stoller R, et al. Reduction by granulocyte colony-stimulating factor of fever neutropenia induced by chemotherapy in patients with small-cell lung cancer. N Engl J Med 1991;315:164–170.

130. Trillet V, Green J, Manegold C, et al. Recombinant granulocyte colony stimulating factor reduces the infectious complications of cytotoxic chemotherapy. Eur J Cancer 1993;29A:319–324.

131. Elias AD. Chemotherapy III–small cell lung cancer. Lung Cancer 1994;11:136–137.

132. Stahel RA, Mabry M, Sabbath K, Speak JA, Bernal SD. Selective cytotoxicity of murine monclonal antibody LAM2 against human small-cell carcinoma in the presence of human complement: possible use for in vitro elimination of tumor cells from bone marrow. Int J Cancer 1985;35:587–592.

133. Postmus PE. Small cell lung cancer and the use of interleukin-3. Lung Cancer 1994;11:189–190.

134. Metcalf D. Thrombopoietin—at last. Nature 1994;369:519–520.

135. Bunn PA, Arriagada R, Choi N, et al. Combined modality therapy in small cell lung cancer. Lung Cancer 1994;10(Suppl 1):S25–S28.

136. Cox J, Ball D, Belani C, et al. Dose intensity in lung cancer treatment. Lung Cancer 1994;10(Suppl 1):S11–S13.

137. Sculier JP, Paesmans M, Bureau G, et al. Multiple-drug weekly chemotherapy versus standard combination regimen in small cell lung cancer—a phase III randomized study conducted by the European Lung Cancer Working Party. J Clin Oncol 1993;11:1858–1865.

138. Miles DW, Earl HM, Souhami RL, et al. Intensive weekly chemotherapy for good-prognosis patients with small cell lung cancer. J Clin Oncol 1991;9:280–285.

139. Miles DW, Fogarty O, Ash CM, et al. Received dose-intensity—a randomized trial of weekly chemotherapy with and without granulocyte colony-stimulating factor in small-cell lung cancer. J Clin Oncol 1994;12:77–82.

140. Murray N. Weekly chemotherapy for small cell lung cancer. Lung Cancer 1994;11:138–139.

141. Murray N, Shah A, Osoba D, et al. Intensive weekly chemotherapy for the treatment of extensive-stage small-cell lung cancer. J Clin Oncol 1991;9:1632–1638.

142. Maurer LH, Tulloh M, Weiss RB, et al. A randomized combined modality trial in small cell carcinoma of the lung/comparison of combination chemotherapy-radiation therapy versus cyclophosphamide-radiation therapy effects of maintenance chemotherapy and prophylactic whole brain irradiation. Cancer 1980;45:30–39.

143. Woods RL, Levi JA. Chemotherapy for small cell lung cancer (SCLC): a randomized study of maintenance therapy with cy-

clophosphamide, Adriamycin and vincristine (CAV) after remission induction with cis-platinum (CIS DDP), VP16-213 and radiotherapy (meeting abstracts). Proc Am Soc Clin Oncol 1984;3:214.
144. Cullen M, Morgan D, Gregory W, et al., and the Midlands Small Cell Lung Cancer Group. Maintenance chemotherapy for anaplastic small cell carcinoma of the bronchus: a randomized, controlled trial. Cancer Chemother Pharmacol 1986;17:157–160.
145. Medical Council Research Lung Cancer Working Party, Gregory W. Controlled trial of twelve versus six courses of chemotherapy in the treatment of small cell lung cancer. Br J Cancer 1989;59:584–590.
146. Spiro SG, Souhami RL, Geddes DM, et al. Duration of chemotherapy in small cell lung cancer: a Cancer Research Campaign trial. Br J Cancer 1989;59:578–583.
147. Byrne MJ, Van Hazel G, Trotter J, et al. Maintenance chemotherapy in limited small cell lung cancer: a randomized controlled clinical trial. Br J Cancer 1989;60:413–418.
148. Ettinger Ds, Finkelstein DM, Abeloff MD, Ruckdeschel JC, Aisner SC, Eggleston JC. A randomized comparison of standard chemotherapy versus alternating chemotherapy and maintenance versus no maintenance therapy for extensive-stage small-cell lung cancer: a phase III study of the Eastern Cooperative Oncology Group. J Clin Oncol 1990;8:230–240.
149. Lebeau B, Chastang CL, Allard P, Migueres J, Boita F, Fichet D, and the Petites Cellules group. Six vs twelve cycles for complete responders to chemotherapy in small cell lung cancer; definitive results of a randomized clinical trial. Eur Respir J 1992;5:286–290.
150. Giaccone G, Dalesio O, McVie GJ, et al., for the EORTC group. Maintenance chemotherapy in small-cell lung cancer: long-term results of a randomized trial. J Clin Oncol 1993;11:1230–1240.
151. Mattson K, Niiranen A, Pyrhönen S, et al. Natural interferon alfa as maintenance therapy for small cell lung cancer. Eur J Cancer 1992;28A:1387–1391.
152. Fishbein GE. Immunotherapy of lung cancer. Semin Oncol 1993;20:351–358.
153. McCraken J, Heilbrun L, White J, et al. Combination chemotherapy, radiotherapy, and BCG immunotherapy in extensive (metastatic) small cell carcinoma of the lung. Cancer 1980;46:2335–2340.
154. Aisner J, Wiernik PH. Chemotherapy versus chemoimmunotherapy for small cell undifferentiated carcinoma of the lung. Cancer 1980;46:2543–2549.
155. Lipson SD, Chretien PB, Makuch R, Kenady DE, Cohen MH. Thymosin immunotherapy in patients with small cell carcinoma of the lung. Correlation of in vitro studies with clinical course. Cancer 1979;43:863–870.
156. Scher H, Chapman R, Shank B, et al. Combination chemotherapy and radiotherapy with and without thymosin in small cell lung cancer (abstract 207). Third World Conference on Lung Cancer, Tokyo, 1982.
157. Jett JR. Is there a role for interferon in the treatment of small cell lung cancer? Lung Cancer 1989;5(4–6):163–168.
158. Clamon G, Herndon J, Perry MC, et al. Interleukin-2 activity in patients with extensive small cell lung cancer: a phase II trial of Cancer and Leukemia Group B. J Natl Cancer Inst 1993;85:316–320.
159. Standford CF. Anticoagulants in the treatment of small cell carcinoma of the bronchus. Thorax 1979;34:113–116.
160. Zacharski LR, Henderson WG, Rickles FR, et al. Rationale and experimental design for the VA Cooperative Study of anticoagulation (warfarin) in the treatment of cancer. Cancer 1979;44:732–741.
161. Gasic GJ, Gasic TB, Murphy S. Antimetastatic effect of aspirin. Lancet 1972;2:932–933.
162. Zacharski LR, Henderson WG, Rickles FR, et al. Effect of warfarin anticoagulation on survival in carcinoma of the lung, colon, head and neck, and prostate. Cancer 1984;53:2046–2052.
163. Lebeau B, Chastang C, Muir JF, Vincent J, Massin F, Fabre C. No effect of an antiaggregant treatment with aspirin in small cell lung cancer treated with CCAVP16 chemotherapy—results from a randomized clinical trial of 303 patients. Cancer 1993;71:1741–1745.
164. Lebeau B, Chastang C, Brechot JM, et al., for the Petites Cellules group. Subcutaneous heparin treatment increases survival in small cell lung cancer. Cancer 1994;74:38–45.
165. Ginsberg RG. Surgery for small cell lung cancer. Lung Cancer 1993;9:275–280.
166. Shields TW, Higgins GA, Matthews MJ, Keehn RJ. Surgical resection in the management of small-cell carcinoma of the lung. J Thorac Cardiovasc Surg 1982;84:481–488.
167. Lad T, Thoms P, Piantadosi S. Surgical resection of small cell lung cancer: a prospective randomized evaluation (abstract). Lung Cancer 1991;7:162.
168. Mitchell JB, Gamson J, Russo A, et al. Chinese hamster pleiotropic multidrug resistant cells are not radioresistant. NCI Monogr 1988;6:187–191.
169. Sklar MD. The ras oncogenes increase the intrinsic resistance of NIH 3T3 cells to ionizing radiation. Science 1988;239:645–647.
170. Wallner K, Li GC. Adriamycin resistance, heat resistance and radiation response in Chinese hamster fibroblasts. Int J Radiat Oncol Biol Phys 1986;12:829–833.
171. Arriagada R, Cosset JM, Le Chevalier T, Tubiana M. The value of adjunctive radiotherapy when chemotherapy is the major curative method. Int J Radiat Oncol Biol Phys 1990;19:1279–1284.
172. Tannock IF. Combined modality treatment with radiotherapy and chemotherapy. Radiother Oncol 1989;16:83–101.
173. Tubiana M, Arriagada R, Cosset JM. Sequencing of drugs and radiation. The integrated alternating regimen. Cancer 1985;55:2131–2139.
174. Tubiana M, Arriagada R, Cosset JM. Optimizing combinations of drugs and radiation. The interdigitated alternating regimen. In: Withers HR, Peters LJ, ed. Innovations in radiation oncology. Berlin: Springer-Verlag, 1988:265–276.
175. Tannock IF. New perspectives in combined radiotherapy and chemotherapy treatment. Lung Cancer 1994;10:S29–S51.
176. Tubiana M. The 1987 Franz Buschke lecture: the role of radiotherapy in the treatment of chemosensitive tumors. Int J Radiat Oncol Biol Phys 1989;16:763–774.
177. Auquier A, Rutqvist LE, Rotstein S, Arriagada R. Post-mastectomy megavoltage radiotherapy: the Oslo and Stockholm trials. Eur J Cancer 1992;28:433–437.
178. DeVita VT. The relationship between tumor mass and resistance chemotherapy: implications for surgical adjuvant treatment of cancer. Cancer 1983;51:1209–1220.
179. Ensley JF, Jacobs JR, Weaver A, et al. Correlation between response to cis-platinum combination and subsequent radiotherapy in previously untreated patients with advanced squamous cell cancers of the head and neck. Cancer 1984;54:811–814.
180. Schwartz JL, Rotmensch J, Beckett MA, et al. X-ray and cis-diamminedichloroplatinum (II) cross-resistance in human tumor cell lines. Cancer Res 1988;48:5133–5135.

181. Rosenthal MA, Tattersall MHN, Fox RM, Woods RL, Brodie GN. Adjuvant thoracic radiotherapy in small cell lung cancer: ten-year follow-up of a randomized study. Lung Cancer 1991;7:235–241.
182. Souhami RL, Geddes DM, Spiro SG, et al. Radiotherapy in small cell cancer of the lung treated with combination chemotherapy: a controlled trial. BMJ 1984;288:1643–1646.
183. Joss R, Alberto P, Bleher E, Kapanci Y, Cavalli F. Combined modality treatment of small cell lung cancer: randomized comparison of three induction chemotherapies followed by maintenance chemotherapy with or without radiotherapy of the chest. In: Proceedings of the Fourth World Conference on Lung Cancer, Toronto, 1985:141.
184. Creech R, Richter M, Finkelstein D. Combination chemotherapy with or without consolidation radiation therapy (RT) for regional small cell carcinoma of the lung (abstract). Proc Am Soc Clin Oncol 1989;7:196.
185. Lebeau B, Chastang C, Brechot JM, Capron F. A randomized trial of delayed thoracic radiotherapy in complete responder patients with small-cell lung cancer. Chest 1993;104:726–733.
186. Brooks BJ Jr, Seifter EJ, Walsh TE, et al. Pulmonary toxicity with combined modality therapy for limited stage small-cell lung cancer. J Clin Oncol 1986;4:200–209.
187. Fu KK. Biological basis for the interaction of chemotherapeutic agents and radiation therapy. Cancer 1985;55:2123–2130.
188. LaGrange JL, Thyss A, Caldani C, Hery M, Schneider M, Bensadoun JR. Toxicity of combination of ABVD chemotherapy and mediastinal irradiation for Hodgkin disease patients with massive initial mediastinal involvement. Bull Cancer 1988;75:801–806.
189. Verschoore J, LaGrange JL, Boublil JL, et al. Pulmonary toxicity of a combination of low-dose doxorubicin and irradiation for inoperable lung cancer. Radiother Oncol 1987;9:281–288.
190. Murray N, Coy P, Pater JL, et al. Importance of timing for thoracic irradiation in the combined modality treatment of limited-stage small cell lung cancer. J Clin Oncol 1993;11:336–344.
191. Nielsen OS, Fode K, Bentzen SM, Schultz HP, Steenholdt S, Palshof T. timing of radiotherapy and chemotherapy in limited stage small cell lung cancer. Final analysis (abstract). Eur J cancer 1991;Suppl 2:S182.
192. Turrisi AT. Considerations on radiotherapy dose intensity for limited small cell lung cancer. Lung Cancer 1994;10(Suppl 1):S167–S173.
193. Turrisi AT. Innovations in multimodality therapy for lung cancer. Combined modality management of limited small-cell lung cancer. Chet 1993;103:S56–S59.
194. Looney WB. Special lecture: alternating chemotherapy and radiotherapy. NCI Monogr 1988;6:85–94.
195. Arriagada R, Le Chevalier T, Baldeyrou P, et al. Alternating radiotherapy and chemotherapy schedules in small cell lung cancer, limited disease. Int J Radiat Oncol Biol Phys 1985;11:1461–1467.
196. Le Chevalier T, Arriagada R, De The H, et al. Combination of chemotherapy and radiotherapy in limited small cell lung carcinoma: results of alternating schedule in 109 patients. NCI Monogr 1988;6:335–338.
197. Johnson DH, Turrisi AT, Chang AY, et al. Alternating chemotherapy and twice-daily thoracic radiotherapy in limited-stage small-cell lung cancer—a pilot study of the Eastern Cooperative Oncology Group. J Clin Oncol 1993;11:879–884.
198. Bleehen N, Girling DJ, Gregor A, et al., on behalf of the Medical Research Council Lung Cancer Working Group. A Medical Research Council phase II trial of alternating chemotherapy and radiotherapy in small-cell lung cancer. Br J Cancer 1991;64:775–779.
199. Bleehen NM, Girling DJ, Machin D, et al. A randomized trial of 3 or 6 courses of etoposide, cyclophosphamide, methotrexate and vincristine or six courses of etoposide and ifosfamide in small cell lung cancer. 1. Survival and prognostic factors. Br J Cancer 1993;68:1150–56.
200. Gregor A, Postmus P, Burghouts J, et al. Combined modality treatment of small cell carcinoma of the bronchus. The EORTC LCCG experience. Lung Cancer 1994;11:175–176.
201. Arriagada R, Le Chevalier T, Baldeyrou P, et al. Alternating radiotherapy and chemotherapy with doxorubicin, etoposide, cyclophosphamide, and cisplatin in limited small cell lung cancer. Cancer Treat Symp 1985;2:115–117.
202. Lebeau B, Chastang C, Brechot JM, et al., and the Petites Cellules group. Limited small cell lung cancer: a randomized comparison of concurrent and alternated thoracic irradiation. Lung Cancer 1994;11:171.
203. Comis RL. Oral etoposide in small cell lung cancer. Semin Oncol 1986;13:75–78.
204. Carney DN, Bryne A. Chemotherapy for the elderly or unfit patient with small cell lung cancer. Lung Cancer 1994;11:140–141.
205. Murray N, Grafton C, Shah A, et al. Abbreviated treatment for elderly and infirm patients with limited stage small cell lung cancer. Lung Cancer 1994;11:171.
206. Johnson DH. Treatment of relapsed small cell lung cancer. Lung Cancer 1994;11:142–143.
207. Faylona E, Loehrer P, Einhorn L, Ansari R, McClean J, Williams S. A phase II study of daily oral VP-16 + ifosfamide + cisplatin for previously treated small cell lung cancer (SCLC): a Hoosier Oncology Group (HOG) trial. Proc Am Soc Clin Oncol 1992;11:307.
208. Arriagada R, Pignon JP, Le Chevalier T. Thoracic radiotherapy in small cell lung cancer: rationale for timing and fractionation. Lung Cancer 1989;5:237–247.
209. Travis EL, Liao Z. Fractionation and volume as factors in radiation injury in the lung. Lung Cancer 1994;11:114–115.
210. Ward WF, Molteni A, Ts'ao C, Taylor JM, Mechanisms and modifiers of radiation pneumotoxicity. Lung Cancer 1994;11:116–117.
211. Gross NJ. Pulmonary effects of radiation therapy. Ann Intern Med 1977;86:81–82.
212. Ward WF, Lin PP, Wong P, et al. Pneumonitis in rats and its modification by the angiotensine-converting enzyme inhibitor captopril evaluated by high-resolution computed tomography. Radiat Res 1993;135:81–87.
213. Marks LB. The pulmonary effects of thoracic irradiation. Oncology 1994;8:89–104.
214. Arriagada R, Pellae-Cosset B, Baldeyrou P, et al. Initial high dose chemotherapy and multifractionated radiotherapy in limited small cell lung cancer (abstract). Lung Cancer 1991;7(Suppl):159.
215. Hellman S, Cligerman MM, Von Essen CF, et al. Sequelae of radical radiotherapy of carcinoma of the lung. Radiology 1964;82:1055–1061.
216. Arriagada R, Cueto Ladron De Guevara J, Mouriesse H, et al. Limited small cell lung cancer treated by combined radiotherapy and chemotherapy: evaluation of a grading system of lung fibrosis. Radiother Oncol 1989;14:1–18.
217. Trask CW, Joannides T, Harper PG, et al. Radiation-induced lung fibrosis after treatment of small cell carcinoma of the lung with very high-dose cyclophosphamide. Cancer 1983;55:57–60.

218. Feld R. Complications associated with the treatment of small cell lung cancer. Lung Cancer 1994;10:S307–S317.
219. Ginsberg SJ, Comis RL. The pulmonary toxicity of antineoplastic agents. Semin Oncol 1982;9:34–51.
220. Arriagada R, Bouhnik H, Sarrazin D. Myélopathie post-radiothérapique tardive. In: Lemerle J, ed. Actualités carcinologiques, Institut Gustave-Roussy. Paris: Masson Publishing 1984:25–33.
221. Johnson BE, Grayson J, Makuch RW, et al. Ten-year survival of patients with small-cell lung cancer treated with combination chemotherapy with or without irradiation. J clin Oncol 1990;8:396–401.
222. Ihde D, Tucker MA. Second primary malignancies in small cell lung cancer: a major consequence of modest success. J Clin Oncol 1992;10:1511–1513.
223. Sagman U, Lishner M, Maki E, et al. Second primary malignancies following diagnosis of small cell lung cancer. J Clin Oncol 1992;10:1525–1533.
224. Heyne KH, Lippman SM, Lee JJ, Lee JS, Hong WK. The incidence of second primary tumors in long term survivors of small cell lung cancer. J Clin Oncol 1992;10:1519–1524.
225. Richardson GE, Tucker MA, Venzon DJ, et al. Smoking cessation after successful treatment of small-cell lung cancer is associated with fewer smoking-related second primary cancers. Ann Intern Med 1993;119:383–390.
226. Pedersen-Bjergaard J, Østerlind K, Hansen M, Philip P, Pedersen P, Hansen HH. Acute non-lymphocytic leukemia, preleukemia and solid tumors following intensive chemotherapy of small cell lung carcinoma of the lung. Blood 1985;66:1393–1397.
227. Johnson DH, Porter LL, List AF, Hande KR, Hainsworth JD, Greco FA. Acute non-lymphocytic leukemia after treatment of small cell lung cancer. am J Med 1986;81:962–968.
228. Arriagada R, Rutqvist LE. Adjuvant chemotherapy in early breast cancer and incidence of new primary malignancies. Lancet 1991;338:535–538.
229. Arriagada R, Le Chevalier T, Borie F, et al. Randomized trials on prophylactic cranial irradiation for patients with small cell lung cancer in complete remission. Lung Cancer 1994;11:177–178.
230. Nicolucci Am, Grilli R, Alexanian AA, Apolone G, Torri V, Liberati A. Quality, evolution, and clinical implications of randomized, controlled trials on the treatment of lung cancer. A lost opportunity formeta-analysis. JAMA 1989;262:2101–2107.
231. Popper KR. Conjectures and refutations. In: The growth of scientific knowledge. 5th ed. London: Routledge Publishing, 1989.
232. Milroy R. A randomized clinical study of verapamil in addition to combination chemotherapy in small cell lung cancer. Br J Cancer 1993;68:813–818.
233. Regnier G, Dhainaut A, Atassi A. New triazine derivatives as potent modulators of multidrug resistance. J Med Chem 1992;35:2481–2496.

22

THERAPEUTIC APPROACH TO DISSEMINATED SMALL CELL LUNG CANCER

Masahiro Fukuoka, Noriyuki Masuda, and Yutaka Ariyoshi

INTRODUCTION

Small cell lung cancer (SCLC) accounts for approximately one fifth of the primary lung cancers (1), and it biologically has different characteristic properties compared with the other types of lung cancer. These include rapid tumor growth, early metastases, and prominent sensitivity to chemotherapy and radiotherapy.

Concerning treatment, surgery or radiotherapy was the major modality for the treatment of SCLC until the end of the 1960s. There were very few long-term survivors, however, because of the early appearance of distant metastases. In fact, by the time the diagnosis of SCLC is established, dissemination to distant organs has occurred in two thirds of patients with SCLC (2). Because of early dissemination, SCLC generally is recognized as a systemic disease. This evidence was first described clearly by autopsy data in patients dying from non–cancer-related causes within 30 days after curative surgical resection of lung cancer (3).

In 1969, a randomized trial by the Veterans Administration Lung Cancer Study Group reported that three courses of cyclophosphamide administration brought more than doubled median survival compared with a placebo-treated control group in disseminated SCLC (4). Consequently, chemotherapy has been the principal therapeutic modality for treatment of this disease, especially in the disseminated stage. This was the starting point of the chemotherapy era for SCLC. Since then, the task of identifying new active agents for SCLC has been initiated. The search for more effective antitumor agents over the past 20 years has led to the discovery of only a few active agents.

Conversely, intensive clinical trials of combination chemotherapy including active agents for SCLC have improved both survival and the control of symptoms. In 1981, the role of chemotherapy for the treatment of SCLC was described in the consensus report of the International Association for the Study of Lung Cancer Workshop (5). However, regrettably, major improvements in survival have not been observed in the last decade. Presently there is a consensus regarding the application of chemotherapy for SCLC (5): (*a*) combination chemotherapy is more effective than single agents; (*b*) combinations should be based on active single agents; and (*c*) treatment should be aggressive for maximal results. But no combination chemotherapy regimens was able to cure a large fraction of patients. Because each single active agent could be the basis for improved therapeutic results in SCLC, development of newer active agents remains the cornerstone of future advances in the treatment of this disease.

In this chapter, therapeutic approaches to the treatment of disseminated SCLC are reviewed and include single-agent chemotherapy, combination chemotherapy, dose intensive chemotherapy, and supportive therapy.

SINGLE-AGENT CHEMOTHERAPY

CHEMOTHERAPEUTIC AGENTS WITH DOCUMENTED ACTIVITY AGAINST SMALL CELL LUNG CANCER

Grant et al. (6) recently reviewed all of the published phase II trials (1970 to 1990) of 57 agents in more than 3,000 patients with SCLC. An agent active against SCLC was defined as one demonstrating a response rate of at least 20% in a trial with more than 14 assessable patients. Eleven of the drugs evaluated were active, and 12 were inactive. The remaining 34 agents were assessed as having uncertain activity because of methodologic problems in the design, conduct, and reporting of the trials. The outcomes of this study is summarized in Table 22.1.

Active agents for SCLC treatment include cyclophosphamide, doxorubicin, hexamethylmelamine, etoposide, vincristine, nimustine, carboplatin, cisplatin, epirubicin, teniposide, and vindesine. Ifosfamide also is considered as a new conventional active agent for SCLC because of the high response rate reported previously in untreated patients with SCLC (7). Etoposide was the drug studied in the greatest number of patients (651 patients in 17 trials). Its response rates ranged from 0% to 81%. According to their analysis this difference depended on criterion of patient eligibility employed in each phase II trial. When etoposide was given to previously untreated patients, a response rate of 40% to 80% could be obtained. Other active agents for SCLC mentioned previously yielded reproducible response rates of more than 30% when they were given to newly diagnosed patients with SCLC. Generally speaking, drugs that are highly active in chemotherapy naive patients may demonstrate only marginal activity (as low as 15%) in previously treated patients, even in SCLC, which is very sensitive to chemotherapy. It is very important to identify whether enrolled patients in clinical phase II trials have been previously treated or untreated. Recently, Ettinger et al. (8) reviewed the justification for evaluating new anticancer drugs in selected untreated patients with extensive-disease SCLC.

Among active agents for SCLC, etoposide, cyclophosphamide, doxorubicin, cisplatin, and vincristine are the most commonly used agents for combination chemotherapy. The optimal dose and schedule of each of these agents have already been investigated. Cyclophosphamide, doxorubicin, and cisplatin usually are administered every 3 to 4 weeks intravenously. For etoposide, however, there is a schedule dependency that optimizes its efficacy. A phase II study suggested that multiday schedules (e.g., days 1 to 5; 1 to 3; or 1, 3, and 5) given every 3 weeks were superior to a once-a-day schedule. Furthermore, Slevin et al. (9) demonstrated that etoposide was more effective when administered over 5 days rather than over 24 hours in continuous infusion. An active single agent for SCLC usually is used as an optional chemotherapy for patients in whom the probability of severe toxicity from intensive combination chemotherapy is high. Elderly or poor-risk patients with extensive disease SCLC are thought to be candidates for single-agent chemotherapy.

TABLE 22.1. Summary of Single-Agent Activity in Small Cell Lung Cancer on Phase II Trials Between 1970 and 1990

AGENTS WITH DEMONSTRATED ACTIVITY[a] (%)	AGENTS DEMONSTRATED AS INACTIVE[b]	AGENTS INADEQUATELY EVALUATED
Carboplatin (6–79)	Amsacrine	Aclacinomycin A[c]
Cisplatin (6–22)	Cytarabine	Fluorouracil[c]
Cyclophosphamide (12–69)	Idarubicin	Lomustine[c]
Doxorubicin (21–23)	Methyl-lomustine	Lonidamine[c]
Etoposide (0–81)	Mitomycin	Prednimustine[d]
Epirubicin[e] (33–50)	Mitoxantrone	Ifosfamide[e]
Hexamethylmelamine (37–42)	Streptozotocin	Iproplatin[d]
Nimustine (11–47)	Vinblastine	Methotrexate[d]
Teniposide (0–90)		Procarbazine[d]
Vincristine (0–42)		Bleomycin[f]
Vindesine (0–33)		Carmustine[f]
		Dacarbazine[f]
		PALA[f]

Numbers in parentheses indicates response rate in ≥14 patients. (From Grant SC, Gralla RJ, Kris MG, Orazem J, Kitsis EA. Single-agent chemotherapy trials in small-cell lung cancer, 1970 to 1990: the case for studies in previously treated patients. J Clin Oncol 1992;10: 484–498.)

[a]≥20% response rate in ≥14 patients.
[b]<10% response rate in ≥29 previously treated patients or a response rate <20% in ≥14 previously untreated patients.
[c]Possibly active because of a 10% to 19% response rate in 14 to 28 previously treated patients.
[d]Possibly inactive because of a <10% response rate in 14 to 28 previously treated patients.
[e]A 48% response rate in 44 previously untreated patients.
[f]Unknown activity because there were ≤14 assessable patients.

NEW CHEMOTHERAPEUTIC DRUGS

Most of the patients with disseminated SCLC respond to the initial chemotherapy with complete remission rates of 30% to 40%. Cures are very rare. To achieve more effective control, the development of new chemotherapeutic agents active for SCLC is essential. Introduced below are some of the promising new agents for SCLC treatment that are still in an investigational phase.

CPT-11

Camptothecin, a plant alkaloid extract from *Camptotheca acuminata* (10), is a potent inhibitor of DNA topoisomerase I (11, 12); it has been shown to have a strong antitumor activity in vitro (13, 14) and in experimental animal tumor systems (15). However, it has not been used clinically because of its low response rates in clinical trials and its high toxicities (15, 16). To improve therapeutic efficacy and reduce toxicities, a water soluble derivative of camptothecin, i.e., irinotecan (CPT-11) has been synthesized. CPT-11 exhibited marked antitumor activity against not only a broad spectrum of experimental tumor models (17, 18), but against pleiotropically drug resistant tumor cell lines (19). Thus, CPT-11 should be recognized as a novel chemotherapeutic agent.

In a phase I study of CPT-11 using a weekly administration schedule, the recommended dose for a phase II study was 100 mg/m^2/day as a 90-minute intraveous influsion; dose-limiting factors (DLFs) included leukopenia and diarrhea. On the basis of these data, phase II trials for SCLC were conducted (20, 21). Negoro et al. (20) have demonstrated that 13 (37%) of 35 patients overall responded, including 33% who had received prior therapy and 50% who had not. Masuda et al. (21) recently reported 16 patients with refractory or relapsed SCLC treated with CPT-11. All 16 patients had been heavily pretreated with cisplatin-based combination chemotherapy. In this study 7 patients (47%) responded to CPT-11 with a median duration of response of 58 days. The major toxicities were myelosuppression (predominantly leukopenia), diarrhea, and pulmonary toxicity. The toxicity profile noted in this trial was similar to that described previously in a phase I trial (22). This treatment schedule was well tolerated. CPT-11 is an active agent against SCLC, and presently further trials of this agent in combination with other drugs such as cisplatin or etoposide are ongoing.

TAXOL (PACLITAXEL)

Taxol (Bristol-Myers Squibb, Princeton, NJ) is a novel diterpene plant product isolated from the Western yew *Taxus brevifolia*. This agent was shown to have a broad antitumor activity in preclinical experimental tumor models such as murine tumors or human xenografts in screening carried out by the U.S. National Cancer Institute (23). The mechanism of cytotoxic action of Taxol is its induction of tubulin polymerization. It also forms extremely stable and nonfunctional microtubules. This unusual stability results in the inhibition of the normal dynamic reorganization of the microtubule network. Because of its impressive antitumor activity and its unique mechanism of action, clinical development of Taxol was anticipated highly.

Phase I trials of many schedules of Taxol were initiated in 1983, but a high incidence of acute hypersensitivity reactions led to the discontinuation of many trials. To prevent this reaction, infusion durations were prolonged from 6 to 24 hours, and premedication with antiallergic regimens—consisting of steroids and H1- and H2-histamine antagonists—was tried. Because of these procedures, the incidence of hypersensitivity was reduced and phase I trials have been completed. The maximum-tolerated dose (MTD) was 30 mg/m^2/day for 5 days every 3 weeks (23, 24) or a single dose of 212 to 250 mg/m^2 every 3 weeks (25–28). Although dose-limiting toxicity varies with the schedule used, significant neutropenia was produced in all trials as a dose-limiting toxicity. Neurotoxicity limited the use of high single and cumulative doses of Taxol.

In phase II trials of Taxol, the most exciting antitumor activity has been observed in advanced ovarian cancer including cisplatin-refractory tumors. Clinical phase II trials of Taxol for extensive disease SCLC also were conducted by the Eastern Cooperative Oncology Group (ECOG) and North Central Cancer Treatment Group (NCCTC). In an ECOG study (29), previously untreated patients with extensive disease SCLC received Taxol at a dose of 250 mg/m^2 administered intravenously over 24 hours every 3 weeks. In this study no enrolled patients had complete responses, and 11 (34%) of 34 evaluable patients had partial responses. The major toxicity was leukopenia. In an NCCTG study (30), previously untreated patients with extensive disease SCLC received Taxol, 250 mg/m^2 via a 24-hour infusion with granulocyte–colony-stimulating factor (G-CSF) support. In 37 evaluable patients, the major response rate was 68%, and the complete response (CR) rate was 0%. In this study leukopenia was the primary toxicity. In conclusion, these two studies showed that Taxol was active against SCLC.

GEMCITABINE

Gemcitabine is a new anticancer drug with novel metabolic properties and mechanisms of action. As a nucleoside analogue, this agent is a prodrug that must be metabolized to its nucleotide forms in the cell. When it is transported into the cell, gemcitabine becomes a substrate for phosphorylation by deoxycytidine kinase. Phosphorylated forms of gemcitabine, such as gemcitabine diphosphate or triphosphate, inhibit the processes required for DNA synthesis.

In preclinical drug screening assays, gemcitabine, the novel pyrimidine antimetabolite, showed high activity against a wide range of human tumor xenografts. These data led to the initiation of clinical trials. Phase I trials were conducted using many schedules—once weekly (31), twice weekly (32), or 5-consecutive-day administration (33). Thus, the MTD of gemcitabine ranged widely, from 9 mg/m^2 to 1300 mg/m^2. These trials suggested that the most favorable schedule was achieved when this agent was administered once weekly for 3 weeks, followed by 1 week of rest. Using this weekly schedule, the MTD identified in previously treated patients was 790 mg/m^2/week (34). In an early phase II study in non–small cell lung cancer (NSCLC), however, it became apparent that 800 mg/m^2 was a conservative dose. Thereafter, 1000 and 1250 mg/m^2/week were employed in phase II trials.

Clinical phase II trials of gemcitabine for extensive disease SCLC also were conducted in Canada and the United States. In the Canadian study (35), among 29 previously untreated patients with extensive disease SCLC enrolled, the first 17 patients received this agent at 1000 mg/m^2/week for 3 weeks, administered intravenously every 4 weeks, and the remainder received 1250 mg/m^2/week. Of 26 evaluable patients, 1 CR and 6 partial responses (PRs) were seen, giving a response rate of 27%. The median response duration was 12.5 weeks. Toxicities including myelosuppression were mild or moderate.

Based on these data, gemcitabine may be active in the treatment of SCLC, but the doses with this schedule were toxic. Further studies evaluating more intense doses and schedules should be performed.

EPIRUBICIN

The anthracyclines are a class of drugs with one of the widest ranges of antitumor activity in human malignancies. Among these, doxorubicin still is thought to be one of the most active agents for SCLC therapy. Epirubicin was developed in the 1970s as part of the search for anthracyclic analogues. In preclinical studies its murine and human xenograft antitumor activity was equivalent to that of doxorubicin, and it had less cardiotoxicity.

In a phase I study, the range of tolerable doses established was 70 to 90 mg/m^2 (36). This dose level is equimyelotoxic to the 60 to 75 mg/m^2 dose range of doxorubicin. Dose escalation became a topic of research interest in chemotherapy in the late 1980s, and clinical trials have been designed to study the issues involved in increasing the epirubicin dose. In an initial dose escalation study of epirubicin, the dose was increased to 120 mg/m^2 (37). The DLF in this trial was mucositis, not myelosuppression.

In a study by Blackstein et al. (38), 40 previously untreated patients with extensive disease SCLC received 120 mg/m^2 of epirubicin as a single agent and showed a response rate of 50%. Nonresponders after two doses of epirubicin received cisplatin and etoposide as a salvage chemotherapy; results compared well with other studies using combination chemotherapy. This finding suggested that if a new agent proves ineffective within two cycles and standard therapy is given quickly thereafter the survival rate may not be affected. In another study, 71 previously untreated patients with extensive disease SCLC received 120 mg/m^2 of epirubicin every 3 to 4 weeks, and an objective response rate of 54% was obtained (39).

The response rates obtained from these clinical trials of epirubicin show that it is active against SCLC.

INVESTIGATION OF NEW SCHEDULES

Investigation of new treatment scheduling of conventional agents is one of the strategies used to improve the results of treatment of extensive stage SCLC. A randomized study by Slevin et al. (9) demonstrated that an intravenous dose of 500 mg/m^2 of etoposide given on a 5-day schedule was superior to the same dose given over 1 day with respect to the response rate (89% versus 10%, respectively; $P = .001$) and median survival time (10.0 months versus 6.3 months, respectively; $P = .01$). Furthermore, there was a trend favoring the response duration and survival for patients with extensive disease SCLC on an 8-day schedule of etoposide administration compared with a 5-day schedule (40). This schedule dependency of etoposide may be the result of the much longer duration of the cytotoxic drug level.

A phase I trial of oral etoposide over a long period (21-day cycle) in patients with several refractory malignancies suggested that the MTD was 50 mg/m^2/day for 21 days, and the DLF was myelosuppression, which usually resolved by days 28 to 35 (41). Based on these data, Johnson et al. (42) and Einhorn (43) have studied etoposide schedule dependency further. In phase II studies, patients with relapsed SCLC were treated with daily oral etoposide at a dose of 50 mg/m^2 on days 1 through 21 every 28 days (43). Overall response rates of these two studies were 46% (42) and 23% (43). Chronic daily administration of oral etoposide was well tolerated and easily administered for refractory SCLC. Keane and Carney (44) conducted a study of 63 elderly patients with SCLC treated using single-agent oral etoposide at a dose of 200 mg/day for 5 days. The overall response rate observed was 76%, with a CR rate of 20%. For all patients, the median survival time was 38 weeks, and the 2-year survival rate was 10%. They have expanded this study to evaluate a combination regimen that includes oral etoposide. Based on these results, Carney et al. (45) commented that a shorter schedule of etoposide administration may be more suitable for elderly or poor-risk patients with extensive disease SCLC because of the significant myelosuppression associated with chronic daily administration. Further studies are required to resolve these conflicting results.

COMBINATION CHEMOTHERAPY

A large number of combination chemotherapy regimens were investigated in the treatment of SCLC during the 1970s and have yielded a high response rate and improved survival. A consensus report in 1981 showed that optimal chemotherapy regimens produced a 75% overall response rate, a 25% CR rate, and a median survival of 7 months in extensive-disease SCLC, although long-term survivors were very rare (5). These results were obtained only through the development of effective combination chemotherapies.

NUMBER OF DRUGS

A few prospective randomized trials compared multidrug combination chemotherapy regimens with single-agent regimens in the 1970s. Two trials compared cyclophosphamide-containing two- or three-drug combination chemotherapy regimens to cyclophosphamide alone (46, 47). These trials confirmed that combination regimens were superior in response rate and overall survival to single-agent chemotherapy. Using drugs of known activity in previously untreated patients with SCLC, Bunn and Ihde (48) demonstrated that the response rates attained with combination chemotherapy were superior to those with single-agent chemotherapy. In this review, there was no evidence to support giving more than three or four drugs simultaneously in the treatment of SCLC.

There are two randomized trials that have evaluated the addition of a third drug to a two-drug combination (49) and of a fourth drug to a three-drug combination (50) in patients with extensive disease SCLC. The first trial compared a two-drug combination of cyclophosphamide and methotrexate and a three-drug combination of cyclophosphamide, methotrexate, and lomustine. A survival benefit was observed in patients treated with the three-drug combination, although there was no significant difference in median survival: 23 weeks versus 33 weeks, respectively; $P = .17$. The second trial was of a three-drug combination of cyclophosphamide, methotrexate, and lomustine versus a four-drug combination of cyclophosphamide, methotrexate, lomustine and vincristine. In this trial, the four-drug combination was significantly superior to the three-drug combination in the median survival observed: 6 versus 7.7 months, respectively; $P < .01$. Another randomized trial demonstrated significantly improved response rates and survival durations in extensive disease patients treated with the three-drug combination of cyclophosphamide, etoposide, and vincristine compared with the two-drug combination of cyclophosphamide and vincristine (51). These results showed convincingly the role of etoposide in the three-drug combination, because the cyclophosphamide was given at double the dose in the two-drug combination.

CAV, CAE, AND CAVE REGIMENS

Although many combination chemotherapy regimens appeared to have similar activity against SCLC, a regimen of cyclophosphamide, doxorubicin, and vincristine (CAV) was used commonly during the 1980s. The CAV regimen has reproducibly yielded high response rates, median survival rates, and long-term survival in both limited- and extensive-stage SCLC patients; thus, it has been considered the standard regimen in the treatment of SCLC.

Etoposide was investigated most extensively in the 1980s and appeared to be one of the most active agents against SCLC. Several randomized trials were conducted to evaluate whether adding etoposide to CAV or substituting it for one of the agents in the CAV regimen was effective (Table 22.2). Three randomized trials compared CAV plus etoposide (CAVE) with CAV alone, keeping drug doses identical (52–54). Two of the three studies demonstrated significantly higher response rates with CAVE, but survival was not improved significantly. A controlled trial comparing standard-dose CAV plus etoposide with higher dose CAV showed no differences in response rates (74% versus 72%, respectively) or survival (42.3 versus 42.1 weeks, respectively) (47). In two randomized trials, survival of patients with extensive disease stage was prolonged when etoposide was substituted for doxorubicin (CEV) (55) or vincristine (CAE) (56) in the CAV regimen. In these studies, the superiority of the etoposide-containing regimen was not proven in patients with limited stage disease. These studies did not provide unequivocal results that etoposide-containing regimens are superior to regimens not containing this drug, although CAVE and CAE are among the acceptable regimens in the treatment of extensive stage SCLC.

ETOPOSIDE AND CISPLATIN

The combination of etoposide and cisplatin (EP) exhibited a synergistic effect in murine tumors (57) and produced a cure rate of approximately 25% in patients with refractory testicular cancer who did not respond to a regimen of cisplatin, vinblastine, and bleomycin (PVB) (58). EP also has produced objective response rates of 50% or more in previously treated SCLC patients (59–61), whereas both single-agent etoposide (62–64) and single-agent cisplatin (65) had response rates of less than 15% in such patients.

This EP combination also was studied as part of first-line chemotherapy for SCLC (Table 22.3) (66–69). Sierocki and his colleagues (66) provided the first report of the use of this two-drug combination in previously untreated SCLC patients. Fifteen (88%) of 17 patients with extensive stage disease had an objective response, with a median survival of 9 months. Evans et al. (67) reported that 5 (29%) CRs and 10

TABLE 22.2. Randomized Trials Testing the Addition or Substitution of Etoposide in a Cyclophosphamide, Doxorubicin, and Vincristine (CAV) Regimen for Treatment of Small Cell Lung Cancer

Author (Reference No.)	Chemotherapy	No. of Patients	CR (%)	Overall Response (%)	Median Survival Months	p Value
Messeih et al. (52)	CAV	49[a]	18	51	8.3	.23
	CAVE	43[a]	44	74	10.3	...
Jackson et al. (53)	CAV	66	12	46	7.8	.084
	CAVE	70	29	70	9.4	...
Jett et al. (54)	CAV	113[b]	57	82	12.1	.13
	CAVE	118[b]	64	84	15.1	...
Lowenbraun et al. (47)	CAV[c]	106	21	72	9.7	.35
	CAVE	108	14	94	9.7	...
Comis et al. (55)	CAV	79	6	NR	7.7	.012
	CEV	66	14	NR	9.1	...
Einhorn et al. (56)	CAV	133	10	45	7.2	<.05
	CAE	130	12	54	9.1	

Abbreviations. CR, complete response; CAV, cyclophosphamide + doxorubicin + vincristine; CEV, cyclophosphamide + etoposide + vincristine; CAE, cyclophosphamide + doxorubicin + etoposide; CAVE, cyclophosphamide + doxorubicin + vincristine + etoposide; NR, not reported.
[a]Limited-disease and extensive-disease patients are included.
[b]All were limited-disease patients who received thoracic radiotherapy after CAV or CAVE.
[c]high-dose CAV.

TABLE 22.3. Phase II Studies of Etoposide and Cisplatin as First-Line Therapy for Extensive Disease Small Cell Lung Cancer

Author (Reference No.)	Dosage (mg/m^2)/day CDDP	Etoposide	No. of Patients	CR (%)	Overall Response (%)	Median Survival (Mo)
Sierocki et al. (66)	60/Day 1	120/Days 4, 6, 8	17	41	78	9.0
Evans et al. (67)	25/Days 1–3	100/Days 1–3	17	29.4	88.2	
Kim and McDonald (68)	75/Day 1	125/Days 1, 3, 5	24	33	88	9.0
Woods and Levi (69)	80/Day 1	80/Days 1–3	98	21	64	NR 11.6[a]

Abbreviations. CR, complete response; NR, not reported; CDDP, cisplatin.

(59%) PRs were achieved in 17 patients with extensive disease SCLC initially treated with the EP combination. The median duration of response was 29 weeks, and the median duration of survival was 39 weeks. Other trials using the EP combination as first-line therapy have resulted in CR rates and overall response rates comparable to those of other combination regimens (68, 69).

Two randomized studies comparing CAV and EP as sole induction chemotherapy regimens have been reported recently (70, 71). In the Japan Lung Cancer Chemotherapy Group study (70), although the response rate for EP (78%) was superior to that for CAV (59%), survival was similar between the two arms in extensive disease patients (median survival, 9 versus 8.3 months, respectively). In the study of the Southeastern Cancer Study Group (SECSG), four cycles of EP was equivalent to six cycles of CAV in the treatment of extensive disease SCLC (response rate, 59% versus 58%, respectively; median survival, 8.8 versus 9.5 months, respectively) (71). In these studies, EP given as a salvage therapy to patients who failed to respond to CAV or who developed disease progression after CAV treatment produced response rates twice as high as those achieved when CAV was given as a salvage therapy after EP. Furthermore, EP was less myelosuppressive than CAV in these studies. Each study also compared these two regimens alone with an alternating regimen of CAV and EP (see Non–Cross-Resistant Alternating Chemotherapy, below). In summary, EP is one of the most effective combination regimens and is used commonly in the treatment of SCLC.

Other Combinations

The substitution of carboplatin for cisplatin in the EP regimen has been studied also. This combination has yielded comparable response rates to those of EP with reduced gastrointestinal toxicity but greater myelosuppression (72–74).

Several studies have evaluated the impact of vincristine or ifosfamide added to the carboplatin/etoposide combination. Gatzemeier et al. (75) have investigated CEV in the treatment of extensive disease SCLC; the results were a CR of 33% and a PR of 53% with a median survival of 9 months. A phase III study has been conducted in 218 patients with extensive disease SCLC comparing the three-drug CEV combination (carboplatin, 300 mg/m^2 on day 1; etoposide, 140 mg/m^2 intravenously on days 1, 2, and 3; and vincristine, 1.4 mg/m^2 on days 1, 8, and 15, every 4 weeks) with the two-drug combination of etoposide and vincristine (EV) (etoposide, 200 mg/m^2 intravenously on days 1, 2, and 3; and vincristine, 1.4 mg/m^2 on days 1 and 8, every 4 weeks) (76). The CEV regimen produced a CR rate of 26.4% and an overall response rate of 79.8%, compared with 14.6% and 59.8%, respectively, for the EV regimen ($P < .001$). No difference in survival was observed between the two groups (survival durations of 10 months for the CEV arm and 9 months for the EV arm; $P = .19$). However, the long-term survival rate showed a significant advantage for patients with good prognostic factors who were treated with CEV. The incidences of leukopenia and thrombocytopenia were higher in the CEV arm than in the EV arm. This trial showed that patients with poor prognostic factors should be treated appropriately with the less aggressive two-drug combination chemotherapy. Smith et al. (77) reported a study of the combination of ifosfamide, carboplatin, and etoposide (ICE). Thirty-two patients (18 with limited disease and 14 with extensive disease) were treated with ifosfamide, 5 g/m^2 on day 1; carboplatin, 400 mg/m^2 on day 1; and etoposide, 100 mg/m^2 intravenously on days 1 through 3, every 4 weeks. The overall response rates were 94% in limited disease patients and 100% in extensive disease patients, with CR rates of 72% and 29%, respectively. The median survival durations were 19 months for limited disease patients and 9.5 months for those with extensive disease. Because of severe myelosuppression, dose reductions of the three drugs were required in 72% of patients.

Large randomized studies are needed to confirm whether carboplatin-containing combinations such as carboplatin/etoposide, CEV, or ICE can improve the median survival, long-term survival, and quality of life.

Recently, new agents active against SCLC have been developed. Such agents include irinotecan, Topotecan (SmithKline Beecham, London, United Kingdom), paclitaxel, docetaxel, gemcitabine, and vinovelbine. Combination chemotherapy with these new agents should be studied aggressively to improve the outcome of patients with extensive disease SCLC.

NON–CROSS-RESISTANT ALTERNATING CHEMOTHERAPY

Several approaches have been explored to overcome the plateau in the outcome of SCLC treatment. Goldie and Coldman (78) have provided a mathematical model of the emergence of drug resistant clones in malignant tumors at a mutation rate proportional to the number of actively dividing tumor cells. They proposed that, if it is impossible to administer all active drugs concurrently at full doses because of overlapping toxic effects, then alternating two non–cross-resistant combinations early in the treatment would lead to maximal eradication of the tumor cell populations (79). A large number of nonrandomized and randomized trials using alternating chemotherapy regimens were used in SCLC treatment in the early 1980s. The duration of remission was prolonged by alternating the chemotherapy regimens in some randomized trials (80, 81); improved survival was seen in other trials (81, 82). However, a consistent survival benefit has not been demonstrated (83).

The Goldie-Coldman hypothesis (79) requires that the combinations employed in alternating chemotherapy regimens should be equally effective and non–cross-resistant. Because the EP combination has been shown to be effective not only as induction therapy but also as salvage therapy (59, 60), it has been considered very suitable for alternating chemotherapy. Several randomized trials evaluating alternating regimens of CAV and EP have been conducted in the treatment of SCLC (70, 71, 84–86). The results of randomized trials in the treatment of extensive disease SCLC are summarized in Table 22.4. The National Cancer Institute of Canada (NCI-C) carried out a comparison of alternating treatment using CAV and EP for six treatment cycles and continuous treatment with CAV for six courses (84) in patients with extensive-stage SCLC. The results in 289 assessable patients demonstrated that the alternating arm was significantly superior in response rate (80% versus 63%), progression free survival, and overall survival (median survivals, 9.6 months on CAV/EP and 8 months on CAV; $P = .03$), although the advantage in median survival was only 6 weeks. The differences in favor of the alternating chemotherapy still remained when adjusted for prognostic factors using a proportional hazards model. In this trial, the question of whether the superiority of the alternating treatment resulted from the alternating strategy or to the fact that EP is superior to CAV remained unanswered. Two recent trials of the Japan Clinical Oncology Group (JCOG) (70) and the SECSG (71) also have addressed this question. These trials

TABLE 22.4. Randomized Trials Evaluating Alternating Chemotherapy in Extensive Disease Small Cell Lung Cancer

Author (Reference No.)	Chemotherapy	No. of Patients	CR (%)	Overall Response (%)	Median Survival Months	P Value
Evans et al. (84)	CAV	144	27.1	63.2	8	.03
	CAV/EP	145	38.6	80	9.6	...
Fukuoka et al. (70)	CAV	46	13	59	8.7	...
	EP	51	9.8	78	8.3	NS
	CAV/EP	40	8	63	9	...
Roth et al. (71)	CAV	146	10.0	50.6	8.3	...
	EP	148	7.1	60.7	8.6	.425
	CAV/EP	143	7.2	59.4	8.1	...

Abbreviations. CR, complete response; CAV, cyclophosphamide + doxorubicin + vincristine; EP, etoposide + cisplatin; CAV + EP: CAV alternating with EP.

compared continuous treatments of CAV or EP with alternating CAV and EP treatments. A JCOG trial including patients with both limited and extensive disease showed that response rates for EP (78%) and CAV/EP (76%) were significantly higher than for CAV (55%) ($P < .01$); overall survival with alternating CAV/EP treatment (median survival, 11.8 months) was superior to that with CAV (9.9 months) ($P = .027$) or EP (9.9 months) ($P < .059$). However, the survival advantage of alternating treatment disappeared when the data were adusted for prognostic factors. In patients with extensive disease, survival was similar among CAV (median survival, 8.7 months), EP (8.3 months), and CAV/EP (9.0 months)–treated patients. The trial of the SECSG (71) evaluating more than 400 patients with extensive disease showed no advantage for the alternating CAV/EP regimen when compared with CAV or EP alone. Overall response rates were 51% for CAV, 61% for EP, and 59% for CAV/EP ($P = .175$), and the median survival durations were 8.3 months on CAV, 8.6 months on EP, and 8.1 months on CAV/EP ($P = .425$).

There are two randomized trials that were confined to patients with limited disease (85, 86). In the NCI-C trial (85), the CAV/EP alternating regimen was not superior to CAV sequentially followed by EP with respect to survival. Another trial from the Southwest Oncology Group (SWOG) (86) compared the CAV/EP alternating treatment with a concurrent four-drug combination CAVE in patients with limited disease patients. In this trial, the response rate and survival did not differ between the two treatment groups. Thoracic radiotherapy also was used in these patients.

The consensus conference in 1989 concluded that randomized phase III trials evaluating alternating chemotherapy showed no major advantage for existing alternating regimens (87). In extensive disease, any combination of CAV, EP, or CAV/EP can be used. However, presently, either EP alone or the CAV/EP alternating regimen is a more reasonable approach, because they were superior to CAV with respect to induction of response or toxicity.

DURATION OF CHEMOTHERAPY AND TREATMENT OF DISEASE PROGESSION

Until the early 1980s, many investigators treated responding patients for up to 2 years because there were few relapses beyond this time. Because prolonged treatment induces both morbidity and mortality, several subsequent nonrandomized trials empirically used a considerably shorter duration of therapy and obtained similar results. Several randomized studies have addressed the optimum duration of chemotherapy in SCLC (8, 88–93). In the Midland Small-Cell Lung Cancer Group study (94), of 211 patients with extensive disease, 61 patients who achieved a CR or good PR after six cycles of CAV treatment were randomized to receive either eight further cycles of CAV or follow-up. This study showed a survival benefit for patients randomized to receive maintenance chemotherapy (median survival, 372 versus 259 days, respectively; $P = .0006$) (89) but no effect on long-term survival. In the Medical Research Council (MRC) trial, all patients with both limited and extensive stage disease were prescribed six courses of cyclophosphamide, etoposide, vincristine, and methotrexate (CEVM) chemotherapy. Patients who obtained a CR or PR by the time of the fifth course were assigned randomly to six more courses of the same chemotherapy or to no chemotherapy. Overall, there was no significant survival advantage in either arm. However, for complete responders, the median survival time from randomization was 42 weeks for the maintenance group and 30 weeks for the no-maintenance patients ($P < .05$). In a Cancer Research Campaign trial (92), patients were randomized initially to receive either four or eight courses of CEV and also upon disease progression to receive either second-line chemotherapy (methotrexate/doxorubicin) or symptomatic treatment only. The median survival of 28 weeks seen in patients given four cycles of CEV only, with no chemotherapy at progression, was significantly worse than that shown in the other three arms (range 34 to 40 weeks). The study showed that four courses of chemotherapy alone in patients with extensive disease produced inferior survival rates, compared with the other three treatments, which were equivalent in outcome. Thus, if only four courses of chemotherapy are given, there is a survival disadvantage unless patients receive chemotherapy at the time of relapse; however, if eight courses are given initially, then there is no survival advantage from giving further chemotherapy at the time of relapse. The study by the ECOG (81) randomized 628 patients with extensive disease to receive CAV or CAV alternat-ing with a hexamethylmelamine, etoposide, and methotrexate (HEM) combination. After six to eight cycles, 110 complete responders were randomized to maintenance or follow-up. Eighty-six complete responders who received the induction chemotherapy could be analyzed for the maintenance step. Although no difference in survival and progression free survival between the maintenance and follow-up arms was observed in patients treated with the alternating regimen, there was a significant prolongation of progression free survival in the maintenance group compared with the follow-up group in CAV-treated patients (24 versus 12 weeks; $P = .015$). The survival benefit was of borderline significance ($P = .09$). This study suggests that if chemotherapy is sufficiently aggressive, there should be no need for maintenance chemotherapy. A significant difference in median time to progression from randomization was found between maintenance and no-maintenance therapy groups ($P = .0038$), but the analysis of survival from randomization showed almost identical curves with an absolute lack of difference, regardless of response to CAE therapy. The study suggests that short-duration combination chemotherapy may be a reasonable choice for standard treatment of SCLC and for attempts to improve the cure rate of this disease. The MRC Lung Cancer Working Party (91) allocated 458 patients with both limited and extensive disease to three chemotherapy regimens. In two regimens, CEVM was given for a total of either three courses or six courses. In the third regimen etoposide and ifosamide were given for six courses. There was no statistically significant survival advantage to any treatment group, although the results do not exclude the possibility of a minor survival advantage with the two 6-course regimens.

The impact of interferon as maintenance therapy on the treatment of SCLC has been evaluated in two trials. Mattson et al. (95) reported a phase III trial that evaluated low-dose natural interferon alfa as a maintenance therapy. Ninety-one patients were randomized to interferon and 87 patients to no further therapy after having responded to four cycles of induction chemotherapy and radiotherapy. There was no significant difference in median survival (interferon, 11 months; control, 10 months); however, a clear difference in 5-year survival (interferon, 11%; control, 2%) favored interferon maintenance therapy. Conversely, in a phase III trial conducted by the North Central Cancer Treatment Group (96), 51 complete responders received recombinant gamma interferon and 49 observation only. The median times to progression with interferon or observation were 7 months and 8 months, respectively, and the median survival from randomization was 13 months with interferon versus 19 months with observation ($P = .15$). The 2-year survival rates were 23% and 34%, respectively. The authors concluded that interferon was not associated with any improvement in survival, but it was associated with significant toxicities.

In summary, chemotherapy in responding patients should be discontinued after four to six cycles, which seems to be a reasonable optimum length of therapy. Several randomized studies of maintenance therapy have shown that chemotherapy beyond an initial four to six cycles does not prolong survival. Treatment should be resumed at recurrence if clinically appropriate.

DOSE INTENSITY

Recently, the importance of dose intensity of chemotherapy in achieving a maximal therapeutic effect has been reported for a variety of responsive tumors (97–102). A high dose intensity of chemotherapy has been achieved by high-dose induction, late intensification with or without autologous bone marrow transplantation (ABMT), and accelerated chemotherapy consisting of standard doses given at shorter intervals.

DOSE INCREASE IN INDUCTION CHEMOTHERAPY

The high rate of systemic relapse has prompted attempts to improve the response rate and survival using higher doses of chemotherapy. In 1977 Cohen et al. (103) first demonstrated that a full dose of cyclophosphamide (1000 mg/m^2) during the initial 6-

week induction therapy was more effective than a relatively low dose (500 mg/m^2), producing a higher CR rate and a longer median and long-term survival in a combination of cyclophosphamide, methotrexate, and lomustine. However, subsequent randomized studies showed that, although higher response rates are achievable, higher doses are not associated with a better outcome within the conventional dose range (Table 22.5) (104–108). A dose intensity meta-analysis of chemotherapy regimens in 60 published studies conducted by Klasa et al. (109) showed that for CAE and CAVE, the relative dose intensity (RDI) of the regimens correlated with the median survival in extensive disease as did the RDI of cyclophosphamide. For CAV and EP, no significant correlations were seen. Thus, no demonstrable effect on response and survival was apparent within the fairly narrow range of dose intensity. Furthermore, there currently are no data to justify further dose escalation supported by ABMT in routine induction chemotherapy (110–112). Several studies have assessed the role of late intensification with very–high-dose chemotherapy and autologous bone marrow support after induction therapy (113–116). In a randomized trial reported by Humblet et al. (117), 45 patients in complete or partial remission after three cycles of standard combination chemotherapy (methotrexate, vincristine, cyclophosphamide, doxorubicin, cisplatin, and etoposide) were assigned randomly to high-dose chemotherapy (cyclophosphamide, carmustine and etoposide) supported by ABMT or the same drugs in a single cycle at a conventional dose. The study showed that late intensification with ABMT increased the CR rate and resulted in a significant increase in the relapse free survival, but it failed to provide an overall survival advantage (68 weeks versus 55 weeks) for the selected population of patients responding to conventional chemotherapy.

WEEKLY DOSE INTENSE REGIMENS

Another recently used method to increase the dose intensity is shortening the interval between chemotherapy cycles. A methotrexate, doxorubicin, cyclophosphamide, vincristine, prednisone, and bleomycin (MACOP-B) regimen, given according to the principles of the Goldie-Coldman hypothesis, has proven beneficial in the treatment of diffuse large cell lymphoma (118). This approach also was tested recently in SCLC (119–124) (Table 22.6). The most encouraging point of these trials has been the high CR rates, ranging from 10% to 48%, which might translate into an improvement in survival. A less selected group of patients was entered onto the study by the SWOG, and the 38% CR rate and 50-week median survival were slightly better than those of other SWOG studies reported over the past decade (119). Although studies by Miles et al. (121) and Murray et al. (122) were performed in highly selected patients, very high 2-year survival rates of 20% to 25% were projected. Perhaps most promising were the results of the cisplatin, vincristine, doxorubicin, etoposide (CODE) regimen (122). The proportion of 5-year survivors (9%) treated with the CODE combination is similar to that of patients with limited stage SCLC treated with standard chemotherapy and late

TABLE 22.5. Randomized Trials Evaluating the Dose of Chemotherapy in Extensive-Disease Small Cell Lung Cancer

Investigators (Reference No.)	Drug and Dose (mg/m^2)	No. of Patients	CR (%)	Overall Response (%)	Median Survival Months	p Value
Hande et al. (104)	M(6000) + A(40) + V(1)	19	21	74	9	...
	C(1000) + E(180 × 3)	...	...	...	...	NS
	M(20) + A(40) + V(1)	21	28	67	9	...
	C(1000) + E(180 × 3)	...	...	...	...	...
O'Donnell et al. (105)	C(2000) + V(2^a) + S(100)	9	5	6	6.7	NR
	C(750) + V(2^a) + S(75)	6	0	17	6	...
Figueredo et al. (106)	C(1560) + A(59) + V(0.9)	36	17	69	7–8	$P = .968$
	C(990) + A(50) + V(1)	33	6	55	7–8	...
Johnson et al. (105)	C(1200) + A(70) + V(1)	101	22	63	6.7	$P > .05$
	C(1000) + A(40) + V(1)	146	12	53	8	...
Ihde et al. (108)	P(135) + E(80 × 5)	39	24	85	12	NS
	P(80) + E(80 × 3)	42	21	81	11	...

Abbreviations. CR, complete response; M, methotrexate; A, doxorubicin; V, vincristine; C, cyclophosphamide; E, etoposide; P, cisplatin; S, methyl-lomustine; NR, not reported
^{a}Mg/kg of body weight.

TABLE 22.6. Weekly Chemotherapy for Extensive-Disease Small Cell Lung Cancer

Author (Reference No.)	Chemotherapy	Treatment (Wk)	No. of Patients	CR (%)	Overall Response (%)	Median Survival (Wk)
Taylor et al. (119)	DCVEPM	16	42	38	81	50
Sculier et al. (120)	DECPVVM	24–40	13	23	92	35
Miles et al. (121)	PE/ID	12	25	48	92	42
Murray et al. (122)	CODE	9–12	48	40	94	61
Wampler et al. (123)	EPVCDM	12	14	36	93	41
Alba et al. (124)	CDVEPM	12	41	10	61	31

Abbreviations. DCVEPM, doxorubicin + cyclophosphamide + vincristine + etoposide + cisplatin + methotrexate; DECPVVM, doxorubicin + etoposide + cyclophosphamide + cisplatin + vindesine + vincristine + methotrexate; PEID, cisplatin + etoposide + ifosfamide + doxorubicin; CODE, cisplatin + vincristine + doxorubicin + etoposide; EPVCDM, etoposide + cisplatin + vincristine + cyclophosphamide + doxorubicin + methotrexate; CDVEPM, cyclophosphamide + doxorubicin + vincristine + cisplatin + etoposide + methotrexate.

TABLE 22.7. Randomized Trials Comparing Standard Therapy with Weekly Intensive Chemotherapy

Investigator (Reference No.)	No. of Patients	Regimen	Response (%)		Median Survival (Wk)
			CR	Overall	
Miles et al. (126)	116	CAV/PE (standard)	18	70	34
		PE/ID (weekly)	24	84	40
Sculier et al. (127)	120	CAE (standard)	NR	61	40
		DECPVVM (weekly)	NR	57	39

Abbreviations. CR, complete response; CAV/PE, cyclophosphamide + doxorubicin + vincristine + cisplatin + etoposide; PE + ID, cisplatin + etoposide + ifosfamide + doxorubicin; CAE, cyclophosphamide + doxorubicin + etoposide; DECPVVM, doxorubicin + etoposide + cyclophosphamide + cisplatin + vindesine / vincristine + methotrexate; NR, no response.

consolidative radiotherapy (125). The regimen consisted of cisplatin, given each week, and doxorubicin and etoposide alternated with vincristine on a weekly basis except for week 1. This regimen is designed to give alternating weekly cycles of myelosuppressive and nonmyelosuppressive drugs. Recently, results of two randomized trials comparing the standard regimen with a weekly regimen were reported (Table 22.7). Miles et al. (126) conducted a randomized trial comparing an every 3-week EP regimen alternating with CAV and a weekly regimen of cisplatin and etoposide/ifosfamide and etoposide. However, no differences in response rate (70% versus 84%) or median survival time (34 weeks versus 40 weeks) were obtained. The comparison of the weekly multidrug combination regimen with a standard chemotherapy regimen by Sculier et al. (127) also failed to show any survival advantage (median survival, 39 weeks versus 40 weeks) in patients with this disease. The CODE regimen has placed particular emphasis on the administration of active agents at full doses rather than on the number of drugs given. Because this strategy makes the CODE regimen differ entirely from other weekly regimens, it seems very promising. However, the definite contribution of the regimen to the care of patients with SCLC must await the results of two randomized trials. One compares a standard regimen (CAV/EP) with the CODE regimen in North America and is being conducted by the NCI-C and SWOG. The other is a trial of CODE with G-CSF versus CAV/EP being conducted by the JCOG.

HEMATOPOIETIC GROWTH FACTORS

Granulocyte-macrophage colony-stimulating factor (GM-CSF) and G-CSF are a group of glycoproteins that regulate the production and maturation of hematopoietic progenitor cells and the function of mature blood cells (128–130). These factors reduce the duration and severity of the leukopenia caused by cytotoxic drugs through the increase in the function and number of granulocytes and macrophages (131–133). Two randomized double-blind placebo-controlled trials (134, 135) demonstrated that the use of G-CSF as an adjunct to CAE chemotherapy led to reductions in the incidence of neutropenic fever and documented infections; in the incidence, duration, and severity of grade 4 neutropenia; and in the total number of days of treatment with intravenous antibiotics and days of hospitalization. They have not been shown to improve response rates, however, Furthermore, no demonstrable improvement in the median survival, time to progression, or mortality rate was observed in the patients receiving G-CSF (134). In a randomized trial of weekly chemotherapy consisting of PE/ID with or without G-CSF conducted by Miles et al. (136) the use of G-CSF significantly decreased dose reductions required because of the development of neutropenia. However, nonhematologic toxicities such as an increased creatinine concentration prevented an increase in the dose intensity in the G-CSF arm. Therefore, administration of G-CSF did not result in a significant increase in the dose intensity (84% of projected in the G-CSF arm versus 82% in the control arm) or the response rate (74% in the G-CSF arm versus 71% in the control arm). The authors stated that the use of G-CSF may not be suitable for weekly regimens in which myelosuppressive drugs are administered with each treatment course. Ardizzoni et al. (137) investigated an accelerated chemotherapy regimen of CAV/PE that was alternated as early as possible. If possible, this regimen was alternated every week with or without GM-CSF in two series of five consecutive patients. With this approach, the average number of days required to recycle was shortened to 10 days with and 13 days without GM-CSF; the standard interval is 20 days. The total treatment duration was shortened to 57 and 73 days, respectively, instead of the usual 107 days. Thus, this approach permitted a twofold or 1.5-fold increase in dose intensity, respectively, compared with a standard regimen given every 21 days. Lastly, Fukuoka et al. (138) conducted a randomized trial of CODE chemotherapy with or without G-CSF. Of 64 patients with extensive stage SCLC enrolled, 53 were fully assessable. Twenty-seven patients receiving G-CSF showed a higher response rate (96% versus 85%), longer median survival (59 weeks versus 35 weeks; $P < .05$), and a lower number of febrile episodes (13 versus 36; $P < .01$). The mean dose intensity delivered for each drug was 85% in the G-CSF group and 76% in the control group ($P < .05$). This preliminary analysis suggested a survival advantage for patients treated with CODE chemotherapy and G-CSF compared with patients treated with chemotherapy alone.

CONCLUSIONS

Significant therapeutic advances have been observed in SCLC. The median survival has increased up to 10 months in patients with extensive disease, although long-term survivors still are quite rare. Whereas many of these advances were made during the 1970s and early 1980s, an apparent plateau in advances with systemic therapy of patients with extensive-stage disease has occurred during the past decade. For example, four cycles of the EP combination appear to be sufficient for treatment of this disease. There is no advantage in providing maintenance chemotherapy beyond the four cycles. With the combination regimens currently available, there is no obvious benefit to the use of a rapidly alternating schedule based on the mathematical model of Goldie and Coldman compared with the use of the EP combination alone. Drug substitutions such as carboplatin for cisplatin also are unlikely to improve outcome substantially. Although the preliminary results with intensive weekly CODE therapy are quite promising, the role of this chemotherapeutic technique should be examined carefully in prospective randomized trials before acceptance as a standard therapeutic regimen.

The identification of new agents active against SCLC remains a high priority for further improving the outcome because chemotherapy remains the mainstay of SCLC treatment. Several new cytotoxic agents with novel mechanisms of action have recently shown high activity against this disease. Among these are CPT-11, Topotecan, Taxol, docetaxel, vinovelbine, and gemcitabine. Further clinical trials are needed to define the optimal use of these agents and their use in combination with other cytotoxic agents already found to have activity against this disease.

REFERENCES

1. Ries LAG, Hankey BF, Miller BA, et al. Cancer statistics review 1973–1988. Bethesda: National Cancer Institute, 1991.
2. Ihde DC. Chemotherapy of lung cancer. N Engl J Med 1992;327:1434–1441.
3. Matthews MJ, Kanhouwa S, Pickren J, Robinette D. Frequency of residual and metastatic tumor in patients undergoing curative surgical resection for lung cancer. Cancer Chemother Rep 1973;4:63–67.
4. Green RA, Humphrey E, Close H, Patno ME. Alkylating agents in bronchogenic carcinoma. Am J Med 1969;46:515–525.
5. Aisner J, Alberto P, Bitran J, et al. Role of chemotherapy in small cell lung cancer: a consensus report of the International Association for the Study of Lung Cancer workshop. Cancer Treat Rep 1983;67:37–43.
6. Grant SC, Gralla RJ, Kris MG, Orazem J, Kitsis EA. Single-agent chemotherapy trials in small-cell lung cancer, 1970 to 1990: the case for studies in previously treated patients. J Clin Oncol 1992;10:484–498.
7. Ettinger D, Finkelstein D, Ritch P, Bonomi P, Blum R. Randomized trial of single agents vs combination chemotherapy in extensive stage cell lung cancer (SCLC) (abstract). Proc Am Soc Clin Oncol 1992;11:295.
8. Ettinger DS, Finkelstein, D, Abeloff MD, et al. Justification for evaluating new anticancer drugs in selected untreated patients with a chemotherapy-sensitive advanced cancer: an ECOG

randomized study (abstract). Proc Am Soc Clin Oncol 1990; 9:224.
9. Slevin ML, Clark PI, Joel SP, et al. A randomized trial to evaluate the effect of schedule on the activity of etoposide in small-cell lung cancer. J Clin Oncol 1989;7:1333–1340.
10. Wall ME, Wani MC, Cook CE, et al. Plant antitumor agents, 1. The isolation and structure of camptothecin, novel alkaloidal leukemia and tumor inhibitor from Camptotheca acuminata. J Am Chem Soc 1966;88:3888–3890.
11. Hsiang YH, Hertzberg R, Hecht S, Liu LF. Camptothecin induces protein-linked DNA breaks via mammalian DNA topoisomerase I. J Biol Chem 1985;260:14873–14878.
12. Andoh T, Ishii K, Suzuki Y, et al. Characterization of a mammalian mutant with a camptothecin-resistant DNA topoisomeraza I. Proc Natl Acad Sci U S A 1987;84:5565–5569.
13. Li LH, Fraser TJ, Olin EJ, Bhuyan BK. Action of camptothecin on mammalian cells in culture. Cancer Res 1972;32:2643–2650.
14. Drewinko B, Freireich EJ, Gottlieb JA. Lethal activity of camptothecin sodium on human lymphoma cells. Cancer Res 1974;34:747–750.
15. Gallo RC, Whang-Peng J, Adamson RH. Studies on the antitumor activity, mechanism of action, and cell cycle effects of camptothecin. J Natl Cancer Inst 1971;46:789–795.
16. Moertel CG, Schutt AJ, Reitemeier RJ, Hahn RG. Phase II study of camptothecin (NSC-100880) in the treatment of advanced gastrointestinal cancer. Cancer Chemother Rep 1972; 56:95–101.
17. Kunimoto T, Nitta K, Tanaka T, et al. Antitumor activity of 7-ethyl-10-[4-(1-piperidino)-1-piperidino] carbonyloxycamptothecin, a novel water-soluble derivative of camptothecin, against murine tumors. Cancer Res 1987;47:5944–5947.
18. Matsuzaki T, Yokokura T, Mutal M, Tsuruo T. Inhibition of spontaneous and experimental metastasis by a new derivative of camptothecin, CPT-11, in mice. Cancer Chemother Pharmacol 1988;21:308–312.
19. Tsuruo T, Matsuzaki T, Matsushita M, Saito H, Yokokura T. Antitumor effect of CPT-11, a new derivative of camptothecin, against pleiotropic drug-resistant tumors in vitro and in vivo. Cancer Chemother Pharmacol 1988;21:71–74.
20. Negoro S, Fukuoka M, Niitani H, Taguchi T. Phase II study of CPT-11, new camptothesine derivative, in small cell lung cancer (SCLC) (abstract). Proc Am Soc Clin Oncol 1991; 10:214.
21. Masuda N, Fukuoka M, Kusunoki Y, et al. CPT-11: a new derivative of camptothecin for the treatment of refractory or relapsed small-cell lung cancer. J Clin Oncol 1992;10: 1225–1229.
22. Negoro S, Fukuoka M, Masuda N, et al. Phase I study of weekly intravenous infusions of CPT-11, a new derivative of camptothecin, in the treatment of advanced non–small-cell lung cancer. J Natl Cancer inst 1991;83:1164–1168.
23. Grem JL, Tutsch KD, Simon KJ, et al. Phase I study of Taxol administered as a short i.v. infusion daily for 5 days. Cancer Treat Rep 1987;71:1179–1184.
24. Legha SS, Tenney DM, Krakoff IR. Phase I study of Taxol using a 5-day intermittent schedule. J Clin Oncol 1986;4:762–766.
25. Donehower RC, Rowinsky EK, Grochow LB, Longnecker SM, Ettinger DS. Phase I trial of Taxol in patients with advanced cancer. Cancer Treat Rep 1987;71:1171–1177.
26. Wiernik PH, Schwartz EL, Einzig A, Strauman JJ, Lipton RB, Dutcher JP. Phase I trial of Taxol given as a 24-hour infusion every 21 days: responses observed in metastatic melanoma. J Clin Oncol 1987;5:1232–1239.
27. Wiernik PH, Schwartz EL, Strauman JJ, Dutcher JP, Lipton RB, Paietta E. Phase I clinical and pharmacokinetic study of Taxol. Cancer Res 1987;47:2486–2493.
28. Kris MG, O'Connell JP, Gralla RJ, et al. Phase I trial of Taxol given as a 3-hour infusion every 21 days. Cancer Treat Rep 1986;70:605–607.
29. Ettinger DS. Overview of paclitaxel (Taxol) in advanced lung cancer. Semin Oncol 1993;20(Suppl 3):46–49.
30. Kirschling RJ, Jung SH, Jett JR, et al. A phase II trial of Taxol and G-CSF in previously untreated patients with extensive stage small cell lung cancer (SCC) (abstract). Proc Am Soc Clin Oncol 1994;13:326.
31. Abbruzzese JL, Grunewald R, Weeks EA, et al. A phase I clinical, plasma, and cellular pharmacology study of gemcitabine. J Clin Oncol 1991;9:491–498.
32. Poplin E, Redman B, Flaherity L. Difluorodeoxycytidine (dFdC): a phase study (abstract). Proc Am Assoc Cancer Res 1989;30:1123.
33. O'Rourke T, Brown T. Hawlin K. Phase I clinical trial of difluorodeoxycytidine (LY 188011) given as intravenous bolus on five consecutive days (abstract). Proc Am Soc Clin Oncol 1989;8:82.
34. Abbruzzese JL, Grunewald R, Weeks EA, et al. A phase I clinical, plasma, and cellular pharmacology study of gemcitabine. J Clin Oncol 1991;9:491–498.
35. Cormier Y, Eisenhauer E, Muldal A, et al. Gemcitabine is an active new agent in previously untreated extensive small cell lung cancer (SCLC). A study of the National Cancer Institute of Canada Clinical Trials Group. Ann Oncol 1994;5:283–285.
36. Bonfante V, Bonadonna G, Villani F, Di Fronzo G, Martini A, Casazza AM. Preliminary phase I study of 4'-epi-Adriamycin. Cancer Treat Rep 1979;63:915–918.
37. Hickish T, Cunningham D, Haydock A, Coombes RC. Experience with intermediate-dose (110–120 mg/m^2) epirubicin. Cancer Chemother Pharmacol 1989;24:61–64.
38. Blackstein M, Eisenhauer EA, Wierzbicki R, Yoshida S. Epirubicin in extensive small-cell lung cancer: a phase II study in previously untreated patients: A National Cancer Institute of Canada Clinical Trials Group study. J Clin Oncol 1990;8: 385–389.
39. Eckhardt S, Kolaric K, Vukas D, et al. Phase II study of 4'-epidoxorubicin in patients with untreated, extensive small cell lung cancer. South-East European Oncology Group (SEEOG). Med Oncol Tumor Pharmacother 1990;7:19–23.
40. Slevin ML, Clark PI, Joes SP, et al. A randomized trial to examine the effect of more extended scheduling of etoposide administration in small cell lung cancer (abstract). Proc Am Soc Clin Oncol 1989;8:236.
41. Hainsworth JD, Johnson DH, Frazier SR, Greco FA. Chronic daily administration of oral etoposide—a phase I trial. J Clin Oncol 1989;7:396–401.
42. Johnson DH, Greco FA, Strupp J, Hande KR, Hainsworth JD. Prolonged administration of oral etoposide in patients with relapsed or refractory small-cell lung cancer: a phase II trial. J Clin Oncol 1990;8:1613–1617.
43. Einhorn LH. Daily oral etoposide in the treatment of cancer. Semin Oncol 1991;18(Suppl 2):43–47.
44. Keane M, Carney DN. Treatment of elderly patients with small cell lung cancer. Lung Cancer 1993;9(Suppl 1):S91–S93.
45. Carney DN, Keane M, Grogan L. Oral etoposide in small cell lung cancer. Semin Oncol 1992; 19(Suppl 14):40–44.

46. Edmonson JH, Lagakos SW, Selawry OS, et al. Cyclophosphamide and CCNU in the treatment of inoperable small cell carcinoma and adenocarcinoma of the lung. Cancer Treat Rep 1976;60:925–932.
47. Lowenbraun S, Birch R, Buchanan R, et al. Combination chemotherapy in small cell lung carcinoma. A randomized study of two intensive regimens. Cancer 1984;54:2344–2350.
48. Bunn PA, Ihde DC. Small cell bronchogenic carcinoma: a review of therapeutic results. The Hague: Martinus Nijhoff, 1981:169–208.
49. Hansen HH, Selawry OS, Simon R, et al. Combination chemotherapy of advanced lung cancer: a randomized trial. Cancer 1976;38:2201–2207.
50. Hansen HH, Dombernowsky P, Hansen M, Hirsch F. Chemotherapy of advanced small-cell anaplastic carcinoma. Superiority of a four-drug combination to a three-drug combination. Ann Intern Med 1978;89:177–181.
51. Hong WK, Nicaise C, Lawson R, et al. Etoposide combined with cyclophosphamide plus vincristine compared with doxorubicin plus cyclophosphamide plus vincristine and with high-dose cyclophosphamide plus vincristine in the treatment of small-cell carcinoma of the lung: a randomized trial of the Bristol Lung Cancer Study Group. J Clin Oncol 1989;7:450–456.
52. Messeih AA, Schweitzer JM, Lipton A, et al. Addition of etoposide to cyclophosphamide, doxorubicin, and vincristine for remission induction and survival in patients with small cell lung cancer. Cancer Treat Rep 1987;71:61–66.
53. Jackson D Jr, Case LD, Zekan PJ, et al. Improvement of long-term survival in extensive small-cell lung cancer. J Clin Oncol 1988;6:1161–1169.
54. Jett JR, Everson L, Therneau TM, et al. Treatment of limited-stage small-cell cancer with cyclophosphamide, doxorubicin, and vincristine with or without etoposide: a randomized trial of the North Central Cancer Treatment Group. J Clin Oncol 1990;8:33–38.
55. Comis RL. Clinical trials of cyclophosphamide, etoposide, and vincristine in the treatment of small-cell lung cancer. Semin Oncol 1986;13(Suppl 3):40–44.
56. Einhorn L, Greco G, Wampler G, Randolph H. Cytoxan, Adriamycin, etoposide versus cytoxan, Adriamycin, vincristine in the treatment of small cell lung cancer (abstract). Proc Am Assoc Clin Oncol 1987;6:168.
57. Schabel F Jr, Trader MW, Laster W Jr, Corbett TH, Griswold D Jr. cis-Dichlorodiammineplatinum(II): combination chemotherapy and cross-resistance studies with tumors of mice. Cancer Treat Rep 1979;63:1459–1473.
58. Hainsworth JD, Williams SD, Einhorn LH, Birch R, Greco FA. Successful treatment of resistant germinal neoplasms with VP-16 and cisplatin: results of a Southeastern Cancer Study Group trial. J Clin Oncol 1985;3:666–671.
59. Evans WK, Osoba D, Feld R, Shepherd FA, Bazos MJ, DeBoer G. Etoposide (VP-16) and cisplatin: an effective treatment for relapse in small-cell lung cancer. J Clin Oncol 1985;3:65–71.
60. Porter LL, Johnson DH, Hainsworth JD, Hande KR, Greco FA. Cisplatin and etoposide combination chemotherapy for refractory small cell carcinoma of the lung. Cancer Treat Rep 1985;69:479–481.
61. Einhorn LH, Crawford J, Birch R, Omura G, Johnson DH, Greco FA. Cisplatin plus etoposide consolidation following cyclophosphamide, doxorubicin, and vincristine in limited small-cell lung cancer. J Clin Oncol 1988;6:451–456.
62. Antman K, Pomfret E, Karp G, Skarin A, Canellos G. Phase II trial of etoposide in previously treated small cell carcinoma of the lung. Cancer Treat Rep 1984;68:1413–1414.
63. Eans WK, Feld R, Osoba D, Shepherd FA, Dill J, Deboer G. VP-16 alone and in combination with cisplatin in previously treated patients with small cell lung cancer. Cancer 1984;53:1461–1466.
64. Issell BF, Einhorn LH, Comis RL, et al. Multicenter phase II trial of etoposide in refractory small cell lung cancer. Cancer Treat Rep 1985;69:127–128.
65. Einhorn LH. Cisplatin plus VP-16 in small-cell lung cancer. Semin Oncol 1986;13(Suppl 3):3–4.
66. Sierocki JS, Hilaris BS, Hopfan S, et al. cis-Dichlorodiammineplatinum(II) and VP-16-213: an active induction regimen for small cell carcinoma of the lung. Cancer Treat Rep 1979;63:1593–1597.
67. Evans WK, Shepherd FA, Feld R, Osoba D, Dang P, Deboer G. VP-16 and cisplatin as first-line therapy for small-cell lung cancer. J Clin Oncol 1985;3:1471–1477.
68. Kim RN, McDonald DB. The combination of VP-16-213 and cis-platinum in the treatment of small cell carcinoma of the lung (abstract). Proc Am Soc Clin Oncol 1982;1:142.
69. Woods RL, Levi JA. Chemotherapy for small cell lung cancer (SCLC): a randomized study of maintenance therapy with cyclophosphamide, Adriamycin and vincristin (CAV) after remission induction with cis-platinum (Cis, DDP), VP-16-213 and radiotherapy (abstract) Proc Am Soc Clin Oncol 1984;3:214.
70. Fukuoka M, Furuse K, Saijo N, et al. Randomized trial of cyclophosphamide, doxorubicin, and vincristine versus cisplatin and etoposide versus alternation of these regimens in small-cell lung cancer. J Natl Cancer Inst 1991;83:855–861.
71. Roth BJ, Johnson DH, Einhorn LH, et al. Randomized study of cyclophosphamide, doxorubicin, and vincristine versus etoposide and cisplatin versus alternation of these two regimens in extensive small-cell lung cancer: a phase III trial of the Southeastern Cancer Study Group. J Clin Oncol 1992;10:282–291.
72. Smith IE, Evans BD, Gore ME, et al. Carboplatin (Paraplatin; JM8) and etoposide (VP-16) as first-line combination therapy for small-cell lung cancer. J Clin Oncol 1987;5:185–189.
73. Bishop JF, Raghavan D, Stuart-Harris R, et al. Carboplatin (CBDCA, JM-8) and VP-16-213 in previously untreated patients with small-cell lung cancer. J Clin Oncol 1987;5:1574–1578.
74. Evans, WK, Eisenhauer E. Hughes P, et al. VP-16 and carboplatin in previously untreated patients with extensive small lung cancer: a study of the National Cancer Institute of Canada Clinical Trials Group. Br J Cancer 1988;58:464–468.
75. Gatzemeier U, Hossfeld DK, Neuhauss R, Reck M, Achterrath W, Lenaz L. Combination chemotherapy with carboplatin, etoposide, and vincristine as first-line treatment in small-cell lung cancer. J Clin Oncol 1992;10:818–823.
76. Gatzemeier U, Pawel JV, Laumen R, Hossfeld DK, Neuhauss R. Etoposide/vincristine–based chemotherapy with or without carboplatin in extensive-stage small cell lung cancer: a prospective randomized phase III trial. Semin Oncol 1994;21(Suppl 6):31–35.
77. Smith IE, Perren TJ, Ashley SA, et al. Carboplatin, etoposide, and ifosfamide as intensive chemotherapy for small-cell lung cancer. J Clin Oncol 1990;8:899–905.
78. Goldie JH, Coldman AJ. A mathematic model for relating the drug sensisitivity of tumors to their spontaneous mutation rate. Cancer Treat Rep 1979;63:1727–1733.
79. Goldie JH, Coldman AJ, Gudauskas GA. Rationale for the use

of alternating non–cross-resistant chemotherapy. Cancer Treat Rep 1982;66:439–449.
80. Østerlind K, Sorenson S, Hansen HH, et al. Continuous versus alternating combination chemotherapy for advanced small cell carcinoma of the lung. Cancer Res 1983;43:6085–6089.
81. Ettinger DS, Finkelstein DM, Abeloff MD, Ruckdeschel JC, Aisner SC, Eggleston JC. A randomized comparison of standard chemotherapy versus alternating chemotherapy and maintenance versus no maintenance therapy for extensive-stage small-cell lung cancer: a phase III study of the Eastern Cooperative Oncology Group. J Clin Oncol 1990;8:230–240.
82. Daniels JR, Chak LY, Sikic BI, et al. Chemotherapy of small-cell carcinoma of lung: a randomized comparison of alternating and sequential combination chemotherapy programs. J Clin oncol 1984;2:1192–1199.
83. Elliott JA, Østerlind K, Hansen HH. Cyclic alternating "non–cross resistant" chemotherapy in the management of small cell anaplastic carcinoma of the lung. Cancer Treat Rev 1984;11:103–113.
84. Evans WK, Feld R, Murray N, et al. Superiority of alternating non–cross-resistant chemotherapy in extensive small cell lung cancer. A multicenter, randomized clinical trial by the National Cancer Institute of Canada. Ann Intern Med 1987;107:451–458.
85. Feld R, Evans WK, Coy P, et al. Canadian multicenter randomized trial comparing sequential and alternating administration of two non–cross-resistant chemotherapy combinations in patients with limited small-cell carcinoma of the lung. J Clin Oncol 1987;5:1401–1409.
86. Goodman GE, Crowley JJ, Blasko JC, et al. Treatment of limited small-cell cancer with etoposide and cisplatin alternating with vincristine, doxorubicin, and cyclophosphamide versus concurrent etoposide, vincristine, doxorubicin, and cyclophosphamide and chest radiotherapy: a Southwest Oncology Group Study. J Clin Oncol 1990;8:39–47.
87. Bunn PA, Curren M, Fukuoka M, et al. Chemotherapy in small cell lung cancer: a consensus report. Lung Cancer 1989;5:127–134.
88. Gregor A, Morgan PGM, Morgan RL, Scadding FH, Turner-Warwick M. Small cell carcinoma: combined approach to treatment. Thorax 1979;34:789–793.
89. Bleehen NM, Fayers PM, Girling, DJ, Stephens RJ. Controlled trial of twelve versus six courses of chemotherapy in the treatment of small-cell lung cancer. Br J Cancer 1989;59:584–590.
90. Giaccone G, Dalesio O, McVie GJ, et al. Maintenance chemotherapy in small-cell lung cancer: long-term results of a randomized trial. European Organization for Research and Treatment of Cancer Lung Cancer Cooperative Group. J Clin Oncol 1993;11:1230–1240.
91. Bleehen NM, Girling DJ, Machin D, Stephens RJ. A randomized trial of three or six courses of etoposide, cyclophosphamide, methotrexate and vincristine or six courses of etoposide and ifosfamide in small cell lung cancer (SCLC) I: survival and prognostic factors. Br J Cancer 1993;68:1150–1156.
92. Spiro SG, Souhami RL, Geddes DM, et al. Duration of chemotherapy in small cell lung cancer: a Cancer Research Campaign trial. Br J Cancer 1989;59:578–583.
93. Splinter TAW, for the EORTC Lung Cancer Cooperative Group. EORTC 08825: induction versus induction plus maintenance chemotherapy in small cell lung cancer. Definitive evaluation (abstract). Proc Am Soc Clin Oncol 1988;7:202.
94. Cullen M, Morgan D, Gregory W, et al. Maintenance chemotherapy for anaplastic small cell carcinoma of the bronchus: a randomized, controlled trial. Cancer Chemother Pharmacol 1986;17:157–160.
95. Mattson K, Niiranen A, Pyrhonen S, et al. Natural interferon alfa as maintenance therapy for small cell lung cancer. Eur J Cancer 1992;28A:1387–1391.
96. Jett JR, Su JQ, Maksymiuk AW. Phase III trial of recombinant interferon gamma (rIFN-γ) in complete responders (CR) with small cell lung cancer (SCC) (abstract). Proc Am Soc Clin Oncol 1992;11:287.
97. Frei E, Canellos GP. Dose: a critical factor in cancer chemotherapy. Am J Med 1980;69:585–594.
98. Hryniuk W, Bush H. The importance of dose intensity in chemotherapy of metastatic breast cancer. J Clin Oncol 1984;2:1281–1288.
99. Hryniuk W, N. LM. Analysis of dose intensity for adjuvant chemotherapy trials in stage II breast cancer. J Clin Oncol 1986;4:1162–1170.
100. Levin L, Hryniuk W. The application of dose intensity to problems in chemotherapy of ovarian and endometrial cancer. Semin Oncol 1987 (Suppl 4);14:12–19.
101. DeVita VT, Hubbard SM, Longo DL. The chemotherapy of lymphomas: looking back, moving forward. The Richard and Hinda Rosenthal Foundation award lecture. Cancer Res 1987;47:5810–5824.
102. DeVita VT, Hubbard SM, Longo DL. Treatment of Hodgkin's disease. J Natl Cancer Inst Monogr 1990;10:19–28.
103. Cohen MH, Creaven PJ, Fossieck BE, et al. Intensive chemotherapy of small cell bronchogenic carcinoma. Cancer Treat Rep 1977;61:349–354.
104. Hande KR, Oldham RK, Fer MF, Richardson RL, Greco FA. Randomized study of high-dose versus low-dose methotrexate in the treatment of extensive small cell lung cancer. Am J Med 1982;73:413–419.
105. O'Donnell MR, Ruckdeschel JC, Baxter D, McNeally MF, Caradonna R, Horton J. Intensive induction chemotherapy for small cell anaplastic carcinoma of the lung. Cancer Treat Rep 1985;69:571–575.
106. Figueredo AT, Hryniuk WM, Strautmanis I, Frank G, Rendell S. Cotrimoxazole prophylaxis during high-dose chemotherapy of small cell lung cancer. J Clin Oncol 1985;3:54–64.
107. Johnson DH, Einhorn LH, Birch R, et al. A randomized comparison of high-dose versus conventional-dose cyclophosphamide, doxorubicin, and vincristine for extensive-stage small-cell lung cancer: a phase III trial of the Southeastern Cancer Study Group. J Clin Oncol 1987;5:1731–1738.
108. Ihde DC, Mulshine JL, Kramer BS, et al. Randomized trial of high vs. standard dose etoposide (VP16) and cisplatin in extensive stage small cell lung cancer (SCLC) (abstract). Proc Am Soc Clin Oncol 1991;10:240.
109. Klasa RJ, Murray N, Coldman AJ. Dose-intensity meta-analysis of chemotherapy regimens in small-cell carcinoma of the lung. J Clin Oncol 1991;9(3):499–508.
110. Souhami RL, Finn G, Gregory WM, et al. High-dose cyclophosphamide in small-cell carcinoma of the lung. J Clin oncol 1985;3:958–963.
111. Marangolo M, Rosti G, Amadori D, et al. High-dose etoposide and autologous bone marrow transplantation as intensification treatment in small cell lung cancer: a pilot study. Bone Marrow Transplant 1989;4:405–408.
112. Souhami RL, Hajichristou HT, Miles DW, et al. Intensive chemotherapy with autologous bone marrow transplantation for small-cell lung cancer. Cancer Chemother Pharmacol 1989;24:321–325.
113. Smith IE, Evans BD, Harland SJ, et al. High-dose cyclophos-

phamide with autologous bone marrow rescue after conventional chemotherapy in the treatment of small cell lung carcinoma. Cancer Chemother Pharmacol 1985;14:120–124.
114. Sculier JP, Klastersky J, Stryckmans P. Late intensification in small-cell lung cancer: a phase I study of high doses of cyclophosphamide and etoposide with autologous bone marrow transplantation. J Clin oncol 1985;3:184–191.
115. Cunningham D, Banham SW, Hutcheon AH, et al. High-dose cyclophosphamide and VP 16 as late dosage intensification therapy for small cell carcinoma of lung. Cancer Chemother Pharmacol 1985;15:303–306.
116. Ihde DC, Deisseroth AB, Lichter AS, et al. Late intensive combined modality therapy followed by autologous bone marrow infusion in extensive-stage small-cell lung cancer. J Clin Oncol 1986;4:1443–1454.
117. Humblet Y, Symann M, Bosly A, et al. Late intensification chemotherapy with autologous bone marrow transplantation in selected small-cell carcinoma of the lung: a randomized study. J Clin Oncol 1987;5:1864–1873.
118. Klimo P, Connors JM. MACOP-B chemotherapy for the treatment of diffuse large-cell lymphoma. Ann Intern Med 1985; 102:596–602.
119. Taylor CW, Crowley J, Williamson SK, et al. Treatment of small-cell lung cancer with an alternating chemotherapy regimen given at weekly intervals: a Southwest Oncology Group pilot study. J Clin Oncol 1990;8:1811–1817.
120. Sculier J-P, Klastersky J, Finet C, Ries F, Sergysels R, Mommen P. Intensive multiple drug induction chemotherapy for small-cell lung cancer a pilot study. Drug Invest 1990;2:99–104.
121. Miles DW, Earl HM, Souhami RL, et al. Intensive weekly chemotherapy for good-prognosis patients with small-cell lung cancer. J Clin Oncol 1991;9:280–285.
122. Murray N, Shah A, Osoba D, et al. Intensive weekly chemotherapy for the treatment of extensive-stage small-cell lung cancer. J Clin Oncol 1991;9:1632–1638.
123. Wampler GL, Ahlgren JD, Schulof RS. A pilot study of intensive weekly chemotherapy for extensive disease small-cell lung carcinoma. Cancer Invest 1992;10:97–102.
124. Alba E, Breton JJ, Alonso L, Paredes G, Belon J, Ballesteros P. Alternating chemotherapy for small-cell lung cancer. A twelve-week schedule of six drugs. Ann Oncol 1992;3:31–35.
125. Murray N, Gelmon K, Shah A, et al. Potential for long-term survival in extensive stage small-cell lung cancer (ESCLC) with CODE chemotherapy and radiotherapy (abstract). Proc Am Soc Clin Oncol 1994;13:338.
126. Miles DW, Souhami RL, Spiro SG, et al. A randomized trial comparing "standard" 3 weekly with weekly chemotherapy (C/T) in patients (pts) with small cell lung cancer (SCLC) (abstract). Proc Am Soc Clin Oncol 1992;11:289.
127. Sculier JP, Paesmans M, Bureau G, et al. Multiple-drug weekly chemotherapy versus standard combination regimen in small-cell lung cancer: a phase III randomized study conducted by the European Lung Cancer Working Party. J Clin Oncol 1993;11:1858–1865.
128. Clark SC, Kamen R. The human hematopoietic colon-stimulating factors. Science 1987;236:1229–1237.
129. Sieff CA. Hematopoietic growth factors. J Clin Invest 1987;79: 1549–1557.
130. Groopman JE, Molina JM, Scadden DT. Hematopoietic growth factors. New Engl J Med 1989;321:1449–1459.
131. Laver J, Moore MAS. Clinical use of recombinant human hematopoietic growth factors. J Natl Cancer inst 1989;81: 1370–1382.
132. Lieschke GJ. Granulocyte colony-stimulating factor and granulocyte-macrophage colony-stimulating factor (first of two parts). New Engl J Med 1992;327:28–35.
133. Lieschke GJ. Granulocyte colony-stimulating factor and granulocyte-macrophage colony-stimulating factor (second of two parts). New Engl J Med 1992;327:99–106.
134. Crawford J, Ozer H, Stoller R, et al. Reduction by granulocyte colony-stimulating factor of fever and neutropenia induced by chemotherapy in patients with small-cell lung cancer. N Engl Med 1991;325:164–170.
135. Trillet-Lenoir V, Green J, Manegold C, et al. Recombinant granulocyte colony stimulating factor reduces the infectious complications of chemotherapy. Eur J Cancer 1993;29A: 319–324.
136. Miles DW, Fogarthy O, Ash CM, et al. Received dose-intensity: a randomized trial of weekly chemotherapy with and without granulocyte colony-stimulating factor in small-cell lung cancer. J Clin Oncol 1994;12:77–82.
137. Ardizzoni A, Sirtoli MR, Corcione A, et al. Accelerated chemotherapy with or without GM-CSF for small cell lung cancer: a non-randomized pilot study. Eur J Cancer 1990;26: 937–941.
138. Fukuoka M, Takada M, Masuda N, et al. Dose intensive weekly chemotherapy (CT) with or without recombinant human granulocyte colony-stimulating factor (G-CSF) in extensive-stage (ES) small-cell lung cancer (abstract). Proc Am Soc Clin Oncol 1992;11:290.

23

Prophylactic Cranial Irradiation

Anna Gregor and Ann Cull

INTRODUCTION

In the last few decades of therapeutic endeavor in lung cancer, few topics have provoked such heated and ongoing controversy as the simple attempt to control one of the most common and frustrating sites of failure, brain metastases. The concept of prophylactic cranial irradiation (PCI), adopted with only minor modifications from the pediatric population with predominantly lymphoproliferative malignancies, has received a markedly changing reception. That spectrum ranged from being hailed in the beginning as the solution to the difficult problem of brain metastases for all patients to an almost total abandonment because of serious reservations about its overall effectiveness and potentially disastrous side effects.

The reasons for these large changes in attitude are multiple. Among them were the initially unrealistic and thus subsequently unfulfilled expectations of the efficacy of low-dose cranial irradiation in permanently controlling small cell lung cancer (SCLC) in the brain, thereby improving long-term survival. In some of the early studies, little regard for well-known potentiators of central nervous system (CNS) toxicity led to serious morbidity. Both of these factors led to disappointment and the reduced popularity of PCI as a treatment concept.

Recent literature reviews (1) have discussed most of these problems, and a number of randomized clinical trials focusing on the main questions of survival and toxicity are in progress (2–11). We can learn from careful analysis of the available data, and some of this experience has been influential in the design and execution of the ongoing next generation of prospective clinical trials. However, as with other elements of the practical management of lung cancer, progress is slow, and significant new therapeutic advances are infrequent.

The paradox of increasing frequency of symptomatic brain metastases with improved duration of survival demands a timely and practical solution. Collaboration and multidisciplinary involvement among radiation oncologists, medical oncologists, respiratory physicians, neurologists, radiologists, clinical psychologists, and neuropathologists is necessary to unravel the complex pattern of tumor behavior, treatment toxicity, and outcome, in terms of both the length and quality of survival. This cooperation will result in a rational and speedier modification of treatment protocols and provide opportunities for better treatment outcome. The need is self-evident, and the solutions are as yet unclear, but a number of presently available strategies show promise.

AVAILABLE EVIDENCE

PCI delays the appearance of symptomatic cerebral metastases and approximately halves the lifetime risk of CNS relapse (12). There are 10 randomized trials (Table 23.1) reported in the literature involving just over 750 patients (13). In addition, three current randomized trials are due to be completed soon and will provide additional information because their design contains a prospective assessment of neurotoxicity and quality of life. The planned size of these trials also allows more reliable evaluation of patterns of failure and their impact on overall survival.

The evaluation of presently available evidence from randomized clinical studies is complicated by many methodologic pitfalls. The published trials summarized in Table 23.1 are individually small in size and span two decades of treatment activity. A large variety of radiation and chemotherapy schedules has therefore been used.

Seven of these chemotherapy schedules included methotrexate (14) or lomustine (15), which each are well known to cause CNS toxicity and would be considered suboptimal regimens by present standards. The radiation doses chosen ranged from 20 Gy in 10 frac-

TABLE 23.1. Randomized Trials of Prophylactic Cranial Irradiation

AUTHOR (REFERENCE NO.)	NO. OF PATIENTS		RADIATION DOSE (GY)	DOSE/ FRACTION (GY)	BRAIN RELAPSE	
	+PCI	−PCI			+PCI (%)	−PCI (%)
Cox et al. (2)	24	21	20	2	17	20
Seydel et al. (3)	111	106	30	3	5	22
Beiler et al. (4)	23	31	24[a]	3	0	16
Maurer et al. (5)	79	84	30	3	4	18
Hansen et al. (6)	55	55	40	2	9	12.5
Aroney et al. (7)	15	14	30	3	0	36
Eagan et al. (8)	15	15	36	3.6	13	73
Jackson et al. (9)	14	15	30	3	0	27
Katsensis et al. (10)	17	18	40	4	12	44
Niranen et al. (11)	25	26	40	2	0	27

Abbreviations. +, with; −, without.
[a]Administered in combination with lomustine (CCNU).

tions to 40 Gy in 20 fractions. For the majority of historical trials, the preferred radiation schedule was 20 to 30 Gy in 8 to 10 fractions; only three trials have used higher radiation doses (6, 10, 11).

Criteria for patient selection was loose and included groups with widely differing prognostic features. Six trials recruited patients with all stages of disease at presentation, and only four restricted entry to those with limited disease.

Seven of the 10 studies reported a statistically significant reduction in rates of brain metastases in the PCI-containing arm. The rates of reported CNS relapse varied from 15% to 73% (mean, 20%) in patients not receiving prophylactic cranial irradiation and from 0% to 17% (mean, 6%) in those treated with radiotherapy. In two large trials (2, 6) and the small study by Aroney et al. (7), the difference in CNS recurrence rates between treated and untreated arms was not statistically significant. Only the Danish trial (6) reported rates for isolated brain relapse that were 4% for both arms regardless of PCI use.

The variability of outcome in all of these trials was further compounded by different observation periods. Follow-up periods were not available for five of the studies (2, 4, 5, 7, 9). In the two largest trials, the median observation period was 18 months (6) and 24 months (3), respectively. One small trial with only 50 patients reported mature data with a minimal 5-year follow-up (11). Although such a long observation period may not be strictly necessary in this aggressive tumor, the rate of detectable brain metastases rises with increasing observation period independently of treatment received. This means that short overall survival will underestimate the CNS relapse rate and favor the relapse rate reduction attributed to PCI.

Other methodologic variables included differing follow-up procedures and evaluation time points. The overall rate of detection is influenced by the thoroughness and frequency of neurologic examinations and the use of routine computed tomography (CT) or magnetic resonance imaging (MRI) in the follow-up of asymptomatic patients.

All of these variables affect the numerical frequency of dynamically changing and time-related events such as CNS relapse and preclude meaningful summation of data from the individual small studies. Comparison within these studies and across the randomization arms is not affected.

Because the potential benefit of reduction in the frequency of cerebral metastases is most apparent in long-term survivors, selection of patients with the best prognostic features should be a logical starting point for future trial design.

Only four of these trials (2, 3, 6, 8) selected patients with limited disease. Only one trial with a very small number of patients ($n = 32$) chose to study only patients achieving complete remission with induction chemotherapy (7).

The proportion of patients achieving major response to chemotherapy cannot be known for the majority of the reported trials. They generally used PCI early (days 1 to 28) in their treatment schedules (2–6, 9–11).

No evidence of survival benefit for PCI was seen in any of the trials. This conclusion is not surprising because brain metastases are the sole cause of death in only a minority of patients (10%) (16). None of these trials was large enough to detect such a difference. Intervening variables of patient-related and tumor-related prognostic factors and the effectiveness of systemic therapy would play a much more important role in determining the survival outcome than would a temporary delay or single-organ relapse.

The discrepancy in the frequency between clinically apparent, symptomatic, brain metastases and the more frequently seen CT or MRI abnormalities is well known (17). The increased frequency of CNS involvement with a longer observation period also is well recognized (12). There is a cumulative risk of CNS involvement of up to 80% at autopsy in patients dying of SCLC (13). Evaluation using a competing risk analysis (18) would be much more informative than a snapshot of the problem at a single time point, but this analysis is sadly not available. Whether these methodologic difficulties can be overcome in the new generation of prospective randomized trials also is unclear.

Of practical relevance is the finding that patients achieving a complete response to chemotherapy appear to have a higher risk of CNS metastases than do those with a lesser degree of tumor chemosensitivity (19). This may be true because responders to chemotherapy live longer than nonresponders and thus have a greater potential risk of developing CNS symptoms during their lifetimes. The other relevant point is the finding that although most randomized trials have shown a reduction of CNS relapse in the irradiated arm, they have not demonstrated the total abolition of brain metastases. Evidence from the review of available data suggests that recurrence after PCI increases with the increasing length of survival and thus follow-up (20).

NEUROPSYCHOLOGIC MORBIDITY

Although the most prominent clinical feature of late radiation damage is impaired mental function, evidence of the extent and degree of neuropsychologic morbidity after PCI remains inconclusive (Table 23.2). As well as differences within and among studies in key clinical treatment variables (e.g., neurotoxic chemotherapy, radiation schedule, timing of PCI relative to chemotherapy), studies also vary in the neurologic function tested, assessment methods used, and timing of the assessments. The number of patients assessed generally is small, and there are no baseline data indicating the patients' level of functioning before the administration of PCI in these cross-sectional studies.

There is a significant methodologic problem in the assessment of patients' higher mental function in this field. Mental state examination is not carried out routinely or reliably and is difficult for clinicians to interpret in the absence of appropriate norms. Neurotoxicity ratings remain inadequate. The common toxicity criteria include only a gross rating of consciousness. Castellanos and Fields (30) proposed more comprehensive neurotoxicity ratings than the original World Health Organization system, but even these signs concentrate on peripheral motor and sensory functions at the expense of higher mental functions.

The Mini-Mental State Examination (31) was intended to meet this need, but it has proved insensitive to all but the grossest impairment; a review of bedside screening instruments for cognitive impairment shows a high false-negative rate to be characteristic of the genre (32).

Of the most widely used quality of life measures, few tap higher mental function. The Rotterdam Symptom Checklist (33) and the European Organization for the Research and Treatment of Cancer Quality of Life Questionnaire–C30 (EORTC QLQ-C30) (34) incorporate items that assess concentration and memory. The more generic Sickness Impact Profile (35) has the most comprehensive scale of cognitive function, but it has not been validated against objective performance.

Several questionnaires have been developed to assess memory failures in everyday life (36, 37), but clearly there is a problem in seeking a reliable and valid account of memory failure by patient self-report alone. These methods generally require cross-referent data from an informant. Lishner et al. (29) (Table 23.2) developed their own questionnaire to record patients' subjective experience of neurotoxicity after cranial irradiation but did not report how well responses correlated with observable deficits.

Objective testing using standardized neuropsychometric assessment procedures offers a cheap, noninvasive, and sensitive method of obtaining useful information about cranial function.

Three studies have included neuropsychometric assessment as an outcome measure (Table 23.2). Twijnstra et al. (26) found no evidence of general intellectual impairment but described an extensive range of neuropsychologic dysfunctions. Without details of the tests used or the scoring method employed, it is difficult to be clear about how deficit was assessed. Although Johnson et al. (25) and Leukkanen et al. (27) had some measures in common, these investigators used different strategies for deriving a summary impairment index, thus making comparison difficult. Abnormalities on mental state examination and CT scan were reflected in abnormal function, but neuropsychometric testing also picked up functional difficulties in three of six patients who had normal CT scans (25).

TABLE 23.2. Assessment of Neurotoxicity After Treatment for Small Cell Lung Cancer

Author (Reference No.)	N[a]	Assessment Method	Findings	Conclusion
Catane et al. (21)	16	CNE, EEG, CT	PCI: 9 of 13 abnormal CT No PCI: 2 of 3 abnormal CT	No contraindication to PCI
Ellison et al. (22)	16	CNE	4 of 10 neurologic problems	PCI + nitrosoureas are associated with neurologic morbidity
Looper et al. (23)	18	I, CNE	14 of 18 neurologic problems	Significant risk of neurologic morbidity
Johnson et al. (24)	20	I, CNE, MSE, NPT, CT	75% neurologic complaints 65% abnormal CNE 60% abnormal MSE 75% abnormal NPT 75% abnormal CT	Neurologic morbidity common More with high-dose chemotherapy More with large radiotherapy factions
Lee et al. (25)	38	CNE, CT	14 of 20 abnormal CT 3 of 20 CNS neurotoxicity	CNS toxicity a problem Higher risk with methotrexate and procarbazine
Twijnstra et al. (26)	21	I, CNE, MSE, NPT	PCI: 12 of 14 memory loss No PCI: no memory loss	PCI is associated with neuropsychiatric morbidity
Laukkanen et al. (27)	12	I, CNE, MSE, NPT, CT	3 dementia 2 neurologic symptoms 7 neuropsychiatric impairment +3 borderline impaired	PCI leads to neuropsychiatric morbidity
Fleck et al. (28)	16	CNE, CT	PCI: 7 of 11 memory deficits	PIC leads to neuropsychiatric morbidity
Lishner et al.(39)	58	Patient self-report Questionnaire (n = 14)	PCI: 9 of 48 neurologic problems (2 dementia) No PCI: 1 neurologic problem 1 of 10 dementia	PCI leads to adverse effects only for minority

Abbreviations. CNE, clinical neurologic examination; 1, interview; MSE, mental state examination; NPT, neuropsychologic testing.
[a]Number of long-term survivors of small cell lung cancer.

Whether this increased sensitivity was a worthwhile return for the lengthy assessment procedure is moot.

Although it is true that the detailed examination of a single patient for clinical reasons requires professional skill and that the input of a trained psychologist is needed for the selection of appropriate methods and the interpretation of results, the rigorous standardization of the administration procedures for most psychologic tests is such that nonpsychologists can readily become competent in administering a battery of measures selected for research purposes. Clearly, this is required if multicenter studies are to incorporate and assess higher mental function in their evaluation of PCI.

The feasibility of this approach was demonstrated recently (38) in an international collaborative review of the outcome for 64 long-term survivors of SCLC (a minimum of 2 years after induction treatment). A battery of four tests was administered by nonpsychologists in the clinic setting. Testing took 20 to 25 minutes and proved sensitive to otherwise undetected deficits of cognitive function. Only 19% of these patients performed at the level expected for their age and intellectual ability on all four tests. Fifty-four percent of patients were impaired on two or more of the tests.

There is a bewildering array of tests available, and professionally guided selection is advisable. Some tests are restricted in their availability to ensure proper professional use. Some general points can be made to facilitate the dialogue between clinicians and psychologists about cognitive testing.

The concept of testing for global organic impairment has given way to a recognition of the validity of profiles in which some functions are compromised while others are preserved. Thus, more than one test is required. Valuable information has been compiled about the nature of damage after brain injury, cerebrovascular disorder, and dementia by developing standardized test procedures; the use of similar methods to trace the effects of CNS poisons or radiation damage would be a logical extension of this approach.

The selection of tests also may be influenced by practical considerations. The choice of measures for the international retrospective review (38) was influenced by the availability of materials that were presented visually, thus avoiding translation difficulties. The selection of instruments for the ongoing United Kingdom Coordinating Committee for Cancer Research (UKCCCR) trial was influenced by the need for parallel forms that allow repeated administration in this prospective study without the problem of learning contaminating the results.

Clinicians sometimes express concern about the acceptability of cognitive testing. This is an important consideration because valid assessment is impossible without the patient's cooperation and motivation. Patients should be informed about the nature and purpose of cognitive assessment and about how the information collected will be used. They have the right to expect some feedback about their performance and, for the patient who is troubled by memory impairment, some coping strategies can be suggested (e.g., use of cues, lists).

It is important to ensure that patients undergoing psychometric testing have whatever aids they may require, e.g., eyeglasses or hearing aid. Uninterrupted time is required, particularly when timed tests or measures of attention or concentration are used.

Cognitive efficiency is impaired by emotional distress, thus it is important to screen for states of anxiety or depression that could lower performance on tests. Brief measures such as the Hospital Anxiety and Depression Scale (39) do not add appreciably to the total testing time and should be included in any testing battery.

Studies have rarely put neuropsychologic morbidity after PCI into the context of patients' lives as a whole, although the impact of side effects of treatment is ultimately very relevant to clinical decision making. Johnson et al. (24) described 12 of 20 long-term survivors who had returned to a lifestyle comparable to that before the diagnosis of SCLC, but 4 of the remaining 8 were hampered in daily living by their intellectual impairment. Of 12 patients in the study of Laukkanen et al. (27), all were capable of self-care and were socially active. Three patients younger than 60 were employed full time, and nine were able to perform complex tasks such as city driving.

There are several advantages of including quality of life assessment in the outcome evaluation. Such testing enables inclusion of other aspects of patients' subjective experience that would otherwise be undetected, or at least unrecorded, and yet that are likely to be relevant to their cognitive efficiency, e.g., fatigue. In one study (38) using the Rotterdam Symptom Checklist, 64% of patients complained of tiredness and 54% had sleeping difficulties. Although clinically recognized as common problems among cancer patients and long-term survivors, these issues are underresearched.

The value of quality of life data assessment as an outcome measure is increasingly being recognized in lung cancer clinical trials, and there are undoubted advantages in building a common database through which studies can be compared and combined. The EORTC QLQ-C30 (34) and the Functional Assessment of Cancer Therapy questionnaires (40) may be particularly useful in this population because they combine a generic multidimensional quality of life measure (for cancer patients generally) with a supplementary module for lung cancer patients.

As concern grows about the need to find a rational basis for resource allocation in health care, there is likely to be an increased effort made to develop and refine methods (e.g., Q-Twist [41], Quality Adjusted Life-Year [42]) of combining quantity and quality of life into a single index to facilitate economic evaluation. To date, there have been few published economic evaluations of lung cancer treatment (43) and none of PCI.

A further reason for including a quality of life assessment comes from investigators exploring the relationship between initial patient-related quality of life and subsequent survival among patients with non–small cell lung cancer (NSCLC) (44, 45) who reported quality of life as an independent prognostic variable for survival in their studies. No comparable data have yet been published for patients with SCLC.

It seems clear that future prospective controlled trials that evaluate the outcome of PCI should include a quality of life assessment. These tests also should include appropriate screening for emotional distress and objective neuropsychometric testing

CONTEMPORARY STUDIES

For durable tumor control, much higher radiation doses may be needed than have been reported thus far in the literature. Realization that higher radiation doses may become necessary if and when the overall survival results of patients with SCLC improves is worrisome in view of the concerns of toxicity, which may preclude the widespread use of high-dose irradiation. Information about the length of time without symptoms of brain metastases and duration of good quality of life as a proportion of the overall survival in patients with SCLC may be the most clinically useful and relevant endpoint.

These data may become available from the current multicenter trials (Federation Nationale des Centres de Lutte Contre le Cancer, Eastern Cooperative Oncology Group, UKCCCR/EORTC). All of these trials share similar design features. They include only patients in complete remission after induction chemotherapy, and some have formal neuropsychometric assessment of CNS toxicity as an intrinsic part of their design.

The UKCCCR/EORTC study contains a separate and optional quality of life protocol as well. The trials have variable treatment schedules, both in terms of induction therapy and radiation parameters, that may complicate their future analysis, however. All have plans to recruit sufficient numbers of patients to achieve an acceptable degree of statistical power.

The British study is a pragmatic multicenter trial now extended into a collaboration with the EORTC Lung Cancer Cooperative Group. Patients with limited disease achieving complete remission from a variety of induction chemotherapy regimens are eligible, and institutions can choose their own radiation schedule from a suggested menu (Table 23.3).

The other multicenter trials include patients of all stages of SCLC who have achieved complete remission. The pragmatic design and heterogeneity of these populations reflect the need for large patient numbers and the relative rarity of long-term survival of patients with this tumor (46). The latter point is particularly relevant when there is a need to retain a meaningful sample size at the point of late toxicity assessment. Despite selecting patients with potentially the best chances of survival, the "fall off" in the first 18 months is considerable, with only one quarter of patients available for the 18- to 24-month assessment. With the long lag time of clinically apparent CNS toxicity, this reduction and the variability of associated clinical and radiologic findings (47) continues to present an important methodologic obstacle in trial design.

One of the two French cooperative trials has recently been completed: 294 evaluable patients were randomized between no PCI and radiation doses of 24 Gy in eight fractions over 12 days. Most of these patients ($n = 240$) had limited disease at presentation, and all had bronchoscopically confirmed complete remission after induction therapy. A significant reduction in overall brain metastasis rate (risk ratio, 0.32) and in the isolated brain metastasis rate (risk ratio, 0.28) at 2 years was seen in the PCI arm (R. Arriagada, personal communication).

Assessment of late morbidity was an intrinsic part of the trial protocol and included neuropsychometric and CT evaluation. A slight increase in CT abnormalities was seen in the patients receiving PCI (11% versus 3%, $P = .06$). Detailed analysis of functional assessments is not yet available.

Another French trial with similar selection and treatment design, but with no psychometric evaluation, is still ongoing. Joint evaluation may provide a more powerful basis for statistical evaluation of survival effects. Taken together these trials would offer a meta-analysis of approximately 1000 patients with complete remission. The PCI trial of the Eastern Cooperative Oncology Group has had considerable recruiting difficulties.

RADIATION MORBIDITY

That ionizing radiation can have detrimental effects on both the function and anatomic structure of the human brain is well known (48). The pathophysiologic mechanisms of radiation-induced brain damage and their functional consequences are not clear, however.

The degree of damage is dependent on the total radiation dose, the radiation fraction size, and the volume of brain irradiated (48). It follows a classical but often unpredictable time course with a lengthy lag period of months or even years preceding the clinical manifestations of late morbidity. As with other radiation side effects, the clinical patterns are divided into early and late (49) depending on their time of onset.

Classic acute CNS radiation reactions are unusual in clinical practice. Large (more than 8 Gy) single radiation dose exposures are needed to produce these effects. Most of the available experience comes from nuclear accidents, and the usual type of dose fractionation schedule used in PCI regiments does not produce similar effects. A mild degree of headache, tiredness, and occasional nausea can occur in a minority of patients during treatment. These effects, together with the inevitable but frequently reversible alopecia, are the only signs of acute toxicity that should be expected (50, 51).

The early delayed reaction of somnolence syndrome is common in the usual PCI radiation dose range. It was first described in children treated for ringworm (52) and became a well-recognized and common syndrome occurring in about 30% of children after cranial prophylaxis for leukemia (53). The features of this syndrome include anorexia, sleepiness, and

TABLE 23.3 Suggested Radiation Dosage for UKCCCR/EORTC PCI Trial

20 Gy in 5 daily fractions
24 Gy in 12 daily fractions
30 Gy in 10 daily fractions
36 Gy in 18 daily fractions
8 Gy single fraction

lethargy for 8 to 10 weeks after cranial irradiation. The effects are self-limiting and do not predict late CNS complications (54). More significant reactions with a similar time course are seen in similar proportions of patients with primary brain tumors treated with therapeutic courses of irradiation (55). These effects seem to be related to the volume of supratentorial brain included in the irradiation field, rather than to the total radiation dose. The underlying pathology is unknown. In the rare cases in which autopsy information is available, edema, perivascular round cell infiltration, and vascular wall changes can be seen. These signs correspond to the area of high radiation dose in phantom reconstructions (56).

The classic hallmark and the most serious and dose-limiting consequences of cerebral irradiation are delayed reactions. Their onset may be from months to several years after irradiation. Pathologically, areas of gliosis affecting predominantly in the white matter are seen (49). A spectrum of clinical findings can be found with characteristic changes on CT or MR imaging (57).

Frank radiation necrosis probably can be omitted from this discussion because it does not occur in the context of PCI. With the low radiation dose (52 Gy in 2-Gy daily fractions) employed by most prophylactic radiation schedules, there is an incidence of necrosis estimated at less than 1% for whole brain radiation (48). Radiation necrosis may become relevant if increasing doses or changing fractionation schedules are used.

The real and more worrisome problem is the progressive, irreversible, and often fatal white matter injury termed leukoencephalopathy This clinical syndrome consists of varying degrees of dementia, ataxia, spasticity, and sometimes seizures. Cognitive impairment often dominates. Most of the available clinical experience comes from the neurooncologic population in which higher radiation doses and additional focal tumor-related deficits complicate the clinical picture. Whole brain irradiation seems particularly prone to causing cognitive impairment. Increased risk has been attributed to supratentorial, large-volume, hemispheric irradiation in the pediatric brain tumor population (58). In adults, the evidence is sparse because the survival of patients with malignant gliomas is poor, and whole brain irradiation generally has been replaced by focal irradiation of the tumor and its immediate vicinity. Comparative data are not available for adults receiving whole brain irradiation and those with apparently normal brain tissue.

An interesting study of 302 consecutive autopsies in patients with leukemia and lymphoma treated with various schemes of radiation and chemotherapy was reported by Budka (59). The majority of these patients had received PCI (24 Gy), and some also had received as systemic therapy the repeated administrations of intrathecal methotrexate. Disseminated necrotizing leukoencephalopathy was seen histologically in two of these patients, both of whom had received PCI and intrathecal methotrexate. No autopsy-proven case of disseminated necrotizing leukoencephalopathy exists in which the patient had not received whole brain irradiation to a dose of at least 20 Gy; however, little neuropathologic information is available for patients with lung cancer. The older age, high frequency of tumor CNS involvement, and different treatment protocols may make this population particularly susceptible to treatment-related CNS toxicity. Furthermore, there is no available information correlating neuropathologic abnormalities with functional deficits.

Neurologic problems are common in patients with SCLC. In a group of 641 patients from Toronto reviewed by Sculier (60), one third developed neurologic problems because of their tumor, most frequently brain metastases.

Radiologic abnormalities characterized by widespread white matter changes secondary to increased intracerebral water content (47) were seen on CT and more readily on MRI. Their predominantly periventricular location is pathognomonic of late radiation-related damage (57).

Interestingly, little is known about the correlation of the presence and severity of radiologic abnormalities and clinical deficits. The severity of CT abnormalities is related to radiation dose, volume of normal brain irradiated, and time since irradiation (57). In most series evidence of radiologic abnormalities is seen in approximately 40% of patients after PCI (47).

Many chemotherapeutic agents produce detrimental effects on the brain (61, 62). Focal coagulation brain necrosis has been described after administration of intravenous vincristine and intrathecal methotrexate. Clinical encephalopathic syndromes characterized by confusion, spasticity, and coma leading to death have been described with high-dose methotrexate (61). Of the drugs regularly incorporated into small cell carcinoma treatment protocols, cisplatin (63), etoposide (VP-16) (64), ifosfamide (65), and, historically, methotrexate, and nitrosourea (15) have been implicated particularly.

The individual neurotoxicity of these drugs can be augmented further by irradiation. The mechanisms both cause sensitization of normal brain tissue to the radiation effects and the pharmacokinetic alteration of drug access caused by temporary disruption of the blood-brain barrier by cerebral irradiation (66). The importance of temporal relationships in the scheduling of systemic chemotherapy and cerebral irradiation and the profound influence on rates and severity of late CNS damage have been described for different routes of methotrexate administration in patients with acute lymphoblastic leukemia (67).

Among the most severely affected adult lung cancer patients reported after PCI, a large number received concurrent or postirradiation chemotherapy and often high doses of potentially neurotoxic drugs (21). The critical evaluation of the relationships between individual chemotherapy and radiation treatment regiments is hampered by the disparity in the schedules and the variety of treatment protocols used in the reported studies.

The poor overall survival of patients with SCLC and consequently the short observation period in most homogeneously treated patient series make further study of these relationships in this clinical situation impossible.

The impact of treatment-induced toxicity must be viewed in the context of symptoms caused by CNS metastases. From several studies (68, 69), brain metastases have been found to have detrimental effects on patients' quality of life and their ability to remain independent. Treatment of established brain metastases with radiation (70) or chemotherapy (71) is far from satisfactory. Effective palliation can be achieved in only about half of the treated patients.

Strategies of close radiologic surveillance using regular CT evaluations also have failed to improve the overall outcome (72).

Although brain metastases frequently are part of a wider spectrum of relapse/recurrent disease and are associated with intrinsically short survival, their specific management is far from satisfactory. Reduction in the number of metastases or delay in their appearance would bring a substantial clinical benefit.

The balance of benefit and toxicity can be evaluated critically only in a prospective randomized trial of PCI. Such a study must consider a variety of endpoints: (a) frequency of brain metastases singly or as a part of wider dissemination, (b) time to brain relapse, and (c) incidence and severity of CNS toxicity and its impact on the control of patients' symptoms and quality of life. Because large numbers of patients will require substantial periods of observation, such a trial will almost certainly require multicenter and multinational cooperation.

PRACTICAL RECOMMENDATIONS

The true value of PCI in patients with small cell and non–small cell lung cancers is unknown at present and needs to be established in prospective randomized trials. If participation in such a clinical assessment is not possible, certain broad recommendations can be followed to minimize the risks of late radiation morbidity and maximize the potential gain for individual patients.

The following recommendations reflect the consensus of two International Association for Study of Lung Cancer (IASLC) workshops on the management of SCLC (16, 73).

Investigators should try to identify patients with the best prognosis. Patients with a good performance status and limited disease at presentation are candidates, particularly if they had a substantial response to induction chemotherapy.

PCI is best done at the end of induction chemotherapy, thus avoiding concurrent chemotherapy or planned courses of subsequent systemic treatment and the use of drugs with known neurotoxic potential. There is no convincing evidence to suggest that delaying PCI until most chemotherapy is completed diminishes its effectiveness or influences the overall outcome.

The optimal radiation dose and fractionation schedule have not been identified. However, for practical purposes total radiation doses between 30 to 40 Gy in less than 3-Gy fractions per day are recommended. Treatment is delivered using a megavoltage apparatus. The patient is treated supine using a custom-made shell as an immobilization device. Two lateral opposing fields encompassing the entire cranial cavity are placed. Particular care should be taken to ensure coverage of the middle fossa and cribriform plate; for this reason use of simulation is recommended. If simulation is not available, then the radiologist should set up the machine using a line from the outer canthus to the lower portion of the tragus to provide a useful baseline. Individual or standardized blocks that shield facial structures are not essential.

Treatment is delivered in daily fractions, and both fields are irradiated daily. The radiation dose is prescribed to the midpoint intersection of the two beams (International Commission on Radiation Units [ICRU] 29).

FUTURE DIRECTIONS

The problem of CNS metastasis is real in all histologic types of lung cancer and is particularly common in small cell, adenocarcinoma, and large cell histologies (74). With improvements in systemic therapy and consequently in survival for patients with small cell and non–small cell carcinomas of the bronchus, the incidence of brain relapse is likely to increase (75). This increase will be seen not only in the overall frequency but also in the incidence of brain metastasis as a sole involvement. In this rare situation, effective prevention may lead to higher overall cure rates.

The only large-scale experience of effects of low-dose whole brain irradiation on cognitive function comes from the pediatric acute lymphocytic leukemia population (76). Findings from this group cannot be used readily in adults, however, and are not comparable with the lung cancer population on the basis of age, differing radiation schedules, and intervening chemotherapy variables. The long latency period of late radiation morbidity and the relatively short survival/observation period of lung cancer patients potentially underestimates the true incidence and degree of late radiation damage to the brain.

Improvement in effectiveness of systemic chemotherapy is unlikely to translate into better control of CNS involvement. The normal brain is protected by a vascular barrier that prevents access of blood-borne agents and toxins into the brain parenchyma. The blood-brain barrier is anatomically formed by nonfenestrated vascular endothelial cells with very tight intercellular junctions (77).

Passage across this phospholipid layer is dependent on the molecular weight, lipid solubility, and ionization state, and most chemotherapeutic agents cannot penetrate it (78). The disruption seen in brain tumor vasculature allows access of water soluble contrast into these specific areas (79) and may be responsible for the chemosensitivity of established brain metastases in SCLC (71). This vascular disruption does not occur in areas with microscopic cellular tumor infiltration.

For the foreseeable future, the use of external beam irradiation by γ-rays or high-energy x-rays will remain the treatment modality of choice. The prolongation of duration or systemic remission and thus the lengthening of the CNS metastases risk period will require higher radiation doses, probably in excess of 40 Gy. Using the experience of treatment of subclinical disease at other sites as an example, the radiation doses necessary for sterilization of micrometastasis of epithelial tumors approaches 50 Gy in 25 fractions over 5 weeks (80). Assessment of intrathoracic control with chemotherapy and irradiation in SCLC suggests that doses in excess of 50 Gy are needed for a more than 80% local control rate (81).

The use of such doses in large (more than 2 Gy) daily fractions is likely to cause significant toxicity. To limit toxicity the strategy of hyperfractionation may be useful. The radiobiologic theory underlying this concept can be simplified as follows. The effects of ionizing radiation on tumors and late-responding normal tissues, of which the brain is a classic example, fortunately are very different. The surviving portion of cells after irradiation is exponentially related to the total irradiation dose (D), number of fractions (n), and thus radiation dose per fraction (d). This relationship can be described by a linear quadratic model (82). Because cell proliferation is absent in the normal brain during irradiation, the equation can be simplified as

$$BED = D \times (1 + d/\alpha/\beta)$$

where BED is the biologically effective dose. The α to β ratios of 1.5:2 are reported for late-reacting tissues of the spinal cord and brain (82). Human tumors have much higher α to β ratios, typically greater than 10 (83). The advantage of using smaller doses per fraction is that a higher total irradiation dose can be given with similar late effects on normal tissues.

When comparing the BED values for conventionally (once-daily) fractionated and hyperfractionated radiotherapy for tumors and late-responding tissues (α to β ratio, 15; and α to β ratio, 2), a therapeutic gain of 24% has been estimated (84). This gain could be useful when tumor radiosensitivity is such that reducing the individual radiation fraction dose will not result in reduced cell kill; the concept is under clinical investigation in pediatric patients with acute lymphoblastic leukemia.

The BED values of commonly used PCI schedules and their relative effects on tumor and normal brain are summarized in Table 23.4. Schedules with the smallest difference between the desirable tumor effects and the unwanted effects on normal brain are best. For example, the 40 Gy in 20 fractions schedule results in a higher BED to the tumor (48), compared with 30 Gy in 10 fractions (39). Both schedules have a similar BED for brain (80 and 75).

Interfraction intervals of 8 hours or more are necessary for adequate repair of sublethal damage in the

TABLE 23.4. BED for Commonly Used Schedules of PCI

No. of Daily Fractions/ Daily Dose (cGy)		α/β^a 2 = Brain	α/β^a 10 = Tumor
3000 cGy	10/300	75	39
2000 cGy	5/400	60	28
3600 cGy	12/240	79	44
4000 cGy	20/200	80	48
2500 cGy	10/250	56	31

^{a}BED = D × (1 + d/α/β). (Formula from Fowler JF. The linear-quadratic formula and progress in fractionated radiotherapy. Br J Radiol 1989;62:679–694.)

CNS. Providing this hiatus is observed, (85) a hyperfractionated schedule of the same total radiation dose will achieve tumor control comparable to conventional treatment with significantly reduced late effects. Conversely, a higher total radiation dose can be delivered safely using a hyperfractionated schedule for a similar level of late normal tissue morbidity. Although these proposals need to be addressed in a prospective, randomized, clinical trial, the experimental and modeling evidence is sufficiently interesting to make this strategy a real possibility.

Other strategies needing prospective assessment include choice of optimal treatment scheduling with avoidance of chemotherapy and irradiation overlap. This separation is particularly important when chemotherapy with neurotoxic potential is used. Brain irradiation disrupts the blood-brain barrier (66) and allows drug access to otherwise protected regions of normal brain. Sensitization properties for cisplatin have been documented both in vitro and in vivo (86). The widespread use of cisplatin in induction protocols of combined modality treatment of SCLC and its nearly universal use in NSCLC make early concurrent PCI therapy in these situations potentially hazardous.

Present clinical evidence suggests that the therapeutic benefit of PCI appears to be greater for patients receiving it early (6 to 8 weeks) in their course of treatment, compared with those treated later (18 weeks) (87). This fact leads to practical problems in patient selection and treatment schedule design. Thus, PCI will need to undergo a careful prospective assessment within the often complex relationship of multidisciplinary therapy.

Strategies addressing the problem of brain metastases are relevant for other types of lung cancer as well. In NSCLC brain metastases are common and just as difficult to treat as in small cell histologic varieties. In 300 consecutive autopsies, the Veteran Administration Lung Group demonstrated that up to half of sufferers of adenocarcinoma and large cell carcinoma had evidence of CNS tumor involvement. For squamous carcinoma histology, this figure, at 25%, was significantly lower (88). It is estimated that approximately 16% of patients with squamous cell carcinoma and 30% with adenocarcinoma and large cell carcinoma histologies will develop symptomatic brain metastasis during the observation period following primary therapy for locally advanced NSCLC (89). Although brain relapse is only rarely the sole cause of death in these patients (88), it has been found to have a profoundly negative impact on patients' quality of life and symptom control. Treatment of established brain metastasis is unsatisfactory. Median survival ranges from 3 to 6 months in different series, and up to 50% of patients die with uncontrolled cerebral involvement despite therapeutic irradiation (90).

A particularly unfortunate scenario is the finding of brain metastasis after apparently successful resection of an early-stage adenocarcinoma (91). The overall risk of brain relapse in this situation approaches 7% but is significantly greater with more advanced tumors. The figures for surgical stages II and III are lower than those for patients with inoperable NSCLC. The brain is the initial site of failure in approximately 20% of patients with adenocarcinoma (89). A similar frequency is seen in patients with residual disease or extensive nodal involvement after resection.

In patients receiving neoadjuvant therapy, similarly high (21%) brain relapse rates were seen by the Lung Cancer Study Group (8). One third of 41 patients receiving neoadjuvant chemotherapy with concurrent chest irradiation in the Memorial Sloan–Kettering study (92) developed brain recurrence as a primary site of failure.

PCI can reduce the lifetime frequency of brain metastasis in patients with NSCLC. The Veterans Administration Lung Group's randomized trial of PCI (20 Gy dose) in all histologic types of inoperable lung cancer produced a significant decrease in the rate of CNS metastasis in patients with adenocarcinoma but with little impact on squamous cell histology (93). A prospective randomized study of 100 patients with locally advanced NSCLC from the M. D. Anderson Hospital showed a significant decrease in the incidence of brain metastases in the irradiated group (4% versus 27%) (94). More recent studies of combined modality treatment incorporating PCI have again confirmed its ability to reduce the clinically apparent relapse rate in the CNS. This conclusion was seen in 18 of 94 randomized patients receiving PCI and 8 of 93 patients not receiving PCI in a study performed by the Radiation Therapy Oncology Group (95). All of these patients were treated with adjuvant mediastinal irradiation.

The Southwest Oncology Group (96) reported a nonrandomized study of 75 patients treated in a phase II study of neutron chest irradiation and postirradiation chemotherapy (platinum, etoposide, and mitomycin). None of the patients completing PCI had developed clinical or radiologic brain metastases. With a median follow-up of 9 months for the whole group and 26 months for eight long-term survivors, one patient developed progressive dementing illness classified as Alzheimer's disease, and one had optic neuritis.

It is likely that relationships between brain irradiation and chemotherapy and the singular late effects of whole brain irradiation in the elderly population would be similar to those in patients with SCLC. The short overall survival in the SCLC population, leading to a limited observation period, is again likely to underestimate both the frequency and degree of these defects.

Although CNS relapse is a common and unpleasant side effect for patients with NSCLC, the poor overall prognosis makes PCI largely irrelevant at the present time. For the 10% or so of surgically resected patients who relapse in the brain, PCI could be useful. The concerns about late morbidity and inability to select prospectively and reliably those individuals at particular risk means that PCI is unlikely to gain general favor in this subgroup of patients. The need to evaluate prospectively the methods that deal effectively with this site of failure and with minimal long-term problems will become particularly useful when effective systemic therapy can produce a reliable number of long-term survivors.

With the continuing problem of access of most active chemotherapeutic agents into the uninvolved brain, the development of a safe and effective radiation schedule remains a priority. The need for tissue penetration and lack of specificity for lung cancer–associated antigens will make antibody-targeted therapy unsuitable as a prophylaxis treatment. The potential cross reactivity of SCLC antibodies with neural tissue (97) may cause a potentially dangerous increase in normal tissue toxicity. The challenge of providing an effective and safe cranial prophylaxis for patients with lung cancer will remain, indicating the continuing need for careful clinical evaluation using appropriate methodology and relevant endpoints. In parallel with the clinical studies, a search for appropriate laboratory models may ease the burden of evaluation and simplify the choice of appropriate schedules for clinical testing.

References

1. Kristjansen PEG, Kristensen CA. The role of PCI in the management of small cell lung cancer. Cancer Treat Rev 1993;19:3–16.
2. Cox JD, Petrovich Z, Paig C, Stanley K. Prophylactic cranial irradiation in patients with inoperable carcinoma of the lung. Cancer 1978;42:1135–1140.
3. Seydel HG, Creech R, Pagano M, et al. Prophylactic versus no brain irradiation in regional small cell lung carcinoma. Am J Clin Oncol 1985;8:218–223.
4. Beiler DD, Kane RC, Bernath AM, Cashdollar MR. Low dose elective brain irradiation in small cell carcinoma of the lung. Int J Radiat Oncol Biol Phys 1979;5:941–945.
5. Maurer LH, Tulloh M, Weiss RB, et al. A randomized combined modality trial in small cell carcinoma of the lung: comparison of combination chemotherapy-radiation therapy versus cyclophosphamide-radiation therapy. Effects of maintenance chemotherapy and prophylactic whole brain irradiation. Cancer 1980;45:30–39.
6. Hansen HH, Doorbernorcky P. Prophylactic irradiation of bronchogenic small cell carcinoma. Cancer 1980;46:279–284.
7. Aroney RS, Aisner J, Wesley MN, et al. Value of prophylactic cranial irradiation given at complete remission in small cell lung carcinoma. Cancer Treat Rep 1983;67:675–682.
8. Eagan RT, Frytak S, Lee RE, Creagan ET, Ingle JN, Nichols WC. A case for preplanned thoracic and prophylactic whole brain radiation therapy in limited small cell lung cancer. Cancer Clin Trials 1981;4:261–266.
9. Jackson DV, Richards F, Cooper MR, et al. Prophylactic cranial irradiation in small cell carcinoma of the lung. A randomized study. JAMA 1983;237(25):2730–2733.
10. Katsensis AT, Karpasitis N, Giannakakis D, Maragoudakis N, Kiparissiadis P. Elective brain irradiation in patients with small-cell carcinoma of the lung: preliminary report. Lung cancer. International Congress Series 558, Exerpta Medica 1982:277–284.
11. Niiranen A, Holsti P, Salmo M. Treatment of small cell lung cancer. Acta Oncol 1989;28:501–505.
12. Nugent JL, Bunn PA Jr, Matthews M, et al. CNS metastases in small cell bronchogenic carcinoma. Increasing frequency and changing pattern with lengthening of survival. Cancer 1979;44:1885–1893.
13. Pedersen AG. Diagnosis of CNS-metastases from SCLC. In: Hansen HH, ed. Lung cancer: basic and clinical aspects. Boston: Martinus Nijhoff Publishers, 1986:153–182.
14. Allen JC, Rosen G, Mehta BM, Horten B. Leukoencephalopathy following high dose IV methotrexate chemotherapy with leucovorin rescue. Cancer Treat Rep 1980;64:1261–1273.
15. Phillips GL, Wolff SN, Fay JW, et al. Intensive 1, 3-bis (2-chloroethyl)-1 nitrosourea (BCNU) mono-chemotherapy and autologous marrow transplantation for malignant glioma. J Clin Oncol 1986:639–645.
16. Pedersen AG, Kristjansen PEG, Hansen HH. Prophylactic cranial irradiation and small cell lung cancer. Cancer Treat Rev 1988; 15:85–103.
17. Bunn PA, Nugent JL, Matthews M. Central nervous system metastases in small cell bronchogenic carcinoma. Semin Oncol 1978;5:314–322.
18. Arriagada R, Kranar A, De Credoux H. Competing events determining relapse free survival in limited small cell lung cancer. J Clin Oncol 1992;10(3):447–451.
19. Østerlind K, Hansen HH, Hansen HS, Dombernowsky P, Hansen M, Rorth M. Chemotherapy vs chemotherapy plus irradiation in limited small cell lung cancer. Results of a controlled trial with 5 years' follow-up. Br J Cancer 1986;54:7–17.
20. Kristjansen PEG. The role of cranial irradiation in the management of patients with small cell lung cancer. Lung Cancer 1989;5:264–274.
21. Catane R, Schwade JG, Yarr I, et al. Follow-up neurological evaluation in patients with small cell lung carcinoma treated with prophylactic cranial irradiation and chemotherapy. In J Radiat Oncol Biol Phys 1981;7:105–109.
22. Ellison N, Bernath A, Kane R, Porter P. Disturbing problems of success: clinical status of long-term survivors of small cell lung cancer (SCLC). Proc Am Soc Clin Oncol 1982;C-579:149.
23. Looper JD, Ginhom LH, Carcia SA, Homback NB, Vincent B, Williams SD. Severe neurological problems following successful therapy for small cell lung cancer. Proc Am Soc Clin Oncol 1984;C-903.
24. Johnson BE, Becker B, Goff WB, et al. Neurologic neuropsychologic and computer cranial tomography scan abnormalities in 2 to 10 year survivors of small cell lung cancer. J Clin Oncol 1985;3:1659–1667.
25. Lee JS, Umswardi T, Lee YY, Barkley HT, Murphy WK, Welch S, et al. Neurotoxicity in long-term survivors of small cell lung cancer. Int J Radiat Oncol Biol Phys 1986;12:313–21.

26. Twijnstra A, Boon PJ, Lormans ACM, Ten Velde GPN. Neurotoxicity of prophylactic cranial irradiation in patients with small cell carcinoma of the lung. Eur J Cancer Clin Oncol 1987;7:983–6.
27. Laukkanen E, Klonoff H, Allan B, Graeb D, Murray N. The role of prophylactic brain irradiation in limited stage small cell lung cancer: clinical neuropsychologic and CT sequelae. Int J Oncol Biol Phys 1988;14:1109–1117.
28. Fleck JF, Ginhom LH, Lauer RC, Schultz SM, Miller ME. Is prophylactic cranial irradiation indicated in small cell lung cancer? J Clin Oncol 1990;8:209–214.
29. Lishner M, Feld R, Payne DG, et al. Late neurological complications after prophylactic cranial irradiation in patients with small cell lung cancer: the Toronto experience. J Clin Oncol 1990;8:215–221.
30. Castellanos AM, Fields WS. Grading of neurotoxicity in cancer therapy. J Clin Oncol 1986;4:1277–1278.
31. Folstein MF, Folstein SE, McHugh PR. Mini-Mental State. A practical method for grading the cognitive state of patients for the clinician. J Psychiatr Res 1975;12:189–198.
32. Nelson A, Fogel S, Faust D. Bedside cognitive screening instruments. J Nerv Ment Dis 1986;2:73–83.
33. de Haes JCJM, Van Knippenberg FCE, Neijt JP. Measuring psychological and physical distress in cancer patients: structure and application of the Rotterdam Symptom Checklist. Br J Cancer 1990;62:1034–1038.
34. Aaronson NK, Ahmedzai S, Bergman B, Bullinger M, Cull A. The EORTC QLQ-C30: A Quality of Life Instrument for Use in International Clinical Trials in Oncology. J Natl Cancer Inst 1993;5:365–76.
35. Bergner M, Bobbitt HRA, Carter WB, Gilson BS. The Sickness Impact Profile: development and final revision of a health status measure. Med Care 1981;19(8):787–805.
36. Broadbent DE, Cooper PF, FItzgerald P, Parkes KR. The Cognitive Failures Questionnaire (CFQ) and its correlates. Br J Clin Psychol 1981;21:1–16.
37. Sunderland A, Harris HE, Gleave J. Memory failures in everyday life following severe head injury. J Clin Neuropsychol 1984;6(2):127–142.
38. Cull A, Gregor A, Hopwood P, et al, Neurological and cognitive impairment in long-term survivors of small-cell lung cancer. Eur J Cancer 1994;30A(8):1067–1074.
39. Zigmond AS, Snaith RP. The Hospital Anxiety and Depression (HAD) Scale. Acta Psychiatr Scand 1983;67:361–370.
40. Cella DF, Tulsky DS, Gray G, et al. The Functional Assessment of Cancer Therapy Scale: development and validation of the general measure. J Clin Oncol 1983;11:570–579.
41. Gelber RD, Godhirsch A, Cole BF. Evaluation of effectiveness: Q-TWIST. Cancer Treat Rev 1993;19(Suppl A):73–84.
42. Speigelhalter DJ, Gore SM, Fitzpatrick R, Fletcher AE, Jones DR, Cox DR. Quality of life measurement in health care III: resource allocation. BMJ 1992;305:1205–1208.
43. Goodwin PJ. Economic factors in cancer palliation—methodologic considerations. Cancer Treat Rev 1993;19(Suppl A):59–65.
44. Kaasa S, Mastekaasa A, Lund E. Prognostic factors for patients with inoperable small cell lung cancer limited disease. The importance of patients' subjective experience of disease and psychosocial well being. Radiother Oncol 1989;15:235–242.
45. Ganz PA, Lee JJ, Siau J. Quality of life assessment. An independent prognostic variable for survival in lung cancer. Cancer 1991;67:3131–3135.
46. Souhami RL, Law K. Longevity in small cell lung cancer. A report to the Lung Cancer Subcommittee of the UK Coordinating Committee for Cancer Research. Br J Cancer 1990;61(4):584–589.
47. Craig JB, Jackson DV, Moody D, et al. Prospective evaluation of changes in computed cranial tomography in patients with small cell lung carcinoma treated with chemotherapy and prophylactic cranial irradiation. J Clin Oncol 1984;2:1151–1156.
48. Sheline GE, William WW, Smith V, et al. Therapeutic irradiation and brain injury. Oncol Intell 1980(6):1215–1228.
49. Leibel SA, Sheline GE. Tolerance of the central and peripheral nervous system to therapeutic irradiation. Lett JT, Altman KI, eds. Advances in radiation biology. New York: Academic Press, 1987:257–288.
50. Perez CA, Einhorn L, Oldham RK, et al. Randomised trial of radiotherapy in limited small cell carcinoma of the lung treated with chemotherapy and prophylactic cranial irradiation. J Clin Oncol 1984;2:1200–1208.
51. Feld R, Clamon GH, Blunn R, Moran E, et al. Short course of prophylactic cranial irradiation for small cell lung cancer. Am J Clin Oncol 1985;8:371–376.
52. Druckmann A. Schlafsucht als folge der Roentgentherapie. Strahlenther Onkol 1929;33:382–384.
53. Freeman JE, Johnston PGB, Voke JM. Somnolence after prophylactic cranial irradiation in children with acute lymphoblastic leukaemia. BMJ 1973;4:523–525.
54. Parker P, Malpas JS, Sandland R, Sheaff PC, Freeman JE, Paxton A. Outlook following somnolence syndrome after prophylactic cranial irradiation. BMJ 1978;4:554–556.
55. Hoffman WF, Levin VA, Wilson CB. Evaluation of malignant glioma patients during the post-irradiation period. J Neurosurg 1979;50:624–628.
56. Almquist S, Dahlgren S, Notter G, Sundbom L. Brain necrosis after irradiation of hypophysis. Acta Radiol 1964;2:179–188.
57. Constine LS, Konski A, Ekholms S, McDonald S, Rubin P. Adverse effects of brain irradiation correlated with MR and CT imaging. Int J Radiat Biol Phys 1988;1(5):319–330.
58. Ellenberg L, McComb JG, Siegel SE, Stowe SS. Factors affecting intellectual outcome in paediatric brain tumour patients. Neurosurgery 1987;21:5 638–644.
59. Budka H. Pathology of encephalopathies induced by treatment or prophylaxis of neoplastic lesions of the nervous system. In: Hilderbrand J, Gangji P, eds. Treatment of neoplastic lesions of the CNS. New York: Pergamon Press, 1980:45–50.
60. Sculier JP, Feld R, Evans WK, et al. Neurologic disorders in patients with small cell lung cancer. Cancer 1987;60:2275–2283.
61. Kaplan RS, Wiemick PH. Neurotoxicity of anti-neoplastic drugs. Semin Oncol 1982;9:103–120.
62. Jellinger K. Pathologic effects of chemotherapy. In: Walker MD, ed. Oncology of the nervous system. Boston: M. Nijhoff, 1983: 285–340.
63. Molman JE. Cisplatin neurotoxicity. N Engl J Med 1990;322: 126–127.
64. Leff RS, Thompson JM, Daly MB, et al. Acute neurologic dysfunction after high-dose etoposide therapy for malignant glioma. Cancer 1988;62:32–35.
65. Pratt CB, Green AA, Horowitz ME, et al. Central nervous system toxicity following the treatment of pediatric patients with ifosfamide/mesna. J Clin Oncol 1986;4:1253–1261.
66. Davella D, Cicciarello R, Albiero F, Mesiti M, Gogliardi ME, Russi E, et al. Quantitative study of blood brain barrier permeability changes after experimental whole brain irradiation. Neurosurgery 1992;30:30–34.
67. Bleyer WA, Griffin TW. White matter necrosis mineralising angiopathy and intellectual abilities in survivors of childhood leukaemia. In: Gilber HA, Kajan AR, eds. Radiation damage to central system. New York: Raven Press, 1980:155–174.

68. Felletti R, Souhami RL, Spiro SG, et al. Social consequences of brain or liver relapse in small cell carcinomas of the bronchus. Radiother Oncol 1985;4:335–339.
69. Lucas CF, Robinson B, Hoskin PJ, Yarnold JR, Smith EI, Ford HT. Morbidity of cranial relapse in small cell lung cancer and the impact of radiation therapy. Cancer Treat Rep 1986;70:565–570.
70. Carmichael J, Crane JM, Bunn PA, Glatstein E, Ihde DC. Results of therapeutic cranial irradiation in small cell lung cancer. Int J Radiat Oncol Biol Phys 1988;14:455–459.
71. Postmus PE, Sleijfer DT, Haaxma-Reiche H. Chemotherapy for central nervous system metastases from SCLC. A review. Lung Cancer 1989;5:254–263.
72. Hardy J, Smith I, Cherryman G, et al. The value of computed tomographic (CT) scan surveillance in the detection and management of brain metastases in patients with small cell lung cancer. Br J Cancer 1990;62:684–686.
73. Arriagada R, Le Chevalier T, Borie F, Tardivon A, Riviere A, et al. Randomised trial of prophylactic cranial irradiation for small cell lung cancer in complete remission. Lung Cancer 1994;11(2): 177–178.
74. Aisner J, Forastiere A, Aroney R. Patterns of recurrence for cancer of the lung and oesophagus. Cancer Treat Symp 1983;2: 87–105.
75. Feld R, Rubinstein LV, Weisenberger TH, et al. Sites of recurrence in resected stage I non–small cell lung cancer: a guide for future studies. J Clin Oncol 1984;2:1352–1358.
76. Mulhern RK, Wasserman AL, Fairclough D, Ochs J. Memory function in disease-free survivors of childhood acute lymphocytic leukemia given CNS prophylaxis with or without 1800 cGy cranial irradiation. J Clin Oncol 1988;6:315–320.
77. Gregoire N. The blood-brain barrier. J Neuroradiol 1989;16: 238–250.
78. Greig NH. Optimising drug delivery to brain tumours. Cancer Treat Rev 1987;14:1–28.
79. Long DM. Capillary ultrastructure and the blood-brain barrier in human malignant brain tumours. J Neurosurg 1970;32:127–144.
80. Fletcher GM. Clinical dose response curves of subclinical aggregates of epithelium. J Radiol Electrol 1972;53:201–206.
81. Arriagada R, Le Chavalier T, Balderyrou P, et al. Alternating radiotherapy and chemotherapy schedules in small cell lung cancer. Limited disease. Int J Radiat Oncol Biol Phys 1985;11: 1461–1467.
82. Fowler JF. The linear-quadratic formula and progress in fractionated radiotherapy. Br J Radiol 1989;62:679–694.
83. Withers HR. Biologic basis of radiation therapy. principles and practice of radiation oncology. Philadelphia: JB Lippincott, 1987:67.
84. Miller-Runkell R, Vijaakuma RS. Therapeutic gain with hyperfractionation in prophylactic cranial irradiation of children with acute lymphoblastic leukaemia. Med Hypotheses 1992;39(4): 384–389.
85. Thames HD, Ng KK, Stewart FA, Wandenschurin. Does complete repair explain apparent failure of the basic LQ model to predict spinal chord and kidney responses to low doses per fraction? Int J Radiat Oncol Biol Phys 1988;54:13.
86. Guchelaar HJ, Uges DRA, De Vries EGE, Oosterhuis J, Mulder NW. Combination therapy with cisplatin: modulation of activity and tumour sensitivity. Clin Oncol 1992;4:388–393.
87. Lee JS, Umsawasdi T, Barclay HJ. Timing of elective brain irradiation: a critical factor for brain metastases free survival in small cell lung cancer. Int J Radiat Oncol Biol Phys 1987;13:697–704.
88. Cox JD, Yesner RA. Adenocarcinoma of the lung: recent results from the Veterans Administration Lung Group. Am Rev Respir Dis 1979;120:1025–1029.
89. Perez CA, Pajak TF, Rubin P, et al. Long term observations of the patterns of failure in patients with unresectable non–oat cell carcinoma of the lung treated with definitive radiotherapy. Cancer 1987;59:1874–1881.
90. Borgelt B, Gelbert R, Kramer S, et al. The palliation of brain metastasis: final results of the first two studies by the Radiation Therapy Oncology Group. Int J Radiat Oncol Biol Phys 1980;6: 1–9.
91. Figlin RA, Piantadosi S, Feld R, et al. Intercranial recurrence of carcinoma after complete surgery resection of stage I, II and III non–small cell lung cancer. N Engl J Med 1988;318:1300–1305.
92. Martini N, Chris MG, Gralla RJ. The effects of pre-operative chemotherapy on resectability of non–small cell lung cancer with mediastinal lymph node metastasis (N2MO). Ann Thorac Surg 1988;45:370–379.
93. Cox JD, Stanley K, Petrovich Z, Paig C, Yesner R. Cranial irradiation in cancer of the lung of all cell types. JAMA 1981;245: 469–472.
94. Umsawarsdi T, Valdivieso M, Chen TT. Role of elective brain irradiation during combined chemo-radiotherapy for limited disease non–small cell lung cancer. J Neurol Oncol 1984;2:253–259.
95. Russell AH, Pajak TE, Selim HM, et al. Prophylactic cranial irradiation for lung cancer patients at high risk for development of cerebral metastasis: results of a prospective randomised trial conducted by the Radiation Therapy Oncology Group. Int J Radiat Oncol Biol Phys 1991;21(3):637–643.
96. Rusch VW, Griffin BR, Livingston RB. The role of prophylactic cranial irradiation in regionally advanced non–small cell lung cancer. A South West Oncology Group study. J Thorac Cardiothorac Surg 1989;98(4):535–539.

24

ISOLATED EXTENSIVE DISEASE

Denise M. Hickey and L. Herbert Maurer

INTRODUCTION

Staging of cancer distinguishes between patients with varying prognoses. Small cell lung cancer can be staged using two distinct systems. The first, the TNM classification, stratifies patients based on the size of the primary tumor, involvement of regional lymph nodes, and the presence of metastases. A revised TNM system for lung cancer, the International Staging System as described by Mountain (1), has been accepted by the American Joint Committee on Cancer (2) and the International Union Against Cancer (3). In addition to prognostic information, this classification identifies patients with non–small cell lung cancer who are candidates for surgical resection.

A second classification system, proposed by the Veterans Administration Lung Group, is used solely to stratify patients with small cell lung cancer (4). In this schema, patients are categorized as having limited or extensive disease. As originally defined, limited disease is restricted to disease involving one hemithorax and regional lymph nodes, and it is able to be encompassed in a single radiation port. Any other disease is considered extensive. Most investigators have considered ipsilateral supraclavicular lymph node involvement as limited disease. Contralateral involvement has been considered limited disease by some investigators, but others have classified it as extensive disease, which does add some confusion in the interpretation of the literature.

Patients with limited stage small cell lung cancer have a significantly better prognosis than patients with extensive disease. In untreated patients the median survival of patients with limited disease was 3 months, and it was less than 2 months in those with extensive disease (5–7). With the advent of chemotherapy, prognosis has improved for both sets of patients but more so for those with limited disease. Several studies report complete response (CR) rates of 40% to 60% and overall response rates of 70% to 90% in patients with limited disease. Patients with extensive disease, in contrast, have CR rates of 10% to 25% and overall response rates of 40% to 75%. The median survival of patients with limited disease is 12 to 21 months versus 7 to 11 months in patients with extensive disease. Approximately 10% to 25% of patients with limited disease survive more than 2 years, whereas only 1% to 4% of those with extensive disease survive more than 2 years (8–24).

There are several complicating factors regarding prognosis. The first is the concept of stage migration (the Will Rogers phenomenon) (25). With more sensitive staging techniques, asymptomatic metastases may be detected. Thus, a patient who had previously been classified as having limited stage disease would now be classified as extensive stage, based on detection of clinically silent metastatic disease. This migration of patients from a lower to a higher disease stage improves the survival of both subsets without changing the overall survival of the whole population.

NUMBER OF METASTATIC SITES

Several investigators have evaluated the prognostic significance of the number of sites of metastatic disease. In a multivariate analysis of 718 patients with extensive disease in Cancer and Leukemia Group B trials, Spiegelman et al. (17) reported a decrease in median survival from 257 days with one site, to 193.5 days with two sites, to 168 days with three sites ($P < .01$). Sheehan and coworkers (26) analyzed 136 patients with extensive disease and found that the number of sites of metastases was an independent predictor of survival. In a study of 106 patients from the National Cancer Institute (NCI), the median survival decreased significantly from 11.5 to 10 to 8 months in patients with 1, 2, and 3 sites of disease, respectively (27). Dearing et al. (28) also found a significant decrease in median survival from 11 to 6 months with an increasing number of sites of disease. However, using a Cox proportional analysis, the number of sites lost its significance, mainly because the number of sites correlated strongly with abnormal biochemical studies. In a Cox analysis of 1217 patients with extensive disease participating in trials by the Southwest Oncology Group (29), the prognostic significance of a single metastatic lesion compared with multiple metastatic sites was confirmed (median survival of 12 months and 6.7 months, respectively). However, these data also were analyzed using a recursive partitioning method. With this method the entire patient population is divided into two groups according to the variable that produced the most significant difference in survival, including laboratory studies. The two groups are then subdivided according to the next most significant variable. Using this method the number of sites of metastatic disease did not define a separate prognostic subgroup. In patients with extensive disease, only the serum lactate dehydrogenase level (normal versus elevated) defined separate subgroups.

SPECIFIC SITES OF ISOLATED EXTENSIVE DISEASE

Brain Metastases

Brain metastases occur in 50% of patients with small cell lung cancer at some point during the course of their disease and are present at the time of diagnosis in 10% of patients. Among those with central nervous system (CNS) involvement at the time of diagnosis, 40% to 50% have brain metastases as the solitary site of disease (30–36).

CNS metastases historically have been considered a marker of poor survival. In a study of 209 patients with small cell lung cancer, the median survival fell from 8 months in patients with extensive disease without CNS involvement to 4 months in patients with CNS involvement (32). Other studies have found median survivals of 2 to 3.5 months in patients with brain metastases (13, 27). In a Cox analysis of 614 patients from the University of Toronto, brain metastases were found to be a poor prognostic factor (37).

However, several studies have challenged this concept. Crane et al. (33) reported a median survival of 9 months in patients with brain metastases versus 11 months for patients with extensive disease without CNS disease. Van Hazel and coworkers (36) reported no significant difference in median survival between patients with limited disease and those with brain metastasis as sole site of extensive disease (13.8 and 15.1, respectively). In contrast, patients with other sites of extensive disease had a median survival of 8 months. Giannone et al. (34) also found no significant difference in survival between patients with limited disease (13 months) and CNS-limited disease (11 months). When a Cox proportional hazards model was used to assess prognostic factors in 411 patients participating in National Cancer Institute trials, brain metastases were not significant predictors of poor outcome in patients with extensive disease (28).

Most investigators agree that the development of brain metastases after diagnosis is a poor prognostic sign (18, 33). In addition, patients with brain metastases are rarely long-term survivors (10, 18, 33, 34).

Liver Metastases

Liver metastases are present in 25% to 35% of patients at the time of diagnosis (10, 27, 38, 39). In 5% to 10% of patients, the liver is the only site of metastatic disease. Several modalities have been used to diagnose liver involvement. In a study of 157 patients with small cell lung cancer, Mulshine and coworkers (39) compared various staging modalities with pathologic staging. Physical examination of the abdomen accurately predicted the presence or absence of liver metastases in only 75% of patients. Bilirubin, serum glutamic–oxaloacetic transaminase (SGOT), alkaline phosphatase, and serum lactate dehydrogenase levels correctly determined liver involvement in 78%, 77%, 62%, and 61% of patients, respectively. Computed tomography (CT), however, was accurate in 85% of patients, whereas radionuclide scans were accurate in 87% of patients. Because most patients have CT scans of the chest and upper abdomen, it no longer is necessary to obtain a radionuclide scan.

Most investigators have found that patients with liver involvement have poor survival rates. Mulshine et al. (39) reported a median survival of patients with extensive disease without liver involvement of 11 months but only 7 months in those with liver involvement. Other investigators found median survival rates of 4.7 to 6 months in patients with liver metastases (13, 27). In a recursive partitioning analysis of 614 patients, the presence of liver metastases identified a subgroup of patients with decreased survival (37).

Pleural Effusions

The staging of patients with small cell lung cancer and pleural effusions as the sole site of metastatic disease has been controversial. Ipsilateral pleural effusions occur in 20% to 25% of patients with small cell lung cancer (5, 10, 37). Isolated pleural effusions occur in 10% of patients (27, 28). Radiographic evidence of pleural effusion has been accepted by many investigators as evidence of malignant disease, regardless of the cytologic analysis (5, 27, 28, 40). In several small series, CT of the chest detected approximately 20% more effusions than chest radiography (41–43). Thus, the radiologic modality used has a major impact on staging. In addition, some investigators have considered unilateral pleural effusion as extensive disease, whereas others have classified it as limited disease.

Livingston and colleagues (40) found that patients with pleural effusions had response rates similar to those of patients with limited disease (CR, 36% versus 41%; overall response rate, 77% versus 79%), whereas other patients with extensive disease had much lower response rates (CR of 16% and overall responses of 58%). In addition, several investigators found that patients with pleural effusions had survival rates similar to those of patients with limited disease, whereas others found that patients with pleural effusions have survival similar to that of patients with extensive disease with one site of metastatic involvement (17, 28, 29, 37). When cytologic studies are done, patients with cytologically positive effusions have the same response rates and survival rates as patients whose effusions are negative (28, 40).

BONE METASTASES

Bone metastases are present in 26% to 38% of patients with small cell lung cancer at the time of diagnosis (27, 28, 37, 44). In 3% to 12% of patients, they are the sole site of metastatic disease (13, 27). The prognostic significance of bony metastases is variable. Sagman and colleagues (37) found that patients with bony involvement had a significantly decreased survival compared with those without it (26 weeks versus 46 weeks). However, several other investigators found that bony metastases were not a significant predictor of survival in patients with extensive disease (26–28). In fact, Maurer and Pajak (13) found that patients with bony involvement had a CR rate of 17%, the best among patients with extensive disease. When this group of patients was analyzed further, it was determined that seven patients had been staged as having extensive disease based solely on the presence of a single defect on a bone scan or radiograph. This subset of patients had a CR rate of 71% and had survival rates similar to those of patients with limited disease (median survival of 12.5 months, 14% long-term survivors). These data are from studies antedating good CT or magnetic resonance imaging (MRI) techniques, and it is possible that these patients did not truly have metastatic disease.

BONE MARROW METASTASES

Bone marrow involvement in small cell lung cancer occurs in 16% to 35% of patients (21, 45, 46). In a study of patients who underwent bilateral bone marrow aspirate studies and biopsies, a higher incidence was found than in studies in which unilateral procedures were done (46). Only 2.3% of patients had bone marrow involvement as the only site of metastatic disease. Other studies confirm that isolated bone marrow involvement is rare, with an incidence of 1% to 5% (47–51).

The significance of bone marrow involvement remains controversial. Some investigators have found that bone marrow involvement is a predictor of poor outcome (47, 49, 51). In a study of 193 patients with extensive small cell lung cancer, patients with bone marrow metastases had a median survival of 149 days (49). Patients without bone marrow metastases had a median survival of 231 days ($P < .01$). Bezwoda and coworkers (47) reported a median survival of 9 weeks in patients with marrow involvement versus 33 weeks in patients without it. However, the negative effect of bone marrow metastases on survival corresponded with an increasing number of other sites of metastases in these patients. In the five patients with isolated bone marrow metastases, survival ranged from 14 to 39 weeks, with three of five patients having a complete response. Holoye et al. (21) also reported a median survival of 42 weeks in 11 patients with isolated bone marrow metastases; 4 of 11 had complete responses, and 5 of 11 had partial responses. Several other investigators have not found a significant difference in either response rates or survival in patients with bone marrow involvement, compared with other patients with extensive disease (27, 45, 46, 50). There are reports of long-term survivors among patients with bone marrow metastases, but this is rare (18, 27).

ADRENAL METASTASES

The adrenal gland is a common site of metastatic disease in patients with small cell lung cancer. With the use of CT, the detection of adrenal metastases has increased. At the time of diagnosis, adrenal metastases are found in 15% to 40% of patients (42, 52–56). Three percent to 8% of patients have adrenal involvement as their sole site of metastatic disease (42, 54).

The diagnosis of adrenal involvement is complicated by several factors. First, a normal adrenal gland visualized by CT does not rule out the presence of metastases. In a study of 24 patients with small cell lung cancer and morphologically normal adrenal glands by CT scan, percutaneous needle biopsies were performed (52). Seventeen percent of these patients were found to have adrenal metastases pathologically. Another study compared autopsy findings in 91 patients with lung cancer and CT scans obtained within 90 days of death (57). A strongly positive CT scan was highly predictive of the presence of adrenal metastases in patients with small cell lung cancer (95% probability of disease). With a negative scan, however, the probability of metastases was still 34%.

The prognostic significance of adrenal metastases, compared with that of other sites of metastatic disease, is uncertain. However, the detection of an adrenal metastasis in a patient who has no other evidence of metastatic disease does change the stage from limited to extensive.

SUMMARY

Because of the significance of any metastasis on decisions for treatment in small cell carcinoma, it is imperative that the physician document the nature of a suspicious single lesion in any organ system. This documentation may need to take the form of further imaging studies such as MRI or direct biopsy. MRI scans have been very useful in detecting metastatic disease in bone marrow and brain. As newer staging techniques are introduced, they continue to add to stage migration in small cell lung carcinoma.

REFERENCES

1. Mountain CF. A new international staging system for lung cancer. Chest 1986;89(Suppl):225S–233S.
2. American Joint Committee on Cancer. Lung. In: Beahrs OH, Hensen DE, Hutter RVP, et al, eds. Manual for staging of cancer. 4th ed. Philadelphia: JB Lippincott, 1992.
3. Mountain CF. Lung cancer staging classification. Clin Chest Med 1993;14:43–51.
4. Zelen M. Keynote address on biostatistics and data retrieval. Cancer Chemother Rep 1973;4:31–42.
5. Abrams J, Doyle LA, Aisner J. Staging, prognostic factors, and special considerations in small cell lung cancer. Semin Oncol 1088;15:261–277.
6. Green RA, Humphrey E, Close H, Patno ME. Alkylating agents in bronchogenic carcinoma. Am J Med 1969;46:516–525.
7. Roswit B, Patno ME, Rapp R, et al. The survival of patients with inoperable lung cancer: a large scale randomized study of radiation therapy versus placebo. Radiology 1968;90:688–697.
8. Crown JPA, Chahinian AP, Jaffrey IS, Glidewell OJ, Kaneko M, Holland JF. Predictors of 5-year survival and curability in small cell lung cancer. Cancer 1990;66:382–386.
9. Davis S, Wright PW, Schulman SF, Scholes D, Thorning D, Hammas S. Long-term survival in small cell carcinoma of the lung: a population experience. J Clin Oncol 1985;3:80–91.
10. Jackson DV, Case LD, Zekan PJ, et al. Improvement of long term survival: I. Extensive small cell lung cancer. J Clin Oncol 1988;6:1161–1169.
11. Livingston RB, Stephens RL, Bonnet JD, Grozea PN, Lehane DE. Long-term survival and toxicity in small cell lung cancer. Am J Med 1984;77:415–417.
12. Maurer LH, Tulloh M, Weiss RB, et al. A randomized combined modality trial in small cell carcinoma of the lung. Cancer 1980;45:30–39.
13. Maurer LH, Pajak TF. Prognostic factors in small cell carcinoma of the lung. A Cancer and Leukemia Group B study. Cancer Treat Rep 1981;65:767–774.
14. Østerlind K, Hansen HH, Hansen M, Dombernowsky P, Andersen PK. Long term disease free survival in small cell carcinoma of the lung: a study of clinical determinants. J Clin Oncol 1986;4:1307–1313.
15. Osterlind K, Andersen PK. Prognostic factors in small cell lung cancer: multivariate model based on 778 patients treated with chemotherapy with or without irradiation. Cancer Res 1986;46:4189–4194.
16. Skarin AT. Analysis of long-term survivors with small cell lung cancer. Chest 1993;103(Suppl):440S–444S.
17. Spiegelman D, Maurer LH, Ware JH, et al. Prognostic factors in small cell carcinoma of the lung: an analysis of 1521 patients. J Clin Oncol 1989;7:344–357.
18. Vogelsang GB, Abeloff MD, Ettinger DS, Booker SV. Long-term survivors of small cell carcinoma of the lung. Am J Med 1985;79:49–56.
19. Morstyn G, Ihde D, Lichter A, et al. Small cell lung cancer 1973–1983. Int J Radiat Oncol Biol Phys 1984;10:515–539.
20. Bunn P, Cohen M, Ihde D, Fossieck EB, Matthews MJ, Minna JD. Advances in small cell bronchogenic carcinoma. Cancer Treat Rep 1977;61:333–342.
21. Holoye P, Samuels M, Lanzotti V, Smith T, Barkley HT. Combination chemotherapy and radiation therapy for small cell carcinoma. JAMA 1977;237:1221–1224.
22. Shepherd FA, Ginsberg RJ, Haddad R, et al. Importance of clinical staging in limited small cell lung cancer. A valuable system to separate prognostic subgroups. J Clin Oncol 1993;11:1592–1597.
23. Johnson DH, Turrisi AT, Chang AY, et al. Alternating chemotherapy and twice-daily thoracic radiotherapy in limited stage small cell lung cancer. J Clin Oncol 1993;11:879–884.
24. Coy P, Hodson I, Murray N, et al. Patterns of failure following loco-regional radiotherapy in the treatment of limited stage small cell lung cancer. Int J Radiat Biol Phys 1993;28:355–361.
25. Feinstein AR, Sosin DM, Wells CK. The Will Rogers phenomenon, stage migration and new diagnostic techniques as a source of misleading statistics for survival in cancer. N Engl J Med 1985;312:1604–1608.
26. Sheehan RG, Balaban EP, Cox JV, Frenkel EP. The relative value of conventional staging procedures for developing prognostic models in extensive stage small cell lung cancer. J Clin Oncol 1990;8:2047–2053.
27. Ihde DC, Makuch RW, Carney DN, et al. Prognostic implications of stage of disease and sites of metastases in patients with small cell carcinoma of the lung treated with intensive combination chemotherapy. Am Rev Respir Dis 1981;123:500–507.
28. Dearing MP, Steinberg SM, Phelps R, et al. Outcome of patients with small cell lung cancer: effect of changes in staging procedures and imaging technology on prognostic factors over 14 years. J Clin Oncol 1990;8:1042–1049.

29. Albain KS, Crowley JJ, LeBlanc M, Livingston RB. Determinants of improved outcome in small cell lung cancer: an analysis of the 2850 patient Southwest Oncology Group data base. J Clin Oncol 1990;8:1563–1574.
30. Hirsch FR, Paulson OB, Hansen HH, Larsen SO. Intracranial metastases in small cell carcinoma of the lung, prognostic aspects. Cancer 1983;51:529–533.
31. Hirsch FR, Paulson OB, Hansen HH, Vraa-Jensen J. Intracranial metastases in small cell carcinoma of the lung, correlation of clinical and autopsy findings. Cancer 1982;50:2433–2437.
32. Nugent JL, Bunn PA, Matthews MJ, et al. CNS metastases in small cell bronchogenic carcinoma. Cancer 1979;44:1885–1893.
33. Crane JM, Nelson MJ, Ihde DC, et al. A comparison of computed tomography and radionuclide scanning for detection of brain metastases in small cell lung cancer. J Clin Oncol 1984;2:1017–1024.
34. Giannone L, Johnson DH, Hande KR, Greco FA. Favorable prognosis of brain metastases in small cell lung cancer. Ann Intern Med 1987;106:386–389.
35. Newman SJ, Hansen HH. Frequency, diagnosis, and treatment of brain metastases in 247 consecutive patients with bronchogenic carcinoma. Cancer 1974;33:492–496.
36. Van Hazel GA, Scott M, Eagan RT. The effect of CNS metastases on the survival of patients with small cell cancer of the lung. Cancer 1983;51:933–937.
37. Sagman U, Maki E, Evans WK, et al. Small cell carcinoma of the lung: derivation of a prognostic staging system. J Clin Oncol 1991;9:1639–1649.
38. Dombernowsky P, Hirsch F, Hansen HH, Hainau B. Peritoneoscopy in the staging of 190 patients with small cell anaplastic carcinoma of the lung with special reference to subtyping. Cancer 1978;41:2008–2012.
39. Mulshine JL, Makuch RW, Johnston-Early, A, et al. Diagnosis and significance of liver metastases in small cell carcinoma of the lung. J Clin Oncol 1984;2:733–741.
40. Livingston RB, McCracken JD, Trauth CJ, Chen T. Isolated pleural effusion in small cell lung carcinoma: favorable prognosis. Chest 1982;81:208–211.
41. Whitley NO, Fuks JZ, McCrea ES, et al. Computed tomography of the chest in small cell lung cancer. AJR Am J Roentgenol 1984;142:885–892.
42. Harper PG, Houang M, Spiro SG, Geddes D, Hodson M, Souhami RL. Computerized axial tomography in the pretreatment assessment of small cell carcinoma of the bronchus. Cancer 1981;47:1775–1780.
43. Lewis E, Bernardino ME, Valdivieso M, Farha P, Barnes PA, Thomas JL. Computed tomography and routine chest radiography in oat cell carcinoma of the lung. J Comput Assist Tomogr 1982;6:739–745.
44. Johnson BE. Management of small cell lung cancer. Clin Chest Med 1993;14:173–187.
45. Ten Velde GPM, Kuypers-Engelen BTMJ, Volovics A, Bosman FT. Examination of bone marrow biopsy specimens and staging of small cell lung cancer. Eur J Cancer 1990;26:1142–1145.
46. Tritz DB, Doll DC, Ringerberg QS, et al. Bone marrow involvement in small cell lung cancer. Cancer 1989;63:763–766.
47. Bezwoda W, Lewis D, Livini N. Bone marrow involvement in anaplastic small cell lung cancer. Cancer 1986;58:1762–1765.
48. Campling B, Quirt I, DeBoer G, Feld R, Shepherd FA, Evans WK. Is bone marrow examination in small cell lung cancer really necessary? Ann Intern Med 1986;105:513–518.
49. Hirsch F, Hansen H. Bone marrow involvement in small cell anaplastic carcinoma of the lung. Cancer 1980;46:206–211.
50. Ihde D, Simms E, Matthews M, Cohen MH, Bunn PA, Minna JD. Bone marrow metastases in small cell carcinoma of the lung. Blood 1978;53:677–686.
51. Zych J, Polowiec Z, Wiatr E, Broniek A, Rowinska-Zakrzewska E. The prognostic significance of bone marrow metastases in small cell lung cancer patients. Lung Cancer 1993;10:239–245.
52. Pagani JJ. Normal adrenal glands in small cell lung carcinoma: CT-guided biopsy. AJR Am J Roentgenol 1983;140:949–951.
53. Jelinek JS, Redmond J, Perry JJ, et al. Small cell lung cancer: staging with MRI imaging. Radiology 1990;177:837–842.
54. Vas W, Zylak CJ, Mather D, Figueredo A. The value of abdominal computed tomography in the pre-treatment assessment of small cell carcinoma of the lung. Radiology 1981;138:417–418.
55. Mirvis SE, Whitley NO, Aisner J, Moody M, Whitacre M, Whitley JE. Abdominal CT in the staging of small cell carcinoma of the lung: incidence of metastases and effect on prognosis. AJR Am J Roentgenol 1987;148:845–847.
56. Hinson JA, Perry MC. Small cell lung cancer. CA Cancer J Clin 1993;43:216–225.
57. Allard P, Yankaskas BC, Fletcher RH, Parker, Halvorsen RA. Sensitivity and specificity for the detection of adrenal metastatic lesions among 91 autopsied lung cancer patients. Cancer 1990;66:457–462.

Section V

Esophageal Cancer

25

Pathology of Esophageal Cancer

Si-Chun Ming

Compared with cancers of the lung, esophageal cancer is uncommon in the United States. The incidence in 1990 was 4.2, and the mortality rate was 3.5 cases per 100,000 population (1). It is estimated that in 1994 esophageal cancer will cause 11,000 new cases and 10,400 deaths (2). Among the esophageal cancers, carcinoma is the most frequent. Because the esophagus is lined almost entirely with squamous epithelium, it is not surprising that squamous cell carcinoma is the principal cancer type. Adenocarcinoma, previously thought to be almost nonexistent, has increased remarkably in recent years, mainly in the distal portion of the esophagus. Other types of malignant tumors are rare. To understand the origin of the carcinoma cells and the reasons for its poor prognosis, the embryologic development and anatomic features of the esophagus are reviewed briefly.

EMBRYOLOGY AND ANATOMIC FEATURES

EMBRYOLOGY

The esophagus develops from the foregut and makes its appearance during the 4th week of embryonic life as a short tube between the pharynx and the stomach. It elongates rapidly as the chest organs expand and the stomach descends. The distal esophagus rotates with the stomach during embryonic life so that its dorsal aspect turns to the left and its ventral aspect turns to the right.

The epithelium is composed initially of columnar cells, which are replaced by ciliated cells in the third month of embryonic life and then by squamous cells beginning during the 14th week. The squamous cells begin to appear in the middle third of the organ and spread to line the entire esophagus during the seventh month. Superficial glands are present in the mucosa by the end of the third month of fetal life. They resemble the cardiac glands of the stomach and secrete neutral mucus. They are referred to as cardiac or gastric glands. The ciliated columnar cells and superficial glands occasionally persist after birth at both ends of the esophagus. The deep esophageal glands are located in the submucosa. They do not appear until late in fetal life and develop mainly after birth.

During the 6th week of fetal life, the mesoderm surrounding the entodermal tube differentiates into muscular and connective tissues that are continuous with those of the stomach without a clear demarcation. Therefore, the lower limit of the esophagus is determined by the squamocolumnar junction.

GROSS ANATOMY

The esophagus in the adult is approximately 25 cm long. Its upper end is about 15 cm from the incisor teeth, and lower end is approximately 2 cm below the diaphragm. The upper esophagus begins in the midline of the neck. It shifts slightly to the left in the upper mediastinum so that it lies left and posterior to the lower trachea; behind the left main bronchus, aortic arch, and heart; and anterior to the descending aorta. It passes through the diaphragm in front of the 10th thoracic vertebra, anterior and slightly to the left of the aorta. Its intimate relationship with the vital thoracic organs plays an important role in both the clinical course and therapy of esophageal cancer.

The luminal surface of the esophagus is lined with pearly white mucosa, which is freely movable and which forms longitudinal folds at the resting state. It is contiguous with the pharyngeal mucosa at the upper end of the esophagus but is sharply demarcated from the pink velvety gastric mucosa at its lower end. This squamocolumnar junction, known as the Z line, serves to define the lower limit of the esophagus. In most people, the Z line is situated below the diaphragm and coincides with the cardiac orifice of the stomach (3).

The esophagus has a sphincter at each end. The upper sphincter is the cricopharyngeus skeletal muscle. The lower sphincter is composed of smooth muscle fibers morphologically similar to those in the adjacent muscularis propria. It is distinct only physiologically, represented by a 5-cm zone of increased pressure in the distal esophagus (4).

The arterial and venous blood vessels of the esophagus are connected with the major vessels of the neighboring organs. The veins have rich anastomoses within the esophageal wall and form a link between the systemic and portal circulation. The lymphatic vessels of the esophagus drain into the paraesophageal, deep cervical, posterior mediastinal, and subdiaphragmatic nodes, depending on the level of their location. The lymphatics of the upper esophagus drain into the cervical nodes, those of the midesophagus into the mediastinal and tracheobronchial nodes, and those of the lower esophagus into the cardiac and perigastric lymph nodes (5).

NORMAL HISTOLOGY

The esophageal wall, like other parts of the digestive tract, is composed of mucosa, submucosa, and muscularis propria. However, it has no serosa. Its outer layer is the adventitia, which contains fibroadipose tissue, corresponding to the subserosa in other segments of the gut. The esophageal mucosa (Fig. 25.1) consists of a thick stratified squamous epithelium, a fibrovascular lamina propria, and a thick muscularis mucosae. The squamous cells are arranged in an orderly pattern. The regenerative cells in the basal zone, occupying less than 20% of the epithelium, are cuboidal and arranged vertically. As they mature toward the luminal surface, they become larger, elliptical, and increasingly horizontal. The cells in the upper half of the epithelium appear clear because of accumulation of glycogen in the cytoplasm. Occasionally, the amount of glycogen is excessive and the cells are enlarged. The affected area may appear pale and elevated. This condition is known as glycogenic acanthosis. The cause is unknown. The nuclei in the superficial cells are small and pyknotic. There is no keratosis, although the cells contain abundant tonofilaments. Endocrine cells and melanocytes may be present in the basal epithelium (6). Rarely, there is sufficient number of melanocytes to cause focal brown pigmentation of the mucosa (7).

The deep esophageal glands are located in the submucosa (Fig. 25.1) and are scattered randomly throughout the length of the esophagus. Their ducts are lined with columnar cells, surrounded by myoepithelial cells. These glands resemble the minor salivary glands and are composed of mucous cells,

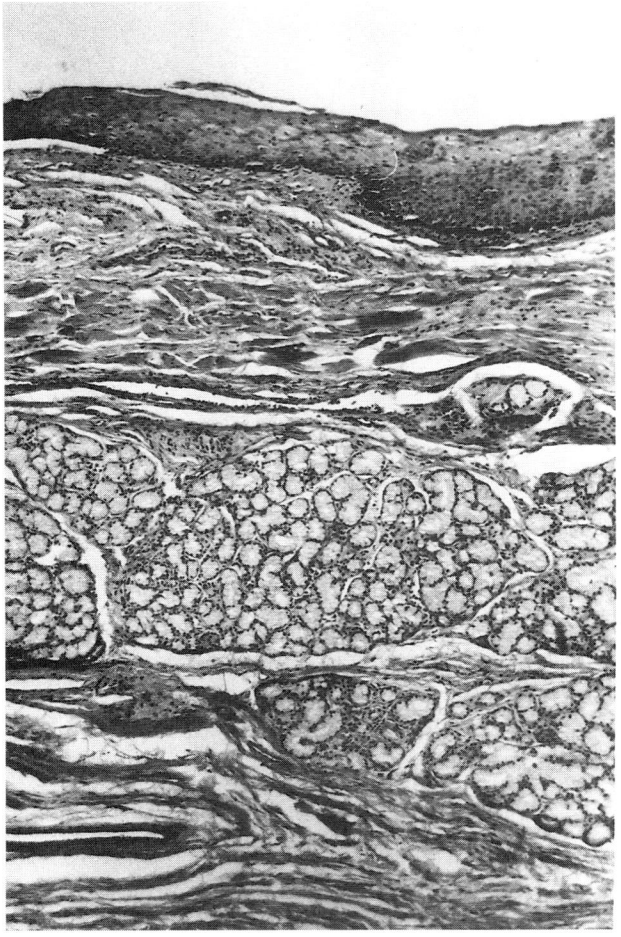

FIGURE 25.1. Normal esophagus showing stratified squamous epithelium and submucosal deep glands. Vascular structures are present in the lamina propria.

which secrete acidic mucin, and occasionally of serous cells.

The lamina propria is composed of fibrous tissue in which blood vessels, lymphatics, and scattered mononuclear inflammatory cells are present. Tongues of lamina propria, called papillae, project into the indentations along the base of the epithelium, for about one quarter of the thickness of the epithelium. The submucosa is composed of fibroadipose tissue that contains blood vessels and lymphatics, but few ganglion cells and nerves.

The muscularis propria in the upper one third of the esophagus is an extension of striated skeletal muscle fibers in the neck. In the lower one third of esophagus, there are two layers of smooth muscle cells that continue into the stomach. In the midesophagus, these two types of muscle cells are intermixed. The distribution of the muscle cells serves as a histologic landmark for different levels of the esophagus.

BARRETT'S EPITHELIUM

Remnants of columnar cells and superficial mucous glands may persist after birth at either end of the esophagus. This condition is called gastric heterotopia. It has been found by endoscopic biopsy in the upper esophagus in 11.8 % of children and 4% of adults (8, 9). In the majority of cases, these glands are identical to the cardiac glands of the stomach. Occasionally, chief and parietal cells, markers of the gastric fundic glands, are also present. Furthermore, intestinal metaplasia may occur in the glands.

All these features are commonly seen in the stomach. The concept that such gastric-type epithelium in the esophagus, regardless of its location and cell type, is congenital was accepted until 1950, when Barrett noted the presence of columnar epithelium in association with peptic ulceration or stricture in the lower esophagus (10). Since then, it has become evident that the columnar epithelium is acquired in most cases, particularly when it is located in the distal esophagus. Such an epithelium is now referred to as Barrett's epithelium, and the portion of esophagus harboring it is called Barrett's esophagus. However, the congenital origin of the glandular mucosa is still accepted for the upper esophagus. Grossly, Barrett's epithelium is pink and velvety, resembling the gastric mucosa, in contrast to the light pearl gray squamous mucosa. The extent of Barrett's epithelium can vary greatly, from a minute focus to diffuse involvement of the esophagus (11).

The pathogenesis and cellular origin of Barrett's epithelium have been studied extensively. First, the squamous epithelium is destroyed due to a variety of injuries, most commonly reflux esophagitis, with or without peptic ulceration or stricture. Then epithelial cells regenerate from several possible sources including residual basal cells of the squamous epithelium, primitive cells from adjacent esophageal or gastric mucosa, or extension of gastric epithelium from the stomach. If Barrett's epithelium originates from the squamous mucosa, it is, by definition, metaplastic, and the lesion may be isolated and surrounded by squamous epithelium. Conversely, if it originates from the gastric cells, Barrett's epithelium is an outgrowth of gastric mucosa and, therefore, must be in continuity with it. In fact, both types of lesions occur, the latter being more frequent.

The composition of Barrett's epithelium is variable and complex. Three types of glands are recognized: cardiac type, fundic type, and specialized type (12). The first two types correspond to those of the same name in the stomach. The specialized type is

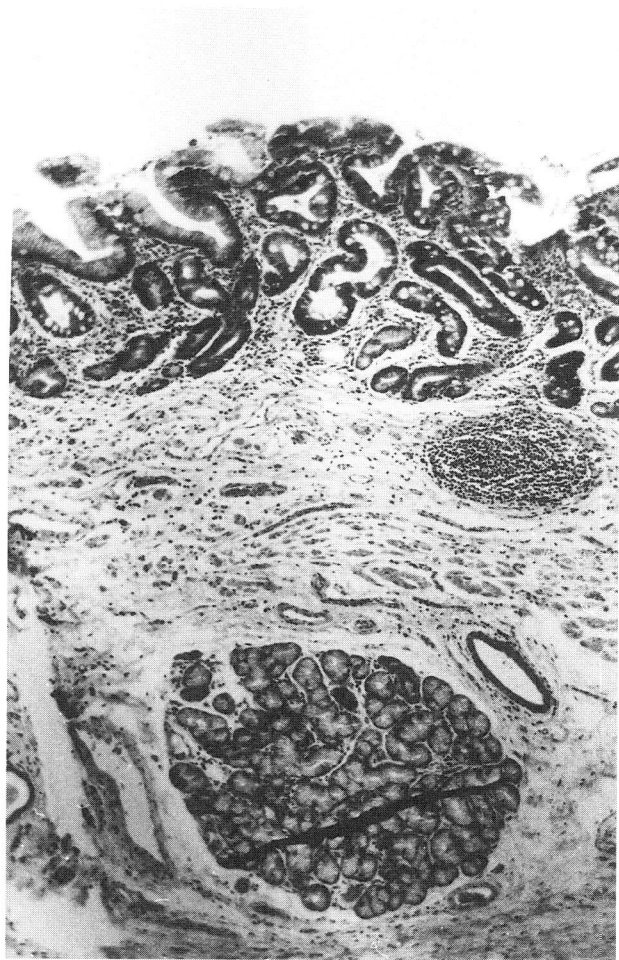

FIGURE 25.2. Barrett's esophagus showing glandular mucosa composed mostly of intestinal-type glands. Gastric-type surface and foveolar mucous cells are shown in the upper left corner. Submucosal glands identify the organ as the esophagus. Lymphocytes are present in the lamina propria.

composed of intestinal-type glands (Fig. 25.2), which are also commonly seen in the stomach as metaplastic tissue. Therefore, the specialized type of Barrett's epithelium should be called intestinal-type epithelium. In addition to goblet cells, Paneth cells and endocrine cells are also present (12–14). Most endocrine cells are argyrophilic, and argentaffin cells are few. Gastrin, as well as pepsinogen, has been found in Barrett's epithelium (15).

As in the stomach, intestinal metaplasia of the Barrett's epithelium may be complete or incomplete (Fig. 25.3). The glands in complete type resemble the glands of normal small intestine or colon and are composed of goblet cells and absorptive cells. The incomplete type has a mixture of goblet cells and intervening columnar cells, resembling the foveolar mucous cells of the stomach. The goblet cells

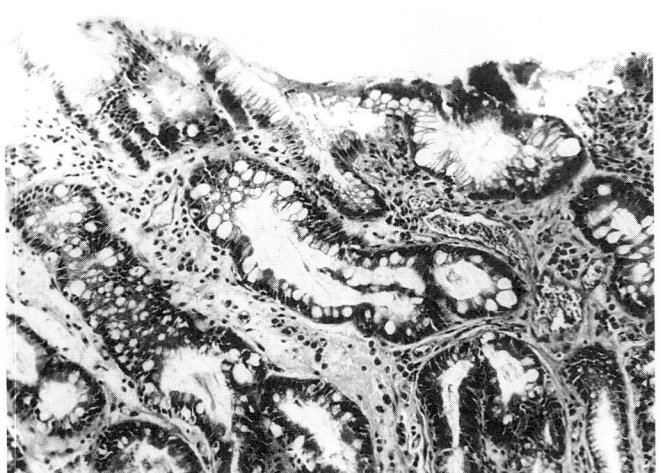

FIGURE 25.3. Barrett's epithelium showing incomplete intestinal metaplasia. The glands are composed of goblet cells and intervening mucous columnar cells.

contain either low acidic sialated mucin, as in the normal small intestine, or strongly acidic sulfomucin, as in the normal colon. Whereas the mucus in the normal stomach has neutral acidity, the mucus in the columnar cells of Barrett's epithelium may be neutral or acidic. Sulfomucin is a marker for precancerous potential (16). The composition of Barrett's epithelium varies from case to case and from area to area. In contrast to the stomach, complete intestinal metaplasia is uncommon in the esophagus, and Paneth cells are only occasionally present (17).

Barrett's esophagus usually follows reflux esophagitis associated with lower sphincter dysfunction or hiatal hernia. The pathologic changes of reflux esophagitis, in order of increasing severity, are: (*a*) the presence of inflammatory cells, including eosinophils, in the epithelium and lamina propria; (*b*) degenerative changes with ballooning or swelling of epithelial cells and hemorrhage in the papillae of lamina propria; (*c*) enhanced regenerative activity of the epithelium with thickening of the basal layer and lengthening of rete pegs and stromal papillae; and (*d*) peptic ulceration and fibrosis with or without stricture. These changes are useful markers for the pathologic diagnosis of Barrett's epithelium. The prevalence of Barrett's epithelium in Western countries is approximately 1% to 2% confirmed by endoscopy for asymptomatic patients and 11% to 13% in patients with symptomatic gastroesophageal reflux (18–20). The prevalence among Asians is considerably lower.

GENERAL PRINCIPLES

CLASSIFICATION AND CELL TYPES OF ESOPHAGEAL CANCERS

Primary esophageal cancers can be classified on the basis of the cell of origin, i.e., epithelial (carcinoma) and nonepithelial (sarcoma) (21). The sarcomas arise from the mesenchymal or supporting stromal tissue and are very rare in the esophagus. Nearly all esophageal cancers are carcinomas, which may arise from any of the epithelial tissues in the esophagus. The types of carcinoma and their possible cell of origin are listed in Table 25.1.

EARLY VERSUS ADVANCED CARCINOMA

The concept of treating early and advanced cancers as separate entities began with gastric cancer in Japan, where it is the most common cause of cancer death. Because of efforts in early diagnosis and treatment, there has been a marked reduction in gastric cancer mortality there. Similar experience with esophageal cancer has been seen in China, where there is a high risk of esophageal cancer. The early carcinoma of the esophagus, as in gastric carcinoma, is defined as a tumor in which the depth of invasion does not extend beyond the submucosa, regardless of the status of lymph node involvement. The advanced carcinoma invades the muscularis propria or beyond. Although metastasis to lymph nodes may occur in early carcinoma, the survival of patients with early carci-

TABLE 25.1. Type and Cell Origin of Esophageal Cancers

TUMOR TYPE	CELL ORIGIN
Squamous cell carcinoma	
Ordinary squamous cell carcinoma	Squamous cell
Verrucous carcinoma	Squamous cell
Basaloid carcinoma	Squamous cell
Spindle cell carcinoma	Squamous cell
Adenosquamous carcinoma	Squamous cell with metaplasia
Carcinosarcoma	Totipotential cell
Adenocarcinoma	
Ordinary adenocarcinoma	Columnar cell
Adenoacanthoma	Columnar cell with metaplasia
Mucoepidermoid carcinoma	Deep esophageal gland duct
Adenoid cystic carcinoma	Deep esophageal gland duct
Choriocarcinoma	Germ cell rest
Small cell carcinoma	Foregut endocrine cell
Carcinoid	Foregut endocrine cell
Malignant melanoma	Melanocyte
Sarcoma	Mesenchymal cell
Lymphoma	Lymphocyte

noma is much better than those with advanced carcinoma. In China, early esophageal carcinoma does not signify cases with lymph node metastasis (22).

DIAGNOSTIC BIOPSY AND CYTOLOGY

Endoscopic biopsy is essential for clinical diagnosis of esophageal cancer. The biopsy specimen should be orientated properly to facilitate the evaluation of tumor invasion. In addition, endoscopically directed and ultrasound-guided fine-needle aspiration cytology and biopsy have been used for invasive tumors (23).

Cytologic examination of endoscopically obtained cells is particularly valuable for suspected but endoscopically indefinite or invisible lesions. The advantage of cytologic examination is that cells from a large area, even the entire length, of the esophagus may be included in one specimen. In China, this technique has been used with considerable success for mass screening. A rubber or plastic catheter with an inflatable balloon attached to the distal end was designed specifically for this purpose (24). It can be inserted easily into the esophagus. After the balloon passes the cardiac opening, it is inflated with air. A cotton mesh net covers the balloon and serves as a scraping device when the inflated balloon is pulled through the esophageal lumen. When the balloon reaches a point 20 cm from the teeth, it is deflated and withdrawn. The cells collected by the net are examined microscopically for malignant as well as dysplastic cells. This simple technique has been used in mass survey and follow-up studies in China.

PATHOLOGIC STUDY

Pathologic examination is used to determine the type of tumor, extent of spread, precursor lesions, and clues for prognosis. To achieve these aims, relevant clinical information is essential. This information is particularly important in dealing with endoscopic biopsies. For the diagnosis of Barrett's epithelium and primary adenocarcinoma of the esophagus, the endoscopic location of the biopsy must be known. Some tumors are heterogeneous. A single, small tissue sample thus may not be representative of the entire tumor. Ulcerated or necrotic tissue is not suitable for diagnosis or special studies, which usually require viable fresh tissue. In this regard, the specimen must be brought to the pathologist as soon as possible, with adequate clinical data and clearly stated specific requests, if any, so that the specimen can be handled properly.

GROSS PATHOLOGY

The surgically resected specimens must be fixed promptly in formalin for a period sufficient to preserve the tissue properly for histologic evaluation. Before it is fixed, however, the specimen should be orientated properly and measured accurately. Samples of fresh tissue may be taken routinely as soon as possible for special studies. Part of the tissue may be quick frozen or placed into appropriate fixative as indicated. Lugol solution may be applied to the mucosal surface to elicit brown staining of glycogen, which is present in normal squamous epithelium but diminished or absent in dysplastic and malignant cells (25). During gross examination, particular attention is paid to the location, size, and shape of the tumor, the depth of invasion, the length of the resection margins, and the evidence of tumor in the lymph nodes and adventitial surface. The number and location of the lymph nodes and the depth of ulceration and fistula tract of the tumor should be recorded. Photographs of the specimen are helpful for later review and orientation.

HISTOLOGIC PATHOLOGY

Histologic examination of the specimen should be guided by the gross observation. Any discrepancy between them must be reevaluated and clarified. The cell type of the tumor, grade of differentiation, extent of invasion, and length of tumor free resection margin should be determined. Tumor permeation of blood vessels and lymphatics is sought. Particular attention should be paid to microscopic foci of tumor extension and metastasis, particularly at or near the resection margin. Each lymph node is examined for the presence of tumor cells. Special stains for tumor cell markers are sometimes necessary to reveal isolated tumor cells or to identify the tumor type. Tumor tissue may be degenerated, necrotic, and hemorrhagic. These features may be exacerbated by therapeutic measures such as radiotherapy and chemotherapy. In such treated cases, the extent of cellular changes may reflect the efficacy of the treatment. Histologic examination of the tissue adjacent to the tumor may reveal precancerous changes that, if present, support the primary nature of the tumor.

HISTOCHEMICAL AND IMMUNOHISTOCHEMICAL STUDIES

Histochemical and immunohistochemical methods are useful in demonstrating specific intracellular substances that in turn may be helpful in confirming or differentiating tumor types. For instance, keratin filaments are present in epithelial cells, S-100 protein in neuroendocrine cells and melanocytes, and desmin and vimentin in mesenchymal tissue. Strongly acidic mucins are more abundant in Barrett's epithelium and adenocarcinoma than in gastric carcinoma and are useful in the differential diagnosis. Cancer-associated antigens and the expression of oncogenes can also be shown by immunohistochemical methods. They are also helpful in the differential diagnosis and evaluation of the prognosis.

OTHER SPECIAL STUDIES

Electron microscopy is useful in revealing cell specific features, such as desmosomes and microvilli in epithelial cells, melanosomes in melanoma, and secretory granules in endocrine cells. Flow or image cytometric analysis of tumor cells for DNA ploidy is now commonly performed for the study of dysplastic cells and for prognostic prediction of tumor behavior (26). Chromosomal analysis (27), as well as cell proliferation and cell cycle studies using cytometry, DNA labeling, or proliferative cell markers (28), can be carried out on excised tumor tissue. The molecular biologic techniques for oncogene mutation and expression studies are valuable in delineating carcinogenic sequences. For these and immunohistochemical studies, fresh or specially fixed tissue samples are essential.

EPIDEMIOLOGY

The epidemiology of esophageal cancer is presented in Chapter 4. However, a brief review of the epidemiology particularly relevant to its pathology should be highlighted. Epidemiologic data from China have been instructive not only in providing insights into possible etiologic factors but also into factors for early diagnosis and survival prospects of patients with this tumor.

GEOGRAPHIC DISTRIBUTION

The incidence and mortality rates of esophageal cancer vary greatly among countries (29). The high-risk regions include parts of Iran along the Caspian Sea and the northern Henan Province of China, where the mortality rate of esophageal cancer exceeds 100 per 100,000 population (30, 31). There is also great regional variation. The region with the highest mortality rate in China is Linxian, where the rate in 1979 was 161.3 in men and 102.9 in women per 100,000 population (32). In Fanxian, about 100 miles from Linxian, the corresponding rates were only 26.5 and 7.5 per 100,000 population, respectively. Such great differences within a short distance clearly support an environmental rather than genetic influence on the development of esophageal cancer. Whereas the mortality rate in the United States has shown a slight increase in recent years (1, 2), it has decreased markedly in China. Largely because of early diagnosis and treatment, the mortality rate in China declined from 31.7 in men and 15.9 in women in 1977 (30) to 17.7 and 10.2, respectively, in 1989 (33).

AGE, SEX, AND RACIAL DISTRIBUTION

Cancer of the esophagus is generally a disease found in older adults. Its incidence increases with age in both low-risk and high-risk countries, more prominently among the high-risk population (33). More esophageal cancers occur in men than in women, but the ratio between the sexes varies among nations. In most countries, the male to female ratio is about 2 or 3 to 1. The sex difference may be related to drinking, smoking, and dietary factors (1).

In the United States, the incidence rate of esophageal cancer among African-Americans is three times higher than that in the white population, 10.8 and 3.3 per 100,000, respectively (1). A similar racial difference, 8.7 versus 2.9, exists for the mortality rate. The survival rate is higher in whites, although the distribution of cases at various cancer stages in both races has been similar at the time of cancer diagnosis.

PREVALENCE AND INCIDENCE OF ADENOCARCINOMA

Adenocarcinomas of the esophagus occur most often in the distal esophagus. Previously, they were often considered extensions of gastric carcinomas. In the past two decades, it has become increasingly accepted that many such tumors are primary esophageal carcinomas, originating mostly in preexisting Barrett's epithelium.

The epidemiology of adenocarcinomas has not been delineated, partly because the true incidence of Barrett's epithelium in the population is unknown. The reported incidence of carcinoma in Barrett's epithelium at the time of initial diagnosis varied from 0% to 46%, with an average of 13.6% (34). It is approximately 30-fold to 40-fold that of the general population. In a few follow-up studies on Barrett's esophagus, carcinoma was diagnosed in an average of 2.4% of patients during follow-up periods of up to 20 years. These reports came mainly from Western countries in which there is a steady increase in the incidence of adenocarcinoma, so that it accounts for up to 50% of all esophageal cancers in some hospitals (35). In the United States, up to one third of esophageal carcinomas are adenocarcinomas (36). Adenocarcinoma in Barrett's esophagus (Barrett's carcinoma) is uncommon in some countries. In a report of 450 esophageal cancers in Taiwan, there was no Barrett's carcinoma or Barrett's epithelium (37). Similarly, among 5481 surgically treated cases in Japan, there were 214 adenocarcinomas at the esophagogastric junction or cardia, but all esophageal carcinomas were of the squamous cell type (38).

Barrett's carcinoma occurs primarily in the elderly, with the mean age being approximately 60 years; however, it has been reported in younger patients (39). Men are more frequently affected than women. In some reports, nearly all patients are men (34, 40). Racially, unlike squamous cell carcinoma, adenocarcinoma affects whites more frequently than blacks, even in places with high black populations (41, 42).

ETIOLOGIC FACTORS

The etiology of esophageal cancer is unknown. Nitrosamines induce esophageal carcinoma in animals and are suspected carcinogenic agents in man. Several factors are known to contribute to the development of esophageal cancer and are discussed briefly.

ALCOHOL AND TOBACCO USE

Heavy alcohol intake and tobacco smoking have long been associated with esophageal cancer (43). They may contribute to the higher incidence of this cancer in blacks than in whites in the United States (1). However, they do not appear to be significant factors in some high-risk regions such as Iran and China. In the case of adenocarcinoma, smoking may play a role in men (44). Carcinogenic substances have been found in alcoholic beverages as well as other drinks (43). They may be more important than alcohol itself in causing the cancer.

DIETARY FACTORS

A low intake of fruits, vegetables, and vitamins A, C, and riboflavin is common in high-risk regions (45). Esophageal cancers are prevalent in areas characterized by low socioeconomic conditions, which have also been incriminated in the high incidence of esophageal cancer in some populations. Levels of trace metals such as molybdenum, magnesium, zinc, and copper are low in the diet as well as in the soil in high-risk areas (45, 46). Low molybdenum in soil may increase the formation of nitrates in plants and possibly of carcinogenic nitrosamine compounds (43).

GENETIC FACTORS

A family history of esophageal carcinoma, particularly in blood relatives, has been reported in some high-risk regions (47). In general, however, genetic factors appear insignificant in esophageal cancer. The only definite genetic predisposition is found in patients with familial tylosis palmaris and plantaris, a rare disease (48). Familial occurrence of Barrett's esophagus and adenocarcinoma was reported recently (49). Six of 24 family members had Barrett's esophagus, 3 of whom had adenocarcinoma. None of the spouses had the disease.

INFECTIOUS AGENTS

Species of fungi, such as *Fusarium*, *Geotrichum*, and *Aspergillus*, found in pickled vegetables and moldy bread in Linxian, China, may produce substances that are carcinogenic to the esophagus (45). These fungi have also been found in corn and wheat (50). Human papilloma virus can induce papillomas in the esophagus (51). DNA of this virus has been found in the squamous cell carcinomas and adjacent precancerous lesions (52).

RADIATION AND THERMAL INJURY

Squamous cell carcinoma may develop in the esophagus many years after radiation therapy to the chest for lymphoma or breast cancer (53). Thermal injury to esophageal mucosa by drinking hot beverages, specifically mate in Brazil (54) and tea in China (55), has been considered a possible contributing factor for esophageal cancer. In both situations, there is a high incidence of esophagitis.

EXPERIMENTAL CARCINOGENESIS

A number of *N*-nitrosamine compounds have been used to induce esophageal carcinoma in experimental animals, mostly rats (56, 57). In these experiments, the induced precancerous lesions progressed first through epithelial hyperplasia and later dysplasia. In some experiments, papillomas were produced in 100% of the animals studied. In China, an interesting natural animal experiment exists. Many rural Chinese families breed chicken in their homes. The chickens roam freely in the house and eat scraps of the same food eaten by the people. In Linxian, the chickens developed carcinomas of the pharynx and upper esophagus, with an incidence rate of 175.8, in contrast to a rate of 18.9 in the lower risk area of Fanxian (30). These rates are comparable to those of esophageal carcinoma in men in these regions.

ASSOCIATED CONDITIONS

The associated conditions are clinical syndromes or local conditions in which esophageal carcinoma occurs in increased frequency. However, the direct link between them and the occurrence of esophageal cancer is not evident.

CHRONIC ESOPHAGITIS

Adenocarcinoma is closely associated with Barrett's epithelium, which in turn is related to reflux esophagitis, with or without chronic peptic ulceration or stricture (58). Squamous cell carcinoma has also been reported in Barrett's epithelium, but only infrequently (59). Nonspecific chronic esophagitis is common. Its etiology is not well understood. Endoscopy and esophagoscopic biopsies in patients in Iran and China showed that its incidence is higher in the high-risk population (60), possibly related to the drinking of hot beverages (55). Some studies, however, did not find an increased incidence in the high-risk population (61).

HIATUS HERNIA

Hiatus hernia is commonly associated with reflux esophagitis and consequently with Barrett's epithelium and adenocarcinoma. Squamous cell carcinoma may develop in the esophagus in approximately 1% of patients with hiatus hernia (62), usually in the squamous epithelium and occasionally in the columnar epithelium (59).

BENIGN STRICTURE

Twenty-two percent of patients with stricture in Barrett's esophagus develop adenocarcinoma (63). Benign esophageal stricture without peptic ulceration is uncommon in adults and is usually seen after a past ingestion of caustic chemicals during childhood. The incidence of esophageal carcinoma in such cases varied from 0% to 4% and occurred primarily in the midesophagus (64).

ACHALASIA

The incidence of esophageal carcinoma in achalasia varies widely. In one report the incidence was 33 times that in the general population (65). The mean interval between the onset of symptoms of achalasia and the diagnosis of carcinoma is 17 years. In patients who had achalasia for 30 years, 12% of the deaths were attributed to esophageal cancer (66).

PLUMMER-VINSON SYNDROME

Patients with Plummer-Vinson syndrome may develop carcinoma in the hypopharynx or upper esophagus, particularly at the postcricoid region. The incidence is about 1.4% (67). This occurrence has been used to explain the relatively high incidence of esophageal cancer in Swedish women (68).

CELIAC DISEASE

Patients with celiac disease have an increased incidence of gastrointestinal carcinoma and lymphoma. Among the carcinomas, esophageal carcinoma is most frequent, seen in approximately 4% to 10% (69, 70).

DIVERTICULUM

Although there are sporadic reports of carcinoma within esophageal diverticulum (71, 72), there is no evidence that it is related to esophageal cancer.

PRECANCEROUS LESIONS

Precancerous lesions are pathologic entities from which cancers may develop from the altered cells.

SQUAMOUS PAPILLOMA

Squamous papillomas are precancerous in animal experiments (56). They are uncommon in humans. Most of these papillomas are located in the distal esophagus, and in some cases they are multiple. Many patients have hiatal hernia, reflux esophagitis, and peptic ulceration (73). Although human papilloma virus DNA has been demonstrated in both papilloma and squamous cell carcinoma (51, 52), dysplastic or malignant changes have not been found in the papillomas.

DYSPLASIA OF SQUAMOUS EPITHELIUM

The squamous epithelium adjacent to an esophageal carcinoma is often dysplastic (74). Histologically,

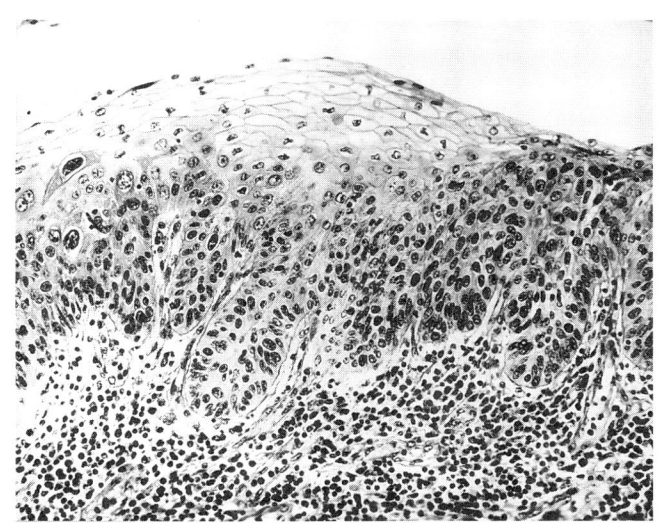

FIGURE 25.4. Moderate dysplasia of squamous epithelium. The epithelial cells have pleomorphic nuclei and reduced cytoplasm. Some cells have large nuclei and nucleoli (*left upper field*). The dysplastic cells extend to the surface area at right, where the cells are more disorganized and compact. The surface cells at the center and left are normal.

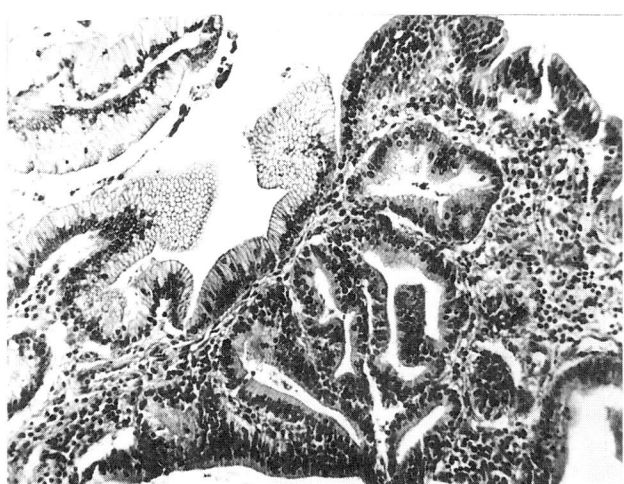

FIGURE 25.5. Adenoma in Barrett's epithelium. The adenoma is composed of immature cells that are low columnar and have reduced or no mucus secretion. The adjoining normal mucous cells in the upper left have basally located nuclei and mucus-filled clear cytoplasm.

the dysplastic changes are usually divided into mild, moderate, and severe grades (Fig. 25.4). In a study in China, they were found in 66.7% of esophagi with early carcinoma (22). In a Japanese study (75), 73 dysplastic foci were found in 32 (20.1%) of 159 carcinomatous esophagi and in continuity with the carcinoma in 42% of cases. The dysplasia was mild in 12 lesions, moderate in 33, and severe in 30. The severity of dysplasia was inversely related to the depth of tumor invasion (75, 76), suggesting coalescence of the foci as the carcinoma progresses.

In a follow-up study of 1 to 12 year's duration (77), 14.9% of esophagi with severe dysplasia and 0.94% of esophagi with only hyperplasia developed cancer. In patients who had only normal esophageal epithelium and who were followed for from 1 to 5 years, no carcinoma developed. Although dysplasia may be reversible (78), the severely dysplastic epithelium must be followed carefully, so that carcinoma may be detected and treated at an early stage.

ADENOMAS

Adenomas, which are composed of immature cells similar to the cells seen in dysplasia, are rare in the esophagus. Adenomas are neoplastic lesions and do not regress. Dysplasia of the flat columnar epithelium is an unstable condition. Its cells show varying degrees of abnormality that may regress. Adenomas may be differentiated from dysplastic lesions by their sharply demarcated and nodular appearance (Fig. 25.5). Some of them have a villous contour and contain foci of carcinoma (14, 79). Adenomas are usually single, but may be multiple (80). In our cases, adenomas were present in 5 of 16 patients with Barrett's esophagi containing adenocarcinoma (81). All of these adenomas were in continuity with the carcinoma (Fig. 25.6).

DYSPLASIA OF BARRETT'S EPITHELIUM

The probability of finding an adenocarcinoma in a Barrett's esophagus is much higher at the time of the initial diagnosis than in later years (34). In follow-up studies, the incidence rate is between 1 in 52 and 1 in 81 patient-years with a mean of 1 in 76 (82). The carcinoma is often accompanied by dysplasia of the adjacent Barrett's epithelium (81, 83) and is seen in all of the cases in some reports (14, 42). It more often affects the intestinal-type epithelium than the gastric-type epithelium (84, 85). Based on the degree of cellular and architectural abnormality, dysplasia of Barrett's epithelium has been divided into low and high grades. High-grade dysplasia includes moderate and severe dysplasia, and low-grade dysplasia is equivalent to mild dysplasia (Fig. 25.7). Flow cytometric studies of high-grade dysplasia often show aneuploid and polyploid cells, and an increased number of cells in S and G2 phases of the cell cycle (86, 87). Furthermore, patients with lesions showing such changes may develop esophageal carcinoma in later years (88). Thus, some investigators consider high-grade dysplasia of Barrett's epithelium a malignant neoplastic lesion encompassing

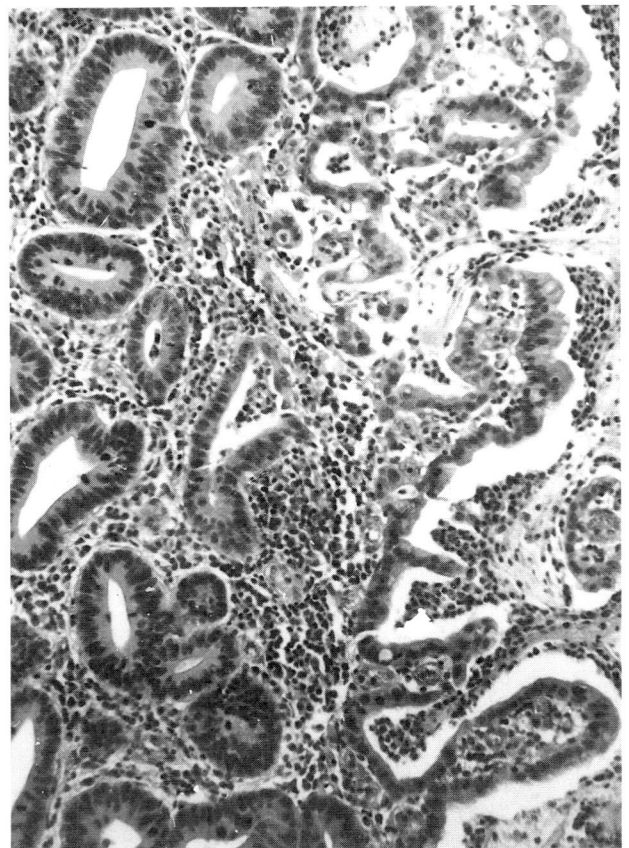

FIGURE 25.6. The interface of an adenoma (*left*) and an adenocarcinoma (*right*). The adenoma is composed of well-formed glands. The carcinoma is composed of irregular branching glands with pleomorphic and depolarized cells.

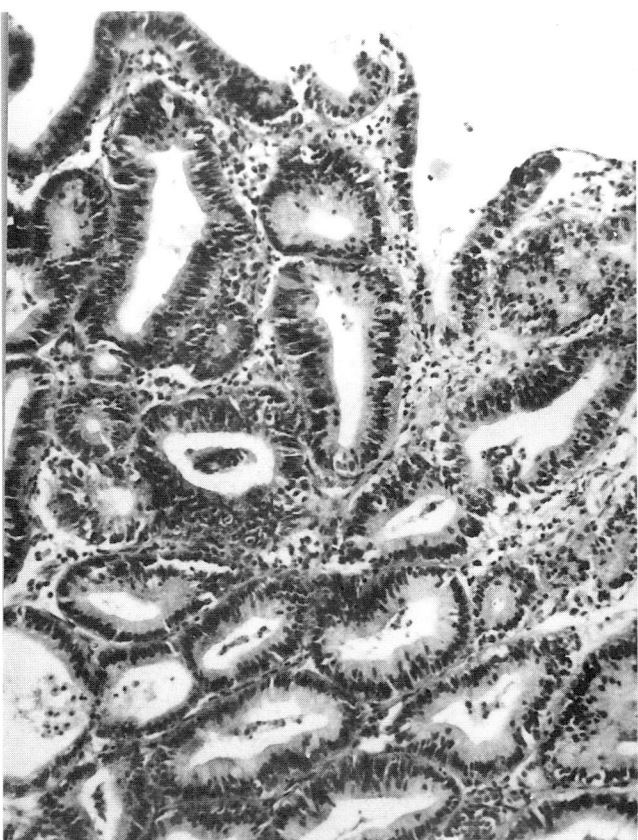

FIGURE 25.7. High-grade dysplasia of Barrett's epithelium. The columnar cells have elongated and irregularly placed nuclei and reduced cytoplasm. Note the similarity between the dysplastic epithelium and the adenoma shown in Figure 24.6.

in situ carcinoma (41, 42, 89). Esophagectomy has been performed in some patients as a result.

In the resected esophagi, invasive adenocarcinoma was present in some, but not all, patients (41, 83, 85). Carcinoma was either absent or occurred infrequently in cases with mild dysplasia (83, 90). In one report, esophagectomy was performed on eight patients, in whom esophageal biopsies showed intramucosal carcinoma in four and high-grade dysplasia in four (91). In the resected esophagi, four carcinomas were confirmed, but the cases with dysplasia showed only dysplasia with no carcinoma identified in the specimen. Two of the eight patients died postoperatively, one died 1 week after the operation, and the other died 9 months after a postoperative stroke. Dysplasia may regress occasionally, more frequently with low-grade lesions (90). Thus, it is important to distinguish high-grade dysplasia from carcinoma, so that unnecessary radical surgery may be avoided. The vigorous endoscopic biopsy protocol adopted by Levine et al. (92) takes this approach. Patients with high-grade dysplasia of Barrett's epithelium should be followed carefully and diligently so that malignant transformation may be discovered early. Because dysplasia and carcinoma may develop anywhere in the Barrett's epithelium (93), multiple biopsies are required for an adequate evaluation.

PATHOLOGY

SQUAMOUS CELL CARCINOMA

LOCATION

The location of squamous cell carcinomas in the esophagus is relatively uniform in most countries. About 40% to 60% of the tumors occur in the middle third of the esophagus, 20% to 40% in the lower third, and 10% to 20% in the upper third (38, 94, 95). Carcinomas at either end of the esophagus are rare. Carcinomas at the postcricoid area occurs mainly in patients with Plummer-Vinson syndrome. Carcinomas at the esophagogastric junction are mostly gastric adenocarcinomas.

EARLY SQUAMOUS CELL CARCINOMA

Through mass screening with the aid of balloon cytology, early carcinoma of the esophagus has been detected in large numbers in China, resulting in a marked improvement in the survival rate after surgical treatment (22, 96). Early esophageal carcinoma is defined in China as a tumor that has not extended beyond the submucosa and that has not metastasized (22). In other reports, the status of lymph node metastasis is not taken into consideration (76, 97, 98).

Four gross types are recognized: occult (7.3%), erosive (33.3%), plaque (51.3%), and papillary (8.0%) (99). The occult carcinoma appears pink and congested in the fresh specimen. After fixation, it is hardly visible. The erosive carcinoma is slightly depressed and has a clearly demarcated margin (Fig. 25.8). The plaque carcinoma is slightly elevated and has a coarse and granular surface. It may be large and circumferential. In spite of its size, it is a mucosal lesion in most cases. The papillary carcinoma has a papillary or polypoid contour and a clear border. Occasionally, the surface is eroded.

Among 150 cases of early esophageal carcinomas analyzed by Liu et al. (22), 148 were situated in the middle and lower portions of the esophagus. The sizes varied from 0.4 cm to 8.5 cm in diameter. Most occult lesions were less than 1 cm in diameter, whereas most other lesions ranged from 1 to 4 cm.

Histologically, the early esophageal carcinomas are divided into intraepithelial (32%), intramucosal (39.3%), and submucosal (28.7%) types (97). All grossly occult tumors are intramucosal, and most erosive tumors remain in the mucosa, whereas nearly one third of the plaque type and more than half of intraluminal tumors involve the submucosa. Intraepithelial carcinoma is also called carcinoma in situ. The tumor is limited by the basement membrane of the epithelium. Dysplasia is often present in the adjacent epithelium. Intramucosal carcinoma has invaded the lamina propria (Fig. 25.9), and submucosal carcinoma has extended into the submucosa. Although lymphatics are present in the lamina propria, lymph node metastasis has not been reported in the intramucosal carcinomas. In contrast, lymph node metastasis may be present in submucosal carcinomas (97, 98).

Intraepithelial carcinoma is often observed at the margins of an invasive carcinoma. In these tumors, there is usually further extension of tumor cells along the base rather than in the superficial portion of the epithelium, and the demarcation between the tumor

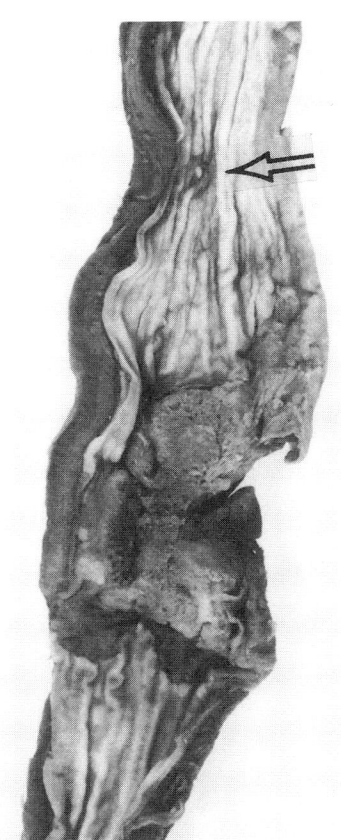

FIGURE 25.8. Early squamous cell carcinoma, erosive type. The 6-mm superficial carcinoma (*arrow*) is slightly depressed. The eroded surface is hemorrhagic. Two centimeters distal to it is an advanced ulcerative squamous cell carcinoma, measuring 5.5 cm × 3 cm.

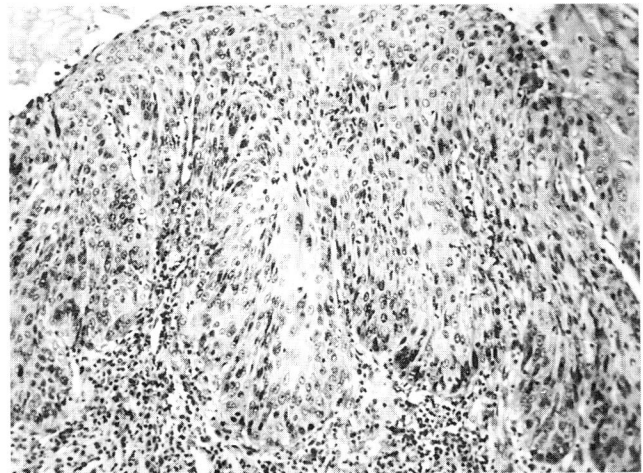

FIGURE 25.9. Intramucosal squamous cell carcinoma. The moderately differentiated tumor cells involve the whole thickness of the squamous epithelium and focally invade the lamina propria at the base.

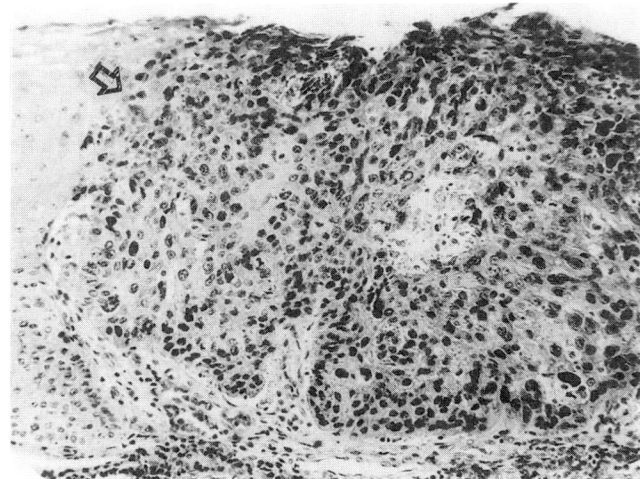

FIGURE 25.10. Intraepithelial invasion of squamous cell carcinoma. Carcinoma cells (*right*) and normal epithelial cells (*left border*) are shown. The demarcation line (*arrow*) is sharply delineated.

and normal epithelium is abrupt (Fig. 25.10). This appearance suggests invasion of malignant cells into the normal epithelium from a neighboring tumor rather than true in situ carcinoma (72).

ADVANCED SQUAMOUS CELL CARCINOMA

At the time of diagnosis, more than half of advanced carcinomas are 5 to 10 cm long, forming prominent protruding and ulcerated masses (38, 94). Based on the relative size of the tumor mass and depth of ulceration, the gross appearance of advanced squamous cell carcinomas can be divided into fungating, ulcerative, and infiltrating types (94).

Fungating Carcinomas

Fungating carcinomas are most common and are found in about 60% of advanced cases. They form large ulcerated masses projecting into the lumen. Some of them have a flat, plaque-like contour with a well-defined border. Others may have a nodular or polypoid appearance (Fig. 25.11). Although large, they are generally not completely annular. A variable strip of uninvolved esophageal wall is usually present between the opposing margins in most cases. Occasionally, an intraluminal carcinoma is polypoid without ulceration. Nevertheless, the surface tissue is clearly cancerous. Such a carcinoma must be differentiated from a submucosal tumor, which is covered by an intact mucosa.

Ulcerative Carcinomas

Ulcerative carcinomas constitute about 25% of advanced cases. Their shaggy surface is flat or de-

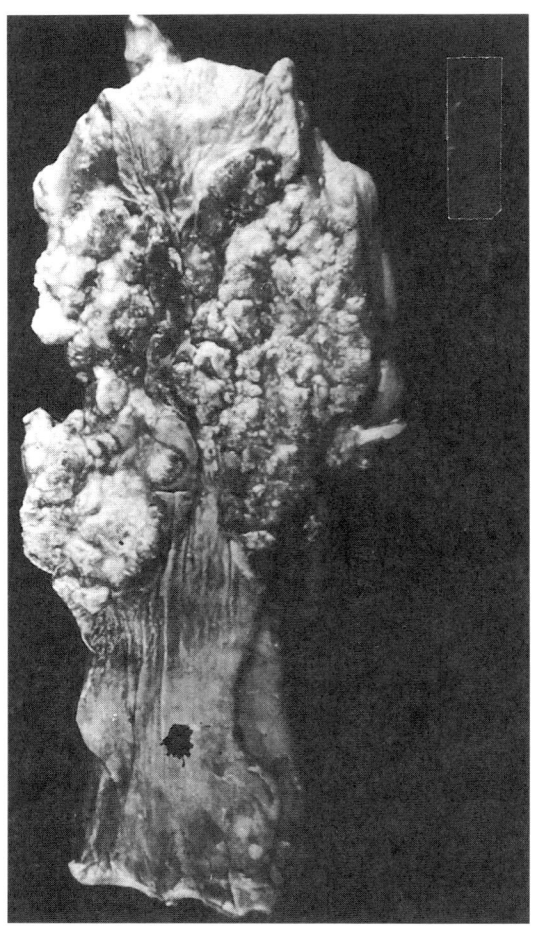

FIGURE 25.11. Advanced squamous cell carcinoma, fungating type. The tumor forms an irregular intraluminal mass measuring 7 cm × 5.5 cm in size. Its surface is nodular.

pressed, but the ulcer margin may be elevated and slightly overhanging (Figs. 25.8 and 25.12). The ulcer sometimes extends into the mediastinum or the neighboring organs. There may be fistulous tracts communicating with trachea or bronchus. Some tumors expand intramurally beneath the intact surrounding epithelium resulting in a nodular or slightly raised, but smooth-surfaced margin. Biopsy of these margins may yield only benign epithelium, missing the deep-seated tumor.

Infiltrating Carcinomas

Infiltrating carcinomas are least common, seen in about 15% of advanced cases. They show extensive intramural growth, without forming a prominent intraluminal mass (Fig. 25.13). They may also burrow under the intact mucosa at its periphery. Less commonly, the tumor spreads superficially. The tumor surface may be ulcerated, but only shallowly. Circumferential involve-

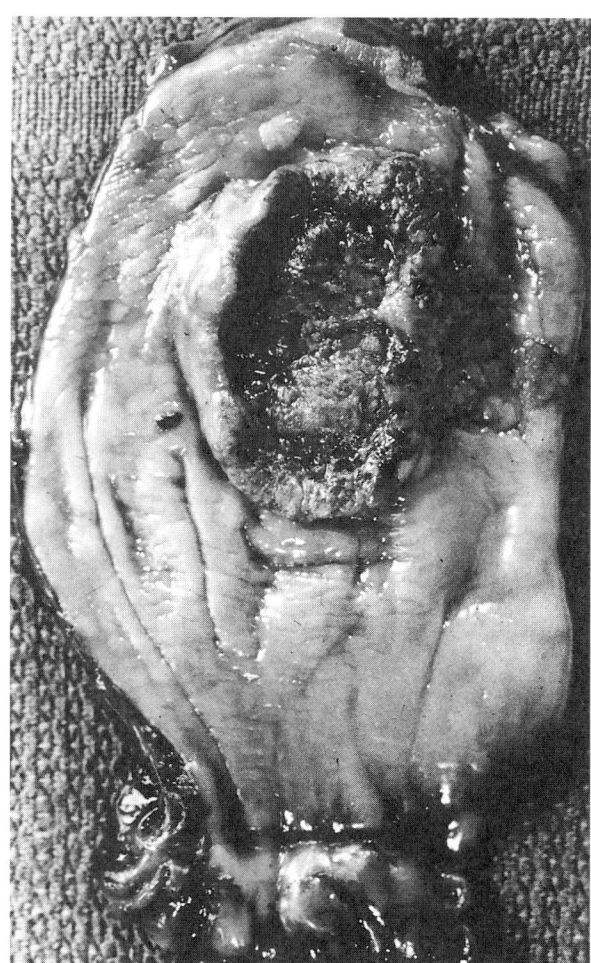

FIGURE 25.12. Advanced squamous cell carcinoma, ulcerative type. The tumor measures 3.5 cm × 2.7 cm. The ulcerated surface is depressed and hemorrhagic, and the ulcer margin is sharply delineated. Submucosal extension of the tumor results in the slightly raised tumor border (*left*), which is covered by an intact mucosa. Note the satellite tumor nodule adjacent to the upper margin of the tumor.

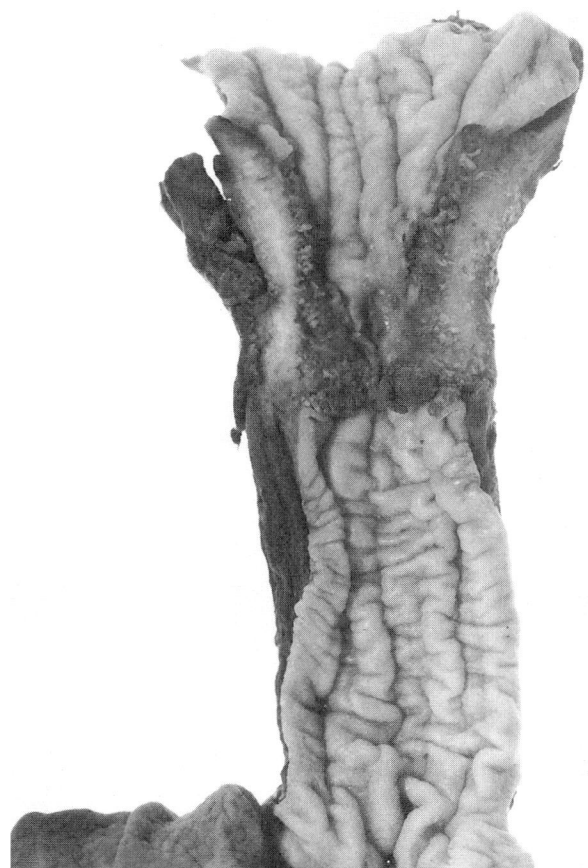

FIGURE 25.13. Advanced squamous cell carcinoma, infiltrative type. The tumor infiltrates circumferentially the whole thickness of esophageal wall without forming an intraluminal mass. The tumor surface is eroded and the lumen of the esophagus narrowed.

ment is common. The tumor-infiltrated segment is rigid and does not contract, causing stenosis and obstruction of the lumen with dilation proximal to it. The upper end of the stenosed segment may be funnel shaped or cup shaped.

Histologically, the invasive tumor is well-differentiated or moderately differentiated in the majority of cases. The well-differentiated tumor cells are oval or polyhedral and contain round or oval nuclei with nucleoli (Fig. 25.14). They show varying degrees of keratinization. The keratotic cells are elongated, arranged in whorls, and contain pyknotic or no nuclei, forming the so-called pearls that are the markers of squamous cell carcinoma. They are usually located in the center of tumor cell groups and are surrounded by nonkeratotic tumor cells.

Moderately differentiated squamous cells are polyhedral and arranged in cords (Fig. 25.15). Mitotic figures are frequent. Undifferentiated carcinoma cells are variable in size. They are polyhedral or round, and some are irregular or spindle shaped (Fig. 25.16). Occasionally, tumor cells are giant sized and bizarre. In some areas, cells adjoining the stroma are arranged in a row, reminiscent of the basal layer of the epidermis. Tumor cells may infiltrate individually or in small groups. When they form large sheets, necrosis is common. Carcinoma composed entirely of undifferentiated cells is rare. Usually, its squamous cell origin may be confirmed readily, because a better differentiated squamous cell pattern can be found in some areas. Rare small cell carcinomas, which once were considered undifferentiated tumors, are now known to be neuroendocrine tumors, similar to the small cell carcinoma of the lung.

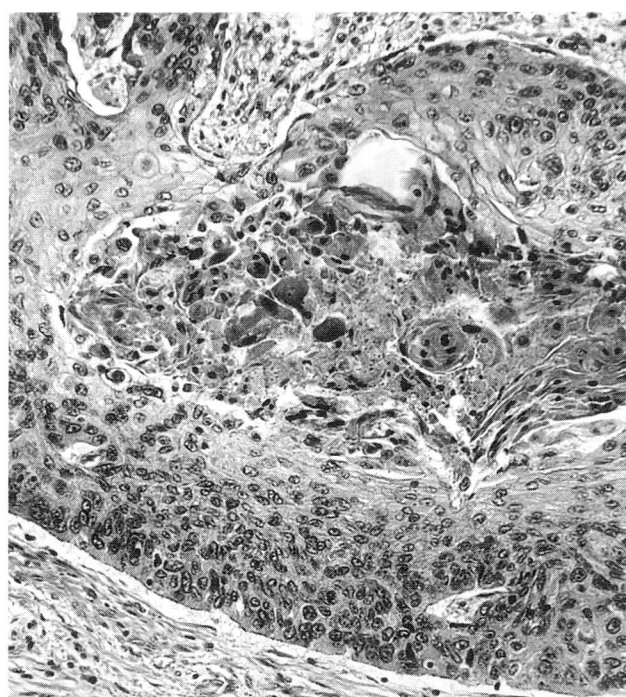

FIGURE 25.14. Squamous cell carcinoma, well differentiated. Invasive tumor cells show progressive differentiation from the periphery toward the center of the patch; the latter contains degenerated keratotic cells. The appearance is reminiscent of dysplastic epithelium.

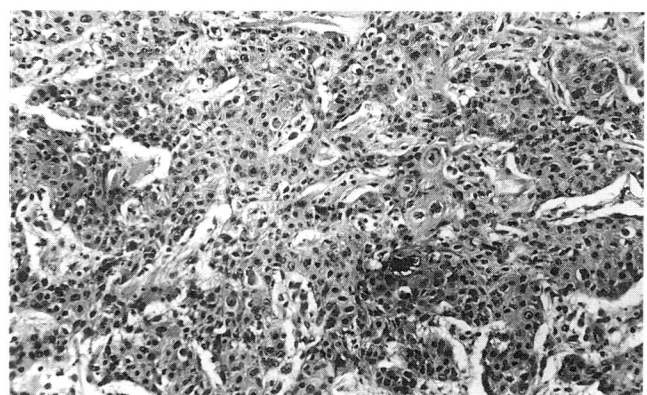

FIGURE 25.15. Squamous cell carcinoma, moderately differentiated. Pleomorphic tumor cells form interconnected irregular patches. Better differentiated cells have abundant cytoplasm (*center right*).

VARIANTS OF SQUAMOUS CELL CARCINOMA

VERRUCOUS CARCINOMA

Verrucous carcinoma is rare in the esophagus (100). It forms an exophytic growth with a papillary surface and is composed of moderately differentiated squamous cells with a prominent intraepithelial com-

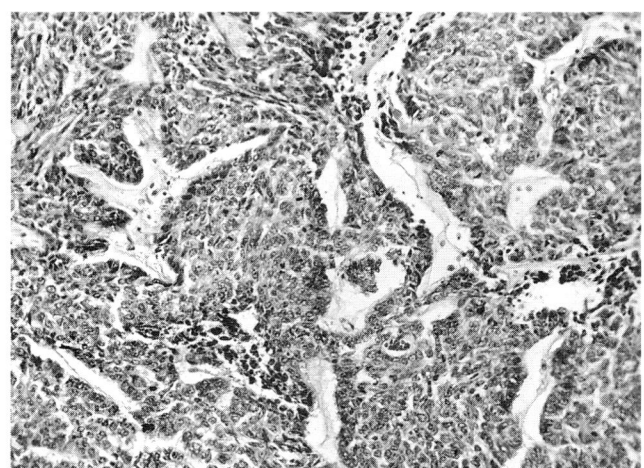

FIGURE 25.16. Squamous cell carcinoma, poorly differentiated. The tumor cells are small and cytoplasm is scanty. Some cells are spindle shaped (*upper center*). Tumor cells next to the stroma are darkly stained and regularly oriented, reminiscent of the basal layer of normal epithelium.

ponent. The papillary fronds have a central fibrous core extending from the lamina propria (Fig. 25.17). The invasive portion of the tumor is similar to that seen in other squamous cell carcinomas. The tumor grows and invades slowly and metastasis is uncommon (101). Nonetheless, the mortality rate, at 67%, is high (102).

BASALOID CARCINOMA

Squamous cell carcinomas may have focal areas showing basaloid features with small nonkeratotic cells at the periphery of tumor cell groups resembling the basal layer of normal epithelium (Fig. 25.16). Such mixed features were found in 6.8% of advanced carcinomas and 16.3% of superficial carcinomas by Tauchi et al. (103). Pure basaloid features, seen in none of the advanced carcinomas, were found among 28.6% of superficial carcinomas. They are characterized by an expanding growth pattern and no lymph node metastases. Some tumors have a cribriform pattern resembling that seen in adenoid cystic carcinoma (104).

SPINDLE CELL CARCINOMA AND CARCINOSARCOMA

Squamous cell carcinoma may contain spindle cells (Fig. 25.16). Rarely, the spindle cells comprise the major portion of the tumor. By electron microscopy and immunohistochemistry, the spindle cells have markers of squamous cells (105, 106). Such a tumor is called spindle cell carcinoma. In some tumors, the

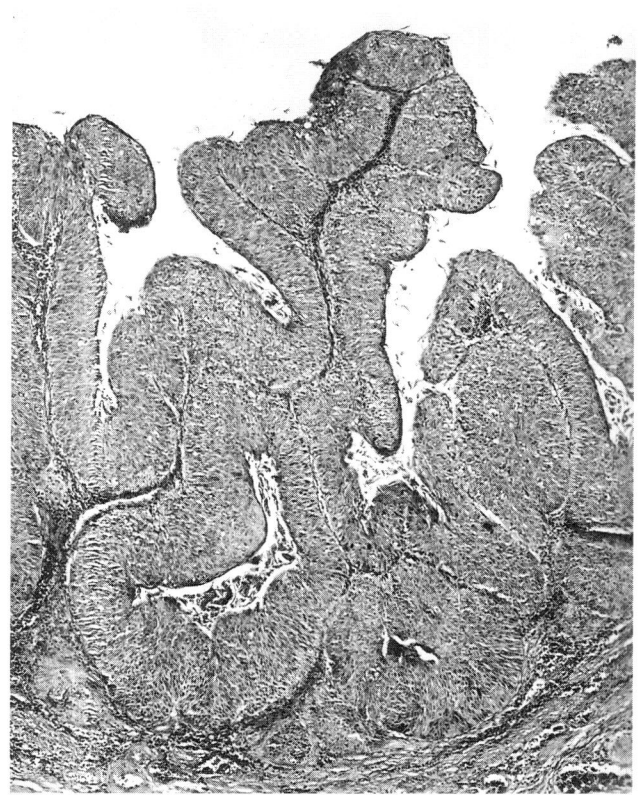

FIGURE 25.17. Verrucous carcinoma. The well-differentiated squamous tumor cells form papillary fronds supported by thin vascular fibrous tissue at the core.

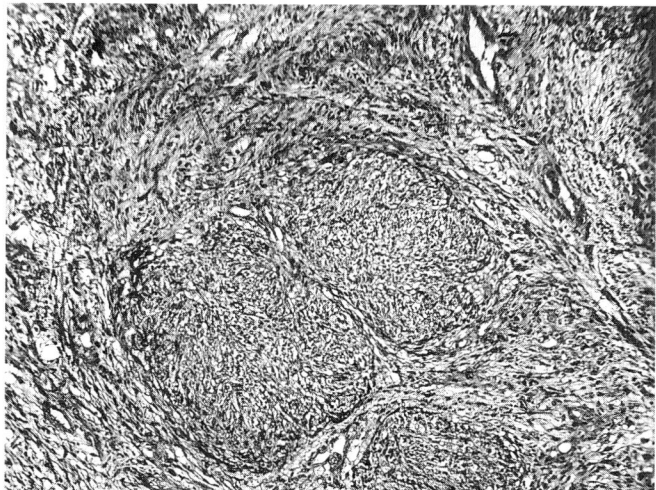

FIGURE 25.18. Carcinosarcoma. The tumor contains both sarcomatous spindle cells and undifferentiated carcinomatous cells.

spindle cells and regular squamous cells coexist, whereas the spindle cells assume a sarcomatous appearance (Fig. 25.18). Osseous, cartilaginous, and muscular tissues may be present. These tumors have been called carcinosarcomas (107, 108). The proportion of different cell types varies. Rarely, the tumor is composed mainly of spindle cells with carcinoma only in the covering or adjacent epithelium. The sarcomatous cells may contain intracellular collagen, intermediate filaments, and vimentin (107, 108), indicating a true sarcomatous nature. Both carcinomatous and sarcomatous components have been found in the metastatic lesions. Rarely, the carcinomatous tissue in the tumor is glandular. One such case occurred in a Barrett's esophagus (109). Whether the mesenchymal cells are metaplastic from squamous cells or whether both epithelial and mesenchymal cells are derived from pluripotential stem cells remain unsettled.

Grossly, regardless of histologic composition, most of these tumors are polypoid and large, up to 15 cm in diameter (110). The tumor surface may be smooth and intact or focally ulcerated. Deeply ulcerative and infiltrative tumors are rare. Thus, spindle cell carcinomas and carcinosarcomas have also been called polypoid carcinomas. However, not all polypoid carcinomas are spindle cell carcinomas or carcinosarcomas. Ordinary squamous cell carcinomas and oat cell or small cell carcinomas may also be polypoid (108). There are no significant differences in the age, sex, and clinical presentations of patients between spindle cell and squamous cell carcinomas (110). The depth of tumor invasion varies. Although most tumors do not extend beyond the esophageal wall, the rate of recurrence, lymph node metastasis, and survival rates are similar to those of the ordinary squamous cell carcinomas.

ADENOCARCINOMA

Adenocarcinomas of the esophagus originate from the columnar epithelium of the mucosa. Tumors arising from the deep glands in the submucosa are mucoepidermoid and adenoid cystic carcinomas, the same type found in the salivary glands.

In recent years, primary esophageal adenocarcinoma has increased remarkably (35, 36). Most of these tumors are Barrett's carcinomas. The origin of an adenocarcinoma may be identified by the nature of the benign epithelium in the vicinity of the tumor. The Barrett's epithelium is grossly evident in most cases (Fig. 25.19). If not, the use of a dissecting microscope has been helpful in the search for any minute focus of Barrett epithelium (14). For tumors at the esophagogastric junction, an esophageal origin is supported if the center of the tumor is located more than 2 cm above the junction. In the lower esophagus, an adenocarcinoma may still be assumed to have arisen in a Barrett's ep-

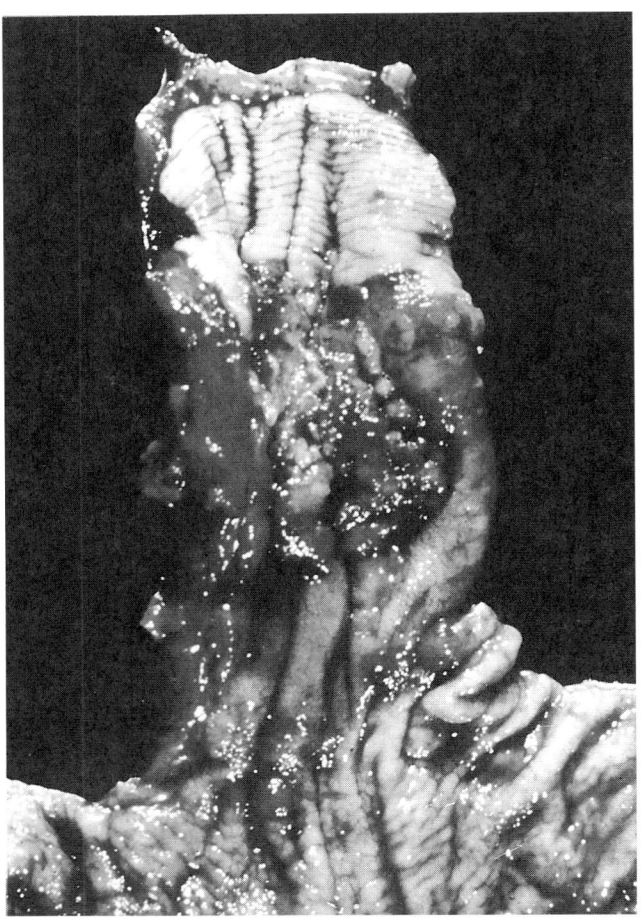

FIGURE 25.19. Adenocarcinoma of Barrett's esophagus. The flat and slightly ulcerated carcinoma is located in the distal esophagus. The columnar mucosa surrounding the tumor resembles the mucosa of the stomach. Proximal to the tumor, the light gray and slightly corrugated mucosa is squamous.

ithelium even if the columnar epithelium is not found. The carcinoma may have destroyed it.

LOCATION

Because the Barrett's epithelium occurs mainly in the distal esophagus, adenocarcinomas arising in it are usually located in the lower third of the esophagus (20) Occasional adenocarcinomas occur in the midesophagus (111, 112). In a recent report, only 11 of 58 cases with adenocarcinoma in midthoracic esophagus were associated with Barrett's epithelium, while the others were extensions from the stomach (113). In another report, the carcinoma developed in the cervical esophagus in a patient with a long history of gastric reflux and extensive Barrett's epithelium (11). The adenocarcinoma in these regions (114, 115) may be associated with congenital remnants of superficial glands or heterotopic gastric epithelium.

GROSS MORPHOLOGY

Regardless of their tissue origin, adenocarcinomas of the esophagus have similar gross and microscopic features. Early adenocarcinomas in the form of intramucosal or submucosal tumors have been detected in patients under endoscopic surveillance (89, 91). They may not be grossly evident. Some early carcinomas are flat. Occasional ones are polypoid and large, up to 4.5 cm in size (116). At the time of diagnosis, most adenocarcinomas are already advanced, with extensive intramural and adventitial involvement (42, 81, 117). Most of the advanced tumors are flat and ulcerated (Fig. 24.19), and about one third are polypoid or fungating. Diffusely infiltrative, in the form of linitis plastica (81, 118), and papillary (119) lesions are rare. The size of the tumors varies, up to 10.5 cm in diameter. Multiple tumors may be present in the same esophagus (42, 117).

The esophageal mucosa surrounding or distal to the tumor is often grossly identifiable as Barrett's epithelium. The normal squamous mucosa, which is pale gray, smooth, and shiny, is present proximal to the tumor or in small patches within the Barrett's epithelium. In some cases, only the squamous mucosa is present. Even in these cases, benign columnar epithelium may be found in histologic sections.

HISTOLOGIC FEATURES

The vast majority of adenocarcinomas are well- or moderately differentiated (Fig. 25.20). Intestinal differentiation of tumor cells with striated cell borders and acidic mucin is common, but gastric differentiation with pepsinogen II and neutral mucus secretion has also been found in about one half of the tumors (120). The mucus is easily seen in the lumen of the glands. However, intracellular mucus goblets are usually few and scattered. Occasionally, mucus pools are

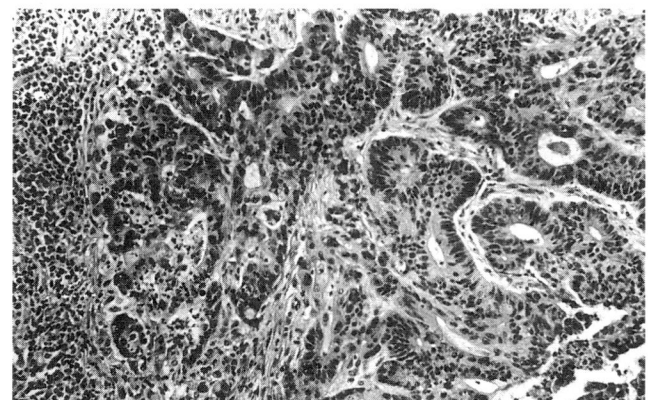

FIGURE 25.20. Adenocarcinoma of Barrett's esophagus. The carcinoma is composed of moderately differentiated glands.

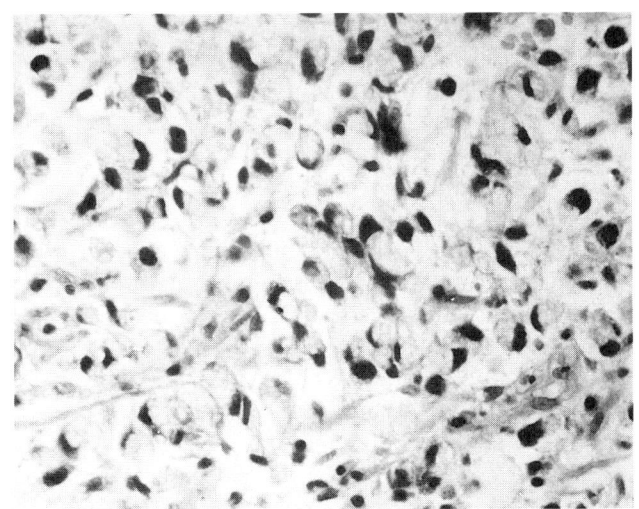

FIGURE 25.21. Signet-ring cell carcinoma of Barrett's esophagus. The tumor cells are round and individually scattered. They contain a large globule of mucus compressing the nucleus to the periphery of the cell.

present. The diffusely infiltrative carcinoma contains signet-ring cells (81, 118) (Fig. 25.21). The tumor may also show infiltration by single glands. These features resemble those of gastric carcinomas. Endocrine cells may be present (121). Vascular and lymphatic invasion are often found. The growth pattern of the tumor is nearly equally divided between expanding and infiltrative types (34). Other tumors occurring in the Barrett's epithelium include squamous cell carcinoma (59, 122), adenoacanthoma, carcinoid, adenocarcinoid, and mucoepidermoid carcinoma (42, 59, 122–124).

The esophageal epithelium adjacent to the carcinoma may show reflux esophagitis and Barrett's epithelium. The size of residual Barrett's epithelium, if present, is variable. Dysplasia and in situ carcinoma are found in many cases (14, 42, 88).

VARIANTS OF ADENOCARCINOMA: ADENOACANTHOMA AND ADENOSQUAMOUS CARCINOMA

Adenoacanthoma and adenosquamous carcinoma are characterized by the presence of both squamous and glandular cells. An adenoacanthoma is essentially a well-differentiated adenocarcinoma with small groups of squamous cells surrounded by glandular cells that are capable of secreting mucus. The squamous cells are most likely metaplastic cells, and the tumor behaves like other adenocarcinomas. Adenoacanthoma probably arises from aberrant columnar epithelium and had been reported in the Barrett's esophagus (42). In another Barrett's adenocarcinoma, squamous cells were recognized in an ultrastructural examination (121). Adenoacanthomas are rare, with one case each being found among 50 superficial and 133 advanced esophageal carcinomas (103).

An adenosquamous carcinoma is essentially a squamous cell carcinoma with occasional glands. This feature was found in 23 of 195 squamous cell carcinomas by Kuwano et al. (125). In a recent report, a polypoid spindle cell carcinoma was found to have adenosquamous elements in addition to squamous cells (126). These features suggest that adenoacanthoma and adenosquamous carcinoma may have originated from the totipotential cells in the squamous epithelium.

Both of these terms have been used interchangeably with mucoepidermoid carcinoma. The latter is a tumor of deep esophageal glands and should be distinguished from them. These tumors should also be differentiated from the squamous cell carcinoma with pseudoglandular degeneration, which has no mucus secretion (94).

CARCINOMA AT THE ESOPHAGOGASTRIC JUNCTION

The vast majority of tumors occurring at the esophagogastric junction are adenocarcinomas. Approximately two thirds originate in the stomach, and one third begin in the esophagus (120, 127). Squamous cell carcinomas of esophageal origin and anaplastic carcinomas comprise only about 10% of the tumors at this site (128). Occasional cases of adenoacanthoma, mucoepidermoid carcinoma, and double carcinomas have also been reported (129).

There is no barrier to carcinomatous invasion at the esophagogastric junction. Carcinoma of one organ can readily invade the other, not only by contiguous intramural expansion but also through lymphatic channels, resulting in the formation of disconnected distant metastatic lesions. In the case of adenocarcinoma, the histologic features of all tumors are essentially the same. It is therefore extremely difficult to determine the tumor origin based on the pathologic features alone. Instead, the differentiation between an esophageal and a gastric adenocarcinoma may rely on circumstantial factors such as the location of the center of the tumor and the landmarks of the respective organs at the tumor site. The landmarks of the esophagus include the submucosal glands, the two-layer structure of muscularis propria, and the absence of serosa on the external surface of the organ. Obviously, these features cannot be applied to a biopsy specimen. In some cases, the presence of incomplete intestinal-type glands in the adjacent mucosa suggests the presence of Barrett's epithelium, and thus an esophageal location of the lesion. In terms of clinical implication, precise knowledge of the tumor origin may not be important because the adenocarcinomas of the distal esophagus, esophagogastric junction, and gastric cardia have many common features pathologically and epidemiologically. They may thus be considered a single entity, different from the squamous cell carcinoma of the esophagus and the adenocarcinoma of the distal stomach (14, 130, 131).

OTHER CARCINOMAS

CARCINOMAS OF DEEP ESOPHAGEAL GLANDS

Two distinct types of carcinoma originate from deep esophageal glands: mucoepidermoid carcinoma and adenoid cystic carcinoma. They are primarily submucosal tumors covered by an intact mucosa (132). Grossly, they are sessile or polypoid, but they may become ulcerated. Adenomas, which are common in the major salivary glands, have not been reported in the esophagus.

MUCOEPIDERMOID CARCINOMA

Mucoepidermoid carcinoma of the esophagus arises from the excretory duct of the deep esophageal gland (133). In two recent reports, approximately 2% of esophageal carcinomas were mucoepidermoid and adenosquamous carcinomas (134, 135). One case developed in a Barrett's esophagus (124). Approximately 50% of the tumors occur in the middle third of the esophagus. Histologically, the tumor is composed of a mixture of squamous, mucous, and intermediate cells in varying proportions. The squamous cells are generally well- to moderately differentiated and show occasional keratotic pearls. The mucous cells are cuboidal or columnar, forming glands or sheets. The amount of mucus varies both intracellularly and intraluminally. Some of the glands may be cystically distended with mucus. Clinically, the patients are mostly male and in their seventh decade. Unlike similar tumors of the salivary glands, mucoepidermoid carcinomas of the esophagus are aggressive tumors. Although most tumors are resectable, extensive invasion and lymph node metastasis are common at the time of surgery. The prognosis is poor, similar to that of squamous cell carcinomas (132, 136), unless the tumor is resected at an early stage when it is still confined to the submucosal layer and there are no lymph node metastases (135).

ADENOID CYSTIC CARCINOMA

Adenoid cystic carcinomas comprise approximately 1.1% to 4.3% of esophageal carcinomas (135, 137). As tumors of deep esophageal glands, they are located primarily in the submucosa and have a smooth surface. Most tumors are polypoid and located in the midesophagus. Histologically, they are characterized by a cribriform pattern with many cystic spaces lined by neoplastic epithelial and myoepithelial cells. Squamous cells may be present. The tumor cells show positive immunohistologic reaction for S-100 protein. Some tumors have a basaloid appearance and may actually be basaloid squamous carcinomas (104). Unlike similar tumors of the major salivary gland, adenoid cystic carcinomas of the esophagus tend to have extensive invasion, lymph node metastases, and a poor prognosis (132, 137). Early tumors without lymph node metastasis have a better prognosis (135). Clinically, the tumors occur about equally among the sexes. Most patients are in the seventh decade. Dysphagia is the primary symptom.

CHORIOCARCINOMA

Only five cases of choriocarcinoma of the esophagus have been reported. Two tumors were pure choriocarcinomas with cytotrophoblasts and syncytiotrophoblasts (138, 139). Three tumors had, in addition to trophoblastic cells, foci of adenocarcinoma in two (140, 141) and undifferentiated carcinoma in one (142). One of the former also showed yolk sac differentiation. The tumors were large and ulcerated. Extensive metastases were common. The favored location was the lower esophagus. All patients were under 50 years of age, and both sexes were affected. Tumor cells showed a positive immunohistochemical reaction for human chorionic gonadotropin and human placental lactogen (139). Serum and urinary gonadotropin levels were increased (140, 142).

PAGET'S DISEASE

A case of Paget's disease was diagnosed in a 60-year-old man with history of dysphagia (143). The resected lower esophagus showed diffuse induration without forming a tumor mass. Histologically, large clear pagetoid cells were found in the squamous epithelium and glandular ducts in the mucosa and submucosa. There was no stromal invasion. In two other cases, similar intraepithelial invasion by pagetoid cells was found in association with an adenosquamous carcinoma in one case (144) and a squamous cell carcinoma in the other (145).

CARCINOID AND SMALL CELL CARCINOMA

Carcinoids and small cell carcinomas of the esophagus are tumors of neuroendocrine cell origin. As tumors of the foregut, they are usually argyrophilic. The argentaffin reaction may be positive in carcinoids (146) but generally are negative in small cell carcinomas (146–148). Immunohistochemical reactions for neuron specific enolase, synaptophysin, S-100 protein, and chromogranin are generally positive and serve as useful diagnostic markers (149).

CARCINOIDS

Carcinoids of the esophagus are rare. They are primarily submucosal tumors and may be covered by an intact epithelium. Most carcinoids are located in the distal esophagus and are composed of uniform round or polygonal cells arranged in trabeculae or solid sheets. In one case, the tumor secreted adrenocorticotropic hormone (150). In another case, the carcinoid developed in Barrett's epithelium and was accompanied by a separate adenocarcinoma (123). Foci of mucus-secreting adenocarcinomatous tissue were present in one carcinoid (146).

SMALL CELL CARCINOMA

Small cell carcinoma is also known as oat cell carcinoma. By 1992, 150 cases of esophageal small cell carcinoma had been reported (151). After the lung, the esophagus is the most common site of these tumors. The reported incidences among carcinomas of the esophagus varied from 0.05% to 7.6% (152–154). The esophageal tumor is similar to the tumor in the lung both structurally and biologically. It is composed mostly of small cells with hyperchromatic nuclei and scanty cytoplasm (Fig. 25.22). Larger intermediate cells are present in about one half of the cases, alone or mixed with small cells (149). Squamous cells and, less commonly, glandular and carcinoid differentiation, are present in some tumors (152). Neurosecretory granules are revealed by electron microscopy (147, 148). Adrenocorticotropic hormone (ACTH) activity is often present (147, 148, 150), but Cushing's syndrome has not been reported. Calcitonin was present in some tumors (148). One patient had inappropriate antidiuretic hormone syndrome, and another had hypercalcemia (152). The origin of these tumors is probably the argyrophilic cells, which are present in the basal portion of normal squamous epithelium (6). The presence of other cell types raises the possibility of tumor origin from the totipotential cells in the squamous epithelium

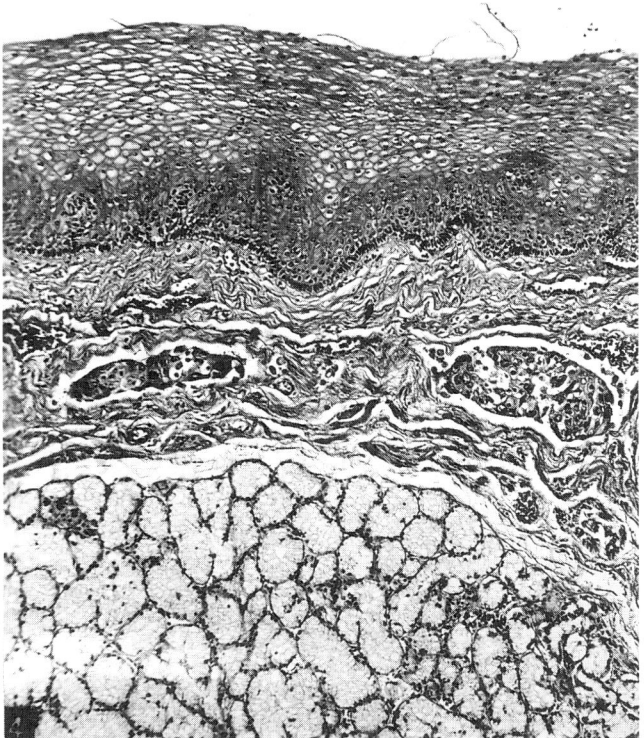

FIGURE 25.22. Small cell carcinoma. The tumor cells are small and hyperchromatic. Cytoplasm is indistinct. They form irregular aggregates randomly scattered within the stroma.

or ducts of the esophageal glands (147), in addition to the argyrophilic cells.

About 90% of the tumors are located in the midesophagus or lower esophagus (154). Most tumors were large and fungating. The polypoid form is rare. Multiple tumors were present in one patient (155). At the time of diagnosis, many tumors are advanced and only one half are resectable. The prognosis is poor, and overall mean survival is only 3.1 months (154).

MALIGNANT MELANOMA

Primary malignant melanoma of the esophagus is rare and accounts for only 0.1% of esophageal cancers (156). It develops from melanocytes normally present in the esophagus (6) and usually is located in the lower esophagus (156, 157). Most tumors are pigmented, polypoid, and large. About 10% of the tumors are amelanotic (158). Multiple tumors may be present (157). Histologically, the tumor is characterized by marked cellularity, frequent mitoses, and the presence of intracellular as well as extracellular melanin pigments. For amelanotic tumors, electron microscopic demonstration of melanosomes and premelanosomes helps to make the correct diagnosis. Tumor cells are positive for neuron specific enolase and S-100 protein. Clinically, most patients are male and are in their 60s and 70s. Distant metastasis is common, and the recurrence rate high (157, 159). Prognosis is poor with a 5-year survival rate of only 4.2% (157).

Melanoma elsewhere may occasionally metastasize to the esophagus. To ascertain the primary nature of the melanoma, efforts should be made to search for junctional changes and increased melanocytes in the adjacent mucosa, which commonly accompany the melanoma (158). In the absence of junctional change, the primary nature of the tumor may be considered after the exclusion of other possible sources.

SARCOMAS

Sarcomas of the esophagus are rare. Among them, leiomyosarcoma is the most common. Rare cases of rhabdomyosarcoma, fibrosarcoma, and Kaposi's sarcoma have been reported. Unusual sarcomas of the esophagus include malignant fibrous histiocytoma (160), liposarcoma (161), synovial sarcoma (162, 163), and malignant schwannoma (163). These tumors grow submucosally. They may be sessile, but most are polypoid.

LEIOMYOSARCOMA

Leiomyomas are relatively common in the esophagus, but leiomyosarcomas are rare. Among 1456 cancers of the esophagus, Goodner et al. (164) found only eight sarcomas—seven leiomyosarcomas and one fibrosarcoma. Men are affected more often than women, and the average age was in the sixth decade (165). Leiomyosarcomas may be found in any part of the esophagus. Grossly, the tumor is often a polypoid intramural mass with a broad base and an intact covering mucosa. Some tumors infiltrate extensively resembling invasive carcinoma, occasionally involving neighboring organs. Microscopically, the tumor is composed predominantly of spindle cells forming interlacing fascicles. Pleomorphism may be marked and giant cells are frequent. Mitoses are always present. At times, the diagnosis of malignancy may be uncertain. In such cases, DNA measurement may be helpful: aneuploidy is indicative of malignancy (166). Metastasis is uncommon. The survival rates are 80% at 1 year, 36% at 5 years, and 30% at 10 years (167). Prognostic factors are histologic grade, mitosis index, size, and location of the tumor.

OTHER SARCOMAS

Rhabdomyosarcoma of the esophagus characteristically contains pleomorphic cells with giant cell forms (168). Immunohistochemical reaction for desmin is positive. Foci of rhabdomyosarcoma may be present in a carcinosarcoma (169). Fibrosarcomas of esophagus were reported in the cervical esophagus many years after radiation to the thyroid (164). Kaposi's sarcoma may involve the esophagus as a part of systemic disease, particularly in patients with acquired immunodeficiency syndrome (AIDS) (170, 171). One patient received immunosuppressive treatment after a renal homograft operation (172).

LYMPHOMA

Mediastinal lymphoma may infiltrate the esophageal wall. Most such patients have Hodgkin's disease (173); primary esophageal lymphomas are usually of the non-Hodgkin's type. Most cases have T-cell lymphoma with diffuse large cells (174, 175). One tumor was composed of small lymphocytic and plasmacytoid cells (176). Grossly, the tumors are polypoid and ulcerated, occasionally diffuse. There is no specific site preference. In one patient, it was submucosal (174). Some patients have AIDS. In one report, two esophageal lymphomas were found among 763 human immunodeficiency virus–seropositive patients (177).

SECONDARY AND METASTATIC TUMORS

Secondary tumors in the esophagus occur in 3% of cancer patients at autopsy (178), mostly from primary tumors of the stomach, lung, or breast (179–181), either by direct invasion or via lymphatic or vascular channels. The hematogenous route appears to be the route of spread in the case of metastatic melanoma to the esophagus (182). Such complications may occur several years after the diagnosis of primary tumor, particularly carcinoma of the breast (180, 181). Secondary tumors resulting from direct extension may mimic a primary tumor with ulceration or stenosis. However, intraluminal masses are rare. The metastatic tumors are generally submucosal. They are small or only microscopic in size and asymptomatic. Surgical resection of the metastatic tumor occasionally results in long survival (183).

MULTIPLE CARCINOMAS

Epithelial dysplasia, intraepithelial carcinoma, and early carcinoma of the esophagus often are found in multiple foci (76, 184). The advanced carcinoma, conversely, is usually single. The dysplastic foci, if present, often are found away from the main invasive lesion rather than in continuity with it (185). These findings suggest that esophageal carcinomas are multicentric in origin. As the tumor foci grow, they coalesce to form a single tumor. In contrast, multiple advanced carcinomas are infrequent in the esophagus. Only 10 (2.5%) of 421 cases of squamous cell carcinoma of the esophagus studied by Moertel and Dockerty (186) had two separate carcinomas. It should be noted that not all separate tumors represent independent lesions. In a histological study, Maeta et al. (187) found 38 separate cancerous foci in 111 resected esophagi. Among them, 27 additional primary early carcinomas were found in 23 specimens and 11 intramural metastatic lesions in 10. The mean distance between the main tumor and another primary lesion was 2.6 cm both proximally and distally, and that between the main tumor and a metastatic lesion was 3.4 cm proximally and 4.6 cm distally. These data emphasize the importance of including a sufficient length of tumor free segment, as determined by histologic examination, in the resected esophagus to reduce local recurrence of the tumor.

Tumors of different types may coexist in the same esophagus. Squamous cell carcinoma (42) and carcinoid (123) may accompany adenocarcinoma of Barrett's epithelium. Paget's disease of the esophagus coexisting with a carcinoma has been reported (144, 145). There also have been reports of benign mesodermal lesions, such as leiomyoma, lipoma, and fibrous polyp, accompanying carcinoma (188).

TUMOR SPREAD AND METASTASIS

INTRAMURAL SPREAD

Intramural spread of esophageal carcinoma may be by direct continuous invasion or via lymphatics (Fig. 25.23). It spreads vertically by penetrating deeply into the esophageal wall and the surrounding tissue, or horizontally along the tissue planes. Intraepithelial expansion of squamous cell carcinoma can be recognized by the sharp demarcation line between the malignant tissue and the normal epithelium (Fig. 25.10). This lesion is associated with invasive carcinoma in the adjacent tissue (74). The term superficial spreading type has been applied to a carcinoma showing horizontal intramucosal extension for 20 mm or more beyond the main lesion (189). The main tumor may be submucosal or advanced. Metastasis to lymph nodes in such tumors occurs in half of the early and all of the advanced cases.

Lateral spread of carcinoma by lymphatics may

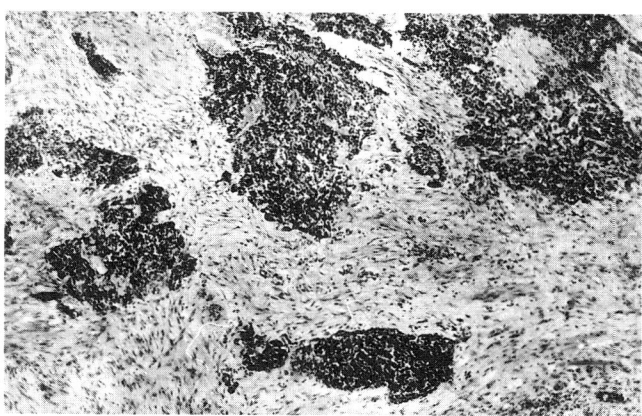

FIGURE 25.23. Lymphatic spread of poorly differentiated squamous carcinoma cells is shown in the lamina propria between the normal squamous epithelium and deep esophageal glands.

result in the formation of isolated nodules resembling separate primary tumors. Intramural metastasis has been found in 12% to 15% of squamous cell carcinomas, usually in the advanced tumors (190, 191). Such cases have higher rates of lymph node and distant organ metastasis and worse survival rates than those without intramural metastasis. Transmural spread of tumor occurs in 60% to 88% of Barrett's carcinomas (88).

CONTIGUOUS INVOLVEMENT OF NEIGHBORING ORGANS

Contiguous extension of esophageal carcinoma into neighboring organs is common. The organs involved depend on the location of the tumor. Tumor extension into periesophageal connective tissue is present in about half of the surgically resected specimens. At autopsy, the neighboring organs are involved in about 34% to 60% of cases (192). Fistulae often develop along the cancerous tissue. Esophagorespiratory fistula is the most common and most life threatening (193, 194). Extensive mediastinitis, pneumonia, and abscess formation are common in these cases. The involved aorta may rupture, resulting in fatal massive bleeding (192).

LYMPH NODE METASTASIS

Intraepithelial and mucosal carcinomas do not show metastases to the lymph nodes. Submucosal early carcinomas, in contrast, have a rather high incidence of lymph node metastases, varying from 22% to 47% (97, 98). The incidence in advanced cases at autopsy is about 60% (224). Most metastatic lesions are limited to the intrathoracic lymph nodes, of which 49% to 62% are mediastinal and 27% are paratracheal and paraesophageal. Abdominal lymph nodes are involved in 29% to 42% of cases. In the surgically resected specimens, metastasis was present in 41% of the cases. In patients with Barrett's adenocarcinoma, lymph node metastasis is present in 55% to 74% (88), even if the tumor does not have deep invasion. The supraclavicular nodes are involved in 22% of patients with squamous cell carcinoma and 10% of patients with adenocarcinoma (195). Sixty-two percent of carcinomas at the esophagogastric junction have lymph node metastasis, mostly intraabdominal (196). Thoracic nodes are involved in 7% of the cases.

HEMATOGENOUS METASTASIS

Venous involvement has not been seen in the intramucosal carcinomas of the esophagus. It is present in 27% of submucosal carcinomas and 63.5% of carcinomas invading the muscularis propria (98). In the surgically resected specimens, venous invasion is present in 76.5%, mostly in those located intramurally (197). Distant metastasis, the result of hematogenous spread, is present in about 5% of the clinical cases (198) and is common in autopsy cases. The most commonly involved organs are liver and lung, each representing approximately 20% to 30% of cases (192).

STAGING OF ESOPHAGEAL CANCERS

The staging of esophageal cancer using the TNM (Primary Tumor, Lymph Node, Distant Metastasis) system as proposed by American Joint Commission on Cancer (199) is listed in Table 25.2. Some investigators use N1 to denote metastasis in one to four regional nodes and N2 in five or more nodes (200). In this staging method, unlike previous systems, the size of the primary tumor and complications such as fistula formation are not considered. The early or superficial carcinoma may be classified as either stage I or stage IIB, depending on the status of regional lymph nodes. Pathologic staging within the TNM system (pTNM) differs from the clinical staging by relying on the histologic diagnosis in determining the status of tumor extent. Therefore, it cannot be applied to conditions not yet studied pathologically, such as lesions detected by diagnostic imaging techniques. Staging does not apply to sarcomas, which begin in the depth of the esophageal wall and may metastasize initially via blood vessels rather than lymphatics.

Iizuka and colleagues (38) reported the percentage of cases in various stages of disease among 4463 surgically treated patients with squamous cell carcinoma: stage I, 5.3%; IIA, 29.3%; IIB, 7.5%; III, 33.3%; and VI, 24.7%. Corresponding data on 60 patients with adenocarcinoma (40) were stage 0, 6.7%; I, 16.7%; II, 28.3%; III, 41.6%; and IV, 6.7%.

SURVIVAL RATES AND PROGNOSTIC FACTORS

Survival Rates

Although metastasis is absent in approximately 40% of autopsy cases (192), the cure rate for esophageal carcinoma is low, even among surgically resectable cases. Muller and associates (201) estimated that among 100 patients, 56 had resectable carcinoma, 7 died postoperatively, 27 survived for 1 year and 10 survived for 5 years. The experience in China has been better. The resectability is 83%, operative mortality is 3.5%, and 5-year survival rate is 30% (96). The reason for better survival may be related to a high number of early carcinomas detected by mass screening. The

TABLE 25.2. TNM Classification of Esophageal Cancer by the American Joint Committee on Cancer

STAGE	PRIMARY TUMOR (T)	LYMPH NODES (N)	DISTANT METASTASIS (M)
0	TIS (carcinoma in situ)	N0 (no metastasis)	M0 (absent)
I	T1 (invasion of lamina propria or submucosa)	N0	M0
IIA	T2 (invasion of muscularis propria)	N0	M0
	T3 (invasion of adventitia)	N0	M0
IIB	T1	N1 (regional lymph node metastasis)	M0
	T2	N1	M0
III	T3	N1	M0
III	T4 (invasion of adjacent structures)	Any N	M0
IV	Any T	Any N	M1 (present)

postoperative 5-year survival rate for stage I carcinoma in China is 90%. There is no significant difference in the survival rates between squamous cell carcinoma and Barrett's adenocarcinoma (42, 202), although some reports have noted longer survival times in patients with Barrett's carcinoma (112).

PROGNOSTIC FACTORS

Prognosis of esophageal carcinoma is not influenced by the gross morphology or histologic grade of the tumor. The pathologic features influencing the outcome of the disease are described below.

STAGE OF CARCINOMA

The stage of esophageal cancer at the time of diagnosis is the most important prognostic factor, i.e., the higher the tumor stage, the lower the survival rate. In the report by Huang et al. (198), the 5-year survival rates of 976 surgically treated patients with stage I, II, III, and IV tumors were 83.3%, 46.3%, 26.4%, and 6.7%, respectively. Similar rates were reported by Iizuka et al. (38): the rate for stage I patients was 64.2%; stage IIA, 40.9%; stage IIB, 24.7%; stage III, 17.2%; and stage IV, 5.4%. Similar results were found in patients with Barrett's adenocarcinoma (45). The 5-year survival rates of patients with early esophageal carcinoma are high, ranging from 64% to 90% for squamous cell carcinoma (23, 96, 99) and from 73% to 85.7% for adenocarcinoma (40, 88). The 5-year survival rate for stage 0 carcinoma was 100% in both types of carcinoma (40, 98).

TUMOR SPREAD AND METASTASIS

Carcinomas with intramural spread have more lymph node metastasis, higher recurrence rates, and lower survival rates than those without it (190, 191). The status of lymph node metastases clearly affects the prognosis. The 5-year survival rate of patients without node metastasis is approximately three times that of patients with metastasis (38, 198). Furthermore, the survival rate decreases as the number of positive nodes increases (203). Among patients with submucosal tumors, the survival rate is 60% without lymphatic or venous involvement and 37.6% with it (98).

LOCATION OF THE CARCINOMA

Contiguous involvement of neighboring organs is an important factor for restricting the resectability of the carcinoma. The effect of this complication is related to the nature of the involved organ, which in turn is dictated by the location of the tumor in the esophagus. For instance, a carcinoma of the midthoracic esophagus may penetrate into the tracheobronchial tree and lung, causing fistula formation and persistent infection, or may invade and rupture the aorta to cause fatal bleeding. Such complications are important causes of death (194).

SIZE OF THE CARCINOMA

The size of the tumor is another factor in determining resectability, which is reduced if the tumor is larger than 7 cm (96). The survival rate is inversely proportional to the size of the tumor. According to Iizuka et al. (38), among patients with tumors of less than 1 cm, the 5-year survival rate was 82.9%. Among those with tumors between 3 and 5 cm, the rate was 27.2%. All 22 patients with tumors larger than 15 cm died within 3 years. Huang et al. (198) reported that the 5-year survival rate of patients with tumors smaller than 3 cm was 48%, whereas the rate of patients with larger tumors was only 28.9%.

PLOIDY OF CARCINOMA CELLS

DNA measurement by flow cytometry has shown that approximately 70% of esophageal carcinomas are aneuploid (204). Aneuploid tumors are associated with decreased survival rates, wide extraesophageal spread, and recurrence of tumor (204, 205). Poor prognosis has also been associated with aneuploidy for adenocarcinomas at the esophagogastric junction (206). However, one study found no relationship between DNA ploidy and prognosis (207).

CLINICOPATHOLOGIC CORRELATION

PATHOLOGIC BASIS OF CLINICAL PRESENTATION AND DIAGNOSIS

Patients with early esophageal cancer are often asymptomatic (99). Only 30% of intramucosal carcinomas and 60% of submucosal carcinomas cause mild esophageal symptoms (208). The diagnosis is often made by cytology from screening procedures (23) or from a follow-up examination for upper gastrointestinal diseases (99). The grossly visible lesions can be visualized readily by endoscopy. For occult lesions, application of Lugol solution is helpful (25). The diagnosis may then be confirmed by brushing cytology and biopsy.

In spite of the narrow caliber of the esophagus, the duration of symptoms is usually rather short, considering the growth rate of the tumor and its large size at the time of diagnosis. Based on the size of the tumor seen on x-ray films, the doubling time of esophageal cancer has been calculated to be 16 ± 7.8 months, and the duration for the tumor's advancement from mucosa to adventitia is 21.1 ± 6.8 months (209). Primary symptoms of dysphagia are related to the gross pathologic type of the tumor and the level of its location. In advanced cases, additional symptoms occur, depending on the extent of tumor invasion and the nature of the complications. These can be detected in most cases by computed tomographic scans and endoscopic ultrasonography. Ultrasound-guided fine-needle biopsy and cytology usually provide pathologic confirmation of the diagnosis (210).

Carcinomas, being epithelial lesions, are readily accessible for endoscopic visualization and biopsy. Most of the tumors are well- or moderately differentiated and therefore are diagnosed easily. Carcinomas arising from deep esophageal glands are located submucosally, thus initially resemble mesenchymal tumors. The most common mesenchymal tumor in the esophagus is leiomyoma, which is characterized clinically as well as pathologically by a well-demarcated and noninvasive appearance. Most of them are small and asymptomatic. Leiomyosarcomas are rare. Histologically, these tumors can be differentiated readily from carcinoma. One possible difficulty is in differentiating a sarcoma from a carcinosarcoma in a biopsy. Additional tissue may be required to show the carcinomatous component in the tumor. Their gross appearances are helpful: carcinosarcoma is usually a polypoid intraluminal tumor, whereas the leiomyosarcoma is a deep-seated intramural mass. Metastatic tumors, mostly carcinomas, are submucosal and asymptomatic. The differentiation between a primary melanoma of the esophagus and a metastatic melanoma relies on the presence of junctional changes adjacent to the primary lesion.

COMPLICATIONS AND CAUSES OF DEATH

Invasion of carcinoma into adjacent tissue and organs not only interferes with adequate eradication of tumor tissue by surgery or radiotherapy, but it also causes serious complications that are the major causes of death. Deep cancer penetration often is accompanied by fistula formation and secondary sepsis. The respiratory system is affected most commonly. One serious complication is fatal hemorrhage caused by the rupture of the aorta. Rarely, symptoms develop from a metastatic lesion. Local recurrence of tumor after surgical resection may be caused by microscopic intramural spread of the tumor. To ensure complete removal of cancerous tissue, frozen section analysis of resection margins of the specimen at the time of operation should be a routine procedure.

TREATMENT-RELATED PATHOLOGIC CHANGES

Esophageal carcinomas are treated with surgery, radiation, or chemotherapy, independently or in combination, depending on the status of the tumor and conditions of the patient. Surgery is curative for early and uncomplicated cases. Operative mortality and postoperative complications such as wound leakage and local recurrence of tumor are primarily technical hazards. Surgery does not produce changes in the tumor tissue itself. Chemotherapy alone is not curative but, together with radiotherapy, is a useful neoadjuvant treatment to improve resectability of the tumor or survival time of the patient (211). Chemotherapy induces degenerative and necrotizing changes of the tumor tissue (212), which can be histologically evaluated to judge the efficacy of the treatment.

Radiotherapy has been used to eradicate or reduce the tumor mass. It is also used as a neoadjuvant treatment (211). Poorly differentiated carcinomas may be radiosensitive, but adenocarcinomas tend to be relatively more resistant. Radiation causes degeneration and necrosis of tumor cells, followed by inflammatory reaction and finally fibrosis (99). Acute cellular changes consist of fragmentation, pyknosis, and disappearance of nuclei and swelling and vacuolation of cytoplasm. Acidophilic bodies and lipid granules may appear in the cytoplasm, and bizarre giant cells may be present. In the postirradiated esophagus, the tumor can show three grades of changes (95). In grade I, there is focal degeneration of the tumor, but the size of the tumor remains unchanged. An inflammatory reaction is prominent. In grade II, the tumor becomes smaller and the border indistinct. Microscopically, only a small number of degenerating tumor cells remain. Foreign body giant cells and neutrophils are present in the granulation tissue. In grade III, tumor cells have disappeared, and the esophageal wall is thin and fibrotic. The degree of these changes is related to the radiation dose. The 5-year survival rate for patients showing grade I changes is 22.3%; grade II, 32.4%; and grade III, 37.8%.

REFERENCES

1. Kessler LG, Brown LM, Kaplan RS. Esophagus. In: Miller BA, Ries LAG, Hankey BF, et al., eds. SEER cancer statistics Re-

view, 1973–1990. Bethesda, MD: National Cancer Institute, NIH Pub 93-2789, 1993;XIII:1–17.
2. Boring CC, Squires TS, Tong T, Montgomery S. Cancer statistics, 1994. CA Cancer J Clin 1994;44:7–26.
3. Botha, GSM. Organogenesis and growth of the gastroesophageal region in man. Anat Rec 1959;133:219–239.
4. Antonioli DA, Madara JL. Functional anatomy of the gastrointestinal tract. In Ming SC, Goldman H, eds. Pathology of the gastrointestinal tract. Philadelphia: WB Saunders, 1992:14–36.
5. Gannon B. The vasculature and lymphatic drainage. In: Whitehead R, ed. Gastrointestinal and oesophageal pathology. Edinburgh: Churchill Livingstone, 1989:117–160.
6. Tateishi R, Taniguchi H, Wada A, Horai T, Taniguchi K. Argyrophil cells and melanocytes in esophageal mucosa. Arch Pathol 1974;98:87–89.
7. De la Pava S, Nigogosyan G, Pickren JW, Cabrera A. Melanosis of the esophagus. Cancer 1963;16:48–50.
8. Rector LE, Connerley ML. Aberrant mucosa in the esophagus in infants and in children. Arch Pathol 1941;31:1285–1294.
9. Jabbari M, Goresky CA, Lough J, Yaffe C, Daly D, Cote C. The inlet patch: heterotopic gastric mucosa in the upper esophagus. Gastroenterology 1985;89:352–356.
10. Barrett NR. Chronic peptic ulcer of the oesophagus and esophagitis. Br J Surg 1950;38:175–182.
11. Goodwin WJ Jr, Larson DL, Sajjad SM. Adenocarcinoma of the cervical esophagus in a patient with extensive columnar cell-lined (Barrett's) esophagus. Otolaryngol Head Neck Surg 1983; 91:446–449.
12. Paull A, Trier JS, Dalton MD, Camp RC, Loeb P, Coyal RK. The histologic spectrum of Barrett's esophagus. N Engl J Med 1976; 295:476–480.
13. Ozzello L, Savary M, Rooethlisberger B. Columnar mucosa of the distal esophagus in patients with gastroesophageal reflux. Pathol Ann 1977;12:41–86.
14. Thompson JJ, Zinsser KR, Enterline HT. Barrett's metaplasia and adenocarcinoma of the esophagus and gastroesophageal junction. Hum Pathol 1983;14:42–61.
15. Mangla JC, Schenk EA, Desbaillets L, Guarasci G, Kubasik NP, Turner MD. Pepsin secretion, pepsinogen, and gastrin in "Barrett's esophagus": clinical and morphological characteristics. Gastroenterology 1976;70:669–676
16. Jass JR. Mucin histochemistry of the columnar epithelium of oesophagus: a retrospective study. J Clin Pathol 1981;34: 866–870.
17. Shreiber DS, Apstein M, Hermos JA. Paneth cells in Barrett's esophagus. Gastroenterology 1978;74:1302–1304.
18. Saubier EC, Gouillat C, Samaniego C, Guillaud M, Moulinier B. Adenocarcinoma in columnar lined Barrett's esophagus. Analysis of 13 esophagectomies. Am J Surg 1985;150:365–369.
19. Schnell T, Sontag S, Wanner J. Endoscopic screening for Barrett's esophagus (BE), esophageal adenocarcinoma (AdCA) and other mucosal changes in ambulatory subjects with symptomatic gastroesophageal reflux (GER) (abstract). Gastroenterology 1985;88:1576.
20. Naef AP, Savary M, Ozzello L. Columnar lined lower esophagus: an acquired lesion with malignant predisposition. Report on 140 cases of Barrett's esophagus with 12 adenocarcinomas. J Thorac Cardiovasc Surg 1975;70:826–834.
21. Watanabe H, Jass JR, Sobin LH. Histological typing of oesophageal and gastric tumours. World Health Organization international classification of tumours. 2nd ed. Berlin: Springer-Verlag, 1990:11–18.
22. Liu FS, Li L, Qu SL. Clinical and pathological characteristic of early esophageal cancer. In: Burghardt E, Holzer E, eds. Minimal invasive cancer (microcarcinoma). Clin Oncol 1982;1: 539–557.
23. Shen Q. Diagnostic cytology and early detection. In: Huang GJ, Wu YK, eds. Carcinoma of the esophagus and gastric cardia, Berlin: Springer-Verlag, 1984:157–190.
24. Layfield LJ, Reichman A, Weinstein WM. Endoscopically directed fine needle aspiration biopsy of gastric and esophageal lesions. Acta Cytol 1992;36:69–74.
25. Mori M, Adachi Y, Matsushima T, Matsuda H, Kuwano H, Sugimachi K. Lugol staining pattern and histology of esophageal lesions. Am J Gastroenterol 1993;88:701–705.
26. Dorman AM, Walsh TN, Droogan O, Curran B, Hourihane DO, Hennessy TP, Leader M. DNA quantification of squamous cell carcinoma of the oesophagus by flow cytometry and cytophotometric image analysis using formalin fixed paraffin embedded tissue. Cytometry 1992;13:886–892.
27. Ming PL. Genetic and cytogenetic aspects. In: Ming SC, Goldman H, eds. Pathology of the gastrointestinal tract. Philadelphia: WB Saunders, 1992:81–97.
28. Reid BJ, Sanchez CA, Blount PL. Levine DS. Barrett's esophagus: cell cycle abnormalities in advancing stages of neoplastic progression. Gastroenterology 1993;105:119–129.
29. World Health Organization 1992 statistics annual. Geneva: World Health Organization, 1993:D4–D345.
30. Liu BQ, Li B. Epidemiology of carcinoma of the esophagus in China. In: Huang GJ, Wu YK, eds. Carcinoma of the esophagus and gastric cardia. Berlin: Springer˜2DVerlag, 1984:1–24.
31. Mahboubi E. Epidemiological study of esophageal carcinoma in Iran. Int Surg 1971;56:68–71.
32. Cancer Prevention, Treatment and Research Center of the Ministry of Health. Research investigation on the mortality from malignant tumors in China (Chinese). Beijing: People's Health Press, Beijing, 1979:96.
33. World Health Organization 1990 statistics annual. Geneva: World Health Organization, 1991:358–369.
34. Ming SC. Adenocarcinoma and other epithelial tumors of the esophagus. In: Ming SC, Goldman H, eds. Pathology of the gastrointestinal tract. Philadelphia: WB Saunders, 1992:459–477.
35. Johnston BJ, Reed PI. Changing pattern of oesophageal cancer in a general hospital in the UK. Eur J Cancer Prev 1991;1: 23–25.
36. Blot WJ, Devesa SS, Kneller RW, Fraumeni JF Jr. Rising incidence of adenocarcinoma of the esophagus and gastric cardia. JAMA 265:1287–1289, 1991.
37. Wang JH, Hsu CP, Chen CY, Chen CL, Lin CT, Wang PY, Kwan PC. Primary adenocarcinoma of the esophagus. Kaohsiung J Med Sci 1991;7:363–368.
38. Iizuka T, Kato H, Watanabe H. One hundred and two 5-year survivors of esophageal carcinoma after resective surgery. Jpn J Clin Oncol 1985;15:369–375.
39. Hassall E, Dimmick JE, Magee JF. Adenocarcinoma in childhood Barrett's esophagus: case documentation and the need for surveillance in children. Am J Gastroenterol 88:282–288, 1993.
40. Streitz JM Jr, Ellis FH Jr, Gibb SP, Balogh K, Watkins E Jr. Adenocarcinoma in Barrett's esophagus. A clinicopathologic study of 65 cases. Ann Surg 1991;213:122–125.
41. Skinner DB, Walther BC, Riddell RH, Schmidt H, Iascone C, DeMeester TR. Barrett's esophagus. Comparison of benign and malignant cases. Ann Surg 1983;198:554–566.
42. Smith RRL, Hamilton SR, Boitnott JK, Rogers EL. The spectrum of carcinoma arising in Barrett's esophagus. A clinicopathologic study of 26 patients. Am J Surg Pathol 1984; 8:563–573.

43. Ming SC. Tumors of the esophagus and stomach, second series. Washington, DC: Armed Forces Institute of Pathology, 1973:24–26.
44. Menke-Pluymers MB, Hop WC, Dees J, van Blankenstein M, Tilanus HW. Risk factors for the development of an adenocarcinoma in columnar-lined (Barrett) esophagus. The Rotterdam Esophageal Tumor Study Group. Cancer 1993;72:1155–1158.
45. Li MX, Cheng SJ. Etiology of carcinoma of the esophagus. In: Huang GJ, Wu YK, eds. Carcinoma of the esophagus and gastric cardia. Berlin: Springer-Verlag, 1984:25–52.
46. Chen F, Cole P, Mi Z, Xing L. Dietary trace elements and esophageal cancer mortality in Shanxi, China. Epidemiology 1992;3:402–406.
47. Ghadirian P. Familial history of esophageal cancer. Cancer 1985;56:2112–2116.
48. Ashworth MT, Nash JR, Ellis A, Day DW. Abnormalities of differentiation and maturation in the oesophageal squamous epithelium of patients with tylosis: morphological features. Histopathology 1991;19:303–310.
49. Jochem VJ, Fuerst PA, Fromkes JJ. Familial Barrett's esophagus associated with adenocarcinoma. Gastroenterology 102: 1400–1402, 1992.
50. Luo Y, Yoshizawa T, Katayama T. Comparative study on the natural occurrence of Fusarium mycotoxins (trichothecenes and zearalenone) in corn and wheat from high- and low-risk areas for human esophageal cancer in China. Appl Environ Microbiol 1990;56:3723–3726.
51. Odze R, Antonioli D, Shocket D, Noble-Topham S, Goldman H, Upton M. Esophageal squamous papillomas. A clinicopathologic study of 38 lesions and analysis for human papillomavirus by the polymerase chain reaction. Am J Surg Pathol 1993;17:803–12.
52. Chang F, Syrjanen S, Shen Q, Wang L, Syrjanen K. Screening for human papillomavirus infections in esophageal squamous cell carcinomas by in situ hybridization. Cancer 1993;72: 2525–2530.
53. Fekete F, Mosnier H, Belghiti J, Uribe M, Sauvanet A. Esophageal cancer after mediastinal irradiation. Dysphagia 1993;8: 289–291.
54. Victora CG, Munoz N, Horta BL, Ramos EO. Patterns of mate drinking in a Brazilian city. Cancer Res 1990;50:7112–7115.
55. Chang-Claude JC, Wahrendorf J, Liang QS, et al. An epidemiological study of precursor lesions of esophageal cancer among young persons in a high-risk population in Huixian, China. Cancer Res 1990;50:2268–2274.
56. Ming SC. Precancerous states of the esophagus and stomach. In: Carter RL, ed. Precancerous states. London: Oxford University Press, 1984:192–229.
57. Wargovich MJ, Imada O. Esophageal carcinogenesis in the rat: a model for aerodigestive tract cancer. J Cell Biochem Suppl 1993;17F:91–94.
58. Ribet ME, Mensier EA. Reflux esophagitis and carcinoma. Surg Gynecol Obstet 1992;175:121–125.
59. Paraf F, Flejou JF, Potet F, Molas G, Fekete F. Esophageal squamous carcinoma in five patients with Barrett's esophagus. Am J Gastroenterol 1992;87:746–750.
60. Monuz N, Crespi M, Grassi A, Qing WC, Quiong S, Cai LZ. Precursor lesions of esophageal cancer in high risk populations in Iran and China. Lancet 1982;1:876–879.
61. Jaskiewicz K, Banach L, Mafungo V, Knobel GJ. Oesophageal mucosa in a population at risk of oesophageal cancer: postmortem studies. Int J Cancer 1992;50:32–35.
62. Kuylenstierna R, Munck-Wikland E. Esophagitis and cancer of the esophagus. Cancer 1985;56:837–839.
63. Moghissi K, Sharpe DA, Pender D. Adenocarcinoma and Barrett's oesophagus. A clinico-pathological study. Eur J Cardiothorac Surg 1993;7:126–131.
64. Hopkins RA, Postlethwait RW. Caustic burns and carcinoma of the esophagus. Ann Surg 1981;194:146–148, 1981.
65. Meijssen MA, Tilanus HW, van Blankenstein M, Hop WC, Ong GL. Achalasia complicated by oesophageal squamous cell carcinoma: a prospective study in 195 patients. Gut 1992;33:155–158.
66. Aggestrup S, Holm JC, Sorensen HR. Does achalasia predispose to cancer of the esophagus? Chest 1992;102:1013–1016.
67. Chisholm M, Ardran GM, Callender ST, Wright R. A follow-up study of patients with postcricoid webs. Quart J Med 1971; 40:409.
68. Wynder EL, Hultberg S, Jacobsson F, Bross IJ. Environmental factors in cancer of the upper alimentary tract, a Swedish study with special reference of Plummer-Vinson (Paterson-Kelly) syndrome. Cancer 1957;10:470–487.
69. Holmes GKT, Stokes PL, Sorahan TM, Prior P, Waterhouse JAH, Cooke WT. Coeliac disease, gluten-free diet and malignancy. Gut 1976;17:612–619.
70. Swinson CM, Slavin G, Coles CE, Booth CC. Celiac disease and malignancy. Lancet 1983;1:111–115.
71. Shah SM, Desai HG. Carcinoma in an oesophageal diverticulum. J Assoc Physicians India. 1992;40:119–120.
72. Philippakis M, Karkanias GG, Sakorafas GH. Carcinoma within an epiphrenic esophageal diverticulum. Case report. Eur J Surg 1991;157:617–618.
73. Carr NJ, Monihan JM, Sobin LH. Squamous cell papilloma of the esophagus: a clinicopathologic and follow-up study of 25 cases. Am J Gastroenterol 1994;89:245–8.
74. Ming SC. Tumors of the esophagus and stomach, second series, supplement. Washington, DC: Armed Forces Institute of Pathology, 1985:S2–S8.
75. Kuwano H, Watanabe M, Sadanaga N, Ikebe M, Mori M, Sugimachi K. Squamous epithelial dysplasia associated with squamous cell carcinoma of the esophagus. Cancer Lett 1993; 72:141–147.
76. Anani PA, Gardiol D, Savary M, Monnier P. An extensive morphological and comparative study of clinically early and obvious squamous cell carcinoma of the esophagus. Pathol Res Pract 1991;187:214–219.
77. Shu YJ, Yuan XQ, Jin SP. Further investigation of the relationship between dysplasia and cancer of the esophagus (Chinese). Chin Med J 1981;6:39–41.
78. Coordinating Group for the Research of Esophageal Carcinoma, Chinese Academy of Medical Sciences and Henan Province. Studies on the relationship between epithelial dysplasia and carcinoma of the esophagus (Chinese). Clin Med J 1975;1:110–116.
79. Stillman AE, Selwyn JI. Primary adenocarcinoma of the esophagus arising in a columnar lined esophagus. Am J Dig Dis 1975;20:577–582.
80. McDonald GB, Brand DL, Thorning DR. Multiple adenomatous neoplasms arising in columnar-lined (Barrett's) esophagus. Gastroenterology 1977;72:1317–1321.
81. Ming SC. Tumors of the esophagus and stomach, supplement, second series. Washington, DC: Armed Forces Institute of Pathology, 1985:S9–S17.
82. Atkinson M, Iftikhar SY, James PD, Robertson CS, Steele RJ. The early diagnosis of oesophageal adenocarcinoma by endoscopic screening. Eur J Cancer Prev 1992;1:327–330.
83. Lee RG. Dysplasia in Barrett's esophagus. A clinicopathologic study of six patients. Am J Surg Pathol 1985;9:845–852.

84. Schmidt HG, Riddell RH, Walther B, Skinner DB, Riemann JF. Dysplasia in Barrett's esophagus. J Cancer Res Clin Oncol 1985;110:145–152.
85. Hameeteman W, Tytgat GN, Houthoff HJ, van den Tweeel JC. Barrett's esophagus: development of dysplasia and adenocarcinoma. Gastroenterology 1989;96:1249–1256.
86. Reid BJ, Haggitt RC, Rubin CE, Rabinovitch PS. Barrett's esophagus: correlation between flow cytometry and histology in detection of patients at risk for adenocarcinoma. Gastroenterology 1987;93:1–11.
87. James PD, Atkinson M. Value of DNA image cytometry in the prediction of malignant change in Barrett's oesophagus. Gut 1989;30:899–905.
88. Reid BJ, Sanchez CA, Blount PL, Levine DS. Barrett's esophagus: cell cycle abnormalities in advancing stages of neoplastic progression. Gastroenterology 1993;105:119–129.
89. Tytgat GN, Hameeteman W. The neoplastic potential of columnar-lined (Barrett's) esophagus. World J Surg 1992;16:308–312.
90. Miros M, Kerlin P, Walker N. Only patients with dysplasia progress to adenocarcinoma in Barrett's oesophagus. Gut 1991;32:1441–1446.
91. Reid BJ, Weinstein WM, Lewin K, et al. Endoscopic biopsy can detect high-grade dysplasia or early adenocarcinoma in Barrett's esophagus without grossly recognizable lesions. Gastroenterology 1988;94:81–90.
92. Levine DS, Haggitt RC, Blount PL, Rabinovitch PS, Rusch VW, Reid BJ. An endoscopic biopsy protocol can differentiate high-grade dysplasia from early adenocarcinoma in Barrett's esophagus. Gastroenterology 1993;105:40–50.
93. McArdle JE, Lewin KJ, Randall G, Weinstein W. Distribution of dysplasias and early invasive carcinoma in Barrett's esophagus. Hum Pathol 1992;23:479–482.
94. Ming SC. Tumors of the esophagus and stomach, second series. Washington, DC: Armed Forces Institute of Pathology, 1973:23–43.
95. Liu FS, Zhou CN. Pathology of carcinoma of the esophagus. In: Huang GJ, Wu YK, eds. Carcinoma of the esophagus and gastric cardia. Berlin: Springer-Verlag, 1984:89–116.
96. Wu YK, Huang GJ. Surgical treatment. In: Huang GJ, Wu YK, eds. Carcinoma of the esophagus and gastric cardia. Berlin: Springer-Verlag, 1984:276–284.
97. Yoshinaka H, Shimazu H, Fukumoto T, Baba M. Superficial esophageal carcinoma: a clinicopathological review of 59 cases. Am J Gastroenterol 1991;86:1413–1418.
98. Kitamura K, Ikebe M, Morita M, Matsuda H, Kuwano H, Sugimachi K. The evaluation of submucosal carcinoma of the esophagus as a more advanced carcinoma. Hepatogastroenterology 1993;40:236–239.
99. Liu FS, Wang QL. Squamous cell carcinoma of the esophagus. In: Ming SC, Goldman H, eds. Pathology of the gastrointestinal Tract. Philadelphia: WB Saunders, 1992:439–458.
100. Agha FP, Weatherbee L, Sams JS. Verrucous carcinoma of the esophagus. Am J Gastroenterol 1984;79:844–849.
101. Meyerowitz BR, Shea LT. The natural history of squamous verrucose carcinoma of the esophagus. J Thorac Cardiovasc Surg 1971;61:646–649.
102. Biemond P, ten Kate FJ, van Blankenstein M. Esophageal verrucous carcinoma: histologically a low-grade malignancy but clinically a fatal disease. J Clin Gastroenterol 1991;13:102–107.
103. Tauchi K, Kakudo K, Machimura T, Makuuchi H, Mitomi T. Superficial esophageal carcinoma. With special reference to basaloid features. Pathol Res Pract 1990;186:450–454.
104. Tsang WY, Chan JK, Lee KC, Leung AK, Fu YT. Basaloid-squamous carcinoma of the upper aerodigestive tract and so-called adenoid cystic carcinoma of the oesophagus: the same tumour type? Histopathology 1991;19:35–46.
105. Battifora H. Spindle cell carcinoma. Cancer 1976;37:2275–2282.
106. Gal AA, Martin SE, Kernen JA, Patterson MJ. Spindle cell carcinoma of the esophagus. An immunohistochemical study. Cancer 1987;60:2244–2250.
107. Hanada M, Nakano K, Ii Y, Yamashita H. Carcinosarcoma of the esophagus with osseous and cartilaginous production. A combined study of keratin immunohistochemistry and electron microscopy. Acta Pathol Jpn 1984;34:669–678.
108. Ooi A, Kawahara E, Okada Y, et al. Carcinosarcoma of the esophagus. An immunohistochemical and electron microscopic study. Acta Pathol Jpn 1986;36:151–159, 1986.
109. Dworak O, Koerfgen HP. Carcinosarcoma in Barrett's oesophagus: a case report with immunohistological examination. Virchows Arch A Pathol Anat Histopathol 1993;422:423–426.
110. Iyomasa S, Kato H, Tachimori Y, Watanabe H, Yamaguchi H, Itabashi M. Carcinosarcoma of the esophagus: a twenty-case study. Jpn J Clin Oncol 1990;20:99–106.
111. Levine MS, Caroline D, Thompson JJ, Kressel HY, Laufer I, Herlinger H. Adenocarcinoma of the esophagus: relationship to Barrett mucosa. Radiology 1984;150:305–309.
112. Haggitt RC, Tryzelaar J, Ellis FH, Colcher H. Adenocarcinoma complicating columnar epithelium lined (Barrett's) esophagus. Am J Clin Pathol 1978;70:1–5.
113. Moghissi K, Papiri N. A clinico-pathological study of the origin of adenocarcinoma of the mid-thoracic oesophagus and results of surgical resection. Chirugie 1992;118:298–303.
114. Christensen WN, Sternberg SS. Adenocarcinoma of the upper esophagus arising in ectopic gastric mucosa. Two case reports and review of the literature. Am J Surg Pathol 1987;11:397–402.
115. Ishii K, Ota H, Nakayama J, et al. Adenocarcinoma of the cervical oesophagus arising from ectopic gastric mucosa. The histochemical determination of its origin. Virchows Arch A Pathol Anat Histopathol 1991;419:159–164.
116. Levine MS, Dillon EC, Saul SH, Laufer I. Early esophageal cancer. AJR Am J Roentgenol 1986;146:507–512.
117. Witt TR, Bains MS, Zaman MB. Adenocarcinoma in Barrett's esophagus. J Thorac Cardiovasc Surg 1983;85:337–34.
118. Chejfec G, Jablokow VR, Gould VE. Linitis plastica carcinoma of the esophagus. Cancer 1983;51:2139–3143.
119. Ming SC, Bullough PG. Coexisting adenocarcinomas of the esophagus and of the esophagogastric junction. Am J Dig Dis 1963;8:439–443.
120. Sarbia M, Borchard F, Hengels KJ. Histogenetical investigations on adenocarcinomas of the esophagogastric junction. An immunohistochemical study. Pathol Res Pract 1993;189:530–535.
121. Banner BF, Memoli VA, Warren WH, Gould VE. Carcinoma with multidirectional differentiation arising in Barrett's esophagus. Ultrastruct Pathol 1983;4:205–217.
122. Resano CH, Cabrera N, Gonzalez-Cueto D, Sanchez-Basse AE, Rubio HH. Double early epidermoid carcinoma of the esophagus in columnar epithelium. Endoscopy 1985;17:73–75.
123. Cary NR, Barron DJ, McGoldrick JP, Wells FC. Combined oesophageal adenocarcinoma and carcinoid in Barrett's oesophagitis: potential role of enterochromaffin-like cells in oesophageal malignancy. Thorax 1993;48:404–405.

124. Pascal RR, Clearfield HR. Mucoepidermoid (adenosquamous) carcinoma arising in Barrett's esophagus. Dig Dis Sci 1987; 32:428–432.
125. Kuwano H, Ueo H, Sugimachi K, Inokuchi K, Toyoshima S, Enjoji M. Glandular or mucus secreting components in squamous cell carcinoma of the esophagus. Cancer 1985;56:514–518.
126. Orsatti G, Corvalan AH, Sakurai H, Choi HS. Polypoid adenosquamous carcinoma of the esophagus with prominent spindle cells. Report of a case with immunohistochemical and ultrastructural studies. Arch Pathol Lab Med 1993;117: 544–547.
127. Potet F, Flejou JF, Gervaz H, Paraf F. Adenocarcinoma of the lower esophagus and the esophagogastric junction. Semin Diagn Pathol 1991;8:126–136.
128. Webb JN, Busuttil A. Adenocarcinoma of the esophagus and of the esophagogastric junction. Br J Surg 1978;65:475–479.
129. Ming SC. Tumors of the esophagus and stomach. 2nd series. Washington, DC: Armed Forces Institute of Pathology, 1973: 44–57.
130. Wang HH, Antoniolli DA, Goldman H. Comparative features of esophageal and gastric adenocarcinoma: recent changes in type and frequency. Hum Pathol 1986;17:482–487.
131. Duhaylongsod FG, Wolfe WG. Barrett's esophagus and adenocarcinoma of the esophagus and gastroesophageal junction. J Thorac Cardiovas Surg 1991;102:36–41.
132. Bell-Thomson J, Haggitt RC, Ellis FH Jr. Mucoepidermoid and adenoid cystic carcinomas of the esophagus. J Thorac Cardiovasc Surg 1979;79:438–446.
133. Woodard BH, Shelburne JD, Vollmer RT, Postlethwait RW. Mucoepidermoid carcinoma of the esophagus: a case report. Hum Pathol 1979;9:352–354.
134. Fegelman E, Law SY, Fok M, Lam KY, Loke SL, Ma LT, Wong J. Squamous cell carcinoma of the esophagus with mucin-secreting component. Mucoepidermoid carcinoma. J Thorac Cardiovasc Surg 1994;107:62–67.
135. Kuwano H, Sugimachi K, Morita M, et al. A consideration of the definition of early esophageal cancer on the basis of clinicopathologic viewpoint (Japanese). J Jpn Surg Soc 1991;92:276–280.
136. Sasajima K, Watanabe M, Takubo K, Takai A, Yamashita K, Onda M. Mucoepidermoid carcinoma of the esophagus: report of two cases and review of the literature. Endoscopy 1990;22: 140–143.
137. Cerar A, Jutersek A, Vidmar S. Adenoid cystic carcinoma of the esophagus. A clinicopathologic study of three cases. Cancer 1991;67:2159–2164.
138. Trillo A, Accettullo LM, Yeiter TL. Choriocarcinoma of the esophagus: histologic and cytologic findings. A case report. Acta Cytol 1979;23:69–74.
139. McKechnie JC, Fechner RE. Choriocarcinoma and adenocarcinoma of the esophagus with gonadotropin secretion. Cancer 1971;27:694–702.
140. Sasano N, Abe S, Satake O. Choriocarcinoma mimicry of an esophageal carcinoma with urinary gonadotropic activities. Tohoku J Exp Med 1970;100:153.
141. Wasan HS, Schofield JB, Krausz T, Sikora K, Waxman J. Combined choriocarcinoma and yolk sac tumor arising in Barrett's esophagus. Cancer 1994;73:514–517.
142. Kikuchi Y, Tsuneta Y, Kawai T, Aizawa M. Choriocarcinoma of the esophagus producing chorionic gonadotropin. Acta Pathol Jpn 1988;38:489–499.
143. Nonomura A, Kimura A, Mizukami Y, Matsubara F, Yagi M. Paget's disease of the esophagus. J Clin Gastroenterol 1993;16: 130–135.
144. Norihisa Y, Kakudo K, Tsutsumi Y, Makuuchi H, Sugihara T, Mitomi T. Paget's extension of esophageal carcinoma. Immunohistochemical and mucin histochemical evidence of Paget's cells in the esophageal mucosa. Acta Pathol Jpn 1988;38:651–658.
145. Yates DR, Koss LG. Paget's disease of the esophageal epithelium. Report of first case. Arch Pathol 1968;86:447–452.
146. Chong FK, Graham JH, Madoff IM. Mucin-producing carcinoid ("composite tumor") of upper third of esophagus: a variant of carcinoid tumor. Cancer 1979;44:1853–1859.
147. Tateishi R, Taniguchi K, Horai T, Iwanaga T, Taniguchi H. Argyrophil cell carcinoma (apudoma) of the esophagus. A histopathologic entity. Virchows Arch A Pathol Anat Histopathol 1976;371:283–294.
148. Mori M, Matsukuma A, Adachi Y, et al. Small cell carcinoma of the esophagus. Cancer 1989;63:564–573.
149. Liu YH. Clinicopathologic and immunohistochemical study on 22 cases of small cell carcinoma of the esophagus (Chinese). Chin Oncol J 1991;13:123–125.
150. Imura H, Matsukura S, Yamamoto H, et al. Studies on ectopic ACTH producing tumors. II. Clinical and biochemical features of 30 cases. Cancer 1975;35:1430–1437.
151. Proctor DD, Fraser JL, Mangano MM, Calkins DR, Rosenberg SJ. Small cell carcinoma of the esophagus in a patient with longstanding primary achalasia. Am J Gastroenterol 1992; 87:664–667.
152. Douherty MA, McIntyre M, Arnott SJ. Oat cell carcinoma of esophagus: a report of six British patients with a review of the literature. Int J Radiat Oncol Biol Phys 1984;10:147–152.
153. Nichols GL, Kelsen DP. Small cell carcinoma of the esophagus. The Memorial Hospital experience 1970 to 1987. Cancer 1989;64:1531–1533.
154. Law SY, Fok M, Lam KY, Loke SL, Ma LT, Wong J. Small cell carcinoma of the esophagus. Cancer 1994;73:2894–2899.
155. Rosenthal SN, Lemkin JA. Multiple small cell carcinomas of the esophagus. Cancer 1983;51:1944–1946.
156. Chalkiadakis G, Wihlm JM, Morand G, Weill-Bousson M, Witz JP. Primary malignant melanoma of the esophagus. Ann Thorac Surg 1985;39:472–475.
157. Sabanathan S, Eng J. Primary malignant melanoma of the esophagus. Scand J Thorac Cardiovasc Surg 1990;24:83–85.
158. Taniyama K, Suzuki H, Sakuramachi S, Toyoda T, Matsuda M, Tahara E. Amelanotic malignant melanoma of the esophagus: case report and review of the literature. Jpn J Clin Oncol 20:286–295, 1990.
159. Sabanathan S, Eng J, Pradhan GN. Primary malignant melanoma of the esophagus. Am J Gastroenterol 84:1475–1481, 1989.
160. Sapi Z, Papp I, Bodo M. Malignant fibrous histiocytoma of the esophagus. Report of a case with cytologic, immunohistologic and ultrastructural studies. Acta Cytol 36:121–125, 1992.
161. Yates SP, Collins MC. Case report: recurrent liposarcoma of the oesophagus. Clin Radiol 1990;42:356–358.
162. Bloch MJ, Iozzo RV, Edmunds LH Jr, Brooks JJ. Polypoid synovial sarcoma of the esophagus. Gastroenterology 1987;92: 229–233.
163. Perch SJ, Soffen EM, Whittington R, Brooks JJ. Esophageal sarcomas. J Surg Oncol 1991;48:194–198.
164. Goodner JT, Miller TR, Watson WL. Sarcoma of the esophagus. AJR Am J Roentgenol 1963;89:132–139.
165. Rainer WG, Brus R. Leiomyosarcoma of the esophagus: review of the literature and report of 3 cases. Surgery 1965;58: 343–350.

166. Chiba W, Konishi T, Sawai S, Hatakenaka R, Matsubara Y, Ikeda S. A resected case of leiomyosarcoma of the esophagus—the diagnosis was supported with DNA content analysis (Japanese). J Jpn Assoc Thorac Surg 1993;41:140–144.
167. Wen J. Biological behavior of smooth muscle tumors of the alimentary tract—a pathological analysis of 501 cases (Chinese). Chin Oncol J 1991;13:217–219.
168. Chetty R, Learmonth GM, Price SK, Taylor DA. Primary oesophageal rhabdomyosarcoma. Cytopathology 1991;2:103–108.
169. Ende N, Pizzolato P, Raider L, Ziskind J. An unusual case of carcinosarcoma of the esophagus. AJR Am J Roentgenol 1951;65:227–231.
170. Bonacini M, Young T, Laine L. Histopathology of human immunodeficiency virus-associated esophageal disease. Am J Gastroenterol 1993;88:549–51.
171. Laine L, Amerian J, Rarick M, Harb M, Gill PS. The response of symptomatic gastrointestinal Kaposi's sarcoma to chemotherapy: a prospective evaluation using an endoscopic method of disease quantification. Am J Gastroenterol 1990;85:959–961.
172. Siegel JH, Janis R, Alper JC, Schutte H, Robbins L, Blaufox MD. Disseminated visceral Kaposi's sarcoma. Appearance after human renal homograft operation. JAMA 1969;207:1493–1496.
173. Ennuyer A, Bataini P, Helary J. Hodgkin's disease of the upper respiratory and digestive tracts. Possible portal of entry of the causal agent of malignant lymphogranuloma. Ann Radiol 1961;4:145–165.
174. Tsukada T, Ohno T, Kihira H, et al. Primary esophageal non-Hodgkin's lymphoma. Intern Med 1992;31:569–572.
175. Bolondi L, De Giorgio R, Santi V, et al. Primary non-Hodgkin's T-cell lymphoma of the esophagus. A case with peculiar endoscopic ultrasonographic pattern. Dig Dis Sci 1990;35:1426–1430.
176. Mengoli M, Marchi M, Rota E, Bertolotti M, Collini C, Signorelli S. Primary non-Hodgkin's lymphoma of the esophagus. Am J Gastroenterol 1990;85:737–741.
177. Cappell MS, Botros N. Predominantly gastrointestinal symptoms and signs in 11 consecutive AIDS patients with gastrointestinal lymphoma: a multicenter, multiyear study including 763 HIV-seropositive patients. Am J Gastroenterol 1994;89:545–549.
178. Abrams HL, Spiro R, Goldstein N. Metastases in carcinoma. Analysis of 1000 autopsied cases. Cancer 1950;3:74–85.
179. Antler AS, Ough, Y, Pitchumoni CS, Donaldson M, Thelmo W. Gastrointestinal metastases from malignant tumors of the lungs. Cancer 1982;49:170–172.
180. Anderson MF, Harell GS. Secondary esophageal tumors. AJR Am J Roentgenol 1980;135:1243–1246.
181. Holyokw ED, Nemoto T, Dao TL. Esophageal metastases and dysphagia in patients with carcinoma of the breast. J Surg Oncol 1979;1:97–107.
182. Caputy GG, Donohue JH, Goellner JR, Weaver AL. Metastatic melanoma of the gastrointestinal tract. Results of surgical management. Arch Surg 1991;126:1353–1358.
183. Oka T, Ayabe H, Kawahara K, et al. Esophagectomy for metastatic carcinoma of the esophagus from lung cancer. Cancer 1993;71:2958–2961.
184. Nagamatsu M, Mori M, Kuwano H, Sugimachi K, Akiyoshi T. Serial histologic investigation of squamous epithelial dysplasia associated with carcinoma of the esophagus. Cancer 1992;69:1094–1098.
185. Kuwano H, Morita M, Matsuda H, Mori M, Sugimachi K. Histopathologic findings of minute foci of squamous cell carcinoma in the human esophagus. Cancer 1991;68:2617–2620.
186. Moertel CG, Dockerty MB, Baggenstoss AH. Multiple primary malignant neoplasms. III. Tumors of multicentric origin. Cancer 1961;14:238–248.
187. Maeta M, Kondo A, Shibata S, Yamashiro H, Murakami A, Kaibara N. Esophageal cancer associated with multiple cancerous lesions: clinicopathologic comparisons between multiple primary and intramural metastatic lesions. Gastroenterol Jpn 1993;28:187–192.
188. Ming SC. Tumors of the esophagus and stomach. 2nd series. Washington, DC: Armed Forces Institute of Pathology, 1973:75–76.
189. Soga J, Tanaka O, Sasaki K, Kawaguchi M, Muto T. Superficial spreading type carcinoma of the esophagus. Cancer 1980;50:1641–1645.
190. Kato H, Tachimori Y, Watanabe H, et al. Intramural metastasis of thoracic esophageal carcinoma. Int J Cancer 1992;50:49–52.
191. Takubo K, Sasajima K, Yamashita K, Tanaka Y, Fujita K. Prognostic significance of intramural metastasis in patients with esophageal carcinoma. Cancer 1990;65:1816–1819.
192. Ming SC. Tumors of the esophagus and stomach, second series. Washington, DC: Armed Forces Institute of Pathology, 1973:54–58.
193. Gschossmann JM, Bonner JA, Foote RL, Shaw EG, Martenson JA Jr, Su J. Malignant tracheoesophageal fistula in patients with esophageal cancer. Cancer 1993;72:1513–1521.
194. Burt M, Diehl W, Martini N, et al. Malignant esophagorespiratory fistula: management options and survival. Ann Thorac Surg 1991;52:1222–1228.
195. van Overhagen H, Lameris JS, Berger MY, et al. Supraclavicular lymph node metastases in carcinoma of the esophagus and gastroesophageal junction: assessment with CT, US, and US-guided fine-needle aspiration biopsy. Radiology 1991;179:155–158.
196. Aikou T, Shimazu H, Takao T, Baba M, Natsugoe S, Simada M. Significance of lymph nodal metastases in treatment of esophagogastric adenocarcinoma. Lymphology 1992;25:31–36.
197. Theunissen PH, Borchard F, Poortvliet DC. Histopathological evaluation of oesophageal carcinoma: the significance of venous invasion. Br J Surg 1991;78:930–932.
198. Huang GJ, Zhang DW, Wang GQ, et al. Surgical treatment of carcinoma of the esophagus. Report of 1647 cases. Chin Med J 1981;94:305–307.
199. Beahrs OH, Henson DE, Hutter RVP, Kennedy BJ. Manual for staging of cancer. 4th ed. Philadelphia: JB Lippincott, 92:57–61.
200. Skinner DB, Skinner KA. Neoplasms of the esophagus. In: Holland JF, Frei E III, Bast RC Jr, Kufe DW, Morton DL, Weichselbaum RR, eds. Cancer medicine. 3rd ed. Philadelphia: Lea & Febiger, 1993:1382–1394.
201. Muller JM, Erasmi H, Stelzner M, Zieren U, Pichlmaier H. Surgical therapy of oesophageal carcinoma. Br J Surg 1990;77:845–857.
202. Oliver SE, Robertson CS, Logan RF. Oesophageal cancer: a population-based study of survival after treatment. Br J Surg 1992;79:1321–1325.
203. Abe S, Tachibana M, Shiraishi M, Nakamura T. Lymph node metastasis in resectable esophageal cancer. J Thorac Cardiovasc Surg 1990;100:287–291.
204. Yu JM, Yang LH, Guo-Qian, et al. Flow cytometric analysis DNA content in esophageal carcinoma. Correlation with histologic and clinical features. Cancer 1989;64:80–82.
205. Walsh TN, Dorman T, Droogan O, et al. DNA ploidy in squamous oesophageal carcinoma. Surg Oncol 1992;1:37–42.

206. Schneeberger AL, Finley RJ, Troster M, et al. The prognostic significance of tumor ploidy and pathology in adenocarcinoma of the esophagogastric junction. Cancer 1990;65:1206–1210.
207. Patil P, Redkar A, Patel SG, Krishnamurthy S, Mistry RC, Deshpande RK, Mittra I, et al. Prognosis of operable squamous cell carcinoma of the esophagus. Relationship with clinicopathologic features and DNA ploidy. Cancer 1993;72:20–24.
208. Adachi Y, Kitamura K, Tsutsui S, Ikeda Y, Matsuda H, Sugimachi K. How to detect early carcinoma of the esophagus. Hepatogastroenterology 1993;40:207–211.
209. Nabeya K, Hanaoka T, Onozawa K, Ri S, Nyumura T, Kaku C. Early diagnosis of esophageal cancer. Hepatogastroenterology 1990;37:368–370.
210. van Overhagen H, Lameris JS, Berger MY, et al. Assessment of distant metastases with ultrasound-guided fine-needle aspiration biopsy and cytologic study in carcinoma of the esophagus and gastroesophageal junction. Gastrointest Radiol 1992;17:305–310.
211. Siewert JR, Holscher AH. Current strategy in surgery for esophageal cancer. Ann Ital Chir 1992;63:13–18.
212. Darnton SJ, Antonakopoulos GN, Newman J, Matthews HR. Effects of chemotherapy on ultrastructure of oesophageal adenocarcinoma. J Clin Pathol 1992;45:979–983.

26

Esophageal Carcinoma: Diagnosis, Evaluation, and Staging

Mark J. Krasna and Rebecca S. Wolfer

Esophageal carcinoma is a relatively uncommon disease in the Western world, but it carries a grim prognosis. In the United States, carcinoma of the esophagus represents approximately 10% of all cancers of the gastrointestinal tract, yet it causes disproportionately more cancer deaths (1). These lesions remain silent during much of their development and rarely present until the later stages of disease and, thus, are associated with a high morbidity and mortality. At the time of initial diagnosis, approximately 95% of patients with malignant lesions of the esophagus present with advanced stage disease. At least 75% have either locoregional tumor invasion or distant metastasis that precludes surgical cure (2).

HISTORICAL PERSPECTIVES

The earliest surgical procedures of the esophagus were limited to the cervical portion, primarily for the removal of foreign bodies. Safe operative procedures on the thoracic portion of the esophagus were very limited until the development of safer anesthetic techniques that permitted opening the thoracic cavity. Resection of the cervical esophagus for carcinoma was first performed successfully by Billroth in 1871 and Czerny in 1877 (3). Mikulitz (4) performed the first resection with reconstruction in 1886. The history of esophageal resection for carcinoma is limited to the 20th century, however. Torek (5) performed the first successful resection of an intrathoracic esophageal carcinoma in 1915. Ohsawa (6) reported the first successful transthoracic esophagectomy with gastroesophageal anastomosis in 1933. This procedure was first accomplished in the United States by Marshall in 1937 and Adams and Phemister in 1938 (7, 8). In the 1940s Sweet (9) and Garlock (10) developed a number of techniques and basic principles that are still used in esophageal surgery today.

ANATOMY

The esophagus is a muscular tube that extends from the cricopharyngeus muscle to the stomach, averages 25 cm (10 inches) in length, and functions as a conduit from the oral cavity to the stomach. It actively transports ingested foodstuffs to the remainder of the digestive system. The esophagus can be divided arbitrarily into four segments: cervical, extending from the pharyngoesophageal junction (the inferior border of the cricoid cartilage) to the suprasternal notch (between 10 and 18 cm from the incisors); upper thoracic, from the suprasternal notch to the bifurcation of the trachea (18 to 24 cm from the incisors); middle thoracic, from the tracheal bifurcation midway to the esophagogastric junction, (between 24 and 34 cm from the incisors); and lower thoracic, from that midpoint to the gastroesophageal junction (from 34 to 44 cm from the incisors). Most thoracic surgeons simply divide the esophagus into three parts according to the relevant surgical approaches: upper (cervical to the thoracic inlet), middle (20 to 34 cm), and lower (distal esophagus and esophageal junction) esophagus (11).

The normal esophagus in the adult is approximately 2.5 cm in diameter. The diameter is not uniform and is characterized by three areas of narrowing. The level of the cricopharyngeus muscle is the narrowest portion of the gastrointestinal tract in the adult, measuring approximately 14 mm in diameter. Two other areas of constriction are at the level at which the esophagus is crossed by the left main stem bronchus and at the esophagogastric junction. These strictures are clinically significant in the study of the esophagus by endoscopic and contrast radiographic techniques (12).

Although the cervical esophagus is midline, it tends to course to the left and posteriorly to the trachea and therefore is more approached easily through a left cervical incision. The thoracic portion of the esophagus lies in the posterior mediastinum and curves toward the left as it passes behind the left main stem bronchus. It deviates slightly to the right in the subcarinal region before passing to the left of the midline and anteriorly to the aorta, passing behind the pericardium. The esophagus enters the abdomen through the esophageal diaphragmatic hiatus, a sling of muscle fibers that arise in approximately 45% of individuals from the right crus at the level of the eleventh thoracic vertebrae.

The esophagus receives its blood supply from the superior and inferior thyroidal arteries in the cervical portion. The major blood supply of the intrathoracic portion is from four to six branches of the aorta. These vessels terminate in fine capillary networks before penetrating the esophageal muscular layer. After penetrating the muscularis propria, the esophageal capillary network courses longitudinally in the submucosa. The distal esophagus and gastroesophageal junction are supplied by the five gastric vascular collaterals. The extensive venous drainage is via the hypopharyngeal, azygos, hemiazygos, and gastric veins.

Histologically, the esophagus is composed of mucosa, submucosa, and muscularis (composed of an inner circular layer and an outer longitudinal layer). It is surrounded by adventitia or mediastinal connective tissue (a layer of loose areolar tissue). Between the two muscular layers is a layer of thin connective tissue that contains blood vessels and ganglion cells of the Meissner's and Auerbach's plexuses.

In the proximal third of the esophagus, the muscularis propria is striated muscle primarily, whereas in the distal two thirds, it is composed primarily of smooth muscle. The mucosal lining is primarily a squamous epithelium, except for the distal 1 to 2 cm, which is primarily columnar epithelium. The submucosa contains an extensive network of lymphatic channels. The esophagus is therefore peculiar in its lack of a serosa.

The esophagus has a rather extensive lymphatic drainage of two lymphatic plexuses, one arising in the mucosa and the other in the muscularis. The mucosal lymphatics may pierce the muscular layer and drain into regional nodes or alternatively may course longitudinally in the esophageal wall before exiting. In general, the flow of lymph in the upper two thirds of the esophagus tends to be upward, whereas the lower third preferentially drains downward.

This lymphatic drainage is not consistent, however, because tumors in the upper third of the esophagus often metastasize to abdominal lymph node groups. Additionally, tumor involvement of lymph nodes may cause obstruction of lymph channels, thus reversing the flow from the usual drainage. Esophageal carcinomas may therefore metastasize to internal jugular, paratracheal, subcarinal, periesophageal, inferior pulmonary ligament, perigastric, and left gastric artery (celiac) lymph nodes. The relatively thick submucosal layer permits considerable mobility of the overlying mucosa. One unique feature of the esophagus is that unlike most of the gastrointestinal tract, it (like the rectum) totally lacks a serosal layer. Perhaps because of this unique histologic feature, early lymphatic spread of esophageal carcinoma is the rule rather than the exception (13) (Fig. 26.1).

EPIDEMIOLOGY

Esophageal carcinoma remains one of the most dismal of all malignancies. In the United States, as in most Western countries, the incidence of this malignancy is low (approximately 3 to 10 cases per 100,000 per year) (1). This incidence tends to be slightly higher in the black population, compared with whites. The increasing incidence of esophageal cancer attests to its being one of the fastest growing tumor groups in the United States (14). The incidence is lower in females, occurring 2 to 5 times more frequently in males. The exception is the incidence of carcinoma of the hypopharynx and cervical esophagus, which occurs with nearly equal frequency in males and females, primarily because of the greater incidence of Plummer-Vinson syndrome in women. Esophageal cancer presents most commonly in the sixth to seventh decades of life. The etiology of esophageal carcinoma remains to be elucidated. Several factors have been associated with the development of esophageal carcinoma, including alcohol consumption in combination with tobacco use, ingestion of nitrosamines, and contamination of foodstuffs with mold and fungus.

In some parts of the world, such as regions in China, the incidence of esophageal carcinoma reaches near epidemic proportions, making it a leading cause of death. When such a variation in incidence and mortality exists with a disease, similarities and differences in geographic, sociologic, nutritional, and other predisposing factors become increasingly evident. An Asian esophageal cancer belt exists and includes Japan, China, southern areas of Russia, Iran, Pakistan, India, the Middle East, and Singapore. The relatively high incidence of this malignancy in these areas has allowed for extensive review of predisposing factors and possible etiologies of this disease (15). Epidemiologic studies in China have suggested that the extraordinarily high incidence of esophageal carcinoma seen there may be related to the presence of large quantities of ni-

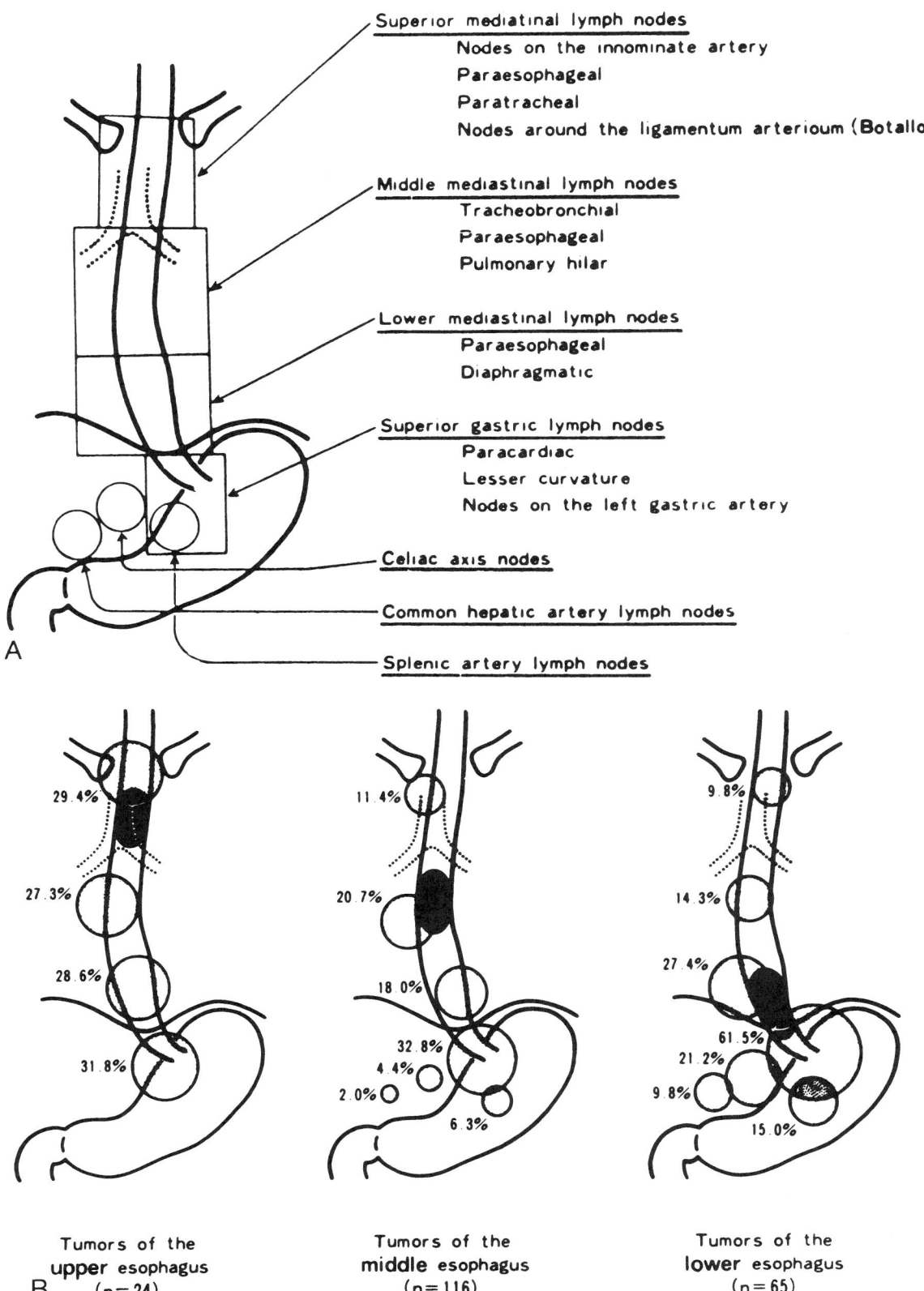

FIGURE 26.1. Lymphatic drainage of the esophagus. A. Involvement of lymph node groups in cancer of the esophagus. B. Involvement of lymph nodes in squamous carcinoma of the esophagus according to location of primary.

trosamines in the soil and contamination of foodstuffs by fungi such as *Geotrichum candidum* and other yeasts. In areas of Iran, ingestion of very hot tea, leading to mucosal injuries by burning, may contribute to the high incidence of this malignancy. In other areas esophageal carcinoma has been linked to the practice of chewing tobacco in combination with ingestion of the betel nut leaf. In the Zulu population, the incidence of esophageal carcinoma has been linked to contamination of food by molds of the *Fusarium* species.

Numerous esophageal lesions have been determined to be premalignant, thus predisposing to esophageal cancer. Achalasia, a disease of disordered esophageal motility and failure of lower esophageal sphincter relaxation, has been associated with a higher incidence of esophageal carcinoma; carcinoma arises in approximately 1% to 10% of individuals who have had symptomatic disease for an average of 15 to 25 years. It has been demonstrated that mucosal irritation as a result of esophagitis is proportional to the duration of disease. This type of tumor most often presents as a squamous cell carcinoma (16). The tumor tends to be located in the middle esophagus in the majority of patients. It also presents in younger individuals than usual. Because it is usually large by the time a diagnosis is made, this tumor carries a poor prognosis and is rarely resectable.

Adenocarcinomas developing in heterotopic gastric epithelium have been reported with increasing frequency. Barrett's esophagus is associated with a 10-fold increase in occurrence. Several studies have indicated that the presence of columnar epithelium in the esophagus is associated with a significant increase in the development of adenocarcinoma of the esophagus (17). Finally, tylosis has been reported to be associated with a 35% incidence of esophageal cancer and is transmitted as an autosomal dominant gene (18).

Radiation esophagitis has been associated with an increased incidence of esophageal carcinoma. A long latent period between exposure and development of carcinoma in the irradiated area is reported (19). There is additional evidence that chemotherapy may have a synergistic effect in the development of esophageal carcinoma in this setting.

Carcinoma of the esophagus has been demonstrated to develop in all forms of esophageal diverticulae, including those of the pharyngeal esophageal junction (Zenker's diverticulum), mid esophageal diverticulae, and epiphrenic locations. These may be related to the development of chronic inflammation because of local stasis. Additional factors that have been associated with an increased incidence of esophageal carcinoma are the Plummer-Vinson syndrome and previous gastric surgery. Nutritional factors that have been implicated in the development of esophageal carcinoma include alcohol, tobacco, zinc deficiency, nitrosamines, malnutrition, dental caries, and ingestion of hot foods and liquids (20) (Table 26.1).

PATHOLOGY

The detailed pathology of esophageal cancer is reviewed in Chapter 25. Esophageal cancer accounts for 2% of all cancers in humans and approximately 7% of all gastrointestinal malignancies. Histologically, the majority of esophageal malignancies are squamous cell carcinomas. Like other squamous cell carcinomas, those of the esophagus arise as an apparent carcinoma in situ. Approximately 50% of these lesions are located in the middle third of the thoracic esophagus, approximately 30% in the distal portion of the esophagus, and the remaining 20% in the proximal third. There are several morphologic variants of early esophageal carcinoma. The most common type in the United States (60%) is a polypoid fungating lesion that protrudes into the lumen of the esophagus. The second most common variant (25%) is a necrotic ulceration that deeply excavates into surrounding tissues. Finally, there is a diffuse infiltrative form that tends to spread within the walls of the esophagus, resulting in a thickened, rigid, narrow lumen, similar to the linitis plastica seen in gastric cancer. These lesions are either poorly or well-differentiated squamous cell carcinoma and may take as long as 4 to 5 years to progress to invasive carcinomas (21).

Approximately 5% to 8% of all primary esophageal carcinomas are adenocarcinomas. These occur most

TABLE 26.1. Factors Associated with Higher than Usual Incidence of Esophageal Carcinoma

Factors associated wtih premalignant lesions
   Barrett's esophagus
   Achalasia
   Plummer-Vinson syndrome
   Diverticulae (?)
   Radiation/chemotherapy (synergistic?)
Geographic/nutritional factors
   Hot tea (Iran)
   Alcohol
   Tobacco
   Zinc deficiency
   Nitrosamines (China)
   Dental caries
   Malnutrition
   Fusarium molds (Zulu)
   Betel nut leaf (Bantu)

frequently in the distal third of the thoracic esophagus, with a male to female ratio of 3:1. This predominance has been associated with one of three predisposing factors: malignant degeneration of Barrett's esophagus, heterotopic islands of columnar mucosa, or esophageal submucosal glands giving rise to adenocarcinoma. Patients with Barrett's esophagus have a 40-fold greater chance of developing adenocarcinoma of the esophagus. Approximately 10% to 15% of all patients with Barrett's esophagus will develop adenocarcinoma. Like its gastric counterpart, adenocarcinoma of the esophagus spreads early to lymphatics and invades local tissues (22).

There are several rare tumors that may present as primary esophageal tumors, including small cell (oat cell) tumors that arise from argyrophilic cells, adenoid cystic tumors, malignant melanomas, and carcinosarcomas. Carcinosarcoma is a tumor with elements of both epithelial cells (squamous carcinomas) and malignant spindle cells (sarcomas) (23).

NATURAL HISTORY

Unfortunately, in the United States only a minority of these lesions are diagnosed at an early stage. Esophageal carcinoma has a reputation for aggressive biologic behavior, resulting in widespread lymphatic involvement, local infiltration, and metastatic hematogenous spread. Tumors in the middle and upper third may extend to invade the aorta, tracheobronchial tree, and left recurrent laryngeal nerve. Lower third lesions have been described to invade the diaphragm, pericardium, and stomach. Local invasion of periesophageal tissues has been described in 70% of all individuals at the time of diagnosis (24).

Up to 75% of all patients diagnosed with esophageal carcinoma have evidence of lymph node involvement at the time of diagnosis. The most commonly involved nodal groups include the mediastinal, supraclavicular, and celiac. Cervical lesions may drain into the deep cervical plexus, paraesophageal nodes, or tracheobronchial nodes. Lower lesions metastasize to the paraesophageal, celiac, and splenic nodal groups (2).

Distant hematogenous spread to the liver and lungs has been demonstrated in approximately 90% of autopsied cases.

CLINICAL PRESENTATION

Esophageal carcinoma often presents insidiously with early carcinomas recognized infrequently. Initially, symptoms include retrosternal discomfort or indigestion. These symptoms together with friction or burning with the passage of food may occur in as many as 90% of patients. These symptoms may be intermittent and may be present for years. As the lesion enlarges, the symptoms may progress to intermittent odynophagia. Many patients note that their pain when swallowing is worse if they swallow large boluses of air or liquid. They often complain that the food gets stuck, and they can point to an area of the chest that correlates generally with the distribution of the esophageal cancer. These symptoms eventually progress, and weight loss, dysphagia, and chest pain predominate. Unfortunately, many patients ignore these symptoms for months and even years until either weight loss is massive or their swallowing becomes so difficult that it precludes even the ingestion of liquids. Significant dysphagia occurs only when approximately two thirds of the esophageal lumen is obstructed. Progressing from intermittent to persistent dysphagia and from solids to soft foods, patients at presentation often are dysphagic 100% of the time to all types of foods.

Patients may present rarely with evidence of an upper gastrointestinal bleed, including hematemesis, hemoptysis, or even melena. Recently, a patient at the University of Maryland Medical Center presented with recurrent episodes of esophageal varices, which proved to be an early-stage esophageal carcinoma with mucosal ulceration. When the tumor has progressed significantly, vomiting and regurgitation associated with aspiration, cough, and even pneumonia can occur. Unfortunately, by the time patients present with these symptoms, the lesion usually is advanced with a high incidence of local invasion and distant metastatic disease. Once the tumor becomes invasive, symptoms usually are reflective of the invaded organs. These signs include hoarseness in patients with invasion of the trachea or recurrent laryngeal nerve, and difficulty swallowing or regurgitation with invasion of the vagus nerve. Evidence of wheezing, hemoptysis, or actual airway obstruction may occur in patients whose tumors are invading the posterior wall of the trachea or the left main bronchus. Hiccups can occur with involvement of the phrenic nerve or direct involvement of the diaphragm. Very rarely, in advanced cases the patient's presenting symptoms may include a tracheoesophageal fistula, actual mediastinitis, or even perforation of the esophagus because of malignancy. Finally, rare cases may present with significant bleeding either from the airway or from the upper gastrointestinal tract from direct invasion of the tumor into the aorta.

Patients should be evaluated for evidence of portal hypertension or supraclavicular cervical lymphadenopathy. The liver should be examined for evidence of metastases, although fewer than 25% of patients actually show clinical signs of metastatic spread. Finally, it must be noted that the nutritional status of the patient must be evaluated because nutrition has been shown in some studies to be an important independent predictor of outcome in patients undergoing esophagectomy. Thus, patients who are severely cachectic with more than a 25% body weight loss at presentation have a much higher risk of morbidity and mortality after esophagectomy (25).

DIAGNOSIS

A barium swallow study or upper esophagoscopy usually demonstrates the esophageal lesion when patients present with clinical symptoms. Brushings or a biopsy of the lesion by esophagoscopy generally confirms the presence of a carcinoma.

In locations where esophageal carcinoma is endemic, such as the Hunan province of China, early diagnosis with cytologic screening of individuals has been performed (26). These studies have demonstrated that with cytologic screening techniques, esophageal carcinoma can be diagnosed accurately in its early stage (see Chapter 25). The treatment of carcinoma in situ of the esophagus, as detected using cytologic screening methods, results in a 5-year survival rate of 85%; lesions identified at a later stage (invasion of the submucosal layer) had 5-year survival rates of 65%. Both of these figures greatly exceed the survival rates of patients with esophageal carcinoma in Western countries in which screening is not performed. In the United States, screening is not feasible because of the relatively low incidence of esophageal cancer.

One of the highest incidences of esophageal carcinoma occurs in areas of north central China. In Linxian county, the crude rates for esophageal cancer per 100,000 are 163 for males and 103 for females (27). In the early 1960s, balloon cytology was devised for the early diagnosis of this disorder. The correct rate for the diagnosis of esophageal cancer was greater than 90%.

It has been demonstrated in studies from Japan that when esophageal carcinoma is diagnosed at an early stage, i.e., either intraepithelial tumors or cancers confined to the muscularis mucosa, the postoperative 5-year survival is 100% and 85.3%, respectively (28). Unfortunately, these lesions usually are not diagnosed in the West. Rarely, lesions can be detected radiologically on a barium swallow study as fine mucosal alterations visualized by double-contrast techniques.

One of the most reliable methods for the diagnosis of esophageal carcinoma is esophagoscopy. Not only does esophagoscopy allow for direct visualization of the lesion, but it also affords the opportunity for biopsy and cytologic studies.

STAGING OF ESOPHAGEAL CARCINOMA

The *Manual for Staging of Cancer of the American Joint Committee on Cancer* (AJCC) (3rd edition) described a new international staging system in 1988 to allow finer discrimination among stages of esophageal carcinoma (29). This new classification is applicable to clinical as well as pathologic criteria and was meant to improve the ability of staging criteria to provide meaningful prognostic stratification. The new system takes into account the extent of tumor invasion, the presence or absence of lymph node involvement, the level of nodal involvement, and the presence of distant metastatic disease.

Esophageal carcinoma is staged preferably using the TNM classification (Table 26.2). The primary tumor is defined by the histologic level of invasion, rather than by tumor size or extent of spread, because neither of the latter variables has been shown to play a significant role in the determination of survival (30). Tumor in situ lesions are those confined to the mucosa (defined as a carcinoma in situ). A T1 lesion invades the lamina propria or the submucosa, a T2 lesion demonstrates invasion through the muscularis propria, whereas a T3 lesion invades the adventitial layer of the esophagus. A new T stage for esophageal carcinoma, reported in the recent edition of the AJCC, is the inclusion of a T4 level to describe lesions that demonstrate invasion, either microscopically or grossly, into adjacent structures of the mediastinum.

The N (lymph node) classification describes the presence or absence of spread to regional lymph node groups, with N0 lesions demonstrating no nodal spread and N1 lesions showing spread to regional nodes. Re-

TABLE 26.2. TNM Staging System for Esophageal Cancer

	STAGE	STAGE FEATURES
Primary tumor		
	TIS	Carcinoma in situ
	T1	Invades submucosa
	T2	Invades muscularis propria
	T3	Invades adventitia
	T4	Invades adjacent tissues
Regional lymph node		
	N0	No lymph nodes involved
	N1	Involved lymph nodes present
Distant metastasis		
	M0	No distant metastases
	M1	Distant metastatic disease present

cent studies have shown both esophageal wall invasion and presence of lymph node metastases to be independent predictors of prognosis (31). Finally, the M (metastatic) classification describes the presence or absence of spread of esophageal carcinoma to distant sites, with lesions grouped as M0 having no distant spread and those graded as M1 showing evidence of distant metastatic disease at the time of diagnosis (Table 26.2).

Esophageal cancer can be grouped into stages I through IV to allow a smaller number of groupings to be considered (Table 26.3). Thus, stage 0 includes tumor in situ lesions (N0, M0) only, and stage I includes T1 lesions only (N0, M0). Stage II is divided into subgroupings of IIA and IIB, in which IIA includes T2 or T3, N0, M0, and IIB includes T1-3, N1, M0. Stage III includes T3, N1, M0, or T4, any N, M0. Stage IV is defined by the presence of metastases (M1). The 5-year survival of stage I tumors is 40% to 50%, stage II is 20% to 30%, stage III is 10% to 20%, and stage IV is 0% (32).

RATIONALE FOR STAGING

Although surgery for esophageal carcinoma presents the best immediate palliation currently available for dysphagia, most lesions of esophageal carcinoma are found at the time of surgery to be full thickness (T3 or T4) or involving lymph nodes (N1) (24). Because of the poor long-term survival with any of the treatment modalities, including surgery, chemotherapy, or radiation therapy, new therapeutic options are being sought. If it were possible to obtain exact preoperative staging in esophageal cancer, patients could be separated prospectively into those most likely to have residual local or lymphatic disease and those thought likely to have curative resections at surgery. This differentiation would enable the physician to allocate modalities such as adjuvant chemotherapy or radiation therapy to the patient populations that would benefit the most, thus limiting the morbidity associated with these treatments.

Staging of esophageal carcinoma is important because individuals with stage I tumors have a 5-year survival approaching 40% and those of higher stages have a minimal 5-year survival. By accurately diagnosing and staging these tumors, patients can be allocated appropriately to treatment groups. Those with low-stage tumors can be offered curative resection, and those with higher stage tumors can be provided palliative treatments.

Several modalities are used in the evaluation and staging of esophageal carcinoma. The most common are plain radiography, barium swallow, esophagoscopy, bronchoscopy, gallium scanning, computed tomography (CT), magnetic resonance imaging (MRI), and endoscopic ultrasound. Recently, thoracoscopic and laparoscopic evaluation of lymph node invasion has been used (33).

Evidence of mediastinal invasion by an esophageal carcinoma precludes safe resection. Precise preoperative evaluation of the extent of disease, showing the presence or absence of distant disease, lymph node invasion, and invasion of local structures, may avoid unnecessary surgical procedures (34). Staging may thus identify those individuals who are candidates for aggressive, palliative, nonsurgical treatment regimens.

The optimal preoperative staging modality should provide an accurate assessment of: (*a*) the extent of tumor invasion, including the precise depth of lesions in the esophageal wall; (*b*) the presence or absence of lymphatic involvement; and (*c*) the extent of extra-esophageal spread of disease.

CHEST RADIOGRAPHY

The plain chest film plays a minimal role in the modern preoperative staging of esophageal carcinoma. It has been reported that pathologically accurate changes were assessed in only 3% to 47% of patients with esophageal or gastroesophageal carcinomas in a retrospective study (35). These changes were seen in cases of lymphatic spread, tumor infiltration of the retroesophageal space, or poststenotic esophageal dilation (Fig. 26.2) (Table 26.4).

BARIUM SWALLOW

In a patient with esophageal carcinoma, a high-quality barium swallow examination is important. The

TABLE 26.3. Stage Groupings by TNM Subset for Esophageal Carcinoma

STAGE	TUMOR (T)	LYMPH NODE (N)	METASTASES (M)
0	is	0	0
I	1	0	0
IIA	2	0	0
	3	0	0
IIB	1	1	0
	2	1	0
III	3	1	0
	4	Any	0
IV	Any	Any	1

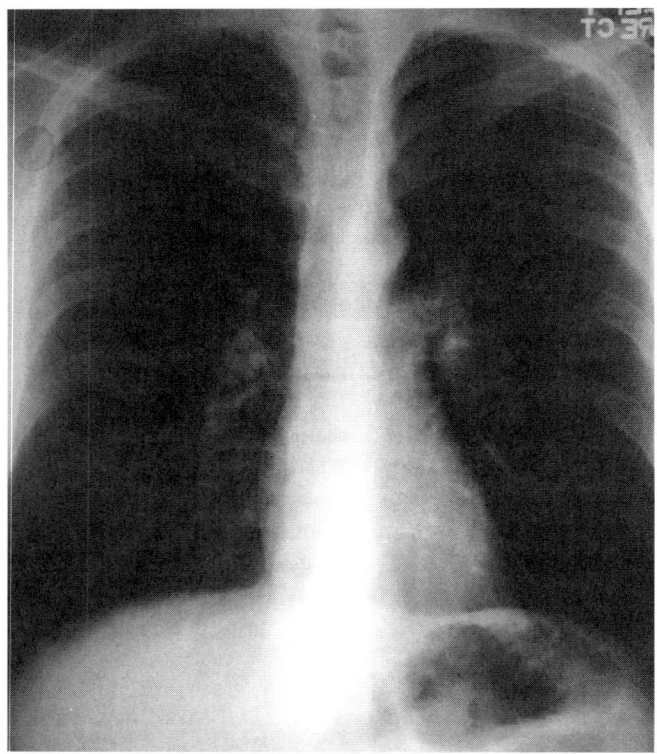

FIGURE 26.2. Chest radiograph in a patient with esophageal cancer showing loss of paraesophageal fat plane.

TABLE 26.4. Signs on Plain Chest Radiograph of Esophageal Malignancy

FINDING	OCCURRENCE (%)
Thickened retrotracheal stripe	11
Anterior tracheal bowing and tracheal impression at the dorsal site or retrotracheal mass	16
Esophageal air-fluid level	5
Deformation or displacement of the trachea	10
Right/lateral deviation of the azygos esophageal line	27
Widened mediastinum	18
Pneumomediastinum to free perforation	Rare
Retrocardiac-retrohilar shadowing	1
Reconfiguration of the stomach	Rare

optimal study includes double contrast with a full column of barium and a mucosal relief. Examination with fluoroscopy helps to analyze the esophageal circumference. Films should be performed in three or four projections, inclined anterior-posterior, lateral, and left/right anterior oblique directions. The double-contrast technique allows for the detection of early lesions that are confined to the mucosa (36). Adequate images are not obtained in as many as 30% of distal lesions and often are not obtained in proximal lesions.

Small lesions also may be detected by cineradiography because the barium bolus passes though the esophagus. Malignant strictures may be detected at an early stage with a solid barium bolus. Because there is a significant incidence of synchronous lesions, the entire esophagus, including the fundus of the stomach, must be visualized during the study.

A barium swallow study may be useful in the determination of tumor length and in evaluating resectability. Yamada (37) considers lesions less than 6 cm in length to potentially be resectable. Lesions longer than 6 cm were found to invade adjacent structures 50% of the time or more. Other investigators suggest that the length of the tumor plays *no* role in determining the depth of tumor invasion because some small submucosal lesions have lymph node metastasis at the time of presentation (38). As noted previously, the length of the esophageal lesion is no longer considered in the TNM staging. Barium swallow examination allows for the determination of deformity of the esophagus, tortuousity, angulation, and deviation. This study thus may permit assessment of resectability (Fig. 26.3). Deformation of the esophageal axis because of tumor fixation and retraction usually is a sign of tumor infiltration of adjacent structures (36). A barium study may show filling defects and help to determine whether the lesion is confined to the epithelium, extends to the submucosa, or extends extramurally. By using air contrast techniques, small lesions confined to the epithelium may be visualized. When viewed tangentially, these tumors tend to show irregularities of the mucosa such as lobulation, nodularity, or ulceration. Lesions invading the submucosa tend to stretch the mucosa and form a filling defect (symmetric or asymmetric) with smooth margins. In tangential views the margins of the tumor appear to form an obtuse angle with the surrounding esophageal wall (Table 26.5).

ESOPHAGOSCOPY

Since the initial attempts to visualize the esophagus by Semelder and Stoerk in 1868, esophagoscopy has played a significant role in the diagnosis of esophageal disease (39). Esophagoscopy provides a reliable assessment of the presence of esophageal carcinoma. The normal esophagus is arranged into four to six longitudinal folds that can normally be eliminated by distension with air insufflation. The epithelium generally is white to pink-gray in appearance with longitudinally arranged blood vessels. The appearance of esophageal carcinomas is distinct. The Japanese Society for Esophageal Disease

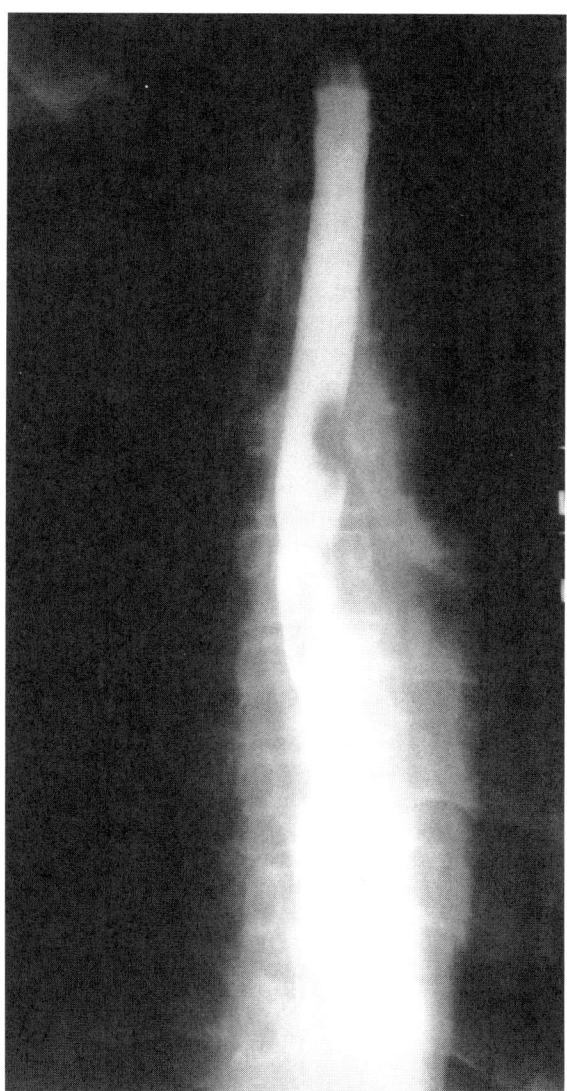

FIGURE 26.3. Barium swallow study showing endophytic mass (*right*) in the mid esophagus.

TABLE 26.5. Appearance of Esophageal Cancer on Barium Swallow Examination

Small lesions (<1.5 cm)
  Mound-like sessile polyps
  Flattened sessile lesions
  Mucosal irregularities
  Flattened areas of decreased compliance
  Smooth tapering
Moderate lesions (1.6 to 3 cm)
  Lobulated, sessile lesions
  Superficial irregularities
  Eccentric ulceration
  Diffuse nodularity
Advanced lesions (>3 cm)
  Overhanging margins
  Irregular narrowed segment
  Bulky endophytic mass
  Large ulcer

Early lesions limited to the mucosa, however, may still be difficult to diagnose by esophagoscopy.

It is known that mucosal color changes often precede surface changes in irregularity. Adequate insufflation can flatten the mucosal folds to determine any slight irregularities in the mucosa (41). In vivo techniques, such as spraying dyes or staining with Lugol's iodine, currently are advocated for the early detection of mucosal lesions. The esophagus is cleaned with a 1% acetic acid solution, with the segment under investigation stained by spraying 1% or 2% Lugol's iodine via a plastic catheter. The stain is rinsed away with water after 10 minutes. Normal mucosa is iodine positive, and carcinoma in situ or invasive lesions are represented by an iodine negative zone. This staining technique may be useful in directing biopsies of suspicious regions (42).

recognizes five distinct patterns at esophagoscopy: superficial, elevated, depressed, stricture, and unclassified (40). The most common presentation is the circumferential "apple core lesion" with mucosal replacement by tumor. Diffusely infiltrating lesions produce thickening and rigidity of the esophageal wall with fixation of the irregularly thickened nodular mucosa to the underlying submucosa. A rare presentation is an exophytic-polypoid type of lesion that is bulky and broad-based in appearance with a coarse, nodular, hemorrhagic surface. Likewise, the tumor may be soft, friable, firm, or irregular with a sarcomatous appearance. The advantage of esophagoscopy is the possibility for tissue diagnosis by biopsy or cytologic means.

BRONCHOSCOPY

Bronchoscopic evaluation in the presence of esophageal lesions can be useful in determining tracheobronchial tree invasion (Fig. 26.4). There are three categories of abnormal bronchoscopic findings (43). In type I no discernible abnormalities are evident. With type II impingement abnormalities are seen, such as bulging of the posterior wall of the trachea or a major bronchus, widening of the carina, or deviation of the trachea or bronchus with or without bronchial narrowing. In type III abnormalities, tumor invasion or a esophageal tracheobronchial fistula is seen. A fistula can be identified when a persistent discharge of fluid or air bubbles arises from a bed of tumor or from the lumen of an airway invaded by tumor.

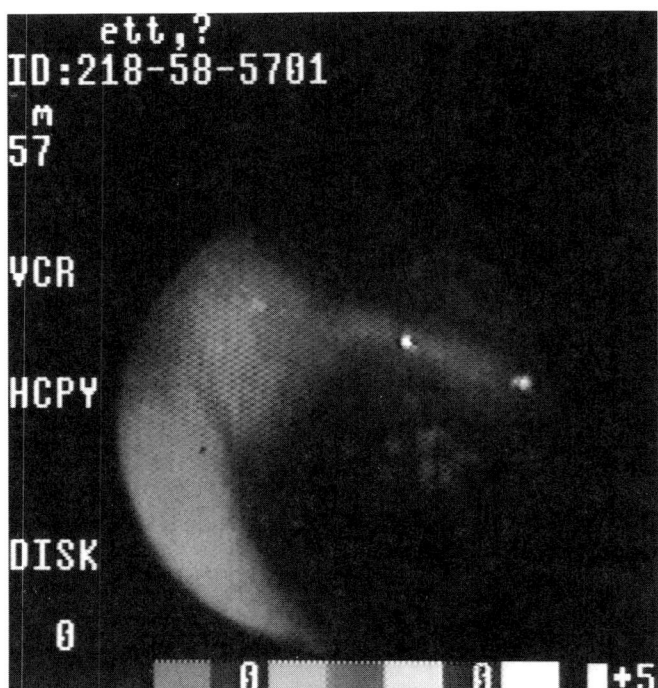

FIGURE 26.4. Bronchoscopy showing invasion into the left main stem bronchus.

LIVER SCANS

Kondo et al. (44) showed that nuclear medicine scans provided only limited information in the preoperative assessment of patients with esophageal cancer. Inculet et al. (45) compared conventional radiologic tomography of the chest, radionuclide scans of the liver, spleen, and bone, and CT of the chest and abdomen in the preoperative assessment of esophageal cancer. They found that CT was the most accurate study, showing an 83% predictive value of local resectability. In their series CT was not as accurate in the preoperative prediction of lymph node involvement. Radionuclide scans did predict bone metastasis not detected by a CT scan, but this result was seen in only one patient (45).

COMPUTED TOMOGRAPHY

CT has long been used to evaluate esophageal disease. The site of the primary tumor does not necessarily indicate which nodal groups will be the site of initial spread (46). Nevertheless, the efficacy of CT in the preoperative staging of esophageal carcinoma varies with the location of the primary lesion (Fig. 26.5). Although it is highly effective in the assessment of thoracic esophageal carcinomas, it is less helpful in the staging of cervical or gastroesophageal junction carcinomas, according to some investigators (47). Esophageal CT should encompass the chest and upper abdomen including the liver, because up to 32% of upper third tumors involve intraabdominal nodes. In 1981 Moss et al. (48) proposed criteria for the CT staging of esophageal carcinoma. Assessment of esophageal carcinoma by CT, however, requires caution in several situations. In the cachectic patient, the lack of normal fat planes between mediastinal structures in the chest and lack of abdominal fat can pose difficulty in the assessment of tumor spread into adjacent structures. Additionally, in patients who have previously undergone esophageal surgery, the tissue planes can be difficult to identify because of scarring and obliteration of normal tissue planes. These findings may be interpreted by an inexperienced radiologist as evidence of mediastinal spread. Furthermore, these tissue planes may be altered by previous chemotherapy or radiation therapy (49) (Table 26.6).

In the normal esophagus, the fatty tissues that interface between the esophagus and the adjacent mediastinal structures are distinct. Blurring or distortion of this fat is an indicator of disease; CT can be effective in delineating these distortions. A CT scan of the normal esophagus shows variable thickness because of the distensibility of the esophageal lumen. Five millimeters is considered the upper limit of normal thickness of the esophageal lumen (50). Although the thickness of the esophageal wall often can be determined, the individual histologic layers of the esophagus cannot. Therefore, T staging by CT is based on total thickness, with T1-2 disease defined as lesions between 5 and 15 mm in thickness, and T3 disease indicated by an esophageal mass thickness greater than 15 mm with an irregular outer mass. T4 disease is represented by apparent invasion of contiguous structures (Table 26.7).

The determination of resectability of esophageal carcinoma by CT is distinguished by several features including aortic, tracheobronchial, or pericardial invasion, and regional or abdominal lymphadenopathy (51). Criteria for CT invasion of local structures include the loss of the normal fat planes between the esophagus and the adjacent mediastinal structures, including the tracheobronchial tree, pericardium, pleura, and aorta. Invasion of the tracheobronchial tree by an upper or middle third lesion carries a grave prognosis (52). Invasion of the tracheobronchial tree may be represented by displacement or bowing of the posterior wall of the trachea or main stem bronchus. In this setting the tumor proves to be invasive in more than 90% of patients (16–18, 53, 54). The usefulness of CT in the assessment of invasion of the tracheobronchial tree is apparent in advanced cases in which there is either a

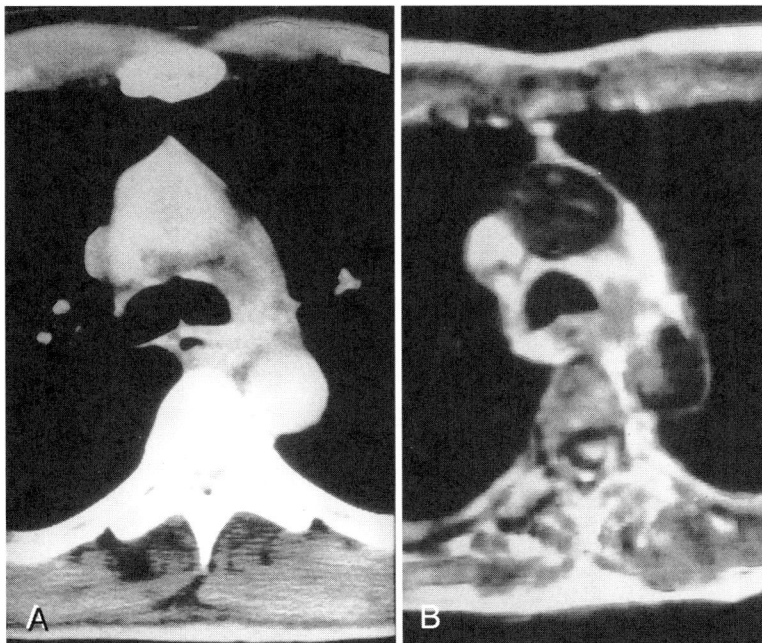

FIGURE 26.5. A. CT scan showing enlarged aortopulmonary window lymph node. B. MRI scan showing the aortopulmonary window.

mass encroaching on the lumen of the airway or a marked airway deformity. Presently, however, CT cannot delineate clearly the membranous portion of the trachea or main stem bronchi and thus cannot distinguish clearly between extrinsic compression and direct invasion.

It has been demonstrated by Postlethwait (55) that 2% of patients dying of esophageal carcinoma have evidence of aortic invasion at the time of autopsy. CT evidence of aortic invasion can be determined by the degree of contact between the esophageal mass and the aorta (56). Aortic invasion often can be difficult to detect by this method because the fat plane between the esophagus and the descending aorta often is absent in normal individuals. Picus et al. (57) claim that invasion may be diagnosed only if the fat plane between these two structures is obliterated over an arc of greater than 90 degrees. If the arc of contact is between 45 and 90 degrees, the result is an indeterminate scan. An arc of contact of less than 45 degrees is considered unlikely to represent aortic invasion (57).

Invasion of the mediastinal fat and pericardium is suggested by visualizing tumor extension into adjacent fat and pericardium or the presence of a pericardial effusion. This identification requires the visualization of multiple CT slices. The loss of the intervening fat planes between the esophagus and the pericardium is taken as direct evidence of invasion (58). When the tumor extends directly into the pericardium without invading the intervening fat plane, the possibility of invasion cannot be ruled out. If this plane is obliterated at one level but not at the preceding and succeeding levels, invasion is highly likely. The accuracy with which CT detects mediastinal invasion ranges from 50% to 100%; detection of aortic invasion, 90% to 96%; tracheobronchial invasion, 88% to 97%; and pericardial invasion, 94% to 97% (59, 60).

Although CT is useful in the determination of the extent of local disease, it is not accurate in the staging of lymph node involvement. The success of CT scanning in predicting positive mediastinal lymph nodes is best exemplified in the 1988 study of lung cancer by Whittlesey (61). In a series of 185 patients with potentially operable lung cancer, CT predictions of mediastinal lymph node invasion were found to be close to the actual size in operative and pathologic findings. Those lymph nodes that were greater than 2 cm were pathologically positive in approximately 70%; those between 1 and 2 cm in size were positive in approximately 32%, and those less than 1 cm were positive for tumor only 10% of the time. The conclusion of this study was that CT was very successful in predicting the size of mediastinal nodes preoperatively, and that it could be used as a screening test for clinical preoperative staging. Subsequent surgical staging of lung cancer is performed using either mediastinoscopy, thoracoscopy, mediastinotomy, or actual operative surgical staging.

No such clear correlations have been published regarding CT for esophageal cancer. CT is of limited use in differentiating between small normal nodes and nodes invaded by tumor but that are small in size. Likewise, it cannot differentiate between hyperplastic

TABLE 26.6. Appearance of Esophageal Malignancy on CT

Focal esophageal wall thickness
Eccentricially positioned enlarged lumen
Large esophageal mass
Obliterated esophageal lumen
Direct extension of esophageal carcinoma into mediastinal structures
Dilation of proximal esophagus

TABLE 26.7. Staging of Esophageal Cancer by CT Appearance

Stage I	Intraluminal mass without wall thickening
Stage II	Mass with esophageal wall thickening (T1, <5 mm; T2-3, 5–15 mm)
Stage III	Evidence of local invasion/lymph node spread
Stage IV	Distant metastatic disease

and neoplastic nodes (60). It has been suggested that mediastinal nodes greater than 1 cm in diameter in the short axis should be classified as abnormal, subdiaphragmatic nodes greater than 8 mm in diameter should be considered abnormal, and nodes between 6 and 8 mm in size should be considered indeterminate. By using these criteria, CT has a sensitivity of 100% but a specificity of only 43% because many invaded lymph nodes are of normal size (60).

CT is very accurate in determining the presence of liver metastases using intravenous contrast. CT accuracy in determining the extent of liver involvement is 94% to 100%, and abdominal lymph node involvement accuracy appears to range from 50% to 87% (59). Although several earlier studies reported favorable results with preoperative staging of esophageal carcinoma using CT, several more recent reports have noted some limitations of its use. In 1981 Moss et al. (48) described the obliteration of the paraesophageal fat space on CT scan as evidence of contiguous disease (T3 and T4 lesions). Thompson et al. (62) and Lea et al. (63) showed the accuracy of CT scanning in predicting the extent of local spread. Predictability of lymph node involvement, however, was poor (less than 69%).

Cross-sectional imaging techniques have been applied to the investigation and staging of esophageal carcinoma since the early 1980s. Earlier studies reported favorable results with CT, whereas later studies were more circumspect about the accuracy of CT in determining the resectability of esophageal carcinoma. All CT studies have employed only conventional CT with 8- or 10-mm image spacing.

In addition to conventional CT, high-resolution CT may have a role in the evaluation of the tumor and involvement of adjacent structures. High-resolution CT involves the use of thin-section (1.5- to 2-mm) scans reconstructed with an edge-enhancing algorithm. This technique may allow better delineation of the tumor, surrounding fat, pericardium, and airways. Spatial resolution improvements also may allow for improved identification of lymph nodes and may decrease the potential for volume-averaging with the adjacent tumor.

MAGNETIC RESONANCE IMAGING

MRI provides considerable benefit in the diagnosis of diseases of the central nervous system. Its role in defining disease in the chest is less well defined, however. Several recent studies have analyzed its usefulness in the staging of esophageal cancers. Maas et al. (64) demonstrated that electrocardiogram-gated MRI could detect most esophageal tumors, although artifacts caused by diaphragmatic motion and the beating heart still caused considerable blurring. Evidence of tumor invasion of surrounding structures, such as the aorta, tracheobronchial tree, and the mediastinum, is similarly based on evidence of loss or invasion of the intervening fat plane by tumor. T1-weighted images allow the best delineation of the neoplasm, whereas T2-weighted images give the worst signal to noise ratios. Because tumor images are increased on T2 images, this "noise" probably diminishes the con-trast between the tumor and the surrounding fat signal (which also is bright). Signal enhancement with gadolinium/diethylenetriamine penta–acetic acid (gadolinium-DPTA), when used, also increases signal in the T1 images, potentially inducing a contrast reduction similar to that seen in T2 images.

The advantage of MRI is its ability to determine tumor length accurately and to image in the coronal and sagittal planes. With CT the tumor length must be estimated indirectly by summing the single slice thicknesses. Additionally, because of its superior contrast of soft tissue, MRI may prove to be superior to CT in determining infiltration of contiguous structures such as the aorta and the tracheobronchial tree (60) (Fig. 26.6).

The literature on MRI of esophageal cancer is limited, and thus far no significant benefit of MRI versus CT has been found (65). All MRI studies reported to date have employed only conventional T1- and T2-weighted spin echo images. Strict radiologic-surgical-pathologic correlation has been lacking in most of these studies. In 1988 Lehr et al. (66) showed the lack of usefulness of MRI in predicting lymph node involvement and found no advantage of MRI over CT.

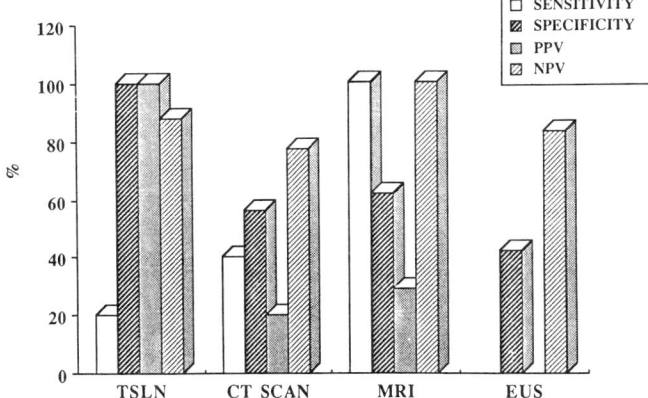

FIGURE 26.6. Sensitivity, specificity, positive predictive value (PPV), and negative predictive value (NPV) of thoracoscopic lymph node staging (TSLN) compared with computed tomography (CT), MRI, and esophageal ultrasound (EUS) in staging of esophageal cancer.

MAGNETIC RESONANCE IMAGING DEFINITIONS

TUMOR INFILTRATION

Criteria for tumor infiltration into surrounding structures include the lack of fat planes around the adjacent tumor or adjacent organ displacement (Fig. 26.7).

AORTIC INFILTRATION

Aortic infiltration has been evaluated by examining the angle of contact that the tumor makes with the circumference of the aorta. When the tumor contacts more than 90 degrees of the aortic circumference, invasion is suggested. Contact of less than 45 degrees makes invasion unlikely, and contact between 45 and 90 degrees is considered indeterminate. These criteria have allowed for an 80% accuracy rate. Other investigators have used the presence of tumor contact with the aorta over at least 3.2 cm (four 8-mm sections) and a transverse contact angle of greater than 60 degrees as diagnostic of aortic invasion.

TRACHEOBRONCHIAL INVASION

Signs of tracheobronchial invasion include tumor extension into the lumen of the airway, displacement of the airways, lack of a fat plane adjacent to the tumor with a visualized fat plane above and below the tumor, and a concave posterior wall of the trachea.

MEDIASTINAL FAT AND PERICARDIUM

Invasion of the fat or pericardium is suggested by visualizing tumor extending into adjacent fat. Pericardial invasion is likewise diagnosed by a lack of intervening fat planes between the tumor and pericardium.

LYMPH NODE INVOLVEMENT

Evaluation of the mediastinal and upper abdominal lymph nodes has met with limited success. The current criterion for positive lymph nodes is enlargement of more than 10 mm in the short transverse axis. Using this definition, small nodes infiltrated by tumor will be

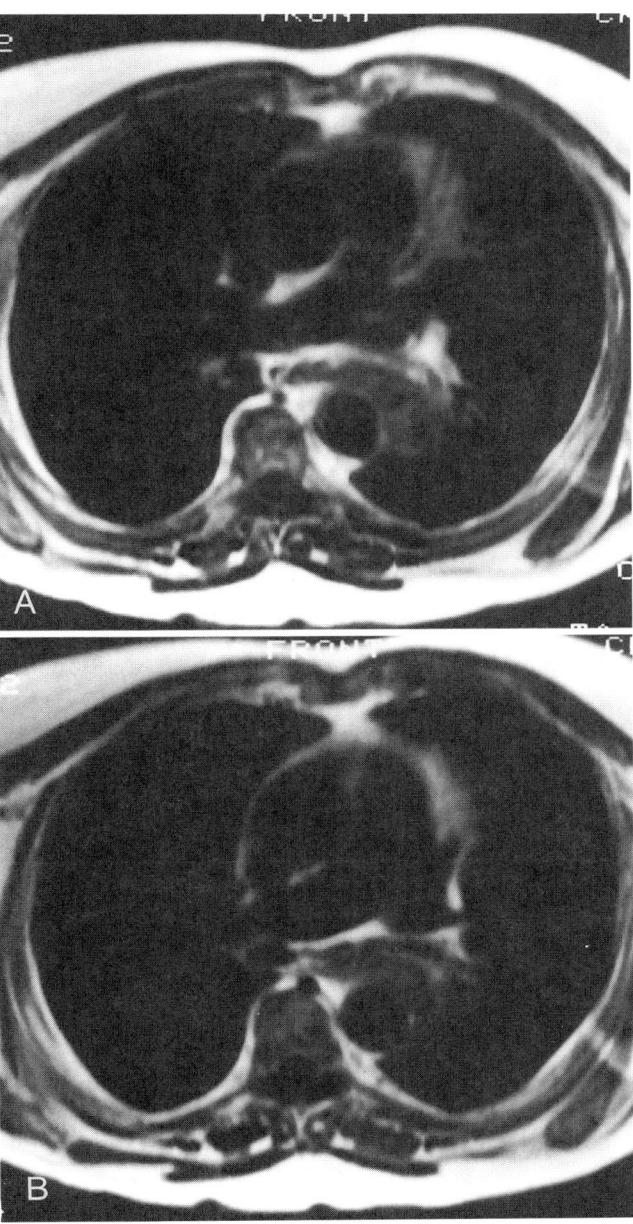

FIGURE 26.7. A. MRI scan showing a clear fat plan between the esophageal tumor and the aorta. B. MRI scan showing loss of the paraesophageal fat plane at the next level.

false-negative, and reactive nodes enlarged more than 10 mm will be false-positive for tumor involvement. Enlarged nodes adjacent to the tumor can be missed because they may be inseparable from the tumor (67).

In addition to the use of standard cardiac-gated (if possible) T1-weighted and T2-weighted axial spin echo images, fat suppression can be employed and T1-weighted images can be evaluated after enhancement with intravenous gadolinium. On standard T1-weighted images, esophageal tumors are isointense to the remaining normal esophagus, and on T2-weighted images the tumor increases (becomes brighter) in signal intensity.

Intravenous gadolinium has been used in other clinical settings to enhance tumors, such as those in the central nervous system. Enhancement of esophageal tumors with gadolinium may allow better delineation of the tumor from surrounding structures, as well as the possible enhancement in tumor-bearing lymph nodes. Theoretically, this enhancement would allow identification of nodes of any size that are tumor bearing and possibly would help to eliminate both false-positive and false-negative diagnoses based on node size alone (68).

Fat suppression techniques decrease the signal from normal fat. This method may be beneficial in differentiating tumor-bearing, abnormally infiltrated fat, which should not suppress the signal, from the normal periesophageal fat (69).

The cartilage rings of the airways can be identified on MRI as areas of low signal intensity, and the interruption of the cartilage ring image could also be evaluated as a sign of tracheobronchial invasion. The pericardium appears as a low-signal–intensity "line" on MRI, and if visible, encroachment of tumor into the pericardium by obliteration of this line can also be evaluated (Table 26.8).

ESOPHAGEAL ULTRASOUND

One of the newest modalities used in the staging of esophageal carcinoma is endoscopic esophageal ultrasound (EUS). Ultrasound is an established imaging modality in many areas of clinical medicine. Using external ultrasound, extensive information can be obtained regarding the site and extent of intraabdominal pathology with minimal risk. Extracorporeal ultrasound has several limitations, however. Examinations may be compromised by overlying bowel or pulmonary gas, bone, or obesity. In addition, the depth of penetration is highly dependent on the placement of the probe and the signal frequency emitted by the probe. In general, high frequencies produce greater clarity of detail but provide little depth of penetration.

TABLE 26.8. MRI Findings in Esophageal Carcinoma

Tumor infiltration
  Obliteration of fat planes
  Organ displacement
Aortic invasion
  Greater than 90-degree contact
  Contact greater than 3.2 mm in length (equivalent to four standard slices)
Airway invasion
  Tumor invasion into lumen
  Displacement/distortion of fat plane
Mediastinal invasion
  Invading adjacent fat
Lymph node invasion
  Greater than 10-mm short axis
  ? Gadolinium enhancement
Pericardial invasion
  Thickened pericardium
  Pericardial effusion
  ? Obliteration of pericardial line on MRI scan

Standard intraluminal endoscopy provides an excellent view of mucosal surfaces; however, mural and submucosal lesions cannot be well visualized. By placing an ultrasound probe on the tip of an esophagoscope, an excellent assessment of mural lesions can be obtained. This technique also avoids interference from bone or abdominal fat and allows close apposition of the probe to the area of interest (70). The probe typically emits a sound wave with a frequency between 1 and 5 million cycles per second (HZ). This frequency allows for superb visualization of all layers of the esophageal wall and gastrointestinal tract. The sound waves are reflected differently depending on the characteristics of the tissues they encounter. This information is then displayed on a screen for viewing and recording. Transmission and reflection depend on the density of tissue encountered. Bone and other calcified tissues have a high reflectivity. Organs and dense tissues transmit sound waves readily, whereas gas and fat impede the transmission of these waves.

Ultrasonic imaging of the gastrointestinal tract shows five distinct layers of alternating echogenicity. The first layer is hyperechoic (light) and corresponds to the superficial mucosa. The next layer is hypoechoic (dark) and represents the remainder of the mucosa and the submucosa. The third layer is hyperechoic, representing the interface between the submucosa and underlying muscularis propria. The fourth layer is echo lucent, representing the muscularis propria. The fifth layer represents the serosa and is hypoechoic. In the chest and mediastinum, the surrounding structures can also be well visualized (71, 72).

It has been demonstrated that EUS is accurate in assessing the depth of tumor invasion in 89% of cases of esophageal cancer by determining alterations in the orderly alignment of the layers of the esophageal wall. It also clearly demonstrates the transition between normal and pathologic esophagus (Fig. 26.8) (73). EUS has rapidly become an important technique in the staging of esophageal cancer. Using EUS different groups have differentiated early from advanced esophageal carcinoma based on the involvement of the muscularis propria. EUS is less accurate in assessing lesions that are stenotic and do not permit passage of the instrument (74).

EUS may be used to identify lymph node metastasis (accuracy, 81%; sensitivity, 95%; and specificity, 50%) (75). There is evidence, however, that EUS is not accurate in differentiating enlarged nonmetastatic from malignant lymph nodes (76). Lymph nodes less than 5 mm on EUS are not likely to be malignant. Aibe et al. (77) reported that lymph nodes greater than 10 mm were malignant 48% of the time. In studies using EUS for preoperative staging of esophageal carcinoma, high sensitivity has been reported (78–81). Botet et al. (50) reported 100% sensitivity for depth of cancer invasion using EUS, compared with 80% for CT and 82% for MRI. EUS also had 89% sensitivity for malignant lymph nodes, compared with 85% for CT and 82% for MRI. Rice et al. (74) used EUS to document response to preoperative chemotherapy and found that EUS predicted the pathologic tumor stage (T) with an accuracy of 82% and the nodes (N) with an accuracy of 73%.

Takemoto et al. (70) described the prediction of correct depth of invasion in 75% of patients. Likewise, assessment of distant metastatic disease is not accurate, probably because of the limited depth of penetration in evaluating the liver (Table 26.9; Fig. 26.6).

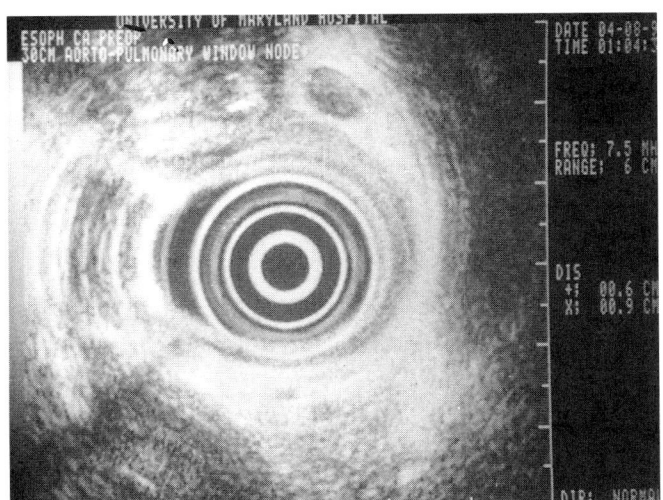

FIGURE 26.8. EUS showing obliteration of the normal layers of the esophagus and enlarged lymph node.

TABLE 26.9. EUS Classification in Accordance with New 1987 TNM Staging

STAGE	
T1	Hypoechoic tumor localized in the mucosa/submucosa
T2	Hypoechoic tumor penetrating the muscularis mucosa
T3	Hypoechoic tumor penetrating the adventitia
T4	Hypoechoic tumor penetrating into adjacent mediastinal structures
N0	Hyperechoic, indistinct nodes
N1	Hypoechoic, clearly delineated nodes or evidence of direct penetration into adjacent nodes
M0	No evidence of celiac nodal metastasis or liver involvement
M1	Celiac nodal or liver metastasis

SURGICAL STAGING

Surgical treatment of esophageal cancer remains controversial. Long-term cures are infrequent despite treatment programs using surgery, radiation therapy, and chemotherapy. In view of the usually advanced stage of this disease at presentation with fragmented submucosal spread, lymph node involvement (seen in 60% of patients at presentation), and extension to surrounding structures (from an organ lacking a serosa), this observation is hardly surprising. Added to these biologic impediments is the lack of any uniformly accepted method of staging esophageal carcinoma preoperatively. The pathologic stage differs from the clinical stage in up to two thirds of cases showing full thickness tumors or lymphatic spread. Huang et al. (82) reported that 51.2% of all esophageal cancer patients had lymph node metastases at the time of resection. Because practically all patients with nonresectable tumors had lymph node spread, the actual incidence is approximately 67%. They found that the 5-year survival without lymph node metastases was 45%, compared with 13% for patients with lymph node spread. Likewise, they found that when more than five lymph nodes were involved, the survival was 0% versus 15% when fewer than five lymph nodes were involved (82).

Akiyama et al. (83) studied lymph node spread in esophageal cancer and found that lymph node metastases commonly occur along the lesser curvature of the stomach and in the celiac axis. In that study tumor spread to distant lymph nodes from all levels of esophageal cancer was noted. Most patients had tumor spread to at least one thoracic lymph node station regardless of the level of tumor.

A recent study by Abe et al. (1) described the pattern of lymph node metastasis in patients with resectable esophageal cancer. This study again emphasized the incidence of spread to mediastinal and celiac nodes in all levels of esophageal cancer. Many other investigators have described the importance of lymph node spread in esophageal cancer. Skinner et al. (84) described the importance of lymph node staging in selecting the type of procedure performed for patients with esophageal cancer. They emphasized that extensive resections should be considered for patients with spread to periesophageal lymph nodes, including all of the structures in the posterior mediastinal compartment, allowing a radical lymphadenectomy. This approach was also adapted successfully by Ide et al. (85). Likewise, Watanabe et al. (86) and Isono et al. (87) have described their results of extended esophagectomy with lymphadenectomy and have shown improved survival with lymphadenectomy in patients with esophageal cancer. In the recent study by Ellis et al. (31), the presence of lymph node metastases in esophageal cancer was noted as an independent predictor of prognosis. In 1993 Hagen et al. (88) reported an improved survival benefit for patients with complete lymphadenectomy associated with esophagectomy for distal third and gastroesophageal junction tumors. These studies must be compared with the excellent results reported by Orringer et al. (89) using combination chemotherapy and radiation therapy followed by transhiatal esophagectomy without radical lymphadenectomy.

One of the major handicaps in allocating and comparing treatment modalities for esophageal cancer is the lack of precise preoperative staging. The CT scan has been cited as the most accurate study in predicting local resectability, but as noted above, the prediction of lymph node involvement is poor. The use of mediastinoscopy in preoperative staging for lung cancer was shown to be highly efficacious by Albertucci et al. (90) in 1987 as well as by Pearson et al. (91) in 1972. The usefulness of this technique suggests a possible role for preoperative surgical staging in esophageal cancer to delineate which patients have advanced disease and which patients, in fact, have early local disease.

Applying the philosophy of pre-resection lymph node staging from lung cancer is an enticing idea. A minimally invasive test that could correctly identify patients with a high risk of failure, such that these patients could be considered for various combined modality studies, would be very appealing.

Preoperative surgical staging in esophageal cancer was first described by Murray et al. in 1977 (92). In this study mediastinoscopy and mini-laparotomy were performed prospectively in 30 patients. In 7 patients positive lymph nodes were found in the mediastinum, and in 16 patients celiac lymph nodes were identified. The investigators considered the lack of access to thoracic lymph nodes the limiting factor. In 1986 Dagnini et al. (93) described the routine use of laparoscopy before undertaking esophagectomy for esophageal cancer. In a series of 369 patients, they found intraabdominal metastases in 14% and celiac lymph node metastases in 9.7%. These findings allowed the investigators to avoid unnecessary resection in these patients. In a recent study from Japan of 209 patients with esophageal cancer, Tachimori et al. (94) described screening using transcervical ultrasound to detect cervical lymph nodes. Twenty-six patients had palpable lymph nodes (9%). Of these 12 went on to resection and radical cervical lymphadenectomy. Ultrasound detected lymph nodes in 18 of 143 patients studied. Of 83 who underwent resection, all had histologically positive lymph nodes. When combined with manual palpation, a diagnostic accuracy of 91.7% was achieved (94).

Diagnostic and therapeutic thoracoscopy for pleural, pulmonary, and pericardial diseases has been reported (95). Recently, thoracoscopic techniques have been used as a complement to mediastinoscopy, replacing the Chamberlain procedure as a preoperative lymph node staging technique (33). Thoracoscopy has been shown thoracoscopy to be a useful means of staging mediastinal lymph nodes, complementing mediastinoscopy. The possible efficacy of thoracoscopic lymph node staging in esophageal cancer was described in another recent study (96). Despite correct thoracic lymph node staging in 14 patients, 2 of 14 had celiac lymph nodes found at the time of esophageal resection. Had laparoscopy been performed, these two patients would have been staged correctly. By combining thoracoscopy and laparoscopy or mini-laparotomy, accurate pre-resection surgical staging may be achieved using minimally invasive methods. Currently, these authors sample all thoracic and abdominal lymph nodes according to the esophageal cancer lymph node map described by Casson et al. (97) (Fig. 26.9).

THORACOSCOPIC TECHNIQUE

After induction of general anesthesia and insertion of a double-lumen endobronchial tube, the patient is placed in the lateral decubitus position similar to that for a posterolateral thoracotomy. The authors generally prefer a right thoracoscopy approach because it allows greater exposure of the esophagus without interference by the aorta (Fig. 26.10). In cases in which preoperative noninvasive staging showed a large aortopulmonary window lymph node, a left thoracoscopic evaluation would be undertaken.

LEFT THORACOSCOPY

Upon entering the chest, inspection may reveal enlarged lymph nodes in the aortopulmonary window

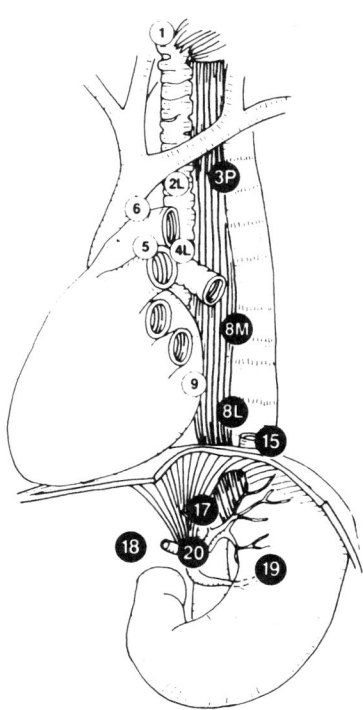

FIGURE 26.9. Lymph node map for staging of esophageal cancer. (From Casson AG, Inculet RI, Zankowicz N, et al. Lymph node mapping for resectable carcinoma of the esophagus. A guide for thoracic surgeons. Princeton, NJ: Bristol-Myers Squibb Company, 1992.)

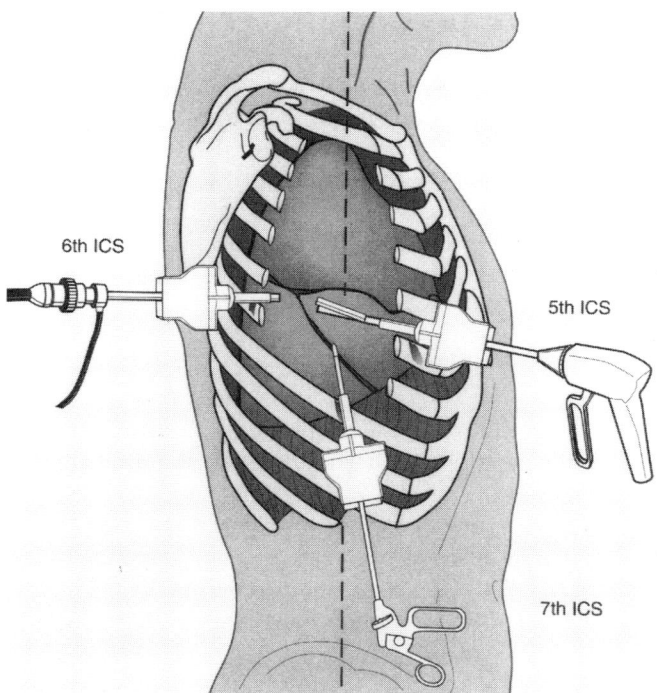

FIGURE 26.10. Patient set-up for thoracoscopic lymph node staging and port placement.

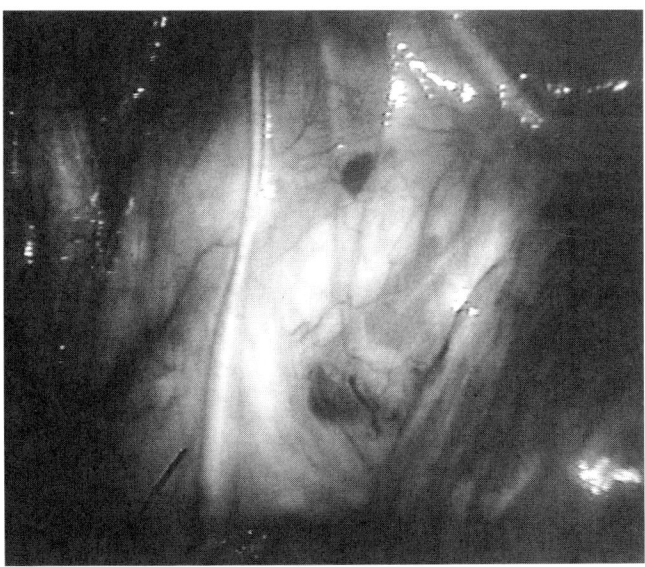

FIGURE 26.11. Exposure of anteroposterior window and lymph nodes at thoracoscopic lymph node staging.

(Fig. 26.11). The remainder of the hemithorax is examined for evidence of gross esophageal tumor extension or metastatic disease to the lung. Two additional incisions are then made in the anterior axillary line, one in the third intercostal space and the other in the seventh interspace. A 5-mm trocar cannula is placed in the upper incision, and a 12-mm cannula is inserted into the lower incision under direct video visualization.

A biopsy grasper is used to elevate the mediastinal pleura overlying the lymph nodes, and a bipolar electrocautery probe is used to incise the pleura. The incision is continued up to the apex of the triangle formed by the phrenic and vagus nerves. Inferiorly, the pleura is incised over the left main pulmonary artery. Lymph nodes in the region are mobilized using a Babcock–Allis–type grasper. The vascular pedicle is ligated with the endoscopic clip applier. The nodes are removed and the area irrigated with saline solution. Additional lymph node biopsies are performed using a similar technique to dissect the inferior pulmonary ligament.

RIGHT-SIDED THORACOSCOPY TECHNIQUE

Right thoracoscopy is performed using one-lung ventilation with the patient in left lateral decubitus position. The telescope is introduced into the sixth intercostal space, posterior axillary line. Two additional trocars are inserted under direct vision. Using CO_2 insufflation and adjusting the position to take advantage of gravity, the lung is collapsed and allowed to fall out of the field. A fourth trocar is inserted into the third intercostal space, anterior axillary line, thus allowing three anterior trocars and one posterior trocar in a so-called "baseball diamond" shape. A lung retractor may help expose the regions of the paraesophageal and inferior pulmonary ligaments.

The mediastinal pleura overlying the upper esophagus is incised (Fig. 26.12), and the incision is continued inferiorly to the level of the azygos vein down to the subcarinal region, and finally to the inferior pulmonary vein (Fig. 26.13). The mediastinal pleura overlying the tracheoesophageal groove is dissected. Biopsies of all nodes are taken using hemoclips for hemostasis.

LAPAROSCOPY TECHNIQUE

The patient is placed in the supine or modified lithotomy position, with the surgeon standing on the patient's left or between the legs, respectively (Fig. 26.14). Both monitors are placed at the head of the table. The abdomen is prepared and draped for a standard laparotomy. The procedure is begun with four operating ports (all 10-mm diameter), although a fifth port may be necessary in the left upper quadrant for retraction of the stomach and placement of tension on the hepatogastric ligament (lesser omentum). An angled laparoscope (30 degrees or greater) is essential for exposure of the operative field.

After thorough exploration of the peritoneal cavity, attention is directed to the upper abdomen. The surface of the liver is inspected, and gross abnormalities are biopsied and sent for frozen section. The liver is then retracted with an expandable fan retractor. The lesser curvature of the stomach is inspected for evidence of grossly abnormal lymph nodes. The lesser sac is entered using sharp dissection through the lesser omentum, just to the right of the esophagus. Identification of the esophagus may be aided by placement of an esophageal dilator or flexible endoscope intraoperatively. The initial dissection is carried cephalad until the right crus of the diaphragm is identified. The undersurface of the esophagus may be exposed with blunt dissection at this time, if necessary. Any abnormal tissue is biopsied. If imaging studies suggested enlarged nodes on the left crus, the peritoneum overlying the esophagus would be opened and the left crus exposed.

After entry into the lesser sac, the lesser omentum is divided in a caudal direction to maximize exposure of the retroperitoneum. Most of this dissection may be performed with electrocautery, but occasionally clips may be necessary. Lymph nodes identified along the lesser curve are biopsied. Pulsations from the

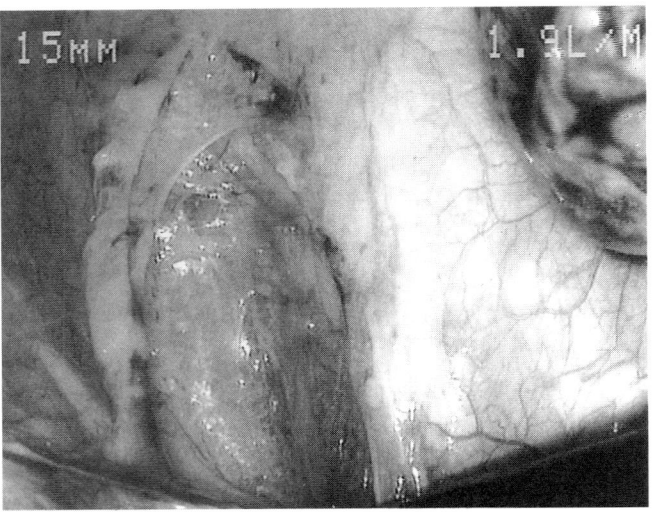

FIGURE 26.12. Thoracoscopic exposure of the upper thoracic esophagus.

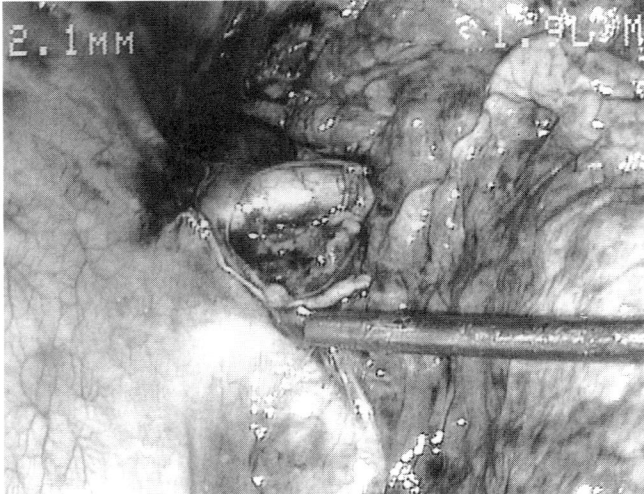

FIGURE 26.13. The subazygous region after dissection of lymph nodes (suction device shown under the vein).

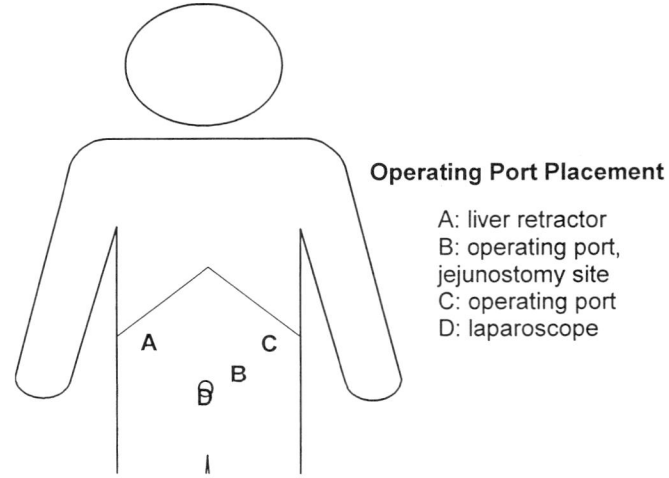

FIGURE 26.14. Patient set-up and port placement for laparoscopic staging.

Operating Port Placement

A: liver retractor
B: operating port, jejunostomy site
C: operating port
D: laparoscope

right gastric artery are visible caudally, and division of the omentum may stop at this point. The superior border of the pancreas is usually visible at this point, and peripancreatic lymph nodes may be obtained if needed. Exposure of the celiac axis is obtained by elevation of the lesser curve of the stomach near the gastroesophageal junction. The left gastric artery is identified by its pulsation as it projects straight up from the celiac axis and enters the posterior wall of the stomach. The areolar tissue can be dissected bluntly from the vessel; this maneuver usually yields several small lymph nodes (Fig. 26.15). The left gastric artery is followed proximally to the origin of the celiac axis. Pulsations from the aorta are obvious at this point, and in thin persons the vessel can sometimes be visualized directly without further dissection.

Usually, there is a substantial amount of fat and areolar tissue containing lymph nodes at the origin of the celiac axis. The tissue is bluntly dissected until the nodes are identified. Further dissection usually allows identification of the vascular pedicle, which may be controlled with surgical clips. Electrocautery should be used with great caution in this area. Efforts should be made to minimize even trivial hemorrhage in the retroperitoneum, because tissue staining with blood makes visualization much more difficult.

After completion of the lymph node harvest, the field is irrigated and the area is inspected for hemostasis. Small bleeding points may be controlled with surgical cellulose and with direct pressure. In cachectic patients the authors generally place a laparoscopic jejunostomy immediately before terminating the procedure. A medical infusion port for chemotherapy also can be placed at this time.

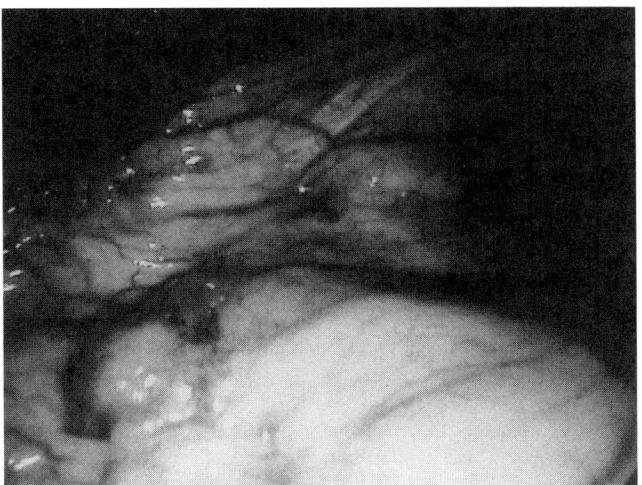

FIGURE 26.15. Celiac lymph node biopsy at laparoscopic lymph node staging.

RESULTS AT UNIVERSITY OF MARYLAND

In a prospective series of cases of esophageal cancer evaluated at the University of Maryland Hospital, preoperative CT, MRI, and EUS were used for noninvasive preoperative staging. A pilot study was undertaken prospectively to evaluate the technical feasibility, safety, and efficacy of thoracoscopic and laparoscopic lymph node staging for patients with endoscopically proven esophageal carcinoma.

CT scans were obtained using oral and intravenous contrast and high-resolution CT when feasible. MRI of the chest and upper abdomen were performed using gadolinium enhancement. EUS was performed from the level of the tumor down to the celiac axis. Bronchoscopy was performed on all patients with tumors adjacent to the carina or bronchi. Studies were excluded from analysis if technically impossible because of obstruction or equipment malfunction.

Thoracoscopy was performed using a standardized technique. After the initial 14 patients were staged through the left chest, thoracoscopy was thereafter performed routinely through the right chest. This approach allowed maximal dissection of paraesophageal lymph nodes, avoiding the aortic arch. One patient with enlarged aortopulmonary window lymph nodes (level 5) preferentially had left-sided exploration. Laparoscopic staging was performed after thoracoscopic staging of lymph nodes was completed.

Forty-five patients underwent attempted thoracoscopic lymph node staging for esophageal cancer. There were 44 males and one female. Forty-one patients had squamous cell carcinoma and four had adenocarcinoma. In four patients thoracoscopy was aborted because of adhesions. There were no deaths. Two patients developed postoperative wound infections. Resections involved either Ivor-Lewis esophagogastrectomy, combined laparotomy-thoracotomy with a neck anastomosis, or a left thoracotomy-esophagogastrectomy. Transhiatal esophagectomy was avoided in this series to assure maximal lymph node sampling.

Forty-one patients completed successful thoracoscopic staging. Of these 41, 33 went on to surgical resection. Three patients were inoperable, because of pulmonary metastasis and one because of portal hypertension. The remaining 5 patients refused surgery. Thirty-three patients with both thoracoscopic staging and surgical resection were therefore assessable for staging corrections.

Of the patients undergoing thoracoscopic lymph node staging, only one was found to have N1 disease. Of the patients who were found to have no positive nodes at thoracoscopy, only one was found to have N1 disease at the time of resection. The sensitivity of thoracoscopy was therefore approximately 80%. The specificity, however, was 100%. The positive predictive value was likewise 100%, and the negative predictive value was approximately 88%. Of nine patients undergoing laparoscopic lymph node staging, four patients had N3 disease (celiac nodes positive). Three of these four patients had no N3 disease at the time of resection after preoperative therapy with chemotherapy and radiation therapy.

Additional information was obtained at thoracoscopy. Three patients thought to be T4 by noninvasive tests were shown to have T3 disease and were therefore able to undergo esophagectomy. Two patients underwent thoracoscopy, which predicted T4 invasion. In two patients thoracoscopy missed T4 lesions. One patient with questionable pulmonary metastasis on CT and MRI was found to have definite pulmonary metastasis with a thoracoscopic lung biopsy.

The precise role of thoracoscopy and laparoscopy in the staging of esophageal cancer remains uncertain at the present time. However, thoracoscopy and laparoscopy offer the potential to stage lymph nodes in esophageal cancer as accurately as mediastinoscopy in lung cancer, thereby defining which patients have early local disease amenable to surgical resection and which have more advanced disease.

The approach of prospectively testing the role of thoracoscopy and laparoscopy for preoperative staging of esophageal cancer has recently been developed as an intergroup study.

REFERENCES

1. Abe S, Tachibana M, Shiraishi M, et al. Lymph node metastasis in resectable esophageal cancer. J Thorac Cardiovasc Surg 1990; 100:287–291.
2. Kirby TJ, Rice TW. The epidemiology of esophageal carcinoma. The changing face of a disease. Chest Surg Clin North Am 1994; 4:217–225.
3. Czerny J. New operations (Neue Operationen). Zentralbl Chir 1877;4:433.
4. Mikulicz J. A case of resection of the esophagus with plastic reconstruction of the excised piece. Praf Med Wochenschr 1886; 11:93.
5. Torek F. The operative treatment of carcinoma of the oesophagus. Ann Surg 1915;61:385.
6. Ohsawa T. The surgery of the esophagus. Arch Jpn Chir 1933; 10:605.
7. Rehn R. Operations on the esophagus in the region of the chest. Verh Dtsch Ges Chir 1898;27:448.
8. Adams WE, Phemister DB. Carcinoma of the lower thoracic esophagus; report of a successful resection and esophagogastrostomy. J Thorac Surg 1938;7:621.
9. Sweet RH. Transthoracic resection of esophagus and stomach for carcinoma; analysis of postoperative complications, causes of death and late results of operations. Ann Surg 1945;121:272.
10. Garlock JH. Reestablishment of esophagogastric continuity following resection of the esophagus for carcinoma of the middle third. Surg Gynecol Obstet 1944;78:23.
11. Ellis FH Jr. Carcinoma of the distal esophagus and esophagogastric junction. Modern Techniques in Cardiaothoracic Surgery 1979;13:1–10.
12. Rothberg R, Demeester TR. Surgical anatomy of the esophagus. In: Shields TW, ed. General thoracic surgery. 3rd ed. Philadelphia: Lea & Febiger, 1989:87–92.
13. Shields TW. Lymphatic drainage of the esophagus. In: Shields TW, ed. General thoracic surgery. 3rd ed. Philadelphia: Lea & Febiger, 1989:76–86.
14. Blot WJ, Devesa SS, Kneller RW, et al. Rising incidence of adenocarcinoma of the esophagus and gastric cardia. JAMA 1991;265: 1287–1289.
15. Duranceau A. Epidemiologic trends and etiologic factors of esophageal carcinoma. International Trends in General Thoracic Surgery 1988;4:3–10.
16. Mathews HR, Pattison CW. Esophageal carcinoma as a complication of achalasia. International Trends in General Thoracic Surgery 1988;4:4–15.
17. Spechler JS, Robbins AH, Rubbins HP, et al. Adenocarcinoma and Barrett's esophagus an over-rated risk? Gastroenterology 1984;54:726.
18. Shine J, Allison PR. Carcinoma of the esophagus with tylosis. Lancet 1966;1:951–953.
19. Sierrif DJ, Grishkin BA, Golal FS, Zajtchuk R, Graeber GM. Radiation associated malignancies of the esophagus. Cancer 1984;54:726.
20. Fong LYY. Environmental carcinogens and dietary deficiencies in esophageal cancer in Asia. In: Pfeiffer CJ, ed. Cancer of the esophagus. Boca Raton, FL: CRC Press, 1982:41–63.
21. Shields TW. Squamous cell carcinoma. In: Shields TW, ed. General thoracic surgery. 3rd ed. Philadelphia: Lea & Febiger, 1989:1044–1059.
22. Murray GF, Rezar GE. Less common malignant tumors of the esophagus. In: Shields TW, ed. General thoracic surgery. 3rd ed. Philadelphia: Lea & Febiger, 1989:1070–1083.
23. Postlethwait RW. Surgery of the esophagus. 2nd ed. Norwalk, CT: Appleton Century Crofts, 1986:443–468.
24. Huang GJ. Natural progression in esophageal carcinoma. International Trends in General Thoracic Surgery 1988;4:87–89.
25. Huang GJ, Wu YK. Clinical diagnosis in carcinoma of the esophagus and gastric cardia. In: Huang GJ, Wu YK, eds. Carcinoma of the esophagus. Berlin: Springer-Verlag, 1984.
26. Shen Q, Wang GQ. Cytologic screening for carcinoma and dysplasia of the esophagus in the People's Republic of China. International Trends in General thoracic Surgery 1988;4:25–31.
27. Blot WJ. Epidemiology of esophageal cancer. In: Roth JA, Ruckdeschel JC, Weisenburger TH, eds. Thoracic oncology. Philadelphia: WB Saunders, 1989:295–304.
28. Nishizawa M, Okada T. Endoscopic diagnosis of early esophageal cancer: establishing an effective detection system. In: Ferguson MK, Little AG, Skinner DB, eds. Diseases of the esophagus: malignant diseases. Mount Kisco, NY: Futura Publishing Company, 1990;I:87–91.
29. American Joint Committee on Cancer, Task Force on Esophagus, Mountain CF (Chairman). Carcinoma of the esophagus. In: Beahrs OH, Meyers M, eds. Manual for staging of cancer. 2nd ed. Philadelphia: JB Lippincott, 1983:61–69.
30. Mountain CF. Rationale in staging of cancer of the esophagus. International Trends in General Surgery 1988;4:73–79.
31. Ellis FH, Watkins E Jr, Krasna, MJ, Heatley GJ, Balogh K. Staging of carcinoma of the esophagus and cardia: a comparison of different staging criteria. J Surg Oncol 1993;52:231–235.

32. Bardini R, Castoro C, Sorrentino P, et al. Prognostic factors for squamous cell carcinoma of the thoracic esophagus after curative resection. In: Ferguson MK, Little AG, Skinner DB, eds. Diseases of the esophagus: malignant diseases. Mount Kisco, NY: Futura Publishing, 1990;I:219–228.
33. Fiocco M, Krasna MJ. Thoracoscopic lymph node dissection. J Laparoendosc Surg 1992;2:111–115.
34. Turnbull ADM, Ginsberg RJ. Options in the surgical treatment of esophageal carcinoma. Chest Surg Clin North Am 1994;42:315–329.
35. Lindell MM Jr, Hill CA, Libshitz HI. Oesophagus cancer: radiographic chest findings and their prognostic significance. AJR Am J Roentgenol 1979;133:461–465.
36. Reeders JW, Bartlsman WM. Radiologic diagnosis and preoperative staging of esophageal malignancies. Endoscopy 1993;25:10–27.
37. Yamada A. Radiologic assessment of resectability and prog-nosis in oesophageal carcinoma. Gastrointest Radiol 1979;4:213–219.
38. Mori S, Kasat M, Watenabe R, et al. Preoperative assessment of resectability for carcinoma of the thoracic oesophagus. Ann Surg 1979;190:100–105.
39. Wong J, Branicki FJ. Esophagoscopy and bronchoscopy. International Trends in General Thoracic Surgery 1988;4:36–44.
40. Japanese Society for Esophageal Diseases. Guidelines for the clinical and pathologic studies for carcinoma of the esophagus. I. Clinical classification. Jpn J Surg 1976;6:69.
41. Monnier P, Savary M, Anani P. Endoscopic morphology of "early" esophageal cancer. In: DeMeester TR, Skinner DB, eds. Esophageal disorders: pathophysiology and therapy. New York: Raven Press, 1985:347–353.
42. Tytgat GN. Non radiological investigation of the esophagus. In: Watson A, Celestin LR, eds. Disorders of the esophagus: advances and controversies. London: Pitman, 1984:24–36.
43. Choi TK, Siu KF, Lam KH, et al. Bronchoscopy and carcinoma of the esophagus. II. Carcinoma of the esophagus with tracheobronchial involvement. Am J Surg 1984;147:760.
44. Kondo M, Ando N, Kosuda S, et al. GA-67 scan in patients with intrathoracic esophageal carcinoma planned for surgery. Cancer 1982;49:103.
45. Inculet RI, Keller SM, Swyer A. Evaluation of non-invasive tests for the preoperative staging of carcinoma of the esophagus. Ann Thorac Surg 1985;40:561–565.
46. Daffner RH, Halber MD, Postlethwait RW, et al. CT of the esophagus II carcinoma. AJR Am J Roentgenol 1979;133:1051–1055.
47. Halvorsen RA Jr, Thompson WM. CT of oesophageal neoplasms. Radiol Clin North Am 1989;27:667–685.
48. Moss AA, Schnuder P, Thoeni RD, et al. Esophageal carcinoma: pretherapy staging by computed tomography. AJR Am J Roentgenol 1981;136:1051–1056.
49. Quint LE, Glazer GM, Orringer MB, et al. Esophageal carcinoma: CT findings. Radiology 1985;155:171–175.
50. Botet JF, Lightdale CJ, Zauber AAG, et al. Preoperative staging of esophageal cancer: comparison of endoscopic ultrasound and dynamic CT. Radiology 1991;181:419–425.
51. Rankin S. The role of computerized tomography in the staging of esophageal carcinoma. Clin Radiol 1990;42:152–153.
52. Schurawitzki H, Kumpan W, Niederie B, et al. Esophageal carcinoma: CT staging of tumor infiltration. Dysphagia 1988;2:170–174.
53. Thompson WM, Halvorsen RA, Foster WL, et al. Computed tomography for staging oesophageal and gastroesophageal cancer: re-evaluation. AJR Am J Roentgenol 1983;141:951–958.
54. Akiyama H, Tsurumaru T, Udagawa H. Imaging techniques. International Trends in General Thoracic Surgery 1988;4:53–68.
55. Postlethwait RW. Squamous cell carcinoma of the oesophagus. In: Surgery of the oesophagus. 2nd ed. Norwalk, CT: Appleton Century Crofts, 1985:369–442.
56. O'Donovan PB. The radiographic evaluation of the patient with esophageal carcinoma. Chest Surg Clin North Am 1994;4:241–256.
57. Picus D, Balfe DM, Koehler RE, et al. Computed tomography in the staging of esophageal carcinoma. Radiology 1980;146:433–438.
58. Rankin S, Manson R. Staging of esophageal carcinoma. Clin Radiol 1992;46:373–377.
59. Lefor AT, Merino MM, Steinberg SM, et al. Computerized tomographic prediction of extraluminal spread and prognostic implications of lesions width in esophageal carcinoma. Cancer 1988;62:1287–1292.
60. Koch J, Halvorsen RA, Thompson WM. Therapy hinges on staging in upper GI tract cancer. Diagn Imaging 1993;Feb:74–81.
61. Whittlesey D. Prospective computed tomographic scanning in the staging of bronchogenic cancer. J. Thorac Cardiovasc Surg 1988;95:876–882.
62. Thompson W, Halvorsen R, Foster W, et al. Computerized tomography for staging esophageal and gastroesophageal cancer. AJR Am J Roentgenol 1983;141:951–958.
63. Lea J, Prager R, Bender H. The questionable role of computed tomography in preoperative staging of esophageal cancer. Ann Thorac Surg 1984;38:479–481.
64. Maas R, Nicholas V, Grimm H, et al. MRI of esophageal carcinoma with ECG gating at 1.5 tesla. In: Ferguson MK, Little AG, Skinner DB, eds. Diseases of the esophagus: malignant diseases. Mount Kisko, NY: Futura Publishing, 1990:145–155.
65. Takashima S, Takeuchi N, Shiozaki H, et al. Carcinoma of the esophagus: CT vs. MRI in determining resectability. AJR Am J Roentgenol 1991;156:297–302.
66. Lehr L, Rupp N, Siewer JR. Assessment of resectability of esophageal cancer by computed tomography and magnetic resonance imaging. Surgery 1988;103:344–350.
67. Quint LE, Glazer GM, Orringer MB. Esophageal imaging by CT and MR. A study of normal anatomy and neoplasms. Radiology 1985;156:727–731.
68. Tempelton PA. Use of gadolinium enhanced MRI to evaluate airway invasion in patients with esophageal carcinoma (abstract). Proceedings of the Radiological Society of North America, 1994.
69. Petrillo R, Balzarini L, Bidoli P, et al. Esophageal squamous cell carcinoma: MRI evaluation of mediastinum. Gastrointest Radiol 1990;15:275–278.
70. Takemoto T, Ito T, Aibe T, et al. Endoscopic ultrasonography in the diagnosis of esophageal carcinoma with particular regard to staging it for operability. Endoscopy 1986;18(Suppl 3):22–25.
71. Rosch T. Endoscopic ultrasonography. Endoscopy 1992;24:144–153.
72. Baker MK, Kopecky KK. Endoscopic US in the staging of esophageal and gastric cancer. Radiology 1991;181:342–343.
73. Zeigler K, Zeitz CS, Friedrich M, et al. Evaluation of endosonography in TN staging of esophageal cancer. Gut 1991;32:16–20.
74. Rice TW, Boyce GA, Sivak MV, et al. Esophageal ultrasound and the preoperative staging of carcinoma of the esophagus. J Thorac Cardiovasc Surg 1991;101:536–544.
75. Tio TL, Cohen P, den Hartog Jager FCA, et al. Preoperative TNM classification of esophageal carcinoma by endoscopy. Hepatogastroenterol 1990;37:376–381.
76. Tio TL, Cohen P, Udding J, et al. Endosonography and computed tomography of esophageal carcinoma. Gastroenterology 1989;96:1478–1486.

77. Aibe T, Ito T, Yoshida T, et al. Endoscopic ultrasonography of lymph nodes surrounding the upper GI tract. Scand J Gastroenterol 1986;12:164–169.
78. Vilgrani V, Mompoint D, Palazo L, et al. Staging of esophageal carcinoma: comparison of results with endoscopic sonography and CT. AJR Am J Roentgenol 1990;155:277–281.
79. Lightdale CJ. Staging of esophageal cancer. Endoscopic ultrasound in gastrointestinal endoscopy. Semin Oncol 1994;21:438.
80. Sallano A, Hamper K, Noar M, et al. Endoscopic ultrasound (EUS) of esophago-gastric cancer: a new requirement of preoperative staging (abstract). Gastrointest Endosc 1988;34:176.
81. Sonquet JC, Valette PJ, Berger F, et al. Endosonography (EUS) compared to computerized tomography (CT) for preoperative staging of esophageal cancer (abstract). Gastrointest Endosc 1990;36.
82. Huang G, Sun KL. Prognostic significance of lymph node metastasis in surgical resection of esophageal carcinoma. Ferguson MK, Little AG, Skinner DB, eds. Diseases of the esophagus: malignant diseases. Mount Kisco, NY: Futura Publishing, 1990.
83. Akiyama H, Tsurumaru M, Kawamura T, et al. Principles of surgical treatment for carcinoma of the esophagus. Ann Surg 1981;194:438–446.
84. Skinner DB, Ferguson MK, Little A, et al. Selection of operation for esophageal cancer based on staging. Ann Thorac Surg. 1986;204:391–401.
85. Ide H, Hanyu F, Murata Y, et al. Extended dissection for thoracic esophageal cancer based on preoperative staging. In: Ferguson MK, Little AG, Skinner DB, eds. Malignant diseases of the esophagus. Mount Kisco, NY: Futura Publishing, 1990:177–186.
86. Watanabe H, Kato H, Tachimori H. A comparative study regarding surgical treatment for thoracic esophageal cancer according to the procedure of lymph node dissection. Ferguson MK, Little AG, Skinner DB, eds. Diseases of the esophagus: malignant diseases of the esophagus. Mount Kisco, NY: Futura Publishing, 1990.
87. Isono K, Okuyama K, Ochiai T. Evaluation of lymphadenectomy of intrathoracic esophageal cancer in terms of patient survival. In: Ferguson MK, Little AG, Skinner DB, eds. Malignant diseases of the esophagus. Mount Kisco, NY: Futura Publishing, 1990.
88. Hagen JA, Peters JH, DeMeester TR. Superiority of extended en bloc esophago-gastrectomy for the lower esophagus and cardia. J Thorac Cardiovasc Surg 1993;106:850–859.
89. Orringer MB, Forastiere AA, Perez-Tamayo C, et al. Chemotherapy and radiation therapy before transhiatal esophagectomy for esophageal carcinoma. Ann Thorac Surg 1990;119:348–355.
90. Albertucci M, DeMeester TM, Golomb HM, et al. Use and prognostic value of staging mediastinoscopy in non–small-cell lung cancer. Surgery 1987;102:652–658.
91. Pearson FG, Nelems JM, Henderson RD, et al. The role of mediastinoscopy in the selection of treatment for bronchial carcinoma with involvement of superior mediastinal lymph nodes. J Thorac Cardiovasc Surg 1972;64:382–390.
92. Murray GF, Wilcox BR, Stared PIK. The assessment of operability of esophageal carcinoma. Ann Thorac Surg 1977;23:393.
93. Dagnini G, Caldironi MW, Marin G, et al. Laparoscopy in abdominal staging of esophageal carcinoma. Gastrointest Endosc 1986;32:400–402.
94. Tachimori Y, Kato H, Watanabe H, Yamaguchi H. Neck ultrasonography for thoracic esophageal carcinoma. Ann Thorac Surg 1994;57:1180–1183.
95. Krasna MJ, McLaughlin JS. Efficacy and safety of thoracoscopy for diagnosis and treatment of intra-thoracic disease. Surg Laparosc Endosc 1994;1:82–188.
96. Krasna MJ, McLaughlin JS. Thoracoscopic lymph node staging for esophageal cancer. Ann Thorac Surg 1993;56:671–674
97. Casson AG, Inculet RI, Zankowicz N, et al. Lymph node mapping for resectable carcinoma of the esophagus. A guide for thoracic surgeons. Princeton, NJ: Bristol-Myers Squibb Company, 1992.

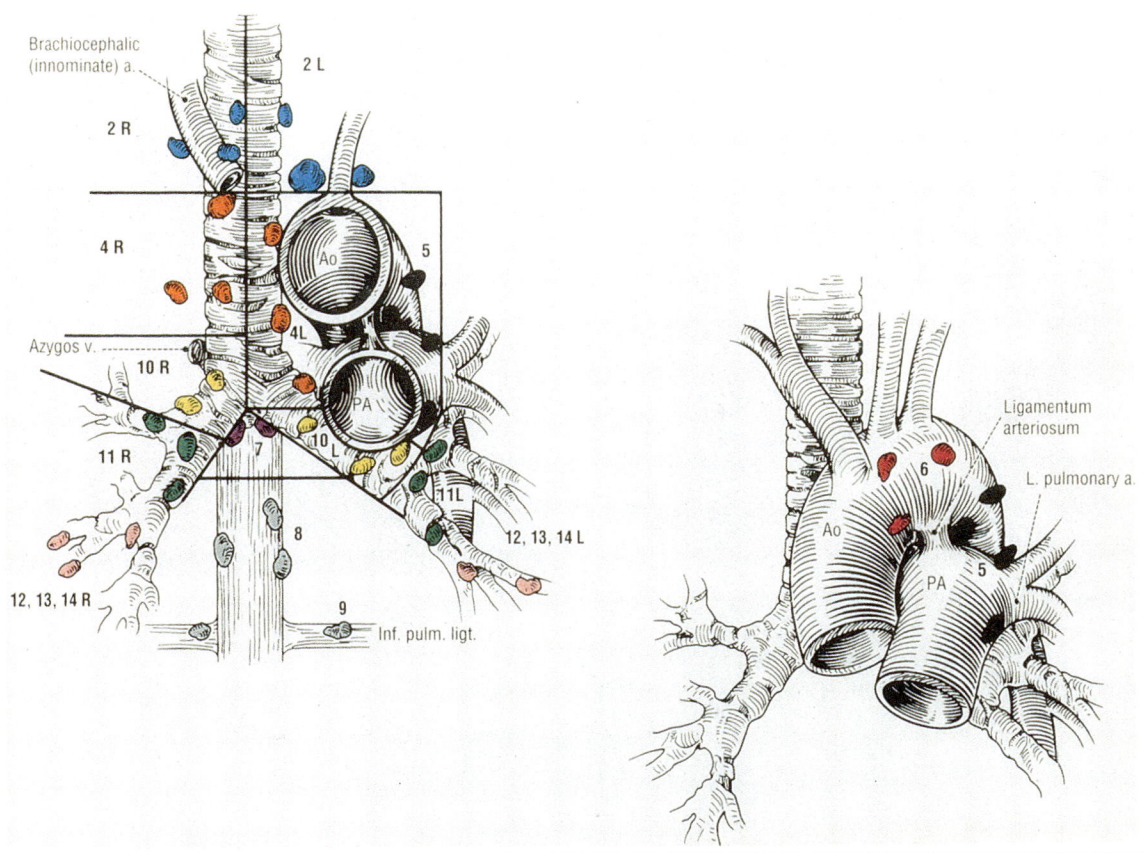

●	2R	Right upper paratracheal nodes	Between intersection of caudal margin of innominate artery with trachea and the apex of the lung (supra-innominate nodes).
●	2L	Upper left paratracheal nodes	Between top of aortic arch and apex of the lung (supra-aortic nodes).
●	4R	Right lower paratracheal nodes	Between intersection of caudal margin of innominate artery with trachea and cephalic border of azygos vein.
●	4L	Left lower paratracheal nodes	Between top of aortic arch and carina (medial to ligamentum arteriosum).
●	10R	Right tracheo-bronchial angle nodes	From cephalic border of azygos vein to origin of RUL bronchus.
●	10L	Left tracheo-bronchial angle nodes	Between carina and LUL (medial to ligamentum arteriosum).
●	5	Aorto-pulmonary nodes	Subaortic and para-aortic nodes lateral to the ligamentum arteriosum (proximal to first branch of left PA).
●	6	Anterior mediastinal nodes	Anterior to ligamentum arteriosum.
●	7	Subcarinal nodes	Caudal to the carina of the trachea.
●	8	Paraesophageal nodes	Dorsal to the posterior wall of the trachea and to the right or left of the midline of the esophagus.
●	9	Pulmonary ligament nodes	Nodes within the inferior pulmonary ligament.
●	11	Interlobar nodes	
●	12	Lobar nodes	
●	13	Segmental nodes	
●	14	Subsegmental nodes	

FIGURE 6.9. Regional nodal stations for lung cancer staging.

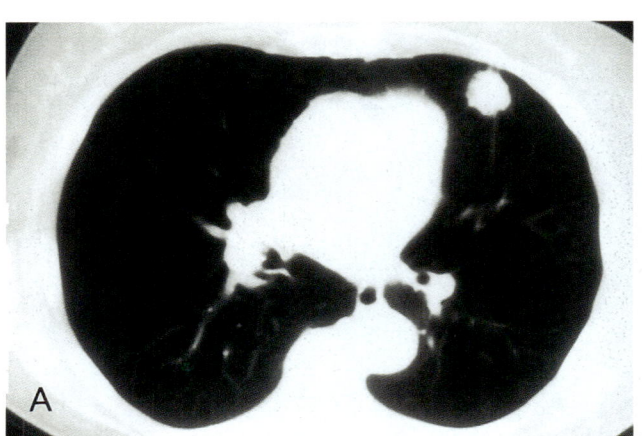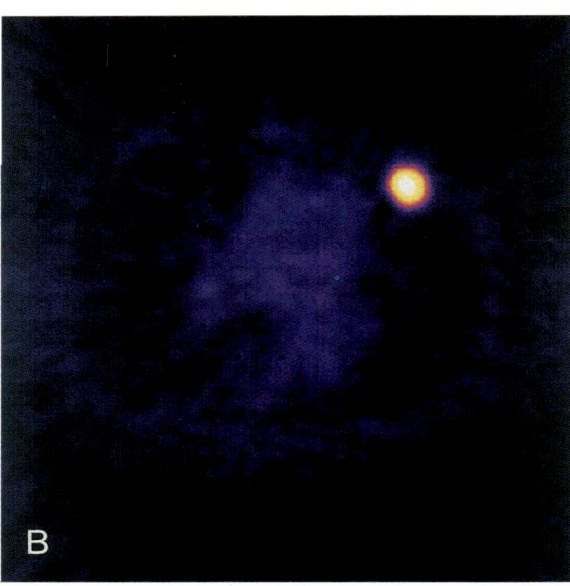

FIGURE 6.15. PET scan of an SPN. **A.** CT scan showing an SPN (*arrow*) in the left lung. **B.** Positron emission tomography (F-18)–2-fluoro-2-deoxy-D-glucose (PET-FDG) scans, showing intense localization in the SPN (*arrow*), which at surgery proved to be lung cancer. The FDG uptake reflects increased metabolic activity, most commonly lung cancer, although granulomas and other processes having metabolic activity may have increased activity on PET scan. (Courtesy of R. Edward Coleman, M.D., Duke University Medical School.)

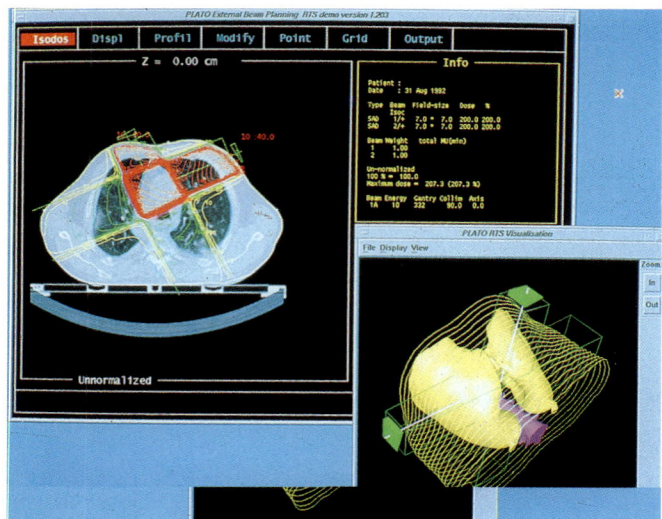

FIGURE 9.12. Example of 3D treatment planning for lung cancer. (Courtesy of Nucletron International, Veanandal, The Netherlands.)

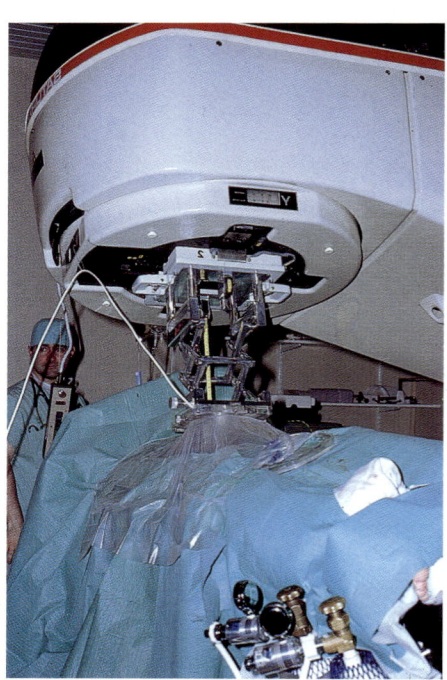

FIGURE 9.16. Intraoperative radiotherapy. The cone is fixed to the linear accelerator through a special device with a sterile drape covering the surgical bed.

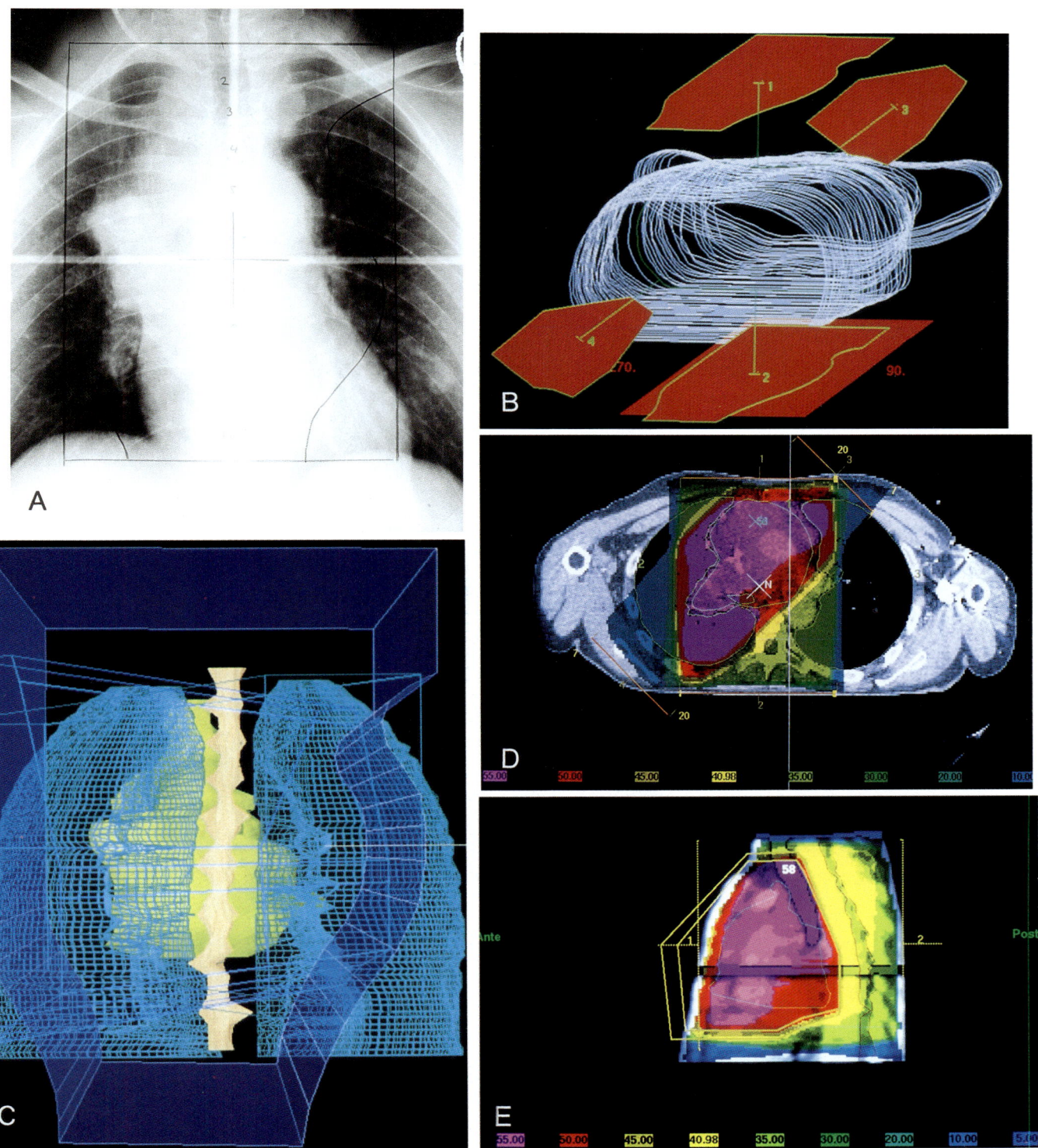

FIGURE 21.5. Radiation technique in the treatment of limited SCLC. A. Anteroposterior beam shaped by the shielding of a fusible alloy at low temperature (MCP70; Mining and Chemical Products, Ltd., Wembley, England), drawn in the prechemotherapy simulator film. B. through G. Tridimensional treatment planning done in a prechemotherapy CT scan for a patient with limited SCLC. B. The patient is treated by anteroposterior fields delivering a total dose of 40 Gy and by oblique fields delivering an additional 15 Gy. C. Lateral fields avoiding the spinal cord. Superimposed tumor and anatomic structures with geometric projects of radiation beams. Lungs, *(green)*, tumor volume *(yellow)*, spinal cord *(beige)*. D. Computed dosimetry in the transverse plane. The tumor volume receives between 50 and 55 Gy. The spinal cord receives 41 Gy.

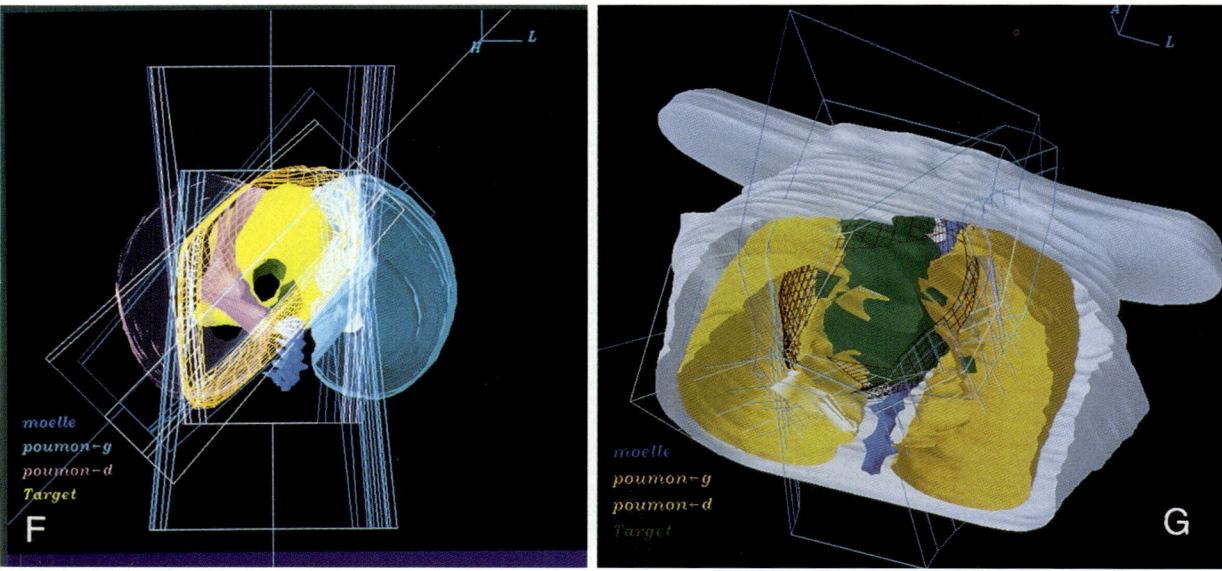

FIGURE 21.5—CONTINUED. **E.** Computed dosimetry in the sagittal plane. The spinal cord receives a homogenous dose of 41 Gy along the treated volume. **F.** Tridimensional view of anatomic structures and tumor volume with geometric projection of radiation beams. Target volume *(yellow)*, left lung *(green)*, right lung *(mauve)*, spinal cord *(blue)*. **G.** Tridimensional view of the treated volume. Lung *(yellow)*, spinal cord *(blue)*, target volume *(green)*, 50% isodose area surrounding target volume *(red grid)*.

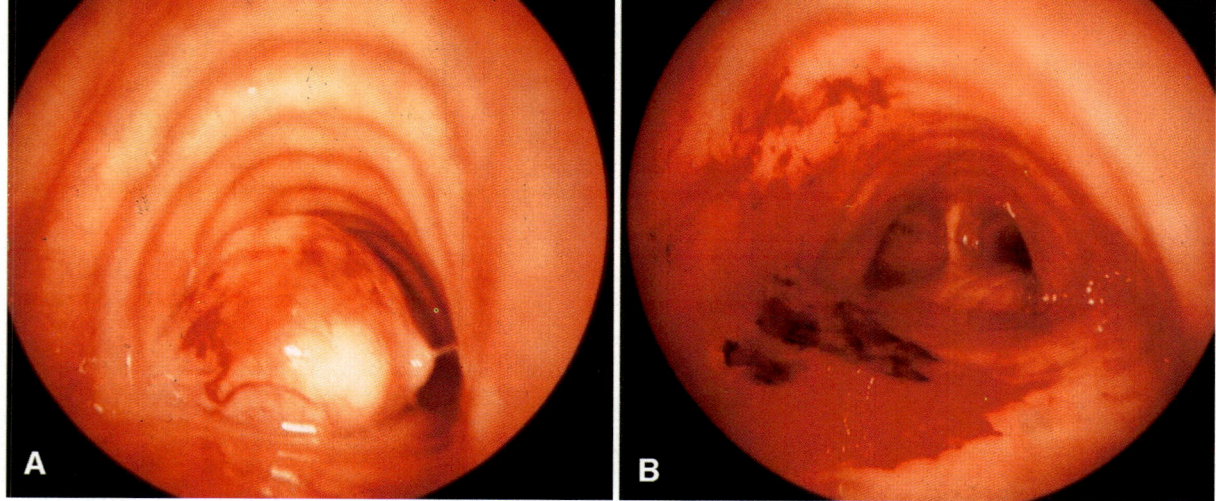

FIGURE 45A.1. **A.** Major intraluminal tracheal obstruction by squamous cell carcinoma. **B.** Trachea after laser resection of intraluminal mass.

FIGURE 45A.2. Moderate extrinsic compression of the origin of the left main bronchus, widened main carina, and Dumon silicone stent in the right main bronchus of a patient with squamous cell bronchogenic carcinoma.

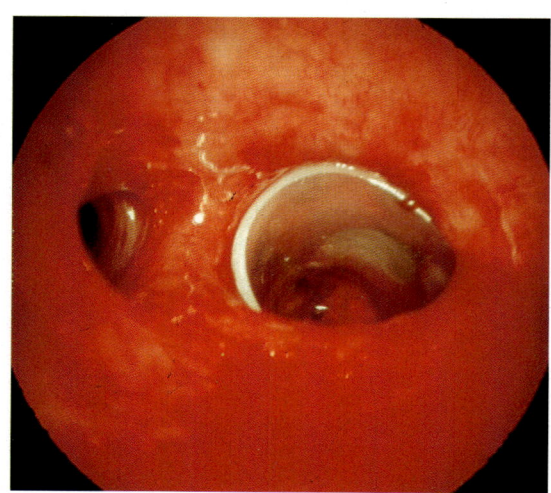

27

Barrett's Esophagus (and Other Premalignant Lesions) and Management of Localized Esophageal Cancer

Nasser K. Altorki

BARRETT'S ESOPHAGUS (AND OTHER PREMALIGNANT LESIONS)

In 1950 Barrett published his original report of a peptic ulcer observed within a tubular intrathoracic stomach drawn cephalad into the thorax by a congenitally short esophagus (1). A few years later Allison and Johnstone (2) provided persuasive anatomic evidence that the segment of the foregut observed by Barrett was actually an esophagus lined with columnar epithelium. They suggested an association with gastroesophageal reflux and proposed the eponym Barrett's esophagus. In 1957 Barrett published a more complete description of the disease and its complications (3). A few years after Barrett's original report, Morson and Belcher (4) reported an esophageal adenocarcinoma arising in association with a columnar-lined esophagus. The premalignant potential of Barrett's esophagus has since been supported by other reports, and a significant association with esophageal adenocarcinoma is now well recognized (5). Barrett's esophagus would have been a disease of little or no consequence had it not been for this dreaded complication. As a result the medical and surgical communities now focus on a disease that Barrett himself initially described as "a condition whose existence is denied by some, misunderstood by others, and ignored by the majority of surgeons" (6).

DEFINITION

Barrett (3) stated that "when the lower esophagus is found to be lined by columnar cells, the abnormally placed mucous membrane extends upwards from the esophagogastric junction in a continuous unbroken sheet." The salient question with respect to a precise definition of Barrett's esophagus is therefore determining where the esophagus ends and the stomach begins. The lack of a serosal coat around the esophagus and the presence of only two layers of muscularis propria clearly differentiate the esophagus from the stomach, which is almost entirely covered in a serosal coat and has three distinct layers of muscularis propria. These anatomic landmarks are valuable only to the surgeon in the operating room or the anatomist in the laboratory. The endoscopically determined squamocolumnar junction normally defines the location of the lower esophageal sphincter. This endoscopic landmark, however, is disassociated from the true anatomic gastroesophageal junction in Barrett's esophagus. Conversely, the lower 1 to 2 cm of the esophagus normally are lined by columnar epithelium and, as such, do not constitute a pathologic entity. Endoscopically, the presence of a hiatal hernia and a patulous cardia, as often occurs, adds to the confusion of a clinical determination of the precise site of the gastroesophageal junction.

The location of the lower esophageal sphincter, determined manometrically, would seem the most logical method of determining the location of the gastroesophageal junction; however, the asymmetry of the sphincter and its frequent profound hypotension may preclude a sharp demarcation of the sphincter from the baseline pressure tracing in the gastric reservoir. Currently, Barrett's esophagus is defined as the presence of columnar epithelium lining at least 3 cm of the distal tubular esophagus, regardless of the presence or absence of a hiatal hernia (7). The tubular esophagus is defined as that part of the foregut that participates in esophageal peristaltic contraction as observed endoscopically, fluoroscopically, or manometrically. Shorter segments of Barrett's esophagus (i.e., less than

3 cm) are diagnosed only when histology shows evidence of intestinal metaplasia, which is not normally encountered in the region of the lower esophageal sphincter. The sheet of columnar epithelium should extend cephalad from the cardia, either as flamelike projections or with a well-circumscribed circumferential edge. Patches of columnar epithelium separated from the cardia with sheets of squamous mucosa are remnants of fetal epithelium and do not represent Barrett's esophagus.

Prevalence

Barrett's esophagus is not the medical rarity or curiosity it was once thought to be. An increased awareness of the condition and use of flexible esophagoscopy resulted in an increased number of clinically diagnosed cases (8). Among all patients undergoing upper gastrointestinal endoscopy, the prevalence of Barrett's esophagus varies between 0.45% to 2.2% (9). The prevalence is about 10% to 20% when only patients with symptomatic gastroesophageal reflux are considered, and it approaches 30% to 50% in patients receiving endoscopy for peptic strictures (10). A large multicenter European study reported nearly 15,000 patients with foregut symptoms undergoing upper gastrointestinal endoscopy (11). Barrett's esophagus was proven histologically in 111 patients. A similar North American study reported data for 51,311 patients undergoing clinically indicated upper gastrointestinal endoscopy (12). Barrett's esophagus without an associated carcinoma was documented histologically in 450 patients with a prevalence of 8.9 per 1000. Barrett's esophagus was twice as prevalent in men. The prevalence increased with age and reached a plateau in the seventh to ninth decade with about half of the final prevalence achieved by age 40. The disease was far more prevalent in whites than in blacks. The prevalence of Barrett's esophagus in the population at large is unknown, but it is presumed to be higher than in symptomatic patients undergoing endoscopy. The known acid insensitivity of Barrett's esophagus lends support to this proposition. Indeed, in one study 40% of patients with biopsy-proven Barrett's esophagus had no evidence of gastroesophageal reflux (11). In a study comparing clinical and autopsy findings, Cameron et al. (12) reported a prevalence of 22.6 cases per 100,000 in patients who required upper endoscopy. Based on that prevalence, 0.19 cases of Barrett's esophagus were expected in 226 autopsies performed in Olmstead County. Four cases were actually observed, corresponding to an estimated prevalence of 376 cases per 100,000 population. Among 7 cases of Barrett's esophagus detected in 733 autopsies in Olmstead and surrounding rural counties, 5 were undiagnosed before death. The likelihood that most subjects with Barrett's esophagus are asymptomatic suggests that the clinically diagnosed cases represent only the tip of a large iceberg. This hypothesis, if proven, is of major epidemiologic and economic impact.

Etiology

The etiology of Barrett's esophagus has been shrouded in controversy. The suggestion by Barrett of a congenital etiology has been challenged by others who proposed an acquired derivation secondary to gastroesophageal reflux (2). Compelling clinical and experimental evidence supports the concept that Barrett's esophagus results from severe gastroesophageal reflux in which the injured esophageal mucosa becomes replaced by the inherently more acid resistant columnar epithelium.

Using a dog model, Bremner et al. (13) was among the first to show experimentally that stripping of the lower esophageal squamous mucosa coupled with surgical creation of gastroesophageal reflux resulted in reepithelialization of the lower esophagus with columnar epithelium. These results have not been reproduced consistently by other investigators, who found that most injuries to the squamous epithelium healed by scarring and stricture formation rather than by metaplastic epithelium (14). The variations in the results of animal experiments may be secondary to species variation or inability to recreate the intraluminal esophageal milieu accurately, thus favoring columnar metaplasia.

Clinical evidence supporting an acquired etiology is more compelling (15, 16). The great majority of patients diagnosed with Barrett's esophagus have severe gastroesophageal reflux. Although there is a bimodal age distribution for Barrett's esophagus, the majority of cases are diagnosed in the fifth or sixth decade of life, with well-documented cases only rarely seen in patients under 10 years of age. Additionally, Goldman and Beckman (17) reported a carefully documented case in which progressive cephalad extension of the metaplastic epithelium was noted in the presence of ongoing severe gastroesophageal reflux. Although similar instances admittedly are quite rare, such observations provide strong support for the acquired theory of Barrett's esophagus. The development of columnar metaplasia also has been noted after esophagogastrectomy and Heller's myotomy, presumably as a result of florid gastroesophageal reflux in the absence of a lower esophageal sphincter. The high association between gastroesophageal reflux and the columnar-lined esophagus supports the theory that Barrett's esophagus is an acquired condition. However, one cannot totally dismiss the possibility of a genetic predisposition. The great majority of patients with gastroesophageal reflux heal their esophageal injury by squamous epithelium and do not develop columnar metaplasia. When metaplasia develops, it is twofold to threefold more common in males, especially whites, and malignant degeneration appears to occur almost exclusively in white men. The rare but definite occurrence of familial clusters of Barrett's esophagus is intriguing. Fahmy and King (18) described four families with strong familial expression of Barrett's/gastroesophageal reflux complex spanning four generations with two to seven affected members per family. Jochem and colleagues (19) reported a family with six cases of Barrett's esophagus in three generations, three of whom developed adenocarcinoma. The pattern of inheritance appears to be autosomal dominant, but it is unclear whether reflux or columnar metaplasia is the transmitted trait. Clearly, there is no satisfactory explanation regarding why some patients develop columnar metaplasia while others do not. At this time Barrett's esophagus and gastroesophageal reflux disease should be considered highly associated disorders without a definite etiologic relationship.

HISTOGENESIS

The cell of origin of Barrett's metaplasia is unknown. Generally, three theories are proposed for metaplastic transformation. Stem cell metaplasia occurs when primordial stem cells differentiate into cells resembling the original cell type of the organ involved. Metaplasia also can occur when a fully differentiated cell undergoes metaplastic transformation, either during cell division (indirect metaplasia) or without cell divison (direct metaplasia).

The columnar metaplasia of Barrett's esophagus has several possible origins. Direct metaplasia or indirect metaplasia can occur in the epithelium normally lining the gastric cardia, the submucosal esophageal glands, or the squamous epithelium of the lower esophagus. The concept of "healing" of erosive esophagitis by upward migration of the epithelium lining the gastric cardia was advanced by Hayward in 1961 (20). Bremner (13) has since produced experimental evidence supporting this concept when similar migration occurred after stripping the lower esophageal squamous membrane in a dog model with iatrogenic gastroesophageal reflux. An alternative theory suggests that the columnar epithelium of the submucosal esophageal gland could also be the source of the metaplastic epithelium. Gillen and colleagues (21) demonstrated in animal experiments that the creation of gastroesophageal reflux in the dog, along with excising a strip of squamous mucosa several centimeters above the cardia, resulted in healing of the denuded area by columnar epithelium. Neither possibility seems to explain readily the morphologic and ultrastructural heterogeneity of Barrett's metaplasia and its differences from the presumed tissue of origin. Using transmission electron microscopy, Levine and coworkers (22) reported ultrastructural features of Barrett's epithelium in 28 patients (134 biopsy specimens) and compared them with biopsy specimens obtained from normal jejunum, normal stomach, esophageal glands, and normal and gastric intestinal metaplasia. Barrett's specialized metaplastic cells included mucous cells resembling those seen in the normal gastric surface or pits, goblet cells similar to those of normal jejunum, and pseudoabsorptive cells with features common to both gastric secretory and jejunal absorptive cells. The subcellular organelles involved in normal mucous synthesis, namely the rough endoplasmic reticulum, glycogen aggregates, Golgi apparatus, and mucus-secreting granules, had features in common with those in mucus-secreting cells in the gastric pits and surface. The remarkable morphologic heterogeneity of Barrett's esophagus suggests a stem cell metaplasia with the gastric mucous neck cell being the likely cell of origin. The location of gastric mucous neck cells in sites close to the origin of Barrett's esophagus, and their ultrastructural similarities to Barrett's metaplastic mucous and some pseudoabsorptive cells, is consistent with that hypothesis. However, the wide spectrum of pseudoabsorptive cells and the presence of intermediate cell types not normally present in the gastrointestinal tract suggest the possibility of various pathways of stem cell differentiation or the presence of a yet unidentified stem cell.

PATHOLOGY

A definite diagnosis of Barrett's esophagus is made only after histologic documentation. Trier (23) recognized that the metaplastic epithelium is clearly distinct from that of the gastric cardia, fundus, or intestinal epithelium. Paull et al. (24) provided a more comprehensive definition of the three types of columnar metaplasia encountered in Barrett's esophagus. The fundic-type mucosa is characterized by the presence of chief and partial cells in the deeper part of the glands in addition to the surface mucus-secreting cells

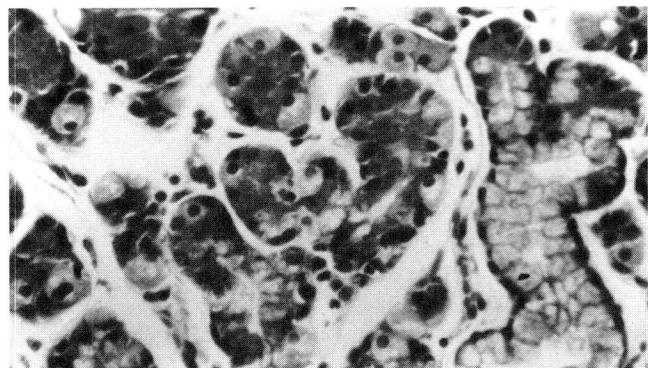

FIGURE 27.1. Fundic-type mucosa exhibits gastric mucous cells as well as parietal and chief cells.

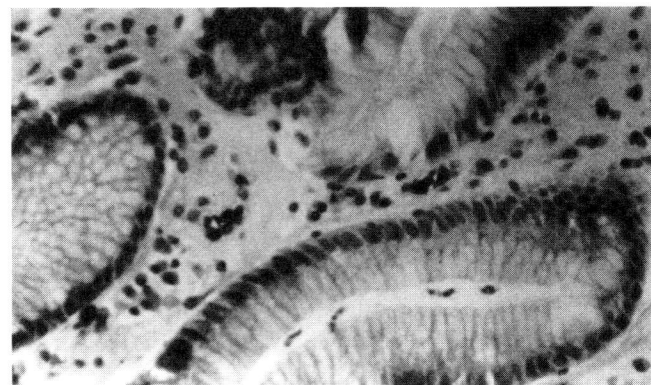

FIGURE 27.2. Junctional-type mucosa are shown in which the glands are lined mainly by mucin-secreting cells.

(Fig. 27.1). The latter usually contain neutral sialomucins and do not stain with Alcian blue, pH 2.5. The junctional type of epithelium resembles that of the gastric cardia and is composed predominately of mucus-secreting cells lining the surface and pits of the glands (Fig. 27.2). The specialized or intestinal type, the distinctive type of epithelium for Barrett's esophagus, is present in virtually all adult cases and is the type most commonly associated with malignant degeneration (Fig. 27.3). The specialized epithelium resembles that of the small bowel with a villiform surface lined by mucus-secreting cells as well as goblet cells that stain positively for acid nonsulfated mucins.

Scanning electron microscopy shows the remarkable topographic heterogeneity of the metaplastic epithelium. Zwas and colleagues (25) reported three different cell types other than goblet cells that were noted on scanning electron microscopy. The gastriclike cell, present in 31% of specimens, resembled normal gastric surface cells and was polygonal in shape with a bulging central core of mucus outlined by a rim of short microvilli. The intestinal-type cells, seen in 40% of specimens, resembled normal surface intestinal cells and were polygonal in shape with a complement of dense microvilli. The variant cell type was encountered most commonly (seen in 80% of specimens) and displayed various topographic subtypes. Variant cells were not encountered in the normal gastrointestinal tract. Interestingly, on light microscopy variant cells usually were classified as intestinal-type metaplasia.

The functional capacity of Barrett's metaplasia is uncertain. The ability of the fundic-type epithelium to secrete acid, particularly after histamine stimulation, has been shown by some investigators (26), but except in rare instances is probably of little clinical significance. Pepsinogen granules also have been demonstrated in chief cells of the fundic-type epithelium both by gel electrophoresis (27) and by immunohistochem-

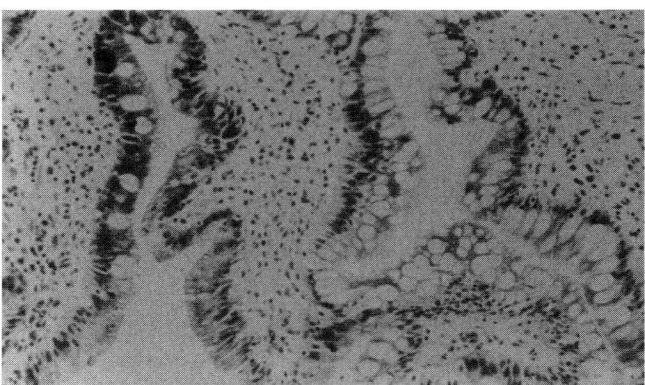

FIGURE 27.3. Intestinal-type (specialized) mucosa is thrown into a villiform pattern with prominent goblet cells.

istry (28); however, they probably are of minimal functional significance. The specialized-type epithelium lacks a well-defined brush border and has low levels of brush border enzymes that do not absorb micellar lipids. A recent immunohistochemical study showed that the specialized epithelium also contained endocrine cells immunoreactive to antiserum against serotonin, glycogen, somatostatin, and pancreatic polypeptide (29).

DYSPLASIA IN BARRETT'S ESOPHAGUS

The exact prevalence of dysplasia among patients with Barrett's esophagus is unknown. In one study epithelial dysplasia was observed in 7 (6.3%) of 111 patients with histologically documented Barrett's esophagus (11). Six patients had low-grade dysplasia and one had high grade, and all seven were found in association with intestinal-type epithelium. In a study of 81 patients with Barrett's esophagus, the prevalence of low-grade dysplasia was 12.5%, and another 12.5% of patients developed low-grade dysplasia after a mean follow-up of 3.6 years (30). From a histopathologic standpoint, dysplasia is defined as unequivocal neoplastic alteration of the epithelium based on both architectural and cytologic changes. Architecturally, the glands show branching and crowding with back-to-back arrangement in some cases. Cytologically, there is prominent cytoplasmic basophilia, and the nuclei are enlarged with an increased nuclear to cytoplasmic ratio. Pleomorphism, hyperchromatism, nuclear stratification, and loss of nuclear polarity also are seen. Dysplastic cells also display diminished mucus secretion. The classification of dysplasia into high-grade (Fig. 27.4), low-grade (Fig. 27.5), and indefinite dysplasia categories is based on a similar classification of dysplasia in inflammatory bowel disease (31). Reactive or regenerative changes usually occur in areas adjacent to ulcerations and represent inflammatory changes that are sometimes difficult to differentiate from low-grade dysplasia and occasionally from high-grade dysplasia.

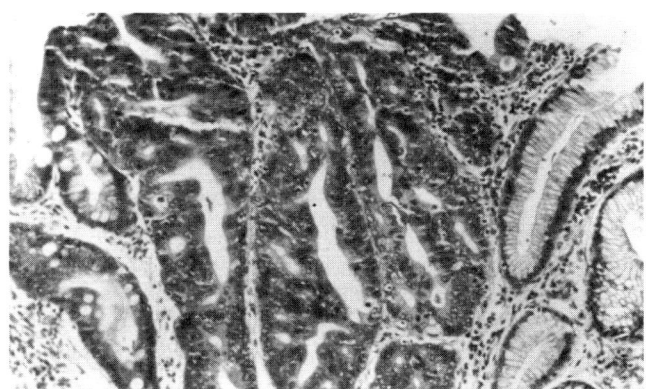

FIGURE 27.4. High-grade dysplasia. Disorganized architecture is apparent with back-to-back crowding of the glands as well as pronounced nuclear atypia and reversal of polarity.

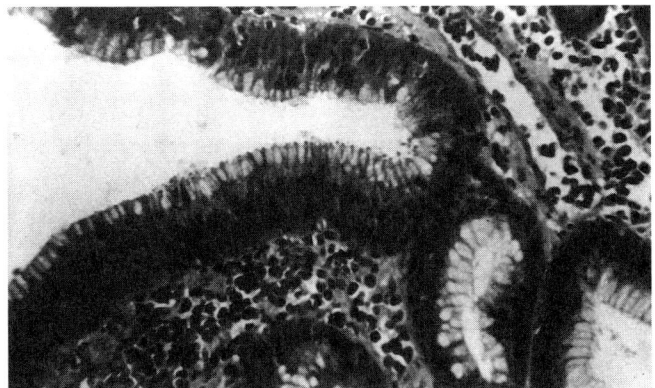

FIGURE 27.5. Low-grade dysplasia. The nuclei are hyperchromatic and stratified, but changes are mainly confined to the basal aspect of the cells.

Such cases often are included in the indefinite category. Interobserver agreement is 86% for high-grade dysplasia, 72% for low-grade dysplasia, and even lower for regenerative epithelial changes (32). Because of this significant interobserver variability and the clinical and prognostic importance of a diagnosis of dysplasia in Barrett's esophagus, biopsies usually are reviewed by more than one experienced cytopathologist before confirming the diagnosis.

DYSPLASIA-CARCINOMA SEQUENCE

Compelling clinicopathologic evidence supports the concept of a dysplasia-carcinoma sequence in the pathogenesis of Barrett's adenocarcinoma. Hamilton and colleagues (33) studied the clinical and pathologic features of adenocarcinoma in Barrett's esophagus in 26 patients. High-grade dysplasia was seen in the adjacent metaplastic epithelium in 89% of resected specimens. Interestingly, the investigators observed two separate adenocarcinomas in three cases: one case of adenocarcinoid tumor, one of adenosquamous, and one of an adenocarcinoma and a separate squamous cell carcinoma arising in an island of squamous epithelium. Schmidt et al. (34) compared the prevalence of dysplasia in Barrett's epithelium in patients with Barrett's adenocarcinoma and those with Barrett's epithelium without associated adenocarcinoma. Dysplasia of various degrees was noted in 18 of 23 specimens with carcinoma, usually in the immediate vicinity of the invasive cancer, whereas in the benign group dysplasia was present in 2 of 38 patients studied. Conversely, in a series of 10 patients resected for high-grade dysplasia without preoperative evidence of carcinoma, invasive carcinoma was found in 5 patients (35). The tumors often were located in sites remote from the location of preoperative biopsies of high-grade dysplasia. Furthermore, two patients had at least two separate foci of invasive carcinoma. The clear association between high-grade dysplasia and adenocarcinoma has been reported by several other investigators (36, 37). However, most studies were done in patients with established carcinoma, and they merely indicate that high-grade dysplasia is highly associated with adenocarcinoma and may be a marker for an associated invasive carcinoma.

Importantly, others have observed the progression from metaplasia to dysplasia and finally to invasive carcinoma. Ried et al. (38) reported 62 patients with Barrett's esophagus, 8 without an associated carcinoma, who were followed prospectively for a mean interval of 34 months. Five patients developed carcinoma over a period of 18 to 60 months. Two patients had high-grade dysplasia upon initial endoscopy and developed invasive carcinoma at 18 and 19 months of follow-up. Two patients initially had low-grade dysplasia and a third had metaplasia without dysplasia, all of whom progressed to high-grade dysplasia and eventually invasive carcinoma over 19 to 55 months of follow-up. Robertson and colleagues (39) followed 56 patients prospectively, 3 of whom developed carcinoma, of which 2 were preceded by worsening dysplasia. Similarly, 5 of 50 patients followed endoscopically by Hameteman and colleagues (40) for 5 years developed carcinoma preceded by high-grade dysplasia. These data clearly support the concept that high-grade dysplasia is a precursor lesion of carcinoma, and they document the metaplasia-dysplasia-carcinoma sequence. The frequency and tempo of that progression remain unclear.

PREVALENCE AND INCIDENCE OF ADENOCARCINOMA

The reported prevalence of Barrett's adenocarcinoma varies between 0% and 46%. The significant variability in prevalence figures is influenced primarily by the nature of referral patterns. Surgical reports are naturally biased toward patients with established carcinoma, whereas series reported from centers with an established interest in Barrett's esophagus may include patients referred with known dysplastic lesions, who thus are not representative of a general community-based practice. Nonetheless, the prevalence of a Barrett's adenocarcinoma is probably in the range of 10% to 15% (41, 42, 43). However, the prevalence rate of an event is the proportion of individuals in a group having the event at one point in time and thus is a static measure of that event. Incidence rates, conversely, measure the frequency of an event over time when:

Incidence = number of events per time period ÷ number of individuals at risk

Defined as such, the incidence of adenocarcinoma in patients with Barrett's esophagus remains controversial. Cameron and coworkers (42) followed 104 patients for an average of 8.5 years, and only 2 patients developed carcinoma for an incidence of 1 of 441 cases per year of follow-up. Spechler et al. (41) followed 105 patients for an average of 3.3 years, and 2 patients developed carcinoma after 5.3 and 8 years, respectively. In one of the few prospective studies evaluating the incidence of adenocarcinoma in Barrett's esophagus, Robertson and colleagues (39) reported an incidence of 1 case in 56 patient-years of follow-up. Compiling data from various reports, the average incidence is approximately 1 in 200 patient-years of follow-up. These figures represent a 30-fold to 40-fold increase in the incidence of carcinoma of the esophagus beyond that expected in adult white males. Assuming an average incidence of 0.5% per year, Spechler (43) estimates the incidence of Barrett's adenocarcinoma to be 500 in 100,000, which exceeds that of lung cancer in white men over 65 years of age. A recent report by Blot et al. (44) stated that the incidence of adenocarcinoma of the esophagus and cardia increased at 10% per year during the 1980s, thus exceeding the increases in incidence of cutaneous melanoma, non-Hodgkin's lymphoma, and lung cancer. By the mid-1980s esophageal adenocarcinoma accounted for 30% to 40% of all esophageal cancers, whereas adenocarcinoma of the cardia accounted for 50% of all gastric cancers. There is persuasive evidence that both of these malignancies are highly associated with Barrett's esophagus. Unfortunately, most incidence reports are retrospective and include only a small number of patients followed for a short period. Furthermore, the dismissal of adenocarcinoma of the cardia as gastric cancer may further underestimate the incidence of Barrett's adenocarcinoma. Hamilton et al. (45) reported that careful pathologic examination of surgically resected specimens of adenocarcinomas of the esophagus and cardia revealed evidence of metaplastic columnar epithelia in 64% of patients, only half of which were recognized preoperatively. Additionally, the epidemiologic and morphologic similarities between carcinomas of the esophagus and the gastric cardia have been well described (46). Both tumors are thus quite likely to be associated with Barrett's esophagus, which on occasion is overgrown totally and replaced by carcinoma.

PATHOPHYSIOLOGY OF ESOPHAGEAL ADENOCARCINOMA

The high prevalence of various degrees of dysplastic lesions, as well as the multiplicity of invasive carcinoma in resected specimens of patients with Barrett's adenocarcinoma, suggests that the entire columnar lining is driven towards malignant transformation. The agents propelling this drive are unknown, but gastroesophageal reflux remains one of the likeliest culprits. The relatively high incidence and prevalence of esophageal adenocarcinoma in patients with Barrett's esophagus is well documented. Skinner and coworkers (7) compared patients with malignant and benign Barrett's esophagus and found that 13 of 20 patients with Barrett's adenocarcinoma had long-standing histories of heartburn and regurgitation; only 3 additional patients with malignant strictures had evidence of severe reflux demonstrated by 24-hour pH testing. Similarly, Harle et al. (47) reported that 59% of patients with Barrett's adenocarcinoma had a prior history of gastroesophageal reflux. Generally, patients with Barrett's adenocarcinoma have a longer duration of reflux symptoms compared with those with benign metaplasia; they are, on average, 5 years older than patients without an associated malignancy. These data imply that long-standing uncontrolled reflux may be an important etiologic agent in the development of carcinoma. The exact component of the refluxate implicated in the process is unknown. Some evidence suggests that patients with increased esophageal alkaline exposure are more prone to develop complications of Barrett's esophagus, such as strictures, ulcers, and carcinoma, compared with patients in whom the refluxate is primarily acidic in composition (48). In a small number of patients studied by hepatobiliary scanning and esophageal pH testing, DeMeester and colleagues (49) showed that 5 of 10 patients with duodenogastric reflux had increased esophageal alkaline exposure as well, whereas none of the patients without duodenogastric reflux had increased esophageal alkaline exposure. Complications of Barrett's esophagus, including strictures, ulcers, and dysplasia, were noted more commonly in patients with increased esophageal alkaline exposure, whereas esophageal acid exposure was similar in patients with or without complications. Dysplasia, specifically, was encountered in 6 (43%) of 14 patients who had abnormal alkaline reflux; however, it also was seen in 20% of patients with normal alkaline exposure. Although the available clinical evidence suggests a possible role of alkaline reflux in the pathogenesis of complications of Barrett's esophagus, including dysplasia, the exact magnitude of its contribution and its interaction with the acid component of the refluxate remains to be clarified.

Experimental evidence derived from animal models also seems to support the role for alkaline reflux in the genesis of esophageal adenocarcinoma. Pera et al. (50) evaluated the influence of esophagojejunostomy on the induction of adenocarcinoma of the distal esophagus in rats receiving subcutaneous injections of 2,6 dimethylnitromorpholine (2,6 DMNM), a known esophageal carcinogen. Among 80 animals without a preexisting esophagojejunostomy who received 2,6 DMNM in two different doses, 15 developed carcinoma of the esophagus, all of which were of the squamous cell type. Adenocarcinoma of the esophagus occurred exclusively in animals receiving the carcinogen following a surgically created esophagojejunostomy. Esophageal adenocarcinoma occurred in the middle and distal thirds of the esophagus in 23 of 74 animals. Histopathologically, these tumors displayed remarkable morphologic similarity to their human counterparts. Interestingly, 11 animals with prolonged reflux esophagitis had foci of glandular metaplasia that probably were the precursors of carcinoma in that model. Using a nearly similar experimental design, Pera et al. (51) examined the separate and combined influences of biliary and pancreatic components of the alkaline refluxate in the induction of esophageal adenocarcinoma. Sprague-Dawley rats with surgically created esophagojejunostomies were treated with subcutaneous injections of 2,6 DMNM. Using surgical diversion techniques, the esophagus was subjected to isolated biliary duodenal juice in one group, pancreatic duodenal juice in another, and combined biliary and pancreatic secretions in a third group. Esophageal adenocarcinoma occurred only in the groups subjected to pancreatic reflux and combined pancreatic and biliary reflux. Thirteen percent of animals in the pancreatic reflux group developed carcinoma, compared with 33% of animals in the combined reflux group. None of the animals receiving the carcinogen and subjected to isolated biliary reflux developed esophageal carcinoma. The clinical relevance of these interesting experiments is unclear at this time. The degree of esophageal injury in control animals (not receiving the carcinogen) with an established esophagojejunostomy is unlike that seen in humans with Barrett's esophagus or erosive esophagitis. Despite the severity of esophageal injury, no carcinoma was found in any of the control animals.

The role of an as yet unidentified carcinogen or a variety of co-carcinogens in the genesis of esophageal adenocarcinoma in humans remains unclear. Peters and coworkers (52) evaluated the level of glutathione and glutathione S-transferase, one of the biotransformation enzymes, in tissue samples obtained at endoscopy from patients with Barrett's esophagus; they compared them with tissue levels in normal esophageal and gastric epithelium. Glutathione levels and glutathione S-transferase activity were significantly lower in Barrett's epithelium compared with normal squamous esophageal epithelium. Deficiency or absence of glutathione S-transferase activity has been correlated with an increased risk of lung cancer in smokers (53), as well as with an increased risk of colon and gastric cancer (54). Biotransformation enzymes such as glutathione transferase serve primarily as detoxifying agents, and their deficiency may result in increased cellular or cytogenetic damage from a variety of noxious agents.

Consumption of alcoholic beverages or tobacco has not been evaluated adequately in patients with Barrett's adenocarcinoma. However, most retrospective analyses suggest a minor contributing role with no significant difference between patients and controls in either alcohol intake or smoking habits. In a case control study evaluating the relationship between tobacco and alcohol and the risk of esophageal adenocarcinoma, 60% of the cases were nonsmokers and 47% were nondrinkers (55). These figures were similar to those of the control group, leading the authors to conclude that there was no apparent relationship between tobacco or alcohol use in the development of esophageal adenocarcinoma.

BIOLOGY OF BARRETT'S ESOPHAGUS

The histologic progression from metaplasia to dysplasia and eventually to carcinoma appears to be mirrored at the cellular and molecular level by corresponding abnormalities in cell cycle, DNA content, and oncogene expression.

DNA ABNORMALITIES

Flow cytometric analysis has shown an increase in the prevalence of aneuploidy in a subset of patients with Barrett's esophagus (56). The incidence of aneuploidy seems to correlate with the increase in severity of the known histologic markers of malignancy. Reid (57) reported 182 patients seen at the University of Washington over several years. The prevalence of aneuploidy was 4% in nondysplastic mucosa, 6% in specimens with low-grade dysplasia, and 63% and 86% in patients with high-grade dysplasia and invasive carcinoma, respectively. Because mucosal biopsies from normal gastric and normal esophageal epithelium are almost always diploid in DNA content, the presence of aneuploidy in a small fraction of patients with metaplasia is especially intriguing. The ability of aneuploid clones to extend over large areas of the esophageal mucosa and to persist for a long period has been well documented (58). Additionally, aneuploidy in patients with metaplasia and those with various degrees of dysplasia is associated with underlying karyotypic abnormalities in the form of chromosomal rearrangement and the presence of marker chromosomes. Raskind et al. (58) reported three patients with cytogenetic abnormalities detected in their metaplastic epithelium who eventually developed either high-grade dysplasia or adenocarcinoma over 5 to 6 years of follow-up. In all three patients the karyotypic abnormalities were present 1 to 4 years before the diagnosis of carcinoma. These abnormal clones were noted in samples obtained over a large area of esophagus, suggesting that in regions of benign histology an abnormal clone may arise, develop a growth advantage, and eventually acquire invasive capacity.

A characteristic feature of aneuploidy in Barrett's esophagus is the multiplicity of abnormal clones commonly seen in patients with high-grade dysplasia and or Barrett's adenocarcinoma. Rabinovitch and coworkers (59) studied abnormalities in DNA content in resected and endoscopic specimens of 14 patients with Barrett's esophagus and an associated adenocarcinoma. Multiple aneuploid populations were noted in 12 patients, including one patient who had 14 overlapping aneuploid populations. The resected specimen of that patient had an intramucosal carcinoma with adjacent dysplasia, both of which were encompassed within a large 4.6 to 4.7 N aneuploid population, suggesting that a subclone contained within that area acquired the malignant phenotype. The multiplicity of abnormal clones suggests a field cancerization effect rendering the entire mucosal surface genetically unstable.

CHROMOSOMAL AND ONCOGENE ABNORMALITIES

Chromosomal abnormalities have been shown to result in activation of protooncogenes or loss of tumor suppressor genes in a variety of hematologic malignancies and solid tumors. A recent cytogenetic study identified a nonrandom chromosomal rearrangement in patients with esophageal adenocarcinoma (60). Rodriguez and coworkers (60) performed cytogenetic analysis on nine adenocarcinomas of the esophagus and gastroesophageal junctions, including three patients with associated Barrett's metaplasia. A specific region of chromosomal rearrangement involving chromosome 11 (11p-13-15) was found in eight tumors, including all three adenocarcinomas associated with Barrett's metaplasia. Abnormalities involving the 11p-13-15 region are commonly found in other solid tumors, and their significance in the neoplastic progression of Barrett's metaplasia is unclear. Cytogenetic analysis of short-term cultures of Barrett's metaplasia identified clonal abnormalities in 9 of 10 patients, including a t(3,6) in one patient, trisomy of chromosome 5 and 7 in one, and loss of the Y chromosome in seven patients (61). Abnormalities involving chromosome 11 were not observed, suggesting that rearrangements involving 11p-13-15 may be a late event in the development of invasive carcinomas. The c-*ras*-Ha-1 protooncogene has been mapped to the 11p-13-15 region, but mutational activation of c-*ras* has not been shown to occur in either Barrett's adenocarcinoma or dysplasia (62). A rearrangement-mediated deregulation may result in c-*ras* activation in such instances. Amplifications of several other protooncogenes have been reported in esophageal adenocarcinoma, including the *erb*B-2 (63) and epidermal growth factor receptor genes (64); however, direct evidence of consistent involvement in the pathogenesis of esophageal adenocarcinoma is still lacking.

Using restriction fragment length polymorphisms, Blount and coworkers (65) showed 17p allelic deletions in 12 (92%) of 13 patients with Barrett's adenocarcinoma. The deletions were seen in early (intramucosal) as well as more advanced tumors and are in keeping with the high prevalence of 17p allelic deletions seen in a variety of other tumors, particularly colon cancer, a tumor with an established dysplasia-carcinoma sequence of progression. The tumor suppressor gene, *p53*, has been mapped to the short arm of chromosome 17 and is the most commonly mutated gene in a variety of human tumors (66). Progression from adenoma to carcinoma in colon cancer has been shown to be associated with a *p53* point mutation that often precedes the development of carcinoma (66). Mutations of *p53* also have been shown to occur in some patients with Barrett's adenocarcinoma. Casson and coworkers (67) identified *p53* mutations in 1 of 14 patients with esophageal adenocarcinoma and in four specimens of Barrett's epithelium present adjacent to invasive adenocarcinoma. *p53* Mutations in Barrett's metaplasia were localized to exon 5 with no mutations detected in the associated adenocarcinoma. Conversely, in the only tumor with *p53* mutations (exon 8) in that series, no mutations were found in the adjoining Barrett's mucosa. Interestingly, specimens of Barrett's mucosa harboring *p53* mutations showed minimal or no dysplasia histologically. Furthermore, identical mutations were identified within separate regions of the same specimen. These observations suggest that *p53* mutations probably (*a*) are early molecular events prompted by dysregulated cellular growth, and (*b*) may confer a growth advantage allowing clonal expansion. Several recent reports have correlated overexpression of the p53 protein product, detected by immunohistochemistry or two-parameter flow cytometry, with increased histologic risk for malignancy (68, 69). Younes et al. (69) reported that p53 protein was not detected by immunohistochemical staining in 53 biopsies without evidence of dysplasia. The probability of positive staining increased to 9% for low-grade dysplasia and 55% for high-grade dysplasia, and it approached 90% with established invasive carcinoma. The value of accumulations of p53 protein in Barrett's mucosa as a biomarker of an increased risk for high-grade dysplasia or carcinoma awaits long-term prospective studies.

CELL CYCLE ABNORMALITIES

Increased cellular proliferation has been shown in at least some patients with Barrett's esophagus since the late 1970s (70). Autoradiographic studies using tritiated thymidine showed an increase in the overall population of proliferative cells in Barrett's metaplasia, particularly the intestinal-type mucosa as well as extension of the proliferative zone from the neck to the rest of the glands. Immunohistochemical studies using antibodies to proliferation-associated antigens, such as Ki67 (71) and proliferative cell nuclear antigen (PCNA) (72), have confirmed the increase in proliferative indices noted by autoradiography. Using an antibody to PCNA, Jankowski et al. (72) showed an extension of the proliferative compartment from the neck to the superficial layers of the gland in specimens with high-grade dysplasia. The PCNA labeling index was highest in adenocarcinoma and high-grade dysplasia (25%), followed by intestinal-type mucosa (20%) and gastric-type metaplasia (12%). A more detailed analysis of cell cycle abnormalities in Barrett's esophagus was offered by Reid and colleagues (71) using Ki67/DNA content multiparameter flow cytometry, a technique developed by his group that allows a correlative assessment of ploidy and cell cycle events. Control specimens obtained from gastric mucosa showed the majority of the cells were in the G0 phase of the cell cycle. In contrast, almost one third of the cells in Barrett's metaplasia with or without dysplasia were cycling in G1. An increase in S phase (DNA synthesis) beyond control levels also was found in Barrett's metaplasia and was more significantly noted in aneuploid populations. Previous work from the same group (73) also showed an increase in the G2 fraction in patients at high risk for developing high-grade dysplasia. These abnormalities suggest that in Barrett's esophagus a substantial fraction of cells are mobilized from G0 to G1 and that, ultimately, in some cells there is loss of control of the G1-/S-phase transition, with an increase in S fraction especially in cells with aneuploid DNA content. The final event is an accumulation of cells in the G2 phase of the cell cycle before mitosis, when failure of DNA reparative mechanisms may allow emergence of abnormal clones.

SURVEILLANCE

Reports of the rising incidence of esophageal adenocarcinoma, as well as the dismal survival rates of patients presenting with carcinoma of the esophagus, have prompted some clinicians to enroll patients with Barrett's esophagus in endoscopic surveillance programs. Controversy persists, however, regarding the value of surveillance in reducing the mortality from esophageal cancer as well as the cost effectiveness of that approach. Some have estimated the cost of detection of one cancer to be $62,000 and 78 days of lost work (74). Missing from such an assessment, however, is the cost of medical care provided to patients presenting with established, often advanced, adenocarcinoma of the esophagus/cardia who undergo a variety of invasive procedures with a substantial number of work days lost. The cost effectiveness of screening programs remains controversial. Clearly, the methods for surveillance, namely endoscopic-directed biopsies, need to be replaced by equally effective and far less expensive techniques. Cytologic screening using abrasive brushing via a nasogastric tube has been used and could represent a major advance in cost containment (75). The question of reduction of cancer-related mortality appears to be answered more readily. Several reports have now confirmed an improved survival rate of patients with esophageal adenocarcinoma detected through a surveillance program (35, 76). Lerut et al. (76) reported a 92% survival rate after esophagectomy, whereas in another experience a survival of 100% was achieved in a group of patients undergoing curative (en bloc) resection for high-grade dysplasia and found to have an associated invasive carcinoma (35).

In our surveillance protocol, patients with Barrett's esophagus undergo endoscopic surveillance with at least two biopsies obtained at 1- to 2-cm intervals throughout the length of the Barrett's segment. A brush cytology is always performed because, occasionally, malignant cells are found with that technique that are not detectable otherwise. In the absence of dysplasia, patients are seen on an annual or biannual basis, and patients with low-grade dysplasia are seen in follow-up every 6 to 12 months. Patients with high-grade dysplasia are seen for repeat endoscopy and rebiopsy immediately, and all biopsy specimens are reviewed by at least two experienced cytopathologists. Confirmation of the diagnosis of high-grade dysplasia should be followed by surgical resection in the absence of a compelling contraindication. The incidence of an associated invasive, often early, carcinoma in such instances approaches 50%.

The interobserver variation in the grading of dysplasia, particularly low grade, has prompted a search for other markers of malignancy. Aneuploidy and an increase in the G2/tetraploid fraction have been evaluated thoroughly and advocated by some groups (72). This technique requires retrieval of large biopsy specimens and an experienced flow cytometry laboratory, both of which may be available only in major medical centers. In one study six out of nine patients who had an increased G2/tetraploid fraction beyond 7% developed carcinoma over a follow-up period of 2 to 5 years (38). However, all six patients developed high-grade dysplasia before the diagnosis of cancer. Other biomarkers for carcinoma under consideration include p53 protein expression (69), increased ornithine decarboxylase activity (77), epidermal growth factor receptor, and transforming growth factor–α expression (78), mucin histochemistry (79), and the presence of nucleolar organizer regions (80).

OTHER PREMALIGNANT LESIONS

ACHALASIA

The first report of esophageal carcinoma associated with achalasia of the cardia was by Fagge in 1872 (81). Several investigators have since confirmed that association, and prevalence rates have varied between 0% and 20% per year. This wide range was probably caused by an initial confusion of incidence and prevalence figures as well as the variability in the length of follow-up periods reported in each study. Ellis (82) reported an "incidence" of 24% among 24 patients seen at the Mayo Clinic between 1944 and 1952, whereas Chuong et al. (83) did not observe a single case of esophageal cancer among 91 patients followed for a period of 6 years. The prevalence of carcinoma of the esophagus in patients with achalasia is probably about 7%. In a recent retrospective analysis of 147 patients who underwent esophagomyotomy, 10 were found to have developed carcinoma of the esophagus over a 23-year period of follow-up (84). In one of the few prospective studies, 195 patients with confirmed achalasia treated by pneumatic dilation were followed by esophagoscopy and biopsy on a biannual basis (85). Three patients developed carcinoma of the esophagus an average of 5.8 years after the diagnosis of achalasia and 17 years after the onset of symptoms. The observed incidence was 33-fold higher than that expected in the general population. Importantly, two of the three patients had early tumors that were resected successfully with long-term disease free survival.

The role of long-standing esophageal obstruction with its attendant retention esophagitis and bacterial overgrowth in the pathogenesis of esophageal carcinoma seems plausible but is as yet unproven. Most studies report patients with advanced achalasia, and it is not possible to assess the influence of early and effective esophageal drainage on the probability of subsequent malignant degeneration. Furthermore, a number of patients develop esophageal carcinoma despite an effective esophagomyotomy or pneumatic dilation and often after many years of follow-up.

Squamous cell carcinoma is the predominant cell type, and the tumor is located primarily in the middle third of the esophagus. The tumors are quite advanced in the majority of patients, primarily because of the insidious nature of the symptoms, which often are indistinguishable from the preexisting symptoms of achalasia. Additionally, the dilated esophagus allows the tumor to grow to a substantial size before producing significant luminal obstruction. Approximately 80% of tumors are thus unresectable at the time of diagnosis with dismal survival rates. Early detection offers the only hope for a meaningful and perhaps curative intervention.

CHRONIC ESOPHAGITIS

Studies in high-risk areas for esophageal cancer such as Central Asia, Northern China, and Iran have consistently indicated a higher prevalence of chronic esophagitis compared with that in low-risk areas, suggesting that it is a precursor lesion for squamous cell carcinoma of the esophagus. Data from limited follow-up studies demonstrated the progression of chronic esophagitis to more advanced lesions such as dysplasia and eventually carcinoma. In the high-risk population of Huixian in Northern China, the prevalence of esophagitis approaches 50% in adults over 35 years old and 40% in younger individuals (86). Interestingly, in neighboring areas with a lower incidence of esophageal cancer, the incidence of chronic esophagitis is only 17% (86). Within the high-incidence areas of esophageal cancer, the occurrence of esophagitis is significantly higher in patients from households with another esophageal cancer patient than in control subjects from households without esophageal cancer. These differences could not be accounted for entirely by dissimilar environmental factors and suggest a degree of familial predisposition. Generally, the presence of chronic esophagitis is positively correlated with the intake of burning hot beverages, and low consumption of fresh fruit and vegetables. A similar epidemiologic study conducted in lower Normandy in France evaluated 134 male volunteers 35 to 64 years old using surveillance endoscopy and biopsy (87). The prevalence of chronic esophagitis, epithelial atrophy, and dysplasia was 63%, 1.6%, and 4.8%, respectively. The prevalence of these lesions was positively correlated with cigarette smoking and frequent consumption of butter. Studies from South America also have associated the presence of esophagitis/dysplasia with cigarette smoking and alcohol consumption as well as mate drinking (88). It appears that whatever the noxious agent the esophageal response to injury is an inflammatory reaction that may progress to various degrees of dysplasia and eventually carcinoma. The concept of a dysplasia-carcinoma sequence in squamous cell carcinoma of the esophagus is supported by indirect as well as direct clinicopathologic evidence. Careful examination of esophagi resected for squamous cell carcinoma reveals at least one focus of carcinoma in situ closely associated with the invasive lesion in the majority of cases, whereas in 14% of cases various degrees of dysplasia are noted throughout the resected specimen (89). Importantly, follow-up studies of 327 Chinese patients with severe dysplasia demonstrated a progression to cancer at a rate of approximately 4% per year (90).

TYLOSIS

Tylosis (Keratopalmar keratosis) is an autosomal dominant, inherited defect of keratinization associated with a very high risk of developing squamous cell carcinoma of the esophagus. The report of Howl-Evans and colleagues (91), in the first detailed description of the disease, estimated the risk of malignant degeneration at 95% by the age of 65. Although hyperkeratosis of the palms and soles clinically characterizes the disease, the esophageal epithelium does not manifest significant abnormalities of keratinization. Ashworth et al. (92) described the morphologic abnormalities in the esophageal epithelium of 29 patients from one of the two original Liverpool families reported by Howl-Evans. All consented to annual esophagoscopy and biopsy, and almost half were found to have acute inflammation, particularly in the middle and lower thirds of the esophagus. Dysplasia was noted in four patients (29%) over a mean follow-up period of 5 years. Fortunately, the disease is rare and accounts for a small fraction of esophageal cancer cases.

PLUMMER-VINSON SYNDROME

Also known as the Patterson-Kelly syndrome, this disease is rare except in northern Scandinavia where it appears predominately in females. The syndrome is characterized by webs of the cervical esophagus, iron deficiency anemia, stomatitis, pharyngitis, and dystrophic nail bed changes (93). An increased incidence of cervical esophageal cancer has been observed and is possibly linked to the various nutritional deficiencies implicated in the pathogenesis of the disorder.

CAUSTIC STRICTURES

The propensity of caustic strictures to undergo malignant degeneration is well recognized. Tumors tend to develop within the esophagus at the site of bronchial bifurcation and are usually of the squamous cell type. A latent period of as long as 40 years occurs between ingestion of lye and the development of carcinoma. Csikos et al. (94) reported 36 patients with scar carcinoma of the esophagus developing after a mean interval of 46 years following ingestion of lye. A 45.6% 5-year survival was attributed to the dense associated scarring that may preclude early direct extension as well as lymphatic permeation. Although this series represented 7.2% of all esophageal cancers seen by the authors, the actual incidence of carcinoma developing after ingestion of lye is unknown. All patients with stricture caused by lye ingestion should undergo endoscopic or cytologic surveillance to detect early tumors. When surgical intervention is required for palliation of dysphagia in patients without an associated carcinoma, serious consideration should be given to the resection of the esophagus and reconstruction rather than simple bypass because a carcinoma can still develop in the excluded portion of the gullet (95).

MISCELLANEOUS DISORDERS

A variety of other disorders have been associated with carcinoma of the esophagus. The spectrum of radiation injury to the esophagus after mediastinal or breast irradiation varies between an acute self-limiting esophagitis to important complications such as stricture, perforation, and occasionally carcinoma (96). Malabsorptive disorders such as idiopathic steatorrhea and celiac disease also have been associated with carcinoma of the esophagus. The associated metabolic and nutritional disturbances may be etiologically important in the development of carcinoma in such patients. Carcinoma also has been found occasionally in association with epiphrenic and pharyngoesophageal diverticula, but a cause and effect relationship is hard to establish.

MANAGEMENT OF LOCALIZED ESOPHAGEAL CANCER

Carcinoma of the esophagus is one of the deadliest neoplasms. Five-year survival rates are generally less than 10% for all patients and range between 15% and 20% for those undergoing surgical resection. Pessimism regarding the outcome of surgically resected patients was reinforced by the critical review of Earlam and Cunha-Melo (97) published in 1980 and comprising more than 80,000 patients. The operative mortality was a formidable 25%, whereas the 5-year survival rate was only 5%. A subsequent review by the same investigators (98) detailing the results of primary radiotherapy revealed an equally bleak outcome. The dilemma of the disease lies primarily in the advanced stages of most tumors at the time of diagnosis. Dysphagia, the universal presenting symptom in the majority of patients, usually occurs in the later stages of the natural history of the disease. As a result most patients have established nodal metastasis at the time of diagnosis, thus compromising their chances of cure by standard modalities of treatment. Some have even postulated that esophageal cancer is a systemic disease at its inception and that attempts at intervention should therefore be directed toward palliation rather than cure (99). In contrast to the dismal survival rates consistently reported in the West, mass screening programs and early detection of esophageal cancer in the Orient have resulted in impressive cure rates after surgical resection (100). The low incidence of squamous cell carcinoma in the Western Hemisphere would render similar attempts economically nonviable. However, the early detection of esophageal adenocarcinoma by periodic surveillance of patients with Barrett's esophagus has resulted in long-term disease free survival approaching 90% in some studies (76). Clearly, early detection of carcinoma is the cornerstone of any attempt to improve survival rates.

The role of more aggressive local therapy, including the type and extent of surgical resection, remains a subject of ongoing debate. The controversy probably will be resolved only by a well-designed study of a significant number of patients properly staged and receiving a standardized method of treatment.

Nonetheless, controversy endures in the literature regarding the likelihood of cure with more advanced, yet potentially resectable, disease. The debate at one end of the spectrum focuses on the extent and technique of surgical resection (limited versus extended), and on the other end it discounts the utility of esophagectomy except as a salvage strategy after failure of chemoradiotherapy. The small number of patients in most studies and the lack of accurate pretreatment staging precludes any meaningful conclusions.

POTENTIALLY CURABLE ESOPHAGEAL CANCER

Although the current TNM staging system adopted by the American Joint Committee on Cancer and the Union Internationale Contre le Cancer represents a definite improvement over previously existing staging criteria, it does not allow for substaging based on the extent of nodal metastases, an important determinant of survival. An all-encompassing N category includes patients with single as well as multiple nodal metastases with no regard to the location or number of involved lymph nodes. Skinner and colleagues (101) reported a multivariate analysis of six prognostic factors after radical esophagectomy in 58 patients. The degree of wall penetration and the presence or absence of nodal involvement emerged as the only independent determinants of survival in the absence of distant metastases. A follow-up study of 100 patients surviving radical (en bloc) resection confirmed these findings as well as a modest but definite survival benefit noted in patients with less than four positive nodes (102). These observations, recently confirmed by other investigators (103), strongly suggest that nodal involvement is not uniformly predictive of disseminated disease. At our institution we define localized or potentially curable esophageal cancer as that in which partial (T1/T2) or complete (T3) mural penetration is associated with no nodal disease or fewer than four positive nodes. More extensive nodal spread substantially reduces the probability of cure by radical resection, and such patients are treated by more standard resection techniques when clinically indicated.

STAGING MODALITIES

A staging protocol should aim to determine not only the pretreatment stage as accurately as possible but also the ability of patients to tolerate major surgical resection. Careful attention is given to assessing nutritional status, and patients with more than 20% weight loss and those with total dysphagia are usually hospitalized for hyperalimentation. Pulmonary function testing is performed routinely, and patients with a forced expiratory volume in 1 second (FEV_1) of less than 1.5 L are not considered candidates for transthoracic esophagectomy. A complete cardiac evaluation also is performed, including coronary angiography if necessary.

Computed tomograms of the chest and upper abdomen are employed routinely. The primary tumor usually is marked by thickening of the esophageal wall. A blurring of the contour of the esophagus in the region of the tumor usually indicates full-thickness wall penetration. Employing this criterion for the T descriptor we were able to predict wall penetration with a 75% accuracy. Prediction of nodal involvement, however, is less reliable with only 50% diagnostic accuracy because of false-negative rates with small nodes. Mediastinal invasion is not detected accurately by computed tomography (CT). Aortic invasion is predictable when the tumor encroaches on more than 90 degrees of the aortic circumference, but the diagnostic accuracy of this sign is poor with lesser degrees of encroachment. CT criteria for gross airway invasion include significant distortion of airway anatomy or an obvious endoluminal extension of the tumor. Nonetheless, CT signs of early invasion of the airway are not reliable uniformly and should not prevent exploration in an otherwise favorable case. Evidence of hepatic or adrenal metastases should be sought diligently. Histologic documentation of isolated metastases usually is obtained by a variety of means, including transcutaneous needle aspiration, mediastinoscopy, laparoscopy, and thoracoscopy.

Over the past decade endoscopic ultrasonography (EUS) has emerged as a useful modality in the clinical staging of esophageal cancer. High-frequency transducers incorporated into the distal end of a fibrescope provide a 360-degree view of the esophageal segment perpendicular to the probe. The five layers of the normal esophageal wall are defined clearly. Esophageal cancer is imaged as a relatively hypoechoic disruption of the normal wall layers. The ability of EUS to determine wall penetration accurately (T stage) approaches 90%. EUS also can detect nodal metastases, even in lymph nodes 2 to 3 mm in size. Lymph nodes that are sharply demarcated, rounded, and hypoechoic are more likely to be malignant, as are larger nodes more than 10 mm in size. The accuracy of nodal involvement by EUS approaches 85%, compared with 50% by CT alone (104).

A major limitation of the currently available EUS instrument is its 13-mm diameter. Inability to pass a malignant stenosis has been reported in 50% to 60% of patients (105). Although wall penetration can be determined, the full extent of nodal involvement, especially the presence of celiac nodal spread (M1), is not possible unless the instrument is passed into the stomach.

SURGICAL THERAPY

The significant advances in perioperative care and the refinement of surgical resection techniques over the last decade have more than halved the hospital mortality after esophagectomy. Nonetheless, an appreciable and consistent survival benefit after surgical resection generally has remained elusive, particularly in the Western Hemisphere. Overall survival rates generally have ranged between 10% and 50%. This variability in survival rates could be attributed to several factors inherent in the current methods of reporting surgical results. Surgical resection procedures vary from limited to extended depending on the expertise and preference of the surgeon. Additionally, limited resection techniques do not allow for full staging of the extent of nodal disease, and thus understaging may be a common problem, precluding a stage-by-stage comparison of survival among various procedures. Indeed, in a recent report the 5-year survival rate for patients without nodal metastasis was 82% after esophagectomy with abdominal, mediastinal, and bilateral cervical node dissection, compared with 55% if lymphadenectomy was limited to the abdomen and mediastinum (106). Finally, terminology such as "curative" or "palliative" add to the confusion because palliation of dysphagia is almost universally accomplished regardless of the "curative" nature of the resection. The International Society of Diseases of the Esophagus proposed an important classification of resections into three groups:

R0, no residual gross or microscopic disease
R1, residual microscopic disease
R2, residual gross disease

The use of the R descriptor may partly resolve some of the confusion in analysis of various reports. The controversy surrounding the extent of resection, however, is unlikely to be resolved in the near future.

SURGICAL APPROACH

Resection of the thoracic esophagus can be accomplished using a variety of surgical approaches. The most commonly used approach worldwide is a right thoracotomy and laparotomy, as initially proposed by Ivor Lewis in 1946. A modification has been proposed since by McKeown: an additional cervical incision allows the anastomosis to be performed in the neck, thus avoiding the potential hazards of an intrathoracic anastomosis. A less commonly used incision for esophageal resection is the left thoracotomy. A peripheral semilunar diaphragmatic incision provides access to the abdominal cavity. The incision thus provides excellent exposure of the lower mediastinum, hiatal tunnel, and left upper quadrant.

Resections of the intrathoracic esophagus also could be accomplished through a transhiatal approach employing an upper abdominal and cervical incision. Special retractors are available that allow adequate exposure of the hiatal tunnel and the lower mediastinum up to the tracheal bifurcation. Surgeons using this approach should be both willing and capable of performing a thoracotomy to deal with the potential, yet quite rare, intrathoracic vascular or tracheal injuries that might occur during esophageal resection.

TRANSHIATAL ESOPHAGECTOMY

This procedure is best suited for resection of carcinoma of the cardia, but it also is used for resections of carcinoma of the intrathoracic esophagus. Perhaps the largest single experience with transhiatal esophagectomy (THE) is that of Orringer (107), who reported 417 patients with carcinoma of the esophagus and cardia resected by this technique over a 15-year interval. The overall hospital mortality was gratifyingly low (5%), and complications were no more significant than those encountered with standard transthoracic resections. The overall 5-year actuarial survival was 27% and did not vary significantly with cell type or tumor location. Predictably, tumor stage was the only significant determinant of survival. Paradoxically, survival for patients with stage IIA disease was worse than that of patients with stage IIB tumors. This may at least partialy result from the acknowledged understaging of mediastinal lymph nodes with THE. Gelfand and colleagues (108) reported 160 patients undergoing transhiatal esophagectomy for carcinoma of the lower esophagus and cardia. The majority of tumors seen were adenocarcinomas with most of these being significantly earlier stage disease. Survival rates at 1, 2, and 5 years were 62%, 40%, and 21%, respectively. Vigneswaran and coworkers (109) reported 131 patients resected by the transhiatal technique with an operative mortality of 2%. The overall 5-year survival was 21%. Five-year survival for stages I, II, and III were 47.5%, 37.7%, and 5.8%, respectively. In the latter study, 5-year survival for adenocarcinoma was 27%, whereas none of the patients with squamous cell carcinoma survived at 5 years of follow-up.

Proponents of THE maintain that overall survival rates are not significantly different with standard transthoracic or even extended resections and that occasional cures are possible only in the few patients with superficial tumors and without nodal metastases (T1-T2, N0). Critics of THE, however, argue that a complete lymphadenectomy is a necessary component of resection for carcinoma, primarily for staging and possibly for curative purposes, at least in some patients with limited nodal metastases. A large body of data indicating the presence of nodal metastases in 30% to 50% of patients in whom the tumor is limited to the submucosa certainly lends some support to the latter argument, particularly because more extensive resections result in 50% to 60% 5-year survival rates in patients with T1-T2, N1 disease (110). The controversy is likely to continue until a well-designed randomized study produces a stage-by-stage comparison of survival rates.

STANDARD TRANSTHORACIC ESOPHAGECTOMY

This procedure is performed through either a right or left thoracotomy, depending on the location of the tumor. When a right thoracotomy is chosen, the chest is entered through the fifth interspace. Because this approach often is used for midesophageal tumors abutting the aortic arch or tracheal bifurcation, the fifth interspace provides excellent exposure of these structures. Mobilization of the esophagus is carried distally to the hiatus and proximally into the prevertebral cervical space with no attempt at a radical mediastinal lymphadenectomy. The stomach is then mobilized through an upper abdominal incision, and the cervical esophagus is exposed through a cervical collar incision. Distal transection of the specimen is performed; the resultant gastric tube is advanced to the neck through the posterior mediastinum, and a hand-sewn, end-to-side esophagogastric anastomosis is performed.

When the procedure is performed through a left thoracotomy, the chest is entered through the sixth interspace. Access to the left upper quadrant is obtained through a semilunar diaphragmatic incision 1 inch away from the chest wall. Extending the incision across the costal margin into the abdomen adds little to the exposure and is not advisable. After mobilization and resection of the proximal stomach and lower half of the thoracic esophagus, reconstruction is performed either in the mediastinum or, preferably, in the neck. If the latter is chosen, then the esophagus is mobilized from underneath the aortic arch and along its course in the supraaortic posterior mediastinum and freed well into the neck. The gastric tube is then passed beneath the aortic arch and attached to the esophageal stump, and both are tucked loosely into the prevertebral cervical space.

Several studies have shown little difference in operative mortality or morbidity between transthoracic and transhiatal esophagectomy (111, 112). Survival rates reported with this technique are essentially identical to those reported after transhiatal resections.

EN BLOC RESECTION

The location of the esophagus deep within the narrow confines of the mediastinum and the lack of a well-defined esophageal mesentery have precluded the application of en bloc resection to the surgical treatment of esophageal cancer; that technique is used in other tumors of the gastrointestinal tract with modest improvement in survival rates. Embryologically, however, the esophagus distal to the aortic arch has a meso-esophagus, the counterpart of which in the adult is the lymphovascular tissue between the esophagus and the spine. This tissue, which includes the azygous vein and the thoracic duct, may be resected en bloc with the tumor-bearing esophagus. The main concept of en bloc resection is the resection of the tumor-bearing esophagus with a wide envelope of tissue, including the posterior meso-esophagus, both pleural surfaces laterally, and the pericardium, where they abut on the esophagus. This technique thus provides excellent local tumor control (Fig. 27.6). In 1961 Logan (113) reported 250 patients with carcinoma of cardia resected by an en bloc technique with a 5-year survival of 16%, the best reported to date. An operative mortality of 21% discouraged wider adoption of the technique. Skinner (114) adopted a similar approach in 1965 and extended its application to carcinoma of the thoracic and cervical esophagus. The technique is practiced in only a few centers in North America and Europe. Collard and colleagues (115) reported 65 patients with esophageal carcinoma resected by an en bloc technique with a 2.4% hospital mortality. Long-term survival was determined by the extent of wall penetration of the primary tumor into the esophageal wall and by the presence or absence of extrathoracic nodal metastases. In his series, the difference between N1 and N2 disease was not the number of involved nodes as originally proposed by Skinner, but rather whether the nodes were intrathoracic (N1) or extrathoracic (N2). Survival of patients without nodal metastases was 58% at 3 years. Patients with intrathoracic nodal spread had a 3-year survival of 32% regardless of the degree of mural penetration.

In an earlier study DeMeester et al. (116) reported an operative mortality of 7% after en bloc resection of carcinoma of the lower esophageal and cardia. The actuarial survival rates were 76%, 66%, and 53% at 1, 2, and 5 years, respectively. A more recent report from the same group compared long-term outcome after esophageal resection for carcinoma of the distal esophagus and cardia in three groups of patients defined by preoperative and intraoperative staging (117). Group 3 patients received a palliative operation because of the presence of extensive disease. Patients in groups 1 and 2 had apparently limited disease and underwent en bloc resection (group 1, $n = 30$), or transhiatal resection (group 2, $n = 16$) based on their ability to withstand transthoracic resection. Overall survival was significantly better after en bloc resection than after transhiatal resection (41% versus 14%, $P < .001$). Specifically, patients resected by the en bloc technique had superior survival to patients of comparable staging (41% versus 21%) subjected to transhiatal resection. Patients with early lesions, defined as intramural tumors (T1 or T2) associated with less than five positive nodes, had a 75% survival following en bloc resection compared with 20% for transhiatal resections. Survival of patients with advanced lesions, i.e., transmural tumors associated with five or more positive nodes, was significantly better after en bloc than transhiatal resections (27% versus 9%).

Lerut et al. (118) reported his experience with 232 patients undergoing resections for carcinoma of the esophagus, excluding those in the cervical esophagus and those located at the gastroesophageal junction. One hundred twenty-nine patients received a curative resection defined as clearance of all gross tumor. Fifty-four patients in the curative resection group were treated with a radical resection (en bloc). Hospital mortality was 7.4% for the curative radical group (en bloc group) and 10.6% for the curative nonradical group. No differences in survival were found between adenocarcinoma and squamous carcinoma nor by the location of tumor in the esophagus. Survival was significantly better in patients treated by curative radical (en bloc) resection versus those receiving a curative nonradical resection (48.5% versus 41%, $P < .002$). This survival advantage was especially evident in patients with nodal metastases rather than negative nodes. The survival advantage was apparent even when only stage III and IV patients treated with curative intent were compared. At 5 years, survival rates were 22% versus 13% in favor of en bloc resections ($P < .05$). Significantly, 5-year survival for patients with stage I disease was 90%, indicating that early lesions are as curable as any other early stage cancer.

THREE-FIELD LYMPHADENECTOMY

The Japanese concept of the surgical treatment of carcinoma of the esophagus always has stressed the need for a subtotal esophagectomy along with resection of the thoracic duct and an extensive mediastinal and upper abdominal lymphadenectomy (two-field lymphadenectomy). Despite the salutary survival rates reported by Japanese investigators (unmatched in the West), large follow-up studies indicated that as many as 30% to 40% of patients developed recurrences in the cervical nodes (119). This result has prompted several esophageal centers in Japan to adopt a three-field lymphadenectomy that included dissection of the cervical, mediastinal, and abdominal nodes for patients with carcinoma of the thoracic esophagus. Isono et al. (120) reported the results of a nationwide study in Japan on three-field lymph node dissection for carcinoma of the thoracic and abdominal esophagus performed at 35 institutions between 1983 and 1989. Despite the enormity of the data generated by this large study, several important points emerge that provide insight into the patterns of nodal spread of squamous cell carcinoma of the esophagus.

1. Metastases to the cervical nodes occurred in almost one third of the 1791 patients treated by three-field lymphadenectomy. Although the incidence of nodal metastases was highest when the tumor was located in the upper third of the thoracic esophagus (42%), almost 20% of patients with cancer of the lower third had cervical nodal metastases.
2. The frequency of nodal metastases increased with the depth of tumor penetration through the esophageal wall. Although none of the patients with carcinoma in situ (intramucosal carcinoma) developed positive nodes, tumor invasion into the submucosa (T1) signaled a 50% probability of nodal metastases. Patients with T2 or T3 tumors had a 60% to 80% probability of nodal involvement. These multiinstitutional data have since been substantiated by subsequent reports and cast doubt on the efficacy of limited resections for the treatment of patients with stage I disease.
3. The cervical nodes most frequently involved with metastatic carcinoma included the chain of nodes along the right and left recurrent nerves as well as the deep cervical nodes along the posterior aspect of the proximal extent of the internal jugular vein. Involvement of the supraclavicular nodes was infrequent and often associated with extensive nodal disease.
4. In the mediastinum, the location of nodal metastases from carcinoma of the thoracic esophagus generally varied with the location of the tumor. Nonetheless, the most commonly involved nodes were those located along the right recurrent nerve, which represented a continuum of nodes into the neck. Additionally, the left paratracheal, periesophageal nodes, subcarinal, and right paratracheal nodes were involved in approximately 20% of the cases.
5. Within the abdomen, nodal metastasis was located predominantly along the cardia, the lesser curvature, the left gastric trunk, and the celiac axis; this pattern was defined by Akiyama in the early 1980s (121).

There is little doubt that the results of three-field lymph node dissection have contributed significantly to our understanding of the pathways and patterns of lymphatic spread in thoracic esophageal cancer. It also is clear that a significant number of patients are staged inaccurately after isolated mediastinal and abdominal lymphadenectomy. Most studies on three-field lymph node dissection have shown a consistent improvement in survival rates beyond those obtained by two-field lymphadenectomy in patients without nodal metastasis. In the study of Isono and colleagues (120) comparing two-field and three-field lymph node dissection, 5-year survival was significantly better in patients without nodal metastases after three-field lymph node dissection (56% versus 45%), suggesting the presence of occult cervical nodal metastases in patients undergoing two-field lymphadenectomy. The impact of extended lymphadenectomy on survival once nodal metastases has occurred has been contested in the West. Nonetheless, the results from the extensive data generated by Japanese surgeons over the last decade are compelling.

Kato et al. (122) reported 79 patients who underwent transthoracic esophagectomy with mediastinal, abdominal, and bilateral cervical lymphadenectomy with an operative mortality of 3.8%. Overall survival for 57 patients with positive nodes was an impressive 33.6% (122). Patients with cervical nodal metastasis had a 30% 5-year survival, suggesting that the cervical nodal basin should be considered a regional (N1) rather than a distant (M1) site of spread. Akiyama and coworkers (106) reported 538 patients of comparable stages treated by either two-field or three-field lymphadenectomy over a 20-year interval. Five-year survival for patients with positive nodes was 42% after three-field dissection compared with 28% after two-field lymphadenectomy. Matsubara et al. (123) reported similar survival data and confirmed previous Japanese and Western data correlating survival with the number of positive nodes. A 5-year survival of 40% to 50% for patients with fewer than seven positive nodes reported by both Akiyama and Matsuhara agrees with similar data reported in the early 1980s.

ADJUVANT RADIOTHERAPY

The local failure rate after standard techniques of esophageal resection varies between 20% and 60%. The theoretical premise underlying postoperative radiotherapy is the eradication of microscopic tumor foci, thus reducing the probabilities of local failure. The potential benefit of this approach has been suggested by several retrospective analyses. In one of the largest studies, Kasai et al. (124) reported an 88% 5-year survival rate among resected node negative patients receiving postoperative radiation. Unfortunately, prospective, randomized studies failed to show any significant impact on overall survival (125). The reduction of the rate of regional recurrence was limited largely to patients without nodal metastases; these patients had a 10% local failure rate after adjuvant radiation, compared with a 35% failure rate after surgical resection alone. This 35% failure rate after resection may reflect an extent of resection that is not compatible with adequate control of local disease. Patients with positive nodes derived no benefit from adjuvant radiotherapy.

COMBINED MODALITY THERAPY

The use of induction therapy or preoperative therapy is prompted by the failure of primary radiotherapy or standard surgical resection to cure localized carcinoma of the esophagus. Although some patients die of the effects of local tumor recurrence, the great majority of patients have disseminated as well as local disease. Induction treatment techniques include preoperative chemotherapy, preoperative radiotherapy, and preoperative chemoradiotherapy.

PREOPERATIVE CHEMOTHERAPY

There are two important advantages of preoperative chemotherapy. Primarily, the physician can assess tumor response objectively and identify patients most likely to respond to postoperative chemotherapy. Secondly, patients are given chemotherapy at a time when they are best able to tolerate the potential toxicity and when the agents are most likely to have an impact on subclinical metastases. Additional potential advantages, such as downstaging of tumors and consequently limiting the extent of surgical resection, are of dubious value. The possibility of dissemination during the course of therapy, although real, is negligible and should not deter utilization of this approach.

Phase II trials have demonstrated that preoperative cisplatin-based combination chemotherapy results in a major response rate in 30% to 60% of patients; a complete pathologic response is seen in approximately 10% of patients. Importantly, preoperative chemotherapy has not affected operative mortality rates adversely. A favorable survival benefit has been suggested by some phase II trials. Three small randomized trials compared various regimens of combination preoperative chemotherapy followed by esophagectomy with surgery alone. Two studies showed no survival advantage (126, 127), whereas the third study demonstrated a trend, albeit statistically insignificant, toward improved survival in patients showing partial or complete response to preoperative chemotherapy (128). A national randomized trial is still in progress, comparing surgical resection with preoperative chemotherapy followed by surgery. Despite the standardization of the chemotherapy regimens, the variety of surgical techniques used nationwide and the insufficient staging requirements may preclude a logical assessment of the surgery arm of the trial.

PREOPERATIVE RADIATION

The rationale for preoperative radiotherapy is the ability to deliver higher doses of radiotherapy to the tumor before the interposition of the esophageal substitute and the consequent dose limitation imposed by its presence in the mediastinum. Additionally, delivery of radiation to oxygenated tumor cells before the surgical interruption of their blood supply enhances radiosensitivity.

Several randomized trials have evaluated the efficacy of preoperative radiotherapy. In general, the dose of radiation varied between 3000 and 6000 cGy followed by a planned surgical resection 3 to 6 weeks later. A few studies delivered 2000 to 3000 cGy in higher fractions followed by surgery in 7 to 10 days. A study by the European Organization for Research on Treatment of Cancer included 208 patients with resectable squamous cell carcinoma of the esophagus (129). Patients were treated with 3000 cGy over 12 days, and esophagectomy was performed 1 week later. Although there was a significant reduction in local recurrences in the combined modality group, there was no difference in resectability, median survival, or 2-year survival. Notably, the operative mortality was 17% for the surgical group and 25% for the combined treatment group. More recently, a randomized trial by Mei and colleagues (130) reported no difference in local failure rate. In another four-arm randomized multicenter trial a survival benefit was reported in patients receiving preoperative radiotherapy; however, almost half of the patients received preoperative chemotherapy as well (126). The 3-year survival in patients receiving only preoperative radiation was 20% and was not statistically different than the 3-year survival in patients treated by esophagectomy alone.

PREOPERATIVE CHEMORADIOTHERAPY

The use of preoperative chemoradiotherapy originally was proposed by the group at Wayne State University (131). Despite an impressive pathologic response rate, the operative mortality was a formidable 27%. Impressively, no survival benefit was noted even among complete responders. The Southwest Oncology Group (SWOG) conducted another phase II trial using preoperative chemoradiotherapy (132). Despite the fact that all patients initially were considered operable, only 63% were operable after induction therapy, and resectability was only 50%. The median survival for all patients was only 12 months. More recently, Naunheim and colleagues (133) reported the results of 47 patients receiving preoperative radiotherapy (3000 to 3600 cGy) with concurrent chemotherapy (5-fluorouracil/cisplatin) followed by esophagectomy. Resection was accomplished in 39 patients with a 5% operative mortality. A complete pathologic response was seen in 20% of patients. The median survival was 23 months with a 40% 3-year actuarial survival rate. Forastiere et al. (134) reported a group of 43 patients treated by a different preoperative regimen comprised of an intensive 21-day course of 5-fluorouracil and cisplatin given by continuous intravenous infusion in addition to vinblastine. Concurrent radiotherapy also was delivered daily during the 21-day treatment program. Transhiatal esophagectomy was performed subsequently in 91% of patients, and the resection was deemed curative in 84%. The operative mortality, pathologically complete response, and 5-year actuarial survival rates were 3%, 24%, and 34%, respectively. There were no significant differences in survival between patients with adenocarcinoma (21) and those with squamous cell carcinoma histologies (22). Presently, a randomized trial is being conducted by the same group comparing preoperative chemoradiotherapy followed by transhiatal esophagectomy with surgery alone.

REFERENCES

1. Barrett NR. Chronic peptic ulcer of the oesophagus and oesophagitis. Br J Surg 1950;38:175–182.
2. Allison PR, Johnstone AS. The oesophagus lined with gastric mucous membrane. Thorax 1953;8:87–101.
3. Barrett NR. The lower esophagus lined by columnar epithelium. Surgery 1957;41:881–894.
4. Morson BC, Belcher JR. Adenocarcinoma of the oesophagus and ectopic gastric mucosa. Br J Cancer 1953;6:127–130.
5. Naef AP, Savary M, Ozzello L, Pearson FG. Columnar-lined lower esophagus. Surgery 1975;70:826–834.
6. Giuli R. The story of a modern disease: In: Barrett N, Lortat-Jacob JL, eds. Diseases of the esophagus. 1992;5:5–19.
7. Skinner DB, Walther BC, Riddell RH, Schmidt H, Iascone C, DeMeester TR. Barrett's esophagus: comparison of benign and malignant cases. Ann Surg 1983;198(4):554–565.
8. Cameron A, Lowboy CT. Barrett's esophagus: age, prevalence and extent of columnar epithelium. Gastroenterology 1992;103:1241–1245.
9. Savary M, Ollyo JB. Frequency and importance of Barrett's esophagus in reflux disease. In: Abstracts: International Esophageal Week. Grafelfing, West Germany: Demeter Verlag, 1986:89.
10. Spechler SJ, Sperber H, Doos WG, et al. The prevalence of Barrett's esophagus in patients with chronic peptic esophageal strictures. Dig Dis Sci 1983;28:769–774.
11. Gruppo Operativo per lo Studio delle Precancerosi delle Esofago (GOSPE). Barrett's esophagus, epidemiological and clinical results of a multicenter survey. Int J Cancer 1991;48:364–368.
12. Cameron AJ, Zinsmeister AR, Ballard DJ, et al. Prevalence of columnar-lined (Barrett's) esophagus: comparison of population-based clinical and autopsy findings. Gastroenterology 1990;99:918–922.
13. Bremner CG, Lynch VP, Ellis FH. Barrett's esophagus: congenital or acquired: an experimental study of esophageal mucosal regeneration in the dog. Surgery 1970;68:209–216.
14. Van de Kerckhof J, Gahagan T. Regeneration of the mucosal lining of the esophagus. Henry Ford Hosp Med Bull 1963;11:129–134.
15. Mossberg SM. The columnar-lined esophagus (Barrett syndrome): an acquired condition? Gastroenterology 1966;50:671–676.
16. Iascone C, DeMeester TR, Little AG, Skinner DB. Barrett's esophagus: functional assessment, proposed pathogenesis, and surgical therapy. Arch Surg 1983;118:543–549.
17. Goldman MC, Beckman RC. Barrett syndrome; case report with discussion about concepts of pathogenesis. Gastroenterology 1960;39:104–110.
18. Fahmy N, King JF. Barrett's esophagus: an acquired condition

with genetic predisposition. Am J Gastroenterol 1993;88(8):1262–1265.
19. Jochem VJ, Fuerst PA, Fromkes JJ. Familial Barrett's esophagus associated with adenocarcinoma. Gastroenterol 1992;102:1400–1402.
20. Hayward J. The treatment of fibrous stricture of the oesophagus associated with hiatal hernia. Thorax 1961;16:45–55.
21. Gillen P, Keeling P, Byrne PJ, et al. Experimental columnar metaplasia in the canine oesophagus. Br J Surg 1988;75:113–115.
22. Levine DS, Rubin CE, Reid BJ, Haggitt RC. Specialized metaplastic columnar epithelium in Barrett's esophagus: a comparative transmission electron microscopic study. Lab Invest 1989;60(3):418–432.
23. Trier J. Morphology of the epithelium of the distal esophagus in patients with midesophageal peptic strictures. Gastroenterology 1970;58:444–461.
24. Paull A, Trier J, Dalton D, et al. The histologic spectrum of Barrett's esophagus. N Engl J Med 1976;295:476–480.
25. Zwas F, Shields HM, Doos WG, Antonioli DA, Goldman H, Ransil BJ, Spechler SJ. Scanning electron microscopy of Barrett's epithelium and its correlation with light microscopy and mucin stains. Gastroenterology 1986;90:1932–1941.
26. Ustach TJ, Tobon F, Schuster MM. Demonstration of acid secretion from esophageal mucosa in Barrett's ulcer. Gastrointest Endosc 1969;16:98–100.
27. Mangla JC, Kim Y, Guarasci G, et al. Pepsinogens in epithelium of Barrett's esophagus. Gastroenterology 1973;65:949–955.
28. Gottfried MR, McClave SA, Boyce HW. Incomplete intestinal metaplasia in the diagnosis of columnar lined esophagus (Barrett's esophagus). Am J Clin Pathol 1989;92:741–746.
29. Feurle GE, Helmstaedter V, Buehring A, Bettendorf U, Eckardt VF. Distinct immunohistochemical findings in columnar epithelium of esophageal inlet patch and of Barrett's esophagus. Dig Dis Sci 1990;35(1):86–92.
30. Miros M, Kerlin P, Walker N. Only patients with dysplasia progress to adenocarcinoma in Barrett's esophagus. Gut 1991;32:1441–1446.
31. Riddell RH, Goldman H, Ransohoff DF. Dysplasia in inflammatory bowel disease: standardized classification with provisional clinical applications. Hum Pathol 1983;14:931–968.
32. Reid BJ, Haggitt RC, Rubin CE, et al. Observer variation in the diagnosis of dysplasia in Barrett's esophagus. Hum Pathol 1988;19:166–178.
33. Hamilton S, Smith R, Cameron J, et al. Prevalence and characteristics of Barrett's esophagus in patients with adenocarcinoma of the esophagus or the esophagogastric junction. Hum Pathol 1988;19:942–948.
34. Schmidt HG, Riddell RH, Walther B, et al. Dysplasia in Barrett's esophagus. J Cancer Res Clin Oncol 1985;110:145–152.
35. Altorki NK, Sunagawa M, Little AG, et al. High-grade dysplasia in the columnar-lined esophagus. Am J Surg 1991;161:97–99.
36. Lee RG. Dysplasia in Barrett's esophagus: a clinicopathologic study of 6 patients. Am J Surg 1985;9:845–852.
37. Pera M, Trastek VF, Carpenter HA, et al. Barrett's esophagus with high-grade dysplasia: an indication for esophagectomy? Ann Thorac Surg 1992;54:199–204.
38. Reid BJ, Blount PL, Rubin CE, et al. Flow-cytometry and histological progression to malignancy in Barrett's esophagus: prospective endoscopic surveillance of cohort. Gastroenterology 1992;102:1212.
39. Robertson CS, Mayberry JF, Nicholson DA, et al. Value of endoscopic surveillance in the detection of neoplastic change in Barrett's esophagus. Br J Surg 1988;75:760–763.
40. Hameteman W, Tygat GNJ, Houthoff HJ, et al. Barrett's esophagus: prevalence and incidence of adenocarcinoma. Arch Intern Med 1991;151:2212–2216.
41. Spechler SJ, Robbins AH, Rubins HB, et al. Adenocarcinoma and Barrett's esophagus: an overrated risk? Gastroenterology 1984;87:927–933.
42. Cameron AJ, Ott BJ, Payne WS. The incidence of adenocarcinoma in columnar-lined (Barrett's) esophagus. N Engl J Med 1985;313:857–859.
43. Spechler SJ. Endoscopic surveillance for patients with Barrett esophagus: does the cancer risk justify the practice? Ann Intern Med 1987;106(6):902–904.
44. Blot WJ, Denesa SS, Kneller RW, et al. Rising incidence of adenocarcinoma of the esophagus and gastric cardia. JAMA 1991;265:1287–1289.
45. Hamilton JW, Thune RG, Morrissey JF. Symptomatic ectopic gastric epithelium in the cervical esophagus: demonstration of acid production with congo red. Dig Dis Sci 1986;31:337–342.
46. Kalish RJ, Clancy PE, Orringer MB, et al. Clinical epidemiologic and morphologic comparison between adenocarcinoma arising in Barrett's esophageal mucosa and in the gastric cardia. Gastroenterology 1984;86:461–467.
47. Harle IA, Finely RJ, Belsheim M, et al. Management of adenocarcinoma in a columnar-lined esophagus. Ann Thorac Surg 1985;40:330–336.
48. Atwood SE, DeMeester TR, Bremner CG, et al. Alkaline gastroesophageal reflux: implications in the development of complications in Barrett's columnar-lined lower esophagus. Surgery 1989;106:764–770.
49. DeMeester TR, Attwood SE, Smyrk TC, et al. Surgical therapy in Barrett's esophagus. Ann Surg 1990;212(4):528–542.
50. Pera M, Cardesa A, Bombi JA, et al. The influence of esophagojejunostomy on the induction of adenocarcinoma of the distal esophagus in Sprague-Dawley rats by subcutaneous injection of 2,6 dimethylnitrosomorphine. Cancer Res 1989;49:6803–6808.
51. Pera M, Trastek VF, Carpenter HA, Fernandez PL, Cardesa A, et al. Influence of pancreatic and biliary reflux on the development of esophageal carcinoma. Ann Thorac Surg 1993;55:1386–93.
52. Peters WH, Roelofs HM, Hectors MP, et al. Glutathione and glutathione S-transferases in Barrett's epithelium. Br J Cancer 1993;67(6):1413–1417
53. van Poppel G, de Vogel N, van Balderen PJ, et al. Increased cytogenetic damage in smokers deficient in glutathione S-transferase isozyme m. Carcinogenesis 1992;13:303–305.
54. Howie AF, Forrester LM, Glancey MJ, et al. Glutathione S-transferase and glutathione peroxidase expression in normal and tumour human tissue. Carcinogenesis 1990;11:451–458.
55. Levi F, Ollyo JB, La Vecchia C, Boyle P, et al. The consumption of tobacco, alcohol and the risk of adenocarcinoma in Barrett's oesophagus. Int J Cancer 1990;45:852–854.
56. Garewal HS, Sampliner RE, Fennerty MB. Flow cytometry in Barrett's esophagus: what have we learned so far? Dig Dis Sci 1991;36:548–551.
57. Reid BJ. Barrett's esophagus and esophageal adenocarcinoma. Gastroenterol Clin North Am 1991;20:817–834.
58. Raskind WH, Norwood T, Levine DS, et al. Persistent clonal areas and clonal expansion in Barrett's esophagus. Cancer Res 1992;52:2946–2950.
59. Rabinovitch PS, Reid BJ, Haggitt RC, et al. Progression to cancer in Barrett's esophagus is associated with genomic instability. Lab Invest 1988;60:65–71.

60. Rodriguez E, Rao PH, Ladanyi M, Altorki NA, et al. 11p13-15 is a specific region of chromosomal rearrangement in gastric and esophageal adenocarcinomas. Cancer Res 1990;50:6410–6416.
61. Garewal HS, Sampliner R, Liu Y, Trent JM. Chromosomal rearrangements in Barrett's esophagus: a premalignant lesion of esophageal adenocarcinoma. Cancer Genet Cytogenet 1989; 42:281–296.
62. Meltzer SJ, Mane SM, Wood PK, Resau JH, et al. Activation of c-Ki-*ras* in human gastrointestinal dysplasia determined by direct sequencing of polymerase chain reaction products. Cancer Res 1990;50:3627–3630.
63. Al-Kasspooles M, Moore JH, Orringer MB, Beer DG. Amplification and over-expression of the EGFR and *erb*B-2 genes in human esophageal adenocarcinomas. Int J Cancer 1993;54: 213–219.
64. Hollstein MC, Smits AM, Galiava C, et al. Amplification of epidermal growth factor receptor gene but no evidence of *ras* mutations in primary human esophageal cancers. Cancer Res 1988;48:5119–5123.
65. Blount PL, Ramel S, Raskind WH, et al. 17p Allelic deletions and p53 protein overexpression in Barrett's adenocarcinoma. Cancer Res 1991;51:5482–5486.
66. Harris CC, Hollstein M. Medical progress: clinical implications of the *p53* tumor-suppressor gene. N Engl J Med 1993;329 (18):1318–1327.
67. Casson AG, Mukhopadhyay T, Cleary KR, et al. *p53* Gene mutations in Barrett's epithelium and esophageal cancer. Cancer Res 1991;51:4495–4499.
68. Ramel S, Reid BJ, Sanchez CA, et al. Evaluation of p53 protein expression in Barrett's esophagus by two-parameter flow cytometry. Gastroenterology 1992;102:1220–1228.
69. Younes M, Lebovitz RM, Lechago LV, Lechago J. p53 Protein accumulation in Barrett's metaplasia, dysplasia, and carcinoma: a follow-up study. Gastroenterology 1993;105: 1637–1642.
70. Herbst JJ, Boynton MM, McCloskey DW, Wiser WC. Cell proliferation in esophageal columnar epithelium (Barrett's esophagus). Gastroenterology 1978;75:683–687.
71. Reid BJ, Sanchez CA, Blount PL, Levine DS. Barrett's esophagus: cell cycle abnormalities in advancing stages of neoplastic progression. Gastroenterology 1993:105(1):119–129.
72. Jankowski J, McMenemin R, Yu C, Hopwood D, et al. Proliferating cell nuclear antigen in oesophageal diseases; correlation with transforming growth factor alpha expression. Gut 1992;33:587–591.
73. Reid BJ, Haggitt RC, Rubin CE, Rabinovitch PS. Barrett's esophagus: correlation between flow cytometry and histology in detection of patients at risk for adenocarcinoma. Gastroenterology 1987;93:1–11.
74. Achkar E, Carey W. The cost of surveillance for adenocarcinoma complicating Barrett's esophagus. Am J Gastroenterol 1988;83:291–294.
75. Dowaltshahi K, Skinner DB, DeMeester TR, et al. Evaluation of brush cytology as an independent technique for detection of esophageal carcinoma. J Thorac Cardiovasc Surg 1985;89: 848–851.
76. Lerut T, Coosemans W, Van Raemdock D, et al. Surgical treatment of Barrett's carcinoma: correlations between morphologic findings and prognosis. J Thorac Cardiovasc Surg 1994; 107:1059–1066.
77. Garewal HS, Gerner EW, Sampliner RE, et al. Ornithine decarboxylase and polyamine levels in columnar upper gastrointestinal mucosae in patients with Barrett's esophagus. Cancer Res 1988;48:3288–3291.
78. Jankowski J, Hopwood D, Wormsley KG. Flow-cytometric analysis of growth regulatory peptides and their receptors in Barrett's oesophagus and oesophageal adenocarcinoma. Scand J Gastroenterol 1992;27:147–154.
79. Haggitt RC, Reid BJ, Rabinovitch PS, et al. Correlation between mucin histochemistry, flow cytometry and histologic diagnosis for predicting increased cancer risk. Am J Pathol 1988;131:53–61.
80. Stuart RC, Nolan N. Nucleolar organizer regions in endoscopic surveillance of Barrett's esophagus. In: Little, Ferguson M, Skinner DB, eds. Diseases of the esophagus. Benign diseases. Mount Kisko, NY: Futura, 1990;2:233–243.
81. Fagge CH. A case of simple stenosis of the oesophagus followed by epithelioma. Guy's Hosp Rep 1872;17:413–421.
82. Ellis FG. The natural history of achalasia of the cardia. Proc R Soc Med 1960;53:663–66.
83. Chuong JJ, DuBovik S, McCallum RW. Achalasia as a risk factor for esophageal carcinoma: a reappraisal. Dig Dis Sci 1984;29(12):1105–1108.
84. Aggestrup S, Holm JC, Sorenson HR. Does achalasia predispose to cancer of the esophagus? Chest 1992;102(4):1013–1016.
85. Meijssen MAC, Tilanus HW, van Blankenstein M, et al. Achalasia complicated by oesophageal squamous cell carcinoma: a prospective study in 195 patients. Gut 1992;33(2):155–158.
86. Chang-Claude JC, Wahrendorf J, Liang QS, et al. An epidemiological study of precursor lesions of esophageal cancer among young persons in a high-risk population in Huixian, China. Cancer Res 1990;50:2268–2274.
87. Jacob JH, Riviere A, Mandard AM, et al. Prevalence survey of precancerous lesions of the oesophagus in a high-risk population for oesophagus in a high-risk population for oesophageal cancer in France. Eur J Cancer Prev 1993;2(1):53–59.
88. Castelletto R, Munoz N, Landoni N, et al. Pre-cancerous lesions of the oesophagus in Argentina: prevalence and association with tobacco and alcohol. Int J Cancer 1992;51:34–37.
89. Mandard AM, Marnay J, Gignoux M, et al. Cancer of the esophagus and associated lesions: detailed pathologic study of 100 esophagectomy specimens. Hum Pathol 1984;15:660–669.
90. Shu YJ, Yang SG, Gin SP. Further studies on the relationship between epithelial dysplasia and carcinoma of the esophagus. Natl Med J China 1980;60:39–41.
91. Howell-Evans W, McConnel RB, Clarke CA, et al. Carcinoma of the oesophagus with keratosis palmaris et plantaris (tylosis). A study of two families. Q J Med 1958;27:413–429.
92. Ashworth MT, Nash JR, Ellis A, et al. Abnormalities of differentiation and maturation in the oesophageal squamous epithelium of patient with tylosis: morphological features. Histopathology 1991;19(4):303–310.
93. Vinson PP: Hysterical dysphagia. Minn Med 1992;5:107–108.
94. Csikos M, Horvath O, Petri A, et al. Late malignant transformation of chronic corrosive oesophageal strictures. Langenbecks Arch Chir 1985;365(4):231–238.
95. Imre J, Kopp M. Argument against long-term conservative treatment of oesophageal strictures due to corrosive burns. Thorax 1972;27:594–598.
96. Goffman TE, McKeen EA, Curtis RE, et al. Esophageal carcinoma following irradiation for breast cancer. Cancer 1983; 52(10):1808–1809.
97. Earlam R, Cunha-Melo JR. Oesophageal squamous cell carcinoma. I. A critical review of surgery. Br J Surg 1980;67:381.
98. Earlam R, Cunha-Melo J. Oesophageal squamous cell carcinoma: II. A critical review of radiotherapy. Br J Surg 1980;67: 457–461.

99. Orringer MB. Ten year survival after esophagectomy for carcinoma: surgical triumph or biologic variation? Chest 1989; 96(5):970–971.
100. Shao LF, Hunag GJ, Zhang DW, et al. Detection and surgical treatment of early esophageal carcinoma. In: Proceedings of the Beijing Symposium on Cardiothoracic Surgery, Beijing. New York: John Wiley, 1981:168.
101. Skinner DB, Dowalatshahi KD, DeMeester TR. Potentially curable cancer of the esophagus. Cancer 1982;50:2571–2575.
102. Altorki NA, Skiner DB. En bloc esophagectomy: the first 100 patients. Hepatogastroenterology 1990;37:360–363.
103. Kato H, Tachimori Y, Watanabe H, et al. Lymph node metastasis in thoracic esophageal carcinoma. J Surg Oncol 1991; 48:106–111.
104. Lightdale CJ, Botet JF, Zauber AG, et al. Endoscopic ultrasonography in the staging of esophageal cancer: comparison with dynamic CT and surgical pathology. Gastrointest Endosc 1990: in press.
105. Yasuda K, Nakajima M, Kawi K. Malignant lesions of the gastrointestinal tract. In: Kawi, ed. Endoscopic ultrasonography in gastroenterology. Tokyo: Igaku-shion, 1988:56.
106. Akiyama H, Tasurumaru M, Udagawa Y, et al. Systemic lymph node dissection for esophageal cancer-effective or not? Dis Esoph 1994;7(1):1–12.
107. Orringer MB, Marshall B, Stiriling MC. Transhiatal esophagectomy for benign and malignant disease. J Thorac Cardiovasc Surg 1993;105(2):265–277.
108. Gelfand GA, Finley RJ, Nelems B, et al. Transhiatal esophagectomy for carcinoma of the esophagus and cardia. Experience with 160 cases. Arch Surg 1992;127(10):1164–1167.
109. Vigneswaran WT, Trasteck VF, Pairolero PC, et al. Transhiatal esophagectomy for carcinoma of the esophagus. Ann Thorac Surg 1993;56(4):838–844.
110. Isono K, Ochiai T, Okuyama K, et al. The treatment of lymph node metastasis from esophageal cancer by extensive lymphadenectomy. Jpn J Surg 1990;20(2):151–157.
111. Tilanus HW, Hop WC, Langenhorst BL, et al. Esophagectomy with or without thoracotomy. Is there any difference? J Thorac Cardiovasc Surg 1993;105(5):898–903.
112. Goldmine M, Maddern G, Le Prise E, et al. Oesophagectomy by a transhiatal approach or thoracotomy: a prospective randomized trial. Br J Surg 1993;80(3):367–370.
113. Logan A. The surgical treatment of carcinoma of the esophagus and cardia. J Thorac Cardiovasc Surg 1963;46:150–161.
114. Skinner DB. En-bloc resection for neoplasms of the esophagus and cardia. J Thorac Cardiovasc Surg 1983;85:59–69.
115. Collard JM, Otte JB, Reynaert M, et al. Feasibility and effectiveness of an bloc resection of the esophagus for esophageal cancer. Results of a prospective study. Int Surg 1991;76:209–213.
116. DeMeester TR, Zaninotto G, Johansson KE, et al. Selective therapeutic approach to cancer of the lower esophagus and cardia. J Thorac Carciovasc Surg 1988;95:42–54.
117. Hagen JA, Peters JH, DeMeester TR. Superiority of extended en bloc esophagogastrectomy for carcinoma of the lower esophagus and cardia. J Thorac Cardiovasc Surg 1993; 106(5):850–858.
118. Lerut T, De Leyn P, Coosemans W, et al. Surgical strategies in esophageal carcinoma with emphasis on radical lymphadenectomy. Ann Surg 1992;216(5):583–590.
119. Isono K, Onoda S, Okuyama K, et al. Recurrence of intrathoracic esophageal cancer. Jpn J Clin Oncol 1985;15:49–60.
120. Isono K, Sato H, Nakayama K. Results of nationwide study on the three-field lymph node dissection of esophageal cancer. Oncology 1991;48:411–420.
121. Akiyma H. Surgery of the esophagus. Curr Probl Surg 1980; 17:55–120.
122. Kato H, Tachimori Y, Watanabe H, et al. Lymph node metastasis in thoracic esophageal carcinoma. J Surg Oncol 1991;48: 106–111.
123. Matsubara T, Mamoru U, Yanagida O, et al. How extensive should lymph node dissection be for cancer of the thoracic esophagus? J Thorac Cardiovasc Surg 1994;107(4):1073–1078.
124. Kasai M, Mori S, Watanabe T. Follow-up results after resection of thoracic esophageal carcinoma. World J Surg 1978;2: 543–551.
125. Fok M, Sham J, Choy D, et al. Postoperative radiotherapy for carcinoma of the esophagus: a prospective, randomized controlled trial. Surgery 1993;113:138–147.
126. Nygaard K, Hagen S, Hansen H, et al. Pre-operative radiotherapy prolongs survival in operable esophageal carcinoma: A randomized, multicenter study of pre-operative radiotherapy and chemotherapy. The second Scandinavian trial in esophageal cancer. World J Surg 1992;16:1104–1110.
127. Shlag P, Hermann R, Fritze E, et al. Pre-operative chemotherapy in localized cancer of the esophagus with cisplatinum, vindesine, and bleomycin, In: Wagner D, Blijhan G, Smeets J, Wils J, eds. Primary chemotherapy in cancer medicine. New York: Alan Liss, 1985:253.
128. Roth J, Pass H, Flanagan M, et al. Randomized trial of pre- and postoperative cisplatin, vindesine, and bleomycin (DVB) chemotherapy in epidermoid carcinoma of the esophagus. In: Ishigami J, ed. Proceedings of the 14th International Congress on Chemotherapy. Tokyo: University of Tokyo, 1985: 1158–1159.
129. Gignoux M, Rousel A, Paillot B, et al. The value of preoperative radiotherapy in esophageal cancer: results of a study of the EORTC. World J Surg 1987;11:426.
130. Mei W, Xian-Zhi G, Weibo Y, et al. Randomized clinical trial on the combination of preoperative irradiation and surgery in the treatment of esophageal carcinoma: report on 206 patients. Int J Radiat Oncol Biol Phys 1989;16:325–327.
131. Steiger Z, Franklin R, Wilson R. Eradication and palliation of squamous cell carcinoma of the esophagus with chemotherapy, radiotherapy, and surgical therapy. J Thorac Cardiovasc Surg 1981;82:713–719.
132. Poplin E, Fleming T, Leichman T, et al. Combined therapies for squamous cell cancer of the esophagus: a Southwest Oncology Group (SWOG 8037) study. J Clin Oncol 1987;5:633.
133. Naunheim K, Petruska P, Roy T, et al. Preoperative chemotherapy and radiotherapy for esophageal carcinoma. J Thorac Cardiovasc Surg 1992;5:887–895.
134. Forastiere A, Orringer M, Perez-Tamayo C, et al. Preoperative chemoradiation followed by transhiatal esophagectomy for carcinoma of the esophagus: final report. J Clin Oncol 1993; 11:1118–1123.

28

THERAPY OF ESOPHAGEAL CANCER

Lee C. Drinkard, Mark K. Ferguson, Arno J. Mundt, and Everett E. Vokes

INTRODUCTION

The 5-year survival rate of patients with esophageal cancer has not changed significantly in the past decade. The primary therapy of early-stage disease has been surgery, when feasible, or radiation therapy. Therapy of more advanced disease has included various combinations of surgery and radiation therapy. Chemotherapy has traditionally been used with palliative intent for metastatic disease. Recently, there has been much interest in the combination of chemotherapy with radiation therapy or surgery, or the use of all three modalities together in locally advanced (nonmetastatic) disease. These multimodality regimens hold promise in improving the dismal prognosis of patients with esophageal cancer.

This chapter discusses the modalities of surgery, radiation therapy, and chemotherapy, individually defining their roles as potentially curative therapy and in the palliation of metastatic disease. It then focuses on combined modality therapy and reviews the results of recent trials in locoregionally advanced esophageal cancer.

SURGICAL THERAPY

Surgical resection is presently the only proven curative single-treatment modality for carcinoma of the esophagus and gastric cardia. Although resection was found to be feasible more than 50 years ago, esophagectomy for carcinoma remains both a technical and intellectual challenge for the surgeon.

SURGERY FOR CURATIVE INTENT

Patient Selection

Esophagectomy is the primary treatment modality for most patients with cancer of the esophagus and gastric cardia. Resection is performed with curative intent in patients with stage I and stage IIA disease. Some physicians also consider it an appropriate means of local control and potential cure for patients with stage IIB and stage III disease, although the results are far less encouraging. In recent years, surgery in these stages increasingly has been performed as a component of multimodality therapy. Selection of patients for resection is based primarily on the results of preoperative clinical staging. Because there is no general agreement regarding what comprises appropriate tests, indications for resection vary widely. The percentage of patients who are surgically explored ranges from 50% to 80%, and the rates of resectability vary from 70% to more than 95% (1–3).

Despite the fact that esophageal cancer is diagnosed predominantly during the seventh and eighth decades of life, advanced age itself is not an absolute contraindication to resection. The higher rates of operative morbidity and mortality found in elderly patients are accounted for primarily by an increased incidence of comorbid factors such as heart, liver, and kidney diseases (4, 5). Excluding operative mortality, long-term disease specific prognosis in elderly patients is similar to that in younger patients.

Cancer of the esophagus and gastric cardia has strong etiologic ties to tobacco and alcohol use, and thus is accompanied by a high incidence of pulmonary, cardiac, and hepatic dysfunction. The likelihood of preoperative pulmonary problems ranges from 20% to 40% and includes both restrictive and obstructive spirometric patterns. Increased operative risk is predicted by the presence of chronic bronchitis, a decreased forced expiratory volume in 1 second (FEV_1), hypercarbia ($PaCO_2$ > 45 mm Hg), and hypoxemia (PaO_2 < 55 mm Hg) (6–9). More than 20% to 30% of patients have cardiovascular disease, including coronary artery disease, with or without prior myocardial infarction. Appropriate preoperative evaluation, including a stress test with scintigraphic imaging, is frequently necessary. With proper perioperative management, most patients can undergo resection without an undue risk of complications. Cirrhosis is not an absolute contraindication to operation when a curative resection can be performed. Although the operative risk is increased, it is acceptable in patients who are in Child's class A and whose prothrombin time is less than 150% of normal (9, 10).

Combined protein-calorie malnutrition is common among patients with carcinoma of the esophagus and gastric cardia. Malnutrition results from the catabolic effects of the cancer as well as from inadequate caloric intake because of loss of appetite and luminal obstruction. Humoral and cellular immune responses are compromised, resulting in an increase in operative complications such as anastomotic leakage, wound dehiscence, infection, and respiratory insufficiency (5, 11). Preoperative nutritional repletion is possible in some patients by enteral or parenteral methods, and it may reduce the incidence of operative complications and mortality (12–15).

SELECTION OF OPERATION

Intelligent selection from among the various surgical options is important in maximizing the potential benefits of resection while minimizing the operative risks. The choice of an operation depends on the individual patient's clinical stage, intraoperative findings, tumor histology and location, and physiologic status, as well as the philosophy and personal preferences of the surgeon. Because clinical staging is relatively inaccurate, a thorough intraoperative exploration of all anatomic regions potentially affected by the cancer is undertaken before beginning a resection.

STANDARD ESOPHAGECTOMY

A standard esophagectomy, the most common method used for both curative and palliative operations, is performed through a transthoracic approach. This technique permits either a partial or subtotal esophageal resection, and provides appropriate exposure for a complete regional lymph node dissection. Most surgeons perform this operation using a modified Ivor Lewis technique using separate laparotomy and right fifth interspace thoracotomy incisions, often with the addition of a cervical incision to permit a proximal esophageal anastomosis (16). For tumors of the lower esophagus and gastric cardia, an exclusive left thoracic approach through the seventh interspace may be used, in which access to the abdomen is provided through a peripheral incision in the diaphragm.

The extent of resection is governed by tumor histology and location as well as by the intended site of reconstruction. Squamous cell cancers are frequently multicentric and are best treated by subtotal esophagectomy. In contrast, adenocarcinomas of the distal esophagus and gastroesophageal junction often spread submucosally, but are rarely multicentric and do not require a subtotal esophagectomy to achieve extirpation of the entire primary tumor. Resection includes, at a minimum, the affected esophagus and 5-cm margins of normal tissue proximally and distally along with the adjacent surrounding soft tissues. All regional lymph nodes are dissected, and any other suspicious lymph nodes are biopsied. Included in routine nodal dissections are paraesophageal, subcarinal, perigastric, and left gastric artery nodal regions (17). For proximal intrathoracic cancers, the paratracheal lymph nodes are dissected, and cervical lymph nodes are biopsied if a cervical anastomosis is performed.

RADICAL EN BLOC ESOPHAGECTOMY

Radical esophagectomy was first described in the early 1960s, but its use initially was not widely accepted because of the high rate of operative mortality (18). The feasibility of this approach has recently been confirmed (19, 20). A variety of technical modifications have been proposed (3, 21, 22). The objective of en bloc esophagectomy is more extensive removal of tissues adjacent to the esophagus accompanied by a more radical lymph node dissection. Advocates of this approach suggest that a more complete cancer resection decreases the likelihood of local recurrence and improves long-term survival without a substantial increase in operative morbidity or mortality. There currently are no data from prospective or randomized studies that support or refute these claims.

Indications for the use of en bloc esophagectomy include: (a) disease that is in an intermediate stage (stages IIA to III); (b) disease that is completely resectable; and (c) a patient whose physiologic status is capable of withstanding the more radical operation. As with the standard esophagectomy, the operative approach is dependent on tumor location and histology. For adenocarcinomas of the distal esophagus or gastric cardia, a left thoracotomy is used, and access to the abdomen is gained through a peripheral phrenotomy. Squamous cell cancers are approached through laparotomy, right thoracotomy, and cervical incisions. The typical resection consists of removal of the affected esophagus with 10-cm margins of normal tissue proximally and distally. The lateral extent of excision includes the azygos vein, thoracic duct, pleura, and, in some patients, posterior pericardium and adjacent right intercostal vessels.

The appropriate extent of lymph node dissection accompanying en bloc radical esophagectomy is controversial. Upper mediastinal lymph nodes are involved by cancer in more than 10% of patients with tumors of the lower esophagus, and 15% to 25% of patients with cancers of the thoracic esophagus have involvement of the cervical lymph nodes. Such findings have prompted the addition of a cervical lymph node dissection in selected patients. Preliminary data indicate that long-term survival may be increased following a three-field (abdominal, thoracic, and cervical) nodal dissection, but that this survival is achieved at the cost of increased operative morbidity (23–27).

TRANSHIATAL ESOPHAGECTOMY

Transhiatal esophagectomy was first described by Denk in 1913 (28) and, following sporadic reports of its use in cancer therapy (29–32), was popularized by Orringer during the 1970s and 1980s (33, 34). Although this technique has become popular for palliative treatment of esophageal cancer, it is used by many surgeons as the definitive surgical procedure for all cancers of the esophagus and gastric cardia. The ability to remove the esophagus completely without performing a thoracotomy is appealing in its potential for reducing postoperative pain and pulmonary morbidity. A contraindication to the use of this technique is direct invasion of the primary cancer into an adjacent mediastinal structure such as the trachea, vertebral column, or aorta. Although much of the operation is performed under direct visualization, the surgeon's ability to resect the soft tissues adjacent to the esophagus is limited compared with a standard esophagectomy; the nodal dissection is likewise compromised. Whether these limitations result in a higher local recurrence rate or decreased long-term survival after potentially curative esophagogastrectomy is not known.

MANAGEMENT OF CERVICAL ESOPHAGEAL CANCER

Resection remains a controversial therapy for cancers of the cervical esophagus. Because these tumors are relatively uncommon, few surgeons have extensive experience with their management. Disappointing postoperative functional results, low rates of long-term survival, and improvements in locoregional therapy, including both radiotherapy and chemoradiotherapy, have generated considerable discussion regarding appropriate selection of treatment. Nevertheless, resection remains a viable option for the primary management of patients with potentially curable cervical esophageal cancer (35)

At operation, exploration is performed to determine whether there is involvement of the larynx or trachea. If such involvement is identified, laryngectomy and tracheostomy are necessary for a curative resection. Bilateral modified neck dissection is performed to remove all regional lymph nodes. If a 5-cm margin of normal esophagus cannot be removed distal to the inferior extent of gross tumor, a total esophagectomy is performed either transthoracically or using a transhiatal technique (36, 37). Some surgeons use this technique routinely to accomplish a more complete excision and lymph node dissection (38, 39). In selected patients a segmental esophagectomy with or without laryngectomy can be performed, and reconstruction is achieved by means of a free jejunal graft with microvascular anastomosis.

COMPLICATIONS

There is an appreciable risk of morbidity and mortality associated with esophagectomy because of the magnitude of the operation and the poor preoperative physiologic condition of many of the patients (Table 28.1) (3, 40–43). The 30-day mortality rate is less than 5% in recent series. This number does not reflect the chronic nature of some operative complications, and a more accurate estimate of operative mortality is best made 3 months postoperatively. The most common causes of operative death are pulmonary insufficiency due to pneumonia or the adult respiratory distress syndrome, and anastomotic leaks.

Nonfatal pulmonary complications develop in more than 20% of patients, and include retained secretions, adult respiratory distress syndrome, and pneumonia. Nursing the patient in a head-elevated position reduces the risk of aspiration, and aggressive pulmonary toilet minimizes problems from retained secretions. The routine use of ventilatory support during the immediate postoperative period is not necessary and can increase the incidence of pulmonary complications.

Esophageal anastomotic leak, a potentially fatal complication, occurs in 5% to 20% of patients. Leaks are more common from cervical than from intrathoracic anastomoses. Cervical anastomotic leaks usually require only local drainage to permit healing. In contrast, intrathoracic leaks often result in severe mediastinitis or empyema, a process that is facilitated by negative intrathoracic pressure and irritation by gastric acid and enzymes. Proper management of an intrathoracic leak

TABLE 28.1. Complications After Esophagectomy

COMPLICATIONS	INCIDENCE (%)
Death	5
Pulmonary	
Pneumonia	10
Respiratory insufficiency	7
Cardiovascular	
Myocardial infarction	3
Arrhythmia	4
Pulmonary embolus	1
Gastrointestinal	
Anastomotic leak	7
Splenic injury	1
Infectious	
Empyema	1
Intraabdominal abscess	1
Wound infection	3
Other	
Recurrent nerve injury	3
Bleeding	1
Chylothorax	1

Data from references: King (40); Mathisen (41); Lozac'h (42); Gelfand (43); Lerut (3.)

typically requires reoperation for appropriate drainage, and diversion of the alimentary tract is sometimes necessary.

RESULTS OF SURGICAL THERAPY

Successful surgery for esophageal carcinoma improves patient lifestyle and often restores the ability to work. Dysphagia is palliated in 80% to 90% of patients (44, 45), and more than half of patients who experience preoperative weight loss regain the weight within the first postoperative year. More than 80% of survivors are able to return to work between 2 and 5 weeks postoperatively (46). Resection reduces the likelihood of local tumor recurrence, esophageal-airway fistula, bleeding, and chronic pain.

Long-term survival is dependent primarily on tumor stage. Whether the technique and extent of resection influences overall outcome is unknown. The tumor characteristics that affect survival include the depth of penetration of the primary tumor, regional lymph node involvement, and distant metastatic spread. Extraesophageal invasion reduces 5-year survival from 50% to 15% (20, 47), and regional lymph node metastases reduce 5-year survival to 10% (48, 49). Tumor location within the esophagus, and whether the tumor is an adenocarcinoma or a squamous cell cancer, does not affect long-term survival. Overall 5-year survival in resected patients is 20% to 25% (35, 41, 48, 50–53)

RADIATION THERAPY

OVERVIEW

Radiation therapy plays an important role in the management of patients with esophageal cancers. In patients undergoing curative treatment, radiation therapy may be used alone, either before or after surgery, or in conjunction with chemotherapy with and without surgery. In addition, radiation therapy may be used for patients who are not eligible for aggressive therapy and in whom the treatment goal is palliation.

The following section outlines the technical aspects of the radiotherapeutic management of patients with esophageal carcinoma and the results of trials using radiation therapy alone with curative intent. The use of radiation as a means of palliation is then discussed.

RADIATION THERAPY TECHNIQUE

The principles of radiation treatment planning for patients with esophageal cancer are similar if radiation therapy is used alone for either curative or palliative intent, or if it is part of combined modality therapy with surgery or chemotherapy. The goal of treatment planning is the uniform irradiation of the gross tumor as well as areas of suspected subclinical disease while limiting radiation dosage to adjacent normal structures such as heart, lung, and spinal cord (54). The treatment volume is dependent on the location of the primary tumor. Tumors in the cervical esophagus require treatment from the laryngopharynx to the midmediastinum with inclusion of the cervical and bilateral supraclavicular lymph nodes (55). Bilateral supraclavicular nodes are often included electively in the treatment of upper esophageal tumors, and the celiac axis is included with middle and lower esophageal tumors (56). Most centers use generous margins above and below the gross tumor (5 to 6 cm) because of the risk of "skip" lesions, and apply 2- to 3-cm margins laterally (57). It is important to use all available clinical and radiographic information to ensure coverage of the gross tumor. Patients should be asked to swallow a radiopaque viscous liquid at the time of simulation to further aid in the localization of the tumor.

Treatment is delivered using high-energy (6 to 24 MV) photons after the delineation of fields at the time of simulation. Initial field arrangements typically consist of equally weighted, opposed, anterior-posterior and posterior-anterior (AP-PA) fields. Figure 28.1 illustrates the initial volume of treatment in a patient with a thoracic esophageal tumor. The use of proper immobilization is essential to enhance day-to-day reproducibility and to minimize treatment setup errors. Patients are typically simulated in the supine position with their arms above their heads. This positioning is necessary if oblique fields are to be used to avoid treatment through the patient's arms. Several authors have demonstrated the dosimetric benefit of prone treatment given the increased distance between the spinal cord and the esophagus (58, 59). It should be noted, however, that many ill and elderly patients are not able to tolerate the prone position. After delineation of the treatment volume, the irradiation of normal adjacent tissues is minimized by using customized cerrobend blocking or multivane collimation. In patients treated with high-dose definitive radiotherapy, the final portion of treatment must be delivered either with a combination of anterior and oblique posterior fields or opposed obliques fields, thus limiting the total dose to the spinal cord to within tolerance. The treatment planning of patients with tumors of the cervical esophagus is more complex. Treatment approaches include the use of lateral fields, oblique fields, anterior wedged pair fields, and three to four field techniques with tissue compensation (55).

The total dose and fractionation scheme depends on whether radiation is used alone or in combination with either chemotherapy or surgery and whether the radiation therapy is being used with curative or palliative intent. Doses of 60 to 70 Gy in 1.8- to 2-Gy fractions are required to control gross disease. Patients treated with combined modality therapy, i.e., with chemotherapy or surgery, have received lower doses in some studies (60, 61). Palliative regimens range from 30 Gy over 2 weeks to 50 to 60 Gy over 5 to 6 weeks. Although numerous centers have suggested the benefits of altered fractionation, i.e., twice-a-day therapy, in head and neck cancer (62), breast cancer (63), and lung carcinoma (64), little information is currently available regarding the treatment of esophageal carcinoma (65). Thus, patients should not be treated with altered fractionation regimens outside of a controlled clinical trial. It is common practice for most radiation oncologists to reduce the daily dose for patients in whom an impending tracheoesophageal fistula is suspected to prevent rapid destruction of the tumor (66). If a fistula develops during therapy, treatment should be discontinued (67).

Recently, there has been an increase in the usage of three-dimensional treatment planning (Fig. 28.2) (68). This approach allows the physician to optimize the selection of beam angles as well as the blocking of normal structures. After simulation and proper immo-

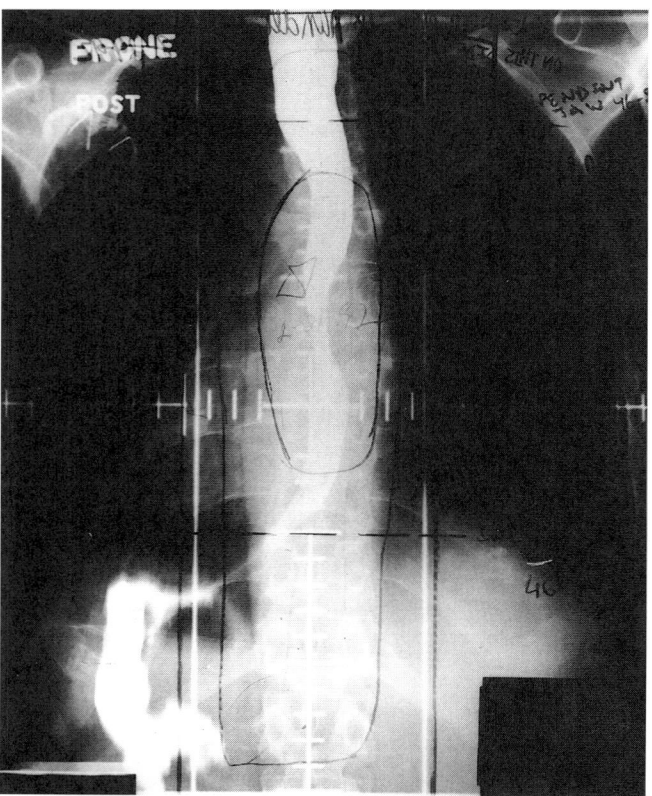

FIGURE 28.1. Initial opposed AP-PA treatment volume of a patient with a mid esophageal carcinoma. Note that the patient is prone. The proximal extent of the tumor is demonstrated by the use of oral contrast.

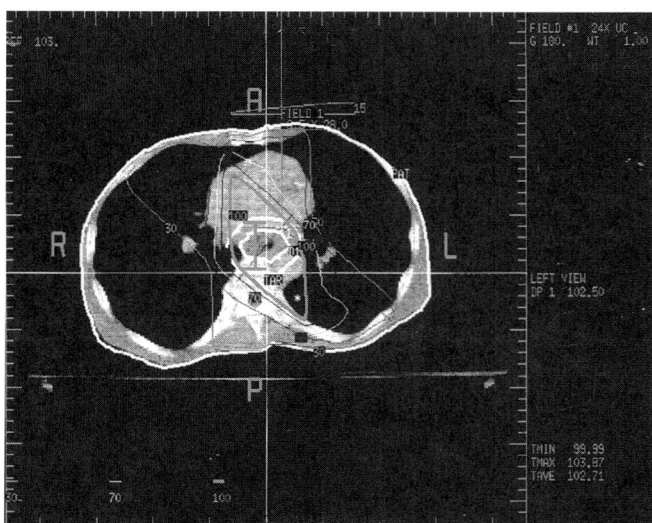

FIGURE 28.2. CT-based treatment plan of a patient with a thoracic esophageal tumor. Isodose curves are overlain on a 0.5-cm CT slice. The tumor is encompassed by the 100% isodose line.

bilization, the patient undergoes CT scanning in the treatment position. The CT images are displayed on a treatment planning computer. The tumor, areas of potential subclinical disease, and adjacent normal structures are then delineated. Optimal beam angles, beam energies, field weighting, and blocking are then determined to provide adequate coverage of the treatment volume while minimizing the radiation dosage to normal adjacent organs (68). Figure 28.2 illustrates a treatment plan generated on the treatment-planning system developed at the University of Chicago.

In addition to external beam radiotherapy, other radiotherapeutic approaches to the treatment of esophageal carcinoma include intracavitary brachytherapy (69–71) and particle beam radiotherapy (72, 73). Intracavitary irradiation may be accomplished with iridium 192 (^{192}Ir) sources or with high-dose–rate techniques, either alone or in combination with external beam radiotherapy (69). Particle beam therapy has been explored with fast neutrons (72) and helium ions (73). No benefit, however, has been demonstrated with particle therapy. Finally, techniques combining hyperthermia and conventional photon irradiation have been explored (74).

CLINICAL TRIALS OF RADIATION THERAPY ALONE

In light of newer approaches combining radiation with chemotherapy or surgery, radiation therapy as a single-treatment modality is used less frequently today as a curative approach in patients with esophageal carcinoma. However, aggressive radiation therapy alone is used in patients who are unfit for or refuse combined modality treatment, and in whom a curative approach seems warranted.

Numerous trials have reported the results of radiation therapy alone for curative intent. Table 28.2 shows the results of trials using radiation therapy alone published since 1975 (75–85, 87, 88). The overall 5-year survival rates range from 0% to 20% with the majority of trials showing figures below 10%. These results are similar to those described by Earlam and Cunho-Melo (89) in their classic review of 8489 patients treated on 49 trials published between 1954 and 1979.

The most favorable group of patients undergoing definitive irradiation are those with tumors sized 5 cm or less. Appelquist and colleagues (81) treated 50 patients, all with tumors measuring 5 cm or less, with definitive irradiation alone and reported a 14% 5-year survival rate. Similarly, Newaishy et al. (83) reported a 5-year survival rate of 12% in patients with tumors less than 5 cm in size. Investigators at Rush University in Chicago noted a 75% local control rate in 12 patients with tumors less than 5 cm in size compared with 36% in patients with larger, more advanced tumors (78).

COMPLICATIONS

Radiation therapy sequelae are subdivided into acute (occurring during or soon after the completion of therapy) or late (developing months to years after treatment). The type as well as the incidence of radiation sequelae depend on a number of factors, including whether radiation is used alone or in combination with surgery or chemotherapy.

Patients treated with radiation therapy alone may experience a variety of acute sequelae including skin irritation, easy fatigability, and nausea commencing in the second or third week of therapy. The most troubling acute sequela, however, is esophagitis. Patients often initially note improvement in their symptoms of dysphagia or odynophagia only to soon complain of recurrent symptoms secondary to esophagitis. Reassurance is necessary because patients may assume this sign represents failure of their treatment. Acute sequelae are generally self-limited but may necessitate treatment breaks.

Several trials using radiation therapy alone have reported high rates of late sequelae including large vessel hemorrhage, tracheoesophageal (TE) fistulae, and stricture. However, many of these complications ascribed to radiation therapy may be secondary to uncontrolled tumor progression. Schuchmann et al. (82) reported an 18.1% rate of TE fistulae and a 10% rate of major vessel hemorrhage in 77 patients treated with radiation therapy alone. Millburn and associates (90) noted a high rate (28%) of severe sequelae in their series of 25 patients. However, only one complication (myelitis) was clearly secondary to irradiation.

The most common late radiation complication is benign stricture. Investigators at the Princess Margaret Hospital reported a 67% rate of esophageal stricture in patients treated with radiation therapy alone. However, 75% of the strictures were shown to be secondary to recurrent tumor (79). Newaishy et al. (83) noted a 43.7% rate of benign stricture in 444 patients treated with radiation alone between 1956 and 1974 at the University of Edinburgh. Seventy-two percent of these patients required dilation. Clearly, any patient developing recurrent symptoms of dysphagia after therapy needs to be evaluated for recurrence of tumor. Other late sequelae secondary to radiation include pneumonitis, pericarditis, myocarditis, and myelitis. These

TABLE 28.2. Radiation Therapy Alone for Esophageal Carcinoma

AUTHOR (REFERENCE NO.)	YEAR	TREATED (NO.)	DOSE	5-YEAR SURVIVAL (%)
Marks et al. (75)	1976	33	60 Gy	6.1
Wara et al. (76)	1976	129	50–60 Gy	7 (3-y)
Pearson (77)	1977	388	50 Gy (230 cGy/fx)	20
Elkon et al. (78)	1979	72	82–126 TDF	11 mo (median survival)
Beatty et al. (79)	1979	176	>40 Gy/<19 fx >45 Gy/<23 fx >50 Gy/<3 mo	0
		168	Less than above	0
Van Andel et al. (80)	1979	120	60–66 Gy	0.9
Appelquist et al. (81)	1979	50	60.3 R	14
Schuchmann et al. (82)	1980	77	>4500 R	0
		50	<4500 R	0
Newaishy et al. (83)	1982	444	50–55 Gy (250–275 cGy/fx)	9
Yin et al. (85)	1983	615	70 Gy	6.2
Morita (87)	1985	119	>50 Gy	11.3[a]
Roussell et al. (88)	1988	...	56.25 Gy (225 cGy/fx)	6

Abbreviations. fx, fraction; TDF, tolerance dose formula.
[a] Patients receiving more than 60 Gy.

sequelae are rare, and their risk can be minimized with careful treatment planning.

PREOPERATIVE RADIATION THERAPY

Numerous investigators have reported the results of radiation therapy administered before surgery in both nonrandomized and randomized trials. The rationale underlying this approach is to increase rates of resectability by "downstaging," i.e., shrinking the size and extent of the tumor.

One uncontrolled trial suggesting that preoperative radiation may be beneficial was reported by Akakura et al. (93). A total of 117 patients were treated with 50 to 60 Gy using conventional fractionation and surgery (no sooner than 14 to 28 days after the completion of radiation therapy). Patients undergoing preoperative irradiation had a higher rate of resectability (65.1% versus 25.8%) and 5-year survival (25% versus 13.6%) when compared with historical controls receiving surgery alone. Moreover, patients treated with preoperative irradiation had a lower rate of tumor extension to the adventitia (30.2% versus 54%) and positive lymph nodes (16.8% versus 22.7%) (93). The results of other nonrandomized trials are shown in Table 28.3.

Although appealing, theoretically, the use of preoperative irradiation has not proven beneficial when tested in two randomized trials comparing preoperative radiation therapy and surgery with surgery alone (Table 28.3). The first trial was conducted by Launois and colleagues (97). One hundred twenty-four patients were randomized to preoperative radiation therapy (39 to 45 Gy over 8 to 12 days) or surgery without radiation. The resectability rates (76% and 70.5%, respectively) and the 5-year survival rates (both 12.5%) were similar for the two treatment arms. Gignoux et al. (98) reported the results of a randomized trial of 208 patients conducted by the European Organization for Research and Treatment of Cancer. Patients were randomized to receive either 33 Gy in 10 fractions before surgery or surgery alone. No differences were seen in median or 5-year survival rates. Furthermore, no improvement in resectability or "downstaging" was noted in the radiation therapy patients. These trials have been criticized, however, because of the dose/fractionation schemes used and the fact that surgery followed within 6 days of the completion of radiation therapy.

A common concern with the usage of preoperative radiation therapy is whether receiving it before radical surgery increases the rate of surgical morbidity and mortality. The results of numerous nonrandomized trials (92–94) and two randomized preoperative trials (97, 98) have not shown a higher rate of complications in patients who received radiation therapy. Launois et al. (97) noted identical rates of postoperative mortality in the two treatment arms. Although Gignoux and colleagues (98) noted a slightly higher incidence of postoperative mortality in the patients receiving preoperative irradiation (24% verses 18%), the difference did not reach statistical significance. Liu

TABLE 28.3. Preoperative Radiation Therapy for Esophageal Carcinoma

AUTHOR (REFERENCE NO.)	TREATED (NO.)	DOSE	RESECTABILITY (%)	OPERATIVE MORTALITY (%)	5-YEAR SURVIVAL (%)
Nonrandomized					
Van Andel et al. (91)	328	60–66 Gy	NS	21	21[a]
Kelsen et al. (92)	76	40–60 Gy	54	12	5
Akakura et al. (93)	117	50–60 Gy	65.1	20.8	25
Liu et al. (94)	74	30–70 Gy	79.7	8.5	60.1
Petrovich et al. (95)	46	4–60 Gy	NS	NS	18
Nakayama and Kinoshita (96)	281	20 Gy (400 cGy/fx)	NS	4.4	37.5
Randomized					
Launois et al. (97)	67 vs. 57	39–45 Gy	76	23	12.5
		No preoperative RT	70.2	23	12.5
Gignoux et al. (98)	102 vs. 106	33 Gy/10 fx	NS	24	10
		No preoperative RT	NS	18	10

Abbreviations. NS, not stated; fx, fraction; RT, radiotherapy.
[a] Only resected patients.

and associates (94) compared the postoperative morbidity of 171 surgery alone patients with 74 patients treated with surgery preceded by 30 to 70 Gy of radiotherapy. They reported similar rates of pulmonary complications (2.4% versus 5.1%), wound dehiscence (4% versus 5.1%), and anastomotic leakage (7.2% versus 10.2%).

POSTOPERATIVE RADIATION THERAPY

The results of studies using radiation therapy after surgery are shown in Table 28.4. The rationale underlying the use of postoperative radiation is to sterilize any residual gross or subclinical disease left behind after surgery. In general, these trials used moderate doses of radiation (50 to 60 Gy over 5 to 6 weeks) and demonstrated that the main advantage of postoperative radiation is the possibility of improving locoregional control. It remains unclear, however, whether postoperative radiation produced an improvement in the rate of survival.

Kasai et al. (100) analyzed the outcome of 111 stage II-III patients treated with radical surgery and either no further therapy or 60 Gy of postoperative radiation over 6 weeks. Local recurrences were less frequent in the patients given postoperative radiation. An improvement in 5-year survival was noted in node negative patients with postoperative radiation (35% versus 16%). However, no improvement in survival was noted in patients with node positive disease.

Two prospective randomized trials were reported recently evaluating the role of postoperative radiation therapy (60, 101). Teniere et al. (60) randomized 221

TABLE 28.4. Postoperative Radiation Therapy for Esophageal Carcinoma

AUTHOR (REFERENCE NO.)	TREATED (NO.)	REGIMEN	MEDIAN SURVIVAL (MO.)	SURVIVAL (%) 3-YEAR–5-YEAR
Nonrandomized				
Gunnlaugsson et al. (99)	14	40–50 Gy	NS	21 35 (No)
Kasai et al. (100)	111	60 Gy	NS	6 (N+)
Randomized				
Fok et al. (101)	60[a]	49 Gy (350 cGy/fx)	NS	22
		vs. No RT	NS	24
	70[b]	52.5 Gy (350 cGy/fx)	NS	0
		vs. No RT	NS	7
Teniere et al. (60)	221	45–55 Gy	18	20
		vs. No RT	18	18

Abbreviations. NS, not stated; No, node negative; N+, node positive; fx, fraction; RT, radiotherapy.
[a]Curative resection.
[b]Palliative resection.

patients with disease in the mid and lower esophagus to surgery alone or surgery plus postoperative irradiation (45 to 55 Gy). No improvement in 5-year survival was seen with the addition of radiation therapy. Moreover, when patients were analyzed by nodal stage, no improvement was evident in either node positive or node negative patients. However, the 5-year locoregional control rate was 95% in the patients receiving postoperative radiation therapy versus 75% in those treated with surgery alone ($P < .02$) (60).

Fok et al. (101) randomized 130 patients to either surgery alone or surgery followed by postoperative radiation therapy. Sixty patients with documented negative margins or microscopically positive lymph nodes were randomized to either observation or 49 Gy in 350-cGy fractions of radiation administered 3 times a week. The remaining 70 patients had either T4 disease or grossly positive lymph nodes and were treated with either no further therapy or 52.5 Gy of administered as above. Patients treated with postoperative radiation had a statistically lower median survival (8.7 months versus 15.2 months) and 3-year survival rate (12% versus 20%). The poorer survival in the patients receiving radiation therapy was due to a high rate of radiation-induced ulceration and fatal hemorrhage.

Severe acute and late sequelae are infrequent with the administration of moderate-dose radiation following radical surgery. Irradiation of the intrathoracic stomach, however, commonly leads to transient symptoms of nausea. The excessively high rate of sequelae seen in the series of Fok and associates (101) is unusual and is possibly due to the unconventional fractionation regimen employed.

CHEMOTHERAPY AND COMBINED MODALITY THERAPY

Chemotherapy has an emerging role in combined modality regimens either as neoadjuvant therapy or as part of concomitant chemoradiotherapy. Chemotherapy has been added to other modalities based on its action alone or in combination in advanced disease, or its ability to synergize the activities of other treatments. This section thus discusses the use of chemotherapy in esophageal cancer, starting with a review of active single agents and combination regimens. The use of chemotherapy as part of a combined modality treatment regimen, either as preoperative therapy or simultaneously with radiation therapy, is then discussed.

SINGLE-AGENT CHEMOTHERAPY

Several single agents used in esophageal cancer reproducibly yield response rates between 15% and 20% when tested in patients with metastatic or recurrent disease. Most single agents have been tested as part of small phase I or II trials in patients with metastatic or advanced disease; frequently, these trials include only patients with squamous cell carcinoma. The single agents tested with the highest activity include: cisplatin, 5-fluorouracil (5-FU), bleomycin, doxorubicin, vindesine, methotrexate, and mitoguazone.

Several investigators have reviewed these single-agent trials in detail (102–104). A summary of single-agent chemotherapy studies and their combined response rates is presented in Table 28.5.

Cisplatin has been studied extensively in patients with esophageal cancer and is incorporated into many multiagent regimens. Table 28.5 reflects the pooled data from a total of seven phase II trials of cisplatin in esophageal cancer (105–111). The highest response rate was reported by Miller et al. (107), who used high-dose cisplatin 120 mg/m^2 on days 1 and 15 as preoperative therapy in 15 patients with squamous cell carcinoma. There were 11 partial responses for a 73% response rate. However, no patient had a pathologically complete response. This high response rate is probably reflective of the chemosensitivity of early-stage disease and perhaps the high dose intensity of cisplatin. This high response rate has not been seen in other trials involving patients with more extensive disease and using less intense doses of cisplatin.

Historically, bleomycin was used in patients with esophageal cancer in trials conducted in the late 1960s and early 1970s (112–119). There have been 80 patients with squamous cell cancer of the esophagus treated in seven different trials. The response rates of these trials range from 0% to 33% with brief response durations. Various schedules of administration have been tested with no schedule being clearly superior to the others.

Three phase II trials of mitomycin have been completed (106, 120, 121). Response rates range from 14% to 42% with the best response rate obtained by Engstrom et al. (105); they administered 20 mg/m^2 every 4 weeks for two cycles then every 6 weeks until disease progression or toxicity occurred.

TABLE 28.5. Active Single Agents in Esophageal Cancer

Drug	Evaluable Patients (No.)	Cell Type	Response Rate[a] (%)	Reference No.
Cisplatin	167	Squamous	32	105–111
Bleomycin	80	Squamous	15	112–118
Mitomycin	58	Squamous	26	105, 119, 120
5-Fluorouracil	39	Both[b]	36	121, 122
Paclitaxel	45	Both[b]	31	123
Methotrexate	70	Squamous	34	118, 124
Mitoguazone	45	Squamous	20	125–127
Vindesine	35	Squamous	17	128
Doxorubicin	33	Squamous	15	121, 129

Adapted from Kelsen D, Atiq OT. Therapy of upper gastrointestinal tract cancers. Curr Probl Cancer 1991;15(Sept–Oct):235–294.
[a]Response rates are pooled response rates of all studies cited.
[b]Studies include patients with either adenocarcinoma or squamous cell carcinoma.

5-FU has been studied in two separate trials (121, 122). Ezdinli et al. (121) gave 5-FU as a bolus injection of 500 mg/m² daily for 5 days with a 15% response rate. Lokich et al. (122) gave 5-FU 300 mg/m² as a continuous 6-week intravenous infusion to 13 patients with both squamous cell and adenocarcinoma histologies. Responses were seen in 11 patients giving an 85% overall response rate (122). This disparity in response rates has no clear explanation. Possible contributing factors include the different administration schedules of 5-FU, differences in disease extent and performance status between the two studies, and the small study cohorts.

Ajani et al. (123) recently completed a phase II trial of the tubulin stabilizing agent paclitaxel (Taxol; Bristol-Meyers Squibb, Princeton, NJ) in advanced esophageal cancer. The trial enrolled 52 patients with either adenocarcinoma or squamous cell carcinoma of the esophagus who received paclitaxel at a dose of 250 mg/m² over 24 hours with granulocyte–colony-stimulating factor support. There was a 34% response rate with no complete responses. The actuarial median survival was 13.2 months.

In summary, single-agent therapy in patients with esophageal cancer results in low overall response rates and brief response durations. These studies must also be interpreted with caution because response evaluation was not uniform, sample sizes were small, and disease extent and performance status varied greatly between studies. Nonetheless, it is clear that esophageal carcinoma is a tumor in which further drug development is needed.

COMBINATION CHEMOTHERAPY

With the observation that several agents have low but reproducible activity in esophageal cancer, attempts at improving response rates have led to the development of multidrug regimens. These regimens have been studied in recurrent or metastatic disease and as preoperative therapy in patients with locally advanced disease. Some trials enrolled patients with both squamous cell carcinoma and adenocarcinoma histologies. The regimens are mostly cisplatin based with small numbers of patients enrolled in any given trial. As with single-agent therapy, responses primarily are partial in extent with brief response durations ranging from 4 to 15 weeks. There are no randomized trials comparing single-agent and combination chemotherapy. Table 28.6 summarizes combined response data of the more active regimens in patients with nonoperable disease.

Cisplatin and bleomycin were combined in two trials. Coonley et al. (130) treated 27 patients with extensive esophageal carcinoma with the combination of 24-hour-infusion bleomycin and cisplatin as part of a 70-patient trial; included were patients with resectable disease, those with recurrent disease who had previous radiation and/or surgery, and those with metastatic disease. There was a 17% response rate in the 27 patients receiving the regimen for advanced disease; median survival was 4 months. In a later trial Marcuelo et al. (131) treated 34 patients with a similar regimen of cisplatin and continuous-infusion bleomycin (given over 18 hours). Objective responses were seen in 15 patients (with an overall response rate of 44%) with locally advanced and metastatic disease. Median survival was not reported.

The three-drug combination of cisplatin, bleomycin, and vindesine was studied by Kelsen et al. (132) and Dinwoodie et al. (133) in two trials of patients with metastatic and nonoperable esophageal carcinoma. The response rates were 33% and 29%, respectively, for a combined response rate of 29% in 51 patients.

The experimental polyamine inhibitor mitoguazone has been added to several different regimens with good overall response rates but low median survivals. Kelsen et al. (134) combined mitoguazone with cisplatin and vindesine in 20 patients with an overall response rate of 40% but a median survival of only 4 months. A similar trial with cisplatin, vinblastine, and mitoguazone yielded a response rate of only 11% with a 3.4-month median survival (135). The four-drug combination of cisplatin, bleomycin, methotrexate, and mitoguazone was used by Vogl et al. (136) in 14 patients with a 64% response rate. Median survival was not reported, but response duration was only 3.4 months.

5-Fluorouracil has been studied extensively in esophageal carcinoma because it is an active agent in squamous cell carcinomas of the head and neck and some gastrointestinal malignancies. The combination of 5-FU (by continuous infusion) with cisplatin has yielded response rates of 35% and 40% in patients with nonoperable disease (Table 28.6). The addition of leucovorin to 5-FU potentiates the drug's antitumor activity by promoting more complete inhibition of the enzyme thymidylate synthase. This combination has been studied in many solid tumors of the aerodigestive tract. The side effects of these combinations are primarily myelosuppression and mucositis. The addition of interferon to a 5-FU–based regimen is based on the observation of increased 5-FU cytotoxicity in the presence of interferon in preclinical experiments (137). Side effects of these regimens include those seen with 5-FU alone (mucositis and skin rashes) in addition to myelosuppression and fatigue. To date the tumor response rates seen in trials incorporating interferon

TABLE 28.6. Active Combination Chemotherapy Programs in Advanced and Metastatic Esophageal Cancer

REGIMEN	PATIENTS (NO.)	RESPONSE RATE (%)	REFERENCE
CDDP-Bleo[a]	51	30	130, 131
CDDP-5-FU	39	40	154
CDDP-5-FU-allopurinol	37	35	133
CDDP-MTX	42	76	138
CDDP-MTX-Bleo	41	32	139, 140
CDDP-MTX-Bleo-MGBG	14	64	136
CDDP-Bleo-VP-16	16	31	141
CDDP-CTX-VDS-CCNU	28	21	142
CDDP-Dox-5-FU	21	33	143
CDDP-5-FU-VP-16	20	65	144
CDDP-5-FU-Bleo	43	53	145
5-FU-LV	35	17	146
CDDP-5-FU-LV[a,b]	56	48	147, 148
CDDP-5-FU-LV-VP-16[a]	38	59	149
5-FU-IFNα[b]	37	27	150
CDDP-5-FU-IFN-α[b]	15	53	151
CDDP-Bleo-VDS	51	29	132, 133
CDDP-VDS-MGBG	20	40	152
CDDP-VBN-MGBG	36	11	153

Abbreviations. CCDP, cisplatin; Bleo, bleomycin; 5-FU, 5-fluorouracil; MTX, methotrexate; MGBG, mitoguazone; CTX, cyclophosphamide; VDS, vindesine; VBN, vinblastine; CCNU, lomustine; VP-16, etoposide; Dox, doxorubicin; LV, leucovorin; IFNα, interferon α 2A.
[a]Therapy was given as part of a combined modality regimen (surgery with radiation) in some patients with locally advanced disease.
[b]Studies included patients with both adenocarcinoma and squamous cell carcinoma.

with 5-FU are similar to those using 5-FU alone (Table 28.6). However, the trials using interferon had more overall toxicity. Interferon thus appears to add very little to chemotherapy in esophageal cancer.

In summary, combination chemotherapy of esophageal cancer produces somewhat higher response rates than single-agent chemotherapy. No direct comparison study of single versus combination therapy has been done. Cisplatin-based regimens are the best studied and appear to produce the highest response rates. Overall survival, however, is still short. Because no randomized phase III trial comparing combination chemotherapy with single-agent chemotherapy or supportive care has been done, it is unclear whether combination chemotherapy confers a survival advantage to patients with nonoperable and metastatic esophageal cancer. A decrease in symptoms in responding patients may be seen, however.

CHEMOTHERAPY AND SURGERY

Preoperative, or induction, chemotherapy has been employed in many different solid tumors (e.g., head, neck, and lung) and has been studied extensively in esophageal carcinoma. The use of preoperative chemotherapy is partially based on the observation in autopsy series that metastasis occurs as an early event (155–158). Neoadjuvant therapy may also shrink lesions, making them more resectable and thus improving local control of tumor. Table 28.7 summarizes the results of pilot studies of neoadjuvant chemotherapy in potentially resectable patients with esophageal cancer. It must be noted, however, that it can be very difficult to measure tumor response radiographically in esophageal cancer, even with both barium esophagram and CT scanning.

The earliest trials of preoperative chemotherapy were conducted at the Memorial Sloan–Kettering Cancer Center. The first trial by Coonley et al. (159) employed one cycle of preoperative cisplatin and bleomycin in 43 patients. The preoperative response rate was 14% with a total of 34 patients undergoing surgery. The median survival was 9.7 months. The second trial by Kelsen et al. (134) employed two cycles of cisplatin, vindesine, and bleomycin given preoperatively to 45 patients. The preoperative response rate was 63% with 34 patients having subsequent resections. The median survival was 16.2 months. A similar regimen was employed by Schlag et al. (160) in a 42-patient trial with a preoperative response rate of 45% (two pathologically complete responses). A total of 40 patients later had surgery, and the median survival was 16 months.

The Memorial group conducted another trial of preoperative chemotherapy with cisplatin and vindesine, substituting the polyamine inhibitor mitoguazone for bleomycin to avoid pulmonary toxicity (161). The trial enrolled 20 patients and yielded a preoperative response rate of 42% with 13 patients going on to surgery. The median survival was only 8.5 months. Forastiere et al. (135) conducted another trial combining mitoguazone with cisplatin and vinblastine for two cycles preoperatively in 29 patients. The preoperative response rate was 44% (one pathologically complete response), and the median survival was 14 months.

Carey et al. (162) conducted a trial with two cycles of preoperative cisplatin (100 mg/m^2 on day 1) with continuous-infusion 5-FU (1000 mg/m^2/day for 4 to 5 days). Cycles were repeated up to 4 times postoperatively. A total of 59 patients were enrolled with a 64% preoperative response rate, a 20-month median survival, and a 29% 5-year actuarial survival. A similar regimen was studied by Kies et al. (163) at Northwestern University where this regimen was given preoperatively for three cycles to 26 patients with a preoperative response rate of 42% and a 17.8-month median survival.

TABLE 28.7. Pilot Studies of Preoperative Chemotherapy

Author (Reference No.)	Regimen	Patients (No.)	Response Rate (%) (CR)	Resectable Patients (No.)	Median Survival (Mo)
Coonley et al. (159)	CDDP–Bleo	43	14	34	9.7
Kelsen et al. (134)	CDDP-VDS-Bleo	45	63	34	16.2
Schlag et al. (160)	CDDP-VDS-Bleo	42	45 (2)	40	16
Kelsen et al. (161)	CDDP-VDS-MGBG	20	42 (1)	13	8.5
Forastiere et al. (135)	CDDP-VBN-MGBG	29	44 (1)	25	14
Carey et al. (162)	CDDP–5-FU	59	64 (1)	NS	20
Kies et al. (163)	CDDP–5-FU	26	42	14	17.8
Ajani et al. (164)	VP-16–CDDP–5-FU	35	49 (1)	32	23
Ajani et al. (165)	VP-16–CDDP–Dox–GM-CSF	27	25	10	12.5
Hoffman et al. (166)	CDDP–5-FU–LV[a]	41	43 (3)	31	12.5

Abbreviations. CR, complete response; NS, not stated; CDDP, cisplatin; Bleo, bleomycin; 5-FU, 5-fluorouracil; MGBG, mitoguazone; VDS, vindesine; VBN, vinblastine; VP-16, etoposide; LV, leucovorin; GM-CSF, granulocyte–macrophage colony-stimulating factor.
[a]Patients received postoperative chemoradiotherapy with 5-FU, hydroxyurea.
[b]Studies included patients with both adenocarcinoma and squamous cell carcinoma.
[c]Therapy was given as part of a combined modality regimen (surgery with radiation) in some patients with locally advanced disease.

Two trials exclusively in patients with adenocarcinoma of the esophagus were conducted by Ajani et al. (164) at the M. D. Anderson Cancer Center. The first trial employed daily cisplatin and 5-FU by continuous infusion for 5 days with etoposide in three daily doses. A total of 35 patients were enrolled with a preoperative response rate of 49% and an 18-month median survival. The second trial employed cisplatin, doxorubicin, and etoposide with granulocyte-macrophage colony–stimulating factor support in 27 patients. Although the preoperative response rate was 50% with 25 patients able to undergo surgery, the median survival was only 12.5 months (165).

Hoffman et al. (166) at the University of Chicago administered cisplatin with 5-FU by continuous infusion for 5 days with oral leucovorin given for two cycles preoperatively to 41 patients with resectable or unresectable disease. This therapy was followed by surgery if feasible and concomitant chemoradiotherapy with radiation therapy given during alternating weeks to a total dose of 5000 to 6000 cGy; 5-FU was administered by continuous infusion for 5 days and oral hydroxyurea for 5 days. A total of 31 patients had resections after induction chemotherapy. The preoperative response rate was 43% with three pathologically complete responses. In a preliminary analysis median survival of all 41 patients was 12.5 months.

The results of these pilot studies of preoperative chemotherapy have shown that this approach is feasible with most patients able to undergo surgery after chemotherapy. The high response rates seen in some of these regimens show that this may be an effective way to debulk tumors before resection and improve complete resection rates.

Several small randomized trials comparing preoperative chemotherapy and surgery with surgery alone have been conducted (Table 28.8). Roth et al. (167) randomized 39 resectable patients to receive either two cycles of preoperative cisplatin, vindesine, and bleomycin followed by surgery and by six cycles of the same chemotherapy postoperatively, or immediate surgery alone. The group receiving preoperative chemotherapy had a 47% overall response rate with one pathologically complete response. Median survival, however, were identical in both groups (9 months). Schlag et al. (168) randomized 46 patients to receive either immediate surgery or three cycles of cisplatin and 5-FU followed by surgery. The preoperative chemotherapy response was 47%, but median survival was 10 months in both groups. There were two toxic deaths in the preoperative chemotherapy group, and this group had more septic and respiratory complications postoperatively.

Kelsen et al. (169) conducted a two-arm randomized study with a crossover design in 96 patients. Patients in the first arm received two cycles of preoperative cisplatin, vindesine, and bleomycin followed by surgery. Radiotherapy was administered if patients' tumors were unresectable or if they were found to have advanced disease (T3 or node positive lesions). Patients on the second arm received preoperative radiotherapy (5500 cGy) followed by surgery. Chemotherapy (cisplatin, vindesine, and bleomycin) was given to patients who were unresectable or who had advanced disease. The preoperative chemotherapy arm had a response rate of 55% compared with

TABLE 28.8. Randomized Trials of Preoperative Chemotherapy

Author (Reference No.)	Regimen	Patients (No.)	Response Rate (%)	Median Survival (Mo)
Roth et al. (167)	CDDP-VDS-Bleo × 2 cycles	39	47	9
	Surgery, CDDP-VDS × 6 cycles	...	...	...
	Surgery	...	...	9
Kelsen et al. (169)	CDDP-VDS-Bleo × 2 cycles	96	55	10.4
	Surgery, then RT if T3 N+ or unresectable			
	RT 5.5 Gy, surgery, then CDDP-VDS-Bleo if T3 N+ or unresectable	64		12.4
Schlag (168)	CDDP, 5-FU × 3 cycles, then surgery vs.	46	47	10
	Surgery alone	...	10	...
Japanese Esophageal Oncology Group (170)	Surgery, then RT (50 GY) vs. surgery, then CDDP-VDS × 2 cycles	25 3	NA ...	NS (2-y, 61%) NS (2-y, 60%)

Abbreviations. CDDP, cisplatin; Bleo, bleomycin; RT, radiotherapy; VDS, vindesine; 5-FU, 5-fluorouracil; NA, not applicable; NS, not stated.

64% in the preoperative radiotherapy group. Median survivals were 10.4 months and 12.4 months, respectively (169). Because the trial employed a crossover design, it is difficult to interpret survival data on either arm.

Postoperative chemotherapy has been compared with postoperative radiation therapy by the Japanese Esophageal Oncology Group (170). In this study 235 evaluable patients were randomized to receive either 5000 cGy of single-fraction radiation therapy given 2 to 4 weeks after, surgery or two cycles of cisplatin (50 mg/m^2) and vindesine (3 mg/m^2) given 2 to 4 weeks postoperatively. Two-year survival rates were not significantly different in either cohort (61% and 60%, respectively; $P = .8601$, log rank test). Myelosuppression was more severe in the chemotherapy arm with one death from neutropenia and sepsis (170).

The question of the benefit of preoperative chemotherapy cannot be answered definitively by these small trials of low statistical power. In the United States there is currently a trial in progress comparing immediate surgery versus three cycles of cisplatin and 5-FU followed by surgery and two cycles of postoperative chemotherapy.

In summary, preoperative chemotherapy incorporating cisplatin is effective in causing tumor shrinkage in as many as 64% of patients, and its use does not preclude subsequent esophagectomy. Small, inconclusive, randomized trials comparing preoperative chemotherapy and surgery with surgery alone have failed to show a significant difference in survival rates. The impact of this strategy on the overall survival of patients with esophageal cancer remains to be determined.

CHEMOTHERAPY AND RADIATION THERAPY

The simultaneous or concomitant administration of a chemotherapeutic agent with radiation therapy has been studied in a number of locally advanced malignancies, including head and neck cancer, limited stage small and non–small cell lung cancer, squamous cell carcinoma of the anus, and esophageal carcinoma (171) Concomitant chemoradiotherapy is aimed at improving local control by overcoming radioresistance and at eradicating distant micrometastasis to decrease systemic failure rates.

Radiation and chemotherapy can combine theoretically in several different ways (172). The first is the independent action of each treatment modality, or "spatial cooperation." The primary site of activity for radiotherapy is within the radiation field; however, the primary site of action of chemotherapy is outside of the radiation field against occult or evident metastasis important in esophogeal cancer, but also is achieved with induction chemotheapy. The combined treatment is "toxicity independent," wherein the specific chemotherapeutic agent and the radiation have different or nonoverlapping toxicities. This allows the two modalities to be administered safely and simultaneously at sufficient doses to produce an antitumor effect but minimizes toxicities and preserves normal tissues. The theoretical outcome is at least additive antitumor activity.

The third mechanism postulates "protection" of normal tissues by the chemotherapeutic agent allowing for higher doses of radiation. Increased efficacy would only result if the tumor were not radioprotected as well. Finally, there can be a positive interaction between the chemotherapeutic agent and radiation, wherein the drug enhances, sensitizes, or potentiates the effect of radiation on tissue. For a truly synergistic therapeutic relationship between chemotherapy and radiotherapy to exist, the enhancing or potentiating effect of the two agents must be higher in the tumor than in the surrounding normal tissues. Otherwise, there is a synergistic interaction but an unchanged therapeutic ratio. In an effort to exploit these principles, there have been several trials of concomitant chemoradiotherapy, with and without surgery, in esophageal cancer.

In 1981 Steiger et al. (173) reported their experience with a regimen consisting of 3000 cGy of radiation given concomitantly with 5-FU, and mitomycin or cisplatin. In this series a total of 42 patients received the regimen before esophagectomy. Thirty-five patients had resections with 13 (37%) having negative resected specimens on pathologic evaluation. The patients who received surgery had an impressive 12-month median survival and a 30% 2-year survival. There was a 30% operative mortality, however. This same group later reviewed their experience with 89 patients treated with combined modality therapy (174). A total of 50 patients had resections whereas 39 patients were unresectable. Median survival in both groups was identical (6 months). With the exception of one patient, all patients without pathologic evidence of tumor in the resected specimen survived at least 30 months. Four patients who did not have esophagectomy were alive 2 to 5 years after treatment. The authors concluded that surgery added no benefit to combined modality therapy and only increased morbidity and mortality. Subsequently, there have been a number of trials incorporating chemotherapy and radiation therapy alone.

The results of several pilot trials using combined chemotherapy and radiation therapy are summarized in Table 28.9. Coia et al. (175) used 5-FU and mitomycin C together with 5000 to 6000 cGy of concurrent radiotherapy in all stages of squamous cell carcinoma of the esophagus. Patients with stage I and II disease had a median survival of 18 months, whereas patients with stage III and IV disease had a median survival of only 8 months. Keane et al. (176) also used 5-FU and mitomycin C with 4500 to 5000 cGy of concomitant radiotherapy to treat 35 patients with esophageal cancer. There was a 78% complete response rate and a 28% 2-year survival. Median survival was not reported. Chan et al. (177) conducted a similar trial in 21 patients with a 13-month median survival.

The combination of mitomycin, bleomycin, cisplatin, and 50 cGy of split-course radiotherapy was studied by Leichman et al. (178) in 20 patients with esophageal cancer. They reported a 22-month median survival. John et al. (179) studied the same chemotherapy regimen using continuous dosing of radiotherapy to 4000 to 5000 cGy and maintenance methotrexate, 5-FU, and leucovorin. They observed a 77% complete response rate and an 11-month median survival in 20 patients.

The combination of cisplatin and 5-FU with radiation has been studied by three groups. Richmond et al. (180) enrolled 27 patients to receive cisplatin, 5-FU, and 5600 to 6000 cGy of concomitant chemoradiation; they showed a 12-month median survival. Herskovic et al. (174) gave 5-FU and cisplatin with 5000 cGy of concurrent radiation therapy to 22 patients and reported a 22-month median survival. Seitz et al. (181) enrolled 35 patients to receive 5-FU, cisplatin, and 4000 cGy of concomitant chemoradiation with a 71% complete response rate and a 17-month median survival.

These encouraging median survival rates have led to larger randomized trials comparing concomitant chemoradiotherapy with radiation therapy alone. These trials are summarized in Table 28.10. The first trial, conducted by Roussel et al. (182), randomized 144 patients to receive either single agent methotrexate with 5600 cGy of radiation therapy or 45 cGy of radiation therapy alone. The difference in median survivals was not statistically significant (9 months and 8 months, respectively). This trial did, however, identify Karnofsky performance status under 70 and weight loss exceeding 10% of body weight as poor prognostic factors.

The second randomized trial by Araujo et al. compared concomitant irradiation (5000 cGy) with 5-FU, mitomycin, and bleomycin versus 5000 cGy of radiation therapy alone (183). There was no statistically significant difference in complete response rate (75% versus 58%, $P = .77$), or 5-year survival rates (16% versus 6%, $P = .29$). The number of patients studied (i.e., 59), however, was too small to detect any but very large differences and may account for the lack of significance between the two treatment arms. Esophagitis and myelosuppression were both more severe in the chemoradiotherapy group.

The Eastern Cooperative Oncology Group randomized 135 patients with stage I and II squamous cell esophageal carcinoma to receive either 4000 cGy of radiation initially, or 4000 cGy with one cycle of bolus mitomycin C (10 mg/m^2) and two cycles of continuous infusion (1000 mg/m^2/day) 5-FU for 4 days. Patients were then considered for resection. Patients not under-

TABLE 28.9. Pilot Trials of Concomitant Chemoradiotherapy

AUTHOR (REFERENCE NO.)	DRUGS	RT DOSE (cGY)	PATIENTS (NO.)	CR (%)	MEDIAN SURVIVAL (MO)
Coia et al. (175)	5-FU–mitomycin	5000–6000	57 (Stages I, II)	NS	18
	5-FU–mitomycin	5000–6000	33 (Stages III, IV)	NS	8
Keane et al. (176)	5-FU–mitomycin	4500–5000	35	78	NS (2-y, 28%)
Chan et al. (177)	5-FU–mitomycin	4000–5000	21	86	13
Leichman et al. (178)	Mitomycin, CDDP-Bleo (split course)	5000	20	NS	22
John et al. (179)	Mitomycin, CDDP-Bleo with MTX–5-FU–LV as maintenance	4500–5000	20	77	11
Richmond et al. (180)	CDDP–5-FU	5600–6000	27	NS	12
Herskovic et al. (174)	CDDP–5-FU	5000	22	NS	22
Seitz et al. (181)	CDDP–5-FU	4000	35	71	17

Abbreviations. CR, complete response; 5-FU, 5-fluorouracil; Bleo, bleomycin; NS, not stated; CDDP, cisplatin; LV, leucovorin.

TABLE 28.10. Randomized Trials of Concomitant Chemoradiotherapy vs. Radiation Therapy

AUTHOR (REFERENCE NO.)	DRUGS	RADIATION (cGY)	PATIENTS (NO.)	RESPONSE (%)	MEDIAN SURVIVAL (MO)
Roussell et al. (182)	MTX vs. control	5600	75	NS	9
		4500	69	NS	8
Araujo et al. (183)	5-FU–mitomycin–Bleo vs. control	5000	28	75	NS (5-y, 16%)
		5000	31	58	NS (5-y, 6%)
Sischy et al. (184)	5-FU–mitomycin vs. control	6000 (split)	65	NS	14.9
		6000 (split)	65	NS	9
Herskovic et al. (185)	5-FU–CDDP vs. control	5000	61	73	12.5
		6400	59	60	8.9

Abbreviations. MTX, methotrexate; NS, not stated; 5-FU, 5-fluorouracil; Bleo, bleomycin.

going surgery received an additional 2000 to 2600 cGy of radiotherapy alone. The median survival in the group treated with concomitant chemoradiotherapy was 14.9 months as compared to 9 months for those given radiotherapy alone ($P = .03$) (184).

In a phase III randomized study conducted by the Radiation Therapy Oncology Group (RTOG), cisplatin and 5-FU by 96-hour continuous infusion with concurrent 5000 cGy of continuous radiotherapy were compared with 64 Gy of radiotherapy alone in locally advanced esophageal carcinoma. Median survivals were 12.5 months in the chemoradiotherapy group as compared with 8.9 months in the radiotherapy group ($P < .001$). Two-year survival was also significantly better in the chemoradiotherapy group (38%) as compared with 10% 2-year survival in those receiving radiotherapy alone ($P < .001$). Local as well as distant failure rates were both significantly lower in the chemoradiotherapy group (185).

These randomized trials support the feasibility of concomitant chemoradiotherapy in esophageal carcinoma with greater but acceptable toxicities than in patients receiving radiation therapy alone. The last two trials by the ECOG and RTOG establish the superiority of concomitant chemoradiotherapy over radiation alone, both in early-stage and locally advanced disease. Future randomized trials should not use radiation alone as a control arm.

CONCOMITANT CHEMORADIOTHERAPY AND SURGERY

The RTOG randomized trial has clearly established concomitant chemoradiotherapy as superior to radiotherapy alone for advanced esophageal cancer. However, the ability of this approach to definitively control tumor locally remains suboptimal because even in the chemoradiotherapy arm of the RTOG study local failures were the most common site of treatment failure (185). This prompted some investigators to include surgery in their regimens in an effort to improve the local control of tumor. Phase II trials incorporating concomitant chemoradiotherapy with esophagectomy have been performed. Concomitant chemoradiotherapy is usually given preceding surgery, except in the trial by Hoffman et al. (166) where chemoradiotherapy was given postoperatively.

Table 28.11 summarizes the results from some of the most significant trials. Steiger et al. (173) were the first to report their experience with mitomycin, 5-FU,

TABLE 28.11. Nonrandomized Trials of Concomitant Chemoradiotherapy with Surgery

AUTHOR (REFERENCE NO.)	DRUGS	RADIATION (cGY)	PATIENTS (NO.)	RESECTIONS	MEDIAN SURVIVAL (MO)
Steiger et al. (173)	5-FU/Mitomycin	3000	30	23	12
Leichman et al. (185)	CDDP–5-FU	3000	21	15	18
Poplin et al. (187)	CDDP–5-FU	3000	113	55	12
Forastiere et al. (189)	CDDP–5-FU–VBN	3750–4500	43	36 (transhiatal)	29
Stewart et al. (188)	CDDP–5-FU–LV–VP-16	3000	24	21	>26
Hoffman et al. (166)	5-FU–Hydroxyurea[a]	5000–6000	41	31	12.5

Abbreviations. 5-FU, 5-fluorouracil; CDDP, cisplatin; VBN, vinblastine; VP-16, etoposide; LV, leucovorin.
[a]Resected patients received chemoradiation postoperatively with preoperative CDDP–5-FU–LV therapy.

and 3000 cGy of radiotherapy showing an impressive survival with a low operative mortality. The unpredictable myelosuppression and pulmonary toxicity seen with mitomycin and the encouraging activity of cisplatin in a variety of solid tumors prompted the investigators to conduct a second trial with cisplatin and 5-FU with 3000 cGy of radiotherapy (185). This trial reported a good resection rate (72%) and an encouraging median survival of 18 months. The mortality was high with 5 treatment-related deaths (24%). The Southwest Oncology Group utilized this regimen in a large phase II trial enrolling 113 patients. Median survival was only 12 months with a 28% 2-year survival. Only 49% of patients were resectable with an 11% protocol mortality. However, there was a 17% pathologically documented complete response rate (187).

A more recent trial was reported by Stewart et al. (188) utilizing preoperative cisplatin, 5-FU, and leucovorin concomitantly with 3000 cGy of radiation therapy in 24 patients. Thirteen of these patients also received etoposide. Complete resections were performed in 21 patients (91%) with six having no evidence of tumor on pathology evaluation (pathologically complete response rate of 23%) and with no treatment deaths. Median survival was greater than 26 months with a 76% 2-year survival.

Forastiere et al. (189) performed the most intensive phase II study to date. A total of 43 patients with locally advanced esophageal cancer were treated with an aggressive preoperative regimen consisting of two cycles of continuous infusion cisplatin and 5-FU with bolus vinblastine given concomitantly, with either 3750 cGy by daily single fractions or 4500 cGy twice daily (hyperfractionated) radiotherapy. A total of 39 patients underwent transhiatal esophagectomy with 10 patients (29%) having no evidence of tumor in the resected specimens on pathologic evaluation. With a median follow-up of 78.7 months, the median survival was 29 months with a 34% 5-year survival. Patients with negative pathologic specimens had a 5-year survival of 60% as opposed to 32% for patients with pathologically positive specimens at resection. There were two treatment-related deaths from sepsis and neutropenia. Poor prognostic factors identified in this study included receiving less than full-dose chemotherapy, and clinically enlarged lymph nodes, but did not include histologic type, age, performance status, or weight loss. This study has prompted the initiation of a randomized trial comparing preoperative chemoradiation and esophagectomy to immediate esophagectomy.

There have been two randomized trials reported comparing preoperative chemoradiotherapy with either radiation and surgery or surgery alone. The results of these trials are summarized in Table 28.12. Andersen et al. (190) randomized a total of 129 patients to receive either concomitant single agent bleomycin with 3000 cGy of radiation therapy prior to esophagectomy versus preoperative radiotherapy (3500 cGy) and esophagectomy. Resection rates were low in both arms (54% and 47%, respectively) with identically low median survivals of 6.5 months. The trial has been criticized for incorporating low doses of radiation and chemotherapy and having lower median survivals than those seen with preoperative radiation therapy.

Another recent study by the European Organization for Research and Treatment of Cancer has been published in abstract form (191). This trial randomized 257 patients with stage I or II squamous cell esophageal cancer to receive either preoperative chemoradiation with two cycles of bolus cisplatin as a single agent and 3700 cGy of radiotherapy followed by esophagectomy or esophagectomy alone. With a median follow-up of 2.7-year median survivals were similar at 20 months for each arm. This survival is in the range of previously reported survivals for locally advanced disease. More follow-up is needed and a full survival and response analysis is pending.

PALLIATIVE THERAPY

Esophageal carcinoma often presents as advanced or metastatic disease that is incurable. There also is a

TABLE 28.12. Randomized Trials of Concomitant Chemoradiotherapy with Surgery

Author (Reference No.)	Drugs	Radiation (cGy)	Patients (No.)	Resections (No.)	Median Survival (Mo)
Andersen et al. (190)	Bleomycin vs.	3000	65	35	6.5
	control	3500	59	28	6.5
Bosset et al. (191)[a]	CDDP vs.	3700	NS	NS	20
	control	...	NS	NS	20

Abbreviations. Bleo, bleomycin; CDDP, cisplatin; NS, not stated.
[a]Data in abstract form only.

very high recurrence rate among patients who were treated originally with curative intent and for whom no curative salvage therapy exists. Some patients with locally advanced disease and poor performance status may also be inappropriate candidates for aggressive, potentially curative regimens but who will need relief of symptoms such as pain and dysphagia. This leaves a significant population that may benefit from palliative therapy.

The goals of palliation are directed at improving the quality of life and specifically include the relief of symptoms such as dysphagia and chest pain. All three modalities of surgery, radiation therapy, and chemotherapy have been used in palliation of this disease. This section will discuss the use of surgery, radiation therapy, and chemotherapy as palliative therapies in esophageal carcinoma.

Surgery As Palliative Therapy

Palliation of dysphagia, pain, and bleeding, and prevention of recurring local problems from esophageal cancer are common indications for esophageal resection. Because long-term survival is not the objective in a palliative intervention, an operative approach under these circumstances is selected that will minimize operative risk and recovery time, typically a transhiatal resection. With continuing improvements in local nonsurgical therapy for esophageal cancer, the incidence of palliative resection is decreasing. As a result, surgical intervention for palliation is more often used to manage specific complications such as obstruction and malignant esophagorespiratory fistula.

Malignant Esophagorespiratory Fistula

About 5% of all patients with carcinoma of the esophagus develop a fistula into the airway (192). Most fistulae involve a main stem bronchus or the trachea, and result in substantial soilage of the tracheobronchial tree with saliva, ingested food, and gastric juices. Although many fistulae develop during or after a course of radiation therapy, nearly 40% occur in the absence of such treatment. This catastrophic complication is associated with a median survival of only 4 to 6 weeks if no definitive treatment is provided (192). Surprisingly, only 20% of patients who have a malignant esophagorespiratory fistula at the time of diagnosis have evidence of distant metastatic disease. Although resection is usually not possible for technical reasons, aggressive intervention may be warranted in selected patients.

Surgical options include bypass, esophageal exclusion, and intubation. The bypass operation involves a substernal pull-up of stomach or colon with a cervical esophageal anastomosis. This permits ingestion of a normal diet and is associated with a median survival of more than 20 weeks. An esophageal exclusion procedure consists of a cervical esophagostomy, ligation of the esophagogastric junction, and placement of an enteral feeding tube. Respiratory symptoms are effectively treated with this technique, but patients are no longer able to eat or drink. Intubation using a pulsion or traction technique can protect the airway from soilage to some extent, but most patients die of continued respiratory problems nevertheless. The high hospital mortality associated with this technique precludes its use except in patients who cannot tolerate more aggressive intervention.

Esophageal Obstruction

Esophageal obstruction is frequently the most disabling symptom of esophageal cancer and often requires palliative intervention. Obstruction is usually secondary to intraluminal growth, but also may be due to extrinsic compression by a primary tumor mass or nodal disease, or to irradiation-induced fibrosis. Therapy is aimed at restoring swallowing function. Endoscopic intervention consists of either laser ablation of endoluminal tumor or esophageal intubation.

Laser therapy has been used in the management of esophageal cancer since 1981, most often employing the neodymium:yttrium aluminum garnet (Nd:YAG) laser. This technique requires dilation of the stenosis to permit passage of an endoscope, followed by retrograde photocoagulation of endoluminal tumor. Restoration of swallowing function is achieved in 80% of patients, and the incidence of complications such as bleeding and perforation is less than 5% (193–196). The likelihood of successful palliation is decreased in patients who have cervical or gastroesophageal junction cancers, tumors that are more than 5 cm in length, or significant extraluminal compression of the esophagus. In patients who experience relief from dysphagia following laser therapy, the median duration of symptomatic improvement is 2 to 3 months in the absence of other interventions.

Photodynamic therapy is a new experimental laser-based technique for managing dysphagia caused by an obstructing cancer. Following intravenous injection of a dihematoporphyrin derivative that is selectively retained in tumor stroma, laser light is used to activate the compound, causing the release of oxygen radicals resulting in selective tumor cell death. Limited clinical experience with this modality suggests that palliation of dysphagia is good and that the incidence of complications such as perforation and dermal photosensitivity is low (197, 198).

Intubation for palliation of dysphagia has been in use since the late 19th century. Endoscopic placement of prosthetic tubes became commonplace during the 1980s, and advances in their design has substantially reduced the morbidity and mortality associated with their placement (199–201). Most current devices are made of polyethylene or silicone rubber and have proximal and distal flanges that anchor them across the obstructing tumor. The use of self-expanding metallic stents has also been described; these may decrease the likelihood of perforation and dislodgment associated with the more traditional stents (202, 203). Hospital mortality is 5% to 15%, reflecting the underlying condition of the patients selected for this therapy, and average survival is 4 to 6 months.

RADIATION THERAPY WITH PALLIATIVE INTENT

Radiation therapy is an effective means of palliation in patients with local symptoms due to tumor recurrence or for advanced incurable disease in patients with poor performance status. Reported rates of partial or complete relief of symptoms in patients treated with esophageal carcinoma range from 50% to 80% (66, 78, 82). Radiation therapy in the palliative setting is often delivered with short courses (30 Gy over 2 weeks), but may delivered with more protracted schedules (50 to 60 Gy over 5 to 6 weeks). In symptomatic terminal patients, however, short courses with high daily fractions are more desirable. An attractive alternative to conventional external beam radiotherapy in the palliative setting is intracavitary brachytherapy using either low-dose–rate ^{192}Ir sources or with high-dose–rate techniques (56, 204).

Wara et al. (76) reported a high rate of palliation (89% response) in a series of 129 patients treated at the University of California at San Francisco. The mean duration of palliation was 3 months. Eleven percent of patients noted no palliative benefit; 66%, improvement lasting less than 2 months; 11%, benefits lasting between 6 and 12 months; and 14%, improvement lasting more than 12 months. Elkon and associates (78) noted a 84% amelioration of symptoms in a series of 72 patients. The likelihood of response was a function of tumor size, with 75% of patients with tumors less than 5 cm in size noting a benefit compared with only 29% of patients with tumors larger than 10 cm (78).

CHEMOTHERAPY AS PALLIATIVE THERAPY

There have been many studies of chemotherapy in esophageal cancer over the last 20 years. Most single-agent and combination agent trials have been in patients with recurrent, nonoperable, or metastatic disease. The endpoint in most of these trials was radiographic response of disease and not palliation of symptoms. Palliation in these studies is often poorly quantified and only given in descriptive terms (Tables 28.5 and 28.6).

There have been very few randomized trials specifically addressing the role of chemotherapy in the palliation of the symptoms of esophageal cancer. In a study by Schmid et al. (205), a total of 127 patients were randomized to receive esophageal intubation alone (46 patients), intubation with 4000 cGy of split-course radiation therapy (41 patients), or intubation with one of three chemotherapeutic agents, trimetrexate, ifosfamide or 5-FU, and leucovorin (40 patients). There was a 20% partial response rate to chemotherapy (all regimens) and a 22% partial response rate to radiation therapy. The median response duration to radiation or chemotherapy treatments was 3 months. There was no reported difference in palliative effect observed among the various regimens. However, the method of assessment of symptoms and severity was not described. The patients who received radiation therapy or chemotherapy had more complications than those who received intubation alone. These side effects included esophagitis, infection, and leukopenia. There was no statistical difference in survival in the three arms (15, 9, and 11 weeks, respectively; $P = .7$) (204). Although this study was small and a detailed analysis of palliation was not performed, it does illustrate the relatively brief and incomplete response durations seen with palliative chemotherapy and radiation therapy with no observed benefit for the addition of either modality to esophageal intubation.

The same group then randomized 20 patients to receive either esophageal intubation or esophageal intubation and concomitant chemoradiotherapy with split-course radiation therapy (4000 cGy) given simultaneously with cisplatin and 5-FU. There were four deaths related to toxicity in the chemoradiotherapy arm. An interim survival analysis showed that patients randomized to intubation had a median survival of 19 weeks, and the patients receiving combined modality therapy had a median survival of 11 weeks ($P = .03$). The trial was then closed (206). Chemotherapy as a single agent or as part of a combined modality regimen when given for a purely palliative intent probably offers very little benefit, but larger trials incorporating quality of life analysis are necessary to define clearly the role of chemotherapy as palliation for patients with incurable esophageal cancer.

Prognostic Factors

Factors predicting outcome in patients with esophageal cancer have not been identified consistently in any study. Roussel et al. (182) identified weight loss exceeding 10% of body weight and a Karnofsky performance status of less than 70% as poor prognostic factors. In a preliminary analysis, Hoffman et al. (166) suggested poorer survival in patients with adenocarcinoma, whereas in the study by Forastiere et al. (189), histology did not affect outcome. Gill et al. (207) identified a significantly poorer survival in patients with adenocarcinoma compared with squamous cell carcinoma (15.6 months versus 26.1 months; $P = .004$). Other poor prognostic factors included failure to respond completely to chemoradiotherapy, and tumor length greater than 5 cm. These prognostic factors remained constant regardless of the type of treatment used. Currently, the identification of prognostic factors in patients undergoing therapy for esophageal carcinoma is very inconclusive and at times contradictory. Larger studies currently in progress will help to clarify this issue.

Summary

Whereas the overall prognosis for esophageal cancer has only recently changed significantly, there is now hope that combined modality therapy may offer significant improvements in survival. Surgery is still considered the mainstay of curative therapy in early-stage disease. Radiation therapy may offer cure in some rare circumstances and may be effective when used before surgery. Both surgery and radiation therapy are effective modalities for the palliation of symptoms of patients with incurable disease.

Chemotherapy, although offering little in terms of palliation, may improve outcome when combined with either or both of the other two modalities. Randomized trials comparing preoperative chemotherapy and surgery with surgery alone are currently under way. Concomitant chemoradiotherapy has been compared with radiation therapy alone as potentially curative therapy in esophageal cancer. Concomitant chemoradiotherapy appears to offer a survival benefit over radiation therapy alone; however, local and distant recurrences are still high. Combined chemoradiotherapy with surgery currently remains investigational and cannot be recommended universally in patients with locoregional esophageal cancer. The results of trials comparing concomitant chemoradiotherapy and surgery with surgery alone are awaited. Prognostic factors in esophageal cancer have not been established clearly, and the roles of tumor histology, response to therapy, and disease stage remain unclear.

References

1. Holscher AH, Schuler M, Siewert R. Surgical treatment of adenocarcinomas of the gastroesophageal junction. Diseases of the Esophagus 1988;1:35–49.
2. Stipa S, Di Giorgio A, Ferri M. Surgical treatment of adenocarcinoma of the cardia. Surgery 1992;111:386–393.
3. Lerut T, De Leyn P, Coosemans W, et al. Surgical strategies in esophageal carcinoma with emphasis on radical lymphadenectomy. Ann Surg, 1992;216:583–590.
4. Kitamura M, Nishihira T, Hirayama K, et al. Surgical treatment for patients 70 years of age or older with carcinoma of the esophagus. In: Siewert JR, Holscher AH, eds. Diseases of the esophagus. Berlin: Springer-Verlag, 1988:261–263.
5. Nishi M, Hiramatsu Y, Hioki K, et al. Risk factors in relation to postoperative complications in patients undergoing esophagectomy or gastrectomy for cancer. Ann Surg 1988;207:148–154.
6. Elman A, Giuli R, Sancho-Garnier H. Risk factors of pulmonary complications following esophagectomy in carcinoma of the esophagus: results of the prospective study conducted by the OESO group. In: Siewert R, Holscher AH, eds. Diseases of the esophagus. Berlin: Springer-Verlag, 1988:224–228.
7. Konder H, Poenitz-Pohl E, Stahlknecht CD, et al. Analysis of cardiopulmonary function in esophageal cancer patients prior to surgery. In: Siewert R, Holscher AH, eds. Diseases of the esophagus. Berlin: Springer-Verlag, 1988:249–252.
8. Chan K-H, Wong J. Mortality after esophagectomy for carcinoma of the esophagus: an analysis of risk factors. Diseases of the Esophagus 1990;3:49–53.
9. Tsutsui S, Moriguchi S, Morita M. Multivariate analysis of postoperative complications after esophageal resection. Ann Thorac Surg 1992;53:1052–1056.

10. Fekete F, Belghiti J, Cherqui D, et al. Results of esophagogastrectomy for carcinoma in cirrhotic patients. Ann Surg 1987; 206:74–78.
11. Muto T, Matsubara Y, Sato N, et al. Appraisal of hyperalimentation and nutritional assessment in esophageal cancer surgery. In: Siewert R, Holscher AH, eds. Diseases of the esophagus. Berlin: Springer-Verlag, 1988:276–280.
12. Burt ME, Gorschboth CM, Brennan MF. A controlled, prospective, randomized trial evaluating the metabolic effects of enteral and parenteral nutrition in the cancer patient. Cancer 1982;49:1092–1105.
13. Nishi M, Hiramatsu Y, Hatano T, et al. Effect of nutritional support as an adjunct to the treatment of esophageal cancer. In: Siewert R, Holscher AH, eds. Diseases of the esophagus. Berlin: Springer-Verlag, 1988:287–290.
14. Daly JM, Massar E, Giacco G, et al. Parenteral nutrition in esophageal cancer patients. Ann Surg 1982;196:203–208.
15. Saito T, Zeze K, Kuwahara A, et al. A prospective study on preoperative parenteral nutrition for patients with esophageal cancer. In: Siewert R, Holscher AH, eds. Diseases of the esophagus. Berlin: Springer-Verlag, 1988:268–271.
16. Lewis I. The surgical treatment of carcinoma of the esophagus with special reference to a new operation for growths of the middle third. Br J Surg 1946;34:18–31.
17. Akiyama H, Tsurumaru M, Kawamura T, Ono Y. Principles of surgical treatment for carcinoma of the esophagus. Ann Surg 1981;194:438–446.
18. Logan A. The surgical treatment of carcinoma of the esophagus and cardia. J Thorac Cardiovasc Surg 1963;46:150–161.
19. Skinner DB. En bloc resection for neoplasms of the esophagus and cardia. J Thorac Cardiovasc Surg 1983;85:59–71.
20. Skinner DB, Little AG, Ferguson MK, Soriano A, Staszak VM. Selection of operation for esophageal cancer based on staging. Ann Surg 1986;204:391–401.
21. Nishihira T, Watanabe T, Ohmori N, et al. Long-term evaluation of patients treated by radical operation for carcinoma of the thoracic esophagus. World J Surg 1984;8:778–785.
22. DeMeester TR, Zaninotto G, Johansson K-E. Selective therapeutic approach to cancer of the lower esophagus and cardia. J Thorac Cardiovasc Surg 1988;95:42–54.
23. Ide H, Hanyu F, Murata Y, et al. Extended dissection for thoracic esophageal cancer based on preoperative staging. In: Ferguson MK, Little AG, Skinner DB, eds. Diseases of the esophagus. Malignant diseases. Mount Kisco, NY: Futura, 1990;I: 177–186.
24. Tsurumaru M, Akiyama H, Udagawa H, et al. Cervical-thoracic-abdominal lymph node dissection for intrathoracic esophageal carcinoma. In: Ferguson MK, Little AG, Skinner DB, eds. Diseases of the esophagus. Malignant diseases. Mount Kisco, NY: Futura 1990;I:187–196.
25. Kato H, Watanabe H, Tachimori Y, et al. Evaluation of neck lymph node dissection for thoracic esophageal carcinoma. Ann Thorac Surg 1991;51:931–935.
26. Nishihira T, Mori S, Hirayama K. Extensive lymph node dissection for thoracic esophageal carcinoma. Diseases of the Esophagus 1992;5:79–89.
27. Peracchia A, Ruol A, Bardini R, et al. Lymph node dissection for cancer of the thoracic esophagus: how extended should it be? Diseases of the Esophagus 1992;5:69–78.
28. Denk W. Zur Radikaloperation des Oesophaguskarzinoms. Zbl Chir 1913;40:1065–1068.
29. Turner GG. Excision of thoracic esophagus for carcinoma with construction of extrathoracic gullet. Lancet 1933;2: 1315–1316.
30. Ong GB, Lee TC. Pharyngogastric anastomosis after oesophagopharyngectomy for carcinoma of the hypopharynx and cervical esophagus. Br J Surg 1960;48:193–200.
31. Akiyama H, Sato Y, Takahashi F. Immediate pharyngogastrostomy following total esophagectomy by blunt dissection. Jpn J Surg 1971;1:225–231.
32. Kirk RM. Palliative resection of oesophageal carcinoma without formal thoracotomy. Br J Surg 1974;61:689–690.
33. Orringer MB, Sloan H. Esophagectomy without thoracotomy. J Thorac Cardiovasc Surg 1978;76:643–654.
34. Orringer MB. Transhiatal esophagectomy without thoracotomy for carcinoma of the esophagus. Ann Surg 1984;200: 282–288.
35. Chakkaphak S, Krishnasamy S, Walker SJ, et al. Treatment of carcinoma of the proximal esophagus. Surg Gynecol Obstet 1989;168:307–310.
36. Kakegawa T, Yamana H, Ando N. Analysis of surgical treatment for carcinoma situated in the cervical esophagus. Surgery 1985;97:150–157.
37. Kasai M, Nishihira T. Reconstruction using pedicled jejunal segments after resection for carcinoma of the cervical esophagus. Surg Gynecol Obstet 1986;163:145–152.
38. Mansour KA, Picone AL, Coleman JJ III. Surgery for high cervical esophageal carcinoma: experience with 11 patients. Ann Thorac Surg 1990;49:597–602.
39. Grillo HC, Mathisen DJ. Cervical exenteration. Ann Thorac Surg 1990;49:401–409.
40. King RM, Pairolero PC, Trastek VF, et al. Ivor Lewis esophagogastrectomy for carcinoma of the esophagus: early and late functional results. Ann Thorac Surg 1987;44:119–122.
41. Mathisen DJ, Grillo HC, Wilkins EW Jr, et al. Transthoracic esophagectomy: a safe approach to carcinoma of the esophagus. Ann Thorac Surg 1988;45:137–143.
42. Lozac'h P, Topart P, Etienne J, et al. Ivor Lewis operation for epidermoid carcinoma of the esophagus. Ann Thorac Surg 1991;52:1154–1157.
43. Gelfand GAJ, Finley RJ, Nelems B, et al. Transhiatal esophagectomy for carcinoma of the esophagus and cardia. Arch Surg 1992;127:1164–1168.
44. Isolauri J, Markkula H, Autio V. Colon interposition in the treatment of carcinoma of the esophagus and gastric cardia. Ann Thorac Surg 1987;43:420–424.
45. Ellis FH Jr, Gibb SP, Watkins E Jr. Esophagogastrectomy. Ann Surg 1983;198:531–540.
46. Sugimachi K, Maekawa S, Koga Y, Ueo H, Inokuchi K. The quality of life is sustained after operation for carcinoma of the esophagus. Surg Gynecol Obstet 1986;162:544–546.
47. Hennessy TPJ, Keeling P. Adenocarcinoma of the esophagus and cardia. J Thorac Cardiovasc Surg 1987;94:64–68.
48. Fekete F, Gayet B, Panis Y. Long-term results of transthoracic esophagectomy for squamous cell carcinoma. Diseases of the Esophagus 1992;5:105–110.
49. Siewert JR, Roder JD. Lymphadenectomy in esophageal cancer surgery. Diseases of the Esophagus 1992;5:91–97.
50. Law SYK, Fok M, Cheng SWK, et al. A comparison of outcome after resection for squamous cell carcinomas and adenocarcinomas of the esophagus and cardia. Surg Gynecol Obstet 1992;175:107–112.
51. Orringer MB, Marshall B, Stirling MC. Transhiatal esophagectomy for benign and malignant disease. J Thorac Cardiovasc Surg 1993;105:265–277.
52. Tilanus HW, Hop WCJ, Langenhorst BLAM, van Lanschot JJB. Esophagectomy with or without thoracotomy. J Thorac Cardiovasc Surg 1993;105:898–903.

53. Ellis FH Jr, Gibb SP, Watkins E Jr. Limited esophagogastrectomy for carcinoma of the cardia. Ann Surg 1988;208:354–361.
54. Dobbs J, Barrett A. Practical radiotherapy planning: Royal Marsden Hospital practice. London: Edward Arnold, 1985.
55. Mendenhall W, Mancuso A, Stringer S, et al. Carcinoma of the cervical esophagus. In: Million R, Cassisi N, eds. Management of head and neck cancer: a multidisciplinary approach. Philadelphia: JB Lippincott, 1994:542.
56. Fisher A, Brady L. Esophagus. In: Perez C, Brady L, eds. Principles and practice of radiation oncology. Philadelphia: JB Lippincott, 1992:859.
57. Miller C. Carcinoma of the thoracic esophagus and cardia. Br J Surg 1962;49:597–580.
58. Vijayakumar S, Muller-Runkel R. Irradiation of the esophagus: prone versus supine treatment positions. Acta Radiol Oncol 1979;18:103–106.
59. Smoron G, O'Brien C, Sullivan C. Tumor localization and treatment technique for cancer of the esophagus. Radiology 1974;111:735–736.
60. Teniere P, Hay J, Fingerhut A, et al. Postoperative radiation therapy does not increase survival after curative resection for squamous cell carcinoma of the middle and lower esophagus as shown by a multicenter controlled trial. Surg Gynecol Obstet 1991;173:123–128.
61. Coia K, Engstrom P, Paul A. Nonsurgical management of esophageal cancer: report of a study of combined radiotherapy and chemotherapy. J Clin Oncol 1987;5:1783–1790.
62. Cox J, Pajak T, Marcial V. Dose-response for local control with hyperfractionated radiation therapy in advanced carcinomas of the upper aerodigestive tracts: preliminary report of the radiation therapy oncology group protocol 83-13. Int. J Radiat Oncol Biol Phys 1990;18:515–521.
63. Barker J, Montague E, Peters L. Clinical experience with irradiation of inflammatory carcinoma of the breast with and without elective chemotherapy. Cancer 1980;45:625–629.
64. Cox J, Azarnia N, Byhardt R. Hyperfractionated radiation therapy (1.2 Gy b.i.d.) with 69.6 Gy total dose increases survival in favourable patients with stage III non–small cell carcinoma of the lung: report of RTOG 83-11. J Clin Oncol 1990;8:1543–1545.
65. Li D. Present status of esophageal cancer in China. Int J Radiat Oncol Biol Phys 1990;18:477–481.
66. Rosenberg J, Franklin R, Steiger Z. Squamous cell carcinoma of the thoracic esophagus: an interdisciplinary approach. Curr Probl Cancer 1981;5:6–52.
67. Stevens K. The esophagus. In: Moss W, Cox J, eds. Radiation oncology: rationale, technique and results. St. Louis: CV Mosby, 1989:30.
68. Weichselbaum R, Hallahan D, Chen G. Biological and physical basis to radiation oncology. In: Holland J, Frei E, Bast R, Kufe D, Morton D, Weichselbaum R, eds. Cancer medicine. Philadelphia: Lea & Febiger, 1993:557.
69. Flores A, Nelems B, Evans K, et al. Impact of new radiotherapy modalities on the surgical management of cancer of the esophagus and cardia. Int J Radiat Oncol Biol Phys 1989;17:937–944.
70. Burt P, Notley H, Stout R. A simple technique for intraluminal irradiation in oesphageal tumors using the high-dose-rate microelectron. Br J Radiol 1989;62:748–750.
71. Fleischman E, Kagan R, Bellotti J, et al. Effective palliation for inoperable esophageal cancer using extensive intracavitary radiation. J Surg Oncol 1990;44:234–237.
72. Laramore G, Davis R, Olson M. RTOG phase I study on fast neutron teletherapy for squamous cell carcinoma of the esophagus. Int J Radiat Oncol Biol Phys 1983;9:465–470.
73. Castro J, Saunders W, Tobias C. Treatment of cancer with heavy charged particles. Int J Radiat Oncol Biol Phys1982;8:2191–2196.
74. Hishikawa Y, Kamikonya N, Tanaka S, et al. Radiotherapy of esophageal carcinoma: role of high-dose–rate intracavitary irradiation. Radiother Oncol 1987;9:13–20.
75. Marks R, Scruggs H, Wallace K. Preoperative radiation therapy for carcinoma of the esophagus. Cancer 1976;38:84–92.
76. Wara W, Mauch P, Thomas A, et al. Palliation for carcinoma of the esophagus. Radiology 1976;121:717–720.
77. Pearson J. The present status and future potential of radiotherapy in the management of esophageal cancer. Cancer 1977;39:882–888.
78. Elkon D, Lee M, Hendrickson F. Carcinoma of the esophagus: sites of recurrence and palliative benefits after definitive radiation therapy. Int J Radiat Oncol Biol Phys 1979;4:615–622.
79. Beatty J, DeBoer G, Rider W. Carcinoma of the esophagus: pretreatment assessment, correlation of radiation treatment parameters with survival, and identification and management of radiation treatment failure. Cancer 1979;43:2254–2267.
80. Van Andel J, Dees J, Dijkhuis C, et al. Carcinoma of the esophagus: results of treatment. Ann Surg 1979;190:684–689.
81. Appelquist P, Silvo J, Rissanen P. The results of surgery and radiotherapy in the treatment of small carcinomas of the thoracic esophagus. Ann Clin Res 1979;11:184–188.
82. Schuchmann G, Heydorn W, Hall R, et al. The treatment of esophageal carcinoma. A retrospective review. J Thorac Cardiovasc Surg 1980;79:67–73.
83. Newaishy G, Read G, Duncan W, et al. Results of radical radiation therapy of squamous cell carcinoma of the oesophagus. Clin Radiol 1982;33:347–352.
84. Smalley SR, Gunderson LL, Reddy EK, Williamson S. Radiotherapy alone in esophageal carcinoma: current management and future directions of adjuvant, curative, and palliative approaches. Semin Oncol 1994;21(4):467–473.
85. Yin W, Zhang L, Miao Y, et al. The results of high-energy electron therapy in carcinoma of the oesophagus compared with telecobalt. Clin Radiol 1983;34:113–116.
87. Morita K, Takagi I, Watanabe M, et al. Relationship between radiologic features of esophageal cancer and local control by radiation therapy. Cancer 1985;55:2668–2676.
88. Roussell A, Jacob J, Haegele P, et al. Controlled clinical trial for the treatment of patients with inoperable esophageal carcinoma: a study of the EORTC Gastrointestinal Tract Cancer Cooperative Group. Rec Results Cancer Res 1988;110:21–29.
89. Earlam R, Cunha-Melo J. Oesophageal squamous cell carcinoma: II. A critical review of radiotherapy. Br J Surg 1980;67:457–461.
90. Millburn L, Faber L, Hendrickson F. Curative treatment of epidermoid carcinomna of the esophagus. AJR Am J Roentgenol 1968;103:291–299.
91. Van Andel J, Dees J, Dijkhuis C, et al. Carcinoma of the esophagus: results of treatment. Ann Surg 1979;190:684–689.
92. Kelsen D, Ahuja R, Hopfan S, et al. Combined modality therapy of esophageal carcinoma. Cancer 1981;48:31–37.
93. Akakura I, Nakamura Y, Kakegawa T, et al. Surgery of carcinoma of the esophagus with preoperative radiation. Chest 1970;57:47–57.
94. Liu G, Huang Z, Rong T, et al. Measures for improving therapeutic results of esophageal carcinoma in stage III: preoperative radiation therapy. J Surg Oncol 1986;32:248–255.

95. Petrovich Z, Lam K, Langholz B, et al. Surgical therapy and radiation therapy for carcinoma of the eosophagus: treatment results in 195 patients. J Thorac Cardiovasc Surg 1989;98:614–617.
96. Nakayama K, Kinoshita Y. Surgical treatment combined with preoperative concentrated irradiation. JAMA 1974;227:178–185.
97. Launois B, Delarue D, Campion J, et al. Preoperative radiation therapy for carcinoma of the esophagus. Surg Gynecol Obstet 1981;153:690–692.
98. Gignoux M, Roussel A, Paillot B, et al. The value of preoperative radiotherapy in esophageal cancer: results of a study of the E.O.R.T.C. World J Surg 1987;11:426–432.
99. Gunnlaugsson G, Wychulis A, Roland A, et al. Analysis of the records of 1657 patients with carcinoma of the esophagus and cardia of the stomach. Surg Gynecol Obstet 1970;130:997–1005.
100. Kasai M, Mori S, Watanabe T. Follow-up results after resection of thoracic esophageal carcinoma. World J Surg 1978;2:543–547.
101. Fok M, Sham J, Choy D, et al. Postoperative radiation therapy for carcinoma of the esophagus: a prospective, randomized controlled study. Surgery 1993;113:138–147.
102. Roth JA, Lichter AS, Putnam JB, et al. Cancer of the esophagus. In: Devita V, Hellman S, Rosenberg S, eds. Cancer, principles & practice of oncology. 4th ed. Philadelphia: JB Lippincott, 1993.
103. Forastiere AA. Treatment of locoregional esophageal cancer. Semin Oncol 1992;19(Suppl 11):57–63.
104. Kelsen D, Atiq OT. Therapy of upper gastrointestinal tract cancers. Curr Probl Cancer 1991;15(Sept–Oct):235–294.
105. Engstrom P, Lavin P, Kalssen D. Phase II evaluation Of mitomycin and cisplatin in advanced esophageal carcinoma. Cancer Treat Rep 1983;67:713–715
106. Panettiere F, Leichman L, Tilchen E, et al. Chemotherapy for advanced epidermoid carcinoma of the esophagus with single agent cisplatin: final report on a Southwest Oncology Group study. Cancer Treat Rep 1984;68:1023–1024.
107. Miller JI, McIntyre MD, Hatcher CR. Combined treatment in surgical management of carcinoma of the esophagus: a preliminary report. Ann Thorac Surg 1985;40:289–293.
108. Murthy SK, Prabhakaran PS, Chandrashekar M, et al. Neoadjuvant cis-DDP in esophageal cancers: an experience at a regional cancer centre. Indian J Surg Oncol 1990;45:173–176.
109. Davis S, Shanmugatheasa M, Kessler W. Cis-dichlordiamine platinum (II): the treatment of esophageal carcinoma. Cancer Treat Rep 1980;64:709–711.
110. Ravry M, Moore M. Phase II pilot study of cisplatin (II) in advanced squamous cell esophageal cancer. Cancer Treat Rep 1985;69:1457.
111. Bleiberg H, Jacob J, Bedenne L, et al. Randomized phase II trial of 5-fluorouracil and cisplatin versus cisplatin alone in advanced esophageal cancer. Proc Am Soc Clin Oncol 1991;10:147.
112. Kolaric K, Moricic Z, Dujmovic I, et al. Therapy of advanced esophageal cancer with bleomycin, irradiation and combination bleomycin and irradiation. Tumori 1976;62:255–262.
113. Clinical Screening Group. Study of the clinical efficiency of bleomycin in human cancer. BMJ 1970;2:643–645.
114. Yagoda A, Mukherji B, Young C, et al. Bleomycin, an antitumor antibiotic: in lymphomas and solid tumors. Ann Intern Med 1972;55:861–870.
115. Bonadonna G, de Lena M, Monfardi S, et al. Clinical trial with bleomycin in lymphomas and in solid tumors. Eur J Cancer 1972;8:205–215.
116. Stephens F. Bleomycin: a new approach in cancer chemotherapy. Med J Aust 1:1277–1283.
117. Ravry M, Moertel CG, Schutt AJ, et al. Treatment of advanced squamous cell carcinoma of the gastrointestinal tract with bleomycin (NSC 125066). Cancer Chemother Rep 1973;57:493–495.
118. Tancini G, Bajetta E, Bonadonna G. Therapy with bleomycin alone or in combination with methotrexate. Epidermoid carcinoma of the esophagus. Tumori 1974;60:65–71.
119. Desai P, Borges E, Vohrs V, et al. Carcinoma of the esophagus in India. Cancer 1969;23:979–989.
120. Whittington R, Close H. Clinical experience with mitomycin-C. Cancer Chemother Rep 1970;54:195–198.
121. Ezdinli E, Gelber R, Desai D, et al. Chemotherapy of advanced esophageal carcinoma: eastern cooperative group experience. Cancer 1980;46:2149.
122. Lokich J, Shea M, Chafey J. Sequential and infusional 5-fluorouracil followed by concomitant radiation for tumors of the esophagus and gastroesophageal junction. Cancer 1987;60:275.
123. Ajani IA, Ilson D, Daugherty R, et al. Activity of Taxol on patients with squamous cell carcinoma and adenocarcinoma of the esophagus. J Natl Cancer Inst 1994;86:1086–1091.
124. Advani S, Saika T, Swaroop S, et al. Anterior chemotherapy in esophageal cancer. Cancer 1985;56:1502.
125. Falkson G. Methyl GAG (NSC 32946) in the treatment of esophageal cancer. Cancer Chemother Rep 1971;55:209.
126. Kelsen DP, Chapman R, Bains M. Methyl-gloxal bis (guanylhydrazone) in the treatment of esophageal cancer: a phase II trial. Cancer Treat Rep 1982;66:1427–1429.
127. Ravry M, Omura G, Hill G, et al. Phase II evaluation of mitoguazone in cancer of the esophagus, stomach and pancreas: a southeastern cancer study group trial. Cancer Treat Rep 1986;60:729.
128. Kelsen DP, Bain MS, Cvitkovic E. Vindesine in the treatment of esophageal carcinoma: a phase II study. Cancer Treat Rep 1979;63:2019–2021.
129. Kolaric K, Maricic Z, Roth A, et al. Adriamycin alone and in combination with radiation therapy in the treatment of inoperable esophageal cancer. Tumori 1977;63:485.
130. Coonley C, Hilaris B, Bains M, et al. Cisplatin and bleomycin in the treatment of esophageal cancer: a final report. Cancer 1984;54:2351–2355.
131. Marcuello E, Alba E, Gomez De Segura G, et a. Cisplatin and intravenous continuous infusion of bleomycin in advanced and metastatic esophageal cancer. Eur J Cancer Clin Oncol 1988;24:633–635.
132. Kelsen D, Hilaris B, Coonley C, et al. Cisplatin, vindesine and bleomycin combination chemotherapy of local-regional and advanced esophageal carcinoma. Am J Med 1983;75:639–52.
133. Dinwoodie W, Bartolucci A, Lyman G. Cisplatin, bleomycin, and vindesine in advanced squamous cell carcinoma of the esophagus. Cancer Treat Rep 1986;70:267–270.
134. Kelsen DP, Hilaris B, Coonley C, et al. Cisplatin, vindesine and bleomycin combination chemotherapy of local-regional and advanced esophageal carcinoma. Am J Med 1983;75:645.
135. Forastiere A, Gennis MK, Orringer M, et al. Cisplatin, vinblastine and mitoguazone chemotherapy for epidermoid and adenocarcinoma of the esophagus. J Clin Oncol 1987;15:1143.
136. Vogl S, Camacho F, Berenzweig M, et al. Chemotherapy for

esophageal cancer with mitoguazone, methotrexate, bleomycin, and cisplatin. Cancer Treat Rep 1983;69:21–23.
137. Schuller J, Caejka M, Schernrhaner G, et al. Influence of interferon alfa-2B with or without folinic acid on pharmacokinetics of fluorouracil. Semin Oncol 1992;19(Suppl 3):45–48.
138. DeBesi P, Chiarion-Sileni V, Salvagno L, et al. Systemic chemotherapy with cisplatin, 5-fluorouracil and allopurinol in the management of esophageal cancer. Cancer Treat Rep 1986;70:909–910.
139. De Besi L, Salvagno L, Endrissi L, et al. Cisplatin, bleomycin and methotrexate in the treatment of advanced oesophageal cancer. Eur J Cancer Clin Oncol 1984;20:743–747.
140. Vogl S, Greenwald B, Kaplan B. Effective chemotherapy for esophageal cancer with methotrexate, bleomycin and cis-daminedichloroplatinum. Cancer 1981;48:2555–2558.
141. Forastiere A, Patel H, Hankins J, et al. Cisplatin, bleomycin, and VP16-213 in combination for epidermoid carcinoma of the esophagus. Proc Am Soc Clin Oncol 1983;2:A127.
142. Spielman M, Kac J, Elias D, et al. Association of vindesine, cyclophosphamide, cisplatin, and CCNU in esophageal squamous cell carcinoma. Bull Cancer (Paris) 1985;72:220–226.
143. Gisselbricht C, Calvo F, Mignot L, et al. Fluorouracil, adriamycin, and cisplatin combination chemotherapy of advanced esophageal carcinoma. Cancer 1983;52:974–977.
144. Preusser, P, Wilke H, Achterath W, et al. Disease oriented phase II study with cisplatin, etoposide, and 5-FU in advanced squamous cell carcinoma of the esophagus. Proc Am Soc Clin Oncol 1988;7:A388.
145. Spielman, M, Guillot T, Kac J, et al. Phase II trial of cisplatin and continuous infusion of bleomycin and 5-fluorouracil in advanced esophageal cancer. Proc Am Soc Clin Oncol 1989;8:A393
146. Alberts A, Schoeman L, Burger W, et al. Phase II trial of 5-fluorouracil in advanced carcinoma of the esophagus. Am J Clin Oncol 1992;15:35–36.
147. Zaniboni A, Simoncini E, Tonini G, et al. Cisplatin, high dose folinic acid and 5-fluorouracil in squamous cell carcinoma of the esophagus. A pilot study. Chemioterapia 1987;6:387–389.
148. Hayashi K, Ide H, Shinoda M, et al. Phase II study of cisplatin plus 5-fluorouracil and leucovorin for squamous cell carcinoma of the esophagus. Proc Am Soc Clin Oncol 1992;11:A526.
149. Wilke H, Stahl M, Preusser P, et al. Phase II trial with 5-FU, folinic acid, etoposide and cisplatin ± surgery in advanced esophageal cancer. Proc Am Soc Clin Oncol 1992;11:A494.
150. Kelsen D, Lovett D, Wong J, et al. Interferon alfa-2A and fluorouracil in the treatment of patients with advanced esophageal cancer. J Clin Oncol 1992;10:269–274.
151. Sigott M, Kelsen D, Johnson B, et al. α-Interferon, 5-fluorouracil, and cisplatin: an active regimen in advanced adenocarcinoma and squamous cancer of the esophagus. Proc Am Soc Clin Oncol 1992;11:A501.
152. Kelsen D, Fein R, Coonley C, et al. Cisplatin, vindesine, and mitoguazone. The treatment of esophageal cancer. Cancer Treat Rep 1986;70:255–259.
153. Chapman R, Fleming T, van Damme J, et al. Cisplatin, vinblastine, and mitoguazone in squamous cell carcinoma of the esophagus: a southwest oncology group study. Cancer Treat Rep 1987;71:1185–1187.
154. Iizuka T, Kakegawa T, Ide H, et al. Phase II evaluation of cisplatin and 5-fluorouracil in advanced squamous cell carcinoma of the esophagus: a Japanese esophageal oncology group trial. Jpn J Clin Oncol 1992;221:172–176.
155. Mandard AM, Chasle J, Marnay J, et al. Autopsy findings in 111 cases of esophageal cancer. Cancer 1981;48:329.
156. Attah E, and Hadju S. Benign and malignant tumors of the esophagus at autopsy. J Thorac Cardiovasc Surg 1980;55:396.
157. Bosch A, Frias Z, Caldwell W, et al. Autopsy findings in carcinoma of the esophagus. Acta Radiol Oncol 1979;18:103.
158. Aisner JA, Forastiere M, Aroney R. Patterns of recurrence for cancer of the lung and esophagus. Cancer Treat Symposia 1983;2:87.
159. Coonley DJ, Bains M, Hilaris B, et al. Cisplatin and bleomycin in the treatment of esophageal carcinoma: a final report. Cancer 1984;54:2341.
160. Schlag P, Herrmenn R, Raeth V, et al. Preoperative (neoadjuvant) chemotherapy in squamous cell cancer of the esophagus. Recent Results Cancer Res 1988;10:14.
161. Kelsen DP, Fein R, Coonley, et al. Cisplatin, vindesine and mitoguazone in the treatment of esophageal cancer. Cancer Treat Rep 1986;70:255.
162. Carey RW, Hilgenberg AD, Wilkins EW, et al. Preoperative chemotherapy followed by surgery with possible postoperative radiotherapy in squamous cell carcinoma of the esophagus: evaluation of the chemotherapy component. J Clin Oncol 1986;4:697.
163. Kies MS, Rosen ST, Tsang TK, et al. Cisplatin and 5-fluorouracil in the primary management of squamous esophageal cancer. Cancer 1987;60:2156–2160.
164. Ajani JA, Roth J Ryan B, et al. Evaluation of pre and postoperative chemotherapy for resectable adenocarcinoma of the esophagus and gastroesophageal junction. J Clin Oncol 1990;8:1231.
165. Ajani JA, Roth J, Ryan B, et al. Intensive preoperative chemotherapy with granulocyte-macrophage colony stimulating factor for resectable adenocarcinoma of the esophagus and gastroesophageal junction. J Clin Oncol 1993;11:22–28.
166. Hoffman PC, Ferguson MK, Haraf DJ, et al. Induction chemotherapy, surgery and concomitant chemoradiotherapy for carcinoma of the esophagus. In: Banzet P, Holland JF, Khayat D, Weil M, eds. Cancer treatment: an update. New York: Springer-Verlag, 1994:386–389.
167. Roth JA, Pass HU, Flanagan MM, et al. Randomized clinical trials of preoperative and postoperative adjuvant chemotherapy with cisplatin, vindesine, and bleomycin for carcinoma of the esophagus. J Thorac Cardiovasc Surg 1988;96:242–248.
168. Schlag P. Randomisierte Studie zur praoperativen chemotherapie beim plattenepithelcarcinom des oesophagus. (abstract in English). Chirurg 1992;63:709–714.
169. Kelsen DP, Minsky B, Smith M, et al. Preoperative therapy for esophageal cancer: a randomized comparison of chemotherapy versus radiation therapy. J Clin Oncol 1990;8:1352–1361.
170. Japanese Esophageal Oncology Group. A comparison of chemotherapy and radiotherapy as adjuvant treatment to surgery for esophageal carcinoma. Chest 1993;104:203–207.
171. Vokes EE, Weichselbaum RR. Concomitant chemoradiotherapy: rationale and clinical experience in patients with solid tumors. J Clin Oncol 1990;8(5):911–934.
172. Steel GG, Peckham MJ. Exploitable mechanisms in combined radiotherapy-chemotherapy: the concept of additivity. Int J Radiat Oncol Biol Phys 1979;5:85–91.
173. Steiger Z, Franklin R, Wilson RF, et al. Complete eradication of squamous cell carcinoma of the esophagus with combined chemotherapy and radiotherapy. Am Surg 1981;47:95–98.
174. Herskovic A, Leichman L, Lattin P, et al. Chemoradiation with and without surgery in carcinoma of the thoracic esophagus: the Wayne State experience. Int J Radiat Oncol Biol Phys 1988;15:655–662.

175. Coia LR, Engstrom PF, Paul AR, et al. Long term results of infusional 5-Fu, mitomycin-C and radiation as primary management of esophageal carcinoma. Int J Radiat Oncol Biol Phys 1991;20:29–36.
176. Keane T, Harwood A, Elhaken T, et al. Radical radiation therapy with 5-fluorouracil infusion and mitomycin-C for oesophageal squamous carcinoma. Radiother Oncol 1985;4:205–210.
177. Chan A, Wong A, Arthur K. Concomitant 5-fluorouracil infusion, mitomycin-C and radical therapy in esophageal squamous carcinoma. Int J Radiat Oncol Biol Phys 1988;16:59–65.
178. Leichman L, Herskovic A, Leichman CG, et al. Nonoperative therapy for squamous-cell cancer of the esophagus. J Clin Oncol 1987;5:365–370.
179. John M, Flam M, Mowry P, et al. Radiotherapy alone and chemoradiation for nonmetastatic esophageal carcinoma: a critical review of chemoradiation. Cancer 1989;63:2397–2403.
180. Richmond J, Seydel H, Bae Y, et al. Comparison of three treatment strategies for esophageal cancer within a single institution. Int J Radiat Oncol Biol Phys 1987;13:1617–1620.
181. Seitz J, Giovanni M, Padaut-Cesana J, et al. Inoperable nonmetastatic squamous cell carcinoma of the esophagus managed by concomitant chemotherapy 95-fluorouracil and cisplatin) and radiation therapy. Cancer 1990;66:214–219.
182. Roussel A, Jacob P, Hegle GM, et al. Controlled clinical trial for the treatment of patients with inoperable esophageal carcinoma: a study of the EORTC gastrointestinal tract cancer cooperative group. Recent Results Cancer Res 1988;110:21–29.
183. Araujo C, Souhami L, Gil R, et al. A randomized trial comparing radiation therapy versus concomitant radiation therapy and chemotherapy in carcinoma of the esophagus. Cancer 1991;67:2258–2261.
184. Sischy B, Ryan L, Haller D, et al. Interim report of EST 1282, phase III protocol for the evaluation of combined modalities the treatment of patients with carcinoma of the esophagus, stage I and II. Proc Am Soc Clin Oncol 1990;9:105.
185. Herskovic A, Martz K, Sarraf M, et al. Combined chemotherapy and radiotherapy compared with radiotherapy alone in patients with cancer of the esophagus. N Engl J Med 1992;326:67–72.
186. Leichman L, Steiger Z, Seydel HG, et al. Preoperative chemotherapy and radiation therapy for patients with cancer of the esophagus: a potentially curative approach. J Clin Oncol 1984;2:75–79.
187. Poplin E, Fleming T, Leichman L, et al. Combined therapies for squamous cell cancer of the esophagus: a Southwest Oncology Group (SWOG 8037) study. J Clin Oncol 1987;5:622–628.
188. Stewart JR, Holf SJ, Johnson DJ, et al. Improved survival with neoadjuvant therapy and resection for adenocarcinoma of the esophagus. Ann Surg 1993;218:571–578.
189. Forastiere AA, Orringer MB, Perez-Tamaya C, et al. Preoperative chemoradiation followed by transhiatal esophagectomy for carcinoma of the esophagus: final report. J Clin Oncol 1993;11:1118–1123.
190. Andersen A, Berdal P, Edsmyr F, et al. Irradiation, chemotherapy and surgery in esophageal cancer: a randomized clinical study. Radiother Oncol 1984;2:179–188.
191. Bosset JF, Gignoux M, Triboulet JP, et al. Randomised phase III clinical trial comparing surgery alone versus pre-operative combined radio-chemotherapy (XRT-CT) in stage I-II epidermoid cancer of the esophagus. Preliminary analysis. A study of the FFCD (French group) No. 8805 and EORTC No. 40881 (abstract). Proc Am Soc Clin Oncol 1994;13:197.
192. Little AG, Ferguson MK, DeMeester TR, et al. Esophageal carcinoma with respiratory tract fistula. Cancer 1984;53:1322–1328.
193. Fleischer D, Kessler F. Endoscopic Nd:YAG laser therapy for carcinoma of the esophagus: a new form of palliative treatment. Gastroenterology 1983;85:600–606.
194. Lightdale CJ, Zimbalist E, Winawer SJ. Outpatient management of esophageal cancer with endoscopic Nd:YAG laser. Am J Gastroenterol 1987;82:46–50.
195. Ahlquist DA, Gostout CJ, Viggiano TR, et al. Endoscopic laser palliation of malignant dysphagia: a prospective study. Mayo Clin Proc 1987;62:867–874.
196. Isaac JR, Sim EKW, Ngoi SS, et al. Safe and rapid palliation of dysphagia for carcinoma of the esophagus. Am Surg 1991;57:245–249.
197. Thomas RJ, Abbott M, Bhathal PS, et al. High-dose photo-irradiation of esophageal cancer. Ann Surg 1987;206:193–199.
198. McCaughan JS, Nims TA, Guy JT, et al. Photodynamic therapy for esophageal tumors. Arch Surg 1989;124:74–80.
199. Richter JM, Hilgenberg AD, Christensen MR, et al. Endoscopic palliation of obstructive esophagogastric malignancy. Gastrointest Endosc 1988;34:454–458.
200. Segalin A, Little AG, Ruol A, et al. Surgical and endoscopic palliation of esophageal carcinoma. Ann Thorac Surg 1989;48:267–271.
201. Liakakos TK, Ohri S, Townsend ER, et al. Palliative intubation for dysphagia in patients with carcinoma of the esophagus. Ann Thorac Surg 1992;53:460–463.
202. Schaer J, Katon RM, Ivancev K, et al. Treatment of malignant esophageal obstruction with silicone-coated metallic self-expanding stents. Gastrointest Endosc 1992;38:7–11.
203. Knyrim K, Wagner H-J, Bethge N, et al. A controlled trial of an expansile metal stent for palliation of esophageal obstruction due to inoperable cancer. N Engl J Med 1993;329:1302–1307.
204. Sur R, Kochhar R, Singh D. High dose rate intracavitary therapy in advanced carcinoma of the esophagus. Indian J Gastroenterol 1991;10:43–45.
205. Schmid EU, Alberts AS, Greeff F, et al. The value of radiotherapy or chemotherapy after intubation for advanced esophageal carcinoma—a prospective randomized trial. Radiother Oncol 1993;28:27–30.
206. Alberts AS, Burger W, Greeff F, et al. Severe complications of 5-fluorouracil and cisplatin with concomitant radiotherapy in inoperable non-metastatic squamous cell oesophageal cancer after intubation—early termination of a prospective randomised trial. Eur J Cancer 1992;28A:1005–1006.
207. Gill PG, Denham JW, Jamieson GG, et al. Patterns of treatment failure and prognostic factors associated with the treatment of esophageal carcinoma with chemotherapy and radiotherapy either as sole treatment or followed by surgery. J Clin Oncol 1992;10:1037–1043.

29

Systemic Therapy in Esophageal Cancer

David H. Ilson and David P. Kelsen

INTRODUCTION

In 1995, 12,000 new cases of esophageal cancer will be diagnosed in the United States and 10,900 patients will die of their disease, representing 1.9% of cancer deaths in America (1). In Western countries an association with abuse of tobacco and alcohol and the development of epidermoid carcinoma of the esophagus is generally accepted (2). Adenocarcinoma of the esophagus, which in the past represented only a small proportion of cases of esophageal cancer, is rapidly overtaking epidermoid carcinoma as the predominant disease histology in the United States. Indeed, esophageal adenocarcinoma poses a potentially daunting health care problem, with cases increasing at an annual rate exceeding that of any other malignancy, including malignant melanoma (3). The epidemiologic factors responsible for the rapid increase in adenocarcinoma incidence have yet to be determined. Although esophageal cancer remains relatively uncommon in the United States, it is a leading worldwide cause of cancer with a particularly high incidence observed in northern China, the Caspian Littoral, and the Transkei province of South Africa (4–6). The epidemiologic factors responsible for the geographic variability in incidence of esophageal cancer, including potential dietary and environmental carcinogens, also remain indeterminate.

The prognosis for esophageal cancer patients treated with the standard approaches of surgery or radiation therapy is dismal. The largest retrospective series of patients treated with either surgery alone or radiotherapy alone, reviewed by Earlam and Cunha-Melo (7, 8), reported equally poor 2-year survival rates of 6% to 8% and 5-year survival rates of 4% to 6%. The operative mortality for surgically treated patients in this review was a sobering 29%. The significant operative mortality has fueled an ongoing debate regarding the relative efficacy of surgery and radiation therapy, although more recent surgical series from single institutions have reported operative mortalities of 5% to 15%, with Muller et al. (9) reporting an overall rate of 12.5% in a review of the surgical literature. Ultimately, the majority of patients treated with either surgery or radiation therapy are destined to die of their disease.

The failure of standard therapy, even in patients with disease clinically limited to the local-regional area prior to treatment, is due both to local regional failure and to early systemic dissemination of disease. Western autopsy series, and a recent autopsy series from Hong Kong, bear out the frequent systemic nature of epidermoid carcinoma, even at or shortly after initial presentation (10–13). Despite the brief duration of illness in these patients, the majority were found at autopsy to have evidence of distant metastatic disease regardless of whether residual local disease was present. Adenocarcinoma of the distal esophagus or gastroesophageal junction appears to have a natural history of disease similar to epidermoid esophageal carcinoma, with equally poor survival after surgical therapy because of a combination of local and systemic disease recurrence (14). The clear need to address the early systemic spread of esophageal carcinoma with systemic treatment has led to the incorporation of chemotherapy into combined modality therapy employing surgery and radiation therapy. Systemic chemotherapy in the treatment of esophageal carcinoma, both in the palliative setting and in the context of combined modality therapy with curative intent, is discussed below.

RESPONSE ASSESSMENT

Chemotherapeutic agents in esophageal cancer were initially studied in patients with either locally advanced, inoperable disease or distant metastatic disease. Metastatic lesions, including lung or liver metastases, lymph nodes, or skin nodules represent bidimensional, measurable disease in which antitumor response to chemotherapy can be assessed readily. The standard objective response criteria, outlined by Miller et al. (15), can be applied easily to these lesions. Local regional disease, in contrast, is evaluable for response by barium esophagram, computed tomography scan, or endoscopy, but it does not have clearly measurable perpendicular tumor diameters. Relief of dysphagia alone, a clinical goal of palliative chemotherapy, may provide a false estimate of the potential antitumor efficacy of chemotherapy because it may occur with even minimal antitumor response seen on barium esophagram. However, reliable assessment of response in the primary lesion has been reported in series of patients in which the radiographic response of the primary tumor to therapy was correlated with response determined endoscopically or pathologically confirmed at surgery (16, 17). Use of the recently available technique of endoscopic ultrasonography may improve the ability to evaluate local regional disease in the esophagus, particularly the degree of local tumor extension by T stage and detection of regional lymph node involvement (18, 19). Evaluation by endoscopic ultrasound is being used increasingly in clinical trials for staging and response evaluation, but at this time assessing response by endoscopic ultrasound should be considered investigational.

SINGLE-AGENT CHEMOTHERAPY

The antitumor activity for single-agent chemotherapy in esophageal carcinoma is summarized in Table 29.1. Nineteen chemotherapeutic agents have undergone evaluation for antitumor response in esophageal cancer, with the majority of studies evaluating only epidermoid carcinoma. Modest antitumor activity for a broad range of chemotherapy drugs is seen in esophageal carcinoma, but the duration of response to single-agent chemotherapy is generally brief and on the order of 4 to 6 months.

Early chemotherapy trials, such as the studies of bleomycin, were performed on small numbers of patients, often in the context of broad phase I–II trials in diverse solid tumors. Such trials also included patients with prior, often extensive, chemotherapy treatment. More recent studies, however, have been larger phase II trials and have generally limited new drug evaluation to patients without prior chemotherapy exposure. Recent studies also have employed a population size large enough to quantify a major antitumor response with some degree of statistical significance. Early chemotherapy trials also evaluated only patients with epidermoid carcinoma, whereas more recent studies have included patients with adenocarcinoma, reflecting the increasing incidence of this disease.

For some single agents, variable response proportions in different trials have been reported. In general, higher response rates for single agents have been observed in patients treated with local regional disease (usually prior to definitive local surgery or radiotherapy) compared with the response in distant metastatic disease. Greater response has also been seen with trials employing chemotherapy-naive patients rather than pretreated patients. In trials employing higher drug doses, higher response rates have also been observed. Despite the disparate response rates for some single agents, the confidence limits of response overlap across different trials in most cases.

The antitumor antibiotics bleomycin, mitomycin C, and doxorubicin have been studied in epidermoid carcinoma of the esophagus with response proportions ranging from 15% to 26% (pooled from multiple clinical trials). Antimetabolites given as single agents, including 5-fluorouracil (5-FU) and methotrexate, also have modest antitumor activity ranging from 10% to 35%. A phase II trial of bolus 5-fluorouracil in patients with metastatic disease, reported by Edzini et al. (20) noted a response rate of 15%. A significantly higher response proportion was observed in the trial reported by Lokich et al. (21) using a continuous intravenous infusion of 5-FU for 6 weeks at a dose of 300 mg/m^2/day. Patients in this study had local regional disease only and were treated prior to definitive radiation therapy. Of 13 patients treated, 11 (85%) had a major response. The high response to continuous infusion 5-FU reported in this one trial, however, has not been confirmed in other studies using continuous infusion 5-FU in combination with surgery or radiotherapy.

Consistent antitumor responses have been observed with the vinca alkaloid vindesine. Response proportions of 20% to 25% have been reported in epidermoid carcinoma (22, 23), and smaller trials have reported similar antitumor activity (24, 25). The epidophyllotoxin etoposide has been studied in adenocarcinoma and epidermoid carcinoma. Kelsen (26) and Coonley et al. (27) reported no activity in 7 patients with adenocarcinoma and no major responses in 20 patients with epidermoid carcinoma, although the majority of these patients had received prior chemotherapy. In a more recent study in previously untreated patients with epidermoid carcinoma, Harstrick et al. (28) observed 5 partial responses in 26 patients (19%) treated with a higher dose of etoposide.

The new antimicrotubule agent paclitaxel, a drug with significant activity in breast and ovarian cancer,

TABLE 29.1. Activity of Single-Agent Chemotherapy

AGENT	HISTOLOGY	PATIENTS (No.)	RESPONSES (No.)	RESPONSE (%)	95% CONFIDENCE INTERVALS (%)	REFERENCE
Antibiotics						
Bleomycin	E	80	12	15	7–23	74, 133–138
Mitomycin	E	58	15	26	15–37	139–141
Doxorubicin	E	38	7	18	5–31	20, 77
Idarubicin	A	16	1	6	0–18	142
Amonafide	E	14	1	7	0–20	143
Antimetabolites						
5-Fluorouracil	E	26	4	15	1–29	20
	A + E	13	11	85	60–100	21
Methotrexate	E	65	23	35	24–47	20, 144
Dichloromethotrexate	E	22	0			145
Trimetrexate	E	20	2	10	1–19	146
Aminothidiazole	E	23	0			147
Plant Alkaloids						
Vindesine	E	86	19	22	14–32	22–25
Etoposide	A + E	27	0			26, 27
	E	26	5	19	4–34	28
Taxol	E	18	5	28	8–48	30
	A	32	11	34	15–51	30
Navelbine	E	24	6	24	8–42	31
Heavy Metals						
Cisplatin	E	152	42	28	20–35	32–35
	A	12	1	8	0–26	36
Carboplatin	E	59	3	5	0–11	37–39
	A	11	1	9	0–26	40
Alkylating Agents						
Ifosfamide	E	22	2	8	1–23	148
Other Drugs						
Lomustine	E	19	3	16	0–32	149
Mitoguazone	E	45	9	20	8–31	150, 151

From Ilson DH, Kelsen DP. Chemotherapy in esophageal cancer. In: Sluyser M, ed. Anti-cancer drugs. Oxford, United Kingdom: Rapid Communications of Oxford, 1993;4:287–299.
Abbreviations. E, epidermoid carcinoma; A, adenocarcinoma.

has been studied recently in epidermoid and adenocarcinoma of the esophagus. First identified by Wani et al. (29), paclitaxel is the first organic compound with a taxane ring to have significant clinical cytotoxic activity. Unlike the vinca alkaloids vincristine and vinblastine, which inhibit microtubular assembly, paclitaxel promotes and stabilizes microtubule assembly. Ajani et al. (30) reported the results of a joint Memorial Sloan-Kettering Cancer Center/M. D. Anderson Cancer Center trial of paclitaxel administered at a dose of 250 mg/m^2 given by 24-hour infusion, recycled every 21 days. Fifty-one patients with unresectable or metastatic esophageal cancer were evaluable for response. Paclitaxel had significant antitumor activity, with 16 major responses seen (32%), including one complete response (2%). Comparable activity was seen for adenocarcinoma and epidermoid carcinoma. Another alkaloid, the semisynthetic vinca alkaloid vinorelbine, has also been reported recently to have significant single-agent activity in epidermoid cancer (31), with responses seen in 25% of previously untreated patients. Surprisingly, neither of the commonly used vinca alkaloids—vinblastine nor vincristine—has had a therapeutic trial as a single agent in esophageal cancer, although vinblastine has been used in combination chemotherapy trials discussed below.

Fairly large Phase II trials with cisplatin have indicated a response proportion of 15% to 20% in metastatic epidermoid carcinoma (32, 33), although one smaller trial had lesser activity (34). One study using single-agent cisplatin as preoperative chemotherapy noted a major response in 55% of patients, with response reported as necrosis of tumor seen at surgery (35). Overall, a major response proportion of 27.6% has been observed in 152 patients with epidermoid carcinoma treated with single-agent cisplatin. A small trial of cisplatin in adenocarcinoma of the esophagus, performed as part of a broad phase II trial of cisplatin in upper gastrointestinal tract malignancies, was reported by Ajani et al. (36). Of 12 patients, only one partial response (8%) was observed.

The cisplatin analogue carboplatin has generated interest in solid tumor clinical trials because of the relative ease of administration and minimal neurologic or renal toxicity compared with cisplatin. Activity for carboplatin in esophageal carcinoma, however, has been disappointing. Three phase II trials of carboplatin have shown little activity for the drug in epidermoid carcinoma (0% to 9%) (37–39). A trial in adenocarcinoma also showed limited antitumor activity, with one major response (9%) observed in 11 patients treated (40).

COMBINATION CHEMOTHERAPY

With modest activity demonstrated for several single chemotherapy agents, combination chemotherapy has also been studied extensively (Table 29.2). In earlier trials, patients with both local regional and metastatic disease were treated on the same protocols, with patients with local regional disease usually undergoing subsequent definitive surgery or radiation therapy. Virtually all studies shared cisplatin as a common agent. Cisplatin-based combination chemotherapy has yielded antitumor activity in metastatic epidermoid carcinoma of the esophagus in the range of 25% to 35%. The response proportion observed in local regional disease has been consistently higher, on the order of 45% to 75%. Despite the higher response rates seen with combination therapy compared with single-agent chemotherapy, the response duration to combination therapy also has been relatively brief, i.e., on the order of 4 to 6 months.

Early trials combined bleomycin with cisplatin and other agents. Coonley et al. (41) reported activity of bleomycin and cisplatin in 61 patients with epidermoid carcinoma, with a major response proportion of only 15%. Comparable response proportions were seen in preoperative patients with local regional disease (given only one cycle of preoperative chemotherapy) and in patients with advanced or metastatic disease. Duration of response in metastatic disease ranged from 5 to 9.5 months. Three other smaller trials showed similar antitumor activity for the combination of bleomycin and cisplatin (42–44). Overall, a response proportion of 25.5% has been observed. Bleomycin in combination with doxorubicin had comparably modest antitumor activity (45).

Cisplatin in combination with vindesine and bleomycin has been studied in three phase II trials and two phase III trials. In the largest phase II trial, reported by Kelsen et al. (46), major responses were seen in 28 (63%) of 44 patients with local regional disease after one to two cycles of preoperative therapy, and 8 (33%) of 24 patients with advanced or metastatic disease. Schlag et al. (47) reported major responses in 45% of patients with epidermoid carcinoma treated preoperatively, with two complete pathologic responses (5%); Dinwoodie et al. (48) reported major responses in 7 (29%) of 27 patients with advanced or metastatic disease. In phase III trials, preoperative cisplatin, vindesine, and bleomycin combination therapy was compared with either surgery alone (49) or preoperative radiotherapy (50), with major responses seen in 47% to 55% of patients and complete pathologic responses in 6% to 8%. Of a total of 192 patients treated with cisplatin, vindesine, and bleomycin, 91 (47%) responded, with consistently different response proportions seen between patients with local regional disease (54%) versus metastatic disease (29%).

Cisplatin in combination with mitoguazone and vindesine or vinblastine was studied in three separate phase II trials, with one trial treating both adenocarcinoma and epidermoid carcinoma (51–53). Overall, 15 (50%) of 30 patients with local regional epidermoid cancer had a major response with 2 pathologically complete responses (7%); 14 (23%) of 60 patients with advanced or metastatic disease had a major response. A lower response proportion was seen in the small number of patients with local regional adenocarcinoma reported by Forastiere et al. (53) with 5 (31%) of 16 patients having a major response. Duration of responses in metastatic disease was brief, lasting a median of 3 to 4 months. Other cisplatin-based combinations have been reported, including combinations with methotrexate and other agents, with response proportions of 20% to 76% in pooled series of patients with metastatic or local regional disease (Table 29.2). One reported preoperative trial of etoposide, adriamycin, and cisplatin in esophageal adenocarcinoma reported a major response in 52% of patients (54).

The combination of cisplatin and 5-FU given by continuous infusion for 4 to 5 days has been studied extensively, based primarily on activity of this regimen with epidermoid carcinoma of the head and neck, and with interest waning in the use of bleomycin-containing regimens because of pulmonary toxicity observed in surgical and radiation therapy protocols. Toxicity observed for the combination of cisplatin and 5-FU, mainly mucositis and myelosuppression, has been substantial but tolerable. Kies et al. (55) reported the first use of 5-FU and cisplatin in local regional epidermoid carcinoma of the esophagus, with 11 (42%) major responses observed in 26 patients treated with three cycles preoperatively. The duration of response was indeterminate because most of the patients underwent resection or later received radiotherapy. Other reports

TABLE 29.2. Activity of Combination Chemotherapy

Drug	Cell Type	Patients (No.)	Responses (No.)	Response (%)	95% Confidence Intervals	Local (L) or Metastatic (M) Disease	Reference
Cisplatin-bleomycin	E	110	28	26	14–37	LM	41–44
Bleomycin-Adriamycin (doxorubicin)	E	16	3	19	1–37	LM	45
Cisplatin-vindesine-bleomycin	E	191	91	47	40–54	LM	46–50
Cisplatin-vindesine/vinblastine-mitoguazone	E	90	29	32	24–40	LM	51–53
	A	16	5	33	8–54	L	53
Cisplatin-methotrexate	E	43	32	76	63–89	L	144
Cisplatin-methotrexate-bleomycin	E	41	13	32	18–46	LM	152, 153
Cisplatin-methotrexate-vincristine	E	28	17	61	43–79	L	154
Cisplatin-methotrexate peplomycin	E	16	9	56	22–70	L	155
Cisplatin-methotrexate-bleomycin-mitoguazone	E	14	9	64	39–89	LM	156
Cisplatin-bleomycin-vincristine–5-fluorouracil	E	10	6	60	30–90	L	157
Cisplatin-bleomycin-etoposide	E	16	5	31	8–54	LM	158
Cisplatin-etoposide	E	15	3	20	0–40	L	159
Cisplatin-cyclophosphamide-vindesine	E	23	8	35	16–54	L	160
Cisplatin-cyclophosphamide-vindesine-lomustine	E	28	6	21	6–35	LM	160
Cisplatin-etoposide-doxorubicin	A	25	13	52	32–72	L	54
Cisplatin vs cisplatin–5-fluorouracil	E	89	NS	11	...	LM	61
			NS	36			
Cisplatin–5-fluorouracil	E	238	116	49	43–55	LM	55–61
Cisplatin–5-fluorouracil–doxorubicin	E	21	7	33	13–53	LM	62
Cisplatin–5-fluorouracil–doxorubicin-etoposide	E	24	17	71	61–81	L	63
Cisplatin–5-fluorouracil–etoposide	E	20	13	65	47–83	LM	68
	A	35	17	49	32–66	L	64
Cisplatin–5-fluorouracil–bleomycin	E	43	23	53	38–68	LM	161
Cisplatin–5-fluorouracil–vindesine	E	32	16	53	36–70	LM	162
5-Fluorouracil–Leucovorin	E	35	6	17	5–29	LM	111
Cisplatin–5-fluorouracil–leucovorin	E	56	27	48.2	37–59	LM	112, 113
Cisplatin–5-fluorouracil–leucovorin-etoposide	E	38	22	58	4–73	LM	70
5-Fluorouracil–interferon	A + E	57	15	26	15–37	LM	117, 118
5-Fluorouracil–interferon-cisplatin	A + E	26	13	50	31–69	LM	119
Carboplatin-vinblastine	E	16	0			LM	163
Carboplatin-cisplatin–5-fluorouracil	A + E	14	10	71	47–95	LM	71

From Ilson DH, Kelsen DP. Chemotherapy in esophageal cancer. In: Sluyser M, ed. Anti-cancer drugs. Oxford, United Kingdom: Rapid Communications of Oxford, 1993;4:287–299.

have noted similar response proportions in patients treated predominantly with local regional disease (56–60). Of 238 patients treated with epidermoid carcinoma, the majority of whom had local regional disease and were treated preoperatively or before local radiotherapy, 116 (48.7%) achieved a major response. Occasional pathologically complete responses have been observed in patients treated preoperatively (14 patients, 7%). In the trials of patients with metastatic or unresectable disease, the response to cisplatin and 5-FU has been lower, ranging from 35% to 40% (58, 61). The addition of doxorubicin (62) or doxorubicin and the epidophyllotoxin etoposide (63) to 5-FU and cisplatin has also been reported in small series of patients, with the 95% confidence limits of the response proportions comparable to 5-FU and cisplatin alone. One preoperative trial in adenocarcinoma using the combination of 5-FU, etoposide, and cisplatin reported a 49% major response rate (64).

Despite the increasingly common use in the community of the combination of 5-FU and cisplatin for the treatment of esophageal carcinoma, only one trial (published only in abstract form [61]) has directly addressed the issue of comparative efficacy of single-agent cisplatin versus the combination of 5-FU and cisplatin. Of 89 patients with unresectable or metastatic epidermoid carcinoma randomly assigned to receive cisplatin alone or the combination of cisplatin and 5-FU, a greater major response proportion was observed for the combination (36% versus 11%, respectively). The greater response for the combination of cisplatin and 5-FU, however, did not result in any significant difference in survival.

Overall, cisplatin-based combination chemotherapy has significant antitumor activity in esophageal cancer. Most studies have evaluated patients with locally advanced disease with epidermoid carcinoma, with response proportions for metastatic disease consistently lower than for local regional disease. Activity for cisplatin-based chemotherapy is also noted for adenocarcinoma, however, the trials have mainly been of preoperative chemotherapy for local, regional resectable disease. The role of cisplatin-based chemotherapy in unresectable or metastatic adenocarcinoma of the esophagus is thus much less well defined.

NEOADJUVANT CHEMOTHERAPY AND RADIOTHERAPY

Clinical trials of systemic chemotherapy given preoperatively in esophagus cancer, also termed neoadjuvant or primary chemotherapy, have been undertaken largely because of the disappointing results achieved with conventional surgery or radiation therapy alone. Such combined modality trials employing chemotherapy have taken one of three approaches: (a) chemotherapy followed by a planned surgical procedure, (b) chemotherapy given concurrently with radiation therapy, followed by surgery, or (c) chemotherapy and radiation therapy without subsequent surgical intervention. The rationale, both preclinical and clinical, for neoadjuvant chemotherapy has been reviewed (65). For esophageal cancer patients, the approach of preoperative chemotherapy offers several potential clinical benefits including enhancing resectability by downstaging the primary tumor. Another potential advantage is the assessment of the response to preoperative chemotherapy directly in the primary tumor, making the endpoint of adjuvant therapy more precise by identifying patients who respond to chemotherapy and who might therefore benefit from further chemotherapy postoperatively. Administering chemotherapy early in the course of the disease also has the advantage of treating subclinical but established micrometastatic disease when chemotherapy is likely to have its greatest impact, given the limited effectiveness of systemic therapy to treat clinically apparent metastatic disease. A disadvantage of preoperative chemotherapy is the delay in achieving local control of disease. The rationale for concomitant chemotherapy and radiation therapy has also been reviewed (66). Concurrent chemoradiotherapy potentially allows the achievement of enhanced local control as well as treatment of systemic micrometastases.

NEOADJUVANT CHEMOTHERAPY

The use of preoperative chemotherapy in locally advanced esophageal carcinoma has been the subject of at least 27 reported clinical trials treating more than 700 patients. Most trials have been single-arm phase II studies evaluating preoperative chemotherapy given from one to up to six cycles, followed by a definitive surgical procedure, with some patients going on to receive postoperative radiation therapy; more recent trials, however, have given chemotherapy both preoperatively and postoperatively.

Preoperative chemotherapy trials used in esophageal cancer have virtually all employed cisplatin-based combination chemotherapy; results of selected phase II and phase III studies are outlined in Table 29.3. Although earlier trials treated predominantly epidermoid carcinoma, with the increased incidence of adenocarcinoma, both histologies have been treated on the same preoperative protocols.

Early trials combined bleomycin with cisplatin and other agents. Coonley et al. (41) treated 34 patients with epidermoid carcinoma with one cycle of cisplatin and bleomycin, followed by surgery, followed by one course of postoperative chemotherapy. Patients with T3 or node-positive lesions at surgery also later received post-treatment radiotherapy. Major antitumor response was seen in only 17% of patients after one cycle of chemotherapy, with no complete responses. All patients were operable after chemotherapy, and resection was possible in 76% of patients. Postoperative mortality was 11%, and the median survival was only 10 months. One patient died of bleomycin-related respiratory failure in the setting of postoperative radiotherapy. Preoperative cisplatin and bleomycin was also studied in the randomized trial by Nygaard et al. (67), which failed to show a survival benefit for preoperative chemotherapy compared with surgery alone.

Because of the marginal antitumor activity observed for cisplatin and bleomycin, Kelsen et al. (46) added the drug vindesine to cisplatin and bleomycin in a subsequent trial in epidermoid carcinoma. Preoperative chemotherapy was again given for only one cycle in the first 21 of 34 patients treated. The observation that patients with metastatic disease achieved maximum tumor regression after two or more cycles of chemotherapy led to the treatment of the final 13 patients on this study

TABLE 29.3. Esophageal Cancer Preoperative Chemotherapy Phase II/III Trials

Author (Reference No.)	Regimen	Histology	Patients (No.)	Operable (%)	Resectable (%)	Operative Mortality (No.)	(%) Major Response /Path CR	Median Survival (Mo.)	5-Year Survival (%)
Phase II Trials									
Coonley (41)	CDDP-Bleo	E	34	100	76	11	17/0	10	6
Kelsen (46)	CDDP-Bleo-V	E	34	100	82	5.6	53/3	16	17.5
Schlag (47)	CDDP-Bleo-V	E	42	90	85	11	45/5	15	25[a]
Kelsen (51)	CDDP-M-Vds	E	14	93	86	7	NS/7	8	NS
Forastiere (53)	CCDP-M-Vlb	A + E	27	86	86	0	44/3	14	21[a]
Kies (55)	CDDP-FU	E	25	54	38	0	42/0	17.8	17
Hilgenberg (56)	CDDP-FU	E	35	89	77	4	57/7	NS	54[b]
Ajani (60)	CDDP-FU	E	18	100	94[c]	6	61/11	28	NS
Ajani (64)	CDDP-FU-VP	A	35	91	90[c]	0	49/4	23	43[d]
Ajani (54)	CDDP-Dox-VP	A	25	NS	60[c]	1	52/0	10	NS
Phase III Trials									
Roth (49)	CDDP-Bleo-V	E	17	89	35[c]	12	47/6	9	25[a, e]
	Surgery		19	95	21[c]	0	...	9	5[a, e]
Schlag (73)	CDDP-FU	E	29	83	71	21	47/NS	8	NS
	Surgery		40	100	77	12	...	9	NS
Nygaard (67)	CDDP-Bleo	E	50	82	58	15	NS	NS	3[a, e]
	Surgery		41	93	69	13	...	NS	9[a, e]
	RT 3500 cGy		48	75	54	11	NS	NS	21[a, e]
	RT/CDDP-Bleo		47	72	66	24	NS	NS	17[a, e]
Kelsen (50)	CDDP-Bleo-Vds	E	48	NS	58	11	55/8	10	20[a, e]
	RT		48	NS	65	14	62/5	12	

Abbreviations. CDDP, cisplatin; Bleo, bleomycin; Vds, vindesine; M, mitoguazone; Vlb, vinblastine; FU, 5-fluorouracil; VP, etoposide; Dox, doxorubicin; NS, not stated; RT, radiotherapy; Path CR, pathologically complete response.
[a] Three-year actuarial survival.
[b] Actuarial survival at 3.5 years.
[c] Curative resection.
[d] Actuarial survival at 2 years.
[e] Not statistically significant.
[f] Survival of all patients.

with two preoperative chemotherapy cycles. Patients with T3 or node-positive lesions received additional postoperative treatment with radiotherapy. A greater antitumor response for the combination of cisplatin, bleomycin, and vindesine was seen in this trial compared with cisplatin and bleomycin, with major responses seen in 53% of patients and a pathologically complete response rate of 3%; 82% of patients were resectable with an operative mortality of 6%. The median survival was 16 months, superior to that of a historical surgically treated control group.

Schlag et al. (47) using a similar chemotherapy regimen with cisplatin, vindesine, and bleomycin reported comparable rates of major antitumor response (45% with 5% complete pathologic responses), resectability (85%), and operative mortality (11%). In two phase III trials employing preoperative cisplatin, bleomycin, and vindesine, similar results were obtained. Roth et al. (49) compared preoperative chemotherapy with surgery alone, reporting a response rate of 47% with 6% pathologically complete responses to preoperative chemotherapy; there were 2 chemotherapy-related deaths in 19 patients (10%). Kelsen et al. (50) reported a phase III trial comparing preoperative cisplatin, vindesine, and bleomycin with preoperative radiotherapy. Major responses to preoperative chemotherapy were seen in 55% of patients with 8% having pathologically complete responses; 58% of patients were resectable, and the operative mortality rate was 11%. Toxicity of preoperative chemotherapy was manageable in these studies and included nausea, vomiting, and pulmonary toxicity, myelosuppression, and peripheral neuropathy.

Given the pulmonary toxicity associated with bleomycin, and the marginal antitumor activity observed for the combination of bleomycin and cisplatin in preoperative therapy and in metastatic disease, other cisplatin-based combinations were studied in phase II preoperative chemotherapy trials. Cisplatin in combination with mitoguazone and vindesine or vinblastine was studied in two phase II trials. The study of

Kelsen et al. (51) evaluated patients with epidermoid carcinoma, and the study of Forastiere et al. (53) treated both adenocarcinoma and epidermoid carcinoma. Major responses to preoperative chemotherapy were reported in 64% of patients with epidermoid cancer in the trial of Forastiere et al. (53) with an overall pathologically complete response rate of 8% reported for epidermoid carcinoma in both trials. In adenocarcinoma, a major response was seen in 31% of patients (53). Resectability rates (86%) and operative mortality (0% to 7%) were comparable to that of earlier trials, and median survival ranged from 8 to 14 months. Postoperative radiotherapy was not given in the trial of Forastiere et al. (53) but was planned for patients with T3 or node-positive disease in the trial of Kelsen et al. (51). Toxicity, mainly nausea, vomiting, and myelosuppression, was substantial but manageable.

The combination of cisplatin and 5-FU given by continuous infusion for 4 to 5 days has been studied extensively in preoperative chemotherapy trials. Kies et al. (55) reported the use of 5-FU and cisplatin in epidermoid carcinoma in a small series of patients, with a major response seen in 42% of patients treated with three cycles preoperatively (42%); 38% of patients were resectable. Hilgenberg et al. (56) reported a larger series of 35 patients with epidermoid carcinoma, with major response seen in 57% with a pathologically complete response rate of 7%; 77% were resectable, and there was one operative death (4%). With a short duration of follow-up, actuarial survival of the 27 resected patients was 54% at 3.5 years. Responding patients were treated with additional postoperative chemotherapy, but only 34% of eligible patients actually received postoperative treatment during this study. Patients with T3 or node-positive disease received radiotherapy postoperatively. In a multivariate analysis, a clinically complete response to chemotherapy, pathologic T stage disease at surgery, and absence of or only microscopic disease present in the resected specimen were identified as significant prognostic factors associated with 3-year survival.

In a recently published study in which from one to six cycles of preoperative 5-FU and cisplatin were delivered, Ajani et al. (60) reported major responses in 66% of 34 patients with epidermoid carcinoma, including 11% pathologically complete responses. The rate of curative resection was 53%, and the median survival was 28 months. In the series by Vignoud et al. (57) 48 patients with local regional disease were treated with a more dose intensive schedule of infusional 5-FU given at a dose of 1 g/m^2/day for 4 days and cisplatin at a dose of 100 mg/m^2 on day 1, recycled every 14 days for three cycles preoperatively. Thirty-two (66%) major responses were seen, including five pathologically complete responses (10%). Ajani et al. (64) reported a preoperative trial of 5-FU, cisplatin, and etoposide in adenocarcinoma of the gastroesophageal junction or of the distal esophagus. Thirty-five patients received two preoperative and three to four postoperative cycles of chemotherapy. Major responses to preoperative chemotherapy were seen in 49% of patients, with 78% undergoing a curative resection. Median survival was 23 months. A univariate analysis identified the percentage of weight loss before diagnosis and the number of chemotherapy cycles delivered as predictive of survival, but only the percentage weight loss remained a significant prognostic factor in the multivariate analysis. A subsequent trial employing preoperative cisplatin, Adriamycin (doxorubicin), and etoposide in esophageal adenocarcinoma noted a similar antitumor response and rate of curative resection (54). Other reported series of patients have been treated with preoperative 5-FU and cisplatin in combination with doxorubicin (62), doxorubicin and etoposide (63), etoposide (68), leucovorin (69), leucovorin and etoposide (70), and carboplatin (71), with the response proportions, resectability, operative mortality, and survival reported all comparable to that of 5-FU and cisplatin alone. Toxicity observed for these trials, mainly mucositis, myelosuppression, and nephrotoxicity, was substantial but tolerable.

Overall, preoperative chemotherapy with cisplatin-based combination chemotherapy achieves a major response in 17% to 66% of patients with pathologically complete responses in 3% to 10%. Operability after chemotherapy has ranged from 50% to 100%, and resectability of operated patients has ranged from 40% to 90%, with operative mortality after preoperative chemotherapy comparable to surgical series alone. These results indicate that the administration of preoperative chemotherapy is safe and without a demonstrable adverse effect on surgical outcome. However, the overall survival of patients treated with preoperative chemotherapy has been disappointing, with a median survival ranging from 10 to 26 months in larger series. The longest follow-up was reported by Kelsen et al. (72) in a series of 34 patients with epidermoid carcinoma treated with cisplatin, vindesine, and bleomycin. After a minimum follow-up of 6 years (median, 7 years), 17.5% of patients were alive and free of disease, and there were no recurrences after 3.5 years; the investigators reported this outcome as a doubling of survival compared with historical surgical controls. An improvement in the percentage of patients achieving long-term survival has been suggested in preoperative chemotherapy trials, with a clear trend toward improved survival in patients manifesting a major objective response to chemotherapy. Whether response to chemotherapy is independent of other favorable prognostic factors is unclear. The duration of chemotherapy delivered in preoperative chemotherapy trials also has evolved: whereas earlier trials administered only one to two cycles of chemotherapy preoperatively without subsequent postoperative therapy, more recent trials have given up to three or more cycles of preoperative therapy and two to three cycles of postoperative chemotherapy. The treatment outcomes of earlier and more recent trials may not be directly comparable, particularly regarding the impact of additional cycles of systemic therapy on systemic recurrence of disease. Postoperative radiation therapy was also delivered in some trials, but with the data from preoperative radiotherapy trials arguing against a survival advantage for preoperative radiotherapy (discussed below), more recent trials have not included postoperative radiotherapy routinely.

The role of preoperative chemotherapy in the treatment of local regional esophageal carcinoma can be defined clearly only in the context of random-assignment trials with a surgery only control arm. Three small randomized trials have compared surgery alone to preoperative chemotherapy followed by surgery, and a fourth trial compared preoperative chemotherapy with preoperative radiotherapy. Roth et al. (49) randomized patients to preoperative chemotherapy with cisplatin, bleomycin, and vindesine versus surgery alone. Schlag (73), reporting in abstract form only, randomly assigned patients to surgery alone or to three cycles of preoperative chemotherapy with 5-FU and cisplatin. Nygaard et al. (67) randomized patients to receive either surgery alone, preoperative chemotherapy with cisplatin and bleomycin, preoperative radiotherapy, or preoperative treatment with sequential chemotherapy and radiotherapy. Kelsen et al. (50) randomly assigned 96 patients to treatment either with preoperative high-dose radiotherapy, 5500 cGy delivered over 5.5 to 6 weeks by a multifield technique, or preoperative chemotherapy with cisplatin, vindesine, and bleomycin. None of these small randomized trials demonstrated a survival advantage for preoperative chemotherapy. In the study of Roth et al. (49), the subgroup of patients responding to chemotherapy showed a trend toward improved survival, compared with surgical controls, that reached statistical significance. A prognostic factor analysis identified percentage weight loss before diagnosis and objective response to chemotherapy as predictive of long-term survival.

Schlag et al. (73) reported no difference in survival for patients receiving 5-FU and cisplatin versus surgery alone. No survival benefit was conveyed by preoperative chemotherapy in the study by Nygaard et al. (67), and, as discussed above, the patients with the poorest survival at 3 years (5%) received preoperative chemotherapy. The use of what was probably a suboptimal chemotherapy regimen may have diminished the effect of chemotherapy in this study. In the trial of Kelsen et al. (50), a survival comparison between the two treatment groups could not be made because the study design permitted a postoperative crossover to the other treatment modality, and most patients received both chemotherapy and radiation therapy. The actuarial survival rate observed for all patients was 20% at 5 years, superior to that of historical controls, with the subgroup of responders to either chemotherapy or radiotherapy showing a trend toward improved survival. Although either preoperative radiotherapy or chemotherapy resulted in regression of local regional disease, the investigators concluded that preoperative chemo-therapy provided the additional opportunity to treat systemic metastases and therefore offered greater promise in future clinical trials, compared with preoperative radiotherapy alone.

Presently, for surgically treated patients surgery alone remains the standard of care, and the use of preoperative chemotherapy outside of an investigational setting cannot be recommended. A conclusive evaluation of preoperative chemotherapy using the best currently available combination regimen awaits the completion of ongoing random assignment clinical trials. Currently, a national intergroup trial is randomizing patients to receive three preoperative and two postoperative chemotherapy cycles with cisplatin and 5-FU versus surgery alone. Completion of accrual to this trial is anticipated in 1995, and entrance on this protocol of patients who are surgical candidates is recommended.

NEOADJUVANT CHEMOTHERAPY AND RADIATION

The intensification of radiotherapy with concurrent chemotherapy used as a radiation sensitizer, either in the preoperative setting or as definitive local therapy, has been the subject of many single-arm phase II studies. More than 35 trials studying in excess of 1400 patients have been reported; phase III trials have been reported recently and are ongoing to clarify the contribution of concurrent chemotherapy and radiation to the treatment of local regional esophageal cancer.

Kolaric et al. (74) performed a series of small trials in which patients with inoperable but localized tumors received either chemotherapy alone or chemotherapy and radiation (45, 74–77). The agents employed included bleomycin, Adriamycin, and the combination of the two. In each study the response rate to combined modality therapy was superior to that of chemotherapy alone, but only a slight increase in survival was noted. In a larger Eastern Cooperative Oncology Group phase III trial, bleomycin with concurrent radiation was tested versus radiation alone. There was no difference in survival outcome (78). Byfield and colleagues (79) reported the first trial of continuous infusion 5-FU therapy used as a radiosensitizer with concurrent radiotherapy in unresectable esophageal cancer; clinically complete responses were seen in this small series of patients. Preoperative radiotherapy alone has been the subject of three randomized trials comparing this approach with surgery alone. None of the trials has demonstrated a survival benefit for preoperative radiotherapy compared with surgery alone (80–82).

More recently, the chemotherapy in most preoperative chemoradiotherapy trials has combined cisplatin or mitomycin C with 5-FU given by continuous infusion. The results of selected phase II and phase III trials are outlined in Table 29.4. The Wayne State University group piloted two regimens in patients with epidermoid cancer: (a) 5-FU and mitomycin C, and (b) 5-FU and cisplatin, administered for two cycles with 3000 cGY of radiotherapy in 15 fractions of 200 cGy given concurrently with the first cycle of chemotherapy, followed by esophagectomy (83, 84). Patients with residual tumor in the esophagus went on to receive an additional 2000 cGy of radiotherapy postoperatively. A total of 51 patients were treated, with operability of patients ranging from 76% to 90%; 71% to 76% of patients were resectable with a substantial operative mortality of 13% to 27%. Toxicity in these studies included leukopenia and pneumonitis. Pathologically complete responses to chemoradiotherapy were seen in 20% to 24% of patients, and the median survival in both studies was 18 months. Long-term follow-up was reported for the patients who achieved a pathologically complete response to treatment with 5-FU, cisplatin, and concurrent radiotherapy; indeed, they were the only patients to survive beyond 3 years. All eventually died of metastatic disease without evidence of local tumor recurrence in the esophagus (85), which raises the question of whether esophagectomy contributed to survival. Evaluation of the Wayne State regimen in a cooperative group setting was performed subsequently by the Southwestern Oncology Group and the Radiation Therapy Oncology Group, based on the initially encouraging results with 5-FU, cisplatin, and radiation in epidermoid cancer. Of the 147 patients with epidermoid cancer evaluated on these trials, operability was 63% to 66% after preoperative therapy and 49% to 66% of patients were resectable, with an operative mortality of 3% to 11% (86, 87). Pathologically complete responses were seen in 17% to 20%. Median survival of all patients was a disappointing 12 to 13 months; the Radiation Therapy Oncology Group study achieved only an 8% three-year survival.

Forastiere and colleagues (88) at the University of Michigan piloted an intensive 21-day preoperative trial

TABLE 29.4. Esophageal Cancer Preoperative Chemoradiotherapy Phase II Trials

Author (Reference No.)	Regimen/RT	Histology	Patients (No.)	Operable (%)	Resectable (%)	Operative Mortality (%)	Major Response/ Path CR (%)	Median Survival (Mo.)	5-Year Survival (%)
Franklin (83)	FU-Mito/3000 cGy	E	30	76	76	13	NS/20	18[b]	30[b,c]
Leichman (84)	FU-CDDP/3000 cGy	E	21	90	71	27	NS/24	18	NS
Poplin (86)	FU-CDDP/3000 cGy	E	113	63	49	11	NS/17	12	16[c]
Seydel (87)	FU-CDDP/3000 cGy	E	41	66	66	4	NS/20	13	8[c]
Forastiere (88,89)	FU-Vlb-CDDP/ 3750–4500 cGy	A + E	43	95	91	2	42/24	29	34
Urba (90)	FU/4900 cGy	A	24	79	79	4	41/8	11	33
Bedenne (91)	FU-CDDP/3000 cGy	E	92	NS	83	9	NS/24	17	NS

Abbreviations. FU, 5-fluorouracil; Mito, mitomycin C; E, epidermoid carcinoma; CDDP, cisplatin; Vlb, vinblastine; NS, not stated; A, adenocarcinoma; RT, radiotherapy; Path CR, pathologically complete response.
[a]Completely resected patients only.
[b]Three-year survival.
[c]Three-year survival.

in which patients with both epidermoid carcinoma and adenocarcinoma were entered on the same treatment protocol. Chemotherapy consisted of 5-FU given by 21-day continuous intravenous infusion, cisplatin given by continuous intravenous infusion on days 1 through 5 and 14 through 19, and vinblastine on days 1 through 4 and 17 through 20. Radiotherapy of 3750 to 4500 cGy was given concurrently over the 21-day treatment program (88). After preoperative chemotherapy and radiation, patients underwent transhiatal esophagectomy. Twenty-two patients had epidermoid carcinoma, and 21 had adenocarcinoma. Operability was 95% with 91% resectable, and 84% were resected for potential cure, with only one postoperative death. Major responses were seen in 42% of patients, with a pathologically complete response rate of 24%. The higher dose of radiotherapy and the change to a twice-daily fractionation schedule during the course of the study did not result in a higher pathologically complete response rate. In a subsequent report of long-term follow-up in these patients, at a median follow-up of 78.7 months (minimum, 58.5 months), the median survival was 29 months with a 5-year survival of 34% (i.e., 34% for adenocarcinoma and 30% for epidermoid carcinoma) (89). The 5-year survival in pathologically complete responders was 60%. Patients with a partial response to preoperative chemoradiotherapy (with residual viable tumor resected at esophagectomy) also achieved a significant 5-year survival of 32%, arguing that esophagectomy contributed to long-term survival in these patients. The failure pattern also was addressed in this study, with no local recurrences (defined as anastomotic recurrence) reported in the resected patients. Regional failure (defined as mediastinal nodal recurrence) occurred in 26% of relapsing patients, and distant failure occurred in 74% of relapsing patients. Toxicity in this trial, in which radiotherapy overlapped all of the chemotherapy delivered, was severe and greater than that seen in earlier trials in which radiotherapy overlapped only the first of two chemotherapy cycles. Grade 3–4 myelosuppression was seen in 93% of patients, with 63% experiencing febrile neutropenia. Nutritional support was required in 79%. Multivariate analysis identified clinically enlarged regional nodes and receipt of less than full-dose cisplatin and vinblastine as poor prognostic indicators for survival.

Based on the encouraging survival results in this phase II study, which the investigators reported as a doubling of survival over institutional historical surgical controls, a random-assignment trial comparing surgery alone with preoperative chemoradiation therapy followed by surgery is now underway at the University of Michigan. A subsequent pilot trial of preoperative chemoradiotherapy in adenocarcinoma of the esophagus by the same group was reported in 1992 by Urba et al. (90). Patients received 5-FU given by 4-day continuous intravenous infusions over 3 weeks and concurrent radiotherapy, using higher dose 350 cGY fractions for 5 days weekly for 14 fractions for a total does of 4900 cGy. Operability and resectability rate were both 79% with an operative mortality of 4%. Major responses were seen in 41% of patients with 8% pathologically complete response. Toxicity attributable to this radiotherapy dose and schedule was severe, including a significant incidence of pericardial and pleural effusions. Median survival was only 11 months, comparable to historical controls treated with surgery alone and inferior to the results reported with cisplatin, 5-FU, and vinblastine.

A recent large series of patients treated with preoperative chemoradiotherapy with 5-FU and cisplatin was reported by Bedenne et al. (91). Ninety-two patients with epidermoid carcinoma received 5-FU and cisplatin on days 1 through 5 and 22 through 26. A total dose of 3000 cGy of radiotherapy was delivered in 300-cGy daily fractions, given as a split course of radiotherapy delivered concurrently only during chemotherapy. The rate of resectability was 83% with an operative mortality of 9.4%. Complete pathologic responses were seen in 24% of patients. Median survival was 17 months. Toxicity was manageable with grade 3 or 4 toxicity observed in 23% of patients.

Other pilot trials have addressed the role of split-course radiotherapy (92) and the contribution of additional chemotherapy agents to preoperative chemoradiotherapy with 5-FU and cisplatin, including etoposide (93), and leucovorin with or without etoposide (94). Comparable rates of resectability, pathologically complete responses, and survival have been observed in preliminary reports of these studies.

CONCURRENT CHEMORADIATION WITHOUT SURGERY

Concurrent chemotherapy and radiation therapy as definitive therapy without esophagectomy has also been the subject of numerous phase II trials, with selected studies outlined in Table 29.5. The Wayne State group piloted a nonoperative trial in 20 patients with epidermoid carcinoma of the esophagus. Esophagectomy after chemoradiotherapy was not planned, based on the operative mortality attributable to esophagectomy in prior Wayne State trials and because the pattern of systemic failure in prior trials questioned the contribution of esophagectomy to long-term survival (85). Patients were treated with 5-FU and cisplatin for

TABLE 29.5. Esophageal Cancer Chemoradiotherapy Nonoperative Phase II/III Trials

Author (Reference No.)	Regimen/RT	Histology	Patients (No.)	Major Response (%)	Treatment Mortality (%)	Median Survival (Mo.)	5-Year Survival (%)
Leichman (85)	FU-CDDP/3000 cGy + Mito-Bleo/2000 cGy	E	20	NS	0	22	NS
Coia (95)	FU-Mito/6000 cGy	A + E	57	NS	4	18	18
John (96)	FU-CDDP-Mito/4140–5040 cGy/FU-LV-MTX	E	30	77	3	15[a]	29[b]
Chan (97)	FU-Mito/4000–5000 cGy	E	21	86	0	13	20[b]
Seitz (99)	FU-CDDP/5600–6000 cGy	E	35	71	3	17	41[b]
Keane (98)	FU-Mito/4500–5000 cGy	E	35	NS	0	NS	28[b]
Richmond (92)	FU-CDDP/4000 cGy	E	25	NS	4	12	37[b]
Phase III Trials							
Sischy (104)	FU-Mito/6000 cGy	E	118	NS	NS	15	NS
	RT	E	118	NS	NS	9	NS
Herskovic (102)	FU-CDDP/5000 cGy	A + E[c]	61	NS	2	12.5	38[b,d]
	6400 cGy	A + E[e]	60	NS	0	8.9	10[b,d]
Araujo (105)	FU-Mito/5000 cGY	E	28	75	0	8	6[f]
	5000 cGy	E	31	58	0	8	16

Abbreviations. FU, 5-fluorouracil; CDDP, cisplatin; Mito, mitomycin C; Bleo, bleomycin; LV, leucovorin; MTX, methotrexate; A, adenocarcinoma; E, epidermoid carcinoma; RT, radiotherapy; NS, not stated.
[a]Median survival in responders only.
[b]Survival at 24 months.
[c]Represents 51 epidermoid cancers and 10 adenocarcinomas.
[d]$p < .001$.
[e]55 epidermoid cancers and 5 adenocarcinomas.

two cycles given concurrently with 3000 cGy of radiotherapy delivered over 3 weeks. Two additional cycles of chemotherapy with mitomycin C and infusional bleomycin were planned after completion of chemoradiotherapy. An additional boost of radiotherapy to 2000 cGy was given on completion of chemotherapy. Median survival in this series was 22 months. Nine patients (45%) had persistence of local regional tumor after treatment. Pulmonary toxicity was prohibitive in this study, leading to the early withdrawal of bleomycin therapy.

Coia et al. (95) reported a 10-year experience in epidermoid carcinomas and adenocarcinomas of the esophagus in 57 patients treated with continuous infusion 5-FU and mitomycin given for two cycles concurrently with higher dose radiotherapy, 6000 cGy over 6 to 7 weeks. Median survival was 18 months with a 18% actuarial disease-free survival at 5 years for clinical stage I–II patients; survival for patients with adenocarcinoma and epidermoid carcinoma were comparable in this series. Local control was reported in 70% of patients. Of the 29 patients with recurrence in this series, local failure occurred in 48% of patients, and 72% had some component of distant failure. Severe toxicities were uncommon in this series, but there were two treatment-related fatalities.

John et al. (96) reported their experience in 30 patients with epidermoid or adenocarcinoma treated with three cycles of infusional 5-FU, mitomycin C, and cisplatin, given concurrently with 4140 to 5040 cGY of radiation in 180 cGy fractions over 4.5 to 8 weeks. Maintenance chemotherapy combining methotrexate, 5-FU, and leucovorin was delivered for three cycles on completion of chemoradiation. A clinically complete response rate of 77% was reported. Actuarial survival was 29% at 2 years, superior to a historical control group treated with radiotherapy alone. Toxicity was manageable, and there was one treatment-related death from respiratory failure.

Other trials using concurrent radiotherapy in doses ranging from 4000 to 6000 cGy, given together with cisplatin or mitomycin in combination with 5-FU, have yielded comparable responses to treatment and survival (92, 97–99). In addition to trials of definitive chemoradiotherapy in local regional esophageal cancer, this approach has also been studied in patients with unresectable disease. Two randomized trials comparing radiotherapy alone and concurrent radiotherapy with single-agent methotrexate or cisplatin failed to show an improvement in survival for combined chemoradiotherapy versus radiotherapy alone in unresectable disease (100, 101); however, the latter trial reported a reduction in local recurrence with chemoradiation versus radiation therapy alone. Evaluation of the combination of 5-FU and cisplatin and concurrent radiotherapy in unresectable disease, compared with radiotherapy alone, continues in an ongoing trial in Europe sponsored by the European Organization for the Research and Treatment of Cancer.

CURRENT ROLE OF CHEMORADIOTHERAPY

Overall, in the trials employing preoperative concurrent chemoradiotherapy, major antitumor responses have been reported in 40% to 80% of patients, and up to 25% pathologically complete responses have been seen consistently at esophagectomy. Overall, median survival in these series has been disappointing, ranging from 11 to 29 months. The contribution of esophagectomy in these trials remains unclear. In the Wayne State University trials, long-term survivors were patients with a complete response to chemoradiotherapy who did not fail locally but died of distant metastatic disease, arguing against the use of esophagectomy. Forastiere and colleagues (89), in contrast, observed that after intensive preoperative chemoradiation therapy, significant 5-year survival was observed both in patients with a pathologically complete response and those with resection of viable tumor, arguing that esophagectomy salvaged partial responders to preoperative chemoradiotherapy. The reason for the divergent results for the Wayne State and University of Michigan trials employing preoperative chemoradiation therapy is unclear. Differences in the trial designs include a higher dose of radiotherapy that overlapped all chemotherapy in the Michigan State trial, as well as a difference in the schedule of 5-FU infusion employing a prolonged 21-day continuous infusion of 5-FU rather than the two interrupted infusions of 5-FU reported in the Wayne State series. However, an increase in radiotherapy from 3000 cGy to 5000 to 6000 cGy, and the overlapping radiotherapy during all cycles of chemotherapy, failed to increase the rate of pathologically complete response in reported preoperative trials. In some trials with cisplatin-based chemotherapy, a higher radiotherapy dose appeared to increase treatment-related toxicity substantially.

Given the promising results with definitive chemoradiation therapy for local regional disease without a planned esophagectomy, a nonsurgical, random-assignment trial in local regional esophageal carcinoma comparing radiation therapy alone with radiation given concurrently with 5-FU and cisplatin was conducted by the Radiation Therapy Oncology Group. The results were published recently by Herskovic et al. (102) (Table 29.5). In this study 60 patients were assigned randomly to treatment with radiation therapy alone, and 61 patients were assigned to receive radiation given with concurrent 5-FU and cisplatin. Patients with both epidermoid and adenocarcinoma were enrolled, although the majority of patients had epidermoid carcinoma. Patients receiving radiotherapy alone were treated with 5000 cGy with a boost of 1400 cGy to a total dose of 6400 cGy, delivered over 7 weeks in 200-cGy fractions. Patients receiving concurrent chemotherapy and radiation received 3000 cGy of radiation with a boost of 2000 cGy delivered over 5 weeks for a total dose of 5000 cGy; chemotherapy consisted of 5-FU given by continuous intravenous infusion for 4 consecutive days on weeks 1, 5, 8, and 11, with cisplatin given on day 1 of each 5-FU treatment course. Radiation therapy, delivered in 200-cGy fractions, overlapped the first two chemotherapy cycles. The chemotherapy design employed two additional cycles of systemic chemotherapy after chemoradiotherapy was completed.

The survival of patients treated with radiotherapy alone or a combination of concurrent chemotherapy and radiotherapy is shown in Figure 29.1. With a median follow-up in these patients of 18 months, a significant median survival benefit was observed for chemoradiation versus radiation therapy alone (12.5 versus 8.9 months). More importantly, 1- and 2-year survival was significantly greater for the combined modality arm, 50% and 38%, respectively, compared with radiotherapy alone, with 1- and 2-year survivals of 33% and 10%, respectively. The results strongly indicate that the combination of chemotherapy and radiation is superior to radiation therapy alone. In a recent update of the survival of patients in this study, 31% of patients treated with chemoradiation were alive at 3 years compared with no patients treated only with radiotherapy alive at 3 years (103). A statistically significant reduction in both local and distant recurrence of disease also was noted, favoring combined chemotherapy and radiation. Nonetheless, a high percentage of patients treated with combined chemotherapy and radiation, 44%, had either persistence or recurrence of local disease at 12 months. The morbidity of chemoradiotherapy was also significantly greater than with radiotherapy alone, with 64% of patients treated with chemoradiotherapy versus 28% of patients treated with radiotherapy experiencing severe or life-threatening toxicity (mainly mucositis and myelosuppression). One patient (1.6%) treated with chemoradiotherapy died from treatment-related toxicity, and there were no deaths in the radiotherapy arm. Because of toxicity, only half of patients treated with combined modality therapy received the final, planned two cycles of systemic therapy. Supportive evidence of

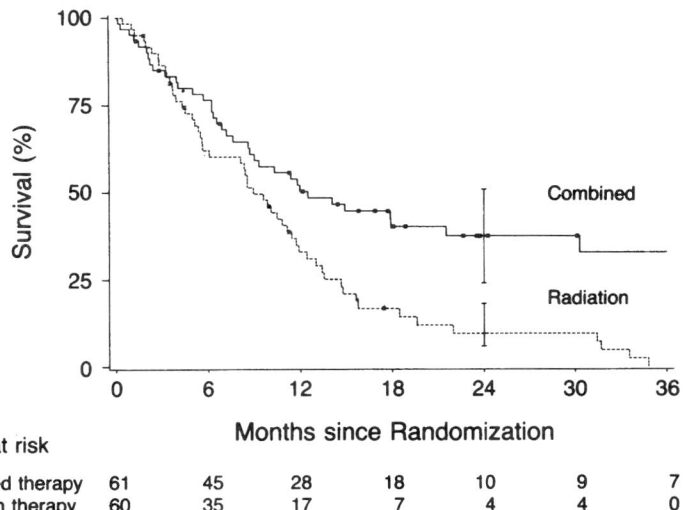

FIGURE 29.1. This survival curve shows that in patients with esophageal carcinoma, combined chemotherapy and radiotherapy is superior to radiotherapy alone in the treatment of local regional esophageal cancer. (From Herskovic A, Martz K, Al-Sarraf M, Leichman L, Brindle J, Vaitkevicius V, Cooper J, et al. Combined chemotherapy and radiotherapy compared with radiotherapy alone in patients with cancer of the esophagus. N Engl J Med 1992;326:1593–1647.)

an improvement in median survival for concurrent chemotherapy and radiation compared with radiotherapy alone also comes from a preliminary report of the trial conducted by Eastern Cooperative Oncology Group comparing radiotherapy alone to radiotherapy with concurrent 5-FU and mitomycin C (104). A small random-assignment trial reported by Araujo et al. (105) also reported a survival advantage for chemoradiotherapy with 5-FU, mitomycin C, and bleomycin compared with radiotherapy alone in patients with epidermoid carcinoma that, however, did not reach statistical significance.

Presently, concurrent chemotherapy given with radiotherapy before an operation remains investigational, and surgery alone is the standard treatment. However, in the nonsurgical setting, recent evidence strongly indicates that concurrent chemotherapy and radiation therapy is superior to radiotherapy alone for locally advanced epidermoid esophageal carcinoma. The role of this approach remains less well established in adenocarcinoma of the esophagus, although recent results have indicated a similar treatment outcome for adenocarcinoma and epidermoid carcinoma treated with preoperative chemoradiation followed by esophagectomy (89, 95, 96). The question of whether esophagectomy is an obligate part of local disease control after combined chemotherapy and radiation therapy must ultimately be asked in the context of a random-assignment trial comparing treatment of local regional disease with surgery or chemoradiotherapy.

SMALL CELL CARCINOMA

Small cell carcinoma of the esophagus is an uncommon histologic subtype of esophageal carcinoma, with fewer than 100 cases reported in the literature. The incidence of small cell carcinoma ranges from less than 1% to 2% to 3% of cases of esophageal cancer diagnosed (106–108). Staging of small cell cancer of the esophagus is similar to that of small cell cancer of the lung, with limited stage disease defined as local regional disease with or without local regional lymph node involvement. Extensive stage disease is defined as distant metastatic disease outside the locoregional area. Like small cell lung cancer, there is a clear association between the development of the disease and tobacco use, and distant metastatic disease is frequently present at diagnosis. Also like small cell lung cancer, the disease appears to be highly responsive to radiotherapy and to a broad spectrum of chemotherapeutic agents (106, 109). The almost universal development of metastatic disease in small cell carcinoma of the esophagus has led to the general acceptance of chemotherapy as part of combined modality therapy in the treatment of small cell carcinoma of the esophagus. However, despite treatment of patients with limited stage disease using a combination of chemotherapy and surgery and/or radiotherapy, the existence of long-term survivors with small cell carcinoma of the esophagus is anecdotal. Median survival of patients with small carcinoma of the esophagus ranges from 3 months to 7.5 months. For local control of disease, it seems more logical to use radiotherapy rather than subject patients to the risks associated with esophagectomy. However, the appropriate role of surgery or radiotherapy for control of the primary tumor remains to be established.

FUTURE DIRECTIONS

Given the limitations of currently used surgical or radiation therapy–based treatment of esophageal cancer, progress in the treatment of this cancer lies in the development of improved systemic therapy, both to treat metastatic disease and to enhance the effectiveness of radiotherapy by radiosensitization. The use of 5-FU and cisplatin in the treatment of esophageal carcinoma has intensified interest in the use of other agents to biomodulate the antitumor activity of 5-FU. Leucovorin, which enhances the cytotoxic activity of 5-FU by potentiating the inhibition of the enzyme thymidylate synthetase, enhances the clinical antitumor response of 5-FU in patients with colorectal carcinoma (110). Leucovorin as a potential biomodulator of 5-FU antitumor activity in esophageal epidermoid carcinoma was recently studied by Alberts et al. (111) using the Mayo Clinic regimen. Of 35 patients with metastatic or locally advanced epidermoid carcinoma, 6 achieved a major response (17%) with a median duration of response of 32 weeks. No improvement was seen in antitumor response over the reported experience with single-agent 5-FU. Cisplatin in combination with infusional 5-FU and leucovorin was studied in 56 patients with locally advanced disease treated preoperatively or with metastatic disease (69, 112–114); of those, 27 patients (48.2%) experienced a major response that was no different from the results achieved without leucovorin (48.7%) (Table 29.2).

Interferon alfa-2a (IFN-α) as a potential biomodulator of 5-FU has been the subject of two recently published phase II trials in esophageal cancer, based on the prior reported activity of the combination of 5-FU and IFN-α in colorectal carcinoma (110). Biomodulation of 5-FU by IFN-α in laboratory studies occurs by inhibiting the cellular expression of thymidylate synthetase (115), and in patients the pharmacokinetics of 5-FU may be altered by the coadministration of IFN-α (116). Kelsen et al. (117) at Memorial Sloan–Kettering Cancer Center studied 5-FU given by continuous infusion for 5 days at a dose of 750 mg/m^2/day, followed by a weekly bolus 5-FU at the same dose given with IFN-α at a dose of 9×10^6 units by subcutaneous injection 3 times per week. Complete and partial responses were seen in 10 (27%) of 37 patients with a median response duration of 6.4 months. Comparable activity was seen for adenocarcinoma and epidermoid carcinoma. Wadler et al. (118) reported a confirmatory trial showing similar activity for the regimen, observing in 20 patients a response proportion of 25%. Ilson et al. (119) subsequently studied the combination of cisplatin, 5-FU, and IFN-α in patients with metastatic or unresectable disease. A preliminary report of this study has shown activity in 50% of patients, suggesting significant activity for this regimen in advanced or metastatic disease. The activity for this regimen in adenocarcinoma was less than that observed in the prior trial of 5-FU and IFN. Greater activity was seen for epidermoid carcinoma than for adenocarcinoma in this trial, with a trend toward improved median survival in epidermoid carcinoma, suggesting a difference in treatment outcome as a function of histology. The study of IFN in esophageal cancer continues, with particular interest engendered by the recent report of significant antitumor activity for the combination of IFN-α and the retinoid cis-retinoic acid in squamous cell carcinomas of the skin and cervix (120, 121). A trial of this non–chemotherapy-containing, biologic response modifier regimen in esophageal cancer is underway. The identification of activity for paclitaxel and vinorelbine has raised interest in combination trials of these drugs, which are currently underway in the United States and Europe.

The search for effective antitumor agents in the treatment of esophageal cancer continues, given the modest activity of currently available agents and the brief duration of antitumor responses observed. Future strategies in the treatment of esophageal carcinoma undoubtedly will be based on advances in the understanding of the biochemistry and molecular biology of the disease. Ongoing studies indicate a potential role for oncogenes and tumor suppressor genes in the mechanism of tumorigenesis, and indicate that these factors may be important biologic prognostic factors predicting eventual clinical outcome. Laboratory studies have revealed evidence of enhanced expression and amplification of the epidermal growth factor (EGF) receptor gene (122, 123), and amplification of the c-*myc* oncogene (123) in esophageal epidermoid carcinoma. Immunohistochemical studies of EGF and EGF receptor protein expression in resected esophageal epidermoid cancers have shown that increased degree of expression of EGF or EGF receptor protein correlates with a worse outcome and poorer survival (124). A high degree of expression of the HER2 receptor also has been demonstrated in esophageal adenocarcinoma and Barrett's esophagus, and like the EGF receptor, HER2 is a tyrosine kinase growth factor receptor (125). The tumor suppressor gene *p53* has been studied in esophageal carcinoma with demonstration of *p53* mutations in epidermoid and adenocarcinoma and in the premalignant lesion of Barrett's epithelium (126, 127). Loss of heterozygosity of the retinoblastoma tumor suppressor gene locus in human epidermoid and adenocarcinoma of the esophagus also has been shown (128). The tumor suppressor genes *APC* (familial polyposis) and *DCC* also have been shown to lose heterozygosity in esophageal epidermoid and adenocarcinoma (129). The *int-2* oncogene, the fibroblast growth factor–related protooncogene, has been shown to be coamplified with the locus *hst*-1; this coamplification correlates with poorer survival and a higher incidence of eventual systemic metastasis in patients with epidermoid carcinoma resected for cure (130). The gene encoding cyclin D, involved in cell cycle regulation, also has been shown to be amplified in esophageal epidermoid carcinoma (131).

A recent model of tumor progression in adenocarcinoma of the esophagus was proposed by Blount et al. (132). Thirty-two patients with Barrett's esophagus were followed with serial endoscopy and biopsy over a 10-year period. These patients ultimately developed either adenocarcinoma, high-grade dysplasia, or both while under endoscopic surveillance. Based on serial cytogenetic and molecular genetic studies on patients, 17p allelic loss (the locus of the *p53* gene) was determined to be an early cytogenetic event, which preceded the development of aneuploidy during neoplastic progression in Barrett's esophagus. Because 17p allelic loss also was associated frequently with mutation of the remaining *p53* gene, the investigators proposed that loss of *p53* was an important early event in neoplastic progression of Barrett's esophagus, leading to genetic instability that results in the development of aneuploidy and ultimately invasive carcinoma.

The ultimate goal in studying potential biochemical perturbation of normal growth factor receptor and growth signal transduction pathways is the identification of novel targets for future chemotherapeutic agents. The challenge to improve the treatment of esophageal cancer lies in advancing the effectiveness of systemic therapy.

REFERENCES

1. Wingo PA, Tong T, Bolden S. Cancer statistics, 1995. CA Cancer J Clin 1995;45:8–26.
2. Rosenberg JC, Lichter AS, Leichman LP. Cancer of the esophagus. In: DeVita VT, Hellman S, Rosenberg SA, eds. Cancer: principles & practice of oncology. Philadelphia: JB Lippincott, 1989:725–764.
3. Blot WJ, Devesa SS, Kneller RW, Fraumeni JF Jr. Rising incidence of adenocarcinoma of the esophagus and gastric cardia. JAMA 1991;265:1287–1289.
4. Wu YK, Huang GJ, Shao LF, Zhang YD, Lin XS. Honored guest's address: progress in the study and surgical treatment of cancer of the esophagus in China, 1940–1980. J Thorac Cardiovasc Surg 1982;84:325–333.
5. Kmet J, Mahoubi E. Esophageal cancer in the Caspian littoral of Iran: initial studies. Science 1972;175:846–853.
6. McGlashan ND. Esophageal cancer and alcoholic spirits in central Africa. Gut 1969;10:643.
7. Earlam R, Cunha-Melo JR. Oesophageal squamous cell carcinoma: I. A critical review of surgery. Br J Surg 1980;67:381–390.
8. Earlam R, Cunha-Melo JR. Oesophogeal squamous cell carcinoma: II. A critical view of radiotherapy. Br J Surg 1980;67:457–461.
9. Muller JM, Erasmi H, Stelzner M, Zieren J, Pichlmaier H. Surgical therapy of oesophageal carcinoma. Br J Surg 1990;77:845–857.
10. Anderson I, Ladd T. Autopsy findings in squamous cell carcinoma of the esophagus. Cancer 1982;50:1587–1590.
11. Bosch A, Frias Z, Pellett JR. Carcinoma of the esophagus: twenty-five years' experience at the University of Wisconsin Hospitals. Wisconsin Medical Journal 1080;79:23–26.
12. Chan KW, Chan EY, Chan CW. Carcinoma of the esophagus. An autopsy study of 231 cases. Pathology 1986;18:400–405.
13. Mandard AM, Chasle J, Marnay J, Villedieu B, Bianco C, Roussel A, Elie H, et al. Autopsy findings in 111 cases of esophageal cancer. Cancer 1981;48:329–335.
14. Nanus DM, Kelsen DP, Niedzwiecki D, Chapman D, Brennan M, Cheng E, Melamed M. Flow cytometry as a predictive indicator in patients with operable gastric cancer. J Clin Oncol 1989;7:1105–1112.
15. Miller AB, Hoogstraten B, Staquet M, et al. Reporting of cancer treatment. Cancer 1981;47:207–214.
16. Kelsen DP, Heelan R, Coonley C, Bains M, Martini H, Hilaris B, Colbey RB. Clinical and pathological evaluation of response to chemotherapy in patients with esophageal carcinoma. Am J Clin Oncol 1983;6:539–546.
17. Agha FP, Orringer MB, Amendola MA. Gastric interposition following transhiatal esophagectomy: radiographic evaluation. Gastrointestinal Radiology 1985;10:17–24.
18. Lightdale CJ, Botet JF. Esophageal carcinoma: pre-operative staging and evaluation of anastomotic recurrence. Gastrointest Endosc 1990;36:S11–S16.
19. Tio T, Cohen P, Coene P, et al. Endosonography and computed tomography of esophageal carcinoma. Gastroenterology 1989;96:1478–1486.
20. Ezdini EZ, Gelber R, Desai DV, Falkson G, Moertel CH, Hahn RG. Chemotherapy of advanced esophageal carcinoma: Eastern Cooperative Oncology Group experience. Cancer 1980;46:2149–2153.
21. Lokich JJ, Shea M, Chaffey J. Sequential infusional 5-fluorouracil followed by concomitant radiation for tumors of the esophagus and gastroesophageal junction. Cancer 1987;60:275–279.
22. Bezwoda WR, Derman DP, Weaving A, Nissenbaum M. Treatment of esophageal cancer with vindesine: an open trial. Cancer Treat Rep 1984;68:783–785.
23. Kelsen DP, Bains MS, Cvitkovic E, Golbey R. Vindesine in the treatment of esophageal carcinoma: a phase II study. Cancer Treat Rep 1979;63:2019–2021.
24. Bedikian A, Valdivieso M, Bodey G, et al. Phase II evaluation of vindesine in the treatment of colorectal and esophageal tumors. Cancer Chemother Pharmacol 1979;2:263.
25. Popkin J, Bromer R, Byrne R, et al. Continuous 48-hour infusion of vindesine in squamous cell carcinoma of the upper aero-digestive tract (abstract 40). Proceedings of the 13th International Cancer Congress, 1983.
26. Kelsen DP, Magill GB, Cheng E, Dukeman M, Sordillo P, Heelan R, Yagoda A. Phase II trial of etoposide in adenocarcinomas of the upper gastrointestinal tract. Cancer Treat Rep 1983;67:509–510.
27. Coonley CJ, Bains M, Heelan R, Dukeman J, Kelsen DP. Phase II study of etoposide in the treatment of esophageal carcinoma. Cancer Treat Rep 1983;67:397–398.
28. Harstrick A, Bokemeyer C, Preusser P, Kohne-Wompner CH, Meyer HJ, Stahl M, Knipp H, et al. Phase II study of single-agent etoposide in patients with metastatic squamous-cell carcinoma of the esophagus. Cancer Chemother Pharmacol 1992;29:321–322.
29. Wani MC, Taylor HL, Wall ME, et al. Plant antitumor agents. VI. The isolation and structure of Taxol, a novel antileukemic

and antitumor agent from *Taxus brevifolia*. J Am Chem Soc 1971;93:2325–2327.
30. Ajani J, Ilson D, Daugherty K, et al. Activity of Taxol in patients with squamous cell carcinoma and adenocarcinoma of the esophagus. J Natl Cancer Inst 1994;86:1086–1091.
31. Conroy T, Etienne PL, Adenis A, et al. Vinorelbine: a promising drug in metastatic epidermoid esophageal carcinoma (abstract). Proc Am Soc Clin Oncol 1993;12:A553.
32. Panettiere FJ, Leichman L, O'Bryan R, Haas C, Fletcher W. Cis-diamminedichloride platinum (II), an effective agent in the treatment of epidermoid carcinoma of the esophagus. A preliminary report of an ongoing Southwest Oncology Group study. Cancer Clin Trials 1981;4:29–31.
33. Ravry MJ, Moore MR, Omura GA, et al. Phase II evaluation of cisplatin in squamous carcinoma of the esophagus: a Southeastern Cancer Study Group trial. Cancer Treat Rep 1985;69:1457–1458.
34. Davis S, Shanmugathasa M, Kessler W. cis-Dichlorodiammineplatinum(II) in the treatment of esophageal carcinoma. Cancer Treat Rep 1980;64:709–711.
35. Murthy SK, Prabhakaran PS, Chandrashekar M, Deshpande R, Doval DC, Copinath KD. Neoadjuvant Cis-DDP in esophageal cancers: an experience at a regional cancer centre, India. J Surg Oncol 1990;45:173–176.
36. Ajani J, Kantarjian H, Kanojia M, Karlin D. Phase II trial of cisplatinum in advanced upper gastrointestinal cancer (abstract). Proc Am Soc Clin Oncol 1984;2:147.
37. Sternberg C, Kelsen D, Dukeman M, Leichman L, Heelan R. Carboplatin: a new platinum analog in the treatment of epidermoid carcinoma of the esophagus. Cancer Treat Rep 1985;69:1305–1307.
38. Mannell A, Winters Z. Carboplatin in the treatment of oesophageal cancer. S Afr Med J 1989;76:213–214.
39. Queisser W, Preusser P, Mross KB, Fritze D, Rieche K, Beyer JH, Achterrath W, et al. Phase II evaluation of carboplatin in advanced esophageal carcinoma. A trial of the Phase I/II Study Group of the Association for Medical Oncology of the German Cancer Society. Onkologie 1990;13:190–193.
40. Einzig A, Kelsen DP, Cheng E, Sordillo P, Heelan R, Winn R, Magill C. Phase II trial of carboplatin in patients with adenocarcinomas of the upper gastrointestinal tract. Cancer Treat Rep 1985;69:1453–1454.
41. Coonley CJ, Bains M, Hilaris B, Chapman R, Kelsen DP. Cisplatin and bleomycin in the treatment of esophageal carcinoma. A final report. Cancer 1984;54:2351–2355.
42. Bosset J, Hurteloup P, Bontemas P, et al. A phase II trial of bleomycin and cisplatin in advanced oesophagus carcinoma (abstract 41). Proceedings of the 13th International Cancer Congress, 1983.
43. Bromer R, Abbruzzese J, Karp D, et al. Ineffectiveness of cisplatin-bleomycin induction chemotherapy for esophageal cancer (abstract). Proc Am Soc Clin Oncol 1984;3:143.
44. Izquierdo MA, Marcuello E, Gomez de Segura G, et al. Unresectable nonmetastatic squamous cell carcinoma of the esophagus managed by sequential chemotherapy (cisplatin and bleomycin) and radiation therapy. Cancer 1993;71:287–292.
45. Kolaric K, Maricic Z, Roth A, Dujmovic I. Combination of bleomycin and Adriamycin with and without radiation on the treatment of inoperable esophageal cancer. A randomized study. Cancer 1980;45:2265–2273.
46. Kelsen D, Hilaris B, Coonley C, Chapman R, Lesser M, Kukeman M, Heelan R, et al. Cisplatin, vindesine, and bleomycin chemotherapy of local-regional and advanced esophageal carcinoma. Am J Med 1983;75:645–652.
47. Schlag P, Herrmann R, Raeth V, Lehner B, Schwarz V, Herfarth C. Preoperative chemotherapy in esophageal cancer. A phase II study. Acta Oncol 1988;27:811–814.
48. Dinwoodie WR, Bartolucci AA, Lyman GH, Velez-Garcia E, Martelo OJ, Sarma PR. Phase II evaluation of cisplatin, bleomycin, and vindesine in advanced squamous cell carcinoma of the esophagus: a Southeastern Cancer Study Group trial. Cancer Treat Rep 1986;70:267–270.
49. Roth JA, Pass HI, Flanagan MM, Graeber GM, Rosenberg JC, Steinberg S. Randomized clinical trial of preoperative and postoperative adjuvant chemotherapy with cisplatin, vindesine, and bleomycin for carcinoma of the esophagus. J Thorac Cardiovasc Surg 1988;96:242–248.
50. Kelsen DP, Minsky B, Smith M, Beitler J, Niedzwiecki D, Bains M, Burt M, et al. Preoperative therapy for esophageal cancer: a randomized comparison of chemotherapy versus radiation therapy. J Clin Oncol 1990;8:1352–1361.
51. Kelsen DP, Fein R, Coonley C, Heelan R, Bains M. Cisplatin, vindesine, and mitoguazone in the treatment of esophageal cancer. Cancer Treat Rep 1986;70:255–259.
52. Chapman R, Fleming TR, Van Damme J, Macdonald J. Cisplatin, vinblastine, and mitoguazone in squamous cell carcinoma of the esophagus: a Southwest Oncology Group study. Cancer Treat Rep 1987;71:1185–1187.
53. Forastiere AA, Gennis M, Orringer MB, Agha FP. Cisplatin, vinblastine, and mitoguazone chemotherapy for epidermoid and adenocarcinoma of the esophagus. J Clin Oncol 1987;5:1143–1149.
54. Ajani J, Roth J, Ryan B, Putnam J, Pazdur R, Gaintuch J, Dumas P, et al. High-dose chemotherapy with GM-CSF for resectable adenocarcinoma of the esophagus (ACE) (abstract). Proc Am Soc Clin Oncol 1991;10:A472.
55. Kies MS, Rosen ST, Tsang TK, Shetty R, Schneider PA, Wallemark CB, Shields TW. Cisplatin and 5-fluorouracil in the primary management of squamous esophageal cancer. Cancer 1987;60:2156–2160.
56. Hilgenberg AD, Carey RW, Wilkins EW Jr, Choi NC, Mathisen DJ, Grillo HC. Preoperative chemotherapy, surgical resection, and selective postoperative therapy for squamous cell carcinoma of the esophagus. Ann Thorac Surg 1988;45:357–363.
57. Vignoud J, Visset J, Paineau J, Le Neel JC, Cuilliere P, Cussac A. Preoperative chemotherapy in squamous cell carcinoma of the esophagus: clinical and pathological analysis, 48 cases (abstract). Ann Oncol 1990;1:45.
58. De Besi P, Sileni VC, Salvagno L, Tremolada C, Cartei G, Fosser V, Paccagnella A, et al. Phase II study of cisplatin, 5-FU, and allopurinol in advanced esophageal cancer. Cancer Treat Rep 1986;70:909–910.
59. Charlois T, Burtin P, Ben-Bouali AK, et al. Predictive factors of response to chemotherapy for esophageal squamous cell carcinoma: study of 60 patients and proposal of a response score. Gastroenterol Clin Biol 1992;16:134–140.
60. Ajani JA, Ryan B, Rich TA, McMurtrey M, Roth JA, DeCaro L, Levin B, et al. Prolonged chemotherapy for localised squamous carcinoma of the oesophagus. Eur J Cancer 1992;28A:880–884.
61. Bleiberg H, Jacob JH, Bedenne L, Paillot B, De Besi P, Lacave A. Randomized phase II trial of 5-fluorouracil (5FU) and cisplatin (DDP) vs DDP alone in advanced esophageal cancer (meeting abstract). Proc Am Soc Clin Oncol 1991;10:A447.
62. Gisselbrecht C, Calvo F, Mignot L, Pujade E, Bouvry M, Danne O, Belpomme D, et al. Fluorouracil (F), Adriamycin (A), and cisplatin (P) (FAP): combination chemotherapy of advanced esophageal carcinoma. Cancer 1983;52:974–977.

63. Bedikian AY, Deniord R, El-Akkak S. Value of pre-op chemotherapy for esophageal carcinoma (meeting abstract). Proc Am Soc Clin Oncol 1987;6:A375.
64. Ajani JA, Roth JA, Ryan B, McMurtrey M, Rich TA, Jackson DE, Abbruzzese JL, et al. Evaluation of pre- and postoperative chemotherapy for resectable adenocarcinoma of the esophagus or gastroesophageal junction. J Clin Oncol 1990;8:1231–1238.
65. Harris DT, Mastrangelo MJ. Theory and application of early systemic therapy. Semin Oncol 1991;18:493–503.
66. Vokes EE, Weichselbaum RR. Concomitant chemoradiotherapy: rationale and clinical experience in patients with solid tumors. J Clin Oncol 1990;8:911–934.
67. Nygaard K, Hagen S, Hansen HS, Hatlevoll R, Hultborn R, Jakobsen A, Mantyla M, et al. Pre-operative radiotherapy prolongs survival in operable esophageal carcinoma: a randomized, multicenter study of pre-operative radiotherapy and chemotherapy. The second Scandinavian trial in esophageal cancer. World J Surg 1992;16:1104–1109.
68. Preusser P, Wilke H, Achterrath W, Pircher W, Meyer J, Blum M, Lenaz L, et al. Disease oriented phase II study with cisplatin (P), etoposide (E), and 5FU (F) (PEF) in advanced squamous cell carcinoma of the esophagus (meeting abstract). Proc Am Soc Clin Oncol 1988;7:A388.
69. Hoffman P, Vokes E, Ferguson M, Haraf D, Krishnasamy S, English C. Induction chemotherapy, surgery and concomitant chemoradiotherapy for carcinoma of the esophagus (meeting abstract). Proc Am Soc Clin Oncol 1992;11:A588.
70. Wilke H, Stahl M, Preusser P, Fink U, Meyer HJ, Achterrath W, Knipp H, et al. Phase II trial with 5-FU (F), folinic acid (L), etoposide (E), and cisplatin (P; FLEP) ± surgery in advanced esophageal cancer (meeting abstract). Proc Am Soc Clin Oncol 1992;11:A494.
71. Cure H, Pezet D, Slim K, et al. High response rate in non-operable esophageal cancer with a neoadjuvant chemotherapy using carboplatin, cisplatin and 5-fluorouracil. Proc Am Soc Clin Oncol 1993;12:A574.
72. Kelsen D. Chemotherapy for local regional and advanced esophageal cancer. In: DeVita VT, Hellman S, Rosenberg SA, eds. Cancer: principles and practice of oncology updates. Philadelphia: JB Lippincott, 1988:1–12.
73. Schlag P. Preoperative chemotherapy in localized squamous cell carcinoma of the esophagus: results of a prospective randomized trial. Eur J Cancer 1991;27:S76.
74. Kolaric K, Maricic Z, Dujmovic I, et al. Therapy of advanced esophageal cancer with bleomycin, irradiation and combination bleomycin and irradiation. Tumori 1976;62:255–262.
75. Kolaric K, Maricic Z, Roth A, Dujmovic I. Chemotherapy versus chemoradiotherapy in inoperable esophageal cancer. Results of three controlled studies. Oncology 1980;37(Suppl 1):77–82.
76. Kolaric K, Maricic Z, Roth A, Dujmovic I. Bleomycin infusions combined with radiotherapy in the treatment of inoperable esophageal cancer. Tumori 1980;66:615–621.
77. Kolaric K, Maricic Z, Roth A, et al. Adriamycin alone and in combination with radiotherapy in the treatment of inoperable esophageal cancer. Tumori 1977;63:485–491.
78. Earle JD, Gelber RD, Moertel CG, Hahn, RG. A controlled evaluation of combined radiation and bleomycin therapy for squamous cell carcinoma of the esophagus. Int J Radiat Oncol Biol Phys 1980;6:821–826.
79. Byfield JE, Barone R, Mendelsohn J, Frankel S, Quinol L, Sharp T, Seagren S. Infusional 5-fluorouracil and x-ray therapy for non-resectable esophageal cancer. Cancer 1980;45:703–708.
80. Gignoux M, Roussel A, Paillot B, Gillet M, Schlag P, Favre JP, Dalesio O, et al. The value of preoperative radiotherapy in esophageal cancer: results of a study of the EORTC. World J Surg 1987;11:426–432.
81. Launois B, Delarue D, Campion JP, Kerbaol M. Preoperative radiotherapy for carcinoma of the esophagus. Surg Gynecol Obstet 1981;153:690–692.
82. Wang M, Huang GJ, Gu XZ et al. Combined preoperative irradiation and surgery versus surgery alone for carcinoma of the midthoracic esophagus: a prospective randomized study in 360 patients. Presented at the Fourth World Congress of the International Society for Diseases of the Esophagus, Rennes, France, 1989.
83. Franklin R, Steiger Z, Vaishampayan G, Asfaw I, Rosenberg J, Loh J, Hoschner J, et al. Combined modality therapy for esophageal squamous cell carcinoma. Cancer 1983;51:1062–1071.
84. Leichman L, Steiger Z, Seydel HG, Dindogru A, Kinzie J, Toben S, MacKenzie G, et al. Preoperative chemotherapy and radiation therapy for patients with cancer of the esophagus: a potentially curative approach. J Clin Oncol 1984;2:75–79.
85. Leichman L, Herskovic A, Leichman CG, Lattin PB, Steiger Z, Tapazoğlou E, Rosenberg JC, et al. Nonoperative therapy for squamous-cell cancer of the esophagus. J Clin Oncol 1987;5:365–370.
86. Poplin E, Fleming T, Leichman L, Seydel HG, Steiger Z, Taylor S, Vance R, et al. Combined therapies for squamous-cell carcinoma of the esophagus, a Southwest Oncology Group Study (SWOG-8037). J Clin Oncol 1987;5:622–628.
87. Seydel HG, Leichman L, Byhardt R, Cooper J, Herskovic A, Libnock J, Pazdur R, et al. Preoperative radiation and chemotherapy for localized squamous cell carcinoma of the esophagus: a RTOG Study. Int J Radiat Oncol Biol Phys 1988;14:33–35.
88. Forastiere AA, Orringer MB, Perez-Tamayo C, Urba SG, Husted S, Takasugi BJ, Zahurak M. Concurrent chemotherapy and radiation therapy followed by transhiatal esophagectomy for local-regional cancer of the esophagus. J Clin Oncol 1990;8:119–127.
89. Forastiere AA, Orringer MB, Perez-Tamayo C, et al. Preoperative chemoradiation followed by transhiatal esophagectomy for carcinoma of the esophagus: final report. J Clin Oncol 1993;11:1118–1123.
90. Urba SG, Orringer MB, Perez-Tamayo C, Bromberg J, Forastiere A. Concurrent preoperative chemotherapy, radiation therapy in localized esophageal adenocarcinoma. Cancer 1992;69:285–291.
91. Bedenne L, Seitz JF, Milan C, et al. Preoperative radiotherapy and chemotherapy in epidermoid oesophageal cancers. Results of a phase II multicenter trial by the French foundation for carcinology of the digestive tract. Proc Am Soc Clin Oncol 1993;12:A587.
92. Richmond J, Seydel HG, Bae Y, Lewis J, Burdakin J, Jacobsen G. Comparison of three treatment strategies for esophageal cancer within a single institution. Int J Radiat Oncol Biol Phys 1987;13:1617–1620.
93. Wilke H, Stahl M, Fink U, et al. High PCR/NED rate with an intensive preoperative combined modality program in patients with esophageal cancer (abstract 649). Proc Am Soc Clin Oncol 1993;12.
94. Butler D, Hoff S, Garrow G, et al. Neoadjuvant therapy with cisplatin, 5-fluorouracil, leucovorin, ±etoposide and radiation

for esophageal cancer. Proc Am Soc Clin Oncol 1993;12:A597.
95. Coia LR, Engstrom PF, Paul AR, Stafford PM, Hands GE. Long-term results of infusional 5-FU, mitomycin-C and radiation as primary management of esophageal carcinoma. Int J Radiat Oncol Biol Phys 1991;20:29–36.
96. John MJ, Flam MS, Mowry PA, Podoksky WJ, Xavier AM, Wittlinger PS, Padmanabhan A. Radiotherapy alone and chemoradiation for nonmetastatic esophageal carcinoma. A critical review of chemoradiation. Cancer 1989;63:2397–2403.
97. Chan A, Wong A, Arthur K. Concomitant 5-fluorouracil infusion, mitomycin C and radical radiation therapy in esophageal squamous cell carcinoma. Int J Radiat Oncol Biol Phys 1989;16:59–65.
98. Keane TJ, Harwood AR, Elhakim T, Rider WD, Cummings BJ, Ginsberg RJ, Cooper JC. Radical radiation therapy with 5-fluorouracil infusion and mitomycin C for oesophageal squamous carcinoma. Radiother Oncol 1985;4:205–210.
99. Seitz JF, Giovannini M, Padaut-Cesana J, Fuentes P, Giudicelli R, Gauthier AP, Carcassone Y. Inoperable nonmetastatic squamous cell carcinoma of the esophagus managed by concomitant chemotherapy (5-fluorouracil and cisplatin) and radiation therapy. Cancer 1990;66:214–219.
100. Roussel A, Bleiberg H, Dalesio O, Jacob JH, Haegele P, Jung GM, Paillot B, et al. Palliative therapy of inoperable oesophageal carcinoma with radiotherapy and methotrexate: final results of a controlled clinical trial. Int J Radiat Oncol Biol Phys 1989;16:67–72.
101. Roussel A, Haegele P, Paillot B, et al. Results of the EORTC-GTCCG Phase III trial of irradiation vs irradiation and CDDP in inoperable esophageal cancer (abstract). Proc Am Soc Clin Oncol 1994;13:A583
102. Herskovic A, Martz K, Al-Sarraf M, Leichman L, Brindle J, Vaitkevicius V, Cooper J, et al. Combined chemotherapy and radiotherapy compared with radiotherapy alone in patients with cancer of the esophagus. N Engl J Med 1992;326:1593–1647.
103. Al-Sarraf M, Pajak T, Herskovic A, et al. Progress report of combined chemo-radiotherapy vs radiotherapy alone in patients with esophageal cancer. Proc Am Soc Clin Oncol 1993;12:580.
104. Sischy B, Ryan L, Haller D, Smith T, Dayal Y, Schutt A, Hinson J. Interim report of EST 1282 phase III protocol for the evaluation of combined modalities in the treatment of patients with carcinoma of the esophagus, stage I and II. Proc Am Soc Clin Oncol 1990;9:105.
105. Araujo CM, Souhami L, Gil RA, Carvalho R, Garcia JA, Froimtchuk MJ, Pinto LH, et al. A randomized trial comparing radiation therapy versus concomitant radiation therapy and chemotherapy in carcinoma of the thoracic esophagus. Cancer 1991;67:2258–2261.
106. Nichols GL, Kelsen DP. Small cell carcinoma of the esophagus. The Memorial Hospital experience 1970 to 1987. Cancer 1989;64:1531–1533.
107. Tateishi R, Taniguchi K, Horai T, et al. Argyrophil cell carcinoma (APUDoma) of the esophagus: a histopathological entity. Virchows Arch A Pathol Anat Histopathol 1976;371:283–294.
108. Saito T, Hikita M, Kohno K, et al. Different sensitivities of human esophageal cancer cells to multiple anti-cancer agents and related mechanisms. Cancer 1992;70:2402–2409.
109. Remick SC, Ruckdeschel JC. Extrapulmonary and pulmonary small-cell carcinoma: tumor biology, therapy, and outcome. Med Pediatr Oncol 1992;20:89–99.
110. Schmoll HJ, Hiddemann W, Rustum Y, eds. Recent developments in biomodulation: second international workshop on gastrointestinal cancer. Semin Oncol 1992;19:1–234.
111. Alberts AS, Schoeman L, Burger W, Greef F, Falkson G. A phase II study of 5-fluorouracil and leucovorin in advanced carcinoma of the esophagus. Am J Clin Oncol 1992;15:35–36.
112. Zaniboni A, Simoncini E, Tonini G, Pezzola D, Farfaglia R, Lancini GP, Marpicata P, et al. Cisplatin, high dose folinic acid and 5-fluorouracil in squamous cell carcinoma of the esophagus. A pilot study. Chemioterapia 1987;6:387–389.
113. Hayashi K, Ide H, Shinoda M, Fukushima M. Phase II study of cisplatin (CDDP) plus 5-fluorouracil (5-FU) and leucovorin (LCV) for squamous cell carcinoma (SCC) of the esophagus (meeting abstract). Proc Am Soc Clin Oncol 1992;11:A526.
114. Ilson D, Kelsen D. Chemotherapy in esophageal cancer. In: Sluyser M, ed. Anti-cancer drugs. Oxford, United Kingdom: Rapid Communications of Oxford, 1993;4:287–299.
115. Wadler S, Schwartz EL. Principles in biomodulation of cytotoxic drugs by interferons. Semin Oncol 1992;19:45–48.
116. Schuller J, Czejka MJ, Schernthaner G, et al. Influence of inerferon alfa-2b with or without folinic acid on pharmacokinetics of fluorouracil. Semin Oncol 1992;19:93–97.
117. Kelsen D, Lovett D, Wong J, Saltz L, Buckley M, Murray P, Heelan R, et al. Interferon alfa-2a and fluorouracil in the treatment of patients with advanced esophageal cancer. J Clin Oncol 1992;10:269–274.
118. Wadler S, Fell S, Haynes H, et al. Treatment of carcinoma of the esophagus with 5-fluorouracil and recombinant alfa-2a-interferon. Cancer 1993;71:1726–1730.
119. Ilson DH, Kelsen DP, Saltz L, Sirott MN, Keretzes R, Dougherty JB. Alfa-interferon (IFN), 5-fluorouracil (FU), and cisplatin (CDDP) in esophageal cancer (ESO): response in epidermoid carcinoma (EPID) is significantly higher than adenocarcinoma (ADENO) (abstract). Proc Am Soc Clin Oncol 1994;13:A563.
120. Lippman SM, Parkinson DR, Loretta MI, et al. 13-Cis-retinoic acid and interferon alfa-2a: effective combination therapy for advanced squamous cell carcinoma of the skin. J Natl Cancer Inst 1992;84:235–241.
121. Lippman SM, Kavanagh JJ, Paredes-Espinoza M, et al. 13-Cis-retinoic acid plus interferon alfa-2a: highly effective systemic therapy for squamous cell carcinoma of the cervix. J Natl Cancer Inst 1992;84:241–245.
122. Hollstein MC, Smits AM, Galiana C, Yamasaki H, Bos JL, Mandard A, Partensky C, et al. Amplification of epidermal growth factor receptor gene but no evidence of ras mutations in primary human esophageal cancers. Cancer Res 1988;48:5119–5123.
123. Lu SH, Hsieh LL, Luo FC, Weinstein IB. Amplification of the EGF receptor and c-myc genes in human esophageal cancers. Int J Cancer 1988;42:502–505.
124. Mukaida H, Toi M, Hirai T, Yamashita Y, Toge T. Clinical significance of the expression of epidermal growth factor and its receptor in esophageal cancer. Cancer 1991;68:142–148.
125. Jankowski J, Coghill G, Hopwood D, Wormsley KG. Oncogenes and onco-suppressor gene in adenocarcinoma of the oesophagus. Gut 1992;33:1033–1038.
126. Casson AG, Mukhopadhyay T, Clear KR, et al. p53 Gene mutations in Barrett's epithelium and esophageal cancer. Cancer Res 1991;51:4495–4499.
127. Hollstein MC, Mewtcalf RA, Welsh JA, et al. Frequent mutation of the p53 gene in human esophageal cancer. Proc Natl Acad Sci U S A 1990;87:9958–9961.
128. Boynton RF, Huang Y, Blount PL, Reid BJ, Raskind WH, Haggitt RC, Newkirk C, et al. Frequent loss of heterozygosity at the retinoblastoma locus in human esophageal cancers. Cancer Res 1991;51:5766–5769.

129. Huang Y, Boynton RF, Blount PL, Silverstein RJ, Yin J, Tong Y, McDaniel TK, et al. Loss of heterozygosity involves multiple tumor suppressor genes in human esophageal cancers. Cancer Res 1992;52:6525–6530.
130. Kitagawa Y, Ueda M, Ando N, Shinozawa Y, Shimizu N, Abe O. Significance of int-2/hst-1 coamplification as a prognostic factor in patients with esophageal squamous carcinoma. Cancer Res 1991;51:1504–1508.
131. Jiang W, Kahn SM, Tomita N, Zhang YJ, Lu SH, Weinstein IB. Amplification and expression of the human cyclin D gene in esophageal cancer. Cancer Res 1992;52:2980–2983.
132. Blount PL, Galipeau PC, Sanchez CA, Neshat K, Levine DS, Yin J, Suzuki H, et al. 17p Allelic losses in diploid cells of patients with Barrett's esophagus who develop aneuploidy. Cancer Res 1994;54:2292–2295.
133. Clinical Screening Group. Study of the clinical efficiency of bleomycin in human cancer. BMJ 1970;2:643–645.
134. Yagoda A, Mukherji B, Young C, et al. Bleomycin, an antitumor antibiotic: clinical experience in 274 patients. Ann Intern Med 1972;77:861–870.
135. Bonadonna G, de Lena M, Monfardini S, et al. Clinical trial with bleomycin in lymphomas and in solid tumors. Eur J Cancer 1972;8:205–215.
136. Stephens F. Bleomycin—a new approach in cancer chemotherapy. Med J Aust 1973;1:1277–1283.
137. Ravry M, Moertel CG, Schutt AJ, et al. Treatment of advanced squamous cell carcinoma of the gastrointestinal tract with bleomycin (NSC 125066). Cancer Chemother Rep 1973;57:493–495.
138. Tancini G, Bajetta E, Bonadonna G. Terapia con bleomycin da sola o in associazione con methodtrexate nel carcinoma epidermoide dell'esofago. Tumori 1974;60:65–71.
139. Desai P, Borges E, Vohrs V, et al. Carcinoma of the esophagus in India. Cancer 1969;23:979–989.
140. Whittington R, Close H. Clinical experience with mitomycin-C. Cancer Chemother Rep 1970;54:195–198.
141. Engstrom PF, Lavin PT, Klaassen DJ. Phase II evaluation of mitomycin and cisplatin in advanced esophageal carcinoma. Cancer Treat Rep 1983;67:713–715.
142. Einzig A, Kelsen D, Cheng E, Sordillo P, Raymond V, Magill G. Phase II study of 4-demethoxydaunorubicin in patients with adenocarcinoma of the upper gastrointestinal tract. Cancer Treat Rep 1984;68:1415–1416.
143. Poplin E, Macdonald J. Phase II study of amonafide in squamous esophageal cancer: a SWOG study (abstract). Proc Am Assoc Cancer Res 1992;33:A1304.
144. Advani SH, Saikia TK, Swaroop S, Ramakrishnan G, Nair CN, Dinshaw KA, Sharma A, et al. Anterior chemotherapy in esophageal cancer. Cancer 1985;56:1502–1506.
145. Bajorin D, Kelsen D. Phase II trial of dichloromethotrexate (dcm) in epidermoid carcinoma of the esophagus (ece) (abstract). Proc Am Assoc Cancer Res 1986;27:187.
146. Brown T, Fleming T, Tangen C, Macdonald J. A phase II trial of trimetrexate in the treatment of esophageal cancer: a Southwest Oncology Group trial (SWOG) (abstract). Proc Am Soc Clin Oncol 1992;11:A479.
147. Engstrom PF, Ryan LM, Falkson G, Haller DG. Phase II study of aminothiadiazole in advanced squamous cell carcinoma of the esophagus. Am J Clin Oncol 1991;14:33–35.
148. Ansell SM, Alberts AS, Falkson G. Ifosfamide in advanced carcinoma of the esophagus: a phase II trial with severe toxicity. Am J Clin Oncol 1989;12:205–207.
149. Moertel C, Schutt A, Reitemeier R, et al. Therapy for gastrointestinal cancer with the nitrosoureas alone in drug combination. Cancer Treat Rep 1976;60:729.
150. Falkson G. Methyl-GAG (NSC 32946) in the treatment of esophageal cancer. Cancer Chemother Rep 1971;55:209–212.
151. Kelsen D, Chapman R, Bains M, Heelan R, Dukeman M, Colbey R. Phase II study of methyl-GAG in the treatment of esophageal carcinoma. Cancer Treat Rep 1982;66:1427–1429.
152. De Besi P, Salvagno L, Endrizzi L, Sileni VC, Fosser V, Cartei G, Paccagnella A, et al. Cisplatin, bleomycin and methotrexate in the treatment of advanced oesophageal cancer. Eur J Cancer Clin Oncol 1984;20:743–747.
153. Vogl SE, Greenwald E, Kaplan BH. Effective chemotherapy for esophageal cancer with methotrexate, bleomycin, and cis-diamminedichloroplatinum II. Cancer 1981;48:2555–2558.
154. Resbeut M, Le Prise-Fleury E, Ben-Hassel M, Goudier MJ, Morice-Rouxel MF, Douillard JY, Chenal C. Squamous cell carcinoma of the esophagus. Treatment by combined vincristine-methotrexate plus folinic acid rescue and cisplatin before radiotherapy. Cancer 1985;56:1246–1250.
155. Kagami Y, Sakurai T, Nishio M, et al. Cisplatin, methotrexate and peplomycin in the treatment of esophageal carcinoma. Gan To Kagaku Ryoho 1986;13:3523–3526.
156. Vogl SE, Camacho F, Berenzweig M, Ruckdeschel J. Chemotherapy for esophageal cancer with mitoguazone, methotrexate, bleomycin, and cisplatin. Cancer Treat Rep 1985;69:21–23.
157. El Akkad S, Amer M, Kerth W. Combination chemotherapy, surgery, and radiotherapy for esophageal cancer. Proceedings of the 13th International Cancer Congress, 40, 1983.
158. Forastiere A, Patel H, Hankins J, et al. Cisplatin, bleomycin and VP-16-213 in combination for epidermoid carcinoma of the esophagus. Proc Am Soc Clin Oncol 1983;2:A127.
159. Burton GV, Wolfe WG, Crocker IR, Medoff JR, Prosnitz LR. Esophageal carcinoma: response to cisplatin and etoposide chemotherapy (abstract). Proc Am Soc Clin Oncol 1986;5:86.
160. Spielman M, Kac J, Elias D, et al. Association of vindesine, cyclophosphamide, cisplatin and CCNU in esophageal squamous cell carcinoma. Bull Cancer (Paris) 1985;72:220–226.
161. Spielmann M, Guillot T, Kac J, Cvitkovic E, Rougier P, Le Chevalier T, Kayitalire L, et al. Phase II trial of cisplatin (P) and continuous infusion (CI) of bleomycin (B) and 5 fluorouracil (F) in advanced esophageal cancer (ESO CA) (abstract). Proc Am Soc Clin Oncol 1989;8:A393.
162. Spielmann M, Kac J, Rougier P, Le Chevalier T, Rouesse J. Phase II study of 5-fluorouracil (FU) infusion, cis-platin (DDP) and vindesine (VDS) in squamous carcinoma of the esophageal (abstract). Proc Am Soc Clin Oncol 1987;6:94.
163. Clovett D, Kelsen D, Eisenberger M, Houston C. A phase II trial of carboplatin and vinblastine in the treatment of advanced squamous cell carcinoma of the esophagus. Cancer 1991;67:354–356.

Section VI

Mediastinal Tumors

30

Thymomas

Philippe Levasseur

Thymoma is the most common tumor of the anterosuperior mediastinum. It is distinguished from other thoracic malignancies by its indolent course and by the very few cases with histologic evidence of malignancy, even when macroscopically invasive.

Many autoimmune diseases are associated with thymoma, the most frequent being myasthenia gravis. Surgery in most cases is the best treatment with good long-term results. Nevertheless, the role of preoperative and postoperative radiotherapy must be discussed as well as that of preoperative adjuvant chemotherapy, especially in the very invasive forms.

EMBRYOLOGY, MORPHOLOGY, AND TOPOGRAPHIC ANATOMY OF THE THYMUS

The thymus is an epithelial gland arising from the third and fourth pairs of pharyngeal pouches; during the early weeks of embryonic development, the right and left thymic portions migrate toward the anterior mediastinum, lose their cervical connection, and finally join but never completely fuse.

The thymus is a very elongated structure with two vertical lobes, joined at variable levels, generally in the superior third. Most frequently, the gland has an H-shaped configuration with two upper horns and two lower horns, but many shapes have been described (e.g., x-shaped thymus, u-shaped, inverted) (1). Unilobar thymus (10%) and trilobed thymus (11%) have also been described (2). Many aberrant islets of thymic tissue have been described, especially around the parathyroid but also in the fatty tissue of the mediastinum. Microscopic examination of the gross fatty tissue surrounding the thymus revealed thymic tissue in 13 of 18 myasthenic patients undergoing excisions of the thymus by means of a median sternotomy (3). Rarely, aberrant thymus may be found in such locations as the neck, eardrum, pulmonary hilum, or posterior mediastinum. Park and MacClure (4) stated that in some cases complete extirpation of the thymus is not possible because thymic tissue can be left anywhere along the embryonic descending pathway of the thymus.

The two upper thymic horns are close to the thyroid gland and connected to the lower part of the thyroid gland through the thyro-thymic ligament, and the dissection is generally easy; the two thymic lobes generally are located in front of the left innominate vein, and the two inferior horns are below the innominate vein in contact with the superior vena cava, pericardium, aortic arch, and pulmonary artery. In approximately 10% of cases, one or two lobes can be located behind the left innominate vein (1).

The arterial blood supply of the thymus comes from several sources: direct branches from the aorta or the brachiocephalic artery, branches from the inferior thyroid arteries, lateral branches from the internal thoracic arteries, and sometimes from the superior phrenic artery. Venous drainage is generally to the left innominate vein at its lower part.

The lymphatic channels of the thymus are generally divided into three groups (5). The superior lymphatic ducts go to lymph nodes near the internal jugular vein; the anterior lymphatic ducts end in lymph nodes behind the sternum and drain into the right and left internal thoracic chains. The posterior lymphatic ducts end in the retro-thymic lymph nodes along the pericardium.

HISTOLOGY AND CLASSIFICATION

Despite numerous studies (7), controversy persists regarding classification of thymic tumors in reference to their histologic characteristics and clinical course.

The first classification was proposed by Levine and Rosai (8). In that classification the term thymoma is restricted to thymic epithelial tumors with minimal or no cytologic atypia. The benign thymomas are well encapsulated and not invasive, whereas malignant thymomas are locally invasive and may be associated with lymphatic or hematogenous spread. Thymic epithelial cells and a variable number of lymphocytes make up thymic tumors, which are divided into predominant lymphocytic, predominant epithelial, and mixed, according to the ratio of lymphocyte to epithelial cells and the shape and size of the epithelial cells. The group of spindle cell thymomas is a special entity with predominant fusiform epithelial cells.

A more descriptive classification, based only on histologic criteria, was proposed by Verley and Hollmann (6) in 1985 and distinguishes four histologic types of increasing malignancy.

Type 1: Spindle and oval cells simulating the epithelium of the resting thymus, regardless of the number of lymphocytes.
Type 2: Lymphocyte rich thymoma, with few small, round, or starlike epithelial cells resembling those of the normal thymus.
Type 3: Differentiated epithelial thymoma with well-differentiated cellular and architectural patterns.
Type 4: Undifferentiated epithelial thymoma, corresponding to thymic carcinoma.

For Verley and Hollmann (7), this histologic typing correlates with invasiveness and is prognostic. Spindle cell thymomas and lymphocyte rich thymomas are benign, whereas differentiated epithelial thymomas are potentially aggressive, and undifferentiated epithelial thymomas are truly malignant. This typing seems useful to the pathologist in establishing a prognosis.

A new histologic classification was proposed by Marino and Müller-Hermelink (9) in 1985, based both on morphology and immunohistochemistry (Table 30.1); three types of thymomas are distinguished by the prevalent epithelial cell type and pattern of lymphoid infiltration:

1. Cortical thymomas derive from the thymic cortex; lymphocytes often have with a blastic appearance and are abundant.

2. Medullary thymomas derive from the medullary epithelial cells; lymphocytes are mature thymocytes and are few in number.
3. Mixed thymomas have both cortical and medullary epithelial cells, associated with a variable number of lymphocytes. Hence, a mixed common type, a mixed cortical predominant, and a mixed medullary predominant represent the three subgroups.

There is an important correlation between the subtype and both the surgical stage of the tumor and the long-term prognosis: the medullary and the mixed types are generally benign and have a good long-term prognosis; the cortical and predominant cortical types are generally invasive and have a poor prognosis. In a recent study (10) using this classification, Pescarmona et al. noted a significant relationship between histologic findings, age, stage of the tumor, and long-term prognosis.

Nomori et al. (11) showed in morphometric studies that the nuclei of the epithelial cells of cortical thymomas are larger than the nuclei of medullary thymomas. This research also observed that cortical thymomas have a higher grade of malignancy than do the medullary and mixed types.

Many studies using flow cytometry and monoclonal antibodies were performed; the most interesting study is that of Ito et al. (12), who identified three types: thymus lymphocyte type (immature thymocyte predominant), peripheral lymphocyte type (mature thymocyte predominant), and intermediate type.

Finally, all of those classifications are somewhat difficult to use and do not characterize the tumor exactly, especially the invasive or noninvasive character of the tumor.

In 1991 Masaoka (13) proposed a staging classification that combined inspection at surgery and histologic findings. This staging is now used extensively and is considered a universal standard (Table 30.2).

The main problem with Masaoka's classification relates to stage III tumors in which no distinction is

TABLE 30.1. Classification of Thymomas by Marino and Müller-Hermelink

Medullary thymoma
Mixed thymoma
Predominantly cortical thymoma
Cortical thymoma
Well-differentiated thymic carcinoma

Classification scheme from Marino M, Müller-Hermelink HK. Thymoma and thymic carcinoma. Relation of thymoma epithelial cells to the cortical and medullary differentiation of the thymus. Virchows Arch A Pathol Anat Histopathol 1985;407:119–149.

TABLE 30.2. Staging of Thymoma

Stage I: Macroscopically completely encapsulated; and microscopically, no capsular invasion
Stage II: Macroscopic invasion into surrounding fatty tissue or mediastinal pleura or microscopic invasion into capsule
Stage III: Macroscopic invasion into neighboring organs (i.e., pericardium, great vessels, or lung)
Stage IVA: Pleural or pericardial dissemination
Stage IVB: Lymphatic or hematogenous metastases

Staging system from Masaoka A, Monden Y, Nakahara K, Tanioka T. Follow-up study of thymomas with special reference to their clinical stages. Cancer 1991;68:1984–1987.

made between totally resected and incompletely resected stage III tumors. The most important, if not the only, prognostic factor reported in all series is the extent and completeness of the resection in invasive thymomas.

Because of these limitations of Masaoka's classification, the Thymic Tumor Study Group proposed in 1982 a modified classification derived from Wilkins and Castleman (14) and Masaoka et al. (13) to allow a common therapeutic protocol (15). The merit of this classification system (Table 30.3) is the separation of invasive tumors by the extent of resection: stage II (total excision) and stage III (incomplete excision or simple biopsy). It also allows stage I to be separated into stage IA, when no postoperative therapy is necessary, and stage IB, when postoperative radiotherapy is recommended.

The gross pathologic appearance of a thymoma typically is a well-circumscribed and encapsulated mass; the tumor may occupy the whole gland or may develop inside a thymic horn. In approximately one third of cases, thymomas are invasive with capsular invasion and invasion of the adjacent structures: mediastinal fat tissue, mediastinal pleura, phrenic nerve, lung, and great vessels (vena cava, left innominate vein). On gross, cross-sectioned specimens, thymomas may be cystic with frequent calcifications in the capsule. Intrathoracic tumorous implants may be present, generally subpleural or pericardial in location; intrapulmonary metastases are uncommon. Metastases generally occur many years after the initial surgery of an invasive thymoma, but in some cases, intrathoracic metastases are present when the thymoma is diagnosed initially.

Extrathoracic metastases are so uncommon that none was reported in 14 cases surveyed by Legg and Brady (16) or the 20 cases reported by Le Golvan and Abell (17). Only 12 such cases were recorded in the literature by Guillan et al. (18) in 1971. In a series reported by Chahinian et al. (19), extrathoracic metastases were present in 11 of 36 patients with invasive thymoma. Since that publication several reports have noted extrathoracic metastases of thymomas including those to bone, supraclavicular lymph nodes, liver, spleen (20), and peritoneum (21).

AGE, SEX, AND FREQUENCY

Thymoma is the most common tumor of the anterosuperior mediastinum and represents about 20% of all mediastinal tumors (22) (Table 30.4). They predominantly occur in adults (25) and rarely are noted in children (23–25). The mean age at diagnosis is 40 to 50 years, and the median age at operation is 47 years (26). The same age distribution is present when myasthenia gravis is associated with a thymoma (27) (Fig. 30.1). When myasthenia gravis is present, the patients

TABLE 30.4. Mediastinal Tumor Distribution

TYPES OF TUMORS	NO. OF TUMORS	% OF TOTAL NO.
Thymomas	142	19
Hematosarcomas	115	15.5
Neurogenic tumors	111	15
Intrathoracic goiters	110	15
Mediastinal cysts	93	12.5
Other malignant tumors	53	7
Other benignant tumors	47	6.5

Data from Levasseur P, Kaswin R, Rojas-Miranda A, N'Guimbous JF, Le Brigand H. Profil des tumeurs chirurgicales du médiastin: A propos d'une série de 742 opérés. Nouvelle Presse Médicale 1976;5:2857–2859.

TABLE 30.3. Thymic Tumor Study Group Classification of Thymoma

Stage IA: Encapsulated, noninvasive tumor; total excision
Stage IB: Apparently encapsulated tumor; total excision but adhesions to mediastinal structures, indicating microscopic invasiveness, seen at surgery
Stage II: Invasive tumor; total excision
Stage IIIA: Invasive tumor; incomplete excision
Stage IIIB: Simple biopsy when performing a mediastinoscopy or thoracotomy
Stage IVA: Subpleural metastases
Stage IVB: Extrathoracic metastases.

Staging system from Bretel JJ. Staging and preliminary results of the thymic tumour study group. Thymic tumors. In: Sarrazin R, Vroussos C, Vincent J, eds. 7th Cancer Research Workshop. Basel: Karger, 1989: 156–164.

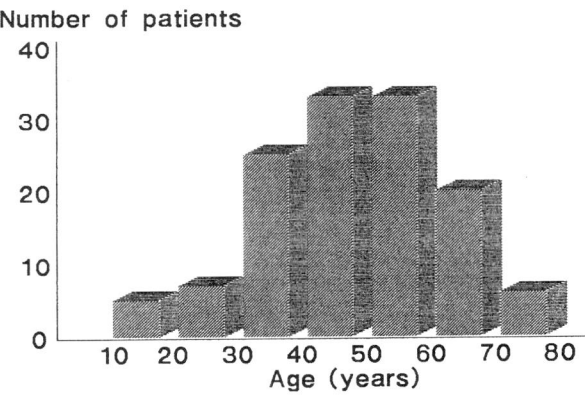

FIGURE 30.1. Age distribution for both thymoma and myasthenia gravis showing ranges. (From Levasseur P, Menestrier M, Gaud C, Dartevelle P, Julia P, Rojas-Miranda A, Navajas M, et al. Thymomes et maladies associées. A propos d'une série de 255 thymomes opérés. Rev Mal Respir 1988;5:173–178.)

are more often female; otherwise, they occur in equal frequency in males and females.

SYMPTOMS

In the series of Kaiser and Martini (26) of 59 thymomas, 19 were asymptomatic. Pain (back or chest) was present in 14 cases, cough in 12, fever and dyspnea in 5, and weight loss in 3. In 6 cases there were myasthenic symptoms (e.g., diplopia, weakness).

In the nonmyasthenic patients, 27 of 49 were asymptomatic (55%), and 22 were symptomatic (45%) (24): the latter included general symptoms (fever, asthenia, weight loss), respiratory symptoms (cough, dyspnea, acute respiratory distress, chest pain), and/or symptoms of mediastinal compression (dysphagia, superior vena cava syndrome).

The presence of myasthenia gravis helped detect the thymoma in all myasthenic patients. The thymoma often was small and well defined, being discovered on computed tomographic (CT) scans. When the thymoma is not associated with any autoimmune disease, 65% of the cases are discovered on routine chest radiographs and 35% by mediastinal compression symptoms: chest pain, cough, dyspnea, dysphagia, hoarseness, or superior vena cava syndrome.

PARANEOPLASTIC SYNDROMES

Many paraneoplastic syndromes, such as autoimmune diseases, are associated with thymoma. Myasthenia gravis is the most common and is present in approximately 40% to 60% of the cases. That rate has been 60% in the author's experience (34) (Tables 30.5 and 30.6).

CLINICAL FEATURES

Myasthenia gravis is classified in five groups:

Group I: Localized, nonprogressive form.
Group II: Generalized, both bulbar and skeletal form. (Group IIA: skeletal form; Group IIB: bulbar and skeletal form.)
Group III: Generalized form with acute fulminating onset and bulbar involvement.
Group IV: Late severe form, developing at least 2 years after onset in group I or II.
Group V: Myasthenia with muscle atrophy; most of these patients are diagnosed as group II.

Muscle weakness and abnormally easy fatigability are characteristics of myasthenia gravis. Muscles commonly are affected first, and the most severely are those innervated by the cranial nerves, producing, for example, ptosis, diplopia, dysphonia, dyspnea, and dysphagia.

TABLE 30.5. Occurrence of Myasthenia Gravis in Patients with Resected Thymoma

STUDY (REFERENCE NO.)	THYMOMAS (NO.)	MYASTHENIA GRAVIS	
		(NO.)	(%)
Maggi et al. (46)	241	180	66
Lewis et al. (72)	283	130	46
Wilkins et al. (53)	85	32	37
Levasseur (34)	255	157	61
Masaoka et al. (13)	96	50	50

TABLE 30.6. Occurrence of Thymomas in Patients with Resected Myasthenia Gravis

STUDY (REFERENCE NO.)	MYASTHENIA GRAVIS (NO.)	THYMOMAS	
		NO.	(%)
Mulder et al. (82)	136	15	(11)
Monden et al. (76)	249	51	(20)
Slater et al. (45)	525	110	(21)
Maggi et al. (46)	642	158	(24)
Levasseur et al. (73)	852	209	(24)

Progressive weakness of truncal and extremity muscles may follow. In many cases there is a very important fluctuation in the severity of symptoms, progressing from fascial muscle weakness to severe generalized weakness that may include respiratory failure. The diagnosis often is clinically apparent; the Tensilon edrophonium chloride test may be useful in confirming the diagnosis when reversing clinically apparent weakness for several minutes; a negative test does not exclude the diagnosis, however. The standard diagnosis uses the electromyogram, which demonstrates a decremental response to supramaximal stimulation of motor nerves with recovery after administration of acetylcholinesterase inhibitors (27).

The detection of circulating antibodies to acetylcholine receptors (ACHR) is highly specific for the diagnosis of myasthenia gravis, because these antibodies are not detected in other neuromuscular or autoimmune disorders. Up to 90% of patients thought to have myasthenia gravis have measurable anti-ACHR antibody titers. The level of ACHR antibodies, however, correlates very poorly with the severity of the myasthenia.

Other paraneoplastic syndromes are less frequent, present in approximately 15% or less of thymomas (Table 30.7). These include hypogammaglobulinemia (28, 29), erythroblastopenic anemia (pure red

TABLE 30.7. Paraneoplastic Syndromes Associated with Thymoma

Syndrome	Occurrence (%)
Myasthenia gravis	61
Other associated diseases	5.9
Hypogammaglobulinemia	1.9
Erythroblastopenic anemia	1.9
Systemic lupus erythematosus	1.9
Gougerot Sjögren syndrome	1
Pemphigus	1
Hemolytic anemia	1

Data from Levasseur P, Menestrier M, Gaud C, Dartevelle P, Julia P, Rojas-Mirando A, Navajas M, et al. Thymomes et maladies associées. A propos d'une série de 255 thymomes opérés. Rev Mal Respir 1988; 5:173–178.

blood cell aplasia) (30, 31), and systematic lupus erythematosus (32, 33). Many other disorders have been reported, with a very low frequency, in association with thymoma: autoimmune hemolytic anemia (34), pemphigus, Gougerot Sjögren syndrome, polymyositis (35), and mucocutaneous candidiasis (36).

Of patients afflicted with paraneoplastic thymic syndromes, approximately one third have two or more syndromes. The most frequent associations are thymoma, myasthenia gravis, erythroblastopenic anemia; and thymoma, myasthenia gravis, hypogammaglobulinemia.

RADIOGRAPHIC FINDINGS

The thymoma generally is located in the anterior mediastinal space (upper and middle) in front of the heart (Fig. 30.2). Initially, in many cases, the thymoma cannot be detected on a posteroanterior chest roentgenogram, but it is well demonstrated on a lateral view. Of course, large thymomas can be detected easily on a posteroanterior chest roentgenogram because a part of the tumor is projected over the hilum. Performance of a lateral chest roentgenogram and a chest CT is recommended as soon as a thymoma is suspected and when a diagnosis of myasthenia gravis is entertained or established. The routine use of the chest CT scan explains why the thymomas of myasthenic patients currently are discovered at a very early stage.

On a CT scan, the thymoma appears as an oval or rounded mass, generally predominant to one side of the anterior mediastinum (Fig. 30.3). Calcification may be present in approximately 10% of cases, and a cystic component often is evident (approximately 30% of cases). A CT scan with contrast is very helpful in distinguishing a thymoma from vascular structures, such as the left innominate vein or superior vena cava.

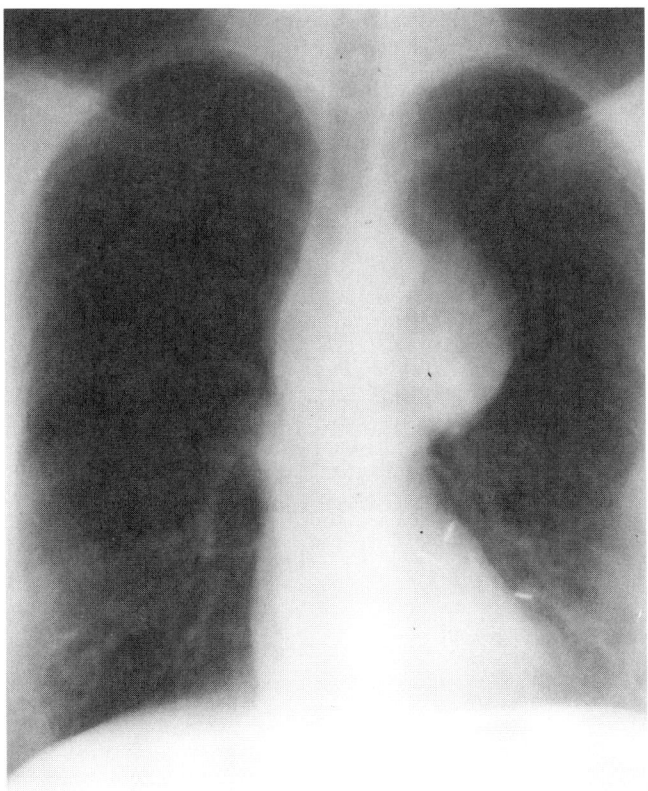

FIGURE 30.2. Conventional roentgenogram showing a thymoma.

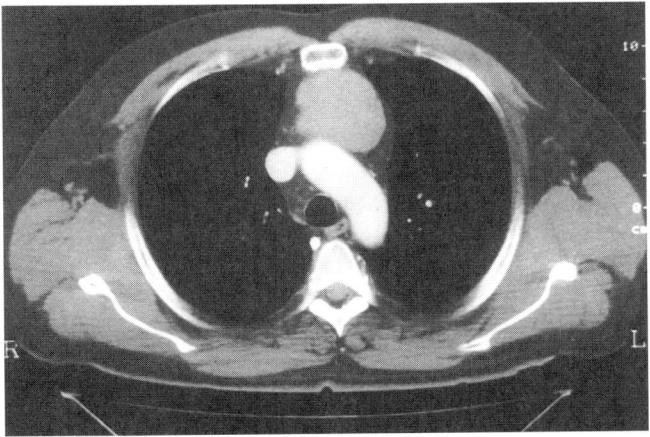

FIGURE 30.3. Thymoma as shown on a CT scan.

Some thymomas are very small (2 or 3 cm in diameter), and in young patients are difficult to distinguish from thymic hypertrophy. Others are very large and may occupy the entire anterior mediastinum and extend into a large part of one hemithorax (Fig. 30.4). Thymomas are generally located in the anterior mediastinum (superior or middle) but may be present at

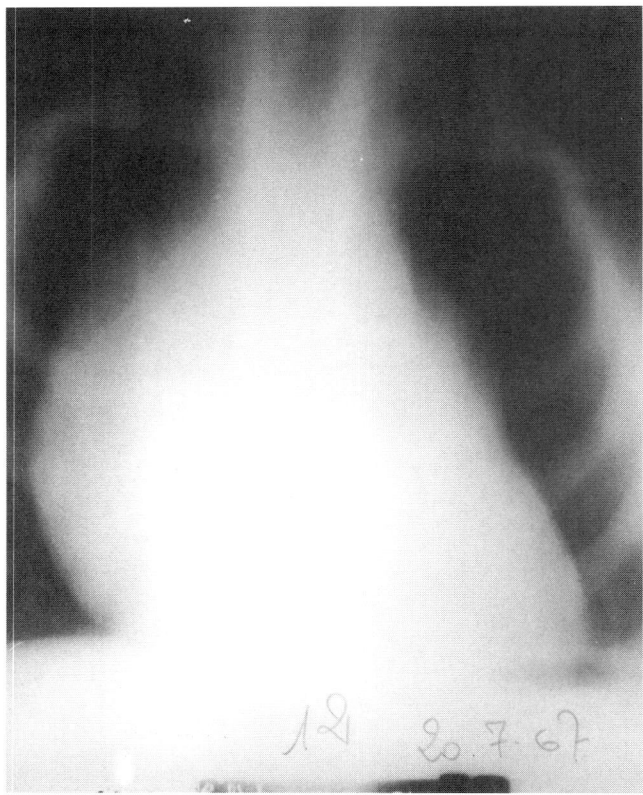

FIGURE 30.4. "Giant" thymoma as seen on a conventional radiograph.

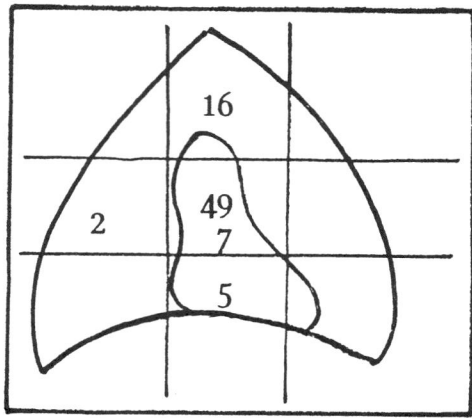

FIGURE 30.5. Diagram showing localization of thymomas in the mediastinum in one series. (From Levasseur P, Rojas-Miranda A, Merlier M, Le Brigand H. Les thymomes réticulothymocytaires. Aspects cliniques et évolutifs a propos de 80 interventions. Ann Chir Thorac Cardiovasc 1971;10(3):329–337.)

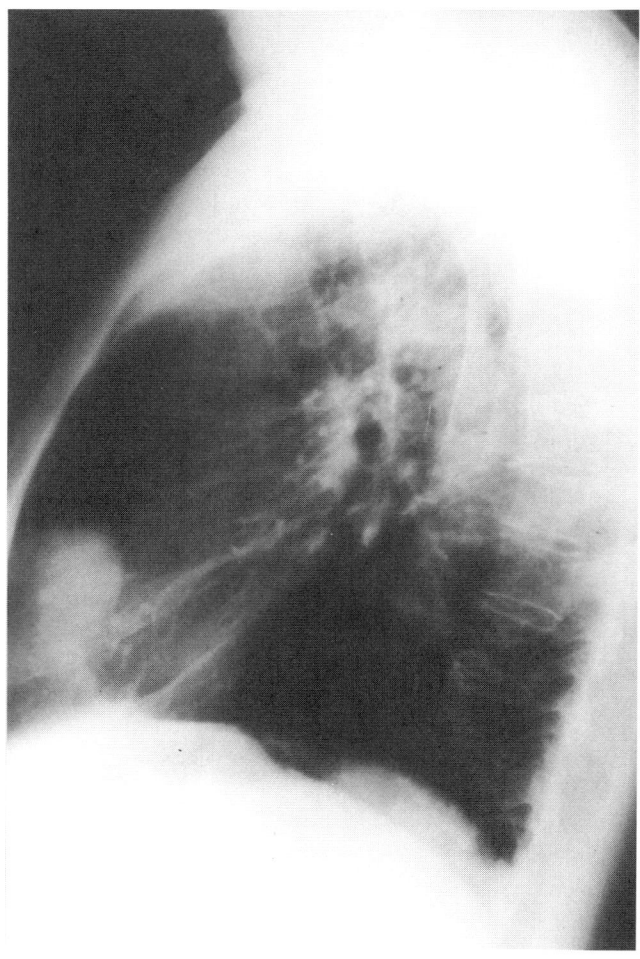

FIGURE 30.6. Ectopic thymoma in the antero–lower mediastinum.

other sites (24, 37). In a review of 80 thymomas (26), 80% were in the anterosuperior or antero–middle mediastinum; five thymomas were in the lower anterior mediastinum and seven between the antero–middle mediastinum and the antero–lower mediastinum. Two giant thymomas were located in all three parts of the anterior mediastinum (upper, middle, and lower), and one thymoma was seen in an axillary position (Figs. 30.5 and 30.6). Cervical thymomas also have been reported (38).

CT scans of the chest may be useful in the assessment of the invasive or noninvasive nature of the tumor, especially invasion of the lung, pericardium, and great vessels (Fig. 30.7); fat planes surrounding the mass suggest lack of invasion. However, in many instances, it is difficult to ascertain invasion preoperatively, and thus surgical exploration is needed to stage the disease adequately.

In some cases pericardial and or pleural metastases of a thymoma are seen on CT scans and are very specific for the presence of such a tumor (Fig. 30.8). Both lungs and especially both subpleural spaces must be evaluated carefully on the CT scan to rule out one or more metastases. Some invasive thymomas can be associated with superior vena cava syndrome; the CT

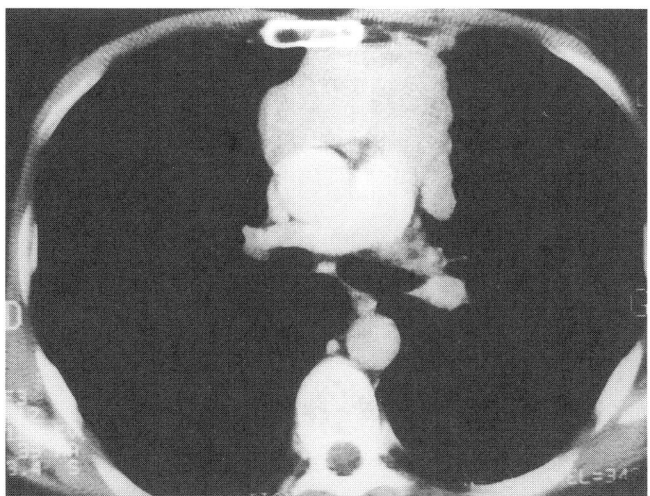

FIGURE 30.7. Invasive thymoma as shown on a CT scan.

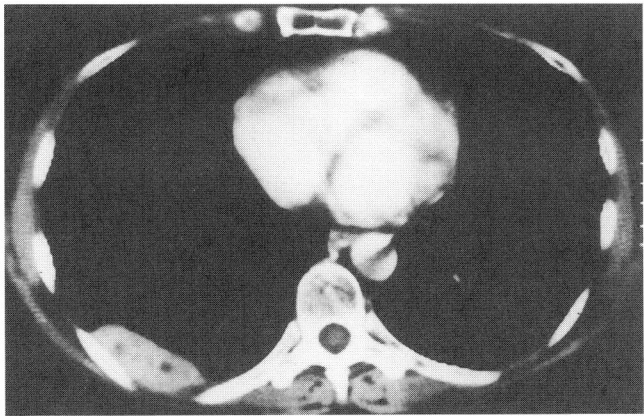

FIGURE 30.8. Typical subpleural metastasis of a thymoma as shown on a CT scan.

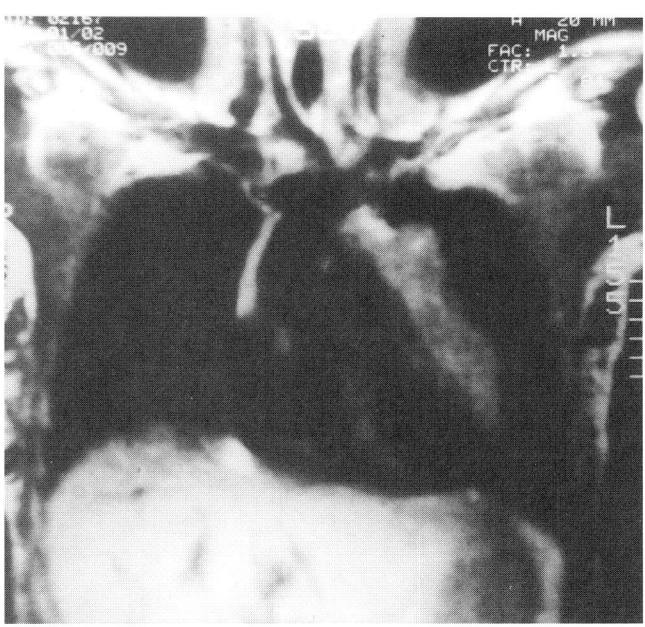

FIGURE 30.9. Invasive thymoma as shown on sagittal MRI.

scan can demonstrate the vena cava invasion. In difficult cases angiography of the superior vena cava may be helpful to assist in planning removal of the thymoma with vena cava resection and reconstruction. Magnetic resonance imaging (MRI) is less accurate and is not as readily available as CT, but it can be useful by imaging in the sagittal plane (Fig. 30.9). Increased signal intensity, when noted on T2-weighted images especially in malignant thymomas, usually corresponds to areas of hemorrhage and cyst formation.

DIAGNOSIS

When autoimmune disease is present (e.g., generally myasthenia gravis but also hypogammaglobulinemia, erythroblastopenic anemia, and lupus erythematosus), a anterior mediastinal mass can be considered a thymoma. Surgery can then be performed without histologic diagnosis.

When there is no clinical or biologic paraneoplastic syndrome, the problem is the differentiation of a thymoma from other anterior mediastinal masses, such as germ cell tumors, lymphomas (Hodgkin's disease and other lymphomas), and thyroid disease.

First, a good clinical examination is necessary; the presence of supraclavicular adenopathy requires a surgical biopsy. Serum marker analyses (e.g., α-fetoprotein and β-human chorionic gonadotrophin) are performed to eliminate non–seminomatous germ cell tumors (choriocarcinomas, embryonal carcinomas, yolk sac tumors). When thyroid disease is suspected, an iodine 133 scintigraphy scan may sometimes be useful, but generally the CT scan can rule out a thyroid pathology. An electromyography is done routinely at Marie Lannelongue Hospital to find a neuromuscular block, even in the absence of clinical myasthenia gravis symptoms (author's unpublished observations).

Finally, in asymptomatic patients and those without biologic abnormalities, it may not be possible to establish the diagnosis of thymoma on CT or MRI. It also may not be possible to differentiate a thymoma from other anterior mediastinal masses without histologic documentation.

A percutaneous fine-needle biopsy or aspiration for cytology is occasionally useful. Percutaneous needle biopsy has been recommended by some with a very good specificity (94%) and good sensitivity (87%) in a series of 33 patients with thymoma (39). A cytologic diagnosis must be substantiated by immunohistochemical and or electron microscopic techniques.

In advanced or nonresectable cases without diagnosis, many surgeons prefer an open biopsy using an anterior mediastinotomy (Chamberlain approach) to confirm the diagnosis of thymoma. Needle aspiration biopsy or open biopsy by mediastinotomy is appropriate for patients with locally extensive thymomas or those with metastases who may benefit from nonsurgical therapy.

Mediastinoscopy is not indicated for thymoma; although thoracoscopy has been used for diagnosis, mediastinotomy is generally preferred if the needle biopsy is unsuccessful (40, 41). Transpleural thoracoscopy is a much more invasive procedure than anterior mediastinotomy because it violates the pleural space.

TREATMENT

Surgery

The most important therapeutic modality for thymoma is complete surgical excision. Surgery without preoperative treatment (radiotherapy or chemotherapy) is ordinarily offered to patients with thymomas that seem on CT to be completely resectable. Surgical resection must realize a total thymectomy (thymoma and all of the thymus). Most patients with recurrent thymomas observed at Marie Lannelongue Hospital (author's unpublished observations) initially had had operations at other institutions, where only the thymoma was resected rather than a total thymectomy performed. When pathologists analyzed the resected thymus, they often found very small incipient thymomas. Because of this fact it is difficult to accept a thoracoscopic resection of a thymoma without a total thymectomy as reported by Landreneau and colleagues (42). The "gold standard" for treatment of such disease is total thymectomy (43).

Operative Approach

The operative approach depends on the surgeon's preference as well as on the location and extent of the tumor. A medial sternotomy is used in most cases and in all median tumors; posterolateral thoracotomy may be used for tumors dominantly located in one pleural space and when the possibility of an associated pneumonectomy is being considered. Although a pulmonary resection may be easier through a posterolateral thoracotomy, a total thymectomy is sometimes very difficult from this approach.

In the case of a very large, bilateral thymoma, bilateral anterolateral fourth interspace thoracotomies with transverse sternotomy provide a very good exposure of both pleural spaces and of all of the mediastinum (44).

For very small thymomas, a cervical approach alone has been proposed (45); a collar incision with a short manubrium split seems more comfortable and safe (46). This approach is especially useful for patients with myasthenia gravis when, occasionally, an unexpected small thymoma is found while performing a transcervical thymectomy.

The use of video-assisted thoracic surgery for small thymomas does not seem to be adequate because extracapsular dissection and total thymectomy are absolutely necessary. Also, for very small stage I thymomas, a cervico-manubrial approach without opening the pleural space is a less invasive, less painful, and more effective for a total thymectomy than a video-assisted transpleural approach. This cervico-manubrial approach is especially valuable for myasthenia gravis patients.

Thus, despite the increasing popularity of video-assisted thoracoscopy, a total or extended resection, if necessary, remains the gold standard for treatment of thymomas. At surgery, an extracapsular dissection must be carried out with total thymectomy and complete resection of all the adjacent structures involved by adherence or invasive thymomas.

Masoaka stage I tumors can easily be completely resected.

Stage II tumors with adherent pleura also are easily resected completely, avoiding injury to the phrenic nerve.

Stage III thymomas benefit from extended resection rather than a total thymectomy. When, on CT scan or MRI, thymomas appear as a very bulky, invasive tumor with a very low possibility of complete surgical removal, preoperative adjuvant therapy is preferred with radiotherapy or chemotherapy administered before surgery. When feasible, excision of the thymoma, the entire thymus gland, and, if necessary, all affected tissues by pleural resection, pericardial resection, lung resection, and vascular resection is preferred over other modes of treatment.

Pleural resection sometimes may require the sacrifice of the phrenic nerve when dissection of the nerve is not possible because of massive invasion by the thymoma. However, if one phrenic nerve has been sacrificed the other one must be preserved.

Pericardial resection is common in stage III thymomas. No prosthesis is necessary to prevent cardiac hernia, except when there is an associated pneumonectomy.

Resectioning of the lung to encompass diseased tissue is important. Generally, a wedge resection with staplers is sufficient, but in some cases a lobectomy and even a pneumonectomy may become necessary to perform a complete resection.

In the experience of Levasseur and colleagues (47), a thymoma resection was extended to the pleura and/or pericardium in 46% of the cases, to lung in 9% (wedge resection, 23; pneumonectomy, 6; and lobectomy, 1), and to one phrenic nerve in 6%.

Resection of the left innominate vein is generally performed without the need for vascular reconstruction. Resection of the vena cava is sometimes partial when using a direct suture or patch (pericardium or synthetic prosthesis), or total with reconstruction using an expanded polytetrafluoroethylene graft having a diameter of 10 to 12 mm with or without rings (Fig. 30.10).

Resection with or without reconstruction of the superior vena cava system was necessary in 6% of cases in one series (47). Shimitzu and coworkers (48), in a series of 84 resected thymomas during the past 27 years, performed a vascular reconstruction in 14 patients (14%), including angioplasty in 4, left brachiocephalic vein reconstruction in 4, and superior vena cava reconstruction in 5. No signs of obstruction of the grafts was observed in any of the 5 patients. Tsubota et al. (49) reconstructed the vena cava in 5 of 15 patients with invasive thymoma and reported that the vascular grafts were patent in 4 patients 1 month after operation; 2 patients survived 4 years. They thought that such an extensive operation may improve the prognosis. Doty and colleagues (50) reported 9 cases of superior vena cava reconstruction with composite spiral vein grafts with long-term satisfactory patency of the graft.

Stage IVA thymomas with pleural or pericardial implants can be resected first if the implants are limited and localized. The thymoma and all implants are removed in the same procedure, followed by external radiotherapy or chemotherapy. If there are many implants, some investigators now prefer a course of preoperative chemotherapy followed by surgery.

Stage IVB thymomas with lymphatic or hematogenous metastases must be treated initially by chemotherapy with or without radiotherapy; surgery is entertained after the neoadjuvant therapy in selected cases.

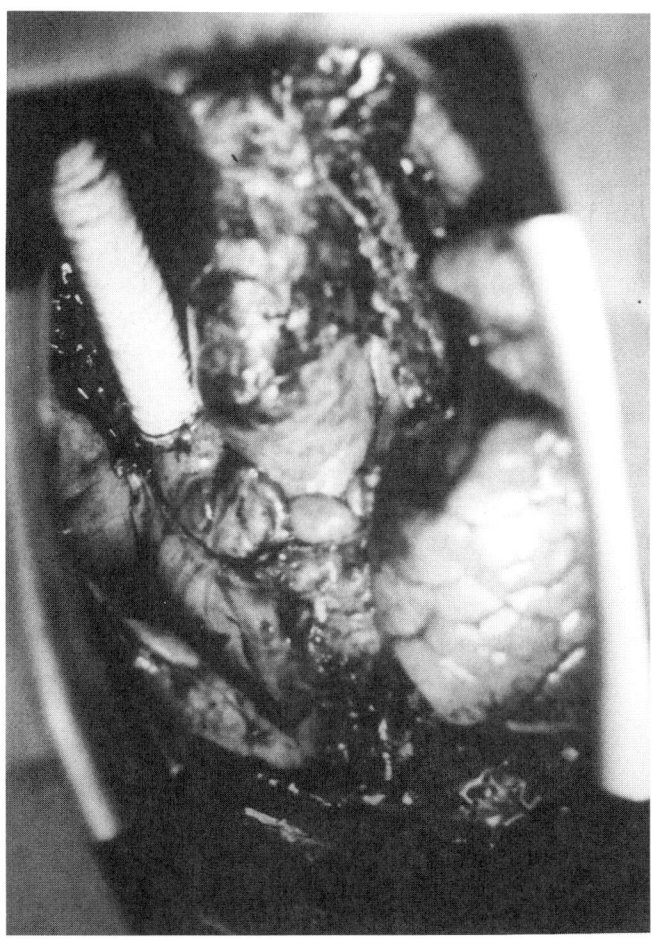

FIGURE 30.10. Resection of an invasive thymoma with vena cava reconstruction (operative view).

THE ROLE OF RADIOTHERAPY

POSTOPERATIVE RADIOTHERAPY: INDICATIONS

Postoperative radiotherapy seems unnecessary in stage I disease but is recommended routinely for all stage II thymomas (51). Recently, Haniuda et al. (52) suggested that radiotherapy prevents recurrence in stage II cases with only fibrous adhesions to the mediastinal pleura. However, for stage II tumors with pleural or mediastinal microscopic invasion and for totally resected stage III tumors, mediastinal irradiation may be insufficient to prevent recurrence, even after complete resection. They suggest that for these patients adjuvant chemotherapy and mediastinal irradiation should be considered.

For many investigators (53–55), postoperative radiation therapy decreases the risk of local recurrence and improves 10-year survival rates. Nakahara and colleagues (56) used postoperative radiotherapy in 48 patients with stage III thymoma; in 35 patients with complete resection, survival rates were 100% at 5 years and 95% at 10 years.

In the experience of Urgesi et al. (54), radiotherapy provided a decreased risk of local recurrence and prolonged survival on resected patients with locally advanced thymoma. However, Cohen and coworkers (57) suggested that complete resection was the most important factor affecting long-term survival. After complete resection of the tumor, no significant difference in survival rates was observed between patients who received postoperative radiotherapy and those who did not.

Radiotherapy also has been proposed for unresectable or incompletely resected stage III thymomas and for stage IV tumors with complete or incomplete resection.

Preoperative Radiotherapy

The role of preoperative irradiation is not yet completely clear. The question of preoperative radiotherapy for bulky malignant thymomas is an intriguing one; however, no large series reported in the literature has addressed this question (26). Urgesi and coworkers (54) report that some thymomas judged not to be resectable at diagnosis were rendered resectable by preoperative radiotherapy.

Maggi et al. (46) initially treated patients with stage III and IVA thymomas with a preoperative radiotherapy dose of 30 Gy when there was clinical or radiologic evidence of invasion. Five patients received preoperative radiotherapy 4 to 6 weeks before their operations. They observed a remarkable reduction in tumor size in all patients that was evident on CT scans. A subtotal resection was performed, followed by another 30 Gy of irradiation. The 5 patients were alive at the last follow-up: the longest survival is 4 years and 7 months.

From a series of 83 resected thymomas, Ribet and colleagues (58) performed 19 resections after radiotherapy (mean dose, 44 Gy), given because of caval obstruction, tracheal compression, dysphonia, or radiologic signs of organ invasion. Surgery was performed 4 to 8 weeks after irradiation. Resections were complete in 10 patients and incomplete in 9. Postoperative radiotherapy was given to 15 patients (mean dose, 31 Gy), and chemotherapy was added for 7 patients. Following preoperative radiotherapy and complete resections, the actuarial survival was 56% ± 16% at 10 years and 42% ± 18% at 20 years.

In those with incomplete secondary resections, no patient survived beyond 5 years. Ribet (59) concluded that if the response to primary radiotherapy were incomplete, it would be better to proceed to the full dose of irradiation; they also noted that incomplete secondary resection gave no better results than combined radiotherapy and chemotherapy.

It is very difficult to prove that preoperative radiotherapy makes excision of an invasive thymoma easier. For most investigators, preoperative radiotherapy does not seem beneficial (60–62), but the number of patients in all the series of preoperative radiotherapy is small and the influence on local control and survival rate are not known. Further studies, preferably randomized and multiinstitutional, are necessary.

Technical Problems

Postoperative Radiotherapy for Stage II Disease

A total dose of 50 Gy seems necessary after resection of stage II thymomas: 40 Gy by anteroposterior fields in 4 weeks (4 fractions of 2.5 Gy/week or 5 fractions of 2 Gy/week) and then 10 Gy by one or two lateral or oblique fields. These fields are used to protect the spinal cord (63).

Postoperative Radiotherapy for Stage III Thymomas

A postoperative dose of 55 to 60 Gy seems necessary in patients with totally or incompletely resected thymomas (64): 40 Gy by two anteroposterior fields and 15 to 20 Gy by one or two lateral fields. High-energy electrons (over 25 MeV) can be useful for irradiating the anterior mediastinum (64).

The Role of Chemotherapy

Systemic chemotherapy for advanced or metastatic thymomas seems worth pursuing, but such treatment has not been studied extensively because thymoma is a relatively rare neoplasm. Nevertheless, there have been several trials showing response to single-agent and combination chemotherapy (65–69).

Good responses were observed with single drugs: cisplatin, doxorubicin, cyclophosphamide, nitrogen mustard, and actinomycin D. Interesting results also were obtained with drug combinations: doxorubicin, lomustine, vincristine, bleomycin; nitrogen mustard, vincristine, procarbazine, vinblastine; and nitrogen mustard, vincristine, procarbazine, prednisone. The most interesting drug combinations seem to be cisplatin, doxorubicin, and cyclophosphamide (CAP); and cisplatin, doxorubicin, cyclophosphamide, and vincristine (ADOC). Loehrer and coworkers (69) obtained a good response in 22 patients (all stage IIIB and IV) with two courses of CAP (70); with the addition of vincristine, they treated 16 patients with invasive thymoma (stage III and IVA) and then performed surgery. Seven patients had a complete remission (43%), and nine patients (57%), a partial remission with an overall complete plus partial remission rate of 100%. After chemotherapy all patients underwent an operation. Radiotherapy or chemotherapy was performed postoperatively based on the postsurgical histologic results. Median survival was 66 months with a 3-year survival of 70%. Loehrer et al. (69) and others think that such a therapeutic approach can be applied to cases of highly invasive stage III thymoma. However, only series with a larger number of patients and a longer follow-up will determine the effectiveness of this approach on long-term survival. The Radiotherapy Oncology Group is currently conducting a study in the United States. This phase II trial of the combination of cisplatin, doxorubicin, cyclophosphamide, and prednisone as a neoadjuvant strategy is being studied with stage III thymoma.

A trial of combined chemotherapy, surgery, and radiotherapy was published by Macchiarini (71) with a small number of patients and a very short postoperative follow-up. Seven patients had chemotherapy first (three courses of the combination of cisplatin, epirubicin, and etoposide), then surgery, and finally postoperative radiotherapy (45 Gy if complete resection and 60 Gy if incomplete resection were performed) delivered in 5 or 6 weeks with 5 fractions each week. All patients showed a partial response of more than 50%. Complete resection was achieved in four of seven patients with a greater than 75% tumor reduction preoperatively; resection was incomplete in three patients. Histologic analysis of the surgical specimens was negative for two patients with completely resected tumors, and it confirmed the initial diagnosis in the other five cases. This study is very interesting, but the follow-up was very short, and the 80% 2-year actuarial survival reported is not significant for thymomas. It is important to remember that in the experience of many other investigators, the 5-year survival rate is approximately 50% for patients with invasive thymomas treated only with a biopsy.

In stage IVA disease, it is not clear whether surgical resection is beneficial. A number of therapies have been used including radiation and chemotherapy followed by surgical resection. Such an aggressive approach is an attractive concept, but there is no proof of its efficacy. In such patients, one must remember the frequently indolent course that these tumors may follow (44).

RESULTS OF TREATMENT

The operative mortality after resection for thymoma is low: 3.1% for Lewis et al. (72) in 227 patients with total resections, 2.5% for Levasseur and colleagues (73), and 6% for Maggi (46) in 241 patients. With improved medical treatment, anesthesia techniques, and intensive care management, the adverse influence of myasthenia gravis on perioperative complications has been essentially eliminated.

LONG-TERM RESULTS

The reported actuarial survival ranges from 53% to 87% at 5 years and 53% to 64% at 10 years (46, 52–54, 72–77) (Table 30.8).

PREDICTORS OF OUTCOME

The usual prognostic factors for survival in thymomas are the presence of myasthenia gravis, clinical stage, extent of resection, histologic type, and postoperative radiotherapy.

Myasthenia gravis as an adverse prognostic factor was found primarily in early series (53), perhaps because of the poor early postoperative and long-term medical control of myasthenia gravis. The prognostic impact of myasthenia gravis on survival is controversial; Maggi et al. (46) found it to be a factor of good prognosis, possibly because of the earlier diagnosis of thymoma and, as a result, the fewer invasive thymo-

TABLE 30.8. Thymomas: Postoperative Long-Term Survival by Stage

STUDY (REFERENCE NO.)	STAGE			
	I	II	III	IV
Masaoka et al. (13) (5 years)	92.6	85.7	69.6	50
Wilkins et al. (14) (5 years)	82	81	23	...
Levasseur et al. (73) (10 years)	80	70	42	28
Haniuda et al. (52) (10 years)	94.1	73.5	68.6	...

mas in this group. For Maggi and colleagues (46), more complete resections were possible in patients with myasthenia gravis (62%) than in those without the disease (43%) ($P = .051$). Monden et al. (76) found a lower recurrence rate in myasthenia gravis patients of the same clinical stage. Levasseur et al. (73) found an equal distribution of the clinical stages of thymoma in myasthenia gravis and non–myasthenia gravis patients and observed similar long-term survival in these two groups. Many other investigators concurred (10, 53, 57, 60).

The analysis of the survival curves in several series showed no significant difference when sex, age, and association with myasthenia gravis were considered as independent predictors (10). Also, multivariate analyses showed that age, sex, and association with myasthenia gravis did not reach statistical significance for prognosis (10, 73).

For Pescarmona et al. (10), clinical stage proved to be a highly significant prognostic factor ($P < .001$). Actuarial survival curves based on both clinical and pathologic stages were also highly significant ($P < .0001$). In all series the 10-year survival rates based on Masaoka's staging are 86% to 100% for stage I, 60% to 84% for stage II, 21% to 77% for stage III, and 26% to 47% for stage IVA (Table 30.8).

The most important prognostic factor seems to be the extent of the resection. Complete resection imparts a more favorable prognosis than does partial resection. In the experience of Levasseur and colleagues (73), the actuarial survival at 10 years was significantly higher ($P < .001$) in the stage III totally resected group than in stage III incompletely resected patients, i.e., 70% versus 28%, respectively (Fig. 30.11).

The following covariables were analyzed by multivariate analysis (73) to assess the independent prognostic impact on survival: extent of resection, Masaoka clinical stage, histologic type, association with myasthenia gravis, and postoperative radiotherapy. Complete thymoma resection was the sole significant prognostic factor ($P < .00001$).

Based on these results and the fact that the most significant prognostic factors were the quality of the resection and the clinical stage, a modified Masaoka classification that includes the extent of the resection is proposed:

Stage I: Noninvasive thymoma.
Stage II A: Thymoma with capsular or pleural invasion.
Stage II B: Totally resected neighboring organs invasive thymomas (lung, pericardium, vessels).
Stage III: Incompletely resected neighboring organs invasive thymoma.
Stage IV: Metastatic thymoma.

RECURRENCES OF THYMOMAS AFTER SURGERY

The mean time from diagnosis to recurrence is approximately 6 years (77). Recurrences have been reported as late as 15 to 20 years after diagnosis. Accordingly, thymomas merit long-term follow-up (60, 72, 78). In the report of Maggi and colleagues (46), local relapse occurred in 8 (4%) of 165 patients.

Fechner (79) reported a recurrence rate of less than 2% in patients with noninvasive thymoma who underwent resection. He described two broad categories based on the type of recurrence: one category with mediastinal recurrence localized in the mediastinum without additional sites of involvement; and the other, pleural metastasis without mediastinal recurrences.

In nonmetastatic and totally resected thymomas, 21 patients (7.5%) had a recurrence (73). These recurrences occurred on average after 6 years (range, 2 to 6 years); their location was mediastinal in 10 patients,

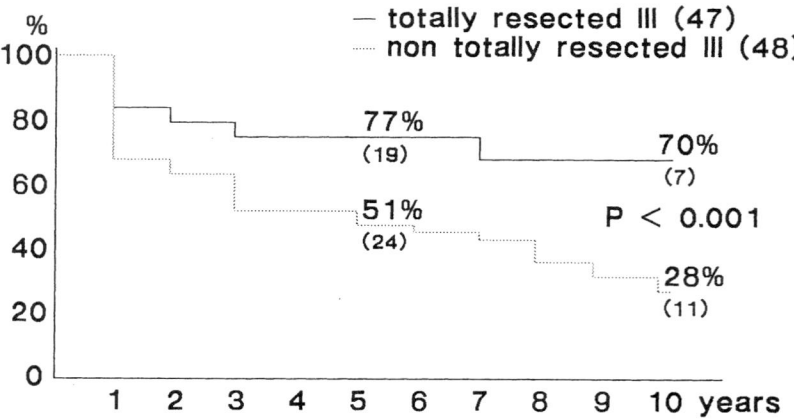

FIGURE 30.11. Actuarial survival based on the quality of the resection in stage III disease (Masaoka classification system). (From Levasseur P, Magdaleinat P, Dromer C. Résultats et facteurs pronostiques des thymomes opérés. In: Lannelonge M, ed. Fourth symposium on thoracic pathology. France: Le Plessis Robinson, 1992.)

pleuropulmonary in 12, and at the sternotomy scar in 1. The observed recurrence rates were 4% (6 patients) in stage I, 10% in stage II, and 15% in totally resected stage III. The differences in the rates of recurrence were significant between stage I and II ($P < .001$) (73).

Reoperation is possible in most cases. Kirschner (78) and Ohmi and Ohuchi (80) recommended performing aggressive surgery for recurrent thymoma on the pleura. In these instances, surgery is easy to perform and extremely effective in improving recurrent myasthenic symptoms. In the Hirst and Robertson (31) series, all of the recurrent thymomas were on the pleura and could be resected. The suspected cause of recurrence was either dissemination of tumor cells resulting from operative manipulation or undetected disseminated foci that existed at the time of the first operation.

Of the 21 patients with recurrence in the series of Levasseur and coworkers (73), 16 were reoperated. The resection was complete in 10 patients and incomplete in 6. In these 16 reoperated patients, the 5- and 10-year actuarial survival rates were 66% and 49%, respectively. For pleural metastases postoperative radiotherapy is used locally after surgical resection.

RESULTS OF SURGERY ON PARATHYMIC SYNDROMES

MYASTHENIA GRAVIS

For many years, it was thought that the presence of a thymoma clearly affected the prognosis of a patient with myasthenia gravis adversely. In 1972, good results were seen in 77% of patients in the absence of thymoma but only in 53% with thymoma (81).

Mulder and colleagues (82) reported that in patients with non–thymomatous myasthenia gravis, the remission rate was 54% as opposed to 37% for patients with thymoma. In recent years this difference has decreased, probably because of the routine use of CT scans in myasthenic patients. CT scans were able to detect many small stage I and II thymomas in these patients.

The good results after 5 years (remissions plus improvements) in patients with myasthenia gravis has increased from 70% to 85%. In the series of Maggi et al. (46), myasthenia gravis was cured in four patients (3.6%), and an improvement was recorded in 69% of the patients. The results have improved steadily in subsequent years. With follow-up periods of more than 9 years in patients with myasthenia and a thymoma, cure can be achieved in up to 33% and improvement in up to 56%.

The same good long-term results (83%) were seen in myasthenic patients with and without thymoma (34). Only Monden et al. (76) found a difference of 10% in the good results between the two series with and without tumor.

Recurrence of myasthenic symptoms or exacerbation of myasthenic symptoms often are associated with recurrence of the thymoma (mediastinal recurrence or subpleural metastases). The resection of the recurrent thymoma typically is easy to perform and improves the myasthenic symptoms.

OTHER PARANEOPLASTIC SYNDROMES

Besides myasthenia gravis, only erythroblastopenic anemia benefits from thymic ablation (31). In all other cases, surgery of the thymic tumor had no benefit on the associated diseases (e.g., hypogammaglobulinemia, disseminated lupus erythematosus) (34).

REFERENCES

1. Sarrazin R, Gabelle P, Dyon JF. Thymic tumors. In: Sarrazin R, Vroussos C, Vincent J, eds. 7th Cancer Research Workshop. Basel: Karger, 1989.
2. Noback GJ. A contribution of the topographic anatomy of the thymus gland with particular references to its changes at birth and in the period of the newborn. Am J Dis Child 1921;22:120.
3. Masaoka A, Nagaoka Y, Kotake Y. Distribution of thymic tissue at the anterior mediastinum. Current procedures in thymectomy. J Thorac Cardiovasc Surg 1975;70(4):747–754.
4. Park EA, McClure RD. The results of thymus extirpation in the dog. Am J Dis Child 1919;18:317.
5. Rouviere H. Anatomie des lymphatiques de l'Homme. In: Masson, ed. Paris, 1974.
6. Verley JM, Hollmann KH. Thymoma: a comparative study of clinical stages, histologic features and survival in 200 cases. Cancer 1985;55:1074–1086.
7. Verley JM, Hollmann KH. Tumors of the mediastinum. Current histo-pathology. Lancaster, UK: Kluwer Academic Publishers, 1992;19.
8. Levine GD, Rosai J. Thymic hyperplasia and neoplasia. A review of current concepts. Hum Pathol 1978;9:495–515.
9. Marino M, Müller-Hermelink HK. Thymoma and thymic carcinoma. Relation of thymoma epithelial cells to the cortical and medullary differenciation of the thymus. Virchows Arch A Pathol Anat Histopathol 1985;407:119–149.
10. Pescarmona E, Rendina EA, Venuta F, Ricci C, Ruco LP, Baroni CD. The prognostic implication of thymoma histologic subtyping: a study of 80 consecutive cases. Am J Clin Pathol 1990;93:190–195.
11. Nomori H, Ishihara T, Torikata C. Malignant grading of cortical and medullary differentiated thymoma by morphometric analysis. Cancer 1989;64:1694–1699.
12. Ito M, Taki T, Miyake M, Mitsuoka A. Lymphocyte subsets in human thymoma studied with monoclonal antibodies. Cancer 1988;61:284–287.
13. Masaoka A, Monden Y, Nakahara K, Tanioka T. Follow-up study of thymomas with special reference to their clinical stages. Cancer 1991;68:1984–1987.

14. Wilkins EW, Castleman B. Thymoma: a continuing survey at the Massachusetts General Hospital. Ann Thorac Surg 1979;28:252–256.
15. Bretel JJ. Staging and preliminary results of the thymic tumour study group. Thymic tumors. In: Sarrazin R, Vroussos C, Vincent J, eds. 7th Cancer Research Workshop. Basel: Karger, 1989:156–164.
16. Legg MA, Brady WJ. Pathology and clinical behaviour of thymomas. A survey of 51 cases. Cancer 1965;18:1131–1144.
17. Le Golvan DP, Abell MR. Thymomas. Cancer 1977;39:2142–2157.
18. Guillan RA, Zelman S, Smalley RL, Iglesias PA. Malignant thymoma associated with myasthenia gravis and evidence of extrathoracic metastases. An analysis of published cases and report of a case. Cancer 1971;27:823–830.
19. Chahinian AP, Bhardwaj S, Meyer RJ, Jaffrey IS, Kirschner PA, Holland JF. Treatment of invasive or metastatic thymoma: report of eleven cases. Cancer 1981;47:1752–1761.
20. Ibrahim NBN, Briggs JC, Jeyasingham K, Owen JR. Metastasing thymoma. Thorax 1982;37:771–773.
21. Lundblad R, Lunde S, Evensen K. A new intra-peritoneal metastasis from thymoma. Eur J Surg Oncol 1988;14(6):697–702.
22. Levasseur P, Kaswin R, Rojas-Miranda A, N'Guimbous JF, Le Brigand H. Profil des tumeurs chirurgicales du médiastin: A propos d'une série de 742 opérés. Nouvelle Presse Médicale 1976;5:2857–2859.
23. Halpern SR, Schoelzel E, Johnson RB. Thymoma in a young child producing symptoms of asthma. Am J Dis Child 1966;111:99–104.
24. Levasseur P, Rojas-Miranda A, Merlier M, Le Brigand H. Les thymomes réticulothymocytaires. Aspects cliniques et évolutifs a propos de 80 interventions. Ann Chir Thorac Cardiovasc 1971;10(3):329–337.
25. Forman WL, Buckley PJ, Green AA, Stokes DC, Chien LT. Thymoma and myasthenia gravis in a 4-year old-child. Case report and review of the literature. Cancer 1985;56:2703–2706.
26. Kaiser LR, Martini N. Clinical management of thymomas. The Memorial Sloan–Kettering Cancer Center experience in thoracic surgery: frontiers and uncommon neoplasms. In: Martini N, Vogt-Moykopf I, eds. International trends in general thoracic surgery. St. Louis: Mosby, 1989;5.
27. Cambier J. La Myasthinia. In: Bailliere JB, ed. Paris: les Cahiers Boillierem, 1968.
28. Saegesser F, Zoupanos G. Thymome et carence acquise en immuno-globuline. Ann Chir Thorac Cardiovasc 1986;7:535–541.
29. Gafni G, Michaeli A, Heller H. Idiopathic acquired agamma-globulinemia with thymoma. N Engl J Med 1960;263:536–537.
30. Fujimura S, Kondo T, Yamauchi A, Handa M, Wakaka T. Experience with surgery for thymoma associated with pure red blood aplasie. Report of three cases. Chest 1986;88:221–225.
31. Hirst E, Robertson TI. The syndrome of thymoma and erythroblastopenic anemiae. A review of 56 cases including 3 case reports. Medicine 1967;46:375–378.
32. Haas C, Riquet M, Hugues FC, Weil J, Carnot F, Rueil M, Lesavre P. Association d'un thymome lympho-épithélial et d'un lupus érythémateux disséminé. Ann Med Interne (Paris) 1985;136:77–78.
33. Simeone JF, MacCloud T, Putnam C. Thymoma and systematic lupus erythematosus. Thorax 1975;30:697–700.
34. Levasseur P, Menestrier M, Gaud C, Dartevelle P, Julia P, Rojas-Miranda A, Navajas M, et al. Thymomes et maladies associées. A propos d'une série de 255 thymomes opérés. Rev Mal Respir 1988;5:173–178.
35. Weiller PJ, Durand JM, Prince-Zuchelli A, Gros D, Poujet J, Pelissier JF, Mongin M. Association polymyosite, myasthenie, thymome: un cas et revue de la littérature. Ann Med Interne (Paris) 1984;135:299–304.
36. Kirkpatrick CH, Windhorst DB. Mucocutaneous candidiasis and thymoma. Am J Med 1979;66:939–945.
37. Good CA. Roentgenographic findings in myasthenia gravis associated with thymic tumor. AJR Am J Roentgenol 1947;57:305–312.
38. Miller WT Jr, Gefter WB, Miller WT. Thymoma mimicking a thyroid mass. Radiology 1992;184:75–76.
39. Herman SJ, Holub RV, Weisbrod GL. Anterior mediastinal masses: utility of transthoracic needle biopsy. Radiology 1991;180:167–170.
40. Kohman LJ. Approach to the diagnosis and staging of mediastinal masses. Chest 1993;103:3285–3305.
41. Mai J, Loddenkemper R, Brandt HJ. Diagnostic thoracoscopy in mediastinal space-occupying lesions. Pneumologie 1989;43:122–125.
42. Landreneau R, Dowling R, Castillo W, Ferson F. Thoracoscopic resection of an anterior mediastinal tumor. Ann Thorac Surg 1992;54:142–144.
43. Pairolero PC. Invited commentary. Ann Thorac Surg 1992;54:144.
44. Patterson GA. Thymomas. Semin Thorac Cardiovasc Surg 1992;4(1):39–44.
45. Slater G, Papatestas A, Kornfeld P, Genkins G. Transcervical thymectomy for thymoma in myasthenia gravis. Am J Surg 1982;144:254–256.
46. Maggi G, Casadio C, Cavallo A, Cianci R, Molinatti M, Ruffini E. Thymoma: results of 241 operated cases. Ann Thorac Surg 1991;51:152–156.
47. Levasseur P, Khalil A, Menestrier M, Gaud C, Regnard JF, Rojas-Miranda A. First intensive radical exeresis surgery in invasive thymomas. Results from a series of 284 operated thymomas. In: Sarrazin R, Vroussos C, Vincent J, eds. Thymic tumors: 7th Cancer Research Workshop. Basel: Karger, 1989.
48. Shimizu N, Moriyama S, Ade M, Nakata M, Ando A, Teramoto S. The surgical treatment of invasive thymoma: resection with vascular reconstruction. J Thorac Cardiovasc Surg 1992;103:414–420.
49. Tsubota N, Yamashita C, Ishii, et al. The results of surgical treatment of invasive thymoma and thymus related tumors. J Thorac Surg 1985;86:752–761.
50. Doty DB, Doty JR, Jones KW. Bypass of superior vena cava: fifteen years experience with spiral vein graft for obstruction of superior vena cava caused by benign disease. J Thorac Cardiovasc Surg 1990;99:889–896.
51. Curran WJ Jr, Kornstein MJ, Brooks JJ, Turrisi AT. Invasive thymoma: the role of mediastinal irradiation following complete or incomplete surgical resection. J Clin Oncol 1988;6:1722–1727.
52. Haniuda M, Morimoto M, Nishimura H, Kobayashi O, Yamanda T, Lida F. Adjuvant radiotherapy after complete resection of thymoma. Ann Thorac Surg 1992;54:311–315.
53. Wilkins EW Jr, Grillo HC, Scannell JG, Moncure AC, Mathisen DJ. Role of staging in prognosis and management of thymoma. Ann Thorac Surg 1991;51:888–892.
54. Urgesi A, Monetti U, Rossi G, Ricardi U, Casadio C. Role of radiation therapy in locally advanced thymoma. Radiother Oncol 1990;273–280.
55. Kersh CR, Eisert DR, Hazra TA. Malignant thymoma: role of radiation therapy in management. Radiology 1985;156:207–209.
56. Nakahara K, Ohno K, Hashimoto J. Thymoma: results with com-

plete resection and adjuvant post-operative irradiation in 141 consecutive patients. J Thorac Cardiovasc Surg 1988;95:1041–1047.
57. Cohen DJ, Ronnigen LD, Graeber GM. Management of patients with malignant thymoma. J Thorac Cardiovasc Surg 1984;87:301–307.
58. Ribet M, Voisin C, Provot FR, Ramon P, Dambrun P. Lympho epithelial thymomas. A retrospective study of 88 resections. Eur J Cardiothorac Surg 1988;2:261–264.
59. Ribet M. Radiothérapie pré-opératoire pour les thymomes lympho-épithéliaux. Ann Chir Thorac Cardiovasc 1983;47(8):766–768.
60. Shamji F, Pearson FG, Todd TRJ. Results of surgical treatment for thymoma. J Thorac Cardiovasc Surg 1984;87:43–47.
61. Ariaratnam LS, Kalnicki S, Mincer F, Botstein C. The management of malignant thymoma with radiation therapy. Int J Radiat Oncol Biol Phys 1978;5:77–80.
62. Simpson WJ. Role of radiotherapy in the treatment of invasive thymomas. In: Sarrazin R, Vroussos C, Vincent J, eds. Thymic tumors: 7th Cancer Research Workshop. Basel: Karger, 1989.
63. Guerin RA. La radiothérapie des thymomes. Rev Mal Respir 1988;5:167–171.
64. Arriagada R, Bretel JJ, Caillaud JM, Garreta L, Guerin RA, Laugier A, Le Chevalier T, Schlienger M. Invasive carcinoma of the thymus: a multicenter retrospective review of 56 cases. Eur J Cancer Clin Oncol 1984;1:69–74.
65. Needles B, Kemeny N, Urmacher C. Malignant thymoma: renal metastasis responding to cis-platinum. Cancer 1981;48:223–226.
66. Coccini G, Boni C, Cuomo A. Long-lasting response to cis-platinum in recurrent malignant thymoma: Case report. Cancer 1982;49:1885–1887.
67. Evans WK, Thomsson DJ, Simpson WJ, Feld R, Phillips MJ. Combination chemotherapy in invasive thymoma: role of COOP. Cancer 1980;46:1523–1527.
68. Hu E, Levine J. Chemotherapy of malignant thymoma. Case report and review of the literature. Cancer 1986;57:1101–1104.
69. Loehrer PJ, Perez CA, Roth LM, Greco FA, Livingston RB, Einhorn LH. Chemotherapy for advanced thymoma: preliminary results of an intergroup study. Ann Intern Med 1990;113:520–524.
70. Rea F, Sartori F, Loy M, Calabro F, Fornasiero A, Daniele O, Altavilla G. Chemotherapy and operation for invasive thymoma. J Thorac Cardiovasc Surg 1993;106:543–549.
71. Macchiarini P, Chella A, Ducci F, Rossi B, Testi C, Bevilacqua G, Angeletti CA. Neo-adjuvant chemotherapy, surgery and post operative radiation therapy for invasive thymoma. Cancer 1981;68:708–713.
72. Lewis JE, Wick MR, Scheithauer BW, Bernatz PE, Paylor WF. Thymoma: a clinico-pathological review. Cancer 1987;60:2727–2743.
73. Levasseur P, Magdaleinat P, Dromer C. Résultats et facteurs pronostiques des thymomes opérés. In: Lannelonge M, ed. Fourth Symposium on Thoracic Pathology, Marie Lannelogue Hospital. France: Le Plessis Robinson, 1992.
74. Etienne T, Deleaval PJ, Spiliopoulos A, Megevand R. Thymoma: prognostic factors. Eur J Cardiothorac Surg 1993;7(9):449.
75. Gamondes JP, Balawi A, Greenland T, Adleine P, Mornex JF, Phang J, Maret G. Seventeen years of surgical treatment of thymoma: factors influencing survival. Eur J Cardiothorac Surg 1991;5(3):124.
76. Monden Y, Nakahara K, Nanjo S, Ohno K, Fujii Y, Hashimoto J, Kitagawa Y, et al. Recurrence of thymoma: clinico-pathologic factors, therapy and prognosis. Ann Thorac Surg 1985;39(2):165.
77. Morgenthaler TI, Brown LR, Colby TV, Harper CM, Coles DT. Symposium on intra-thoracic neoplasms. Part 9: thymoma. Mayo Clin Proc 1993;68:1110–1123.
78. Kirschner PA. Reoperation for thymoma: report of 23 cases. Ann Thorac Surg 1990;49:550–555.
79. Fechner RE. Recurrence of noninvasive thymomas: report of five cases and review of literature. Cancer 1969;23:1423–1427.
80. Ohmi M, Ohuchi M. Recurrent thymoma in patients with myasthenia gravis. Ann Thorac Surg 1990;50:243–247.
81. Levasseur P, Noviant Y, Rojas-Miranda A, Merlier M, Le Brigand H. Thymectomy for myasthenia gravis. Long term results in 74 cases. J Thorac Cardiovasc Surg 1972;64:1–5.
82. Mulder DG, Herrmann C, Buckberg GD. Effect of thymectomy in patients with myasthenia gravis. A 16 years experience. Am J Surg 1974;128:202–206.

31

MEDIASTINAL GERM CELL TUMORS

George J. Bosl and Teresa Murray Law

INTRODUCTION

Germ cell tumors (GCT) of the mediastinum are relatively rare and account for only 10% to 25% of all mediastinal tumors (1). Several histologic subtypes comprise this entity, including seminoma, mature teratoma, embryonal cell carcinoma, yolk sac tumor, and choriocarcinoma. The prognosis and management of patients with mediastinal GCT are directed by the histologic subtype. In general, patients with seminoma have a more favorable prognosis than patients with nonseminomatous GCT (NSGCT). Primary therapeutic modalities include surgery for teratoma, chemotherapy or radiation for seminoma, and chemotherapy plus surgery for NSGCT.

INCIDENCE AND EPIDEMIOLOGY

GCTs account for approximately 1% of all malignancies occurring in men, with the testis being the most common site of origin (2). In adults, the anterior mediastinum is the most frequent extragonadal site of origin and is second to the sacrococcygeal site in children (1, 3). Other sites of origin include the retroperitoneum and the pineal gland (1, 3).

GCT represents a greater proportion of mediastinal tumors occurring in children compared with adults (1). In a review of 702 adults with primary anterior mediastinal tumors, thymic lesions (benign or malignant thymoma) were the most frequent tumors followed by lymphoma, endocrine tumors, and GCT (1). In children, GCT is the second most frequent anterior mediastinal tumor with lymphoma being more prevalent (1). Mature teratoma is the most frequent histology and occurs with approximately equal sex distribution (1, 4–6). The mean age of presentation is 28 years with a range of 7 months to 65 years (5). In contrast, malignant GCT (including seminoma and nonseminoma) is less common and occurs predominantly in men during their third decade of life (1, 6, 7). The median age of presentation of patients with seminoma is somewhat older than that of patients with NSGCT: 34 years versus 28 years, respectively (6).

ETIOLOGY

The origin of extragonadal GCT (including mediastinal GCT) is not well understood. Clinical studies and autopsy series of patients with extragonadal GCT have shown that a primary testis tumor is found in up to two thirds of patients with tumors of retroperitoneal origin (8–10). Therefore, some cases of GCT of the retroperitoneum may represent a metastatic site of an occult testis primary tumor. Primary testis tumors have been suspected in patients with mediastinal tumors because of the rare occult tumor or scar formation (possibly representing a prior focus of carcinoma) found at pathologic examination of the testis (11, 12). In these patients, retroperitoneal and mediastinal adenopathy occurred simultaneously and represented metastatic sites of a primary testis tumor (10, 11). Most studies of mediastinal tumors report neither retroperitoneal nor primary testis cancer upon clinical or pathologic examination (8, 9, 12–14). Therefore, the majority of mediastinal GCTs do not represent a metastatic disease site. It has been hypothesized that mediastinal GCT arises from nests of primordial germ cells that remain in the region of the anterior mediastinum at the time of migration along the gonadal ridge during embryogenesis (3, 15, 16). During migration, the primordial cells pursue a dorsal route (3). The anterior mediastinum (ventral in location), however, is the most frequent location of these tumors. Furthermore, cephalad migration has not been observed, and thus the origin of pineal GCT does not fit this model (15–17). Additionally, normal germ cells have not yet been identified in the thymus or pineal gland (17). Another theory of histogenesis suggests that these tumors originate in somatic cells, which acquire the capacity to differentiate (17, 18). Studies of the biology of extragonadal GCT may increase our understanding of the histogenesis of both gonadal and extragonadal GCT.

CLINICAL PRESENTATION AND EVALUATION

CLINICAL PRESENTATION

More than 80% of patients with mediastinal seminoma or NSGCT present with symptoms (Table 31.1) (1, 6, 7, 19, 20). Pain and cough are the most common symptoms, occurring in about one half and one third of patients, respectively (4–7, 19, 20). Other common complaints include dyspnea, weight loss, and fever (7, 19, 20). Fewer than 10% of patients were diagnosed after presentation with superior vena cava (SVC) syndrome, lymphadenopathy, hemoptysis, gynecomastia (related to the production of human chorionic gonadotropin by tumor cells), pericarditis, pleural effusion, or tracheobronchial fistula (1, 6, 7, 19, 20). In contrast, approximately 50% of patients with mature teratoma (previously considered a benign lesion) presented with no symptoms: rather, the tumors were found incidentally on chest radiographs done for other reasons (Table 31.2) (1, 5, 6). Cough productive of hair indicates the presence of a tracheobronchial fistula and is virtually diagnostic of teratoma (5).

The physical examination at presentation is often normal but may suggest one of the above syndromes.

TABLE 31.2. Clinical Presentation of Patients with Mature Teratoma

CLINCAL PRESENTATION	AUTHOR (REFERENCE NO.) AND % OF PATIENTS		TOTAL[c,d] (%)
	COURAUD (6) N = 219[a]	LEWIS (5) N = 86[b]	
No symptoms	107 (50%)	31 (36%)	138/305 (45%)
Chest pain	50 (23%)	33 (38%)	88/305 (29%)
Cough	60 (27%)	15 (18%)	75/305 (25%)
Dyspnea	50 (23%)	17 (20%)	67/305 (22%)
Pleural effusion	20 (9%)	N/A	20/219 (9%)
SVC	3 (1%)	N/A	3/219 (1%)

Abbreviations. SVC, superior vena cava syndrome; N/A, not available.
[a]Mean age at presentation, 28 years.
[b]Mean age at presentation, 28 years.
[c]Total number of patients for whom data were available presenting with the specified symptom.
[d]Mean age at presentation, 28 years.

Careful examination of the testes including ultrasonography is required to rule out the presence of a primary tumor. If an occult gonadal tumor is found, an inguinal orchiectomy is required as part of the overall patient management. A history of developmental delay, and the presence of skeletal deformities or hypogonadism on the physical examination, may suggest Klinefelter's syndrome, which can be associated with NSGCT of the mediastinum (see Tumor Biology, below) (21).

TABLE 31.1. Clinical Presentation of Patients with Malignant GCT (Seminoma and Nonseminoma)

CLINICAL PRESENTATION	AUTHOR (REFERENCE NO.) AND NO. OF PATIENTS (%)				TOTAL[b] (%)
	COURAND (6) N = 157[a]	KNAPP (7) N = 56[c]	WRIGHT (19) N = 48[d]	KAY (20) N = 12[f]	
Pain	74 (47%)	22 (39%)	31 (65%)	8 (66%)	135/273 (49%)
Cough	N/A	15 (26%)	23 (48%)	4 (33%)	42/116 (36%)
Dyspnea	N/A	8 (14%)	14 (29%)	4 (33%)	26/116 (22%)
SVC	12 (8%)	8 (14%)	N/A	1 (8%)	21/225 (9%)
Pleural effusion	9 (6%)	N/A	N/A	N/A	9/157 (6%)
Lymph nodes	5 (3%)	7 (12%)	3	N/A	15/261 (6%)
Pericarditis	6 (4%)	N/A	N/A	N/A	6/157 (4%)
Gynecomastia	8 (5%)	N/A	2 (4%)	3 (25%)	13/217 (6%)
Weight loss	N/A	10 (18%)	6 (13%)	N/A	16/104 (15%)
Hemoptysis	N/A	4 (7%)	7 (15%)	N/A	11/104 (11%)
Fever	N/A	N/A	14 (29%)	N/A	14/48 (29%)
Lethargy	N/A	N/A	N/A	5 (42%)	5/12 (42%)
No Symptoms	33 (21%)	8 (14%)	N/A	N/A	41/213 (19%)
Other	1[b]	N/A	2 (4%)[e]	N/A	3/205 (1%)

Abbreviations. N/A, not available; SVC, superior vena cava syndrome.
[a]Median age at presentation, 27 years.
[b]The total number of patients for whom data were available presenting with the specified symptom.
[c]Median age at presentation, 29 years.
[d]Median age at presentation, 27 years.
[e]One patient with Klinefelter's syndrome.
[f]Median age at presentation, 29 years.

LABORATORY EVALUATION

Specific laboratory tests are important diagnostic tools and are useful in assessing response to therapy in specific GCT histologic subtypes. A complete blood cell count may suggest the presence of a hematologic malignancy that may occur in association with NSGCT of the mediastinum (see Tumor Biology, below) (22, 23). Serum concentrations of lactate dehydrogenase (LDH), and of the oncofetal tumor markers human chorionic gonadotropin (HCG) and α-fetoprotein (AFP), can be elevated; the pattern of elevation of these serum markers is dependent on the histology of the tumor (Table 31.3) (24–26). LDH is ubiquitous, and elevated levels are observed in many malignancies including GCT, Hodgkin's and non-Hodgkin's lymphomas, and other carcinomas. HCG, classically produced by syncytiotrophoblasts, is secreted in GCT with choriocarcinoma and, less commonly, with pure seminoma. Yolk sac (endodermal sinus) tumors produce AFP. Embryonal carcinoma may produce either marker protein.

Patients with pure seminoma may have elevations of serum concentrations of either HCG or LDH. Among 168 patients with advanced gonadal or mediastinal seminoma, 45 (27%) had elevated serum HCG concentrations at diagnosis (6, 25). The serum AFP concentration is not elevated in patients with seminoma. A pathologic diagnosis of seminoma with an elevation in serum AFP concentration implies the presence of NSGCT, and the patient should be managed as though they have NSGCT. In contrast, neither AFP nor HCG concentrations are elevated in the serum of patients with pure mature teratoma.

Seventy percent to 80% of patients with NSGCT of any site of origin have elevated concentrations of LDH, HCG, and/or AFP (24). Patients with NSGCT of the mediastinum more frequently have elevations in serum AFP (approximately 75%) compared with those with NSGCT of the testis or of retroperitoneal origin (26). This result corresponds to the more frequent finding of yolk sac tumor in mediastinal NSGCT (26, 27).

RADIOGRAPHIC EVALUATION AND DIAGNOSIS

Radiographic evaluation of patients with mediastinal GCT usually begins with a chest radiograph. Calcification occurs in approximately 25% of mature teratomas (5). GCTs arise in the anterior mediastinum and can invade local structures such as the great vessels (causing superior vena cava syndrome), the pericardium, or the pleura (1, 4, 6, 7). A computed tomography (CT) scan of the chest better defines the exact location of the tumor mass and its relationship to contiguous structures (4, 28, 29). A magnetic resonance imaging scan (MRI) can differentiate vascular from nonvascular structures in patients who are unable to tolerate contrast material, but its use is not indicated in most cases (4, 28, 29).

Patients also must be evaluated with a CT scan of the abdomen and pelvis to assess retroperitoneal adenopathy and liver metastases. Sonography of the testes is necessary to evaluate an occult primary gonadal tumor. The likelihood of finding a primary testis tumor is greater if retroperitoneal adenopathy exists because the first site of metastasis of a primary testis carcinoma is often the retroperitoneum. In patients with mediastinal GCT who present with metastatic disease, the most common sites are the lung, liver, bone, lymph nodes, and retroperitoneum (7, 26, 30). In contrast, mature teratoma presents as a solitary or cystic mediastinal mass (5). Bone scans, CT of the brain, or other imaging studies should be performed to evaluate a specific complaint in an individual patient, but these tests generally are not required. The extent of disease defined by these radiographic scans is helpful in planning therapeutic interventions and serves as a baseline measurement against which posttreatment evaluations are compared.

Establishing the diagnosis of mediastinal GCT and its pathologic subtype (mature teratoma, seminoma, nonseminoma, or mixed GCT) and differentiating it from other mediastinal tumors can be challenging. A core needle biopsy may not yield sufficient tissue to perform the routine hematoxylin and eosin analysis as well as the immunohistochemical stains and/or molecular studies needed to establish a diagnosis in difficult cases. Therefore, mediastinotomy, mediastinoscopy, or thoracotomy is often required (4, 28, 29).

When considering the differential diagnosis of mediastinal tumors, certain clinical characteristics are

TABLE 31.3. Serum Tumor Marker Elevation in Germ Cell Tumors

HISTOLOGY	AFP	HCG	LDH
Seminoma	−	±	+
Yolk sac tumor	+	−	+
Choriocarcinoma	−	+	+
Embryonal carcinoma	+	+	+
Mature teratoma	−	−	−

Data from Bosl et al. (24), Mencel et al. (25), and Toner et al. (26).
Abbreviations. AFP, α-fetoprotein; HCG, human chorionic gonadotropin; LDH, lactate dehydrogenase; −, negative—staining absent; +, positive—staining present.

helpful. Thymoma most commonly presents in the fifth or sixth decade, and a proportion of patients have associated myasthenia gravis at presentation (31–33). Patients with Hodgkin's and non-Hodgkin's lymphomas can present during the third decade of life with symptoms similar to those of patients with mediastinal GCT (3). A sufficient amount of tumor must be obtained to perform the pathologic evaluation, which can distinguish between the hematologic malignancies, mediastinal GCT, and other mediastinal tumors (see Pathology, below). Serum tumor markers alone should not be used to diagnose GCT except perhaps in the most life-threatening circumstances.

PATHOLOGY

The pathologic diagnosis ultimately directs the primary treatment choice and the sequence in which combined modality therapies are delivered. Therefore, it is critical to distinguish GCT from other mediastinal tumors and to differentiate NSGCT from seminoma. Occasionally, immunohistochemical stains and/or molecular studies are required in addition to the routine histologic analysis.

SEMINOMA

Pure seminoma must be distinguished from lymphoma, both of which appear as monomorphic round cell neoplasms. It must also be distinguished from seminoma mixed with nonseminomatous elements because patients with "mixed tumors" must be treated as though they have NSGCT (3, 34). In general, classic seminoma stains negatively for cytokeratin, AFP, and the type 1 precursor to blood group antigens (BG-1), but it expresses placental-like alkaline phosphatase (Table 31.4) (3, 35, 36). Syncytiotrophoblastic-like giant cells give rise to the expression of HCG in seminoma (34). The serum concentration of AFP and immunohistochemical stains for AFP are negative in classic seminoma, and their presence suggests a yolk sac component to the tumor (34). In contrast, NSGCT usually expresses both cytokeratin and BG-1 (3, 35, 36). Tumor expression of leukocytic common antigen is consistent with a hematologic malignancy such as lymphoma (3).

A subtype of seminoma, "atypical seminoma," is characterized by an increased mitotic index, increased nuclear to cytoplasmic ratio, and nuclear pleomorphism (25). Unlike classic seminoma, it is positive for BG-1 (Table 31.4) (35, 36). Like classic seminoma, it generally does not express cytokeratin (35, 36). Atypical seminoma appears to have a more aggressive clinical course than classic seminoma and may be associated with elevated serum concentrations of AFP and/or HCG in patients who have refractory disease (25). It is possible that seminoma expressing BG-1 represents an early transformation to NSGCT rather than a variant seminoma morphology (25).

MEDIASTINAL NSGCT

NSGCT is usually of mixed histology and includes the extraembryonic tissues of yolk sac tumor (also referred to as endodermal sinus tumor) and choriocarcinoma, and of embryonal cell carcinoma. Yolk sac tumor (pure or mixed with other elements) is the most common histology of mediastinal NSGCT, found in 40% to 45% of tumors (26, 27). When the serum concentrations of AFP and/or HCG are elevated, they are useful in assessing response to therapy and in detecting recurrent disease.

Pure choriocarcinoma or pure embryonal cell carcinoma of the mediastinum is relatively uncommon. These patterns are usually a component of mixed histologies (3, 7, 26). Choriocarcinoma is often accompanied by hemorrhage and necrosis that may obscure the detection of the malignant cells (3). Embryonal cell carcinoma is the most undifferentiated GCT morphology and has the potential to differentiate into extraembryonic (choriocarcinoma and endodermal sinus tumor) or somatic (mature teratoma consisting of endoderm, mesoderm and ectoderm) cell types (34). Therefore, embryonal cell carcinoma can produce either AFP or HCG or both markers, and can express multiple immunohistochemical markers (Table 31.4) (3). Cytogenetic studies have identified an isochromosome of the short arm of chromosome 12, (i[12p]), which is found in approximately 80% of GCT with an abnormal karyotype; it is diagnostic for GCT when

TABLE 31.4. Immunohistochemical Stains in the Pathologic Diagnosis of Mediastinal Tumors

HISTOLOGY	CTK	LCA	AFP	PLAP	BG-1
Nonseminoma GCT	+	−	+	±	+
Seminoma: classical	−	−	−	+	−
Seminoma: atypical	−	−	−	±	+
Lymphoma	−	+	−	−	−
Thymoma	+	−	−	−	N/A

Data from Dehner (3), Cooper et al. (35), and Mozer et al. (36).
Abbreviations. CTK, cytokeratin; LCA, leukocyte common antigen; AFP, α-fetoprotein; PLAP, placental-like alkaline phosphatase; BG-1, precursor to the type 1 blood group antigen; N/A, data not available; + positive—staining present; −, negative—staining absent.

routine and immunohistochemical stains are unable to provide a diagnosis (see Tumor Biology, below) (37).

TERATOMA

Mature teratoma contains elements of all three germ cell lines (endoderm, mesoderm, and ectoderm) and is often classified as a benign tumor because it represents the most differentiated GCT morphology (3). However, it must be treated as a malignant tumor because the presence of mature teratoma implies that the totipotential precursor, embryonal carcinoma, gave rise to it (38). Common differentiated tissues present include skin and neuroglia (ectoderm), bone, cartilage, muscle and adipose tissue (mesoderm), and gastroenteric mucosa and respiratory epithelium (endoderm) (3, 5). Further malignant differentiation of these "adult" tissues occurs and does so more frequently in the mediastinum than at other sites (7, 12, 39, 40). The most common non–germ cell malignancies associated with mature teratoma are sarcoma and adenocarcinoma (7, 12, 39, 40). In one retrospective review of 580 pathology reports of GCT patients, 17 cases of malignant transformation occurred (39). Fifteen cases of mesodermal differentiation (sarcoma) and nine cases of endodermal differentiation (adenocarcinoma) were observed. In seven cases both sarcoma and carcinoma were present (39). In another series of 32 patients with mediastinal NSGCT, four patients had non–germ cell malignancies concurrent with mature teratoma at diagnosis (7). Thus, benign teratoma is a misnomer, and aggressive management of these tumors is required for patients to achieve long-term disease free status (see Therapy, below).

Teratoma may present pathologically as mature teratoma, as mature teratoma with malignant transformation, or as mature teratoma mixed with embryonal carcinoma, choriocarcinoma, yolk sac tumor, or seminoma. When teratoma is associated with other germ cell elements, it is classified as mixed NSGCT or seminoma with teratoma. Rarely, teratoma has fetal tissue present and is then referred to as immature teratoma (3).

UNDIFFERENTIATED (POORLY DIFFERENTIATED) TUMORS OF UNCERTAIN HISTOGENESIS

Undifferentiated tumors of uncertain histogenesis that present in the mediastinum and other midline structures represent a group of neoplasms in which a primary site cannot be determined by routine pathologic examination (41). Through the identification of i(12p) in resected tumor specimens, it is now recognized that some of these patients (usually young men) with poorly differentiated midline carcinomas have unrecognized GCT, and that they can benefit from treatment directed toward GCT (see Tumor Biology, below) (37, 41).

PROGNOSIS OF MEDIASTINAL GERM CELL TUMORS

Treatment strategies of GCT have evolved substantially as lessons have been learned from a series of clinical trials conducted in patients with all types of GCT. These studies have looked at prognostic factors, and the efficacy, schedule, and toxicity of chemotherapy regimens. They have observed the following: (a) 70% to 80% of patients with advanced GCT are cured of their disease with cisplatin-based chemotherapy (42); (b) the pretreatment clinical features, including the serum concentrations of LDH, AFP, HCG, and the number and sites of metastatic disease at presentation, have prognostic significance in primary GCT (43–45); (c) pure seminoma histology, regardless of the site of origin, imparts a favorable prognosis (25, 43); (d) primary mediastinal NSGCT imparts a very unfavorable prognosis regardless of the extent of disease or biochemical marker values found (26, 27, 43); (e) surgery after chemotherapy to resect viable carcinoma and/or residual mature teratoma in those patients with NSGCT and normal tumor markers is necessary to maximize the complete response (CR) proportion (46–48); and (f) effective salvage regimens are available for the minority of patients whose tumors are refractory to the initial cisplatin-based chemotherapy or who relapse from therapy (49–52).

PROGNOSTIC FACTORS AND RISK ASSIGNMENT IN GCT

Considerable effort has been directed toward developing satisfactory algorithms that predict treatment outcome to cisplatin-containing chemotherapy regimens and that can be used to allocate patients to specific therapy. For the patients predicted to have a more favorable outcome (i.e., "good risk"), the goals of clinical trials have been to maintain the high cure rate while reducing the treatment-related toxicity. In "poor-risk" patients (i.e., those predicted to have an unfavorable outcome), treatment efforts have been directed toward improving the CR proportion with tolerable treatment-related toxicity.

Using pretreatment clinical characteristics, several multivariate analyses have been performed to define a prognostic model predictive for CR and overall survival that was both sensitive and specific. Various investigators have found different prognostic features to be predictive for CR in GCT patients (Table 31.5) (43–45, 53–57). These clinical features include the primary site of disease, extent of disease (measured either as the total number of metastatic sites of disease, sites of metastatic disease, and/or size of the tumor[s] at a particular site), and increased concentration of the serum tumor markers LDH, HCG, and/or AFP (measured as discrete or continuous variables using different techniques and normal values). In one study patients treated for advanced GCT were assigned retrospectively to various good-risk and poor-risk criteria to compare patients' response to therapy based on the different risk criteria (Table 31.6) (58). Although patients assigned to good-risk status did uniformly well, the initial CR proportions for poor-risk patients ranged from 38% to 62% depending on the specific criteria used to allocate the patients (58). Thus, the criteria used to allocate patients to good- and poor-risk studies vary considerably. Despite differences in risk stratification, most investigators agree that patients with pure seminoma, regardless of the primary site, have a uniformly good prognosis based on their excellent survival with cisplatin-based chemotherapy (25, 43, 59). Furthermore, patients with primary mediastinal NSGCT have a uniformly poor prognosis based on their low CR proportion, high relapse rate, and poor survival observed in clinical trials (26, 27, 43, 60–62).

TABLE 31.6. Comparison of Risk Criteria and Initial Complete Response to Therapy in 118 Patients with Advanced GCT

STUDY	RISK CRITERIA	
	GOOD RISK	POOR RISK
MSKCC	77/81 (95%)	14/37 (38%)[a]
IU	65/74 (88%)	23/44 (52%)[b]
NCI	57/60 (95%)	31/58 (53%)[c]
EROTC[d]	43/46 (93%)	45/72 (62%)[e]

Data from Bajorin D, Katz A, Chan E, Geller N, Vogelzang, N, Bosl GJ. Comparison of criteria for assigning germ cell tumor patients to "good risk" and "poor risk" studies. J Clin Oncol 1988;6:786–792.
Abbreviations. MSKCC, Memorial Sloan–Kettering Cancer Center; IU, Indiana University; NCI, National Cancer Institute; EORTC, European Organization for the Research and Treatment of Cancer.
[a]Median survival in poor-risk group, 11.5 months.
[b]Median survival in poor-risk group, 15 months.
[c]Median survival in poor-risk group, 15 months.
[d]The EORTC criteria have been modified since this analysis. Therefore, the current EORTC/MRC criteria do not pertain to this analysis.
[e]Median survival in poor-risk group, 23 months.

SERUM TUMOR MARKERS

The rate of decrease of serum concentrations of AFP and HCG has also been analyzed as a predictive marker. After surgical resection the half-life clearance of AFP and HCG have been shown to be less than 5 to 7 days and 18 to 48 hours, respectively (63, 64). Using this information several investigators evaluated the prognostic value of posttreatment decreases in the serum concentration of AFP and/or HCG (63–66). When evaluating posttreatment decreases in serum tumor marker concentrations, serial measurements must be obtained to determine the clearance time accurately and to monitor for the posttreatment "surge" that can occur soon after treatment (67). In one retrospective study of 198 patients, a prolonged clearance of AFP or HCG ($t_{1/2}$ of more than 7 days for AFP or $t_{1/2}$ of more than 3 days for HCG) measured during the initial two cycles of chemotherapy correlated with eventual treatment failure in both good-risk and poor-risk groups (Table 31.7) (63). Two other studies showed similar results with HCG (65) and AFP (66). Therefore, a prolonged postchemotherapy decrease in the serum tumor marker of AFP or HCG may serve as an unfavorable prognostic factor. This factor could be used in se-

TABLE 31.5. Pretreatment Prognostic Factors (Determined by Multivariate Analyses) Used to Allocate GCT Patients to "Good-Risk" Versus "Poor-Risk" Therapy

Study (Reference No.)	Extent of Metastatic Disease	Serum Tumor Markers
MSKCC (44)	Number of sites	LDH (Log_{10} U/L)
		HCG (Log_{10} ng/ml)
IU (53, 57)	Number of metastases	Markers not used to
	Bulk of disease	assess risk status
	Sites of disease	
MRC (45, 54)	Number of metastases	HCG, >1000 IU/L
	Bulk of disease	AFP, >1000 kU/L[a]
	Sites of disease	
NCI (55, 56)	Number of metastases	HCG, >10,000
	Bulk of disease	mIU/ml
	Sites of disease	AFP, >2000 ng/ml[b]

Note. Bulk of disease usually referred to specific tumor measurements that differed by investigator among the sites of disease.
Abbreviations. MSKCC, Memorial Sloan–Kettering Cancer Center; IU, Indiana University; MRC, Medical Research Council Working Party on Testicular Tumours; NCI, National Cancer Institute; LDH, lactate dehydrogenase; HCG, human chorionic gonadotropin; AFP, α-fetoprotein.
[a]Data from MRC, i.e., Mead et al. (45).
[b]Data from NCI, i.e., Ozols et al. (55).

TABLE 31.7. Correlation of Serum Tumor Marker Decline (AFP or HCG) with Response Proportion to Chemotherapy

Tumor Marker Decrease by Half-Life	No. of Patients		
	Total	Complete Response (%)	Incomplete Response (%)
Appropriate[a]	156	139 (89%)	17 (11%)
Prolonged[b]	42	12 (29%)	30 (71%)

Data from Toner GC, Geller NL, Tan C, Nisselbaum J, Bosl GJ. Serum tumor marker half-life during chemotherapy allows early prediction of complete response and survival in nonseminomatous germ cell tumors. Cancer Res 1990;50:5904–5910.
[a]Appropriate serum tumor marker decrease by half-life ($T_{1/2}$) for HCG, ≤3 days; $T_{1/2}$ for AFP, ≤7 days.
[b]Prolonged serum tumor marker decrease by $T_{1/2}$ for HCG, >3 days; $T_{1/2}$ for AFP, >7 days.

lected cases to direct an early treatment change to more intensive therapy.

THERAPY

MEDIASTINAL SEMINOMA

Historically, radiation therapy has been the primary treatment modality of localized mediastinal seminoma, based on its efficacy in achieving high cure rates in early stage seminoma of testis origin (68). In patients with mediastinal seminoma, long-term survival after radiation therapy has ranged from 50% to 100% because the studies have varied in the number of patients treated and the total radiation dose delivered (Table 31.8) (7, 14, 69–73). Three small studies, of six patients each, showed long-term survival proportions of 66% to 100% (14, 69, 71). Two series of patients showed that disease free survival (DFS) was approximately 50% (7, 70). Common sites of relapse included the thorax (mediastinum and lung), adjacent lymph nodes, and distant sites (bone, brain, and liver) (7, 70). The time from diagnosis to metastasis of the disease is usually less than 12 months (7). Thus, radiation therapy is an option for the treatment of mediastinal seminoma. However, it does not achieve a uniformly high long-term DFS because of the occurrence of local and distant relapses. Therefore, chemotherapy has been evaluated extensively during the past 15 years.

Cisplatin-based chemotherapy as a first-line treatment has resulted in excellent long-term DFS (25, 59, 74, 75). One early study of 21 patients with extragonadal seminoma showed that those who received cisplatin-based chemotherapy followed by surgical resection had a better DFS compared with those treated with surgical resection plus radiation therapy and non–cisplatin-based chemotherapy (91% versus 50%, respectively) (75). In the largest series of seminoma patients reported to date, 142 patients with advanced gonadal or mediastinal seminoma were treated with cisplatin-based regimens (25). The chemotherapy regimens included both etoposide and earlier non–etoposide regimens in conjunction with high-dose cisplatin (100 to 120 mg/m^2 per cycle) (42, 76, 77). Ninety-three percent of patients achieved a favorable response (CR or progression free partial response with negative tumor markers), and 86% were alive without progression at a median follow-up of 43 months (25). Among the 19 patients with mediastinal primary tumors, all achieved a CR, and 95% (18 of 19 patients) remained disease free (Table 31.8) (25). Similar results have been reported in other series in which cisplatin-based chemotherapy was used as the primary treatment (59, 74, 78, 79). In addition, patients who received their initial cisplatin-based therapy at the time of relapse (after radiation therapy) had an inferior treatment outcome and experienced more severe hematologic toxicity than those who received chemotherapy as first-line treatment (25, 79). Therefore, cisplatin-based chemotherapy is preferred as the first treatment in patients who present with advanced gonadal or extragonadal seminoma. Lastly, patients with mediastinal seminoma should be considered a good risk for the purpose of treatment assignment because the cure rate is high after cisplatin-based chemotherapy.

The role of adjunctive surgery in patients with seminoma is not as well defined as for patients with NSGCT (Table 31.9). Studies have shown that the incidence of viable cancer in resected tumor specimens from seminoma patients ranged from 10% to 42% (59, 80, 81). For patients with a residual radiographic mass less than 3 cm in maximum diameter, the likelihood of finding malignancy in the resected tumor is very low, and close observation is recommended (59, 81). In patients with a postchemotherapy mass of at least 3 cm, viable tumor at surgery has been encountered (81). If viable cancer is found at resection, additional therapy (chemotherapy or radiation) is required.

MEDIASTINAL NONSEMINOMATOUS GCT

Patients with mediastinal NSGCT are considered to have poor-risk disease and have a much lower likelihood of achieving a CR to combined modality therapy (26). In addition, they more often require surgical resection of residual masses to achieve a disease free state when compared with patients with NSGCT of testis or retroperitoneal origin (26, 27).

Prior to the availability of cisplatin-based chemotherapy, patients with mediastinal NSGCT were treated

TABLE 31.8. Treatment of Mediastinal Seminoma

STUDY (REFERENCE NO.)	NO. OF PATIENTS	PRIMARY TREATMENT	CR (%)	LONG-TERM SURVIVAL[e] (%)
Cox (14)	6	Radiation	6 (100%)	4 (66%)
Raghavan et al. (69)	6[a]	Radiation (4 pts) Radiation + CT (2 pts)	5 (83%)	4 (67%)
Bush et al. (70)	13	Radiation	N/A	7 (54%)
Lee and Jackson (71)	6[b]	Radiation	6 (100%)	6 (100%)
Martini et al. (73)	10[b]	Surgery (2 pts) Radiation ± CT, SUR (8 pts)	N/A	4 (40%)
Knapp et al. (7)	24	Radiation (21 pts)	N/A	12 (50%)
Loehrer et al. (79)	9	Chemotherapy[c]	7 (78%)	N/A
Mencel et al. (25)	19	Chemotherapy[d]	19 (100%)	18 (95%)
Total	93		43/46 (93%)	55/84 (65%)

Abbreviations. CR, complete response; CT, chemotherapy; N/A, not available; pts, patients; SUR, surgery.
[a]One patient relapsed at 2 months requiring additional radiotherapy to achieve disease free status; one patient receiving therapy at the time of publication achieved long-term disease free status for more than 7 years (update of original publication, personal communication, Dr. Alan Horwich, June 29, 1994).
[b]One patient relapsed requiring additional therapy to achieve disease free status.
[c]Chemotherapy was second-line treatment in some patients (cisplatin based).
[d]Chemotherapy was first-line therapy (cisplatin or carboplatin based).
[e]Usually, at least 24 months with disease free status.

TABLE 31.9. Postchemotherapy Histology of Resected Mediastinal Tumor Masses

HISTOLOGY	PATIENTS WITH NONSEMINOMA[a] N = 17	PATIENTS WITH SEMINOMA[b] N = 9
Necrosis	7 (41%)	7 (78%)
Teratoma	7 (41%)	0
Malignancy	3 (18%)	2 (22%)

[a]Data from Toner et al. (99).
[b]Data from Motzer et al. (81).

with surgery, radiation therapy, and/or non–cisplatin-containing chemotherapy regimens; they had a uniformly dismal prognosis with a median survival of less than 10 months (13, 14, 73). With the introduction of cisplatin-based chemotherapy and the recognition of the need for aggressive, combined modality therapy, the CR proportion (with or without adjunctive surgery) has increased to between 30% to 58%, and the long-term survival at 2 years is as high as 48% (Table 31.10) (20, 26, 27, 30, 61, 62, 82, 83).

The optimal chemotherapy regimen for patients with poor-risk disease (including mediastinal NSGCT) continues to evolve. Several trials have studied various schedules and combinations of high-dose cisplatin-containing regimens with etoposide, vinblastine, and/or bleomycin (42, 84–90). The durable CR proportion in these studies ranged from 26% to 85% depending on the criteria used to allocate patients to poor-risk status and on the specific treatment regimen. Currently, the combination of cisplatin, etoposide, and bleomycin (PEB) for four cycles is the usual, standard, first-line chemotherapy for poor-risk GCT patients (86, 89).

For patients who relapse from CR or are refractory to initial cisplatin-based chemotherapy, effective salvage therapy is available (91). Ifosfamide, an oxazophosphorine related to cyclophosphamide, was shown to have efficacy in the treatment of patients with refractory GCT (49, 92). Cisplatin plus ifosfamide–based regimens are now considered part of first-line salvage therapy with a 33% to 69% CR proportion: of those CRs approximately one half are durable (49, 52, 91, 93). Furthermore, ifosfamide/cisplatin regimens are being studied as initial therapy for untreated poor-risk patients (94, 95). However, one randomized trial failed to show a significant benefit for ifosfamide plus cisplatin as induction therapy compared with standard etoposide plus cisplatin–based therapy (94).

High-dose chemotherapy is one new approach being investigated in poor-risk patients. High-dose chemotherapy (HDCT) with autologous bone marrow transplant (ABMT) was investigated initially in heavily pretreated patients with refractory GCT (51). Between 15% and 25% of patients were cured despite their failure to respond to previous chemotherapy, but they suffered considerable treatment-related toxicity (51). Subsequently, HDCT plus ABMT as part of first-line treatment has been studied (96–98). In these series durable CR proportions ranged from 46% to 64% (96–98). In one study of untreated poor-risk patients,

TABLE 31.10. Results of Multimodality Therapy (Chemotherapy/Surgery/Radiation) in the Treatment of Patients with Mediastinal NSGCT

STUDY/YEAR (REFERENCE NO.)	NO. OF PATIENTS	FIRST-LINE CHEMOTHERAPY[a]	PRIOR THERAPY	CR (%)	LONG-TERM SURVIVAL (%)[b]
Feun et al./1980 (82)	7	CDDP-based	3: XRT	0	0
Vogelzang et al./1982 (61)	12	7: CDDP-based 5: Non-CDDP	6: XRT 2: SUR	7 (58%)	4 (33%)
Kuzur et al./1982	10 (All YST)	8: CDDP-based 2: Non-CDDP	3: XRT	3 (30%)	1 (10%)
Garnick et al./1983 (83)	8	CDDP-based	None	3 (38%)	1 (12%)
Truong et al./1986 (30)	7 (All YST)	5: CDDP-based 2: Non-CDDP	5: SUR	N/A	2 (29%)
Kay et al./1987 (20)	12	CDDP-based	2: SUR	7 (58%)	4 (33%)
Nichols et al./1990 (27)	31	CDDP-based	None	18 (58%)	15 (48%)
Toner et al./(1991) (26)	32	27: CDDP-based 5: Carbo-based	None	12 (38%)	12 (38%)
Total	119	...	...	50/112 (44%)	39/119 (33%)

Abbreviations. CT, chemotherapy; XRT, radiation therapy; SUR, surgery; YST, yolk sac histology; CR, complete response to CT only, CT + SUR, CT + XRT, or CT + XRT + SUR; CDDP, cisplatin; Carb, carboplatin-based.
[a]Number of patients treated with CDDP, non-CDDP, and carboplatin-based chemotherapy regimens.
[b]Long-term survival, at least 2 years of disease free status in most series.

28 patients received two cycles of standard cisplatin-based chemotherapy (96). If a prolonged clearance of either AFP or HCG was observed, then two cycles of high–dose carboplatin and etoposide with ABMT were administered. Alternatively, patients with appropriate rates of decrease in serum tumor markers completed three cycles of standard chemotherapy (96). Compared with their prior results, i.e., a median survival of 13.3 months in poor-risk patients, this study suggested a survival benefit, with 53% of patients alive at 21 months ($P = .07$) (96). A randomized trial to evaluate the therapeutic benefit of HDCT with ABMT is currently ongoing. Patients are randomized to receive either four cycles of PEB or two cycles of PEB followed by two cycles of HDCT with stem cell rescue. All patients with poor-risk GCT, including patients with mediastinal GCT, are candidates for this trial. Currently, HDCT with ABMT is not considered a standard initial treatment option for these patients.

Adjunctive surgery in all patients with NSGCT is important to evaluate the response to chemotherapy and to resect residual teratoma or viable GCT. Recent series of mediastinal GCT patients undergoing postchemotherapy resection of residual masses show that 38% to 50% of patients required both treatment modalities to achieve a disease free status (26, 27). Additionally, adjunctive surgery has shown that resected tumor specimens may contain necrotic debris, teratoma, or viable cancer (Table 31.9) (99). Resection of either necrotic debris or teratoma requires no further therapy. However, patients with viable GCT at resection require additional chemotherapy because of the high rate of relapse (47). Finally, resection must be performed at all sites of residual tumor because the histology is not uniform at all sites of resection in a given patient (99).

NSGCT of the mediastinum has an unfavorable prognosis. These patients should be referred to a center that specializes in the treatment of these tumors. The standard treatment for patients with mediastinal NSGCT is chemotherapy with cisplatin, etoposide, and bleomycin, although ifosfamide plus cisplatin–based chemotherapy would be considered reasonable. An inappropriately slow decrease by half-life of AFP and/or HCG may represent resistance to standard cisplatin-based chemotherapy. All patients achieving a marker negative status should be evaluated for postchemotherapy adjunctive surgery. Patients with resected tumors that contain viable GCT require additional chemotherapy.

MATURE TERATOMA OF THE MEDIASTINUM

Similar to teratoma of other sites, primary mediastinal teratoma can be cured with complete surgical resection (5, 6). Complete resection of the teratoma is mandatory for two reasons. The unresected teratoma progresses slowly and can invade adjacent structures (growing teratoma syndrome) (100). Also, malignant transformation of the teratoma can occur with sarcomatous or carcinomatous differentiation presenting in the primary tumor or at a metastatic site (7, 12, 39,

40). Malignant transformation of the teratoma is refractory to cisplatin-based chemotherapy and portends a poor prognosis (12, 39).

TUMOR BIOLOGY
ISOCHROMOSOME 12P

The chromosomal abnormality most commonly associated with GCT is an isochromosome of the short arm of chromosome 12 (i[12p]) (37, 101). An extensive evaluation of cytogenetic abnormalities in 171 GCT histologic specimens showed that an abnormal karyotype was identified in 101 (59%) of them (37). The most frequent abnormality, i(12p), was found in 79% and occurred more commonly in NSGCT (81%) than in seminoma (30%) (37). The frequency of i(12p) implies an important role for one or more 12p genes in the malignant transformation of germ cells. Furthermore, it has been observed only rarely in other tumors, implying that it can be used to determine diagnosis and lineage (102). In addition to i(12p), a 12q deletion is also a consistent finding in GCT.

Karyotype analysis requires short-term tissue culture and is a time-consuming and specialized process. Fluorescence in situ hybridization (FISH) can detect i(12p) accurately during both metaphase and interphase (103). In 47 tumor specimens with i(12p) detected by conventional karyotype analysis, the abnormality also was detected by the FISH technique (37). Furthermore, among tumor specimens in which i(12p) is not detected by conventional analysis, i(12p) can be detected by FISH analysis in approximately 25%.

MIDLINE TUMORS OF UNCERTAIN HISTOGENESIS

The possibility of unrecognized GCT presenting as a poorly differentiated midline carcinoma of an unknown primary site has been reported (41, 102). Unlike most patients with carcinomas of an unknown primary site, a minority of these patients with midline tumors of uncertain histogenesis achieved long-term DFS with cisplatin-based chemotherapy (41). Either i(12p) or 12q deletion can be identified by cytogenetic or molecular genetic analysis in approximately 25% of midline tumors of uncertain histogenesis (37). When such a tumor has a GCT cytogenetic marker, a high likelihood of response to therapy has been reported, whereas an absence of a GCT genetic marker was associated with only rare significant responses (37). Genetic studies can also identify other malignancies, including neuroepithelioma and lymphomas, indicating the potential importance of genetic studies in the identification of tumors of uncertain histogenesis (102). The routine use of genetic markers in this setting awaits adaptation to use in tissue sections.

ASSOCIATED HEMATOLOGIC MALIGNANCIES

A unique feature of mediastinal GCT is its association with hematologic malignancies. These hematologic disorders include acute leukemia (megakaryoblastic, monoblastic, myeloid, and mixed-lineage subtypes) and myelodysplastic syndrome (22, 23, 104–106). Some reports of malignant histocytosis associated with mediastinal GCT have now been reclassified as a specific type of non-Hodgkin's lymphoma known as Ki-1 lymphoma because of their expression of the Ki-1 antigen (CD 30) (104). These hematologic disorders are unrelated to prior chemotherapy because they may occur concurrently with, or subsequent to, the diagnosis of mediastinal GCT (usually within 12 months). The i(12p) marker has been identified in both the primary GCT and the associated leukemic cell, indicating a common clonal origin for these malignancies (107).

ASSOCIATION WITH KLINEFELTER'S SYNDROME

Klinefelter's syndrome (KFS), characterized by an XXY karyotype, presents with hypogonadism, infertility, gynecomastia, developmental delay, and musculoskeletal abnormalities including brachyclinodactyly (hypoplasia of the middle phalanges of the fifth digit) and limitation of pronation and supination of the forearms (108). The incidence of KFS is 0.2% in males in the United States (108). Several case reports and series have documented the association of KFS with mediastinal NSGCT (21, 109–112). In a retrospective review of 19 mediastinal GCT patients at one institution, four (21%) had KFS (21). In a prospective karyotypic analysis of patients presenting with primary mediastinal GCT, 5 of the 22 patients (22%) had associated KFS (109). All patients in both series had NSGCT and presented at a younger median age, i.e., 15 to 16 years old, compared with the median age of 27 to 28 years for all patients with mediastinal GCT (21, 109).

SUMMARY

Many histologic subtypes comprise mediastinal GCT. Accurate diagnosis by immunohistochemistry and molecular genetics, and the appropriate management of these complex tumors, is imperative to optimize the treatment outcome of these patients. Complete surgical resection of mature teratoma is mandatory to avoid the growing teratoma syndrome and the malignant transformation to a non–germ cell malignancy. Evaluation for associated entities, such as malignant transformation and hematologic malignancies, is sometimes necessary, and an accurate assessment of pretreatment prognostic features is required. Cisplatin-based chemotherapy is the mainstay of systemic management. Patients with mediastinal seminoma have good-risk disease and achieve a uniformly high long-term DFS with cisplatin-based chemotherapy. Patients with NSGCT have poor-risk disease and should be entered into clinical trials whenever possible to increase the proportion of patients who are rendered free of disease.

REFERENCES

1. Mullen B, Richardson JD. Primary anterior mediastinal tumors in children and adults. Ann Thorac Surg 1986;42:338–345.
2. Boring CC, Squires TS, Tong T, Montgomery S. Cancer statistics, 1994. CA Cancer J Clin 1994;44:7–26.
3. Dehner LP. Germ cell tumors of the mediastinum. Semin Diagn Pathol 1990;7:266–284.
4. Davis RD, Oldham HN, Sabiston D. Primary cysts and neoplasms of the mediastinum: recent changes in clinical presentation, methods of diagnosis, management, and results. Ann Thorac Surg 1987;44:229–237.
5. Lewis BD, Hurt RD, Payne WS, Farrow GM, Knapp RH, Muhm JR. Benign teratomas of the mediastinum. J Thorac Cardiovasc Surg 1983;86:727–731.
6. Couraud L, Martigne C, Michaud JL, Al-Qudah AH. Primary germ cell tumors of the mediastinum. In: Martini N, Vogt-Moykopf I, eds. Thoracic surgery: frontiers and uncommon neoplasms. St. Louis: Mosby, 1989:226–232.
7. Knapp RH, Hurt RD, Payne WS, et al. Malignant germ cell tumors of the mediastinum. J Thorac Cardiovasc Surg 1985;89:82–89.
8. Daugaard G, von der Masse H, Olsen J, Rorth M, Skakkebaek NE. Carcinoma-in-situ testis in patients with assumed extragonadal germ-cell tumors. Lancet 1987;528–530.
9. Bohle A, Studer UE, Sonntag RW, Scheidegger JR. Primary or secondary extragonadal germ cell tumors? J Urol 1986;135:939–943.
10. Friedman NB. The comparative morphogenesis of extragenital and gonadal teratoid tumors. Cancer 1951;4:265–276.
11. Luna MA, Valenzuela-Tamariz J. Germ-cell tumors of the mediastinum, postmortem findings. Am J Clin Pathol 1976;65:450–454.
12. Aliotta PJ, Castillo J, Englander LS, Nseyo UO, Huben RP. Primary mediastinal germ cell tumors. Cancer 1988;62:982–984.
13. Oberman HA, Libcke JH. Malignant germinal neoplasms of the mediastinum. Cancer 1964;17:498–507.
14. Cox JD. Primary malignant germinal tumors of the mediastinum. Cancer 1975;36:1162–1168.
15. Witschi E. Migration of the germ cells of human embryos from the yolk sac to the primitive gonadal folds. Contr Embryol Carnegie Inst 1948;32:67–80.
16. Chiquoine AD. The identification, origin, and migration of the primordial germ cells in the mouse embryo. Anat Rec 1954;118:135–146.
17. Rosai J, Parkash V, Reuter VE. On the origin of mediastinal germ cell tumors in males. Int J Pathol 1994: in press.
18. Watanabe K. Multipotentiality in differentiation of the pineal as revealed by cell culture. Curr Top Develop Biol 1986;20:89–97.
19. Wright CD, Kesler KA, Nichols CR, et al. Primary mediastinal nonseminomatous germ cell tumors. Results of a multimodality approach. J Thorac Cardiovasc Surg 1990;99:210–217.
20. Kay PH, Wells FC, Goldstraw P. A multidisciplinary approach to primary nonseminomatous germ cell tumors of the mediastinum. Ann Thorac Surg 1987;44:578–582.
21. Dexeus FH, Logothetis CJ, Chong C, Sella A. Genetic abnormalities in men with germ cell tumors. J Urol 1988;140:80–84.
22. Dement SH, Eggleston SC, Spivac JL. Association between mediastinal germ cell tumors and hematologic malignancies: report of two cases and review of literature. Am J Surg Pathol 1985;9:23–30.
23. Nichols CR, Hoffman R, Einhorn LH, Williams SD, Wheeler LA, Garnick MB. Hematologic malignancies associated with primary mediastinal germ-cell tumors. Ann Intern Med 1985;102:603–609.
24. Bosl GJ, Geller NL, Cirrincione C, et al. Serum tumor markers in patients with metastatic germ cell tumors. A 10-year experience. Am J Med 1983;75:29–35.
25. Mencel PJ, Motzer RJ, Mazumdar M, Vlamis V, Bajorin DF, Bosl GJ. Advanced seminoma: treatment results, survival, and prognostic factors in 142 patients. J Clin Oncol 1994;12:120–126.
26. Toner GC, Geller NL, Lin SY, Bosl GJ. Extragonadal and poor risk nonseminomatous germ cell tumors. Survival and prognostic features. Cancer 1991;67:2049–2057.
27. Nichols CR, Saxman S, Williams SD, et al. Primary mediastinal nonseminomatous germ cell tumors. A modern single institution experience. Cancer 1990;65:1641–1646.
28. Kohman LJ. Approach to the diagnosis and staging of mediastinal masses. Chest 1993;103:328S–330S.
29. Mark JBD. Management of anterior mediastinal tumors. Semin Surg Oncol 1990;6:286–290.
30. Truong LD, Harris L, Mattioli C, et al. Endodermal sinus tumor of the mediastinum. Cancer 1986;58:730–739.
31. Maggi G, Giaccone G, Donadio M, et al. Thymomas. Cancer 1986;58:756–776.
32. Rosenow EC, Hurley BT. Disorders of the thymus. Arch Intern Med 1984;144:763–770.
33. Monden Y, Uyama T, Taniki T, et al. The characteristics of thymoma with myasthenia gravis: a 28 year experience. J Surg Oncol 1988;38:151–154.
34. Ulbright TM, Roth LM. Recent developments in the pathology of germ cell tumors. Semin Diagn Pathol 1987;4:304–319.
35. Cooper K, Cordon-Cardo C, Motzer RJ, et al. Blood group antigens and intermediate filaments in differentiating germ cell tumors (abstract). Proc Am Assoc Cancer Res 1989;30:226.
36. Motzer RJ, Reuter VE, Cordon-Cardo C, Bosl GJ. Blood group-related antigens in human germ cell tumors. Cancer Res 1988;48:5342–5347.
37. Bosl GJ, Ilson DH, Rodriguez E, Motzer RJ, Reuter V, Chaganti RSK. Clinical relevance of the i(12p) marker chromosome in germ cell tumors. J Natl Cancer Inst 1994;86:349–355.
38. Chaganti RSK, Rodriguez E, Bosl GJ. Cytogenetics of male germ cell tumors. Urol Clin North Am 1993;20:55–66.
39. Ahmed T, Bosl GJ, Hajdu SI. Teratoma with malignant transformation in germ cell tumors in men. Cancer 1985;56:860–863.

40. Ulbright TM, Michael H, Loehrer PJ, Donohue JP. Spindle cell tumors resected from male patients with germ cell tumors. Cancer 1990;65:148–156.
41. Hainsworth JD, Johnson DH, Greco FA. Cisplatin-based combination chemotherapy in the treatment of poorly differentiated carcinoma and poorly differentiated adenocarcinoma of unknown primary site: results of a 12-year experience. J Clin Oncol 1992;10:912–922.
42. Bosl GJ, Gluckman R, Geller NL, et al. VAB-6: an effective chemotherapy regimen for patients with germ-cell tumors. J Clin Oncol 1986;4:1493–1499.
43. Bajorin DF, Mazumdar M, Vlamis V, Motzer RJ, Bosl GJ. Factors predictive of response to platin-based chemotherapy in germ cell tumors (GCT): a multivariate analysis in 773 patients (abstract). Proc Am Soc Clin Oncol 1993;12:234.
44. Bosl GJ, Geller NL, Cirrincione C, et al. Multivariate analysis of prognostic variables in patients with metastatic testicular cancer. Cancer Res 1983;43:3403–3407.
45. Mead GM, Stenning SP, Parkinson MC, et al. The second Medical Research Council study of prognostic factors in nonseminomatous germ cell tumors. J Clin Oncol 1992;10:85–95.
46. Einhorn LH, Williams SD, Mandelbaum I, Donohue JP. Surgical resection in disseminated testicular cancer following chemotherapeutic cytoreduction. Cancer 1981;48:904–908.
47. Fox EP, Weathers T, Williams SD, et al. Outcome analysis for patients with persistent nonteratomatous germ cell tumor in postchemotherapy retroperitoneal lymph node dissections. J Clin Oncol 1993;11:1294–1299.
48. Brenner J, Vugrin D, Whitmore WF. Cytoreductive surgery for advanced nonseminomatous germ cell tumors of testis. Urology 1982;19:571–575.
49. Motzer RJ, Cooper K, Geller NL, et al. The role of ifosfamide plus cisplatin-based chemotherapy as salvage therapy for patients with refractory germ cell tumors. Cancer 1990;66:2476–2481.
50. Motzer RJ, Bosl GJ. High-dose chemotherapy for resistant germ cell tumors: recent advances and future directions. J Natl Cancer Inst 1992;84:1703–1709.
51. Nichols CR, Tricot G, Williams SD, et al. Dose intensive chemotherapy in refractory germ cell cancer: a phase I/II trial of high-dose carboplatin and etoposide with autologous bone marrow transplantation. J Clin Oncol 1989;7:932–939.
52. Einhorn EH, Weathers T, Loehrer P, Nichols C. Second line chemotherapy with vinblastine, ifosfamide, and cisplatin after initial chemotherapy with cisplatin, VP-16 and bleomycin (PVP16B) in disseminated germ cell tumors (GCT): long term followup (abstract). Proc Am Soc Clin Oncol 1992;11:196.
53. Birch R, Williams S, Cone A, et al. Prognostic factors for favorable outcome in disseminated germ cell tumors. J Clin Oncol 1986;4:400–407.
54. Medical Research Council Working Party on Testicular Tumours. Prognostic factors in advanced non-seminomatous germ-cell testicular tumours: results of a multicentre study. Report from the Medical Research Council Working Party on Testicular Tumours. Lancet 1985;1:8–11.
55. Ozols RF, Ihde D, Jacob J, Ostchega A, Linehan M, Young RC. Poor prognosis nonseminomatous testicular cancer: mature results of a randomized trial of PVeBV (high dose [HD] cisplatin [P], vinblastine [Ve], bleomycin [B], VP-16 [V]) vs PVeB (abstract). Proc Am Soc Clin Oncol 1987;6:107.
56. Ozols RF, Diesseroth AB, Javadpour N, et al. Treatment of poor prognosis non-seminomatous testicular cancer with a "high dose" platinum combination chemotherapy regimen. Cancer 1983;51:1803–1807.
57. Einhorn LH. Treatment of testicular cancer: a new and improved model. J Clin Oncol 1990;8:1777–1781.
58. Bajorin D, Katz A, Chan E, Geller N, Vogelzang N, Bosl GJ. Comparison of criteria for assigning germ cell tumor patients to "good risk" and "poor risk" studies. J Clin Oncol 1988;6:786–792.
59. Schultz SM, Einhorn LH, Conces DJJ, Williams SD, Loehrer PJ. Management of postchemotherapy residual mass in patients with advanced seminoma: Indiana University experience. J Clin Oncol 1989;7:1497–1503.
60. Logothetis CJ, Samuels ML, Selig DE, et al. Cyclic chemotherapy with cyclophosphamide, doxorubicin, and cisplatin plus vinblastine and bleomycin in advanced germinal tumors. Results with 100 patients. Am J Med 1986;81:219–228.
61. Vogelzang NJ, Raghavan D, Anderson RW, Rosai J, Levitt SH, Kennedy BJ. Mediastinal nonseminomatous germ cell tumors: the role of combined modality therapy. Ann Thorac Surg 1982;33:333–339.
62. Kuzur ME, Cobleigh MA, Greco FA, Einhorn LH, Oldham RK. Endodermal sinus tumor of the mediastinum. Cancer 1982;50:766–774.
63. Toner GC, Geller NL, Tan C, Nisselbaum J, Bosl GJ. Serum tumor marker half-life during chemotherapy allows early prediction of complete response and survival in nonseminomatous germ cell tumors. Cancer Res 1990;50:5904–5910.
64. Lange PH, Vogelzang NJ, Goldman A, Kennedy BJ, Fraley EE. Marker half-life analysis as a prognostic tool in testicular cancer. J Urol 1982;128:708–711.
65. Picozzi VJJ, Freiha FS, Hannigan JFJ, Torti FM. Prognostic significance of a decline in serum human chorionic gonadotropin levels after initial chemotherapy for advanced germ-cell carcinoma. Ann Intern Med 1984;100:183–186.
66. Horwich A, Peckham MJ. Serum tumour marker regression rate following chemotherapy for malignant teratoma. Eur J Cancer Clin Oncol 1984;20:1463–1470.
67. Vogelzang NJ, Lange PH, Goldman A, Vessela RH, Fraley EE, Kennedy BJ. Acute changes of alpha-fetoprotein and human chorionic gonadotropin during induction chemotherapy of germ cell tumors. Cancer Res 1982;42:4855–4861.
68. Thomas GM, Rider W, Dembo AJ, et al. Seminoma of the testis: results of treatment and patterns of failure after radiation therapy. Int J Radiat Oncol Biol Phys 1982;8:165–174.
69. Raghavan D, Barrett A. Mediastinal seminoma. Cancer 1980;46:1187–1191.
70. Bush SE, Martinez A, Bagshaw MA. Primary mediastinal seminoma. Cancer 1981;48:1877–1882.
71. Lee YM, Jackson SM. Primary seminoma of the mediastinum. Cancer 1985;55:450–452.
72. Kersh CR, Constable WC, Hahn SS, et al. Primary malignant extragonadal germ cell tumors. Cancer 1990;65:2681–2685.
73. Martini N, Golbey RB, Hajdu SI, Whitmore WF, Beattie EJ. Primary mediastinal germ cell tumors. Cancer 1974;33:763–768.
74. Paz-Ares L, Lianes P, Rivera F, Lopez-Brea M, Hitt R, Cortes-Funes H. Long-term results in advanced seminoma treated with cisplatin chemotherapy. Ann Oncol 1992;3(Suppl):166.
75. Jain KK, Bosl GJ, Bains MS, Whitmore WF, Golbey RB. The treatment of extragonadal seminoma. J Clin Oncol 1984;2:820–827.
76. Bosl GJ, Geller NL, Bajorin D, et al. A randomized trial of etoposide + cisplatin versus vinblastine + bleomycin + cisplatin + cyclophosphamide + dactinomycin in patients with good-prognosis germ cell tumors. J Clin Oncol 1988;6:1231–1238.
77. Bajorin DF, Sarosdy MF, Pfister DG, et al. Randomized trial of

etoposide and cisplatin versus etoposide and carboplatin in patients with good-risk germ cell tumors: a multiinstitutional study. J Clin Oncol 1993;11:598–606.
78. Logothetis CJ, Samuels ML, Selig DE, et al. Chemotherapy of extragonadal germ cell tumors. J Clin Oncol 1985;3:316–325.
79. Loehrer PJS, Birch R, Williams SD, Greco FA, Einhorn LH. Chemotherapy of metastatic seminoma: the Southeastern Cancer Study Group experience. J Clin Oncol 1987;5:1212–1220.
80. Freidman EL, Garnick MB, Stomper PC, et al. Therapeutic guidelines and results in advanced seminoma. J Clin Oncol 1985;3:1325–1332.
81. Motzer R, Bosl G, Heelan R, et al. Residual mass: an indication for further therapy in patients with advanced seminoma following systemic chemotherapy. J Clin Oncol 1987;5:1064–1070.
82. Feun LG, Samson MK, Stephens RL. Vinblastine, bleomycin, cis-diamminedichloroplatinum in disseminated extragonadal germ cell tumors. Cancer 1980;45:2543–2549.
83. Garnick MB, Canellos GP, Richie JP. Treatment and surgical staging of testicular and primary extragonadal germ cell cancer. JAMA 1983;250:1733–1741.
84. Bosl GJ, Geller NL, Vogelzang NJ, et al. Alternating cycles of etoposide plus cisplatin and VAB-6 in the treatment of poor-risk patients with germ cell tumors. J Clin Oncol 1987;5:436–440.
85. Motzer RJ, Cooper K, Geller NL, et al. Carboplatin, etoposide, and bleomycin for patients with poor-risk germ cell tumors. Cancer 1990;65:2465–2470.
86. Williams SD, Birch R, Einhorn LH, Irwin L, Greco FA, Loehrer PJ. Treatment of disseminated germ-cell tumors with cisplatin, bleomycin, and either vinblastine or etoposide. N Engl J Med 1987;316:1435–1440.
87. Ozols RF, Ihde DC, Linehan WM, Jacob J, Ostchega Y, Young RC. A randomized trial of standard chemotherapy v a high-dose chemotherapy regimen in the treatment of poor prognosis nonseminomatous germ-cell tumors. J Clin Oncol 1988;6:1031–1040.
88. Horwich A, Brada M, Nicholls J, et al. Intensive induction chemotherapy for poor risk non-seminomatous germ cell tumours. Eur J Cancer Clin Oncol 1989;25:177–184.
89. Einhorn LH, Williams S, Loehrer P, et al. Phase III study of cisplatin dose intensity in advanced germ cell tumors: a Southeastern and Southwestern Oncology Group protocol (abstract). Proc Am Soc Clin Oncol 1990;9:132.
90. Stoter G, Kaye S, Sleyfer DT, et al. Preliminary results of BEP (bleomycin, etoposide, cisplatin) versus and alternating regimen of BEP and PVB (cisplatin, vinblastine, bleomycin) in high volume metastatic (HVM) testicular nonseminomas. An EORTC study (abstract). Proc Am Soc Clin Oncol 1986;5:106.
91. Murphy BA, Motzer RJ, Bosl GJ. Chemotherapy for cisplatin-resistant germ cell tumors. Problems in Urology 1994;8:127–140.
92. Loehrer PJS, Lauer R, Roth BJ, Williams SD, Kalasinski LA, Einhorn LH. Salvage therapy in recurrent germ cell cancer: ifosfamide and cisplatin plus either vinblastine or etoposide. Ann Intern Med 1988;109:540–546.
93. Harstrick A, Schmoll HJ, Wilke H, et al. Cisplatin, etoposide, and ifosfamide salvage therapy for refractory or relapsing germ cell carcinoma. J Clin Oncol 1991;9:1549–1555.
94. Einhorn LH, Elson P, Williams SD, et al. Phase III study of cisplatin (P) plus etoposide (VP16) with either bleomycin (B) or ifosfamide (I) in advanced stage germ cell tumors (GCT): an intergroup trial (abstract). Proc Am Soc Clin Oncol 1993;12:261.
95. Lewis C, Fossa SD, Mead GM, et al. BOP/VIP: a new platinum-intensive chemotherapy regimen for poor prognosis germ cell tumours. Ann Oncol 1991;2:203–211.
96. Motzer RJ, Mazumdar M, Gulati SC, et al. Phase II trial of high-dose carboplatin and etoposide with autologous bone marrow transplantation in first-line therapy for patients with poor-risk germ cell tumors. J Natl Cancer Inst 1993;85:1828–1835.
97. Biron P, Brunat-Hentigny M, Bayle JY, et al. Cisplatin VP-16 and ifosfamide (VIC) + autologous bone marrow transplantation (ABMT) in poor prognostic nonseminomatous germ cell tumors (NSGCT) (abstract). Proc Am Soc Clin Oncol 1989;8:148.
98. Droz JP, Pico JL, Ghosn M, et al. High complete remission (CR) and survival rates in poor prognosis (PP) non seminomatous germ cell tumors (NSGCT) with high dose chemotherapy (HDCT) and autologous bone marrow transplantation (ABMT) (abstract). Proc Am Soc Clin Oncol 1989;8:130.
99. Toner GC, Panicek DM, Heelan RT, et al. Adjunctive surgery after chemotherapy for nonseminomatous germ cell tumors: recommendations for patient selection. J Clin Oncol 1990;8:1683–1694.
100. Logothetis CJ, Samuels ML, Trindade A, et al. The growing teratoma syndrome. Cancer 1982;50:1629–1635.
101. Bosl GJ, Dmitrovsky E, Reuter VE, et al. Isochromosome of the short arm of chromosome 12: clinically useful marker for male germ cell tumors. J Natl Cancer Inst 1989;81:1874–1878.
102. Motzer RJ, Rodriguez E, Reuter VE, et al. Genetic analysis as an aid in diagnosis for patients with midline carcinomas of uncertain histologies. J Natl Cancer Inst 1991;83:341–346.
103. Mukherjee AB, Murty VVVS, Rodriguez E, et al. Detection and analysis of origin of i(12p), a diagnostic marker of human germ cell tumors, by fluorescent in situ hybridization. Genes Chromosom Cancer 1991;3:300–307.
104. Dement SH. Association between mediastinal germ cell tumors and hematologic malignancies: an update. Hum Pathol 1990;21:699–703.
105. Domingo A, Romagosa V, Callis M, Vivancos P, Guionnet N, Soler J. Mediastinal germ cell tumor and acute megakaryoblastic leukemia. Ann Intern Med 1989;111:539.
106. Nichols C, Roth B, Heerema NA, et al. Hematologic neoplasia associated with primary mediastinal germ cell tumors. N Engl J Med 1990;322:1425–1429.
107. Ladanyi M, Samaniego F, Reuter VE, et al. Cytogenetic and immunohistochemical evidence for the germ cell origin of a subset of acute leukemias associated with mediastinal germ cell tumors. J Natl Cancer Inst 1990;82:221–227.
108. Gerald PS. Current concepts in genetics: sex chromosome disorders. N Engl J Med 1976;294:706–710.
109. Nichols CR, Heerema NA, Palmer C, Loehrer PJS, Williams SD, Einhorn LH. Klinefelter's syndrome associated with mediastinal germ cell neoplasms. J Clin Oncol 1987;5:1290–1294.
110. McNeil MM, Leong A, Sage RE. Primary mediastinal embryonal carcinoma in association with Klinefelter's syndrome. Cancer 1981;47:343–345.
111. Lee MW, Stephens RL. Klinefelter's syndrome and extragonadal germ cell tumors. Cancer 1987;60:1053–1055.
112. Hasle H, Jacobsen BB, Asschenfeldt P, Andersen K. Mediastinal germ cell tumour associated with Klinefelter syndrome. Eur J Pediatr 1992;151:735–739.

32

TUMORS OF THE HEART AND PERICARDIUM

Todd L. Demmy

Because of their rarities, cardiac tumors have been reported primarily by pathologic reviews, mostly from institutions that had large numbers of patient referrals. These reviews, especially those from McAllister and Fenoglio (1), defined the literature. Then, progressive improvement in medical technology increased the ability to detect and treat these tumors. The most notable improvements were the development of echocardiography to allow diagnosis, and the evolution of heart surgery to allow the removal or palliation of most cardiac neoplasms. Better treatment of non–cardiac primary malignancies also allowed more patients to survive until their tumors metastasized to the myocardium. This changed the relative incidence of these tumors from that reported previously. Also recognized was an increased incidence of benign tumors and a relative increase in the number of myxomas compared with that reported in the older literature (2). An autopsy rate for cardiac tumors of 0.28% or less was cited commonly (1). Today, the more appropriate way to report the incidence of primary cardiac tumors is by large cardiac surgical series, in which the incidence has ranged from 0.11% to 0.29% (3–5). Because of these issues, this chapter primarily reviews current reports of cardiovascular tumors. The median ending year of the compiled studies surveyed in this chapter is 1988.

OVERVIEW
HISTORY

Probably, the first report of a primary cardiac tumor was in 1559 by Columbus (6). The first diagnosis of a cardiac tumor in a living person was by Barnes in 1934, when a primary cardiac sarcoma was detected (6). The first tumors removed were an intrapericardial teratoma in 1942 and a pericardial hemangioma in 1950 (6, 7). It was not until 1951 that the first epicardial neoplasm was resected successfully by Mauer (6). In 1952, the preoperative diagnosis of a myxoma was made by Goldberg using angiocardiography (6). In 1954, the first successful intraluminal tumor excision was performed by Crafoord at the Karolinska Institute (8). During his first use of extracorporeal circulation, Crafoord successfully removed a large left atrial myxoma from a 40-year-old woman, and the patient lived until the age of 82. The following year, a similar tumor was removed from a patient suspected preoperatively of having mitral stenosis (7). These landmark cases occurred during the infancy of open heart surgery. As technology improved, the number of cardiac tumors treated surgically rose steadily.

SYMPTOMS

The symptoms of cardiac tumors are diverse and simulate typical manifestations of other cardiac maladies. The most common symptoms are those that manifest impaired cardiac performance, such as congestive heart failure or shortness of breath. Symptoms of impaired cardiac function are from myocardial replacement by tumor or from the extrinsic effects of pericardial neoplastic disease. In addition, cardiac arrhythmias or systemic emboli from intraluminal cardiac neoplasms are common. The patient also may have cardiac pain from neoplasm-induced myocardial necrosis or acute ischemia from a coronary artery tumor embolus (9).

The next most common group of symptoms are those considered "constitutional." Some of these systemic symptoms result from autoimmune disease, possibly from the alteration of serum proteins or release of tumor degradation products by the neoplasm (6). A compilation of these symptoms with their relative frequency is presented in Table 32.1. Malignant tumors and certain types of benign cardiac tumors have a higher rate of presentation with atypical chest pain. An asymptomatic presentation occurs in about 12% of patients (10). Unfortunately, there are few historical

TABLE 32.1. Symptoms and Physical Findings

Sign	Combined Series[a]	Myxoma Only[b]	Specific Cardiac Tumors[c]	Malignant Tumors[d]	Total Excluding Duplicates
Dyspnea	881	506	72	117	1576
Palpitations	662	...	...	5	667
Congestive heart failure	517	380	40	87	1024
Syncope	210	43	6	5	264
Hemoptysis	80	1	7	6	94
Embolic	75	265	...	1	340
CVA	12	28	...	0	40
Extremity ischemia	5	8	...	0	13
MI	1	0	1	1	3
Pulmonary infarction	1	0	...	0	1
Atypical chest pain	49	69	29	41	188
"Constitutional"	47	89	5	18	159
Fever	15	50	4	10	79
Fatigue	7	5	4	4	20
Weight loss	17	31	3	14	65
Night sweats	0	11	2	2	15
Murmur	38	40	1	0	79
Arrhythmia	28	47	9	4	88
Sudden death	...	...	12	3	15
Pericardial effusion	7	...	13	11	31
Paroxysmal nocturnal dyspnea	7	45	...	...	52
Cyanosis	2	...	...	...	2
SVC syndrome	1	...	1	1	3
Pericarditis	1	...	...	...	1
Dizziness	...	3	...	...	3
Pulmonary edema	...	6	...	...	6
Seizures	...	4	1	...	5
Peripheral edema	...	3	...	...	3
Pleuritis	...	1	2	...	3
Asymptomatic	12	17	19	13	61

Abbreviations. CVA, cerebral vascular accident; MI, myocardial infarction; SVC, superior vena cava syndrome.
[a]Data from Moggio et al. (3), Silverman (6), van de Wal et al. (11), Fyfe et al. (12), Mundinger et al. (24), Dapper et al. (27), Selzer et al. (46), Murphy et al. (47), Moriyama et al. (154), Sugimoto et al. (155), Guang-ying (156), Curtis et al. (157), and Verkkala et al. (158).
[b]Data from Miralles et al. (2), McGarry et al. (13), Ferrans and Roberts (14), Badui-Dergal et al. (15), Hanson et al. (17), Bulkley and Hutchins (18), Larsson et al. (19), Saint John Sutton (22), Blondeau (29), Lazzara et al. (37), Bortolotti et al. (38), Fang et al. (40), Shimono et al. (48), Burke et al. (76), and Mohandas et al. (149).
[c]Data from Curtsinger et al. (16), Burke et al. (76), Brizard et al. (79), Reece et al. (80), Geha et al. (94), Burke et al. (98), Herrmann et al. (104), Roller et al. (116), and Burke and Virmani (119).
[d]Data from Miralles et al. (2), Fyfe et al. (12), Curtsinger et al. (16), Mundinger et al. (24), Dapper et al. (27), Burke et al. (98), Putnam et al. (100), Herrmann et al. (104), Roller et al. (116), and Burke and Virmani (119).

clues and no pathognomonic symptoms or signs for cardiac tumors. One higher risk group is women older than age 40; these women have a 4 times greater rate of primary cardiac tumors (10). The duration of symptoms ranges from 4 to 93 months (median, 15 months) for benign tumors and an average of 5.2 months for malignant neoplasms (2, 10–19).

PHYSICAL FINDINGS

Physical findings in cardiac tumors are also related to problems with cardiac function or the systemic complications related to these neoplasms. Pericardial disease may yield signs of tamponade or constriction, or may be relatively subtle with a pericardial friction rub being the only abnormal finding (20). One of the most common manifestations of a cardiac tumor is atrial fibrillation, atrial flutter, or, if atrial-ventricular conduction tissue is invaded, heart block (20, 21). Besides the pericardial and myocardial physical manifestations, endocardial tumors potentially cause valve obstruction or insufficiency and have characteristic murmurs. This insufficiency may cause rales or other signs of congestive heart failure (20). Approximately 20% to 40% of patients with obstruction of their atrial ventricular valves have a late diastolic sound or "tumor plop" (10, 22). Some of these heart murmurs wax or wane with the effect of gravity on the intraluminal tumor. A pulsus alternans may be present (20). Finally, physical examination may reveal signs of embolic disease, such as retinal infarcts as well as limb, visceral, or central nervous system ischemia from larger tumor emboli. These findings are similar to the embolic complications seen in endocarditis. Other physical findings are also listed in Table 32.1.

LABORATORY FINDINGS

Laboratory tests usually are not helpful in establishing the diagnosis of a cardiac tumor. Approximately half of adults or children in two series had some abnormal finding on their chest roentgenogram (22, 23). Some of these findings were an enlarged left atrium, enlarged ventricle, generalized cardiomegaly, diversion of blood to the upper lobes, and right or left atrial calcifications. The electrocardiogram (EKG) commonly shows an atrial arrhythmia. More often, there is evidence of atrial enlargement or nonspecific electrocardiographic wave segment (ST) changes. If there is valvular dysfunction from cardiac tumors, there may be evidence of right or left ventricular hypertrophy (22). Examination of the patient's blood may show anemia, particularly if the tumor is causing hemolysis. There may be an increase in the erythrocyte sedimentation rate or an alteration in the serum or plasma protein content (22).

Echocardiography is by far the most common screening test used to diagnosis a cardiac tumor (24). This study is accomplished using either a transthoracic or transesophageal technique. Transesophageal echocardiography seems to have advantages over the transthoracic technique, particularly in identifying extracardiac tumors or masses in the upper right atrium (25). Also, the transesophageal technique more clearly identifies thrombi or the point of attachment of atrial tumors.

Angiocardiography was the primary method of diagnosis between its first demonstration of a myxoma in 1952 and the advent of two-dimensional echocardiography (26). Angiocardiography, or coronary angiography, is not needed to supplement a satisfactory echocardiographic study. However, this study is required to confirm the clinical suspicion of concomitant cardiac problems, such as coronary artery disease (27).

To a lesser extent, computed tomographic (CT) scanning has become more popular, particularly as scanning speed has increased. Magnetic resonance imaging (MRI) scans offer the advantage of limiting radiation exposure. They also allow for use of a wide variety of imaging planes and tissue density enhancement by changing the weighting of relaxation times (28).

Comparing the different diagnostic modalities, echocardiography was the most popular in the series reported in this chapter. The relative usage rates and sensitivities are listed in Table 32.2. Although early reports of false-negative rates were as high as 16% to 33% for angiocardiography and 8% for echocardiography, the sensitivities shown in Table 32.2 are similar to those in a recent study comparing radiographic techniques for the demonstration of heart tumors (22, 24, 29). In that study investigators also found a usage rate of 80% for echocardiogram, 58% for angiocardiogram, 7% for CT scan, and 2.5% for MRI in patients with cardiac tumors. Although MRI has a higher false-negative rate as a screening test, it is considered helpful, particularly if the tumor is extracardiac (24). In one study MRI found an extrinsic mass in four of seven patients in whom a transthoracic echocardiogram suggested a left atrial mass (two hiatal hernias, one bronchogenic cyst, and one ectatic aorta) (28). The MRI also is helpful in diagnosing the tissue densities found in myxomas, lipomas, or vascular tumors (28). No technique differentiates neoplasm from thrombus well (24).

DIFFERENTIAL DIAGNOSIS

Before echocardiography, primary cardiac tumors were diagnosed clinically in only 8% to 37% of patients (12, 18, 22, 30). Most cases were misdiagnosed as mitral valve disease, and less commonly as congestive heart failure, infectious endocarditis, collagen vascular disease, atrial fibrillation, myocarditis, pericardial effusion, pulmonary embolus, stroke, or other intracardiac defects (18). Before 1970 reports describe an accurate preoperative diagnosis in only 53% of cases; after 1970 this rate rose to 94% for patients with primary cardiac tumors (10). Without the aid of contemporary imaging technology, accurate preoperative diagnosis would still be unusual; however, certain findings should lead a physician to suspect intracavitary tumor rather than a disease like mitral stenosis. These include a lack of history of rheumatic fever, a change in position that alters the symptoms or heart murmur of a patient, syncope, a rapid increase in the patient's symptomatology, or marked cardiac failure refractory to medical management (7). One should consider a cardiac tumor such as

TABLE 32.2. Diagnostic Modalities

MODALITY	UTILIZATION[a] PATIENTS RESPONDING/ TOTAL PATIENTS (%)	SENSITIVITY PATIENTS RESPONDING/ TOTAL PATIENTS (%)
Echocardiography	289/617 (46.8)	73/75 (97)
Angiocardiography	243/617 (39.4)	57/74 (77)
Both	178/617 (28.8)	21/21 (100)
MRI	5/617 (0.8)	
CT scan	25/617 (4.1)	
Intraoperative	10/617 (1.6)	

Data from Moggio et al. (3), Nassar et al.(4), Silverman (6), McGarry et al. (13), Badui-Dergal et al. (15), Hanson et al. (17), Larsson et al. (19), Saint John Sutton et al. (22), Dapper et al. (27), Castells et al. (36), Lazzara et al. (37), Bortolotti et al. (38), Fang et al. (40), Snyder et al. (44), Murphy et al. (47), Shimono et al. (48), Mosodorf et al. (102), Awang and Sallehuddin (159), Carranza-Rebollar et al. (160), and Chen (161).
[a]Reflects results of older studies. Echocardiography is predominant in more recent reports.

myxoma in patients who develop spontaneous atrial flutter before the age of 20 (27). Also, it is important to consider that larger cardiac tumors tend to cause symptoms by obstruction, and smaller tumors are usually asymptomatic, except when they embolize (27). If the diagnosis of an intracardiac neoplasm is considered, the other differential diagnoses that may simulate a cardiac tumor should be excluded. These include luminal, tumorlike masses such as thrombi, ectopic calcification, or endocarditis vegetations. Also, extracardiac causes, such as intrathoracic hematomas, vascular compressions, hiatal hernias, or pericardial tumors, are possible (31).

TREATMENT AND RESULTS

The treatment of most primary cardiac tumors is surgical. Surgery typically requires the use of cardiopulmonary bypass for all intraluminal and mural cardiac tumors and possibly for some epicardial and pericardial tumors. Separate cannulation of the superior and inferior vena cavae allows total diversion of blood from the heart. This technique yields a relatively bloodless field in all cardiac chambers once the heart is cross-clamped and arrested with cardioplegia (Fig. 32.1) (26). Although details of the various surgical techniques are beyond the scope of this chapter, the different approaches are guided by careful preoperative planning and occasionally by intraoperative imaging such as transesophageal echocardiography. Basically, the surgical technique involves removing all the obstructing cardiac tumor with as large a margin as ap-

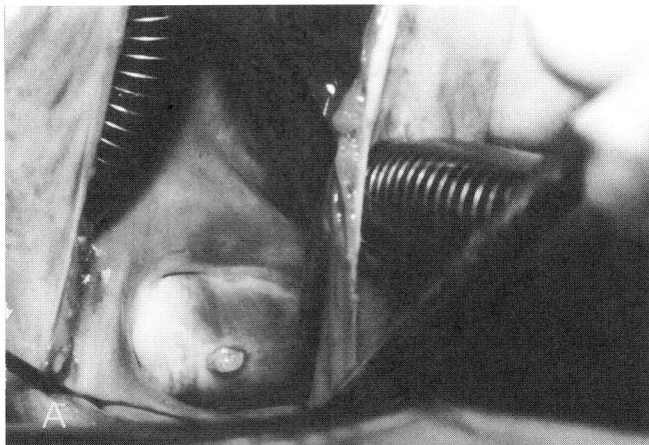
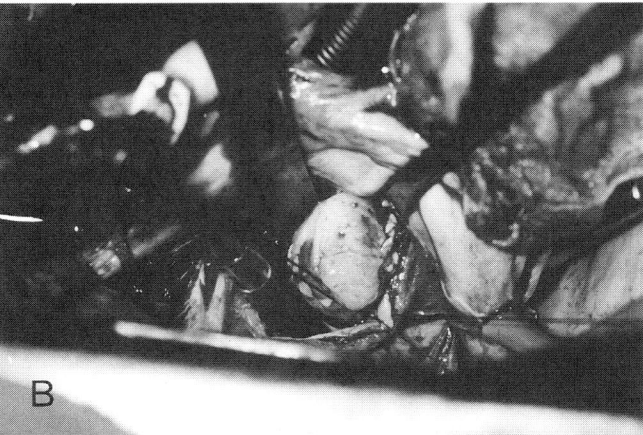

FIGURE 32.1. Operative exposure. A. Intraoperative photograph showing a right atriotomy and split caval cannulation. The smaller end of a dumbbell shaped bi-atrial myxoma was penetrating the fossa ovalis. B. Intraoperative photograph of a myxoma diagnosed by studies in Figure 32.2 delivered through a left atriotomy after excising the tumor from atrial septum.

propriate or possible for the particular histologic type. Because most myxomas do not penetrate deeply beneath the endocardium, a narrow surgical margin is probably adequate. For inoperable tumors, long-term survival is enhanced by "debulking" certain benign tumors, and short-term palliation is obtained by debridement of certain malignant tumors (10). More recent technical advances allow treatment of larger cardiac tumors that were unresectable previously. One such technique involves explantation of the entire heart, removal of tumor on the "bench," and autotransplantation of the reconstructed heart (26). Cardiomyoplasty and orthotopic cardiac transplantation also have been used to treat patients who could not survive the loss of functioning heart muscle required to remove the entire tumor (32, 33). The addition of chemotherapy and radiation therapy have been tried for patients with malignant cardiac tumors; unfortunately, the results were disappointing (10, 34).

Results of surgical therapy are summarized in Table 32.3. Data show a rather consistent mortality rate for benign disease, i.e., 5% for both perioperative mortality and late mortality, with surveillance lasting as long as 20 years. For most of the late fatalities, death was not caused by tumor recurrences. In fact, the recurrence rate was approximately 1% to 2%, with the majority coming from the myxoma group. Deaths occurred in nearly 100% of patients with malignant cardiac tumors, with most fatalities occurring within the first 6 to 18 months. Whereas many of these patients received postoperative adjuvant radiation or chemotherapy with little benefit, promising advances in treatment of extracardiac soft tissue sarcomas warrant further attempts at treatment of this group with an otherwise dismal prognosis (35).

Some operations performed to treat a cardiac tumor are extended to treat an additional cardiac problem, such as coronary disease, or to repair damage done by the cardiac neoplasm. Of 13 reported series, the incidence of concomitant operations ranged from 3% to 36%, with an average of 11.4% (2–5, 10, 17, 22, 24, 34, 36–39). These operations included 21 mitral valve replacements, 15 coronary artery bypasses, 12 mitral valve repairs with or without annuloplasty, 6 closures of an atrial septal defect, 5 tricuspid valve replacements, and 2 aortic valve replacements.

SPECIFIC PRIMARY CARDIAC TUMORS

Primary cardiac tumors are either benign and malignant; the benign category is further subdivided into those common in adults and those common in children. Lastly, metastatic, valvular, and pericardial tumors are considered.

BENIGN ADULT CARDIAC TUMORS

A compilation of benign cardiac tumors appears in Table 32.4. This table is divided into single institution reports of all primary cardiac tumors and other series that describe only myxomas, only pediatric cases, and neoplasms other than myxomas. Cardiac myxomas are the most common of all tumors described, making up more than 90% of the cases listed in Table 32.4. Although the myxoma is the most common adult tumor, rhabdomyomas are reported more than twice as often as other pediatric cardiac tumors. Whereas myxomas occur primarily in the atrium, nonmyxomas usually arise in the ventricles (29). Information on the reported cardiac sites of origin in specific benign and malignant cardiac neoplasms is compiled in Table 32.5.

MYXOMA: SPORADIC

Cardiac myxomas are found most commonly in adult females with a median age at presentation of 49 years. In series from Oriental nations, the female to male ratio is 2:1; whereas in western countries the ratio is reported to be 3:1 (40). Myxoma incidence peaks during the 40- to 59-year age group; in one large study only eight patients younger than 20 years and three older than 90 years of age were diagnosed with these tumors (41). Although up to 25% of these tumors were reported to occur in the right atrium, the relative ratio found in this review was 10 times greater for left atrial myxomas (6). These tumors usually occur without any predisposing genetic disorder and are considered sporadic cases. In a recent study, multiple cardiac myxomas occurred in 16% of the patients (37).

SYMPTOMATOLOGY

The symptoms common to patients with myxoma are summarized in Table 32.1. These complaints are often subtle or misleading, and consequently patients in one series went up to 14 years without diagnosis (10). Symptoms are related primarily to one of three

TABLE 32.3. Results

RESULT	COMBINED SERIES[a] NO. OF PATIENTS/ TOTAL PATIENTS(%)	MYXOMA ONLY[b] NO. OF PATIENTS/ TOTAL PATIENTS(%)
Hospital or operative mortality	30/595 (4.3%)	29/662 (4.4%)
Later death, benign	10/232 (4.3%)	27/540 (5%)
Mean follow-up time	4.5–15 years	5.5–20 years
Late death, malignant	88/100 (88%)	...
Mean follow-up time	Less than 3–48 mo	...
Benign recurrences	3/232 (1.3%)	15/540 (2.2%)

[a]Data from Miralles et al. (2), Moggio et al (3), Silverman (6), Larrieu et al. (10), Badui-Dergal, et al. (15), Bauer et al. (34), Murphy et al. (46), Chen et al. (52), Mosodorf (102), Poole et al. (135), Sugimoto et al. (155), Awang and Sallehuddin (159), Yin (162), and Hake et al. (163).
[b]Data from Nassar et al. (4), McGarry et al. (13), Ferrans and Roberts (14), Hanson, et al. (17), Bulkley and Hutchins (18), Larsson et al. (19), Saint John Sutton et al. (22), Blondeau (29), Nomeir et al. (30), Castells et al. (36), Lazzara et al. (37), Bortolotti et al. (38), Fang et al. (40), Shimono et al. (47), Mishra et al. (90), Carranza-Rebollar et al. (160), and Hake et al. (163).

TABLE 32.4. Numbers of Patients with Benign Cardiac Tumors

	SERIES OF ALL PRIMARY TUMORS[a]	SERIES OF MYXOMA TUMORS[c]	SERIES OF BENIGN TUMORS OTHER THAN MYXOMA[d]	PEDIATRIC TUMORS[e]	TOTAL EXCLUDING DUPLICATES
Myxoma	1831	988	...	6	2304
Fibroma	57	...	17	9	73
Rhabdomyoma	42	...	13	25	72
Lipoma	36	...	15	1	42
Papillary fibroelastoma	24	...	3	...	25
Purkinje cell tumor	17	...	...	...	17
Hamartoma	16	...	5	...	17
Hemangioma	16	...	8	5	22
Teratoma	4	...	...	7	11
Mesothelioma of AV node	2	...	...	...	2
Lymphangioma	2	...	...	...	2
Lipofibroma	2	...	...	...	2
Hydated cyst	2	...	...	...	2
Thyroid	2	...	2	...	2
Lipomatous hypertrophy	1	...	1	...	2
Paraganglioma	1	...	36	...	37
Neurofibroma	1	...	...	...	1
Granular cell tumor	1	...	...	...	1
Pseudomyxoma	1	...	...	...	1
Varix	1	...	...	...	1
Glomangioma	1	...	...	...	1
Unknown	3	...	...	1	4
Total	2046	988	100	54	2643
Male:female ratio	635:948	303:542	...	10:13	...
Age range	46–54[b]	32–55[b]	49[b]	1 day–16 years[f]	...

[a] Data from Miralles et al. (2), Moggio et al. (3), Wiatrowska et al. (5), Silverman (6), Larrieu et al.(1), van de Wal et al. (11), Abbott et al. (21), Mundinger et al. (24), Cooley (26), Dapper et al. (27), Blondeau (29), Bauer et al. (34), Molina et al. (41), Selzer et al. (46), Murphy et al. (47), Tazelar et al. (50), Chen et al. (52), Mosodorf et al. (102), Poole et al. (135), Moriyama et al. (154), Sugimoto et al. (155), Guang-ying (156), Curtis et al. (157), Awang and Sallehuddin (159), Yin (162), Hake et al. (163), Sutsch et al. (164), and Zie (165).
[b] Represents reported median ages.
[c] Data from Nassar et al. (4), Wiatrowska et al. (5), McGarry et al. (13), Ferrans and Roberts (14), Hanson et al. (17), Bulkley and Hutchins (18), Larsson et al. (19), Saint John Sutton et al. (22), Blondeau (29), Nomeir et al. (30), Castells et al. (36), Lazzara et al. (37), Bortolotti et al. (38), Shimono et al. (48), Ashar and van Hoeven (68), Mishra et al. (90), Bisel et al. (138), Carranza-Rebollar et al. (160), and Chen (161).
[d] Data from Wiatrowska et al. (5), Blondeau (29), Reece et al. (80), Jebara et al. (81), Orringer et al. (83), and Carbi et al. (166).
[e] Data from Roux et al. (23), Arcinegas et al. (78), Bertolini et al. (86), Schmaltz and Apitz (87), Curtis et al. (157), and Biancaniello et al. (167).
[f] Represents actual age range.

major categories: the hemodynamic effects of the tumor, embolism, or constitutional symptoms (19). The hemodynamic effects are caused by valve obstruction or destruction by the tumor. Symptoms of dyspnea occur when pulmonary venous blood entering the left heart is obstructed by a left atrial tumor. Right atrial myxomas also cause cardiomegaly, shortness of breath, and even massive pulmonary emboli (42–44). Systemic embolism occurs from tumors of any size without associated obstructive cardiac symptomatology. The symptoms of pulmonary hypertension result from chronic pulmonary artery occlusion by right heart myxomatous emboli and mitral valve obstruction by left atrial cardiac myxomas. Finally, cardiac myxomas produce generalized systemic effects, i.e., "constitutional" symptoms (45). Theories explaining systemic symptoms postulate production of active substances by the neoplasm, microembolism of small tumor fragments from the myxoma, or a systemic autoimmune reaction to shed myxoma cells (43). Finally, the patient may be symptomatic from cardiac arrhythmias, such as atrial fibrillation, that improve after removing the tumor (4, 40).

Physical findings. The physical findings in patients with cardiac myxoma are typically as unhelpful as the patient's history in making the diagnosis. Signs mimic a wide variety of mitral valve diseases. Manifestations of peripheral or pulmonary edema are present occasionally (17). Heart sounds may disclose a late diastolic tumor plop of a mass obstructing the mitral

TABLE 32.5. Sites of Tumors

SERIES	SITE OF TUMOR					TOTAL	MALE:FEMALE RATIO	MEAN AGE (YEARS)
	LA	RA	RV	LV	COMBINATION/ COMPLEX			
Combined series[a]	190	35	9	20	1	255	635:948	46–54
Myxoma only[b]	1506	117	22	13	29	1687	303:542	49
Nonmyxoma[c]	4	7	3	9	4	27	36:33	21–54
Rhabdomyoma[d]	0	2	3	8	7	20	14:3	5.3 months
Hemangioma[e]	0	2	4	3	2	11	16:17	23
Fibroma[f]	0	4	1	0	0	5	21:15	3.3–14.2
Lipoma[g]	1	2	1	3	1	8	6:6	49–60
Papillary fibroelastoma[h]	0	0	0	1	6	7	4:3	7
Hamartoma[i]	0	0	0	1	0	1	4:9	12.6 months
Angiosarcoma[j]	3	43	4	1	10	61	22:8	44–53
Leiomyosarcoma[k]	16	3	1	1	3	24	3:2	18–26
Osteosarcoma[l]	9	...	...	...	...	9	3:6	38
Myosarcoma[m]	3	0	0	0	0	3	1:3	...
Fibrosarcoma[n]	1	1	0	4	0	6	3:4	26–37
MFH[o]	4	1	1	0	0	6	5:3	29.5–43
Synovial sarcoma[p]	1	0	1	0	0	2	1:1	30
Neurofibrosarcoma[q]	0	1	0	0	0	1	1:1	48
Undifferentiated sarcoma[r]	6	8	5	3	5	27	10:10	5–37
Total	1763	222	51	56	72	2144	...	...

Abbreviations. MFH, malignant fibrous histiocytoma; LV, left atrium; RA, right atrium; RV, right ventricle; LV, left ventricle; Combination/ Complex, tumor involving cardiac valve or multiple chambers.
[a]Data from Silverman (6), Abbott (21), Selzer et al. (46), Chen et al. (52), Cham et al. (54), Mosodorf et al. (102), Poole (135), Mohandas (149), and Sugimoto et al. (155).
[b]Data from Miralles et al. (2), Moggio et al. (3), Nassar et al. (4), Wiatrowska et al. (5), McGarry et al. (13), Ferrans and Roberts (14), Hanson et al. (17), Bulkley and Hutchins (18), Larsson et al. (19), Saint John Sutton et al. (22), Dapper et al. (27), Nomeir et al. (30), Castells et al. (36), Lazzara et al. (37), Bortolotti et al. (38), Fang et al. (40), Shimono et al. (48), Tazelar et al. (50), Garah (64), Ashar and van Hoeven (68), Mosodorf et al. (102), Guang-ying (156), Carranza-Robollar et al. (160), Chen (161), and Loire and Delaye (168).
[c]Data from Miralles et al. (2), Wiatrowska et al. (5), Dapper et al. (37), and Reece et al. (80).
[d]Data from Burke and Virmani (89).
[e]Data from Burke et al. (76) and Brizard et al. (79).
[f]Data from McAllister and Fenoglio (1).
[g]Data from Murphy et al. (47) and Tazelar et al. (50).
[h]Data from Tazelar et al. (50).
[j]Data from Burke et al. (98), Putnam et al. (100), and Herrmann et al. (104).
[k]Data from Fyfe et al. (12) and Putnam et al. (100).
[l]Data from Burke et al. (98).
[m]Data from Burke et al. (98) and Burke and Virmani (119).
[n]Data from Burke et al. (98).
[o]Data from Murphy et al. (47) and Burke et al. (98).
[p]Data from Burke et al. (98).
[q]Data from Burke et al. (98).
[r]Data from Dapper et al. (27), Murphy et al. (47), and Burke et al. (98).

valve. In addition, there are occasional physical findings of hypertrophic subaortic stenosis, mitral regurgitation, or pulmonary hypertension. If the tumor is right sided, there may be a delayed pulmonary systolic ejection murmur from obstruction of the right ventricular outflow tract (44). A pulse examination may show diminished peripheral circulation that leads to an arteriogram and embolectomy. Any embolic material should be sent for pathologic examination. However, absence of myxoma on pathologic examination does not exclude the presence of the cardiac myxoma. Tumor emboli are common and occurred in 40% of patients in one report (6).

NONDIAGNOSTIC LABORATORY TESTS

Several routine laboratory observations frequently are abnormal in patients with cardiac myxomas; however, they are not specific enough to suggest the diagnosis (22). Routine chest roentgenogram findings are abnormal as commonly as 87% of the time (19, 40). Twenty-five percent of patients with right atrial myxomas have polycythemia from a right to left shunt through a patent foramen ovale (22). An elevated erythrocyte sedimentation rate, anemia, or abnormal serum protein fractions, specifically elevated γ-globulin, occur in 33% to 50% of patients (13, 17, 38, 46). Patients undergoing right and left heart catheterization have elevations of pulmonary artery pressures, pulmonary capillary wedge pressures, and mean transvalvular gradients (17). In a series of 39 patients, pulmonary hypertension occurred in 70% (47). This tumor-related pulmonary hypertension can be quite severe, with 70% of patients having pulmonary vascular resistances greater than 600 dyne-second/cm^5 (46).

CONFIRMATORY TESTS AND DIFFERENTIAL DIAGNOSIS

The invention of diagnostic imaging changed the clinical picture of atrial myxomas from a disease with a correct premortem diagnosis rate of only 50% to one in which most or all preoperative patients have the correct diagnosis (14, 17, 37). Preoperative diagnostic accuracy for cardiac myxomas increased from 33% before 1970 to more than 87% after 1970 (2, 29). Diagnostic tests of choice are usually echocardiography and angiocardiography (Table 32.2 and Fig. 32.2). Coronary or cerebral angiography is recommended if patients have concomitant cardiac symptoms, such as angina or symptoms of cerebrovascular disease (19). Although echocardiography usually leads to a correct preoperative diagnosis, it still is unusual to have a correct clinical suspicion before this test. For instance, the diagnosis of myxoma was suspected in only 8% of the patients in one series before the imaging studies were obtained (40). The major incorrect diagnoses were any type of mitral valve disease, infectious endocarditis, and cardiomyopathy (45). Patients' clinical findings depend on the sites of their myxomas. Left atrial myxomas are confused most commonly with mitral stenosis, and right atrial myxomas can simulate tricuspid stenosis. Right ventricular myxomas may cause right ventricular hypertrophy (20, 42, 44). Also, tricuspid valves may be more prone to damage by right atrial myxomas and their "wrecking ball" effect (20). Finally, patients with right atrial and ventricular myxomas tend to be younger than patients with left atrial myxomas because right heart tumors are more commonly familial or syndrome related (38).

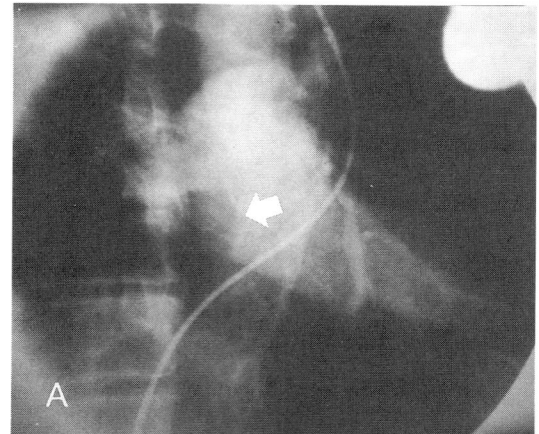

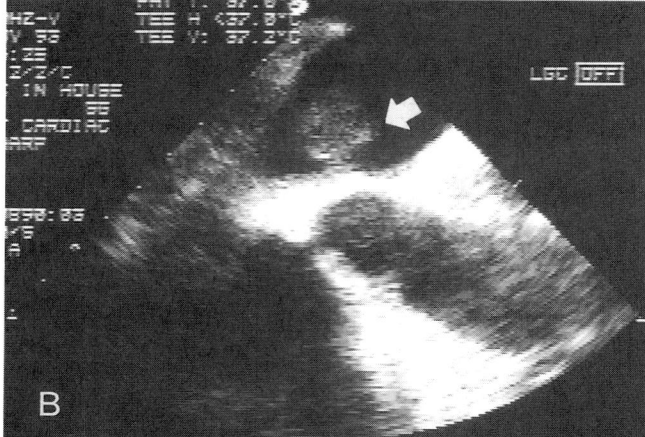

FIGURE 32.2. Preoperative diagnostic imaging. **A.** Angiocardiogram showing contrast in the left atrium, left ventricle, and aortic outflow tract. Note the outline of an atrial myxoma (*white arrow*). **B.** Transesophageal echocardiogram showing the same tumor within the left atrium. Note the tumor mass (*white arrow*). (Courtesy of Darla Hess, M.D., University of Missouri, Columbia.)

HISTOPATHOLOGY

Cardiac myxomas comprise more than 50% of benign heart tumors in pathologic reviews; their sizes range from less than 1 cm to more than 15 cm (mean size, 5.6 cm) (26). Their growth rate probably is rapid (17). Seventy-five percent to 88% of these tumors are pedunculated with a narrow 1- to 2-cm base, and 76% originate near the fossa ovalis (17, 18, 22, 26). Grossly, they are categorized into two types: tumors with a gelatinous appearance and others that resemble a round, firm mass (Fig. 32.3) (48). Microscopy may show extreme calcification or findings that occasionally are similar to those of thrombi (45, 49). A varied cellularity of eosinophilic vascular myxoid stroma contains polygonal or stellate cells with lymphocytes and plasma cell infiltrates (14, 50). Electron microscopy shows myxoma cells, smooth

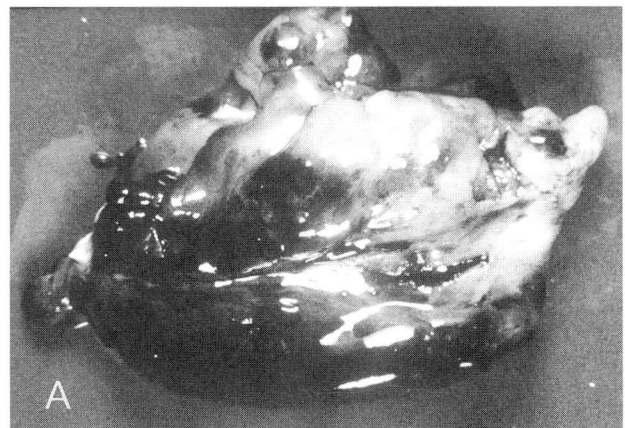

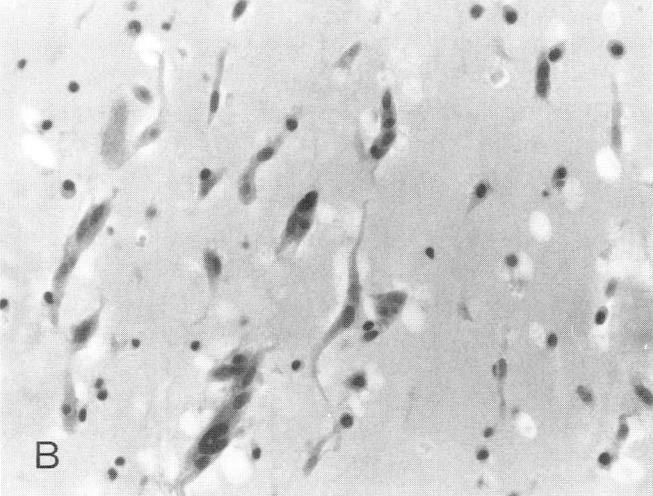

FIGURE 32.3. Myxoma pathology. A. Gross appearance of a friable atrial myxoma. B. Photomicrograph of an atrial myxoma at 2000× magnification, showing prominent myxoid stroma with interspersed round to stellate primitive-appearing mesenchymal cells, as well as scattered mononuclear inflammatory cells. (Courtesy of Ann Havey, M.D., University of Missouri, Columbia.)

muscle cells, endothelial cells, macrophages, and cytoplasmic filaments. The origin of these tumors is thought to be from a multipotential mesenchymal cell similar to that seen in the umbilical cord. This hypothesis is supported by the finding of rests of similar type cells in the hearts of 80% of infants less than 1 month old (51). It is not clear what may trigger the neoplastic proliferation of these cells. For instance, there is a well-documented case of a tumor arising at the site of an atrial septal puncture used to perform balloon dilation of the mitral valve in a 74-year-old patient (39). This puncture led to the development of a typical 3 × 2 cm myxoma within 12 months. Histologically, these tumors rarely penetrate deeper than the endocardium. This fact accounts for the high degree of success in resections with only a moderate margin of normal tissue.

TREATMENT AND RESULTS

Treatment of atrial myxomas is surgical excision. Different investigators report similar good results with their particular preferences for the conduct of the operation. Some recommend incising the atrial septum through a right atriotomy, and others open only the left atrium and excise the myxoma accordingly. Regardless of the technique, most surgical series have a 4% to 5% operative mortality and a similar late mortality for survivors of the operation (Table 32.3). If the patient is not a candidate for cardiac surgery, death is expected within 2 years of the time that congestive heart failure develops (36). Death occurs from arrhythmias (sudden death) or congestive heart failure (52).

After this operation, patients have an average 1-cm reduction in the size of their left atrium by echocardiography (38). Postoperative complications typically are atrial fibrillation or flutter. On occasion, patients have low cardiac output resulting from problems with myocardial protection or associated cardiac conditions (37). Also, when atrial excision is extensive, a permanent pacemaker may be necessary to restore normal atrial-ventricular synchrony. A pacemaker was needed in 16% of patients in one study (37).

After surgery, cases were followed for up to 20 years with a greater than 90% survival (38). For those patients who died, the cause usually was not related to recurrent tumor. A simple excision of these tumors with a small "button" of atrium around the stalk of the tumor was enough to prevent recurrence (6). If recurrence happened, it was more likely to occur in patients with multiple myxomas (33%), myxoma syndrome (21%), or familial myxomas (10%) rather than in patients with sporadic myxoma (1% to 3%) (36). Recurrence was attributed to inadequate resection, multicentricity, embolization, and implantation of tumor shed during excision (17).

Besides recurrence at the area of resection or a different cardiac site, the myxoma may spread to another part of the body as a benign metastatic lesion. In two studies these metastases had histologically benign features, occurred up to 10 years after the original cardiac tumor removal, and were reported most commonly in the brain (37, 53).

In summary, the finding of an atrial myxoma by echocardiography or other test is an indication for urgent surgery because of potential life-threatening complications. Patients require long-term surveillance because of the incidence of recurrence. Although most recurrences surface within the first 5 years, longer reported intervals justify more protracted follow-up (54). Associated familial or hereditary syndromes should be considered, particularly in patients with multiple-chamber myxomas. Therefore, testing of family members is appropriate.

SYNDROMES AND FAMILIAL CARDIAC MYXOMAS

The tendency of myxomas to run in families was described in several studies (37, 55–62). Patients with the syndrome of atrial myxoma tend to present at a younger age than do those with the sporadic form, 25 compared with 56, respectively, and the female to male ratio is 1.8:1 compared with 2.7:1, respectively (57). Whereas the sporadic cases are uniformly atrial tumors, patients with the syndrome have a 13% incidence of myxomas outside the atrium, usually in the ventricular cavities. The myxoma syndrome, first described by Atherton in 1980, was then called the nevi, atrial myxoma, mucinosis, endocrine (NAME) overactivity syndrome (55, 56). It also was called "Lamb syndrome" (for lentigines, atrial myxomas, mucocutaneous blue nevi) (56). More recently, it was called Carney's complex, an autosomal dominant syndrome in which patients have myxomas in multiple areas besides the heart as well as spotty pigmentation and endocrine overactivity (55). This complex also was called Swiss syndrome (58). Along with cardiac myxomas, patients with Carney's complex have mammary or cutaneous myxomas, a variety of pigmented skin lesions, and overactivity of the adrenal or testicular glands, or pituitary tumors (55). Approximately half of the children of patients with this syndrome will have the disorder (55). In general, 72% of patients with Carney's complex will have one or more atrial myxomas (56).

Familial occurrences have been noted in patients without Carney's complex. In the series by von Gelder et al. (59), there were 17 families afflicted with atrial myxomas since the first family was identified in 1971. Patients typically are younger, with a mean age of 27 years, and 22% have multicentric tumors that are located in the left atrium only 61% of the time. They also have a 10% recurrence rate (59).

Generally, patients should be suspected as having one of these syndromes if they present with myxomas in any site other than the left atrium. Patients should be tested for signs of endocrine, specifically adrenal, overactivity, even though not clinically manifested. If cases with familial myxomas are followed prospectively, two thirds are expected to have disease recur as early as 4 years after resection (64).

Patients with familial or multiple atrial myxomas may require multiple tumor excisions or need subsequent operations to deal with recurrences; however, their mortality is not higher than patients with similar risk factors who have sporadic atrial myxomas. Because these patients have a propensity for tumors outside the typical left atrial location, care should be taken to explore all potential tumor sites during the operation and to search for all possible tumors identified preoperatively. Intraoperative transesophageal echocardiography is invaluable in this search.

Intraoperative echocardiography makes it possible to find tumors not visualized by standard preoperative testing. In addition, echocardiography should be used to observe patients for recurrence postoperatively, and family members should be screened for possible asymptomatic atrial myxoma. In a recent study, 10.5% of isolated atrial myxoma patients without a known familial syndrome had family members with an undiagnosed myxoma (64). Although this finding is interesting, it may not be sufficient to warrant screening all family members of patients with myxomas. Patients who are younger, have atypical heart chamber myxomas, or recurrences of previous myxomas are statistically more likely to need greater surveillance of their families and themselves.

Generally, patients with familial atrial myxomas have history, symptoms, and physical findings similar to those of the sporadic myxomas. In addition, they or their family members may have a history or symptoms suggestive of a myxoma syndrome. For instance, one patient presented with a history of three operations for recurrent left ventricular myxomas during the preceding 6 years (60). Patients with myxomas that have a tendency to recur or run in families are diagnosed by methods similar to those used for sporadic atrial myxomas. However, examination of the myxoma DNA pattern by flow cytometry identifies a higher incidence of abnormal patterns for recurrent tumors than in those with nonrecurrent tumors (65). This work was duplicated by other investigators who found that myxoma tumors with a greater proliferative cell fraction had a higher risk for recurrence or embolus. Also, an aneuploid pattern on the flow cytometry study predicted recurrence (62).

Recurrent myxomas need to be differentiated from other tumors with myxoid elements that behave quite differently. These include histologically malignant tumors, such as myxosarcoma or fibromyxosarcoma; tumors that are histologically benign but behave like malignancies, such as angiomyxoma and fibromyxoma; and those that are histologically benign but tend to be aggressive and recurrent, such as a myxoma with mitral valve invasion, pulmonary vein invasion, multiple sites of myocardial involvement, or extracardiac spread to the brain or elsewhere (66).

LIPOMA AND LIPOMATOUS HYPERTROPHY

Lipomas of the heart have been reported as commonly as 10% of primary cardiac tumors (67). They are rare and only 63 such tumors were reported, with an age range from birth to 77 years (67). There is no sex predilection, and most of the patients are asymptomatic (67). Symptoms, if present, are caused by enlargement of the tumor, thus decreasing ventricular function and leading to fatigue, dyspnea, and syncope (67). Although lipomas as small as 14 mm were reported, they have grown to 4.8 kg and led to sudden death (68). Approximately half of the tumors are subepicardial, with the remainder divided evenly among tumors within the myocardium and those that are subendocardial. The epicardial tumors tend to be larger (67).

Lipomas typically arise in the left ventricle and the right atrium, and appear histologically like lipomas elsewhere in the body (6). Imaging studies with CT and MRI scans are uniformly accurate and can occasionally predict whether coronary arteries are involved, a finding that means that the tumor is less likely to be resectable (67).

Treatment of these tumors is surgical with good expectation for recovery and long-term survival. This entity is different from the more common lipomatous hypertrophy of the heart. The latter entity was described in a series of 91 patients found to have atrial septa larger than 2 cm by fatty infiltration (69). In this study, as the thickness of the atrial septum enlarged, the risk of atrial arrhythmias increased. However, because the average age of these patients and the associated coronary artery disease also increased, the fatty infiltration may not be causal. This tumor does not represent a true neoplasm and does not require surgical therapy.

PAPILLARY FIBROELASTOMA

Papillary fibroelastomas occur in the majority of patients with primary cardiac valvular tumors and are responsible for more than 70% of these cases (70). They have an incidence at autopsy of approximately 7% to 8% of all cardiac tumors. Patients with these tumors usually present later in life at ages between 21 and 77 years (70–74). The most common clinical presentation for these patients is an embolic event, such as a stroke or transient ischemic attack, that leads to a test that discloses the cardiac tumor. Many times the patient is asymptomatic, and the tumor is found incidentally. Papillary fibroelastomas originating in the mitral valve have the lowest association with symptoms (73). Less commonly, patients have symptoms of chest tightness, angina, or sudden death (70, 73).

Physically, these patients have normal cardiac auscultatory and other physical findings except for signs of systemic embolization. The gross pathology of these tumors shows multiple fronds resembling a sea anemone (71, 72). Histologically, the fronds has a dense central core of collagen surrounded by a peripheral myxomatous layer, and a layer of hyperplastic endothelial cells. These tumors are small, rarely being larger than 4 cm. Because they are found in areas of previous valvular disease, one investigator thought that the etiology of this tumor was chronic trauma to the endocardium (72).

Others think these tumors represent true neoplasms (71, 73). In one recent series, 32% of the cases had papillary fibroelastomas not related to cardiac valvular tissue (74). The relative incidence is highest in the aortic valve, followed by the tricuspid, pulmonary, and mitral valve, each of which has a frequency approximately half that of the aortic valve (71). Fifteen percent of the time, the tumor occurred in one of the other chambers (71). Because of their similarity to normal chordae tendineae, and occasionally to other cardiac tumors, they were called fibromas, myxomas, or, occasionally, giant Lambl's excrescences (71).

The treatment of these neoplasms is surgical excision because of the increased risk of embolic complications associated with them. Many times, concomitant valvular repair or replacement is necessary. Long-term prognosis after adequate surgical excision is excellent (71).

HEMANGIOMA

Hemangioma is the most common vascular tumor of the heart (6). In some reports this type makes up 10% of benign lesions (76). Symptoms associated with hemangiomas are related primarily to the location of the tumor. If the tumor is close to the epicardium, there is a greater chance of pericardial effusion and symptoms (76). Of all benign tumors, hemangiomas are the most likely to be accompanied by pericardial effusion (77). If the tumor is smaller and located within the ventricle, it tends to be asymptomatic. Symptoms of hemangioma can range from no signs to symptoms of sudden death (76). These symptoms are similar to those of specific cardiac tumors (Table 32.1). In one series approximately 40% of the patients were asymptomatic (76).

Physical findings may be present if the tumor is obstructing cardiac blood flow. In general, there are no specific laboratory findings to suggest hemangioma. Seventy-four percent of patients with cardiac hemangioma have an abnormal chest roentgenogram finding at the time of the initial evaluation (78).

Because of the lack of diagnostic features for hemangiomas, many patients were undiagnosed before their operations. The incidence of correct diagnoses before surgery ranged from 0% to 34% (76, 78). Of common diagnostic tests, coronary angiography has a 90% chance of disclosing the tumor, whereas echocardiography has 81% chance of disclosing the mass, and cardioangiography only a 33% sensitivity (78). Because of the ability of these tumors to enhance with CT or MRI imaging, both tests are recommended. Of interest, one such tumor was detected while the patient was in utero (76).

Hemangiomas are located in any chamber, occurring in the lateral wall of the left ventricle in 21% of the patients, anterior right ventricle in 21%, multiple occurrences in 30%, and septa in 17% (76, 78). These tumors have variable histologic appearances. The cavernous type, showing dilated thin wall vessels, is the most common (6, 76). The next most common varieties are the capillary type, with nests of smaller capillaries, and the arteriovenous hemangioma, which has dysplastic arteries and veins (76). These neoplasms may be difficult to distinguish from low-grade angiosarcomas, and indices such as lack of mitotic activity, a solid growth pattern, and necrosis within the tumor predict benign behavior (76). These tumors can occur in the Kasabach-Merritt syndrome, which is diagnosed by multiple systemic hemangiomas, recurrent thrombocytopenia, and a consumptive coagulopathy (79). Treatment of this tumor is surgical exploration with resection when possible (80). Patients who have only a partial resection frequently have a good long-term prognosis without evidence of recurrence (76, 78). Although radiation may be useful in other sites, it is not effective for cardiac hemangiomas (6). Approximately half of the patients who undergo resection will require cardiopulmonary bypass, and approximately half will have a total resection. Of the remaining patients, approximately 40% will undergo incomplete resection, and 60% will be unresectable. It is important to avoid bleeding from the tumor bed when resecting these tumors because postoperative arterial venous fistulas have been reported when hemostasis was incomplete (79).

PHEOCHROMOCYTOMAS

Pheochromocytomas, often known as paragangliomas, can occur solely in the chest and represent only 1% to 2% of all such cases (81). Cardiac pheochromocytomas comprise less than 2% of this small thoracic paraganglioma group. To date, 30 to 40 cases of cardiac pheochromocytoma have been reported; patients present most commonly with hypertension, headache, palpitations, sweating, and a duration of symptoms of from 2 months to 22 years. There was no sex predilection, and the mean age of patients with this tumor was 37.4 years. In this large review, 5 patients were found to have a concomitant chemodectoma of the carotid body. A diagnosis was confirmed with angiocardiography in 7 patients, echocardiography in 5, and CT scan in only 1 patient. An attempt to find a tumor in the abdomen was required in 17 patients. In 81% of patients, a metaiodo-benzylguanidine (mIBG) scan positively identified the tumor in the heart (82). Along with the findings of the tests described, there are increased levels of serum catecholamines or vanillylmandelic acid in the urine.

Two thirds of these tumors occurred in the left atrium, with the remainder in the atrial septum or the anterior surface of the heart. The gross pathology is that of a soft, fleshy, easily compressed mass that is closely related to the coronary arteries and that intimately involves the atrial wall. The cell origin is most likely a branchial arch–derived structure such as a great vessel or coronary artery paraganglium (83). As in other reports of extraadrenal pheochromocytomas, there is a 15% to 20% incidence of multiple tumors. This disease is the cause of 0.1% to 0.01% of hypertension in patients (83). In 25 patients who were offered operations, 20 were cured and the remainder died of hemorrhagic or other postoperative complications.

OTHER ADULT BENIGN CARDIAC TUMORS

Other unusually rare tumors are neurofibroma, granular cell tumor, or Lambl's excrescence (6, 84, 85). This neurofibroma is an extremely rare tumor with only one case found in this recent review of cardiac tumors. This case was a 4 × 4 cm solid mass in the left ventrical apex of a male patient. It was removed successfully with cardiopulmonary bypass and did not recur (84).

Granular cell tumors have a neuroendocrine origin by histologic staining and electron microscopic findings. The noncardiac form of this tumor is found most frequently in the tongue. These tumors may be asymptomatic, but they were found in the perineural conduction tissue of patients who died of sudden death. They usually are unifocal but sometimes are multifocal; fewer than 2% of granular cell tumors are malignant (four reported cases) (85). Usually, the benign tumors are found in atrial or epicardial tissue.

Lambl's excrescence is a papillary lesion that can resemble myxoma of the aortic valve in adults or myxoma of the tricuspid valve in children. Rarely, this tumor can cause valve dysfunction and require surgical therapy (6). Generally, this finding was a curiosity in previous autopsy series of primary cardiac tumors.

BENIGN CARDIAC TUMORS IN CHILDREN

Cardiac tumors were found in 0.08% of all pediatric patients and 0.027% of pediatric autopsies (78, 86). Considerations regarding diagnostic imaging, physical findings, and treatment are generally the same as for adult tumors. Depending on the age of the child, symptoms are difficult to obtain; 42% of children are asymptomatic (87). Pediatric patients usually present with signs of rhythm disturbance, cardiac outflow obstruction causing CHF, or cyanosis from blood shunting through a patent foramen ovalis (86). Many childhood cardiac tumors arise from the interventricular septum (78).

RHABDOMYOMA

Rhabdomyomas are the most common childhood cardiac neoplasm described in recent reviews (6, 41, 46, 48, 78, 80, 88, 89). These tumors occur in young children, two thirds of whom are under the age of 3 years (6, 78). The mean age of these children is 5 months, and up to 40% have tuberous sclerosis. The oldest patient with such a tumor was 26 years of age (41). There is a male predominance, and many of the patients have recurrent tachyarrhythmias that relate to symptoms such as sudden death. They also present with CHF and cardiac murmurs (90). Because most patients are quite young, the primary symptom usually is failure to thrive; diagnoses are made with a combination of physical examination and echocardiography (78). There may be cardiomegaly, irregular cardiac rates, or ejection murmurs in these children if there are obstructions to ventricular outflow (6, 88).

The histopathology of rhabdomyomas suggests a hamartoma of atypical Purkinje-type cells (48, 89). Therefore, rhabdomyomas are considered to be hamartomas more often than true neoplasms. They are grouped into three categories: those associated with tuberous sclerosis, those that are congenital, and those that are sporadic (89). Patients with tumors associated with tuberous sclerosis have a poor prognosis, and most die from arrhythmias within 6 months of diagnosis. Those of congenital origin are associated with other cardiac defects such as hypoplastic left heart syndrome, transposition of the great arteries, ventricular septal defect, or endocardial fibroelastosis. This group also has a high 6-month mortality (89). The sporadic type of rhabdomyoma has a better prognosis, with a larger number of these children eligible for surgical excision. Because these tumors are hamartomas, there have been reports of spontaneous resolution. Patients with tuberous sclerosis have associated findings that include familial transmission, mental retardation, convulsions, skin lesions, and other hamartomatous nodules in the brain, kidney, pancreas, and sebaceous glands (78). Typically, these tumors are multicentric and therefore are difficult to remove (6).

The treatment of rhabdomyomas causing severe cardiac compromise is surgery. Aggressive surgical therapy is recommended at a young age before patients suffer complications of ventricular outflow obstruction or recurrent tachyarrhythmias (Fig. 32.4). The nonoperative mortality is 60% by 1 year (80). For the patients who underwent surgery, there was an approximate 75% survival (89).

FIBROMA

Fibromas are pediatric tumors in 83% of reported cases, and 25% of the primary cardiac tumors in children are fibromas (91). Presently, there are at least 95 reported cases; the average age at presentation was 4.3 years (45, 80, 92), a statistically significantly higher age than patients with rhabdomyoma (80). The first accurate case description was in 1955 by Luschka (93, 94). Seventy percent of the cases have symptoms (6, 78), and these usually relate to congestive heart failure (91). Fibromas are associated with sudden death from supraventricular or ventricular tachycardias, which occur in 26% to 30% of patients.

Problems with diagnoses of these tumors are encountered frequently. In a recent study, only 7% of preoperative patients were diagnosed correctly (94). For instance, one of the few surviving adults with this problem is a 31-year-old man who was misdiagnosed for several years with mitral valve disease (93). He underwent the first successful partial excision as an adult.

The histopathology of fibromas is usually that of fibrous stroma with calcification. The tumors are solitary, and multiple fibromas are reported only rarely (80). Besides being unifocal, the tumors often are intramural and arise either from free wall, interventricular septum, or both (91). The tumor displaces, but does

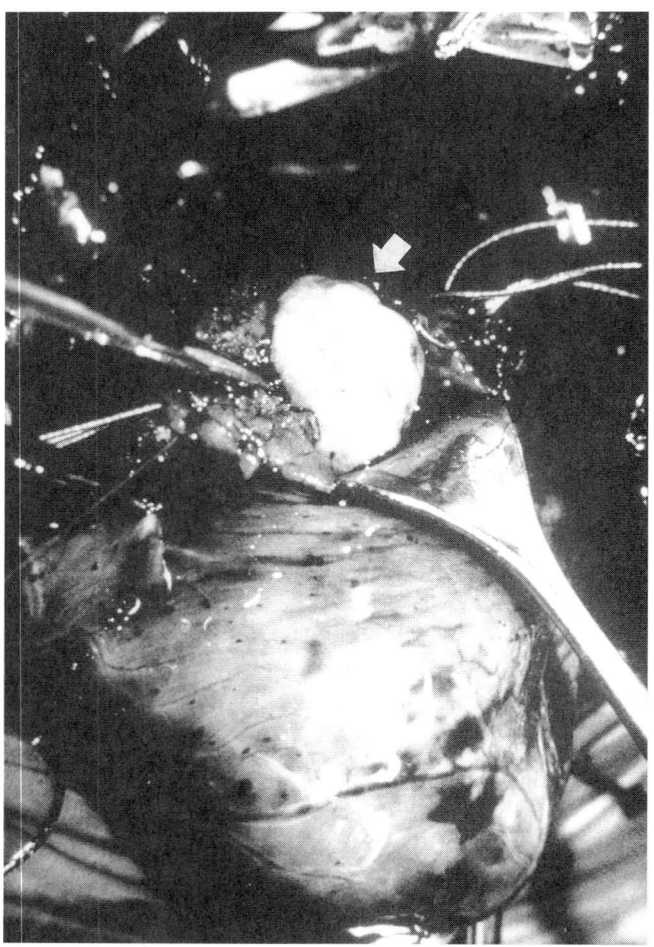

FIGURE 32.4. Rhabdomyoma. Photograph of right ventricle in neonate with outflow tract opened. Note the rhabdomyoma obstructing the ventricular outflow tract (*white arrow*). (Courtesy of Jack Curtis, M.D., University of Missouri, Columbia.)

not replace, the cardiac tissue, making excision somewhat easier. Their origin is thought to be of mesenchymal origin (94). In some instances the fibroma is associated with the so-called Gorlin syndrome. This syndrome is associated with nevoid basal cell carcinoma, neurofibromatosis, tuberous sclerosis, familial myxoma, characteristic facies, ocular hypertelorism, bifid ribs, and unilateral renal agenesis. Eighty-nine percent of the diagnoses are made before the age of 12 and 38% before the age of 1 year. It is an autosomal dominant syndrome with complete penetrance but variable expressibility. The most frequent signs in newborns are bifid ribs, vertebral abnormalities, and a large head (95).

Treatment of this tumor is surgical, and many of the tumors can be enucleated (78, 91). If total excision is not possible, partial excision is indicated. In a large series, excision was attempted in 41 cases, and 30 were successful (92). Results of surgery are poor for patients with huge biventricular masses, severe congestive heart failure, or recurrent ventricular tachyarrhythmias. In patients with congestive heart failure or arrhythmias, death is inevitable without resection, thus surgery should be attempted. At the time of operation, every attempt should be made to remove the tumor completely. Patients who survive surgery have done well long term (92).

TERATOMA

Teratomas are rare cardiac tumors: only 12 cases reported (26, 96). All but two of these cases were in children. All occurred in the right heart or interventricular septum. Their histopathology is similar to that of teratomas in other parts of the body, demonstrating elements from embryonic mesoderm, endoderm, and ectoderm. Although these tumors can attain a size of 4.5 cm and cause cardiac obstruction, the usual cause of mortality and morbidity is fatal arrhythmias (26, 48, 96). Treatment of teratomas is surgical resection, and recurrence has not been reported. The prognosis is satisfactory even if incompletely resected (26, 41, 96).

MESOTHELIOMA OF THE ATRIOVENTRICULAR NODE

Mesothelioma of the atrioventricular (AV) node is an uncommon neoplasm described as the "smallest cardiac tumor that can lead to sudden death" (6). Most were compiled in earlier reports in which there was a slight female predominance. More than 50% of the patients were younger than 5 years old (1). Most patients with this problem died and were found to have small tumors in the region of their atrioventricular node (1, 6, 41). These patients had varying degrees of AV conduction block for which AV cardiac pacing was required.

The gross pathologic findings of these tumors were poorly circumscribed nodules in the atrial septum. Microscopically, there were nests of polygonal cells in a dense fibrous stroma (1). Even with cardiac pacing, many patients died of ventricular fibrillation that was attributed to accessory conduction pathways. Because of this, patients who have this problem probably should undergo treatment with antiarrhythmic medication or have electrophysiologic studies. Resection of these small tumors is not indicated because of the permanent heart block that would result (6).

LYMPHANGIOMA

Lymphangioma is one of the rarest primary benign tumors, with only three reported cases. This tumor was first reported in 1911 in a 10-year-old boy with a 5 × 3 cm left atrial tumor mass (97). Histopathology showed mature mesenchymal elements. Other lymphangiomas present during childhood and develop in areas of primitive lymph sacs. Only one tumor was removed successfully, and the patient was symptom free on follow-up 5 years later (97).

PRIMARY CARDIAC MALIGNANCIES

Primary cardiac malignancies have accounted for approximately 17% of cardiac neoplasms in pathologic series, and the rate of malignancy in surgically excised cardiac tumors is approximately 10% (6, 29, 41). A compilation of malignant primary cardiac tumors found in this review is shown in Table 32.6. Angiosarcoma is the most common primary malignant tumor; malignant tumors are extremely rare in the pediatric population.

Symptoms of primary malignant tumors are shown in Table 32.1. As with other primary malignant tumors, dyspnea and symptoms of congestive heart failure are common because of the obstructive nature of these neoplasms. There also is a slightly higher rate of atypical chest pain in patients with primary cardiac malignancies. Other typical findings in the preoperative evaluation of these patients include cardiomegaly in more than 50%, pericardial effusion in 21%, lung nodules in 13%, and phrenic nerve paralysis in 3% (98). Also, 50% of these patients have an abnormal EKG interpretation, with sinus arrhythmia, decreased voltage, and right ventricular hypertrophy being common (98). Physical findings and definitive diagnostic studies in these patients are similar to those described in benign cardiac tumors. Of the definitive tests, echocardiography yields a diagnosis of a mass in 70% of cases (98). A pericardial effusion is present in 20% of cases.

These malignancies tend to spread by direct extension, by lymphatics to mediastinal lymph nodes, or hematogenously to other organs (6). Imaging of thoracic structures, notably the lungs, is important to ex-

TABLE 32.6. Malignant Primary Tumors

	ALL PRIMARY TUMORS[a]	SINGLE SERIES[b]	PEDIATRIC PRIMARY TUMORS[c]	TOTAL
Angiosarcoma	74	6	...	80
Fibrosarcoma	36	...	...	36
Rhabdomyosarcoma	27	...	...	2
Malignant fibrous histiocytoma	20	...	...	20
Leiomyosarcoma	20	10	...	30
Myxosarcoma (malignant myxoma)	18	...	...	18
Sarcoma (NOS)	18	...	...	18
Lymphoma	10	...	...	10
Osteosarcoma	10	...	...	10
Liposarcoma	7	...	...	7
Mesothelioma	8	...	...	8
Synovial sarcoma	5	...	...	5
Spindle cell sarcoma	4	...	...	4
Fibromyxosarcoma	3	...	...	3
Thymoma	2	...	...	2
Neurofibrosarcoma	1	...	...	1
Malignant teratoma	1	...	1	2
Round cell sarcoma	1	...	...	1
Mesenchymal sarcoma	1	...	...	1
Reticulum cell sarcoma	1	...	...	1
Malignant histiocytoma	1	...	...	1
Endothelioblastoma	1	...	...	1
Immunocytoma	1	...	...	1
Angioendothelioma	1	...	...	1
Hemangiosarcoma	1	...	1	2
Small cellular sarcoma	...	...	1	1
Total	272	16	3	291

Notes. Male to female ratio of patients in all series, 53:43. Mean age of patients in all series, 39.
For *All Primary Tumors* series, data from Lazzara et al. (37), Attum et al. (66), Burke et al. (98), Putnam et al. (100), and Verkkala et al. (158).
For *Single* series, data from Fyfe et al. (12), Herrmann et al. (104), Burke (119), and Volk et al. (132). For *Pediatric Primary Tumors* series, data from Burke et al. (98) and Putnam et al. (100).
Abbreviations. NOS, not otherwise specified.

clude metastatic disease. In fact, 26% of patients with primary cardiac malignancy have metastases to the pulmonary parenchyma at the time of diagnosis (41). Sarcomas are the most common malignancy, and 80% of patients have distant metastases when diagnosed (6). These sites of metastases from a series of 31 patients were: lung, 19; lymph nodes, 3; pleural, 2; chest wall, 3; bone, 4; liver, 4; skin, 3; spleen, 1; testes, 1; kidney, 1; and adrenal, 1.

TREATMENT

The optimal treatment of cardiac malignancies may be categorized by their presentations. For small, localized, solid cardiac malignancies without evidence of metastases, complete surgical resection may be curative. Coronary angiography may be helpful before such a resection to determine the tumor's blood supply. For other tumors that are sensitive to chemotherapy and have undergone a potentially curative resection, adjuvant treatment is considered. These tumors are angiosarcoma, undifferentiated sarcoma, myxosarcoma, rhabdomyosarcoma, osteogenic sarcoma, leiomyosarcoma, and liposarcoma. Adjuvant therapy is important for rhabdomyosarcoma, which seems to metastasize particularly early (99). For patients with distant metastases, resections of the primary malignant cardiac tumors are unlikely to extend the patient's survival and generally are not recommended. If a neoplasm cannot be resected totally, tumor debridement may provide effective palliation if the malignancy is causing congestive heart failure from intraluminal obstruction. Several studies had up to a 75% complete resection rate for malignant cardiac tumors. The remaining 25% were partially resected or underwent only biopsy (2, 41, 46, 98, 99, 100). Adjuvant therapy included chemotherapy and, occasionally, radiation therapy in more than half of patients who had undergone resection (98).

Chemotherapy for cardiac sarcomas was based on combined agent programs such as doxorubicin, vindesine, dacarbazine, cyclophosphamide, and cisplatin (99, 101). Other regimens included the combination of doxorubicin, actinomycin D, methotrexate, cisplatin, and dacarbazine (98). Postoperative radiotherapy is considered for some cardiac tumors. Although radiation to the heart is avoided because of its high (30%) incidence of constrictive pericarditis, one study reported patients with prolonged survival (2, 99). The dosage of the radiation was in the range of 25 Gy. Radiation and chemotherapy can be initial therapy for primary cardiac lymphoma (99). Systemic chemotherapy is the treatment of choice for primary cardiac malignancy that has metastasized. There is one case in which the primary cardiac sarcoma and its metastases responded completely but recurred after 16 months (101).

Unfortunately, results even with aggressive treatment are still poor. As noted in Table 32.3, there is an almost 90% long-term mortality rate after resection of cardiac malignancies. Findings correlated with improved survival are the lack of histologic necrosis in the malignancy, the ability of the patient to undergo surgery, chemotherapy, or radiation therapy, and the location of the primary cardiac malignancy within the left heart rather the right heart (98). The presence of relatively low numbers of mitoses (fewer than 10 mitoses per high power field), and either medical or surgical treatments of the tumor are the major predictors of 1-year survival by multivariate analysis (98).

The majority of primary cardiac malignancies occur in the left atrium with the exception of angiosarcoma, which has a predilection for the right atrium (Table 32.5). In addition, angiosarcomas have a male predominance, and the remaining tumors have equal sex distribution.

Tumors in the left heart may yield symptoms earlier and thus lead to an earlier diagnosis and an improved survival (98). The ability to perform a complete resection leads to a statistically significantly improved 24-month median survival compared with an 11-month survival for unresectable patients (100). In that particular study, adjuvant chemotherapy did not influence survival. Also, cell type may affect prognosis. One report showed a 2.14-year survival with angiosarcoma versus a 0.75-year survival with fibrosarcoma (29).

In summary, surgery is the treatment of choice for patients with primary cardiac malignancy if possible; however, few studies show a median survival longer than 6 months. The cause of death is cardiac failure from progressive tumor growth or postoperative complications (98, 100). Two-year survivors are quite rare, and data showing improved survival with adjuvant chemotherapy and radiation are anecdotal and not found in larger descriptive series (102). Nevertheless, there are few data on the response of cardiac malignancy to newer chemotherapeutic regimens that were effective in other soft tissue sarcomas (35). Therefore, many investigators continue to recommend a multimodality treatment approach for patients with cardiac malignancy (2, 41, 46, 98, 100, 101).

ANGIOSARCOMA

Angiosarcoma was described first in 1888 and is the most frequent primary malignant cardiac tumor (80). There is an 80% occurrence rate in the right atrium, a male predominance, and a mean patient age of 40 (103). The tumor is less common in surgical series because it usually is unresectable by the time of diagnosis (50). The symptoms of this tumor are related to a bloody pericardial effusion, right-sided heart failure, or pleuritic chest pain. Cough, weakness, and fever are also common presenting symptoms (80, 103–105). There is an increased incidence of blood flow obstruction or extracardiac invasion in almost half of the patients. Approximately one fourth of the patients have a hemopericardium or pericardial spread of the tumor. Anemia occurs in some patients (104). Preoperative chest roentgenograms commonly show cardiomegaly, and other laboratory and radiographic tests demonstrate metastases in 89% of the patients. The most common sites are lung (75%), liver (35%), lymph nodes (17%), bone (17%), adrenal glands (8%), central nervous system (24%), and spleen (16%) (103). The ability of this tumor to enhance on CT or MRI scan secured a diagnosis in half of the patients in a recent study (Fig. 32.5) (104). This diagnosis can be confirmed in the operating room with biopsy or excision of the primary tumor. Because of improved surgical and imaging techniques, 70% of the diagnoses since 1986 were made before death.

Pathology of this tumor reveals a hemorrhagic tumor that often replaces the right atrium (103). Histology can be confusing and ranges from a pattern that looks benign (like a regular hemangioma), to a pattern of vascular spindle cell elements so malignant in appearance that it can be confused with other sarcomas (103). Many times, there is a sinusoidal pattern in the arrangement of vascular channels. The benign hemangioma with which this can be confused is the histiocytoid type (103). Commonly, there are cutaneous metastases by this tumor.

Optimal treatment is surgical excision, which is possible for only approximately 50% of patients (103). For those on whom surgery was attempted unsuccessfully, survival was only 4.2 months from the onset of symptoms (103). In this series, patients in whom surgery was attempted sustained a 33% operative mortality rate. For the patients who survived their operation, life expectancy increased to approximately 10 months. The majority of patients received radiation therapy with or without chemotherapy postoperatively. Chemotherapy improved survival in one series (80).

There was one 36-month patient survival with resection and adjuvant radiation therapy (104). In addition, there was a patient with a complete primary tumor response from 60 Gy (small volume) of radiation therapy for an unresectable angiosarcoma. When this patient developed pulmonary metastases, combined agent chemotherapy with vincristine, doxorubicin, platinum, actinomycin D, and cyclophosphamide was added and yielded a 20-month survival, the second longest for a patient with this tumor. For the radiation therapy, a 45- to 50-Gy dose was recommended for an extended field, with upwards of 60 Gy for smaller volumes (105). The prognosis for patients with angiosarcoma is poor. Causes of death include pulmonary hemorrhage, thoracic metastases, and hemopericardium (104). Anecdotal reports of increased survival may warrant aggressive treatment with multimodality therapy in selected patients.

FIBROSARCOMA AND MALIGNANT FIBROUS HISTIOCYTOMA

Although they have histologic features that allow them to be distinguished, fibrosarcoma and malignant fibrous histiocytoma (MFH) often are considered together because of their probable common cell origin and uniformly poor prognosis. In a recent study, ages of patients ranged from 3 to 76 years, 83% were women, and 75% had surgical treatment. Fibrosarcomas typically present in middle-aged women (49 years) with symptoms or physical findings suggesting cardiac disease, such as murmurs, atypical chest pain, or congestive heart failure (75). Fibrosarcomas also cause generalized symptoms of cough, weakness, and fever. They are locally invasive and lead to tumor emboli (80). These tumors can arise in any chamber, but they typically occur in the left atrium or interatrial septum. They are closely associated with mitral valve structures. Therefore, they typically are not diagnosed outside of the operating room (1, 75). The histopathology

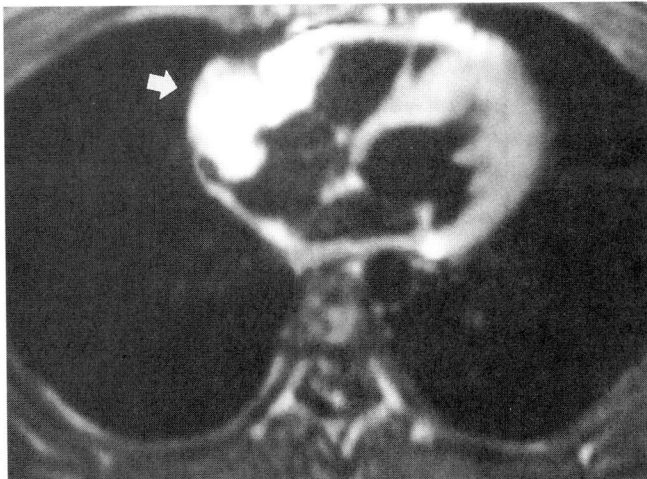

FIGURE 32.5. MRI of right atrial angiosarcoma. Note the vascular involvement by the tumor (*white arrow*). (From Churchill RJ. CT of the heart. In: Haaga JR, ed. Computed tomography of the whole body. 3rd ed. St. Louis: Mosby, 1994:838.)

of fibrosarcoma and MFH are similar, with the differentiation based on the presence of giant cells and a certain pattern of spindle cells in the latter (1). Grossly, the tumors are soft, white, and have an appearance of "fish flesh" from hemorrhage and necrosis (48). Although usually rare, this tumor represented approximately 25% of the primary cardiac malignancies in one report (106).

Treatment of fibrosarcomas is surgical. Typically, there is a 33% or greater incidence of metastases at the time of presentation (75). Even if the tumor is resected successfully, the patient usually dies of metastatic disease within 6 to 8 months (75, 107). Radiation and chemotherapy were tried in 50% of postoperative patients, and the results were inconsistent to poor (75). One patient received good palliation from an unresectable multiloculated MFH with a radiation dose of 5580 cGy (100 cGy doses over 6 weeks) using shrinking complex customized fields. After the tumor recurred at 15 months, the patient received a partial response to salvage chemotherapy consisting of etoposide, ifosfamide, and mesna (75).

RHABDOMYOSARCOMA

Rhabdomyosarcoma is the third most common malignant primary tumor of the heart. In one series, approximately 46 tumors were reported, and only 25% occurred in patients less than 20 years old (108). Typically, patients present with symptoms, such as cough, fever, and fatigue, that suggest a generalized malignancy more than a cardiac problem (1, 109). Approximately 50% of the patients have an abnormal cardiac murmur, and almost all patients have cardiomegaly on chest roentgenograms. Tumors may be demonstrated by echocardiography as well as by MRI, and there does not appear to be a propensity for occurrence in any one chamber (1). Histologically, this tumor has spindle cells that appear straplike and have cross-striations (48). There is usually pleomorphism and anaplasia. There also can be contractile elements on electron microscopy. Grossly, the tumor is nodular, soft, and necrotic (1, 48, 109). Treatment of this tumor is surgical excision whenever possible. Many times, because of their extensive involvement of ventricular myocardium, resections are not possible, and the diagnoses are established with open or transvenous biopsy techniques (41, 108, 109). Two studies have reported a favorable response with a combination chemotherapy using vincristine, actinomycin D, and cyclophosphamide. There was one complete echocardiographic regression of the tumor after the first course of chemotherapy, with remission of symptoms for 7 months and survival of 11 months (109). Other studies reported using a combination of 35 Gy of radiation with chemotherapy (108). Despite these interventions, prognosis is generally poor, and many patients die within the first year from progressive local disease.

MALIGNANT MYXOMA (MYXOSARCOMA)

Malignant myxomas represent approximately 6% of primary malignant tumors. Patients' ages ranged from 16 to 65 years (110). These tumors resemble benign myxomas; however, they have a propensity to metastasize early to multiple sites. Although "benign" myxomas can metastasize, malignant myxomas do so much earlier, usually at the time of diagnosis (51). In addition, myxosarcomas have aggressive local traits uncharacteristic of benign cardiac myxomas. Surgery offers the best palliation. For cases in which the malignant myxoma was resected, patients died $3\frac{1}{2}$ and 5 years later; without resection, the patients died within 2 months. In these few patients, postoperative chemotherapy was ineffective (41).

LEIOMYOSARCOMA

Leiomyosarcoma is another rare tumor that can lead to prolonged symptoms of chest pain, cough, and great vessel obstruction such as jugular venous distention and pulmonary artery occlusion (80). Patients develop cachexia and have a cardiac murmur. When the ventricular outflow is obstructed, there are findings of ventricular hypertrophy by EKG and cardiomegaly by chest roentgenogram (12, 23). Only 30% to 44% of leiomyosarcomas were diagnosed before the patients' death, typically during an operation (12, 111). These tumors can grow quite large, and there often are diagnostic findings on CT scan, MRI, and even displacement of the esophagus on barium swallow examinations (12, 111). The neoplasms have an increased prevalence for the left atrium, occurring there 70% of the time. The right ventricle is the next most common site (30%) (112). Histopathologic findings reveal spindle cells, and smooth muscle origin is confirmed by special stains or electron microscopy (112). Treatment of this tumor is surgery; however, long-term prognosis is poor because of death from local recurrence and occasionally from metastases (12, 113, 114). Although death can be rapid after attempted surgical excision, some investigators find no use for adjuvant radiation or chemotherapy (114). However, favorable responses were obtained in two patients using combination chemotherapy that included doxorubicin, dacarbazine, ifosfamide, etoposide, and carboplatin (113). One patient received chemotherapy after an incomplete resection, and the other after a 5-month tumor recurrence. Each achieved a 2-year survival. This survival compares favorably with that of patients with similar scenarios, in whom death usually occurred in less than 1 year (113).

MALIGNANT LYMPHOMA

Malignant lymphoma occurs as a primary cardiac tumor in only 1% of cardiac neoplasms (16). The typical age ranges between 3 and 80, and it has equal sex distribution. This is in contrast to metastatic heart involvement that occurs in 16% to 20% of extracardiac lymphomas. It is increasing in frequency in elderly or immunocompromised patients, who tend to have high-grade B cell lymphomas. Typical presentations of primary cardiac lymphomas include congestive heart failure, hemopericardium, superior vena cava syndrome, arrhythmias, and EKG changes. For establishing the diagnosis, MRI scanning appears to have higher accuracy than CT scanning (115). The usual preoperative diagnostic tests, such as echocardiography, are useful in demonstrating the tumor and may show a pericardial effusion that can yield malignant cells if tapped. In reviews of this unusual tumor, only 13% of cases had the diagnosis made before their death. The histopathology of these tumors is similar to reports of other extracardiac lymphomas. This tumor has a near equal distribution among every cardiac chamber (16). Occasionally, the diagnosis can be made by endomyocardial biopsy using a transvenous bioptome (116). The size of the tumor masses can vary, but a 7-cm lymphoma in the right atrium was reported (117).

Treatment involved the use of radiation therapy and steroid administration but, more commonly, multiagent chemotherapy (115–118). Regimens include the combination of cyclophosphamide, doxorubicin, vincristine, and prednisone, which has achieved a 75% reduction in the size of a cardiac tumor. Although there were 60% mortality rates for patients treated with radiation therapy and steroids, there were longer survival times in patients undergoing chemotherapy (115). There also was one reported case of aggressive resection of a malignant cardiac lymphoma followed by postoperative chemotherapy using etoposide, prednisone, and pirarubicin. The patient died 234 days after the operation of a fungal infection (117).

EXTRASKELETAL OSTEOSARCOMA

Ten cases with extraskeletal osteosarcomas have been identified. They typically have a left atrial mass that is confused with a myxoma on echocardiography. History and physical findings are similar to those of other patients with malignant primary cardiac tumors. The chest roentgenogram shows cardiomegaly, but no abnormal calcification is seen (119). They characteristically have atypical echocardiographic findings that include extension into the pulmonary veins. The extent of these invasions and hence the tumor's resectability may not be predicted by preoperative echocardiograms (63). Of interest, 10% of all primary malignant heart tumors have histology similar to that of osteosarcomas. Also, primary bone osteosarcomas commonly metastasize to the heart hematogenously. Therefore, several criteria are helpful in classifying these tumors properly. Many metastatic tumors appear in the right heart, but primary osteosarcomas of the heart tend to be left atrial and mitral valve neoplasms. The histopathology of these tumors is somewhat diverse, with portions showing findings typical of cardiac myxoma. If the histology shows large amounts of bone formation without myxomatous features, the tumor is probably osteosarcoma. These tumors are no longer thought to arise from calcified atrial myxomas.

Complete surgical resection is successful in 89% of patients (119). Osteosarcomas are as aggressive as other primary cardiac malignancies, and all patients died of a recurrent tumor or from metastases. Regimens of postoperative chemotherapy including doxorubicin, methotrexate, and cisplatin were attempted in several cases (63, 119). There were some adequate responses with combined chemotherapy and radiation, yielding 30- and 67-month survivors (119).

LIPOSARCOMA

Although liposarcoma is one of the most common soft tissue sarcomas, there have been only 10 reported primary cardiac liposarcomas in the literature. The typical extracardiac liposarcoma occurs in males aged 40 to 60 years. In contrast, cardiac liposarcomas occur in equal sex distribution, and patients have a mean age of 53 years with a range of 30 to 70 years. Patients present with congestive heart failure in 80% of cases and arrhythmia in 20%. Six of the 10 reported cases were diagnosed before the death of the patient. There was equal distribution of these tumors between the right and left atria. Two patients had adjuvant radiation and chemotherapy. Metastatic disease occurred frequently in the bone. Median survival, like that with other cardiac sarcomas, was poor, i.e., 8.3 months (120).

NEUROGENIC SARCOMAS

Primary malignancies of the heart arising from nerve elements are extremely rare and have been reported in only four patients (1, 121). All were male, and their ages ranged from 9 to 60 years. One case was attributed to possible environmental exposure to dioxin (121). Their origin is from the cardiac neural plexus or vagal fibers. After 1 year, all patients were either dead or had recurrent disease. Unfortunately, chemotherapy and radiation therapy were not effective.

MALIGNANT TERATOMA

Malignant teratoma is another extremely rare malignant cardiac tumor that occurs when one of the components of its benign counterpart undergoes malignant change. Only four reported cases have occurred. All were in children, the group most likely to develop a benign cardiac teratoma. All four of these patients had congestive heart failure with nausea and vomiting. Unfortunately, all the tumors were nonresectable, and death usually occurred within 3 months of the onset of symptoms (1).

THYMOMA

Thymomas can arise from an embryologic rest of thymic tissue in the pericardium, usually as it reflects onto the base of the heart. These tumors may cause compression of the heart or other vascular structures that leads to superior vena cava syndrome (122). There have been approximately 5 cases reported in the literature, with one tumor growing into the lumen of the heart. Most patients were women, and they had symptoms of congestive heart failure that led to their presentation (1). Surgical excision is the preferred treatment; however, a favorable response rate using chemotherapy for advanced stage noncardiac thymoma was reported recently (123).

MESENCHYMOMA

Mesenchymomas are tumors that have a female predominance; only 14 have been reported. The common symptoms were dyspnea and fatigue, and diagnostic and physical findings were similar to those of other malignant tumors. The histopathology of this entity shows two or more cellular types derived from primitive mesenchyme. The tumors tend to grow rapidly, recur, and metastasize frequently, and arise in a variety of cardiac locations. For instance, one reported tumor reached the size of 7 × 5 × 3 cm, obstructed the right ventricular outflow tract, and contained fibrosarcoma, chondrosarcoma, and mesenchymoma elements (124). These tumors are likely to show the echocardiographic signs of malignancy, which include rapid growth, lack of a stalk, a combined mural and intracavitary location, and extension into the pulmonary veins (125). Tumors metastasize frequently, with 40% of these to the lung. Prognosis is poor with a survival of 5 to 48 months. The patients die from obstruction of blood flow and local extension into other vital structures. Treatment is surgical excision if possible. Although some patients were treated with chemotherapy or radiation, the benefit was not established clearly.

SYNOVIAL SARCOMA

There have been only three well-documented cases of synovial sarcoma of the heart. One of these later turned out to be from a metastatic sarcoma (126). The tumor seems to behave like other cardiac tumors, presenting with symptoms of congestive heart failure. Of the three synovial sarcomas reported, none had metastases and one grew to the size of 10 × 15 cm (1). Death in all patients was caused by local recurrence. Treatment of this tumor is similar to that of other cardiac tumors. In one patient, cardiac transplantation was performed but was unsuccessful because of tumor recurrence 2 months later (1, 32, 126).

CARDIAC VALVE TUMORS

Cardiac valve tumors are less aggressive than other cardiac tumors and are generally papillary fibroelastomas. In a recent large series, 56 patients with this problem were identified (Table 32.7). The patients

TABLE 32.7. Cardiac Valve Tumors

CLASSIFICATION	NO. OF PATIENTS
Symptoms	
Asymptomatic	36
Dyspnea	14
CHF	14
CVA	8
Sudden death	4
Site	
MV	15
TV	12
PV	13
AV	16
Benign	
Papillary fibroelastoma	41
Myxoma	5
Fibroma	4
Hemangioma	1
Hamartoma	1
Malignant	
Sarcoma NOS	2
MFH	1
Undifferentiated carcinoma	1

Notes. $n = 53$. Male:female ratio, 42:14. Age range, 2 to 88 years; mean, 52 years.
Data from Edwards et al. (74).
Abbreviations. CHF, congestive heart failure; CVA, cerebral vascular accident; MV, mitral valve; TV, tricuspid valve; PV, pulmonic valve; AV, aortic valve; MFH, malignant fibrous histiocytoma; NOS, not otherwise specified.

were likely to be asymptomatic, but if they did have symptoms, the tumors were generally on the left side of the heart. A common symptom was sudden death, which occurred in patients with left-sided cardiac valve tumors (74). These tumors ranged from 3 mm to 7 cm, and 93% were benign. Malignant tumors occurred only on the mitral valve, pulmonary valve, or tricuspid valve, and were 10 times more common in females. Otherwise, valve tumors are more common in men, less common in children, have a lower rate of malignancy, and a higher rate of asymptomatic status compared with nonvalvular cardiac tumors (74).

METASTATIC MALIGNANCY TO THE HEART

Cardiac metastases occur much more commonly than primary cardiac tumors (Table 32.8). Secondary cardiac tumors are found in 0.24% to 6.54% of all autopsies, compared with rates as low as 0.0017% of autopsies showing primary cardiac tumors (127, 128). Classically, they were encountered 20 to 40 times more commonly than primary cardiac tumors (129). When secondary cardiac tumors occur, other intrathoracic metastases are present in 63% to 93% of patients, compared with a rate of only 36% in patients without cardiac metastases (130). When the number of metastatic sites in the body goes from four to five, 50% of the patients will have cardiac spread (128, 131). The first description of a cardiac metastasis was in 1700, and it was first diagnosed before death in 1913 (130). Usually, cardiac metastasis is a late manifestation of carcinoma, and it occurs in 34% of patients with leukemia and 27% of patients with lymphoma. Half of the patients are between the age of 57 and 60 (54). There has been a reported increase in the incidence of cardiac metastases (132). This was attributed to an increased incidence in cancer, increase in longevity of patients with cancer because of better treatment, increased frequency of tumors prone to cardiac metastases, and better diagnostic imaging to establish the diagnosis (132).

SYMPTOMS

Most patients with cardiac metastases are asymptomatic. In fact, only 13% to 17% have symptoms, and without them no evaluation for cardiac metastases is indicated. The common symptoms are dyspnea (73%), palpitations (7%), orthopnea (5%), dizziness (5%), and weakness (5%) (54). These metastases are grouped conveniently based on how the tumor invades the heart.

TABLE 32.8. Secondary Cardiac Tumors

LOCATION	CARDIAC[a]	PERICARDIAL[b]
Lung	145	214
Lymphoma	68	19
Breast	54	84 37[c]
Leukemia	40	54
Melanoma	29	26
Sarcoma (NOS)	25	21
Mesothelioma	8	2
Adrenal	1	0
Gastrointestinal		
Stomach	18	2
Esophagus	8	1
Pancreas	8	3
Tongue	6	0
Liver	5	0
Colon	4	1
Rectum	4	14
Jejunum	1	1
Gallbladder	1	0
Genitourinary		
Kidney	9	12
Ovary	8	9
Cervix	7	20
Bladder	3	2
Penis	3	0
Miscellaneous		
Thyroid	0	17
Thymoma	0	4
Teratoblastoma	0	8
Other	33	29
Total	485	617

Abbreviations. NOS, not otherwise specified.
[a]Data from Murphy et al. (46), Abraham et al. (128), Prichard (129), Hanfling (130), Karwinski and Svendsen (131), and Tamura et al. (134).
[b]Data from Cham et al. (54), Hanfling (130), Karwinski and Svendsen (131), Skhvatsabaja (133), Tamura et al. (134), Bisel et al. (138), Celermajer et al. (152), and Wiener et al. (153).
[c]Report did not differentiate between lymphoma and leukemia.

The three major groups are tumor invading the pericardium, the epicardium/myocardium, or the endocardium. In each group most patients present without symptoms, but the highest asymptomatic rate is seen with pericardial involvement alone. Clues for this type of involvement are symptoms or signs of pericarditis, effusion, or constriction. When the tumor is invading the epicardium or myocardium, there may be a change in heart rate or rhythm on EKG. Other findings consist of heart failure, angina, or sudden death. Endocardial tumors may cause heart failure when symptomatic, and may induce murmurs or sudden death.

The sizes of the metastases are important as well. Fifty-two percent of the patients have micronodular metastases that tend be nonobstructive and lead to symptoms of congestive heart failure by globally replacing functioning heart muscle. Thirty percent of patients have extension of tumors into the cardiac lumen, giving 74% of them persistent chest pain and 28% symptomatic superior vena cava syndrome. The least common are macronodular metastases, which occur in 18% of patients. These may lead to cardiac enlargement, up to 2.4 kg, and may cause murmurs or symptoms of flow obstruction (133).

Finally, the patients' symptomatology can be classified by specific manifestations of the metastases. When superior vena cava syndrome occurs, 75% are from lung cancer, and 10% are from lymphoma metastases. To diagnosis this entity, most well-planned biopsy techniques are safe, including mediastinoscopy. Patients also may present with dilated abdominal veins, lower extremity edema, paroxysmal nocturnal dyspnea, syncope, decreased pulses, and heart murmurs from tumors that invade the heart through the inferior vena cava, such as renal cell carcinomas and hepatocellular carcinoma. Patients with lung cancers have direct metastatic extensions through the pulmonary veins; these usually are asymptomatic but do increase the risk of thromboembolism. Pulmonary artery metastases are common in patients with lung carcinoma, and left ventricular outflow tract obstruction can occur with some intrapericardial tumors such as synovial sarcoma. Symptoms of myocardial infarction can be produced by hematogenous metastases to the coronary arteries, as well as endocardial or myocardial hematogenous metastases.

Physical Findings and Diagnostic Tests

Physical findings of cardiac metastases are pleural effusion, 42%; paradoxical pulse, 23%; congestive heart failure, 13%; arrhythmias, 10%; and cardiac rubs, 5%. Seventy-nine percent of patients have an enlarged heart shadow on chest roentgenogram, 50% have low-voltage EKGs, and more than 50% have a hemorrhagic pericardial effusion (54). Patients with coronary artery emboli or macronodular invasion have EKG changes consistent with myocardial infarction.

Diagnosis

The diagnosis of cardiac metastases can be confirmed with echocardiography (84% effectiveness) as well as the other diagnostic imaging techniques mentioned previously. The diagnosis can be suspected clinically by an unexplained rapid cardiac enlargement, and symptoms resulting from cardiac compression, cardiac failure, or various arrhythmias (48).

Histopathology

Metastases to the heart occur by three major methods: direct extension, lymphatic spread, or hematogenous spread (Fig. 32.6) (99, 134). These metastases lead to three major types of cardiac invasion: epicardial and pericardial (most common), myocardial involvement, and intracavitary involvement (least common) (99). Although any tumor with metastatic potential can spread to the heart, lung cancer, breast cancer, melanomas, and sarcomas, particularly leukemia and lymphoma, are found most frequently. Metastases to the heart are usually small and firm, and resemble the primary lesion grossly and histologically (130). Lung cancer represents the most common metastatic tumor of the heart, occurring in up to 10.7% of patients with this disease (131). The metastatic pathways of lung cancer, in addition to direct extension, are hematogenous and multiple lymphatic pathways. These lymphatic pathways are through the hilar lymph nodes, or other direct mediastinal lymph nodes by way of the superior vena cava, the pulmonary arteries, and the left atrium through subcarinal lymph nodes (134). Lung cancer makes up 40% of secondary cardiac tumors, with 90% involving a combination of pericardium or epicardium (133). Only 10% have myocardial involvement alone; 3.5% of all other cancers have cardiac involvement including mesothelioma, which never involves the myocardium without involving the pericardium; melanoma, which can involve myocardium and pericardium but rarely involves pericardium alone; and breast, which typically involves pericardium with occasional myocardial extension but never the myocardium alone (131).

Sites of intracardiac metastasis vary among different reports. One study reported a higher incidence in the right heart, whereas in others the metastases were distributed evenly (129). It is unclear whether lymphatic invasion for some tumors is as important as direct extension or hematogenous spread.

There has been a recent increase in cardiac metastases, possibly because of better treatment of the primary tumor with radiation therapy rather than chemotherapy (except for leukemia and lymphomas) (135). Besides an increase in the number of cardiac metastases diagnosed, there has been a shift in their sites, with 20% of the patients presenting with both epicardial and pericardial involvement between 1981 and 1987, compared with only 7.5% presenting with this characteristic between 1974 and 1980 (128). Time from diagnosis of the original primary tumor to the

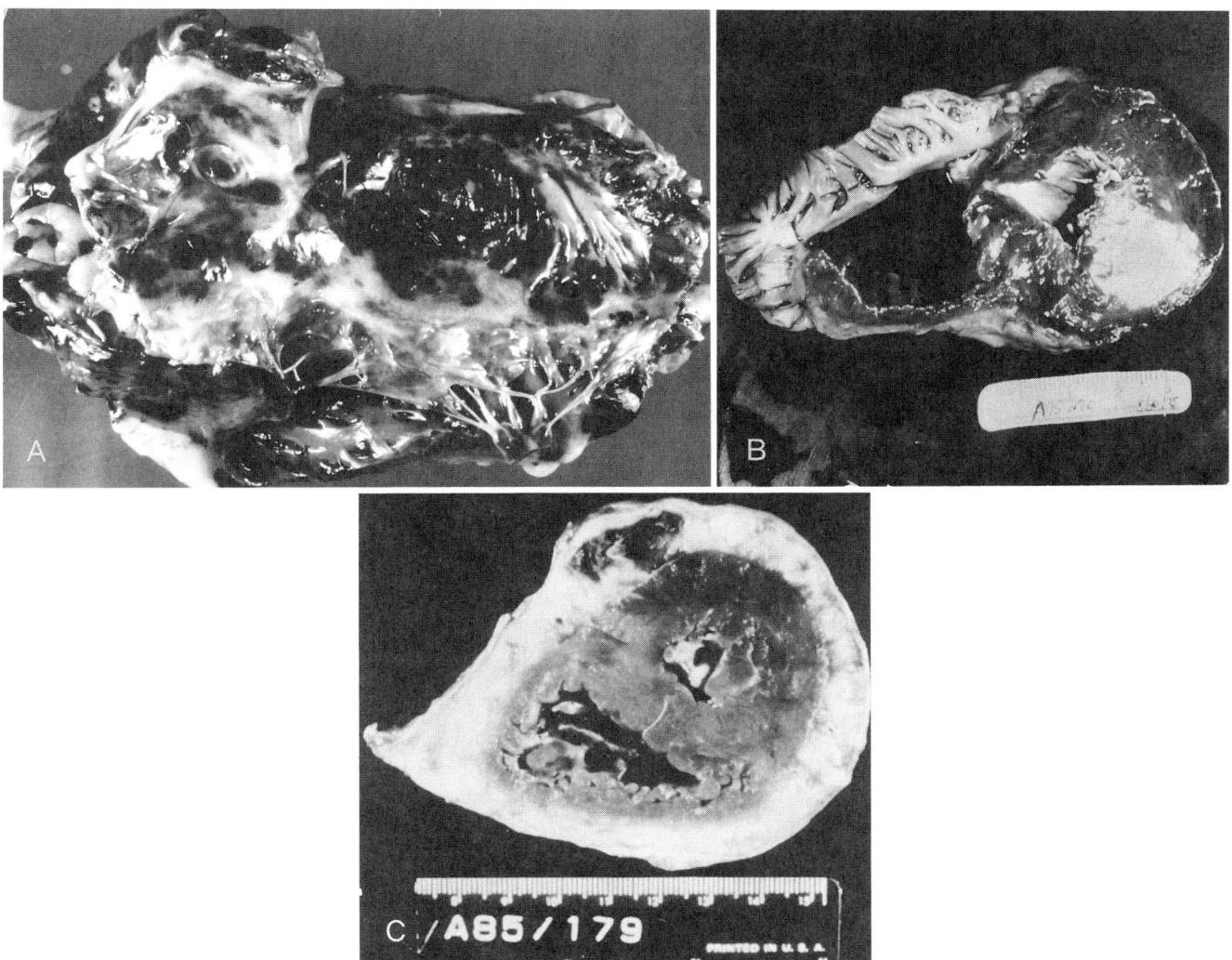

FIGURE 32.6. Selected types of cardiac metastases. A. Section of right atrium opened longitudinally. Gross replacement of myocardium with hematogenously spread melanoma. B. Macronodular metastasis of pulmonary adenocarcinoma to lateral wall of left ventricle. C. Transverse section of heart encased by pericardial lymphoma. (Courtesy of Ann Havey, M.D., University of Missouri, Columbia.)

onset of symptoms is 5.5 years for breast, approximately 2 months for lung, 25 months for lymphomas and leukemias, and 17 months for the group of miscellaneous tumors (54). With the many other sites to which cancers metastasize, the heart appears comparatively resistant. This resistance has been attributed to the "kneading action" of the heart. The general resistance of muscle to metastases, and the rapid blood flow through cardiac blood vessels and lymphatics, may also explain this phenomenon (136).

TREATMENT AND RESULTS

Selected patients with metastatic tumors of the heart can be offered surgery. In a study of 19 patients, 13 survived hospitalization. Eight of those 13 died months after leaving the hospital, and only 5 were alive at a mean of 3.2 years. The next preferred method of treatment is chemotherapy if the tumor is responsive to drugs, or radiation therapy if it is a radiosensitive tumor. Radiation therapy is usually given at a dosage of 25 to 35 Gy during a 3- to 4-week period, and leads to palliation in 61% of patients. The dose is typically greater than 3000 cGy over 4 weeks for carcinomas and sarcomas, and greater than 1500 cGy for 1½ weeks for leukemias and lymphomas (54). The patients' symptomatic improvements are malignancy dependent, with 69% of breast carcinoma patients receiving palliation for 2 to 36 months. Twenty-nine percent of lung cancer patients received palliation for 1 to 9 months, and 86% of lymphoma or leukemia patients had palliation for 2 to 4 months before recurrence of symptoms. Specific problems, such as superior vena cava syndrome, were treated with higher doses of radiation therapy (up to 5000 cGy) for non–small cell cancers with chemotherapy for small cell malignancies. Pericardial metastases can be treated with a pericardial window and possibly pericardial sclerosis (99, 137). Death in most patients with this type of malignancy results from generalized carcinomatosis rather than cardiac failure because these tumors do not generally displace, deform, or obstruct the heart (5). The cause of death in 51 patients was pneumonia (17), tumor burden (7), cardiac tamponade (6), anasarca (6), myocardial infarction (6), congestive heart failure (3), pulmonary embolus (5), or peritonitis (3) (127).

SELECTED SECONDARY CARDIAC MALIGNANCIES

ACUTE LEUKEMIA AND LYMPHOMA

Cardiac involvement was reported in 44% of patients dying with leukemia and 20% of patients with lymphoma (138). This rate was higher than a recent autopsy series showing only three cardiac leukemias and four cardiac non-Hodgkin's lymphomas in 103 patients who died of lymphoproliferative disease (127). The higher rates reflect inclusion of patients with only microscopic invasion of the myocardium and no gross cardiac involvement. Both sides of the heart are involved equally with systemic lymphoma, and acute myocardial infarction can occur. Time to death from onset of congestive heart failure is approximately 2 months, and only one case of prolonged survival with radiation therapy was reported (139).

MELANOMA

Approximately 44% of patients dying of melanoma have cardiac involvement (138), thus this is a relatively common metastatic cardiac tumor despite the lower incidence of the primary tumor compared with other malignancies. Patients with cardiac metastases from melanoma present with acute pericarditis, pericardial effusion with cardiomegaly, cardiac tamponade, atrial tachycardia, second- or third-degree heart block, congestive heart failure, and a history of previous melanoma. Pathology reveals a "charcoal" heart with involvement of both the pericardium and myocardium in diffuse fashion (140). Survival, as with other forms of widely metastatic melanoma, has not been reported.

PULMONARY CARCINOMA

Metastatic lung carcinoma to the heart was discussed previously. Bronchogenic carcinoma in the heart causes a malignant pericardial effusion in 93% of patients with lymphatic metastases, and 78% of patients have myocardial spread from lymphatic metastases. Hematogenous metastases lead to pericardial metastases in 7% of patients and myocardial metastases in 22% (134). Symptoms include myocardial infarction in 7% and cardiac arrhythmias in 35%. The metastases generally enter the heart through the hilar and subcarinal lymph nodes found on the dorsal side of the pericardium.

BREAST

Breast carcinoma may lead to cardiac metastases, primarily pericardial metastases, up to 5 years after the presentation of the primary tumor. Symptoms include fatigue and dyspnea on exertion. Chemotherapy and radiation may provide palliation (132).

TUMORS THAT INVADE THE HEART THROUGH THE INFERIOR VENA CAVA

HYPERNEPHROMA

Four percent to 10% of the 15,000 to 17,000 reported renal carcinomas had extension to the heart through the inferior vena cava. Patients with this disease have hematuria (42%), flank pain and fullness (23%), lower extremity swelling (10%), and a palpable mass (26%). The preoperative workup includes a CT scan, MRI, chest roentgenogram, and, if these tests are inadequate, venography and echocardiography. Surgical excision is the mainstay of therapy. Radiation or chemotherapy yields poor results (141). The operation's complexity is dependent on the extent to which tumor has invaded the heart. The abdominal approach is usually adequate to reach a tumor that has extended only to the infrahepatic level. For tumors that have reached the retrohepatic region or above, a combination of a thoracoabdominal incision or a median sternotomy with cardiopulmonary bypass may be necessary. Overall, the postoperative mortality is 3.4%, with a 31% morbidity. Patients with greater extension into the heart or lymph node metastases have a higher incidence of postoperative death from metastatic disease (141). For patients whose hypernephroma had not extended into the right atrium, the metastatic disease occurred less frequently, in only 20% to 30% of patients (141).

WILMS' TUMOR

Wilms' tumor with an extension into the right heart occurred in 21 of more than 2300 patients. This tumor is a disease of childhood with a mean patient age of 3.5 to 5.6 years and a male to female ratio of approximately 3:2 (142). The incidence of cardiac symptoms is low. The majority of the symptoms and signs are abdominal mass, hypertension, hematuria, ascites, abdominal pain, hepatomegaly, hypotension, and murmur. In a series of 15 patients with cardiac involvement, the tumor was not suspected to involve the heart preoperatively in 9. The correct diagnoses were made preoperatively by CT of the chest and abdomen, and ultrasound of the abdomen (142). Patient survival is good if there is a favorable histology. There is an 86% 2-year survival with a combination of radiation therapy plus actinomycin, doxorubicin, or cyclophosphamide. There appears to be a better survival with even more aggressive chemotherapy (143).

PERICARDIAL TUMORS

The majority of primary pericardial tumors are malignant and predominately are mesotheliomas and angiosarcomas in adults and teratomas in children (Table 32.8). Patients present with shortness of breath, cardiac tamponade, and occasionally pleural effusion. The paroxysmal nocturnal dyspnea and orthopnea occurring in these patients is less severe than in patients with typical congestive heart failure (144). Physical findings show tachycardia, decreased heart sounds, increased jugular venous distention, and pulsus paradoxus. Useful tests include EKG (which shows low voltage or electrical alternans), CT or MRI scanning, or echocardiogram. The echocardiogram is the most consistent and often shows diastolic right ventricle collapse or tumor implants. The histopathologies of these tumors are related to some of the metastatic malignancies discussed in the preceding section. If there is heart encasement, usually it is from a mesothelioma or lymphoma. When symptomatic pericardial effusion exists, treatment of these tumors requires drainage and/or sclerosis with an agent such as doxycycline. Other local chemotherapeutic agents such as thiotepa, bleomycin, cisplatin, and vinblastine have been used, as well as immunotherapy or radiation therapy (144).

SELECTED PRIMARY PERICARDIAL TUMORS
MALIGNANT PERIPHERAL NERVE TUMOR

Malignant peripheral nerve tumors can arise in the pericardium, either from neural rests within the pericardium or from the phrenic nerve (Fig. 32.7). Histologically, malignant schwannoma and perineurial cell tumors have been described (145, 146). Treatment is surgical excision, with radiation therapy or chemotherapy as adjuvant therapy.

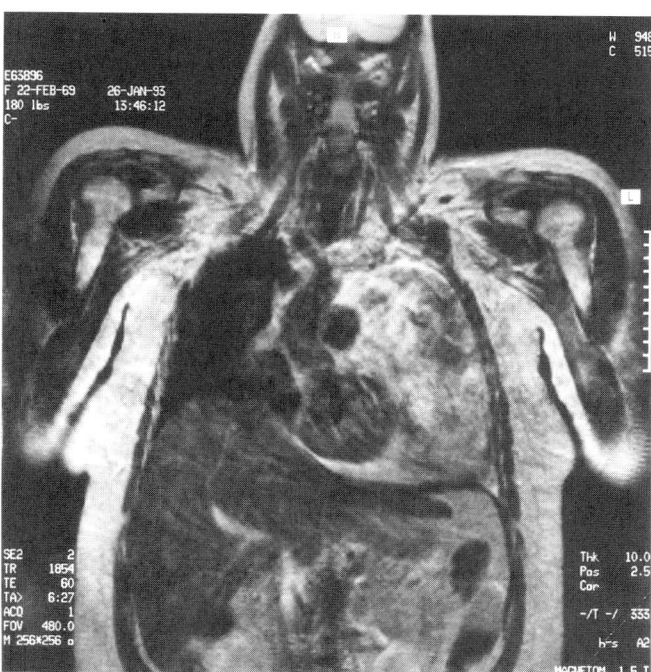

FIGURE 32.7. MRI scan of pericardial tumor. Coronal section shows evidence of a large pericardial perineurioma involving left ventricle and mediastinal structures.

MESOTHELIOMA

Mesothelioma is an extremely rare pericardial tumor, occurring in fewer than 0.0022% of 500,000 autopsies. The diagnosis typically was made after death, with patients having symptoms of a nonspecific or effusive pericarditis, cardiac tamponade, or cardiac constriction (147). The tumor was either localized to the pericardium or encased the heart. There was no relationship shown to asbestos exposure. The histologic subtypes are epithelial, spindle cell, or mixed. Classifying these tumors by cytology of the aspirated fluid can be difficult and is sometimes aided by the finding of increased hyaluronic acid in the fluid. Mesothelioma represents fewer than 4% of primary pericardial tumors and is thought to arise from immature pluripotent cells within the lining of the pericardium. Although surgical excision is ideal, the tumor is often unresectable, and the patient dies of tamponade, venal caval occlusion, or heart failure in less than 6 months despite palliative surgery or radiation therapy (147, 148).

SMALL CELL TUMOR

A primary tumor infiltrating the pericardium that showed small round cells by histology was described recently in an 18-year-old female. A review of similar rare tumors showed that small cell tumor typically occurs in the second decade, has a female predilection, and is treated by surgery. Radiation and chemotherapy

LIPOSARCOMA

Liposarcoma is an extremely rare tumor, last reported in a 22-year-old male who presented with chest pain. Ordinary liposarcomas tend to metastasize late, but pericardial liposarcomas (like cardiac liposarcomas) metastasize early. The patient was found to have metastases in his brain, lung, liver, and kidney (150). Therapy is similar to that for cardiac liposarcomas.

TERATOMA

In a recent review of 61 cardiac teratomas, there were only three pure pericardial teratomas reported. Seventy-five percent of cardiac teratomas occur in patients aged 15 years or younger. Partial or complete excision generally gives good long-term results (151).

OTHER PERICARDIAL TUMORS

Granular cell tumor, carcinosarcoma, plasmacytoma, chondrosarcoma, MFH, and myxosarcoma have been reported rarely as primary pericardial tumors. Specific symptoms and treatments of these rare tumors are not well known.

METASTATIC PERICARDIAL TUMORS

Secondary pericardial malignancies are found in 10% of patients who die of carcinoma. Lung cancer is the most common primary malignancy, accounting for one third of the cases; breast cancer is the second most common, accounting for one quarter of the cases; hematologic malignancies are the third most common, representing 15% of cases; and melanoma accounts for fewer than 5% of all pericardial malignancies. However, 50% of patients dying from melanoma have pericardial spread (152). Pericardial effusions in patients are generally out of proportion to the amount of intrapericardial tumor discovered. Lymphatic drainage from the pericardium is through the visceral pericardium at the root of the aorta. Tumor burden there can block drainage easily and lead to a rapid accumulation of pericardial fluid. Ninety-four percent of patients with pericardial metastatic malignancies are dyspneic on presentation, and the majority have fatigue, malaise, and anorexia. In addition, pulsus paradoxus or hypotension is found in 72% of patients, and another 8% present with pedal edema. The diagnosis of malignancy can be secured with pericardial cytologic examination, which is positive in 66% of cancer patients with pericardial effusion (153). In patients who present with pericardial effusion and a history of lung or breast cancer, approximately 71% have positive cytologic results. The presence of chronic inflammation can lead to a suspicious result or a false-positive cytologic interpretation. Also, 43% of some cancer patients with a negative cytologic examination had pericardial tumors found at autopsy.

Time from diagnosis to presentation of effusion is 44 months in breast cancer and approximately 8 months for other tumors. When a pericardial effusion occurs, 83% of patients will have intrathoracic tumors, and 25% will have metastases elsewhere. Treatment of a symptomatic malignant pericardial effusion is a pericardiocentesis. The pericardial drainage catheter is allowed to remain to perform sclerosis, or a pericardial window operation is performed. Use of this technique leads to success in 77% of patients (152). Using tetracycline sclerosis is more effective if done at the initial tap, yielding a 11% recurrence rate versus 57% if it is tried subsequently. Tetracycline or doxycycline at a dose of 275 to 550 mg is used. Besides sclerosis, a pericardial window can be made between the pericardium and the preperitoneal space or either pleural space. Survival after this therapy is approximately 10 months for breast cancer, 2 months for lung cancer, 12 months for leukemia, and approximately 2 to 6 months for other tumors.

ACKNOWLEDGMENTS

I wish to thank Elizabeth Doyle for her assistance in preparation of this manuscript as well as Drs. Jack Curtis, Ann Havey, Robert Churchill, and Darla Hess for their graphical contributions.

REFERENCES

1. McAllister HA Jr, Fenoglio JJ. Tumors of the cardiovascular system. In: Atlas of tumor pathology, second series, fascicle 15. Washington, DC: Armed Forces Institute of Pathology, Washington, D.C., 1978.
2. Miralles A, Bracamonte L, Soncul H, et al. Cardiac tumors: clinical experience and surgical results in 74 patients. Ann Thorac Surg 1991;52:886–895.
3. Moggio RA, Pucillo AL, Schechter AG, Pooley RW, Sarabu MR, Reed GE. Primary cardiac tumors: diagnosis and management in 14 cases. N Y State J Med 1992;92:48–52.
4. Nassar TK, Nasser WK, Slack JD, et al. Cardiac myxoma: the Indiana Heart Institute experience. Indiana Med 1990;83:644–647.
5. Wiatrowska BA, Walley VM, Masters RG, Goldstein W, Keon WJ. Surgery for cardiac tumors: the University of Ottawa Heart Institute experience 1980–91. Can J Cardiol 1993;9:65–72.
6. Silverman NA. Primary cardiac tumors. Ann Surg 1980;191:127–138.
7. Scannel JG, Grillo HC. Primary tumors of the heart. J Thorac Surg 1958;35:23–36.
8. Chitwood WR Jr. Clarence Crafoord and the first successful resection of a cardiac myxoma. Ann Thorac Surg 1992;54:997–998.

9. Bloor CM, O'Rourke RA. Cardiac tumors: clinical presentations and pathologic correlations. Curr Probl Cardiol 1984;9:1–48.
10. Larrieu AJ, Jamieson WRE, Tyers GFO, Burr LH, Munro AI, Miyagishima RT, Gerein AN, et al. Primary cardiac tumors: experience with 25 cases. J Thorac Cardiovasc Surg 1982;83:339–348.
11. van de Wal HJ, Fritschy WM, Skotnicki SH, Lacquet LK. Primary cardiac tumors. Acta Chir Belg 1988;88:74–78.
12. Fyfe AI, Huckell VF, Burr LH, Stonier PM. Leiomyosarcoma of the left atrium: case report and review of the literature. Can J Cardiol 1991;7:193–196.
13. McGarry KM, Jugdutt BI, Rossall RE. The modern diagnosis of cardiac myxoma: role of the two-dimensional echocardiography. Clin Cardiol 1983;6:511–518.
14. Ferrans VJ, Roberts WC. Structural features of cardiac myxomas. Histology, histochemistry and electron microscopy. Hum Pathol 1973;4:111–146.
15. Badui-Dergal E, Cordero E, Soberanis N, Verdin R, Arquero R. Cardiac myxoma: a report of 23 cases. Gac Med Mex 1992;128:245–252.
16. Curtsinger CR, Wilson MJ, Yoneda K. Primary cardiac lymphoma. Cancer 1989;64:521–525.
17. Hanson EC, Gill CC, Razavi M, Loop FD. Clinical experience and late results in 33 patients. J Thorac Cardiovasc Surg 1985;89:298–303.
18. Bulkley BH, Hutchins GM. Atrial myxomas: a fifty year review. Am Heart J 1979;97:639–643.
19. Larsson S, Lepore V, Kennergren C. Atrial myxomas: results of 25 years' experience and review of the literature. Surgery 1989;105:695–698.
20. Harvey W. Clinical aspects of cardiac tumors. Am J Cardiol 1968;21:328–343.
21. Abbott OA, Warshawski FE, Cobbs BW. Primary tumors and pseudotumors of the heart. Ann Surg 1963;155:855–572.
22. Saint John Sutton MG, Mercier LA, Giuliani ER, Lie JT. Atrial myxomas: a review of clinical experience in 40 patients. Mayo Clin Proc 1980;55:371–376.
23. Roux PM, Ghorayeb G, Touati G, et al. Tumors of the heart in newborn infants. Apropos of 5 cases. Ann Pediatr (Paris) 1990;37:323–326.
24. Mundinger A, Gruber HP, Dinkel E, et al. Imaging in cardiac mass lesions. Diagn Radiol 1992;10:135–140.
25. Matsumura M, Takamoto S, Kyo S, Yokote Y, Omoto R. Advantages of transesophageal color Doppler echocardiography in diagnosis and surgical treatment of cardiac masses. J Cardiol 1990;20:701–714.
26. Cooley DA. Surgical treatment of cardiac neoplasms: 32 year experience. Thorac Cardiovasc Surg 1990;38:176–182.
27. Dapper F, Gorlach G, Hoffman C, Fitz H, Marek P, Scheld HH. Primary cardiac tumors: clinical experiences and late results in 48 patients. Thorac Cardiovasc Surg 1988;36:80–85.
28. Menegus MA, Greenberg MA, Spindola-Franco H, Fayemi A. Magnetic resonance imaging of suspected atrial tumors. Am Heart J 1992;123:1260–1268.
29. Blondeau P. Primary cardiac tumors: French studies of 533 cases. Thorac Cardiovasc Surg 1990;38:192–195.
30. Nomeir AM, Watts LE, Seagle R, Joyner CR, Corman C, Prichard RW. Intracardiac myxoma: twenty-year echocardiographic experience with review of the literature. J Am Soc Echocardiogr 1989;2:139–150.
31. Salcedo EE, Cohen GI, White RD, Davison MB. Cardiac tumors: diagnosis and management. Curr Probl Cardiol 1992;17:77–137.
32. Siebenmann R, Jenni R, Makek M, Oelz O, Turina M. Primary synovial sarcoma of the heart treated by heart transplant. J Thorac Cardiovasc Surg 1990;99:567–568.
33. Carpentier A, Chachques JC. Myocardial substitution with a stimulated skeletal muscle: first successful clinical case. Lancet 1985;1:1267.
34. Bauer EP, von Segesser LK, Carrel T, Laske A, Turina MI. Early results following surgical treatment of heart tumors. Schweiz Med Wochenschr 1991;121:255–258.
35. Antman K, Crowley J, Balcerzak S, et al. An intergroup phase III randomized study of doxorubicin and dacarbazine with or without ifosfamide and mesna in advanced soft tissue and bone sarcomas. J Clin Oncol 1993;11:1276–1285.
36. Castells E, Ferran V, Octavio de Toledo MC, et al. Cardiac myxomas: surgical treatment, long-term results and recurrence. J Cardiovasc Surg 1993;34:49–53.
37. Lazzara RR, Park SB, Magovern GJ. Cardiac myxomas: results of surgical treatment. J Cardiovasc Surg 1991;32:824–827.
38. Bortolotti U, Maraglino G, Rubino M, et al. Surgical excision of intracardiac myxomas: a 20-year follow-up. Ann Thorac Surg 1990;49:449–453.
39. Nolan J, Carder PJ, Bloomfield P. Atrial myxoma: tumor or trauma? Br Heart J 1992;67:406–408.
40. Fang BR, Chiang CW, Hung JS, Lee YS, Chang CS. Cardiac myxoma: clinical experience in 24 patients. Int J Cardiol 1990;29:335–341.
41. Molina JE, Edwards JE, Ward HB. Primary cardiac tumors: experience of the University of Minnesota. Thorac Cardiovasc Surg 1990;38:183–191.
42. Sakakibara S, Osawa M, Konno S, et al. Myxoma of the right ventricle of the heart. Report of a case with successful removal and review of the literature. Am Heart J 1965;69:382–391.
43. Gonzalez A, Altieri PI, Marquez E, Cox R, Castillo M. Massive pulmonary embolism associated with a right ventricular myxoma. Am J Med 1980;69:795–798.
44. Snyder SN, Smith DC, Lau FYK, Turner AF. Diagnostic features of right ventricular myxoma. Am Heart J 1976;91:240–248.
45. Heath D. Pathology of cardiac tumors. Am J Cardiol 1968;21:315–327.
46. Selzer A, Sakai FJ, Popper RW. Protean clinical manifestations of primary tumors of the heart. Am J Med 1972;52:9–18.
47. Murphy MC, Sweeney MS, Putnam JB, et al. Surgical treatment of cardiac tumors: a 25-year experience. Ann Thorac Surg 1990;49:612–618.
48. Shimono T, Komadaa T, Kusagawa H, et al. Left atrial myxomas: clinical characteristics, evolution, and considerations in classifying tumors. Nippon Kyobu Geka Gakkai Zasshi 1992;40:1060–1066.
49. Lie JT. Petrified cardiac myxoma masquerading as organized atrial mural thrombus. Arch Pathol Lab Med 1989;113:742–745.
50. Tazelar HD, Locke TJ, McGregor CGA. Pathology of surgically excised primary cardiac tumors. Mayo Clin Proc 1992;67:957–965.
51. Budzilovich G, Aleksic S, Greco A, Fernandez J, Harris J, Finegold M. Malignant cardiac myxoma with cerebral metastasis. Surg Neurol 1979;11:461–469.
52. Chen HZ, Jiang L, Rong WH, et al. Tumors of the heart. An analysis of 79 cases. Chin Med J (Engl) 1992;105:153–158.
53. Seo IS, Warner TFCS, Colyer RA, Winkler RF. Metastasizing atrial myxoma. Am J Surg Pathol 1980;4:391–399.
54. Cham WC, Freiman AH, Carstens PHB, Chu FCH. Radiation therapy of cardiac and pericardial metastases. Radiology 1975;114:701–704.

55. Carney JA, Hruska LS, Beauchamp GD, Gordon H. Dominant inheritance of the complex of myxomas, spotty pigmentation, and endocrine overactivity. Mayo Clin Proc 1986;61:165–172.
56. Koopman RJJ, Happle R. Autosomal dominant transmission of the NAME syndrome (nevi, atrial myxoma, mucinosis of the skin, and endocrine overactivity). Hum Genet 1991;86:300–304.
57. Chaudron JM, Jacques JM, Heller FR, Cheran P, Luwaert R. The myxoma syndrome: unusual entity: a family study. Eur Heart J 1992;13:569–573.
58. Meyer BJ, Weber R, Jenzer HR, Jenni R, Conen D, Turina M. Rapid growth and recurrence of atrial myxomas in two patients with Swiss syndrome. Am Heart J 1990;120:220–222.
59. von Gelder HM, O'Brien DJ, Staples ED, Alexander JA. Familial cardiac myxoma. Ann Thorac Surg 1992;53:419–424.
60. Soma Y, Ogawa S, Iwanaga S, et al. Multiple primary left ventricular myxomas with multiple intraventricular recurrences. J Cardiovasc Surg 1992;33:765–767.
61. Grauer K, Grauer MC. Familial atrial myxoma with bilateral recurrence. Heart Lung 1983;12:600–602.
62. Kotylo PK, Kennedy JE, Waller BF, Sample RB. DNA analysis of atrial myxomas. Chest 1991;99:1203–1207.
63. Seidal T, Wandt B, Lundin SE. Primary chondroblastic osteogenic sarcoma of the left atrium. Scand J Thorac Cardiovasc Surg 1992;26:233–236.
64. Farah MG. Familial cardiac myxoma: a study of relatives of patients with myxoma. Chest 1994;105:65–68.
65. McCarthy PM, Schaff HV, Winkler HZ, Lieber MM, Carney JA. Deoxyribonucleic acid ploidy pattern of cardiac myxomas: Another predictor of biologically usual myxomas. J Thorac Cardiovasc Surg 1989;98:1083–1086.
66. Attum AA, Johnson GS, Masri Z, Girardet R, Lansing AM. Malignant clinical behavior of cardiac myxomas and "myxoid imitators." Ann Thorac Surg 1987;44:217–222.
67. Hananouchi GI, Goff WB. Cardiac lipoma: six-year follow-up with MRI characteristic, and a review of the literature. Magn Reson Imaging 1990;8:825–828.
68. Ashar K, van Hoeven KH. Fatal lipoma of the heart. Am J Cardiovasc Pathol 1992;4:85–90.
69. Shirani RJ, Roberts WC. Clinical, electrocardiographic and morphologic features of massive fatty deposits ("lipomatous hypertrophy") in the atrial septum. J Am Coll Cardiol 1993;22:226–238.
70. Gallo R, Kumar N, Prabhakar G, Awada A, Maalouf Y, Duran CMG. Papillary fibroelastoma of mitral valve chorda. Ann Thorac Surg 1993;55:1576–1577.
71. Gorton ME, Soltanzadeh H. Mitral valve fibroelastoma. Ann Thorac Surg 1989;47:605–607.
72. Fishbein MC, Ferrans VJ, Roberts WC. Endocardial papillary elastofibromas. Histologic, histochemical, and electron microscopical findings. Arch Pathol 1975;99:335–341.
73. Shub C, Tajik AJ, Seward JB, et al. Cardiac papillary fibroelastomas: two-dimensional echocardiographic recognition. Mayo Clin Proc 1981;56:629–633.
74. Edwards FH, Hale D, Cohen A, Thompson L, Pezzella AT, Virmani R. Primary cardiac valve tumors. Ann Thorac Surg 1991;52:1127–1131.
75. Stevens CW, Sears-Rogan P, Bitterman P, Torrisi J. Treatment of malignant fibrous histiocytoma of the heart. Cancer 1992;69:956–961.
76. Burke A, Johns JP, Virmani R. Hemangiomas of the heart: a clinicopathologic study of ten cases. Am J Cardiovasc Pathol 1990;3:283–290.
77. Scully RE, Mark EJ, McNeely BU. Case records of the Massachusetts General Hospital: weekly clinicopathological exercises. N Engl J Med 1983;308:206–214.
78. Arcinegas E, Hakimi M, Farooki ZQ, Truccone NJ, Green EW. Primary cardiac tumors in children. J Thorac Cardiovasc Surg 1980;79:582–591.
79. Brizard C, Latremoville C, Jebara VA, et al. Cardiac hemangiomas. Ann Thorac Surg 1993;56:390–394.
80. Reece IJ, Cooley DA, Frazier OH, Hallman GL, Powers PL, Montero CG. Cardiac tumors: clinical spectrum and prognosis of lesions other than classical benign myxomas in 20 patients. J Thorac Cardiovasc Surg 1984;88:439–446.
81. Jebara VA, Uva MS, Farge A, et al. Cardiac pheochromocytomas. Ann Thorac Surg 1992;53:356–361.
82. Abad C, Jimenez P, Santana C, et al. Primary cardiac paraganglioma. J Cardiovasc Surg 1992;33:768–772.
83. Orringer MB, Sisson JC, Glazer G, et al. Surgical treatment of cardiac pheochromocytomas. J Thorac Cardiovasc Surg 1985;89:753–757.
84. Gotah S, Orita H, Shimanuki T, Fukasawa M, Masaoka T, Washio M. A case of primary neurofibroma of the left ventricle. Nippon Kyobu Geka Gakkai Zasshi 1992;40:1010–1015.
85. Wang J, Kragel AH, Friedlander ER, Cheng JT. Granular cell tumor of the sinus node. Am J Cardiol 1993;71:490–492.
86. Bertolini P, Meisner H, Paek SU, Sebening F. Special considerations on primary cardiac tumors in infancy and childhood. Thorac Cardiovasc Surg 1990;38:164–167.
87. Schmaltz AA, Apitz J. Primary heart tumors in infancy and childhood: report of four cases and review of the literature. Cardiology 1981;67:12–22.
88. Rees AH, Elbl FE, Minhas KV, Solinger RE. Echocardiographic evidence of left ventricular tumor in a neonate. Chest 1978;73:433–435.
89. Burke AP, Virmani R. Cardiac rhabdomyoma: a clinicopathologic study. Mod Pathol 1991;4:70–74.
90. Mishra RC, Khanna SK, Gupta BK, et al. Surgical management of cardiac myxomas. Indian Heart J 1991;43:367–371.
91. Ceithmal EL, Midgley FM, Perry LW, Dullum MK. Intramural ventricular fibroma in infancy: survival after partial excision in 2 patients. Ann Thorac Surg 1990;50:471–472.
92. Yamaguchi M, Hosokawa Y, Ohashi H, Imai M, Oshima Y, Minamiji K. Cardiac fibroma. Long-term fate after excision. J Thorac Cardiovasc Surg 1992;103:104–105.
93. Reul GJ, Howell JF, Rubio PA, Peterson PK. Successful partial excision of an intramural fibroma of the left ventricle. Am J Cardiol 1975;36:262–265.
94. Geha AS, Weidman WH, Soule EH, McGoon DC. Intramural ventricular cardiac fibroma: successful removal in two cases and review of the literature. Circulation 1967;36:427–440.
95. Coffin CM. Congenital cardiac fibroma associated with Gorlin syndrome. Pediatr Pathol 1992;12:255–262.
96. Swalwell CI. Benign intracardiac teratoma. A case of sudden death. Arch Pathol Lab Med 1993;117:739–742.
97. Pasaoglu I, Dogan R, Ozme S, Kale G, Bozer AY. Cardiac lymphangioma. Am Heart J 1991;121:1821–1824.
98. Burke AP, Cowan D, Virmani R. Primary sarcomas of the heart. Cancer 1992;69:387–395.
99. Loffler H, Grille W. Classification of malignant cardiac tumors with respect to oncological treatment. Thorac Cardiovasc Surg 1990;38:173–175.
100. Putnam JB, Sweeney MS, Colon R, Lanza LA, Frazier OH, Cooley DA. Primary cardiac sarcomas. Ann Thorac Surg 1991;51:906–910.

101. Vergnon JM, Vincent M, Perinetti M, Loire R, Cordier JF, Burne J. Chemotherapy of metastatic primary cardiac sarcomas. Am Heart J 1985;110:682–684.
102. Mosodorf R, Scheld HH, Hehrlein FW. Tumors of the heart: experiences at the Giessen University Clinic. Thorac Cardiovasc Surg 1990;38:208–210.
103. Janigan DT, Husain A, Robinson NA. Cardiac angiosarcomas: a review and a case report. Cancer 1986;57:852–859.
104. Herrmann MA, Shakerman RA, Edwards WD, Shub C, Schaff HV. Primary cardiac angiosarcoma: a clinicopathologic study of six cases. J Thorac Cardiovasc Surg 1992;103:655–664.
105. Potter R, Baumgart P, Greve H, Schnepper E. Primary angiosarcoma of the heart. Thorac Cardiovasc Surg 1989;37:374–378.
106. Knobel B, Rosman P, Kishon Y, Husar M. Intracardiac primary fibrosarcoma. Case report and literature review. Thorac Cardiovasc Surg 1992;40:227–230.
107. Linder J, Woodard BH. Primary cardiac fibrosarcoma. S Med J 1985;78:607–608.
108. Orsmond GS, Knight L, Dehner LP, Nicoloff DM, Nesbitt M, Bessinger FB. Alveolar rhabdomyosarcoma involving the heart. An echocardiographic, angiographic, and pathologic study. Circulation 1976;54:837–842.
109. Satoh M, Horimoto M, Sakurai K, Funayama N, Igarashi K, Yamashiro K. Primary cardiac rhabdomyosarcoma exhibiting transient and pronounced regression with chemotherapy. Am Heart J 1990;120(6):1458–1460.
110. Todo T, Usui M, Nagashima K. Cerebral metastasis of malignant cardiac myxoma. Surg Neurol 1992;37:374–379.
111. Takamizawa S, Sugimoto K, Tanaka H, Sakai O, Arai T, Saitoh A. A case of primary leiomyosarcoma of the heart. Intern Med 1992;31:265–268.
112. Segesser LV, Cox J, Gross J, et al. Surgery in primary leiomyosarcoma of the heart. Thorac Cardiovasc Surg 1986;34:391–394.
113. Antunes MJ, Vanderdonck KM, Andrade CM, Rebelo LS. Primary cardiac leiomyosarcomas. Ann Thorac Surg 1991;51:999–1001.
114. Dossche K, Wellens F, Goldstein JP, Deferm H. Pulmonary homograft replacement for primary leiomyosarcoma of the pulmonary artery. J Thorac Cardiovasc Surg 1992;104:844–846.
115. Nand S, Mullen GM, Lonchyna VA, Moncada R. Primary lymphoma of the heart. Prolonged survival with early systemic therapy in a patient. Cancer 1991;68:2289–2292.
116. Roller MB, Manoharan A, Lvoff R. Primary cardiac lymphoma. Acta Haematol 1991;85:47–48.
117. Takagi M, Kugimiya T, Fujii T, et al. Extensive surgery for primary malignant lymphoma of the heart. J Cardiovasc Surg 1992;33:570–572.
118. Zaharia L, Gill PS. Primary cardiac lymphoma. Am J Clin Oncol 1991;14:142–145.
119. Burke AP, Virmani R. Osteosarcomas of the heart. Am J Surg Pathol 1991;15:289–295.
120. Paraf F, Bruneval P, Balaton A, Deloche A, Mikol J, Maitre F, Scholl JM, et al. Primary liposarcoma of the heart. Am J Cardiovasc Pathol 1990;3:175–180.
121. Erikson M, Hardell L. Employment in pulp mills as a possible risk factor for soft tissue sarcoma: a case report. Br J Ind Med 1991;48:288.
122. Missault L, Duprez D, DeBuyzere M, Cambier B, Adang L, Clement D. Right atrial invasive thymoma with protrusion through the tricuspid valve. Eur Heart J 1992;13:1726–1727.
123. Rea F, Sartori F, Loy M, et al. Chemotherapy and operation for invasive thymoma. J Thorac Cardiovasc Surg 1993;106:543–549.
124. Ceretto WJ, Miller ML, Shea PM, Gregory CW, Vieweg WVR. Malignant mesenchymoma obstructing the right ventricular outflow tract. Am Heart J 1981;101:114–115.
125. McKenney PA, Moroz K, Haudenschild CC, Shemin RJ, Davidoff R. Malignant mesenchymoma as a primary cardiac tumor. Am Heart J 1992;123:1071–1075.
126. Tak T, Goel S, Chandrasoma P, Colletti P, Rohimtoola SH. Synovial sarcoma of the right ventricle. Am Heart J 1991;121:933–936.
127. MacGee W. Metastatic and invasive tumours involving the heart in a geriatric population: a necropsy study. Virchows Arch A Pathol Anat Histopathol 1991;419:183–189.
128. Abraham KP, Reddy V, Gattuso P. Neoplasms metastatic to the heart: review of 3314 consecutive autopsies. Am J Cardiovasc Pathol 1990;3:195–198.
129. Prichard RW. Tumors of the heart. Arch Pathol 1951;51:98–128.
130. Hanfling SM. Metastatic cancer to the heart: review of the literature and report of 127 cases. Circulation 1960;22:474–483.
131. Karwinski B, Svendsen E. Trends in cardiac metastasis. APMIS 1989;97:1018–1024.
132. Volk MJ, Carbone PP, Pozniak MA, Rahko PS. Cardiac involvement in metastatic breast cancer. Wis Med J 1990;89:56–60.
133. Skhvatsabaja EV. Secondary malignant lesions of the heart and pericardium in neoplastic disease. Oncology 1986;43:103–106.
134. Tamura A, Matsubara O, Yoshimura N, Kasuga T, Akagawa S, Aoki N. Cardiac metastases of lung cancer. A study of metastatic pathways and clinical manifestations. Cancer 1992;70:437–442.
135. Poole GV, Breyer RH, Holliday RH, et al. Tumors of the heart: surgical considerations. J Cardiovasc Surg 1984;25:5–11.
136. Smith C. Tumors of the heart. Arch Pathol Lab Med 1986;110:371–374.
137. Weinberg BA, Conces DJ, Waller BF. Cardiac manifestations of non-cardiac tumors. Part II: direct effects. Clin Cardiol 1989;12:347–354.
138. Bisel HF, Wroblewski F, LaDue JS. Incidence and clinical manifestations of cardiac metastasis. JAMA 1953;153:712–715.
139. Gelman KM, Ben-Ezra JM, Steinschneider M, Dutcher JP, Keefe DL, Factor SM. Lymphoma with primary cardiac manifestations. Am Heart J 1986;111:808–811.
140. Canver CC, Lajos TZ, Bernstein Z, DuBois DP, Mentzer RM Jr. Intracavitary melanoma of the left atrium. Ann Thorac Surg 1990;49:312–313.
141. Suggs WD, Smith RB, Dodson TF, Salam AA, Graham SD. Renal cell carcinoma with inferior vena caval involvement. J Vasc Surg 1991;14:413–418.
142. Thompson WR, Newman K, Seibel N, et al. A strategy for resection of Wilms' tumor with vena cava or atrial extension. J Pediatr Surg 1992;27:912–915.
143. Nakayama DK, deLorimier AA, O'Neill JA, Norkool P, D'Angio GJ. Intracardiac extension of Wilms' tumor: a report of the national Wilms' tumor study. Ann Surg 1986;204:693–697.
144. Hancock EW. Neoplastic pericardial disease. Cardiol Clin 1990;8:673–682.
145. Hirose T, Sumitoms M, Kudo E, et al. Malignant peripheral nerve sheath tumor (MPNST) showing perineurial cell differentiation. Am J Surg Pathol 1989;13:613–620.
146. Woodruff JM. The pathology and treatment of peripheral nerve

tumors and tumor-like conditions. CA Cancer J Clin 1993; 43:290–308.
147. Nambiar CA, Tareif E, Kishore KU, Ravindran J, Banerjee AK. Primary pericardial mesothelioma: one-year event-free survival. Am Heart J 1992;124:802–803.
148. Fazekas T, Ungi I, Tiszlavicz L. Primary malignant mesothelioma of the pericardium. Am Heart J 1992;124:227–231.
149. Mohandas KM, Chinoy RF, Merchant NH, Lotliker RG, Desai PB. Malignant small cell tumor (Askin-Rosai) of the pericardium. Postgrad Med J 1992;68:140–142.
150. Can C, Arpaci F, Celason B, Gunhan B, Finci R. Primary pericardial liposarcoma presenting with cardiac tamponade and multiple organ metastases. Chest 1993;103:328.
151. Meissner A, Kirch W, Regensburger D, Mayer-Eichberger S, Ohnhaus EE. Intrapericardial teratoma in an adult. Am J Med 1988;84:1089–1090.
152. Celermajer DS, Boyer MJ, Bailey BP, Tattersall MHN. Pericardiocentesis for symptomatic malignant pericardial effusion: a study of 36 patients. Med J Aust 1991;154:19–22.
153. Wiener HG, Kristensen IB, Haubek A, Kristensen B, Baandrup U. The diagnostic value of pericardial cytology. An analysis of 95 cases. Acta Cytol 1991;35:149–153.
154. Moriyama Y, Saigenzi H, Shimokawa S, et al. Surgical treatment of primary cardiac tumors. Nippon Kyobu Geka Gakkai Zasshi 1993;41:367–371.
155. Sugimoto T, Ogawa K, Asada T, et al. Surgical treatment of primary cardiac tumors. Nippon Kyobu Geka Gakkai Zasshi 1992;40:1847–1852.
156. Guang-ying L. Incidence and clinical importance of cardiac tumors in China: review of the literature. Thorac Cardiovasc Surg 1990;38:205–207.
157. Curtis JJ, Deese L, Walls JT, Boley TM, Schmaltz RA, Demmy TL. A 36-year experience with primary cardiac tumors. American College of Chest Physicians 59th Annual International Scientific Assembly in Orlando, FL, October 24–28, 1993.
158. Verkkala K, Kupari M, Maamies T, et al. Primary cardiac tumors: operative treatment of 20 patients. Thorac Cardiovasc Surg 1989;37:361–364.
159. Awang Y, Sallehuddin A. Surgical experience with cardiac tumors at the General Hospital, Kuala Lumpur. Med J Malaysia 1991;46:28–34.
160. Carranza-Rebollar A, Ochoa-Ramirez E, Ponce de la Garza L, de la Fuente Magallanes FJ, Rodriquez-Gonzalez H, Angulano-Cardenas R. The surgical treatment of cardiac myxomas: 10 years of experience. Arch Inst Cardiol Mex 1992;62:121–126.
161. Chen ZD. Diagnosis and treatment of 52 cases of cardiac myxoma. Chung Hua Wai Ko Tsa Chih 1991;29:233–4270–1.
162. Yin BL. Surgical treatment of primary tumor in the right heart. Chug Hua Wai Ko Tsa Chih 1992;29:755–756, 798.
163. Hake V, Iverson S, Schmid FX, Erbel R, Oelert H. Urgent indications for surgery in primary or secondary cardiac neoplasm. Scand J Thorac Cardiovasc Surg 1989;23:111–114.
164. Sutsch G, Jenni R, von Segesser L, Schneider J. Heart tumors: incidence, distribution, diagnosis. Exemplified by 20,305 echocardiographics. Schweiz Med Wochenschr 1991;121:621–629.
165. Xie S. Cardiac tumors: clinical and echocardiographic diagnosis of 65 cases. Chung Hua Hsin Hsueh Kuan Ping Tsa Chih 1990;18:17–19, 61.
166. Corbi P, Jebara V, Fabiani JN, et al. Benign tumors of the heart (excluding myxoma). Experience with 9 surgically treated cases. Ann Cardiol Angeiol (Paris) 1990;39:433–436.
167. Biancaniello TM, Meyer RA, Gaum WE, Kaplan S. Primary benign intramural ventricular tumors in children: pre- and post-operative electrocardiographic, echocardiographic, and angiocardiographic evolution. Am Heart J 1982;103:852–857.
168. Loire R, Delaye J. Myxoma of the right atrium. Apropos of 10 surgically treated cases. Ann Cardiol Angeiol (Paris) 1992;41:177–183.

33

Posterior Mediastinal Tumors

David R. Jones and Geoffrey M. Graeber

The posterior mediastinum is defined as the space anterior to the vertebral column and posterior to the esophagus. Some include the esophagus as a posterior mediastinal structure, but it is preferable to classify the esophagus as part of the visceral or middle mediastinum. Structures contained within the posterior mediastinum include the intercostal nerves, proximal portion of the anterior ramus, sympathetic ganglia, paraganglia, and connective and lymph tissue.

Primary tumors of the posterior mediastinum are usually neurogenic and are divided into two groups based on their tissue of origin. Tumors of neural sheath origin are usually benign. Tumors of neuroendocrine tissue may be benign or malignant. This classification of neurogenic tumors is somewhat arbitrary because all of these tumors arise from the embryonic neural crest.

The incidence of posterior mediastinal tumors relative to all tumors of the mediastinum is 23% to 30% (1, 2). In a review of more than 1840 mediastinal tumors, the incidence of neurogenic tumors was 19% (3). Benign tumors predominate in the adult population, whereas malignant tumors are more common in infants and children. Advances in imaging, diagnostic biopsy techniques, and immunocytochemical analysis have enhanced the physician's ability to treat these lesions effectively. Perhaps the most important advances in the understanding of tumors of neural crest origin has been the further elucidation of the molecular and tumor biology of these lesions.

Posterior mediastinal tumors are encountered in every thoracic surgeon's practice. Thus, a working knowledge of the clinical presentation, available imaging techniques, staging systems, tumor biology, and treatment of these tumors is mandatory.

EMBRYOLOGY OF NEUROGENIC TUMORS

All neurogenic tumors arise from the neural crest. At day 14 of embryonic life, a thickened plate of ectoderm forms the neural plate. The edges of this plate become the neural folds, and, at the junction of these neural folds and the neural groove, a group of cells appears. These are the neural crest cells. The cells coalesce and form an intermediate zone between the surface ectoderm and neural tube. This zone then migrates caudally to form the sensory ganglia or dorsal root ganglia of the spinal and cranial nerves.

In addition to forming the sensory ganglia, the cells of the neural crest develop into Schwann cells, melanocytes, neurons, the adrenal medulla, and other endocrine tissues. Neural crest tissues in the thorax give rise to peripheral nerves, including the sympathetic ganglia, paraganglia, and Schwann cells.

Tumors of nerve sheath origin include neurilemoma and neurofibroma. Neuroblastoma, ganglioneuroma, paraganglioma, and pheochromocytoma arise from a neuronal cell origin (Table 33.1).

NERVE SHEATH TUMORS

NEURILEMOMA

Neurilemoma and neurofibroma constitute 60% to 65% of all posterior mediastinal tumors in adults. Neurilemomas (also called schwannomas) arise from Schwann cells, which sheath the peripheral nerve fibers as they exit from the spinal canal through the intervertebral foramen until their termination in the periphery. These tumors rarely occur in children and with equal rarity exhibit malignant degeneration.

CLINICAL PRESENTATION

The majority of these lesions occur in young or middle-aged adults and have a female predilection (4). The most common presentation is of an asymptomatic mass on chest roentgenogram. These tumors grow slowly and do not cause pressure symptoms until late in their course (5). Symptoms may include chest pain,

TABLE 33.1. Neurogenic Tumors of the Posterior Mediastinum

Nerve sheath origin
   Neurilemomas (schwannoma)
   Neurofibroma
   Melanotic schwannoma
   Malignant schwannoma
Autonomic ganglia
   Neuroblastoma
   Ganglioneuroblastoma
   Ganglioneuroma
Paraganglionic system
   Pheochromocytoma
   Chemodectoma
   Paraganglioma
Neuroepithelioma (Askin tumor)

cough, dyspnea, or radicular pain relating to the affected nerve. Neurilemomas are usually solitary but may be multiple, especially when associated with von Recklinghausen's disease. The majority of tumors associated with von Recklinghausen's disease are neurofibromas, but 18% of neurilemomas are also associated with the syndrome (6). In fact, there may be admixtures of neurofibroma and neurilemoma in the same patient (7).

Akwari et al. (8) demonstrated that 10% of benign nerve sheath tumors may extend through the intervertebral foramen into the spinal canal. In addition, 30% to 40% of these patients may be asymptomatic at the time. Love and Dodge (9) in 1952 first described these as dumbbell tumors. The importance of preoperative identification and management of the dumbbell tumor is discussed below.

RADIOGRAPHIC FEATURES

The characteristic plain radiograph usually shows a solitary, smooth mass that lies in the upper third to half of the posterior mediastinum. These tumors are more common on the right, 65% to 75% (10).

Computed tomography (CT) is the next diagnostic study used to delineate the mass from surrounding structures and to evaluate for possible intraspinal extension. If the CT scan suggests extension into the spinal canal, myelography can be performed to determine the extent of the lesion within the canal. Ricci et al. (11) found magnetic resonance imaging (MRI) with its coronal and sagittal planes to be very accurate in investigating suspected dumbbell tumors (Fig. 33.1). In addition, MRI has been shown to correlate with the histopathologic findings of neurilemomas (12). The inhomogeneous high-intensity T2-weighted MR images correspond to the cystic degeneration with the surrounding collagenous fibrous tissue, a finding that is compatible with the Antoni type B histologic classification (Fig. 33.2).

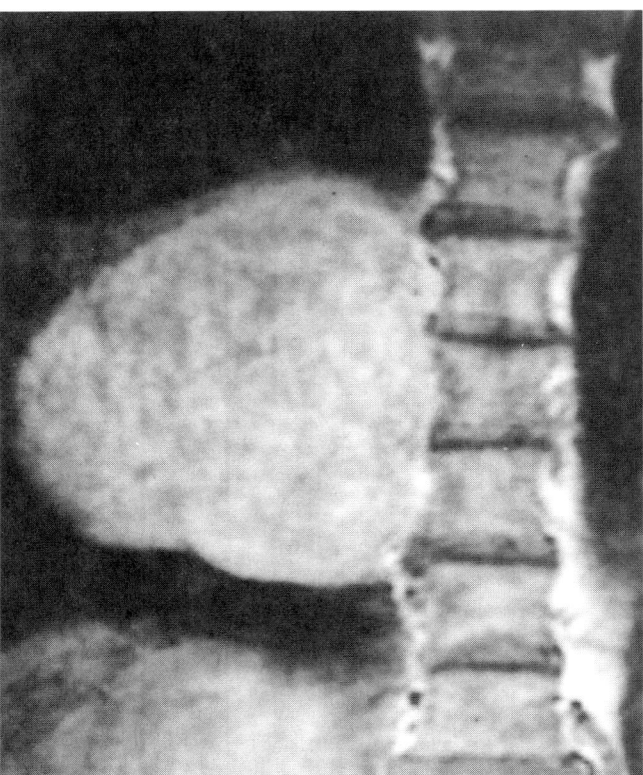

FIGURE 33.1. This MRI scan was performed after a CT scan suggested intraspinal neurilemoma extension. No intraspinal extension is seen in this coronal view. (Courtesy of Dr. Orlando Ortiz, West Virginia University School of Medicine, Morgantown, WV.)

Shields and Reynolds (7) suggested that if a paravertebral tumor occurs in the lower half of the thorax and extends into the spinal canal, the site of origin and course of the artery of Adamkiewicz, one of the sources of the anterior spinal artery, can be shown by angiography. This study may allow intraoperative protection of this vessel when the tumor is being removed.

PATHOLOGY

Neurilemoma is an encapsulated benign tumor that occurs not only in the mediastinum, but also in the flexor surfaces of the extremities, neck, retroperitoneum, and cerebellopontine angle (13). These tumors grow slowly and have a high frequency of regressive change that consists of fatty degeneration, hemorrhage, and cystic formation. In fact, some neurilemomas may become completely cystic.

Two different histologic patterns are seen in this tumor (Fig. 33.3). The Antoni type A histology usually is seen in smaller tumors and comprises highly cellu-

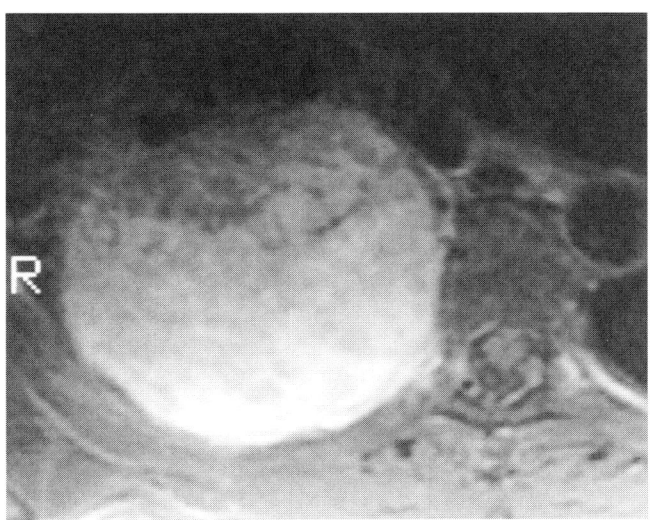

FIGURE 33.2. A T2-weighted MRI axial view of a neurilemoma shows cystic degeneration anteriorly with adjacent collagenous fibers posteriorly. The inferior vena cava, esophagus, and aorta are seen from right to left. (Courtesy of Dr. Orlando Ortiz, West Virginia University School of Medicine, Morgantown, WV.)

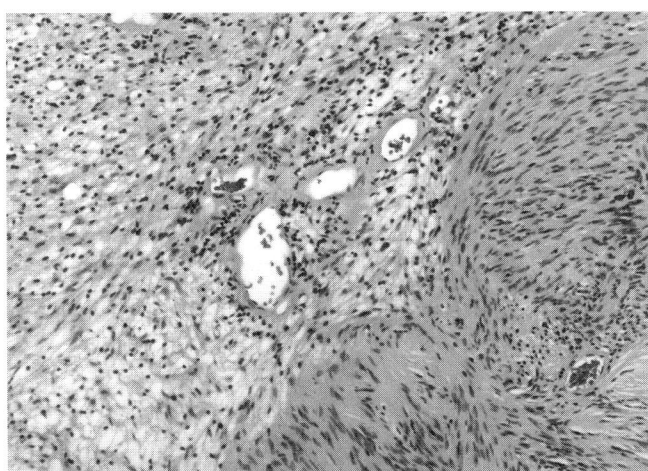

FIGURE 33.3. The Antoni A palisading, spindle cell, histologic pattern of neurilemoma is seen on the right. The Antoni B pattern of cells separated by cystic spaces is seen on the left (40×). (Courtesy of Dr. Sidney Shochet, West Virginia University School of Medicine, Morgantown, WV.)

lar, spindlelike cells arranged in palisading fashion. This palisading array of cells forms whorls that can make differentiation from sarcoma quite difficult. Despite their marked cellularity, there is little to no mitotic activity, which normally is seen in a malignancy (14). The Antoni type B pattern is one characterized by tumor cells separated by fluid-filled cystic spaces. Frequently, there are bizarre hyperchromatic nuclei that are of no particular significance. Antoni type B lesions also may have prominent blood vessels that simulate a vascular tumor.

Neurilemomas arise from Schwann cells and thus have positive S-100 immunoreactivity. The S-100 protein helps identify nerve sheath tumors (e.g., neurilemoma, some neurofibromas) from tumors of nerve cell origin (15). Keratin, desmoplakin, and neurofilaments are not expressed in these tumors (16).

TREATMENT

Treatment of a neurilemoma is excision with clear resection margins. Landreneau and colleagues (17) successfully resected a posterior mediastinal neurilemoma using video-assisted thoracoscopy. This technique has potential application for tumors in which preoperative studies show no evidence of intraspinal extension. The tumor does not recur locally, and the prognosis is excellent.

NEUROFIBROMA

Neurofibroma is a benign tumor most commonly associated with von Recklinghausen's disease. von Recklinghausen's disease is an autosomal dominant disorder characterized by cafe-au-lait hyperpigmentation of the skin, neurofibromas, and Lisch nodules (pigmented iris hamartomas) (18). Neurofibromas account for 8% of benign posterior mediastinal masses in children and 25% in adults (1, 19). These tumors are thought to arise from cells of neural crest origin and to result from a neurocristopathy (20). Neurofibromas can occur as solitary masses or be associated with other lesions as part of von Recklinghausen's disease.

PATHOLOGY

Neurofibromas are usually nonencapsulated tumors in anatomic locations other than the mediastinum. In the mediastinum, however, these tumors may be encapsulated, thus making the differentiation between neurilemoma and neurofibroma difficult. These tumors generally have a softer consistency than neurilemomas and may be very large. They usually arise from the intercostal nerves but may originate from the spinal or vagus nerves. When the peripheral nerves are enlarged and distorted diffusely by a large tumor mass, these lesions are designated as plexiform neurofibromas. Plexiform neurofibromas are associated with von Recklinghausen's disease.

Microscopically, neurofibromas are formed by a combined proliferation of Schwann cells, fibroblasts, perineural cells, and a thick tissue matrix (14). The Schwann cell is the predominant cell and can be demonstrated by neuron specific enolase (NSE) or acetylcholinesterase stains (21).

CLINICAL FEATURES AND TREATMENT

Neurofibromas most frequently are identified as an incidental finding on chest roentgenogram. They have smooth borders on radiographs and can be very large (Fig. 33.4). Presenting symptoms usually are related to compression effects or chest wall pain. As with all posterior mediastinal tumors, a CT or MRI scan should be obtained to rule out intraspinal extension and to define the borders of the tumor better.

Treatment of these lesions is surgical excision with histologically tumor negative margins. Plexiform neurofibromas may be impossible to resect because of invasion of the brachial plexus or contiguous structures. These plexiform neurofibromas may be very aggressive but do not metastasize unless transformation to a malignant schwannoma occurs (22).

MALIGNANT SCHWANNOMA

Schwannoma is a rare malignancy of nerve sheath origin that accounts for less than 1% to 2% of all posterior mediastinal tumors (7). These tumors usually arise in patients with von Recklinghausen's disease but can occur de novo. Ducatman and Scheithauer (23) described an association between malignant schwannoma and therapeutic or occupational radiation exposure. The tumor usually occurs after a 15- to 20-year latency period.

The diagnosis is made after the histologic examination of the tumor shows the presence of irregularly shaped Schwann cells in a matrix of reticulum fibers with stellate zones of necrosis. This epithelial histologic pattern is seen most commonly with the malignant transformation of a benign neurilemoma or with de novo formation arising in a patient with von Recklinghausen's disease (22). If a diffuse epithelial histologic pattern is seen, then these tumors may respond to chemotherapy (22). The majority of these tumors react with S-100 protein but are NSE nonimmunoreactive.

Malignant schwannoma is associated with von Recklinghausen's disease in 40% of cases (24). Metastases are most common to the lung, liver, skin, bone, and abdomen (24). Approximately 4% of patients with von Recklinghausen's disease develop malignant schwannomas (25).

Treatment is complete surgical excision if possible. Incomplete surgical resection predisposes to local recurrence and the development of metastatic disease. Sordillo et al. (24) suggested that patients with von Recklinghausen's disease who develop malignant schwannoma have a worse prognosis than patients with de novo tumor formation. They attribute this prognosis to the central location of von Recklinghausen tumors, which makes them more difficult to resect (24). Adjuvant radiotherapy is usually not advantageous (24), and the role of chemotherapy is as of yet undefined.

MELANOTIC SCHWANNOMA

Primary malignant melanoma of the mediastinum is very rare. Melanotic schwannomas have been identified as arising from the intercostal nerves; most of these tumors are benign. They very rarely arise from sympathetic ganglia; most of these tumors are malignant. The presence of melanin in these tumors is expected because both Schwann cells and melanocytes arise from the neural crest (26, 27). Thus, tumors in which both cell types are present could derive from a neoplastic proliferation of these undifferentiated cells (27). An alternative explanation for the presence of both cell types is that these tumors may arise from Schwann cells by aberrant differentiation of monocytes

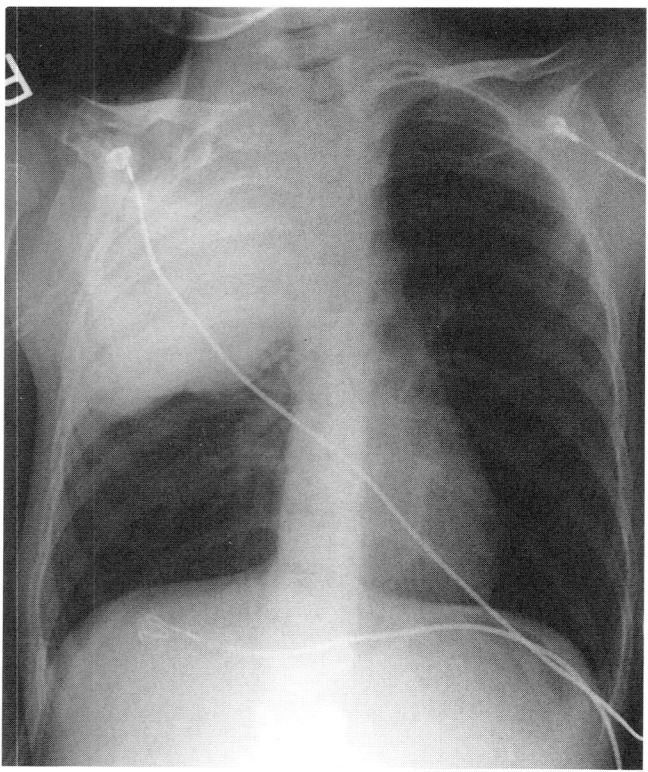

FIGURE 33.4. A large neurofibroma in a patient whose chief complaint was chest wall pain. Notice the slight scoliosis of the thoracic spine. (Courtesy of Dr. Herbert E. Warden, West Virginia University School of Medicine, Morgantown, WV.)

in the course of the neoplastic proliferation of the nerve sheath cells (27).

Grossly, the tumor is usually a well-circumscribed lesion with microscopic interdigitation with the nerve of origin. Histopathologically, the tumor is composed of elongated spindlelike cells that frequently are arranged in a palisading fashion, similar to that of the Antoni type A classification for neurilemomas (26). Mitotic activity usually is absent. Intracytoplasmic brown-black pigmented granules are seen and alternate with areas showing no pigmentation.

The treatment of melanotic schwannomas of the spinal nerve roots is excision of the tumor (26). Postoperative radiation has been reported; however, its efficacy is difficult to assess because of the small number of patients identified who have this tumor.

Melanotic schwannomas of the sympathetic ganglia are also very rare (27, 28). These tumors are more likely to be malignant than their peripheral nerve counterparts. The majority of these tumors arise in the thorax. There are reports, however, of their presence in the lumbar and cervical sympathetic ganglia. The clinical presentation of these tumors is related to their size and proximity to adjacent structures. CT and MRI studies are very helpful in evaluating the extent of the tumor and the actual tumor size.

Histopathologically, these tumors are very hypercellular with cellular pleomorphism and spindle cells arranged in palisading fashion. Immunostaining with the S-100 protein and NSE are both positive, suggesting that these tumors are of neural sheath origin (27). The degree of differentiation of the melanotic schwannomas of the sympathetic ganglia is determined ultrastructurally by the amounts and continuity of basement membrane production (29). In addition, the tumor's mitotic activity, necrosis, and any invasive characteristics noted at the time of operation correlate with the tumor's aggressiveness (28).

Treatment for melanotic schwannomas of the sympathetic ganglion is total surgical excision. Adjuvant therapy is not well established and probably should be made on an individual basis, depending on the tumor's gross and histologic characteristics.

NEURONAL CELL TUMORS

NEUROBLASTOMA

Neuroblastoma, a tumor arising from the embryonic neural crest, is another expression of the malignancies of a neurocristopathy. Neuroblasts generally differentiate into aggregates of small, round cells that become paravertebral or prevertebral ganglia and the postganglionic cells of the adrenal medulla. Primary presentation of these tumors within the mediastinum occurs in 10% to 20% of cases, with the majority presenting as intraabdominal malignancies (30–36). Neuroblastoma is a malignancy of childhood with a mean age at diagnosis of less than 2 years. The diagnosis and management of neuroblastoma have been evaluated by many clinical trials, most of which have not differentiated thoracic neuroblastoma from all other sites. This lack of differentiation occurs despite the fact that thoracic neuroblastoma has a better prognosis than abdominal neuroblastoma. The current management of thoracic neuroblastoma begins with the thoracic surgeon; thus it is imperative that these specialists have a complete understanding of the tumor biology, staging systems, and adjuvant treatment.

TUMOR BIOLOGY

Neuroblastoma is a tumor resulting from an arrest in differentiation of, or in the dedifferentiation of, neuroblasts to sensory or autonomic ganglia, Schwann cells, and other cell types. Because in vitro cell lines derived from neuroblastoma respond to modifiers of differentiation similar to the in vivo response, several studies have attempted to alter neuroblast maturation (36, 37). Biologic response modifiers including papaverine, nerve growth factor, phosphodiesterase inhibitors, and retinoic acid have been used to simulate maturation of neuroblastoma cells (34). These agents are thought to raise intracellular levels of cyclic adenosine monophosphate, which in turn accelerate nucleotidase degradation, inhibit membrane transport of the neuroblastoma cell, and accelerate maturation. Clinical application of papaverine and retinoic acid with combined chemotherapy for stage IV tumors has not altered disease progression or improved survival (38).

Several tumor markers are clinically useful in diagnosing neuroblastoma and predicting prognosis. In addition to the urinary catecholamine metabolites, NSE, and ganglioside G_{D2} have become very important diagnostic aids (39, 40). NSE antibodies are usually positive in neuroblastic tissue and may be found in the serum of patients with advanced disease. Ganglioside G_{D2} is a complex lipid molecule that is shed into the bloodstream from tumors of neuroectodermal origin. It appears to inhibit normal lymphoproliferative responses. A decrease in the circulating level of G_{D2} has been associated with remission in neuroblastoma patients (41, 42).

Vanillylmandelic acid (VMA) and homovanillic acid (HVA) are catecholamine metabolites secreted by the neuroblastoma tumor. Eight-five percent to 90% of all patients have elevated urinary VMA and HVA levels, whereas only 75% of patients with thoracic neuroblastoma have increased levels (34, 43). If the tumor originates in the dorsal root ganglia, there usually is no production of catecholamines, thus emphasizing the importance of other tumor markers, such as NSE and ganglioside G_{D2}, in making the diagnosis (44). Mass screening attempts using urine spot VMA during infancy have discovered neuroblastoma in 1 of 17,600 infants and improved the age at diagnosis, earlier stage at diagnosis, and improved survival, compared with infants who did not have the test (45).

Vasoactive intestinal peptide (VIP) is a nonspecific neural tumor marker that rarely is found in the serum of patients with neuroblastoma (46). These patients have severe, watery diarrhea and may respond symptomatically to somatostatin. Interestingly, increased secretion of VIP has been correlated with an improved outcome, presumably because VIP is secreted by more well-differentiated tumors (47).

MOLECULAR BIOLOGY AND IMMUNOLOGY

A deletion of the short arm of chromosome 1 and of the long arm of chromosome 11 are the most common chromosomal abnormalities found in neuroblastoma (48). In fact, 80% of neuroblastomas exhibit chromosomal abnormalities that may result in loss of tumor suppresser gene products (36).

Analysis of neuroblastoma cell lines by flow cytometry has shown that aneuploid tumors have a more favorable prognosis than diploid tumors (49). DNA aneuploid tumors have a better response to therapy compared with the diploid tumors, especially those with a high percentage of cells in the S phase. It also appears that DNA diploid tumors are associated with advanced stages of disease and unfavorable histology (49). For these reasons flow cytometric analysis of tumor cell DNA content is performed in all patients with neuroblastoma; thus, DNA content is a prognostic indicator for this malignancy.

Further understanding of the molecular biology of neuroblastoma came when the oncogene N-*myc* was found to be amplified in the tumor (50). N-*myc* is a nuclear-controlling factor for tumor growth and differentiation. Amplification of the N-*myc* oncogene has been associated with poorly differentiated, aggressive tumors in advanced stages of malignancy. Seeger et al. (51) demonstrated the estimated progression free survival at 18 months to be 70%, 30%, and 5% for patients with tumors having 1, 3 to 10, and 11 or more N-*myc* copies, respectively. This finding strongly suggests that genomic amplification of N-*myc* determines aggressiveness of the tumor and prognosis of the patient. Patients with unresectable hyperdiploid neuroblastomas have a much better response to chemotherapy than patients with diploid tumors (52). This fact implies that cellular DNA content may be a response predictor to chemotherapy in patients with later stage neuroblastoma. Unfortunately, DNA diploidy and N-*myc* amplification have not been found to correlate, suggesting that other biologic modifiers also play a role in determining tumor aggressiveness (53).

Because neuroblastoma tumors can and do undergo spontaneous regression, particularly the Evans stage IV-S tumor, much research has centered on the body's immunologic response to the tumor. Chung et al. (54) showed evidence of a cell-mediated immune influence and found circulating immune complexes in patients with neuroblastoma. Tracy and Weber (36) summarize the most important immunologic facets of neuroblastoma: (*a*) the cellular surface expresses G_{D2}, (*b*) the neuroblastoma cell surface proteins do not interfere with complement activation, and (*c*) the natural killer cells kill neuroblastoma cells. These findings suggest that monoclonal antibody–targeted immunotherapy and imaging will be possible in the future. In fact, murine monoclonal antibody 3F8 has been administered to patients with neuroblastoma with complete and partial responses observed (36, 55).

CLINICAL FEATURES

Neuroblastoma is a neoplasm of infancy and early childhood. The median age of presentation for nonthoracic neuroblastoma is 1.8 years and for thoracic neuroblastoma is 0.9 years (43). The majority of children (50%) with thoracic neuroblastoma present with symptoms of an upper respiratory tract infection or as an incidental chest roentgenogram finding (Figs. 33.5 and 33.6). Other presenting symptoms include acute respiratory distress (14%), neurologic symptoms (16%), or metastatic disease (10%) (43). Patients who present with acute respiratory distress are usually less than 1 year old and require emergency intervention, but they have an excellent overall survival rate. Neurologic symptoms of thoracic neuroblastoma are focal paresis or paralysis secondary to spinal cord compression and Horner's syndrome. Intraspinal extension of the neuroblastoma is found in 17% of posterior mediastinal tumors, and 45% of these patients are asymptomatic (43). The management and diagnosis of neuroblastoma dumbbell tumors are discussed below. Finally, an opsomyoclonus syndrome may precede discovery of a tumor mass (46). These symptoms are not related to the presence of brain metastasis and usually are controlled with steroids.

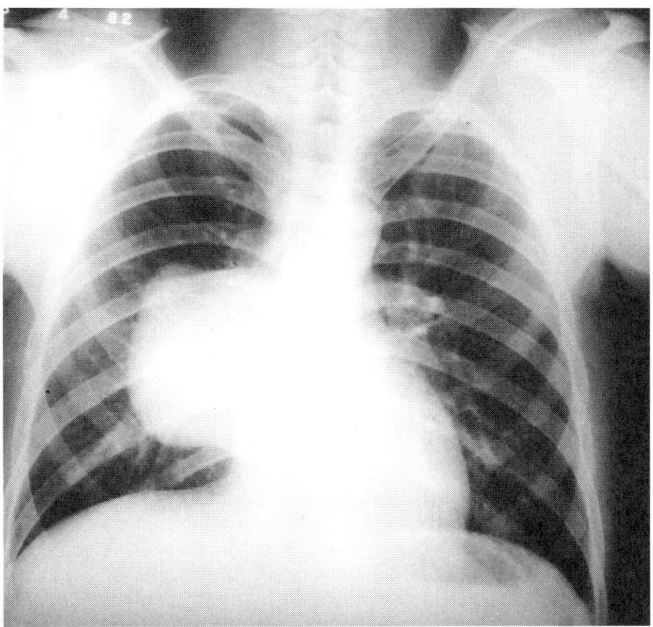

FIGURE 33.5. A posteroanterior (PA) chest roentgenograph showing an incidental mediastinal mass. The histology was compatible with neuroblastoma. (Courtesy of Dr. Orlando Ortiz, West Virginia University School of Medicine, Morgantown, WV.)

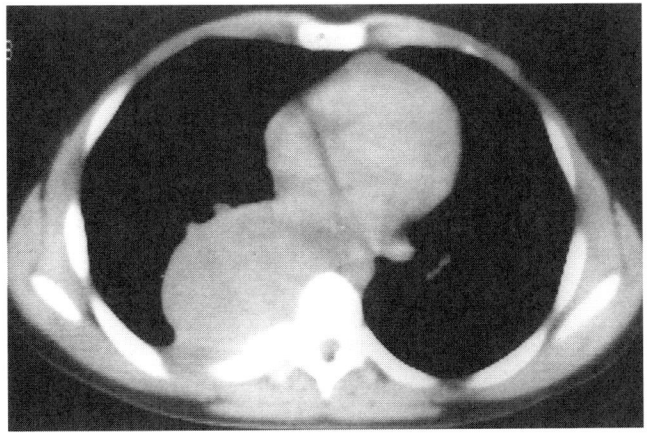

FIGURE 33.6. CT scan of the same patient shows no intraspinal extension. (Courtesy of Dr. Orlando Ortiz, West Virginia University School of Medicine, Morgantown, WV.)

Neuroblastoma is associated with several syndromes, including von Recklinghausen's disease, multiple endocrine neoplasias, Hirschsprung's disease, fetal hydantoin syndrome, and Beckwith-Wiedemann syndrome. There also have been reported cases of familial occurrence of neuroblastoma that follow an autosomal dominant pattern of inheritance (36).

In a patient with a suspected neuroblastoma of the posterior mediastinum, a complete blood cell count should be obtained to evaluate the possibility of bone marrow involvement. Liver and renal function tests also should be obtained to evaluate for metastatic disease. Urine should be screened for catecholamines, not only to aid in diagnosis but also as a baseline for follow-up therapy. In thoracic neuroblastoma, Young (31) reported that patients with normal levels of urinary VMA/HVA had more deaths than those with elevated levels. A chest roentgenogram and skeletal bone survey should also be obtained.

In addition, a radioisotope bone scan may be obtained to evaluate for bone metastasis. Recently, the utility of the bone scan has been questioned and metaiodo-benzylguanidine (mIBG)–iodine 123 (^{123}I) imaging has been proposed as a better study (56). mIBG is concentrated in most neuroblastomas with an imaging sensitivity of greater than 90% and a specificity of nearly 100% (56). Gelfand (57) proposes that the bone scan underestimates the true extent of metastatic bone disease and that areas remain positive on the bone scan after therapy because of delayed healing. mIBG imaging in Gelfand's hands has correctly identified 99% of bone metastases. Another potential advantage of mIBG imaging is using mIBG-^{131}I as initial therapy followed by chemotherapy in patients with advanced stages of neuroblastoma (57, 58).

Confirmation of the diagnosis can only be made by histologic examination of the tissue. Complete excision of the tumor is preferred, but incisional biopsies and partial resections (debulking) may be required, depending on the tumor location and involvement with adjacent organs.

PATHOLOGY

Neuroblastomas are soft, grayish-colored, and relatively well-circumscribed tumors. It is common to find focal areas of calcification, hemorrhage, or necrosis. Microscopically, there is a collection of small, oval-shaped cells with dark-staining nuclei. There usually is very little cytoplasm, and one can see Homer Wright's rosettes (tumor cells collected around fibrinous material) in 25% of cases (Fig. 33.7). Electron microscopy of this fibrinous material confirms the presence of neurites. These neurites develop spontaneously over 24 hours if exposed to retinoic acid during in vitro maturation.

Immunocytochemical analysis of neuroblastoma cells shows immunoreactivity for NSE, VIP, neurofilaments, and other related antigens. Because neuroblastoma can be confused with other small cell tumors, such as rhabdomyosarcoma or Ewing's sarcoma, these immunocytochemical studies are very important in differentiating the tumors.

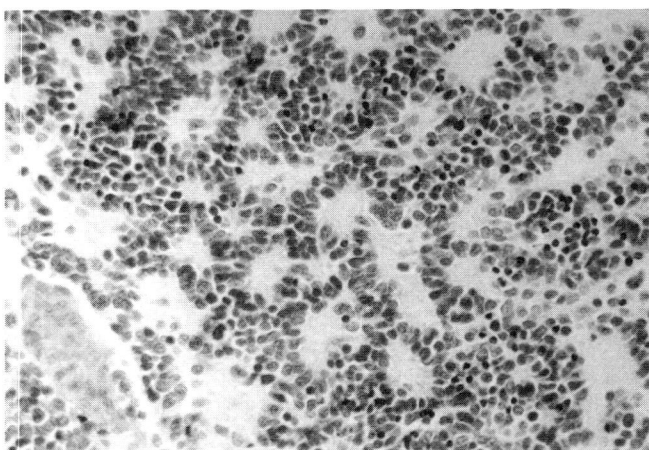

FIGURE 33.7. Representative photomicrograph of a neuroblastoma shows the small, oval-shaped cells with dark nuclei arranged in Homer-Wright rosette formation (40×). (Courtesy of Dr. Sidney Shochet, West Virginia University School of Medicine, Morgantown, WV.)

Histopathologic classification of neuroblastoma into stroma rich and stroma poor subgroups by Shimada et al. (59) has been shown to have prognostic value (Table 33.2). The Shimada histologic grading system of neuroblastoma has demonstrated that stroma rich tumors, in general, have a more favorable prognosis than stroma poor tumors. Thoracic neuroblastomas are more likely to have a stroma rich histopathologic pattern than neuroblastomas from other sites.

Neuroblastoma rarely can progress to a ganglioneuroma, a benign tumor. This progression has been suggested to occur in tumors that are well-differentiated and in patients with neuroblastomas as they age (32).

STAGING

The staging of neuroblastoma, like that of most tumors, has undergone revision, and several staging classifications have been proposed. The Evans classification is used by the Children's Cancer Study Group (60). This classification focuses on tumor resectability, distant metastasis, and tumor extension across the midline. The Evans staging system has been very accurate in categorizing patients into prognostic groups. It also identified a subgroup of stage IV tumors, called stage IV-S, that are ipsilaterally localized tumors with metastatic disease in the liver and bone marrow. Patients with stage IV-S disease are usually younger than 6 months old, and their tumors disappear without treatment in 6 to 18 months in 75% to 85% of cases. The Evans system has been criticized for its upstaging of mediastinal tumors. Mediastinal neuroblastoma is a

TABLE 33.2. Shimada Histologic Grading System for Neuroblastoma

I. STROMA POOR GROUPS

Characterized by a diffuse growth of neuroblastic cells irregularly separated by thin septa of fibrovascular tissue. Corresponds to classic neuroblastoma and diffuse ganglioneuroblastoma in other terminologies. Tumors of this group are further subdivided by grade of differentiation and nuclear morphology of the neuroblastic cells.

Grade of Differentiation

Undifferentiated histology: Composed almost entirely of immature neuroblasts with less than 5% of differentiating population. The differentiating population is characterized by nuclear enlargement, cytoplasmic eosinophilia and enlargement with distinct border, and cell processes that are clearly evident in routinely stained sections.

Differentiated histology: Composed of a mixture of neuroblastic cells with various degrees of maturity with at least 5% or more of the differentiating population. If in doubt about defining the 5% differentiation limit, one would err on the side of undifferentiation.

Nuclear Morphology

Mitosis and karyorrhexis is quantified as an index (MKI). The total of both mitosis and karyorrhexis in 500 cells in randomly selected fields is counted and divided into three categories.

Low MKI: less than 100 per 5000 cells have mitosis or karyorrhexis.

Intermediate MKI: 100 to 200 per 5000 cells have mitosis or karyorrhexis.

High MKI: more than 200 per 5000 cells have mitosis or karyorrhexis.

II. STROMA RICH GROUPS

Well Differentiated

Composed of a dominating mature ganglioneuromatous tissue with only a few randomly distributed immature neuroblastic cells. These cells aggregate but do not make distinct nests interrupting the stroma.

Intermixed

Composed of ganglioneuromatous tissue studded with scattered, variably differentiated neuroblastic cell nests. These neuroblastic cell foci are sharply defined and "make a space" in the stroma and are without apparent capsule.

Nodular

Characterized by the presence of one or a few grossly discrete masses of stroma poor neuroblastoma tissue trapped in mature matrix. The nodule is usually appreciable grossly as a hemorrhagic focus and microscopically has a sharp pushing margin or an encapsulated edge. In some areas, the capsule may be broached by apparent outward invasion by the malignant cells.

From Shimada H, Chatten J, Newton WA, et al. Histopathologic prognostic factors in neuroblastic tumors. definition of subtypes of ganglioneuroblastoma and an age-linked classification of neuroblastomas. J Natl Cancer Inst 1984;73:405–416.

midline tumor, thus making it a stage III lesion by the Evans classification (60). As will be discussed later, thoracic neuroblastoma frequently is cured by total resection, and a classification of stage III mandates chemotherapy, which may be unnecessary.

The Pediatric Oncology Group (POG) uses a modification of the St. Jude classification system that emphasizes lymph node involvement, residual tumor after resection, and hepatic involvement (61). This staging system avoids the issue of tumor extension across the midline, which is important for abdominal but not for thoracic neuroblastoma. Using this classification 68% of thoracic neuroblastomas are POG stage A or B, and only 16% are stage D at the time of diagnosis (43).

Recently, an international staging system for neuroblastoma (INSS) was proposed that attempts to maintain the stages on which agreement exists and to change the other stages to reflect current knowledge of tumor behavior (36, 62). The INSS gives prognostic weight to lymph node status, degree of resectability (complete or partial), and midline violation by the tumor. Midline tumors such as mediastinal or pelvic neuroblastomas, which cross the midline but do not invade contiguous structures, are considered stage II. It is hoped that this new staging system will be used by clinicians and investigators, but the older, more well-established classifications certainly will continue to be used as well (Table 33.3).

The importance of the thoracic surgeon in correctly staging neuroblastoma cannot be overemphasized. Most posterior mediastinal neuroblastomas can be resected totally. A wide sampling of lymph nodes adjacent to the tumor, as well as distant nodes if possible, should be performed. Although contralateral lymph node involvement is important in abdominal neuroblastoma, contralateral lymph nodes do not require assessment in thoracic neuroblastoma. The surgeon's impression of the lymph nodes intraoperatively aids in prognostication as well. If the surgeon states that there is no nodal involvement or that no nodes are seen, patients do much better (86%), compared with those whose nodes were said to be positive (66%) (63).

PROGNOSTIC FACTORS

The prognosis of children with neuroblastoma is dependent on many factors—demographic, anatomic, histologic, and molecular biologic characteristics of the tumor. Evaluation of these prognostic indicators has helped, in part, to explain why patients do well or poorly independent of the stage of their disease.

Children younger than 2 years who are diagnosed with neuroblastoma generally have a better prognosis than children older than 2 years (35). Age, however, is not as applicable as a prognostic indicator in thoracic neuroblastoma as it is in abdominal neuroblastoma because the median age at presentation for thoracic neuroblastoma is less than 1 year (43). Four-year survival for thoracic neuroblastoma is 96% for children diagnosed before 1 year of age and 80% for those who presented after their first birthday (43).

TABLE 33.3. Pediatric Oncology Group (POG) and International Staging System for Neuroblastoma (INSS) Classification for Neuroblastoma

STAGE	POG
A	Complete surgical excision of the primary tumor, histologically negative or positive margins; nonadherent intracavitary lymph nodes histologically negative for tumor; liver negative for tumor in abdominal and pelvic primary tumor
B	Incomplete surgical resection of primary tumor; lymph nodes histologically negative for tumor as in stage A
C	Complete or incomplete surgical resection of primary tumor; nonadherent intracavitary lymph nodes histologically positive for tumor; liver histologically negative for tumor
D	Disseminated disease beyond intracavitary nodes (i.e., bone marrow, bone, liver, skin, or lymph nodes beyond the cavity of the primary tumor)
DS	Localized primary tumor with dissemination limited to liver, skin, and/or marrow (no evidence of bone metastasis)

STAGE	INSS
I	Localized tumor confined to the area of origin; complete gross excision without microscopic residual disease; identifiable ipsilateral and contralateral lymph nodes negative microscopically
IIA	Unilateral tumor with incomplete gross excision; identifiable ipsilateral and contralateral lymph nodes negative microscopically
IIB	Unilateral tumor with complete or incomplete gross excision; positive ipsilateral regional lymph nodes; identifiable contralateral lymph nodes negative microscopically
III	Tumor infiltrating across the midline with or without regional lymph node involvement; or unilateral tumor with contralateral regional lymph node involvement; or midline tumor with bilateral regional lymph node involvement
IV	Dissemination of tumor to distant lymph nodes, bone, bone marrow, liver, or other organs (except as defined in stage IVS)
IVS	Localized primary tumor as defined for stage I or IIA with dissemination limited to liver, skin, or bone marrow

The Shimada histologic classification of favorable or unfavorable histology is a strong independent predictor of survival. All studies of neuroblastoma prognostic factors show the Shimada classification to correlate with prognosis.

The stage of the tumor is a prognostic indicator in thoracic neuroblastoma. Four-year survival by the POG staging classification for thoracic neuroblastoma is stage A, 100%; stage B, 89%; stage C, 92%; and stage D, 56% (43). This rate is contrasted with that of nonthoracic neuroblastoma, which has a 2-year survival of 31% for all stages (Fig. 33.8) (34). It also is interesting to note that thoracic neuroblastoma presents as POG stage A or B in 68% of cases, whereas nonthoracic neuroblastoma presents as stage A or B in only 19% of cases (Table 33.4) (43).

Other negative prognostic indicators of survival in neuroblastoma are an abnormally high level of tissue or serum NSE, increased serum ferritin levels (less than 150 mg/mL), and a VMA:HVA ratio of less than 1 (64). Lymph node involvement carries a worse prognosis in most neuroblastomas, although POG stage C thoracic neuroblastomas have excellent survival rates (43, 61). Finally, if flow cytometry shows an aneuploid tumor DNA content, this finding is a significant positive prognostic indicator (49). Diploid tumors have a much worse prognosis. Amplification of the N-*myc* oncogene is associated with a worse prognosis (51).

Clinical application of these prognostic indicators usually is limited by the availability of the facilities needed to perform these studies. With respect to thoracic neuroblastoma, age, stage, Shimada histologic classification, urinary catecholamine concentrations, and serum ferritin level have been found to be easy to perform and helpful as prognostic indicators.

TREATMENT OF NEUROBLASTOMA

The treatment for thoracic neuroblastoma centers around removal of the tumor and appropriate lymph node dissection and sampling by the thoracic surgeon. Because thoracic neuroblastoma is not as common as nonthoracic neuroblastoma, large clinical

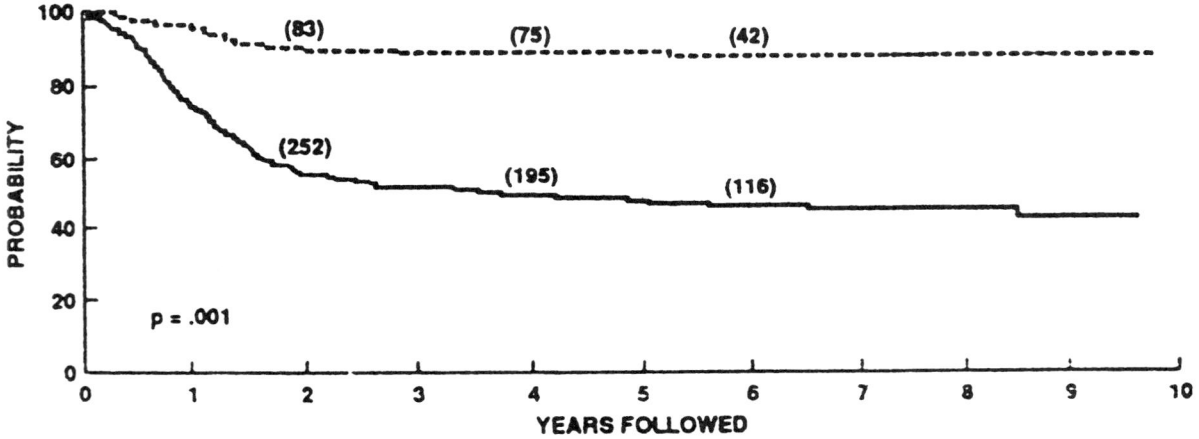

FIGURE 33.8. (From Adams GA, Shochat SJ, Smith EI, et al. Thoracic neuroblastoma: a pediatric oncology group study. J Pediatr Surg 1993;28:372–378.)

TABLE 33.4. Stage and Age at Presentation

| POG STAGE | THORACIC | | | NONTHORACIC | | |
| | AGE | | | AGE | | |
	<1 YR (No.)	>1 YR (No.)	TOTAL (%)	<1 YR (No.)	>1 YR (No.)	TOTAL (%)
A	27	19	46 (48)	30	30	60 (12)
B	11	8	19 (20)	18	14	32 (7)
C	6	7	13 (13)	26	44	70 (15)
D	6	10	16 (17)	46	229	275 (58)
DS	2	0	2 (2)	38	0	38 (8)
Total	52	44	96	158	317	475[a]

Note. Difference in stage between thoracic and nonthoracic tumors is significant ($P < .001$).
From Adams GA, Shochat SJ, Smith EI, et al. Thoracic neuroblastoma: a Pediatric Oncology Group study. J Pediatr Surg 1993;28:372–378.
[a]One patient unclassified as to stage.

trials of adjuvant or neoadjuvant chemoradiation therapy have not been performed relative only to thoracic neuroblastoma. For this reason, thoracic neuroblastoma adjuvant therapy follows similar protocols for all neuroblastoma tumors.

The treatment for neuroblastoma, POG stages A and B or Evans stage I and II, is surgical excision of the tumor with histologically tumor free margins of resection. This resection is accomplished through a posterolateral thoracotomy with liberal use of electrocautery. The tumor may invade the chest wall or the intervertebral foramina. Formal chest wall resection or dangerous intraoperative maneuvers to remove an intraspinal extension of tumor should be avoided. Because of the excellent prognosis of thoracic neuroblastomas, radical procedures do not increase survival rates (30, 32, 43). Chemotherapy or radiotherapy does not increase survival rates in Evans stage I and II tumors and only contributes to morbidity (65). If a child had a stage II tumor with several negative prognostic indicators (e.g., high serum ferritin, diploid tumor), then chemotherapy should be considered, preferably as part of a clinical trial.

Treatment for Evans stage III or POG stage C lesions begins with tumor debulking and adequate lymph node sampling. After the tumor has been debulked, chemotherapy and rarely radiotherapy are used to eradicate the remaining tumor. If there is a suggestion of residual tumor on standard imaging studies, a follow-up operation can be performed and may improve survival (66). An alternative to initial debulking of the tumor is neoadjuvant chemotherapy and radiotherapy to shrink the tumor and increase the chances for resection (67). A biopsy, usually CT-guided, is performed to establish the initial diagnosis. Standard chemotherapy requires the use of vincristine and cyclophosphamide as the main agents, with other drugs added in efforts to increase the efficacy (Table 33.5).

GANGLIONEUROMA AND GANGLIONEUROBLASTOMA

Ganglioneuromas are fully differentiated neuroendocrine tumors that are found most commonly in the paravertebral sulci or the retroperitoneum. These tumors arise from the sympathetic ganglia and are uniformly benign. They are the most common benign mediastinal tumor in children, occurring in 33% to 66% of cases (68, 69). Roughly 50% of cases occur in adolescents and young adults.

Radiographically, these tumors may be large and have focal areas of calcification (Fig. 33.9). They have an edematous appearance on T2-weighted MRI scans (Fig. 33.10). In contrast to ganglioneuroblastomas or neuroblastomas, these tumors rarely have intraspinal extension.

The tumor is frequently a large, encapsulated mass with a firm consistency on palpation. Microscopically, the appearance is similar to that of a neurofibroma except for the presence of mature ganglion cells (Fig. 33.11). Thorough sampling should be done to confirm the absence of friable, hemorrhagic areas, which are suspicious for malignancy.

The treatment for ganglioneuromas is surgical excision. The prognosis is excellent and recurrence is uncommon.

Ganglioneuroblastoma is a transitional tumor of sympathetic cell origin that contains elements of a benign ganglioneuroma interspersed between islands of malignant neuroblastoma (Fig. 33.12). These tumors are more common in children less than 3 years old (50%) and are not associated with von Recklinghausen's disease or family history (70). There is no sex predilection, and whites are affected more often than blacks. The majority of these tumors are incidental roentgenographic findings, but they can present with airway symptoms, paraplegia, or chest wall pain (70).

Diagnostic workup should proceed with CT or MRI scanning of the chest and urinary catecholamine evaluation. Adams and Hochholzer (70) reported a 12.5% incidence of elevated urinary VMA and HVA in 40 patients. This rate had no prognostic significance. An intravenous pyelogram or abdominal CT scan should be done to rule out metastatic adrenal neuroblastoma. A modified Evans staging system is used in which stage I is an encapsulated, noninvasive tumor; stage II is an ipsilateral locally invasive tumor in which lymph nodes may be positive; stage III is a tumor that crosses the midline; and stage IV is metastatic disease.

Treatment for stage I lesions should be surgical excision. Radiation and chemotherapy offer no survival advantage in stage I disease. If there is incomplete excision of the tumor, or a composite histologic pattern is identified, radiation may be considered. Zajtchuk et al. (71) documented a 44% incidence of skeletal deformity in children who received adjuvant radiation. They suggest that if radiation is used, it should be limited to 20 Gy and encompass both sides of the vertebral column. Stage II and III lesions should be resected if possible, but they may respond to vincristine or cyclophosphamide–based chemotherapy and radiation therapy. All patients with stage IV tumors in the series of Adams and Hochholzer (70) died with widespread metastatic disease.

Prognostic factors include age (younger patients do much better), degree of differentiation, and the presence of a diffuse histologic pattern. Malignant recurrences usually are seen only in older patients. Five-

TABLE 33.5. Pediatric Oncology Group Stage-Related/Age-Related Treatment Regimens for Neuroblastoma

STAGE: AGE (YEAR)	PRIMARY INDUCTION THERAPY	MAINTENANCE THERAPY	CROSSOVER/ RELAPSE THERAPY
A: ≤1 and >1	None	None	CYC/ADR
B: ≤1 and >1	CYC/ADR × 5	None	PLAT/VM
C: ≤1	CYC/ADR × 5	None	PLAT/VM
C: >1	CYC/ADR × 5 ± XRT	CYC/ADR × 2 and PLAT/VM × 2	PLAT/VM
D: ≤1	CYC/ADR × 5	None	PLAT/VM
D: >1 (1981–1984)	CYC/ADR × 5 vs. PLAT/VM × 5	CYC/ADR × 3 PLAT/VM × 3	None
D: >1 (1984–1987)	CECA × 5	CECA × 3	None

Abbreviations. CYC/ADR, cyclophosphamide (150 mg/m^2 PO, days 1 to 7), adriamycin (35 mg/m^2 IV, day 8); XRT, radiation therapy; PLAT/VM, cisplatin (90 mg/m^2 IV, day 1), VM26 (100 mg/m^2 IV, day 3); CECA, cisplatin (90 mg/m^2 IV, day 1), VM26 (100 mg/m^2 IV, day 3), cyclophosphamide (150 mg/m^2 PO, days 7 to 13), adriamycin (35 mg/m^2 IV, day 14).

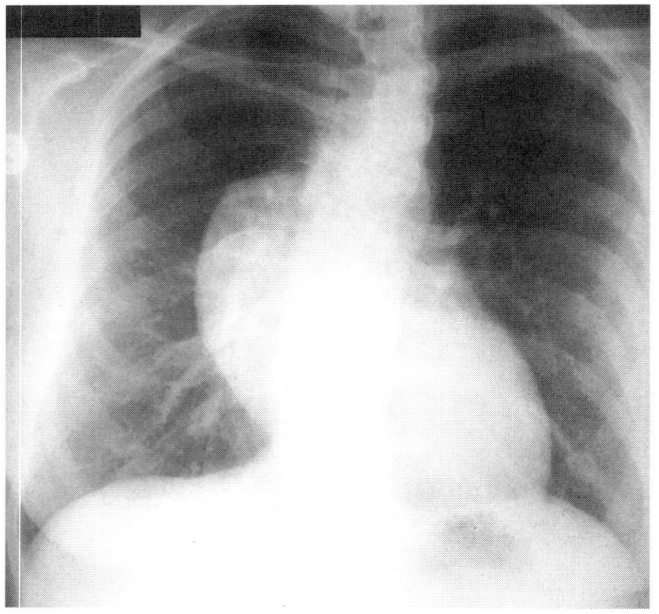

FIGURE 33.9. PA chest roentgenograph shows a large ganglioneuroma with resultant scoliosis. (Courtesy of Dr. Orlando Ortiz, West Virginia University School of Medicine, Morgantown, WV.)

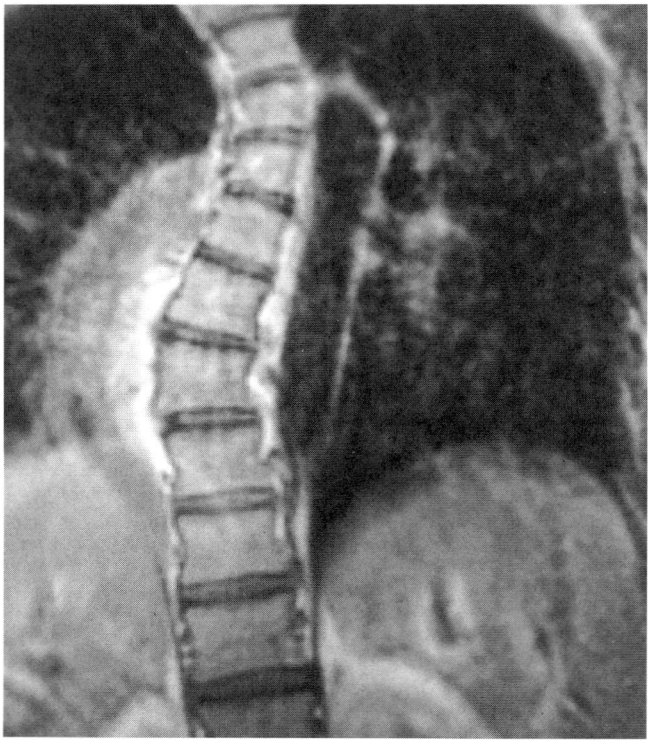

FIGURE 33.10. T2-weighted MRI scan shows edematous changes characteristic of a ganglioneuroma. (Courtesy of Dr. Orlando Ortiz, West Virginia University School of Medicine, Morgantown, WV.)

year actuarial survival for posterior mediastinal ganglioneuroblastoma is 88% for all cases (68). This survival rate compares favorably with a 3-year survival rate of 65% reported for 20 patients with tumor in all locations (72).

PARAGANGLIOMA

The paraganglia are small collections of cells having a common neural crest origin. These paraganglia are distributed symmetrically and segmentally in the paraaxial regions of the trunk and in the vicinity of the ontogenetic gill arches (73). Locations of the paraganglia include the adrenal medulla, aorta, blood vessel walls, heart, and mediastinum. The majority of mediastinal paragangliomas are biologically inactive and are called nonfunctioning paragangliomas. These tumors may involve the parasympathetic chemoreceptor tissues of the carotid body, aorticopulmonary glomus, or vagal body; when they do they are called chemodec-

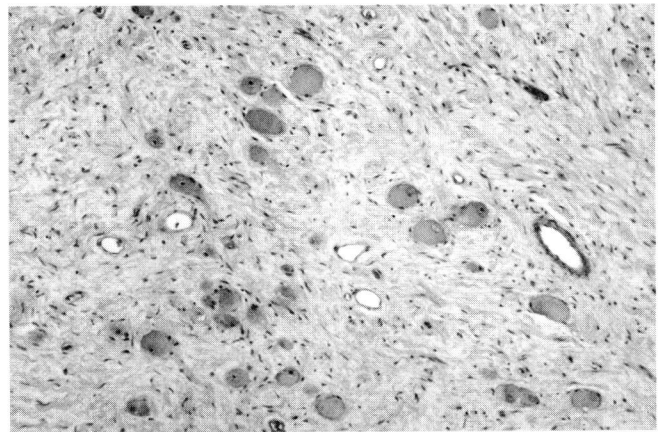

FIGURE 33.11. Photomicrograph of a ganglioneuroma shows mature ganglion cells in a fibrous matrix. (Courtesy of Dr. Sidney Shochet.)

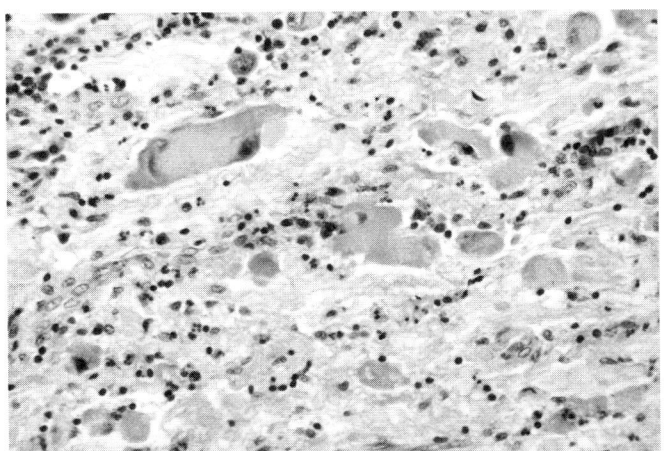

FIGURE 33.12. Photomicrograph of a ganglioneuroblastoma shows malignant neuroblastoma cells surrounded by mature ganglion cells and occasional mitotic figures. (Courtesy of Dr. Sidney Shochet.)

tomas (74). The majority of chemodectomas and nonfunctioning paragangliomas are benign, although they can become malignant (73, 75, 76). Mediastinal paragangliomas that become biologically active are called extraadrenal pheochromocytomas. These lesions are discussed in the following section.

In 1974 Glenner and Grimley (77) categorized the extraadrenal paraganglia into four groups based on their anatomic location, innervation, and microscopic appearance. The branchiomeric paraganglia are the orbital, jugulotympanic, carotid, subclavian, laryngeal, aorticopulmonary, coronary, and pulmonary paraganglia. The other three groups are the intravagal, aorticosympathetic, and visceral-autonomic paraganglia. Posterior mediastinal paragangliomas are classified as intravagal or aorticosympathetic in most cases.

CLINICAL FEATURES

Nonfunctioning paragangliomas are found incidentally on chest roentgenograms in 50% of patients (75, 78). Patients who have symptoms usually complain of chest wall pain or symptoms related to mass effect, including coughing, superior vena cava syndrome, dyspnea, and hemoptysis (75, 76). There is a slight male preponderance for posterior mediastinal paragangliomas, and the mean age at diagnosis is 40 years with a range of 16 to 64 years (75).

Malignancy in a paraganglioma is very rare and has been reported in only five cases (76). These tumors are more common in males (6:1) and usually involve the right second to fourth costovertebral sulcus. These patients either present with metastatic disease or develop it shortly after their initial diagnosis. The most common sites of metastasis include the lung and bone; other sites include the liver, heart, and kidneys (76).

The radiographic diagnosis of paraganglioma has been facilitated by MRI. Axial T1-weighted images reveal a mass with nonhomogeneous intermediate signal intensity. The T2 images show the same high signal intensity seen with other mediastinal tumors (79). Preoperative angiography has been suggested by Drucker et al. (80) to help define the vascular supply to the tumor. Angiographic features of paragangliomas include hypervascularity; multiple, large feeding vessels; and early draining veins (80, 81). MRI is an excellent alternative noninvasive imaging technique to determine tumor vascularity. Rapid blood flow in vessels is manifested as flow void by MRI. Mediastinal tumors with high vascularity are limited to Castleman's disease, hemangioma, goiter, and paraganglioma (80). mIBG-131I imaging is not very useful in the identification of nonfunctioning paragangliomas (82).

PATHOLOGY

The tumors are soft and irregular and occasionally have a fibrous capsule. Microscopically, these tumors show marked hypervascularity with tumor cells arranged in a striking, nested, organoid (Zellballen) pattern. The nuclei are oval with prominent nucleoli, and eosinophilic cytoplasm is abundant. Cellular pleomorphism is seen routinely, but mitotic figures are rare (73, 75).

Immunohistochemical analysis demonstrates immunoreactivity with the S-100 protein. Vimentin, neurofilament, and *leu*-enkephalin are also immunoreactive (73, 75).

No specific histologic feature in the tumor has proven to be a reliable determinant of malignancy potential (76). Evidence of local invasion or metastasis of the paraganglioma at operation appears to be the most significant determinant of aggressive behavior (75, 76).

TREATMENT

The treatment of the nonfunctioning paraganglioma is extirpation. Because the tumors can be quite vascular, there should be adequate intravenous access and several units of blood available. A posterolateral thoracotomy is the usual surgical approach. If the tumor invades contiguous structures or is infiltrative at the time of operation, the surgeon should have a high index of suspicion of malignancy. Resection of the entire tumor in this setting may be impossible, but debulking of the mass should be done. Radiotherapy and chemotherapy have been used for these aggressive tumors, but their usefulness remains unproved (76).

PHEOCHROMOCYTOMA

Extraadrenal pheochromocytoma occurs in 10% of all cases, and less than 2% of these occur within the chest (83). The extraadrenal pheochromocytoma also is referred to as a functioning paraganglioma. Ninety percent of these lesions are benign, and in 10% of cases there are multiple tumors. If another lesion is present in addition to an intrathoracic pheochromocytoma, this finding should raise the suspicion of Carney's syndrome. This nonfamilial syndrome describes an association among gastric epithelial leiomyosarcoma, pulmonary chondroma, and extraadrenal pheochromocytoma (84). Gastric tumors usually occur first, followed by the chondroma and pheochromocytoma, but any order of presentation is possible. Survival in patients with Carney's triad is good (81%), but 55% of patients are alive with residual disease. If a pheochromocytoma is present, the prognosis is worse (85). A comparison between features of mediastinal and adrenal pheochromocytomas shows that multicentricity occurs more frequently (43% versus 13%), malignancy is more common (43% versus 20%), and diploid tumors with a malignant course are more common (43% versus 0%) (83).

CLINICAL PRESENTATION

The majority of patients experience sweating, tachycardia, and headaches. They are almost always hypertensive, which can be paroxysmal. Compressive signs secondary to the tumor may occur and include paralysis, Horner's syndrome, dysphagia, or dyspnea. Pheochromocytomas, in general, are associated in about 10% of cases with familial neurocristopathic syndromes. These include multiple endocrine neoplasia (MEN)–2a, MEN-2b, Von Hippel-Lindau disease, and von Recklinghausen's disease. Finally, these tumors may be identified as an incidental chest roentgenogram finding. Both sexes are affected equally and at all ages.

Biochemical diagnosis of a mediastinal pheochromocytoma is made initially by urine catecholamine measurements of VMA, normetanephrine, and metanephrine. Engelman and Hammond (86) suggested that if urinary epinephrine or its metabolites are elevated, the tumor is most likely adrenal rather than extraadrenal. Plasma and platelet catecholamine measurements may also be diagnostic (84). If these biochemical assays are equivocal, a clonidine suppression test may be performed. Clonidine reduces sympathetic tone and catecholamine secretion through a central α-agonist pathway. Pheochromocytomas do not have a nerve supply; thus, serum catecholamine levels do not decrease in response to clonidine.

Preoperative localization of the tumor and its relationship to contiguous structures is very important. An abdominal CT should be performed first to rule out an adrenal pheochromocytoma. A CT or MRI study of the chest should be performed if the lesion is suspected to be intrathoracic by chest roentgenogram or if the patient's symptoms are complex. If the tumor has not been localized, mIBG scintography is the procedure of choice. This radiopharmaceutical is concentrated in the storage granules of chromaffin cells derived from the embryonic neural crest. mIBG-^{131}I positive scans have been reported for neuroblastoma, carcinoid, and medullary thyroid carcinoma (82). Shapiro et al. (87) reported a 99% specificity and 87% sensitivity for pheochromocytoma localization in all cases. The importance of this study in mediastinal pheochromocytomas localization is threefold: (*a*) It can identify multiple pheochromocytomas, which are more common with mediastinal pheochromocytomas than with adrenal lesions. (*b*) Localization to the chest may allow better definition of the mass by high-resolution CT scan, MRI, or angiography. (*c*) mIBG scanning can provide useful information for follow-up of recurrence after resection.

PATHOLOGY

Grossly, the tumor is soft, reddish-brown in color, and quite vascular. Microscopically, there are collections of pheochromocytes, which show brown cytoplasmic staining with chromic salts. These cells are usually very pleomorphic with nuclear atypia.

Electron microscopy shows an abundance of cytoplasmic granules and mitochondria (88). All tumors have immunoreactivity with NSE. Flow cytometry has shown that with mediastinal pheochromocytomas all benign tumors were diploid or tetraploid, whereas all aneuploid DNA patterns were malignant (83).

TREATMENT

Once the tumor has been localized to the mediastinum, the only chance for cure is surgical excision. Preparation of the patient for surgery begins first with α-adrenergic blockade. Phenoxybenzamine is the drug of choice and is started 10 to 14 days before surgery and is increased daily until a normotensive state is reached (89). This drug should be stopped 2 days before surgery because postoperative hypotension has been reported secondary to the drug's long half-life (84). Other drugs that have been used successfully for α-blockade include prazosin, labetalol, and phentolamine.

Once adequate α-blockade is established, β-blockade may be needed for persistent tachycardia. β-Blockade should not precede α-blockade because antagonism of β-mediated vasodilator effects with unopposed α-mediated vasoconstriction precipitates a hypertensive crisis (89). In addition, β-blockade can precipitate cardiac failure with pulmonary edema.

Patients with pheochromocytoma are intravascularly volume depleted, but this condition usually is corrected with adequate α-blockade. Aggressive preoperative intravenous volume expansion has been associated with congestive heart failure (90).

Anesthetic management of these patients is beyond the scope of this discussion, but Hull offers an excellent review of the subject (89).

Pheochromocytomas are approached through a posterolateral thoracotomy. Usually, they are removed easily because most are noninvasive and benign. If they invade the intervertebral foramina or involve one of the spinal nerves, they may need to be approached using techniques described for the management of dumbbell tumors. These lesions are often very vascular, and paying attention to large vessels entering or surrounding the tumor can prevent extensive blood loss. Intraoperative hypertensive crisis is rare provided an adequate preoperative pharmacologic blockade has been done.

Once the tumor is removed and plasma catecholamine levels decrease, there may be a precipitous decrease in blood pressure. This decrease in pressure should be anticipated and volume loading instituted with normal saline solution, based on central venous pressure recordings. In addition, blood sugar levels should be checked frequently after tumor removal because decreased catecholamine levels cause a surge in insulin production with resultant hypoglycemia (89).

Postoperatively, the blood pressure is usually normal, but serum catecholamine levels do not return to normal for 1 to 2 weeks (74). Residual mild hypertension after return of catecholamine levels to normal is most likely caused by microvascular damage to the kidney from long-standing hypertension (74). Failure of the blood pressure to return to near normal levels suggests the presence of incomplete resection, metastases, or a second primary tumor. mIBG scanning is very useful in determining the specific cause.

Malignant pheochromocytomas within the chest are relatively uncommon relative to all pheochromocytomas, and no prospective randomized trials of adjuvant therapy have been undertaken. The diagnosis of malignancy is made only if there is demonstrable metastatic disease because there are no histologic or immunocytochemical differences between benign and malignant tumors. Resection, if possible, is the treatment of choice for metastatic disease. The 10-year survival of patients with resected malignant tumors is roughly 50% (83). If the tumor is unresectable, debulking may make subsequent pharmacologic management easier. The tumors are radiosensitive, and radiotherapy to decrease local recurrence or to treat bony metastases may be effective (89, 91). In a nonrandomized trial, combination chemotherapy with cyclophosphamide, vincristine, and dacarbazine produced a complete or partial clinical response rate of 57% and a biochemical response rate of 79% in patients with malignant pheochromocytoma (92). This regimen was used because of its effectiveness in treating neuroblastoma, a tumor that is embryologically similar to pheochromocytoma. Recently, high-dose ^{131}I-mIBG has been suggested as a therapeutic agent for malignant pheochromocytomas (91, 93, 94). Because ^{131}I-mIBG is concentrated in these tumors, radiation doses of 2000 cGy can be delivered to the tumor (93). Patients with rapidly growing tumors and soft tissue metastases (but not bone metastasis) appeared to respond best to this form of treatment. Finally, embolization of the tumor has been performed for abdominal pheochromocytomas (95).

NEUROEPITHELIOMA

In 1979 Askin et al. (96) described a small, malignant, round cellular tumor of the thoracopulmonary region that was histologically similar to rhabdomyosarcoma, Ewing's sarcoma, and neuroblastoma. The Askin tumor was discovered after a 13-year retrospective review from three major universities identified 20 cases. It is now thought to be much more common, perhaps because surgeons and pathologists are aware of its existence. Ultrastructural studies, immunocytochemical analysis, and DNA analysis all suggest that this tumor has a neuroectodermal origin (96–98). The possibility of cervical or thoracic sympathetic ganglion origin for the posterior mediastinal location of these tumors is unlikely because they do not secrete any detectable catecholamines (97). A more likely origin for Askin's tumor is the intercostal nerves because many have been reported there (97, 98). Investigators now consider Askin's tumor to be a thoracic presentation of a peripheral neuroepithelioma.

MOLECULAR BIOLOGY

A chromosome translocation rcp (11;22) (q24:q12) is commonly found in neuroepitheliomas. This chromosomal abnormality confirms the different cellular origins of the neuroepithelioma and neuroblastoma but not the Ewing's sarcoma, which has the same translocation (99). Ultrastructural analysis via electron microscopy shows more cell-to-cell attachments, the presence of irregular microtubular processes, and a filamentous cytoskeleton in the neuroepithelioma in contrast to Ewing's sarcoma (97). In addition, neuroepitheliomas do not make cartilage or bone, which is seen occasionally in Ewing's tumors.

Neuroepitheliomas exhibit significant immunoreactivity to NSE (97). Although NSE immunostaining is common to both neuroblastoma and neuroepithelioma tumors, there is a conspicuous absence of catecholamine synthesis enzymes in neuroepitheliomas (98). In contrast to neuroblastoma, there are high levels of acetylcholine synthetic enzymes in the neuroepithelioma (98).

Protooncogene expression in neuroepithelioma is similar to that of neuroblastoma in that c-*src* protein kinase activity and the pattern of c-*sis* and c-*myb* expression are constant (98). Neuroblastoma, however, has high levels of N-*myc* expression, whereas the cell lines of neuroepitheliomas invariably have only a single copy of N-*myc* (100). Neuroepithelioma expresses high levels of the c-*myc* oncogene whereas neuroblastoma does not (98). The altered protooncogene regulation seen in neuroepithelioma is an area of intense research because protooncogenetic expression may be useful as a tumor marker or as an intermediate biomarker of treatment.

PATHOLOGY

Grossly, the tumor is a gray-white lobulated mass that is circumscribed but not encapsulated. There may be focal areas of hemorrhage and necrosis.

Histologically, there are compact sheets of small round cells alternating with a nesting pattern of cells and necrotic tissue (96). Classic Homer-Wright pseudorosettes are not seen, but pseudorosettes around a fibrous band are frequently present. There usually is a moderate degree of mitotic activity.

Ultrastructural analysis demonstrates prominent cytoplasmic processes and occasional neurosecretory granules. There is no collection of thick and thin microfilaments forming Z-bands like those characteristically seen in rhabdomyosarcoma.

CLINICAL FEATURES

Neuroepithelioma occurs as a posterior mediastinal tumor in 10% of cases. Other more common locations for neuroepithelioma include the chest wall, lung, or pleura. It presents between the ages of 4 months and 20 years with a mean age at diagnosis of 14.5 years (96). It more commonly affects females (male to female ratio, 1:3) (96).

Patients with neuroepithelioma as a posterior mediastinal mass usually complain of dyspnea, posterior chest wall pain, or unexplained fever with generalized malaise (96, 101). Radiographic findings of this tumor are that of a paravertebral mass, which may be rather large. Calcification of the mass is rare, but adjacent rib destruction or pleural effusions are common (96). Serum ferritin and urine catecholamine levels are not elevated in neuroepitheliomas in contrast to elevated levels seen in neuroblastoma.

TREATMENT

Because neuroepithelioma has only recently been diagnosed as a entity separate from other small cell tumors, large clinical trials comparing treatment modalities do not exist. These tumors have a tendency for locoregional recurrence and rarely metastasize to the liver, adrenals, distant bone, or lymphatics (96).

The median survival for patients with neuroepithelioma is poor (8 months in the study of Askin et al. [96]). Therefore, treatment involves a multimodality approach with wide excision of the lesion if possible. The tumors are radiosensitive, and local control of unresectable, partially resected, or recurrent tumors can be achieved using radiation doses of 35 to 50 Gy.

Chemotherapy consists of a combination of cyclophosphamide, actinomycin D, and vincristine. Methotrexate, 5-fluorouracil, doxorubicin, and dacarbazine have also been used with some success (96). Miser et al. (102) reported an aggressive multimodality approach in which remission is induced with chemotherapy and local control of the tumor is obtained with excision and/or radiation. After remission occurs, marrow ablative chemotherapy as well as total body irradiation with autologous bone marrow reimplantation is performed (22, 102). Long-term results of this approach are not available but are promising. At present, patients with a neuroepithelioma should probably be enrolled in a clinical trial if at all possible.

MANAGEMENT OF DUMBBELL TUMORS

Dumbbell tumors are neurogenic tumors of the posterior mediastinum that have an intraspinal extension through the intervertebral foramen (Fig. 33.13).

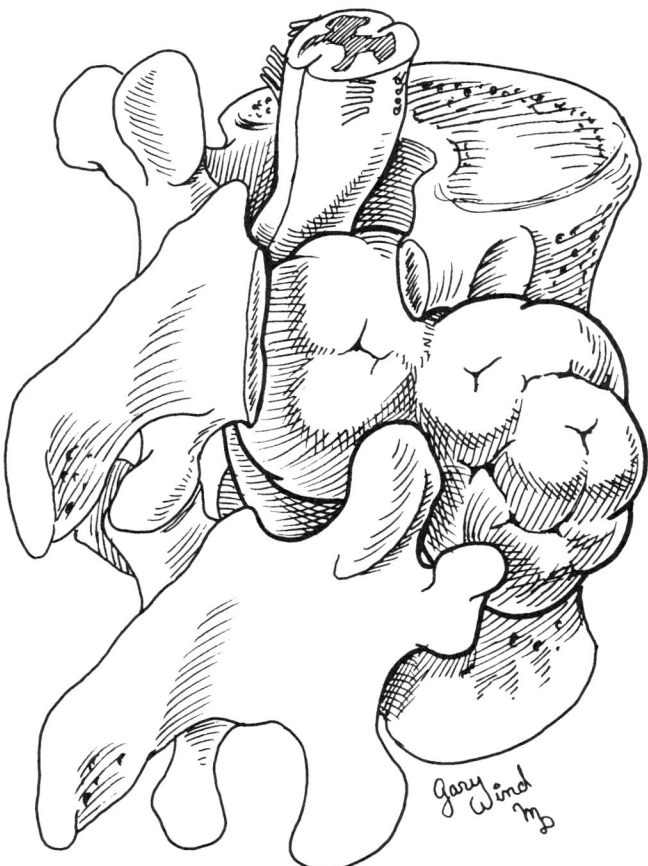

FIGURE 33.13. This illustration shows the dumbbell extension of a paravertebral tumor through the intervertebral foramen. Notice the spinal cord compression caused by the tumor.

These tumors are also called hourglass tumors. Akwari et al. (8) reported an incidence of 9.8% of dumbbell tumors among 706 posterior mediastinal neurogenic tumors. In their series, 60% of patients had symptoms related to the intraspinal component of their tumor, whereas 40% were asymptomatic at initial presentation. The clinical presentation of a dumbbell tumor, if symptomatic, may involve motor weakness, sensory loss, paresthesias, chest wall pain, or fecal or urinary incontinence (8, 103). Tumors with a large intrathoracic component can produce shortness of breath or cough.

Roentgenograms of the chest, both posterior-anterior and lateral views, and of the thoracic spine are the first diagnostic radiographic studies that should be performed. There are several findings on plain radiography that are suggestive of the presence of intraspinal extension of the tumor. If the intervertebral foramen is widened with evidence of smooth erosion of the surrounding pedicles, this finding strongly suggests a dumbbell tumor (8, 103, 104). Other radiographic findings include scalloping of the posterior vertebrae, overgrowth of the pedicles, increased interpediculate distance, and rib thinning with increased distance between the ribs (104). If any of these findings is present on plain roentgenograms, or if the physician has a clinical suspicion of the presence of a dumbbell tumor, further studies are warranted.

CT scans of the thorax are a routine part of the workup of posterior mediastinal tumors. CT imaging provides a very clear delineation between the mass and surrounding tissues, but it is limited by axial plane imaging only. In the past, dumbbell tumors were evaluated by CT and myelography (8, 103, 104). Myelography accurately determines the length of tumor extension within the spinal canal, but it is an invasive procedure with associated risks. Ricci et al. (11) and others (105) stressed the use of MRI in the evaluation of dumbbell tumors (11, 105). MRI axial views have less definition than CT, but the images on the coronal and sagittal views allow precise evaluation of the intraspinal extension of the tumor (Figs. 33.14 and 33.15) (11). Use of MRI to evaluate dumbbell tumors in the pediatric population is especially useful because intrathecal contrast material is avoided (105). Currently, chest and spine roentgenograms and a CT scan or MRI are recommended to evaluate the posterior mediastinum. If a dumbbell tumor is suspected, MRI is currently the diagnostic modality of choice (Fig. 33.16).

The histology of dumbbell tumors in pediatric patients is usually a neuroblastoma or ganglioneuroblastoma (104). In adults neurilemomas, neurofibromas,

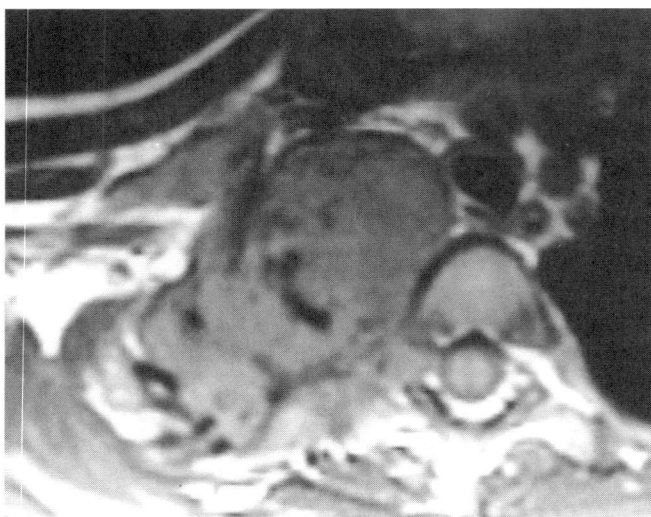

FIGURE 33.14. Axial MRI view shows intraspinal extension with pedicle erosion of this large neurofibroma. (Courtesy of Dr. Orlando Ortiz.)

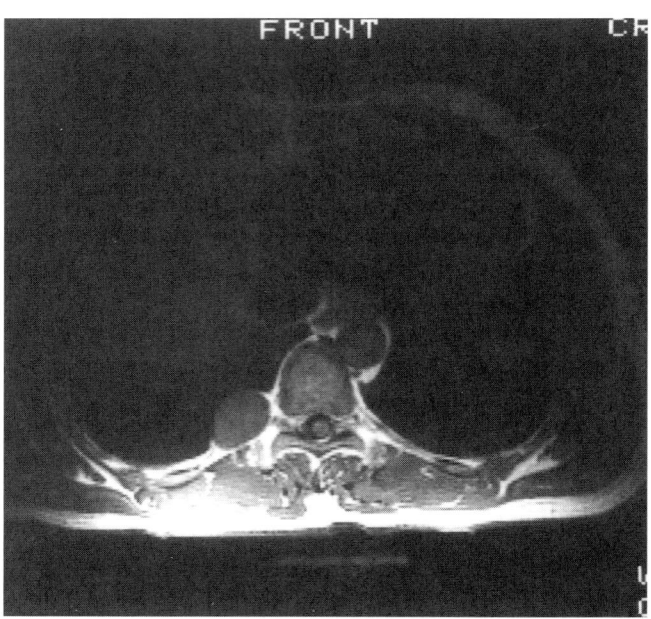

FIGURE 33.16. A CT scan suggested the presence of a dumbbell tumor, but this MRI scan shows no intraspinal extension of the neuroblastoma. (Courtesy of Dr. Deborah Granke, West Virginia University School of Medicine, Morgantown, WV.)

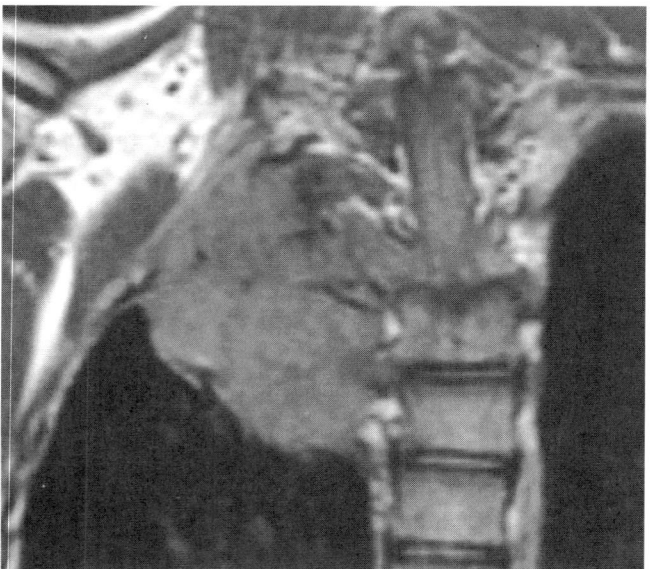

FIGURE 33.15. Coronal MRI view shows intraspinal extension of this large right paravertebral tumor. (Courtesy of Dr. Orlando Ortiz.)

and rarely paragangliomas are found to have intraspinal extension of the tumor (5).

Once the diagnosis of a dumbbell tumor is made, a surgical approach is planned in consultation with a neurosurgeon. The goal is the removal of the entire tumor. Akwari et al. (8) in 1978 performed a two-stage procedure, a laminectomy followed by a thoracotomy at a later date, in 9 of 16 patients. Thirty-three percent of these patients required urgent surgery for epidural hematomas and formation of a pseudomeningocele after the laminectomy portion of the procedure. The remaining 7 patients in this series had combined laminectomy and thoracotomy as a single procedure with good results (8). If a thoracotomy is performed first and the intrathoracic component of the tumor is removed, there can be bleeding into the intraspinal portion of the tumor that can cause spinal cord compression.

Grillo and colleagues (103) popularized the combined approach to dumbbell tumors in 1983. The thoracotomy is performed first by raising a skin and subcutaneous tissue flap over the muscular fascia. The thorax is entered beneath this flap with reference given to the intercostal space nearest the involved foramen (Fig. 33.17). The intrathoracic portion of the tumor is mobilized so that it is attached only at its intraforaminal portion. The laminectomy portion of the procedure is then performed. A large majority of these tumors are extradural and can be dissected free relatively easily. If there are intradural projections of the tumor, the dura is opened laterally over the tumor and dissected from the spinal cord with microsurgical techniques. The nerve root entering the tumor is divided. Radicular arterial branches may enter the intervertebral foramen to supply the spinal cord; every attempt should be made to preserve these arteries. If the artery must be sacrificed to remove the tumor completely, neurologic compromise is rarely seen. Depending on the size, the foramen may need to be enlarged to remove the tumor.

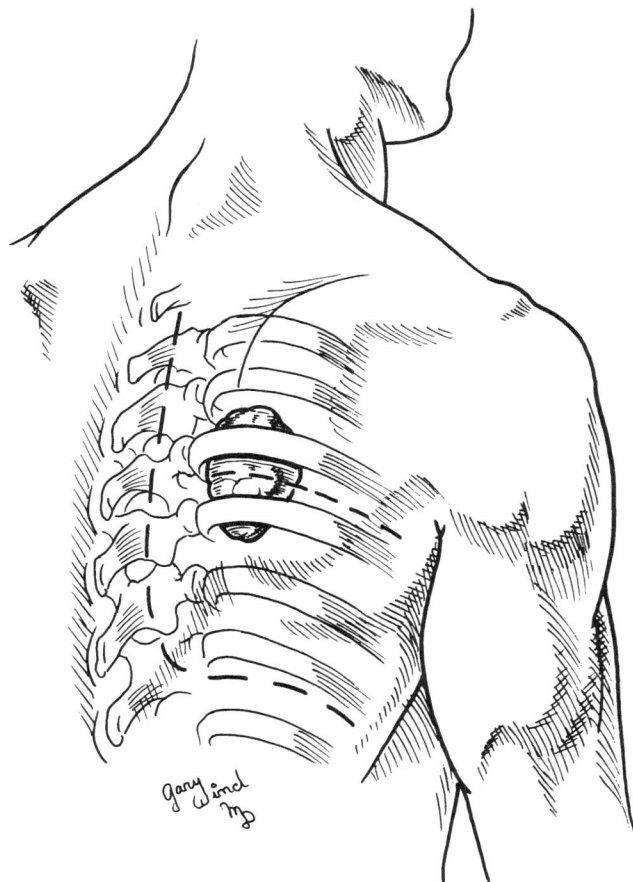

FIGURE 33.17. Operative technique for excision of a dumbbell tumor. A thoracotomy incision is made, and a flap of skin and subcutaneous tissue is raised. The interspace directly overlying the tumor is opened and mobilization of the tumor is begun.

If the dura was opened, it should be closed to prevent a cerebrospinal-pleural fistula. The closure should be buttressed with a pleural flap, pericardial fat graft, or intercostal muscle (103).

Special mention of the dumbbell tumor in the pediatric patient is relevant. The majority of dumbbell tumors in children are neuroblastomas or ganglioneuroblastomas. Adams et al. (43) reported the Pediatric Oncology Group experience, in which 16.6% of patients with neuroblastoma had a dumbbell tumor. These tumors may involve several foramina while destroying the adjacent bone. Aggressive attempts to resect these tumors do not improve the survival and only increase the morbidity (30, 34). Residual thoracic neuroblastoma responds well to chemotherapy and to localized radiotherapy for bone involvement. Extensive resection of the vertebral bodies or pedicles in a child predisposes to kyphoscoliosis and later spine stabilization procedures.

MISCELLANEOUS TUMORS

Although the majority of posterior mediastinal tumors have been described above, there are other less common tumors. Aisner et al. (106) reported granular cell tumors of the posterior mediastinum. These tumors appear to have a Schwann cell origin as demonstrated by S-100 immunoreactivity. Treatment of these lesions is excision, and recurrence is very rare.

Only 29 cases of intrathoracic tumors of the vagus nerve, referred to as nerve sheath tumors, have been reported (107). Both neurilemoma and neurofibroma may arise from the vagal nerve fibers. The majority of these patients are asymptomatic, and the mass is identified on incidental chest roentgenogram. Most of these tumors occur in the left vagus nerve because the proximal intrathoracic vagal trunk is large on that side (107). Treatment is incision of the epineurium and dissection of the tumor away from the nerve fibers. If the tumor encompasses the nerve fibers or invades contiguous structures, a more extensive resection should be done.

Posterior mediastinal goiter occurs in 1.4% of all goiters (108). These tumors result from a downward displacement of the thyroid from its normal cervical location. The goiter is found on the right side in two thirds of cases because of the position of the aortic arch and descending aorta on the left side. The most common clinical manifestations are dyspnea, cough, stridor, or dysphagia (108). Ninety-five percent of these tumors can be removed by a cervical approach, but a few require an anterior thoracotomy through the third intercostal space in addition to the cervical incision. A sternal splitting incision does not usually aid in removal of the posterior mediastinal goiter. The anterior thoracotomy is made on the side of extension of the tumor into the mediastinum, thus allowing for protection of the recurrent laryngeal nerve, control of the inferior thyroid vessels, and bimanual extraction of the tumor (108).

Finally, thoracic lymphoma generally occurs in the middle mediastinum but can present as a posterior mediastinal mass or adenopathy (109). A CT scan can identify enlarged lymph nodes in this area and can help stage the lymphoma. Thoracoscopy may have a role in biopsying and staging these lesions.

REFERENCES

1. Davis RD Jr, Oldham HN Jr, Sabiston DC Jr. Primary cysts and neoplasms of the mediastinum: recent changes in clinical presentation, methods of diagnosis, management and results. Ann Thorac Surg 1987;44:220–237.
2. Teixeira JP, Bibas RA. Surgical treatment of tumors of the mediastinum: the Brazilian experience. In: Delarue NC, Escha-

passe H, eds. International trends in general thoracic surgery. Thoracic surgery: frontiers and uncommon neoplasms. St. Louis: Mosby, 1989;5.
3. Hoffman OA, Gillespie DJ, Aughenbaugh GL, Brown LR. Primary mediastinal neoplasms (other than thymoma). Mayo Clin Proc 1993;68:880–891.
4. Reed JC, Hallett KK, Feigin DS. Neural tumors of the thorax: subject review from the AFIP. Radiology 1978;126:9–17.
5. Gale AW, Jelihovsky T, Grant AF, Leckie BD, Nicks R. Neurogenic tumors of the mediastinum. Ann Thorac Surg 1974;17:434–443.
6. Stout AP. The peripheral manifestations of specific nerve sheath tumor (neurilemoma). Am J Cancer 1935;24:751–796.
7. Shields TW, Reynolds M. Neurogenic tumors of the thorax. Surg Clin North Am 1988;68:645–668.
8. Akwari OE, Payne WS, Onofrio BM, Dines DM, Muhm JR. Dumbbell neurogenic tumors of mediastinum: Diagnosis and management. Mayo Clin Proc 1978;53:353–358.
9. Love JG, Dodge HW Jr. Dumbbell (hourglass) neurofibromas affecting the spinal cord. Surg Gynecol Obstet 1952;94:161–172.
10. Rosenberg JC. Neoplasms of the mediastinum. In: Devita VT, Hellman S, Rosenberg SA, eds. Cancer: principles and practice of oncology. 2nd ed. Philadelphia: JB Lippincott, 1985:599–620.
11. Ricci C, Rendina EA, Venuta F, Pescarmona EO, Gagliardi F. Diagnostic imaging and surgical treatment of dumbbell tumors of the mediastinum. Ann Thorac Surg 1990;50:586–589.
12. Sakai F, Sone S, Kiyono K, et al. Intrathoracic neurogenic tumors: MR-pathologic correlation. AJR Am J Roentgenol 1992;159:279–283.
13. Oberman HA, Sullenger G. Neurogenous tumors of the head and neck. Cancer 1967;20:1992–2001.
14. Rosai J. Soft tissues. In: Rosai J, ed. Ackerman's surgical pathology. 7th ed. St. Louis: Mosby, 1989:1547–1633.
15. Weiss SW, Langloss JM, Ensinger FM. Value of S-100 protein in the diagnosis of soft tissue tumors with particular reference to benign and malignant Schwann cell tumors. Lab Invest 1983;49:299–308.
16. Gould VE, Moll R, Moll I, Lee I, Schwechheimer K, Franke WW. The intermediate filament complement of the spectrum of nerve sheath neoplasms. Lab Invest 1986;55:463–474.
17. Landreneau RJ, Dowling RD, Ferson PF. Thoracoscopic resection of a posterior mediastinal neurogenic tumor. Chest 1992;102:1288–1290.
18. Riccardi VM. von Recklinghausen neurofibromatosis. N Engl J Med 1981;305:1617–1627.
19. King RM, Telander RL, Smithson WA, Banks PM, Han MT. Primary mediastinal tumors in children. J Pediatr Surg 1982;512–520.
20. Bolande RP. Neurofibromatosis: the quintessential neurocristopathy: pathogenic concepts and relationships. Adv Neurol 1981;29:67–75.
21. Kamata Y. Study on the ultrastructure and acetylcholinesterase activity in von Recklinghausen's neurofibromatosis. Acta Pathol Jpn 1978;28:393–410.
22. Cohen PS, Israel MA. Biology and treatment of thoracic tumors of neural crest origin. In: Roth JA, Ruckdeschell JC, Weisenburger TH, eds. Thoracic oncology. Philadelphia: WB Saunders, 1989:520–540.
23. Ducatman BS, Scheithauer BW. Postirradiation neurofibrosarcoma. Cancer 1983;51:1028–1033.
24. Sordillo PP, Helson L, Hadju SI, et al. Malignant schwannoma: clinical characteristics, survival, and response to therapy. Cancer 1981;47:2503–2509.
25. Sorensen SA, Mulvihill JJ, Nielsen A. Long-term follow-up of von Recklinghausen neurofibromatosis. Survival and malignant neoplasms. N Engl J Med 1986;314:1010–1015.
26. Lowman RM, Livolsi VA. Pigmented (melanotic) schwannomas of the spinal canal. Cancer 1980;46:391–397.
27. Krausz T, Azzopardi JG, Pearse E. Malignant melanoma of the sympathetic chain with a consideration of pigmented nerve sheath tumors. Histopathology 1984;8:881–894.
28. Abbott AE Jr, Hill RC, Flynn MA, McClure S, Murray GF. Melanotic schwannoma of the sympathetic ganglia: pathological and clinical characteristics. Ann Thorac Surg 1990;49:1006–1008.
29. Kayano H, Katayama I. Melanotic schwannoma arising in sympathetic ganglion. Hum Pathol 1988;19:1355–1358.
30. Catalano PW, Newton WA Jr, Williams TE Jr, Clatworthy HW Jr, Kilman JW. Reasonable surgery for thoracic neuroblastoma in infants and children. J Thorac Cardiovasc Surg 1978;76:459–464.
31. Young DG. Thoracic neuroblastoma/ganglioneuroma. J Pediatr Surg 1983;18:37–41.
32. Goon HK, Cohen DH, Harvey JG. Review of thoracic neuroblastoma. Aust Pediatr J 1984;20:17–21.
33. Caradin R, Campbell PE, Kent M. Thoracic neural crest tumors. A clinical review. Cancer 1983;51:949–954.
34. Grosfield JL, Baehner RL. Neuroblastoma: an analysis of 160 cases. World J Surg 1980;4:29–38.
35. Thomas PRM, Lee JY, Fineberg BB, et al. An analysis of neuroblastoma at a single institution. Cancer 1984;53:2079–2082.
36. Tracy T Jr, Weber TR. Current concepts in neuroblastoma. Surg Annu 1992;24:227–245.
37. Tsokos M, Ross RA, Triche TJ. Neuronal, schwannian and melanocytic differentiation of human neuroblastoma cells in vitro. Proc Clin Biol Res 1984;175:55–69.
38. Berthold F, Brandeis WE, Campert F. Neuroblastoma: diagnostic advances and therapeutic results in 370 patients. Monogr Paediatr 1986;18:206–224.
39. Tsokos M, Linnoila RI, Triche TJ, et al. Neuron specific enolase as an aid to the diagnosis of primitive small round cell tumors of neuronal origin. Hum Pathol 1984;15:575–584.
40. Zeltzer PM, Parma AM, Dalton A, et al. Raised neuron-specific enolase in serum of children with metastatic neuroblastoma. Lancet 1983;2:361–363.
41. Ladisch S, Wu ZL. Detection of a tumor-associated ganglioside in plasma of patients with neuroblastoma. Lancet 1985;1:136–138.
42. Floutsis G, Ulsh L, Ladisch S. Immunosuppressive activity of human neuroblastoma tumor gangliosides. Int J Cancer 1989;43:6–9.
43. Adams GA, Shochat SJ, Smith EI, et al. Thoracic neuroblastoma: a pediatric oncology group study. J Pediatr Surg 1993;28:372–378.
44. Voute PA, Van Patten WJ, Burgers JMV. Tumors of the sympathetic nervous system. In: Bloom HJC, Lemerle J, Neidhart MK, et al., eds. Cancer in children: clinical management. New York: Springer-Verlag, 1975.
45. Sawada T, Hirayama M, Nakata T, et al. Mass screening for neuroblastoma in infants in Japan. Lancet 1984;2:271–273.
46. Williams TH, House RF, Burgert EO, et al. Unusual manifestations in neuroblastoma: chronic diarrhea, polymyocloniaopso-

clonus and erythrocyte abnormalities. Cancer 1972;29:475–480.
47. Mendelsohn G, Eggleston JC, Olson JL, Said SI, Baylin SB. Vasoactive intestinal peptide and its relationship to ganglion cell differentiation in neuroblastic tumors. Lab Invest 1979;41:144–149.
48. Brodeur GM, Green AA, Hayes FA, Williams KJ, Williams DL, Tsiastis AA. Cytogenetic features of human neuroblastomas and cell lines. Cancer Res 1981;41:4678–4686.
49. Gansler T, Chatten J, Varello M, Bunin GR, Atkinson B. Flow cytometric DNA analysis of neuroblastoma: correlation with histology and clinical outcome. Cancer 1986;58:2453–2458.
50. Brodeur GM, Seeger RC, Schwab M, Varmus HE, Bishop JM. Amplification of N-myc in untreated human neuroblastomas correlates with advanced disease stage. Science 1984;224:1121–1124.
51. Seeger RC, Brodeur GM, Sather H, et al. Association of multiple copies of the N-myc oncogene with rapid progression of neuroblastomas. N Engl J Med 1985;313:1111–1116.
52. Look AT, Hayes FA, Nitschke R, McWilliams NB, Green AA. Cellular DNA content as a predictor of response to chemotherapy in infants with unresectable neuroblastoma. N Engl J Med 1984;311:231–235.
53. Cohn SL, Rademaker AW, Salwen HR, et al. Analysis of DNA ploidy and proliferative activity in relation to histology and N-myc amplification in neuroblastoma. Am J Pathol 1990;136:1043–1052.
54. Chung HS, Higgins GR, Siegel SE, et al. Abnormalities of the immune system in children with neuroblastoma related to neoplasm and chemotherapy. J Pediatr 1977;90:548–554.
55. Cheung NKV, Lazarus H, Miraldi FD, et al. Ganglioside (G_{D2}). specific monoclonal antibody 3F8: a phase I study in patients with neuroblastoma and malignant melanoma. J Clin Oncol 1987;5:1430–1440.
56. Lambroso JD, Guermazi F, Hartmann O, et al. Meta–iodobenzylguanidine (mIBG) scans in neuroblastoma: sensitivity and specificity, a review of 115 scans. Prog Clin Biol Res 1988;271:689–705.
57. Gelfand MJ. Meta-iodobenzylguanidine in children. Semin Nucl Med 1993;23:231–242.
58. Mastrangelo R, Lasorella A, Iavarone A, et al. Critical observations on neuroblastoma treatment with 131-I-metaiodobenzylguanidine at diagnosis. Med Pediatr Oncol 1993;21:411–415.
59. Shimada H, Chatten J, Newton WA Jr., et al. Histopathologic prognostic factors in neuroblastic tumors: definition of subtypes of ganglioneuroblastoma and an age-linked classification of neuroblastomas. J Natl Cancer Inst 1984;73:405–416.
60. Evans AE, D'Angio GJ, Randolph J. A proposed staging for children with neuroblastoma. Cancer 1971;27:374–378.
61. Hayes FA, Green A, Husto HO, et al. Surgicopathologic staging of neuroblastoma: prognostic significance of regional lymph node metastases. J Pediatr 1983;102:59–62.
62. Brodeur GM, Seeger RC, Barrett A, et al. International criteria for diagnosis, staging and response to treatment in patients with neuroblastoma. J Clin Oncol 1988;6:1874–1881.
63. Evans AE, D'Angio GJ, Sather HN, et al. A comparison of four staging systems for localized and regional neuroblastoma: a report from the children's cancer study group. J Clin Oncol 1990;8:678–688.
64. Evans AE, D'Angio GJ, Propert K, Anderson J, Hann HL. Prognostic factors in neuroblastoma. Cancer 1987;59:1853–1859.
65. Evans AE, Albo V, D'Angio GJ, et al. Cyclophosphamide treatment of patients with localized and regional neuroblastoma: a randomized study. Cancer 1976;36:655–660.
66. Koop CE, Schnaufer L. The management of intraabdominal neuroblastoma. Cancer 1975;35:905–909.
67. Smith EI, Krous HF, Tunnell WF, et al. The impact of chemotherapy and radiation therapy on secondary operations in neuroblastoma. Ann Surg 1980;19:561–569.
68. Saenz NC, Schnitzer JJ, Eraklis AE, et al. Posterior mediastinal masses. J Pediatr Surg 1993;28:172–176.
69. King RM, Telander RL, Smithson WA, Banks PM, Han MT. Primary mediastinal tumors in children. J Pediatr Surg 1982;17:512–520.
70. Adams A, Hochholzer L. Ganglioneuroblastoma of the posterior mediastinum: a clinicopathologic review of 80 cases. Cancer 1981;47:373–381.
71. Zajtchuk R, Bowen TE, Seyer AE, Brott WH. Intrathoracic ganglioneuroblastoma. J Thorac Cardiovasc Surg 1980;80:605–612.
72. Hassenbusch S, Kaizer H, White JJ. Prognostic factors in neuroblastic tumors. J Pediatr Surg 1976;11:287–297.
73. Assaf HM, Al-Momen AA, Martin JG. Aorticopulmonary paraganglioma: a case report with immunohistochemical studies and literature review. Arch Pathol Lab Med 1992;116:1085–1087.
74. Shapiro B, Orringer MB, Gross MD. Mediastinal paragangliomas and pheochromocytomas. In: Shields TW, ed. Mediastinal surgery. Malvern, PA: Lea & Febiger, 1991:254–271.
75. Moran CA, Suster S, Fishback N, Koss MN. Mediastinal paragangliomas: a clinicopathologic and immunohistochemical study of 16 cases. Cancer 1993;72:2358–2364.
76. Odze R, Begin LR. Malignant paraganglioma of the posterior mediastinum. Cancer 1990;65:564–569.
77. Glenner GC, Grimley PM. Tumors of the extra-adrenal paraganglion system (including chemoreceptors). In: Firminger HI, ed. Atlas of tumor pathology. Washington, DC: Armed Forces Institute of Pathology, 1974:13.
78. Seemayer TA. Paragangliomas. In: Sternberg SS, ed. Diagnostic surgical pathology. New York: Raven Press, 1989:467–477.
79. Tanaka F, Kitano M, Tatsumi A, et al. Paraganglioma of the posterior mediastinum: value of magnetic resonance imaging. Ann Thorac Surg 1992;53:517–519.
80. Drucker EA, McLoud TC, Dedrick CG, Hilgenberg AD, Geller SC, Shepard JO. Mediastinal paraganglioma: radiologic evaluation of an unusual vascular tumor. AJR Am J Roentgenol 1987;148:521–522.
81. Castanon J, Gil-Aguado M, de la Llana R, O'Conner F, Alswies A, Kowacevich T. Aortopulmonary paraganglioma, a rare aortic tumor: a case report. J Thorac Cardiovasc Surg 1993;106:1232–1233.
82. Hoefnagel CA, Voute PA, de Kraker J, Marcuse HR. Radionuclide diagnosis and therapy of neural crest tumors using iodine-131 metaiodobenzylguanidine. J Nucl Med 1987;28:308–314.
83. Herrera MF, van Heerden JA, Puga FJ, Hogan MJ, Carney JA. Mediastinal paraganglioma: a surgical experience. Ann Thorac Surg 1993;56:1096–1100.
84. Carney JA. The triad of gastric epithelioid leiomyosarcoma, functioning extra-adrenal paraganglioma, and pulmonary chondroma. Cancer 1979;43:374–382.
85. Argos MD, Ruiz A, Sandrez F, Garcia C, Gaztambide J. Gastric leiomyoblastoma associated with extra-adrenal paraganglioma

and pulmonary chondroma: a new case of Carney's triad. J Pediatr Surg 1993;28:1545–1549.
86. Engelman K, Hammond WG. Adrenaline production by an intrathoracic pheochromocytoma. Lancet 1968;1:609–611.
87. Shapiro B, Copp JE, Sisson JC, Eyre PL, Wallis J, Beierwaltes WH. Iodine-131 metaiodobenzylguanidine for the locating of suspected pheochromocytoma: experience in 400 cases. J Nucl Med 1985;26:576–585.
88. Ogawa J, Inoue H, Koide S, Kawada S, Shohtsu A, Hata J. Functioning paraganglioma in the posterior mediastinum. Ann Thorac Surg 1982;33:507–510.
89. Hull CJ. Phaeochromocytoma. Diagnosis, preoperative preparation and anesthetic management. Br J Anaesth 1986;58:1453–1468.
90. Pinaud M, Desjars P, Tasseau F, Cozian A. Preoperative acute volume loading in patients with pheochromocytoma. Crit Care Med 1985;13:460–463.
91. Scott HW Jr, Reynolds V, Green N, et al. Clinical experience with malignant pheochromocytomas. Surg Gynecol Obstet 1982;154:801–818.
92. Averbuch SD, Steakley CS, Young RC, et al. Malignant pheochromocytoma: effective treatment with a combination of cyclophosphamide, vincristine, and dacarbazine. Ann Intern Med 1988;109:267–273.
93. Sisson JC, Shapiro B, Beierwaltes WH, et al. Radiopharmaceutical treatment of malignant pheochromocytoma. J Nucl Med 1984;24:197–206.
94. Cornford EJ, Wastie ML, Morgan DAL. Malignant paraganglioma of the mediastinum: a further diagnostic and therapeutic use of radiolabelled mIBG. Br J Radiol 1992;65:75–78.
95. Timmis JB, Brown MJ, Allison DJ. Therapeutic embolization of phaeochromocytoma. Br J Radiol 1981;54:420–422.
96. Askin FB, Rosai J, Sibley RK, Dehner LP, McAlister WH. Malignant small cell tumor of the thoracopulmonary region in childhood. Cancer 1979;43:2438–2451.
97. Linnoila RI, Tsokos M, Triche TJ, Marangos PJ, Chandra RS. Evidence of neuronal origin and PAS-positive variants of the malignant small cell tumor of thoracopulmonary region (Askin tumor). Am J Pathol 1986;10:124–133.
98. Thiele CJ, McKeon C, Triche TJ, Ross RA, Reynolds CP, Israel MA. Differential proto-oncogene expression characterizes histopathologically indistinguishable tumors of the peripheral nervous system. J Clin Invest 1987;80:804–811.
99. Turc-Carel C, Philip I, Berger MP, et al. Chromosomal translocations in Ewings sarcoma. N Engl J Med 1983;309:497–498.
100. Whang-Peng J, Triche TJ, Knutsen T, et al. Cytogenic characterization of selected small round cell tumors of childhood. Cancer Genet Cytogenet 1986;21:185–208.
101. Hashimoto H, Enjoji M, Nakajima T, et al. Malignant neuroepithelioma (peripheral neuroblastoma): a clinicopathologic study of 15 cases. Am J Surg Pathol 1983;7:309–318.
102. Miser JS, Steis PS, Longo DL, et al. Treatment of newly diagnosed high risk sarcoma and primitive neuroectodermal (PNET) in children and young adults. Proc Am Soc Clin Oncol 1985;4:240.
103. Grillo HC, Ojemann RG, Scannell JG, Zervas NT. Combined approach to "dumbbell" intrathoracic and intraspinal neurogenic tumors. Ann Thorac Surg 1983;36:402–407.
104. Holgersen LO, Santulli TV, Schullinger JN, Berdon WE. Neuroblastoma with intraspinal (dumbbell) extension. J Pediatr Surg 1983;18:406–411.
105. Siegel MJ, Jamroz GA, Glazer HS, Abramson CL. MR imaging of intraspinal extension of neuroblastoma. J Comput Assist Tomogr 1986;10:593–595.
106. Aisner SC, Chakravarthy AK, Joslyn JN, Coughlin TR. Bilateral granular cell tumors of the posterior mediastinum. Ann Thorac Surg 1988;46:688–689.
107. Dabir RR, Piccione W Jr, Kittle CF. Intrathoracic tumors of the vagus nerve. Ann Thorac Surg 1990;50:494–497.
108. DeAndrade MA. A review of 128 cases of posterior mediastinal goiter. World J Surg 1977;1:789–797.
109. North LB, Libshitz HI, Lorigan JG. Thoracic lymphoma. Radiol Clin North Am 1990;28:745–762.

Section VII

Mesothelioma

34

Mesothelioma: Causes and Fiber-Related Mechanisms

Jean Bignon, Patrick Brochard, and Jean-Claude Pairon

INTRODUCTION

Diffuse carcinoma of the pleura was first described by Wagner (1) in the 19th century, but it was only in 1931 that the term mesothelioma was coined (2). This term is now used for all diffuse malignant primary tumors that develop from the mesenchyma, whether mesothelial or fibroblasticlike submesothelial cells (3).

Malignant mesothelioma of the pleura is a comparatively rare disease, accounting for no more than 2% to 3% of all pleural malignancies. Peritoneal and pericardial malignant mesothelioma are much less common.

The causal relationship between asbestos and malignant mesothelioma was discovered by Wagner et al. in 1960 (4), 5 years after Doll (5) had demonstrated the link between asbestos exposure and lung cancer. These fundamental discoveries were followed by many others that confirmed the fibrogenic and carcinogenic potential of asbestos fibers for the lung and pleura. However, during this period, tons of asbestos accumulated in our environment, carrying a risk of asbestos-related diseases, both for exposed workers (6) and for rural and urban populations subjected to possible environmental exposure (7), such as that found in buildings with sprayed asbestos or other asbestos-containing materials (ACMs) (8–10).

Initially, the definition of asbestos included different naturally occurring fibrous minerals that in fact had different mineralogical properties and probably different biologic activity. The main commercial types of asbestos are Chrysotile, Crocidolite, and Amosite. Chrysotile accounts for some 95% of the total asbestos marketed in the world. It is a fibrous hydrated magnesium–layered silicate made up of bundles that may split into very thin flexible fibrils, 30 nm in diameter.

The other two commercial varieties belong to the amphibole group. They both have rectilinear fibers, which have diameters of 0.13 mm for Crocidolite and 0.5 mm for Amosite. Three other fiber types—anthophyllite, tremolite, and actinolite (the so-called ATA)—also are amphiboles but have no commercial significance; all forms may be responsible for mesothelioma in humans and animals.

There are many other naturally occurring minerals with a fibrous shape that are considered nonasbestos minerals. These are described as asbestiform, a term applied to all crystals with an elongated shape along parallel planes, forming long, threadlike fibers with aspect ratios ranging from 20:1 to 100:1 or even higher. In contrast, nonasbestiform minerals have crystals with multidirectional growth patterns, characterized by prismatic cleavage fragments (7, 11). This distinction is related to the carcinogenic potential of the elongated minerals (see Comprehensive Mechanisms of Fiber-Related Carcinogenesis, below).

The study of the relationship between inhalation of asbestos or other natural or synthetic fibers and malignant mesothelioma depends on the accuracy of diagnosis and the measurement of exposure dose. The mechanisms by which fiber-related mesothelial carcinogenesis is produced and the possible role of host factors also are considered.

IMPROVEMENTS IN THE ACCURACY OF EARLY DIAGNOSIS

DIAGNOSIS OF DISEASE

The diagnosis of malignant mesothelioma, relying on pathology, is difficult and often is made only at an advanced stage of the disease when the prognosis is poor. Nevertheless, diagnosis must be precise, both for epidemiologic studies and for the evaluation of new therapies (12).

Malignant mesothelioma develops silently within the enclosed cavities of the pleural and peritoneal serosa, typically resulting in a long latency period between exposure and the appearance of the first symptoms. There is a further delay between the appearance of initial symptoms and the definite diagnosis. This delay, in fact, was estimated at 3.5 months in a retrospective study of 332 cases of malignant mesothelioma (13). The median survival for malignant mesothelioma, for which there is no standard treatment available, is 9 to 12 months; if the prognosis is to be improved, it is vital to reduce significantly the time lag before diagnosis.

Although an insidious pleural effusion is the most frequent initial clinical presentation, the diagnosis of the tumor is seldom ascertained before it has reached an advanced stage. Thoracoscopy is the best available tool for early diagnosis of malignant mesothelioma, and its use is indicated in all forms of chronic exudative pleurisy of unknown etiology. It enables direct visualization of the gross aspects of a pleural tumor and makes possible the removal of multiple, large biopsies (14). It also makes staging more accurate, following the classification of Butchart (15) or its recent modification (16). This staging provides the earliest identification of malignant mesothelioma from gross aspects while it still is restricted to the ipsilateral parietal pleura, including diaphragmatic pleura, with no involvement of the visceral pleura (TIa), or to both ipsilateral parietal and visceral pleura (TIb).

Definite diagnosis of malignant mesothelioma depends on an accurate histologic examination of large tissue samples by experienced pathologists (17). The histologic features of malignant mesothelioma are extremely variable, with some tumors exhibiting a biphasic pattern in which both mesenchymal and epithelial components are associated (mixed histology). However, a metastatic epithelial tumor, particularly an adenocarcinoma, often mimics mesothelioma. Diagnosis usually is based on a battery of histochemical and immunohistochemical markers. For example, keratin and vimentin antigens are both present in malignant mesothelioma, whereas carcinoembryonic antigen usually is absent (18). In contrast, in metastatic adenocarcinoma malignant cells are usually positive for keratin antigen and carcinoembryonic antigen but negative for vimentin antigen. A recent immunocytochemical study of human mesothelioma cell lines confirms the constancy of these phenotypic markers, which indicate the mesenchymal origin of this tumor (19). The commercial availability of monoclonal antibodies that are specific for cell membrane antigens of malignant mesothelioma, such as ME1 (20) or thrombomodulin (21), may make it possible to discriminate even more certainly between malignant mesothelioma and the so-called pseudomesothelioma carcinoma. The latter corresponds to peripheral lung adenocarcinoma mimicking malignant mesothelioma by a widespread invasion of the pleura (22, 23). Electron microscopy often is used as a reference technique for diagnosis. A panel of expert pathologists may still be necessary for the unequivocal identification of disputable diagnoses (24). The pathology of mesothelioma is reviewed in detail in Chapter 35 by Corson and Renshaw.

The accuracy of diagnosis must be questioned in some epidemiologic studies, because in a number of retrospective investigations, the original pathologic diagnoses were shown to have been overestimated (25–27) or underestimated. When the histologic slides were reviewed, a significant percentage of misdiagnoses was revealed (28).

PRECLINICAL STAGES OF DEVELOPMENT OF ASBESTOS-INDUCED MESOTHELIOMA

A major clinical issue concerns the extent to which the different nonmalignant, clinicopathologic forms of asbestos-related pleural diseases might predispose to malignant mesothelioma and eventually be predictive of this malignancy.

Asbestos exposure can cause subacute recurrent exudative pleuritis, most often associated with some degree of asbestosis (29–31). The diagnosis of the benign condition is difficult, particularly when there has been a history of asbestos exposure. Biopsies are essential for an accurate diagnosis, with clear differentiation between benign asbestos-related pleuritis and a pleural effusion symptomatic of malignant mesothelioma.

Pleural plaques are focal fibrohyaline areas, more or less calcified and mainly localized at the level of the parietal and diaphragmatic pleura. Usually, they do not involve the visceral pleura (32, 33). There are often proliferative aspects on the periphery of pleural plaques, but their malignant transformation is exceedingly rare (3). Pleural plaques can be associated with all types of asbestos, but they appear to be observed more frequently in association with exposure to amphibole fiber types; this association is particularly obvious for environmental exposure to Anthophyllite in Finland (34). The lag time (median) between initial exposure to asbestos and radiographic diagnosis of pleural plaques is approximately 15 years, but this is less than half the mean latency period for malignant mesothelioma, which is nearly 40 years (13).

Although malignant mesothelioma in humans often seems to develop on the parietal side of the pleura, where there are pleural plaques, the plaques cannot be considered premalignant lesions (3). Preliminary results obtained in our clinical department on 40 pleural malignant mesothelioma cases indicate that pleural plaques were detected by CT scan in only approximately 5% of the cases on the opposite side of the malignant mesothelioma, even in those associated with past exposure to asbestos (unpublished data). Other studies, however, have claimed that pleural plaques were predictive both of asbestos-related lung carcinoma and pleural mesothelioma (35); however, this conclusion has been challenged because it was based on inaccurate asbestos exposure data (36). In fact, it is better to consider pleural plaques indicators of past exposure to asbestos rather than preneoplastic lesions, although often they are associated with a low lung fiber burden. For example, in one autopsy study (33), the lung fiber burden in up to 50% of patients with pleural plaques was in the range of the control population. Another study, in which levels of asbestos bodies in bronchoalveolar lavage fluid (BALF) were measured, showed no significant increase in 60% of the subjects with circumscribed pleural plaques (37).

Other asbestos-related benign pleural changes seem to be associated mainly with asbestosis. One such example is diffuse pleural thickening with blunting of the costodiaphragmatic angle, usually associated with adhesive fibrothorax, either as a consequence of asbestos-associated pleuritis, a subpleural asbestos-related alveolitis (38), or rounded atelectasis (39, 40). These different pathologic inflammatory-fibrous pleural and subpleural changes have no obvious relationship with malignant mesothelioma.

For subjects at risk of developing mesothelioma, it would be invaluable if biologic markers could be identified that indicated an early stage of mesothelioma, thus justifying the decision to perform a thoracoscopy. Serum markers, such as hyaluronan (41, 42) or tissue peptide antigen (43), are not sufficiently specific and sensitive to make an early diagnosis possible. Cytogenetic analysis of pleural cells from a chronic pleural effusion could theoretically have a useful predictive value for the possible development of malignant mesothelioma. A recent case report suggested that the cytogenetic follow-up of exfoliated cells in the pleural fluid from a patient with past exposure to asbestos showed karyotypic changes in chromosomes 1, 14, 21, and 22. These changes were linked retrospectively to malignant mesothelioma, which developed 4 years later and which demonstrated even more extensive karyotypic abnormalities (44).

EPIDEMIOLOGY

INCIDENCE OF MALIGNANT MESOTHELIOMA

METHODOLOGIC PROBLEMS

Mortality data on the occurrence of mesothelioma is obtained from death certificates and incidence data from cancer registries. Because a definite diagnosis of malignant mesothelioma requires the opinions of trained clinicians and pathologists, it is probable that estimates from death certificates do not match those obtained from cancer registries. For example, in France the incidence rates of pleural mesothelioma in Ile de France—the region that includes Paris, with approximately 12 million inhabitants—were estimated for 1987–1990 from data obtained from a hospital-based case control study. When these data were compared with mortality data based on death certificates recorded by the French National Institute for Health and Medical Research (INSERM) for the same period (45), the results were discordant. The average annual incidence rate for males was 7.5 per million and for females, 1.6 per million. The average annual mortality rates for primary pleural malignancies, classified as 163 in the World Health Organization/International Classification of Diseases (WHO/ICD 163, 9th revision), as indicated on death certificates, were 25.2 per million in males and 8.9 per million in females, considerably higher than the rates estimated from the case control study. This discrepancy has prompted a study in those areas of France where the case control study is operating as a means of comparing mortality data from death certificates (WHO/ICD 163) and incidence data from this case control study.

Discrepancies also have been reported from other industrialized countries where both registry-based incidence data and mortality data were available (46). In different studies based on incidence registers (25, 27, 47–49), the variations in the percentage of histologically confirmed diagnoses of malignant mesothelioma ranged from 26% to 96% (45). On the other hand, the accuracy of cause of death as established on the death certificate varied from 23% (50) to 76% (25). The discrepancies between mortality data and incidence data based on a case control study in France (which reported the highest malignant mesothelioma mortality in Europe compared with other European countries, even those using much more asbestos during World War II, such as Great Britain [25, 51] or The Netherlands [52]) may stem from two main reasons: (a) category 163 of the ICD-WHO may, in fact, include malignant tumors other than pleural mesothelioma; and (b) incomplete recording of cases, which obviously leads to an underestimation of the true incidence. The latter reason probably explains the very low incidence rates in the case control study in the Ile de France region.

VARIATIONS IN INCIDENCE RATES

Incidence rates of malignant mesothelioma vary by country, region, and city. The background level of mesothelioma is estimated at 1 to 2 per million per year for a population with no a priori asbestos exposure (53). Higher incidence rates have been observed in the general population (including occupationally exposed workers) of former Crocidolite-producing countries: 33 per million in South Africa (54) and 28.3 per million among males in Australia (55). In Europe the mortality rate in Great Britain was 17.5 per million (51) and in The Netherlands, 20.9 per million (52). Moreover, an increasing trend in disease occurrence has been demonstrated, particularly in males, but more recently also in females in several industrialized countries, including Great Britain (51), Canada (53), South Africa (54), Australia (55), and the United States (50). A prospective mortality study in the United States suggests that this increase should reach a peak around the year 2010 (56), with differences among industrialized countries, depending on their asbestos industry histories. Recently, Peto et al. (57) claimed that the peak of mesothelioma mortality in males in Great Britain will be observed in 2020. An accurate follow-up of the incidence of malignant mesothelioma in general populations is particularly important to determine the epidemiologic impact of exposure to low doses of both natural and synthetic fibers as a possible cause of observed progressions of malignant mesothelioma.

DOSE-RESPONSE RELATIONSHIPS OF ASBESTOS EXPOSURE WITH MALIGNANT MESOTHELIOMA

METHODOLOGIC PROBLEMS

EFFECT ASSESSMENT

Dose-response relationships usually are established from industrial cohorts for which mortality data are obtained from death certificates, the reliability of which has been questioned. A study by Selikoff and Seidman (28) illustrates the variation in mortality rates for malignant mesothelioma, i.e., when the number has been established from original death certificate data or recomputed using best evidence diagnosis obtained by revision of pathologic material. Best evidence diagnosis allowed identification of many more mesothelioma cases than the exclusive use of death certificates. Thus, it was shown that an error of 1% caused by a misclassification of malignant mesothelioma as a lung cancer would lead to an underestimation of malignant mesothelioma by 50% in a population in which the ratio of lung cancer to malignant mesothelioma was 100:1 (28).

DOSE ASSESSMENT

Ideally, the effective exposure dose should be reconstituted from cohorts of asbestos workers who have been followed for several decades and who, if possible, had been exposed to only one asbestos fiber type, either Chrysotile, Crocidolite, or Amosite. Such ideal cohorts, which are very rare, are presented in Table 34.1. In most historical cohorts of asbestos workers, moreover, there have been inconsistencies in the assessment of fiber concentrations to which subjects have been exposed.

Three complementary approaches can be used to obtain the best quantitative retrospective evaluation of exposure: (a) the collection of existing data of the measurements of fiber concentrations in air samples; (b) the reconstitution of asbestos exposure history, which presents many difficulties and uncertainties, especially in view of the long latency period; and (c) the quantitative measurement (biometrology) of lung fiber burden.

RETROSPECTIVE EVALUATION OF ASBESTOS DUST CONCENTRATION DATA MEASURED IN AIR SAMPLES

The ideal situation would require an exact assessment of the cumulative concentrations of respirable dusts, including both particles and fibers, inhaled by each worker during his working life. This determination is very nearly achievable for current exposure, but 20 to 40 years ago the techniques used for dust measurement were very imprecise. However, the latter period represents the exposure responsible for the asbestos-related diseases now being observed. These insurmountable methodologic difficulties in assessing doses of exposure justify a general agreement that the levels of asbestos fiber concentrations in workplaces used for most cohort studies of asbestos workers entailed major underevaluation (58). At a time when air sampling techniques were not available, doses usually were assessed by duration of work in the exposed area; however, even when historical airborne particle measurements were available in some cohorts, discrepancies in sampling strategies and analytical procedures

TABLE 34.1. Proportional Mortality Ratio for Mesothelioma Cohorts of Workers Exposed to Mineral Fibers

FIBER TYPES	TYPE OF INDUSTRIES	NOS. OF DEATHS		MESOTHELIOMA PROPORTIONAL MORTALITY (PER 1000)	REFERENCE NO.
		ALL	MESOTHELIOMA		
Chrysotile	Mining	3500	11	3.1	88, 89
	Manufacturing	2136	2	0.9	90–94
Amphiboles	Mining	1640	55	33.5	95–100
	Manufacturing	892	36	33.6	101–105
Asbestos mixture	Manufacturing	8751	176	20.1	61, 106–119
	Insulation	2749	238	86.1	
	Shipyard	1517	39	25.7	
Zeolite-erionite	Environmental	141	29	205	120
Manmade vitreous fiber	Manufacturing	9000	5	0.5	121, 122
General population 1989 (France)	Exposures to any kind of fibers	529,283	809	1.5	123

Data from McDonald AD, McDonald TC. Epidemiology of malignant mesothelioma. In: Antman K, Aisner J, eds. Asbestos related malignancy. London: Grune & Stratton, 1987:31–56.

prevented any meaningful assessment of cumulative exposure indexes.

Several attempts have been made to convert previous measurements of particles expressed in millions of particles per cubic foot, with no quantification of fibers into an equivalent number per milliliter of fibers corresponding to the WHO classification: length of less than 5 μm, diameter of less than 3 μm, and length to diameter ratio of less than 3 (59). The use of such conversion factors has been the subject of numerous discussions (60), with the observation that values vary by fiber types and/or industry studied. More accurate approaches have used conversion factors, obtained by comparing the two methods of measurement on samples collected simultaneously in the same industrial setting, such as in the asbestos textile industry (61) or Canadian Chrysotile mines and mills (62).

RECONSTITUTION OF ASBESTOS EXPOSURE HISTORY BY QUESTIONNAIRE AND JOB EXPOSURE MATRIX

Because of the difficulties and inaccuracies entailed in the reconstitution of doses of exposure, exposure assessments have been obtained by extrapolation from similar situations. However, even within the same type of asbestos industries, there are extremely wide ranges of exposure level, with variations of more than four orders of magnitude between different periods or different plants (58, 63). These difficulties may have led to important exposure misclassifications within retrospective and historical cohorts. For this reason, two approaches have been proposed for the retrospective assessment of asbestos exposure: modeling of past exposure (64) and use of job exposure matrices (65).

BIOMETROLOGY OF LUNG FIBER BURDEN

When retrospective data on occupational exposure to asbestos are lacking or unreliable, the quantification of asbestos fibers retained in the lung can be a useful method of assessing previous asbestos exposure. This assessment includes the counting of asbestos bodies (ABs) by optical microscopy and/or the evaluation of asbestos fibers by analytical transmission electron microscopy (ATEM) or scanning electron microscopy (66, 67). The most pertinent lung samples are parenchymal tissue and BALF (68), but ABs may also be quantified in sputum.

Coated fibers, such as typical ferruginous bodies, are counted as ABs (69). A significant correlation has been reported between AB concentrations in BALF and lung parenchyma, and it has been possible to determine threshold values indicative of a nontrivial asbestos exposure, compared with the general population (70), of 1 AB per milliliter of BALF and 1000 ABs per gram of dry lung tissue (68). Good correlation has been reported between the count of ATEM-sized fibers, which are mainly amphiboles, and ABs in patients with various asbestos-related diseases (71–76). However, the counting of uncoated fibers by ATEM or scanning electron microscopy may still be justified, despite the expense, because it provides valuable information on the number of fibers, their bivariate lengths and diameters, and their types, whether amphibole, Chrysotile, or other fiber. In fact, it has been shown that most ABs isolated from human lungs have an amphibole asbestos core. This finding suggests that counting ABs using optical microscopy may fail to identify previous exposure to pure Chrysotile. Electron microscopy techniques thus may be recommended for such patients as a further means of studying Chrysotile exposure.

Two questions remain: (a) What is the significance of asbestos retention at a nontrivial concentration in a biologic sample obtained from subjects with a history of asbestos exposure 30 to 40 years ago? Although ABs are known to remain in lung parenchyma for decades, Chrysotile fibers have low biologic durability (see Comprehensive Mechanisms of Fiber-Related Carcinogenesis, below) and are poorly associated with the formation of ABs; thus, neither light nor electron microscopic methods may be able to detect retention of ABs in some Chrysotile-exposed workers. (b) Do fibers migrate from the lung compartment to the pleura and, particularly, to the parietal mesothelial tissue in which mesothelial cell transformation usually begins? Few studies have documented a translocation of asbestos fibers to the parietal pleura, and these were either short microfibrils of Chrysotile (77) or longer amphibole fiber types (78).

EXPOSURE KINETICS

Whatever the method used to assess the fiber exposure, the risk of respiratory cancers has been computed in cohort studies using cumulative asbestos exposure indices. A very important issue in the assessment of past exposure to asbestos is the significance of peak or discontinuous exposure. Historical cohorts with high and continuous exposures were not at issue; however, it becomes critical for cases associated with the low-level exposures observed today. It has been shown that in cohorts exposed continuously to a fiber aerosol, the ratio of benign pleural abnormalities to small parenchymal opacities was much higher than in cohorts with discontinuous exposure (79).

In animal studies, however, no differences in lung biopersistence were observed among experiments in which a given number of fibers were administered to rats by a unique intratracheal instillation and one in which fibers were administered by a continuous inhalation (5 hours/day, 5 days/week, over a period of 3 months) (80, 81). These apparently anomalous results require further studies to test the effect of the flow rate of exposure dose. No data are available concerning fiber migration to the pleura in these experiments.

RISK ASSESSMENT USING MATHEMATICAL MODELS

Large populations, including school children, have been or still are being exposed to low concentrations of asbestos fibers in buildings with ACMs; it is essential to determine if these populations are at increased risk of asbestos-related malignancies, including lung cancer and malignant mesothelioma (8–10). A few scattered cases of malignant mesothelioma have already been attributed to such exposure (82, 83), but the evidence is not entirely convincing. There presently is great uncertainty about the effects of exposure to low doses of asbestos fibers, and the exact form of the corresponding dose-response curve for respiratory malignancies is not known. A mathematical downward extrapolation has been attempted to model a low-dose–response curve based on the curves obtained from mortality occupational epidemiologic studies (84), but this result may not represent an exact model, which would be difficult to establish. Indeed, the number of subjects necessary for the evaluation of the potential risk of cancer associated with an exposure to low doses of asbestos is so large that it could not be attained in a single study (85). Moreover, the asbestos fibers, either Chrysotile or amphibole, recovered in most buildings with ACMs often are associated with other particulate matter that is not usually taken into account. In a recent study, however, the in vitro cytotoxicity and DNA damage to rat pleural mesothelial cells of air samples from buildings with ACMs was attributed primarily to the total number of associated suspended particles (including asbestos), not specifically to the asbestos fibers (86). For example, silicates, metallic compounds, fly ash, and welding fume particles were detected in certain samples. Because outdoor airborne particulate matter contains more than 500 chemical compounds (87), it is not surprising to find many of these compounds in indoor air.

ROLE OF FIBER TYPE

PLEURAL CARCINOGENIC POTENTIAL OF DIFFERENT ASBESTOS FIBER TYPES

It generally is agreed that there is a gradient of carcinogenicity among different fiber types when inhaled by humans. The comparative analysis of the proportional mortality ratios of several cohorts of asbestos workers indicates that exposure to commercial amphiboles (Crocidolite, Amosite, and Anthophyllite) or to a mixture of amphiboles and Chrysotile was associated with a high proportional mortality ratio for deaths from pleural or peritoneal mesothelioma (20 to 86 per thousand), compared with the much lower proportional mortality ratios for workers exposed to pure Chrysotile. For the cohort exposed in Chrysotile manufacturing industries, the proportional mortality ratio was 0.9 per thousand and for the cohort in the Quebec mines and mills, 3.1 per thousand (Table 34.1). In several mortality studies of workers exposed to pure Chrysotile, mesothelioma has been shown to be rare or absent (Table 34.1), but lung cancer mortality was the same as for those exposed either to amphiboles or to amphiboles plus Chrysotile (61, 88–119). This is well illustrated by the recent follow-up of mortality in the cohort of Quebec Chrysotile miners and millers: of the 33 deaths from malignant mesothelioma, 28 had been miners or millers, representing 0.4% of deaths from all causes; in contrast, among the employees of a small asbestos products factory in which commercial amphiboles had been used, five deaths from malignant mesothelioma were observed, representing 2.5% of all deaths.

Exposure to tremolite appears to be associated with a higher risk of malignant mesothelioma. This association is exemplified by the comparison of the frequency of malignant mesothelioma among workers in the mines and mills of Thetford, Quebec, where there is heavy contamination with tremolite, and workers employed in the mine at Asbestos, Quebec, where tremolite contamination is much lighter (124). Correlating with this observation, measurements of fiber types found in the lungs of ex-workers from the Thetford mine show that tremolitic amphibole fibers were more numerous than Chrysotile fibers (125).

The proportional mortality ratios related to exposure to other fiber types are shown in Table 34.1: the highest ever observed of 205 per thousand for environmental exposure to erionite in Turkey (120), compared with a low of 0.5 per thousand for exposure to manmade vitreous fibers (MMVFs). The data were derived from a cohort study of about 9000 workers in the United States and Europe where there were five cases of malignant mesothelioma (121, 122). For comparison, the proportional mortality ratios for the general population of France based on death certificate data is approximately 1.5 per thousand (123).

Moreover, case control studies of asbestos lung fiber burden have shown that pulmonary retention of amphibole fiber types (tremolite) was at significantly higher concentrations in mesothelioma than in lung cancer (126, 127).

Tremolite is a ubiquitous mineral in the earth's crust, and it may take an asbestiform form, being released as long, thin fibers in both outdoor and indoor air in many rural areas, where it has been found to cause both pleural plaques and malignant mesothelioma. These areas included Greece (128), Cyprus (129), Corsica (130), and more recently New Caledonia (131) and Afghanistan (132). Tremolite is often present in commercial mineral deposits, such as in Chrysotile mines in Quebec (125) and vermiculite mines in Montana (133), where tremolite fibers are considered the main determinants of malignant mesothelioma observed among the miners and ex-miners.

The Chrysotile Paradox

Although amphibole fiber types certainly appear to be associated strongly with malignant mesothelioma, the disease is observed less frequently in the follow-up of cohorts exposed to Chrysotile. However, this observation does not imply that Chrysotile is non-carcinogenic for the mesothelium, but rather that it is a dose dependent effect. At high concentrations Chrysotile can induce malignant mesothelioma in humans, even in the absence of any amphibole contaminant (134). The paradox remains: in cases of exposure to Chrysotile, is the most important parameter for malignant mesothelioma induction a high level of exposure to pure Chrysotile, or a lower level of Chrysotile contaminated with a small proportion of tremolite fibers?

Fiber Types Other than Asbestos

Among natural asbestiform minerals, erionite, a volcanic fibrous zeolite (Table 34.1), is the most potent mesothelial carcinogen, both in man and in rodents; it is responsible for the dramatic incidence of malignant mesothelioma in Karain, a small village in Capadoccia in Turkey. Villagers there have been exposed since childhood to low concentrations of erionite in the environment (135). In the rat model, exposure to erionite by inhalation resulted in an occurrence rate of malignant mesothelioma of up to 100% (136).

Currently, a major concern is the possible toxicity of synthetic fibers now available commercially in different forms, known collectively as MMVFs (137). European and North American mortality studies (Table 34.1) of several cohorts of workers engaged in the manufacture of mineral wools thus far have been unable to relate the five suspected cases of malignant mesothelioma to a specific exposure to MMVFs, because a possible associated exposure to asbestos could not be excluded definitely (121, 138, 139). Regardless, these cohort studies involved only workers exposed to glass wool, slag wool, and rock wool fibers. Presently, there are no epidemiologic data concerning exposure to any other synthetic fiber types, because their industrial development is relatively recent. There are data, however, from inhalation experiments in which rodents were exposed to thin (diameter of less than 1 μm), durable synthetic fibers, such as ceramic fibers. Both malignant mesothelioma and lung tumors were induced in these rodents (140, 141). Thus, it is evident that physicians must remain vigilant if a repetition of the problems associated with asbestos is to be avoided in the MMVF industry.

PROBLEMS OF RISK ASSESSMENT RELATED TO LOW-DOSE EXPOSURE TO ASBESTOS

The discovery of ancestral mesothelioma related to environmental exposures to tremolite and erionite has raised a general fiber-related health problem, i.e., the risk of malignant mesothelioma for the general population in modern society (7). It is not known whether a low level of indoor and outdoor air pollution by asbestos or any other fiber types, either natural or synthetic, is responsible for an increased incidence of malignant mesothelioma. The primary risk of malignant mesothelioma would result from exposure of building occupants, including children, to asbestos fibers released from friable sprayed asbestos and from ACMs; thus far, epidemiologic studies have reported only morbidity data for different categories of building occupants, especially maintenance and custodial workers (142, 143). Only one study has reported morbidity data for general building occupants, and this study showed no difference in asbestos-related diseases between the exposed group and the controls (144). Even though a panel of experts appointed by the Health Effects Institute–Asbestos Research (U.S. Congress) has reached rather optimistic conclusions on this major issue (10), the mathematical method used to extrapolate risk assessment at low doses has serious limitations (84). Indeed, the assumed linear model may be wrong, and the response of children may well be different from that of healthy workers in asbestos industries (145).

DETECTION OF CAUSAL FACTORS OTHER THAN FIBERS

The finding of a French study in the 1980s—that there was no definite evidence of exposure to mineral fibers for 30% of malignant mesothelioma cases, and that the lung burden of asbestos bodies or fibers was low (146)—led to the search for other possible etiologic factors in humans (147). Thoracic irradiation for the treatment of lymphomas has been reported as the causal factor in sporadic cases. Many chemicals by different routes of administration and at different doses have been shown to induce mesothelial tumors in experimental animals (148). Moreover, it has been shown that benzo(a)pyrene was capable of transforming rat pleural mesothelial cells in vitro without any synergy with asbestos (149). In addition, rat pleural mesothelial cells exhibit some cytochrome P450 activity necessary to metabolize chemical compounds such as benzo(a)pyrene (150). Despite this finding, no chemical has been identified definitively as a possible cause of malignant mesothelioma in humans.

There have been recent suggestions of a possible role for the monkey virus SV40, which could have been transmitted in SV40-contaminated polio vaccines (151), because wild-type SV40 administered by intrapleural injection induced pericardial and pleural mesothelioma in 100% of Syrian hamsters (152). Apart from this possibility, no other co-factor (including tobacco smoking) has been identified epidemiologically in the pathogenesis of malignant mesothelioma in humans.

These findings provide sufficient grounds to justify the maintenance of an accurate epidemiologic surveillance of the background incidence rates of malignant mesothelioma in the general population.

COMPREHENSIVE MECHANISMS OF FIBER-RELATED CARCINOGENESIS WITH IMPLICATIONS FOR MESOTHELIOMA

FIBER PARAMETERS INVOLVED IN CARCINOGENICITY

The biologic effects of fibers pertain not only to asbestos but also are valid for all fibrous minerals, both natural (the so-called asbestiforms) and synthetic. All of these fibers are capable of developing biologic activities responsible for fibrogenesis and/or carcinogenesis, provided they fulfill the conditions of dose, dimension, and durability (153). The significance of each of these important issues is analyzed in detail below.

GEOMETRY

The three-dimensional shape of particulate matter plays a major role in carcinogenesis, thus it is important to characterize the geometry of elongated particles before deciding on their carcinogenic potential. Recent animal experiments in which pure tremolite samples were administered by intraperitoneal injection in rats have shown that the nonasbestiform cleavage fragments of tremolite did not induce mesothelioma, whereas fibrous asbestiform tremolite was highly carcinogenic (154). Moreover, in vitro incubation of rat pleural mesothelial cells with different particles demonstrates that genotoxic responses are observed only with fibrous particles, not with platy particles such as talc (155) or anatase, or with globular particles such as vitreous beads (156).

SIZE

The pioneering work of Stanton and coworkers (157, 158) showed that three size parameters of fibrous particles—length, diameter, and aspect ratio—were the main factors for inducing cancer after intraserosal inoculation. Extensive experiments were carried out in rats by intrapleural implantation of various types of respirable mineral particles of a wide variety of chemical compositions and structures. Results showed that for particles with a fibrous shape, the probability of pleural malignant mesenchymal neoplasms correlated well with the number of fibers having diameters of 0.25 μm or less and lengths of more than 8 μm. Subsequent studies in other laboratories either by intraperitoneal (159) or intrapleural injections of various fibrous materials in rats (160–163) supported the Stanton hypothesis. However, the results indicated that a risk of mesothelial tumors could also exist for thicker size ranges, i.e., diameters up to 1 μm, if the fibers were long enough.

The role of fiber size and particularly length in carcinogenesis also has been demonstrated in rats when dust was inhaled. One series of experiments showed that fibers more than 20 μm long had the greatest carcinogenic potential (162, 164); in another series it was shown that shortening extremely carcinogenic erionite fibers totally suppressed the carcinogenic response after inhalation in rats (165).

BIOPERSISTENCE

A large amount of magnesium can be leached from Chrysotile fibers under acidic conditions, using a weak organic acid such as oxalic acid, thus resulting in a dramatic decrease in their carcinogenic potential after intrapleural injection (161, 163). This finding would indicate that the persistence of Chrysotile might be decreased in an acidic biologic milieu, such as that found in the alveolar macrophage phagolysosome (166). Amphiboles, in contrast, were resistant to acidic treatment (163).

Recently, the term biopersistence was coined to designate the in vivo durability of mineral fibers in lung tissue (167). This term refers to the result of the complex mechanisms to which respirable fibers are subjected when they are deposited on the surface of the alveolar spaces. Biopersistence includes clearance, translocation to other sites such as lymph nodes and pleura, and physicochemical modifications of thickness and fragmentation related to the dissolution or leaching of different cations (168). All of these parameters, still insufficiently assessed, have to be considered in evaluating the critical dose responsible for an effect at the site of the target cells. Thus, the balance of biopersistence versus biosolubility appears to be the crucial in vivo determinant for the carcinogenic potency of fibers, particularly at the level of the pleura. Some asbestiform fibers, such as Chrysotile and wollastonite, have been shown to be cleared rapidly and/or to be more or less dissolved, whereas amphiboles have long durability in the lung. This dramatic difference between Chrysotile and amphiboles was demonstrated both in animal experiments (169) and in humans (170).

Biopersistence also depends on the fiber size parameters of length and diameter, which significantly influence the retention time and clearance pathways of inhaled fibers in the lung and their subsequent potency for inducing lung cancer and mesothelioma. Fiber length seems to be a very important parameter, determining the pulmonary retention of fibers, with those as long as 10 or even 20 μm being retained for a longer time both within human lung tissue (171) and in animals (172). The higher durability of long fibers must be related to the inability of alveolar macrophages to ingest fully those fibers longer than 10 μm, whereas short fibers are more easily phagocytized and can be dissolved rapidly at the intralysosomal pH. However, depending on their chemical composition, natural and synthetic fibers have a different optimal pH for dissolution. Considering asbestos fibers, amphiboles are resistant to dissolution, but Chrysotile is leached easily at an acidic pH of 4 to 5 (161, 163, 166). This difference may explain how a highly durable amphibole fiber could be more carcinogenic for the human pleura than the less durable Chrysotile, which during the long human life-span could undergo a progressive long-term dissolution.

Actually, one may question whether the biopersistent fibers recovered from lung tissue samples at the time of diagnosis of mesothelioma are the most significant indicators for assessing a dose-response relationship. Indeed, the early events, including direct hits on mesothelial cells by fibers translocated to the pleura, are probably more crucial to the induction of genotoxicity and cell transformation. Conversely, the time necessary for the translocation of fibers to the pleura might, in part, also explain the long latency period of mesothelioma. However, there also is the possibility that fibers located in subpleural alveolar spaces might stimulate the mitotic process of mesothelial cells (173) and stimulate the release of growth factors (Fig. 34.1).

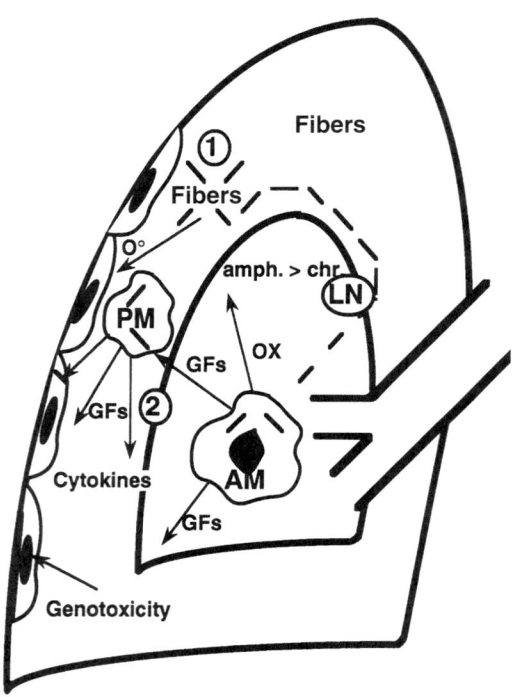

FIGURE 34.1. Fibers can induce mesothelioma by two hypothetic mechanisms: 1, direct hit to mesothelial cells: fibers reach the pleural space (PS) and penetrate into mesothelial cells of the parietal pleura, hitting the DNA material. Moreover, they also translocate to mediastinal lymph nodes (LN), whose role is not understood. 2, indirect mechanisms: fibers are taken up by alveolar macrophages (AM) and pleural macrophages (PM). Activated macrophages release growth factors (GFs), cytokines, and oxyradicals (Ox).

CHEMISTRY

The global chemical composition of fibers must be an important parameter in the solubility of both natural and synthetic fibers. Among MMVFs, glass wool, for example, is soluble at a neutral pH, whereas rock wool is soluble at an acidic pH. There is a decreasing rate of in vitro dissolution of fibers in acellular solutions, mimicking either the lysosomal acidic pH or the neutral pH of the interstitial fluid: soluble glass wool less than rock wool less than Chrysotile less than ceramic fibers less than insoluble amphibole fibers. Among MMVFs, those with a higher proportion of alkaline earth elements seem to be more soluble in vitro in Gamble's solution, whereas components such as alumina render the fibers less soluble (174).

Among chemical elements, iron seems to be an important constituent in the production of the reactive oxygen species often evoked as factors in asbestos-induced cell toxicity and genotoxicity (see Comprehensive Mechanisms of Fiber-Related Carcinogenesis, below). The best example is represented by Crocidolite, wherein the iron content may be as high as 30% by weight, about half being Fe^{2+} and the other half, Fe^{3+} ions. It has been shown that this fiber type is capable of catalyzing a Fenton-type reaction, generating hydroxy radicals in the presence of hydrogen peroxide ($Fe^{2+} + H_2O_2 \rightleftharpoons Fe^{3+} + OH^- + OH° + O$) and then reducing oxygen to generate the superoxide anion ($Fe^{2+} + O_2 = Fe^{3+} + O_2°^-$) (175–178). However, iron is not present in Chrysotile nor in other asbestiforms, such as erionite and tremolite, both of which are potent carcinogens for the mesothelium. Neither is it found in many synthetic fibers, such as ceramic or organic fibers (137).

INCONSISTENCIES BETWEEN ANIMAL AND HUMAN DATA

Several inconsistencies remain between human and animal data relating to the potential of fibers to induce lung tumors and mesothelioma (179).

DOSE RESPONSE

In inhalation experiments in the rat, asbestos concentration and cumulative doses usually were much higher than those to which workers might have been exposed (162, 164, 170). An overload effect, therefore, may at least partly have been responsible for the carcinogenic response in rats, making any extrapolation to humans difficult. Conversely, in reviewing recent experiments carried out in rats by nose only exposure to size-selected fibers (140, 141), questions have been raised because the numerical concentrations and total doses of inhaled MMVFs were approximately one or two orders of magnitude less than the concentration of asbestos fibers used as positive controls. This may explain the apparently conflicting results obtained in inhalation experiments, in which the dose-response relationship for lung tumors—both adenomas and carcinomas—induced by ceramic fibers was compared with that of Chrysotile. Results suggested that ceramic fibers were the more potent for inducing lung tumors. One fiber, refractory ceramic fiber 1, induced 13% of tumors, and the other refractory ceramic fiber 3, 15.7%, for a fiber concentration of 234 fibers per cubic centimeter in the aerosol; Chrysotile, however, which was used as a positive control, induced 18.5% of tumors, for a fiber concentration of 10,200 fibers per cubic centimeter. This difference may be explained by the relatively lower proportion of long fibers in the Chrysotile controls, for which the arithmetic mean length was only 2.2 + 3.0 μm, compared with 22.3 + 17 μm for refractory ceramic fiber 1.

MESOTHELIOMA INDUCTION AND SPECIES VARIATIONS

In most inhalation experiments in rats with a variety of fiber types, no more that 1% to 2% of pleural mesotheliomas were observed (140, 162, 164, 169), with the exception of erionite, which produced 27 mesotheliomas in 28 rats (136). However, there are no conclusive experimental data to support the hypothesis that inhaled Chrysotile fibers pose relatively little, if any, risk of malignant mesothelioma. Actually, it may depend on the dose inhaled.

The species effect is another important issue. In principle the carcinogenic potency of any new substance must be tested in two different species; for fibers there was a major discrepancy between the incidence of asbestos-related pleural mesotheliomas induced in rats and in hamsters. After inhalation experiments with Crocidolite or Chrysotile in rats, approximately 1% of pleural malignant mesotheliomas were observed compared with a malignant lung tumor rate as high as 30%. This finding contrasts with a recent experiment in hamsters (140) exposed to long-term inhalation of RCF1 ceramic fiber: 42% of animals developed pleural malignant mesothelioma. When rats were exposed under the same conditions, only 1.6% developed malignant mesothelioma. The reasons for this species specificity are not known.

The low percentage of pleural mesothelioma induced in rats might be explained by the short life span of these rodents compared with humans and primates. This argument does not explain the results in hamsters. In baboons with a longer life span, higher percentages of pleural and peritoneal malignant mesotheliomas were obtained after inhalation of Amosite at very high doses, i.e., approximately 1000 fibers per milliliter over several months (180).

COMPREHENSIVE CELL MECHANISMS OF FIBER-RELATED CARCINOGENESIS

GENERAL OBSERVATIONS

When encountering pulmonary cells, natural or synthetic fibers induce two types of biologic reactions (Fig. 34.1). (*a*) The first are early responses, corresponding mainly to inflammatory reactions initially involving alveolar macrophages and polymorphonuclear leukocytes, and then affecting interstitial cells and tracheobronchial epithelial or mesothelial cells. When activated, all of these cells are prone to releasing reactive oxygen species, cytokines, and mediators, some of which are fibrogenic; others possibly are clastogenic for the cell DNA and cell growth stimulators. (*b*) The second type are late responses at the level of lung parenchyma and pleura that are responsible for the endpoint diseases of lung and pleural fibrosis and, later, pulmonary or pleural malignancies (9, 121, 153).

The initial event in fiber carcinogenesis involves a physical or chemical hit on the genomic material responsible for mutagenic or clastogenic changes of cells. Subsequently, neoplastic transformation and full development of cancer evolve in successive steps, involving the proliferation of the mutated cell clone and thus increasing the population of initiated cells. The promotion steps correspond to successive epigenetic events that, under the effect of durable carcinogenic agents such as mineral fibers, permit an increase in the rate of expression of the cancer cell phenotype in a given tissue. All of these events involve mutation, rearrangement, amplification, or deletion of specific genes, either suppressor genes or oncogenes. Tumor progression then is characterized by a series of permanent phenotypic changes, probably related to the microenvironment of the cells.

In asbestos-related respiratory cancers, the issue is the determination of which of these consecutive molecular events is mainly involved in lung carcinoma rather than mesothelioma. Indeed, from epidemiologic studies (181, 182), the estimate of respiratory cancer risk caused by asbestos exposure, and possibly by all types of fibers, could be based on different statistical models according to the site of origin. For lung cancer the relative risk increased proportionally to cumulative asbestos exposure, and the effects of asbestos and cigarette smoking were multiplicative (183, 184). This finding suggests that asbestos might work more as a promotor, acting only at a late stage in bronchial carcinogenesis, for which the main causal factor probably is tobacco smoking. In vitro studies on tracheobronchial epithelium support this hypothesis (185, 186). In contrast, in the epidemiologic study of Peto et al. (181), the incidence of mesothelioma was found to increase proportionally to the cumulative exposure and to the third or fourth power of time since the first exposure, even after exposure has ceased, independently of age at the first exposure and history of smoking. Thus, at the level of the serosal cavities, asbestos fibers seem to work either as initiators or as complete carcinogens. Indeed, in vitro studies on rat pleural mesothelial cells have provided convincing data supporting the hypothesis that asbestos must act as a complete carcinogen for mesothelioma, by mechanisms implying that fibers must hit mesothelial cells directly. (187–189).

Presently, this distinction in mechanisms, in fact, is not so strict because the cancer phenotype corresponds to an immortalization of cells capable of expressing genes normally repressed in tissue as a result of the interaction of both genetic and epigenetic events. However, it is probable that asbestos-related carcinogenesis follows different pathways: for lung cancer, the major carcinogens are provided by tobacco smoke, which facilitates the intraepithelial penetration of fibers (190), whereas for mesothelioma the initial hit would have happened long before the clinical expression of the tumor in an enclosed serosal cavity. As mentioned previously (Fig. 34.1), there is some evidence favoring asbestos fiber migration to the pleural cavity and particularly to the parietal pleura, the usual site of initiation of mesothelioma (77, 78). It is possible that long and durable fibers, like amphiboles, accumulate at the level of the lymphatic pores of the parietal pleura (191)

Genotoxicity of Fibers

Chromosomal Aberrations in Malignant Mesothelioma

In human mesothelioma specific nonrandom karyotypic abnormalities have been described extensively (192–196). These chromosomal alterations are often difficult to interpret in humans, because at the stage of diagnosis, the tumor progression usually is already far advanced.

Among the numerous nonrandom numerical and structural abnormalities described in a cytogenetic study of more than 100 cases of malignant mesothelioma in humans, attention focused particularly on deletions and rearrangements of chromosomes 1, 3, 5, 7, 9, 11, 14, 21, and 22 (197). However, it seems appropriate to distinguish two types of chromosomal abnormalities: on the one hand, karyotypic losses involving chromosomes 1, 14, 21, and 22, which might correspond to primary changes induced by fibers; and on the other hand, trisomy 7, 7p, and 11 and monosomy or partial monosomy of chromosomes 3 and 9, which could correspond to secondary changes accompanying tumor progression (197).

Actually, the nonrandom abnormalities observed in human mesothelial cells in culture exposed to asbestos have indicated that chromosome 1 was involved more often than other chromosomes (198). Interestingly, a break point at 1p11-22, which was a frequent abnormality in malignant mesothelioma, has been found in association with a high fiber burden (194). In contrast, some karyotypic markers currently observed in advanced malignant mesothelioma were lacking in human mesothelial cells treated in vitro with asbestos, particularly those concerning chromosome 3 (198). These successive steps toward full cancerization of mesothelial cells have been confirmed by Lechner et al. (199), who succeeded in transforming normal human mesothelial cells in vitro under the action of asbestos, which is associated with major chromosomal changes, either numerical or structural. The numerical changes involved either hypodiploidy (loss of chromosomes 11 and 21) or hyperdiploidy. The structural changes involved dicentric, double minute, long chromosomes with repetitive bands. Nevertheless, these cells were not tumorigenic in nude mice because apparently they had not yet reached a sufficiently advanced stage of phenotypic cancer differentiation. These successive karyotypic modifications during tumoral progression are illustrated in the case of malignant mesothelioma reported by Hansteen et al. (44).

Similarly, several chromosome modifications have been observed in asbestos-induced mesothelioma in rodents, particularly chromosome 1 in rats and chromosome 3 in hamsters (197).

In Vitro Genotoxicity of Fibers

Based on the numerous karyotypic abnormalities observed in malignant mesothelioma in humans and rodents, a number of in vitro studies were conducted on different cell systems to understand the successive genotoxic steps leading to DNA alterations, chromosome structural aberrations, and ploidy abnormalities. Most of the published data have been reviewed extensively (187, 189), but this discussion will focus on the available results concerning human and rat mesothelial cells.

DNA Damage

Most studies have been unable to detect point mutations resulting from the action of asbestos fibers in various prokaryote and eukaryote cell systems. However, the induction of mutations of human and hamster cell hybrids under the action of Chrysotile has been achieved recently (200). No such data have been described thus far for human mesothelial cells.

DNA single-strand breaks have not been observed in mammalian mesothelial cells treated with asbestos. However, the exploration of DNA damage by the indirect method of unscheduled DNA repair has made it possible to identify an increased unscheduled DNA synthesis in rat pleural mesothelial cells under the action of different fibers (201, 202). It seems that such responses could be dependent on the nature of the cell used because different cell types probably have different repair efficiencies (189). The induction of DNA strand breaks in cells exposed to Crocidolite has been demonstrated using the technique of nick translation (203).

CHROMOSOMAL ABNORMALITIES

Two previously quoted studies (198, 199), in which chromosome abnormalities were obtained in normal human mesothelial cells in culture under the action of asbestos, suggest that such structural and numerical aberrations may have been induced by a direct hit of fibers on chromosomal material, particularly during mitosis. Indeed, it has been shown that fibers phagocytosed by Syrian hamster cells (204) or by rat pleural mesothelial cells (205) enter into direct contact with the genetic material during mitosis, suggesting that they could be responsible for chromosomal damage and mis-segregation of chromatids. Thus, fibers have been observed interfering mechanically with the chromatids during the different phases of mitosis, and this interference would be capable of inducing sister chromatid exchanges (155) and chromosomal aberrations such as aneuploidy, abnormal anaphases with lagging chromatin, bridges, and multipolar segregations (189). All these karyotypic events can play a role in inducing mutations or modifications of tumor suppressor genes, oncogenes, or genes controlling growth factor that might contribute to cell transformation and tumor progression (206). Indeed, these numerical or structural chromosomal abnormalities have been observed in vitro in different cell types—including Syrian hamster embryo cells (204), rat pleural mesothelial cells (207–209), and human mesothelial cells (198, 199)—during their transformation under the action of asbestos and MMVFs.

Whatever the mechanism, damage to the genetic material and chromosome mis-segregation and probably other chromosomal aberrations appear to be related directly to the fibrous form of particles, because it is not observed with nonfibrous particles such as anatase (156). However, size parameters of fibers seem to be the major factors, because the highest proportions of abnormal anaphases were observed when rat pleural mesothelial cells were treated in vitro with the longest and thinnest asbestos fibers based on Stanton's criteria (length, less than 8 μm; diameter, less than 0.25 μm). However, fiber type also is important because Crocidolite was more efficient than Chrysotile in inducing abnormal anaphases (209), which may be related to the release of reactive oxygen species.

INDIRECT MECHANISMS THROUGH OXIDATIVE PROCESSES

It is commonly thought that the production of reactive oxygen species under the action of asbestos must play a role in fiber cytotoxicity and genotoxicity. Indeed, different oxygen derivatives (hydroxy and oxy radicals) can be generated either by cells exposed to fibers or by the fibers themselves, particularly those containing iron (210–213). The inhibition of cell responses by iron chelation (desferrioxamine) or by antioxidants (catalase and superoxide dismutase) suggests the important part played by these mediators as well as the possible role of iron (214).

Thus, two factors can cooperate in the production of free radicals: (a) The phagocytic cells themselves can produce them after internalization of asbestos fibers (210, 215–217). It has been shown that oxygen species were released in a dose dependent manner by alveolar macrophages exposed to different asbestiform fibers (Crocidolite, Chrysotile, erionite, glass fibers, whereas nonfibrous analogues (riebeckite, glass beads) caused less striking responses at comparable concentrations (218). It has also been shown that mesothelial cells in culture behaved similarly, confirming the importance of the fibrous shape for the release of O_2 by phagocytic cells (219). (b) Iron-containing fibers themselves, such as Crocidolite, which are able to produce $OH°$ by Fe (II) present at the surface. However, the fact that proteins have been shown to have the same protective effect as two antioxidants (catalase and superoxide dismutase) against the asbestos-induced cytotoxicity and genotoxicity on rat pleural mesothelial cells in culture suggests a nonspecific protection against oxygen derivatives, probably by adsorption of proteins at the surface of the fibers, thus reducing cell-fiber interaction (220). Moreover, experiments in vitro comparing the cytotoxic effects on mesothelial cells of oxidants versus Amosite fibers showed that Amosite, which contains iron, did not induce direct oxidant-type injury to human mesothelial cells (219, 221).

Arising from these contradictory results concerning the generation of reactive oxygen species by fibrous and nonfibrous mineral particles with different iron content, it is postulated that different forms of iron could be involved in fiber toxicity and carcinogenicity. There is no doubt that iron reactivity is unrelated to the total iron content of fibers, but it appears that not only Fe (II) (177) but also Fe (III) can potentially be reactive, as suggested by the inhibitory action of desferrioxamine and by scavengers of reactive oxygen species (210, 219, 222–224). Moreover, active forms of iron (particularly Fe [II]) at the surface of the fibers would be more reactive than those buried in the core (177, 225, 226). Mobilized iron also could play an important role, as suggested by the increased production of OH° or DNA breaks under the action of ethylenediamine–tetraacetic acid (EDTA), a chelator of iron (223, 227, 228).

CLASTOGENIC FACTORS

As a subsidiary effect of chromosome aberrations observed in rat pleural mesothelial cells exposed in vitro to Chrysotile fibers, it has been found that some clastogenic factors must be involved, because these effects persisted even when fibers were removed from the media (229). The exact nature of clastogenic factors with a molecular weight between 1000 and 10,000 has not yet been identified, but it seems that superoxide radicals are involved both in the formation and action of clastogenic factors, as suggested by the constant inhibitory effect of superoxide dismutase (230). Such hypothetic clastogenic factors could be phospholipid peroxidation–derived products, e.g., 4-hydroxynonal, which is clastogenic at concentrations of 0.1 mmol or below. However, clastogenic factors have not yet been characterized definitely. Whatever the mechanisms, antioxidants may theoretically be protective both as anticlastogens and as anticarcinogens.

HOST FACTORS

IMMUNE CELL IMBALANCES INDUCED BY ASBESTOS FIBERS

Several published studies describe immune imbalances in subjects exposed to asbestos, some of whom subsequently developed lung cancer or mesothelioma (231). However, among the different aspects of immune dysfunction, it is difficult or even impossible to discriminate between the effect of the direct toxicity of asbestos fibers on the immune system and the effect related to smoking and underlying infraclinical asbestosis. Considered are some of the in vivo and in vitro studies focusing on immune dysfunction apparently related directly to asbestos, which might be responsible for a marked immune defense depression and consequently with an increased risk of developing asbestos-related respiratory malignancies.

The interpretation of immune system impairment by asbestos fibers is complicated in humans by the fact that fibers always induce a subacute or chronic alveolitis with its characteristic immune reaction, e.g., the activation of macrophages releasing mediators and cytokines (232). Nevertheless, a substantial amount of data comparing immune cells in peripheral blood (PB) and in BALF suggests that asbestos exposure, with or without lung or pleural fibrosis, usually is associated with immune cell imbalance. Concerning T lymphocytes, the main characteristics are an increase of helper-inducer T-cell CD4 subsets, both in PB and in BALF, whereas the cytotoxic/suppressor T-cell (CD8) subsets are correspondingly depressed in the lung, with a significantly enhanced CD4 to CD8 ratio in BALF (233–235).

The data concerning number, proportion, and activity of natural killer (NK) cells in the PB of asbestos-exposed individuals were inconsistent, or were related more to smoking than to asbestos exposure in the majority of the publications (233, 236–238). In most of these studies, NK cells identified by the CD16 (Leu-11a) antibody were reduced in absolute number in subjects exposed to asbestos, compared with a control group. This result is consistent with the hypothesis that asbestos fibers suppress NK cell activity. An in vitro study also showed that all types of asbestos suppressed NK cell activities against human mesothelioma cell lines, which could be restored by interleukin-2 (239). In a study on another anticancer immune defense, a significant depression of lymphokine-activated killer cells has been reported in asbestos-exposed individuals, compared with non–asbestos-exposed controls (240).

FAMILIAL PREDISPOSITION

In the industrial cohorts, only a few of the workers with the same level of occupational exposure to asbestos contract mesothelioma, suggesting that there is some individual predisposition to develop this tumor. The role of human leukocyte antigen (HLA) type in susceptibility to mesothelioma has been investigated rarely. Studies in which an increase was found in HLA-Bwzi, contrasting with a decrease in HLA-A11 (241), were not significant, nor were they confirmed by others (242).

There are several cases, in which several members of the same family died of the disease, that document a possible genetic or at least a familial predisposition to malignant mesothelioma (243). In the most extraordinary family reported, the father, three sons, and a daughter died of malignant mesothelioma (244). Other familial aggregations of malignant mesothelioma concern two or three members of a family, either two brothers or one brother and one sister (146), or one parent and one child.

These observations suggest that malignant mesothelioma might happen more often in cancer prone families—as noted previously for lung cancer—and suggest a possible genetic predisposition to develop this malignant tumor, either alone or more probably in conjunction with an environmental factor. Indeed, in the majority of cases, asbestos exposure probably was present and was confirmed in one case by an abnormally high AB count in the lung (245). Exposure was sometimes related to contact within the household of several members of the family with a parent who was exposed to asbestos occupationally (246, 247). The indoor asbestos concentrations in the houses of such families were not known.

In any case there are several arguments supporting the role of a genetic factor or at least an individual predisposition to the development of mesothelioma: (a) Few cases are observed in which there has been no asbestos exposure, even when other members of the same family have been exposed. This was true in the case of the daughter in the family mentioned previously (244). Furthermore, two cases of mesothelioma have been observed in a brother and sister in a family in which there was neither domestic nor environmental asbestos exposure (146). (b) Mesothelioma has occurred in identical twin brothers who developed the disease at the same age and who had been exposed to asbestos when doing the same job (242). (c) When there is a family history of cancer, even in sites other than the pleura or peritoneum, there is a higher risk of malignant mesothelioma. Forty-three of 63 mesothelioma patients had a positive history of a primary invasive cancer of all types in one or more first-degree relatives, the proportion of cases being identical in males and females (243). Even though reporting of true familial malignant mesothelioma remains rather anecdotal, a familial predisposition seems to be possible and would justify the development of a research program aimed at identifying predisposing gene(s) to this type of cancer.

CONCLUSION

Mesothelioma is still a relatively new disease, its real history having started approximately 30 years ago with Wagner's discovery of its strong association with asbestos exposure, both occupationally and environmentally. Presently, this serosal malignancy causes considerable concern because incidence rates are still increasing in most industrialized countries, and they may be expected to follow the same trend into the first two decades of the 21st century (57).

Asbestos exposure has been widespread in many Western countries and is still an important factor in Europe and in developing countries. At the same time, the exposure-related risk levels for malignant mesothelioma are still not yet determined. Emphasis, therefore, must be placed on programs of screening, education, and prevention of exposure, and serious consideration should be given to banning the use of amphiboles.

The extensive use of new synthetic fibers may provide an alternative, but it is one that will require the closest surveillance. As research progresses, particularly in the mechanism of fiber carcinogenesis at the cellular level, it should become feasible to develop standard in vitro tests for biologic activity of new fibers that may permit valid hazard and risk assessments to be made before production begins.

Efforts also must be made to discover the other causes or predisposing factors for malignant mesothelioma, because in approximately one third of malignant mesothelioma cases, there has been no evidence of a history of asbestos exposure. With both epidemiologic research and in vitro studies of mechanisms of fiber carcinogenesis, progress is being made, but there still are gaps to fill. Epidemiologic studies are hampered by inadequate reporting of cases and insufficient recording of past exposures to asbestos.

Presently, neither early detection nor treatment of malignant mesothelioma is successful. Much greater efforts thus are needed to strengthen research into the etiologic factors and mechanisms of fiber toxicology.

Acknowledgments

The authors express their gratitude to Walter Davis, who did his best to convert their Franglais into American English without disturbing their science, and to Joan Beaurain, whose careful and conscientious typing produced the text in its present readable form.

References

1. Wagner E. Das tuberklahnliche Lymphadenom (der cytogene oder reticuloite Tuberkel). Arch Heilk (Leipzig) 1870;11:497.
2. Klemperer P, Rabin CB. Primary neoplasms of the pleura: report of five cases. Arch Pathol 1931;11:385–412.
3. Craighead JE. Current pathogenic concepts of diffuse malignant mesothelioma. Hum Pathol 1987;18:544–557.
4. Wagner JC, Sleggs CA, Marchand P. Diffuse pleural malignant mesothelioma and asbestos exposure in the North Western Cape Province. Br J Ind Med 1960;17:260–271.
5. Doll R. Mortality from lung cancer in asbestos workers. Br J Ind Med 1955;12:81–86.
6. Becklake MR. Asbestos-related diseases of the lung and other organs: their epidemiology and implications for clinical practice. Am Rev Respir Dis 1976;114:187–227.
7. Bignon J. Mineral fibers in the non-occupational environment. In: Bignon J, Peto J, Saracci R, eds. Non-occupational expo-

sure to mineral fibers. Lyon: International Agency for Research on Cancer Scientific Publication No 90, 1989:3–29.
8. Sébastien P, Bignon J, Martin M. Indoor airborne asbestos pollution: from the ceiling to the floor. Science 1982;216:1410–1412.
9. Mossman BT, Bignon J, Corn M, Seaton A, Gee JBL. Asbestos: scientific developments and implications for public policy. Science 1990;247:294–301.
10. HEI-AR. Asbestos in public and commercial buildings: a literature review and synthesis of current knowledge. Cambridge, MA: Health Effects Institute—Asbestos Research, 1991.
11. Langer AM, Nolan RP, Addison J. Distinguishing between amphibole asbestos fibers and elongate cleavage fragments of their non-asbestos analogues. In: Brown RC, Hoskins JA, Johnson NF, eds. North Atlantic Treaty Organization ASI series: mechanisms in fiber carcinogenesis. New York: Springer-Verlag, 1991;223:253–268.
12. Bignon J, Brochard P, De Cremoux H, Nebut M, Jaurand MC. Contribution of epidemiology and biology to the comprehension of causes and mechanisms of mesothelioma. In: Deslauriers J, Lacquets LK, eds. Thoracic surgery: surgical management of pleural diseases. Toronto: Mosby, 1990;6:327–335.
13. Ruffie P, Feld R, Minkin S, et al. Diffuse malignant mesothelioma of the pleura in Ontario and Quebec: a retrospective study of 332 patients. J Clin Oncol 1989;7:1157–1168.
14. Boutin C, Rey F. Thoracoscopy in pleural malignant mesothelioma: a prospective study of 188 patients. Part 1: diagnosis. Cancer 1993;72:389–393.
15. Butchart EG, Ashcroft T, Barnsley WC, Holden MP. Pleuropneumonectomy in the management of diffuse malignant mesothelioma of the pleura. Thorax 1976;31:15–24.
16. Boutin C, Rey F, Gouvernet J, Viallat JR, Astoul P, Ledoray V. Thoracoscopy in pleural malignant mesothelioma: a prospective study of 188 patients. Part 2: prognosis and staging. Cancer 1993;72:394–404.
17. Craighead JF, Abraham JL, Churg A, et al. The pathology of asbestos-associated diseases of the lungs and pleural cavities: diagnostic criteria and proposed grading schema. Arch Pathol Lab Med 1982;106:544–596.
18. Sheibani K. Immunopathology of malignant mesothelioma. Editorial. Hum Pathol 1994;25:219–220.
19. Zeng L, Fleury-Feith J, Monnet I, Boutin C, Bignon J, Jaurand, MC. Immunocytochemical characterization of cell lines from human malignant mesothelioma. Hum Pathol 1994;25:227–234.
20. Stahel RA, O'Hara CJ, Waibel R, et al. Monoclonal antibodies against mesothelial membrane antigen discriminate between malignant mesothelioma and lung adenocarcinoma. Int J Cancer 1988;41:218–223.
21. Collins CL, Schaefer R, Cook CD, et al. Thrombomodulin expression in malignant pleural mesothelioma and pulmonary adenocarcinoma. Eur Respir Rev 1993;3:59–60.
22. Dessy E, Pietra GG. Pseudomesotheliomatous carcinoma of the lung. An immunohistochemical and ultrastructural study of three cases. Cancer 1991;68:1747–1753.
23. Harwood TR, Gracey DR, Yokoo H. Pseudomesotheliomatous carcinoma of the lung: a variant of peripheral lung cancer. Am J Clin Pathol 1976;65:159–167.
24. Bignon J, Sébastien P, Di Menza L, Nebut M, Payan H. French mesothelioma register. Ann N Y Acad Sci 1979;330:455–466.
25. Greenberg M, Lloyd Davies TA. Mesothelioma register 1967–68. Br J Ind Med 1974;31:91–104.
26. Kannestein M, Churg J. Functions of mesothelioma panels. Ann N Y Acad Sci 1979;76:143–149.
27. Wright WE, Sherwin RP, Dickson EA, Bernstein L, Fromm JB, Henderson B. Malignant mesothelioma: Incidence, asbestos exposure, and reclassification of histopathology. Br J Ind Med 1984;41:39–45.
28. Selikoff I, Seidman H. Use of death certificates in epidemiological studies, including occupational hazards: variations in discordance of different asbestos-associated diseases on best evidence ascertainment. Am J Ind Med 1992;22:481–492.
29. Gaensler EA, Kaplan AI. Asbestos pleural effusion. Ann Intern Med 1971;74:178–191.
30. Chahinian P, Hirsch A, Bignon J, et al. Les pleurésies asbestosiques non tumorales. Rev Fr Mal Respir 1973;1:5–39.
31. Hillerdal G, Özesmi M. Benign asbestos pleural effusion: 73 exudates in 80 patients. Eur J Respir Dis 1987;71:113–121.
32. Hillerdal G. Non-malignant asbestos pleural disease. Thorax 1981;36:669–675.
33. Churg A. Asbestos fibers and pleural plaques in a general autopsy population. Am J Pathol 1982;109:88–96.
34. Meurmann L. Asbestos bodies and pleural plaques in a Finnish series of autopsy cases. Acta Pathol Microbiol Scand 1966;181(Suppl):7–107.
35. Hillerdal G. Pleural plaques and risk for bronchial carcinoma and mesothelioma. A prospective study. Chest 1994;105:144–150.
36. Smith DD. Plaques, cancer, and confusion (editorial). Chest 1994;105:8–9.
37. Orlowski E, Pairon JC, Ameille J, et al. Pleural plaques, asbestos exposure, and asbestos bodies in bronchoalveolar lavage fluid. Am J Ind Med 1994;26:349–358
38. Stephens M, Gibbs AR, Pooley FD, Wagner JC. Asbestos induced diffuse pleural fibrosis: pathology and mineralogy. Thorax 1987;42:583–588.
39. Mintzer RA, Cugell DW. The association of asbestos induced pleural disease and rounded atelectasis. Chest 1982;81:457–460.
40. Hillerdal G. Rounded atelectasis. Clinical experience with 74 patients. Chest 1989;95:836–841.
41. Frebourg T, Lerebours G, Delpech B, et al. Serum hyaluronate in malignant mesothelioma. Cancer 1987;59:2104–2107.
42. Lindqvist U, Chichibu K, Delpech B, et al. Seven different assays of hyaluronan compared for clinical utility. Clin Chem 1992;38:127–132.
43. Pluygers E, Baldewyns P. Tissue polypeptide antigen (TPA) as a biomarker of the mesothelial cell and of mesothelioma. Eur Respir Rev 1993;3:47–46.
44. Hansteen IL, Hilt B, Lien JTH, Skaug V, Haugen A. Karyotypic changes in the preclinical and subsequent stages of malignant mesothelioma. A case report. Cancer Genet Cytogenet 1993; 70:94–98.
45. Iwatsubo Y, Pairon JC, Archambault de Beaune C, Chamming's S, Bignon J, Brochard P. Pleural mesothelioma: a descriptive analysis based on a case-control study and mortality data in Ile-de-France, 1987–1990. Am J Ind Med 1994;26: 77–88.
46. McDonald AD, McDonald JC. Epidemiology of malignant mesothelioma. In: Antman K, Aisner J, eds. Asbestos related malignancy. London: Grune & Stratton, 1987:31–56.
47. Zielhuis RL, Versteeg JPL, Planteydt HT. Pleural mesothelioma and exposure to asbestos: A retrospective case-control study in Nederlands. Int Arch Occup Environ Health 1975;36: 1–18.
48. McDonald AD, McDonald JC. Malignant mesothelioma in North America. Cancer 1980;46:1650–1656.

49. Ferguson DA, Jelihovsky T, Andreas SB, et al. The Australian Mesothelioma Surveillance Program 1979–1985. Med J Aust 1987;147:166–172.
50. Connelly RR, Spirtas R, Myers MH, Percy Cl, Fraumeni JF. Demographic patterns for mesothelioma in the United States. J Natl Cancer Inst 1987;78:1053–1060.
51. Jones RJSP, McLoud T, Rockoff SD. Mesothelioma in Great Britain in 1958–1983. Scand J Work Environ Health 1988;14:145–152.
52. Meijers JMM, Planteyd HT, Slangen JJM, Swaen GMH, Vilet CV, Sturmans F. Trends and geographical patterns of pleural mesothelioma in Netherlands 1970–1987. Br J Ind Med 1990;47:775–781.
53. McDonald JC. Health implications of environmental exposure to asbestos. Environ Health Perspect 1985;62:319–328.
54. Zwi AB, Reid G, Landau SP, Kiekowski D, Sitas F, Becklake MR. Mesothelioma in South Africa, 1976–84: Incidence and case characteristics. Int J Epidemiol 1989;18:320–329.
55. Leigh J, Corvalan CF, Grimwood A, Berry G, Ferguson DA, Thompson R. The incidence of malignant mesothelioma in Australia 1982–1988. Am J Ind Med 1991;20:643–655.
56. Nicholson WJ, Perkel G, Selikoff IJ. Occupational exposure to asbestos: population at risk and projected mortality—1980–2030. Am J Ind Med 1982;3:259–311.
57. Peto J, Hodgson JT, Matthews FE, Jones JR. Continuing increase in mesothelioma mortality in Britain. Lancet 1995;345:535–539.
58. Wikeley NJ. Measurement of asbestos dust levels in British asbestos factories in the 1930s. Am J Ind Med 1993;24:509–520.
59. Dement JM, Harris RL, Symons MJ, Shy C. Estimates of dose-response for respiratory cancer among Chrysotile asbestos workers. Ann Occup Hyg 1982;26:869–887.
60. Doll R, Peto J. Asbestos effects on health of exposure to asbestos. A report to the Health and Safety Commission. London: Her Majesty's Stationery Office, 1985:1–58.
61. Peto J, Doll R, Hermon C, Binns W, Clayton R, Goffe T. Relationships of mortality to measures of environmental asbestos pollution in an asbestos textile factory. Ann Occup Hyg 1985;29:305–355.
62. McDonald JC, Liddell FDK, Dufresne A, McDonald AD. The 1891–1920 birth cohort of Quebec Chrysotile miners and millers: mortality 1976–1988. Br J Ind Med 1993;50:1073–1081.
63. Liddell D. Asbestos in the occupational environment. In: Liddell D, Miller K, eds. Mineral fibers and health. Boca Raton, Ann Arbor, Boston: CRC Press, 1991:80–87.
64. Krantz S, Cherrie JW, Schneider T, Ohberg I, Kamstrup O. Modelling of past exposure to MMMF in the European rock-slag wool industry. Arbete Och Halsa 1991;1:1–41.
65. Ahrens W, Jöckel KH, Brochard P, et al. Retrospective assessment of asbestos exposure. 1. Case control analysis in a study of lung cancer: efficiency of job specific questionnaires and job exposure matrices. Int J Epidemiol 1993;22:S83–S95.
66. Sebastien P, Fondimare A, Bignon J, Monchaux G, Desbordes J, Bonnaud G. Topographic distribution of asbestos fibers in human lung in relation with occupational and non-occupational exposure. In: Walton WH, McGovern B, eds. Inhaled particles and vapors. IV, Part 2. New York: Pergamon, 1977:237–246.
67. Roggli VL, Pratt PC, Brody AR. Analysis of tissue mineral fiber content. In: Roggli VL, Greenberg SD, Pratt PC, eds. Pathology of asbestos-associated diseases. Boston: Little Brown, 1992:299–346.
68. Sebastien P, Armstrong B, Monchaux G, Bignon J. Asbestos bodies in bronchoalveolar lavage fluid and in lung parenchyma. Am Rev Respir Dis 1988;137:75–78.
69. Churg AM, Warnock ML. Analysis of the cores of ferruginous (asbestos) bodies from the general population. I. Patients with and without lung cancer. Lab Invest 1977;37:280–286.
70. Churg AM, Warnock ML. Analysis of the cores of ferruginous (asbestos) bodies from the general population. III. Patients with environmental exposure. Lab Invest 1979;40:622–626.
71. Dodson RF, Williams MG, O'Sullivan MF, Corn CJ, Greenberg SD, Hurst GA. A comparison of the ferruginous body and uncoated fiber content in the lungs of former asbestos workers. Am Rev Respir Dis 1985;132:143–147.
72. Roggli VL, Pratt PC, Brody AR. Asbestos content of lung tissue in asbestos associated diseases: a study of 110 cases. Br J Ind Med 1986;43:18–28
73. Warnock ML. Lung asbestos burden in shipyard and construction workers with mesothelioma: comparison with burdens in subjects with asbestosis or lung cancer. Environ Res 1989;50:68–85.
74. Dodson RF, Garcia JGN, O'Sullivan M, et al. The usefulness of bronchoalveolar lavage in identifying past occupational exposure to asbestos: a light and electron microscopy study. Am J Ind Med 1991;19:619–628.
75. Murai Y, Kitagawa M. Asbestos fiber analysis in 27 malignant mesothelioma cases. Am J Ind Med 1992;22:193–207.
76. Tuomi T, Oksa P, Anttila S, et al. Fibres and asbestos bodies in bronchoalveolar lavage fluids of asbestos sprayers. Br J Ind Med 1992;49:480–485.
77. Sébastien P, Janson X, Bonnaud G, Riba G, Masse R, Bignon J. Translocation of asbestos fibers through respiratory tract and gastrointestinal tract according to fiber and size. In: Lemen R, Dement J, eds. Dusts and disease. Park Forest South, IL: Pathotox Publishers, 1979:65–85.
78. Dodson RF, Williams MG, Corn CJ, Brollo A, Bianchi C. Asbestos content of lung tissue, lymph nodes, and pleural plaques from former shipyard workers. Am Rev Respir Dis 1990;142:843–847.
79. Becklake M. Asbestos and other fiber related diseases of the lungs and pleural. Distribution and determination in exposed population. Chest 1990;100:248–54.
80. Bernstein DM, Mast R, Anderson R, et al. An experimental approach to the evaluation of the biopersistence of respirable synthetic fibers and minerals. In: Bignon J, Saracci R, Touray J, eds. Biopersistence of respirable synthetic fibers and minerals. Environ Health Perspect 1994;102(Suppl 5):15–18.
81. Muhle H, Bellmann B, Pott F. Comparative investigations of the biodurability of mineral fibers in the rat lung. In: Bignon J, Saracci R, Touray J, eds. Biopersistence of respirable synthetic fibers and minerals. Environ Health Perspect 1994;102(Suppl 5):163–168.
82. Stein RC, Kitajewska JY, Tait JB, Sinha G, Rudd RM. Pleural mesothelioma resulting from exposure to Amosite asbestos in a building. Respir Med 1989;83:237–239.
83. Anderson HA, Hanrahan LP, Schirmer J, Higgins D, Sarow P. Mesothelioma among employees with likely contact with in-place asbestos-containing materials. Ann N Y Acad Sci 1991;550–572.
84. Hughes JM, Weill H. Asbestos exposure: quantitative assessment of risk. Am Rev Respir Dis 1986;133:5–15.
85. Valleron AJ, Bignon J, Hughes JM, et al. Low dose exposure to natural and man-made fibers and the risk of cancer: towards a collaborative European epidemiology. Br J Ind Med 1992;49:606–614.

86. Dong H, Saint-Etienne L, Renier A, Billon Galland MA, Brochard P, Jaurand MC. Air samples from a building with asbestos-containing material: asbestos content and in vitro toxicity on rat pleural mesothelial cells. Fundam Appl Toxicol 1994;22:178–185.
87. Crebelli R, Fuselli S, Meneguz A, et al. In vitro and in vivo mutagenicity studies with airborne particulate extracts. Mutat Res 1988;204:564–575.
88. McDonald JC, Liddell FDK, Gibbs GW, Eyssen G, McDonald AD. Dust exposure and mortality in Chrysotile mining 1910–75. Br J Ind Med 1980;37:11–24.
89. Rubino GF, Piolatto G, Newhouse ML, Scancetti G, Aresini GA, Murray R. Mortality of Chrysotile asbestos workers at the Balangero mine, northern Italy. Br J Ind Med 1979;36:187–194.
90. McDonald AD, Fry JS, Woolley AJ, McDonald JC. Dust exposure and mortality in an American Chrysotile friction products plant. Br J Ind Med 1984;41:151–157.
91. McDonald AD, Fry JS, Woolley AJ, McDonald JC. Dust exposure and mortality in an American Chrysotile textile plant. Br J Ind Med 1983;40:368–374.
92. Hughes JM, Weill H, Hammad YY. Mortality of workers employed in two asbestos cement manufacturing plants. Br J Ind Med 1987;44:161–174.
93. Weiss W. Mortality of a cohort exposed to Chrysotile asbestos. J Occup Med 1977;19:737–740.
94. Ohlson CG, Hogstedt C. Lung cancer among asbestos cement workers. A Swedish cohort study and a review. Br J Ind Med 1985;42:397–402.
95. Liddell IJ. Epidemiological observations on mesothelioma and their implications for non-occupational exposure to asbestos. In: Spengler JD, Ozkaynak H, McCarthy JF, Lee H, eds. Health effects of exposure to asbestos in buildings. 1989.
96. Armstrong BK, DeKlerk NH, Musk AX, Hobbs MST. Mortality in miners and millers of Crocidolite in Western Australia. Br J Ind Med 1988;45:5–13.
97. McDonald JC, McDonald AD, Armstrong B, Sébastien P. Cohort study of mortality of vermiculite miners exposed to tremolite. Br J Ind Med 1986;43:436–444.
98. Meurman LO; Kiviluoto R, Hakama M. Mortality and morbidity among the working population of Anthophyllite asbestos miners in Finland. Br J Ind Med 1974;31:105–112.
99. Brown DP, Dement JM, Wagoner JK. Mortality patterns among miners and millers occupationally exposed to asbestiform talc. In: Lemen R, Dement JM, eds. Dust and diseases. Park Forest South, IL: Pathotox, 1979:317–324.
100. Kleinfeld M, Messite J, Zaki MH. Mortality experiences among talc workers: a follow up study. J Occup Med 1974;16:345–349.
101. McDonald AD, McDonald JC. Mesothelioma after Crocidolite exposure during gas mask manufacture. Environ Res 1978;17:340–346.
102. Seidman H, Selikoff IJ, Gelb SK. Mortality experience of Amosite asbestos factory workers: dose-response relationships 5 to 40 years after onset of short-term work exposure. Am J Ind Med 1986;10:479–514.
103. Acheson ED, Gardner MJ, Winter PD, Bennett C. Cancer in a factory using Amosite asbestos. Int J Epidemiol 1984;13:3–10.
104. Hilt B, Langard S, Andersen A, Rosenberg J. Asbestos exposure, smoking habits and cancer incidence among production and maintenance workers in a electrochemical plant. Am J Ind Med 1985;8:565–577.
105. Finkelstein MM. Analysis of mortality patterns and workers' compensation awards among asbestos insulation workers in Ontario. Am J Ind Med 1989;16:523–528.
106. McDonald AD, Fry JS, Woolley AJ, McDonald JC. Dust exposure and mortality in an American Chrysotile textile plant. Br J Ind Med 1983;40:361–367.
107. Thomas HF, Benjamin IT, Elwood PC, Sweetnam PM. Further follow up study of workers from an asbestos cement factory. Br J Ind Med 1982;39:273–276.
108. Newhouse ML, Berry G, Wagner JC. Mortality of factory workers in East London 1933–1880. Br J Ind Med 1985;42:4–11.
109. Finkelstein malignant mesothelioma. Mortality among employees of an Ontario asbestos-cement factory. Am Rev Respir Dis 1984;129:754–761.
110. Albin M, Jacobsson J, Attewell R, et al. Mortality and cancer morbidity in cohorts of asbestos cement workers and referents. Br J Ind Med 1990;47:602–610.
111. Raffin E, Lynge E, Juel K, Koorsgard B. Incidence of cancer and mortality among employees in the asbestos cement industry in Denmark. Br J Ind Med 1989;46:90–96.
112. Enterline PE, Hartley J, Henderson V. Asbestos and cancer: a cohort followed up to death. Br J Ind Med 1987;44:396–401.
113. McDonald AD, Fry JS, Woolley AJ, McDonald JC. Dust exposure and mortality in an American factory using Chrysotile, Amosite and Crocidolite in mainly textile manufacture. Br J Ind Med 1983;40:368–378.
114. Magnani C, Terracini B, Bertolone GP, et al. Mortalita per tumori e altre malattie del sistema respiratorio tra i lavoratori del cemento-amianto a Cassale Monferrato. Uno studio di coorte storico. Med Lav 1987;78:441–453.
115. Selikoff IJ, Hammond EC, Seidman H. Mortality experience of insulation workers in the United States and Canada 1943–1976. Ann N Y Acad Sci 1979;330:91–116.
116. Elmes PC, Simpson MJC. Insulation workers in Belfast. A further study of mortality due to asbestos exposure (1940–75). Br J Ind Med 1977;34:174–180.
117. Kleinfeld M, Messite J, Kooyman O. Mortality experience in a group of asbestos workers. Arch Environ Health 1967;15:177–180.
118. Kolonel LN, Yosnizawa CN, Hirohata T, Myers BE. Cancer occurrence in shipyard workers exposed to asbestos in Hawaii. Cancer Res 1985;45:3924–3928.
119. Rossiter CE, Coles RM, Dockyard HM. Devonport: 1947 mortality study. In: Wagner JC, ed. Biological effects of mineral fibers. Lyon: International Agency for Research on Cancer, 1980;2:713–721.
120. Gardner MJ, Saracci R. Effects on health of non occupational exposure to airborne mineral fibers. In: Bignon J, Peto J, Saracci R, eds. Non-occupational exposure to mineral fibers. Lyon: International Agency for Research on Cancer, Scientific Publication No. 90, 1989:375–397.
121. Doll R. Overview and conclusions. Symposium on MMMF, Copenhagen, October 1986. Ann Occup Hyg 1987;31:805–819.
122. Simonato L, Fletcher AC, Cherrie JW et al. The International Agency for Research on Cancer historical cohort study of MMMF production workers in seven European countries: extension of the follow-up. Ann Occup Hyg 1987;31:603–623.
123. Lion J, Hatton F, Maguin P, Manjol L, Pavillon G. Statistiques des causes de décès. Paris: Editions INSERM, 1989.
124. McDonald JC, Liddell FDK, Dufresne A, McDonald AD. The 1891–1920 birth cohort of Quebec Chrysotile miners and millers: mortality 1976–88. Br J Ind Med 1993;50:1073–1081.
125. Sebastien P, McDonald JC, McDonald AD, Case B, Harley R.

Respiratory cancer in Chrysotile textile and mining industries/exposure inferences from lung analysis. Br J Ind Med 1989;46:180–187.
126. Gaudichet A, Janson X, Monchaux G, et al. Assessment by analytical microscopy of the total lung fibre burden in mesothelioma patients matched with four other pathological series. Ann Occup Hyg 1988;32(Suppl 1):213–223.
127. Rogers AJ, Leigh J, Berry G, Ferguson DA, Mulder HB, Ackad M. Relationship between lung asbestos fiber type and concentration and relative risk of mesothelioma. A case-control study. Cancer 1991;67:1912–1920.
128. Constantopoulos SH, Goudevenos JA, Saratzis N, et al. Metsovo lung: pleural calcification and restrictive lung function in northwestern Greece. Environmental exposure to mineral fiber as etiology. Environ Res 1985;38:319–331.
129. McConnochie K, Simonato L, Mavrides P, Pooley FD, Wagner JC. Mesothelioma in Cyprus: the role of tremolite. Thorax 1987;42:342–347.
130. Rey F, Viallat JR, Boutin C, et al. Les mésothéliomes environnementaux en Corse du Nord-est. Rev Mal Respir 1993;10:339–345.
131. Goldberg M, Goldberg P, Leclerc A, et al. A 10 year incidence survey of respiratory cancer and a case-control study within a cohort of nickel mining and refining workers in New Caledonia. Cancer Causes Control 1994;5:15–25.
132. Voisin C, Marin I, Brochard P, Pairon JC. Environmental airborne tremolite asbestos pollution and pleural plaques in Afghanistan. Chest 1994;106:974–976.
133. Amandus HE, Wheeler R, Amstrong BG, McDonald AD, McDonald JC, Sébastien P. The morbidity and mortality of vermiculite miners and millers exposed to tremolite-actinolite. Am J Ind Med 1987;11:15–26.
134. Churg A, Wright JL. Fiber content of lung in amphibole and Chrysotile induced mesothelioma: implications for environmental exposure. In: Bignon J, Peto J, Saracci R, eds. Non-occupational exposure to mineral fibers Lyon: International Agency for Research on Cancer, Scientific Publication No 90, 1989:314–318.
135. Baris Y I, Saracci R, Simonato L, Skidmore JW, Artvingli M. Malignant mesothelioma and radiological chest abnormalities in two villages in central Turkey. Lancet 1981;2:984–987.
136. Wagner JC, Skidmore JW, Hill RJ, Griffiths DM. Erionite exposure and mesothelioma in rats. Br J Cancer 1985;51:727–730.
137. Thermal Insulation Manufacturing Association. Man-made vitreous fibers: nomenclature, chemical and physical properties. Stanford, CA: Thermal Insulation Manufacturing Association, 1991.
138. Saracci R, Simonato L, Acheson ED, et al. Mortality and incidence of cancer of workers in the man made vitreous fibres producing industry: an international investigation at 13 European plants. Br J Ind Med 1984;41:425–436.
139. Enterline PE, Marsh GM, Callahan C. Mortality update of a cohort of US man-made mineral fibre workers. Ann Occup Hyg 1987;31:625–656.
140. Bunn WB, Bender JR, Hesterberg TW, Chase GR, Konzen JL. Recent studies of man-made vitreous fibers. Chronic animal inhalation studies. J Occup Med 1993;35:101–113.
141. Hesterberg TW, McConnell EE, Chevalier J, Hadley J, Thevenaz P, Anderson E. Chronic inhalation toxicity of size separated glass fibers in Fischer 344 rats. Fundam Appl Toxicol 1993;20:464–476.
142. Balmes JR, Daporte A, Cone JE. Asbestos related disease in custodial and building maintenance workers from a large municipal school district. In: Landrigan PJ, Kazemi H, eds. The third wave of asbestos disease: exposure to asbestos in place. Ann N Y Acad Sci 1991:540–549.
143. Oliver LC, Sprince NL, Gree RE. Asbestos related radiographic abnormalities in public school custodians. Toxicol Ind Health 1990;6:629–636.
144. Cordier S, Lazar P, Brochard P, Bignon J, Ameille J, Proteau J. Epidemiologic investigation of respiratory effects related to environmental exposure to asbestos inside insulated buildings. Arch Environ Health 1987;42:303–309.
145. Sterling TD, Collett CW, Rosenbaum WL, Weinkam JJ. Comments on the Health Effects Institute–Asbestos Research (HEI-AR) report: "asbestos in public and commercial buildings," with emphasis on risk assessment methods used. Am J Ind Med 1993;24:767–787.
146. Hirsch A, Brochard P, De Cremoux H, et al. Features of asbestos-exposed and unexposed mesothelioma. Am J Ind Med 1982;3:413–422.
147. Peterson JT, Greenberg SD, Bufler PA. Non asbestos related malignant mesothelioma. Cancer 1984;54:951–960.
148. Ilgren EB. Mesotheliomas of animals. A comprehensive, tabular compendium of the world's literature. London: CRC Press 1993;1:1–356.
149. Paterour MJ, Bignon J, Jaurand MC. In vitro transformation of rat pleural mesothelial cells by Chrysotile fibres and/or benzo(a)pyrene. Carcinogenesis 1985;6:523–529.
150. Buard A, Beaune PH, Renier A, Jaurand MC, Bignon J, Laurent P. Expression of cytochrome P 450 in rat pleural mesothelial cells in secondary cultures. J Cell Physiol 1994;160:176–184.
151. Carbone M. Simian virus 40-like DNA sequences in human pleural mesothelioma. Oncogene 1994;9:1781–1790.
152. Cicala C, Pompetti F, Carbone M. SV40 induces mesotheliomas in hamsters. Am J Pathol 1993;142:1524–1533.
153. Donaldson K, Brown RC, Brown GM. Respirable industrial fibres: mechanisms of pathogenicity. Thorax 1993;48:390–395.
154. Davis JMG, Addison J, McIntosh C, Miller BG, Niven K. Variations in the carcinogenicity of tremolite dust samples of differing morphology. Ann N Y Acad Sci 1991;643:473–489.
155. Endo-Capron S, Renier A, Janson X, Kheuang L, Jaurand MC. In vitro response of rat pleural mesothelial cells to talc samples in genotoxicity assays (sister chromatid exchanges and DNA repair). Toxicology in Vitro 1993;7:7–14.
156. Yegles M. Cytotoxicité et ségrégations anormales de chromosomes produites sur des cultures de cellules mésothéliales pleurales de rat par des fibres minérales. Importance des caractéristiques dimensionnelles des fibres. Paris: University of Paris, Ph.D. Thesis VII 18/07/1994.
157. Stanton MF, Layard M, Tegeris A, Miller E, May M, Kent E. Carcinogenicity of fibrous glass: pleural response in the rat in relation to fiber dimension. J. Natl Cancer Inst 1977;58:587–603.
158. Stanton MF, Layard M, Tegeris A, et al. Relation of particle dimension to carcinogenicity in amphibole asbestos and other fibrous minerals. J. Natl Cancer Inst 1981;67:165–175.
159. Pott F, Friedrichs KH. Tumours in rats after intraperitoneal injection of asbestos dusts. Naturwissenschaften 1972;59:318.
160. Wagner JC, Berry G, Timbrell V. Mesotheliomas in rats after inoculation with asbestos and other materials. Br J Cancer 1973;28:173–185.
161. Monchaux G, Bignon J, Jaurand MC, et al. Mesothelioma in rats following inoculation with acid-leached asbestos and other mineral fibers. Carcinogenesis 1981;3:229–236.
162. Davis JMG, Addison J, Bolton RE, Donaldson K, Jones AD,

Smith T. The pathogenicity of long versus short fiber samples of amosite administered to rats by inhalation and intraperitoneal injection. Br J Exp Pathol 1986;67:415–430.
163. Jaurand MC, Fleury J, Monchaux G, Nebut M, Bignon J. Pleural carcinogenic potency of mineral fibres (asbestos, attapulgite) and their cytotoxicity on cultured cells. J Natl Cancer Inst 1987;79:797–804.
164. Davis JMG. Information obtained from fiber-induced lesions in animals. In: Liddell D, Miller K, eds. Mineral fibers and health. London: CRC Press, 1991:249–263.
165. Wagner JC. Significance of the fiber size of erionite (abstract). Proceedings of the VIIth International Pneumoconioses Conference, NIOSH-ILO, Pittsburgh, PA, August 23–26, 1988, 1:158.
166. Jaurand MC, Gaudichet A, Halpern S, Bignon J. In vitro biodegradation of Chrysotile fibres by alveolar macrophages and mesothelial cells in culture: comparison with a pH effect. Br J Ind Med 1984;41:389–395.
167. Bignon J, Saracci R, Touray JC. Introduction: INSERM-IARC-CNRS Workshop on Biopersistence of Respirable Synthetic Fibers and Minerals. Environ Health Perspect 1994;102(Suppl 5):3–5.
168. McClellan RO, Hesterberg JW. Role of biopersistence in the pathogenicity of man-made fibers and methods for evaluating biopersistence: a summary of two roundtable discussions. Environ Health Perspect 1994;102(Suppl 5):277–283.
169. Wagner JC, Berry G, Skidmore W, Timbrell V. The effects of the inhalation of asbestos in rats. Br J Cancer 1974;29:252–269
170. Sébastien P, Begin R, Case BW, McDonald JC. Inhalation of Chrysotile dust. Accomplishments in oncology. In: Wagner JC, ed. The biological effects of Chrysotile. 1986;1:19.
171. Churg A. Deposition and clearance of Chrysotile asbestos. Ann Occup Hyg 1994;38:625–633.
172. Morgan A, Holmes A, Davison W. Clearance of sized glass fibers from the rat lung and their solubility in vivo. Ann Occup Hyg 1982;25:317–331.
173. Adamson IYR, Babowska J, Bowden DH. Mesothelial cell proliferation after instillation of long or short asbestos fibers into mouse lung. Am J Pathol 1993;142:1209–1216.
174. De Meringo A, Morscheidt C, Thelohan S, Tiesler H. In vitro dynamic solubility test: influence of various parameters. In: Bignon J, Touray JC, Saracci R, eds. Biopersistence of respirable synthetic fibers and minerals. Environ Health Perspect 1994;102(Suppl 5):47–53.
175. Weitzman SA, Graceffa P. Asbestos catalyses hydroxyl and superoxide radical generation from hydrogen peroxide. Arch Biochem Biophys 1984;228:337–376.
176. Eberhardt MK, Roman-Franco AA, Quiles MR. Asbestos induced decomposition of hydrogen peroxide. Environ Res 1985;37:287–292.
177. Zalma R, Bonneau L, Guignard J, Pézérat H. Formations of oxy-radicals by oxygen reduction arising from the surface activity of asbestos. Can J Chem 1987;65:2338–2341.
178. Adachi S, Yoshida S, Kawamura K, et al. Inductions of oxidative DNA damage and mesothelioma by Crocidolite, with special reference to the presence of iron inside and outside of asbestos fiber. Carcinogenesis 1994;15:753–758.
179. Bignon J, Brochard P. Inconsistencies and limitations. In: Liddell D, Miller K, eds. Mineral fibers and health. London: CRC Press, 1991;197–210.
180. Webster I, Goldstein B, Coetzee FSJ, Van Sittert GCH. Malignant mesothelioma induced in baboons by inhalation of amosite asbestos. Am J Ind Med 1993;24:659–666.
181. Peto J, Seidman H, Selikoff IJ. Mesothelioma mortality in asbestos workers: implications for models of carcinogenesis and risk assessment. Br J Cancer 1982;45:124–135.
182. Peto J. Fiber carcinogenesis and environmental hazards. In: Bignon J, Peto J, Saracci R, eds. Non-occupational exposure to mineral fibers. Lyon: International Agency for Research on Cancer, Scientific Publication No. 90, 1989;457–470.
183. Selikoff IJ, Hammond EC, Churg J. Asbestos exposure, smoking and neoplasia. JAMA 1968;204:106–112.
184. Saracci R. Asbestos and lung cancer: an analysis of the epidemiological evidence on the asbestos-smoking interaction. Int J Cancer 1977;20:323–331.
185. Mossman BT, Gee JBL. Pulmonary reactions and mechanisms of toxicity of inhaled fibers. In: Gardner DE, Crapo JD, Massaro EJ, eds. Toxicology of the lung. 2nd ed. New York: Raven Press, 1993:371–387.
186. Heintz NH, Janssen YM, Mossman BT. Persistent induction of c-fos and c-jun expression by asbestos. Proc Natl Acad Sci U S A 1993;90:3299–3303.
187. Jaurand MC. Particulate-state carcinogenesis: a survey of recent studies on the mechanisms of action of fibers. In: Bignon J, Peto J, Saracci R, eds. Non-occupational exposure to mineral fibers. Lyon: International Agency for Research on Cancer, Scientific Publication No. 90, 1989:54–73.
188. Jaurand MC, Saint Etienne L, Van Der Meeren A, Endo-Capron S, Renier A, Bignon J. Neoplastic transformation of rodents cells. In: Harris CC, Lechner JF, Brinkley BR, eds. Cellular and molecular aspects of fiber carcinogenesis: current communications in molecular biology. Cold Spring Harbor, NY: Cold Spring Harbor Laboratory Press, 1991;131:122–147.
189. Jaurand MC. Mechanisms of fiber genotoxicity. In: Brown RC, Hoskins JA, Johnson NF, eds. Mechanisms in fiber carcinogenesis. New York: Plenum Press, 1992:287–306.
190. Hobson J, Gilks B, Wright J Churg A. Direct enhancement by cigarette smoke of asbestos fiber penetration and asbestos-induced epithelial proliferation in rat tracheal explants. J Natl Cancer Inst 1988;80:518–521.
191. Wang NS. The preformed stomas connecting the pleural cavity and the lymphatics in the parietal pleura. Am Rev Respir Dis 1975;111:12–20.
192. Gibas Z, Li FP, Antman KH, et al. Chromosome changes in malignant mesothelioma. Cancer Genet Cytogenet 1986;20:191–201.
193. Stenman G, Olofsson K, Mansson T, et al. Chromosomes and chromosomal evolution in human mesotheliomas as reflected in sequential analyses of two cases. Hereditas 1986;105:233–239.
194. Popescu NC, Chahinian AP, DiPaolo JA. Nonrandom chromosome alterations in human malignant mesothelioma. Cancer Res 1988;48:142–147.
195. Tiainen M, Tammilehto L, Rautonen J, et al. Chromosomal abnormalities and their correlation with asbestos exposure and survival in patients with mesothelioma. Br J Cancer 1989;60:618–626.
196. Hagemeijer A, Versnel MA, Van Drunen E, et al. Cytogenetic analysis of malignant mesothelioma. Cancer Genet Cytogenet 1990;47:1–28.
197. Jaurand MC, Barrett JC. Neoplastic transformation of mesothelial cells. In: Jaurand MC, Bignon J, eds. The mesothelial cell and mesothelioma. Lung biology in health and disease series. New York: Marcel Dekker, 1994:207–222.
198. Olofsson K, Mark J. Specificity of asbestos-induced chromosomal aberrations in short-term cultured human mesothelial cells. Cancer Genet Cytogenet 1989;41:33–39.

199. Lechner JF, Tokiwa T, Laveck MA, et al. Asbestos-associated chromosomal changes in human mesothelial cells. Proc Natl Acad Sci U S A 1985;82:3884–3888.
200. Hei TK, Piao CP, He ZY, Vannais D, Waldren CK. Chrysotile fiber is a strong mutagen in mammalian cells. Cancer Res 1992;52:6305–6309.
201. Jaurand MC, Kheuang L, Magne L, Bignon J. Chromosomal changes induced by chrysotile fibres and benzo-3,4-pyrene in rat pleural mesothelial cells. Mutat Res 1986;169:141–148.
202. Renier A, Levy F, Pillière F, Jaurand MC. Unscheduled DNA synthesis in rat pleural mesothelial cells treated with mineral fibres. Mutat Res 1990;241:361–367.
203. Libbus BL, Illeneye SA, Craighead JE. Induction of DNA strand breaks in cultured rat embryo cells by Crocidolite asbestos as assessed by nick translation. Cancer Res 1989;49:5713–5718.
204. Hesterberg TW, Barrett JC. Induction by asbestos fibers of anaphase abnormalities: mechanism for aneuploidy induction and possibly carcinogenesis. Carcinogenesis 1985;6:473–475.
205. Wang NS, Jaurand MC, Magne L, et al. The interactions between asbestos fibers and metaphase chromosomes of rat pleural mesothelial cells in culture. Am J Pathol 1987;126:343–349.
206. Barrett JC. Mechanisms of multistep carcinogenesis and carcinogen risk assessment. Environ Health Perspect 1993;100:9–20.
207. Jaurand MC, Bastier Sigeac I, Bignon J, Stoebner P. Effect of chrysotile and Crocidolite on the morphology and growth of rat pleural mesothelial cells. Environ Res 1983;30:255–269.
208. Achard S, Perdriset M, Jaurand MC. Sister chromatid exchanges in rat pleural mesothelial cells treated with Crocidolite, attapulgite or benzo-3,4-pyrene. Br J Ind Med 1987;44:281–283.
209. Yegles M, Saint-Etienne L, Renier A, Janson X, Jaurand MC. Induction of metaphase and anaphase/telophase abnormalities by asbestos fibers in rat pleural mesothelial cells in vitro. Am J Respir Cell Mol Biol 1993;9:186–191.
210. Goodlick LA, Kane AB. Cytotoxicity of long and short Crocidolite asbestos fibers in vitro and in vivo. Cancer Res 1986;46:5153–5163.
211. Turver CJ, Brown RC. The role of catalytic iron in asbestos induced lipid peroxidation and DNA-strand breakage in C3H10T1/2 cells. Br J Cancer 1987;56:133–136.
212. Mossman BT, Masch JP. Evidence supporting a role for active oxygen species in asbestos induced toxicity and lung disease. Environ Health Perspect 1989;81:91–94.
213. Kamp DW, Graceffa P, Pryor WA, Weitzman SA. The role of free radicals in asbestos induced diseases. Free Radic Biol Med 1992;12:292–315.
214. Walker C, Everitt J, Barrett JC. Possible cellular and molecular mechanisms for asbestos carcinogenicity. Am J Ind Med 1992;21:253–273.
215. Kamp DW, Dunne M, Weitzman SA, Dunn MM. The interaction of asbestos and neutrophils injures cultured human pulmonary epithelial cells: role of hydrogen peroxide. J Lab Clin Med 1989;114:604–612.
216. Leanderson P, Tagesson C. Hydrogen peroxide release and hydroxyl radical formation in mixtures containing mineral fibres and human neutrophils. Br J Ind Med 1992;49:745–749.
217. Vallyathan V, Mega JF, Shi X, Dalal NS. Enhanced generation of free radicals from phagocytes induced by mineral dusts. Am J Respir Cell Mol Biol 1992;6:404–413.
218. Hansen K, Mossman BT. Generation of superoxide ($O_2^{\bullet-}$) from alveolar macrophages exposed to asbestiform and non fibrous particles. Cancer Res 1987;47:1681–1686.
219. Dong HY, Buard A, Renier A, Saint-Etienne L, Jaurand MC. Role of oxygen derivatives in the cytotoxicity and DNA damage produced by asbestos on rat pleural mesothelial cells in vitro. Carcinogenesis 1994;15:1251–1255.
220. Chao CC, Aust AE. Effect of long-term removal of iron from asbestos by desferrioxamine B on subsequent mobilization by other chelators and induction of DNA single-strand breaks. Arch Biochem Biophys 1994;308:64–66.
221. Gabrielson EW, Rosen GM, Drafstrom RC, Strauss E, Harris CC. Studies on the role of oxygen radicals in asbestos-induced cytopathology of cultured human lung mesothelial cells. Carcinogenesis 1986;7:1161–1164.
222. Kinnula VL, Allto K, Raivio KO, Walles S, Linnainmaa K. Cytotoxicity of oxidants and asbestos fibers in cultured human mesothelial cells. Free Radic Biol Med 1994;16:169–176.
223. Garcia JGN, Dodson RF, Callahan KS. Effect of environmental particulates on cultured human and bovine endothelium, cellular injury via an oxidant dependent pathway. Lab Invest 1989;61:53–61.
224. Shatos MA, Doherty JM, Marsh JP, et al. Prevention of asbestos induced cell death in rat lung fibroblasts and alveolar macrophages by scavengers of active oxygen species. Environ Res 1987;44:103–116.
225. Ghio AKJ, Zhang J, Piantadosi CA. Generation of hydroxyl radical by Crocidolite asbestos is proportional to surface [Fe^{3+}]. Arch Biochem Biophys 1992;298:646–650.
226. Fubini B. The possible role of surface chemistry in the toxicity of inhaled fibers. In: Warheit D, ed. Fiber toxicology. San Diego: Academic Press, 1993:223–257.
227. Lund LG, Aust AE. Iron mobilization from Crocidolite asbestos greatly enhances Crocidolite-dependent formation of DNA single-strand breaks in phiX174 RFI DNA. Carcinogenesis 1992;13:637–642.
228. Gulumian M, Bhoolia DJ, Dutoit RSJ, et al. Activation of UICC Crocidolite. The effect of conversion of some ferric ions to ferrous ions. Environ Res 1993;60:193–206.
229. Emerit I, Jaurand MC, Saint Etienne L, Levy A. Formation of a clastogenic factor by asbestos treated rat pleural mesothelial cells. Agents Actions 1991;34:410–415.
230. Emerit I. Reactive oxygen species, chromosome mutation, and cancer: possible role of clastogenic factors in carcinogenesis. Free Radic Biol Med 1994;16:99–109.
231. Robinson BWS. Immunobiology and immunotherapy of malignant mesothelioma. In: Jaurand MC, Bignon J, eds. The mesothelial cell and mesothelioma. Lung biology in health and disease series. New York: Marcel Dekker, 1994:253–268.
232. Rom W, Travis WD, Brody AR. Cellular and molecular basis of the asbestos-related diseases. Am Rev Respir Dis 1991;143:408–422.
233. Tsang PH, Chu FN, Fischbein A, Bekesi JG. Impairments in functional subsets of T-suppressor (CD8). Lymphocytes, monocytes and natural killer cells among asbestos-exposed workers. Clin Immunol Immunopathol 1988;47:323–332.
234. Wallace JM, Oishi JS, Barbers RG, Batra P, Aberle DR. Bronchoalveolar lavage cell and lymphocyte phenotype profiles in healthy asbestos exposed shipyard workers. Am Rev Respir Dis 1989;139:33–38.
235. Sprince NL, Oliver LC, McLoud TC, Eisen EA, Christiani DC, Ginns LC. Asbestos exposure and asbestos related pleural and parenchymal disease: associations with immune imbalance. Am Rev Respir Dis 1991;143:822–828.
236. Ginns LC, Ryu JH, Rogol PR, Prine NL, Oliver LC, Larsson CJ. Natural killer cell activity in cigarette smokers and asbestos workers. Am Rev Respir Dis 1985;131:831–834.

237. Lew F, Tsang P, Holland JF, Warner N, Selikoff IJ, Bekesi JG. High frequency of immune dysfunction in asbestos workers and in patients with malignant mesothelioma. J Clin Immunol 1986;6:225–233.
238. Al Jarad N, Macey M, Uthayakumar S, Newland AC, Rudd RM. Lymphocyte subsets in subjects exposed to asbestos: changes in circulating natural killer cells. Br J Ind Med 1992;49:811–814.
239. Manning L, Bowman RV, Darby SB, Robinson BWS. Lysis of human malignant mesothelioma cells by natural killer (NK) and lymphokine activated killer (LAK) cells. Am Rev Respir Dis 1989;139:1369–1374.
240. Robinson BWS. Asbestos and cancer: human natural killer cell activity is suppressed by asbestos fibres but can be restored by recombinant interleukin-2. Am Rev Respir Dis 1989;139:897–901.
241. Wagner MM, Darke C, Coles RM, Evans CC. HLA-A and B antigen frequencies and mesothelioma in relation to asbestos exposure. Br J Cancer 1983;48:727–730.
242. Martenson G, Hagmar B, Zettergren L. Diagnosis and prognosis in malignant pleural mesothelioma: a prospective study. Eur J Respir Dis 1984;65:169–178.
243. Lynch HT, Anton-Culver H, Kurosaki T. Is there a genetic predisposition to malignant mesothelioma. In: Jaurand MC, Bignon J, eds. The mesothelial cell and mesothelioma. Lung biology in health and disease series. New York: Marcel Dekker, 1994:47–69.
244. Risberg B, Nickels J, Wagermark J. Familial clustering of malignant mesothelioma. Cancer 1980;45:2422–2427.
245. Hammar SP, Bockus D, Remington F, Freidman S, Lazerte G. Familial mesothelioma: a report of two families. Hum Pathol 1989;20:107–112.
246. Lillington GA, Jamplis RW, Differding JR. Conjugal malignant mesothelioma. N Engl J Med 1974;291:583–584.
247. Anderson H, Lilis R, Daum SM, Fischbein A, Selikoff IJ. Household contact asbestos neoplastic risk. Ann N Y Acad Sci 1976;271:311–323.

35

Pathology of Mesothelioma

Joseph M. Corson and Andrew A. Renshaw

PATHOLOGY OF MESOTHELIOMA

INTRODUCTION

Diffuse malignant mesothelioma (or simply, mesothelioma) has increased in frequency in the last several decades, resulting in pathologists having greater familiarity with its gross and histologic features. Nonetheless, diagnostic pitfalls remain. Accurate diagnosis usually requires careful coordination of clinical, radiologic, and operative findings with skilled histologic evaluation, as well as the application of ancillary techniques. These include histochemical, immunohistochemical, and/or electron microscopic examination. In addition, other modalities, such as flow cytometry, image analysis, and cytogenetics, although largely still investigational, show promise of diagnostic utility. This chapter describes the morphologic features of pleural mesothelioma and evaluates ancillary techniques that may be helpful in the pathologic appraisal and differential diagnosis of mesothelioma. The much less common primary tumor of the pleura, designated a solitary fibrous tumor of the pleura but sometimes referred to as localized fibrous mesothelioma, is considered under Differential Diagnosis, below.

MORPHOLOGY

The gross and microscopic features of mesothelioma are considered in this section.

GROSS PATHOLOGY

Mesothelioma of the pleura is characterized by local growth and invasion of contiguous structures and by relatively late spread to distant organs. Recent studies provide evidence that pleural mesothelioma begins in the parietal layer and subsequently spreads to involve the visceral pleura (1, 2). Pleural effusion usually is present and may contain desquamated malignant cells detectable by cytologic examination. Early lesions may mimic nonspecific pleuritis, forming fine granulations 1 to 2 mm in diameter (1) with minimal thickening of the serosa, or tiny gray plaques or seedlings may coat the pleura (Fig. 35.1) (3, 4). Proliferation of mesothelioma cells and accompanying stromal elements form firm, gray nodules that subsequently coalesce. The pleura gradually thickens, especially over the basal two thirds of the lung and the diaphragmatic aspect, and its layers fuse into a rind that envelops and constricts the lung. Pockets of hemorrhagic, viscid effusion may persist between the thickened pleural layers. Tumor extends into major fissures, but penetration of lung parenchyma usually is delayed until late in the course (Fig. 35.2). However, at that time the tumor may form one or more large parenchymal masses, suggestive of primary or metastatic carcinoma (Fig. 35.3).

Invasion of fibrofatty tissues of the pleura may be followed by invasion of muscle of the chest wall, diaphragm, and pericardium, and envelopment of vessels, airways, and esophagus within the mediastinum. In addition, extension along needle-biopsy tracts into the skin may occur. Contiguous or lymphatic spread may lead to involvement of the contralateral pleura and lung and to extension through the diaphragm into the peritoneal cavity. The parietal peritoneum and serosa of abdominal organs may be invaded, or peritoneal involvement may be so extensive that it leads one to question the primary site (5).

Exceptional instances of malignant mesothelioma of the pleura presenting as a solitary, localized mass have been described recently (6), and a single case of an apparently reactive, cystic mesothelial proliferation has been observed in the pleura (7). The pathologic features in the latter were identical to previously reported multicystic "mesotheliomas" of the peritoneum.

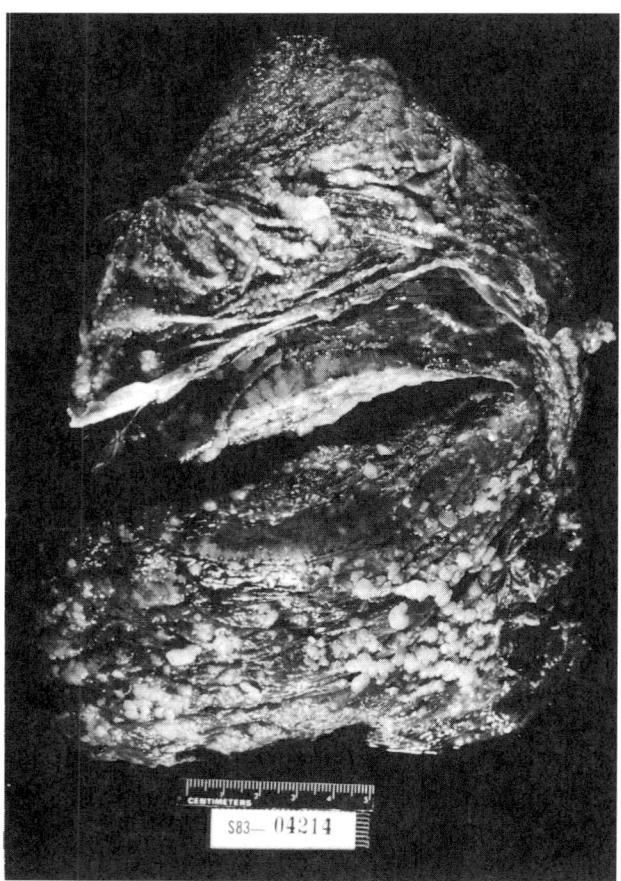

FIGURE 35.1. Lung and pleura with mesothelioma. The pleura is studded with innumerable small plaques and nodules. The parietal pleura (overlying the upper lobe in the upper portion of the photograph) has been removed from the lower portion of the lung to reveal the involvement of the visceral pleura. Fusion of the pleural layers and of the major fissure has not yet occurred.

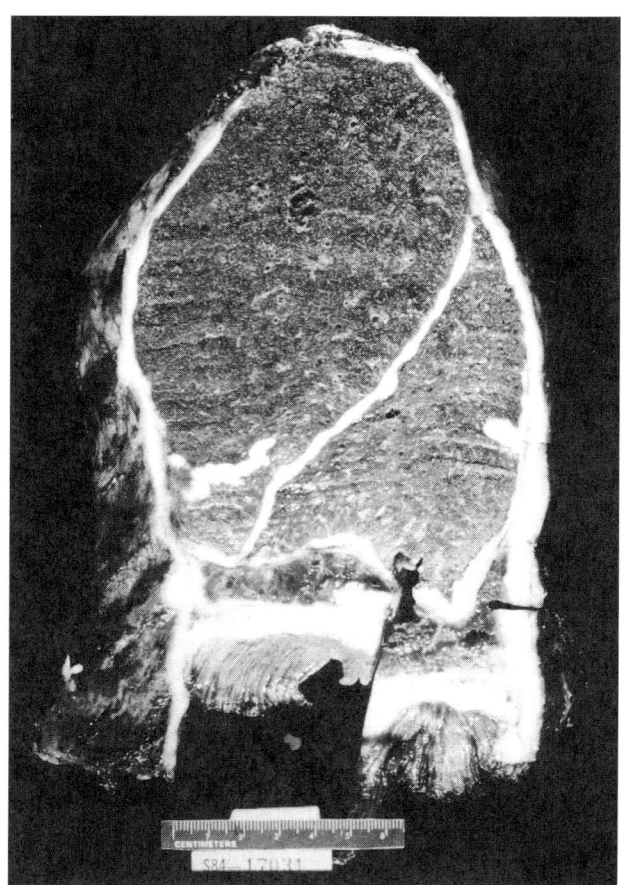

FIGURE 35.2. Sectioned surface of lung with pleura and hemidiaphragm. Mesothelioma thickens the pleura and encases the lung. The tumor has grown into the major fissure and focally into several minor fissures, but it has not invaded the parenchyma. The visceral diaphragmatic pleura is separated from the greatly thickened parietal layer by an organizing, hemorrhagic effusion.

Metastases to thoracomediastinal lymph nodes may occasionally be the initial manifestation of mesothelioma (8) in patients selected for multimodality therapy. Their presence in regional lymph nodes portends a worse prognosis than those without lymph node involvement (9). In late stages of mesothelioma, spread to regional lymph nodes is common. This spread is present in about half of mesotheliomas at autopsy (10, 11). Hematogenous metastases may be seen in one third to one half of cases, but they usually only occur late in the disease (10, 11). The most common sites are contralateral lung, liver, kidney, adrenal, and bone. Involvement of the brain is seen only rarely (12). Infrequently, early metastases, such as those to the lungs (13) or bone (14), lead to unexpected clinical findings.

MICROSCOPIC PATHOLOGY

Microscopically, mesotheliomas exhibit diverse architectural patterns, although an individual case often maintains surprising cytologic uniformity. Mesotheliomas traditionally have been classified as epithelial, sarcomatoid, and mixed, or as biphasic types containing both epithelial and sarcomatoid elements. In one series of 819 cases, the proportions of each type were 50%, 34%, and 16%, respectively (15). Most series report significantly longer survival for the epithelial type than for the sarcomatoid type, with the mixed type having survival intermediate between the two (2, 9, 11, 15, 16). Several modifications to the above classification have been introduced in recent years (3, 5, 17). Recognizing the difficulty in distinguishing between poorly differentiated epithelial and sarcomatoid types, a transitional (undifferentiated) type has been introduced (3, 17) (Table 35.1). Mesotheliomas with extensive fibrosis have been described as desmoplastic (18–20). Desmoplastic mesotheliomas constitute about 5% to 10% of pleural mesotheliomas and are predominantly sarcomatoid, although a small proportion are of mixed or

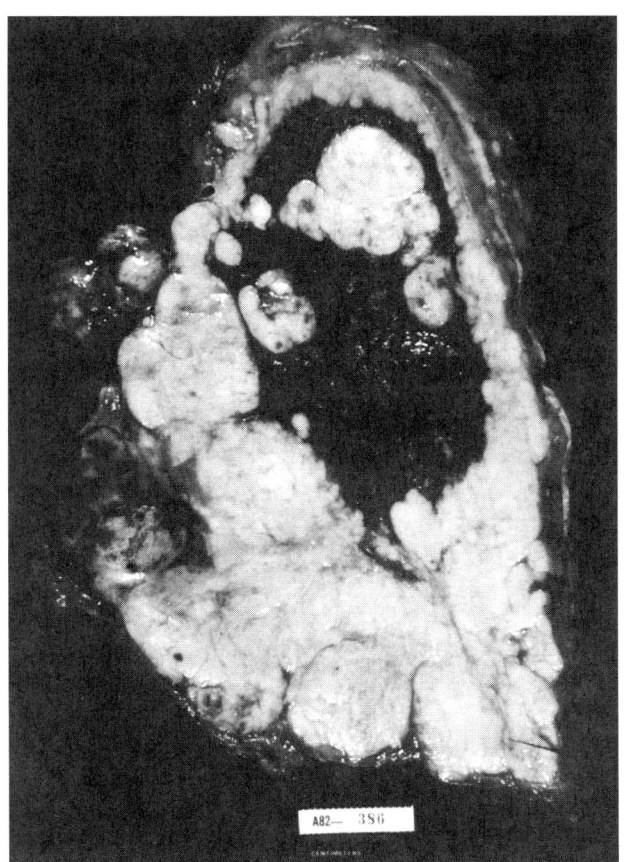

FIGURE 35.3. Mesothelioma late in its course. Sectioned surface of the lung reveals greatly thickened and fused pleura that encases and constricts the parenchyma. Bulky, coalescent tumor nodules invade the lung.

TABLE 35.1. Histologic Types of Mesothelioma

Epithelial
Sarcomatoid
Mixed (biphasic)
Transitional (undifferentiated)

evenly dispersed chromatin and a small nucleolus. Mitoses are uncommon. In the less frequent poorly differentiated forms, nuclear pleomorphism and hyperchromatism, conspicuous nucleoli and frequent mitoses are seen. Necrosis usually is confined to poorly differentiated types and is seldom as conspicuous as that seen in carcinomas. The stroma is quite variable. It usually is comprised of moderately cellular, loose, fibrous tissue; however, it may be so highly cellular that it mimics a sarcoma, or it may be myxoid, densely collagenous, or inflammatory. Inflammatory areas may exhibit exudation of fibrin and neutrophils or an infiltrate of lymphocytes and a few plasma cells. Psammoma bodies may be seen, notably in papillary types, but these are rarely conspicuous.

Various types of epithelial mesotheliomas have been identified based on architectural or cytologic features (3, 17, 21); these features are useful for histologic recognition but have no known prognostic value. They include the common tubulopapillary, epithelioid, and solid types, and the rare microcystic, adenoid cystic, giant cell, small cell (3, 22), signet cell, and clear cell (17) types (Figs. 35.4 through 35.8).

The sarcomatoid type—also termed sarcomatous, spindle cell, or fibroblastic mesothelioma—is comprised of spindle cells arranged in sheets or fascicles or occasionally in a true storiform pattern (Figs. 35.9 and 35.10). The cytoplasm varies from eosinophilic to amphophilic, and cell borders are often poorly defined. Nuclei are spindle shaped, oval, or sometimes round. Nuclear pleomorphism and mitotic activity are common. Stroma varies as in the epithelial type, but hyalinization is more common. Well-differentiated epithelial type. Some investigators classify desmoplastic mesotheliomas as a subtype of sarcomatoid mesothelioma, and others classify them as a separate entity (17). Survival is often short in desmoplastic mesotheliomas; mean survival from onset of symptoms is only 5.8 to 6.18 months in cases of the purely sarcomatoid type (19, 20).

In epithelial mesotheliomas, cells are usually cuboidal, polygonal, or round, but occasionally they are flat or columnar. Well-defined borders circumscribe abundant, eosinophilic cytoplasm. Cells with vacuolated cytoplasm or even clear cytoplasm may be present. In the well-differentiated form, nuclei are placed centrally, and are round and uniform with fine,

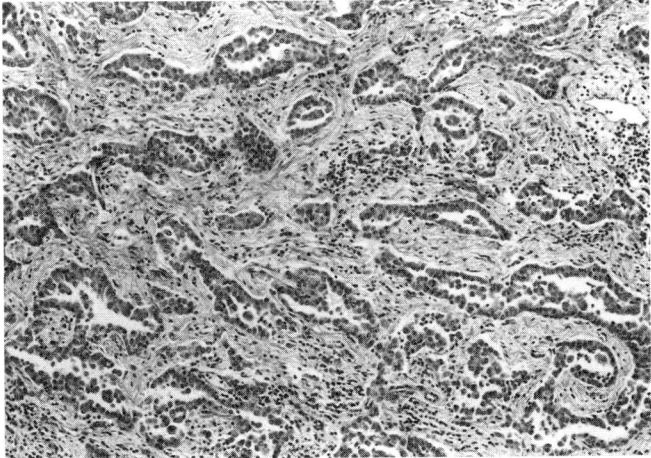

FIGURE 35.4. Epithelial mesothelioma, tubular subtype. The tumor forms irregular tubular profiles within a fibrous stroma that contains a modest lymphocytic infiltrate (hematoxylin and eosin–stained histologic section, as are subsequent figures except those identified otherwise).

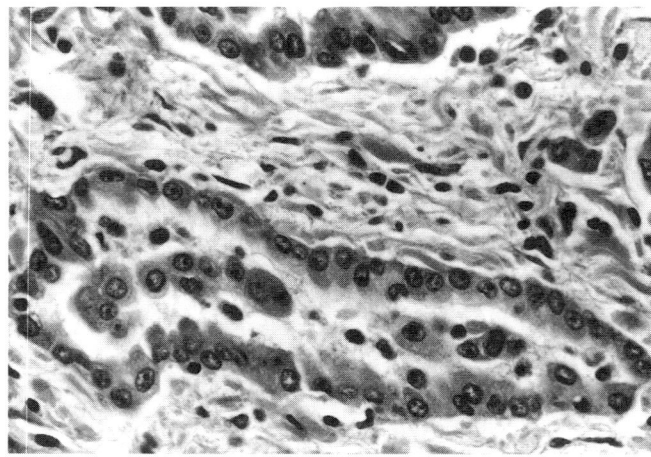

FIGURE 35.5. In this higher magnification of a tubular subtype of epithelial mesothelioma, a single layer of cuboidal cells lines the tubule. Tumor cells have desquamated into the lumen, and a few are seen among the collagen fibers of the stroma. The cytology is characteristic of a mesothelioma. Cells are cuboidal. Nuclei are round to oval and uniform. Many have a solitary, prominent nucleolus. Cytoplasm is relatively abundant.

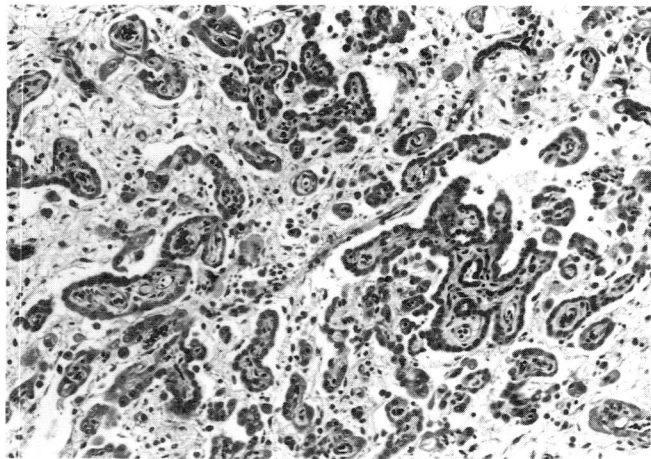

FIGURE 35.6. Papillary growth pattern in an epithelial mesothelioma. Papillae are comprised of an outer layer of uniform cuboidal mesothelial cells and an inner highly vascular connective tissue core.

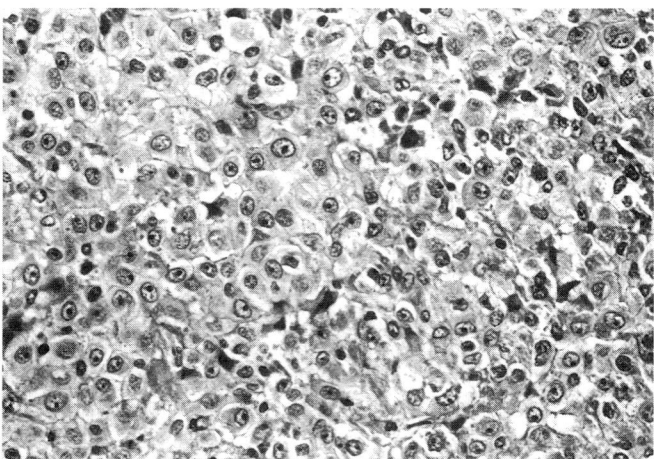

FIGURE 35.7. Solid growth of an epithelial mesothelioma. Tumor cells are "epithelioid." They are polygonal or round with nuclear features similar to those in Figure 35.5. Some carcinomas and melanomas may have a similar appearance.

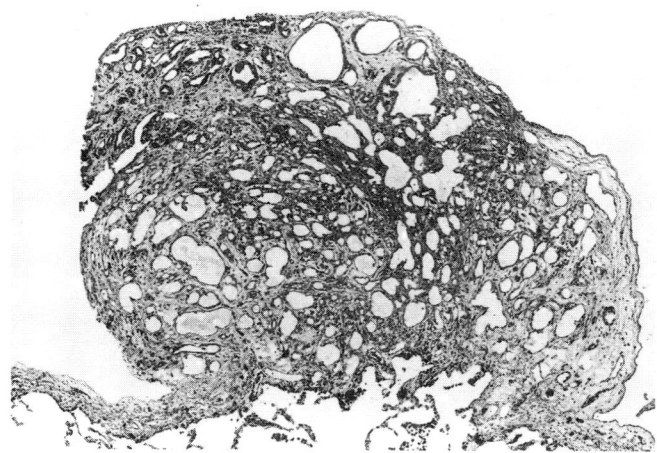

FIGURE 35.8. Cystic subtype of mesothelioma. Spaces are lined by epithelial mesothelioma cells. The tumor, which is sessile and polypoid, was one of many projecting from the visceral pleura into the pleural space.

forms may be difficult to distinguish from fibrosing pleuritis (Fig. 35.11), and poorly differentiated cases require separation from sarcomas involving the pleura or chest wall (see Differential Diagnosis, below). In addition to the desmoplastic variant, a number of rare variants of sarcomatoid mesothelioma have been noted. The intense inflammatory infiltrate of the lymphohistiocytic variant may lead to an erroneous diagnosis of lymphoma (23). Osteoblastic (24), chondroblastic (25), and rhabdomyoblastic (5) types have been described.

The mixed, or biphasic, type of mesothelioma is composed of epithelial and sarcomatoid elements in variable proportions. Both elements definitely should be malignant before classifying the mesothelioma as mixed (3). Identification of the second element may require multiple blocks and a prolonged search. Cells intermediate in appearance between epithelial and sarcomatous types are often seen in the mixed type, both on light microscopic and ultrastructural examination.

CYTOLOGY

Most patients with pleural mesothelioma seek medical attention because of chest pain and/or dysp-

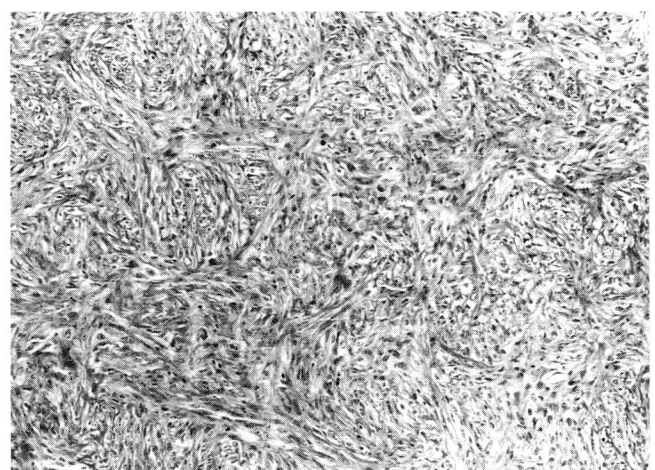

FIGURE 35.9. Sarcomatoid type of mesothelioma. Spindle-shaped tumor cells are grouped into fascicles that appear to radiate from a central core in a so-called storiform pattern.

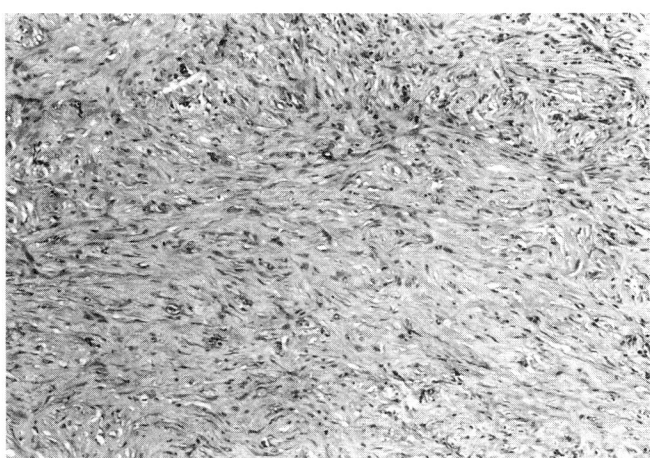

FIGURE 35.11. Cellular fibrous tissue of chronic, fibrosing pleuritis. Although suggestive of sarcomatoid mesothelioma, extensive sectioning and careful scrutiny failed to reveal the hyperchromatism, nuclear pleomorphism, and necrosis usually present in sarcomatoid mesotheliomas.

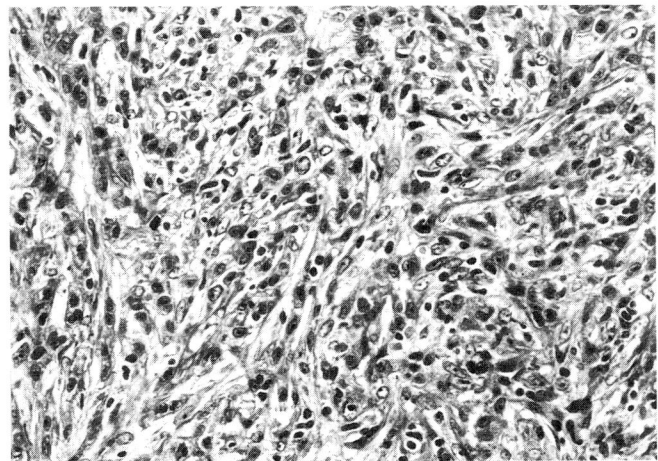

FIGURE 35.10. Higher magnification of a sarcomatoid mesothelioma. Tumor cells dominate the field with their spindled to round, hyperchromatic, pleomorphic nuclei. The smaller, dense nuclei are those of small lymphocytes.

nea. The majority of those with epithelial mesothelioma have a large pleural effusion (26). Features commonly found in epithelial mesothelioma on cytologic examination are cell aggregates, often of 50 to 200 cells, with a knobby external border; dense, homogeneous cytoplasm with gradation from red-orange surrounding the nucleus to green at the periphery in Papanicolaou-stained smears; brush borders, occasionally with blebs; close apposition of cell borders often with cytoplasmic "windows" separating adjacent cells; and multinucleation (27–29). Cytologic examination of the effusion in pleural mesotheliomas has yielded positive signs of mesothelioma in 5% to 93% of cases (28, 29). In the last decade, the examination of multiple

rather than single specimens, the careful attention to details of processing, and the interpretation of cytologic preparations by experienced observers generally have led to sensitivity in the range of 60% to 80% for malignant mesotheliomas (28, 29).

Two challenges are encountered in the examination of cytologic material: first, differentiating reactive cells from malignant mesothelial cells; and secondly, differentiating mesothelioma cells from other tumors, particularly adenocarcinomas.

Differentiating reactive from malignant epithelial mesothelial cells may be difficult. The usual criteria of malignancy apply: nuclear enlargement with an increased nuclear/cytoplasmic ratio, nuclear irregularity, and hyperchromasia. These criteria are often present in only a few of the cells, or they are completely absent in the malignant mesothelial cell population, and one is obligated to seek other criteria (29). The presence of more cells, larger cells, and larger, three-dimensional cell clusters (often in knobby, papillary clusters) favors mesothelioma (3). In a recent study employing stepwise logistic regression analysis, four cytologic features were noted to favor malignant over reactive mesothelial cells with a high level of accuracy: nuclear pleomorphism, macronucleoli, cell-in-cell engulfment, and lack of cell monolayers (30).

Epithelial mesothelioma cells may on occasion be quite difficult to distinguish from metastatic adenocarcinomas and certain other malignancies. A combined approach is generally favored, using cytologic examination of smears and histologic examination of cell blocks prepared from the fluid. In a logistic regression analysis, five parameters favored mesothelioma over adenocarcinoma: true papillary aggregates, multinucleation with atypia, cell-to-cell apposition, and the absence of acinuslike structures and balloonlike vacuolation (30).

In malignant pleural effusions that are not clearly adenocarcinomas based on the clinical history, cytology, and routine cell block examination, most investigators recommend the application of histochemistry and immunohistochemistry sections from cell blocks to aid in the distinction (see Histochemistry and Immunohistochemistry, below).

Reactivities of mesothelioma cells and adenocarcinoma cells generally are similar to those seen in tissue sections (29, 31). Antibodies to epithelial membrane antigen (EMA) have been observed to stain cell membranes of malignant epithelial mesothelial cells. Strong membrane staining of most cell clusters, or of most mesothelial cells in the absence of clusters, is said not to occur in benign cells and to signify malignant mesothelioma (29). Moreover, strong staining for EMA of the periphery of mesothelioma cell clusters and the circumference of individual mesothelioma cells in a "thick" membrane pattern is held to reflect the staining of long microvilli on the surface of mesothelioma cells and to distinguish mesotheliomas from adenocarcinomas (32, 33). Electron microscopy of cell sediments of pleural fluids also may be helpful in distinguishing adenocarcinomas and mesotheliomas (33–35).

In contrast to epithelial mesotheliomas, effusions in sarcomatoid mesotheliomas are present less often, and tumor cells desquamate less frequently. Thus, none, or only a few tumor cells, may be present in the examined material. Moreover, the spindle cells that comprise sarcomatoid mesotheliomas often are difficult to distinguish from reactive spindle cells and to differentiate from sarcomas and other tumor types (27, 29).

ANCILLARY TECHNIQUES

Currently accepted ancillary techniques in the diagnosis of mesothelioma include histochemistry, immunohistochemistry, and electron microscopy applied to tissue or cytology specimens. These techniques are valuable in distinguishing mesotheliomas from other tumors, specifically adenocarcinomas, sarcomas, melanomas, and lymphomas. With a rare exception (i.e., EMA), they are not of value in distinguishing benign from malignant proliferations. Investigational techniques include flow cytometry, image analysis, and cytogenetics. These studies have been employed in attempts to distinguish mesotheliomas from other malignant tumors and from benign proliferations.

HISTOCHEMISTRY

Mucins, which also have been designated mucosubstances, mucopolysaccharides, glycosaminoglycans, and more recently, glycoconjugates (36), may be detected in tissues by relatively simple histochemical procedures using light microscopic observation of conventional histologic sections of formalin-fixed, paraffin-embedded tumor tissue. Histochemical methods that identify mucins in neoplastic cells are useful in distinguishing epithelial mesotheliomas from adenocarcinomas. In a positive histochemical reaction, mucins aggregating in cytoplasmic vacuoles of the tumor cells or secreted into the lumen of neoplastic ducts or tubules are stained distinctively. Regardless of the staining method, they appear morphologically similar except for color, which reflects the stain used in the procedure (Fig. 35.12). Staining of the cell surface or the stroma may be seen in many tumors and does not constitute a positive reaction. The histochemical procedures are based on differences in the mucins secreted by epithelial mesotheliomas and adenocarcinomas. Epithelial mesotheliomas elaborate acid mucins, principally hyaluronic acid, whereas adenocarcinomas produce mainly neutral mucins and lesser amounts of acid mucins.

The mucicarmine stain, which identifies neutral and weakly acidic mucins, is the simplest of the three methods generally employed in pathology laboratories

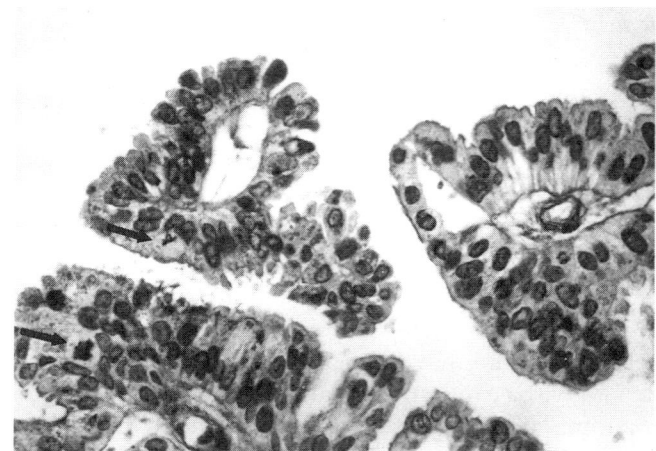

FIGURE 35.12. Papillary adenocarcinoma stained with d-PAS. Stratification and columnar cells suggest adenocarcinoma. Mucin-filled secretory vacuoles in the cytoplasm of the tumor cells stained a vivid purple with d-PAS (*arrows*) and confirmed the diagnosis. In this black and white photomicrograph, dense, irregular material representing contracted secretory product (purple in the d-PAS stain) is seen within clear vacuoles.

TABLE 35.2. Histochemical Findings

STAIN	MESOTHELIOMA (% POSITIVE)	ADENOCARCINOMA (% POSITIVE)
Mucicarmine	3–5	50–60
d-PAS	Occasional	60
Alcian blue with hyaluronidase digestion	30–50	Rare

Abbreviation. d-PAS, diastase–periodic acid Schiff.

for the identification of mucins. Approximately 50% to 60% of adenocarcinomas are mucicarmine positive (Table 35.2), including those of the lung, breast, and gastrointestinal tract, whereas mesotheliomas are routinely negative (31, 37). However, adenocarcinomas of a few organs, such as the kidney, thyroid, and prostate, are only rarely mucicarmine positive. About 3% to 5% of mesotheliomas may be focally positive. This false-positive mucicarmine staining may be eliminated by preincubation of tissue sections with hyaluronidase (17, 38–40).

The diastase–periodic acid Schiff (d-PAS) reaction stains neutral mucins. It is positive in up to 60% of adenocarcinomas (Table 35.2) (31, 41–43) and is routinely negative in mesotheliomas. Close attention must be directed to microscopic examination of the structural features of the material that is PAS positive after diastase digestion and to the negative and positive controls. Glycogen, present in many mesotheliomas, is removed by diastase digestion. However, inadequate digestion leaves PAS positive glycogen granules that may be misinterpreted as mucins. Structures that regularly resist diastase digestion and that may yield a false-positive result include PAS positive lysosomes, which are often present as small cytoplasmic granules, and basement membranes, which may be interposed between tumor cells. Rarely, d-PAS positivity of a mesothelioma has been attributed to crystallized hyaluronic acid (44), and occasionally it may represent true mucin deposition in epithelial mesotheliomas.

Both Alcian blue and colloidal iron stain acid mucins that are elaborated by mesotheliomas and adenocarcinomas. Hyaluronic acid is the major mucin elaborated by mesotheliomas. Preincubation of tissue sections with the appropriate hyaluronidase results in digestion of hyaluronic acid and an absence or marked reduction in mucin positivity after Alcian blue (pH, 2.5) or colloidal iron staining. In contrast, adenocarcinomas produce acid mucins in which hyaluronic acid is only a minor component. In these tumors digestion with hyaluronidase results in little or no reduction in Alcian blue or colloidal iron staining. A positive reaction (digestion of acid mucins with hyaluronidase) strongly supports a diagnosis of mesothelioma, whereas a negative reaction strongly favors an adenocarcinoma. Sensitivity is low, however, because only one third to one half of mesotheliomas yield a positive reaction (Table 35.2) (3, 41, 45, 46). Technical factors such as the choice of hyaluronidase, incubation conditions, and monitoring with appropriate controls (5, 47) may contribute to positive reactions reported in some adenocarcinomas (48). Conversely, the production by tumor cells of dominant acid mucins other than hyaluronic acid in mesotheliomas (49, 50), or the crystallization of hyaluronic acid (44), may rarely lead to a negative reaction in mesotheliomas.

IMMUNOHISTOCHEMISTRY

Since their introduction in the early 1980s, immunohistochemical procedures have become valuable adjuncts in the identification of malignant mesotheliomas. In addition to the factors cited below, the observed immunoreactivity of tumors is affected by technical factors such as tissue fixation, antibody dilution, and incubation conditions. Their standardization in each laboratory using appropriate tissue controls is essential to minimize variation in immunoreactivity. Immunoreagents commonly employed in the distinction of mesotheliomas and adenocarcinomas and their reactivity for these tumors are listed in Table 35.3.

INTERMEDIATE FILAMENTS

Antibodies to keratin protein are now a routine component of the immunohistochemical examination of mesotheliomas (5, 17, 51). Keratin proteins, one of a family of five intermediate cytoplasmic filaments (10-nm diameter), are widely distributed in normal and neoplastic epithelial cells. They form a family of at least 20 polypeptides ranging in molecular weight from 40 to 67 kd (52–54). Since their demonstration in

TABLE 35.3. Immunohistochemical Findings

	MESOTHELIOMA	ADENOCARCINOMA	
	% POSITIVE	NONPULMONARY (% POSITIVE)	PULMONARY (% POSITIVE)
Keratin	100	100	100
CEA	9–11	50–100	93
Leu-M1	0–8	58	69–100
EMA	84–100	91	100
HFMG-2	0–75	85	91–100
B72.3	0–44	30–40	75–96
Ber-EP4	1–20	83–87	100

Abbreviations. CEA, carcinoembryonic antigen; EMA, epithelial membrane antigen.

mesotheliomas in 1980 (55), many immunohistochemical studies have confirmed their presence in mesotheliomas (43, 56, 57). Essentially all mesotheliomas, including sarcomatoid and mixed types as well as the epithelial type, are keratin positive if the tissue sample is adequate and appropriately preserved, the formalin-fixed tumor is subjected to protease digestion to uncover binding sites (58, 59), and the appropriate keratin antibodies are employed (60, 61).

Numerous attempts have been made to distinguish epithelial mesotheliomas from adenocarcinomas using antibodies to keratin proteins of different molecular weights. This approach has not yet proved fruitful (62), however, an antibody to keratin 5 (MW 58,000) preserved in frozen tissues recently has been reported reactive with epithelial and biphasic mesotheliomas and unreactive with pulmonary adenocarcinomas (63).

Different localization patterns of keratin proteins have been observed in epithelial mesotheliomas and adenocarcinomas (5, 56, 64, 65). However, this distinction is controversial because a number of experienced observers have not confirmed the observation (60–62). Diffuse cytoplasmic and perinuclear, ringlike staining in epithelial mesotheliomas that contrasts with the cytoplasmic staining and peripheral (membrane) accentuation of adenocarcinomas has been noted (Figs. 35.13 and 35.14) (4, 66). A small percentage of mixed and indeterminate patterns has been observed (66). This distinction has been found to be reliable with all of the various monoclonal and polyclonal keratin antibodies tested and has been used routinely

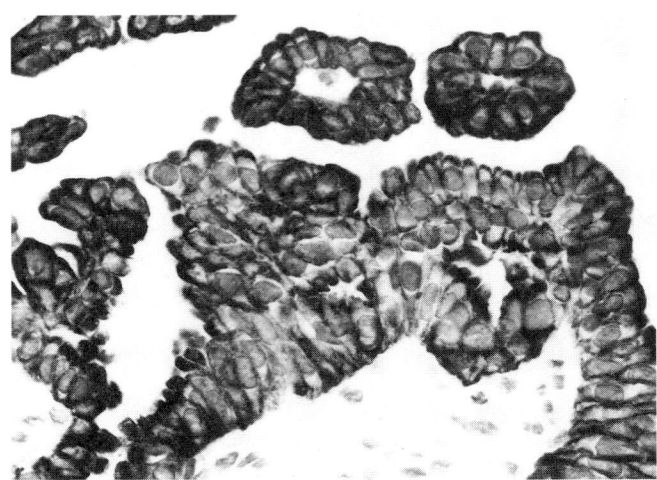

FIGURE 35.14. Papillary adenocarcinoma stained by an immunoperoxidase method for AE1/AE3 keratin proteins. Intense black staining of the periphery of the cell and generally weak or absent cytoplasmic staining is well seen. This localization pattern is characteristic of most adenocarcinomas.

in our assessment of epithelial mesotheliomas. Important technical considerations include good fixation and optimal digestion with trypsin (58).

Vimentin, another intermediate filament, is widely expressed in normal and neoplastic mesenchymal tissues. It has been suggested that coexpression of keratin and vimentin strongly favors mesothelioma over adenocarcinoma (67); however, these results have not been supported by others (60, 68). The principal use of vimentin in assessment of mesotheliomas is as a control to assure that antigenicity has not been destroyed during tissue processing (61).

GLYCOPROTEINS

Numerous membrane-bound glycoproteins have been employed in efforts to distinguish epithelial mesotheliomas from adenocarcinomas.

Carcinoembryonic Antigen. Using an immunofluorescence method, the carcinoembryonic antigen (CEA), a membrane-bound glycoprotein, was shown in the cytoplasm of neoplastic cells of tissue sections of adenocarcinomas of the lung and its absence noted in mesotheliomas in 1979 (69). This report was followed quickly by studies applying immunoperoxidase methods to formalin-fixed, paraffin-embedded tissues. These studies also demonstrated differential CEA reactivity of adenocarcinomas and mesotheliomas (Fig. 35.15) (41, 56, 70). Subsequently, many studies of CEA have confirmed its utility in the distinction of epithelial mesotheliomas and adenocarcinomas (41, 43, 57, 68, 71–78)

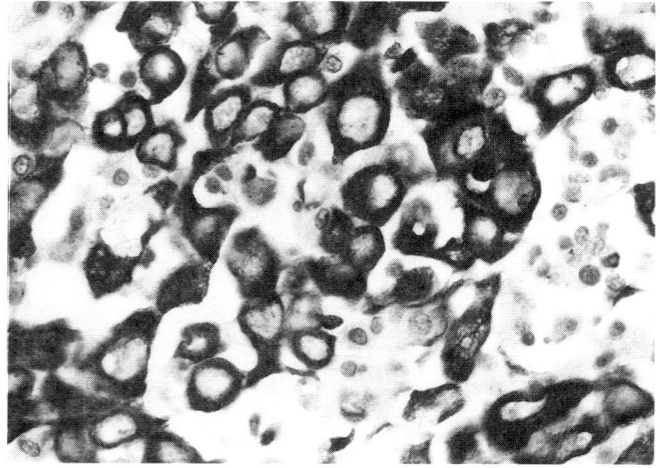

FIGURE 35.13. Immunoperoxidase staining for AE1/AE3 keratin proteins in an epithelial mesothelioma. Nuclei appear as round, hollow areas, and they are surrounded by black cytoplasmic staining (in the photomicrograph) representing perinuclear and cytoplasmic localization of keratin proteins, highly characteristic of mesothelial cells.

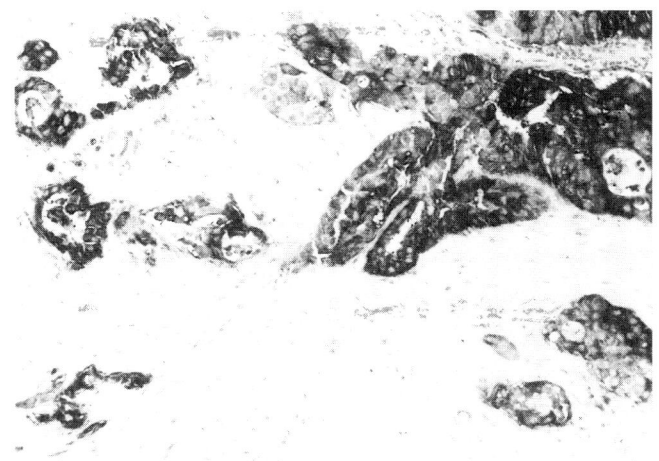

FIGURE 35.15. CEA-immunoperoxidase staining of adenocarcinoma of the lung. The cells forming the irregular ducts of this adenocarcinoma stain strongly for CEA, whereas the stroma is unstained. CEA reactivity is seen in most adenocarcinomas. Although mesotheliomas may sometimes be CEA positive, staining is usually focal and weak. Staining of this degree, which is frequent in adenocarcinomas, is seen very rarely in mesotheliomas.

Currently, CEA is a member of most antibody panels developed to distinguish epithelial mesotheliomas from adenocarcinomas, and some regard it as the best of the antibodies available for this purpose. CEA was immunoreactive in 93% of primary adenocarcinomas of the lung and in 84% of adenocarcinomas of various sites in a compilation of 40 reports (77). CEA positivity of adenocarcinomas of other organs that may be the source of metastases to the pleura is estimated as 75% to 100% for the gastrointestinal tract, 60% to 75% for breast, and 50% for ovarian carcinomas (Table 35.3). Adenocarcinomas of the kidney, prostate, and thyroid are rarely CEA positive. In contrast to most adenocarcinomas, epithelial mesotheliomas are usually negative. An analysis of 621 literature cases revealed 11% positive with the polyclonal CEA antibody and 9% positive with the monoclonal antibody (77). Positive reactions are usually only weak and focal.

Variability in the proportion of adenocarcinomas of a given organ site and of mesotheliomas immunoreactive for CEA occurs and may be caused by a number of factors. CEA is a member of a relatively large gene member family of glycoproteins and shares epitopes with other glycoproteins of the family (77, 79). Both monoclonal and polyclonal antibodies to CEA with varying specificity and cross-reactivity are used in the immunohistochemical assessment of tumors. Monoclonal antibodies to CEA recognize at least five major epitope clusters (80). Comparison of polyclonal and monoclonal antibodies and of various monoclonal antibodies to CEA is an area under active investigation. Recent studies report differences in specificity and sensitivity among the various CEA antibodies (81, 79). Much of the nonspecificity encountered with polyclonal antibodies is readily monitored by examination of the staining of neutrophils and macrophages. It may be avoided by adsorption of the antibody with spleen powder (82). Nonspecific staining also is associated with necrotic areas and with the high content of hyaluronic acid definable by its abrogation when sections are incubated with hyaluronidase before exposure to the CEA antibody (40). An unusual false-positive reaction to a monoclonal CEA has been observed in 5 of 45 mesotheliomas (83). Reactivity was coarsely granular, unlike the pattern usually seen in CEA-reactive epithelia, and had features suggesting localization to the Golgi region.

Monoclonal Antibody Leu-M1. Leu-M1—a monoclonal antibody, that is one of a large family of similar antibodies designated CD15, directed against membrane glycoproteins—has been established as useful in the distinction of adenocarcinomas from epithelial mesotheliomas (60). First described as recognizing an antigen present on myelomonocytic cells, it was later detected in non-Hodgkin's lymphomas and in Reed-Sternberg cells as well as in adenocarcinomas, but it was not observed in mesotheliomas (84). In five large series, Leu-M1 immunoreactivity has been reported in a total of 192 (84%) of 228 cases of pulmonary adenocarcinomas (range, 69% to 100%) (43, 57, 68, 78, 85); epithelial mesotheliomas have been positive in only 3 (2%) of 158 cases (range, 0% to 8%). In adenocarcinomas of diverse origin, 105 (58%) of 179 have been Leu-M1 positive (Table 35.3)(84).

Milk Fat Globules. A number of antibodies to high-molecular-weight glycoproteins derived from milk fat globules have been developed.

The monoclonal EMA antibody reacts with 91% to 100% of adenocarcinomas, but also with 84% to 100% of epithelial mesotheliomas (43, 57, 86).

Another monoclonal antibody to milk fat globules, HFMG-2, displays immunoreactivity in 91% to 100% of pulmonary adenocarcinomas (57, 72, 74, 76, 78, 85) and in 85% to 100% of adenocarcinomas from diverse sites (74); however, it stains from 0% to as much as 47% to 75% of epithelial mesotheliomas (Table 35.3) (57, 72, 74, 76, 78, 85). Some controversy surrounds its use in distinguishing adenocarcinomas from epithelial mesotheliomas. Some workers report strong cytoplasmic staining in adenocarcinomas, but they note that reactivity in mesotheliomas, if present, primarily is membranous and that cytoplasmic staining usually is confined to less than 3% of the neoplastic cells (60, 74, 85). They include the antibody in their antibody panel to distinguish mesotheliomas and adenocarcinomas.

Monoclonal Antibody B72.3. Monoclonal antibody B72.3 binds to a high-molecular-weight glycoprotein (designated TAG-72) derived from a membrane-enriched fraction of a metastatic mammary carcinoma. Immunoreactivity of B72.3 with 19 of 22 pulmonary adenocarcinomas and with 0 of 20 epithelial mesotheliomas was observed (87). However, positivity was set at more than 10%. Eight mesotheliomas with 1% and one with 5% immunoreactive tumor cells were regarded as negative. Subsequent studies report 75% to 96% of pulmonary adenocarcinomas to be positive (43, 68, 78), but sensitivity for adenocarcinomas of only 30% to 40% is the experience of others (60). In some large series, no immunoreactive mesotheliomas were observed (43, 68); however, 16 (44%) of 36 epithelial mesotheliomas were positive in one study (78), and others note occasional weak reactivity in mesotheliomas (Table 35.3) (60).

Monoclonal Antibody Ber-EP4. Ber-EP4, a monoclonal antibody directed to 34- and 39- kilodalton (kd) glycoproteins of human epithelia (88), has shown initial promise in distinguishing adenocarcinomas from epithelial mesotheliomas. It has immunoreactivity for 83% to 87% of adenocarcinomas from various sites and for 100% of pulmonary adenocarcinomas (89, 90). Only 1 of 115 epithelial mesotheliomas was immunoreactive for Ber-EP4 (89) in one study; however, 10 (20%) of 49 were reactive in another (90). The reason for the discrepancy is not apparent. In an examination of cell blocks of malignant pleural effusions and fine-needle aspirates, 13 (57%) of 23 pulmonary adenocarcinomas and 32 (80%) of 40 nonpulmonary metastatic adenocarcinomas were Ber-EP4 positive (Table 35.3)(91).

OTHER IMMUNOHISTOCHEMICAL REAGENTS

A number of lectins, antibodies to blood group antigens, and other substances have been reported to be reactive with adenocarcinomas. Because they have little or no reactivity for mesotheliomas, they thus are useful in distinguishing between these tumor types. In general, however, they have been less widely used than those described above (92–97).

Although highly desirable, a useful antibody reactive with mesotheliomas but not with adenocarcinomas has not been reported. A number of antibodies have been observed to react preferentially with epithelial mesotheliomas, but they have not gained general acceptance for a variety of reasons, including the requirement for frozen tissue (98–100), commercial unavailability (60, 101), and lack of independent confirmation (68, 102–104).

ULTRASTRUCTURE

Extensive ultrastructural examinations of reactive and neoplastic pleural disorders in several excellent reviews (5, 17, 35, 105, 106) have confirmed and extended early observations (107, 108) that epithelial mesotheliomas exhibit characteristic ultrastructural features that may be valuable in distinguishing them from adenocarcinomas. Sarcomatoid mesotheliomas contain fibroblastlike spindle cells and may display focal evidence of epithelial differentiation that aids in their distinction from other tumors, whereas mixed type mesotheliomas share features common to both epithelial and sarcomatoid mesotheliomas.

Epithelial mesotheliomas typically possess numerous long, thin, curved microvilli that project from the cell surface and interdigitate with those of adjacent tumor cells (Fig. 35.16). They also possess readily detected tonofilaments, often concentrated around the nucleus and desmosomes as well as other cell-cell junctions (Table 35.4) (5, 35, 109). Adenocarcinomas usually have short, blunt microvilli (Fig. 35.17) and fewer tonofilaments without predilection for perinuclear areas. Certain structures, such as filamentous glycocalyx-coating microvilli, microvillous core rootlets, mucin granules, and myelin figures, typify adenocarcinomas and ex-

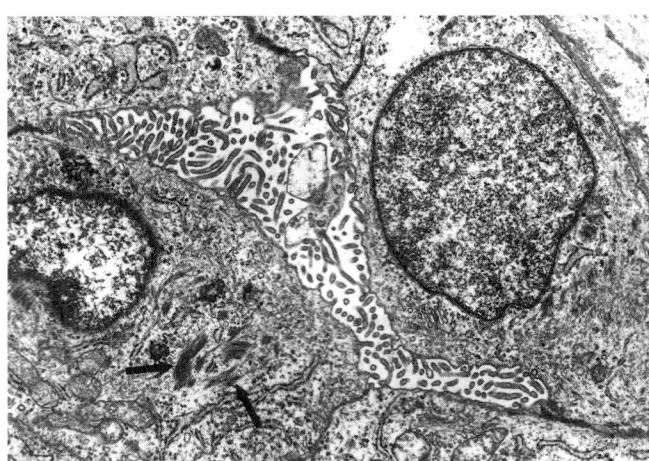

FIGURE 35.16. Electron micrograph of an epithelial mesothelioma. Tumor cells with round to ovoid nuclei are separated by a space into which many long, thin, curved microvilli project. Occasional branching is seen, and microvilli interdigitate with those of opposing cells. Compare these with the microvilli of the adenocarcinoma in Figure 35.17. Keratin intermediate filaments, which laterally aggregate to form tonofilaments in the cytoplasm of the cell, are well seen in the lower left portion of the photomicrograph (*arrows*). These filaments are characteristic of epithelial mesotheliomas, but they do not distinguish them from adenocarcinomas.

TABLE 35.4. Electron Microscopic Findings

	EPITHELIAL MESOTHELIOMA	ADENOCARCINOMA
Microvilli	Long	Short
	Thin	Thick
	LDR >5	LDR <10
	Branched	Unbranched
	Curved	Straight
	Interdigitating	Single
Mucin granules	None	±
Myelin figures	None	±
Microvillus	...	...
Core rootlets	None	±
Glycocalyx	None	±

Abbreviation. LDR, length to diameter ratio; ±, indicates that a structure may or may not be present.

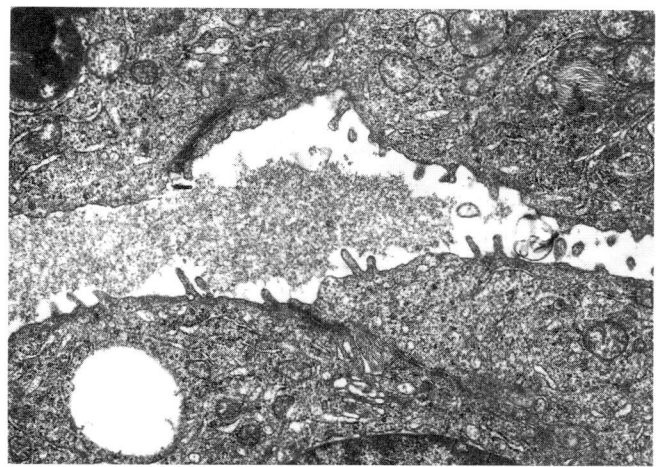

FIGURE 35.17. Electron micrograph of an adenocarcinoma. Several tumor cells are separated by an elongated space containing electron-dense granular material. Of note are the sparse, short, stubby microvilli that project from the cell surface into the intercellular space. They contrast sharply with those seen in epithelial mesotheliomas.

clude mesothelioma (Table 35.4). Initially, the association of microvilli with extracellular collagen was noted in virtually all mesotheliomas but not in any adenocarcinomas (105, 110). Subsequent studies, however, have shown the association in up to 21% of adenocarcinomas (111, 112). The single most important ultrastructural feature in distinguishing epithelial mesotheliomas and adenocarcinomas is the character of the microvilli. The importance of considering all characteristics of the microvilli, such as the profusion of interlacing, curved, and branching microvilli in meso-theliomas, has been emphasized (106). A useful quantitative measure of microvilli is their length to diameter ratio (LDR) (109, 113–115). Values of 15 or more are highly suggestive of mesothelioma, whereas adenocarcinomas usually have an LDR of 10 or less (106). However, the microvillous LDR of some adenocarcinomas, especially those of ovarian or endometrial origin (116), may overlap with mesotheliomas. Moreover, microvilli in poorly differentiated epithelial mesotheliomas, or in poorly differentiated areas of well-differentiated mesotheliomas, are sparse and short (117) with an LDR of less than 10.

INVESTIGATIONAL ANCILLARY TECHNIQUES

FLOW CYTOMETRY

Flow cytometry has been used to compare the DNA content and proliferation rate in mesotheliomas with that of nonmesothelial tumors, particularly pulmonary carcinomas, and with reactive mesothelial proliferations. Most studies compare mesotheliomas to pulmonary adenocarcinomas. Virtually all these studies involve paraffin-embedded tumors. Most mesotheliomas are diploid (65% to 86%) (118–120), whereas most pulmonary carcinomas are aneuploid (75% to 88%) (118–120). However, two studies report the majority of mesotheliomas (53% to 61.4%) to be aneuploid (121, 122). Hence, the presence of aneuploidy does not distinguish mesotheliomas from adenocarcinomas reliably (60). However, the majority of aneuploid mesotheliomas have a relatively low DNA index, with a mean of approximately 1.5 and a maximum of approximately 2.0 (118–120). In contrast, in pulmonary adenocarcinomas both the mean and maximum DNA index of the aneuploid tumors were generally higher than that of aneuploid mesotheliomas (118–120). Again, the overlap in DNA indexes remains considerable (118–120). Thus, although the DNA index of pulmonary carcinomas is more often aneuploid and generally higher than mesotheliomas, the significant amount of overlap limits the use of this index as an aid in distinguishing these two tumors.

Measurement of proliferation rates, particularly S-phase fraction, has been performed, but there has not been a consistent difference between mesothelioma and pulmonary carcinomas (118–120).

When mesotheliomas have been compared to benign mesothelial cells, mesotheliomas were found to be diploid 45% of the time in biopsy specimens (121) and 75% of the time in effusions (123). Reactive mesothelial cells generally were found to be diploid. The mean DNA index of mesotheliomas was higher than that of benign cells, but there was significant overlap (121, 123). These studies do not support a role for flow cytometry in distinguishing mesotheliomas and reactive mesothelial hyperplasia.

Overall, the lack of standardization in flow cytometry makes interpretation and comparison of studies difficult. Determination of diploid DNA content has been done using a variety of standards. Cut-offs for acceptable coefficients of variation of DNA peaks have varied considerably, DNA content has been reported in various forms, and criteria for the elimination of noise, a crucial step in determining S-phase fractions, vary widely. The method and duration of fixation has been observed to affect ploidy sufficiently to preclude the use of any standard but adjacent normal tissue processed exactly as the tumor (124). In the future careful standardization of methods, including stringent guidelines for interpretation of histograms, should help assure consistent results and elucidate the role of flow cytometry in the evaluation of mesotheliomas (124).

IMAGE ANALYSIS

Image analysis refers to the use of automated and semiautomated methods of measuring cytologic features. Most systems use a computer to help in obtaining and/or analyzing the data. Most of the work with mesotheliomas has been with effusions and has focused on distinguishing benign from malignant mesothelial cells, and, less commonly, mesotheliomas from other malignancies such as carcinoma. Much of this work was done in the mid 1980s when the systems were not fully automated, necessitating significant operator interpretation (and bias), e.g., selecting which cells to measure. There also was an interest in using cases as training sets to create an algorithm to distinguish benign and malignant cells. In some instances the same cases were then used as part of the test group.

Initial studies demonstrated that malignant mesothelial cells had larger nuclear and cytoplasmic areas than benign mesothelial cells in pleural effusions (125). Later studies confirmed this observation in biopsy specimens as well as in pleural effusions, but there was significant overlap (126, 127). Examination of ultrastructural nuclear features revealed that adenocarcinoma nuclei were generally more irregular than mesothelioma nuclei, but the difference was not significant. In addition, no significant difference was seen between benign and malignant mesothelial cells (128).

Later studies used Feulgen-stained slides to measure DNA content by image analysis. Other investigators (129) showed that malignant mesotheliomas generally had higher DNA content than reactive mesothelial cells. However, the results of this study showed a very high percentage of aneuploid mesotheliomas (approaching 90%), which does not correlate with flow data. One possible reason for this discrepancy was that every mesothelioma case selected was diagnostic by conventional cytology. Perhaps this reflects a population of mesotheliomas with significant increases in DNA content. Others (130) have also looked at Feulgen-stained slides of tissue sections. They also found a high percentage of aneuploid mesotheliomas but were again unable to distinguish benign and malignant cells consistently because of a significant overlap of values.

Currently, image analysis remains an investigational tool in the appraisal of mesotheliomas.

CYTOGENETICS

Cytogenetics involves the harvesting of proliferating cells in metaphase and the analysis of specific chromosomal structural aberrations. Although some tumors have been found to have characteristic, simple, chromosomal abnormalities, such has not been the case for mesothelioma. Examinations have been performed on established mesothelioma cell lines and on cells after short- or long-term culture. Early studies of effusions found most mesotheliomas to have complex chromosomal abnormalities (131). Studies of cell lines derived from surgical specimens have revealed complex chromosomal abnormalities, but also nonrandom alterations of chromosomes (132) and numerous complex structural abnormalities (133). Karyotyping (134, 135) of 34 mesotheliomas cultured for from 2 hours to several months revealed clonal abnormalities in 25 with a complex karyotype in most cases, but with no characteristic clonal abnormality. In a study of 40 mesotheliomas karyotyped after 1 to 3 days or 1 to 4 weeks in culture, the majority had complex chromosomal abnormalities (136). Nevertheless, the authors were able to characterize two groups with nonrandom abnormalities. The larger had losses of chromosomes 4, 22, 9p, and 3p, and the smaller had gains of chromosomes 7, 5, 20 and deletions or rearrangements of 3p. In a recent study successful tumor growth in short-term culture (1–7 days) was achieved in 27 of 29 consecutive malignant mesotheliomas. Each of the 27 cultured tumors contained clonal chromosomal aberrations; however, no single aberration was common to all tumors. Frequently deleted regions (70% to 36%), in order of decreasing frequency, were 3p, 1p, 22q, 9p, 6q, and 13q (137, 138).

Cytogenetics does not yet have an established role in the diagnosis of mesothelioma. However, some observations suggest that it could be useful in pathologic diagnosis. For example, clonal aberrations have been described in many of the mesotheliomas but not in nonneoplastic mesothelial proliferations. Therefore, cytogenetics may prove helpful in distinguishing reactive from neoplastic mesothelial proliferations (137). Cytogenetic analysis has aided in rare instances in the distinction of mesotheliomas from tumors with characteristic, established, cytogenetic abnormalities such as synovial sarcoma (139).

DIFFERENTIAL DIAGNOSIS

Mesothelioma of the pleura has a broad differential diagnosis that is closely related to the histologic type of the mesothelioma (Table 35.5).

Epithelial mesotheliomas must be distinguished from mesothelial hyperplasia and adenocarcinomas. Mesothelial hyperplasia is a reactive proliferation that may be associated with a variety of inflammatory and other processes, including tumors and other lesions that involve the subpleural parenchyma (3, 4, 17). The mesothelial nature of the hyperplastic cells usually is readily apparent in Papanicolaou-stained smears and hematoxylin and eosin–stained sections, but the mesothelial cells are frequently cytologically atypical. Although these atypical cells may closely resemble mesothelioma cells both in effusions and in tissue sections, they can usually be distinguished from them by their cytologic features (3, 30, 33). Cytologic features favoring malignancy are nuclear pleomorphism, hyperchromatism, and nuclear membrane irregularity in the malignant cells. However, all of these features may be absent in well-differentiated mesotheliomas.

Of considerable interest is the recent introduction of the concept of mesothelioma in situ (140). The investigators reported seven cases and proposed histologic and other criteria for their distinction from reactive hyperplasia and from invasive epithelial mesothelioma.

In tissue sections, frank invasion, when present, establishes a malignant diagnosis, but minimal invasion must be distinguished from entrapped, hyperplastic mesothelial cells. Invasion is characterized by irregular, elongate, penetrating tubules, whereas entrapped reactive mesothelial cells are arranged in rounded, discrete pseudoacini within the stroma (141). Of the special methods, immunohistochemistry is reported to be helpful because the strong staining of mesothelial cells for epithelial membrane antigen in a membrane pattern is supportive of a diagnosis of malignancy (5, 29). Although the methodology is not widely available, detection of clonality by cytogenetic methods may aid in identifying malignant epithelial mesothelial cells in effusions or in tissues (137, 138).

The need to distinguish epithelial mesotheliomas from both primary adenocarcinomas of the lung involving the pleura and metastatic adenocarcinomas from distant sites is well recognized and may be difficult. Their similarity is embodied in the term pseudomesotheliomatous adenocarcinoma (142–144). The difficulty in obtaining agreement, even among experts in this field, is attested to in a recent report of the United States–Canadian mesothelioma panel (62). Nonetheless, this problem has been greatly ameliorated over the past decade. This progress is attributed to the increasing firsthand familiarity of pathologists with the histologic appearance of mesotheliomas and especially to the widespread use of ancillary techniques, particularly immunohistochemistry. The most common primary site of adenocarcinoma metastasis to the pleura is the lung, followed by the breast and stomach (145), and less commonly, the ovary, colon, pancreas, kidney, prostate, and thyroid (145–149). Although many of the cytologic and architectural features of epithelial mesothelioma and adenocarcinoma overlap, the presence of marked nuclear pleomorphism, frequent mitoses, extensive necrosis,

TABLE 35.5. Differential Diagnosis of Mesothelioma

HISTOLOGIC TYPE	DIFFERENTIATING CHARACTERISTICS
Epithelial type	
Atypical mesothelial hyperplasia	Histology, EMA
Adenocarcinomas	
Lung	Mucin stains, keratin pattern, CEA, Leu-M1, Ber-EP4, EM
Kidney	Keratin pattern
Prostate	PSA, PAP
Thyroid	Thyroglobulin
Melanoma	Keratin, S-100, HMB-45, EM
Lymphoma	Keratin, CD3, CD19, CD20, CD45, UCHL1
Epithelioid	
Hemangioendothelioma	Factor VIII, CD34
Sarcomatoid type	
Chronic pleuritis	Histology
SFTP	Keratin, CD34
Most sarcomas	Keratin
Synovial sarcoma, monophasic	Histology, cytogenetics
Lymphoma	Keratin, CD3, CD19, CD20, CD45, UCHL1
Melanoma	Keratin, S-100, HMB-45, EM
Spindle cell carcinoma	Clinical, EM

Abbreviations. SFTP, solitary fibrous tumor of the pleura; EMA, epithelial membrane antigen; CEA, carcinoembryonic antigen; EM, electron microscopy; PSA, prostatic specific antigen; PAP, prostatic acid phosphatase.

and/or many columnar cells is more suggestive of adenocarcinoma. Histochemical procedures still are used routinely by many experienced workers to help distinguish epithelial mesotheliomas from metastatic adenocarcinomas of the pleura. In addition, panels of immunohistochemical reagents (including antibodies to keratin proteins, CEA, and Leu-M1) are now in general use (5, 17, 47, 51, 60, 61).

Electron microscopy is valuable and sometimes critical in the distinction, but its application is limited by availability, cost, and turnaround time. At Brigham and Women's Hospital, the following tests are used routinely: histochemical stains (mucicarmine, d-PAS, and in selected cases, hyaluronidase–Alcian blue), an immunohistochemical panel (AE1/AE3 and callus keratins with characterization of the keratin localization pattern, adsorbed polyclonal CEA, Leu-M1, and occasionally EMA, B72.3, Ber-EP4, and ME-1, the latter restricted to frozen sections), and electron microscopy.

Metastatic adenocarcinomas that often are negative with the mucin stains and unreactive with antibodies to CEA and other antibodies to glycoproteins include those from the kidney, prostate, and thyroid, as well as some poorly differentiated adenocarcinomas. Renal adenocarcinomas often have a prominent clear cell component that is rarely seen in mesotheliomas. If pathologic findings suggest a renal primary site, radiologic studies of the kidneys should be sought to evaluate this possibility. Prostatic adenocarcinomas occasionally metastasize to the pleura, although rarely when the primary site is occult. They may be histologically indistinguishable from an epithelial mesothelioma, particularly in a small specimen. Immunohistochemistry with prostatic specific antigen and prostatic acid phosphatase stains should provide a definitive diagnosis. Metastatic papillary adenocarcinoma of the thyroid may closely simulate a papillary mesothelioma of the pleura. Both may contain psammoma bodies. Immunoreactivity for thyroglobulin is diagnostic. Poorly differentiated adenocarcinomas may be quite difficult to distinguish from poorly differentiated epithelial mesotheliomas. A careful clinical history for a possible occult primary site, generous biopsies providing well-fixed tissue, careful histologic examination for differentiated areas, and application of ancillary techniques offer the greatest possibility for distinguishing the two entities. Of note when making the distinction is the recent report of concurrent mesothelioma and adenocarcinoma of the lung in a patient with asbestosis (150).

Rarely, tumors other than metastatic adenocarcinoma enter into the differential diagnosis. These include metastatic amelanotic melanoma, large cell lymphoma, epithelioid hemangioendothelioma (151, 152), and epithelioid sarcoma. Again, immunohistochemistry may be of considerable help. Antibodies to S-100 protein, the monoclonal antibody HMB-45, and a low-molecular-weight keratin antibody comprise a panel that usually is definitive in distinguishing metastatic melanoma from mesothelioma. Large cell lymphomas are almost always keratin negative and usually are reactive with antibodies to leukocyte common antigen (CD45) and the generic markers for B cells (CD19, CD20) or T cells (CD3, UCHL1). Epithelioid hemangioendotheliomas may be keratin positive, but usually the reactivity is limited to a small proportion of the tumor cells, whereas immunoreactivity for some or all of the endothelial markers (factor VIII–related antigen, CD34, CD31, and Ulex europaeus) is more prominent. Of these, factor VIII has the greatest specificity but the least sensitivity (unpublished observations). Epithelioid sarcomas rarely may metastasize to the pleura. This tumor is strongly keratin positive. CEA was reported to be negative in the 15 cases examined in one study (153). A history of a primary tumor in soft tissues is the most helpful clue in its distinction from epithelial mesothelioma.

The differential diagnosis of sarcomatoid mesotheliomas includes fibrosing pleuritis, sarcomas, solitary fibrous tumor of the pleura, and, occasionally, other tumors such as sarcomatoid carcinoma, or carcinosarcoma and melanoma.

Chronic pleuritis with fibrosis may lead to extensive pleural thickening that closely simulates desmoplastic forms of malignant mesothelioma radiologically and on gross examination. Nodular or gray translucent areas in a background of dense, white, fibrous tissue may signify the presence of lesional mesothelioma and should be sought carefully in problem cases. On occasion, extensive pleural resection and widespread sampling are necessary to establish or exclude a diagnosis of sarcomatoid mesothelioma. Features that favor the diagnosis of sarcomatoid mesothelioma include increased cellularity, hyperchromatism and nuclear pleomorphism of the spindle cells, disorderly arrangement of collagen bundles in storiform or twisted patterns, areas of bland necrosis, usually with a stellate or geographic outline, and invasion of fat or skeletal muscle of the chest wall (3, 5, 19). In contrast, fibrosing pleuritis often has a fibrinous exudate, proliferating capillaries perpendicular to the pleural surface, and maturation from loose to dense fibrosis from the surface toward chest wall. Both fibrosing pleuritis and desmoplastic sarcomatoid mesothelioma are characterized by the proliferation of spindle cells that are keratin positive (65, 154–156).

Pleural plaques, seen in 21 of 200 biopsy specimens of malignant mesothelioma in one series (47), are greatly thickened pleura (Fig. 35.18) comprised of paucicellular, dense, collagenous tissue with a basket-weave pattern in which collagen bundles are parallel and are separated by uniform, ovoid, clear spaces (Fig. 35.19). Fibrosing pleuritis or sarcomatous mesothelioma may fuse with or invade such plaques, and the presence of plaques does not favor either entity.

Solitary fibrous tumor of the pleura (SFTP), also called a localized fibrous tumor of the pleura or a localized fibrous mesothelioma, is usually distinguishable by virtue of its presentation as a solitary, often pedunculated, mass arising from either visceral or parietal pleura (Fig. 35.20) (157, 158). Small biopsy specimens and/or incomplete information regarding gross features of the tumor from radiologic examination or surgical procedures may create difficulties in distinguishing such tumors from sarcomatoid mesotheliomas. A panel of keratin and CD34 antibodies can be helpful (Fig. 35.21

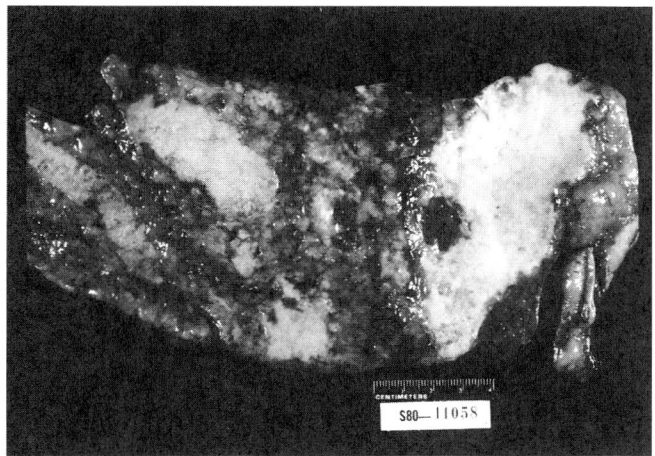

FIGURE 35.18. Gross photograph of parietal pleura containing irregular, large, flat, white plaques. They were 2- to 5-mm thick and quite firm. Mesothelioma also is present. It forms many small, white nodules that coalesce in the pleura adjacent to the plaques.

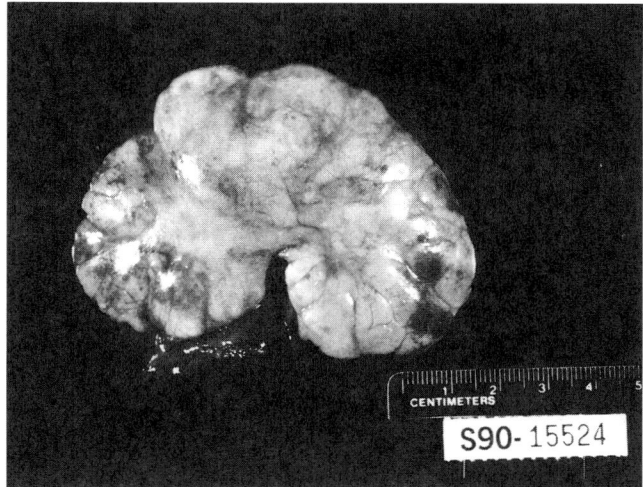

FIGURE 35.20. Gross photograph of hemisected solitary fibrous tumor of the pleura. The tumor was 8 cm in greatest dimension, polypoid, and well circumscribed. It projected into the pleural space; a small piece of the underlying lung and visceral pleura from which it arose are visible below the peripheral indentation.

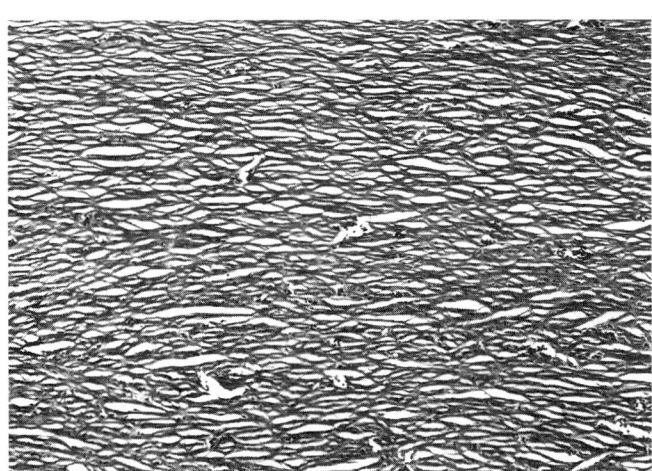

FIGURE 35.19. Pleural plaque. The plaque is hypocellular and composed of a dense array of collagen fibers. The parallel, linear spaces, which are artifactual, are characteristic of pleural plaque and help to distinguish plaques from desmoplastic mesotheliomas. In the latter the dense fibrous tissue often has a twisted, or storiform, pattern.

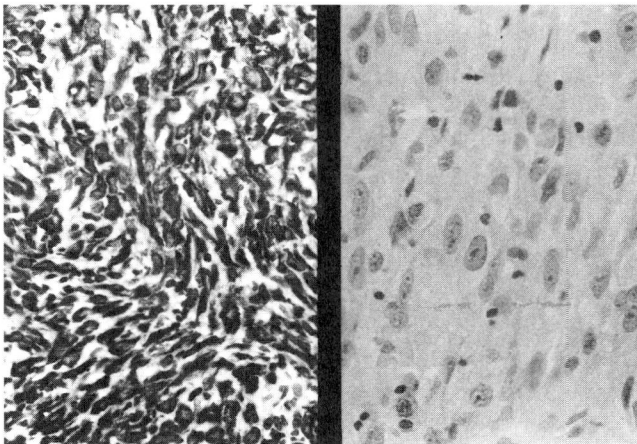

FIGURE 35.21. Immunoperoxidase staining of sarcomatoid mesothelioma for AE1/AE3 keratin proteins (*left*, strongly positive) and CD34 (*right*, negative). This pattern of immunoreactivity contrasts with that of solitary fibrous tumor of the pleura.

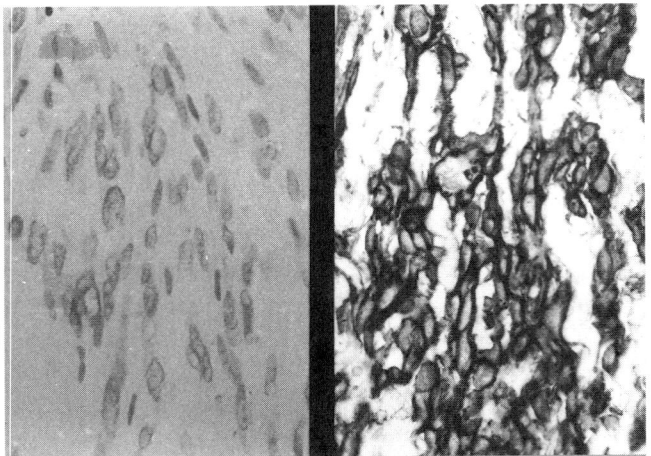

FIGURE 35.22. Immunoperoxidase staining of solitary fibrous tumor of the pleura. The pattern of keratin protein negativity (*left*) and CD34 positivity (*right*) helps to distinguish this tumor from sarcomatoid mesothelioma and other tumors of the pleura and chest wall.

and 35.22). Sarcomatoid mesotheliomas are nearly always immunoreactive for keratin proteins, and most of the tumor cells of positive tumors are reactive (154–156, 159, 160, 161). In contrast, benign SFTPs are uniformly keratin negative (158, 161–163), and although some malignant SFTPs may contain keratin reactive tumor cells, the percentage of reactive cells has been small (less than 1% to 20%) (161). Conversely, CD34 antibodies have been found to stain both benign and malignant SFTPs (161, 164) and only rarely to stain mesotheliomas (161). With one CD34 antibody (QBEND), 16 of 16 SFTPs were positive and 20 of 20 sarcomatoid mesotheliomas were negative (161).

The architectural patterns formed by the proliferating spindle cells of sarcomatoid mesotheliomas may suggest the diagnosis of a number of other sarcomas, including fibrosarcoma, malignant fibrous histiocytoma, malignant schwannoma, malignant hemangiopericytoma, leiomyosarcoma, angiosarcoma, and monophasic spindle cell synovial sarcoma. In most cases the anatomic distribution of the tumor as defined in radiologic studies and by the surgeon at thoracotomy is quite important. The presence of a solitary mass together with the absence of abnormality of pleura apart from the mass are strong evidence against the diagnosis of mesothelioma.

Careful gross examination of the pleura at thoracotomy or thoracoscopy, and biopsies of any suspicious areas of thickening and other suspicious abnormalities of the pleura apart from the mass, may be valuable in evaluating possible subtle, early foci of diffuse malignant mesothelioma. Immunohistochemically, keratin reactivity excludes most sarcomas except monophasic synovial sarcoma, which is usually keratin positive. In these cases monophasic synovial sarcoma can usually be recognized by its histologic features, the relative paucity of keratin reactive tumor cells, and the identification of the characteristic X:18 translocation.

Several other tumors may occasionally enter into the differential diagnosis of sarcomatoid mesothelioma, including lymphoma, malignant melanoma, and spindle cell variants of metastatic carcinoma (sarcomatoid renal cell or pulmonary carcinoma). Immunohistochemical panels for lymphoma and melanoma help to identify most of these entities. Sarcomatoid carcinomas can be keratin positive, and careful clinical evaluation to identify a primary mass often is necessary to exclude them.

The differential diagnosis of the mixed type of malignant mesothelioma includes mainly carcinosarcoma and biphasic synovial sarcoma. The presence of a dominant mass with sparing of pleura sways one heavily toward a nonmesothelial neoplasm; however, primary carcinosarcomas of the lung may rarely present as diffuse pleural thickening (165). Histology often is sufficiently different to avoid confusion; special procedures also may be helpful. Carcinosarcomas and synovial sarcomas share a proclivity for keratin (166) and epithelial membrane immunoreactivity (167, 168) with mesotheliomas, but they differ in that they may be CEA positive or positive for other glycoprotein markers that usually are negative in mesotheliomas. Electron microscopy may reveal differences in microvillous structure. Cytogenetics may be helpful for identifying synovial sarcoma.

APPROACH TO DIAGNOSIS

To assure a high level of accuracy in the diagnosis of mesothelioma, pathologists usually require knowledge of the clinical and radiologic features. Although a careful history of asbestos exposure is important in patients suspected of mesothelioma, the presence or absence of occupational asbestos exposure should not influence the pathologic diagnosis of malignant mesothelioma because it has no value in the individual case and because up to 40% or more of mesotheliomas are unassociated with an established history of asbestos exposure (5).

Certain features may render the diagnosis of mesothelioma less likely or highly unlikely (4). Clinically detected distant metastases, such as those in bone, liver, kidney, and brain early in the course of a tumor, i.e., at a time when there is minimal thickening of the pleura, are highly unusual in mesothelioma as are a high serum level of CEA and local invasion of rib, sternum, or thoracic vertebra. Absence of thickening of the pleura remote from a pleural-based mass radiologically and at thoracoscopy or thoracotomy should cause one to seriously question the diagnosis of mesothelioma. The corollary is that these features should be evaluated carefully and recorded by the surgeon or others directly viewing the pleura in situ. The gross characteristics and extent of abnormalities of both the parietal and visceral pleura should be defined and recorded.

Frozen section examination of tissue biopsies has a limited role in the diagnosis of mesothelioma. Difficulty in the distinction of epithelial mesothelioma from adenocarcinoma and mesothelial hyperplasia precludes routine use of this approach to diagnosis. Conversely, examination by frozen section to establish the adequacy of the biopsy or to evaluate the presence of recurrent/residual tumor in known cases is usually reliable. Moreover, examination in the frozen section room may assure appropriate division of tissue for pathologic studies, prompt fixation for ultrastructural study, and sterile tissue for cytogenetic or other special studies.

In earlier years an autopsy often was required to assure an accurate diagnosis of mesothelioma. However, with the application of multimodal approaches to pathologic diagnosis, it has become possible to achieve an accurate diagnosis of pleural mesothelioma with much smaller premortem specimens. Some conclude that an accurate diagnosis of mesothelioma can be made by cytologic examination of serous fluids alone (30, 33). Others favor examination of cytology specimens coupled with needle biopsy of the pleura (5, 17). This study yields positive findings in up to 80% of mesotheliomas (5). Thoracoscopy provides excellent samples for histologic studies and abets early diagnosis (1). Open thoracotomy usually is best reserved for cases not yielding a diagnosis by less invasive means. However, thoracotomy is frequently required to establish a diagnosis, especially in cases of desmoplastic mesothelioma, or to rule out mesothelioma in fibrosing pleuritis.

Accuracy of diagnosis with smaller samples, including effusions, has been abetted by the application of multiple modalities, specifically histochemical, immunochemical, and ultrastructural methods (4, 5, 17, 47, 51, 61). Immunohistochemical studies are the most powerful, but histochemical and ultrastructural approaches are also of established value. Although other newer techniques are still largely investigational, some, such as cytogenetics, have already achieved utility in special circumstances (139).

Autopsy examination is especially valuable in patients suspected of having pleural mesothelioma in whom the diagnosis of mesothelioma has not been established and in cases of adenocarcinoma metastatic to the pleura in which the primary site is unknown. The limitation of the autopsy is the delay in fixation of tissues, which may impede immunohistochemical and ultrastructural examinations. The proclivity of mesotheliomas late in their course to form large parenchymal masses or distant hematogenous metastases needs to be considered before excluding a diagnosis of mesothelioma. An added value of the autopsy is that it provides lung tissue for quantitative asbestos fiber analysis.

CONCLUSION

In the last decade, the application of a multimodal approach has made possible the diagnosis of mesothelioma on small tissue samples obtained by needle biopsy or thoracoscopy, or even on cytologic specimens, although open thoracotomy is still required for diagnosis in some cases. Evaluation of clinical and morphologic findings, coupled with the judicious application of histochemical, immunohistochemical, and electron microscopic methods now leads to a high level of diagnostic accuracy. Antibodies to glycoproteins aid greatly in excluding metastatic adenocarcinomas of the pleura, but still awaited is a monoclonal antibody with specificity for a mesothelioma antigen that is preserved in formalin-fixed, paraffin-embedded tissue. Distinction of mesothelial hyperplasia from mesothelioma is still based largely on morphologic criteria and may be difficult, necessitating extensive tissue sampling for diagnosis. Other modalities, including flow cytometry, image analysis, and cytogenetics, have been tested for their utility in diagnosis and prognosis, but additional studies are needed to define their role in the pathologic diagnosis and clinical management of pleural mesothelioma.

REFERENCES

1. Boutin CRF. Thoracoscopy in pleural malignant mesothelioma: a prospective study of 188 consecutive patients. Part 1: diagnosis. Cancer 1993;72:389–393.
2. Boutin C, Rey F, Gouvernet J, Viallat J, Astoul P, Ledoray V. Thoracoscopy in pleural malignant mesothelioma: a prospective study of 188 consecutive patients: Part 2: prognosis and staging. Cancer 1993;72:394–404.

3. McCaughey W, Kannerstein M, Churg J,. Tumors and pseudotumors of the serous membranes. 2nd ed. Washington, DC: Armed Forces Institute of Pathology, 1985.
4. Corson J. Pathology of malignant mesothelioma. In: Antman K, Aisner J, eds. Asbestos-related malignancy. New York: Grune & Stratton, 1987:179–199.
5. Henderson D, Shilkin KB, Whitaker D, et al. The pathology of malignant mesothelioma, including immunohistology and ultrastructure. In: Henderson D, Shilkin KB, Langlois S, Whitaker D, eds. Malignant mesothelioma. New York: Hemisphere Publishing, 1992:69–139.
6. Crotty T, Myers JL, Katzenstein ALA, Tazelaar HD, Swenson SJ, Churg A. Localized malignant mesothelioma: a clinicopathologic and flow cytometric study. Am J Surg Pathol 1994;18:357–363.
7. Ball M, Urbanski SJ, Green FHY, Kieser T. Pleural multicystic mesothelial proliferation. Am J Surg Pathol 1990;14:375–378.
8. Sussman J, Rosai J. Lymph node metastasis as the initial manifestation of malignant mesothelioma. Am J Surg Pathol 1990;14:819–828.
9. Sugarbaker D, Strauss G, Lynch T, et al. Node status has prognostic significance in the multimodality therapy of diffuse, malignant mesothelioma. J Clin Oncol 1993;11:1172–1178.
10. Roberts G. Distant visceral metastases in pleural mesothelioma. Br J Dis Chest 1976;70:246–250.
11. Elmes P, Simpson MJC. The clinical aspects of mesothelioma. Quart J Med 1976;179:427–449.
12. Falconieri G, Grandi G, DiBonito L, Bonifacio-Gori D, Giarelli L. Intracranial metastases from malignant pleural mesothelioma. Arch Pathol Lab Med 1991;115:591–595.
13. Uri A, Schulman E, Steiner R, Scott R, Rose L. Diffuse contralateral pulmonary metastases in malignant mesothelioma. Chest 1988;93:433–434.
14. Machin T, Mashiyama ET, Henderson JAM, McCaughey WTE. Bony metastases in desmoplastic pleural mesothelioma. Thorax 1988;43:155–156.
15. Hillerdal G. Malignant mesothelioma 1982: review of 4710 published cases. Br J Dis Chest 1983;77:321–343.
16. Manzini V, Brollo A, Franceschi S, De Matthaeis M, Talamini R, Bianchi C. Prognostic factors of malignant mesothelioma of the pleura. Cancer 1993;72:410–417.
17. Hammar S. Pleural diseases. In: Dail D, Hammar SP, eds. Pulmonary pathology. 2nd ed. New York: Springer-Verlag, 1994:1463–1579.
18. Kannerstein M, Churg J. Desmoplastic diffuse malignant mesothelioma. Prog Surg Pathol 1980;2:19–29.
19. Cantin R, Al-Jabi M, McCaughey WTE. Desmoplastic diffuse mesothelioma. Am J Surg Pathol 1982;6:215–222.
20. Wilson G, Hasleton PS, Chatterjee AK. Desmoplastic malignant mesothelioma: a review of 17 cases. J Clin Pathol 1992;45:295–298.
21. McCaughey W. Primary tumors of the pleura. J Pathol Bacteriol 1958;76:517–529.
22. Mayall F, Gibbs AR. The histology and immunohistochemistry of small cell mesothelioma. Histopathology 1992;20:47–51.
23. Henderson D, Attwood HD, Constance TJ, Shilkin KB, Steele RH. Lymphohistiocytoid mesothelioma: a rare lymphomatoid variant of predominantly sarcomatoid mesothelioma. Ultrastruct Pathol 1988;12:367–384.
24. Yousem S, Hochholzer L. Malignant mesotheliomas with osseous and cartilaginous differentiation. Arch Pathol Lab Med 1987;111:62–66.
25. Donna A, Betta PG. Differentiation towards cartilage and bone in a primary tumour of pleura. Further evidence in support of the concept of mesodermoma. Histopathology 1986;10:101–108.
26. Antman K, Corson JM. Benign and malignant mesotheliomas. In: Moosa A, Schimpff SC, Robson, MC, eds. Comprehensive textbook of oncology. 2nd ed. Baltimore: Williams & Wilkins, 1991:774–784.
27. Whitaker D, Shilkin KB. The cytology of malignant mesothelioma in western Australia. Acta Cytol 1978;22:67–70.
28. Sherman M, Mark EJ. Effusion cytology in the diagnosis of malignant epithelioid and biphasic pleural mesothelioma. Arch Pathol Lab Med 1990;114:845–851.
29. Whitaker D, Shilkin KB, Sterrett GF. Cytological appearances of malignant mesothelioma. In: Henderson DW, Shilkin KB, Langlois SLP, Whitaker D, eds. Malignant mesothelioma. New York: Hemisphere Publishing, 1992:167–182.
30. Stevens M, Leon AS, Fozzalari NC, Dawling KD, Henderson DW. Cytopathology of malignant mesothelioma: a stepwise regression analysis. Diagn Cytopathol 1992;8:333–341.
31. Cibas E, Corson J, Pinkus GS. The distinction of adenocarcinoma from malignant mesothelioma in cell blocks of effusions. Hum Pathol 1987;18:67–74.
32. Leong A, Parkinson R, Milios J. "Thick" cell membranes revealed by immunocytochemical staining: a clue to the diagnosis of mesothelioma. Diagn Cytopathol 1989;5:58–62.
33. Leong A, Stevens MW, Mukherjee TM. Malignant mesothelioma: cytologic diagnosis with histologic, immunohistochemical and ultrastructural correlation. Semin Diagn Pathol 1992;9:141–150.
34. Kobzik L, Antman KH, Warhol MJ. The distinction of mesothelioma from adenocarcinoma in malignant effusions by electron microscopy. Acta Cytol 1985;29:219–225.
35. Warhol M. Electron microscopy in the diagnosis of mesothelioma with routine biopsy, needle biopsy, and fluid cytology. In: Antman K, Aisner J, eds. Asbestos-related malignancy. New York: Grune & Stratton, 1987:201–221.
36. Cook H. Carbohydrates. In: Bancroft J, Stevens A, eds. Theory and practice of histological techniques. 3rd ed. New York: Churchill Livingstone, 1990:177–213.
37. Kannerstein M, Churg J, Magner D. Histochemistry in the diagnosis of malignant mesothelioma. Ann Clin Lab Sci 1973;3:207–211.
38. Triol J, Conston AS, Chandler SV. Malignant mesothelioma. Cytopathology of 75 cases seen in a New Jersey Community Hospital. Acta Cytol 1984;:37–45.
39. Triol J. Distinguishing adenocarcinoma from mesothelioma in effusions (letter). Hum Pathol 1987;18:969.
40. Robb J. Mesothelioma versus adenocarcinoma: false-positive CEA and Leu-M1 staining due to hyaluronic acid (letter). Hum Pathol 1989;20:400.
41. Kwee W, Veldhuizen RW, Golding RP, et. al. Histologic distinction between malignant mesothelioma, benign pleural lesion and carcinoma metastasis. Virchows Arch A Pathol Anat 1982;397:287–299.
42. Warnock M, Stoloff A, Thor A. Differentiation of adenocarcinoma of the lung from mesothelioma. Am J Pathol 1988;133:30–38.
43. Wick M, Loy T, Mills S, Legier J, Manivel C. Malignant epithelioid pleural mesothelioma versus peripheral pulmonary adenocarcinoma. Hum Pathol 1990;21:759–766.

44. MacDougall D, Wang S, Zidar B. Mucin-positive epithelial mesothelioma. Arch Pathol Lab Med 1992;116:874–880.
45. Griffiths M, Riddell RJ, Xipell JM. Malignant mesothelioma: a review of 35 cases with diagnosis and prognosis. Pathology 1980;12:591–603.
46. Kannerstein M, McCaughey WTE, Churg J, Selikoff I. A critique of the criteria for the diagnosis of diffuse malignant mesothelioma. Mt Sinai J Med 1977;44:485–494.
47. Roggli V, Sanfilippo F, Shelburne JD. Mesothelioma. In: Roggli V, Greenberg SD, Pratt PG, eds. Pathology of asbestos-associated diseases. Boston: Little, Brown, 1992:109–164.
48. Loosli H, Hurlimann J. Immunohistological study of malignant diffuse mesotheliomas of the pleura. Histopathology 1984;8:793–803.
49. Iozzo R, Goldes J, Chen W, Wight T. Glycosaminoglycans of pleural mesothelioma. Cancer 1981;48:89–97.
50. Nakano T, Fojii J, Tamura S, et al. Glycosaminoglycan in malignant pleural mesothelioma. Cancer 1986;57:106–110.
51. Bedrossian C, Bonsib S, Moran C. Differential diagnosis between mesothelioma and adenocarcinoma: a multimodal approach based on ultrastructural and immunocytochemistry. Semin Diagn Pathol 1992;9:124–140.
52. Moll R, Franke WW, Schiller DL, Geiger B, Krepler R. The catalog of human cytokeratins: patterns of expression in normal epithelia. Cell 1982;31:11–34.
53. Moll R, Lowe A, Laufer J, Franke W. Cytokeratin 20 in human carcinomas. Am J Pathol 1992;140:427–447.
54. Miettinen M. Keratin immunohistochemistry: update of applications and pitfalls. In Rosen PP, Fechner, RE, eds. Pathology annual. Norwalk, CT: Appleton & Lange, 1993;28(Part 2):113–143.
55. Schlegel R, Banks-Schlegel S, Pinkus GS. Immunohistochemical localization of keratin in normal human tissues. Lab Invest 1980;42:91.
56. Corson J, Pinkus GS. Mesothelioma: profile of keratin proteins and carcinoembryonic antigen. Am J Pathol 1982;108:80–87.
57. Ordonez N. The immunohistochemical diagnosis of mesothelioma. Am J Surg Pathol 1989;13:276–291.
58. Pinkus G, O'Connor E, Etheridge C, Corson J. Optimal immunoreactivity of keratin proteins in formalin-fixed, paraffin-embedded tissue requires preliminary trypsinization. J Histochem Cytochem 1985;33:465–473.
59. Battifora H, Kopinski M. The influence of protease digestion and duration of fixation on the immunostaining of keratins. A comparison of formalin and ethanol fixation. J Histochem Cytochem 1986;34:1095–1100.
60. Sheibani K, Esteban JM, Ailey, A, Battifora H, Weiss L. Immunopathologic and molecular studies as an aid to the diagnosis of malignant mesothelioma. Hum Pathol 1992;23:107–116.
61. Battifora H. The pleura. In: Sternberg S, ed. Diagnostic surgical pathology. 2nd ed. New York: Raven, 1994:1095–1123.
62. McCaughey W, Colby T, Battifora H, et al. Diagnosis of diffuse malignant mesothelioma: experience of a US/Canadian mesothelioma panel. Mod Pathol 1991;4:342–353.
63. Moll R, Dhouailly D, Sun, T. Expression of keratin 5 as a distinctive feature of epithelial and biphasic mesotheliomas. Virchows Arch B Cell Pathol 1989;58:129–145.
64. Corson J. Keratin protein immunohistochemistry in surgical pathology practice. In: Sommers S, Rosen PP, Fechner RE, eds. Pathology annual. Norwalk, CT: Appleton-Century-Crofts, 1986;21(Part 2):47–81.
65. Kahn H, Thorner P, Yeger H, Bailey D, Baumal R. Distinct keratin patterns demonstrated by immunoperoxidase staining of adenocarcinomas, carcinoids, and mesotheliomas using polyclonal and monoclonal anti-keratin antibodies. Am J Clin Pathol 1986;86:566–574.
66. Corson J, Pinkus G. Cellular localization patterns of keratin proteins in pleural mesotheliomas and metastatic adenocarcinomas: a diagnostic discriminant. Lab Invest 1991;114A.
67. Mullink H, Henzen-Logmans SC, Alons-Van Kordelaar JJM, Tadema TM, Meiter CJLM. Simultaneous immunoenzyme staining of vimentin and cytokeratins with monoclonal antibodies as an aid in the differential diagnosis of malignant mesothelioma from pulmonary adenocarcinoma. Virchows Arch A Pathol Anat 1986;52:55–65.
68. Brown R, Clark G, Tandon A, Allred C. Multiple-marker immunohistochemical phenotypes distinguishing malignant pleural mesothelioma from pulmonary adenocarcinoma. Hum Pathol 1993;24:347–354.
69. Wang N, Huang S, Gold P. Absence of carcinoembryonic antigen-like material in mesothelioma. Cancer 1979;44:937–943.
70. Whitaker D, Sterrett GF, Shilkin KB. Detection of tissue CEA-like substance as an aid in the differential diagnosis of malignant mesothelioma. Pathology 1982;14:255–258.
71. Said J, Nash G, Tepper G, Banks-Schlegel S. Keratin proteins and carcinoembryonic antigen in lung carcinoma. Hum Pathol 1983;14:70–76.
72. Marshall R, Herbert A, Braye SG, Jones DB. Use of antibodies to carcinoembryonic antigen and human milk fat globule to distinguish carcinoma, mesothelioma, and reactive mesothelium. J Clin Pathol 1984;37:1215–1221.
73. Holden J, Churg A. Immunohistochemical staining for keratin and carcinoembryonic antigen in the diagnosis of malignant mesothelioma. Am J Surg Pathol 1984;8:277–279.
74. Battifora H, Kopinski MI. Distinction of mesothelioma from adenocarcinoma. Cancer 1985;55:1679–1685.
75. Pfaltz M, Odermatt B, Christen B, Ruttner JR. Immunohistochemistry in the diagnosis of malignant mesothelioma. Virchows Arch A Pathol Anat Histopathol 1987;411:387–393.
76. Otis C, Carter D, Cole S, Battifora H. Immunohistochemical evaluation of pleural mesothelioma and pulmonary adenocarcinoma. Am J Surg Pathol 1987;11(6):445–456.
77. Mezger J, Lamerz R, Permanetter W. Diagnostic significance of carcinoembryonic antigen in the differential diagnosis of malignant mesothelioma. J Thorac Cardiovasc Surg 1990;100:860–866.
78. Wirth P, Legier J, Wright GL. Immunohistochemical evaluation of seven monoclonal antibodies for differentiation of pleural mesothelioma from lung adenocarcinoma. Cancer 1991;67:655–662.
79. Esteban J, Paxton R, Mehta P, Battifora H, Shively J. Sensitivity and specificity gold types 1 to 5 anti-carcinoembryonic antigen monoclonal antibodies. Hum Pathol 1993;24:322–328.
80. Hammarstrom S, Shively JE, Paxton RJ, et al. Antigenic sites in carcinoembryonic antigen. Cancer Res 1989;49:4852–4858.
81. Dejmek A, Hjerpe A. Carcinoembryonic antigen-like reactivity in malignant mesothelioma. Cancer 1994;73:464–469.
82. Primus F, Clark CA, Goldenberg DM. Immunohistochemical detection of carcinoembryonic antigen. In: DeLellis R, ed. Diagnostic immunohistochemistry. New York: Masson Publishing USA, 1981:263–277.
83. Stirling J. Unusual granular reactivity for carcinoembryonic antigen in malignant mesothelioma. Hum Pathol 1990;21:678–679.

84. Sheibani K, Battifora H, Burke JS, Rappaport H. Leu-M1 antigen in human neoplasms. Am J Surg Pathol 1986;10:227–236.
85. Sheibani K, Battifora H, Burke JS. Antigenic phenotype of malignant mesotheliomas and pulmonary adenocarcinomas. Am J Pathol 1986;123:212–219.
86. Pinkus G, Kurtin P. Epithelial membrane antigen: a diagnostic discriminant in surgical pathology. Hum Pathol 1985;16:929–940.
87. Szpak C, Johnston WW, Roggli V, et al. The diagnostic distinction between malignant mesothelioma of the pleura and adenocarcinoma of the lung as defined by a monoclonal antibody (B72.3). Am J Pathol 1986;122:252–260.
88. Latza U, Niedobitek G, Schwarting R, Nekarda H, Stein H. Ber-EP4: new monoclonal antibody which distinguishes epithelia from mesothelia. J Clin Pathol 1990;43:213–219.
89. Sheibani K, Shin SS, Kezirian J, Weiss LM. Ber-EP4 antibody as a discriminant in the differential diagnosis of malignant mesothelioma versus adenocarcinoma. Am J Surg Pathol 1991;15:779–784.
90. Gaffey M, Mills SE, Swanson PE, Zarbo RJ, Shah AR, Wick MR. Immunoreactivity for BER-EP4 in adenocarcinomas, adenomatoid tumors, and malignant mesotheliomas. Am J Surg Pathol 1992;16:593–599.
91. Maguire B, Whitaker D, Carrello S, Spagnolo D. Monoclonal antibody Ber-EP4: its use in the differential diagnosis of malignant mesothelioma and carcinoma in cell blocks of malignant effusions and FNA specimens. Diagn Cytopathol 1994;10:130–134.
92. Lee I, Radosevich JA, Chejfec G, et al. Malignant mesotheliomas. Am J Pathol 1986;123:497–507.
93. Kawai T, Greenberg SD, Truong LD, Mattioli CA, Klima M, Titus JL. Differences in lectin binding of malignant pleural mesothelioma and adenocarcinoma of the lung. Am J Pathol 1988;130:401–410.
94. Noguchi M, Nakajima T, Hirohashi S, Akiba T, Shimosato Y. Immunohistochemical distinction of malignant mesothelioma from pulmonary adenocarcinoma with anti-surfactant apoprotein, anti-Lewis[a], and anti-Tn antibodies. Hum Pathol 1989;20:53–57.
95. Jordon D, Jagirdar J, Kaneko M. Blood group antigens, Lewis[x] and Lewis[y] in the diagnostic discrimination of malignant mesothelioma versus adenocarcinoma. Am J Pathol 1989;135:931–937.
96. Koukoulis G, Radosevich JA, Warren WH, Rosen ST, Gould VE. Immunohistochemical analysis of pulmonary and pleural neoplasms with monoclonal antibodies B72.3 and CSLEX-1. Virchows Arch B Cell Pathol 1990;58:427–433.
97. Spagnolo D, Whitaker D, Carrello S, Radosevich JA, Rosen ST, Gould VE. The use of monoclonal antibody 44-3A6 in cell blocks in the diagnosis of lung carcinoma, carcinomas metastatic to lung and pleura, and pleural malignant mesothelioma. Am J Clin Pathol 1991;95:322–329.
98. Stahel R, O'Hara CJ, Waibel R, Martin A. Monoclonal antibodies against mesothelial membrane antigen discriminate between mesothelioma and lung adenocarcinoma. Int J Cancer 1988;41:218–223.
99. O'Hara C, Corson JM, Pinkus GS, Stahel RA. ME1: a monoclonal antibody that distinguishes epithelial-type malignant mesothelioma from pulmonary adenocarcinoma and extrapulmonary malignancies. Am J Pathol 1990;136:421–428.
100. Chang K, Pai LH, Pass H, et al. Monoclonal antibody K1 reacts with epithelial mesothelioma but not with lung adenocarcinoma. Am J Surg Pathol 1992;16:259–268.
101. Donna A, Betta PG, Jones JS. Verification of the histologic diagnosis of malignant mesothelioma in relation to the binding of an antimesothelial cell antibody. Cancer 1989;63:1331–1336.
102. Anderson T, Holmes EC, Kosaka CJ, Cheng L, Saxton RE. Monoclonal antibodies to human malignant mesothelioma. J Clin Immunol 1987;7:254–261.
103. Hsu S, Hsu PL, Zhao X, et al. Establishment of human mesothelioma cell lines (MS-1, -2) and production of a monoclonal antibody (anti-MS) with diagnostic and therapeutic potential. Cancer 1988;48:5228–5236.
104. Collins C, Ordonez NG, Schaefer R, et al. Thrombomodulin expression in malignant pleural mesothelioma and pulmonary adenocarcinoma. J Pathol 1992;141:827–833.
105. Coleman M, Henderson DW, Mukherjee TM. The ultrastructural pathology of malignant pleural mesothelioma. In: Rosen PP, Fechner RE, eds. Pathology annual. Norwalk, CT: Appleton & Lange, 1989;24(Part 1);303–353.
106. Henderson D. Transmission electron microscopy of malignant mesothelioma. Microsc Soc Am Bull 1993;23:288–297.
107. Wang N. Electron microscopy in the diagnosis of pleural mesothelioma. Cancer 1973;31:1046–1054.
108. Suzuki Y, Churg J, Kannerstein M. Ultrastructure of human malignant diffuse mesothelioma. Am J Pathol 1976;85:241–262.
109. Warhol M, Hickey WF, Corson JM. Malignant mesothelioma: ultrastructural distinction from adenocarcinoma. Am J Surg Pathol 1982;6:307–314.
110. Dewar A, Valente M, Ring NP, Corrin B. Pleural mesothelioma of epithelial type and pulmonary adenocarcinoma: an ultrastructural and cytochemical comparison. J Pathol 1987;152:309–316.
111. Carstens H. Contact between abluminal microvilli and collagen fibrils in metastatic adenocarcinoma and mesothelioma. J Pathol 1992;166:179–182.
112. Ghadially F, McCaughey WTE, Perkins DG, Rippstein P, Jeans D. Morphogenesis and frequency of microvillus-matrix associations in mesotheliomas and adenocarcinomas. Microsc Soc Am Bull 1993;23:281–287.
113. Burns T, Greenberg SD, Mace ML, Johnson EH. Ultrastructural diagnosis of epithelial malignant mesothelioma. Cancer 1985;56:2036–2040.
114. Roggli V, Kolbeck J, Sanfilippo F, Shelburne JD. Pathology of human mesothelioma: etiologic and diagnostic considerations. In: Rosen PP, Fechner, RE, eds. Pathology annual. Norwalk, CT: Appleton & Lange, 1987;22(Part 2):91–131.
115. Jandik W, Landas SK, Bray CK, Lager DJ. Scanning electron microscopic distinction of pleural mesotheliomas from adenocarcinomas. Mod Pathol 1993;6:761–764.
116. Warhol M, Hunter NJ, Corson JM. An ultrastructural comparison of mesotheliomas and adenocarcinomas of the ovary and endometrium. Int J Gynaecol Pathol 1982;1:125–134.
117. Dardick I, Jabi M, McCaughey WTE, Deodhare S, van Nostrand AWP, Srigley JR. Diffuse epithelial mesothelioma: a review of the ultrastructural spectrum. Ultrastruct Pathol 1987;11:503–533.
118. Burmer G, Rabinovitch PS, Kulander BG, Rusch V, McNutt MA. Flow cytometric analysis of malignant pleural mesotheliomas. Hum Pathol 1989;20:777–783.
119. El-Naggar A, Ordonez NG, Garnsey L, Batsakis JG. Epithelioid pleural mesotheliomas and pulmonary adenocarcinomas. Hum Pathol 1991;22:972–978.

120. Esteban J, Sheibani K. DNA ploidy analysis of pleural mesotheliomas: its usefulness for their distinction from lung adenocarcinomas. Mod Pathol 1992;5:626–630.
121. Frierson H, Mills SE, Legier JF. Flow cytometric analysis of ploidy in immunohistochemically confirmed examples of malignant epithelial mesothelioma. Am J Clin Pathol 1988;90:240–243.
122. Dazzi H, Thatcher N, Haselton PS, Chatterjee AK, Lawson RAM. DNA analysis by flow cytometry in malignant pleural mesothelioma: relationship to histology and survival. J Pathol 1990;162:51–55.
123. Croonen A, van der Valk P, Herman CJ, Lindeman J. Cytology, immunopathology and flow cytometry in the diagnosis of pleural and peritoneal effusions. Lab Invest 1988;58:725–732.
124. Esteban J, Sheibani K, Owens M, Joyce J, Bailey A, Battifora H. Effects of various fixatives and fixation conditions on DNA ploidy and analysis. Am J Clin Pathol 1991;95:460–466.
125. Kwee W, Veldhuizen RW, Alons CA, Morawetz F, Boon ME. Quantitative and qualitative differences between benign and malignant mesothelial cells in pleural fluid. Acta Cytol 1982;26:401–406.
126. Marchevsky A, Gil J, Caccamo D. Computerized interactive morphometry. A study of malignant mesothelioma and mesothelial hyperplasia in pleural biopsy specimens. Arch Pathol Lab Med 1985;109:1102–1105.
127. Marchevsky A, Hauptman E, Gil J, Watson C. Computerized interactive morphometry as an aid in the diagnosis of pleural effusions. Acta Cytol 1987;31:131–136.
128. Dardick I, Butler EB, Dardick AM. Quantitative ultrastructural study of nuclei from exfoliated benign and malignant mesothelial cells and metastatic adenocarcinoma. Acta Cytol 1986;30:379–384.
129. Hafiz M, Becker RL, Mikel UV, Bahr GF. Cytophotometric determination of DNA in mesotheliomas and reactive mesothelial cells. Acta Cytol 1988;10:120–126.
130. Tierney G, Wilkinson MJ, Jones JSP. The malignancy grading method is not a reliable assessment of malignancy in mesothelioma. J Pathol 1990;160:209–211.
131. Gibas Z, Li FP, Antman KH, Bernal S, Stahel R, Sandberg AA. Chromosome changes in malignant mesothelioma. Cancer Genet Cytogenet 1986;20:191–201.
132. Popescu N, Chahinian AP, DiPaolo JA. Nonrandom chromosome alterations in human malignant mesothelioma. Cancer Res 1988;48:142–147.
133. Pelin-Enlund K, Husgafvel-Pursiainen K, Tammilehto L, et al. Asbestos-related malignant mesothelioma: growth, cytology, tumorigenicity and consistent chromosome findings in cell lines from five patients. Carcinogenesis 1990;11:673–681.
134. Tiainen M, Tammilehto L, Mattson K, Knuutila S. Nonrandom chromosomal abnormalities in malignant pleural mesothelioma. Cancer Genet Cytogenet 1988;33:251–274.
135. Tiainen M, Tammilehtol L, Rautonen J, Tumoi T, Mattson K, Knoulita S. Chromosomal abnormalities and their correlations with asbestos exposure and survival in patients with mesothelioma. Br J Cancer 1989;60:618–626.
136. Hagemeijer A, Versnel MA, Van Drunen E, et al. Cytogenetic analysis of malignant mesothelioma. Cancer Genet Cytogenet 1990;47:1–28.
137. Fletcher J, Cibas E, Granados R, et al. Consistent chromosome aberrations and genetic stability in malignant mesotheliomas (MM): diagnostic relevance (abstract). Lab Invest 1991;64:114A.
138. Fletcher J, Kozakewich HP, Hoffer FA, et al. Diagnostic relevance of clonal cytogenetic aberrations in malignant soft-tissue tumors. N Engl J Med 1991;324:436–443.
139. Karn C, Socinski MA, Fletcher JA, Corson JM, Craighead JE. Cardiac synovial sarcoma with translocation (X:18) associated with asbestos exposure. Cancer 1994;73:74–78.
140. Whitaker D, Henderson DW, Shilkin KB. The concept of mesothelioma in-situ: implications for diagnosis and histogenesis. Semin Diagn Pathol 1992;9:151–161.
141. Whitaker D, Shilkin KB. Diagnosis of pleural malignant mesothelioma in life: a practical approach. J Pathol 1984;143:147–175.
142. Harwood T, Gracey DR, Yokoo H. Pseudomesotheliomatous carcinoma of the lung: a variant of peripheral lung cancer. Am J Clin Path 1976;65:159–167.
143. Dessy E, Pietra GG. Pseudomesotheliomatous carcinoma of the lung. Cancer 1991;68:1747–1753.
144. Koss M, Travis W, Moran C, Hochholzer L. Pseudomesotheliomatous adenocarcinoma: a reappraisal. Semin Diagn Pathol 1992;9:117–123.
145. Chernow B, Sahn SA. Carcinomatous involvement of the pleura: an analysis of 96 patients. Am J Med 1977;63:695–702.
146. Whitwell F, Rawcliffe RM. Diffuse malignant pleural mesothelioma and asbestos exposure. Thorax 1971;26:6–22.
147. Taylor D, Page W, Hughes D, Varghese G. Metastatic renal cell carcinoma mimicking pleural mesothelioma. Thorax 1987;42:901–902.
148. Merino M, Kennedy SM, Norton JA, Robbins J. Pleural involvement by metastatic thyroid carcinoma "tall cell variant": an unusual occurrence. Surg Pathol 1990;3:59–64.
149. Mizukami Y, Michigishi T, Nonomura A, et al. Distant metastases in differentiated thyroid carcinomas. Hum Pathol 1990;21:283–290.
150. Cagle P, Wessels R, Greenberg SD. Concurrent mesothelioma and adenocarcinoma of the lung in a patient with asbestosis. Mod Pathol 1993;6:438–441.
151. Yousem S, Hochholzer L. Unusual thoracic manifestations of epithelioid hemangioendothelioma. Arch Pathol Lab Med 1987;111:459–463.
152. Battifora H. Epithelioid hemangioendothelioma imitating mesothelioma. Appl Immunocytochem 1993;1:220–222.
153. Meis J, Mackay B, Ordonez NG. Epithelioid sarcoma: an immunohistochemical and ultrastructural study. Surg Pathol 1988;1:13–31.
154. Bolen J, Hammar SP, McNutt MA. Reactive and neoplastic serosal tissue. Am J Surg Pathol 1986;10:34–47.
155. Montag A, Pinkus GS, Corson J. Keratin protein immunoreactivity of sarcomatoid and mixed types of diffuse malignant mesothelioma. Hum Pathol 1988;19:336–342.
156. Cagle P, Truong LD, Roggli VL, Greenberg SD. Immunohistochemical differentiation of sarcomatoid mesotheliomas from other spindle cell neoplasms. Am J Clin Pathol 1989;92:566–571.
157. Briselli M, Mark EJ, Dickersin GR. Solitary fibrous tumors of the pleura. Cancer 1981;47:2678–2689.
158. England D, Hochholzer L, McCarthy MJ. Localized benign and malignant fibrous tumors of the pleura. Am J Surg Pathol 1989;13:640–658.
159. Epstein J, Budin RE. Keratin and epithelial membrane antigen immunoreactivity in nonneoplastic fibrous pleural lesions. Hum Pathol 1986;17:514–519.
160. Carter D, Otis CN. Three types of spindle cell tumors of the pleura. Am J Surg Pathol 1988;12:747–753.

161. Renshaw A, Pinkus GS, Corson JM. CD34 and AE1/AE3. Appl Immunohistochem 1994;2:94–102.
162. Said J, Nash G, Banks-Schlegel S, Sassoon A, Shintaku IP. Localized fibrous mesothelioma. Hum Pathol 1984;15:440–443.
163. Dervan P, Tobin B, O'Connor M. Solitary (localized) fibrous mesothelioma: evidence against mesothelial cell origin. Histopathology 1986;10:867–875.
164. Westra W, Gerald WL, Rosai J. Two novel observations on solitary fibrous tumor: consistent CD34 immunoreactivity and occurrence in the orbit. 1994;18:992–998.
165. Mayall F, Gibbs AR. "Pleural" and pulmonary carcinosarcomas. J Pathol 1992;167:305–311.
166. Corson J, Weiss LM, Banks-Schlegel SP, Pinkus GS. Keratins proteins and carcinoembryonic antigen in synovial sarcomas. Hum Pathol 1984;15:615–621.
167. Fisher C. Synovial sarcoma: ultrastructural and immunohistochemical features of epithelial differentiation in monophasic and biphasic tumors. Hum Pathol 1986;17:996–1008.
168. Ordonez N, Soheir MM, Mackay B. Synovial sarcoma: an immunohistochemical and ultrastructural study. Hum Pathol 1990;21:733–749.

36

DIAGNOSIS, STAGING, AND NATURAL HISTORY OF PLEURAL MESOTHELIOMA

Joseph Aisner

INTRODUCTION

Malignant pleural mesothelioma is a rare tumor that was brought to epidemiologic and clinical attention in 1959 when it was linked to asbestos exposure in the workplace (1). In the past, mesothelioma was often difficult to identify, and, consequently, patients were diagnosed late in the natural history of the tumor. Many pathologists thought that the diagnosis could only be made by exclusion of other primary tumors, and the presence of this disease as a discrete entity was debated well into this century (2). Because mesothelioma often was included with lung cancers, the incidence of mesothelioma has been difficult to determine. Recently, it has been estimated that there are 3000 cases seen annually in the United States, and the number of cases is expected to increase because of the large number of individuals who have potentially been exposed to asbestos in the workplace, at home, or in the general environment.

With the recognition of an at-risk population and the identification of specific pathologic criteria for establishing the diagnosis (3–5), many patients now are diagnosed with an earlier presentation or stage of disease. This earlier presentation has allowed for the development of many diagnostic and therapeutic approaches, some of which offer promising outcomes. For afflicted individuals to benefit from the newer approaches, it is necessary to understand the various presentations of this disease, identify the disease, and obtain appropriate diagnostic materials. Because mesothelioma remains a rare tumor and controlled trials comparing diagnostic methods and treatments are unlikely, it is necessary to understand the natural history of the disease. Such an understanding could allow for a relative perspective about the outcomes of current interventions.

PRESENTATION

In the formation of mesotheliomas and other asbestos-related cancers, it generally is thought that thin, small, needlelike asbestos fibers are inhaled and make their way to the terminal alveoli (6). The fibers then migrate through the alveolar wall distally to the pleural surfaces, where they generate an inflammatory response (7). The fibers may be engulfed anywhere in the course of their migration by macrophages that are damaged in the process of ingesting the fibers, thus leaking cytokines, oxidants, and other bioactive substances (8). The fibers also may carry absorbed carcinogens, enhancing the formation of various cancers. Lung cancer, head and neck cancers, gastrointestinal cancers, and lymphoproliferative tumors also have been reported to occur at higher than expected rates among asbestos-exposed individuals (9–12).

Because of the association with workplace exposure, pleural mesothelioma occurs 5 to 10 times more frequently among men than women. The median age of presentation is approximately 60 years, reflecting the relatively long latency period, but there is a wide age range. Younger individuals and women often have household exposures. Because of the pleural reactions described previously, signs and symptoms associated with pleural effusion (e.g., dyspnea, shortness of breath or nonpleuritic chest pain) most often bring the patients to medical attention. Examination at this stage usually demonstrates dullness at one lung base, and chest roentgenograms show a large, unilateral, freely moveable effusion. Right-sided involvement is more common than left by a ratio of 3 to 2, and bilateral involvement is unusual. The chest roentgenogram shows pleural plaques, pleural or diaphragmatic calcifications, and other signs of asbestosis in only a minority of patients. Sputum cytology specimens may show ferruginous bodies (also known as asbestos bodies) in a higher percentage of cases. Computed tomography (CT) scans and pathologic specimens, however, show a much higher percentage of such asbestos exposure features.

Fever, sweats, weight loss, and declining performance status are common presenting complaints (13), although they tend to indicate more advanced disease and are associated with a shortened survival. Occasionally, asymptomatic patients are found by incidental findings on a routine chest roentgenogram (14). Thrombocytosis (15, 16), disseminated intravascular coagulation, thrombophlebitis, pulmonary emboli, and Coomb's positive hemolytic anemia also have been reported (17). The coagulation disturbances are seen more often with peritoneal than with pleural mesothelioma, however. Hypercalcemia with a parathormone-like activity has been reported as well (18).

Diagnostic studies such as CT scans can show pleural effusion, thickened pleura or a pleural rind, pericardial thickening, and loss of lung volume. With more advanced disease, the lung becomes fixed, and there can be chest wall contraction and scoliosis.

DIAGNOSTIC METHODS AND TECHNIQUES

Chest roentgenograms are usually the first diagnostic test performed on patients presenting with signs of disease. Such roentgenograms show evidence of asbestos exposure, such as pleural plaques or calcifications in the diaphragm, in only approximately 20% of cases. Findings of asbestosis can be very helpful in raising the index of suspicion for mesothelioma. However, asbestosis is a sufficient, although not a necessary, precondition for the formation of mesothelioma, i.e., patients with minimal asbestos exposure can develop malignant mesothelioma.

The use of CT scans in preoperative assessment has been well defined. A CT scan of the chest provides the best preoperative assessment in defining the extent of disease (19), and it is an important tool in defining therapeutic options. Common CT findings include thickening of the pleura and intralobar fissure, large effusions, atelectasis, and pericardial thickening (20–25). Pleural and diaphragmatic calcifications are seen on CT scans in only 20% to 50% of patients. There remains a large differential diagnosis for pleural effusions and pleural thickening, including benign inflammatory diseases, metastatic tumor, and primary pleural tumors. Although a CT scan may suggest a malignant etiology for the pleural disease, it does not distinguish between a primary and a metastatic etiology.

Magnetic resonance imaging (MRI) scans also have been studied to define more accurately the extent of disease preoperatively. In some cases, MRI scans using coronal images were very useful in demonstrating the extent of tumor invasion into adjacent structures such as the pericardium, diaphragm, chest wall, and vertebral bodies (26, 27). This technique has permitted a better assessment of potential operability. MRI thus may be useful as an adjunct to CT scaning when surgery is contemplated. Overall, however, the role of MRI scanning as a routine method of staging has not been well established.

To confirm the presence of mesothelioma and to distinguish it from metastases to the pleura, more invasive techniques are needed to obtain tissue. Most patients undergo repeated thoracenteses that usually fail to establish the diagnosis. Fine-needle aspirates and core-needle biopsies also typically fail to yield diagnostic material because of the small specimens obtained. Immunocytochemistry and electron microscopy of cytology preparations have been used successfully by a few laboratories in establishing the diagnosis (28–30). Most pathologists, however, usually require larger tissue samples to perform the special histochemistry and electron microscopy needed to make the diagnosis (3–5). Thoracoscopy and pleuroscopy have been used with considerable success in obtaining adequate amounts of tissue for diagnosis (31, 32). Boutin et al. (31, 33) showed that thoracoscopy was nearly 95% as accurate as open thoracotomy for obtaining a diagnosis of mesothelioma. With thoracotomy and thoracoscopy, discreet nodules and coalescent plaques are seen on the visceral and parietal pleura in early disease. As the disease progresses, the nodules coalesce and form a thick pleural rind.

On histologic evaluation, three subtypes of mesothelioma usually are identified: an epithelial, a sarcomatous, and a mixed type (34, 35). The epithelial subtype is seen most commonly, accounting for one half to two thirds of all cases. The sarcomatous form is the least frequent subtype. The mixed or biphasic form demonstrates both epithelial and sarcomatous elements. The finding of both elements is virtually diagnostic of malignant mesothelioma. The epithelial form needs to be distinguished from adenocarcinoma metastatic from the lung, breast, ovary, stomach, kidney, or prostate. Today, there are excellent criteria for the pathologic diagnosis of mesothelioma, as discussed in Chapter 35 (36).

NATURAL HISTORY

Early in the course of the disease, one costophrenic angle becomes blunted by an early pleural effusion. At this time patients rarely are symptomatic, and according to Boutin et al. (37), pleuroscopy is likely to show only parietal pleural involvement. The pleural effusions accumulate, and the pleura thickens to form a rind of tumor that progressively encases the lung as it grows (38). The pleural rind fixes the lung and diaphragmatic and intercostal muscles, producing a so-called frozen chest. Clinically, there is no chest or intercostal muscle movement, and physical examination shows considerable dullness to percussion, mediastinal shift, and bulging masses. Chest contraction and scoliosis can occur. Growth of the mesothelioma continues locally until late in the natural history; metastases are seen unusually premortem but occur in up to 30% at autopsy (39). Dysphagia, chest pain, cord compression, plexopathy, Horner's syndrome, or superior vena cava syndrome can arise from extension into the esophagus, ribs, vertebrae, nerves, and superior vena cava (13, 14, 30, 40).

A unique feature of this tumor is its propensity to grow out of surgical scars, and drainage and thoracotomy tracts (38, 31–43). Extension into the pulmonary parenchyma, chest wall, mediastinum, and diaphragm are common as the disease progresses (Figs. 36.1 through 36.3). Symptomatically, the patient may complain of fatigue and dyspnea with the dyspnea being out of proportion to the roentgenographic findings. This

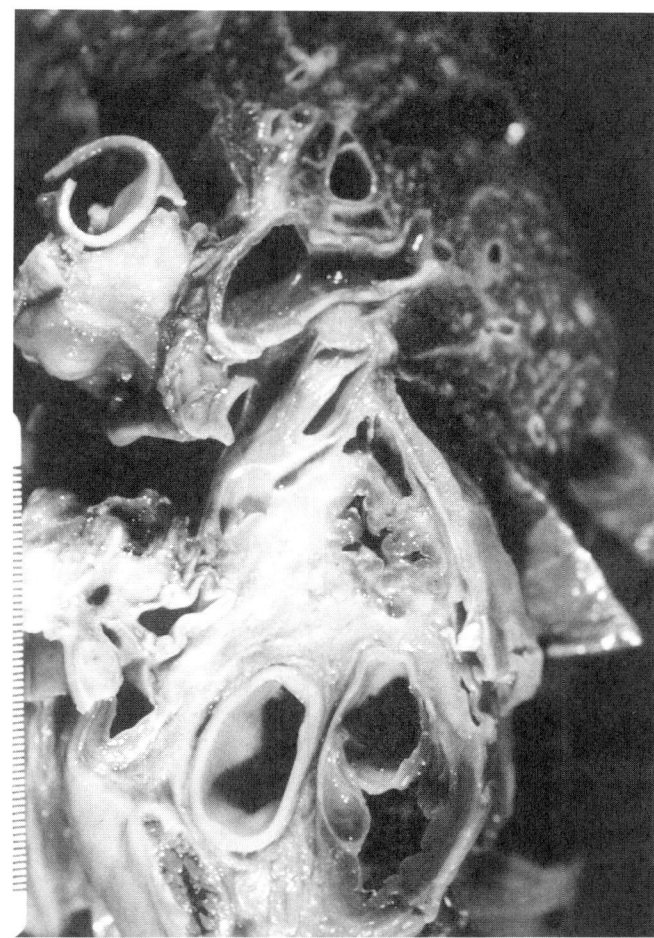

FIGURE 36.2. Mediastinal infiltration of mesothelioma involving the superior vena cava and base of heart. Complete blockage occurred with cardiopulmonary failure. (From Aisner J, Antman KH, Belani CP. Tumors of the pleura and mediastinum. In: Abeloff MA, Armitage J, Lichter AS, eds. Science of clinical oncology. New York: Churchill Livingstone, 1995.)

excessive dyspnea probably is caused by the significant atrioventricular shunting of poorly aerated blood in the trapped lung. Invasion into the mediastinum can produce cardiopulmonary failure (Fig. 36.2). If the disease penetrates the diaphragm, the disease can spread easily throughout the peritoneal cavity, producing a variety of problems such as malabsorption syndromes and bowel obstruction (Fig. 36.3).

The median duration of survival has been reported to range from 4 to 18 months, with most reports suggesting a less than 2-year survival for all patients. Anecdotal reports of prolonged survival, with and without therapy, have confounded the interpretation of the literature. Part of the difficulty in defining the natural history rests in an incomplete understanding of the biology and behavior of this tumor. Few series have sufficient numbers of patients to allow performance of the necessary statistical regressions to identify the impor-

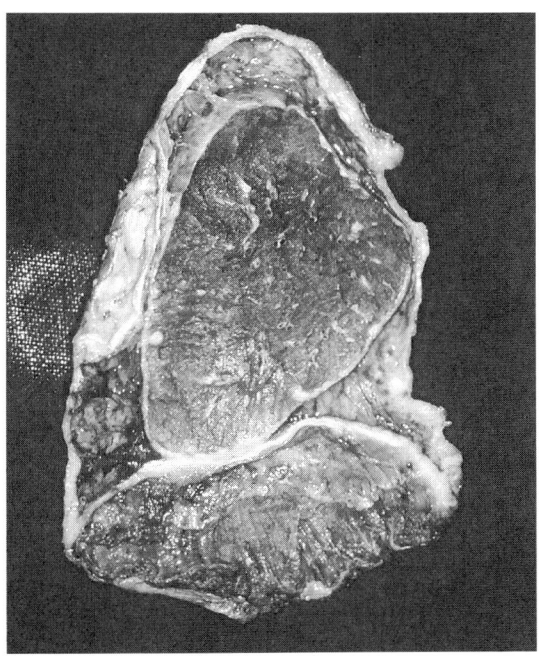

FIGURE 36.1. Resected lung showing thick rind of tumor encasing entire lung and trapping its expansion. Also illustrated is the extension of the pleural tumor into adjacent lung from the visceral pleura. Attempts to remove the visceral pleura would obviously leave residual tumor on the pulmonary surface. (From Aisner J, Antman KH, Belani CP. Tumors of the pleura and mediastinum. In: Abeloff MA, Armitage J, Lichter AS, eds. Science of clinical oncology. New York: Churchill Livingstone, 1995).

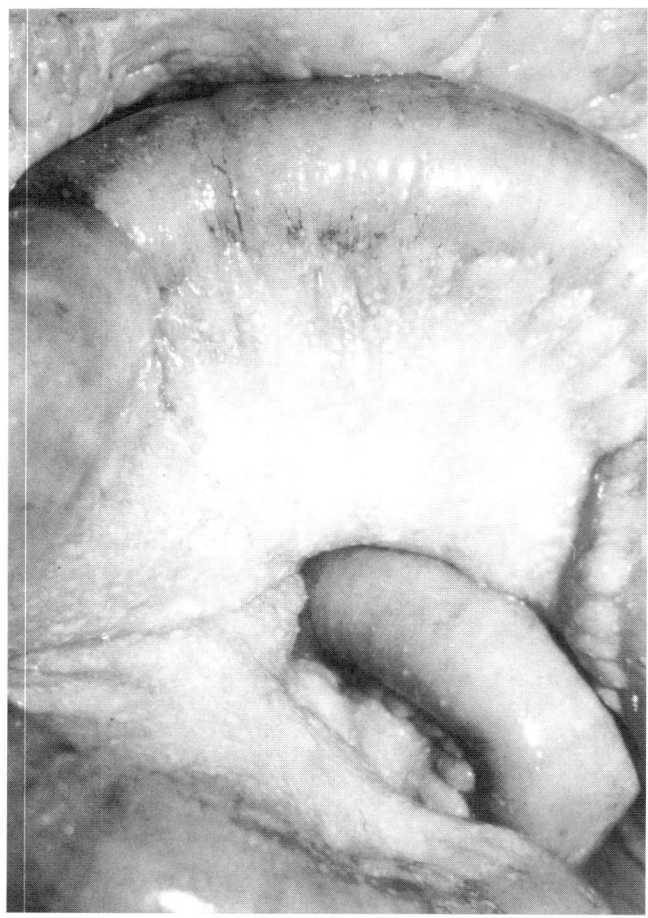

FIGURE 36.3. Invasion of pleural mesothelioma through the diaphragm and invading the mesentery, producing bowel obstruction. (From Aisner J, Antman KH, Belani CP. Tumors of the pleura and mediastinum. In: Abeloff MA, Armitage J, Lichter AS, eds. Science of clinical oncology. New York: Churchill Livingstone, 1995.)

TABLE 36.1. Butchart Staging Classification

STAGE	
I	Tumor confined within the capsule of the parietal pleura, involving only ipsilateral pleura, lung, pericardium, and diaphragm
II	Tumor invading chest wall or involving mediastinal structures, such as esophagus, heart, or opposite pleura
III	Tumor penetrating diaphragm to involve peritoneum; involvement of opposite pleura Lymph node involvement outside the chest
IV	Distant blood-borne metastases

tant prognostic factors. From some reports, better survival appears to correlate with younger age (43, 44), good performance status (28), early stage (45), epithelial histology (43, 46), lack of chest pain (43, 47), and a normal platelet count (43–46). Further study of the prognostic factors from large single-institution experiences or cooperative databases using multivariate regression analyses may allow some suggestions about the important pretreatment prognostic factors.

STAGING

Ideally, a staging system should define different categories of disease that can discriminate among potential outcomes and help decide between therapeutic options. The Butchart staging system (48), illustrated in Table 36.1, was the first to define a staging system based on a surgical series, and it currently is the most widely used for staging pleural mesothelioma. Unfortunately, the Butchart staging system does not discriminate adequately among some of the stages in predicting survival outcomes. For example, this staging system, although identifying a group of potential candidates for surgery, does not offer an adequate description of known prognostic factors such as lymph node involvement (49) or the degree of chest wall invasion. Mattson (50) developed a modification of the Butchart staging system, but it too lacked the descriptors that discriminate clinical outcome. To deal with these potential shortcomings, Chahinian (51) and subsequently the International Union Against Cancer (UICC) (52) developed a tumor, node, metastasis (TNM)–based staging system. The latter is shown in Table 36.2. The Chahinian and UICC staging systems included the extent of local invasion and the involvement of regional lymph nodes. To simplify the UICC system, the TNM categories were then collapsed into numerical stages, I through IV, using criteria similar to those used for non–small cell lung cancer (Table 36.2).

Despite the staging system proposals, there are few prospective trials to validate the clinical predictive value of the UICC or other staging systems. Although this paucity of trials in part results from the rarity of the tumor, the lack of a uniform staging system retards the potential comparisons of outcomes. To meet the need for an internationally accepted staging system, the International Mesothelioma Interest Group (IMIG)—composed of pulmonary physicians, thoracic surgeons, medical and radiation oncologists, radiologists, pathologists, and laboratory researchers with an interest in mesothelioma—met in Colorado Springs in 1994 during the VIIth International Lung Cancer Congress. The purpose of the meeting was to compare group and individual institutional experiences in staging and treatment of pleural mesothelioma. Based on a consensus from that meeting, a new staging system was proposed recently (53); it reconciles prior systems,

TABLE 36.2. UICC Staging of Mesothelioma

DEFINITIONS

T—Primary tumor and extent
- TX Primary tumor cannot be assessed
- T0 No evidence of primary tumor
- T1 Primary tumor limited to ipsilateral parietal and/or visceral pleura
- T2 Tumor invades any of the following: ipsilateral lung, endothoracic fascia, diaphragm, pericardium
- T3 Tumor invades any of the following: ipsilateral chest wall muscle, ribs, mediastinal organs or tissues
- T4 Tumor extends to any of the following: contralateral pleura or lung by direct extension, peritoneum or intraabdominal organs by direct extension, cervical tissues

N—lymph nodes
- NX Regional lymph nodes cannot be assessed
- N0 No regional lymph node metastases
- N1 Metastases in ipsilateral bronchopulmonary or hilar lymph nodes
- N2 Metastases in ipsilateral mediastinal lymph nodes
- N3 Metastases in contralateral mediastinal internal mammary, supraclavicular, or scalene lymph nodes

M—Metastases
- MX Presence of distant metastases cannot be assessed
- M0 No (known) distant metastases
- M1 Distant metastasis present

STAGE	TNM CLASSIFICATION
I	T1, N0, M0
	T2, N0, M0
II	T1, N1, M0
	T2, N1, M0
III	T3, N0, M0
	T3, N1, M0
	T1, N2, M0
	T2, N2, M0
	T3, N2, M0
IV	Any T, N3, M0
	T4, any N, M0
	Any T and N, M1

Note. Staging solely on clinical measures is designated cTNM. Staging that can be done on pathologic information is designated pTNM.

TABLE 36.3. International Mesothelioma Interest Group Staging System

DEFINITIONS

T—Primary tumor and extent
- TX Primary tumor cannot be assessed
- T0 No evidence of primary tumor
- T1a Tumor limited to ipsilateral plema parietal with or without involvement of mediastinal pleura and/or diaphragmatic pleura; no involvement of the visceral pleura
- T1b Tumor involving the ipsilateral pleura with or without mediastinal involvement of pleura and/or diaphragmatic pleura; tumor also involves the visceral pleura
- T2 Tumor involving each of the ipsilateral pleural surfaces (parietal, mediastinal, diaphragmatic, and visceral) with at least one of the following features: involvement of the underlying ipsilateral lung or diaphragmatic muscle
- T3 Tumor is locally advanced but potentially resectable. Tumor involves all of the ipsilateral pleural surfaces and invades at least one of the following: endothoracic fascia, mediastinal fat, isolated segment of ipsilateral chest wall, pericardium but not transmural pericardium
- T4 Unresectable local tumor. Tumor involves all of the ipsilateral pleural surfaces and extends to at least one of the following: diffuse extension or multifocal masses on the chest wall with or without rib destruction, direct trans-diaphragmatic extension of tumor to the peritoneum, direct extension to the contralateral pleura or lung, extension through the internal surface of the pericardium with or without an effusion; or involvement of the myocardium.

N—Lymph nodes
- NX Regional lymph nodes cannot be assessed
- N0 No regional lymph nodes metastases
- N1 Metastases in ipsilateral bronchopulmonary or hilar lymph nodes
- N2 Metastases in subcarinal or ipsilateral mediastinal lymph nodes including the ipsilateral internal mammary nodes
- N3 Metastases in contralateral mediastinal internal contralateral internal mammary, ipsilateral or contralateral supraclavicular, or scalene lymph nodes

M—Metastases
- MX Presence of distant metastases cannot be assessed
- M0 No (known) distant metastases
- M1 Distant metastasis present

STAGE	TNM CLASSIFICATION
I	T1a, N0, M0
	T1b, N0, M0
II	T2, N0, M0
III	Any T3, M0
	Any N1, M0
	Any N2, M0
IV	Any T4
	Any N3
	Any M1

uses nomenclature similar to that employed in other solid tumors, and considers recent data regarding the influence of T and N status on potential survival. The new IMIG staging system proposal is shown in Table 36.3.

The new IMIG staging system, similar to the earlier systems, remains unvalidated. For example, the distinction between T1a and T1b is based on the thorascopic observations by Boutin et al. (37). Their experience in 66 patients suggests that the tumor arises in the parietal pleura and then extends to the visceral surfaces. Patients with T1a tumors had a median survival of 32.7 months, whereas those with T1b tumors showed a median survival of only 7 months. Although there appears to be an adquate distinction of outcome by T1a and T1b, the survival differences between patients with T1 and T2 tumors are less well defined, however. T1 tumors are found less often in the United States. Complete removal of all disease (at least T2) may require an extrapleural pneumonectomy because of the extension into the pulmonary parenchyma. In more locally advanced disease, the difference between T3 and T4 lesions has potential implications for surgical resection. For T4 tumors the prognosis is dismal, with median survival durations of 6 months or less (37, 54).

The impact of lymph node involvement has only recently been appreciated fully. For patients undergoing uniform preoperative staging, surgery, and postoperative therapies in a study by Sugarbaker et al. (49), those with mediastinal lymph node involvement had a significantly worse survival than patients without such involvement. Among 89 patients reviewed by Rusch (53), those with mediastinal lymph node involvement had a 9.4-month median survival, whereas those with N0 tumors had an 18.3-month median survival. The use of N0, N1, and N2 is similar to that used in other intrathoracic tumors, but it still needs confirmation, because the anatomic arrangement makes it possible for N2 tumors to occur as the initial spread to the lymph nodes. N1 and N2 thus are grouped together with stage III. The numerical groupings of stage are the greatest departure from prior staging systems. The IMIG staging system separates the subsets with early potentially resectable tumors. Further use of the staging system with surgical specimens will be needed to resolve any distinctions between T1b and T2, N0 tumors.

None of the staging systems acknowledges the impact of well-defined prognostic factors that can influence survival. The most important of these appears to be histology. Patients with epithelial histology exhibit a survival superior to those with the sarcomatous form, and the mixed form appears to produce an intermediate survival (38, 43, 45, 46, 48, 49, 55–63). Recognizing the dismal outcome for at least the sarcomatous form, it may be appropriate to consider these cases separately and to avoid surgical procedures at present. These findings are somewhat similar to those found in soft tissue sarcomas, in which the histologic grade is an important feature of prognosis and staging. Future studies are needed to define the need for histologic determination as part of the staging system for mesothelioma.

REFERENCES

1. Wagner JC, Sleggs EA, marchand P. Diffuse pleural mesothelioma and asbestos in the North Western Cape Province. Br J Ind Med 1960;17:260–271.
2. Robertson HE. Endothelioma of the pleura. Cancer Res 1924; 8:317–375.
3. Kannerstein M, Churg J, Magner D. Histochemistry in the diagnosis of malignant mesothelioma. Ann Clin Lab Sci 1973;3:207–211.
4. Corson J, Pinkus G. Cellular localization patterns of keratin proteins in pleural mesothelioma and metastatic adenocarcinomas: a diagnostic discriminant. Lab Invest 1991;64:114A.
5. Suzuki Y, Churg C, Kannerstein M. Ultrastructure of human malignant diffuse mesothelioma. Am J Pathol 1976;85:241–262.
6. Stanton MF, Layard M, Tegeris A, et al. Carcinogenicity of fibrous glass: pleural response in relation to fiber dimension. J Natl Cancer Inst 1977;58:589–603.
7. Warheit DB, George G, Hill LH, et al. Inhaled asbestos activates a complement-dependent chemoattractant for macrophages. Lab Invest 1985;52:505–514.
8. Rom WN, Travis WD, Brody AR. Cellular and molecular basis of the asbestos-related diseases. Am Rev Respir Dis 1991;143:408–422.
9. Smith Ah, Handley MA, Wood R. Epidemiological evidence indicates asbestos causes laryngeal cancer. J Occup Med 1990;32: 499–507.
10. Selikoff, IJ, Churg J, Hammond EC. Asbestos exposure and neoplasia. JAMA 1964;188:22–26.
11. Ross R, Nichols P, Wright W, et al. Asbestos exposure and lymphomas of the gastrointestinal tract and oral cavity. Lancet 1982;2:1118–1119.
12. Newhouse M. Epidemiology of asbestos-related tumors. Semin Oncol 1981;8:250–262.
13. Antman KH. Clinical presentation and natural history of benign and malignant mesothelioma. Semin Oncol 1981;8:313–320.
14. Antman KH. Malignant mesothelioma. N Engl J Med 1980;303: 200–202.
15. Wojtukiewicz MZ, Zacharaski RL, Memoli VA, et al. Absence of components of coagulation and fibrinolysis pathways in situ in mesothelioma. Thromb Res 1989;55:179–84.
16. De Pangher, Manzini V, Brollo A, et al. Thrombocytosis in malignant pleural mesothelioma. Tumori 1990;76:576–8.
17. Antman K, Pomfret E, Aisner J, et al. Peritoneal mesothelioma: natural history and response to chemotherapy. J Clin Oncol 1983;1:386–91.
18. McAuley P, Asa SL, Chiu B, et al. Parathyroid hormone-like peptide in normal and neoplastic mesothelial cells. Cancer 1990; 66:1975–9.
19. Mirvis S, Dutcher JP, Haney PJ, et al. CT of malignant pleural mesothelioma. AJR Am J Roentgenol 1983;140:665–670.
20. Kawashima A, Libshitz HI, Lukeman JM. Radiation-induced malignant pleural mesothelioma. Can Assoc Radiol J 1990;41:384–386.
21. Cohen BA, Efremidis A, Chahinian AP, et al. Computed tomography of the chest of diffuse malignant pleural mesothelioma. Am Rev Respir Dis 1981;123:131–139.
22. Alexander E, Clark R, Colley D, et al. CT of malignant pleural mesothelioma. AJR Am J Roentgenol 1981;137:287–291.

23. Kreel L. Computed tomography in mesothelioma. Semin Oncol 1981;8:302–312.
24. Grant DC, Seltzer SE, Antman KH, et al. Computer tomography of malignant pleural mesothelioma. J Comput Assist Tomogr 1983;7:626–632.
25. Leung AN, Muller NL, Miller RR. CT in differential diagnosis of diffuse pleural disease. AJR Am J Roentgenol 1990;154:487–92.
26. Lorigan JG, Libshitz HI. MR imaging of malignant pleural mesothelioma. J Comput Assist Tomogr 1989;13:617–20.
27. Patz EF Jr, Shaffer K, Piwnico-Worm DR, et al. Malignant pleural mesothelioma: value of CT and MRi imaging in predicting resectability. Am J Radiol 1992;159:961–966.
28. Said J, Nash G, Lee M. Keratin proteins and carcinoembryonic antigen in lung carcinoma. An immunoperoxidase study of 54 cases with ultrastructural correlations. Hum Pathol 1983;14: 70–76.
29. Corson JM, Pinkus GSS. Mesothelioma: profile of keratin proteins and carcinoembryonixc antigen; an immuno-peroxidase study of 20 cases and comparison with pulmonary adenocarcinomas. Am J Pathol 1982;108:80–88.
30. Corson JM. Pathology of malignant mesothelioma. In: Aisner J, Antman KH, eds. Asbestos related malignancy. Orlando: Grune & Stratton, 1986:179–199.
31. Boutin C, Rey F. Thoracoscopy in pleural malignant mesothelioma: a prospective study of 188 patients. Part 1: diagnosis. Cancer 1993;72:389–393.
32. Geroulanos S, Lampe P, Hafner F, et al. Malignant pleural mesothelioma: diagnosis, therapy and prognosis. Schweiz Rundsch Med Prax 1990;79:261–367.
33. Boutin C, Viallat JR, Zandwijk NV, et al. Activity of intrapleural recombinant gamma-interferon in malignant mesothelioma. Cancer 1991;67:2033–2037.
34. Kannerstein M, Churg J, Magner D. Histochemistry in the diagnosis of malignant mesothelioma. Ann Clin Lab Sci 1973;3:207–211.
35. Kannerstein M, Churg J. A critique of the criteria for the diagnosis of diffuse malignant mesothelioma. Mt Sinai J Med 1977;44: 485–497.
36. Corson JM, Renshaw AA. Pathology of mesothelioma. In: Aisner J, Arriagada R, Green M, Martini N, Perry MC, eds. Comprehensive textbook of thoracic oncology. Baltimore: Williams & Wilkins, 1996.
37. Boutin C, Nussbaum E, Monnet I, et al. Intrapleural treatment with recombinant gamma interferon in diffuse malignant mesothelioma. Cancer 1994;74:2460–2467.
38. Elmes PC, Simpson M. The clinical aspects of mesothelioma. Q J Med 1976;45:427.
39. Roberts GH. Distant visceral metastases in pleural mesothelioma. Br J Dis Chest 1976;70:246–250.
40. Aisner J. Current approach to malignant mesothelioma of the pleura. Chest 1995;107(Supp):332S–344S.
41. Boutin C, Irrisson M, Rathelot P, Petite JM. L'extension parietale des mesotheliomas pleuraux malins diffus apres biopsies: prevention par radiotherapie locale (letter). Presse Med 1983;12:1823.
42. Gordon W, Antman K, Breenberger J, et al. Radiation therapy in the management of patients with mesothelioma. Int J Radiat Oncol Biol Phys 1982;8:19–25.
43. Chahinian AP, Pajak T, Holland J, et al. Diffuse malignant mesothelioma: prospective evaluation of 69 patients. Ann Intern Med 1982;96:746–755.
44. Antman K, Shemin R, Ryan L, et al. Malignant mesothelioma: prognostic variables in a registry of 180 patients, the Dana-Farber Cancer Institute and Brigham and Women's Hospital experience over two decades 1965–1985. J Clin Oncol 1988;6:147–153.
45. Ruffie P, Feld R, Minkin S, et al. Diffuse malignant mesothelioma of the pleura in Ontario and Quebec: a retrospective study of 332 patients. J Clin Oncol 1989;7:1157–1168.
46. Schildge J, Kaiser D, Henss H, et al. [Prognostic factors in diffuse malignant mesothelioma of the pleura.] Penumologie 1989;43: 660–664.
47. Hulks G, Thomas JS, Waclawski E. Malignant pleural mesothelioma in Western Glasgow 1980–86. Thorax 1989;44:496–500.
48. Butchart EG, Ashcroft T, Barnsley WC, et al. Pleuro-pneumonectomy in the management of diffuse malignant mesothelioma of the pleura: experience with 29 patients. Thorax 1976;31:15–24.
49. Sugarbaker DJ, Strauss GM, Lynch TJ, et al. Node status has prognostic significance in the multimodality therapy of diffuse, malignant mesothelioma. J Clin Oncol 1993;11:1172–1178.
50. Mattson K. Natural history and clinical staging of malignant mesothelioma. Environ J Respir Dis 1982;63(Suppl 124):87.
51. Chahinian AP. Therapeutic modalities: malignant pleural mesothelioma. In: Chretien J, Hirsch A, eds. Diseases of the pleura. New York: Masson, 1983:224–236.
52. Rusch VS, Ginsberg RJ. New concepts in the staging of mesotheliomas. In: Deslauriers J, Lacquet K, eds. International trends in general thoracic surgery. St. Louis: Mosby, 1990:336–343.
53. Rusch V. A new international TNM staging system for malignant pleural mesothelioma: report of the International Mesothelioma Interest Group. Chest; in press.
54. Tammilehto L. Malignant mesothelioma: prognostic factors in a prospective study of 98 patients. Lung Cancer 1992;8:175–184.
55. Boutin C, Viallat JR, Rey F. Thoracoscopy in diagnosis, prognosis, and treatment of mesothelioma. In: Aisner J, Antman KH, eds. Asbestos related malignancy. Orlando: Grune & Stratton, 1986:301–321.
56. Wanebo HJ, Martini N, Melamed MR, et al. Pleural mesothelioma. Cancer 19876;38:2481–2488.
57. Martini N, McCormach PM, Baines MS, et al. Pleural mesothelioma. Ann Thorac Surg 1987;43:113.
58. Griffiths MH, Riddell RJ, Xippell JM. Malignant mesothelioma. A review of 35 cases with diagnosis and prognosis. Pathology 1980; 12:591–603.
59. Law MR, Hodson Me, Heard BE. Malignant mesothelioma of the pleura: Relation between histologic type and clinical behavior.
60. Oels HC, Harrison EG, Carr DT, et al. Diffuse malignant mesothelioma of the pleura: a review of 37 cases. Chest 1971;60:564–570.
61. Stirtas R, Connelly RR, Tucker MA. Survival pattern for malignant mesothelioma: the SEER experience. Int J Cancer 1988; 41:525–530.
62. Rusch VW, Piantadosi S, Holmes EC, et al. The role of extrapleural pneumonectomy in malignant pleural mesothelioma. J Thorac Cardiovasc Surg 1991;102:1–9.
63. Allen KB, Faber LB, Warren WH, et al. Malignant pleural mesothelioma: extrapleural pneumonectomy and pleurectomy. Chest Surg Clin North Am 1994;4:113–126.
64. Aisner J, Antman KH, Belani CP. Tumors of the pleura and mediastinum. In: Abeloff MA, Armitage J, Lichter AS, eds. Science of clinical oncology. New York: Churchill Livingstone, 1995.

37

THERAPEUTIC APPROACHES FOR MALIGNANT PLEURAL MESOTHELIOMA

David J. Sugarbaker and Michael J. Liptay

Malignant pleural mesothelioma (MPM) is a rare but deadly malignancy for which no standard therapy has been successful. In 1994 nearly 3000 patients (1, 2) will have been diagnosed with the diffuse spreading type of MPM, and a combination of therapies will have been used to combat this relentless killer.

In the less common presentation of mesothelioma, a focal lesion may be seen invading a confined area of the pleura. In this unusual circumstance, wide surgical excision may be curative. Unfortunately, much more commonly the patient with mesothelioma presents with obvious involvement of the entire pleural surface in one hemithorax. MPM is a relentless invasive malignancy with the majority of patients dying of local thoracic complications. Until recently the role of surgery in this setting has been limited to biopsy for diagnosis with occasional pleurodesis for palliation.

Because of the rarity of this malignancy and its relentless fatal progression despite the implementation of often heroic regimens, many physicians have developed a nihilistic approach to its treatment. Recently, with the cooperation of multimodality and often multi-institutional study groups, new prognostic indicators are being identified that may aid in the careful selection of subgroups of patients who may benefit from intensive multimodality therapy. This chapter provides an overview of prognostic factors and reviews current therapeutic options in resectable malignant pleural mesothelioma.

EPIDEMIOLOGY

Asbestos exposure was clearly established in 1960 by Wagner and associates (3) as a risk factor for the development of MPM. Since then, widespread efforts to reduce human exposure to asbestos have been ongoing in the United States and elsewhere. The relationship between duration or intensity of exposure and risk of MPM has been more difficult to ascertain. There appears to be a long latency period (often several decades) between exposure to asbestos and development of MPM. This delay would account for the gradual rise in cases diagnosed during the past decade despite reduced asbestos exposure over the past 30 years.

Mesothelioma most often occurs in the sixth decade of life. Males have an incidence rate 5 times that of females (1.5 cases per 100,000 versus 0.3 cases per 100,000). Although the interaction of asbestos with cigarette smoking clearly is synergistic regarding the risk of primary lung cancer, the same does not appear to be true for mesothelioma. Cigarette smoking has not been shown to increase the likelihood of a diagnosis of MPM (4).

HISTOPATHOLOGY/TUMOR BEHAVIOR

Malignant, diffuse, spreading mesothelioma arises from the pluripotent mesothelial cells lining the pleural surface of the lungs. The two major histologic subtypes are epithelial and sarcomatoid. Often, both types are present in a mixed setting. The epithelial type appears to be the most common, occurring in more than 84% of 819 cases reviewed recently (5). Of these, the pure epithelial cell type occurred in 50% of the cases, whereas mixed tumors and the sarcomatous variety occurred in 34% and 16% of the cases, respectively.

The precise histologic diagnosis of MPM can be difficult. Cytologic examination from pleural fluid is often insufficient for definitive diagnosis, and a thoracoscopic or open pleural biopsy is most often needed for confirmation. Mesothelioma can often be confused with the more commonly occurring metastatic or locally invasive adenocarcinomas from either a primary lung cancer or elsewhere. Before the wide use of immunohistochemistry and electron microscopy to confirm histologic diagnoses, the distinction was often impossible. Current immunohistochemical techniques facilitate differential diagnosis and cell type definition. Mesothelioma always stains negatively for carcinoembryonic antigen, whereas up to 75% of adenocarcinomas express the antigen to some degree. Mesotheliomas stain positively for low-molecular-weight cytokeratins, allowing differentiation from sarcomas. Vimentin staining, a marker of cells with a mesenchymal origin, is positive in most cases of MPM and negative in adenocarcinoma (6, 7). Electron microscopy also is useful in distinguishing cells of mesothelial origin from adenocarcinoma. On electron microscopy mesothelial cells have long microvilli with a length to diameter ratio of greater than 10:1, whereas adenocarcinomas exhibit much shorter and thicker microvilli (Table 37.1).

Obtaining a sufficient amount of tissue is critical to the definitive diagnosis of MPM. To assure adequate tissue sampling, several investigators have recommended open or thoracoscopic biopsy of these lesions (8–10). This procedure can be performed with minimal morbidity and should be done before planning therapy in all but the most advanced presentations.

The therapeutic approach to diffuse spreading mesothelioma differs significantly from that of locally advanced or metastatic adenocarcinoma. Despite the propensity of MPM to track along the skin incisions and thoracoscopy tracts, the information confirming the diagnosis and, to a lesser degree, the tumor cell type and degree of differentiation are critical in planning treatment. Definitive surgical therapy is not compromised if the incisions are well placed along subsequent areas of resection. Pre-resection thoracoscopy or open pleural biopsy should be performed in all protocol settings to assure meaningful interpretation of outcomes with respect to tested therapies.

CLINICAL PRESENTATION

The clinical presentation of diffuse spreading malignant mesothelioma is most often related to the local spread of the tumor. In the earlier phase of the disease, dyspnea is the most common complaint. This symptom usually is secondary to a pleural effusion. As the tumor progresses, it invades the chest wall musculature and intercostal nerves, leading to unrelenting, severe chest pain. Worsening dyspnea often is noted, which is related to restrictive lung disease secondary to tumor encasement.

PROGNOSTIC FACTORS ASSOCIATED WITH CLINICAL PRESENTATION

In an attempt to identify prognostic factors in the clinical presentation of MPM, several centers have reviewed their series of patients and performed univariate and multivariate analyses of characteristics that may be predictors of survival (Table 37.2). As in most other malignancies and diseases encountered today, age and performance status at diagnosis were both independent predictors of survival in most of the series reviewed (11–18). Those who presented at a younger age (usually less than 55 years) had improved survival. Performance status of 0 to 1 (Eastern Cooperative Oncology Group scale) or a Karnofsky status of more than 80% also had a positive effect on survival and was the most reproducible clinical prognostic factor in the communications reviewed. Several studies found female sex to be an independent predictor of survival (12, 14, 19). The explanations offered for this finding included the presumed greater cumulative exposure to asbestos of males, who are more likely to have experienced occupational exposure.

Another constitutional sign at presentation found to influence survival in some series was weight loss. The presence of a greater than 10% weight loss before diagnosis of MPM was associated with a decreased sur-

TABLE 37.1. Pathologic Diagnosis of Mesothelioma

TECHNIQUE	MPM	ADENOCARCINOMA
Periodic acid Schiff stain	Negative	Positive
Mucicarmine stain	Negative	Positive
Alcian Blue stain (detects hyaluronic acid)	Positive (20%)	Negative
CEA antibody	Negative	Positive (75%)
Cytokeratin antibody (low molecular weight)	Positive	Negative (also in sarcomas)
Vimentin	Positive	Negative
Electron microscopy	Long microvilli	Short microvilli

Abbreviation. MPM, malignant pleural mesothelioma.

TABLE 37.2 Prognostic Factors for Improved Survival in MPM

CLINICAL
Age less than 55 years
Female sex
Performance status of 0 to 1 (Zubrod or ECOG scale)
No significant weight loss (less than 10%)
Dyspnea without chest pain
Symptoms present for more than 6 months

DIAGNOSTIC
No malignant cells found in pleural fluid
Stage I disease
Epithelial predominant cell type
No lymph node invasion

vival, regardless of other factors, in a recent review of 301 patients from Heidelberg, Germany (11).

The presence of chest pain at the time of diagnosis was identified as a negative predictor of survival (11, 12, 15, 20). This result has been explained by the localized chest pain being a sign of chest wall invasion by the tumor similar to T3 lesions involving the chest wall in lung cancer. A series of 188 MPM patients examined thoracoscopically showed that involvement of only the parietal pleura without extension to the visceral pleura was a marker of improved prognosis (21).

Interestingly, several series have identified the duration of symptoms before diagnosis as predictors of survival. In particular, those patients who had a duration of symptoms longer than 6 months before the diagnosis of MPM had an improved survival rate over those whose symptoms were present for a shorter period before diagnosis (14, 15). This finding is believed to relate to the variability in tumor aggressiveness and differing growth patterns.

PLEURAL FLUID

The presence of pleural effusion is one of the most common initial findings. It is associated with dyspnea in nearly 80% of MPM patients at presentation (17, 20). Evaluation of the pleural fluid from 80 patients subsequently diagnosed with MPM demonstrated a slightly improved prognosis for patients in whom no malignant cells were found (13). A small study evaluated pleural fluid from 26 patients and found a statistically decreased mean survival correlating with a lower pleural fluid pH (no more than 7.30) (22). With the growing use of diagnostic thoracoscopy, these studies may be shown only to document the effects seen with increased pleural tumor bulk.

PLATELET COUNT

Thrombocytosis has been reported in up to 40% of cases. A platelet count greater then 400,000 appears to have a negative effect on survival (17, 18). Interestingly, thrombocytosis does not appear to be related to an increase in thromboembolic phenomena. It remains unclear whether the thrombocytosis is secondary to a systemically elaborated factor or a generalized leukemoid reaction to the tumor (23).

PATHOLOGIC ASSOCIATIONS
EPITHELIAL HISTOLOGY

Once the diagnosis of MPM has been established, several series have demonstrated a clearly improved prognosis with the purely epithelial subtype (9, 17, 18, 24, 25). For this reason it is critical to obtain an adequate tissue sample to assess the presence of sarcomatoid cells in the tumor accurately because the mixed variety and sarcomatous type have worse prognoses with all treatment plans reported to date.

In a series addressing prognostic indicators at the Dana-Farber Cancer Institute and Brigham and Women's Hospital (17), 136 patients with pleural MPM treated over a 20-year period were reviewed. A mean survival of 17 months for patients with the pure epithelial cell type was shown, versus a 13-month survival for those with mixed tumors and a 7-month survival for patients with sarcomatoid lesions when all stages were considered. A more recent publication from the same center (9) reported 52 patients who underwent multimodality treatment including extrapleural pneumonectomy for Butchart stage I disease. The 1-, 2-, and 3-year survival rates of the 32 patients with pure epithelial tumors were 77%, 50%, and 42%, respectively. The remaining 20 patients with the mixed or sarcomatoid cell type had 1- and 2-year survival rates of 45% and 7.5%, respectively. No patient with the mixed or sarcomatoid type had a survival longer than 25 months (Fig. 37.1).

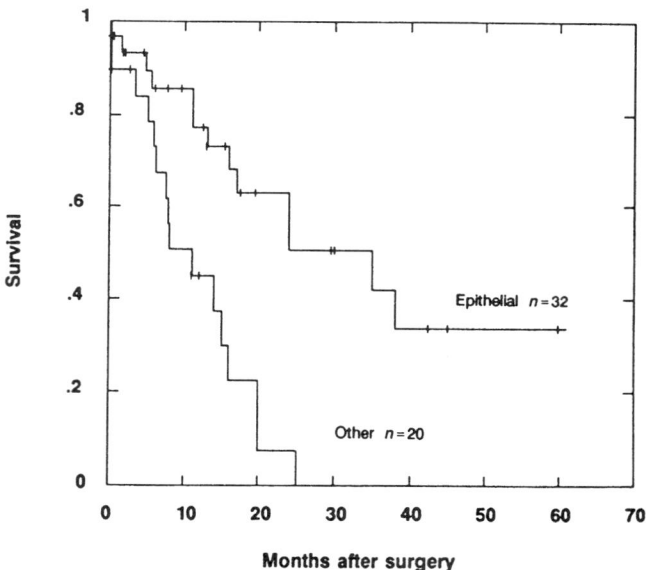

FIGURE 37.1. Kaplan-Meier survival curve of 52 patients treated with multimodality therapy at the Dana-Farber Cancer Institute/Brigham and Women's Hospital. Comparison is made between all patients with epithelial tumors and those with nonepithelial (sarcomatoid and mixed) cell types. Those with the nonepithelial cell type had the poorer survival (P < .05). (From Sugarbaker DJ, Strauss GM, Lynch TJ, et al. Node status has prognostic significance in the multimodality therapy of diffuse, malignant mesothelioma. J Clin Oncol 1993;11:1172–1178.)

The improved survival with the epithelial cell type has been reproduced in several series with divergent treatment protocols. The epithelial cell type appears to be one of the most reliable predictors of outcome found to date. These findings highlight once again the importance of accurate pretreatment assessment of cytologic features and cell type.

The uniformly bad prognosis of the sarcomatoid cell type also has been reproducible, and this fact calls into question the aggressive treatment of patients with this cell type. Until better treatment is available (probably in the form of more active chemotherapeutic regimens), the role of aggressive treatment of sarcomatoid cell type MPM is unclear.

NODAL STATUS

Mesothelioma has long been known to be a disease of local-regional spread leading to the death of the patient, often with no evidence of significant spread outside of the thorax. For this reason little attention has been paid to the contribution nodal spread may make to potential curative treatment and ultimate survival. Nodal staging in nearly all other solid tumors has been found to be a major (and often the most important) predictor of survival. The use of surgical staging in the form of mediastinoscopy and thoracoscopy has gained much-deserved prominence in the planning of therapy in lung cancer. For MPM the presence of positive lymph nodes in the chest is considered stage II disease by the Butchart staging system. However, until recently little if any data have been available correlating the effect of nodal spread with outcome in MPM. Fifty-two patients underwent a multimodality treatment approach to MPM between 1980 and 1992 at Brigham and Women's Hospital/Dana-Farber Cancer Institute. All of these patients underwent extrapleural pneumonectomy before adjuvant chemotherapy and radiation (9). Thirteen patients (25%) had positive mediastinal lymph nodes at resection. Positive mediastinal nodes were associated with a poorer survival than were negative lymph nodes (Fig. 37.2). Nodal status was found to be an independent predictor of survival in this group, regardless of tumor cell type or whether gross residual disease was left after extrapleural pneumonectomy. These results, although based on a small single-site study, raise the possibility that further pretherapy staging may be possible with the use of mediastinoscopy or thoracoscopy before resection. Information on the nodal status may allow for better stratification of patients when considering aggressive treatment protocols.

MOLECULAR BIOLOGY

Great interest has surrounded the study of the biologic behavior of mesothelioma cells from tumor blocks and cell lines. The most widely accepted theories of tumorigenesis center around the carcinogenic influence of asbestos, which leads to loss of chromosomal heterozygosity and tumor suppressor genes. Inactivation of tumor suppressor genes is found commonly with chromosomal deletions, many of which have been found consistently with MPM. In a study of 25 MPM tumors, 24 had a deletion on chromosome 3p most often centered around 3p21 (26). In another study of 23 MPM tumors, loss of heterozygosity of chromosomes 1p and 9p was found in two thirds of the cases, whereas deletions at 3p21 were present in 13 of the 23 cases studied (27). Deletions on the short arm of chromosome 9 (9p) are common in MPM as well as in non–small cell lung cancer (28). MPM also is associated with deletions on chromosome 6q and 22q, as well as with the complete loss of chromosomes 14, 16, 18, and 22 (27). The significance of many of these chromosomal abnormalities has yet to be elucidated.

One of the most intensively researched tumor suppressor genes is *p53*. There have been mixed reports regarding its role in the pathogenesis of MPM. After early reports of deletions and mutations present near its locus on chromosome 17p (29), several studies have not been able to reproduce findings consistent with *p53* being significant in mesothelioma (30–32). Similarly, Kirsten-*ras* and HER2*neu* have not been found to play significant roles in MPM (30, 32).

Chromosomal number was found to be a predictor of survival in one study (33). In a review of 34 cases of MPM, normal mean chromosomal number correlated with a mean survival of 31 months, whereas tumors with a mean chromosomal number of either less than or greater than 46 had mean survivals of 26 and 13 months, respectively.

Although DNA ploidy patterns have been useful prognostic instruments in other tumors, similar attempts have not been as effective in predicting survival in MPM. One study compared 23 epithelial cell type mesotheliomas with 41 primary lung adenocarcinomas and found 78% of the mesotheliomas to be diploid and 88% of the adenocarcinomas to be aneuploid (34). An association was seen between aneuploidy and shorter survival time in one series of 37 MPM patients (35), but another group observed no correlation of aneuploidy to survival in 70 cases (36).

Fifty-one cases of MPM were analyzed by one group for the presence of an elevated S-phase frac-

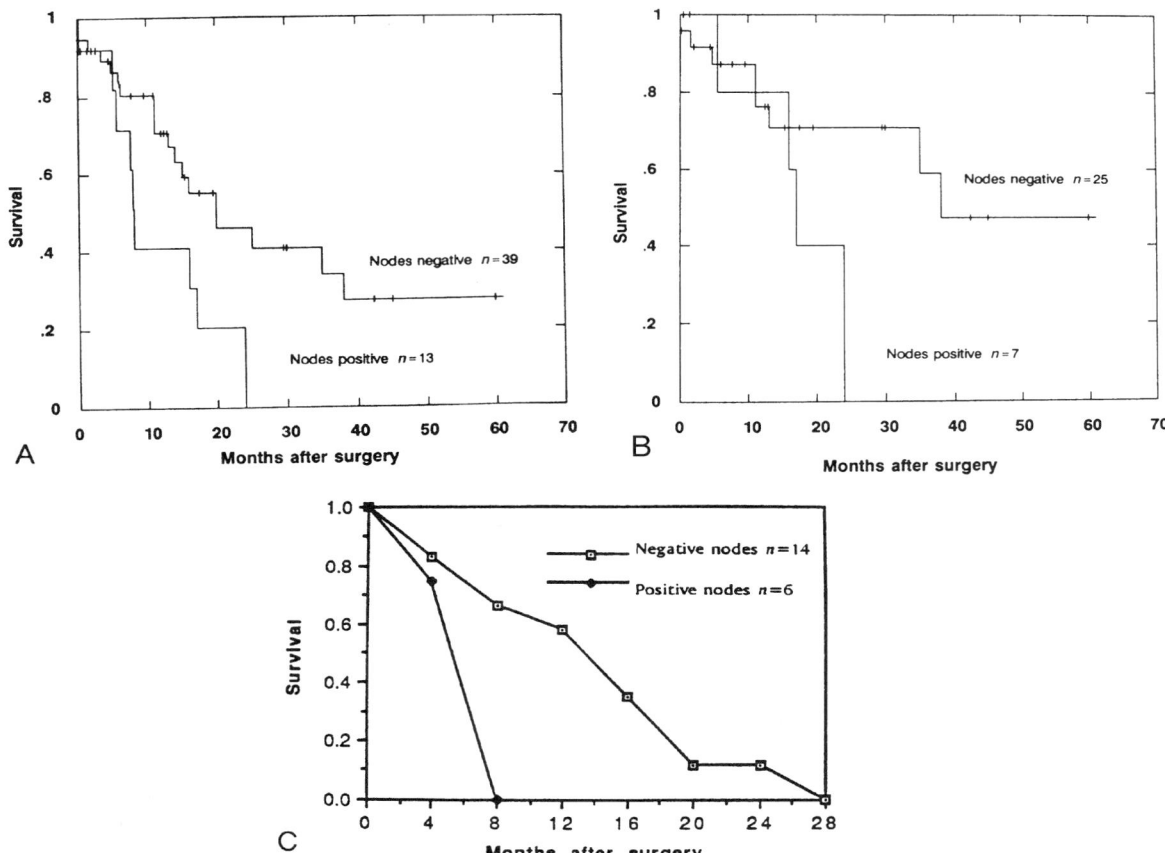

FIGURE 37.2. Kaplan-Meier survival curves of 52 patients treated with multimodality therapy including extrapleural pneumonectomy at the Dana-Farber Cancer Institute/Brigham and Women's Hospital. Comparison is made between: **A.** all patients with node positive and node negative pathologic specimens; **B.** epithelial cell type; and **C.** mixed and sarcomatoid cell types. Node positive patients had a poorer survival regardless of cell type (P < .05). (From Sugarbaker DJ, Strauss GM, Lynch TJ, et al. Node status has prognostic significance in the multimodality therapy of diffuse, malignant mesothelioma. J Clin Oncol 1993;11:1172–1178.)

tion. They found a significant negative correlation between a high S-phase fraction and survival. This finding was independent of the presence of aneuploidy, which was not found to predict outcome in this cohort (36).

The presence of increased levels of several growth factors and their receptors has been found. Platelet-derived growth factor and elevations of its β-receptor have been found in 10 of 16 mesotheliomas examined in one study (37). These findings suggest the possibility of an autocrine loop effect with local growth factor secretion and specific receptors on mesothelioma cells leading to tumor proliferation (38).

The biologic role of these findings in disease development and progression remains unclear and is the subject of intense research.

STAGING

The first and still most widely used staging system for MPM was proposed in 1976 by Butchart and colleagues (39). Because of the rarity of this tumor and its propensity for extensive local invasion before any evidence of distant metastasis, this initial staging affords a relatively crude assessment of extent of disease (Table 37.3) (39). Stage I MPM is described as disease confined to the "capsule" of the parietal pleura without obvious invasion of vital mediastinal structures or lymph nodes. Patients presenting with clinical stage I disease had a better long-term survival in nearly all series reviewed (16). Even with the use of modern noninvasive staging techniques (computed tomography [CT] scan and magnetic resonance imaging [MRI]), 70% of

TABLE 37.3. Butchart Staging System for Malignant Pleural Mesothelioma

Stage I	Within the "capsule" of the parietal pleura: ipsilateral pleura, lung, pericardium, diaphragm
Stage II	Invading chest wall or mediastinum: esophagus, heart, opposite pleura Positive lymph nodes within the chest
Stage III	Through diaphragm to the peritoneum. Opposite pleura Positive lymph nodes outside the chest
Stage IV	Distant blood-borne metastases

Adapted from Patz EF Jr, Shaffer K, Piwnica-Worms DR, et al. Malignant pleural mesothelioma: value of CT and MR imaging in predicting resectability. AJR AM J Roentgenol 1992;159:961–966.

TABLE 37.4. Proposed UICC International Staging System

T—Primary Tumor and Extent

T_x	Primary tumor cannot be assessed
T_0	No evidence of primary tumor
T_1	Primary tumor limited to ipsilateral parietal and/or visceral pleura
T_2	Tumor invades any of the following: ipsilateral lung, endothoracic fascia, diaphragm, pericardium
T_3	Tumor invades any of the following: ipsilateral chest wall muscle, ribs, mediastinal organs or tissues
T_4	Tumor extends to any of the following: contralateral pleura or lung by direct extension, peritoneum or intraabdominal organs by direct extension, cervical tissues

N—Lymph Nodes

N_x	Regional lymph nodes cannot be assessed
N_0	No regional lymph node metastases
N_1	Metastases in ipsilateral bronchopulmonary or hilar lymph nodes
N_2	Metastases in ipsilateral mediastinal lymph nodes
N_3	Metastases in contralateral mediastinal, internal mammary, supraclavicular, or scalene lymph nodes

M—Metastases

M_x	Presence of distant metastases cannot be assessed
M_0	No (known) distant metastasis
M_1	Distant metastasis present

Mesothelioma Staging System[a]

T_1, N_0, M_0	I
T_2, N_0, M_0	
T_1, N_1, M_0	II
T_2, N_1, M_0	
T_3, N_0, M_0	III
T_3, N_1, M_0	
T_1, N_2, M_0	
T_2, N_2, M_0	
T_3, N_2, M_0	
Any T, N_3, M_0	IV
T_4, any N, M_0	
Any T, any N, M_1	

From Rusch VW, Ginsberg RJ. New concepts in the staging of mesothelioma: invited comment to chapter 26. In: Deslauriers J, Lacquet LK, eds. Thoracic surgery: surgical management of pleural diseases. International trends in general thoracic surgery. St. Louis: Mosby, 1990;6:336–343.
[a]Staging solely on clinical measures is designated cTNM. Staging that can be done on clinical pathologic information is designated as pTNM. Clinical and pathologic groups are identical.

patients are diagnosed before treatment with clinical stage I disease. Despite this fact the median survival for all patients after the diagnosis of MPM is reported as between 5 and 14 months.

Traditionally, surgical resection has been offered only to those with Buchart stage I disease. To allow for appropriate selection of patients with treatable (if not curable) disease, the need for a more rigorous staging philosophy has emerged. In 1990 the Lung Cancer Study Group proposed the use of a Union Internationale Contre le Cancer (UICC) tumor, node, metastasis (TNM) classification system (Table 37.4) (40) analogous to the one used for lung cancer (41). Although insufficient data are available to support a survival difference between every parameter, the availability of more precise staging (both noninvasive and surgical) allows for better stratification of patients to potentially beneficial therapy or the avoidance of needless morbidity in more advanced cases. The TNM staging system is intuitively hard to grasp in a malignancy that is so diffusely spreading, however, and the prognostic value of separating N1 from N2 or N3 disease is unclear. Thus, a system has been proposed that is similar to Butchart's in description but that also accounts for the recently appreciated negative prognostic influence of positive nodes (Table 37.5) (9).

THERAPEUTIC APPROACHES FOR MPM

Single-modality treatment of mesothelioma has yielded disappointing results. No single mode of treatment (surgery, chemotherapy, or radiotherapy) has been able to impact significantly on the progression of MPM and its ultimate lethality. Each modality has its limitations in efficacy. Attempted complete resection of the tumor often is hindered by positive resection margins and the many vital structures adjacent to the tumor. Radiation dosages are limited by the vast surface area of tumor involvement and the proximity of

TABLE 37.5. BWH/DFCI Proposed Staging System

Stage	Description
Stage I	Disease confined to within the "capsule" of the parietal pleura: ipsilateral pleura, lung, pericardium, diaphragm, or chest wall disease limited to previous biopsy sites
Stage II	All of stage I with positive intrathoracic (N1 or N2) lymph nodes
Stage III	Local extension of disease into the chest wall or mediastinum; heart; or through the diaphragm, peritoneum; with or without extrathoracic or contralateral (N3) lymph node involvement
Stage IV	Distant metastatic disease

From Sugarbaker DJ, Strauss GM, Lynch TJ, et al. Node status has prognostic significance in the multimodality therapy of diffuse, malignant mesothelioma. J Clin Oncol 1993;11:1172–1178.

radiosensitive organs (e.g., heart, lung, liver). Single-agent or combination chemotherapy has yielded response rates of only 15% to 20% (42).

These poor results have led many physicians to adopt a nihilistic approach to the treatment of MPM. Others have adopted combined or multimodality treatment approaches in an attempt to improve local control and survival.

CHEMOTHERAPY

Treatment of MPM with chemotherapy alone has not yielded encouraging results. The average response rate to any single-agent therapy was reviewed in 21 trials consisting of 552 patients. Only 13% of the 552 patients responded to single-agent chemotherapy (25). The response rates with combination chemotherapy have not been much better. A large intergroup trial compared results in patients with advanced MPM for doxorubicin and cyclophosphamide and dacarbazine, doxorubicin, and cyclophosphamide in a total of 85 patients. The response rates were 11% and 10%, respectively (43). Despite these discouraging numbers, chemotherapy has improved survival in selected series as a part of multimodality treatment. The search for more efficacious chemotherapeutic agents continues. The most recent Cancer and Leukemia Group B (CALGB) protocol (9234) involved paclitaxel (Taxol; Bristol-Myers Squibb Oncology Division, Princeton, NJ) in a phase II setting. Preliminary results were analyzed in 18 patients receiving 250 mg/m² over 24 hours every 3 weeks and granulocyte colony stimulating factor for myelosuppression rescue. Two patients had a partial response, five patients had stable disease, and eight had progression of their disease (44). Three patients refused to be reevaluated. The study was reopened, and further analysis is pending.

IMMUNOCHEMOTHERAPY

The use of systemically administered immunotherapy for MPM has been studied for interferons (α-, β-, and γ-interferon) and interleukin-2 with or without lymphocyte-activated killer cells. In small phase I pilot trials, single-agent partial response rates have varied from 0% to 16% for these agents (45, 46).

Trials involving the intrapleural administration of biologic response modifiers such as interleukin-2 and γ-interferon have yielded mixed results. Intrapleural administration of interleukin-2 was examined in 14 patients with a partial response noted in 3 patients. The addition of lymphocyte-activated killer cells to this regimen in four patients resulted in significant systemic toxicity with no perceived increase in efficacy (47). In a phase I trial, 22 patients were treated with multiple doses of intrapleural γ-interferon over a 2-month period (48). Response was assessed by thoracoscopy and CT scans. An overall response rate of 56% was reported, easily the highest associated with any single biologic agent.

The difficulties with intrapleural administration are twofold. First, there appears to be variable systemic absorption of the agent, often leading to toxicity. Secondly, for adequate response the pleural space must be free and contiguous to allow for full distribution. This favorable scenario only exists in early-stage disease, which has a more favorable outlook regardless of therapy.

RADIATION THERAPY

Of the three modalities used alone to combat MPM, radiotherapy appears to be the least effective. The data on radiation therapy as the sole treatment for mesothelioma are sparse; usually, radiation treatment is part of a combined approach. Its effectiveness is limited both by difficulties encountered with adequate dosing secondary to pulmonary and mediastinal toxicity and by the large field needed to include the entire hemithorax. With the administration of curative doses ranging from 50 to 65 Gy, the development of radiation pneumonitis is almost certain (49). To avoid toxicity to the underlying lung, several groups have employed postoperative radiation therapy after extrapleural pneumonectomy. This technique allows for the deliverance of higher doses of radiation (50 to 55 Gy) to the hemithorax as well as for boost dosing to residual tumor areas marked at resection with radiopaque clips.

SURGICAL OPTIONS

PREOPERATIVE EVALUATION FOR EXTRAPLEURAL PNEUMONECTOMY

Surgical approaches described in the literature include extrapleural pneumonectomy, pleurectomy with decortication and debulking of gross tumor, and diagnostic biopsy with palliative pleurodesis. The high perioperative mortality reported in earlier series of extrapleural pneumonectomy (15% to 31%) has precluded its practical application for curative or palliative intents (18, 39). The inclusion of extrapleural pneumonectomy in a treatment protocol requires a thorough preoperative evaluation to allow for maximal benefit while limiting treatment-related morbidity.

After the diagnosis of MPM has been established, noninvasive evaluation of the extent of disease with CT and chest MRI are undertaken. Sagittal MRI views add much useful information regarding invasion of mediastinal structures, including the heart, aorta, vena cavae, esophagus, and trachea (50). Patients with involvement of these vital mediastinal structures or documented transdiaphragmatic extension have not experienced long-term survival.

Another tool used to evaluate the mediastinum is echocardiography. Using this procedure one can assess pericardial invasion as well as ventricular function preoperatively and establish a baseline before administration of doxorubicin-based adjuvant chemotherapy. All patients being evaluated for surgery receive pulmonary function testing with dynamic spirometry, functional oxymetry, and arterial blood gas measurement. In borderline cases in which the initial forced expiratory volume in 1 second (FEV_1) is less than 2 L or the predicted postoperative FEV_1 is less than 1.2 L, a quantitative ventilation/perfusion scan is obtained.

Patients with a left ventricular ejection fraction of less than 45% on echocardiogram, a predicted postoperative FEV_1 of less than 1 L, a room air arterial carbon dioxide tension greater than 44 mm Hg, or an oxygen tension of less than 65 mm Hg are not offered extrapleural pneumonectomy (Table 37.6).

Bone scans or head CT scans are not obtained routinely preoperatively because the asymptomatic occurrence of occult metastases is exceedingly rare.

TABLE 37.6. Selection Criteria for Extrapleural Pneumonectomy

Left ventricular ejection fraction, >45%
Predicted postoperative FEV_1, >1 L
Preoperative pCO_2, <44 mm Hg
Preoperative pO_2, >65 mm Hg
Disease confined to hemithorax

OPERATIVE TECHNIQUE FOR EXTRAPLEURAL PNEUMONECTOMY

If curative resection is contemplated and any question of transdiaphragmatic spread of the tumor remains, a laparoscopy or minilaparotomy is performed before the thoracic procedure. Any evidence of spread below the hemidiaphragm precludes thoracic resection.

Once the presence of peritoneal spread has been ruled out, the patient is then placed in the lateral decubitus position. A detailed description of the operative technique for extrapleural pneumonectomy has been published elsewhere (51). Briefly, a standard extended thoracotomy incision is made, and the sixth rib is completely resected to allow for wide exposure (Fig. 37.3) (51). The plane of dissection is through the chest wall external to the parietal pleura (Fig. 37.4) (51). The dissection proceeds toward the apex initially. Great care is taken to achieve meticulous hemostasis along with preservation of the pleural envelope. Continuing the apical dissection in the extrapleural fat plane allows for removal of the parietal pleura from the subclavian and internal mammary vessels. Avoidance of avulsion of these vessels from their origins is critical to the safe conduction of the procedure. The dissection proceeds circumferentially around the edges of the diaphragm to the anterior pericardium. To preserve the pleural envelope, the diaphragm is resected en bloc with the speci-

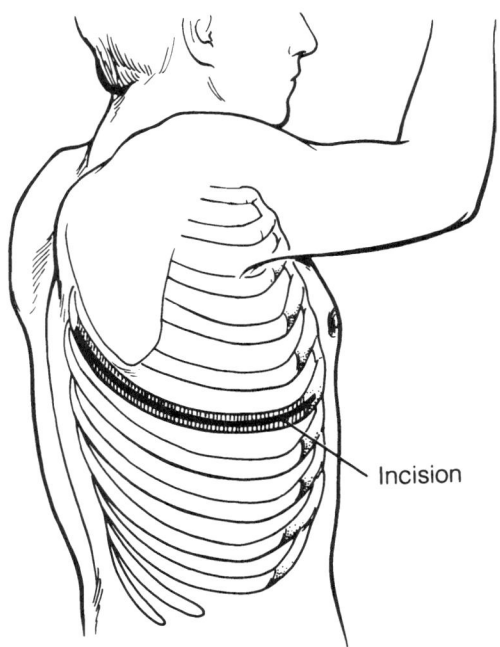

FIGURE 37.3. The extended right thoracotomy incision demonstrating resection of the sixth rib. (From Sugarbaker DJ, Mentzer SJ, Strauss G. Extrapleural pneumonectomy in the treatment of malignant pleural mesothelioma. Ann Thorac Surg 1992;54:941–946.)

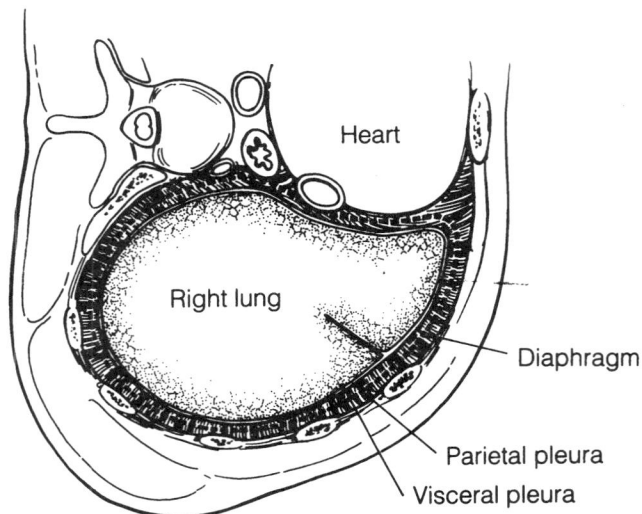

FIGURE 37.4. Cross-sectional view of plane of resection (*dotted line*) for right extrapleural pneumonectomy. (From Sugarbaker DJ, Mentzer SJ, Strauss G. Extrapleural pneumonectomy in the treatment of malignant pleural mesothelioma. Ann Thorac Surg 1992; 54:941–946.)

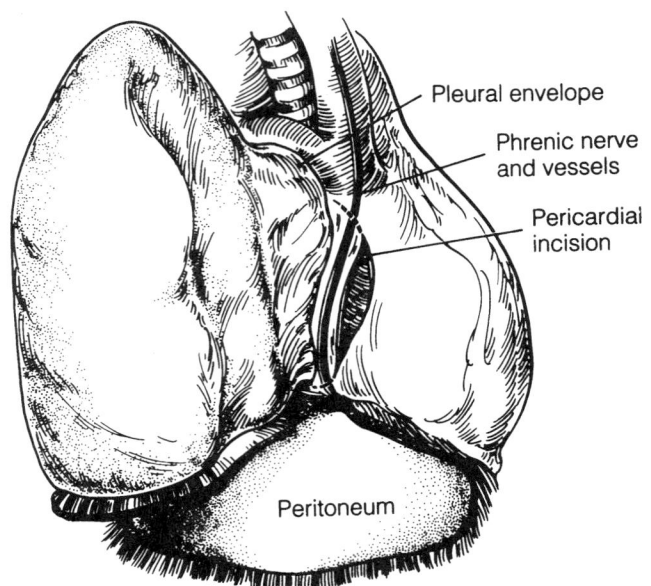

FIGURE 37.5. Resection of the lung and pleural envelope includes the diaphragm, lateral pericardium, and phrenic nerve. (From Sugarbaker DJ, Mentzer SJ, Strauss G. Extrapleural pneumonectomy in the treatment of malignant pleural mesothelioma. Ann Thorac Surg 1992;54:941–946.)

men (Fig. 37.5) (51). The pericardium is entered anteromedially, and the phrenic nerve is sacrificed after division of the vascular structures and main bronchus. The specimen is then removed en bloc, and a frozen section analysis of the resection margins is completed. Unresectable gross disease or areas found to have positive margins on frozen section are outlined with radiopaque clips to facilitate tailored postoperative radiotherapy. On occasion, unresectable residual disease has been treated with the intraoperative application of radioactive seeds.

After the resection, attention is directed to reconstruction of the pericardial and diaphragmatic defects. A fenestrated prosthetic patch is used to prevent cardiac herniation. The fenestrations are important in the prevention of postoperative tamponade. This patch is needed in all cases on the right side, whereas in left-sided resections pericardial reconstruction it can often be omitted. The routine repair of the diaphragmatic defect with an impermeable prosthetic patch is important for two reasons. The watertight seal prevents the acute postoperative accumulation of peritoneal fluid in the thorax that may result in cardiorespiratory embarrassment secondary to tamponade or mediastinal shift. Secondly, the diaphragmatic reconstruction prevents migration of abdominal contents into the hemithorax postoperatively, because the superior displacement of the liver or bowel may limit the amount of adjuvant radiotherapy to the involved hemithorax.

Every attempt is made to perform a complete resection with clear margins. However, because of the nature of the diffuse spread of the tumor, in which margins are often vital structures not amenable to excision, microscopic or gross tumor is left in up to 60% of patients. Clear surgical margins have not been shown conclusively to predict survival, and the benefits of maximal cytoreduction with extrapleural pneumonectomy are well established (9, 18, 52).

Previously reported series of patients treated with extrapleural pneumonectomy have demonstrated operative mortality rates often far worse than those seen with traditional pneumonectomy for primary lung cancer (5% to 10%). Our present series (9), as well as another recent review (56), have shown that this operation can be performed with an operative mortality similar to that reported with standard pneumonectomy (Table 37.7).

PLEURECTOMY/DECORTICATION

Many patients are unable to tolerate extrapleural pneumonectomy because of performance status, limited pulmonary reserve, or other comorbid factors. In patients with disease limited to the hemithorax who can tolerate an operation with general anesthesia, pleurectomy with decortication allows for tumor debulking and control of the pleural effusion, often with significant palliation (54).

The procedure consists of removal of all grossly involved pleura, often including portions of the di-

TABLE 37.7. Select Series of Extrapleural Pneumonectomy in the Treatment of Pleural Mesothelioma

Author (Reference)	Year	No. of Patients	Adjuvant Therapy	2-Year Survival	5-Year Survival[a]	Operative Mortality
Worn (53)	1974	62	None	37%	10%	Not stated
Butchart (54)	1976	29	None	10%	4%	31%
Rusch (18)	1991	20	None	33%	NA	15%
Sugarbaker (9)	1993	52	EP + CAP 4–6 cycles, then 55 Gy XRT	17% (overall) 50% (epithelial) 8% (other types)	4% 45%[a] 0%	6%
Allen (55)	1994	40	EP + CAP	23%	10%	8%
		56	Pleur + CAP	9%	5%	5%

Abbreviations. EP + CAP, extrapleural pneumonectomy followed by adjuvant cyclophosphamide, Adriamycin, and cisplatin chemotherapy; CAP, cyclophosphamide, Adriamycin, and cisplatin chemotherapy; XRT, radiotherapy; Pleur, pleurectomy; NA, not available.
[a]5-year survival for patients with epithelial histology and no positive mediastinal nodes at resection.

aphragm and pericardium in the resection, while leaving the lung parenchyma. This approach is feasible only as a form of complete resection in very early stages of the disease, and it requires a free pleural space without a thick constricting growth of tumor encasing the lung. In most instances gross tumor is left behind. Operative mortality has been reported to be between 1.5% and 5% (54–56).

PLEURODESIS

In debilitated patients with advanced disease who are not candidates for major surgery, pleurodesis, either with thoracoscopic assistance or through a minithoracotomy, has been shown to improve quality of life in several series. It also has provided effective palliation of recurrent pleural effusion–induced dyspnea (10, 23).

MULTIMODALITY THERAPY

Several series have demonstrated that surgical treatment, either extrapleural pneumonectomy or pleurectomy/decortication, of mesothelioma applied alone does not significantly alter the expected dismal long-term survival (18, 57). This finding has led to the development of several combined modality approaches based on initial surgical therapy followed by various adjuvant chemotherapy, radiation, or biologic modifiers. These aggressive protocols have yielded promising results, and the combined modality approach forms the basis of the future treatment of MPM.

To improve the local control and survival attained with pleurectomy/decortication, several additional combinations of therapies have been implemented and reported. From 1976 to 1982, 41 patients with epithelial cell type mesotheliomas were treated with pleurectomy. Patients received perioperative interstitial brachytherapy with either iodine 125 or iridium 192 for gross residual disease and diffuse residual disease, respectively, as needed. In addition, external beam radiation therapy was given (45 Gy) to the pleural surface using mixed beam therapy over 4.5 weeks postoperatively. Median survival of the group was reported as 21 months with no operative deaths (58). An update of this series in 1988 reported 105 patients who underwent pleurectomy. A median survival of 12.6 months was attained for all patients with MPM regardless of cell type (59).

Postoperative radiation therapy is limited by toxicity to the underlying lung parenchyma and mediastinal structures, prohibiting the administration of curative doses (50 to 60 Gy) with the native lung in place.

A retrospective analysis of pleurectomy followed by variable systemic chemotherapy regimens (currently cyclophosphamide, Adriamycin, and cisplatin) was reported in 56 patients undergoing operation between 1958 and 1993. A 2-year survival of 9% and an operative mortality of 5% were observed for the reviewed cohort (56).

The pharmacokinetics of intrapleurally administered chemotherapy after pleurectomy/decortication was studied in 12 patients (60). Cisplatin (100 mg/m^2) and mitomycin (8 mg/m^2) were administered intrapleurally immediately after pleurectomy for MPM. Pleural fluid and plasma samples were collected and demonstrated appropriately elevated intrapleural drug levels and plasma levels near those attained with systemic administration.

A phase II trial of 28 patients who underwent pleurectomy/decortication and the aforementioned intrapleural chemotherapy regimen was conducted. There was one postoperative death (4%), and two patients sustained grade 4 renal toxicity after the intrapleural chemotherapy. Systemic chemotherapy consisting of cisplatin and mitomycin was administered to

FIGURE 37.6. Protocol for resectable malignant mesothelioma at the Dana-Farber Cancer Institute/Brigham and Women's Hospital. (From Sugarbaker DJ, Taklitsch MT, Liptay MJ. Mesothelioma and radical multimodality therapy: who benefits? Chest 1995;107:345.)

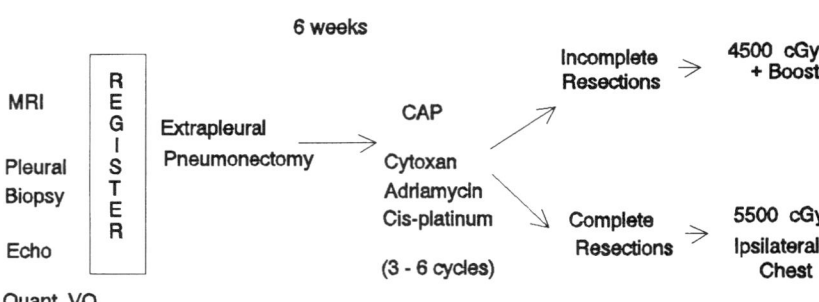

23 patients with no grade 3 or 4 toxicities observed. The median survival was 17 months, and the overall 1- and 2-year survival rates were 68% and 40%, respectively (55).

Photodynamic therapy involves the use of a light-activated photosensitizing drug typically given intravenously 24 to 48 hours before the administration of laser light beamed at the pleural surface of the tumor. The drug, Photofrin II (Quadra Logic Technologies, Vancouver, BC), a hematoporphyrin derivative, has been shown to sensitize and destroy human mesothelial cell lines in vitro and in mice with the addition of 630 nm of laser light (61, 62)

Fifty-four patients with thoracic malignancies (including 31 with MPM) were treated at the National Cancer Institute with photodynamic therapy in a phase I trial beginning in 1990 (63). The maximum tolerated dose was found to be 30 J/cm^3 with a 24-hour dosing interval. Survival data are lacking for this new approach, and a randomized phase III trial comparing surgical resection with or without photodynamic therapy followed by systemic immunotherapy with cisplatin, interferon-α, and tamoxifen is currently underway at the National Cancer Institute. Local toxicity suffered by nearby organs (heart, lungs, esophagus) must be controlled while administering tumoricidal doses of photodynamic therapy before this therapy can become a standard treatment option for patients with MPM.

The trade-off of an increased operative mortality with extrapleural pneumonectomy compared with pleurectomy/decortication is the superior local cytoreduction and greater likelihood of complete resection, even in more advanced disease that has encased the involved lung with a thickened tumor peal. For multimodality treatment that includes postoperative radiation therapy to the involved hemithorax, the absence of underlying lung on that side aids in the ability to deliver maximal doses of radiation to the field.

At Brigham and Women's Hospital and the Dana-Farber Cancer Institute in Boston, an aggressive trimodality approach in selected patients with MPM has been used since 1985 (9, 64). This approach consists of extrapleural pneumonectomy with sequential adjuvant chemotherapy (cyclophosphamide, doxorubicin, and cisplatin for 4 to 6 cycles) and up to 55 Gy of radiation therapy to the postoperative hemithorax.

In a series from 1980 to 1992, 52 patients were treated with extrapleural pneumonectomy, adjuvant chemotherapy (four to six cycles of cisplatin [70 mg/m^2], cyclophosphamide [600 mg/m^2], and doxorubicin to a cumulative dose of 450 mg/m^2), and 55 Gy of adjuvant radiotherapy (Fig. 37.6) (65). The median survival was 16 months; patients having the epithelial variant survived a median of 24 months. Five-year survival for those with epithelial histology and no involved lymph nodes at resection was 45%.

Presently available therapies have not meaningfully improved survival for the majority of patients with malignant pleural mesothelioma. The prolonged survival attained in selected aggressively treated patients provides encouragement for the future use of multimodality therapy in this rare but deadly disease. Further progress is rooted in the development of new combinations of innovative therapies coupled with a better understanding of the biology of mesothelioma.

REFERENCES

1. Connelly RR, Spirtas R, Myers MH, Percy CL, Fraumeni JF Jr. Demographic patterns for mesothelioma in the United States. J Natl Cancer Inst 1987;78:1053–1060.
2. Walker AM, Loughlin JE, Freidlander ER, Rothman KJ, Dreyer NA. Projections of asbestos-related disease 1980–2009. J Occup Med 1983;25:409–425.
3. Wagner JC, Sleggs EA, Marchand P. Diffuse pleural mesothelioma and asbestos exposure in the North Western Cape Province. Br J Ind Med 1960;17:260–271.
4. Selikoff IJ, Churg J, Hammond EC. Asbestos exposure and neoplasia. JAMA 1964;188:142–146.

5. Hillerdal G. Malignant mesothelioma 1982: review of 4710 published cases. Br J Dis Chest 1983:77:321.
6. Churg A. Immunohistochemical staining for vimentin and keratin in malignant mesothelioma. Am J Surg Pathol 1985;9:360–365.
7. Duggan MA, Masters CB, Alexander F. Immunohistochemical differentiation of malignant mesothelioma, mesothelial hyperplasia and metastatic adenocarcinoma in serous effusions, utilizing staining for carcinoembryonic antigen, keratin and vimentin. Acta Cytol 1987;31:807–814.
8. Wakabayashi A. Expanded applications of diagnostic and therapeutic thoracoscopy. J Thorac Cardiovasc Surg 1991;102:721–723.
9. Sugarbaker DJ, Strauss GM, Lynch TJ, et al. Node status has prognostic significance in the multimodality therapy of diffuse, malignant mesothelioma. J Clin Oncol 1993;11:1172–1178.
10. Boutin C. Thoracoscopy in malignant mesothelioma. Pneumologie 1989;43:61–65.
11. Branscheid D, Krysa S, Bauer E, et al. Diagnostic and therapeutic strategy in malignant pleural mesothelioma. Eur J Cardiothorac Surg 1991;5(9):466–472.
12. Boutin C, Viallat JR, Rey F, et al. Diagnosis and prognosis of malignant mesothelioma (French). Rev Prat 1990;40(20):1846–1850.
13. Manzini V, Brollo A, Franceschi S, et al. Prognostic factors of malignant mesothelioma of the pleura. Cancer 1993;72(2):410–417.
14. Alberts AS, Falkson G, Vorobiof DA, Van der Merwe CA. Malignant pleural mesothelioma: a disease unaffected by current therapeutic maneuvers. J Clin Oncol 1988;6(3):527–535.
15. Sridar KS, Doria R, Raub WA, Thurer RJ, Saldana M. New strategies are needed in diffuse malignant mesothelioma. Cancer 1992;70(12):2969–2979.
16. Antman KH, Blum RH, Greenberger JS, Flowerdew G, Skarin AT, Canellos GP. Multimodality therapy for malignant mesothelioma based on a study of natural history. Am J Med 1980;68:356–362.
17. Antman K, Shemin R, Ryan L, et al. Malignant mesothelioma: prognostic variables in a registry of 180 patients, the Dana-Farber Cancer Institute and Brigham and Women's Hospital experience over two decades, 1965–1985. J Clin Oncol 1988;6:147–153.
18. Rusch VW, Piantadosi S, Holmes EC. The role of extrapleural pneumonectomy in malignant pleural mesothelioma. A Lung Cancer Study Group trial. J Thorac Cardiovasc Surg 1991;102:1–9.
19. Tammilehto L, Tuomi T, Tiainen M., et al. Malignant mesothelioma: clinical characteristics, asbestos mineralogy and chromosomal abnormalities of 41 patients. Eur J Cancer 1994;28A(8–9):1373–1379.
20. Achatzy R, Beba W, Ritschler R, et al. The diagnosis, therapy and prognosis of diffuse malignant mesothelioma. Eur J Cardiothorac Surg 1989;3(5):445–448.
21. Viallat JR, Boutin C, Rey F, Astoul P, Farisse P. Malignant mesothelioma: study of prognostic factors of 188 cases (French). Arch Anat Cytol Pathol 1993;41(5–6):205–211.
22. Gotterer A, Taryle DA, Reed CE, Sahn SA. Pleural fluid analysis in malignant mesothelioma. Prognostic implications. Chest 1991;100(4):1003–1006.
23. Ruffie P, Feld R, Minkin S, et al. Diffuse malignant mesothelioma of the pleura in Ontario and Quebec: a retrospective study of 332 patients (abstract). J Clin Oncol 1989;7:1157–1168.
24. Fusco V, Ardizzoni A, Merlo F, Cinquegrana A, Faravelli B, et al. Malignant pleural mesothelioma. Multivariate analysis of prognostic factors on 113 patients. Anticancer Res 1994;13(3):683–689.
25. Rice TW, Adelstein DJ, Kirby TJ, et al. Aggressive multimodality therapy for malignant pleural mesothelioma. Ann Thorac Surg 1994;58:24–29.
26. Lu YY, Jhanwar SC, Cheng JQ, Testa JR. Deletion mapping in the short arm of chromosome 3 in human malignant mesothelioma. Genes Chromosom Cancer 1994;9(1):76–80.
27. Taguchi T, Jhanwar SC, Siegfried JM, Keller SM, Testa JR. Recurrent deletion of specific sites in 1p, 3p, 6q, and 9p in human malignant mesothelioma. Cancer Res 1993;53(18):4349–4355.
28. Center R, Lukeis R, Dietzsch E, Gillespie M, Garson OM. Molecular deletion of 9p sequences in non–small cell lung cancer and malignant mesothelioma. Genes Chromosom Cancer 1993;7(1):47–53.
29. Elahi A, Gerdes H, Chen Q, Saad A, Jhanwar SC. Abnormalities of chromosome 17 and the *p53* locus in malignant mesothelioma (abstract). Proc Ann Meet Am Assoc Cancer Res 1992;33:A2275.
30. Chang K, Ding IY, Chang X, et al. Heterogeneous expression of *p53* is a common feature of human malignant mesothelioma (abstract). Proc Ann Meet Am Assoc Cancer Res 1992;33:A2280.
31. Metcalf RA, Welsh JA, Bennett WP, Seddon MB, Lehman TA, et al. *p53* And Kirsten-*ras* mutations in human mesothelioma cell lines. Cancer Res 1992;52(9):2610–2615.
32. Kishimoto T. The distribution of various types of oncogenes products in the tumor tissue of malignant mesothelioma. Jpn J Thorac Dis 1991;29(9):1168–1173.
33. Tiainen M, Rautonen J, Pyrhonen S, Tammilehto L, Mattson K, Knuutila S. Chromosome number correlates with survival in patients with malignant pleural mesothelioma. Cancer Genet Cytogenet 1992;62(1):21–24.
34. el-Naggar AK, Ordonez NG, Garnsey L, Batsakis JG. Epithelioid pleural mesotheliomas and pulmonary adenocarcinomas: a comparative DNA flow cytometric study. Hum Pathol 1991;22(10):972–978.
35. Dejmek A, Stromberg C, Wikstrom B, Hjerpe A. Prognostic importance of the DNA ploidy pattern in malignant mesothelioma of the pleura. Anal Quant Cytol Histol 1992;14(3):217.
36. Pyrhonen S, Laasonen A, Tammilehto L, Rautonen J, Anttila S, Mattson K, Holsti LR. Diploid predominance and prognostic significance of S-phase cells in malignant mesothelioma. Eur J Cancer 1991;27(2):197–200.
37. Pgrebniak HW, Lubensky IA, Pass HI. Differential expression of platelet derived growth factor-B in malignant mesothelioma. Surg Oncol 1993;2:235–240.
38. Versnel MA, Claesson-Welsh L, Hammacher A, et al. Human malignant mesothelioma cell lines express PDGF beta receptors whereas cultured normal mesothelial cells express PDGF-alpha receptors. Oncogene 1991;6:2005–2011.
39. Butchart EG, Ashcroft T, Barnsley WC, Holden MP. Pleuropneumonectomy in the management of diffuse malignant mesothelioma of the pleura. Experience with 29 patients. Thorax 1976;31:15–24.
40. Rusch VW, Ginsberg RJ. New concepts in the staging of mesothelioma: invited comment to chapter 26. In: Deslauriers J, Lacquet LK, eds. Thoracic surgery: surgical management of pleural diseases. International trends in general thoracic surgery. St. Louis: Mosby, 1990;6:336–343.
41. Mountain CF. A new international staging system for lung cancer. Chest 1986;89(Suppl):225S–233S.
42. Vogelzang NJ. Malignant mesothelioma: diagnostic and management strategies for 1992. Semin Oncol 1992;19(4):64–71.
43. Samson MK, Wasser LP, Borden EC, et al. Randomized comparison of cyclophosphamide, imidazole carboxamide, and Adri-

amycin versus cyclophosphamide and Adriamycin in patients with advanced stage malignant mesothelioma: a sarcoma intergroup study. J Clin Oncol 1987;5:86–91.
44. Vogelzang NJ, Herndon J, et al. Paclitaxel (Taxol) for malignant mesothelioma (MM): a phase II study of the Cancer and Leukemia Group B (CALGB 9234). Proc Am Soc Clin Oncol 1994;13:405.
45. Von Hoff DD, Metch B, Lucas JG, et al. Phase II evaluation of interferon-beta in patients with diffuse mesothelioma: a Southwest Oncology Group study. J Interferon Res 1990;10:531–534.
46. Christmas TI, Musk AW, Robinson BWS. Phase II study of recombinant human alpha interferon therapy in malignant pleural mesothelioma. Proc Am Assoc Cancer Res 1990;31:283.
47. Stoter G, Coey SH, Slingerland R, et al. Intrapleural interleukin-2 (IL-2) in malignant pleural mesothelioma: a phase I-II study (abstract). Proc Am Assoc Cancer Res 1990;31:275.
48. Boutin C, Viallat JR, Van Zandwijk N, et al. Activity of intrapleural recombinant gamma-interferon in malignant mesothelioma. Cancer 1991;67:2033–2037.
49. Maasilta P. Deterioration in lung function following hemithorax irradiation for pleural mesothelioma. Int J Radiat Oncol Biol Phys 1990;20:433.
50. Patz EF Jr, Shaffer K, Piwnica-Worms DR, et al. Malignant pleural mesothelioma: value of CT and MR imaging in predicting resectability. AJR Am J Roentgenol 1992;159:961–966.
51. Sugarbaker DJ, Mentzer SJ, Strauss G. Extrapleural pneumonectomy in the treatment of malignant pleural mesothelioma. Ann Thorac Surg 1992;54:941–946.
52. Sugarbaker DJ, Heher EC, Lee TH, et al. Extrapleural pneumonectomy, chemotherapy, and radiotherapy in the treatment of diffuse malignant pleural mesothelioma (discussion). J Thorac Cardiovasc Surg 1991;102:10–14.
53. Mentzer SJ, Filler RM, Phillips J. Limited pulmonary resections for congenital cystic adenomatoid malformation of the lung. J Pediatr Surg 1992;27:1410–1413.
54. McCormack PM, Nagasaki F, Hilaris BS, Martini N. Surgical treatment of pleural mesothelioma. J Thorac Cardiovasc Surg 1982;84:834–842.
55. Rusch V, Saltz L, Venkatraman E, et al. A phase II trial of pleurectomy/decortication followed by intrapleural and systemic chemotherapy for malignant pleural mesothelioma. J Clin Oncol 1994;12(6):1156–1163.
56. Allen KB, Faber LP, Warren WH. Malignant pleural mesothelioma: extrapleural pneumonectomy and pleurectomy. Chest Surg Clin North Am 1994;4:113–126.
57. Alberts AS, Falkson G, Goedhals L, Vorbiof DA, van der Merwe CA. Malignant pleural mesothelioma: a disease unaffected by current therapeutic maneuvers. J Clin Oncol 1988;6:527–535.
58. Hilaris BS, Nori D, Kwong E, Kutcher GJ, Martini N. Pleurectomy and intraoperative brachytherapy and postoperative radiation in the treatment of malignant pleural mesothelioma. Int J Radiat Oncol Biol Phys 1984;10:325–331.
59. Mychalsak BR, Nori D, Armstrong JG, et al. Results of treatment of malignant pleural mesothelioma with surgery, brachytherapy, and external beam irradiation. Endocurie Hypertherm Oncol 1989;5:245.
60. Rusch VW, Niedzwiecki D, Tao Y, et al. Intrapleural cisplatin and mitomycin for malignant mesothelioma following pleurectomy: pharmacokinetic studies. J Clin Oncol 1992;10:1001–1006.
61. Feins RH, Hilf R, Ross H, et al. Photodynamic therapy of human malignant mesothelioma in the nude mouse. J Surg Res 1990;49:311.
62. Keller SM, Taylor DD, Weese JL. In vitro killing of human malignant mesothelioma by photodynamic therapy. J Surg Res 1990;48:337.
63. Pass HI, Delaney TF, Tochner Z, et al. Intrapleural photodynamic therapy: results of a phase I trial. Ann Surg Oncol 1994;1:28–37.
64. Antman KH, Shemin RJ, Corson JM. Malignant pleural mesothelioma: a combined modality approach. In: Kittle CF, ed. Current controversies in thoracic surgery. Philadelphia: WB Saunders, 1986:68–75.
65. Sugarbaker DJ, Taklitsch MT, Liptay MJ. Mesothelioma and radical multimodality therapy: who benefits? Chest 1995;107:345.

38

Current Therapeutic Approaches to Unresectable (Primary and Recurrent) Disease

Sin-Tiong Ong and Nicholas J. Vogelzang

Although malignant pleural mesothelioma is a relatively rare tumor and accounts for only about 1500 cancer deaths per year in the United States, epidemiologic studies show the incidence rates have increased by as much as 50% since the mid-1970s (1). Because the latency period, i.e., the period from exposure to clinical diagnosis, can be 30 or more years, this rising rate suggests either that the benefits of legislation to reduce asbestos exposure in the workplace have not yet taken effect, or that asbestos exposure during the 1960s was more widespread than previously believed. Mesothelioma remains a difficult and frustrating disease to treat, with no conclusive studies to date demonstrating any significant impact of surgery, radiotherapy, chemotherapy, or combined modality treatment on survival. A number of studies have compared treated with untreated patients and claimed that median survival has been unaffected by therapy; no prospective phase III studies comparing treatment with no treatment have been performed because of the rarity of the disease and the unimpressive results to date of phase II trials. However, the clinician managing a patient with an unresectable primary or recurrent mesothelioma in a non-clinical trial setting often is obliged to offer some form of therapy.

Because there is currently no consensus on the most appropriate treatment, clinicians are left with a number of unanswered questions: (*a*) When should chemotherapy be used? (*b*) Which agents should be used? (*c*) Should they be combined or used singly? (*d*) Should combined modality therapy (in the form of chemotherapy or radiotherapy) be given? (*e*) Is there a role for debulking surgery as part of combined modality treatment? (*f*) Is there a role for adjuvant therapy? The clinician also must address the therapeutic options available for palliating symptoms of recurrent or nonresponsive local disease, which is often the most distressing aspect of managing these patients.

Before discussing treatment, certain aspects of the natural history of mesothelioma should be highlighted to provide a thorough understanding of the impact of therapy on the seemingly relentless progression of this disease. The role of chemotherapy (single-agent, combination, and intrapleural) with an emphasis on the peculiar problems of conducting and interpreting trials in mesothelioma is reviewed. Finally, there is a review of the role of radiotherapy, either alone or combined with surgery and/or chemotherapy.

NATURAL HISTORY

Pleural mesotheliomas, mainly found in males with a ratio of 3.6:1 in the largest review to date (2), occur most commonly in the fifth to seventh decade of life. The tumor tends to be locally invasive and encases the lung by growing along the pleural space, resulting in a tumor "rind" that may be several centimeters thick. With advancing disease local structures become involved. Pleural effusions become loculated and difficult to drain, and eventually the pleural space becomes obliterated, resulting in a nonfunctioning lung. Autopsy findings in one series of 92 patients showed the presence of lymphatic and hematogenous metastases in 50% of cases, liver in 33%, contralateral lung in 16%, kidney in 13%, adrenal in 12%, and bone in 10% (3). This high incidence of metastatic disease is supported further by another series of 40 autopsies in which the percentage of cases with involvement of the mediastinal lymph nodes was 35%; liver, 33%; contralateral lung, 27%; hilar nodes, 22%; adrenal glands, 22%; bone, 22%; heart, 20%; spleen, 15%; and kidney and peritoneum, 10% each (4). Death usually is caused by respiratory failure or pneumonia, or in 10% of cases by pericardial/myocardial involvement. Ascites and small bowel obstruction secondary to transdiaphragmatic tumor spread also contribute to morbidity.

The median survival for patients with diffuse malignant pleural mesothelioma has been reported to be between 4 and 18 months. There are at least eight studies describing the median survival of untreated patients (Table 38.1). The variation in quoted median survival probably results from differences in tumor biology, host response to tumor, detection bias, and lead-time bias. Because no studies were randomized, differences in survival between treated and untreated patients cannot be statistically valid. In this setting ad hoc treatment decisions were commonly made. It also follows that the median survival of the untreated patients can only be used for historical comparisons if the prognostic factors of the untreated group are taken into account. Unfortunately, prognostic data for survival were largely incomplete. The often quoted study by Law et al. (12) demonstrating an 18-month survival among 64 untreated patients is particularly striking, but it also illustrates the problem of extrapolating the results of one trial to others. In the calculations of Law et al. (12), median survival was determined from the onset of symptoms, rather than from the time of diagnosis, and symptoms may precede diagnosis by 6 months or more (8).

Prognostic factors that improve median survival include a good performance status, stage I disease, absence of chest pain, age less than 50 years, epithelial histology, female sex, longer duration of symptoms, and uninvolved mediastinal lymph nodes (13). Retrospective and prospective phase II studies, regardless of treatment modality, thus are unlikely to provide meaningful conclusions about better survival among treated patients. It thus is apparent that a large number of the available studies recommending a particular therapeutic approach are inconclusive and potentially misleading.

ASSESSMENT OF CLINICAL TRIALS IN MESOTHELIOMA

The rarity of pleural mesotheliomas precludes the luxury of large comparison trials, and therefore the therapeutic advances in mesothelioma will necessarily rely on trials with limited numbers. This restriction does not prevent the possibility of a major therapeutic breakthrough, illustrated by the example of fludarabine in hairy cell leukemia. The drug was almost discarded from further clinical trials because of its toxicity and the search discontinued because this leukemia was a relatively rare malignancy. As for mesothelioma trials, the presence of the following factors strengthens the validity of the studies and will permit the practicing physician to make an independent assessment of a given mesothelioma trial: (*a*) multiinstitutional study; (*b*) the provision of adequate tissue for diagnosis by histochemistry, supplemented by immunohistochemistry and electron microscopy in atypical cases; (*c*) accurate pretreatment staging and response to treatment at least by computed tomography (CT) scanning and possibly magnetic resonance imaging; and (*d*) adequately described protocols including information on any previous treatment that may influence chemotherapeutic response (14). In both phase II and comparison trials, stratification by these prognostic criteria will be an important consideration.

ASSESSMENT OF DISEASE AND RESPONSE PARAMETERS

The most important aspect of assessment of disease at diagnosis is the determination of isolated hemithorax disease that may be potentially curable

TABLE 38.1. Studies of Median Survival in Untreated Patients with Malignant Mesothelioma

Study (Reference No.)	Patients Treated	Patients Untreated	Median Survival (Mo)	Comments
Antman et al., 1980 (5)	35	5	4.2	
Lewis et al., 1980 (6)	36	10	9.1	
Brenner et al., 1982 (7)	123	18	10.0	
Chahinian et al., 1982 (8)	69	21	11.3	
Antman et al., 1988 (9)	19	117	13.0	
Chailleux et al., 1988 (10)	167	69	7.0	Treated group included patients treated with talc poudrage only
Ruffie et al., 1989 (3)	332	176	6.8	
DePangher-Manzini et al., 1993 (11)	24	56	13.0	

Note: All trials were retrospective, except that of Chahinian et al. (8), and had median survivals calculated from the time of diagnosis.

with surgical resection, i.e., Butchart stage I disease confined within the capsule of the parietal pleura, involving only the ipsilateral lung, pericardium, and diaphragm. In practice this would involve CT evaluation of the chest because CT has a more than 90% sensitivity for detecting resectable disease (15). CT also is the most reliable method of assessing disease response parameters after therapy, which was not possible with chest radiographs in areas such as the paravertebral gutters, mediastinal pleural reflections, and diaphragmatic surfaces, especially in the presence of loculated pleural effusions.

However, even with CT it is not always possible to tell accurately the difference between asbestosis (the presence of pleural thickening, pleural plaques and calcification, and pleural effusions with a history of asbestos exposure) and malignant mesothelioma, both at the time of diagnosis and after therapy. Because of the poor prognosis of mesothelioma, an unequivocal tissue diagnosis is mandatory and usually is best accomplished by thoracoscopy or thoracotomy. When thoracoscopy is performed, multiple biopsies should be taken because of the diffuse nature of the disease, together with a lung biopsy of unaffected lung for the counting of asbestos fibers. Subsequent surgery should encompass the thoracoscopy tract because of the high incidence of tumor seeding along such tracts.

ROLE OF CHEMOTHERAPY

SINGLE-AGENT CHEMOTHERAPY

A wide variety of agents has been evaluated in malignant mesothelioma, both in the setting of single-agent and combination chemotherapy. Table 38.2 lists the results of single-agent chemotherapy studies in which at least 15 patients were treated. Smaller trials were omitted because they are statistically less reliable, and review articles were omitted as the result of both publication bias and possible duplication of results.

DOXORUBICIN

The most widely used single agent is doxorubicin, and a number of reviews (16, 17) have cited a response rate of approximately 20%. These reviews included data from old trials, some of which were broad phase II studies that may have been biased by a trend toward publishing positive results. If the individual trials are assessed carefully, the results are less clear. For example, the largest series using doxorubicin reported a response rate of 7 (14%) of 51 with two complete responses (lasting 38 and 52 weeks) (18). This was a retrospective study, however, in which results from three different trials were compiled, using different doses and schedules of administration. These included doxorubicin given at 20 mg/m^2 for 3 days every 3 weeks, 70 mg/m^2 every 3 weeks, and 20 mg/m^2 for 3 days followed by 15 mg/m^2 every week. Furthermore, neither the response criteria nor the methods of assessing response were stated clearly. The median survival of doxorubicin-treated patients was 7.5 months. In a randomized prospective trial (19) comparing doxorubicin with cyclophosphamide, 15 patients received doxorubicin at 60 mg/m^2 every 3 weeks, and 16 received cyclophosphamide. At disease progression patients were crossed over to the other arm of the study. Patients had not received any prior chemotherapy. None of the patients showed any response to either agent, and all had progressive disease. Neither the duration of disease free survival nor overall survival was given, and patients were assessed for response only on the basis of plain chest roentgenograms. Caution should be exercised in concluding from this trial that doxorubicin has no activity in mesothelioma, because any antitumor effect resulting in stable disease on the chest radiograph would not have been detected easily. In another trial (20) that included 11 patients treated with doxorubicin after progression on 5-fluorouracil, there was one partial response of 34 months' duration. The other 10 patients had progression within 6 months. Response was assessed by physical examination and chest roentgenograms only. The poor results of doxorubicin should again be interpreted cautiously because it has been shown that response to doxorubicin in mesothelioma is influenced by prior chemotherapy.

Doxorubicin thus appears to have some activity with at least two complete responses reported in the literature. However, activity is probably no greater than 15% in terms of either partial or complete response. It also should be appreciated that antitumor effect producing stable disease may be underestimated in the published trials of single-agent doxorubicin because such trials were small and noncontrolled; they also were conducted before the widespread availability of CT scanning as an accurate measure of tumor response.

OTHER ANTHRACYCLINES

A number of other anthracyclines have been tested, including detorubicin, pirarubicin, epirubicin, and mitoxantrone (an anthracycline analogue). Thirty-five patients were given detorubicin at 40 mg/m^2 for 3 days every 3 weeks for up to five cycles (21). Two pa-

TABLE 38.2. Series of at Least 15 Patients with Malignant Mesothelioma Treated with Single-Agent Chemotherapy

AGENT	STUDY (REFERENCE NO.)	NO. OF PATIENTS	NO. OF RESPONSES (%)
Doxorubicin	Lerner et al., 1983 (18)	51	7 (14)
Doxorubicin	Sørensen et al., 1985 (19)	15	0 (0)
Detorubicin	Colbert et al., 1985 (21)	35	9 (26)
Pirarubicin	Kaukel et al., 1987 (22)	35	8 (22)
Epirubicin	Magri et al., 1991 (25)	21	1 (5)
Epirubicin	Mattson et al., 1992 (26)	48	7 (15)
Mitoxantrone	Eisenhauer et al., 1986 (27)	28	2 (7)
Mitoxantrone	van Breukelen et al., 1991 (28)	34	1 (3)
Cisplatin	Mintzer et al., 1985 (29)	24	3 (13)
Cisplatin	Zidar et al., 1988 (30)	35	5 (14)
Carboplatin	Mbidde et al., 1986 (36)	17	2 (12)
Carboplatin	Raghavan et al., 1990 (37)	31	5 (16)
Carboplatin	Vogelzang et al., 1990 (38)	40	3 (7)
Vindesine	Kelsen et al., 1983 (34)	17	1 (6)
Vindesine	Boutin et al., 1987 (40)	21	0 (0)
Vincristine	Martensson et al., 1989 (41)	23	0 (0)
Vinblastine	Cowan 1988 (42)	20	0 (0)
Paclitaxel	Vogelzang et al., 1994 (43)	15	2 (13)
Cyclophosphamide	Sørensen et al., 1985 (19)	16	0 (0)
Ifosfamide	Alberts et al., 1988 (45)	17	4 (24)
Ifosfamide	Zidar et al., 1992 (46)	26	2 (8)
Ifosfamide	Falkson et al., 1992 (47)	40	1 (3)
Mitomycin C	Bajorin et al., 1987 (48)	19	2 (21)
Methotrexate	Solheim et al., 1992 (49)	60	22 (37)
Trimetrexate	Vogelzang et al., 1994 (52)	51	6 (12)
Edatrexate	Belani et al., 1994 (53)	20	5 (25)
CB3717	Cantwell et al., 1986 (54)	18	1 (6)
5-Fluorouracil	Harvey et al., 1984 (20)	20	1 (5)
5-Dihydroazacytidine	Harmon 1991 (55)	42	7 (17)
Amsacrine	Falkson et al., 1980 (58)	19	1 (5)
Diazquone (AZQ)	Eagan et al., 1986 (59)	20	0 (0)
Bacille Calmette-Guérin	Webster et al., 1982 (60)	30	Not evaluable
Acivicin	Alberts et al., 1988 (61)	19	0 (0)
Alpha interferon	Christmas et al., 1993 (62)	25	3 (12)
Beta interferon	von Hoff et al., 1990 (64)	14	0 (0)
Interleukin-2[a]	Eggermont et al., 1991 (82)	17	4 (24)
Gamma interferon[a]	Boutin et al., 1991 (83)	22	5 (23)

[a] Agent was administered as intrapleural therapy for early-stage disease.

tients (6%) achieved a complete response, whereas seven (20%) achieved a partial response, although the methods of response assessment were not described. Interestingly, 8 of 15 patients with chest pain (53%) were found to have complete relief of the pain. Median survival was 19 months after diagnosis, which was significantly longer than in most published series of both treated and untreated patients. The activity of pirarubicin, another anthracycline with supposedly less cardiotoxicity than doxorubicin, also has been reported in three trials (22–24). These trials, which reported response rates between 9% and 38%, used CT scans in evaluating response.

Two trials have been published using epirubicin (25, 26). The initial trial of 21 patients published in 1991 (25) resulted in one partial response, but it used a dose of 75 mg/m2 compared with 110 mg/m^2 in the more recent trial with 63 previously treated and untreated patients (26). In the latter study, 7 of 48 assessable patients (15%) (95% confidence intervals, 6.1% to 27.8%) showed a partial response according to World Health Organization criteria, i.e., tumor shrinkage more than 50% (product of two diameters) with no new tumor manifestations appearing during therapy. Notably, one patient was alive and well 4 years after the start of chemotherapy, although this patient had prior surgery and subsequent radiotherapy. With the higher dose, side effects of cardiotoxicity were observed with left ventricular ejection fraction reductions; none of the patients had clinical cardiac failure. A third related drug in the class of anthracyclines is mitoxantrone. Two phase II trials (27, 28) have been conducted with this agent. Both trials used essentially similar doses and schedules of 12 mg/m^2 and 14 mg/m^2 given every 3 weeks in 28 and 34 previously untreated evaluable patients, respectively. They used the same response criteria and CT scan assessments. Both studies concluded that mitoxantrone showed minimal activity against mesothelioma, although there was one complete response of 8 months' duration in the trial by Eisenhauer et al. (27).

In summary, the activity of doxorubicin, epirubicin, and the anthracyclines is in the range of 15%, although no modern single-agent trials have been conducted using doxorubicin. Two sequential trials with pirarubicin at 75 mg/m^2 and 110 mg/m^2 suggest a possible dose-response relationship for that drug. There have been no trials of doxorubicin at a dose of at least 90 mg/m^2 given every 3 weeks that have had significant statistical power. Thus, a dose-response relationship for doxorubicin cannot be estimated. The high response rate (26%) attributable to detorubicin in one unconfirmed study conducted before the availability of routine CT scanning assessment should be confirmed. Mitoxantrone had minimal activity in two well-conducted trials.

PLATINUM COMPOUNDS

There have been only two phase II trials using cisplatin that have enrolled more than 15 patients. In the first study by Mintzer et al. (29), 24 evaluable patients were treated with cisplatin at 120 mg/m^2 given every 4 weeks for two doses and then every 6 weeks. Seven patients had received prior chemotherapy. There were three partial responses, lasting a median of 5 months, giving a 13% response rate with 95% confidence limits of 4% to 31%. Unfortunately, the use of CT scans for assessment was not uniform. All of the responders were chemotherapy naive. The largest trial, performed by the Southwest Oncology Group (30), included 35 patients who received 100 mg/m^2 of single-agent cisplatin. There were five partial responses, and the medial survival was 7.5 months. The other reports of cisplatin involve either small numbers of patients treated in early, nontumor specific trials using unspecified doses of cisplatin (31, 32), or they were trials including fewer than 15 patients (33). Dabouis et al. (33), for example, reported a single complete response in nine patients. Of interest is a recent small trial by Planting and coworkers (34) using high-dose cisplatin at 80 mg/m^2 given weekly for six courses. Thus far nine patients have been treated with four (44%) partial responses. Toxicities included grade 3 thrombocytopenia and grade 3 leukopenia in three patients each. Further accrual is ongoing.

There are four well-conducted trials (35–38) of carboplatin in pleural mesothelioma. All used doses of 400 mg/m^2 to 450 mg/m^2 every 4 weeks. Patient characteristics were similar, and tumor response was assessed by CT scans. The first trial by Cantwell et al. (35) enrolled nine patients (three with prior chemotherapy) who received a median of three courses of carboplatin at 400 mg/m^2 every 3 weeks. Two of the nine had a 50% decrease in tumor volume, thus giving a response rate of 22% with 95% confidence intervals of 2.8% to 60.0%. In the trial by Mbidde et al. (36), 17 patients received carboplatin at 300 mg/m^2 to 400 mg/m^2 every 4 weeks. One patient with peritoneal mesothelioma achieved a complete response that lasted 15 months, and one patient with pleural mesothelioma achieved a partial response of 11 months. Their overall response rate was 12%. Raghavan et al. (37) published a trial of 31 evaluable patients with mesothelioma (including two patients with peritoneal disease) treated with carboplatin at 150 mg/m^2 for 3 days repeated every 4 weeks. Five (16%) achieved a partial response. The largest phase II trial was that of Vogelzang et al. (38), who treated 40 chemotherapy naive patients, all of whom were evaluable. Carboplatin was administered at 400 mg/m^2 every 4 weeks. Two partial responses and one with regression of evaluable disease were observed. A median of two doses was given. In these four studies toxicity was mild, and there were no treatment-related deaths. Because the study parameters, i.e., patient selection, drug dosages and intervals, response parameters, and techniques of assessment, were essentially the same, it is reasonable to combine their results: a partial response was seen in 12 (12%) of 97 patients treated with carboplatin. The mild toxicities observed may allow further dose escalation in subsequent trials.

PLANT DERIVATIVES

VINCA ALKALOIDS

The vinca alkaloids have been evaluated in a small number of trials and have been found to be largely inactive. Vindesine, in two phase II studies, has been given at 3 mg/m^2 weekly (39) and also at 2 mg/m^2 for 2 days every 2 weeks (40). Responses were seen in 1 of 17 evaluable patients at the former schedule and in none of the 21 patients treated with the latter. Both trials, however, used plain chest radiographs for assessment. Equally disappointing results have been reported with vincristine: no responses were seen in 23 patients treated at a dose of 1.3 mg/m^2 every 4 weeks (41) and also with vinblastine, again with no responses seen in 20 patients receiving a 5-day infusion of 1.4 mg/m^2 every 4 weeks (42). The new vinca alkaloid, Navelbine, has not yet been tested in phase II trials.

TAXOL

This plant derivative (Taxol; Bristol-Myers Squibb, Princeton, NJ) is being tested in an ongoing phase II trial of the Cancer and Leukemia Group B (CALGB). Eighteen patients have been enrolled in the trial, which administers paclitaxel at 250 mg/m^2 over 24 hours every 3 weeks, with filgrastim support. Among the initial 15 evaluable patients, there were two documented regressions, giving a response rate of 13% (43). Toxicity was mild except for one patient who was taken off study because of cardiac arrhythmias. Another common toxicity was a painful peripheral neuropathy seen in three patients by day 5, which resolved by day 14. According to the design of this trial, responses in the initial cohort require further accrual with larger numbers. The final response rate awaits completion of the study.

The plant alkaloids of the camptothecin class have not yet been evaluated in mesothelioma, although the North Central Cancer Treatment Group opened a study of single-agent topotecan in August 1993 using a dose of 1.5 mg/m^2/day for 5 days (44).

ALKYLATING AGENTS

Cyclophosphamide and ifosfamide have both been evaluated in clinical trials. However, only one trial mentioned previously (19) tested cyclophosphamide in a phase II-III setting that randomized patients to either doxorubicin or cyclophosphamide, and then crossed patients over to the other arm at disease progression. There were no responses among the 16 patients treated initially with cyclophosphamide at 1500 mg/m^2 every 3 weeks, nor among the six patients who had failed initial treatment with doxorubicin. Other reviews (16) have quoted response rates as high as 28%, but these have been calculated on the basis of combined results from case reports, a method that tends to overrepresent responding patients and that thus may explain the disparate response rates seen in the literature.

Ifosfamide and mesna have been evaluated in three phase II studies. In the South African series (45), 17 patients were treated with ifosfamide at either 1.2 g/m^2 or 1.5 g/m^2 on days 1 to 5 every 21 days. There were four (24%) partial responses with a median response duration of 7 months. Overall median survival was 9 months. CT scanning was used when plain radiographs or clinical examination was unable to assess disease. In a later study by the Southwest Oncology Group (46), 26 patients received 2 g/m^2 by continuous infusion over 24 hours for 4 days, with mesna. There were two (8%) patients who demonstrated a partial response as assessed by CT scans. Myelotoxicity was significant: 42% of patients had grade 4 granulocytopenia (less than 250 per microliter), and 20% had at least grade 2 thrombocytopenia (less than 75,000 per microliter). In the largest trial using ifosfamide, conducted by the Eastern Cooperative Oncology Group (47), 40 patients were treated with ifosfamide at 1.5 g/m^2 for 5 days every 21 days. Only 1 partial response lasting 6.3 months was observed, with 2 patients dying of treatment-related toxicity and more than 50% having at least one episode of severe or life-threatening toxicity.

Mitomycin, an antitumor antibiotic that functions in part as an alkylator, has been found to have a response rate of 21% in a single phase II trial, but at the cost of significant pulmonary toxicity (48). In 19 evaluable patients treated with mitomycin at 10 mg/m^2 every 4 weeks for three cycles and then with subsequent cycles every 6 weeks, four patients (21%) achieved a partial response lasting a median of 5.25 months. Two of the four responders had drug-related pulmonary toxicity. Future trials of mitomycin C should limit the cumulative dose to 40 mg/m^2. In a recent report the addition of cisplatin to mitomycin C did not improve that response rate (see Combination Chemotherapy, below).

The other alkylating agents, such as thiotepa, melphalan, nitrogen mustard, and the nitrosureas, have not been evaluated in sufficiently large clinical trials to make meaningful conclusions about their activity.

Among the alkylating agents, ifosfamide is seen to have modest activity against pleural mesothelioma but at the risk of potentially life-threatening myelotoxicity. Cyclophosphamide may have a higher response rate, but this level of activity has not been confirmed in contemporary phase II trials. Mitomycin appears moderately active but produces significant toxicity.

ANTIMETABOLITES

ANTIFOLATES

Among the antifolates high-dose methotrexate has the highest response rate. In one recent well-conducted trial by Solheim et al. (49) of 63 patients, 60 were evaluable for tumor response to high-dose methotrexate at a 3-g total dose administered over 16 hours. The first four infusions were given at 10-day intervals, and response was evaluated 3 weeks later by CT scan. Responding patients were treated with four additional infusions at 21-day intervals. Twenty-one patients (35%) showed a partial response using the parameters of either a 50% reduction in the thickness of two sections or a 30% reduction of three sections. One patient (2%) showed a complete response. The overall response rate, using these unique response criteria, was 37%. Three patients showed delayed methotrexate excretion that was attributed to delayed renal clearance rather than to accumulation in the pleural fluid, although the evidence for the latter was not elaborated. One death caused by toxicity was seen secondary to pneumonitis after a second infusion of methotrexate. The patients with epithelial histology had a longer survival than those with sarcomatous histology, but the former did not show any difference in response to therapy. Confirmation of this high response rate in another trial is important. Interestingly, in a trial conducted in 1982 (50), three of nine patients treated with high-dose methotrexate at 1.5 gm/m^2 over 16 hours with 2 mg of vincristine had complete remissions defined as "disappearance of all clinically detectable malignant disease for at least four weeks with normalization of radiographs, sonograms and biochemical profile (52)"; three had partial responses. Similarly, a trial reported by Djerassi et al. in 1985 (51) showed an appreciable response rate (four of nine responders) to high-dose methotrexate. Some of the patients then also received small doses of cisplatin, and the final response was eight of nine. The small numbers and complexity of the therapy precluded definitive statements about the activity of the high-dose methotrexate.

Other antifolates that have been evaluated include trimetrexate, edatrexate, and dideazafolic acid (CB3717). Trimetrexate, which appears to have delayed clearance from pleural effusions and may therefore have enhanced efficacy, has been tested recently by the CALGB in a cohort of 51 evaluable patients with chemotherapy naive malignant mesothelioma (52). Two (12%) of 17 patients in the group treated at 6 mg/m^2 for 5 days every 3 weeks had a partial response; 4 (12%) of the 34 patients treated at the 10 mg/m^2 dose level had either a partial response or regression. There was one toxicity-related death from sepsis, and a 12% rate of grade 4 thrombocytopenia and granulocytopenia was observed. The overall survival in the two treatment groups was 5 and 8.9 months in the 6 mg/m^2 and 10 mg/m^2 dose groups, respectively. Because the study was not designed to evaluate the response to different dosage levels, the apparent dose-response relationship must be confirmed. However, it is promising enough, especially considering the high response rates seen in high-dose methotrexate, to warrant further assessment of higher doses of trimetrexate.

Edatrexate, another folate antagonist that undergoes polyglutamation and retention within tumor cells, has also been evaluated recently (53). Twenty previously untreated patients were given edatrexate at 80 mg/m^2 weekly. There was one complete response, two partial responses, and two regressions of evaluable disease, for an overall response rate of 25% (95% confidence intervals of 9% to 49%). However, there was significant toxicity with three treatment-related deaths. A subsequent trial, being conducted by the CALGB, of the same dose with leucovorin rescue may result in less toxicity.

Lastly, among the antifolates, dideazafolic acid (CB3717) was evaluated in 18 patients (56). One patient had a partial response lasting 7 months for a response rate of 6% (95% confidence limits of 0.1% to 27.3%). However, dose-response relationships were not explored.

OTHER ANTIMETABOLITES

Other antimetabolites that have been evaluated include 5-fluorouracil, 5-azacytidine, and dihydro-5-azacytidine. Only one trial (20) has evaluated 5-fluorouracil in a phase II setting. Twenty patients were given the drug at 10 mg/kg or 15 mg/kg for 5 days, repeated monthly. One partial response was seen as assessed by CT scan. 5-Azacytidine has undergone limited trials in mesothelioma (8). A water soluble analogue of 5-azacytidine, 5-dihydroazacytidine (DHAC), which causes pleuritis and serositis, has been evaluated by the CALGB in 42 patients (55). Among these patients there was one complete response that was continuing at 2 years, three partial responses, and three regressions. The overall response rate was 17%. Toxicity was significant with chest pain occurring in 52% and requiring cessation of treatment in 18%. In contrast, a smaller trial by Dhingra et al. (56) of 14 evaluable patients treated at 5 g/m^2 every 28 days showed no response. More recently, the same drug was given with cisplatin to 36 patients at the same dose of 1500 mg/m^2 for 5 days every 3 weeks (57). A response rate similar to that of single-agent DHAC (13%) was observed, but there was increased myelosuppression because of the addition of cisplatin. Other antimetabolites, such as hydroxyurea and gemcitabine, have not been tested.

Thus, among the antimetabolites, high-dose methotrexate given with leucovorin rescue has the highest response rate (37%), including one complete response in a single, large, recent phase II trial. The new antifolate, edatrexate, also appears to be very promising, with response rates of 25% reported in the first series. The other antimetabolites appear less active, although the 5-azacytidine analogue, dihydro-5-azacytidine, has a 17% response rate in one trial that includes one complete response. 5-Fluorouracil has minimal activity.

MISCELLANEOUS DRUGS

Other agents tested in single phase II trials include cycloleucine, amsacrine, diaziquone, bacille Calmette-Guérin vaccine, acivicin, and both alpha interferon (α-INF) and beta interferon (18, 58–62, 64). None of these agents showed a greater than 5% response rate, except for α-INF, which produced a 12% response in 25 patients treated with 3×10^6 units (U) daily (62). In a preliminary report by Pogrebniak et al. (63), 25 patients were treated with one to three cycles of immunochemotherapy consisting of α-INF at a dose of 5 million units per meter squared (MU/m^2) given 3 times a week, tamoxifen 20 mg orally twice daily for 35 days, and cisplatin at 25 mg/m^2 weekly for four doses. Four (16%) partial responses were observed, with mild toxicity (grade 2 or less) seen in 24% of patients. The Memorial Sloan–Kettering Cancer Center is currently conducting a study of α-INF plus carboplatin in malignant mesothelioma, and the National Cancer Institute is conducting a phase II trial of α-INF plus cisplatin and tamoxifen (44).

SUMMARY OF SINGLE-AGENT TRIALS

To date, there are no drugs that have consistently induced response rates much greater than 20%. Higher response rates in single trials have been seen with detorubicin, high-dose methotrexate, and edatrexate, i.e., 26%, 37%, and 25%, respectively, but these have yet to be confirmed. As a class the antimetabolites appear to be the most promising therapeutic agents in mesothelioma, and confirmatory trials are awaited eagerly. The use of higher dose trimetrexate also warrants further investigation. Agents producing responses in 10% to 20% of patients include doxorubicin, epirubicin, mitomycin, cyclophosphamide, ifosfamide, cisplatin, and carboplatin. The often-quoted higher response rates for the older agents, such as doxorubicin (28% to 44%) and cyclophosphamide (28%), are compromised by institution, selection, or positive data publication biases. Indeed, the disappointing response rates of combination chemotherapy trials using doxorubicin and cyclophosphamide suggest that their true activity as single agents is probably no higher than 15%.

COMBINATION CHEMOTHERAPY

Thus far there have been at least 15 trials, dating from 1978 onward, enrolling more than 15 patients using combination chemotherapy in malignant pleural mesothelioma (Table 38.3). The majority have employed two agents and have used combinations of an antitumor antibiotic (doxorubicin, epirubicin, rubidazone, mitomycin, or pirarubicin), and an alkylating agent (cyclophosphamide or ifosfamide) or a platinum compound (cisplatin or carboplatin). Different combinations also have been compared (doxorubicin and cyclophosphamide with or without imidazole carboxamide, and cisplatin with either mitomycin or doxorubicin), but they have not demonstrated any significant relative superiority.

Doxorubicin has been included most often, and there have been four trials using it in combination with either cyclophosphamide or ifosfamide (65–68, 71). In a multiinstitutional, randomized, controlled trial (65), 36 patients received doxorubicin at 50 $mg/m2$ and cyclophosphamide at 500 mg/m^2 every 3 weeks, whereas 40 received the same combination with the addition of imidazole carboxamide (DTIC)–dacarbazine at 250 mg/m^2 from days 1 to 5. Partial responses of 11% and 13% were seen in each arm, respectively, with median survivals of 30 and 25 weeks. Unfortunately, the methods of assessment were not described clearly. It was concluded that the addition of cyclophosphamide or DTIC to doxorubicin produced no higher response than that expected from single-agent doxorubicin. The low response rate to the doxorubicin, cyclophosphamide, and the dacarbazome combination contrasts with the 25% level reported by Dhingra et al. in 1983 (66), in which higher doses of both doxorubicin (60 mg/m^2 to 90 mg/m^2 for 4 days) and cyclophosphamide (600 mg/m^2 to 900 mg/m^2) were used with DTIC at 1 g/m^2 for 4 days every 3 weeks. However, this was a single-institution study without the benefit of routine CT assessment, and it has been published thus far only in abstract form.

Doxorubicin in combination with ifosfamide appears to produce similar response rates. Carmichael et al. (67) used doxorubicin at 40 mg/m^2 and ifosfamide at 5 gm/m^2 given every 3 weeks, resulting in two partial responses among 16 patients for a 12.5% response rate.

TABLE 38.3. Series of at Least 15 Patients with Malignant Mesothelioma Treated with Combination Chemotherapy

AGENT	STUDY (REFERENCE NO.)	NO. OF PATIENTS	NO. OF RESPONSES (%)
Doxorubicin + cyclophosphamide	Samson et al., 1987 (65)	36	4 (11)
Doxorubicin + DTIC + cyclophosphamide	Samson et al., 1987 (65)	40	5 (13)
Doxorubicin + cyclophosphamide + DTIC	Dhingra et al., 1983 (66)	20	5 (25)
Doxorubicin + ifosfamide	Carmichael et al., 1989 (67)	16	2 (12.5)
Doxorubicin + cisplatin	Ardizzoni et al., 1991 (69)	24	6 (25)
Doxorubicin + cisplatin	Chahinian et al., 1993 (70)	35	5 (14)
Mitomycin + cisplatin	Chahinian et al., 1983 (70)	35	9 (26)
Doxorubicin + cisplatin + cyclophosphamide	Shin et al., 1993 (71)	23	6 (26)
Epirubicin + ifosfamide	Magri et al., 1992 (72)	17	1 (6)
Rubidazone + DTIC	Zidar et al., 1983 (73)	23	0 (0)
5-Dihydroazacytidine + cisplatin	Samuels et al., 1994 (52)	30	4 (13)
Mitomycin + bleomycin + cisplatin + doxorubicin	Breau et al., 1991 (74)	25	11 (44)
Cisplatin + etoposide	Eisenhauer et al., 1988 (75)	26	3 (12)
Pirarubicin + cisplatin	Koschel et al., 1991 (24)	39	6 (15)
Doxorubicin + 5-azacytidine	Chahinian et al., 1982 (8)	36	8 (22)

Abbreviation. DTIC, imidazole carboxamide.

Alberts et al. (68), in a small study of only 10 patients employing a higher dose (60 mg/m^2) of doxorubicin, achieved a 30% response.

Anthracycline/platinum compound combinations have been studied less widely. Ardizzoni et al. (69) reported a 25% response rate to the doxorubicin and cisplatin combination, whereas the CALGB reported only a 14% response rate (5 of 35 patients) to the same combination (70). The median survival was 8.8 months. In the same study, the CALGB also randomized patients to cisplatin with mitomycin. In the mitomycin arm, there were two complete responses, three partial responses, and four regressions of evaluable disease in 35 patients, with a median survival of 7.7 months. The overall response rates and median survivals were similar in the doxorubicin and mitomycin groups. Because this was a recent, multiinstitutional study with significant numbers of patients, the response rates generated have external validity and are probably near the true response rates that would be seen in a community setting. Importantly, no treatment-related deaths were recorded among the 79 patients (which included some with peritoneal mesothelioma), with generally good tolerance (except for one patient with pulmonary toxicity secondary to mitomycin, which resolved after discontinuing therapy and instituting treatment with corticosteroids). The higher response rates reported by Ardizzoni et al. (69) for doxorubicin plus cisplatin, compared with those of the CALGB, may relate to the inconsistent use of CT evaluation and the high percentage of patients with Butchart stage I disease (50%) in the Italian study.

Similar rates—6 (26%) of 23 partial responses—were seen with the addition of cyclophosphamide to a doxorubicin and cisplatin combination regimen in a trial by Shin et al. (71). Three cycles of induction chemotherapy (cyclophosphamide, 500 mg/m^2, day 1; doxorubicin, 50 mg/m^2, day 1; cisplatin, 50 mg/m^2, day 1) were given with subsequent cisplatin doses at 50 mg/m^2 every 3 to 4 weeks.

Other combinations that have been tested include epirubicin plus ifosfamide; rubidazone plus DTIC; 5-dihydroazacytidine plus cisplatin; doxorubicin, cisplatin, bleomycin, and mitomycin; cisplatin plus etoposide; cisplatin plus pirarubicin; and doxorubicin plus 5-azacytidine (8, 24, 57, 72–75). In general, the response rates range from 0% to 22%, and they represent no advantage over single-agent studies. The highest response rate (44%) was seen in the trial with doxorubicin, cisplatin, bleomycin, and mitomycin by Breau et al. (74), but this study remains unconfirmed.

CURRENT RECOMMENDATIONS FOR SYSTEMIC CHEMOTHERAPY

At this time combination chemotherapy cannot be recommended over single-agent treatment on a noninvestigational basis. The drug of first choice would be high-dose methotrexate on the basis of a well-conducted modern study by Solheim et al. (49) and similarly high responses recently reported to related drugs such as edatrexate. Confirmatory trials are needed urgently. Other reasonable alternatives would be single-agent doxorubicin, epirubicin, ifosfamide, and the platinum analogues.

INTRAPLEURAL THERAPY

Malignant mesothelioma tends to remain confined to the thoracic cavity, and death from this disease tends in most patients to result from intrathoracic causes. Thus, it is reasonable to attempt local control of the disease with intrapleural therapy. Earlier trials of intrapleural therapy aimed merely for control of pleural effusions. However, it was not until the relatively recent acceptance of intraperitoneal chemotherapy of both ovarian cancer and peritoneal mesothelioma that interest in intrapleural therapy was rekindled. Numerous studies have investigated the use of intrapleural therapy in either malignant mesothelioma or malignant pleural effusions caused by a variety of other solid tumors (76–81).

Pharmacokinetic studies by Rusch et al. (79, 80) have demonstrated the pharmacologic advantage of intrapleural treatment: they showed a threefold to fivefold advantage on a logarithmic scale for pleural to plasma areas under the curve for cisplatin (100 mg/m^2) and mitomycin (8 mg/m^2). They also showed that the half-life of both drugs was significantly prolonged in pleural fluid relative to plasma; however, it should be remembered that this group of patients had treatment immediately following pleurectomy, which would be expected to influence drug uptake into the systemic circulation.

Even before the pharmacologic advantage of intrapleural therapy with cisplatin was proven, a number of small trials demonstrated the feasibility of such treatment in patients. Markman et al. (78) treated eight patients with cisplatin at a dose of 90 mg/m^2 weekly for 3 weeks followed by a 3-week break. Patients who responded were given a total of six cycles. One patient showed a reduction in volume of the pleural effusion and a decrease in the thickening of the pleura that lasted for 5 months. The investigators suggested that future trials include more patients with less bulky disease. Theoretically, intrapleural therapy would lend itself well to the adjuvant setting in patients with no residual macroscopic disease after surgical resection, or as part of combined modality therapy after debulking surgery.

In another trial Aitini et al. (81) administered intrapleural cytosine arabinoside and cisplatin to five patients with pleural mesothelioma. The drug doses were 100 mg each. Three complete responses were achieved, and survival was 51, 26, and 25+ months in these patients. Unfortunately, neither prognostic factors in their patients nor the methods of assessment of response were reported.

Other agents also have been used intrapleurally and include interleukin-2 (82) and gamma interferon (83). The response rate in the study using interleukin-2 doses of 5×10^3 to 6×10^6 U/day was 24%. The drug was given over 14 days via an indwelling intrapleural catheter at 2-week intervals. The use of gamma interferon appeared to be particularly useful in patients with stage I disease and nodules less than 5 mm in diameter. Four of nine such patients had complete responses as assessed by posttreatment thoracoscopy and biopsy.

The results of intrapleural treatment in these early trials are interesting enough to justify further studies using this method of drug delivery. Future trials should answer the question of the role of such treatment in both adjuvant and combined modality settings. However, the usefulness of intrapleural therapy, which relies on achieving high local concentrations of drug, may be limited to those patients with Butchart stage I and IIA disease, and those patients with small-volume disease that allows adequate uptake or diffusion into the tumor. New combinations of drugs also should be tried. Combinations of cytotoxic drugs and cytokines may be useful as suggested by studies showing synergy between these two types of agents (84).

RADIOTHERAPY ALONE AND COMBINED MODALITY TREATMENT IN UNRESECTABLE DISEASE

For tumors that are Butchart stage III or IV and deemed incompletely resectable, a number of studies have investigated the value of radiotherapy given alone or radiotherapy combined with chemotherapy.

RADIOTHERAPY ALONE

Most series (85–90) employing radiotherapy alone have not shown any survival benefit over supportive care. However, there appear to be benefits in terms of symptomatic improvement with alleviation of pain, dyspnea, and sustained regression of recurrent pleural effusions. For example, in the series from the Royal Marsden (86, 87), two such patients of 12 treated with radiotherapy alone experienced control of their previously recurrent pleural effusions until their deaths; no significant prolongation in survival was observed. The lack of any effect on survival was emphasized again in a South African series (61) in which 13 patients received 200 cGy/day for 5 days every 6 weeks, or 150 cGy/day for 10 doses. All had either stage I or II disease and a good performance status, but they had a median survival of only 7.8 months. For those patients in whom noncurative radiotherapy is being considered, short-course treatment with 2000 cGy in five fractions in 1 week may give comparable palliation, compared with the more prolonged courses (3000 to 4000 cGy in 10 to 15 fractions) suggested by an Australian study (91). Radiotherapy also may be used in prevention of seeding of biopsy tracks and surgical wounds. In a French series (92), 2100 cGy in three fractions was successful in preventing such occurrences in 24 patients, a significant improvement over the 61% seeding rate seen in 33 previous patients not given prophylactic radiotherapy.

Before embarking on a course of radiotherapy, especially in a palliative setting, the very real risks of causing significant pulmonary toxicity, hepatitis, carditis, and even myelitis, because of the large areas being irradiated, must be addressed. Patients should be evaluated carefully with lung function tests, assessment of liver position, and cardiac function tests. Thus, the role of radiotherapy alone as curative therapy for mesothelioma is limited by the extent of disease and by normal tissue tolerances. As palliative treatment it appears to be effective in some patients who have recurrent pleural effusions and chest pain, and it also is helpful in preventing seeding of biopsy tracks.

RADIOTHERAPY AND CHEMOTHERAPY

The role of combined treatment with radiotherapy and chemotherapy has not been investigated extensively because neither modality applied individually appears to offer a consistently good response. Of the studies published, no survival extension has been demonstrated clearly. Among 31 patients described by Vogelzang et al. (93), the survival of patients treated with radiotherapy alone and radiotherapy combined with chemotherapy was not significantly different from those treated with chemotherapy alone. Similar results were achieved by South African (61) and Finnish groups (94). In the retrospective South African study, patients received radiotherapy with either doxorubicin, cyclophosphamide, or procarbazine, and they had median survivals of 22.6, 10.8, and 10.9 months, respectively. The doxorubicin group, however, included a higher percentage (40%) of female patients with early-stage disease. The risks of combined therapy were well illustrated in the Finnish study in which 100 patients received varying doses of radiotherapy (between 2000 and 5500 cGy) and also combination or single-agent chemotherapy with either mitoxantrone, epirubicin, or etoposide. Patients who were able to complete the therapy had prolongation of median survival from 8 to 12 months, with progressive disease being the invariable outcome in all patients. Radiation pneumonitis was significant. In the group treated with 5500 cGy in a split-course regimen, damage to the irradiated lung at 12 months was almost total, whereas in patients who received 7000 cGy, no normal lung tissue was present by 4 to 6 months after treatment in irradiated areas.

It thus is apparent that high-dose radiotherapy has risks that outweigh most survival benefits. Furthermore, there is little support for the use of high-dose treatment in the palliative setting when lower dosages may be given with equal effectiveness for relief of pain, dyspnea, and recurrent pleural effusions. At lower doses radiotherapy may also be given alone in patients who cannot receive chemotherapy or who are likely to have tumor seeding along surgical incisions or biopsy tracks.

COMBINED MODALITY THERAPY AFTER DEBULKING SURGERY

Previous series (94, 95) employing adjuvant chemotherapy with or without radiotherapy have concentrated on patients with early-stage disease who are potentially curable, i.e., those who have had gross removal of all disease. However, in reality, even those patients who undergo radical surgery with extrapleural pneumonectomy often have microscopic disease at resection margins, as reported in 23 of 25 patients treated with the technique who had no residual gross disease (95). Therefore, it is not surprising that extrapleural pneumonectomy as a single modality has not been shown to influence overall survival significantly. Patients with gross residual disease would be expected to have an even poorer outcome. These results have stimulated interest in the use of intraoperative photodynamic therapy, in which a photosensitizer (meso-tetra-[hydroxphenyl]-chlorin) is given preoperatively, retained by tumor tissue, and when activated intraoperatively by an argon dye laser, results in cytotoxicity. This technique has been found to work best in residual tumors of less than 5 mm in depth (96). Presently, the National Cancer Institute is conducting such a trial with patients undergoing either debulking surgery with photodynamic therapy and chemoimmunotherapy with cisplatin, α-INF, and tamoxifen, or surgery with chemoimmunotherapy alone (44). If local control can be achieved, this form of therapy may produce good palliation. If combined with an effective systemic agent, it conceivably may result in significant improvements in overall survival.

Conclusions and Future Directions

The successful treatment of unresectable pleural mesothelioma awaits the discovery of active agents against this highly chemoresistant tumor. The recent trials of high-dose methotrexate and related antifolates, such as edatrexate, offer a glimmer of hope that effective agents have been discovered, but these trials need confirmation. Newer agents such as topotecan are under evaluation in specific mesothelioma trials. Other agents such as suramin also should be evaluated in phase II trials. Combination chemotherapy has no definite advantage over single-agent therapy, and future trials should test combinations that include newer active agents. Intrapleural therapy offers pharmacologic advantages that appear promising, and its role in combined modality treatment after surgery with pleurectomy, followed by postoperative systemic chemotherapy, is being investigated. High-dose radiotherapy with curative intent should be avoided, but lower doses should be considered for palliation of symptoms, such as pain and dyspnea caused by pleural effusions. Debulking surgery has no proven role, unless perhaps it leaves residual disease of less than 5 mm depth that can be eradicated by photodynamic therapy or combinations of radiation and chemotherapy.

There is a growing armamentarium of treatment approaches that may be adopted in this challenging disease. Thus far, however, mesothelioma has eluded any significant impact of such therapy on overall survival. Future breakthroughs will depend on the combination of basic laboratory work that seeks to elucidate the mechanisms of chemoresistance in this tumor, and perseverance in the search for effective agents against local and systemic disease within the setting of phase II trials.

Acknowledgments

This study is supported in part by National Institutes of Health/National Cancer Institute grant CA41287-09.

References

1. Connelly RR, Spirtas R, Myers MH, Percy CL, Fraumeni JF. Demographic patterns for mesothelioma in the United States. J Natl Cancer Inst 78:1053, 1987.
2. Hillerdal G. Malignant mesothelioma 1982: review of 4710 published cases. Br J Dis Chest 1983;77:321–43.
3. Ruffie P, Feld R, Minkin S, et al. Diffuse malignant mesothelioma of the pleura in Ontario and Quebec: a retrospective study of 332 patients. J Clin Oncol 1989;7:1157–1168.
4. Hulks G, Thomas SJ, Waclawski E. Malignant pleural mesothelioma in Western Glasgow. Thorax 1989;44:496–500.
5. Antman KM, Blum RH, Greenberger JS, Flowerdew G, Skarin AT, Canellos GP. Multimodality therapy for malignant mesothelioma based on a study of natural history. Am J Med 1980;68:356–362.
6. Lewis RJ, Sisler GE, Mackenzie JW. Diffuse, mixed malignant pleural mesothelioma. Ann Thorac Surg 1981;31:53–60.
7. Brenner J, Sordillo PP, Magill G, Golbey RB. Malignant mesothelioma of the pleura, review of 123 patients. Cancer 1982;49:2431–2435.
8. Chahinian AP, Pajak TF, Holland JF, Norton L, Ambinder RM, Mandel EM. Diffuse malignant mesothelioma: prospective evaluation of 69 patients. Ann Intern Med 1982;96(1):746–755.
9. Antman K, Shemin R, Ryan L, et al. Malignant mesothelioma: prognostic variables in a registry of 180 patients, the Dana-Farber Cancer Institute and Brigham and Women's Hospital experience over two decades, 1965–1985. J Clin Oncol 1988;6:147–153.
10. Chailleux E, Dabouis G, Pioche D, et al. Prognostic factors in diffuse malignant pleural mesothelioma, a study of 167 patients. Chest 1988;93:159–162.
11. DePangher-Manzini V, Brollo A, Franceschi S, DeMatthaeis M, Talamini R, Bianchi C. Prognostic factors of malignant mesothelioma of the pleura. Cancer 1993;72(2):410–417.
12. Law MR, Gregor A, Hodson ME, Bloom HJG, Turner-Warwick M. Malignant mesothelioma of the pleura: a study of 52 treated and 64 untreated patients. Thorax 1984;39:255–259.
13. Sugarbaker DJ, Strauss GM, Lynch TJ, et al. Node status has prognostic significance in the multimodality therapy of diffuse, malignant mesothelioma. J Clin Oncol 1993;11:1172–1178.
14. Sridhar KS, Doria R, Raub WA, Thurer RJ, Saldana M. New strategies are needed in diffuse malignant mesothelioma. Cancer 1992;70:2969–2979.
15. Patz EF, Shaffer K, Piwnica-Worms DR, et al. Malignant pleural mesothelioma: value of CT and MR imaging in predicting resectability. Am J Radiol 1992;159:961–966.
16. Antman KH, Li FP, Pass HI, Corson J, Delaney T. Benign and malignant mesothelioma. In: DeVita V, Hellman S, Rosenberg SA, eds. Cancer principles and practice of oncology. Philadelphia: JB Lippincott, 1993:1486–1508.
17. Aisner J, Sigman LM. The role of chemotherapy in the treatment of malignant mesothelioma. In: Antman K, Aisner J, eds. Asbestos-related malignancy. Orlando, FL: Grune & Stratton, 1986:385–401.
18. Lerner HJ, Schoenfeld DA, Martin A, Falkson G, Borden E. Malignant mesothelioma. The Eastern Cooperative Oncology Group (ECOG) experience. Cancer 1983;52:1981–1985.
19. Sørensen PG, Bach F, Bork E, Hansen HH. Randomized trial of doxorubicin versus cyclophosphamide in diffuse malignant pleural mesothelioma. Cancer Treat Rep 1985;69:1431–1432.
20. Harvey VJ, Slevin ML, Ponder BAJ, Blackshaw AJ, Wrigley PFM. Chemotherapy of diffuse malignant mesothelioma: phase II trials of single agent 5-fluorouracil and Adriamycin. Cancer 1984;54:961–964.
21. Colbert N, Vannetzel JM, Izrael V, et al. A prospective study of detorubicin in malignant mesothelioma. Cancer 1985;56:2170–2174.
22. Kaukel E, Koschel G, Gatzemeyer U, Salewski E. A phase II study of pirarubicin in malignant pleural mesothelioma. Cancer 1990;66:651–654.
23. Sridhar KS, Hussein AM, Feun LG, Zubrod CG. Activity of pirarubicin (4′-0-tetrahydropyranyladriamycin) in malignant mesothelioma. Cancer 1989;63:1084–1091.

24. Koschel G, Calavrezos A, Kaukel E, et al. Phase III randomized comparison of pirarubicin vs. pirarubicin and cisplatin for treatment of pleural mesotheliomas. Proceedings of the Sixth European Congress Against Cancer, 1991.
25. Magri MD, Veronesi A, Foladore S, et al. Epirubicin in the treatment of malignant mesothelioma: a phase II cooperative study. Tumori 1991;77:49–51.
26. Mattson K, Giaccone G, Kirkparick A., et al. Epirubicin in malignant mesothelioma: a phase II study of the European Organization for Research and Treatment of Cancer Lung Cancer Cooperative Group. J Clin Oncol 1992;10:824–828.
27. Eisenhauer EA, Evans WK, Raghavan D, et al. Phase II study of mitoxantrone in patients with mesothelioma: a National Cancer Institute of Canada Clinical Trials Group Study. Cancer Treat Rep 1986;70:1029–1030.
28. van Breukelen FJM, Mattson K, Giaccone G, et al. Mitoxantrone in malignant pleural mesothelioma: a study by the EORTC Lung Cancer Cooperative Group. Eur J Cancer 1991;27:1629–1633.
29. Mintzer DM, Kelsen D, Frimmer D, et al. Phase II trial of high dose cisplatin in patients with malignant mesothelioma. Cancer Treat Rep 1985;69:711–712.
30. Zidar BL, Green S, Pierce HI, Roach RW, Balcerzak SP, Militello L. A phase II evaluation of cisplatin in unresectable diffuse malignant mesothelioma: a Southwest Oncology Group Study. Invest New Drugs 1988;6:223–226.
31. Hayes M, Cvitkovic E, Golbey RB, et al. High-dose cisplatinum diamine dichloride-amelioration of renal toxicity by mannitol diuresis. Cancer 1977;39:1372–81.
32. Rossoff AH, Slayton RE, Perlia CP. Preliminary clinical experience with cis-diamine dichloroplatinum (II) (NSC 1198875). Cancer 1972;30:1451–1456.
33. Dabouis G, Le Mevel B, Covoller J. Treatment of diffuse pleural malignant mesothelioma by cis-dichlorodiamine platinum in nine patients. Cancer Chemother Pharmacol 1981;5:209–210.
34. Planting A, Goey H, Verweij J. Phase II study of six weekly courses of high dose cisplatin (CDDP) in mesothelioma (abstract). Proc Am Assoc Cancer Res 1991;32:194.
35. Cantwell BMJ, Franks CR, Harris AL. A phase II study of the platinum analogues JM8 and JM9 in malignant pleural mesothelioma. Cancer Chemother Pharmacol 1986;18:286–288.
36. Mbidde EK, Harland SJ, Cavert AH, Smith IE. Phase II trial of carboplatin (JM8) in treatment of patients with malignant mesothelioma. Cancer Chemother Pharmacol 1986;18:284–285.
37. Raghavan D, Gianoutsos P, Bishop J, et al. Phase II trial of carboplatin in the management of malignant mesothelioma. J Clin Oncol 1990;8:151–154.
38. Vogelzang NJ, Goutsou M, Corson JM, et al. Carboplatin in malignant mesothelioma: a phase II study of the Cancer and Leukemia Group B. Cancer Chemother Pharmacol 1990;27:239–242.
39. Kelsen D, Gralla R, Cheng E, Martini N. Vindesine in the treatment of malignant mesothelioma: a phase II study. Cancer Treat Rep 1983;67:821–822.
40. Boutin C, Irisson M, Guerin JC, et al. Phase II trial of vindesine in malignant pleural mesothelioma. Cancer Treat Rep 1987;71:205–206.
41. Martensson G, Sorenson S. A phase II study of vincristine in malignant mesothelioma—a negative report. Cancer Chemother Pharmacol 1989;24:133–134.
42. Cowan JD, Green S, Lucas J, et al. Phase II trial of five day intravenous infusion vinblastine sulfate in patients with diffuse malignant mesothelioma: a Southwest Oncology Group Study (letter). Invest New Drugs 1988;6:247–248.
43. Vogelzang NJ, Herndon J, Clamon GH, Mauer AM, Cooper MR, Green MR. Paclitaxel (Taxol) for malignant mesothelioma (MM): a phase II study of the Cancer and Leukemia Group B (CALGB 9234) (abstract). Proc Am Soc Clin Oncol 1994;13:405.
44. Berg CD, Carlson JA, Gorrell C, Grayson J, Haller DG, Kaplan RS, Kramer BS, et al. Current clinical trials: oncology. National Cancer Institute. Green Brook, NJ: Pyros Education Group, 1994;1(2).
45. Alberts AS, Falkson G, Zyl LV. Malignant pleural mesothelioma: phase II pilot study of ifosfamide and mesna. J Natl Cancer Inst 1988;80:968–700.
46. Zidar BL, Metch B, Balcerzak SP, et al. A phase II evaluation of ifosfamide and mesna in unresectable diffuse malignant mesothelioma: a Southwest Oncology Group study. Cancer 1992;70:2547–2551.
47. Falkson G, Hunt M, Borden EC, Hayes JA, Falkson CI, Smith TJ. An extended phase II trial of ifosfamide plus mesna in mesothelioma. Invest New Drugs 1992;10:337–343.
48. Bajorin D, Kelsen D, Mintzer DM. Phase II trial of mitomycin in malignant mesothelioma. Cancer Treat Rep 1987;71:857–858.
49. Solheim OP, Saeter G, Finnanger AM, Stenwig AE. High-dose methotrexate in the treatment of malignant mesothelioma of the pleura. A phase II study. Br J Cancer 1992;65:956–960.
50. Dmitrov NV, Egner J, Balcueva E, Suhrland CG. High-dose methotrexate with citrovorum factor and vincristine in the treatment of malignant mesothelioma. Cancer 1982;50:1245–1247.
51. Djerassi I, Kim JS, Kassarov L, et al. Response of mesothelioma to large doses of methotrexate with rescue (HDMTXCF) used alone or with cis platinum. Proc Am Soc Clin Oncol 1985;4:191.
52. Vogelzang NJ, Weissman LB, Herndon JE, et al. Trimetrexate in malignant mesothelioma: a CALGB phase II study. J Clin Oncol 1994;12:1436–1442.
53. Belani CP, Herndon J, Vogelzang NJ, Green MR. Edatrexate for malignant mesothelioma: a phase II study of the Cancer and Leukemia Group B, 9131 (abstract). Proc Am Soc Clin Oncol 1994;13:329.
54. Cantwell BMJ, Earnshaw M, Harris AL. Phase II study of a novel antifolate, $_N$10-propargyl-5,8 dideazafolic acid (CB3717), in malignant mesothelioma. Cancer Treat Rep 1986;70:1335–1336.
55. Harmon D, Vogelzang NJ, Roboz J, et al. Dihydro-5-azacytidine (DHAC) in malignant mesothelioma (Meso) using serum hyaluronic acid (SHA) as a tumor marker: a phase II trial of the CALGB (abstract). Proc Am Soc Clin Oncol 1991;10:351.
56. Dhingra HM, Murphy WK, Winn RJ, Raber MN, Hong WK. Phase II trial of 5,6-dihydro-5-azacytidine in pleural malignant mesothelioma. Invest New Drugs 1991;9:69–71.
57. Samuels BL, Herndon J, Vogelzang NJ, et al. Dihydro-5-azacytidine (DHAC) and cisplatin (DDP) in mesothelioma (CALGB 9031) (abstract). Proc Am Soc Clin Oncol 1994;13:402.
58. Falkson G, Vorobiof DA, Lerner JH. A phase II study of M-AMSA in patients with malignant mesothelioma. Cancer Chemother Pharmacol 1980;4:135.
59. Eagan R, Frytak S, Richardson R, et al. Phase II trial of diaziquone in malignant mesothelioma. Cancer Treat Rep 1986;70:429.
60. Webster I, Cochrane JWC, Burkhardt KR. Immunotherapy with BCG vaccine in 30 cases of mesothelioma. S Afr Med J 1982;61:277.
61. Alberts AS, Falkson G, Goedhals L, et al. Malignant pleural mesothelioma: a disease unaffected by current therapeutic maneuvers. J Clin Oncol 1988;6:527–535.

62. Christmas TI, Manning LS, Garlepp MJ, Musk AW, Robinson BW. Effect of interferon-alpha 2a on malignant mesothelioma. J Interferon Res 1993;13:9–12.
63. Pogrebniak H, Kranda K, Steinberg S, Temeck B, Feuerstein I, Pass H. Cisplatin, interferon-α, and tamoxifen (CIT) for malignant pleural mesothelioma (abstract). Proc Am Soc Clin Oncol 1993;12:398.
64. von Hoff DD, Metch B, Lucas JG, Balcerzak SP, Grunberg SM, Rivkin SE. Phase II evaluation of recombinant interferon-beta (IFN-beta Ser) in patients with diffuse mesothelioma: a Southwest Oncology Group study. J Interferon Res 1990;10:531–534.
65. Samson M, Wasser L, Borden EC, et al. Randomized comparison of cyclophosphamide, DTIC and Adriamycin vs. cyclophosphamide and Adriamycin in patients with advanced stage malignant mesothelioma: a sarcoma intergroup study. J Clin Oncol 1987;5:86–91.
66. Dhingra H, Valdivieso M, Tannir N, et al. Combined modality treatment for mesothelioma with Cytoxan, Adriamycin, and DTIC (CYADIC) and adjuvant surgery (abstract). Proc Am Soc Clin Oncol 1983;2:205.
67. Carmichael J, Cantwell BM, Harris AL. A phase II trial of ifosfamide/mensa with doxorubicin for malignant mesothelioma. Eur J Cancer Clin Oncol 1989;25:911–912.
68. Alberts AS, Falkson G, van Zyl L. Ifosfamide and mensa with doxorubicin have activity in malignant mesothelioma. Eur J Cancer 1990;26:1002.
69. Ardizzoni A, Rosso R, Salvati F, et al. Activity of doxorubicin and cisplatin combination chemotherapy in patients with diffuse malignant pleural mesothelioma. An Italian Lung Cancer Task Force (FONICAP) phase II study. Cancer 1991;67:2984–2987.
70. Chahinian AP, Antman K, Goutsou M, et al. Randomized phase II trial of cisplatin with mitomycin or doxorubicin for malignant mesothelioma by the Cancer and Leukemia Group B. J Clin Oncol 1993;11:1559–1565.
71. Shin DM, Fossella FV, Putnam JB, Murphy WK, Mortensen TG, Chasen MH, McMurtrey MJ. Phase II study of combination chemotherapy with Cytoxan (C), Adriamycin (A), and cisplatin (P) for unresectable or metastatic malignant pleural mesothelioma (MPM) (abstract). Proc Am Soc Clin Oncol 1993; 12:398.
72. Magri MD, Foladore S, Veronis A, et al. Treatment of malignant mesothelioma with epirubicin and ifosfamide, a phase II comparative study. Ann Oncol 1992;3:237–238.
73. Zidar BL, Benjamin RS, Frank J, Lane M, Baker LH. Combination chemotherapy for advanced sarcomas of bone and mesothelioma utilizing rubidazone and DTIC: a Southwest Oncology Group study. Am J Clin Oncol 1983;6:71–74.
74. Breau JL, Boaziz C, Morere JJF, Sadoun D, Israel L. Combination chemotherapy with cisplatinum, Adriamycin, bleomycin and mitomycin C, plus systemic and intra-pleural hyaluronidase in 25 consecutive cases of stages II, III pleural mesothelioma. Presented at the First International Mesothelioma Conference, Paris, 1991:5.
75. Eisenhauer EA, Evans WK, Murray N, Kocha W, Wierzbicki R, Wilson K. A phase II study of VP-16 and cisplatin in patients with unresectable malignant mesothelioma. An NCI Canada clinical trials group study. Invest New Drugs 1988;6:327–329.
76. Markman M, Howell S, Green MR. Combination intra-cavitary chemotherapy for malignant pleural disease. Cancer Drug Delivery 1984;1:333–336.
77. Markman M, Cleary S, King M, et al. Cisplatin and cytarabine administered intra-pleurally as treatment of malignant pleural effusions. Med Pediatr Oncol 1985;13:191–193.
78. Markman M, Cleary S, Pfeifle C, Howell SB. Cisplatin administered by the intra-cavitary route as treatment for malignant mesothelioma. Cancer 1986;58:18–21.
79. Rusch V, Figlin R, Godwin D, Piantadosi S. Intra-pleural cisplatin and cytarabine in the management of malignant pleural effusions: a Lung Cancer Study Group trial. J Clin Oncol 1991;9: 313–319.
80. Rusch V, Niedzwiecki D, Tao Y, et al. Intra-pleural cisplatin and mitomycin for malignant mesothelioma following pleurectomy: pharmacokinetic studies. J Clin Oncol 1992;10:1001–1006.
81. Aitini E, Pasquini E, Cavazzini G, Fattori P, Smerieri F. Local treatment of malignant pleural mesothelioma with intra-cavitary cytosine-arabinoside and cisplatin. Ann Oncol 1992;3:771–774.
82. Eggermont AMM, Goey SH, Slingerland R, et al. Clinical and immunological evaluation of intrapleural (IPL) interleukin-2 (IL-2) in malignant pleural mesothelioma: a phase I-II study. Proc Am Soc Cancer Res 1991;32:206.
83. Boutin C, Viallat JR, Van-Zandwijk N, et al. Activity of intrapleural recombinant gamma-interferon in malignant mesothelioma. Cancer 1991;67:2033–2037.
84. Sklarin NT, Chahinian AP, Fever E, Lahman LA, Szrajer L, Holland JF. Augmentation of activity of cisplatin and mitomycin C by interferon in human malignant mesothelioma xenografts in nude mice. Cancer Res 1988;48:64–67.
85. Ehrenhaft JL, Sensenig DM, Lawrence MS. Mesotheliomas of the pleura. J Thorac Cardiovasc Surg 1960;40:393–409.
86. Law MR, Hodson ME, Turner-Warick M. Malignant mesothelioma of the pleura: clinical aspects and symptomatic treatment. Eur J Respir Dis 1984;65:162.
87. Law MR, Gregor A, Hodson ME, Bloom HJG, Turner-Warwick M. Malignant mesothelioma of the pleura: a study of 52 untreated patients. Thorax 1984;39:255–259.
88. Gordon W, Antman K, Breenberger J, Weichselbaum R, Chaffey J. Radiation therapy in the management of patients with mesothelioma. Int J Radiat Oncol Biol Phys 1982;8:19.
89. Eschwege F, Schlienger M. La Radiotherapie des mesotheliomes pleuraux malins: a propos de 14 cas irradies a dose elevees. J Radiol Electrol 1973;54:255–259.
90. Dobelbower RR, Strubler KA, Vaisman I. Clinical applications of high energy electron beams: the pancreas, pleura, and spine. In: Zuppinger A, Bataini JP, Irigaray JM, Chu F, eds. High energy electrons in radiation therapy. Berlin: Springer-Verlag, 1980:91–97.
91. Ball DL, Cruickshank DG. The treatment of malignant mesothelioma of the pleura: review of a 5-year experience, with special reference to radiotherapy. Am J Clin Oncol 1990;13:4–9.
92. Boutin C, Irrisson M, Rathelot P, Petite JM. L'extension parietale des mesotheliomas pleuraux malins diffus apres biopsies: prevention par radiotherapie locale. Press Med 1983;12:1823.
93. Vogelzang NJ, Schultz SM, Iannucci AM, Kennedy BJ. Malignant mesothelioma. The University of Minnesota experience. Cancer 1984;53:377–383.
94. Mattson K, Holsti LR, Tammilehto L, et al. Multimodality treatment programs for malignant pleural mesothelioma using high-dose hemithorax irradiation. Int J Radiat Oncol Biol Phys 1992;24:643–650.
95. Sugarbaker DJ, Heber EC, Lee TH, et al. Extrapleural pneumonectomy, chemotherapy, and radiotherapy in the treatment of diffuse malignant pleural mesothelioma. J Thorac Cardiovasc Surg 1991;102:10–15.
96. Ris HB, Altermatt MJ, Inderbitzi R, et al. Photodynamic therapy with chlorins for diffuse malignant mesothelioma: initial clinical results. Br J Cancer 1991;64:1116–1120.

Section VIII

Other Malignancies

39

Malignant Nonepithelial Neoplasms of the Lungs and Pleural Surfaces

Jane C. Huang, Jon H. Ritter, and Mark R. Wick

Primary malignant neoplasms of the lung that lack epithelial differentiation are uncommon. By an overwhelming majority, tumors showing mesenchymal or hematopoietic lineage are proven to be secondary lesions when they involve the pulmonary parenchyma and tracheobronchial tree.

Indeed, it is because of the rarity of noncarcinomatous malignancies in the lungs that relatively little has been written about such proliferations from morphologic or clinical perspectives. Therefore, it is not surprising that clinical physicians, radiologists, and pathologists all may be subject to considerable uncertainty and anxiety when confronted with mesenchymal pulmonary malignancies.

This chapter provides a summary of the clinicopathologic data pertaining to such cases. Attention is paid primarily to malignant lesions, inasmuch as virtually all benign mesenchymal tumors and pseudotumors of the lung are surgical lesions curable by conservative excision. However, some of the latter proliferations—as well as selected other pulmonary neoplasms—are mentioned in reference to the differential diagnosis of malignant noncarcinomatous lesions. Entities discussed are arranged in order of frequency of occurrence.

TUMORS OF THE LUNG

SARCOMATOID CARCINOMA

Sarcomatoid carcinoma (SC) of the lung is an epithelial proliferation. It must be discussed before any true mesenchymal tumors can be considered, however, because sarcomalike neoplasms are encountered in the thorax far more often than true sarcomas. In fact, one can assert that a malignant pleuropulmonary tumor having the appearance of a sarcoma morphotype should be regarded as epithelial in nature until proven otherwise by rigorous pathologic examination (1). The histogenesis of SC has been a subject of much debate, which is reflected in part by the various terms that have been used to refer to it, including carcinosarcoma, metaplastic carcinoma, spindle cell carcinoma, and pseudosarcoma. The current concept of SC is that of an epithelial neoplasm whose primitive characteristics result in pleomorphism, poor intercellular adhesion, and a sarcomatoid appearance. Moreover, partial divergent differentiation—into mesenchymal tissues having histologic characteristics of muscle, bone, fat, cartilage, or endothelial tissue—also is part of the morphologic repertoire of pulmonary SC (2).

It is because of the latter point that electron microscopic analyses, immunohistochemical studies, or both are mandatory before assigning a diagnosis of true mesenchymal malignancy in the lung. Ultrastructural features of epithelial differentiation (e.g., intercellular junctional complexes and cytoplasmic tonofilaments) and immunoreactivity for epithelial protein products (such as keratin and epithelial membrane antigen) usually are observed in the mesenchymoid components of SC (1, 3–6). This is true regardless of whether the tumor is morphologically indeterminate or, whether it simulates the appearance of specialized mesenchymal tissues. Thus, it should be apparent that there were many erroneous reports of pulmonary sarcoma made before the advent of adjunctive pathologic screening. This fact, in turn, confounds our ability to predict confidently the clinical behavior and response to therapy of true mesenchymal malignancies of the lung, because it is likely that the aggregate groups of all such lesions reported in the literature have been contaminated by SC cases.

CLINICAL SUMMARY

Pulmonary SC represented 0.2% of all lung cancers seen at the Mayo Clinic from 1971 to 1982 (7), and it accounted for approximately 1% of all such neoplasms seen at Washington University Medical Center over a 12-year period. This tumor is seen principally in adults, with a peak incidence in the sixth decade of life. Men predominate, with a male to female ratio of 5:1 (2, 7). Most patients have a history of cigarette smoking, and they present with recurrent pneumonia, cough, hemoptysis, dyspnea, and chest pain. Radiographic examination of the chest shows a single discrete mass (Fig. 39.1), most often in the upper lobes, that may demonstrate extrapulmonary extension into the chest wall if it is located peripherally. SCs may be either endobronchial or intraparenchymal. They are relatively well circumscribed and range from 1.5 to 15 cm in greatest dimension (7).

PATHOLOGIC FINDINGS

Histologically, some lesions in this category betray their epithelial lineage by showing small but discrete foci of obviously carcinomatous growth that may include any of the recognized morphotypes of conventional lung cancer. Other examples of SC lack all traces of epithelial architecture, and consist instead of nondescript sheets and fascicles of spindled and pleomorphic cells like those observed in soft tissue sarcomas (Fig. 39.2). As mentioned above, morphologically specialized cell lines that mimic pure mesenchymal neoplasms (e.g., rhabdomyosarcoma, angiosarcoma) may be part of the latter tumors as well. To reiterate, the identity of such SCs is discernible only after specialized pathologic studies have been done.

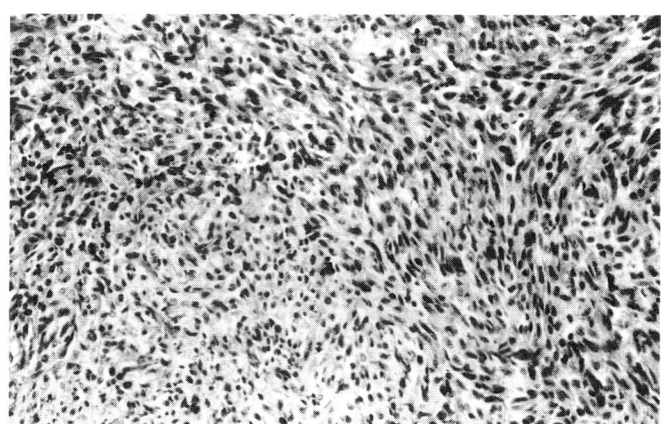

FIGURE 39.2. A sarcomatoid carcinoma is composed of sheets and vague fascicles of oval to spindled cells, without evidence of epithelial differentiation.

THERAPY AND PROGNOSIS

Most pulmonary SCs are deemed resectable; indeed, 17 of 21 such lesions treated at Washington University Medical Center were stage I or II tumors using the criteria established by the American Joint Committee on Cancer (8). Despite these characteristics, the overall prognosis is grim for patients with surgically treated pulmonary SC. The median survival of those in the Mayo Clinic series was 1 year (7), and all but two of the individuals treated at Washington University died within 22 months of diagnosis (8). These neoplasms, like conventional lung cancers, show a tendency to metastasize to intrathoracic and supraclavicular lymph node groups, contralateral lung, adrenal glands, liver, brain, and bone. To date, the efficacy and optimal constitution of adjuvant radiation therapy and chemotherapy protocols for pulmonary SC have not been determined in any concerted prospective analysis. Empirically, the lesions are best treated in a manner similar to that of other undifferentiated carcinomas of the lung, except that stage should be regarded as a relatively unimportant factor in planning the nonsurgical management of SC cases.

KAPOSI'S SARCOMA

The recent natural history of Kaposi's sarcoma (KS) is a sad testimony to the global impact of the acquired immunodeficiency syndrome (AIDS). Before the 1980s KS was a relatively rare neoplasm outside of Africa and the Mediterranean basin. Moreover, with relatively uncommon exceptions, this lesion was a cutaneous proliferation that uncommonly involved the viscera (9). However, with particular regard to the in-

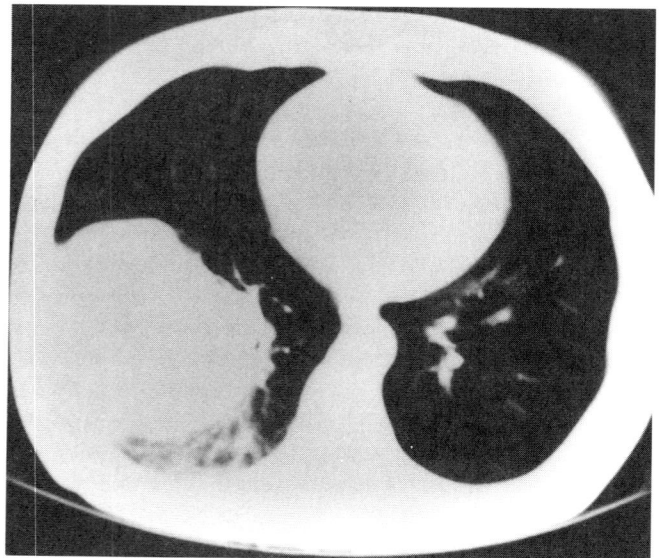

FIGURE 39.1. CT scan of a sarcomatoid carcinoma shows a large, circumscribed mass that extends to the chest wall.

trathoracic organs, KS now is the most common pulmonary sarcoma found in most large metropolitan areas worldwide (10). Whereas initial presentation of this tumor in the bronchopulmonary tract was an almost-unknown phenomenon before the advent of AIDS, it currently is a well-recognized variation of that disease (11).

CLINICAL SUMMARY

In this context, most patients with KS of the lung are homosexual men (11–14), and more uncommonly they include others from high-risk groups for AIDS such as intravenous drug abusers. Most individuals with KS generally have other symptoms and signs of AIDS, such as weight loss, fever, night sweats, fatigue, lymphadenopathy, and opportunistic infections. However, fever may be caused directly by KS in the lungs. There has been a case report of an AIDS patient with persistent pyrexia for which no source of infection was found but which finally resolved after radiation therapy (15). Cutaneous KS usually is detected early in its clinical evolution, but identical tumors of the bronchial mucosa and lung parenchyma typically have grown to a volume sufficient to produce symptoms, and thus are relatively advanced at the time of diagnosis (16). Presenting complaints specific to the neoplasm include dyspnea, stridor (when endobronchial lesions are present), cough, and hemoptysis, which may be massive (11).

On bronchoscopic examination, nodular or flat bluish red discoloration is seen in the mucosa, some of which may be bleeding actively. This bronchoscopic appearance usually is considered diagnostic, and endobronchial lesions generally are not biopsied. The diagnostic yield of transbronchial biopsies usually is quite low, and unless they are deep enough, KS of the lung is missed because the mucosa usually is uninvolved (17). In addition, bronchoscopy is necessary to exclude other causes of pulmonary infiltrates, especially infections. Open lung biopsies are diagnostically more productive, but they are not absolutely sensitive.

Radiographic findings on chest radiographs may be nonspecific, showing only ill-defined interstitial infiltrates (Fig. 39.3). An alveolar filling pattern is usually evident only if the patient has suffered hemoptysis and aspirated blood, but pleural effusions or pneumothorax may be seen when the lesion involves the serosal surfaces as well as the lung parenchyma (18, 19). Mediastinal adenopathy is not common, but if it is present, this sign can be very helpful in differentiating KS from *Pneumocystis carinii* infection because the latter does not cause adenopathy. Computed tomographic scans

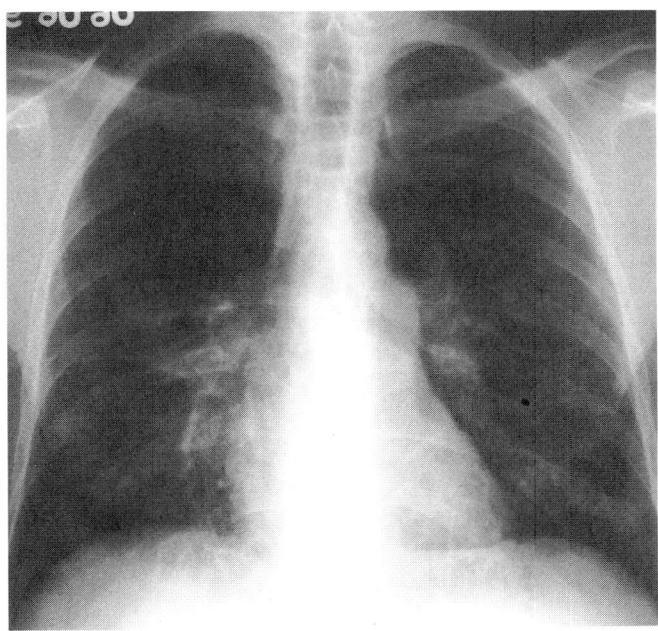

FIGURE 39.3. Chest radiograph of Kaposi's sarcoma with bilateral nodular opacities in a patient with AIDS.

and magnetic resonance (MR) images generally provide no more information than the chest radiographs. In summary, the presence of bilateral pleural effusions and bilateral interstitial infiltrates with ill-defined nodularity is suggestive of pulmonary KS, especially in a patient with known tumor elsewhere (12, 13).

PATHOLOGIC FINDINGS

It is distinctly uncommon for the pathologist to be able to make a definitive diagnosis of KS of the lung on a transbronchial biopsy specimen. Usually, a wedge biopsy is necessary, obtained using video-guided thoracoscopy or a limited thoracotomy (17). On gross examination, this type of specimen exhibits numerous hemangiomatoid or ecchymosislike zones of bluish red discoloration in the parenchyma, with ill-defined borders.

In the lung KS shows a tendency to grow along preexisting fibrous intrapulmonary septa, and it also concentrates around small tubular airways and blood vessels (Fig. 39.4). The tumor is composed of a mixture of ectatic, thin-walled blood vessels that dissect or push through the pulmonary interstitial collagen, together with haphazardly arranged fascicles of spindle cells that show only modest nuclear atypia and may contain cytoplasmic vacuoles (11, 17). Extravasated erythrocytes and hemosiderin pigment are common in and around the tumor masses. Pleural KS layers itself over the submesothelial mantle of connective tissue, thus effacing the mesothelium itself.

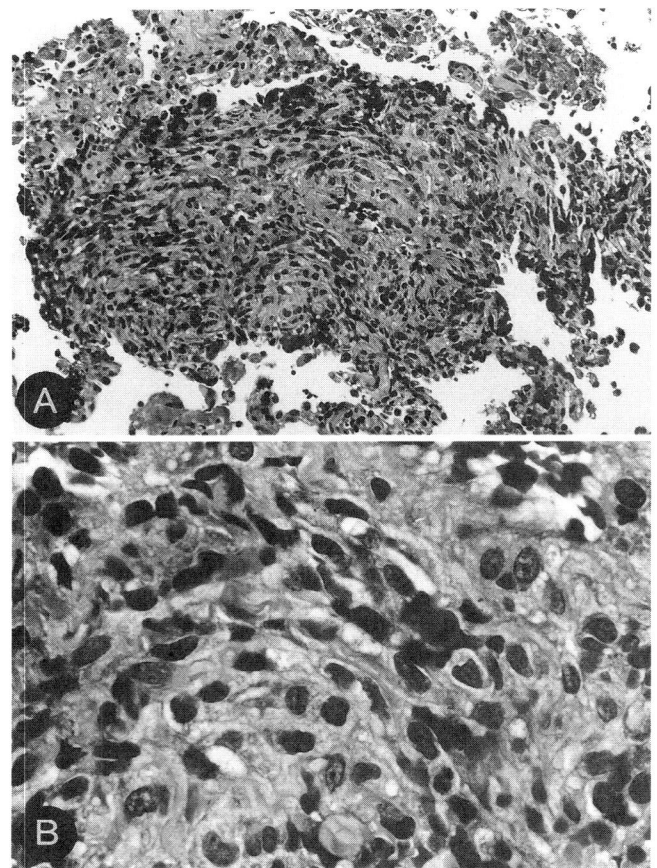

FIGURE 39.4. A. Kaposi's sarcoma expands and widens the interstitium and surrounds blood vessels. B. The tumor cells are oval to spindled and contain intracytoplasmic vacuoles.

Mitotic activity is variable in primary KS of the lung, but it usually is detectable. If it is present at all, necrosis is limited in scope and visible only on microscopy.

THERAPY AND PROGNOSIS

Regardless of its occurrence in AIDS or in non–human immunodeficiency virus (HIV)–related cases, the presence of KS in the lung is prognostically ominous. Virtually all patients with visceral disease die within 2 years, from infection if not from KS itself (10). Because of the multiplicity of KS lesions, surgical resection is not a realistic option in the management of patients with this neoplasm. Chemotherapy is considered the treatment of choice, with a relatively good response rate and relatively rapid improvement within 2 to 4 weeks (20). Chemotherapy regimens in the few published therapeutic trials designed specifically for pulmonary KS have included primarily Adriamycin, bleomycin, and vincristine (11, 21, 22). Gill et al. (21) reported an 85% response with combination chemotherapy in a group of 13 patients. Patients who benefited from this treatment included those who achieved at least partial responses. Complete response is defined by the following criteria: (a) direct bronchoscopy revealing complete disappearance of KS lesions in the tracheobronchial tree, (b) a normal chest radiograph, and (c) resolution of all other sites of disease. A partial response is characterized by the same points except that the degree of resolution is not total (20, 21).

Despite fairly good results with combination chemotherapy, patients with pulmonary KS do not survive long. In the trial reported by Gill et al. (21), the median survival for responders was slightly but significantly longer than that of nonresponders (10 versus 6 months, respectively). However, considerable overlap between the two groups was present.

Other more experimental (and inconclusive) approaches have included the administration of zidovudine, interferon, and other antiviral compounds (9). Radiotherapy may provide palliation of symptoms but is noncurative. The most important piece of information in prognosticating cases of KS of the lung is the serologic HIV status of the patient, inasmuch as AIDS is currently a uniformly lethal illness.

FIBROSARCOMA

Primary fibrosarcoma of the lung, like its soft tissue counterpart, is defined as a fibroblastic spindle cell neoplasm without evidence of specialized cellular differentiation. Although it has been cited, along with leiomyosarcoma, as the most common primary pulmonary sarcoma (23), fibrosarcoma of the lung was, and probably remains, overdiagnosed (24). Two separate studies from the Mayo Clinic cited two time dependent incidence figures for fibrosarcoma of the lung. From 1950 to 1978, it constituted 50% of all primary pulmonary sarcomas (25) but only 20% in the decade 1980 to 1990 (26). It is our belief that the great majority of pulmonary fibrosarcomas thus are actually sarcomatoid carcinomas. Only those tumors subjected to rigorous and specialized pathologic examination should be accepted as bona fide examples of this rare sarcoma variant.

CLINICAL SUMMARY

Guccion and Rosen (23) studied 13 cases of fibrosarcoma of the lung, dividing them into endobronchial and intrapulmonary types. This classification scheme was said to have clinical and prognostic importance. In conjunction with a review of 48 reported cases in the literature, these authors found that the majority of endobronchial fibrosarcomas of the lung occurred in children and young adults, whereas parenchymal tumors predominated in middle-aged and elderly patients. In contrast, Pettinato and associates (27) reported parenchymal tumors in two newborns and a 6-month-old infant. There was roughly an equal distribution by gender among endobronchial lesions; however, most intraparenchymal neoplasms occurred in men. All endobronchial fibrosarcomas of the lung in a series reported by the Armed Forces Institute of Pathology (AFIP) (23) produced symptoms of cough, hemoptysis, or chest pain; some of the parenchymal cases did so as well, but others were asymptomatic. Thoracic imaging studies of fibrosarcoma of the lung usually show discrete, homogenous masses. However, one pulmonary fibrosarcoma reported by Goldthorn et al. (28) simulated a bronchogenic cyst clinically and radiographically.

PATHOLOGIC FINDINGS

Endobronchial fibrosarcomas are smaller than microscopically similar tumors in the parenchyma; the former variants usually measure less than 3 cm, and the latter range from 3.5 to 23 cm in greatest dimension. Parenchymal masses are typically well delimited and lobulated with frequent areas of necrosis and hemorrhage.

Fibrosarcoma of the lung is histologically identical to its soft tissue counterparts, and it characteristically shows sheets and intertwining fascicles of spindle-shaped cells with a typical herringbone growth pattern and discernible stromal collagenogenesis (Figs. 39.5 and 39.6). The tumor cells contain oval to elon-

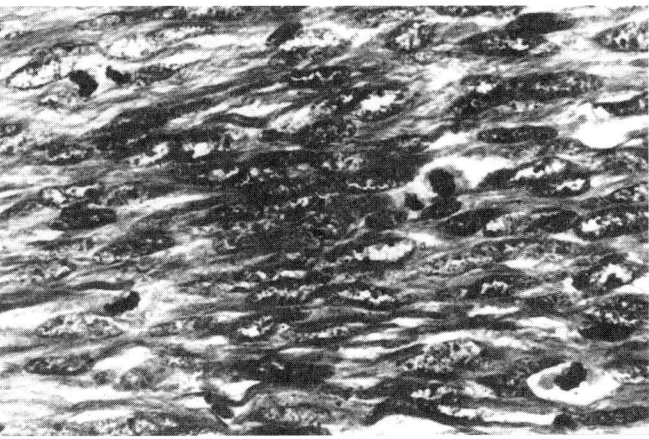

FIGURE 39.6. Fibrosarcomas are mitotically active with four mitotic figures seen in this field. Collagen fibers in the stroma surround the tumor cells. (From Wick MR, Manivel JC. Primary sarcomas of the lung. In: Williams CJ, Krikorian JG, Green MR, Raghavan D, eds. Textbook of uncommon cancer. New York: John Wiley, 1988: 335–381.)

gated, hyperchromatic nuclei and scant amphophilic cytoplasm with ill-defined cellular borders. In addition, some areas may have a slightly epithelioid appearance, in which the tumor cells are more ovoid than spindled, and others may show significant pleomorphism that merges with the image of malignant fibrous histiocytoma. Mitotic activity is variable.

Electron microscopic and immunohistochemical studies are required to confirm the fibroblastic nature of these neoplasms. The tumor cells in fibrosarcoma of the lung are characterized by abundant rough endoplasmic reticulum and free ribosomes, as well as the production of extracellular collagen fibers that may be aligned at right angles to the tumor cell membranes. There should be no detectable myofilaments, pericellular basal lamina, or intercellular junctions in lesions thought to represent fibrosarcoma of the lung. Because there are no specific immunologic markers for fibroblasts, the diagnosis of fibrosarcoma is one of immunohistologic exclusion. Tumor cells in fibrosarcoma of the lung generally stain only for vimentin, a primitive intermediate filament protein, and they lack all myogenous, neural, and endothelial markers (27, 29).

THERAPY AND PROGNOSIS

Although resection is the treatment of choice, many surgically treated fibrosarcomas of the lungs do recur, and survival after this event is short with death of the patient usually within 2 years (23). Three cases seen at the Mayo Clinic between 1980 and 1990 occurred in young women whose lesions all recurred within 15 months after surgical excision (26). In con-

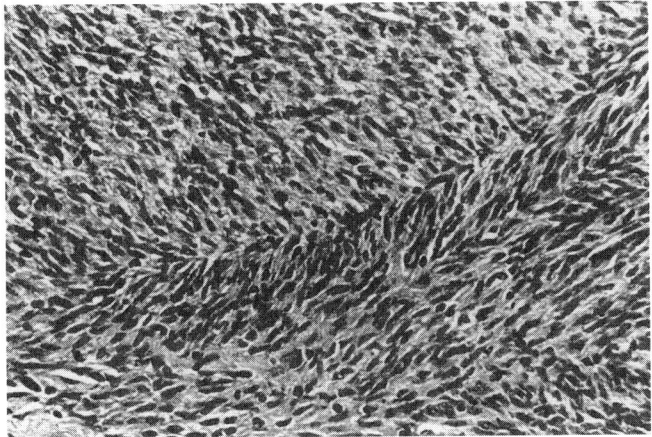

FIGURE 39.5. Fibrosarcoma demonstrates a herringbonelike arrangement of atypical spindle cells. (From Wick MR, Manivel JC. Primary sarcomas of the lung. In: Williams CJ, Krikorian JG, Green MR, Raghavan D, eds. Textbook of uncommon cancer. New York: John Wiley, 1988:335–381.)

trast, primary bronchopulmonary fibrosarcomas in children appear to have a relatively favorable prognosis and behave only as low-grade malignancies (27, 28). The five patients with pediatric fibrosarcoma of the lung reported by Pettinato et al. (27) had complete surgical removal of their tumors, and four were disease free after 4 to 9 years. The fifth case in that series had insignificant follow-up. The efficacy of adjunctive chemotherapy and irradiation has not yet been proven.

Primary Pulmonary Leiomyosarcoma

The most common anatomic locations for leiomyosarcomas in general are the uterus, gastrointestinal tract, and soft tissue, in order of relative frequency. Primary pulmonary leiomyosarcomas (PPLMSs) are extremely uncommon and presumably take their origins from bronchial or pulmonary vascular smooth muscle. Only three cases of leiomyosarcoma were found among roughly 10,000 primary malignancies of the lung at one large American medical center between 1980 and 1990 (26). Because secondary pulmonary involvement by malignant smooth muscle tumors is a relatively frequent event, the diagnosis of PPLMS absolutely requires exclusion of an occult extrathoracic neoplasm presenting with a single herald metastasis to the lung.

Clinical Summary

A series of 19 patients with PPLMS seen at the AFIP was divided into neoplasms that were predominantly endobronchial and others that were intraparenchymal, analogous to the typing of pulmonary fibrosarcomas (23). The majority of these tumors in children are endobronchial in nature (30, 31), whereas those in adults are not. In contrast to leiomyosarcomas of the soft tissue, which occur most commonly in women, patients in the AFIP report were almost exclusively males. However, another survey that reviewed 92 cases of PPLMS in the literature found a male to female ratio of 2.5, suggesting that the AFIP study was biased demographically by its affiliation with the armed services (32). In contrast to carcinoma of the lung, leiomyosarcoma is not associated with cigarette smoking or other potential inhaled carcinogens. Most patients with PPLMS (particularly its endobronchial form) are symptomatic, often complaining of cough, hemoptysis, or chest pain. However, intraparenchymal lesions may be discovered incidentally on chest radiographs. Roentgenographically, PPLMS usually takes the form of a discrete mass, sometimes with cavitation or cyst formation that is best seen by computed tomography (CT) of the thorax (23, 33).

Pathologic Findings

Parenchymal tumors range from 3 to 15 cm in maximum dimension (Fig. 39.7); they are well circumscribed, white to yellowish tan in color, and variably firm. Cut surfaces of these neoplasms commonly show hemorrhagic and necrotic areas. Endobronchial tumors often are smaller than the intraparenchymal lesions, presumably because of confinement by the bronchial walls.

Microscopy discloses histologic features that mirror those of leiomyosarcomas elsewhere in the body. On low-power magnification, there are interlacing fascicles of spindled cells that are arranged haphazardly, yielding a whorled appearance. The neoplastic cells have cigar-shaped nuclei with blunt ends, a moderate amount of cytoplasm, and indistinct cell borders (Fig. 39.8). Fascicles cut in cross-section demonstrate characteristic intracellular perinuclear lucencies.

The differential diagnosis of PPLMS includes fibrosarcoma and malignant schwannoma, as well as sarcomatoid carcinoma. Electron microscopy and immunohistochemistry are again helpful in confirming the smooth muscle nature of a spindle cell neoplasm (34). Ultrastructural features of leiomyogenous differentiation include cytoplasmic dense bodies punctuating skeins of thin filaments, subplasmalemmal dense plaques, plasmalemmal pinocytotic vesicles, and pericellular basal lamina. Immunoreactivity for desmin, muscle specific actin, or smooth muscle actin also is characteristic of the tumor cells in PPLMS.

Therapy and Prognosis

The natural history of PPLMS and its responses to various therapeutic regimens are difficult to predict because of the rarity of this neoplasm. However, there generally is a consensus that surgical resection is the treatment of choice (32, 35, 36) and that it produces a

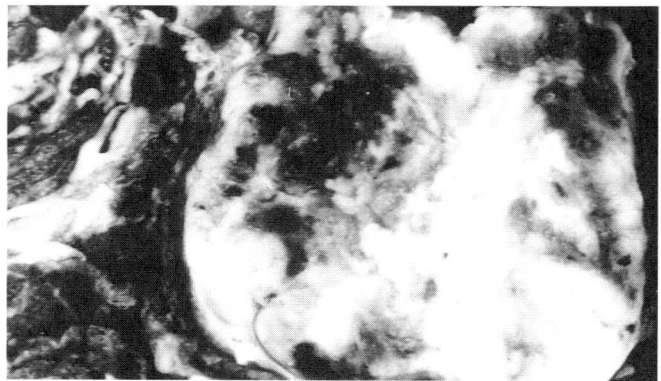

FIGURE 39.7. Primary pulmonary leiomyosarcoma. A discrete mass in the parenchyma adjacent to large airways is mostly solid with hemorrhagic areas.

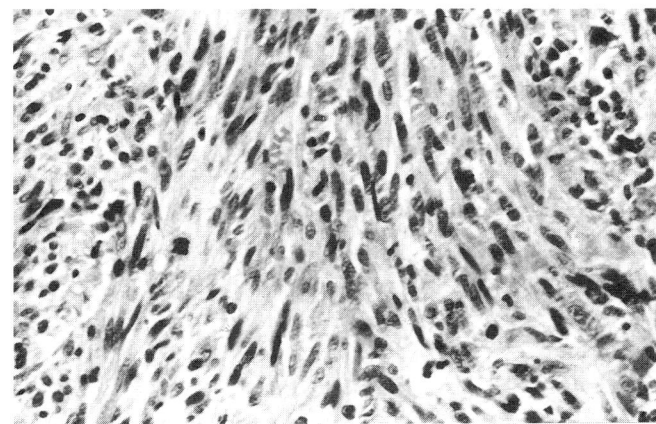

FIGURE 39.8. Leiomyosarcoma. Spindled cells show characteristic cigar-shaped nuclei.

survival rate of 45% to 50% at 5 years' follow-up. Survival for as long as 15 to 30 years has been documented in PPLMS cases (23, 25). However, pulmonary leiomyosarcomas appear to be resistant to irradiation and chemotherapy (32, 37). Various prognostic variables have been discussed in connection with these lesions (23, 25). Endobronchial tumors are thought to be less aggressive than parenchymal neoplasms, largely because the former tend to be smaller and are diagnosed earlier. It follows, therefore, that tumor size is an important indicator of biologic behavior for all pulmonary leiomyosarcomas. The scope of mitotic activity may affect prognosis as well. In an AFIP series on PPLMS (23), a mitotic rate of 8 or less per 10 high-power fields was associated with infrequent metastasis and a generally favorable clinical outcome.

EPITHELIOID HEMANGIOENDOTHELIOMA

In 1975 Dail and Liebow (38) reported the first cases of an unusual pulmonary neoplasm that they called intravascular bronchioloalveolar tumor (IVBAT). This name reflected their original hypothesis that the lesion was an epithelial tumor, specifically, a bronchioloalveolar carcinoma variant showing prominent vascular invasion (39). In 1979, Corrin et al. (40) alternatively proposed an endothelial origin for this tumor based on the results of ultrastructural studies. Subsequent evaluations by other investigators have confirmed the vascular histogenesis of the IVBAT. Indeed, in 1982 Weiss and Enzinger (41) described a series of soft tissue tumors that were histologically identical to IVBAT, coining the term epithelioid hemangioendothelioma (EH) for these lesions to emphasize their distinctively epithelioid (or histiocytoid) cytologic features. In addition to the lungs and soft tissues, EH also commonly occurs in the bone and liver.

CLINICAL SUMMARY

EH of the lung is a neoplasm that arises predominantly in female patients who account for roughly 80% of all cases (39, 42). It primarily occurs in young adults with approximately 50% being younger than 40 years; only 10% are older than 50 years at diagnosis (43). Many affected persons are asymptomatic, and their tumors are detected incidentally on chest radiographs (Fig. 39.9). Patients who have tumor-related complaints usually present with pleuritic pain, dyspnea, and cough. One case report also has documented alveolar hemorrhage as a presenting sign of pulmonary EH (44). Chest radiographs commonly show numerous, small nodular lesions throughout both lung fields. Therefore, EH enters the roentgenographic differential diagnosis of multiple pulmonary nodules in asymptomatic young women, together with metastatic germ cell tumors, chondroid pulmonary hamartomas, multiple arteriovenous malformations of the lung, deposits of benign metastasizing leiomyoma, and malignant lymphoma (45).

PATHOLOGIC FINDINGS

The pathologic diagnosis of EH is almost always made by open lung biopsy, inasmuch as transbronchial

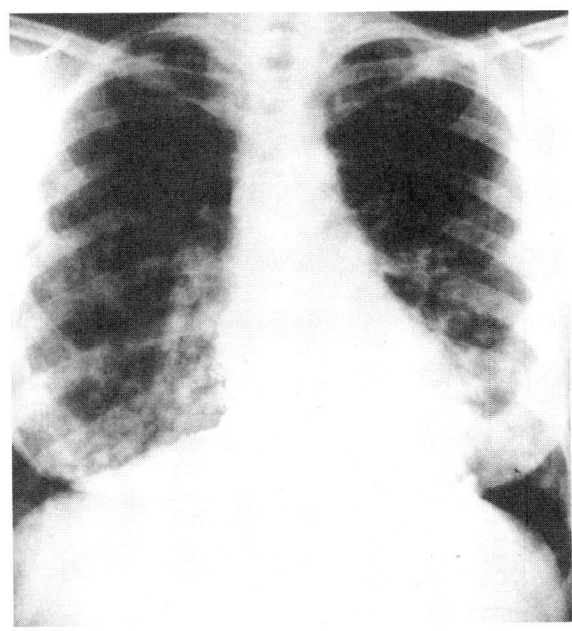

FIGURE 39.9. A characteristic radiograph of EH depicts multiple small nodules throughout both lungs. (From Dail DH, Liebow AA, Gmelich JT, et al. Intravascular, bronchiolar, and alveolar tumor of the lung [IVBAT]. Cancer 1983;51:452–464.)

biopsy is usually ineffective because of sampling constraints. Most nodules of EH are discrete and usually measure less than 2 cm. They are grayish white to tan in color and have a chondroid macroscopic consistency. More nodules typically are seen on histologic examination than are apparent grossly. Microscopically (39, 42), EH is typified by multiple oval or round nodules with hypocellular, sclerotic, or necrotic centers (Fig. 39.10). These are surrounded by rims of viable, more cellular tissue that is associated with a myxohyaline fibrous stroma. The neoplastic cell population is composed of plump, epithelioid cells that are the histologic hallmark of EH. They have centrally located, round to oval nuclei and ample amounts of eosinophilic cytoplasm. Often, intracytoplasmic vacuoles are evident, which should raise the possibility of endothelial differentiation on light microscopy. Tumoral involvement of arterioles, venules, and lymphatics is variable within the tumor nodules as well as other distant sites. EH commonly shows an intraalveolar pattern of growth secondary to tumor extension through the pores of Kohn, and surgical margins thus are difficult to ascertain on gross examination if a resection of the lesion is attempted.

Ultrastructural examination and immunohistochemical evaluation can assist greatly in confirming the endothelial origin of EH (40, 42, 46, 47). Briefly, ultrastructural features of this tumor include cytoplasmic vacuoles, Weibel-Palade bodies, cell membranous pinocytotic vesicles, and pericellular basal lamina. Histochemical and immunologic markers of endothelial differentiation, such as anti–von Willebrand factor, Ulex europaeus I lectin, anti-CD31, and anti-CD34, are helpful in labeling the neoplastic cells in virtually all examples of EH.

THERAPY AND PROGNOSIS

Surgery usually is not feasible as effective treatment for EH because of its tendency to show intrapulmonary multicentricity. Unfortunately, irradiation and chemotherapy likewise have been of little benefit (39, 42). Nevertheless, EH is generally an indolent neoplasm that is classified as a borderline malignancy. It is associated with a protracted clinical course and potential survival of several years after diagnosis (46). Most patients do eventually die of respiratory failure secondary to progressive parenchymal replacement resulting from the tumor. Adverse prognostic factors that predict a more rapid decline in pulmonary function include prominent symptoms at the time of presentation, and radiographic demonstration of extensive intravascular, endobronchial, or pleural spread of the tumor (39).

The general predilection of EH in women, a reported association of primary hepatic EH with oral contraceptives, and the lack of effective therapy for this tumor have prompted some investigators to explore the possibility of treatment involving hormonal modulation. These tumors have been examined for possible expression of estrogen and progesterone receptor proteins, as well as other estradiol-binding moieties. Ohori et al. (48) analyzed five cases of pulmonary EH for steroid hormone receptors by immunohistochemical methods, using paraffin-embedded material. Only one case showed apparent binding of estradiol. Experience at Washington University Medical Center (unpublished observations) with the immunohistologic characteristics of pulmonary EH has disclosed no reactivity with monoclonal antibodies against estrogen and progesterone receptor proteins. Thus, hormonal therapies are unlikely to produce significant results in this setting.

HEMANGIOPERICYTOMA

As first described in 1942 by Stout and Murray (49), hemangiopericytoma is an uncommon, potentially malignant neoplasm that shows apparent differentiation towards the phenotype of pericytes. These are cells with long cytoplasmic processes that surround capillaries and serve a vasoregulatory function. Hemangiopericytoma occurs most commonly in the deep muscles of the thigh, the pelvic fossa, and the retroperitoneum. However, 5% to 10% of all hemangiopericytomas are said to present as primary pul-

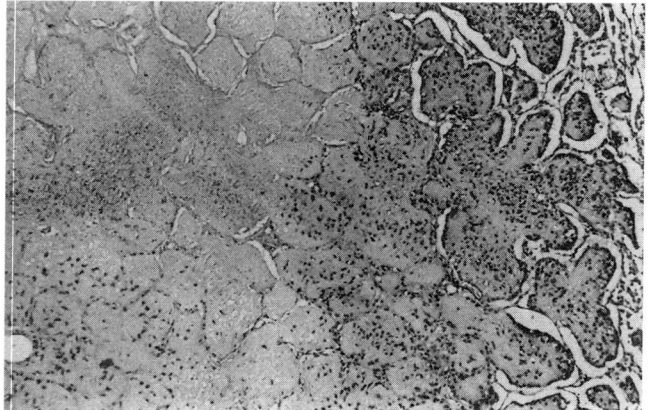

FIGURE 39.10. A nodule of EH contains a necrotic center. The tumor shows an intraalveolar growth pattern with more cellular areas at the edge. (From Dail DH, Liebow AA, Gmelich JT, et al. Intravascular, bronchiolar, and alveolar tumor of the lung [IVBAT]. Cancer 1983;51:452–464.)

monary tumors (50). It must be remembered that the lungs and the bones are the anatomic sites that most frequently harbor metastases of hemangiopericytoma (51), and therefore a primary extrapulmonary tumor must be excluded before a diagnosis of a primary hemangiopericytoma can be rendered safely.

CLINICAL SUMMARY

Pulmonary hemangiopericytoma affects men and women equally and most commonly arises in middle adulthood. The peak incidence of this lesion is in the fifth decade of life, although individuals as young as 4 years and as old as 73 years have been reported (52, 53). Some tumors are detected incidentally on radiographic studies without causing pulmonary symptoms; 6 of 18 cases in one series fit this scenario (54). Alternatively, presenting symptoms may include hemoptysis, chest pain, cough, and dyspnea, and, more rarely, pulmonary osteoarthropathy (54).

Various radiographic imaging studies have been utilized in studying this neoplasm. Although angiography usually has not been performed, vascular contrast studies of hemangiopericytoma generally show a characteristic intralesional blush (55). No other pathognomonic features are evident in chest roentgenograms, CT scans, and MR images of hemangiopericytomas of the lung (53, 56). Plain film radiographs typically show a discrete, homogeneously dense mass with lobulated contours. On CT images, however, hemangiopericytoma is heterogeneous. Central low-density areas are evident, corresponding to necrotic foci, and an apparent capsule may be seen at the interface with surrounding lung parenchyma. MR imaging also shows intratumoral heterogeneity with respect to tissue density, and it apparently is more sensitive in depicting intralesional hemorrhage. MR images were found to be the most useful in delineating the potential plane of surgical separation between a hemangiopericytoma and surrounding soft tissue in one report (57). In summary, a radiologic diagnosis of pulmonary hemangiopericytoma may be suspected in a middle-aged person lacking pulmonary symptoms but in whom radiographic imaging studies reveal a large, lobulated, sharply marginated, variably dense mass that does not cause compression atelectasis (56).

PATHOLOGIC FINDINGS

Hemangiopericytomas of the lung can attain large sizes, and lesions measuring up to 18 cm have been documented. The typical gross appearance of this tumor is that of a well-circumscribed, yellow to tan-brown mass with a pseudocapsule, and areas of internal necrosis and hemorrhage. Histologic sections typically show a relatively monomorphic cellular proliferation (Fig. 39.11) that surrounds thin-walled, anastomosing vascular channels lined by a single endothelial layer. These blood vessels often (but not always) assume gaping, staghorn, or antlerlike configurations (Fig. 39.12). The population of neoplastic cells is uniform, with oval compact nuclei and ill-defined cytoplasm. Mitotic activity and areas of necrosis and hemorrhage are noted frequently. Vascular invasion of large pulmonary vessels, however, is uncommon. With regard to the latter features, some pathologists, in the past, rendered a diagnosis of benign hemangiopericytoma if necrosis, hemorrhage, and mitoses were absent. This assumption is dangerous, because cases of

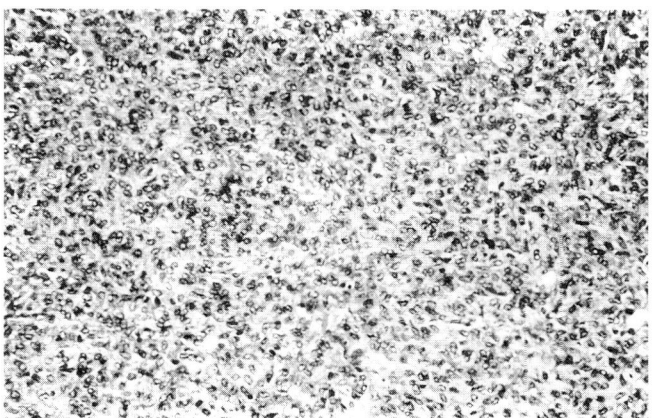

FIGURE 39.11. Tumor cells of a hemangiopericytoma are relatively uniform in appearance.

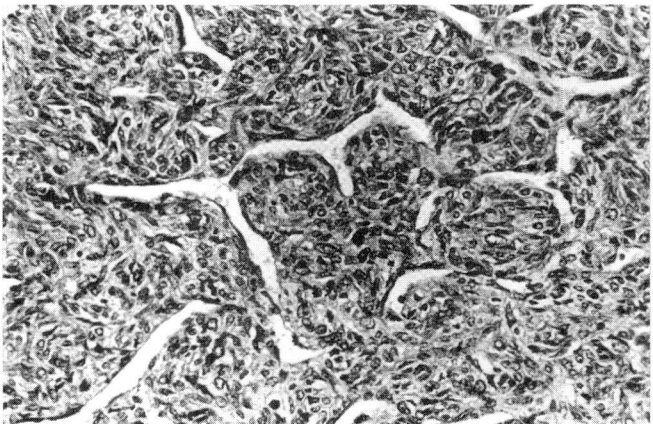

FIGURE 39.12. Hemangiopericytoma cells grow around blood vessels of various calibers and shapes, some of which assume a staghorn configuration. (From Wick MR, Manivel JC. Primary sarcomas of the lung. In: Williams CJ, Krikorian JG, Green MR, Raghavan D, eds. Textbook of uncommon cancer. New York: John Wiley, 1988:335–381.)

pulmonary hemangiopericytoma have been seen with exceedingly bland histologic profiles in which metastasis nonetheless supervened. Accordingly, it is advisable that each report on this tumor carry the statement that hemangiopericytoma is at least potentially malignant behaviorally (51, 54).

Pulmonary hemangiopericytoma has sometimes been overdiagnosed because other neoplasms may show foci that resemble it. Pathologists should remember that in their seminal report Stout and Murray (49) admonished others to make the diagnosis of hemangiopericytoma by exclusion. The histologic differential diagnosis includes synovial sarcoma, pleuropulmonary fibrous tumors, fibrous histiocytomas, and mesenchymal chondrosarcoma (51); distinctions between these neoplasms are best made by ancillary studies. Electron microscopy can confirm the pericytic nature of hemangiopericytoma through the demonstration of polygonal cells with cytoplasmic processes, pinocytotic vesicles, basal lamina, and a paucity of other organelles (29, 51). Hemangiopericytoma is a neoplasm that is devoid of most immunohistochemical markers except vimentin, collagen type IV, and Leu-7 (29). Endothelial stains, such as Ulex europaeus and factor VIII–related antigen, highlight the lining of intralesional vascular spaces, but they do not label the surrounding tumor cells.

THERAPY AND PROGNOSIS

As in the management of soft tissue hemangiopericytoma, complete surgical excision is the mainstay of therapy for primary pulmonary tumors of this type. However, it is known that intraoperative rupture of pulmonary hemangiopericytoma is prone to occur (especially those that are adherent to the chest wall); as expected, this complication results in early local recurrence, as reported by Van Damme et al. (53), and it thus should be avoided at all costs. Chemotherapy and irradiation have not been shown to be consistently effective adjuvant modalities, but they may have some role in management. Adriamycin appears to be the most effective chemotherapeutic agent (58). A study by Jha et al. (59) on the general role of radiation therapy in treating hemangiopericytoma showed that postoperative irradiation was useful for local tumor control, salvage therapy after local recurrence, and palliation. A dosage of more than 25 Gy is recommended, and tumors less than 5 cm in maximum dimension exhibit a better response than those larger than 10 cm (60).

Hemangiopericytomas generally are well known for their unpredictable biologic behavior. Postoperative survival has ranged from 10 weeks to 18 years (53, 61).

Even with apparently complete surgical resection, hemangiopericytoma recurs locally in approximately 50% of cases within 2 years (54, 57, 61), and later recurrences are common. Clinical and histologic features cited as prognostically useful (51, 52, 57) include the presence of symptoms at presentation; mitotic activity of at least four mitoses per 10 high-power microscopic fields; spontaneous tumor necrosis; vascular invasion; and tumor size of more than 5 cm. In one series metastases were seen in one third of tumors measuring more than 5 cm and in two thirds of those larger than 10 cm (52). However, Yousem and Hochholzer (54) did not find any single histologic or clinical feature that was statistically significant in reliably predicting the clinical course of pulmonary hemangiopericytoma.

MALIGNANT FIBROUS HISTIOCYTOMA

Malignant fibrous histiocytoma is a common, extensively studied, soft tissue sarcoma of older adults that develops most frequently in the extremities and the retroperitoneum. In a series of 200 cases by Weiss and Enzinger (62), the lungs were the most common site of metastases. Thus, exclusion of an occult soft tissue tumor is once again necessary before a diagnosis of primary pulmonary malignant fibrous histiocytoma (PPMFH) can be made. A recent review of Mayo Clinic cases found only 4 examples among 10,134 tumors arising in the lung (26). Currently, there are fewer than 40 reported cases of PPMFH in the English-language literature (62–68).

CLINICAL SUMMARY

In general, malignant fibrous histiocytoma is a neoplasm of patients who are in late middle age, with a median of 54 years. However, its occurrence in adolescents and young adults also has been reported (63, 69). No consistent predilection for either gender is seen. Previous irradiation is a pathogenetic risk factor for tumors arising in soft tissue, and the literature similarly contains one case report of a PPMFH presenting in a patient who had received radiation therapy for malignant lymphoma 7 years previously. Clinical and radiographic features of this tumor are nonspecific, and a distinction from the much more common epithelial tumors of the lungs absolutely requires tissue examination. The majority of patients present with symptoms of cough, chest pain, hemoptysis, or dyspnea. Chest radiographs generally show a solitary mass with a nondescript appearance and a relatively homogeneous density on CT or MR imaging studies.

PATHOLOGIC FINDINGS

Most examples of PPMFH are intraparenchymal, but occasional endobronchial lesions also have been observed (63). There is apparently no predilection for any particular lobe of either lung. These tumors are usually large, ranging up to 25 cm in maximum dimension (69), with an average size of 6 to 7 cm. They are well circumscribed, lobular, and white-tan in color, and they commonly contain central necrosis or cavitation on macroscopic examination.

Histologically, PPMFH is characterized by three basic cell types that are arranged in storiform, fascicular, or medullary patterns. As the term malignant fibrous histiocytoma implies, this tumor was thought to be composed of malignant fibroblastlike and histiocytoid cells; however, it now appears that there is little if any relationship between the neoplastic elements and true histiocytes. Fusiform tumor cells contain elongated nuclei and relatively scant cytoplasm, and histiocytoid cells have round to oval nuclei with a moderate quantity of amphophilic cytoplasm. A hallmark of most lesions in this category is the presence of large, bizarre, often multinucleated cells with irregular contours (Fig. 39.13). Mitoses, including atypical forms, are found easily and number from 5 to 30 per 10 high-power microscopic fields (29).

The differential diagnosis of PPMFH by light microscopy may include primary or secondary pleomorphic sarcomas (dedifferentiated leiomyosarcoma and pleomorphic rhabdomyosarcoma), metastatic malignant melanoma, and sarcomatoid carcinoma. Immunohistochemical and electron microscopic studies can be employed to separate these pathologic entities (64–69). Briefly, PPMFH shows fibroblastic and histiocytelike differentiation ultrastructurally, with abundant rough endoplasmic reticulum, numerous lysosomes, and a variable number of small cytoplasmic lipid droplets. Desmosomes, tonofibrils, elongated cell processes, myogenous filament skeins, and cytoplasmic dense bodies are absent. PPMFH expresses vimentin, but on immunohistologic analyses it is devoid of other specialized markers of myogenous, neural, or epithelial differentiation.

THERAPY AND PROGNOSIS

The rarity of PPMFH again serves as an impediment to assessments of optimal treatment for this tumor. Surgical resection is currently the recommended treatment of choice, even if the lesion shows limited extrapulmonary spread to the intrathoracic great vessels or soft tissue (70). Adjunctive chemotherapy and irradiation have not proven to be effective in the few published cases of PPMFH in which these treatments were employed (63, 69). In a series of 22 cases (63), 7 of 15 patients who underwent radical surgical resection suffered relapses and died of metastatic disease. There was recurrence in the lungs and pleura, as well as metastasis to the liver and brain; almost all of these events occurred within 12 months of diagnosis. However, survival periods of as long as 5 to 10 years have been documented in a few patients with PPMFH (63, 65).

Potential adverse prognostic factors include an advanced clinical or pathologic stage at presentation (with mediastinal, chest wall, or carinal involvement), prominent symptoms at diagnosis, incompleteness of excision, and tumor recurrence. Histologic findings have not been found to affect behavior.

RHABDOMYOSARCOMA

For practical purposes primary rhabdomyosarcoma of the lung is a tumor that is confined to the pediatric population. In adults tumors resembling rhabdomyosarcoma almost invariably are examples of sarcomatoid carcinoma (1), and this fact should be considered in interpreting all but the most recent literature on this topic. Moreover, this tumor is another sarcoma type that much more commonly arises outside of the lungs, and the probability that one is dealing with metastasis to the pulmonary parenchyma is therefore important to remember.

CLINICAL SUMMARY

To date, there are fewer than 10 well-documented examples of bona fide intrapulmonary rhabdomyosarcoma in the pertinent literature. They all occurred in patients who were in the first two decades of life, and most were in children under 10 years old (71). Symp-

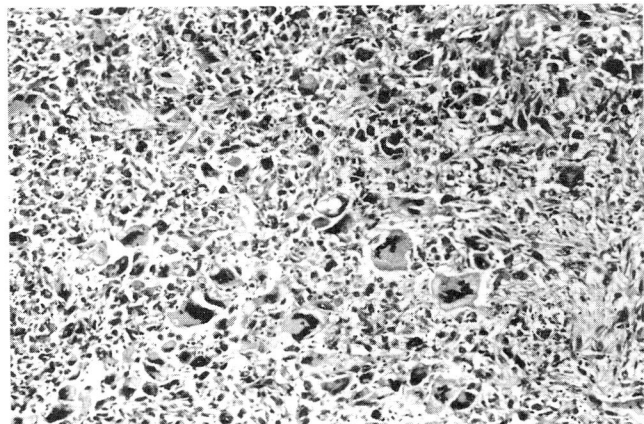

FIGURE 39.13. Malignant fibrous histiocytoma consists of pleomorphic cells including multinucleated, bizarre, giant cells.

toms and signs of pulmonary rhabdomyosarcoma may be nonspecific, including cough, wheezing, and dyspnea, or the patient may present with spontaneous pneumothorax (72). The latter relates to a peculiar tendency of pulmonary rhabdomyosarcoma to associate itself with cystic lesions of the lungs (73). When these cysts rupture, pneumothorax results. The underlying lesions in such cases of pulmonary rhabdomyosarcoma have included congenital cystic adenomatoid malformations and peripheral bronchogenic cysts (73).

Roentgenographic studies may demonstrate a single, nondescript, intraparenchymal mass that is homogeneous on CT or MR imaging analyses, or they may reveal the presence of a mass in the wall of a cyst (Fig. 39.14). The latter scenario is much more likely to result in a correct diagnosis by the radiologist.

PATHOLOGIC FINDINGS

Pulmonary rhabdomyosarcoma may be associated with preexisting cysts of the lung, such as congenital cystic adenomatoid malformations or intrapulmonary bronchogenic cysts. Thus, the latter lesions should always be examined—at least cursorily—for a malignant component, despite the extreme rarity of that complication.

Pulmonary rhabdomyosarcomas have most often assumed an embryonal or alveolar growth pattern, although pleomorphic tumors, which usually are encountered in the soft tissues of adult patients, have been reported in the lung (74). These neoplasms typically are composed of small round cells configured in one of three ways: (*a*) solid sheetlike clusters with no further distinguishing morphologic attributes; (*b*) dyscohesive groups with internal pseudolumina or alveoli; and (*c*) botryoid proliferations in which a polypoid lesion (usually within a bronchial lumen) shows a zonation into hypocellular and hypercellular cellular strata (so-called Cambium layers) (75) (Fig. 39.15). In contradistinction to other small round cell tumors of children, pulmonary rhabdomyosarcoma demonstrates a moderate degree of cellular pleomorphism and anisonucleosis. Nuclear chromatin is usually coarse and clumped; cytoplasm is scanty and amphophilic or eosinophilic; and mitoses and apoptotic cells are found easily. Small foci of spontaneous necrosis also are present.

Particularly in lesions having an embryonal solid appearance histologically, special pathologic studies are nearly always necessary to make a definitive diagnosis. Moreover, these analyses should also be done in *all* putative cases in adults, for the reasons mentioned above. Histochemical stains show that striated muscle tumors contain abundant glycogen, determined using the periodic acid–Schiff method with and without diastase digestion. Electron microscopically, rhabdomyosarcoma is characterized by the focal presence of intermediate filament whorls in the cytoplasm, sometimes with the addition of thick filaments in aggregates that resemble primitive muscular Z bands. Furthermore, cytoplasmic glycogen is present, and pericellular basal lamina can be visualized. This constellation of fine structural attributes excludes other small cell tumors from diagnostic consideration (76). By immunohistology, pulmonary rhabdomyosarcoma

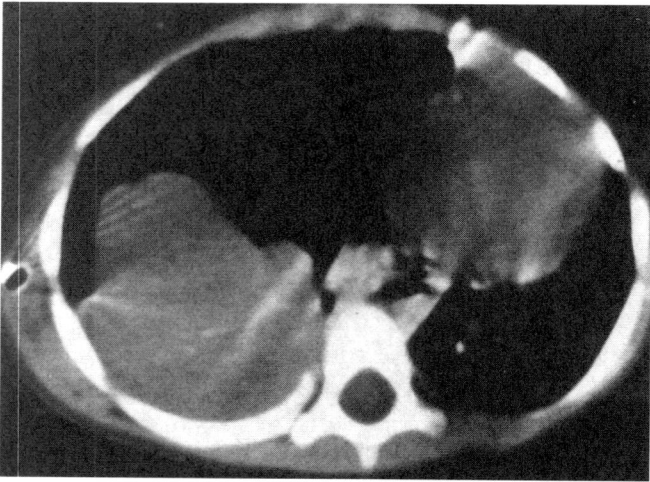

FIGURE 39.14. CT of intrapulmonary rhabdomyosarcoma. (From Dehner LP. Soft tissue, peritoneum, and retroperitoneum. In: Pediatric surgical pathology. 2nd ed. Baltimore: Williams & Wilkins, 1987:869–938.)

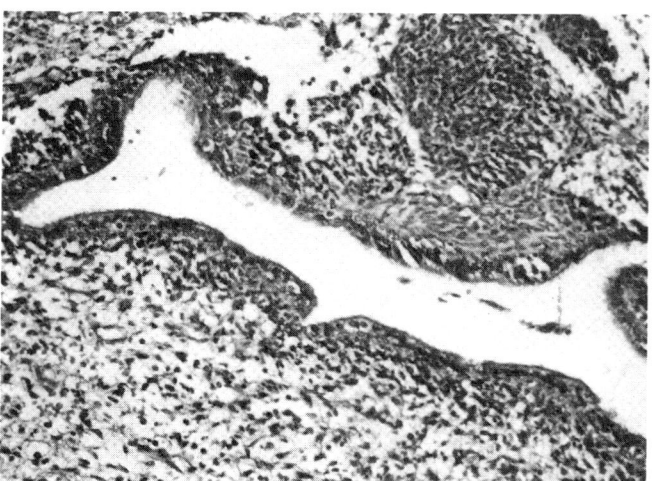

FIGURE 39.15. Typical small, round to oval tumor cells of a rhabdomyosarcoma focally surround an airway, simulating the appearance of a cambium layer. (From Dehner LP. Soft tissue, peritoneum, and retroperitoneum. In: Pediatric surgical pathology. 2nd ed. Baltimore: Williams & Wilkins, 1987:869–938.)

is found to express one or more myogenous determinants, such as desmin, tropomyosin, muscle specific actin, or Z-band protein (77). Vimentin also is found uniformly, but markers of epithelial differentiation, such as keratin and epithelial membrane antigen, must be *absent* in order to make the diagnosis.

THERAPY AND PROGNOSIS

The great majority of reported cases of pulmonary rhabdomyosarcoma have been treated surgically, with the usual addition of postoperative irradiation and standard chemotherapy, such as that used by the InterGroup Rhabdomyosarcoma Study (71–74). However, there have been no controlled studies to determine whether this protocol is the optimal approach to management. Once again, the extreme rarity of the lesion interferes with the design of the most efficacious therapeutic regimen.

Prognostically, the fact that the pulmonary version is a visceral manifestation of rhabdomyosarcoma is an adverse clinical variable, along with the probability that such tumors may attain a size of several centimeters before coming to clinical attention. Pathologic features associated with unfavorable tumoral behavior include the focal or global presence of an alveolar growth pattern and the existence of areas that resemble adult-type pleomorphic rhabdomyosarcoma (78).

CHONDROSARCOMA OF THE RESPIRATORY TRACT

Chondrosarcomas are uncommon but well documented in the supporting tissues of both the upper and lower airways. Indeed, although cartilaginous malignancies usually are observed in the proximal long bones of adults, visceral lesions of this type have been reported in a variety of locations. As one would expect, there are few if any examples of primary pulmonary chondrosarcoma (PPCS) that involve the most distal portion of the respiratory tract, because cartilaginous support for the bronchi ends at the level of the subsegmental bronchi (79). Accordingly, most PPCSs affect the trachea and major bronchial divisions (80, 81), and chondrosarcomas seen in the peripheral lung fields should be examined radiologically to make certain that they are not extensions of contiguous bony lesions in the sternum, vertebral bodies, or ribs.

In contrast to statements pertaining to most other sarcomas of the lung, it is virtually unknown for chondroid malignancies to metastasize while they are still occult in peripheral osseous or soft tissue sites. Thus, once a pathologic diagnosis of chondrosarcoma has been established for a lesion that clearly involves the airway, it may safely be considered to have arisen at that location.

CLINICAL SUMMARY

Patients with PPCS are adults, and there is no predilection of the tumor for either gender. Tumors may present with slowly evolving stridor, wheezing, cough, vague chest pain, or episodes of hemoptysis (80). Systemic complaints are not encountered. Tracheobronchoscopy usually demonstrates a smooth, nodular, glistening mass that stretches and attenuates the overlying mucosa but that does not ulcerate it. Attempted biopsy of the mass through the bronchoscope is usually unsuccessful because of the general difficulty of sampling submucosal lesions (79).

Radiographically, there may be no visible abnormalities on plain films if the neoplasm is predominantly or exclusively intraluminal in a large airway. Other examples of PPCSs are manifest simply as sharply circumscribed, peripheral, lobulated masses that may contain flecks of central calcification or cystic change. The latter findings are more graphically displayed in CT or MR imaging studies (80).

PATHOLOGIC FINDINGS

Chondrosarcomas of the lung differ significantly from pulmonary chondroid hamartomas microscopically. The latter lesions typically entrap small tubular airways and are composed of extremely well-differentiated chondrocytes. In contrast, PPCS exhibits at least modest nuclear pleomorphism, nuclear crowding, and cellular binucleation, and it does not contain respiratory epithelial profiles (79) (Fig. 39.16). Despite these characteristics, most chondrosarcomas of the lung are well-differentiated tumors. Thus, a striking degree of nondescript spindle cell growth or cellular anaplasia in

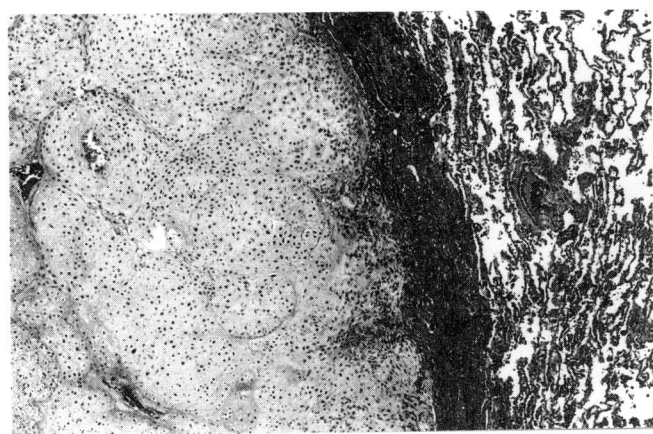

FIGURE 39.16. A pulmonary chondrosarcoma is composed of hypercellular lobules of chondrocytes that exhibit mild pleomorphism.

a cartilage-forming tumor should invoke concerns over a probable diagnosis of sarcomatoid carcinoma with divergent chondroid areas (1).

With these caveats in mind, there are few other differential diagnostic considerations in cases of PPCS. Thus, special histochemical, ultrastructural, and immunohistochemical assessments usually are not needed to establish a diagnosis confidentially.

THERAPY AND PROGNOSIS

Primary chondrosarcomas of the airway are best treated by surgical ablation. Because these are slow-growing and generally low-grade malignancies, such intervention carries with it a good chance of long-term survival if the tumor can be extirpated completely (80). Chemotherapy and irradiation are ineffectual in treating PPCS, and they probably incur more morbidity than is acceptable in the treatment of an indolent sarcoma.

Extrapolating from bone tumor pathology, there are only two features that correlate with a risk of recurrence or metastasis of chondrosarcoma. These include a tumor size of more than 5 cm and vascular invasion by the neoplastic cells. There is no evidence that adjuvant treatment of patients with these risk factors in any way improves the clinical outlook. Indeed, reoperation to remove any recurrent masses is the most sensible approach to patient management in this context.

OTHER PRIMARY PULMONARY SARCOMAS

There are four other sarcoma morphotypes that may be encountered in the lungs. These include liposarcoma (82), angiosarcoma (83, 84), malignant schwannoma (85), and osteosarcoma (86). Fewer than 10 cases each of these neoplasms have been documented in the literature, making it impossible to present their clinicopathologic attributes as if they were thoroughly studied and well characterized.

However, a few generalizations do appear to be appropriate. First, liposarcomas and malignant schwannomas of the lung have been documented primarily as tumors having an endobronchial component, potentially producing airway obstruction. In contrast, this feature is not part of the profile of either angiosarcoma or osteosarcoma. Secondly, both angiosarcomalike and osteosarcomalike epithelial neoplasms are vastly more common in the respiratory tract than are true sarcomas with those respective microscopic patterns (1, 87). Thus, the pathologist must be certain to address the likelihood of sarcomatoid carcinoma under such circumstances. Finally, therapy for those rare lesions in this category that have proven to be primary in the lungs is completely anecdotal and has been based on extrapolation from the treatment used for histologically similar neoplasms in osseous and soft tissue sites.

TUMORS OF THE PULMONARY BLOOD VESSELS

SARCOMAS OF THE PULMONARY ARTERIAL TRUNK

Although technically it is not part of the respiratory tract, the pulmonary arterial trunk is an appropriate topic for a discussion centering on intrathoracic mesenchymal malignancies. For more than 70 years, it has been known that this vascular segment may serve as the point of origin for sarcomas with diverse histologic features and clinical manifestations that are just as variable (88). To date, approximately 125 cases of pulmonary trunk sarcoma (PTS) have been documented.

CLINICAL SUMMARY

Patients with PTS are adults in middle life or beyond; there is no predilection for either gender. They present with a panoply of potential symptoms and signs, the most common of which simulate the findings of right-sided cardiac failure or pulmonary thromboembolic disease. Patients often complain of intractable cough, progressive dyspnea, and dull chest pain that may increase with exertion. Neck veins may be distended, a loud precordial systolic heart murmur may be audible at the upper left sternal border, and the patient may manifest the complete clinical scenario of anasarca (89, 90). However, cardiac imaging studies demonstrate no evidence of ventricular hypokinesis or perfusion abnormalities (91).

In the era before modern angiography, echocardiography, CT, and specialized radionuclide scans, the diagnosis of PTS usually was made for the first time at autopsy (88). However, current imaging modalities now are capable of revealing the tumor rather easily (91). It takes the form of a partially obstructing, endoluminal mass at or above the level of the right ventricular outlet, and it may extend over a span of several centimeters (Fig. 39.17). Attachment of the lesion to the arterial wall is variable in character, and the lesion may be either sessile or pedunculated. The neoplasm generally is somewhat heterogeneous in density and greatly variable in size.

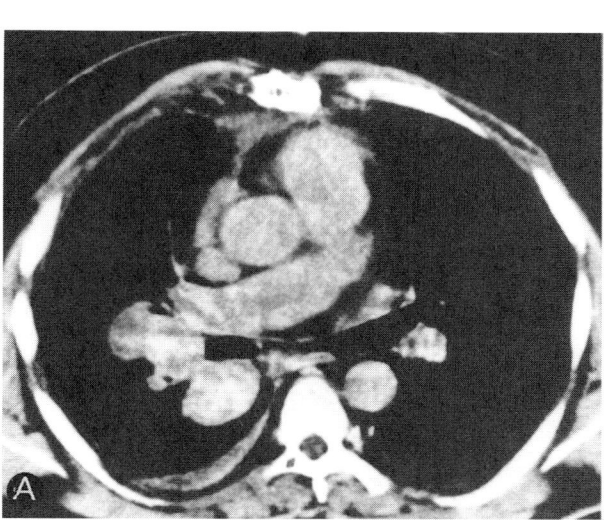
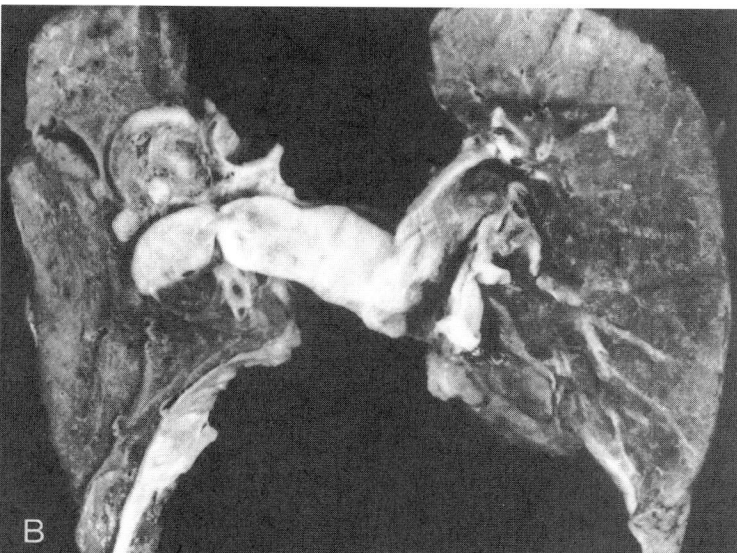

FIGURE 39.17. Gross specimen and CT scan at the level of the outlet of the great vessels. A. Tumor fills the main pulmonary artery and extends to the right and left pulmonary artery. B. Correlation of tumor in gross specimen. (From McGlennen RC, Manivel JC, Stanley SJ, et al. Pulmonary artery trunk sarcoma: a clinicopathologic, ultrastructural, and immunohistochemical study of four cases. Mod Pathol 1989;2:486–494.)

PATHOLOGIC FINDINGS

The preoperative diagnosis of PTS typically is one that may not involve the pathologist, inasmuch as biopsy of an intravascular mass in the right ventricular outlet is a challenging procedure. Thus, a pathologist's first encounter with such lesions may be in the frozen section laboratory during a definitive surgical procedure. In this context it is important to realize that a firm diagnosis of a particular sarcoma type (or even of a malignancy) may not be easy. Some PTSs take the form of rather paucicellular myxoid proliferations with surprisingly bland cytologic characteristics, whereas others are wildly anaplastic tumors that defy easy classification under the microscope (88). The proffered pathologic interpretations in the literature on PTS include such diagnoses as undifferentiated sarcoma, angiosarcoma, leiomyosarcoma, rhabdomyosarcoma, fibromyxosarcoma, fibrosarcoma, chondrosarcoma, osteosarcoma, hemangioendothelioma, malignant fibrous histiocytoma, and malignant mesenchymoma (90) (Fig. 39.18). What one can glean from this apparently confusing list is that the histologic spectrum and pathologic grades of PTS are distributed broadly, such that no two lesions look quite the same under the microscope. Beyond that, pathologists have speculated widely on the mechanistic reasons for this diversity, but this issue admittedly has little clinical import at the present time.

With respect to differential diagnosis, the majority of PTSs have the characteristics of high-grade spindle cell or pleomorphic sarcomas, which, in current parlance, would usually be grouped together under the rubric of malignant fibrous histiocytoma. However, some low-grade fibromyxoid variants can closely simulate an intracardiac myxoma or organizing mural thrombus (88). Close attention to cytologic detail is the only certain method for distinguishing between such possibilities.

THERAPY AND PROGNOSIS

Because of the dominance of autopsy reports in the earliest literature on PTS, the recommended therapy for this tumor must still be considered evolutionary. Presently, provided that a firm radiologic diagnosis can be made or a frozen section interpretation of sarcoma can be rendered, the surgeon may perform an en bloc resection of the pulmonary trunk and its luminal tumor contents, followed by interposition of a synthetic graft (92). This technique probably is the most definitive approach to operative therapy, because it is difficult to determine the boundaries of intramural tumor growth by visual inspection. The latter point makes more limited vascular resections and reconstructions a tenuous enterprise.

Extension of the tumor through the wall of the pulmonary artery is the single most important piece of pathologic information in cases of PTS, because histologic grading does not appear to correlate with tumor behavior consistently (88, 90). In addition, the surgeon's or radiologist's estimation of whether the lesion is pedunculated or sessile has considerable importance. Tumors with a narrow stalk tend to flutter in the

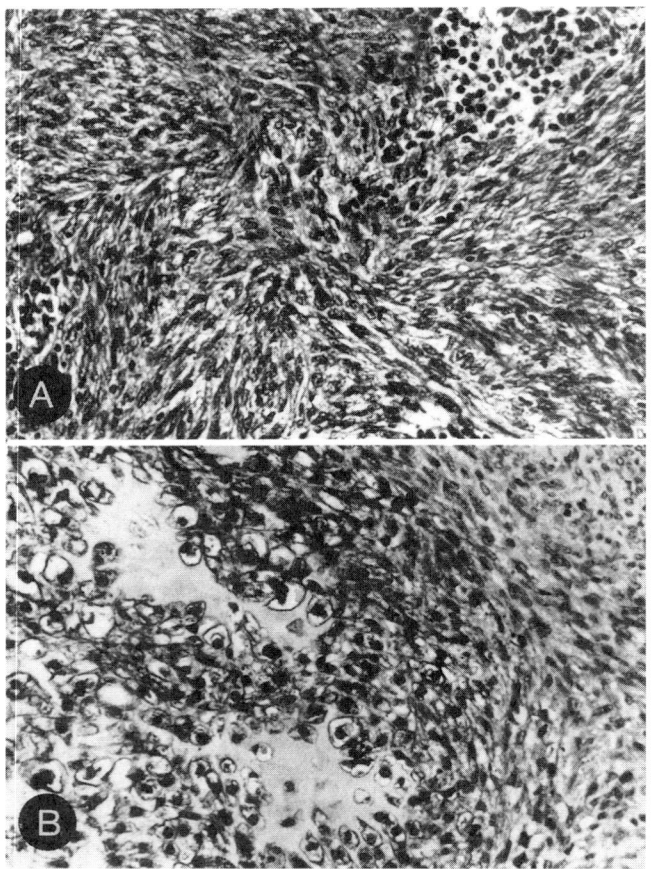

FIGURE 39.18. Histologic variability of pulmonary trunk sarcomas, ranging from **A.** undifferentiated spindle cells in a whorled configuration to **B.** differentiated areas with chondrosarcomalike features. (From McGlennen RC, Manivel JC, Stanley SJ, et al. Pulmonary artery trunk sarcoma: a clinicopathologic, ultrastructural, and immunohistochemical study of four cases. Mod Pathol 1989;2:486–494.)

stream of ejected blood in the ventricular outflow tract, and pieces of the neoplasm may be embolized into the lungs (93). This phenomenon is not as common with lesions assuming a broadly based sessile macroscopic growth pattern.

Cases demonstrating metastasis or obvious extravascular spread of PTS may be managed with irradiation or chemotherapy. However, there are no unified recommendations for the use of these treatments, and their implementation has produced discouraging results thus far.

TUMORS OF THE PLEURA

Sarcomas are as rare in the pleura as they are in the lungs. Most neoplasms that take the generic appearance of malignant mesenchymal tumors in the serosae of the thorax are actually epithelial lesions. However, rather than representing sarcomatoid carcinomas, they are variants of malignant mesotheliomas (94). In addition to the latter (considered in detail in Chapter 35), there are only a limited number of definable clinicopathologic entities to consider in this specific anatomic location. These include fibrosarcoma, malignant solitary fibrous tumor of the pleura, Askin's malignant thoracopulmonary small round cell tumor, pleuropulmonary blastoma, KS, EH, and angiosarcoma. Extraordinarily rare examples of granulocytic sarcoma (extramedullary tumefactive acute myeloid leukemia), malignant schwannoma, and extraosseous osteosarcoma have been documented as apparently primary pleural tumors (95–97), but information on such lesions is only anecdotal and is not recounted here.

PLEURAL FIBROSARCOMA AND MALIGNANT SOLITARY FIBROUS TUMOR

A review of the literature on serosal neoplasms reveals few examples of well-documented primary pleural fibrosarcoma (PPFS) (98). The latter is arbitrarily distinguished from malignant solitary fibrous tumor (MSFT) of the pleura by its clinical growth pattern, which is diffuse rather than localized. However, in other respects these two tumor entities are virtually identical; in fact, some examples of PPFSs have apparently evolved from solitary fibrous tumors of the pleura (99). Although some authors prefer to separate malignant fibrous tumors of the pleura into true fibrosarcoma and malignant fibrous histiocytoma (MFH)–like tumors (100), all of these lesions are considered here as a single group because of their closely similar clinicopathologic attributes.

CLINICAL SUMMARY

Pleural fibrosarcoma and MSFT arise in adult patients over a wide range of ages (15 to 75 years), with a male to female ratio of 3:1. They may be associated with dull or pleuritic chest pain, dyspnea, cough, systemic flulike symptoms, and digital clubbing (100, 101). In addition, a small proportion of patients may manifest paraneoplastic hypoglycemia because of the production of an insulinlike peptide by the tumor cells (101). It appears that pleural sarcomas have no association with prior asbestos exposure (in contradistinction to many malignant mesotheliomas) (99). Other potential etiologies of these lesions are unsettled at the present time, but some authors have reported a putative pathogenetic linkage to chronic tuberculous pleuritis and prior pyothorax (102, 103).

Radiographic studies in cases of PPFS commonly demonstrate the presence of a unilateral pleural effusion, which may be massive (101, 104). In addition, a dominant mass and diffuse but irregular thickening of the pleura are usually evident, and they are especially well seen with CT or MR imaging studies (104). Based on clinical data, it is not possible to distinguish PPFS from diffuse malignant mesothelioma, and tissue procurement is necessary for this purpose. Conversely, MSFTs typically are well-circumscribed, pleural-based masses on chest radiographs (Fig. 39.19); they usually show rounded contours but may occasionally be lobulated (101). Most measure between 1 and 10 cm in maximal dimension. In contrast to benign solitary fibrous pleural tumors, MSFTs are less often pedunculated and usually attain a larger size. Moreover, the latter lesion has a higher likelihood of involving the parietal pleura or mediastinum, or of demonstrating inverting growth into the subjacent lung parenchyma (101, 104).

PATHOLOGIC FINDINGS

The macroscopic appearance of PPFS is virtually identical to that of diffuse malignant mesothelioma, i.e., as a rind of solid tissue that encases the lung and restricts its movement. These tumors commonly extend into interlobar fissures and intrapulmonary interstitial septa as well (98, 101, 104, 105). MSFTs are sessile or pedunculated localized masses that most often are seen in the upper portions of either hemithorax (Fig. 39.20). They have bosselated, fleshy, tan-gray cut surfaces, usually with foci of spontaneous necrosis and hemorrhage (101, 105).

Microscopically, one sees a dense proliferation of spindle cells with high nuclear to cytoplasmic ratios, coarse chromatin, nuclear irregularity, and prominent nucleoli. Mitotic activity typically is brisk, and foci of

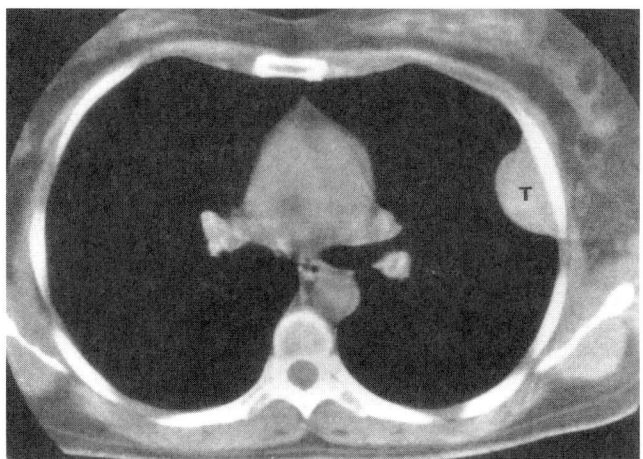

FIGURE 39.19. A typical CT scan of a malignant solitary fibrous tumor, presenting as a circumscribed mass in the pleura that abuts the chest wall. (From England DM, Hochholzer L, McCarthy MJ. Localized benign and malignant fibrous tumors of the pleura. Am J Surg Pathol 1989;13:640–658.)

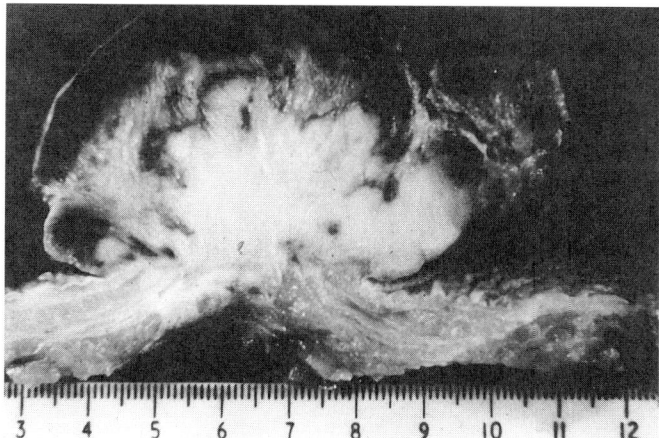

FIGURE 39.20. Malignant solitary fibrous tumor. A discrete, sessile mass is attached to the underlying thickened pleura.

spontaneous hemorrhage and necrosis may be evident as well. The neoplastic cells may be arranged in a storiform fashion and show moderately to markedly pleomorphic cytologic features, calling to mind the histologic attributes of MFH (98, 101) (Fig. 39.21). In other cases they are aligned in a fascicular herringbone configuration, such as that occurring in pulmonary fibrosarcomas. The subjacent lung is involved by tumor only if it extends downward from the pleura via the intrasegmental fibrous septa, and there is no association with pleural fibrohyaline plaques, the presence of intraparenchymal asbestos fibers, or asbestosis. MSFTs may contain areas resembling benign solitary fibrous pleural tumors, in which more bland spindle cell aggregates are enmeshed in hyalinized, keloidal-type collagen (101). A staghorn stromal vascular pattern is common in such areas as well.

Electron microscopy shows only primitive, fibroblastlike characteristics of the neoplastic cells. They are loosely apposed and surrounded in part by collagen fibers; cytoplasmic contents are rudimentary and include the basic metabolic organelles as well as abundant free polyribosomes and rough endoplasmic reticulum (105). There is no ultrastructural evidence of epithelial or myogenous differentiation. Similarly, immunohistologic assessment of PPFSs and MSFTs demonstrates reactivity for vimentin alone, to the exclusion of actin, desmin, keratin, and epithelial membrane antigen (98, 101). In contrast, true mesotheliomas (including sarcomatoid variants) uniformly express epithelial markers (106).

THERAPY AND PROGNOSIS

PPFS is not often treatable by surgical means, owing to its diffuse nature. The only operative procedure that can be attempted in such circumstances is extrapleural pneumonectomy, which generally is as-

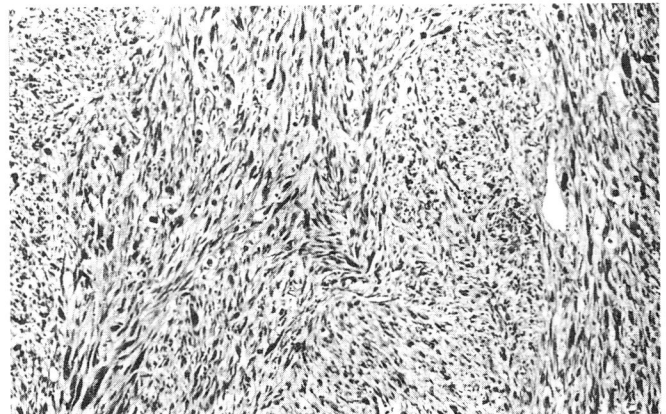

FIGURE 39.21. Malignant solitary fibrous tumor/pleural fibrosarcoma. Spindled hyperchromatic cells are arranged in a storiform/fascicular pattern.

sociated with a very high level of morbidity and mortality. Radiotherapy and chemotherapy (including intrapleural instillation of pharmaceuticals) may play a role in palliation of symptoms, but unfortunately they are not curative. Death is caused by progressive respiratory compromise, and PPFS also may involve the pericardium and produce cardiac embarrassment (107). Actuarial 1-year survival was only 39% in one series in which multimodality therapy was employed (100).

MSFT, conversely, is amenable to complete surgical resection in a high proportion of cases; in a series from the AFIP (101), 45% of such lesions were cured by excision alone. Most of these were pedunculated, well-localized masses that involved only a small area of the pleural surface, and the authors thus suggested that resectability was the single most favorable prognostic feature in MSFT cases. Lesions that ultimately cause recurrence may involve the contralateral pleura, lung parenchyma, and other viscera. Interestingly, relapses often still take the form of localized masses rather than dissemination along the pleural surface, and even patients with persistent tumor may survive for extended periods (99). Irradiation and chemotherapy do not appear to offer any benefits in this setting, and they may even shorten the survival of patients with MSFT (101).

Askin's Tumor (Peripheral Neuroepithelioma)

In 1979 Askin and colleagues (108) described a peculiar thoracic neoplasm that was seemingly limited to children, adolescents, and young adults. This lesion arises from the pleura or the extrapleural intercostal soft tissue and originally was named malignant small cell tumor of the thoracopulmonary region. It now is known more simply as Askin's tumor; alternatively, because the neoplasm has been shown to exhibit neuroepithelial differentiation, it is called thoracopulmonary peripheral neuroepithelioma (TPNE) (109, 110). Prior to its seminal description, this lesion probably was included among cases of Ewing's sarcoma of the thorax or peripheral neuroblastoma (111).

CLINICAL SUMMARY

Askin's tumor demonstrates a peak incidence during the second decade of life (mean age, 15 years) and shows a slight male predilection. Isolated cases of TPNE in infants and in older adults also have been documented (112–114). This neoplasm may present as an asymptomatic mass in the chest wall or by producing symptoms of cough, unilateral chest pain, and dyspnea or tachypnea. Pleural effusion is a common complication, and it may be detected on physical examination or by radiography of the thorax (109). Although it has been confused with classic neuroblastoma in some reports, Askin's tumor is not associated with elevations of catecholamine metabolite levels in the urine or blood, nor does it produce the opsoclonus-myoclonus syndrome (108, 112).

Chest radiographs and other imaging studies typically show a large mass that may be pleural based or centered in the thoracic soft tissue (Fig. 39.22), with secondary extension into the pleural space. TPNE often reaches a size of more than 10 cm at the time of initial diagnosis, and it demonstrates ill-defined interfaces with the subjacent lung or surrounding tissues (115).

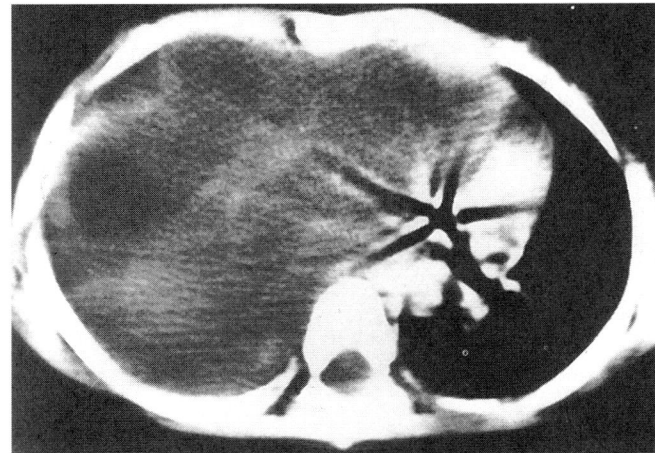

FIGURE 39.22. CT scan shows an Askin's tumor, presenting as a huge, bulky mass that compresses the lungs and shifts the mediastinum. (From Dehner LP. Soft tissue, peritoneum, and retroperitoneum. In: Pediatric surgical pathology. 2nd ed. Baltimore: Williams & Wilkins, 1987:869–938.)

PATHOLOGIC FINDINGS

Askin's tumor is one of the prototypical small round cell neoplasms of children, and it may be confused with several other tumor entities by the pathologist (76). At a macroscopic level, TPNE is lobulated with fleshy, relatively soft, tan-gray cut surfaces that may show foci of hemorrhage and necrosis (108). Microscopically, it exhibits a high degree of cellular monomorphism with round to oval nuclei, even distribution of chromatin, indistinct nucleoli, and variable mitotic activity. Stromal blood vessels are numerous and form a discernible network within the tumor mass; small blood lakes also may be manifest (108–115). One of the most characteristic findings of TPNE on conventional microscopy is the presence of neural-type cellular rosettes, wherein tumor cells are disposed radially around small virtual tissue space (108, 109) (Fig. 39.23). Histochemically, Askin's tumor may or may not contain abundant glycogen with the periodic acid–Schiff method, although in the original series on this lesion, only periodic acid–Schiff negative neoplasms were accepted to facilitate differentiation from classic Ewing's sarcoma.

Special studies of biopsy or resection specimens are mandatory to recognize TPNE properly and exclude other diagnostic possibilities. Along with other peripheral neuroepitheliomas, Askin's tumor demonstrates a characteristic 11;22 chromosomal translocation that is shared only with Ewing's sarcoma (109). By electron microscopy it demonstrates blunt cytoplasmic processes that contain dense core granules or microtubules; these characteristics are seen in classic neuroblastoma as well but not in other small round cell tumors (76). Immunohistochemically, TPNE differs from Ewing's tumor in that it shows reactivity for synaptophysin (a neural synaptic protein) (77). Moreover, Askin's tumor may be distinguished from classic neuroblastoma by immunologic means as well; the former lesion is reactive for β–2-microglobulin and the MIC-2 (p30-32) glycoprotein (116), whereas the latter tumor is not.

THERAPY AND PROGNOSIS

The most important prognostic procedure in cases of TPNE is accurate staging. Using a scheme devised by the National Cancer Institute, stage I tumors are defined as those measuring more than 5 cm in maximum diameter that can be completely excised; stage II lesions are smaller than 5 cm in maximum dimension and are grossly resectable but show positive microscopic margins; stage III neoplasms are more than 5 cm in maximum dimension and are nonresectable; and stage IV Askin's tumors have metastasized to extrapleural sites (109). Low stage has shown a direct correlation with long-term survival after surgical removal and intensive cyclical postoperative treatment with irradiation and chemotherapy, using protocols similar to those employed for Ewing's sarcoma (110, 117). Stage III and IV Askin's tumors are probably best managed nonsurgically, because there are no data to support a role for debulking surgery in such circumstances (109).

A sobering aspect of the therapy for TPNE is that it undeniably subjects survivors to the risk of a second malignancy. Intensive radiation to the chest wall may be followed years later by a postradiation sarcoma in approximately 1% of cases, and Farhi et al. (118) have described several examples of postchemotherapy myelodysplastic syndrome and acute leukemia in this context.

PLEUROPULMONARY BLASTOMA

Until 1988 a group of anaplastic mesenchymal tumors of the peripheral lung and pleura in children had been grouped under the rubric of pediatric pulmonary blastoma. Nonetheless, Manivel et al. (119) showed that such lesions differed from typical pulmonary blastomas in adults, which probably comprise a subset of sarcomatoid carcinomas. The childhood tumors were found more often to be primary in the pleura; they also showed a histologic resemblance to soft tissue sarcomas. Because of these important points of difference from adult pulmonary blastomas, the pediatric lesions were reclassified as pleuropulmonary blastomas (PPBs).

CLINICAL SUMMARY

Pleuropulmonary blastomas arise most often in the first decade of life, without a distinct preference for

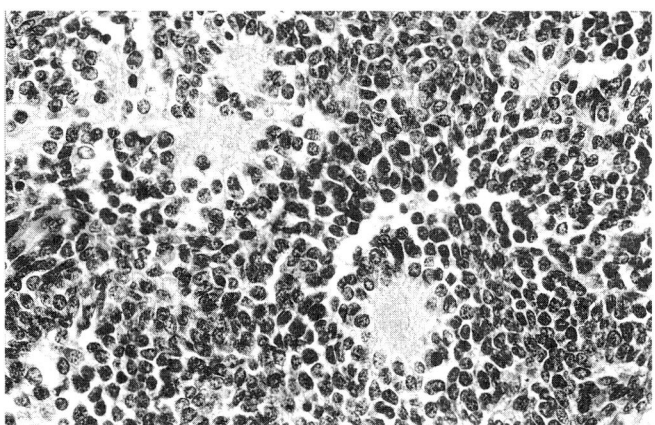

FIGURE 39.23. Small, round to oval tumor cells of an Askin's tumor are arranged radially around small spaces, forming rosettelike structures.

males or females. However, examples have been reported of this tumor in patients as old as 30 years (119–121). Cough, chest pain, weight loss, and dyspnea or tachypnea are the most common presenting complaints of PPB (119). Evidence of a pleural effusion also may be found on physical examination. It appears that this neoplasm may be part of certain cancer families, in which other soft tissue sarcomas, variants of Wilms' tumor, and cystic nephromas may be seen in other family members (122).

Radiologic studies typically demonstrate the presence of a large, irregularly outlined mass in the thorax, which may have its epicenter in the pleura, the mediastinal soft tissue, or the peripheral lung parenchyma (Fig. 39.24). These lesions can be massive, sometimes effacing an entire hemithorax, and they demonstrate internal variation in density on CT or MR imaging studies. Some examples may show focal internal calcification (119).

PATHOLOGIC FINDINGS

PPB is grossly fleshy and tan-pink or gray in color on prosection, with frequent foci of internal hemorrhage and punctate necrosis. Chondroid areas may be apparent on macroscopic examination of the mass, and areas of calcification may be manifested as grittiness encountered when sectioning the lesion.

Microscopically, one sees a heterogeneous mixture of growth patterns admixed with one another in various regions of the tumor. Some foci resemble MFH (Fig. 39.25), others take a rhabdomyosarcomatous appearance, and still others have the features of fibrosarcoma, liposarcoma, chondrosarcoma, or osteosarcoma (119, 121). Some observers may apply the term malignant mesenchymoma to PPB, but this designation has generally fallen from favor in current nosology. Importantly, epithelial foci are absent in PPB, in contrast to their dominance in adult pulmonary blastoma (119, 121). Immunohistochemical and ultrastructural studies demonstrate findings that agree with the microscopic features noted previously, and they again fail to reveal epithelial characteristics in these lesions (119).

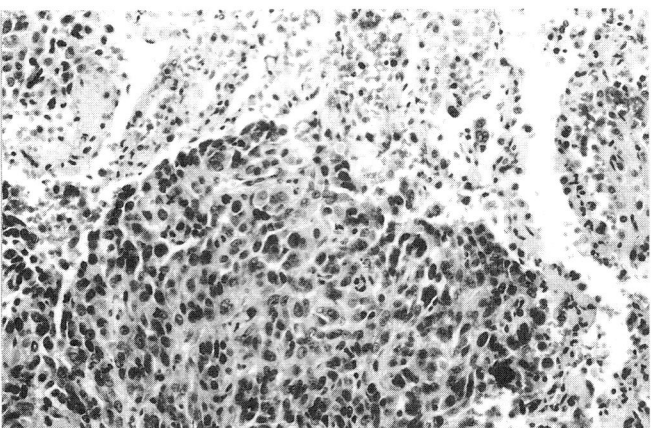

FIGURE 39.25. Pleomorphic, undifferentiated cells of a pleuropulmonary blastoma with abundant mitotic figures. Unlike a pulmonary blastoma in adults, there is no evidence of epithelial differentiation.

THERAPY AND PROGNOSIS

PPB is a relatively rare tumor; therefore, no organized protocol studies of therapy have been applied to its management. In general, however, it is obvious that this neoplasm is a highly aggressive lesion that requires intensive irradiation and chemotherapy. Because of the histologic characteristics of the tumor, which are like those of de novo soft tissue sarcomas, it would seem appropriate to employ drug combinations that are directed toward the various histologic components of PPB (e.g., rhabdomyosarcoma, MFH, osteosarcoma). Surgical debulking of the tumor mass is of unproven benefit at present, but it should be considered in individual cases in which complete resection is not thought to be feasible. Five-year, disease free survival in PPB cases is relatively uncommon. In the seminal series of Manivel et al. (119), 7 of 11 patients died within 2 years of diagnosis. Similarly, 5 of 7 cases reported by Hachitanda and associates (121) proved fatal.

VASCULAR SARCOMAS OF THE PLEURA

As mentioned previously, angiosarcoma, KS, and EH may originate in the pleura as well as in the pul-

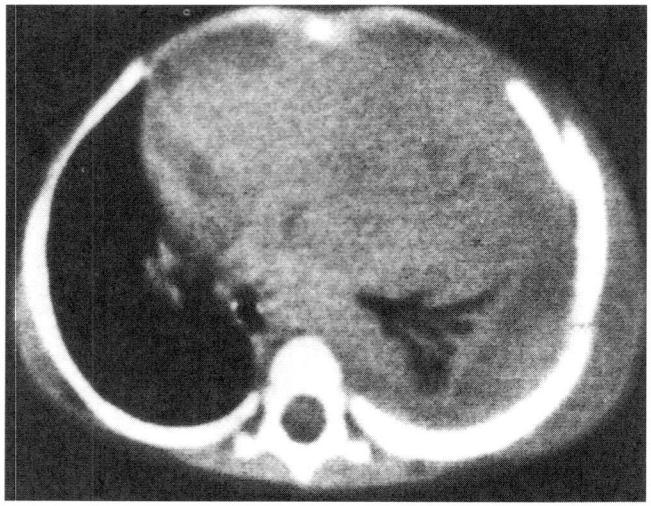

FIGURE 39.24. CT of a pleuropulmonary blastoma in a 2-year-old girl, presenting as a large mass filling the entire right hemithorax. (From Dehner LP. Pleuropulmonary blastoma is *the* pulmonary blastoma of childhood. Semin Diagn Pathol 1994;11:144–151.)

monary parenchyma. The general clinical attributes of these lesions have been described above. It is notable that the most common initial sign of angiosarcoma and KS of the pleura is the presence of a bloody pleural effusion (18, 83). Gross examination at thoracotomy shows multiple soft, hemorrhagic, red-violet, nodular, pleural implants in examples of angiosarcoma and KS tumors. However, EH is virtually identical to malignant mesothelioma at a macroscopic level, and pathologic study is necessary to distinguish between them (123). As is true of their intrapulmonary counterparts, KS and angiosarcoma of the pleura are associated with a dismal prognosis, whereas patients with EH may survive for prolonged periods (123).

LYMPHOPROLIFERATIVE PULMONARY DISEASES

The lung is a relatively uncommon site of primary malignant lymphomas. As summarized expertly by Koss (124), pulmonary lymphoproliferative disease is, in itself, a heterogeneous group of disorders that have been given a variety of diagnostic designations. The constraints of space do not permit consideration of the attributes of putatively benign lymphoproliferations in the lung, and these are mentioned only in the specific context of discussions centering around selected non-Hodgkin's lymphomas (NHLs). Likewise, it is certainly beyond the scope of this discussion to elaborate on the molecular biology of hematopoietic diseases in general. Thus, the following sections present synopsized data only on those primary malignant lymphoproliferative disorders encountered most commonly in the pulmonary parenchyma.

As reviewed by Koss (124), there has been no uniform agreement on the criteria necessary for a diagnosis of primary pulmonary NHL. He preferred the stipulation that there be biopsy-proven disease only in the lung, pleura, or both, with the only additional site of permissible spread being the regional intrathoracic lymph nodes. Other authors have included patients with concomitant extrathoracic lymphoma in their series of primary pulmonary lymphoproliferative disease, if the lung was judged to be the dominant site at presentation (125–127). The former (more restrictive) approach to this issue is preferred. Therefore, a diagnosis of NHL in the lung mandates radiologic examination of the viscera and pathologic assessment of the bone marrow, so that a proper tumor stage can be determined.

SMALL LYMPHOCYTIC PROLIFERATIONS

Proliferations of small lymphoid cells are perhaps the most diverse subset of hematopoietic disorders that are potentially primary in the lung. They include the entities known as small lymphocytic (well-differentiated lymphocytic) lymphoma (SLL), mantle cell lymphoma, intermediately differentiated lymphocytic lymphoma (IDLL), small cleaved follicular center cell (poorly differentiated lymphocytic) lymphoma (SCCL), and Waldenstrom's macroglobulinemia (SLL with plasmacytoid features).

Some authors still make a distinction between lymphoid interstitial pneumonia (LIP) or nodular lymphoid hyperplasia and SLL (128), but there is so much sharing of clinicopathologic attributes between these disease entities that the maintenance of strictly defined nosologic partitions is not realistic. Colby (129) has stressed that the advent of current technology has shown many (if not all) examples of LIP and pseudolymphoma to consist of monotypic populations of lymphocytes, reflecting a neoplastic character for these conditions. However, these are indolent processes that tend to remain confined to the lung for extended periods, thus separating them from more conventional forms of NHL.

CLINICAL SUMMARY

The majority of lymph nodal small cell NHLs occur in patients who are in middle age or beyond, and those with such tumors in the lung are no exception. There is minor variation in the median patient age attached to SLL versus mantle cell lymphoma versus SCCL, but generally individuals with primary pulmonary disease in these categories are older than 45 years (130, 131). There is no compelling difference in occurrence between the sexes.

It is true that certain other diseases tend to be associated more often with particular forms of small cell NHL in the lung. For example, LIP is linked to preexisting rheumatoid arthritis, Sjögren's syndrome, myasthenia gravis, systemic lupus erythematosus, and other autoimmune conditions in middle-aged or elderly patients (130), whereas it is part of the Epstein-Barr virus (EBV)–driven spectrum of lymphoproliferations in young individuals with AIDS or other causes of profound immunosuppression (132). Similarly, some cases of small cell NHL (approximately 20% to 35%), including LIP, show a monoclonal paraprotein in the serum or urine (usually of the IgM or IgA class) or an absolute lymphocytosis in the peripheral blood (124). In the latter scenario, a distinction from chronic lymphocytic leukemia is academic.

As many as 75% of patients with small cell pulmonary NHL lack symptoms at the time of diagnosis, which is made radiographically (131). When present, complaints may include dyspnea, cough, vague chest pain, and hemoptysis (133). Regardless of the histologic type of lymphoma in this subgroup, chest radiographic findings are similar. These most often take the form of a solitary nodule in the peripheral lung fields, followed in relative order by a regional interstitial-alveolar infiltrate, or multiple nodules or infiltrates that may be confluent with one another (124). CT or MR imaging studies demonstrate a uniform density within the lesions and may show that they have indistinct interfaces with the surrounding parenchyma. One quarter of all cases show a pleural effusion (126).

Bronchoscopically, approximately one fourth of cases show nodular irregularity of the bronchial mucosa, with or without accompanying stenosis of the airway lumen (134). In these instances transbronchial biopsy provides diagnostic tissue. However, in the remaining cases of small cell NHL, open lung biopsies are necessary to procure suitable pathologic specimens.

PATHOLOGIC FINDINGS

The hallmark of small cell lymphomas of the lung is their permeative quality with respect to the interstitial septa and the intrabronchial tissues (124–126) (Fig. 39.26). Sheets of lymphoid cells expand and widen the septal connective tissue, sometimes with focal formation of germinal centers or large nodules that efface the normal lung. In the bronchial wall, neoplastic lymphocytes surround plates of bronchial cartilage and splay the submucosal bronchial glands without destroying them (124). The mucosa is commonly infiltrated as well, yielding a shotgun configuration of intraepithelial lymphocytes (so-called lymphoepithelial complexes).

These architectural patterns featuring abnormal lymphoid density are all that one has to identify cases of SLL, in that the cytologic characteristics of the neoplastic population are generally those of mature lymphocytes. More nuclear irregularity is progressively apparent in SLL with plasmacytoid features, IDLL, and mantle cell lymphoma, although it may be relatively subtle (125, 129). As its name suggests, small cleaved cell lymphoma (SCCL) is comprised by lymphocytes with notched, cleaved, or folded nuclear membranes. It typically forms rudimentary neoplastic follicles of relatively uniform sizes and lacks germinal centers; IDLL may exhibit this tendency as well. Mitotic activity is generally sparse in all forms of small cell NHL in the lung. Some cases may show an admixture of noncaseating granulomas throughout the tumor, in the absence of microorganisms (124). This finding presumably represents a peculiar host response to the neoplastic cells.

With regard to microscopic attributes that can be employed to distinguish benign from well-differentiated malignant lymphoid infiltrates, Koss and associates (131) found that there were few, if any, such findings. Germinal centers may be seen clearly in both categories of lesion, as may infiltration of bronchial cartilage and parietal pleura. Thus, one is left with the need to demonstrate immunohistochemical light-chain immunoglobulin restriction to confirm the presence of a B-cell NHL, or alternatively to document the presence of immunoglobulin heavy chain gene rearrangements by Southern blot or polymerase chain reaction technology (135). These procedures are best done on frozen tissue; thus, the clinician is well advised to be certain that a portion of each wedge biopsy in suspected lymphoma cases is saved in the fresh state for such analyses. If this provision has not been made, the demonstration of an aberrant B-cell immunophenotype (e.g., coexpression of CD20 and CD43) and a proliferating cell nuclear antigen index of more than 30% in paraffin sections of small cell lymphoproliferations both correlate with the presence of malignancy (136). Immunostains for EBV latent membrane protein may be of etiologic interest, but they are potentially positive in both benign and malignant lymphoid infiltrates. Electron microscopy has no role in the differential diagnosis of small cell NHL.

THERAPY AND PROGNOSIS

Paradoxically, the recommended first-line treatment for localized primary small cell NHL of the lung is surgical excision of the affected tissue (124). If this is not feasible because of bilaterality or multifocality, chemotherapy (using cyclophosphamide, vincristine, and prednisone) is suggested. The latter interventions are most often utilized in IDLL and SCCL, which have

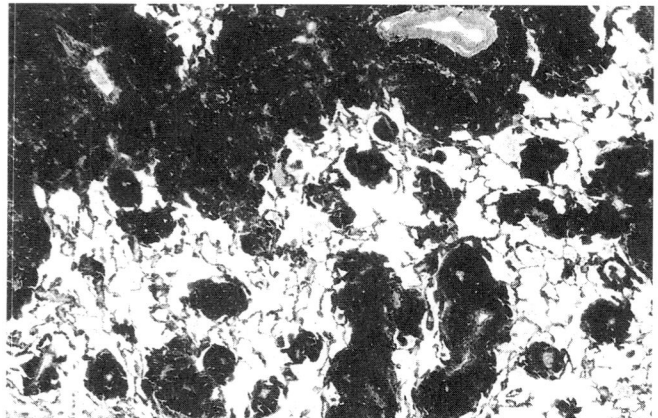

FIGURE 39.26. Small cell lymphoma expands the interstitial septae and forms confluent areas of tumor in the upper part of the figure.

the greatest potential for adverse behavior in this subset of NHLs (133). A legitimate case can be made in examples of primary pulmonary SLL, with or without plasmacytoid differentiation, for withholding treatment altogether, providing the patient is asymptomatic. In one large series on these diseases, only 13% of individuals died of their tumors after follow-up periods of as long as 15 years (131). The 5-year survival is 90%, and the median survival for patients with this group of tumors is more than 16 years (124).

MIXED AND LARGE CELL NON-HODGKIN'S LYMPHOMAS

Mixed small and large cell and pure large cell NHLs are somewhat less common as primary pulmonary lesions, compared with the occurrence of small cell lymphoproliferative diseases. Nosologically, the former neoplasms include mixed small cell and large cell follicular center cell NHL of both diffuse and nodular varieties; diffuse or nodular large cell NHL of cleaved or noncleaved cell types; and diffuse immunoblastic large cell lymphoma.

CLINICAL SUMMARY

In contrast to small cell lymphomas of the lung, most mixed and large cell tumors produce symptoms. Potential complaints include cough and dyspnea, and systemic manifestations such as fever, weight loss, and extreme malaise are seen much more often in patients with large cell NHL (124, 125, 129). A subset of patients with immunoblastic lymphoma of the lung have HIV infection and AIDS. On average, patients with mixed or large cell lymphomas are younger, by one to three decades, than those with small cell NHL (133).

Radiographically, mixed and large cell lymphomas are most likely to show multiple large nodular lesions throughout both lung fields (Fig. 39.27), often with central cavitation. If the tumors are centered on bronchi, air bronchograms may be seen (124). As such, various infectious processes and metastatic neoplasms may be considered in the radiologic differential diagnosis.

As with small cell lymphoid tumors, transbronchial biopsies are effective in obtaining diagnostic tissue only in cases of mixed or large cell lymphoma that directly involve the large airways. Otherwise, open lung biopsy is required.

PATHOLOGIC FINDINGS

The growth pattern of mixed and large cell NHLs mirrors its radiographic appearance, in that it typically

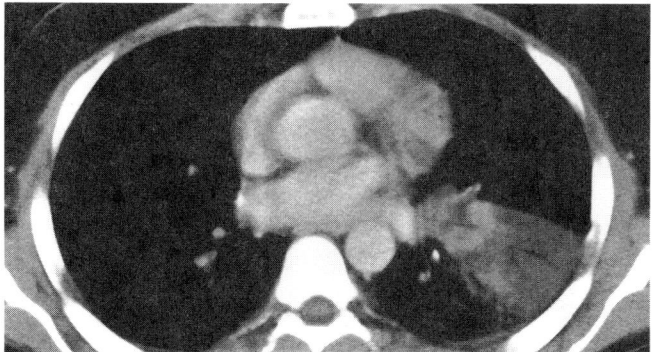

FIGURE 39.27. CT of a large cell lymphoma demonstrates a well-defined mass in the left lower lobe that is not a typical presentation of large cell lymphomas of the lung.

forms large destructive nodules in the pulmonary parenchyma that compress and displace the surrounding tissue (129). Mixed cell tumors contain large cells that may comprise between 10% and 30% of the lesions and may demonstrate cleaved or rounded nuclear profiles. The small cells in these lesions may likewise simulate those seen in either SLL or SCCL. Large cell lymphomas are dominated by large atypical cells that in selected instances may be extremely pleomorphic and yield the microscopic profile of anaplastic lymphoma. The latter variant is commonly immunoreactive for CD30 and manifests an aggressive biologic potential (137). Other large cell NHLs are composed of monomorphous sheets of polygonal cells with vesicular nuclei, uniformly prominent nucleoli, and numerous mitoses, and these represent immunoblastic lesions. These similarly are of high grade behaviorally. All varieties of large cell lymphoma have a greater tendency to involve regional lymph nodes than do small cell tumors; the former lesions do so in roughly 50% of cases (124).

Pathologic differential diagnosis in mixed cell NHL is principally that of Hodgkin's disease (HD), as discussed subsequently. These two histologic entities are best distinguished by immunohistochemical means; however, occasional cases may require gene rearrangement studies for this separation to be made definitively (138). In contrast, large cell NHL is confused principally with primary or metastatic carcinoma or malignant melanoma. In this context immunostaining positivity for CD45 is diagnostic of lymphoma (Fig. 39.28).

THERAPY AND PROGNOSIS

Mixed cell and large cell NHLs are higher grade lesions than most small cell lymphoproliferations. Accordingly, treatment must be more aggressive and is

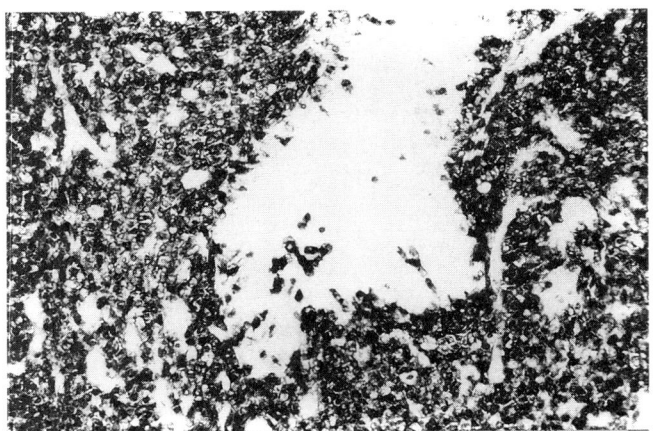

FIGURE 39.28. The large lymphoma cells show diffuse strong membrane staining with antibody against leukocyte common antigen (CD45). The central lucent area is unlabelled stroma.

usually predicated on polycyclic, multiagent chemotherapy directed at the specific lineage (i.e., B cell or T cell) of the proliferating cells (133, 134). Staging has a strong bearing on long-term survival in this setting. Non–small cell lymphomas that are restricted to the lung and that respond to therapy have a rate of recurrence of under 10%, whereas those with extrapulmonary involvement relapse in almost half of cases (124). Data generated by Koss et al. (131) also suggest that patients who attain complete remissions that are sustained for 3 years are unlikely to have subsequent recurrences.

LYMPHOMATOID GRANULOMATOSIS (ANGIOCENTRIC MALIGNANT LYMPHOMA OF THE LUNG)

Lymphomatoid granulomatosis (LYG), also known as angiocentric immunoproliferative disease, is a systemic lymphoid disorder that predominantly involves the lungs. However, it also affects the skin, central and peripheral nervous systems, and kidneys. LYG was first described in 1972 by Liebow, Carrington, and Friedman (139) and was defined initially as an angiocentric and angiodestructive proliferative lymphoreticular and granulomatous disease. This entity was thought to share some features of Wegener's granulomatosis and malignant lymphoma, resulting in the diagnostic designation applied. The true biologic nature of this disorder has been the subject of considerable debate, which to some extent continues to this date. It is included in this discussion because of the authors' belief that this condition represents a lymphoid malignancy.

CLINICAL SUMMARY

LYG has been reported in patients ranging in age from 7 to 85 years, with a mean of 48 years. Men are more likely to be affected than women, by a ratio of 3:2. Other concomitant disease processes in these patients have included autoimmune disorders (e.g., juvenile rheumatoid arthritis, Hashimoto's thyroiditis) and immunodeficiency states associated with organ transplantation, AIDS, and unrelated hematolymphoid malignancies (140–142). Most patients with LYG present with cough, dyspnea, chest pain, or systemic symptoms such as fever and weight loss.

Up to 40% of individuals with pulmonary LYG also have skin lesions that take the form of maculopapular eruptions or violaceous subcutaneous nodules. Of these patients, approximately 27% developed cutaneous lesions before chest radiographic abnormalities were detected (140). In addition, the skin is a common site of recurrent disease. Approximately 30% of cases show neurologic abnormalities, including seizures, ataxia, hemiparesis, trigeminal neuralgia, Bell's palsy, and peripheral neuropathies (140). Although the kidneys have been affected in one third of autopsied cases, renal involvement usually is clinically silent (140).

The upper respiratory tract, including the nasopharynx, nose, and paranasal sinuses, may be involved by LYG as well. Primary LYG in the latter sites has been known in the otolaryngologic literature as polymorphic reticulosis, lethal midline granuloma of Stewart, and malignant midline reticulosis (143, 144). DeRemee et al. (143) first drew attention to the histologic and clinical similarities between LYG and polymorphic reticulosis and concluded that they were probably reflections of the same disease process.

Chest radiographs show bilateral disease in 80% of LYG cases, with multiple nodular lesions throughout both peripheral lung fields. Spirometric testing generally shows a restrictive pattern of abnormality. The diagnostic procedure of choice is open lung biopsy; the rate of success with transbronchial biopsies is 30% at most (141).

PATHOLOGIC FINDINGS

Lymphomatoid granulomatosis of the lungs is characterized by a prominent lymphoid infiltrate that invades the walls of pulmonary arteries and veins, commonly producing luminal thrombosis. In turn, this results in extensive infarctive-type necrosis of the subserved pulmonary parenchyma. The cellular infiltrate is polymorphous, consisting of mature lymphocytes, plasma cells, histiocytes, and a variable number of large, atypical lymphoid cells with vesicular, irregular nuclei and prominent nucleoli. LYG shares these angiocentric and angiodestructive lesions (Fig. 39.29) and geographic necrosis with Wegener's granulomatosis; however, true granulomatous inflammation with multinucleated giant cells and epithelioid histiocytic aggregates is lacking in LYG. Some cases of LYG show an almost pure population of highly atypical lymphoid cells, resembling type ordinaire NHL of the large cell type.

Histologic grading schemes have been proposed to encompass the spectrum of potential microscopic observations in LYG. Teams including both Jaffe and Katzenstein (142, 145, 146) have used a tripartite grading system based on the degree of cytologic atypia and the type of cellular infiltrate. Grade I disease has been likened to pure LYG, with a polymorphous inflammatory infiltrate that lacks appreciable cytologic atypia. Grade II lesions are represented by predominantly polymorphous infiltrate but with small foci of admixed atypical lymphoid cells. In grade III LYG, the cellular infiltrate consists almost exclusively of monomorphous, atypical, lymphoid cells that generally warrant the diagnosis of malignant lymphoma.

In addition to Wegener's granulomatosis and other vasculitides, the histopathologic differential diagnosis of LYG also includes HD and pulmonary involvement by other forms of NHL. A polymorphous inflammatory infiltrate is common to low-grade LYG and HD, but diagnostic Reed-Sternberg cells and their mononuclear variants in the latter condition serve to separate these two entities. Secondary pulmonary involvement by other lymphomas may demonstrate focally vasodestructive growth, but, unlike LYG, these tumors also feature prominent septal and interstitial infiltrates of atypical lymphoid cells.

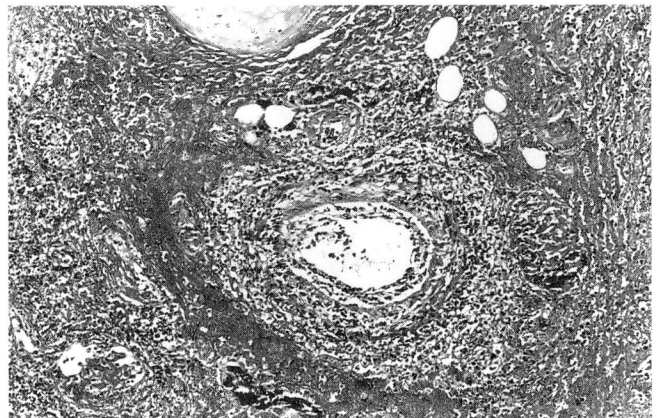

FIGURE 39.29. Lymphomatoid granulomatosis. The tumor cells concentrate around blood vessels and diffusely infiltrate the vascular walls. The surrounding parenchyma is necrotic.

There are two basic schools of thought regarding the cellular nature of LYG. Jaffe et al. (145) coined the term angiocentric immunoproliferative lesion (AIL) as a proposed replacement for lymphomatoid granulomatosis. This new designation breaks from the concept that LYG is related to vasculitis and granulomatous inflammation, and rather emphasizes its lymphoproliferative character. Some authors (142, 146) do not consider all AILs to be lymphomas at the outset of the disease process; in their view only grade III lesions are equated with overt malignancies. An opposing philosophy is that LYG does represent a peculiar form of lymphoma.

Unlike the case in B-cell lymphomas, monoclonality in T-cell proliferations cannot be proven by immunohistochemical means. It can only be suggested by the demonstration of an aberrant T-lymphoid immunophenotype. However, molecular genetic studies requiring frozen tissue are capable of providing definitive evidence of monoclonality by demonstrating rearrangements of T-cell receptor genes. Most cases of LYG have been shown by immunohistology to possess a T-cell phenotype (144, 145, 147–149). Some analyses have shown that AILs of grades I and II have a mature T-cell immunophenotype without aberrancy; but the cells of grade III lesions most commonly show an abnormal immunologic profile with loss of pan–T-cell antigens (145, 147). Likewise, there are examples of the disease that appear to lack T-cell gene rearrangements by Southern blot evaluations (148–150), whereas others (especially grade III lesions) do manifest such changes (144, 145). The former data have been used to support the contention that low-grade AILs are nonneoplastic; however, the clinical behavior of such proliferations is indeed potentially aggressive, and the authors respectfully demur with the latter premise on that basis.

The spectrum of histologic features in LYG has been compared with that observed in posttransplantation lymphoproliferative disorders (PTLDs). In fact, histologically typical LYG has been reported in renal transplant recipients (146). In this context it is germane to note that genomic integration of the EBV into lymphoid cells of the host is thought to be responsible for posttransplantation lymphoproliferative disorders. These observations led Katzenstein and Peiper (146) to analyze 29 cases of pulmonary LYG for their content of nucleic acid segments of EBV, using the polymerase chain reaction technique on paraffin-embedded tissue. Among all cases 72% (including lesions of all three grades) contained EBV genomes (146). EBV genomes also have been detected in lesions of LYG by Southern blot analyses and in situ hybridization techniques. In contrast to the latter results, Medeiros et al. (147) were able to detect the nucleic acid of EBV only in grade III lesions. Despite this finding the results of molecular pathologic evaluations sufficiently confirm the contention that the grades of LYG/AIL simply represent various faces of a single disease entity.

In the same study by Medeiros et al. (147), double-labeling studies showed that the majority of EBV positive cells were also T cells with positive staining by Leu-22. However, Guinee et al. (151) found that the large, atypical cells that correlate with the prognosis and grade of lesion were actually B cells, and that the latter were EBV infected. These investigators, therefore, hypothesized that LYG is a B-cell lymphoproliferative process that is associated with EBV. Their hypothesis was supported further by the presence of immunoglobulin gene rearrangements in 60% of cases and the absence of T-cell receptor gene rearrangements in three of the cases tested.

THERAPY AND PROGNOSIS

In a study of 152 patients by Katzenstein et al. (140), treatment for LYG ranged from simple symptomatic relief or administration of antibiotics to therapy with a combination of steroids and cytotoxic agents. In that analysis the prognosis was found to be poor regardless of treatment modality. Almost two thirds of the patients died, with a median survival period of only 14 months reported. Twelve percent had progression of disease, with subsequent development of obvious nodal NHL.

Fauci et al. (152) found that combination chemotherapy with cyclophosphamide and prednisone was effective in slightly more than 50% of LYG patients. Likewise, Jaffe and colleagues (145) reported that grade I lesions responded completely to a regimen of steroid and cyclophosphamide. If untreated, a large percentage of grade I and grade II lesions progressed to malignant lymphomas that were thereafter refractory to chemotherapy. In contrast, most grade III lesions responded to aggressive chemotherapy, and seven of eight patients in this subgroup were alive with no evidence of disease up to 12 years after diagnosis. These investigators concluded that grade I AIL should be treated conservatively with prednisone and cyclophosphamide, but that grade II and grade III lesions must be managed aggressively with additional chemotherapy (145). Letendre and associates (153) were able to achieve remission in three of four patients by using a combination of doxorubicin, vinblastine, bleomycin, and dacarbazine. It also has been shown that radiation therapy may be effective in treating localized LYG, such as that seen in the skin or the upper airway in polymorphic reticulosis (143).

Poor prognostic factors in LYG cases include bilaterality of disease, the presence of neurologic symptoms, and large numbers of anaplastic lymphoid cells in histologic material (140). Achievement of an initially complete response to therapy is the best predictor of long-term survival in this disease (145).

HODGKIN'S DISEASE

Similarly to non-Hodgkin's lymphomas, secondary pulmonary involvement by HD is much more common, by several orders of magnitude, than primary disease in the lungs. Available information on primary pulmonary HD consists principally of case reports. A recent review by Radin (154) documents 61 such examples in the English-language literature. Accepted criteria for the diagnosis of bona fide primary pulmonary HD (PPHD) include pathologic confirmation of the process and limitation of the lesions to the lung parenchyma (or at most minimal extrapulmonary involvement of regional lymph nodes) (155).

CLINICAL SUMMARY

The age at diagnosis of PPHD is greatly variable, ranging from 12 to 82 years. A series of 15 cases reported by Yousem et al. (156) showed a bimodal age distribution with one peak in young adulthood and another in patients older than 60 years of age. These findings are similar to incidence data generated on nodal HD. Females predominate in PPHD, and most patients present with respiratory complaints. In addition, systemic symptoms including fever, night sweats, and weight loss are relatively common. Chest radiographs of PPHD usually show single or multiple nodules in the upper lobes, and lesional cavitation is seen in roughly one third of cases (154, 157).

PATHOLOGIC FINDINGS

Wedge biopsies of the lung have typically been necessary to obtain a firm diagnosis of PPHD. The histologic criteria used in these circumstances are identical to those pertaining to nodal HD and include a polymorphous infiltrate of lymphoid cells, plasma cells, histiocytes, and eosinophils, along with classic Reed-Sternberg cells and their mononuclear variants (Fig. 39.30). The nodular sclerosing variant of HD is the most common one encountered in the lung, but detailed histopathologic typing of this process does not

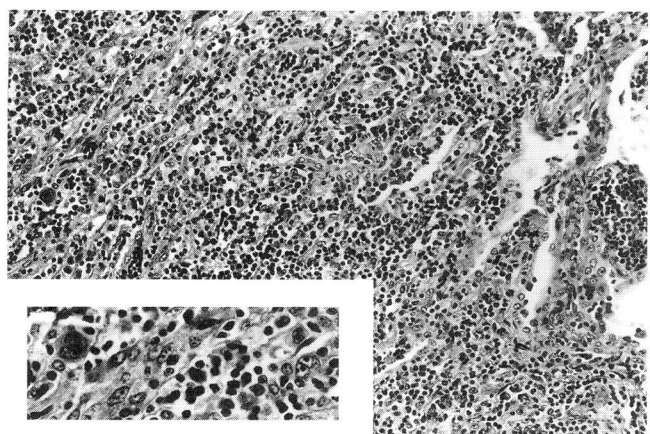

FIGURE 39.30. Hodgkin's disease is composed of a polymorphous mixture of cells admixed with the characteristic Reed-Sternberg cells and variants (*inset*).

appear to provide clinically meaningful information (156, 158).

THERAPY AND PROGNOSIS

Because of the rarity of PPHD, the most effective therapy for this disorder has not been determined systematically. Before the 1960s the therapy of choice was surgical resection, with or without adjuvant radiation therapy (155). Since then various chemotherapeutic regimens have been administered (154). In one account (156), 9 of 14 patients relapsed (most commonly in the lung), and 6 of those individuals (66%) later died of HD. Adverse prognostic factors included the presence of systemic symptoms, multifocal or bilateral lung involvement, pleural extension, cavitation, and clinical relapse (154, 156).

PULMONARY INTRAVASCULAR LYMPHOMATOSIS

Intravascular lymphomatosis (IVL)—formerly known as angioendotheliomatosis proliferans systemisata, malignant angioendotheliomatosis, angiotropic lymphoma, and neoplastic angioendotheliosis—is a rapidly fatal, systemic lymphoproliferative disorder that manifests with an exclusively intravascular growth pattern. Because of this peculiar anatomic distribution, IVL was originally thought to represent an endothelial malignancy. Several studies appeared to confirm this contention, with reports of focal immunoreactivity for factor VIII–related antigen and ultrastructural demonstration of Weibel-Palade bodies in putatively neoplastic cells (159–162).

However, subsequent analyses have disproven such theories and have shown that IVL is actually a lymphoid malignancy (161, 162). Apparent immunostaining for factor VIII–related antigen was explained subsequently by adsorption of this moiety from fibrin-platelet aggregates in which the neoplastic cells were enmeshed (161). Likewise, the presumed presence of Weibel-Palade bodies in the tumor was explained by trapping of nonneoplastic endothelial cells in the lesion.

CLINICAL SUMMARY

IVL is a systemic disorder that begins most commonly with involvement of the skin and central nervous system; however, this disease can affect virtually any organ in the body, including the adrenal glands, lungs, heart, gastrointestinal tract, prostate, and uterine cervix. Paradoxically, the reticuloendothelial system (liver, spleen, lymph nodes, and bone marrow) is involved only late in the clinical course, if at all (160–162).

Primary involvement of the lungs by IVL is rare, but Yousem and Colby (159) have reported a series of four such cases, and another case has been documented by Demirer and colleagues (163). Patients ranged in age from 40 to 60 years, as noted also in other reports on IVL (161, 162, 164–166), and there is no preference for either gender. Most patients with primary pulmonary IVL presented with the clinical profile of an interstitial pulmonopathy, whereas one case was initially thought to represent thromboembolic disease. All of these individuals developed progressive respiratory insufficiency, and bilateral reticulonodular infiltrates were apparent on chest radiographs. Two of them also had concomitant neurologic manifestations simulating multiinfarct dementia, but none had skin lesions. The latter usually take the form of multiple, painless, erythematous plaques and nodules on the trunk and extremities (161).

PATHOLOGIC FINDINGS

Open lung biopsies were required diagnostically in four reported cases of pulmonary IVL, whereas its characteristic morphologic features were visible by transbronchial biopsy in the fifth patient (159, 163). All specimens showed patchy interstitial widening secondary to distention and occlusion of arterioles, venules, and capillaries by large, dyscohesive, atypical cells (Fig. 39.31). These contained vesicular or clumped chromatin and prominent nucleoli, and they often were entrapped in intraluminal fibrin-platelet thrombi. This basic histologic appearance is common to all involved organs in IVL.

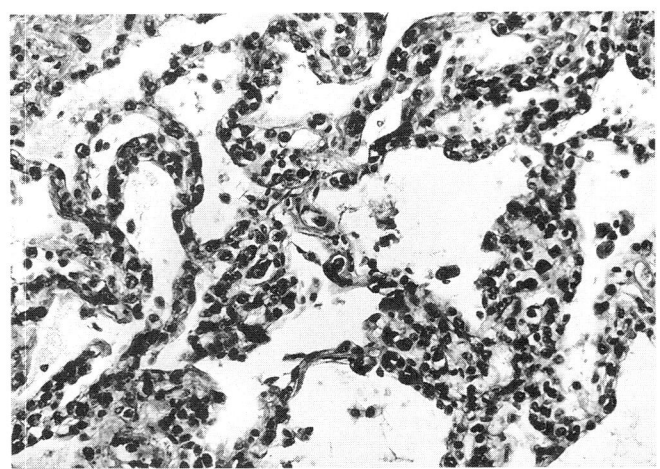

FIGURE 39.31. Intravascular lymphomatosis in lung is demonstrated by widened interstitial septae with lymphoma cells within blood vessels.

Immunohistochemical studies confirm that IVL is a lymphoid process; it demonstrates uniform positivity for CD45 (leukocyte common antigen). The great majority of cases of IVL show B-cell differentiation (160, 162), but there have been a few published reports of lesions that apparently were T-cell lymphomas (165, 166). Studies based on Southern blot analyses have supported the monoclonality of IVL by showing rearrangement of immunoglobulin heavy chain genes or T-cell receptor genes (166, 167).

Differential diagnosis of pulmonary IVL includes metastatic intravascular carcinoma, malignant melanoma, and acute leukemia. Immunohistologic studies and examination of the peripheral blood are capable of distinguishing among these disorders.

THERAPY AND PROGNOSIS

All reported patients with primary pulmonary IVL have received systemic chemotherapy, usually with cyclophosphamide, doxorubicin, vincristine, and prednisone (163). Two died of disease at 6 and 9 months after diagnosis; one was alive with persistent disease; and two were alive and disease free at the last clinical contact (163). Untreated IVL typically is rapidly fatal; virtually all patients die within 2 years (160, 162, 164). Early and aggressive chemotherapy thus is recommended.

OTHER MALIGNANT LYMPHOMAS

Other high-grade lymphomas, particularly including lymphoblastic and small noncleaved cell (Burkitt's) tumors, only rarely present in the pulmonary parenchyma. If they involve the lungs at all, it is by direct extension from the mediastinum or in the context of disseminated spread. Regardless, these lesions are biologically aggressive and require heroic chemotherapy for patients to have any chance of sustained complete remission.

PRIMARY PLASMACYTOMA OF THE LUNG

The occurrence of plasma cell tumors outside of the bones has been well documented. In the aggregate literature reviewed by Joseph et al. in 1993 (168), there are reports on more than 300 extramedullary plasmacytomas. However, only 20 of these apparently arose primarily in the lungs (169–172).

CLINICAL SUMMARY

Patients with primary pulmonary plasmacytoma (PPP) were divided equally between the sexes, with a median age of 42 years (168). The latter is notable, in that it is substantially younger than the age at which multiple myeloma (osseous plasmacytoma) typically occurs (170). Virtually all of these tumors were found on routine chest radiographs taken for other reasons, and they had not produced symptoms. Only 17% of patients were found to have a monoclonal paraprotein in studies of the blood and urine, as assessed after the diagnosis had been made pathologically (168).

Chest radiographs demonstrated discrete masses in all instances, with no particular distinguishing features (Fig. 39.32). Most were thought to represent granulomatous disease or bronchogenic carcinoma. By

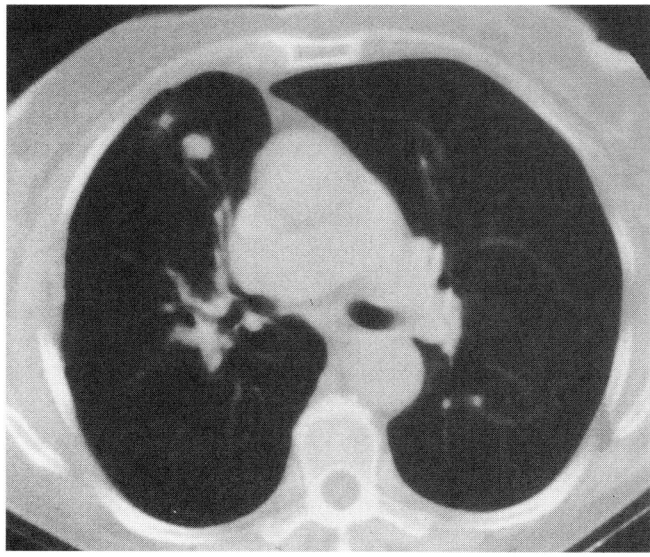

FIGURE 39.32. CT scan of a pulmonary plasmacytoma shows a circumscribed nodule.

definition, bone lesions were not seen in plain-film skeletal survey studies or radionuclide scans.

Fine-needle aspiration biopsy was performed in five cases, yielding a definitive diagnosis in two (173). The diagnosis in the remaining examples was obtained via thoracotomy and excisional biopsy.

PATHOLOGIC FINDINGS

PPP is a well-defined, solitary mass that effaces normal pulmonary architecture and shows a relatively sharp interface with the surrounding lung tissue (Fig. 39.33). It is composed of a pure culture of monomorphic plasma cells in close apposition to one another, with minimal supporting stroma (168) (Fig. 39.34). Some examples of this tumor do, however, contain intralesional deposits of amyloid (170). Occasional binucleated or multinucleated cells may be part of the neoplastic cell population, and scattered mitotic figures may be seen. Nuclear chromatin in the proliferating cells is distinctive, in that it assumes a clock face distribution and is clumped coarsely. The cytoplasm is eccentric and amphophilic, often with a perinuclear clear zone.

Differential diagnosis includes neuroendocrine tumors of the lung, large cell lymphomas, and plasma cell granulomas (inflammatory pseudotumors). Immunostains for κ– and λ–light-chain immunoglobulins are useful in the recognition of PPP, in that they demonstrate cytoplasmic monotypism for one or the other of these proteins. However, malignant lymphomas may do so as well, and they must be distinguished from plasmacytomas on the basis of cytologic features alone. In contrast, only neuroendocrine carcinomas are immunoreactive for keratin in this context, and inflammatory pseudotumors contain abundant hyalinized fibrous tissue that is lacking in PPP and neuroendocrine tumors.

THERAPY AND PROGNOSIS

The majority of PPPs have been treated by complete surgical excision, with or without adjunctive irradiation (168). In contrast to other hematopoietic lesions, it appears that very limited doses of radiotherapy (less than 100 Gy) are successful in eradicating this lesion in most instances. Joseph et al. (168) rightly question whether surgery is necessary in cases in which fine-needle aspiration biopsy provides a firm diagnosis. Only one tumor recurred locally among all the reports on PPP (174), but 3 of 19 patients went on to develop systemic multiple myeloma during the follow-up period. Thus, careful surveillance, studies of the blood and urine for paraproteins, and restaging procedures at regular intervals are recommended in all cases.

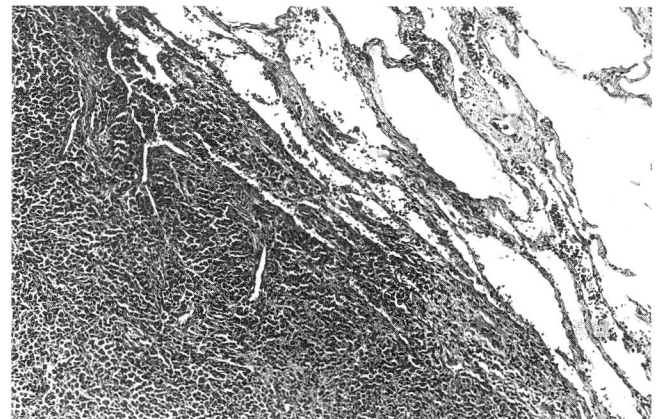

FIGURE 39.33. Pulmonary plasmacytoma forms a discrete interface with nonneoplastic parenchyma.

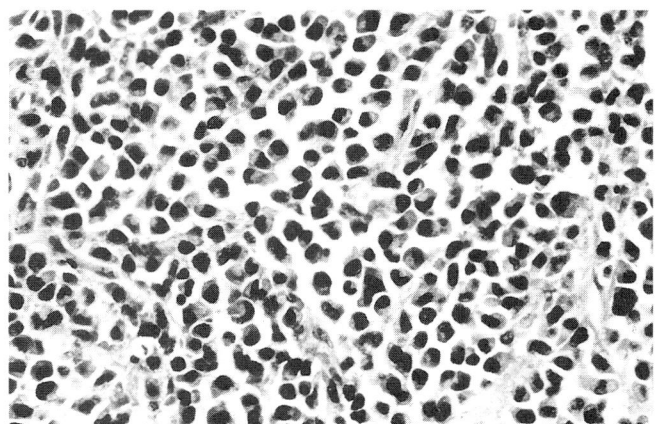

FIGURE 39.34. Plasmacytoma is comprised of sheets of plasma cells with eccentric nuclei.

PRIMARY MALIGNANT MELANOMA OF THE LUNG

Melanomas arising primarily in the lung are extraordinarily rare; the literature contains only a handful of case reports on this topic. The largest series is from the Mayo Clinic, consisting of three cases seen over a 10-year period (26). Although rigorous criteria have been proposed for primary malignant melanoma of the lung (PMML), this interpretation cannot be established with absolute certainty because of the well-known capacity for spontaneous regression of primary melanomas in mucosal or cutaneous sites. To consider a diagnosis of PMML seriously, there obviously must be no prior history of a potentially malignant pigmented tumor of the skin or ocular uveal tract. Moreover, clinical examination for possibly occult melanomas in the integument, nail beds, eyes, nasal cavity, paranasal sinuses, oral cavity, esophagus, anus, rectum, vulva, and leptomeninges should not show any extrapulmonary lesions. In fact, some authors have suggested that a case of PMML can be regarded as bona fide only retrospectively, after a postmortem examination has excluded another source of a primary melanoma (175, 176). Thus, it is evident that this diagnosis can never be considered irrefutable during the lifetime of the patient.

Regarding the fundamental question of the origin of primary melanoma in the respiratory tract, some have stressed that the tracheobronchial tree is in fact of endodermal derivation, similar in origin to that of the oral cavity and esophagus, in which well-documented primary melanomas have originated (176). Nonetheless, these tumors generally are thought to be neuroectodermal, and their presence in endodermal or mesodermal sites therefore is problematic with reference to classic histogenetic theory. The recommended interpretation is the stem cell theory of neoplasia, wherein embryologic constructs are essentially irrelevant as an explanation of the phenomenon of the origin of primary melanoma.

CLINICAL SUMMARY

The ages of reported patients with PMML have ranged from 29 to 80 years. Because of the rarity of this lesion, no meaningful statements can be made regarding gender-related incidence. Some patients with bronchopulmonary melanoma have been asymptomatic, whereas others have presented with hemoptysis, dyspnea, or cough (175–181). Plain-film radiographic examinations generally have shown abnormalities only if the tumors were in the pulmonary parenchyma; in other words, endobronchial tumors are visible only on CT or MR imaging studies.

PATHOLOGIC FINDINGS

In several reported cases of PMML, the lesions have been centered in large airways, including the trachea and major bronchi (176, 177, 179, 180, 182). Grossly, these tumors are generally polypoid, endoluminal masses that are partially or completely obstructing, or they present as nodules within the lung parenchyma ranging from 1 to 4.5 cm in greatest dimension. In addition, they are characteristically colored in shades of brown or black.

Histologically, PMMLs are composed of heterogeneously pigmented and variably pleomorphic cells that range from epithelioid to fusiform in configuration with occasional gigantiform figures. An important histologic feature that further supports a primary origin in the respiratory tract is the presence of a cytologically atypical in situ melanocytic proliferation in adjacent bronchial mucosa that may be metaplastic (176). Electron microscopic studies showing the presence of cytoplasmic premelanosomes, or immunohistochemical negativity for keratin and labeling for S100 protein, HMB-45 antigen, or NK1/C3 are useful in confirming the presence of melanocytic differentiation.

THERAPY AND PROGNOSIS

Most patients with documented PMML have fared extremely poorly, with the majority dying within 1 year of diagnosis (176–178, 180). Reid and Mehta (179) reported one individual who survived 11 years after surgery; however, there was no mention in that study of clinical evaluations designed to exclude other primary sites of origin, and no in situ melanocytic proliferation was found in the pulmonary resection specimen. Thus, this case is doubtful as a verifiable example of PMML. Most patients have undergone surgical resections of their tumors, although a few have received irradiation or chemotherapy (26, 180). In extension of therapeutic results obtained in cases of other primary melanomas of the viscera, it must be concluded that long-term survival of patients with PMML is an idiosyncratic and highly unlikely event.

REFERENCES

Sarcomatoid Carcinoma

1. Nappi O, Wick MR. Sarcomatoid neoplasms of the respiratory tract. Semin Diagn Pathol 1993;10:137–147.
2. Cabarcos A, Gomez-Dorronsoro M, Lobo-Beristain JL. Pulmonary carcinosarcoma: a case study and review of the literature. Br J Dis Chest 1985;79:83–94.
3. Ro JY, Chen JL, Ordonez NG, Ayala AG. Sarcomatoid carcinoma of the lung: immunohistochemical and ultrastructural studies of 14 cases. Cancer 1992;69:376–386.
4. Wick MR, Swanson PE. Carcinosarcomas: current perspectives and an historical review of nosological concepts. Semin Diagn Pathol 1993;10:118–127.
5. Cupples J, Wright J. An immunohistological comparison of primary lung carcinosarcoma and sarcoma. Pathol Res Pract 1990;186:326–329.
6. Humphrey PA, Scroggs MW, Roggli VL, et al. Pulmonary carcinoma with a sarcomatoid element. Hum Pathol 1988;19:155–165.
7. Davis MP, Eagan RT, Weiland LH, Pairolero PC. Carcinosarcoma of the lung: Mayo Clinic experience and response to chemotherapy. Mayo Clin Proc 1984;59:598–603.
8. Nappi O, Glasner SD, Swanson PE, Wick MR. Biphasic and monophasic sarcomatoid carcinomas of the lung. Am J Clin Pathol 1994;102:331–340.

Pulmonary Kaposi's Sarcoma

9. Wick MR. Kaposi's sarcoma unrelated to the acquired immunodeficiency syndrome: a review. Curr Opin Oncol 1991;3:377–383.
10. Ognibene FP, Shelhamer JH. Kaposi's sarcoma. Clin Chest Med 1988;9:459–465.

11. Garay SM, Belenko M, Fazzini E, Schinella R. Pulmonary manifestations of Kaposi's sarcoma. Chest 1987;91:39–43.
12. White DA, Matthay RA. Noninfectious pulmonary complications of infection with the human immunodeficiency virus. Am Rev Respir Dis 1989;140:1763–1787.
13. Meduri GU, Stover DE, Lee M, Myskowski PL, Caravelli JF, Zaman MB. Pulmonary Kaposi's sarcoma in the acquired immune deficiency syndrome: clinical, radiographic, and pathologic manifestations. Am J Med 1986;81:11–18.
14. Purdy LJ, Colby TV, Yousem SA, Battifora H. Pulmonary Kaposi's sarcoma: premortem histologic diagnosis. Am J Surg Pathol 1986;10:301–311.
15. Bach MC, Bagwell SP, Fanning JP. Primary pulmonary Kaposi's sarcoma in the acquired immunodeficiency syndrome: a cause of persistent pyrexia. Am J Med 1988;85:274–275.
16. Hanno R, Owen LG, Callen JP. Kaposi's sarcoma with extensive silent internal involvement. Int J Dermatol 1979;18:718–721.
17. Gal AA, Koss MN, Hartmann B, Strigle S. A review of pulmonary pathology in the acquired immune deficiency syndrome. Surg Pathol 1988;1:325–346.
18. O'Brien RF, Cohn DL. Serosanguineous pleural effusions in AIDS-associated Kaposi's sarcoma. Chest 1989;96:460–466.
19. Floris C, Sulis ML, Bernascani M, et al. Pneumothorax in pleuropulmonary Kaposi's sarcoma related to acquired immune deficiency syndrome. Am J Med 1989;87:123–124.
20. Ireland-Gill A, Espina BM, Akil B, Gill PS. Treatment of acquired immunodeficiency syndrome–related Kaposi's sarcoma using bleomycin-containing combination chemotherapy regimens. Semin Oncol 1992;19(Suppl 5):32–37.
21. Gill PS, Akil B, Colletti P, et al. Pulmonary Kaposi's sarcoma: clinical findings and results of therapy. Am J Med 1989;87:57–61.
22. Ognibene FP, Steis RG, Macher AM, et al. Kaposi's sarcoma causing pulmonary infiltrates and respiratory failure in the acquired immunodeficiency syndrome. Ann Intern Med 1985;102:471–475.

Primary Pulmonary Fibrosarcoma

23. Guccion JG, Rosen SH. Bronchopulmonary leiomyosarcoma and fibrosarcoma: a study of 32 cases and review of the literature. Cancer 1972;30:836–847.
24. Enzinger FM, Weiss SW. Fibrosarcoma. In: Soft tissue tumors. 2nd ed. St. Louis: Mosby, 1988:201–222.
25. Nascimento AG, Unni KK, Bernatz PE. Sarcomas of the lung. Mayo Clin Proc 1982;57:355–359.
26. Miller DL, Allen MS. Rare pulmonary neoplasms. Mayo Clin Proc 1993;68:492–498.
27. Pettinato G, Manivel JC, Saldana MJ, Peyser J, Dehner LP. Primary bronchopulmonary fibrosarcoma of childhood and adolescence: reassessment of a low-grade malignancy. Hum Pathol 1989;20:463–471.
28. Goldthorn JF, Duncan MH, Kosloske AM, Ball WS. Cavitating primary pulmonary fibrosarcoma in a child. J Thorac Cardiovasc Surg 1986;91:932–934.
29. Wick MR, Manivel JC. Primary sarcomas of the lung. In: Williams CJ, Krikorian JG, Green MR, Raghavan D, eds. Textbook of uncommon cancer. New York: John Wiley, 1988:335–381.

Primary Pulmonary Leiomyosarcoma

30. Beluffi G, Bertolotti P, Mietta A, Manara G, Luisetti M. Primary leiomyosarcoma of the lung in a girl. Pediatr Radiol 1986;16:240–244.
31. Jimenez JF, Uthman EO, Townsend JW, Gloster ES, Seibert JJ. Primary bronchopulmonary leiomyosarcoma in childhood. Arch Pathol Lab Med 1986;110:348–351.
32. Yellin A, Rosenman Y, Lieberman Y. Review of smooth muscle tumours of the lower respiratory tract. Br J Dis Chest 1984;78;337–351.
33. Lillo-Gil R, Albrechtsson U, Jakobsson B. Pulmonary leiomyosarcoma appearing as a cyst: report of one case and review of the literature. Thorac Cardiovasc Surg 1985;33:250–252.
34. Enzinger FM, Weiss SW. Leiomyosarcoma. In: Soft tissue tumors. 2nd ed. St. Louis: Mosby, 1988:402–421.
35. Morgan PGM, Ball J. Pulmonary leiomyosarcomas. Br J Dis Chest 1980;74:245–252.
36. Wick MR, Scheithauer BW, Piehler JM, Pairolero PC. Primary pulmonary leiomyosarcomas: a light and electron microscopic study. Arch Pathol Lab Med 1982;106:510–514.
37. Chaudhuri MR. Primary leiomyosarcoma of the lung. Br J Dis Chest 1973;67:75–80.

Pulmonary Epithelioid Hemangioendothelioma

38. Dail DH, Liebow AA. Intravascular bronchioloalveolar tumor (abstract). Am J Pathol 1975;78:6a.
39. Dail DH, Liebow AA, Gmelich JT, et al. Intravascular, bronchiolar, and alveolar tumor of the lung (IVBAT). Cancer 1983;51:452–464.
40. Corrin B, Manners B, Millard M, Weaver L. Histogenesis of so-called intravascular bronchioloalveolar tumour. J Pathol 1979;128:163–167.
41. Weiss SW, Enzinger FM. Epithelioid hemangioendothelioma: a vascular tumor often mistaken for a carcinoma. Cancer 1982;50:970–981.
42. Weiss SW, Ishak KG, Dail DH, Sweet DE, Enzinger FM. Epithelioid hemangioendothelioma and related lesions. Semin Diagn Pathol 1986;3:259–287.
43. Rock MJ, Kaufman RA, Lobe TE, Hensley SD, Moss ML. Epithelioid hemangioendothelioma of the lung (intravascular bronchioloalveolar tumor) in a young girl. Pediatr Pulmonol 1991;11:181–186.
44. Carter EJ, Bradburne RM, Jhung JW, Ettensohn DB. Alveolar hemorrhage with epithelioid hemangioendothelioma: a previously unreported manifestation of a rare tumor. Am Rev Respir Dis 1990;142:700–701.
45. Ross GJ, Violi L, Friedman AC, Edmonds PR, Unger E. Intravascular bronchioloalveolar tumor: CT and pathologic correlation. J Comput Assist Tomogr 1989;13:240–243.
46. Bhagavan BS, Murthy MSN, Dorfman HD, Eggleston JC. Intravascular bronchiolo-alveolar tumor (IVBAT): a low-grade sclerosing epithelioid angiosarcoma of lung. Am J Surg Pathol 1982;6:41–52.
47. Corrin B, Harrison WJ, Wright DH. The so-called intravascular bronchioloalveolar tumour of lung (low grade sclerosing angiosarcoma). Diagn Histopathol 1983;6:229–237.
48. Ohori NP, Yousem SA, Sonmez-Alpan E, Colby TV. Estrogen and progesterone receptors in lymphangioleiomyomatosis, epithelioid hemangioendothelioma, and sclerosing hemangioma of the lungs. Am J Clin Pathol 1991;96:529–535.

Primary Pulmonary Hemangiopericytoma

49. Stout AP, Murray MR. Hemangiopericytoma: a vascular tumor featuring Zimmerman's pericytes. Ann Surg 1942;116:26–33.
50. Meade JB, Whitwell F, Bickford BJ, Waddington JKB. Primary haemangiopericytoma of lung. Thorax 1974;29:1–15.
51. Enzinger FM, Weiss SW. Hemangiopericytoma. In: Soft tissue tumors. 2nd ed. St. Louis: Mosby, 1988:596–613.

52. Shin MS, Ho KJ. Primary hemangiopericytoma of lung: radiography and pathology. AJR Am J Roentgenol 1979;133:1077–1083.
53. Van Damme H, Dekoster G, Creemers E, Hermans G, Limet R. Primary pulmonary hemangiopericytoma: early local recurrence after perioperative rupture of the giant tumor mass (two cases). Surgery 1990;108:105–109.
54. Yousem SA, Hochholzer L. Primary pulmonary hemangiopericytoma. Cancer 1987;59:549–555.
55. Yaghmai I. Angiographic manifestations of soft-tissue and osseous hemangiopericytomas. Radiology 1978;126:653–659.
56. Halle M, Blum U, Dinkel E, Brugger W. CT and MR features of primary pulmonary hemangiopericytomas. J Comput Assist Tomogr 1993;17:51–55.
57. Rusch VW, Shuman WP, Schmidt R, Laramore GE. Massive pulmonary hemangiopericytoma: an innovative approach to evaluation and treatment. Cancer 1989;64:1928–1936.
58. Wong PP, Yagoda A. Chemotherapy of malignant hemangiopericytoma. Cancer 1978;41:1256–1260.
59. Jha N, McNeese M, Barkley HT, Kong J. Does radiotherapy have a role in hemangiopericytoma management? Report of 14 new cases and a review of the literature. Int J Radiat Oncol Biol Phys 1987;13:1399–1402.
60. Mira JG, Chu FCH, Fortner JG. The role of radiotherapy in the management of malignant hemangiopericytoma: report of eleven new cases and review of the literature. Cancer 1977;39:1254–1259.
61. Hansen CP, Francis D, Bertelsen S. Primary hemangiopericytoma of the lung: case report. Scand J Thorac Cardiovasc Surg 1990;24:89–92.

Primary Pulmonary Malignant Fibrous Histiocytoma

62. Weiss SW, Enzinger FM. Malignant fibrous histiocytoma: an analysis of 200 cases. Cancer 1978;41:2250–2266.
63. Yousem SA, Hochholzer L. Malignant fibrous histiocytoma of the lung. Cancer 1987;60:2532–2541.
64. McDonnell T, Kyriakos M, Roper C, Mazoujian G. Malignant fibrous histiocytoma of the lung. Cancer 1988;61:137–145.
65. Lee JT, Shelburne JD, Linder J. Primary malignant fibrous histiocytoma of the lung: a clinicopathologic and ultrastructural study of five cases. Cancer 1984;53:1124–1130.
66. Bedrossian CW, Verani R, Unger KM, Salman J. Pulmonary malignant fibrous histiocytoma: light and electron microscopic studies of one case. Chest 1979;75:186–189.
67. Kern WH, Hughes RK, Meyer BW, Harley DP. Malignant fibrous histiocytoma of the lung. Cancer 1979;44:1793–1801.
68. Chowdhury LN, Swerdlow MA, Jao W, Kathpalia S, Desser RK. Postirradiation malignant fibrous histiocytoma of the lung: demonstration of alpha-1-antitrypsin–like material in neoplastic cells. Am J Clin Pathol 1980;74:820–826.
69. Juettner FM, Popper H, Sommersgutter K, Smolle J, Friehs GB. Malignant fibrous histiocytoma of the lung: prognosis and therapy of a rare disease: report of two cases and review of the literature. Thorac Cardiovasc Surg 1987;35:226–231.
70. Higashiyama M, Doi O, Kodama K, et al. Successful surgery of malignant fibrous histiocytoma in the lung with gross extension into the right main pulmonary artery. Thorac Cardiovasc Surg 1993;41:73–76.

Primary Pulmonary Rhabdomyosarcoma

71. McDermott VG, MacKenzie S, Hendry GM. Case report: primary intrathoracic rhabdomyosarcoma: a rare childhood malignancy. Br J Radiol 1993;66:937–941.
72. Allan BT, Day DL, Dehner LP. Primary pulmonary rhabdomyosarcoma of the lung in children: report of two cases presenting with spontaneous pneumothorax. Cancer 1987;59;1005–1011.
73. Murphy JJ, Blair GK, Fraser GC, et al. Rhabdomyosarcoma arising within congenital pulmonary cysts: report of three cases. J Pediatr Surg 1992;27:1364–1367.
74. Lee SH, Rengaciary SS, Paramesh J. Primary pulmonary rhabdomyosarcoma: a case report and review of the literature. Hum Pathol 1981;12:92–96.
75. Eriksson A, Thunell M, Lundquist G. Pedunculated endobronchial rhabdomyosarcoma with fatal asphyxia. Thorax 1982;37:390–391.
76. Triche TJ, Askin FB, Kissane JM. Neuroblastoma, Ewing's sarcoma, and the differential diagnosis of small round blue cell tumors. In: Finegold M, ed. Pathology of neoplasia in children and adolescents. Philadelphia: WB Saunders, 1986:145–195.
77. Wick MR, Swanson PE, Manivel JC. Immunohistochemical analysis of soft tissue sarcomas: comparisons with electron microscopy. Appl Pathol 1988;6:169–196.
78. Dehner LP. Soft tissue, peritoneum, and retroperitoneum. In: Pediatric surgical pathology. 2nd ed. Baltimore: Williams & Wilkins, 1987:869–938.

Primary Pulmonary Chondrosarcoma

79. Sun CCJ, Kroll M, Miller JE. Primary chondrosarcoma of the lung. Cancer 1982;50:1864–1866.
80. Morgan AD, Salama FD. Primary chondrosarcoma of the lung: case report and review of the literature. J Thorac Cardiovasc Surg 1972;64:460–466.
81. Fallahnejad M, Harrell D, Tucker J, et al. Chondrosarcoma of the trachea: report of a case and five-year followup. J Thorac Cardiovasc Surg 1973;65:210–213.

Other Sarcomas of the Lung

82. Sawamura K, Hashimoto T, Nanjo S, et al. Primary liposarcoma of the lung. J Surg Oncol 1982;19:243–246.
83. Yousem SA. Angiosarcoma presenting in the lung. Arch Pathol Lab Med 1986;110:112–115.
84. Segal SL, Lenchner GS, Cicchelli AV, et al. Angiosarcoma presenting as diffuse alveolar hemorrhage. Chest 1988;94:214–216.
85. Bartley TD, Arean VM. Intrapulmonary neurogenic tumors. J Thorac Cardiovasc Surg 1965;50:114–123.
86. Reingold IM, Amromin GD. Extraosseous osteosarcoma of the lung. Cancer 1971;28:491–498.
87. Nappi O, Swanson PE, Wick MR. Pseudovascular adenoid squamous cell carcinoma of the lung: clinicopathologic study of three cases and comparison with true pleuropulmonary angiosarcoma. Hum Pathol 1994;25:373–378.

Pulmonary Trunk Sarcoma

88. McGlennen RC, Manivel JC, Stanley SJ, et al. Pulmonary artery trunk sarcoma: a clinicopathologic, ultrastructural, and immunohistochemical study of four cases. Mod Pathol 1989;2:486–494.
89. Sethi GK, Slaven JE, Kepes JJ. Primary sarcoma of the pulmonary artery. J Thorac Cardiovasc Surg 1972;63:587–596.
90. Baker PB, Goodwin RA. Pulmonary artery sarcoma. Arch Pathol Lab Med 1985;109:35–40.
91. Hynes JK, Smith HC, Holmes DR. Pulmonary artery sarcoma: preoperative diagnosis noninvasively by two-dimensional echocardiography. Circulation 1983;67:459–477.
92. Lyerly HK, Reves JG, Sabiston DC. Management of primary sarcomas of the pulmonary artery and reperfusion intra-

bronchial hemorrhage. Surg Gynecol Obstet 1986;163:291–298.
93. Bleisch VR, Kraus FT. Polypoid sarcoma of the pulmonary trunk. Cancer 1980;46:314–321.

Pleural Sarcomas

94. Andrion A, Mazzucco G, Bernardi P, Mollo F. Sarcomatous tumor of the chest wall with osteochondroid differentiation: evidence of mesothelial origin. Am J Surg Pathol 1989;13:707–712.
95. Lee MJ, Grogan L, Meehan S, Breatnach E. Pleural granulocytic sarcoma: CT characteristics. Clin Radiol 1991;43:57–59.
96. Stark P, Smith DC, Watkins GE, Chun KE. Primary intrathoracic extraosseous osteogenic sarcoma: report of three cases. Radiology 1990;174:725–726.
97. Verhaven E, Van Betten F, Vanden Houte K, et al. Malignant schwannoma: a case report and review of the literature. Arch Orthop Trauma Surg 1989;108:394–396.
98. Moran CA, Suster S, Koss MN. The spectrum of histologic growth patterns in benign and malignant fibrous tumors of the pleura. Semin Diagn Pathol 1992;9:169–180.
99. Carter D, Otis CN. Three types of spindle cell tumors of the pleura: fibroma, sarcoma, and sarcomatoid mesothelioma. Am J Surg Pathol 1988;12:747–753.
100. Myoui A, Aozasa K, Iuchi K, et al. Soft tissue sarcoma of the pleural cavity. Cancer 1991;68:1550–1554.
101. England DM, Hochholzer L, McCarthy MJ. Localized benign and malignant fibrous tumors of the pleura. Am J Surg Pathol 1989;13:640–658.
102. Theegarten D, Meisel M. Malignant fibrous histiocytoma of the thoracic wall in the area of a tuberculous pleural callosity. Pneumonologie 1993;47:458–460.
103. Watanabe S, Hitomi S, Nakamura T, et al. A clinical study of six surgically treated patients with malignant tumors arising from chronic pleuritis and pyothorax. Nippon Kyobu Geka Gakkai Zasshi 1989;37:281–286.
104. Saiffudin A, DaCosta P, Chalmers AG, et al. Primary malignant localized fibrous tumors of the pleura: clinical, radiological, and pathological features. Clin Radiol 1992;45:13–17.
105. Briselli M, Mark EJ, Dickersin GR. Solitary fibrous tumors of the pleura. Cancer 1981;47:2678–2689.
106. Cagle PT, Truong LD, Roggli VL, Greenberg SD. Immunohistochemical differentiation of sarcomatoid mesotheliomas from other spindle cell neoplasms. Am J Clin Pathol 1989;92:566–571.
107. Toochika H, Kiminok K, Tagawa Y, et al. Malignant fibrous histiocytoma of the chest cavity: report of four resected cases. Nippon Kyobu Geka Gakkai Zasshi 1990;38:647–653.

Askin's Tumor

108. Askin FB, Rosai J, Sibley RK, et al. Malignant small cell tumor of the thoracopulmonary region in childhood. Cancer 1979;43:2438–2451.
109. Israel MA. Peripheral neuroepithelioma. In: Williams CJ, Krikorian JG, Green MR, Rhagavan D, eds. Textbook of uncommon cancer. New York: John Wiley, 1988:683–690.
110. Jurgens H, Bier V, Harms D, et al. Malignant peripheral neuroectodermal tumors. Cancer 1988;61:349–357.
111. Dehner LP. Soft tissue sarcomas of childhood. Natl Cancer Inst Monogr 1981:56:43–59.
112. Sarkar MR, Bahr R. The Askin tumor. Chirurg 1992;63:973–976.
113. Contesso G, Llombart-Bosch A, Terrier P, et al. Does malignant small round cell tumor of the thoracopulmonary region (Askin tumor) constitute a clinicopathologic entity? Cancer 1992;69:1012–1020.
114. Takahashi K, Dambara T, Uekusa T, et al. Massive chest wall tumor diagnosed as Askin tumor: successful treatment by intensive combined modality therapy in an adult. Chest 1993;104:287–288.
115. Fitzgibbons JF, Feldhaus SJ, McNamara LF, Langdon RM Jr. Diagnostic features and treatment of the Askin tumor—malignant small cell tumor of the thoracopulmonary region: a case report. Nebr Med J 1993;78:2–6.
116. Dehner LP. Peripheral neuroectodermal tumor and Ewing's sarcoma. Am J Surg Pathol 1993;17:1–13.
117. Miser JS, Kinsella TJ, Triche TJ, et al. Treatment of peripheral neuroepithelioma in children and young adults. J Clin Oncol 1987;5:1752–1758.
118. Farhi DC, Odell CA, Shurin SB. Myelodysplastic syndrome and acute myeloid leukemia after treatment for solid tumor of childhood. Am J Clin Pathol 1993;100:270–275.

Pleuropulmonary Blastoma

119. Manivel JC, Priest JR, Watterson J, et al. Pleuropulmonary blastoma: the so-called pulmonary blastoma of childhood. Cancer 1988;62:1516–1526.
120. Cohen M, Kaschula RO. Primary pulmonary tumors in childhood: a review of 31 years' experience and the literature. Pediatr Pulmonol 1992;14:222–232.
121. Hachitanda Y, Aoyama C, Sato JK, Shimada H. Pleuropulmonary blastoma in childhood: a tumor of divergent differentiation. Am J Surg Pathol 1993;17:382–391.
122. Delahunt B, Thomson KJ, Ferguson AF, et al. Familial cystic nephroma and pleuropulmonary blastoma. Cancer 1993;71:1338–1342.

Vascular Sarcomas of the Pleura

123. Dail DH. Uncommon tumors. In: Dail DH, Hammar SP, eds. Pulmonary pathology. 2nd ed. New York: Springer-Verlag, 1994:1279–1461.

Lymphoproliferative Disorders of the Lung

124. Koss MN. Lymphoproliferative disorders of the lung. In: Marchevsky AM, ed. Surgical pathology of lung neoplasms. New York: Marcel Dekker, 1990:433–486.
125. Colby TV, Carrington CB. Lymphoreticular tumors and infiltrates of the lung. Pathol Annu 1983;18:27–70.
126. Kennedy JL, Nathwani BN, Burke JS, Hill LR, Rappaport H. Pulmonary lymphomas and other pulmonary lymphoid lesions. Cancer 1985;56:539–552.
127. Weiss LM, Yousem SA, Warnke RA. Non-Hodgkin's lymphoma of the lung. Am J Surg Pathol 1985;9:480–490.
128. Glickstein M, Kornstein MJ, Pietra GG, et al. Non-lymphomatous lymphoid disorders of the lung. AJR Am J Roentgenol 1986;147:227–237.
129. Colby TV. Lymphoproliferative disease. In: Dail DH, Hammar SP, eds. Pulmonary pathology. 2nd ed. New York: Springer-Verlag, 1994:1097–1122.
130. Koss MN, Hochholzer L, Langloss JM, et al. Lymphoid interstitial pneumonitis: clinicopathologic and immunopathological findings in 18 cases. Pathology 1987;19:178–185.
131. Koss MN, Hochholzer L, Nichols PW, Wehunt WD, Lazarus AA. Primary non-Hodgkin's lymphoma and pseudolymphoma of the lung: a study of 161 patients. Hum Pathol 1983;14:1024–1038.
132. Andiman WA, Eastman R, Martin K, et al. Opportunistic lymphoproliferations associated with Epstein-Barr viral DNA in infants and children with AIDS. Lancet 1985;2:1390–1393.

133. Vath RR, Alexander CB, Fulmer JD. The lymphocytic infiltrative lung diseases. Clin Chest Med 1982;3:619–634.
134. LeTourneau A, Audoin J, Garbe L, et al. Primary pulmonary malignant lymphoma: clinical and pathological findings, immunocytochemical, and ultrastructural studies in 15 cases. Hematol Oncol 1983;1:49–60.
135. Ratech H. The uses of molecular biology in hematopathology. Am J Clin Pathol 1993;99:381–384.
136. Ritter JH, Wick MR. Cutaneous lymphoid infiltrates: paraffin section immunohistology as an adjunct to morphologic diagnosis. Mod Pathol 1993;6:36A.
137. Close PM, Macrae MB, Hammand JM, et al. Anaplastic large-cell Ki-1 lymphoma: pulmonary presentation mimicking miliary tuberculosis. Am J Clin Pathol 1993;99:631–636.
138. Harris NL. The relationship between Hodgkin's disease and non-Hodgkin's lymphoma. Semin Diagn Pathol 1992;9:304–310.

Lymphomatoid Granulomatosis

139. Liebow AA, Carrington CB, Friedman PJ. Lymphomatoid granulomatosis. Hum Pathol 1972;3:457–558.
140. Katzenstein A-LA, Carrington CB, Liebow AA. Lymphomatoid granulomatosis: a clinicopathologic study of 152 cases. Cancer 1979;43:360–373.
141. Pisani RJ, DeRemee RA. Clinical implications of the histopathologic diagnosis of pulmonary lymphomatoid granulomatosis. Mayo Clin Proc 1990;65:151–163.
142. Katzenstein A-LA, Askin FB. Primary lymphoid lung lesions. In: Surgical pathology of non-neoplastic lung disease. Philadelphia: WB Saunders, 1990:290–320.
143. DeRemee RA, Weiland LH, McDonald TJ. Polymorphic reticulosis, lymphomatoid granulomatosis: two diseases or one? Mayo Clin Proc 1978;53:634–640.
144. Gaulard P, Henni T, Marolleau J, et al. Lethal midline granuloma (polymorphic reticulosis) and lymphomatoid granulomatosis: evidence for a monoclonal T-cell lymphoproliferative disorder. Cancer 1988;62:705–710.
145. Jaffe ES, Lipford EH, Margolick JB, Longo DL, Fauci AS. Lymphomatoid granulomatosis and angiocentric lymphoma: a spectrum of post-thymic T-cell proliferations. Semin Respir Med 1989;10:167–172.
146. Katzenstein A-LA, Peiper SC. Detection of Epstein-Barr virus genomes in lymphomatoid granulomatosis: analysis of 29 cases by the polymerase chain reaction technique. Mod Pathol 1990;3:435–441.
147. Medeiros LJ, Jaffe ES, Chen Y-Y, Weiss LM. Localization of Epstein-Barr viral genomes in angiocentric immunoproliferative lesions. Am J Surg Pathol 1992;16:439–447.
148. Bleiweiss IJ, Strauchen JA. Lymphomatoid granulomatosis of the lung: report of a case and gene rearrangement studies. Hum Pathol 1988;19:1109–1112.
149. Vergier B, Capron F, Trojani M, et al. Benign lymphocytic angiitis and granulomatosis: a T-cell lymphoma? Hum Pathol 1992;23:1191–1194.
150. Donner LR, Dobin S, Harrington D, Bassion S, Rappaport ES, Peterson RF. Angiocentric immunoproliferative lesion (lymphomatoid granulomatosis): a cytogenetic, immunophenotypic, and genotypic study. Cancer 1990;65:249–254.
151. Guinee D, Jaffe E, Kingma D, et al. Pulmonary lymphomatoid granulomatosis: evidence for a proliferation of Epstein-Barr virus infected B-lymphocytes with a prominent T-cell component and vasculitis. Am J Surg Pathol 1994;18(8): 753–764.
152. Fauci AS, Haynes BF, Costa J, Katz P, Wolff SM. Lymphomatoid granulomatosis: prospective clinical and therapeutic experience over 10 years. N Engl J Med 1982;306:68–74.
153. Letendre L. Treatment of lymphomatoid granulomatosis: old and new perspectives. Semin Respir Med 1989;10:178–181.

Primary Pulmonary Hodgkin's Disease

154. Radin AI. Primary pulmonary Hodgkin's disease. Cancer 1990;65:550–563.
155. Kern WH, Crepeau AG, Jones JC. Primary Hodgkin's disease of the lung: report of 4 cases and review of the literature. Cancer 1961;12:1151–1165.
156. Yousem SA, Weiss LM, Colby TV. Primary pulmonary Hodgkin's disease: a clinicopathologic study of 15 cases. Cancer 1986;57:1217–1224.
157. Wood NL, Coltman CA. Localized primary extranodal Hodgkin's disease. Ann Intern Med 1973;78:113–118.
158. Burke JS. Hodgkin's disease: histopathology and differential diagnosis. In: Knowles EM, ed. Neoplastic hematopathology. Baltimore: Williams & Wilkins, 1992:497–533.

Intravascular Lymphomatosis in the Lungs

159. Yousem SA, Colby TV. Intravascular lymphomatosis presenting in the lung. Cancer 1990;65:349–353.
160. Wick MR, Mills SE. Intravascular lymphomatosis: clinicopathologic features and differential diagnosis. Semin Diagn Pathol 1991;8:91–101.
161. Wick MR, Mills SE, Scheithauer BW, Cooper PH, Davitz MA, Parkinson K. Reassessment of malignant angioendotheliomatosis: evidence in favor of its reclassification as intravascular lymphomatosis. Am J Surg Pathol 1986;10:112–123.
162. Ferry JA, Harris NL, Picker LJ, et al. Intravascular lymphomatosis (malignant angioendotheliomatosis): a B-cell neoplasm expressing surface homing receptors. Mod Pathol 1988;1:444–452.
163. Demirer T, Dail DH, Aboulafia DM. Four varied cases of intravascular lymphomatosis and a literature review. Cancer 1994;73:1738–1745.
164. Glass J, Hochberg FH, Miller DC. Intravascular lymphomatosis: a systemic disease with neurologic manifestations. Cancer 1993;71:3156–3164.
165. Sheibani K, Battifora H, Winberg CD, et al. Further evidence that malignant angioendotheliomatosis is an angiotropic large-cell lymphoma. N Engl J Med 1986;314:943–948.
166. Sepp N, Schuler G, Romani N, et al. Intravascular lymphomatosis (angioendotheliomatosis): evidence for a T-cell origin in two cases. Hum Pathol 1990;21:1051–1058.
167. Otrakji CL, Voigt W, Amador A, Mehrdad N, Gregorios JB. Malignant angioendotheliomatosis—a true lymphoma: a case of intravascular malignant lymphomatosis studied by southern blot hybridization analysis. Hum Pathol 1988;19:475–478.

Plasmacytoma of the Lung

168. Joseph G, Pandit M, Korfhage L. Primary pulmonary plasmacytoma. Cancer 1993;71:721–724.
169. Favis EA, Kerman HD, Schildecker W. Multiple myeloma manifested as a problem in the diagnosis of pulmonary disease. Am J Med 1960;28:323–327.
170. Sekulich M, Pandola G, Simon T. A solitary pulmonary mass in myeloma. Dis Chest 1965;48:100–103.
171. Romanoff H, Milwidsky H. Primary plasmacytoma of the lung. Br J Dis Chest 1962;56:139–143.
172. Roikjaer O, Thomsen JK. Plasmacytoma of the lung. Cancer 1986;58:2671–2674.
173. Amin R. Extramedullary plasmacytoma of lung. Cancer 1985;56:152–156.
174. Childress WG, Adie GC. Recurrent plasmacytoma of lung. J Thorac Surg 1955;29:480–487.

Primary Pulmonary Melanoma

175. Jensen OA, Egedorf J. Primary malignant melanoma of the lung. Scand J Respir Dis 1967;48:127–135.
176. Salm R. A primary malignant melanoma of the bronchus. J Pathol Bacteriol 1963;85:121–126.
177. Bagwell SP, Flynn SD, Cox PM, Davison JA. Primary malignant melanoma of the lung. Am Rev Respir Dis 1989;139:1543–1547.
178. Carstens PHB, Kuhns JG, Ghazi C. Primary malignant melanomas of the lung and adrenal. Hum Pathol 1984;15:910–914.
179. Reid JD, Mehta VT. Melanoma of the lower respiratory tract. Cancer 1966;19:627–631.
180. Robertson AJ, Sinclair DJM, Sutton PP, Guthrie W. Primary melanocarcinoma of the lower respiratory tract. Thorax 1980;35:158–159.
181. Reed RJ, Kent EM. Solitary pulmonary melanomas: two case reports. J Thorac Cardiovasc Surg 1964:48:226–231.
182. Gephardt GN. Malignant melanoma of the bronchus. Hum Pathol 1981;12:671–673.
183. Dehner LP. Pleuropulmonary blastoma is *the* pulmonary blastoma of childhood. Semin Diagn Pathol 1994;11:144–151.

40

Bronchial Carcinoids

Victor F. Trastek

Bronchial carcinoids were first described by Laennec (1) in 1831 and constitute approximately 5% of all primary lung cancers. Initially, they were thought to be benign and were known as bronchial adenomas (2, 3). However, it is now clear that they are malignant neoplasms that can develop nodal and distant blood-borne metastases, thus the term bronchial adenoma is no longer relevant.

PATHOPHYSIOLOGY

The etiology of bronchial carcinoids remains unclear and has been difficult to prove. They have not been associated with environmental factors or exposure to known carcinogens. Possible etiologic cells include amine precursor uptake and decarboxylation (APUD) cells that migrate from the neural crest (4, 5); Kulchitsky cells (KCC), the argentaffin-containing cells located within the bronchial mucus glands (6, 7); and, more recently, undifferentiated epithelial stem cells that originate from the bronchial lining (8).

All classification systems used for bronchial carcinoids take into account this spectrum of disease and include the evolution of a more normal histologic process (typical carcinoid or KCC-I) through a transition phase (atypical carcinoid or KCC-II) to a highly undifferentiated group of cells (small cell carcinoma of the lung or KCC-III). Although it is thought that all of the phases may come from the same cell type, a description of the progression has been much less clear. It has been noted by Paladugu et al. (9) that the progression of KCC-II (atypical carcinoid) to KCC-III (small cell carcinoma) has occurred in up to 10% of patients.

Typical carcinoid tumors represent well-differentiated, organized cells with abundant eosinophilic or clear cytoplasm and round organized nuclei with fine granular chromatin (Fig. 40.1). They can be characterized as groupings of cells in nests with ribbonlike structures or broad sheets, producing a glandular appearance (10). There is an orderly arrangement of the cells in which stromal tissue is separated by septa. There is no increased mitotic activity, and they are richly vascular. Ultrastructurally, they have been described as closely packed cells with small but well-formed desmoid cells (6). Grossly, they are highly vascularized, reddish tumors, covered by intact epithelium. They may be polypoid with a stalk located within the bronchial tree, or they can occur as peripheral nodules. Approximately 5% of typical carcinoids metastasize.

Atypical carcinoids were first described by Engelbreth-Holm (11) in 1944 and constitute approximately 10% of all bronchial carcinoids (12). They are high-grade neoplasms with some of the same features of architecture noted previously but with increasing degrees of nuclear and cytologic pleomorphism, increased mitotic activity, and even areas of hemorrhage or necrosis (Fig. 40.2) (12). Up to 50% of these tumors are located peripherally, and there is a much greater ability to metastasize to lymph nodes in 50% to 75%. They may be difficult to differentiate from small cell carcinoma.

An unusual presentation associated with the carcinoid was noted in 1955 by Whitwell (13), who first described carcinoid tumorlets of the lung (Fig. 40.3). These nodules of bland neuroendocrine cells currently are thought to be hyperplastic abnormalities rather than malignant neoplasms (14).

Immunohistochemical techniques reported by Wain et al. (15) have been used more recently to differentiate tumors in the carcinoid line, particularly from lung cancers or lymphoproliferative disorders (Table 40.1). Included in the analysis were markers such as neuron specific enolase, Leu-7, chromogranin, cytokeratins, neurofilaments, and immunoglobulins. It also has been shown that the DNA content displays a spectrum of change as one progresses through the carcinoid line (9, 16).

Many investigators have noted that carcinoid tumors can produce neuroendocrine abnormalities because they can secrete a variety of chemical substances. Initially, in 1928, Brown (17) first noted an

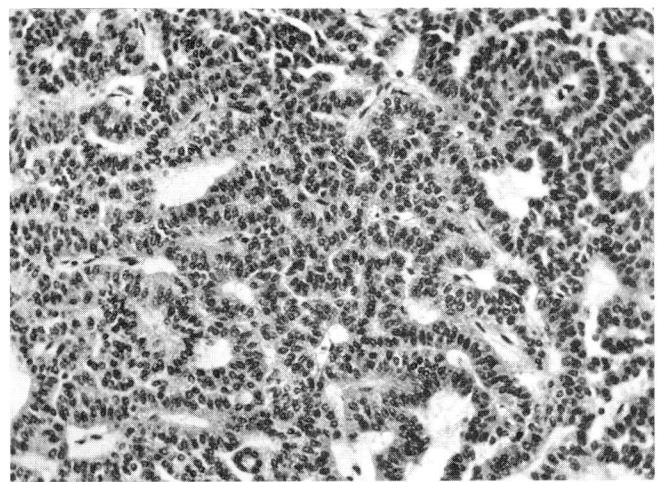

FIGURE 40.1. Typical bronchial carcinoid showing larger cells with a prominent glandular and ribbonlike pattern. (Hematoxylin-eosin stain; original magnification ×200). (From Okike N, Bernatz PE, Woolner LB. Carcinoid tumors of the lung. Ann Thorac Surg 1976;22:270–277.)

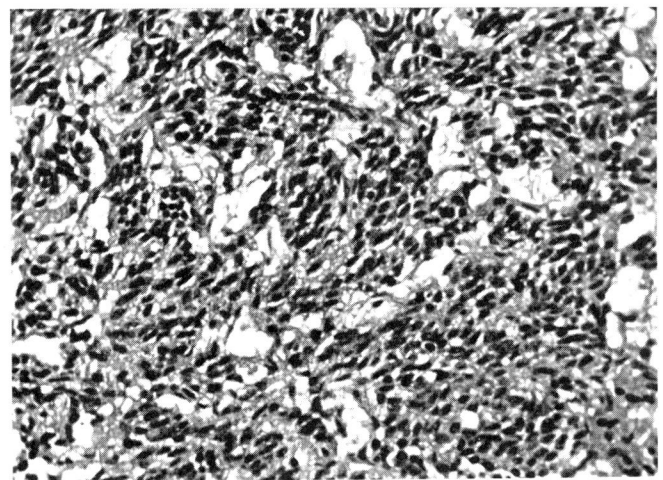

FIGURE 40.2. Atypical bronchial carcinoid. Highly atypical histology showing spindle cells, hyperchromatism, and prominent mitotic activity. (Hematoxylin-eosin stain; original magnification ×200). (From Okike N, Bernatz PE, Woolner LB. Carcinoid tumors of the lung. Ann Thorac Surg 1976;22:270–277.)

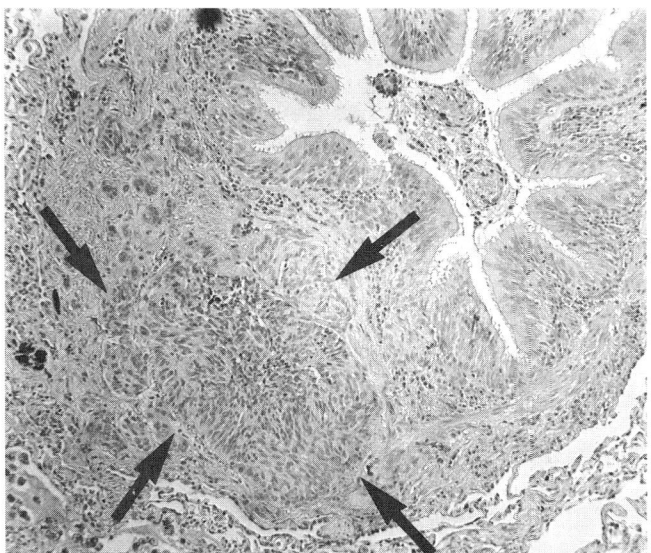

FIGURE 40.3. Histologic appearance of carcinoid tumorlet. Microscopic nodule of bland neuroendocrine cells (*arrows*) is present adjacent to a bronchiole. (Hematoxylin-eosin stain; ×160). (From Davila DG, Dunn WF, Tazelaar HD, Pairolero PC. Bronchial carcinoid tumors. Mayo Clinic Proc 1993;68:795–803.)

TABLE 40.1. Immunohistochemical Staining of Pulmonary Neoplasms

	KULCHITSKY CELL CANCERS	NON–SMALL CELL CANCERS	LYMPHO-PROLIFERATIVE DISORDERS
Cytokeratins	+	+	−
Neurofilaments	+[a]	−	−
Immunoglobulins	−	−	+
Neuron specific enolase	+	−	−
Chromogranins	+	−	−
Leu-7	+	−	+[b]

From Wain JC Jr, Pak SHY, Benfield JR. Immunohistochemistry and new trends in the diagnosis of carcinoids. In: Martini N, Vogt-Moykopf I, eds. Thoracic surgery: frontiers and uncommon neoplasms. St. Louis: Mosby, 1989:249–257.
[a] Variable.
[b] On natural killer cells.

association between small cell lung cancer and Cushing's syndrome; however, Hamperl (18) may have been the first to note that bronchial carcinoids also had endocrine properties.

CLINICAL FINDINGS

Bronchial carcinoids account for 0.5% to 1% of all bronchial tumors and occur equally in men and women, usually peaking in the fifth decade of life. The estimated age-adjusted incidence for both sexes is 0.21 new cases per 100,000 population (19).

Most carcinoid tumors arise in major bronchi with 10% in the main stem bronchi and approximately 75% in the lower bronchi (10, 12). The remaining 15% originate in the periphery of the lung. Extrabronchial extensions can be found in 10% of patients, and combined regional lymph node metastasis is found in both typical and atypical forms in approximately 15% (10, 12). Distant metastasis occurs rarely, but when found is located in the liver, bone, and adrenal glands, much as with carcinoma of the lung.

Presentation of symptoms depends on location. Central tumors can grow and obstruct the bronchi, producing symptoms of cough, wheezing, and recurrent infection (Fig. 40.4). It is not uncommon for a patient to be treated for asthma for an extended period before making the diagnosis of carcinoid tumor. Hemoptysis also is characteristic of these tumors and can be a presenting symptom in many patients. It could be said that these tumors frequently masquerade as other diseases, particularly asthma, bronchitis, bronchiectasis, and carcinoma of the lung. Peripheral carcinoids basically are asymptomatic and are found incidentally on chest radiographs done for other reasons.

Although it was first reported in 1956 (20), carcinoid syndrome is much more common with gastrointestinal carcinoids and rarely is related to bronchial carcinoids. Fewer than 5% of patients with bronchial carcinoids present with carcinoid syndrome. It would appear that patients with atypical carcinoids have a higher potential for developing this syndrome. Because of their location in the lung, carcinoids producing carcinoid syndrome may be associated with valvular disease on the left side of the heart, unlike gastrointestinal tumors with liver metastasis, which involve the right side of the heart. The cardiac abnormalities include valvular lesions with deposits of fibrous tissue on the normal valve, resulting in stenosis of the orifice.

One percent of Cushing's syndrome cases is caused by ectopic production of corticotropin or releasing enzyme (21, 22), both of which have been isolated from bronchial carcinoid tumors (23, 24). Although Cushing's syndrome, because of ectopic adrenocorticotropic hormone (ACTH) production, has most often been caused by bronchial carcinomas, recent reports indicate that bronchial carcinoid tumors may be the most common cause (22, 25). In the report by Jex et al. (25), 7 (28%) of 25 patients with ectopic ACTH-producing tumors were bronchial carcinoids. Limper and associates (26) reported that occasionally Cushing's syndrome may be diagnosed and treated with the patient displaying a normal radiograph. Computed tomography (CT) can be very helpful in detecting small, occult carcinoids that can be the site of the production of the ACTH (Fig. 40.5) (27).

Short of a histologic review of a biopsy, there is no single laboratory or radiologic examination that is sufficiently accurate to diagnosis a bronchial carcinoid.

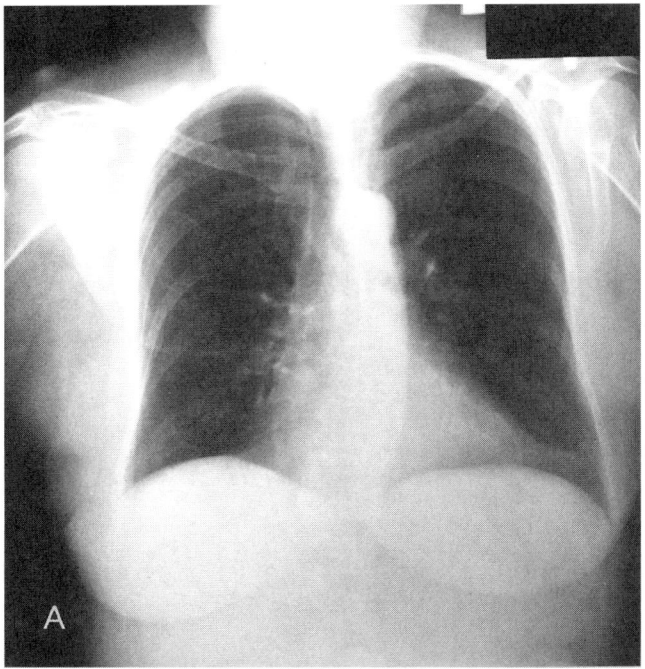
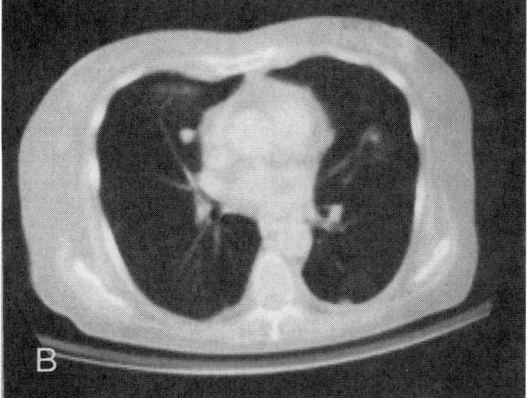

FIGURE 40.5. CT in detecting radiographically occult bronchial carcinoid tumors. A. Standard chest radiograph failed to localize any abnormality in this patient presenting with Cushing's syndrome. B. A CT scan of the same patient showing an intrathoracic nodule of the right middle lobe that proved to be a typical bronchial carcinoid tumor. (From Limper AH, Carpenter PC, Scheithauer B, Staats BA. The Cushing syndrome induced by bronchial carcinoid tumors. Ann Intern Med 1992;117:209–214.)

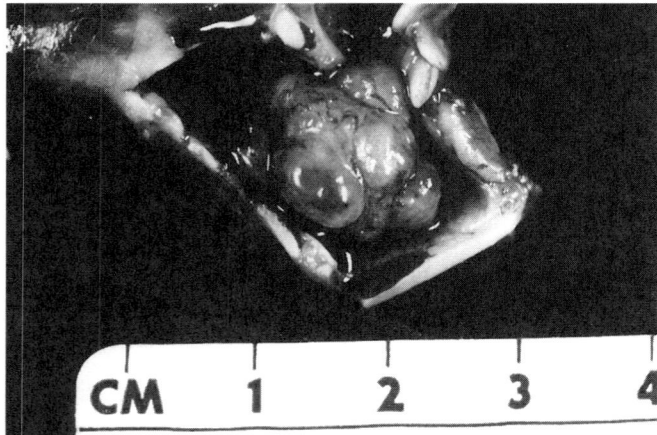

FIGURE 40.4. Postsurgical specimen showing endobronchial typical carcinoid tumor obstructing the airway.

Sputum cytology and fine-needle aspiration are seldom helpful, primarily because of the lack of cells and the inability on many occasions to differentiate a higher state of malignancy such as atypical or, more importantly, small cell carcinoma. Screening patients for serotonin or metabolites such as 5-hydroxindole acetic acid has essentially no role because of the low rate of occurrence.

Conventional chest roentgenograms may demonstrate abnormal findings in approximately 75% of patients and can consist of either a peripheral abnormality in 15% of patients or a central mass with resulting obstructive symptomatology (10, 12, 28, 29). As previously noted, CT can be extremely helpful in the diagnosis of bronchial carcinoids, particularly if they are occult. Magnetic resonance imaging has not been thought to be superior to CT and probably does not have a role in the diagnosis of this particular disease.

Bronchoscopy remains the gold standard for diagnosing carcinoid tumors if they are central and for providing tissue for histologic review. The risk of bleeding on biopsy of these tumors has been described. Bleeding more likely was caused by the large size of the biopsy forceps used and the lack of recognition of the possibility of the event. Today, with flexible bronchoscopy and the ability to inject epinephrine, the biopsy of carcinoid tumors can be done safely (30). Because of the possibility of small cell carcinoma, obtaining an adequate amount of tissue is important. It is imperative that the differentiation between a carcinoid tumor and small cell carcinoma can be made. It should be noted that normal biopsies do not exclude the diagnosis of a carcinoid tumor because it is possible to have an intact mucus membrane overlying the submucosal tumor, causing a false-negative biopsy. A high index of clinical suspicion remains important. Because of the extremely low rate of lymph node involvement, a preoperative mediastinoscopy is seldom indicated.

TREATMENT

The treatment of a bronchial carcinoid is surgical resection (3, 10, 12, 31, 32). Goals of the procedure include complete removal of the neoplasm with preservation of as much normal lung tissue as possible. Currently, for peripheral carcinoids, a lobectomy remains the accepted standard; a segmentectomy for peripherally located tumors is acceptable if the patient has limited pulmonary reserve. Wedge resection, either performed via thoracotomy or video-assisted thoracoscopy, is not recommended for treatment unless the patient absolutely cannot tolerate a segmentectomy or lobectomy. Resection of central, main stem, or more central bronchial tumors can be accomplished by sleeve resection; frozen section margins of 0.5 cm are sufficient. This margin allows for preservation of pulmonary parenchyma. Mediastinal lymph node staging should always be performed. Pneumonectomy is rarely indicated; however, it may be needed for very central tumors that are not amenable to some type of sleeve or bronchoplasty maneuver.

The role of endoscopic resection, whether by forceps or laser, is limited to palliative situations only. Resection for cure is not realistic because this technique can leave tumor behind and provides no nodal staging. Preoperative laser dissection, though, may be useful to open the airway in preparation for a future resection.

Radiation therapy has little role in the treatment of bronchial carcinoids because they tend to be resistant. Despite this fact, there have been reports (33) that have shown some response in a few inoperable patients. Also, postoperative radiation may be considered for atypical carcinoids with lymph node metastasis if complete resection has not been possible.

Similarly, chemotherapy has little effect and probably has no role in the primary treatment of bronchial carcinoids, although it has been used adjunctively for atypical carcinoids. Etoposide and cisplatin have response rates of up to 67% in patients with atypical carcinoids. Combination therapy has been shown to be effective in a limited number of patients (34, 35).

RESULTS

Bronchial carcinoids have been shown to be slow growing and to have a prolonged natural history. Therefore, the long-term prognosis tends to be excellent. Survival depends on the grade, type of carcinoid tumor, and stage at the time of resection. In general, because most bronchial carcinoids of the typical variety are without lymph node metastasis, 90% of patients are alive at 5 years (Table 40.2). Patients with stage I typical carcinoids have been shown to have a 5-year survival of 94% and a 25-year survival of 66% (10). If lymph nodes are involved, the 5-year survival is decreased but is still 71% (12). Patients with atypical carcinoids have a poorer survival with only 57% alive at 5 years.

CONCLUSIONS

Bronchial carcinoids are malignant tumors of the lung with a controversial cell of origin. Despite the potential for invasion and distant metastasis, the long-term survival is excellent if treated adequately. Presentation can be occult, and a high index of suspicion remains important for early diagnosis. Bronchoscopy

TABLE 40.2. Survival for Resected Typical Carcinoid Tumors

INSTITUTION	YEAR	NO. OF PATIENTS	SURVIVAL (%) 5-YR	SURVIVAL (%) 10-YR
National Survey (NCI)	1974	151	96	...
Mayo Clinic	1976	190	94	87
University of Chicago	1980	13	96	...
Toronto	1980	65	65	...
Massachusetts General	1984	111	90	82
Middlesex (London)	1984	79	96	94
Memorial Sloan–Kettering	1985	95	92	77
Los Angeles County Registry	1985	115	95	...
Denmark Tumor Registry	1985	82	89	85
Emory/State of Iowa	1987	96	96	...
Lund, Sweden	1987	91	93	...
Essen-Heidhausen, FRG	1990	210	97	95
Present series	1992	106	93	90

From Harpole DH Jr, Feldman JM, Buchanan S, Young WG, Wolfe WG. Bronchial carcinoid tumors: a retrospective analysis of 126 patients. Ann Thorac Surg 1992;54:50–55.

remains the gold standard for diagnosis, and surgical resection is the only acceptable treatment.

REFERENCES

1. Laennec RTH. Traite de l'auscultation mediate et des maladies des poumons et du coeur. 3rd ed. Paris: Chaude, 1831:1.
2. Kramer R. Adenoma of bronchus. Ann Otol Rhinol Laryngol 1930;39:689–695.
3. Alp M, Ucanok K, Dogan R, et al. Surgical treatment of bronchial adenomas: results of 29 cases and review of the literature. Thorac Cardiovasc Surg 1987;35:290–294.
4. Pearse AGE. The cytochemistry and ultrastructure of polypeptide hormone-producing cells of the APUD series and the embryologic, physiologic and pathologic implications of the concept. J Histochem Cytochem 1969;17:303–313.
5. Pearse AGE. The diffuse neuroendocrine system and the APUD concept: related "endocrine" peptides in brain, intestine, pituitary, placenta, and anuran cutaneous glands. Med Biol 1977;55:115–125.
6. Bensch KG, Gordon GB, Miller LR. Electron microscopic and biochemical studies on the bronchial carcinoid tumor. Cancer 1965;18:592–602.
7. Payne WS, Fontana RS, Woolner LB. Bronchial tumors originating from mucous glands: current classification and unusual manifestations. Med Clin North Am 1964;48:945–960.
8. Gould VE, Linnoila RI, Memoli VA, Warren WH. Neuroendocrine components of the bronchopulmonary tract: hyperplasias, dysplasias, and neoplasms. Lab Invest 1983;49:519–537.
9. Paladugu RR, Benfield JR, Pak HY, Ross RK, Teplitz RL. Bronchopulmonary Kulchitsky cell carcinomas. A new classification scheme for typical and atypical carcinoids. Cancer 1985;55:1303–1311.
10. Okike N, Bernatz PE, Woolner LB. Carcinoid tumors of the lung. Ann Thorac Surg 1976;22:270–277.
11. Engelbreth-Holm J. Benign bronchial adenomas. Acta Chir Scand 1944–45;90:383–409.
12. Arrigoni MG, Woolner LB, Bernatz PE. Atypical carcinoid tumors of the lung. J Thorac Cardiovasc Surg 1972;64:413–421.
13. Whitwell F. Tumourlets of the lung. J Pathol Bacteriol 1955;70:529–541.
14. Cutz E, Chan W, Kay JM, Chamberlain DW. Immunoperoxidase staining for serotonin, bombesin, calcitonin, and Leu-enkephalin in pulmonary tumorlets, bronchial carcinoids, and oat cell carcinomas. Lab Invest 1982;46:16A.
15. Wain JC Jr, Pak SHY, Benfield JR. Immunohistochemistry and new trends in the diagnosis of carcinoids. In: Martini N, Vogt-Moykopf I, eds. Thoracic surgery: frontiers and uncommon neoplasms. St. Louis: Mosby, 1989:249–257.
16. DeCaro LF, Paladugu R, Benfield JR, Lovisatti L, Pak H, Teplitz RL. Typical and atypical carcinoids within the pulmonary APUD tumor spectrum. J Thorac Cardiovasc Surg 1983;86:528–536.
17. Brown WH. A case of pluriglandular syndrome: "diabetes of bearded women." Lancet 1928;2:1022–1023.
18. Hamperl H. Uber gutartige bronchialtumoren (cylindrome und carcinoide). Virchows Arch Pathol Anat 1937;300:46–88.
19. Godwin JD II, Brown CC. Comparative epidemiology of carcinoid and oat-cell tumors of the lung. Cancer 1977;40:1671–1673.
20. Kincaid-Smith P, Brossy JJ. A case of bronchial adenoma with liver metastasis. Thorax 1956;11:36–40.
21. Melmon KL, Sjoerdsma A, Mason DT. Distinctive clinical and therapeutic aspects of the syndrome associated with bronchial carcinoid tumors. Am J Med 1965;39:568–581.
22. Leinung MC, Young WF Jr, Whitaker MD, Scheithauer BW, Trastek VF, Kvols LK. Diagnosis of corticotropin-producing bronchial carcinoid tumors causing Cushing's syndrome. Mayo Clin Proc 1990;65:1314–1321.
23. Mason AMS, Ratcliffe JG, Buckle RM, Mason AS. ACTH secretion by bronchial carcinoid tumours. Clin Endocrinol 1972;1:3–25.
24. Zarate A, Kovacs K, Flores M, Moran C, Felix I. ACTH and CRF-producing bronchial carcinoid associated with Cushing's syndrome. Clin Endocrinol 1986;24:523–529.
25. Jex RK, van Heerden JA, Carpenter PC, Grant CS. Ectopic ACTH syndrome. Am J Surg 1985;149:276–281.
26. Limper AH, Carpenter PC, Scheithauer B, Staats BA. The Cushing syndrome induced by bronchial carcinoid tumors. Ann Intern Med 1992;117:209–214.
27. Davila DG, Dunn WF, Tazelaar HD, Pairolero PC. Bronchial carcinoid tumors. Mayo Clin Proc 1993;68:795–803.
28. Hurt R, Bates M. Carcinoid tumours of the bronchus: a 33 year experience. Thorax 1984;39:617–623.
29. Harpole DH Jr, Feldman JM, Buchanan S, Young WG, Wolfe WG. Bronchial carcinoid tumors: a retrospective analysis of 126 patients. Ann Thorac Surg 1992;54:50–55.
30. Rozenman J, Pausner R, Lieberman Y, Gamsu G. Bronchial adenoma. Chest 1987;92:145–147.
31. Stamatis G, Freitag L, Greschuchna D. Limited and radical resection for tracheal and bronchopulmonary carcinoid tumour: report on 227 cases. Eur J Cardiothorac Surg 1990;4:527–532.
32. Martensson H, Bottcher G, Hambraeus G, Sundler F, Willen H, Nobin A. Bronchial carcinoids: an analysis of 91 cases. World J Surg 1987;11:356–363.
33. Baldwin JN, Grimes OF. Bronchial adenomas. Surg Gynecol Obstet 1967;124:813–818.
34. Moertel CG, Kvols LK, O'Connell MJ, Rubin J. Treatment of neuroendocrine carcinomas with combined etoposide and cisplatin: evidence of major therapeutic activity in the anaplastic variants of these neoplasms. Cancer 1991;68:227–232.
35. Marsh HM, Martin JK Jr, Kvols LK, et al. Carcinoid crisis during anesthesia: successful treatment with a somatostatin analogue. Anesthesiology 1987;66:89–91.

41

TRACHEAL TUMORS

Douglas J. Mathisen

Experience with tracheal tumors is limited because they occur at a rate of approximately three new cases per 1 million people. Experience has been gained from a few institutions with a special interest in airway surgery, but long-term follow-up is limited. Randomized trials comparing different forms of treatment obviously are not available. Rough guidelines for management have been established, however, based on this limited experience.

The rarity of this tumor and the apparently normal chest radiograph associated with it account for the difficulty in initial diagnosis. The benign and low-grade malignant tumors grow at a slow rate and are associated with the insidious onset of symptoms. Because of the apparently normal radiographs, patients often are treated for other illnesses, sometimes for many months, before the diagnosis of a tracheal tumor is established. It is common for these patients to have undergone the full gamut of asthma treatment, including high-dose steroid therapy. Squamous carcinoma of the trachea is much more aggressive, and patients usually present earlier with symptoms of hemoptysis, stridor, or paralyzed vocal cords. The key to successful management is a high degree of suspicion in patients with atypical airway symptoms being considered for a diagnosis of adult onset asthma.

The surgical management of these tumors requires an in-depth knowledge of airway surgery. The surgeon must be familiar with the indications and contraindications for surgery, techniques of airway management, techniques of resection and reconstruction, release maneuvers to reduce anastomotic tension, perioperative care, and indications and timing of postoperative adjuvant treatment.

The experience at the Massachusetts General Hospital exceeds 200 patients (1), the largest reported series, and it allows certain inferences to be made. Even these data are somewhat inconclusive, however.

TUMOR CLASSIFICATION

Approximately two thirds of primary tracheal tumors are of two histologic types: squamous cell carcinoma and adenoid cystic carcinoma, formally called cylindroma. These two types occur in about the same numbers (1–6). The remaining third of the tumors are distributed widely among a heterogeneous group of tumors, both malignant and benign. A variety of secondary tumors involve the trachea. These include carcinomas of the larynx, thyroid, lung, and esophagus. Rarely, tumors such as carcinoma of the breast and mediastinal lymphoma may metastasize to the submucosa of the trachea or to the mediastinum, with secondary invasion of the trachea.

In the Massachusetts General Hospital series, 70 of the 198 patients had primary squamous cell carcinoma of the trachea or carina (36% of the series), 80 had adenoid cystic carcinomas (40%), and the remaining 48 (24%) had a variety of benign and malignant lesions (1). (Table 41.1).

Squamous cell carcinomas may be either exophytic or ulcerative. They may also be multiple and scattered over a considerable length of trachea. The tumor metastasizes to the regional lymph nodes and, in its more aggressive and late forms, invades mediastinal structures. Its progress appears to be relatively rapid, compared with that of adenoid cystic carcinoma. Forty percent of patients had either a prior squamous carcinoma of the aerodigestive tract or subsequently developed one. Careful screening and follow-up of these patients is indicated.

Adenoid cystic carcinoma often has a very prolonged symptomatic period, sometimes extending for years. After treatment, many years may pass before a recurrence is noted. Adenoid cystic carcinoma may extend over long distances submucosally in the airways as well as perineurally. It spreads to regional lymph

TABLE 41.1. Other Primary Tracheal Tumors

TYPE	NO. OF PATIENTS
Benign	
Squamous papillomata	
Multiple	4
Solitary	1
Pleomorphic adenoma	2
Granular cell tumor	2
Fibrous histiocytoma	1
Leiomyoma	2
Chondroma	2
Chondroblastoma	1
Schwannoma	1
Paraganglioma	2
Hemangioendothelioma	1
Vascular malformation	2
Intermediate	
Carcinoid	10
Mucoepidermoid	4
Plexiform neurofibroma	1
Pseudosarcoma	1
Malignant	
Adenocarcinoma	1
Adenosquamous carcinoma	1
Small cell carcinoma	1
Atypical carcinoid	1
Melanoma	1
Chondrosarcoma	1
Spindle cell sarcoma	2
Rhabdomyosarcoma	1

nodes, although less characteristically than does squamous cell carcinoma. Although it may invade the thyroid or the muscular coats of the esophagus by contiguity, adenoid cystic carcinoma that has not been treated surgically frequently displaces mediastinal structures before actually invading them. Metastases to the lungs are common. These may grow very slowly over a period of many years and remain asymptomatic until they are huge. Metastases to bone and other organs occur.

The group of tumors other than squamous cell and adenoid cystic carcinoma, although representing only about one third of the series, was composed of several tumor types and varying degrees of malignancy (Table 41.1), including both epithelial and mesenchymal neoplasms. Multiple squamous papillomas were not resected but were removed by cryotherapy, electrocoagulation, or laser treatment, depending on technology available at the time. One of the patients with pleomorphic adenoma had had a similar tumor excised from a salivary gland years before. There had been no evidence of other metastases, and the lesion thus was classified as a primary tracheal tumor. A patient with rhabdomyosarcoma had an isolated pedunculated lesion without extratracheal penetration; however, he had a cervical rhabdomyosarcoma treated by a radical operation and intensive irradiation 6 years earlier without evidence of local recurrence. No other foci developed. This lesion may well have been a secondary site. The plexiform neurofibroma and the two paragangliomas were inextricably involved with the airway wall and appeared to have originated there. The vascular malformations involved arterial and venous components throughout the neck and mediastinum but had localized intraluminal obstructing protrusions. The small cell carcinoma was confined to the trachea, without any involvement or adherence of lung. The melanoma appeared to be solitary, without any previous known skin lesions and without evidence of retinal or other primary tumor. Additional patients with tumors of apparent mediastinal origin were excluded.

SEX

Squamous cell carcinoma occurred predominantly in men (52 men, 17 women). The distribution was similar to that of squamous carcinoma of the lung. Every patient with primary squamous carcinoma of the trachea was a cigarette smoker. In contrast, the male to female ratio of adenoid cystic carcinoma was essentially even (41:39). Smoking history of these patients appeared to be incidental. The distribution of the other tumors was fairly even, with 26 male and 22 female patients represented.

AGE INCIDENCE

Age incidence is shown in Table 41.2. Squamous cell carcinoma predominated in patients in their sixth or seventh decade. This finding is similar to the incidence of squamous cell carcinoma of the lung. Adenoid cystic carcinoma, in contrast, was distributed between patients aged 20 and 69 years, with a slight peak in the

TABLE 41.2. Incidence of Primary Tracheal Tumors by Age

	NO. OF TUMORS		
AGE (YR)	SQUAMOUS	ADENOID CYSTIC	OTHER
1–10	. . .	. . .	4
11–19	. . .	. . .	8
20–29	1	13	11
30–39	1	16	9
40–49	9	19	5
50–59	29	15	6
60–69	24	13	4
70–79	6	5	1

fifth decade. Other tumors showed a scattered distribution because of their variety of types.

Secondary tumors involving the trachea have been noted. Both papillary and follicular carcinoma of the thyroid and mixed varieties of the two may invade the trachea primarily, usually at the level of the isthmus (7). Thus, a patient presenting initially with hemoptysis may have carcinoma of the thyroid. Invasion of the trachea by thyroid carcinoma is best managed by resection with airway reconstruction. Localized extension of tumor also may require partial esophageal resection or radical resection, including laryngectomy with mediastinal tracheostomy. More commonly, invasion is seen after thyroidectomy for carcinoma, in cases in which the surgeon was aware that the tumor was being shaved off of the trachea. In such cases, concurrent or early resection of the involved trachea should be considered.

SIGNS AND SYMPTOMS

Tracheal tumors may present insidiously. Their most common symptoms are cough (37%), hemoptysis (41%), and signs of progressive airway obstruction, including shortness of breath on exertion (54%), wheezing and stridor (35%), and, less commonly, dysphagia or hoarseness (7%) (Table 41.3). Wheezing, in particular, may cause diagnostic errors. It is not commonly appreciated that wheezing for a prolonged period may be a predominant symptom of a tracheal tumor. A standard chest radiograph usually shows clear lung fields, and on this basis the physician assumes that no organic mass lesion is present. Patients often are treated for adult onset asthma. Hemoptysis also may not be pursued aggressively in the face of an apparently normal chest radiograph. Another presentation is with unilateral or bilateral recurrent attacks of pneumonitis that may respond to antibiotic treatment but then recur.

Signs and symptoms may vary with the type of tumor. Hemoptysis is prominent in patients with squamous cell carcinoma and usually leads to earlier diagnosis. The presence of hoarseness as an early symptom may signify advanced disease. Adenoid cystic carcinoma more often presents with wheezing or stridor as a predominant symptom, leading to a delay in diagnosis. Only a little more than one quarter of these patients have hemoptysis early in the course of their disease. Dyspnea, however, may be prominent. In one study the mean duration of symptoms prior to diagnosis in patients with squamous cell carcinoma of the trachea was only 4 months, whereas in those with adenoid cystic carcinoma it was 18 months (4). In some benign or low-grade malignant tumors of the trachea, the mean duration of an incorrect diagnosis was up to 4 years. The mean duration of symptoms of miscellaneous malignant tumors was 11 months.

DIAGNOSIS

Diagnosis long after the symptoms commence is the rule rather than the exception. Many patients present initially with troublesome cough, dyspnea on exertion, and, eventually, wheezing and stridor. The presence of normal lung fields on chest radiographs usually lulls the physician into a sense of security. The patient is frequently misdiagnosed as asthmatic and treated as such. Only when hemoptysis or recurrent focal pneumonia occurs is bronchoscopy done. In a few patients, flow-volume curves demonstrate the loss of peaks, and findings suggest upper airway obstruction. If tumor is suspected, simple radiologic studies, avoiding contrast medium, usually show the location and extent of the tumor (8). It is as important to outline the extent of the grossly uninvolved airway remaining for reconstruction as it is to define precisely the extent of the tumor. The functioning of the larynx also is studied fluoroscopically. Bronchoscopy may be done cautiously as a separate procedure if it is especially indicated. If the tumor appears to be highly obstructing or exceedingly vascular, then biopsy should not be performed until arrangements have been made for a definitive surgical approach under the same anesthesia.

Definitive bronchoscopy, when done at the time of a projected resection, must assume the availability of accurate frozen section diagnosis. The flexible bronchoscope is used to look beyond a very extensive tumor, especially at the carinal level, to check for the possibility of distal infiltration, which occurs with an

TABLE 41.3. Symptoms of Tracheal Tumors in 84 Patients

SYMPTOM	NO. OF CASES
Dyspnea	44
Hemoptysis	28
Cough	22
Wheeze	16
Dysphagia	13
Change in voice, hoarseness	13[a]
Stridor	12
Pneumonia	10

Data from Weber AL, Grillo HC. Tracheal tumors: a radiological, clinical, and pathologic evaluation of 84 cases. Radiol Clin North Am 1987; 16:227.
[a]Eight of 13 patients had vocal cord paralysis.

adenoid cystic carcinoma. Caution must be exercised in using flexible bronchoscopy in the outpatient setting when dealing with tumors producing high-grade obstruction. Secretions, bleeding, or swelling may precipitate sudden airway obstruction. The patient may die if adequate facilities are not available to secure the airway. Careful measurements are crucial and are best done by rigid bronchoscopy. Such measurements are needed to determine the extent of involvement and amount of remaining airway. The important measurements are the carina, bottom of the tumor, top of the tumor, and vocal cords. Approximately half of the trachea in an adult can be removed and reconstructed with appropriate release maneuvers. Of course, this amount varies with body habitus, the age of patient, and prior operations. Half of the length of the trachea should be considered the upper limit of safe resection. Esophagoscopy is mandatory if esophageal symptoms persist or radiologic evaluation suggests involvement.

RADIOLOGIC EVALUATION

The primary diagnostic techniques for identifying tracheal abnormalities are radiologic study and bronchoscopy. All too often a plain chest radiograph considered to be normal shows an abnormality of the tracheal air column. Relatively simple radiologic techniques, without the use of contrast media, will delineate tracheal pathology (8). The location of the lesion, its linear extent, extratracheal involvement, and, of particular importance to the surgeon, the amount of airway uninvolved by the process can be determined. In addition to standard views of the chest in various projections, centered high enough to show tracheal detail, anteroposterior filtered tracheal views of the entire airway (from the larynx to the carina) are obtained. A lateral neck view, using soft tissue technique with the patient swallowing and the neck hyperextended to bring the trachea up above the clavicles, is useful in defining pathology in the upper trachea. Fluoroscopy demonstrates functional asymmetry of the vocal cords if present and also provides additional information about the extent of the lesion. Spot films usually are all that are required. In some cases polytomography (anteroposterior and lateral views) gives additional detail, particularly of mediastinal involvement. Barium esophagography is useful in defining esophageal involvement by extrinsic compression or invasion. Computed (axial) tomography (CT) offers little information over that provided by standard radiologic techniques, except to define an extratracheal component. The exact role of magnetic resonance imaging (MRI) has yet to be defined. Sagittal and coronal views, however, have been helpful in certain cases and may give more accurate detail than standard radiographic techniques.

AIRWAY MANAGEMENT

Crucial to the management of all problems of the trachea is the ability to control the airway. Tracheal tumors may present as emergency obstructive airway problems. Endotracheal intubation may be impossible and even dangerous because it may lead to complete airway obstruction, especially in patients with high tracheal lesions. Simple maneuvers to elevate the head of the patient, administration of cool mist and oxygen, and careful sedation may allow control of the airway in an elective manner. Control is best accomplished in the operating room, where an assortment of rigid bronchoscopes, dilators, biopsy forceps, and instruments to perform emergency tracheostomy are available (9). Anesthesia, as in elective tracheal operations, is best accomplished by inhalation technique (10, 11). It requires patience on the part of the anesthesiologist and surgeon to allow the patient to become anesthetized adequately. Induction of anesthesia deep enough to allow rigid bronchoscopy may take as long as 20 minutes. Paralyzing agents should not be used because of the potential for the lethal combination of airway obstruction and apnea.

The initial evaluation should be done with a rigid bronchoscope carefully inserted through the vocal cords, stopping just proximal to the level of the obstruction. Rigid telescopes can be used to assess the obstruction. Most tumors, even those causing nearly total obstruction, allow a rigid bronchoscope to be passed beyond them. After the status of the distal airway has been assessed, the tumor can be removed partially with biopsy forceps to determine its consistency and vascularity. For most tumors the tip of the rigid bronchoscope can be used to "core out" most of the tumor. The tumor can then be grasped with biopsy forceps and removed. If bleeding ensues, the bronchoscope may be passed into the distal airway for ventilation. The bronchoscope serves to tamponade the bleeding. Direct application of epinephrine-soaked pledgets helps to control any persistent oozing. Very rarely the surgeon may have to resort to direct cautery (with insulated electrodes) in these situations. The use of the laser is time consuming, costly, and rarely advantageous, compared with the cautery technique.

Endotracheal removal of malignant tumors, mechanically or by laser, is only a temporary measure. The use of these techniques in emergency situations enables more thorough evaluation of the patient and allows surgery to be performed electively. Having been treated for refractory asthma, many patients with low-grade tumors are on high doses of steroids at the time of presentation. By establishing an airway the steroids may be tapered and discontinued, and a subsequent operation can be performed without the threat of impaired healing. Repeat core-out of the tumor may be required during the interval of steroid tapering.

These maneuvers are also sometimes used at the time of elective surgery if the patient has presented with a stable airway. Core-out of the tumor allows assessment of the distal airway, placement of an endotracheal tube, and provision of an adequate lumen to prevent CO_2 accumulation early in the procedure. At the time of tracheal resection, this tube can be pulled back or removed and a sterile cuffed endotracheal tube (Tovell tube; Rusch, Inc., Duluth, GA) inserted into the distal airway. Sterile connecting tubing is passed to the anesthesiologist and connected to allow ventilation of the patient. The Tovell tube can be removed whenever necessary for suctioning or placement of sutures. At the conclusion of the operation, the original endotracheal tube is advanced into the distal airway and sutures are tied. The patient should be breathing spontaneously at the end of the procedure so that extubation can be performed in the operating room. High-frequency ventilation has been used with equal success intraoperatively. High-frequency ventilation is useful in certain complex carinal reconstructions.

ANESTHESIA

Anesthesia for tracheal reconstruction, especially when there is a high degree of airway obstruction distally, is best administered by Ethane (Anaquest, Inc., Liberty Corner, NJ) inhalation (10, 11). A slow induction may be necessary if there is a high degree of airway obstruction. This technique is preferable and safer than paralysis of respiration with a consequent urgent need to establish an airway. The surgeon should have available an array of rigid bronchoscopes from pediatric to adult sizes as the induction commences. The residual airway through which the patient is breathing may measure as little as 2 or 3 mm in diameter. In most cases tumors are not circumferential. After bronchoscopy a small endotracheal tube can often be insinuated past a highly obstructive tumor. In other cases the tube is left above the tumor. This technique contrasts with the circumferential stenoses seen in some inflammatory lesions. In rare cases it may be necessary to nibble away bits of tumor with biopsy forceps to enlarge the channel for passage of a tube.

The patient should be extubated and able to breathe spontaneously at the conclusion of the procedure. Particularly when the trachea has been shortened greatly, it is desirable that not even a low pressure cuff lie in contact with the anastomosis for any time. Cardiopulmonary bypass has been found to be unnecessary even in complex carinal reconstructions, and it is of no use whatsoever in upper tracheal resections.

SURGICAL TECHNIQUES

The patient must be positioned so there is full access to whatever operative field may be necessary. A cervical collar incision is employed for relatively limited tumors that present in the upper half of the trachea. Partial sternal division through a vertical midline extension provides greater access to the upper mediastinum (Fig. 41.1). If the larynx must be exposed, this can be done either from beneath the upper flap of the collar incision or through a second short horizontal incision above the hyoid. If the tumor appears to be somewhat longer or of a type that may prove to be more extensive, such as in adenoid cystic carcinoma, the patient must be positioned for potential further extension of the incision into the right fourth interspace

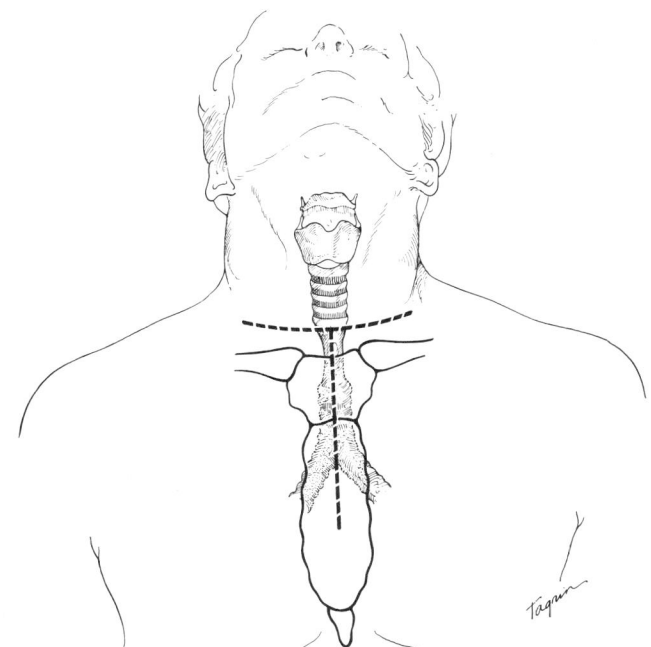

FIGURE 41.1. Incisions for tracheal resection. Most tracheal operations are done through a low-collar incision. For very low lesions, a T incision is made and a partial upper sternotomy performed to give exposure to the distal trachea. (A full sternotomy is not required.)

to the posterior axillary line. For this reason the right arm is best draped and kept within the field so that it can be moved back and forth.

The preferred approach to tumors of the lower trachea and carina is through a high right posterolateral thoracotomy. Again, the right arm is draped and kept in the operative field. The field includes the entire neck for access to the hyoid region, larynx, and trachea for possible cervical mobilization and laryngeal release.

In rare cases individual incisions are designed. For example, in a case involving a subtotal removal of the trachea or if a laryngotracheectomy may be necessary, a long, somewhat lower, horizontal incision is used. In this way a vertical incision is avoided to preserve the possibility of mediastinal tracheostomy (12). The latter is rarely needed but must be planned for in advance.

In the dissection of the tumor, an effort is made to take as much tissue as possible from around the level of the tumor, limited as this may be. The trachea is approached above and below the lesion, and these areas are cleared first. If the primary tumor is a malignancy of the thyroid gland, it may be necessary to include strap muscles en bloc, sometimes accompanied by a partial neck dissection. With other primary tumors of the upper trachea, resection of one or both lobes of the thyroid on the side in which the tumor is based is done simply to avoid the possibility of exposing tumor that may have invaded the tracheal wall at that point. Each of these situations must be individualized and approached with caution.

The surgical approach used for tumors contrasts with the approach to the trachea in benign disease, in which dissection is kept close to the trachea and possibly scar-encased recurrent laryngeal nerves are not visualized. With surgery for tumors, the nerves are identified at a distance from the location of the tumor and followed toward the area of tumor. Sometimes it is necessary to sacrifice a recurrent nerve because of its involvement with tumor, even when no functional paralysis is evident. Special care must be exerted in the right transthoracic approach not to injure the left recurrent nerve because the aortic surface is approached from the right side. Adjacent lymph nodes are included with the dissection. Only a limited node dissection may be done, however, without endangering the blood supply of the trachea (13). This blood supply enters segmentally, principally from the branches of the inferior thyroid artery above and the bronchial arteries below. Contributions also arise from the internal mammary artery, the highest intercostal artery, and other esophageal branches. It is critically important not to dissect around the trachea for any great distance if that portion of trachea is to be left in the patient. As a matter of safety, it is best not to free circumferentially more than 1 or 2 cm of tracheal length if the tissue is to remain in the patient. Devascularization leads to later necrosis and stenosis.

The entire pretracheal plane is freed bluntly to the carina and, often, part way down the anterior surface of the right and left main bronchi. Care is taken to spare the lateral pedicles, which contain the blood supply described. Once the apparent lower level of the tumor has been identified, lateral traction sutures (2-0 Vicryl; Ethicon, Inc., Piscataway, NJ) are placed through the full thickness of the tracheal wall in the midline on either side at a distance estimated to be one or more centimeters distal to the eventual line of transection. A flexible, sterile endotracheal tube is prepared in advance to be available in the field along with sterile connecting anesthesia tubing.

The trachea is opened horizontally opposite to the lower margin of the tumor, and the lumen is inspected cautiously. If the incision is not sufficiently distal to the tumor, a lower level is selected. The trachea is then transected cleanly and horizontally. Intubation is carried out across the operative field. A small sliver of tissue may be taken from the distal resection margin at the point closest to the tumor and sent for immediate frozen section analysis to determine if the distal margin is adequate. The anesthesia tube from above is withdrawn at this point. If the line of resection in the trachea is close to the cricoid, it is advisable to suture a catheter to the tip of the endotracheal tube so that, if the tube is withdrawn above the vocal cords, it can be pulled back down again later with ease. An assistant is assigned the tasks of stabilizing the endotracheal tube in the distal trachea, assuring that the tip does not pass into the right main bronchus, and seeing that blood that puddles above the cuff is suctioned away constantly. Blood seeping past the cuff into the distal tracheobronchial tree may produce shunting postoperatively.

The divided end of the trachea may then be grasped with forceps and placed on tension, and the specimen may be further dissected upward. On occasion, if the location of the tumor is slightly lower, it is better to do the transection above the tumor and leave the tumor in place with an endotracheal tube passed beyond it to provide a reasonable handle until a clean line for transection can be established below the tumor. Lateral traction sutures also are placed in the airway above the level of transection, as they were below it. If the transection is high, the sutures may be placed in the larynx rather than in the trachea. Occasionally, it has been necessary to bevel, obliquely, a portion of the lower larynx, i.e., half (or sometimes more) of the cricoid cartilage. If the esophageal wall is involved, as demonstrated by preoperative barium swallow, esophagoscopy, or, more often, observation in the operative field, a partial-thickness or full-thickness resection of the anterior or anterolateral esophageal wall may be necessary. The esophagus may be reconstructed with layers of interrupted 4-0 silk sutures over an in-laying nasogastric tube. A pedicled strap muscle may sometimes be useful for further reinforcement.

After removal of the specimen and establishment of negative transection margins at either end, reconstruction may be approached (Fig. 41.2). The surgeon and assistant draw together the tracheal traction sutures (2-0 Vicryl) on their respective sides, while the anesthetist tentatively flexes the neck. The chin is brought down in an arc toward the sternum. Gentle traction on the lateral sutures should now approximate the two ends. There is no definitive rule about how much trachea may be taken out and how much approximation may be achieved in this relatively simple fashion. In young, relatively thin, supple patients, even 60% of the trachea may be resected and a simple end-to-end anastomosis done without excessive tension. In an older, heavy-set patient, in whom the angle of the trachea is different, it may be impossible to bring the ends together in this way even after only 3 cm of trachea has been resected. When excessive tension is applied, the likelihood of separation or stenosis increases markedly in the adult. Tension is even less well tolerated in pediatric patients. Intraoperative clinical appraisal of tension is essential in determining the extent of the resection.

If further relaxation is needed, a variety of maneuvers can be used. Suprahyoid laryngeal release or the Montgomery maneuver is particularly effective, especially after resections of the proximal trachea (14). A length of 1 to 2.5 cm may be obtained, primarily anteriorly, where the length is needed most.

Anastomosis is performed with fine, strong, absorbable suture material (4-0 Vicryl), preferably coated (Fig. 41.2). Its use has reduced to zero the incidence of suture-line granulomas—in sharp contrast with prior experience.

All sutures are placed individually in circumferential fashion beginning posteriorly and working anteriorly, first on one side and then on the other (Fig. 41.2). These sutures are placed at approximately 4-mm intervals 3 mm back from the cut edge of the trachea. Anterolaterally, they pass through cartilage. No effort is made to pass sutures submucosally. The sutures are clipped carefully to the drapes so they will not become confused, the endotracheal tube is removed from across the operative field, and the proximal endotracheal tube is readvanced distally. The patient's head and neck are supported securely in the flexed position. The lateral traction sutures are tied to approximate the tracheal ends without telescoping them. The anastomotic sutures are tied from front to back on both sides, and the ends of each are cut as they are tied. The lateral traction sutures are withdrawn. Saline is placed in the wound, the endotracheal tube cuff is deflated, and the anastomosis is tested for air-tightness. Occasionally, the thyroid isthmus is sutured over a high anastomosis, or other tissues are placed over it. If the innominate artery has not been dissected bare deliberately, there is no particular need for interposition of muscle between it and the operative field. If there is any question, it may be better to interpose a pedicled strap muscle or other tissue. Closure is made in the usual fashion, wiring the sternum if it has been divided partially and closing the other tissues in layers after insertion of soft suction drains. If possible, the patient is extubated on the operating table.

If the tumor involves the carina, various reconstructive techniques are used (Fig. 41.3). Unless the tumor is very small, it is rarely adaptable to reconstruction by approximating the right and left main bronchus to form a new carina and then attaching it to

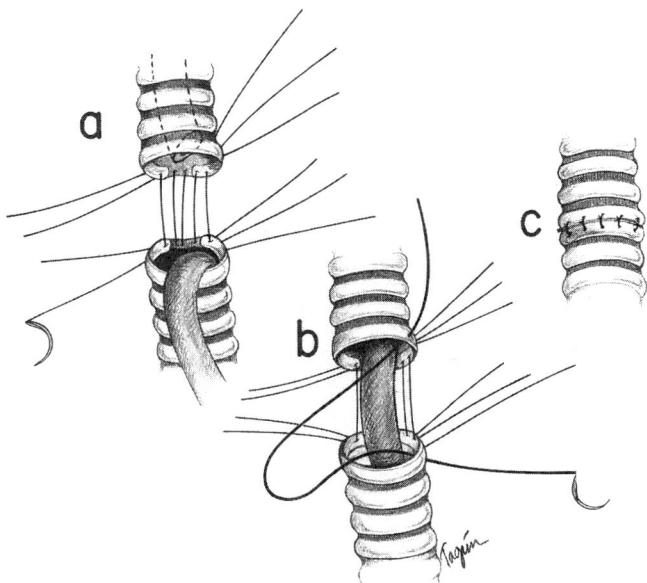

FIGURE 41.2. Once the pathologic segment of trachea is removed, reconstruction begins. A. Lateral traction sutures of 2-0 Vicryl are placed in the mid-lateral position of the proximal and distal trachea. B. Interrupted sutures of 2-0 Vicryl are carefully placed in an open fashion circumferentially. C. The traction sutures are approximated and tied. The individual sutures are tied and the anastomosis completed.

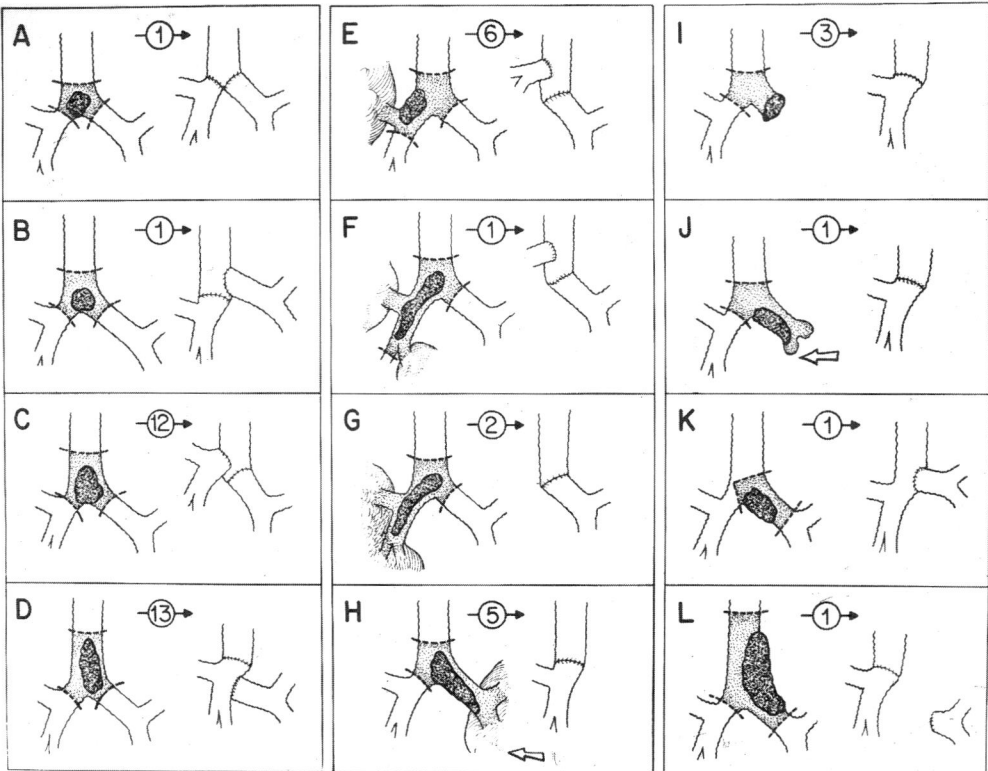

FIGURE 41.3. Modes of carinal resection and reconstruction used. Circled numbers indicate the number of patients. Open arrows indicate the side of approach when not conventionally right sided. A. A limited resection permits carinal restitution. B. Technique used in initial carinal resection; technique in Figure 41.3A would then be used. C. More extensive resection. D. Greater length of trachea. Technique of Barclay and coworkers (10). E. Involvement of right main bronchus and right upper lobe bronchus requires right upper lobectomy. F. Middle lobe also is removed. The right lower lobe bronchus may be anastomosed to left main bronchus. G. Right carinal pneumonectomy. H. Left carinal pneumonectomy. I. Resection of carina after previous left pneumonectomy. J. Resection of carina with extra-long stump. K. Wedge removal of left main bronchus from the right. L. Tracheocarinal resection with long segment of the left main bronchus. Exclusion of remaining left lung from the right. Left pneumonectomy also through bilateral thoracotomy.

the trachea (Fig. 41.3A). Such suturing anchors the carina very low in the mediastinum, and, if more trachea has been excised, approximation is not possible. More commonly, either the right or left main bronchus is sutured to the trachea, and a lateral anastomosis of the other bronchus to the lower portion of the tracheal wall is performed above the initial anastomosis.

The principles and techniques of anastomosis are exactly as described previously for tracheal resection. Management of the airway intraoperatively is more difficult and requires close cooperation with the anesthesiologist. Jet ventilation has been useful in some of the more complicated reconstructions. All intrathoracic anastomoses are covered with a second layer of either pedicled pleura or pericardial fat pad, just as in sleeve lobectomy. It is important to interpose tissue between the airway suture line and adjacent pulmonary vessels. Omentum is used only when prior irradiation is a factor.

If a recurrent laryngeal nerve is involved by tumor, the nerve is sacrificed. Usually the nerves are identified and carefully saved whenever possible. Local paratracheal lymph nodes are excised with the specimen if possible. Extensive lymph node dissection cannot be done for fear of destroying the blood supply to the residual trachea.

Resection usually is controlled with frozen sections to be certain that the margins are clear. Adenoid cystic carcinoma, in particular, may extend for distances that may make total resection of microscopic tumor impossible. Irradiation for positive microscopic margins is effective in preventing local recurrence.

TREATMENT RESULTS

One hundred forty-seven of the 198 tumors were resected by the following modes: (*a*) resection and reconstruction of trachea or carina; (*b*) laryngotracheal resection, with or without cervicomediastinal exenteration; or (*c*) staged reconstruction with excision of the tumor in the hope of restoring airway continuity with cervical cutaneous tubes (Table 41.4). Eleven patients

TABLE 41.4. Primary Tracheal Tumors

VARIABLE	SQUAMOUS	ADENOID CYSTIC	OTHER	TOTAL
Number of lesions	70	80	48	198
Percentage of total	36	40	24	100
Surgical treatment	50	65	43	158
Excised	44	60	43	147
Percentage of type	63	75	90	74
Explored	6	5	0	11
Resection with reconstruction	41	50	41	132
Trachea	32	22	28	82
Carina	9	28	13	50
Laryngotracheal	1	4	2	7
Staged procedure	2	6	0	8

TABLE 41.5. Surgical Approach to Resection and Reconstruction of Primary Tracheal Tumors

APPROACH	SQUAMOUS	ADENOID CYSTIC	OTHER	TOTAL
Trachea				
Cervical	6	8	12	26
Cervicomediastinal	11	3	6	20
Transthoracic	12	10	10	32
Transpericardial	3	1	0	4
Carina				
Transthoracic	9	25	13	47
Bilateral transthoracic	...	3	...	3
Total	41	50	41	132

underwent exploration only, with or without institution of a tracheostomy or T tube. This report focuses on the 132 patients who had resection and primary reconstruction and does not include those who simply underwent coring out of tumor, placement of a T-tube, or tracheostomy. Seven underwent removal of the larynx and trachea because tumor involved the larynx to the degree that it could not be salvaged functionally. Eight patients underwent staged reconstruction. These procedures were performed when the extent of possible surgical resection was being explored. Because of their complications, high mortality, and the small number of patients who could be carried to completion, the procedure was abandoned. These patients, however, are included in this review as part of the total experience. Most unresected patients received radiotherapy.

Approximately equal numbers of patients with squamous cell carcinoma, adenoid cystic carcinoma, and other types of tumor were amenable to primary resection and reconstruction (41, 50, and 41 patients, respectively). However, the number of patients in each category subjected to tracheal resection, as distinct from carinal resection, varied markedly. Although approximately one third (37%) of patients who had primary reconstruction underwent carinal resection, in the case of adenoid cystic carcinoma, more than half were so treated. Only 9 of 41 patients with squamous carcinoma had carinal resection, reflecting the differing distribution of the tumors.

SURGICAL APPROACH

Operations were planned flexibly so that the approach would be adequate if unexpectedly longer lengths of trachea than anticipated were involved by tumor (Table 41.5). Upper tracheal tumors were explored through a cervical collar incision, with the options to extend exposure through the upper sternum. For mid-tracheal tumors, the option was kept open to extend the incision through a full median sternotomy with the possibility of a a transpericardial approach or through a trapdoor incision through the right fourth interspace. Lower tracheal tumors were most often approached through a right thoracotomy. The earliest operations were performed electively through a trapdoor incision, which allows access to the entire trachea. Median sternotomy with transpericardial approach was used but offers less adequate exposure for extensive tumors (Table 41.6).

Carinal resection was approached principally through a right posterolateral thoracotomy, through a left thoracotomy in a few patients, and through a bilateral thoracotomy in three patients in whom carinal reconstruction with combined left pneumonectomy was anticipated. The modes of reconstruction are diagrammed in Figure 41.3.

TECHNICAL FEATURES

In nine patients (one with squamous, three adenoid cystic, and six with other tumors), laryngoplasty (partial resection of the larynx) was necessary to establish adequate margins around a tumor. Each case was individualized. The trachea was tailored appropriately to mortise into the irregular defect thus created in the larynx. Careful attention was paid to the recurrent laryngeal nerve and its functional state. This type of resection has been described in detail for management of secondary invasion of the airway by thyroid carcinoma (7).

Adjunctive procedures, in addition to pretracheal dissection and cervical flexion, were used to lessen tension on the anastomosis. Laryngeal release was performed in seven patients undergoing tracheal resection and in five undergoing carinal resection. Surgeons at Massachusetts General Hospital have since concluded on the basis of clinical observation, supported by experimental evidence, that laryngeal release does not generally translate into relaxation after carinal resection. It may be useful, however, in patients undergoing extensive resection of the mid trachea as well as the carina. Hilar release, which at least involves a U-shaped incision in the pericardium beneath the inferior pulmonary vein or a complete circumcision of the pericardium around the hilum, was performed in 12 of 32 patents undergoing transthoracic tracheal resection and in 23 of the 50 patients undergoing carinal resections. In addition, 4 patients with adenoid cystic carcinoma undergoing carinal resection had both laryngeal and hilar releases.

Ten patients had varying amounts of thyroidectomy performed to encompass tumors. Seven patients with tracheal tumors, and two with carinal tumors, underwent lateral removal of the esophageal wall, either muscularis alone or the full thickness of the wall. The recurrent laryngeal nerve was deliberately sacrificed in four tracheal resections and in one carinal resection because of tumor involvement. Three patients with squamous carcinoma and one patient with sarcoma had omental pedicles brought up substernally for reinforcement of the suture line. All of these patients had received high-dose irradiation previously.

In two patients with tracheoesophageal fistula caused by adenoid cystic carcinoma, in whom prolonged survival was possible, colon esophageal bypass with exclusion of the fistula was performed.

TABLE 41.6. Results of Surgical Treatment of Primary Tracheal Tumors

VARIABLE	SQUAMOUS	ADENOID CYSTIC	OTHER	TOTAL
Number of tumors resected	44	60	43	147
Operative deaths (resection)	3	8	1	12
Resection, reconstruction				
Trachea	1	0	0	1
Carina	1	4	1	6
Percentage (resection, reconstruction)	5%	8%	2%	5%
Laryngotracheal	0	0	0	0
Staged procedures	1 of 2	4 of 6	0	5
Exploration only	2 of 6	1 of 3	0	3
Survival (resected tumors)				
Dead				
Of tumor	13	7	3	23
Of other cause	6	5	1	12
Alive				
With tumor	0	1	0	1
Without tumor	20	39	35	94
Lost to follow-up	2	0	3	5

OPERATIVE COMPLICATIONS

Anastomotic stenosis developed in two patients undergoing tracheal resection; in one of them the stenosis occurred after a transient air leak had developed (15). The second patient was operated on while still receiving high-dose steroids. Both patients later underwent re-resection successfully. Stenosis developed in four patients after carinal resection. Two patients who had undergone pneumonectomy with carinal resection underwent re-resection successfully, one through a cervical incision because the anastomosis was so high. Two others required upper lobectomy of the reimplanted right lung with reattachment of the bronchus intermedius or lower lobe. Both procedures were successful. Three air leaks were handled conservatively with success. Four patients developed suture line granulomas in the era before absorbable sutures were used. These were managed bronchoscopically. One patient in whom laryngoplasty had been performed showed an elevation of the posterior mucosal flap, which healed in place after brief intubation. One esophageal fistula occurred after transthoracic tracheal resection with extensive full-thickness resection of the esophageal wall. A small fistula healed spontaneously.

Vocal cord paralysis, reversible over time in some cases, occurred in eight patients undergoing tracheal or carinal resection for squamous carcinoma and in three patients undergoing tracheal or carinal resection for adenoid cystic carcinoma. Six patients experienced aspiration on deglutition, principally after laryngeal release necessitated by extended resection. Most resolved over time, although, rarely, a temporary gastrostomy was required. One patient had a small empyema, treated by drainage, after a transthoracic tracheal resection. One patient developed Guillain-Barré syndrome.

Two patients developed acute pulmonary edema after carinal resection with right pneumonectomy. Three others had pneumonia. One patient who underwent carinal resection with anastomosis of the right main bronchus and exclusion of the left lung had hypoxemia. The pulmonary artery had not been ligated. Later, left pneumonectomy was required to remove the nonfunctioning but shunting lung.

OPERATIVE DEATHS

There were 7 operative deaths in the 132 patients undergoing primary resection and reconstruction (5%) (Table 41.7). One death occurred in the group of 82 tracheal reconstructions (1%), but 6 occurred among the 50 carinal reconstructions (12%). The highest mor-

TABLE 41.7. Survival After Resection of Tracheal Carcinoma

VARIABLE	SQUAMOUS	ADENOID CYSTIC
Operative deaths	3	8
Alive without carcinoma		
>10 yr	3 (9)[a]	5 (11)[a]
5–10 yr	4 (10)[a]	11 (12)[a]
3–5 yr	3 (6)[a]	10 (11)[a]
0–3 yr	10 (11)[a]	13 (13)[a]
Died of carcinoma		
>10 yr	0	4
5–10 yr	0	1
3–5 yr	5	2
0–3 yr	8	0
Died without carcinoma; lost to follow-up		
>10 yr	1	0
5–10 yr	3	0
3–5 yr	1	1
0–3 yr	3	4
Alive with carcinoma	0	1

[a]The number in parentheses indicates the original number of survivors of the operation, exlcuding those who later died of other causes later.

tality (4 patients) occurred in carinal resections of adenoid cystic carcinoma, probably because of excessive tension after extended resection for this infiltrating disease (2). One death after tracheal resection and reconstruction resulted from anastomotic leakage followed by pneumonia. Of patients who underwent carinal resection and reconstruction, respiratory failure developed in 2 after leakage of the anastomosis; 1 patient had respiratory failure after development of postoperative pulmonary edema; and 1 had a sudden massive hemorrhage on the ninth postoperative day, presumably from the pulmonary artery.

No deaths occurred in the seven patients with laryngotracheal tumors (with or without cervicomediastinal exenteration). Mortality was unacceptably high in the patients undergoing staged reconstruction (five of eight patients), and the procedure has been abandoned. Three of nine patients who underwent exploration alone died. In one patient death after exploration resulted from hemorrhage of the innominate artery after establishment of a mediastinal tracheostomy in continuity; in two others death was the result of respiratory failure. The deaths after staged reconstruction were the result of anastomotic separation in two patients, respiratory failure in one hemorrhage from the innominate artery in one; one patient died because of hypoxemia related to the use of cardiopulmonary bypass with extensive manipulation of the right middle and lower lobe (to accomplish reconstruction in a patient with only a left upper lobe on the opposite side).

Two additional deaths were the result of technical failure of the operation, although they occurred many months later in other jurisdictions. One patient had undergone a carinal resection with reconstruction, and the other had a staged resection. Stenosis developed in both, and one probably also was having continued aspiration from laryngeal malfunction. Further treatment would have been advisable in both cases.

ONCOLOGIC RESULTS

Of the 147 patients who underwent resection of tumor (including patients with primary reconstruction and those without), 135 survived the operation. Seventy percent of these are currently alive without tumor. Forty-nine percent of patients with squamous cancer, 75% of patients with adenoid cystic tumors, and 83% of the other patients are alive and disease free. Table 41.7 shows the number of patients in each category who have died of tumor or other causes as well as the number who are alive with known carcinoma. Interpretation of these figures is difficult because the cases are spread over many years. Because more patients have been referred for treatment in the last 10 years, and especially in the last 5 years, this distribution reflects favorably on the number of patients living without known disease. Nonetheless, the figures appear to be encouraging.

If patients who had squamous cell carcinoma and are living without known disease are considered, 10 were operated on more than 3 years ago; another 4 died of other disease and had been followed for 5, 7, 8, and 15 years disease free (Table 41.7). Thus, 14 patients probably were cured of their cancer. An additional 10 are free of disease but were treated within the last 3 years. This interval is clinically significant for squamous cancer of the trachea, which tends to recur early, in approximately the same time frame as squamous carcinomas of the lung.

The first patient who underwent a resection (of the carina) for adenoid cystic carcinoma in this series was disease free until recurrence at the suture line 17 years later. Because her resection margins and lymph nodes had been negative, no irradiation had been given. Bronchoscopic follow-up had been terminated after 10 years. Because this type of tracheal carcinoma has such proclivity for a long clinical course and late recurrence, it is more difficult to interpret results of its resection. Sixteen patients are living without evidence of recurrent disease 5 or more years after surgery. Twenty-three additional patients who had undergone resection are living without known disease. The long-term outlook with adenoid cystic carcinoma is less clear (Table 41.7). Five patients operated on more than 10 years ago are living without disease, but 4 died of late metastases or recurrence after 10 years. Conversely, 3 have died of recurrence of metastasis within 3 to 10 years, whereas 21 are alive for between 3 and 10 years without evidence of recurrent disease. These figures emphasize the sharp decrease in the number of patients free of squamous carcinoma after 3 years with little further decrease thereafter. Patients with adenoid cystic carcinoma, in contrast, remain disease free for many years but appear to be threatened by late recurrence.

As might be expected in the heterogeneous group of other tumors, statistical results are good, because many of these tumors were benign or of low-grade malignancy. One of the 11 carcinoids was highly atypical and had metastasized to regional lymph nodes in a highly malignant fashion. All mucoepidermoid tumors behaved benignly. Adenocarcinoma occurred in a child in the membranous wall of the carina in the base of a cyst. This tumor has not recurred in more than $3\frac{1}{2}$ years. The single patient with adenosquamous carcinoma had a tumor that involved the larynx to such an extent that it could not be saved. The patient died of metastasis $4\frac{2}{3}$ years later. A single patient with small cell carcinoma confined to the trachea had subsequent chemotherapy and radiation because of the histologic appearance of the tumor. He is without recurrence $3\frac{2}{3}$ years after resection. The single patient with melanoma has no history of previous cutaneous lesions and no current cutaneous or retinal lesions, but the follow-up has been brief. No other metastatic disease has been detected, and it is thought that this is indeed a primary lesion of the airway. The patient with pseudosarcoma remains disease free 19 years later. Several patients reported with this disease in the era before extended tracheal resection died of strangulation because of local growth without metastasis. The chondrosarcoma was of low grade, but the patient died of pulmonary metastases slightly more than 5 years after resection. The patient with rhabdomyosarcoma died of osteogenic sarcoma, probably because of irradiation treatment received for his previous cervical rhabdomyosarcoma in early childhood. The remaining death from tumor was that of a patient who had a spindle cell sarcoma of the carina.

Five patients with other tumors had operations for the same tumor before referral. Three had carcinoids removed incompletely, with recurrence from 10 to 14 years later. An 8-year-old child with malignant fibrous histiocytoma had a previous incomplete resection by a local bronchoplastic procedure at the carina. She remained disease free for 3 years after carinal resection but has been lost to follow-up. A 19-year-old patient with a fibrous tumor of the carina underwent prior pneumonectomy with residual tumor left at the carina. He remains disease free nearly 2 years after carinal resection. Two patients were lost to follow-up: 1 had a low-grade spindle cell sarcoma and was followed for 10 years, and the other had a solitary squamous papilloma and was followed for 7 years, both without recurrence. One patient with granular cell tumor high in the trachea involving the lower posterior larynx was later found to have a concurrent granular cell tumor of the bronchus intermedius, which was removed by sleeve resection.

EFFECT OF TUMOR AT RESECTION MARGINS AND IN LYMPH NODES

The finding of tumor at the resection margins, even by frozen section during operation, has particular importance in airway reconstruction. Because of the requisites for reconstruction, it is sometimes impossible to resect more airway without endangering the safety of the anastomosis by creating excessive anastomotic tension. Furthermore, extensive regional lymph node dissection may destroy the blood supply to the trachea. Loss of blood supply can lead to necrosis at the anastomosis, followed by irreparable stenosis. Therefore, only immediately adjacent regional lymph nodes are blocked out with the specimen. Others may be sampled for prognostic information. Table 41.8 shows the distribution of involved lymph nodes and margins for both squamous cell carcinoma and adenoid cystic carcinoma in two critical groups of patients: those who died with cancer and those who are alive

TABLE 41.8. Effect on Survival of Tumor at Margins and in Lymph Nodes at Resection

	NO. OF PATIENTS	
VARIABLE	DIED WITH CANCER	ALIVE, NO CANCER
Squamous cell carcinoma	13	22
Nodes positive	6	2
Margins positive		
Invasive	4	1
In situ	0	6
Nodes, margins negative	3	12
Adenoid cystic carcinoma	7	38
Nodes, margins positive	3	16
Nodes, margins negative	4	22

Note. Almost all patients received postoperative radiotherapy.

without known cancer. The clinical significance of the findings appears to differ in the two types of carcinoma.

Positive lymph nodes in squamous cell carcinoma were found more commonly in patients who later died with cancer than in those who survived without cancer. The 6 patients with positive nodes are from a total of 13 who died of cancer. Only 2 of the 20 disease free patients had positive nodes. Invasive carcinoma at the resection margin is of graver consequence than in situ carcinoma; 4 of 5 patients with invasive carcinoma died. In contrast, all 6 patients with in situ disease are disease free. Essentially all of these patients have undergone radiotherapy in doses ranging from 4500 to 6500 cGy. Because irradiation was administered in many centers, it was impossible to control dosage or portals. With adenoid cystic carcinoma accompanied by positive margins, lymph nodes, or both, little effect appears evident, compared with patients having negative margins and nodes. Because of the proclivity of this tumor to extend for long distances submucosally and perineurally, the finding of malignant cells distant from the gross tumor is all too common. The surgeon often must compromise total resection for safety. All of these patients now receive postoperative irradiation. Suture line recurrence thus far has been rare. Late recurrence has been in the lung, bone, liver, or brain. In contrast, irradiation of unresected tumor is all but uniformly characterized by local recurrence in 3 to 5 years, despite early good response.

OTHER SQUAMOUS CELL CARCINOMA

Sixteen (40%) of 40 patients who had a resection of squamous carcinoma of the trachea had either a previous history, concurrent finding, or later occurrence of squamous cell carcinoma in the respiratory tract. One had concurrent squamous cell carcinoma of the tongue. One patient had carcinoma of the larynx treated before tracheal resection, and a second patient later had carcinoma of the larynx. In 1 patient, previously noted, a second primary carcinoma of the trachea developed at a different level. Seven patients had received prior treatment for squamous carcinoma of the lung by lobectomy or pneumonectomy, and in 5 of them, squamous cell carcinoma of the lung developed later. Of these 12 patients, 2 of whom had two primary squamous carcinomas of opposite lungs at wide time intervals, 3 died of recurrent tracheal carcinoma, 1 died of recurrence of prior carcinoma of the lung, 1 died of a later carcinoma of the lung, and 1 is expected to die soon of a second primary carcinoma of the lung, with a tracheal resection occurring between the two pulmonary episodes. Four patients who underwent lung resection either preceding or subsequent to the tracheal resection were living without disease from $2\frac{1}{2}$ to 15 years after the tracheal episode.

ROLE OF IRRADIATION

Because of the narrow margins often obtainable in tracheal resection, even when the margins and lymph nodes are histologically negative, it is deemed prudent to use postoperative irradiation for both squamous cell and adenoid cystic carcinoma of the trachea. Both, particularly adenoid cystic carcinoma, are sensitive to irradiation. After recurrence of adenoid cystic carcinoma in a nonirradiated patient 17 years after resection, it appeared wise to use irradiation subsequent to operation. Irradiation alone has been argued to be appropriate primary treatment for carcinoma of the trachea. In an effort to clarify this question, patients who underwent resection (with or without subsequent radiotherapy) were compared with those who received radiotherapy alone as primary treatment. A few also underwent exploration. Admittedly, the principal reason for assigning patients to the radiotherapy category was the extent of tumor. This extension, however, was frequently longitudinal and did not necessarily indicate a large bulk of neoplasm. Table 41.9 lists the number of patients dead of disease and those alive without disease for more than 1 year for each type of tracheal carcinoma and each treatment method (operation and irradiation versus irradiation alone). The spectrum of patients is scattered over a broad time scale, thus the comparison is not precise.

Of patients with squamous cell carcinoma of the trachea who underwent what is considered optimal therapy—surgical resection followed by radiotherapy—11 patients have nonetheless died of carcinoma of the trachea. Eighteen remain alive for periods of more

TABLE 41.9. Treatment of Tracheal Tumor: Resection Versus Irradiation

	NO. OF PATIENTS	
TUMOR TYPE	DEAD OF CARCINOMA	ALIVE (>1 YR) WITHOUT DISEASE
Squamous		
Resection(± irradiation)	11	18
Irradiation (± exploration)	16	1
Adenoid cystic		
Resection (± irradiation)	7	38
Irradiation (± exploration)	9	3

Abbreviation. ±, with or without.

than 1 year without evidence of disease. In marked contrast, 16 patients for whom radiotherapy was essentially the only treatment are dead of carcinoma. One remains alive approximately 7 years after treatment.

Patients with adenoid cystic carcinoma have been divided into those who died of their carcinoma and those who are alive without known disease. Analysis is more difficult in the latter patients because the disease may have long periods of apparent control after either operation or irradiation. Of patients treated with operation (and usually postoperative radiotherapy), 7 are dead of carcinoma and 38 are alive without known disease. With irradiation alone, 9 are dead of carcinoma and only 3 are alive without evidence of disease.

Survival of patients with squamous carcinoma receiving one or the other treatment but who nonetheless died of carcinoma has been examined. This effort was made to determine whether there is palliative benefit to patients who undergo operation, given its risks, in combination with radiotherapy, compared with radiotherapy alone. Table 41.10 shows the number of surviving patients in 12-month periods. The results of radiotherapy alone are much like those obtained for squamous carcinoma of the lung, with most patients showing recurrence within 2 years. In contrast, resection with radiotherapy provides 2 to 4 years of survival. Because the course of adenoid cystic carcinoma is such a prolonged one, similar treatment groups with the same endpoint (death from disease) have been examined, both for squamous and adenoid cystic carcinoma. Table 41.11 compares the median and average survival in months for these patients. Resection combined with irradiation, given the limits of this nonrandomized comparison, provides a tripled survival time for squamous cell carcinoma and at least a tripled survival time for adenoid cystic carcinoma.

The analysis of this 26-year experience with surgical management of primary tumors of the trachea appears to confirm and extend conclusions based on previously reported experiences. Eschapasse (3) collected,

TABLE 41.10. Palliative Value of Operation and Irradiation for Squamous Cell Tracheal Carcinoma

TIME TO DEATH FROM CARCINOMA (MO)	NO. OF PATIENTS	
	IRRADIATION ONLY	RESECTION + IRRADIATION
<12	5	1
12–24	3	2
24–36	1	4
36–48	0	4
>48	1	0

TABLE 41.11. Duration of Survival: Irradiation Versus Operation With or Without Irradiation

VARIABLE	SURVIVAL (MO)	
	MEDIAN	AVERAGE
Squamous carcinoma		
Irradiation only	10	11
Resection (± irradiation)	34	31
Adenoid cystic carcinoma		
Irradiation only	28	39
Resection (± irradiation)	118	107

Abbreviation. ± with or without.

from multiple teams in France and the U.S.S.R., information about 152 patients with primary tracheal tumors. In 1974 he reported 121 patients treated surgically, of whom 75 had reconstruction after cylindrical resection and anastomosis (47 patients) or carinal resection (28 patients). There were 13 deaths in 121 operations. Five of 19 patients with adenoid cystic tumors were alive and free of disease for 3 to 9 years, and 11 of 27 patients with squamous carcinoma were alive and free of disease for from 7 months to 16 years. In 1987 Perelman and Koroleva (16) reported a 20-year experience (1963 to 1983) with 116 open operations in 135 patients; 41 were treated by sleeve resection and 34 by carinal resection, with 11 deaths. Overall survival for squamous cell carcinoma was 27% at 3 years and 13% at 5 and 10 years; for adenoid cystic carcinoma, overall survival was 71% at 3 years, 66% at 5 years, and 56% at 10 and 15 years. Pearson and colleagues (4) also reported surgical treatment of 44 patients between 1963 and 1983. Twenty-nine patients underwent reconstruction, including 16 sleeve resections and 13 carinal resections, with 2 deaths. Nine patients with adenoid cystic carcinoma were alive without disease at from 1 to 20 years after operation, 3 had died of other disease within 6 to 18 years, and 2 were alive with disease. Four of 6 patients with squamous carcinoma who underwent resection were alive at from 6 to 56 months.

Several therapeutic recommendations appear to be justified by the Massachusetts General Hospital experience and the data of other studies. First, benign primary tumors of the trachea and tumors of intermediate aggressiveness are best treated by surgical resection with reconstruction of the airway. Second, primary squamous cell carcinoma and adenoid cystic carcinoma of the trachea are best treated by resection when primary reconstruction can be accomplished safely. Resection should be followed by full-dose mediastinal irradiation in most cases. Third, malignant primary tracheal tumors of other types should also be resected if such resection will permit safe primary reconstruction.

The surgical mortality and morbidity described in this report undoubtedly will be improved upon in the years ahead on the basis of experience obtained over the last quarter century. It appears prudent that extensive tracheal reconstruction, in particular that of the carina, continue to be performed in centers specializing in this type of surgery.

References

1. Grillo HC, Mathisen DJ. Primary tracheal tumors. Ann Thorac Surg 1990;49:69–77.
2. Grillo HC. Carinal reconstruction. Ann Thorac Surg 1982;34:356–373.
3. Eschapasse H. Les tumeurs tracheales primitives. Traitement chirurgical. Ref Fr Mal Respir 1974;2:425–430.
4. Pearson FG, Todd TRJ, Cooper JD. Experience with primary neoplasms of the trachea. J Thorac Cardiovasc Surg 1984;88:511–518.
5. Perelman JI, Koroleva N. Surgery of the trachea. World J Surg 1974;18:16–25.
6. Xu LT, Sun ZF, Li ZJ, Wu LH, Shang ZY, Yu XQ. Clinical and pathologic characteristics in patients with tracheobronchial tumors: report of 50 patients. Ann Thorac Surg 1987;43:276–278.
7. Grillo HC, Suen HC, Mathisen DJ, Wain JC. Resectional management of thyroid carcinoma invading the trachea. Ann Thorac Surg 1992;54:3–10.
8. Weber AL, ed. Symposium on the larynx and trachea. Radiol Clin North Am 1978;16(2).
9. Mathisen DJ, Grillo HC. Endoscopic relief of malignant airway obstruction. Ann Thorac Surg 1989;48:469–475.
10. Wilson RS. Tracheostomy and tracheal reconstruction. In: Kaplan JA, ed. Thoracic anesthesia. New York: Churchill Livingstone, 1983:421–445.
11. Wilson RS. Tracheal resection. In: Marshall BE, Longnecker DE, Fairley HB, eds. Anesthesia for thoracic procedures. Boston: Blackwell Scientific, 1988:415–432.
12. Grillo HC, Mathisen DJ. Cervical exenteration. Ann Thorac Surg 1990;49:401–409.
13. Salassa JR, Pearson BW, Payne WS. Gross and microscopical blood supply of the trachea. Ann Thorac Surg 1977;24:100–107.
14. Montgomery WW. Suprahyoid release for tracheal anastomosis. Arch Otolaryngol 1974;99:255–260.
15. Grillo HC. Complications of tracheal operations. In: Cordell AR, Ellison RG, eds. Complications of intrathoracic surgery. Boston: Little, Brown, 1979:287–288.
16. Perelman MI, Koroleva NS. Primary tumors of the trachea. In: Grill HC, Eschapasse H, eds. International trends in general thoracic surgery. Philadelphia: Saunders, 1987:91.

42

Tumors of the Chest Wall

Patricia M. McCormack

The chest wall consists of multiple tissue layers, each uniquely suited to its role in maintaining and preserving respiration and hemodynamics. Each layer can give rise to tumors, and benign tumors usually have a malignant counterpart. A classification of chest wall tumors is given in Table 42.1. Metastases from other primary sites also occur. Mammary malignancies as well as lung or thymic malignancies may invade the chest wall directly.

Primary chest wall tumors are rare, and half of them are malignant. These tumors constitute only 5% of thoracic malignancies. A palpable mass or a mass seen on a chest radiograph is the usual presentation. Nearly three quarters produce no symptoms, even when malignant. Pain occurs when normal structures are compressed or invaded and can be present even if the tumor is benign.

Judicious use of computed tomography (CT) scans and magnetic resonance imaging (MRI) provides a very clear delineation of a chest wall tumor. Cystic masses can be separated from solid ones, and invasion of the chest wall can be outlined more clearly. MRI sagittal and coronal planes have replaced plain tomography. Diagnostic bronchoscopy is used when a primary lung cancer invades the chest wall to determine operability for the lung primary tumor. It is not indicated for any other chest wall tumor.

Biopsy of the mass is necessary for tissue diagnosis. Careful planning of type and site of the biopsy is essential. Tumors smaller than 5 cm that can be excised completely without major reconstruction should be treated by a planned excisional biopsy.

If the CT or MRI scan confirms a soft tissue tumor, a core needle biopsy should yield a diagnostic sample. In bony tumors an open biopsy is needed. Careful planning places the biopsy scar in a position where it and all contaminated tissue can be encompassed by the subsequent surgical resection.

BENIGN TUMORS
SUPERFICIAL TUMORS

Cutaneous nevi include the junctional nevus. This pigmented variant can be distinguished from a melanoma only by pathologic determination. Complete resection is sufficient treatment.

Fat cells give rise to lipomas. These very common tumors are well circumscribed, thin walled, and very soft. They are composed of mature adipose tissue. Variants with spindle cell features can occur in the shoulder area. Deeper lipomas may infiltrate muscle. If resected, a wider excision is required and recurrence is common (1). These tumors can usually be diagnosed clinically, and resection is indicated only for cosmetic reasons or if the true nature of the tumor is in doubt.

Lymphangiomas are found commonly in the neck. These poorly circumscribed tumors can grow downward and present as a chest wall tumor, usually in the thoracic inlet. Complete excision is sufficient to prevent recurrence.

Hemangiomas when superficial are called birthmarks. Cosmesis dictates the need for treatment of these blemishes. Cavernous hemangiomas and arteriovenous malformations cause problems as they increase in size. Surgical excision should be done at a time when contraindications are minimal (2). One type of hemangioma involving the trunk can be difficult to distinguish from a hemangiosarcoma on histology (3).

DEEP TUMORS

Fibromas rarely occur on the chest wall. They present as firm, slowly growing masses. They usually grow near joints but can occur anywhere in the soft tissue. Clinically, a diagnosis is secured by the history of a slow growth pattern and lack of local infiltration on

TABLE 42.1. Classification of Tumors of Chest Wall Tumors

PRIMARY TUMORS

Benign	Malignant
Skin nevus	Melanoma
Lipoma	Squamous cell
Hemangioma	Liposarcoma
Fibroma	Hemangiopericytoma
Lymphangioma	Fibrosarcoma
Rhabdomyoma	Lymphangiosarcoma
Neurofibroma	Rhabdomyosarcoma
Fibrous dysplasia	Neurofibrosarcoma
Chondroma	Fibrosarcoma
Osteoblastoma	Chondrosarcoma
Plasmoma	Osteosarcoma
Radiation fibrosis	Multiple myeloma
	Radiation-induced sarcoma

CONTIGUOUS TUMORS
Breast carcinoma
Lung carcinoma
Thymic carcinoma

METASTATIC TUMORS
　Renal
　Breast
　Colon
　Lung
　Sarcoma

CT scan. Resection is required only for symptomatic relief or cosmesis.

Rhabdomyoma is a rare muscle tumor. Any mass arising in a muscle should be biopsied. A slow growth pattern confirms the benign pathology. Its malignant counterpart can be virulent, making a biopsy mandatory. If the tumor interferes with the function of the muscle, it may be excised. Resection must be complete to prevent recurrence locally.

Neurofibromas usually present as multiple lesions associated with von Recklinghausen's multiple neurofibromatosis (Elephant man syndrome). Most lesions are benign. Pain or an enlarging mass heralds degeneration into a malignant neurofibrosarcoma, and resection is indicated. Needle biopsy may be inconclusive, thus complete excision is recommended. The occurrence of the tumors near the vertebral body raises the possibility of a dumbbell tumor with extension via the neural foramen inside the spinal canal. A CT or MRI scan delineates this growth clearly. Neurosurgical consultation is indicted for combined resection of these tumors, whether benign or malignant.

Desmoid tumors are considered benign or malignant depending on the report of the pathologist. They arise from the deep fascia and connective tissue of muscles, and present as slowly enlarging masses that invade locally. Pain caused by pressure is a common presenting symptom. No report of metastasis has been recorded, but the local recurrence rate is very high.

Treatment is wide local excision (4). The presence of clear surgical resection margins does not preclude recurrence. The addition of radiation therapy, either external beam or brachytherapy, is recommended after resection. This therapy has been reported to decrease the recurrence rate (5).

BONY TUMORS

Fibrous dysplasia tumors constitute 30% of benign chest wall tumors. They usually present as a solitary rib mass but may be multiple. Originating from the lateral or posterior rib surface, they grow very slowly and remain asymptomatic until the size infringes on an adjacent structure or the rib fractures. Classically, on radiographs an expansile lesion is seen with a translucent center. Malignant degeneration is very rare, and complete resection is curative.

Chondromas commonly occur in young adults between the ages of 20 and 40 years. They arise at the costochondral or chondrosternal junction. The radiographic appearance shows a medullary mass thinning the bony cortex. Marcove and Huvos (6) state that a lesion of less than 4 cm is benign. Size is the only parameter distinguishing a chondroma from its malignant counterpart. Biopsy cannot always make this distinction, thus these tumors should be resected completely when diagnosed.

Osteochondroma and osteoblastoma are very rare benign tumors of bone. They grow from the bony rib cortex and have a stalk and a cartilaginous cover. Growth may be inward, and detection is by radiograph alone. A palpable mass occurs when growth is outward. Rarely do they become malignant, thus a complete resection is the treatment of choice.

MALIGNANT TUMORS
SUPERFICIAL TUMORS

Basal cell tumors require complete resection for control. Recurrence can lead to the need for major chest wall resection when removal is incomplete.

Malignant melanoma is the most common malignant skin tumor. Occurrences on the chest wall are treated in the same fashion as melanomas growing elsewhere on the body.

DEEP TUMORS

Liposarcoma is a rare malignancy of the chest wall. Resection with clear margins is effective treatment.

Angiosarcoma is usually seen in a lymphedematous arm secondary to chest wall or axillary radiotherapy (7).

Fibrosarcoma, neurofibrosarcoma, and rhabdomyosarcoma are the same when growing on the chest wall as when they occur elsewhere in the body. The most characteristic feature is a rapidly growing painful mass. Diagnosis followed by complete resection yields the best results. Wide resection is recommended, and a CT scan of the lungs to check for metastases is mandatory. Placement of the skin incision depends on whether the tumor has invaded the skin. If no invasion is present, skin flaps can be raised and used for coverage after en bloc resection of the entire tumor with clear margins. Dissection of en bloc muscles follows the guidelines for resection of any sarcoma invading muscle. Dissection occurs one tissue plane away from the tumor; the tissue plane is never visualized or violated during its removal (Fig. 42.1). If clear margins require including ribs in the resection, this should be done. Resection techniques are described below.

BONY TUMORS

Chondrosarcomas represent the most common malignant tumor occurring in the chest wall. They occur most commonly on the front of the chest at the anterior costochondral junctions and sternum. Pathologic grading based on histology is very important for prognosis. Grade I tumors have good survival, whereas grade II or III tumors have a higher rate of metastases and local recurrence. The survival rate in patients with grade II or III disease is shorter (8).

Surgical resection is the treatment of choice, with a wide margin of normal tissue preserved, including 5-cm soft tissue margins, one normal rib above and below, and adequate margins on the sternum. When the tumor has not crossed the anastomotic junctions of the manubrium or xiphoid process of the sternum, these may be retained for reconstruction. Specific reconstruction techniques are described below.

A report from the Mayo Clinic (1) included 96 patients with chondrosarcoma of the bony chest wall. The 10-year survival rate was 14% when palliative resection was done, 65% when limited resection was carried out, and 96% when a wide resection was performed. The local recurrence rate correlated well with the type of resection: the recurrence rate was only 14% in those resected widely versus 60% when a limited resection was done (1). No grading was reported.

Marcove (6) reported 27 patients with rib chondrosarcomas. Local excision yielded a prompt local recurrence. Histologic grading and survival is shown in Table 42.2. Marcove stressed that adequate resection required removal of a normal rib above and below the tumor, a 5-cm margin all around, and removal of the underlying parietal pleura.

Osteogenic sarcoma is found most commonly in young adults, primarily occurring in the long bones—the femur, tibia, and humerus. Tumor originating in the ribs is less common. This tumor is much more virulent than chondrosarcoma, and it metastasizes earlier. Most metastatic lesions are found in the lungs exclusively. A CT scan of the lungs is necessary before definitive treatment of the primary tumor is planned. Osteosarcoma is responsive to both chemotherapy and radiation therapy.

The current approach for a primary tumor that can be resected with a limb-sparing operation is the administration of two cycles of chemotherapy while the patient's prosthesis is being made. A limb-sparing resection is performed with immediate placement of the prosthesis. After the wound has healed, additional chemotherapy is given to obliterate microscopic disease.

When there is simultaneous presentation of the primary tumor and the lung metastases, chemotherapy is administered first. One regimen consists of vincristine, Adriamycin, and high-dose methotrexate as described by Marcove and Rosen (9). Depending on the response, surgery is then planned for both areas. Results showed a 15% to 25% 5-year survival with this regimen. If amputation is required for the primary tumor, the residual lung metastases are resected first. If the metastases cannot be resected, then the primary tumor is treated with a less aggressive approach.

Ewing's sarcomas of the chest wall are very rare. A rapidly growing painful mass occurs most often in male adolescents. Malaise, fever, and leukocytosis are common, supporting the theory that Ewing's sarcoma is a systemic disease at diagnosis.

A review of 62 patients treated over a period of 40 years at Memorial Sloan–Kettering Cancer Center was reported by Burt (10). Thirty-four patients (55%) had rib tumors, 21 (34%) had tumors arising from the scapula, and 5 (8%) had tumors arose in the clavicle and 2 (3%) in the sternum. Survival was 48% at 5 and 10 years. Twenty-three percent presented with synchronous distant metastases, the most significant factor in survival. Forty-five patients (73%) received chemotherapy with surgery and/or radiation therapy. The remainder had local therapy only. Patients who developed metastases had a 28% 5-year survival rate. Chemotherapy, therefore, must be combined with local radiation or surgery to achieve good results with this tumor. Multiple-agent therapy is recommended by various authors (11–15).

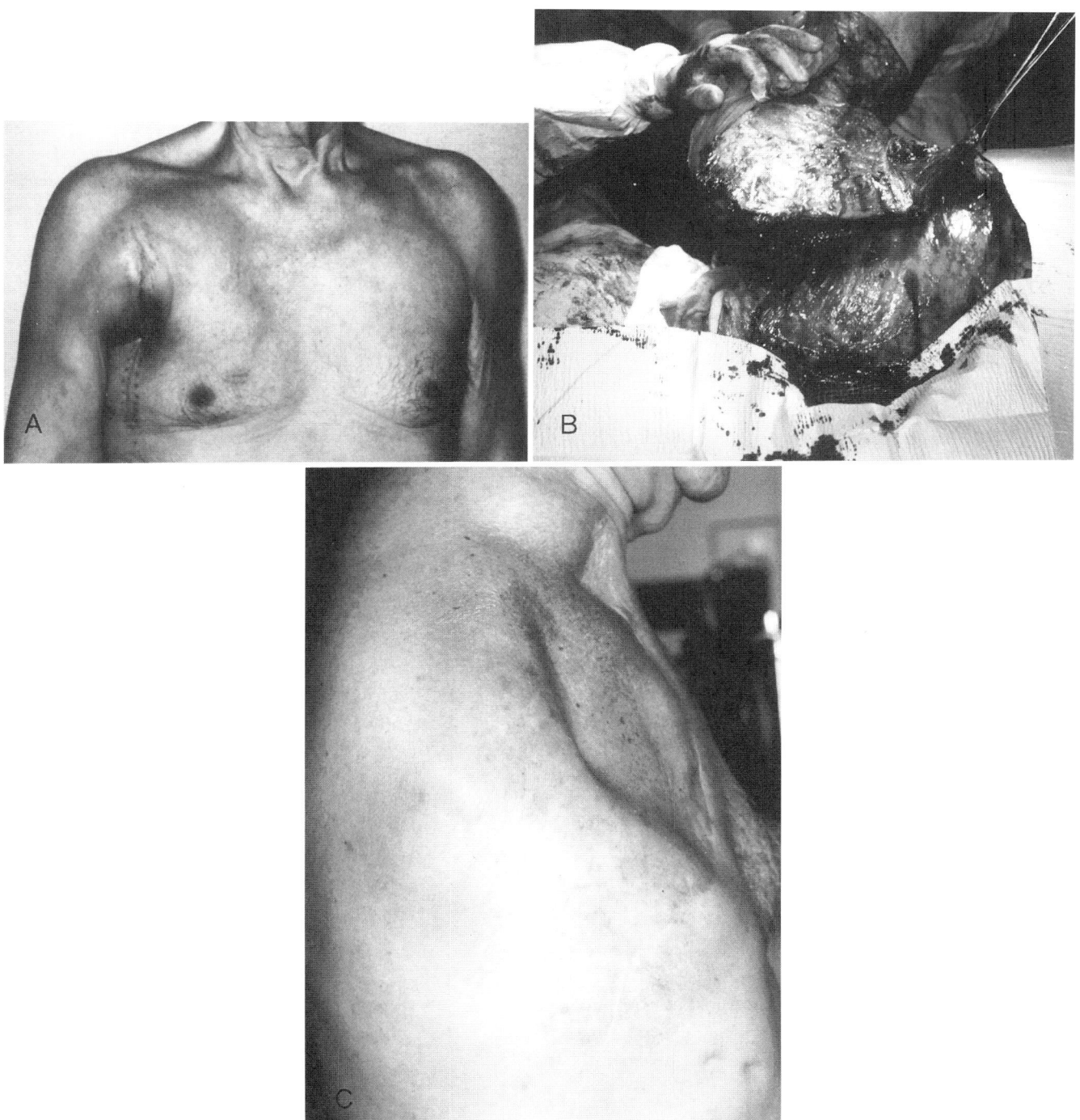

FIGURE 42.1. A. Sarcoma of the right axilla, which at biopsy could not be resected locally. B. Surgical specimen included a right forequarter amputation with en bloc chest wall. C. Exterior chest 2 months post operation.

Myelomatous tumors of the thorax are most likely just a manifestation of multiple myeloma, a systemic disease. They occur most commonly in adults in the sixth and seventh decades and account for 20% of chest wall malignancies. A positive diagnosis can be made by the presence of a monoclonal protein in serum or urine (Bence Jones proteinuria) confirmed on immunoelectrophoresis with a bone marrow biopsy showing more than 10% plasma cells. Systemic chemotherapy can be supplemented with radiation therapy for painful lesions.

The solitary variant is termed a plasmacytoma. Of 24 patients reported by Burt (1) over a 40-year span, 75% later developed multiple myeloma. This find-

TABLE 42.2. Five-Year Survival Rate in Resected Lung and Chest Wall

Depth of Invasion	No. of Patients	5-Yr Survival (%)
Completely resected patients	70	40
Number of lymphatic metastases	45	56
Parietal pleura only	54	48
Rib invasion, negative nodes	10	35

ing confirms the premise that systemic therapy should be combined with local treatment even when the presentation is of a solitary tumor.

PRIMARY CARCINOMA OF LUNG

Invasion of the chest wall by a primary bronchogenic carcinoma occurs in just 5% of lung cancers. This feature by itself does not denote nonresectability or a dismal prognosis. Of far greater significance is the presence of metastatic disease, either in mediastinal lymph nodes or outside of the chest, or with contiguous spread to the spinal column or mediastinal structures. The stage of disease is paramount in ascertaining the prognosis (16).

A report from Memorial Sloan–Kettering Cancer Center (20) included a 10-year analysis of 1252 patients seen for lung cancer (excluding Pancoast tumors). One hundred twenty-five of these had neoplastic invasion of the chest wall. In 70 patients the tumor invaded parietal pleura, in 43 it extended through muscle to the rib, and in the remaining 12 patients, the vertebral body was invaded as well. Fourteen of these 125 patients had no parenchymal resection but had iodine 125 radioactive seeds implanted into the tumor. Postoperatively, they also received external radiotherapy. These patients survived a median of 7 months.

The 111 remaining patients had resection of both the lung and the involved chest wall. In 66 (60%), extension was to the parietal pleura only; the remaining 45 (40%) patients required chest wall resection to ensure clear margins. In a third of the patients, defects smaller than 5 cm precluded the need for reconstruction. The other two thirds had chest wall reconstruction with implantation of a prosthesis.

One operative death was reported secondary to respiratory failure secondary to refractory bronchopneumonia. There was a 62% complete resection rate. Survival rates are shown in Table 42.2.

Piehler (17) and Grillo (18) reported their results in treating T3 tumors. They thought that when adherence to parietal pleura is found at surgery, a complete full-thickness chest wall resection should be done in all cases. They reported 22 patients with rib resection, for whom the 5-year survival rate was 75%. The survival rate for those "who had parietal pleurectomy only" dropped to 28%.

Survival in these patients depends primarily on the completeness of the resection (19). The use of radiation therapy to sterilize positive margins is controversial. McCaughan (20) reports a median survival of just 9 months, but Patterson (21) reports an improved survival with adjunctive radiation. The most reliable technique involves beginning the extrapleural dissection 3 to 5 cm distant from the point of tumor invasion. This plane is then developed with a finger dissection. If the plane separates easily from the ribs, there usually is no deeper tumor penetration. This depth can be verified by frozen section biopsy of the involved area. If positive, the chest wall can be resected secondarily without jeopardizing survival. When dissection does not proceed easily, the en bloc resection is begun at this point. This en bloc resection must include one rib above and below the palpable tumor spread and a 5-cm margin laterally.

The intercostal neurovascular bundle is identified and clipped after the rib is cut; then all other soft tissues are cut. The piece of chest wall is then resected with the pulmonary lobe(s). Frozen section analysis of suspicious margins can be made at this time. A mediastinal lymph node dissection is then carried out to complete the staging.

Spinal invasion, similar to mediastinal invasion, precludes a complete resection in most instances. Twelve patients in the report of McCaughan et al. (20) lived a median of just 10 months after resection with spinal invasion. A palliative resection of all tumor, including the vertebral body with immediate reconstruction, as described by Sundareson and colleagues (22), can achieve a similar duration of survival.

INVASION BY BREAST CARCINOMAS

Breast cancer is the second most common malignancy in women and results in chest wall invasion in a small number of cases. Invasion usually occurs in large neglected tumors or in recurrence after resection with or without radiotherapy (Fig. 42.2). Chest wall involvement also occurs when the internal mammary chain of lymph nodes is the site of metastatic tumor. These nodes can grow quite large (Fig. 42.3) and require resection of the sternum and ribs for cure. McCormack and coworkers (23, 24) reported 35 patients undergoing chest wall resection for recurrent breast cancer. Survival results are related directly to the stage of the

TUMORS METASTATIC TO THE CHEST WALL

CARCINOMAS

When metastases are multiple, it is common to have rib or chest wall soft tissue involvement. The role of surgery in these instances is diagnostic only. However, a solitary metastasis can occur. Mammary, renal, colon, and salivary glands are the most frequent primary sites. If a diligent search for other disease is fruitless, a chest wall resection should be offered to the patient. The presence of subsequent disease is prognostically the most significant factor in survival. In the two groups (23, 24), 15 (23%) patients receiving resection for metastatic carcinoma had a survival of 5 years.

SARCOMAS

Sarcomas are the rarest of all chest wall tumors. Burt et al. (10) reported 36 of 317 chest wall tumors over a 20-year period. Confirmation by needle biopsy and a search for other disease is mandatory before resection. The results show that 7 of the 36 patients survived 5 years with this clinical presentation (19%).

TECHNIQUES FOR CHEST WALL RESECTION

Surgical guidelines include a 2- to 3-cm soft tissue clear margin and removal of one normal rib above and below the involved ribs. A 2-cm margin on the sternum is sufficient. An intact tissue plane around the tumor precludes violation of the cancer. If the tumor is entered, spread through the operative site is inevitable, preventing a good outcome. Full-thickness chest wall resection includes removal of the parietal pleura. Contiguous structures invaded by tumor are resected if possible. Overlying skin should always be taken if it is adherent to the tumor, or if it is the site of a previous biopsy.

If the tumor arises in or near the thoracic inlet, an MRI scan can be very helpful in delineating vascular or neural involvement. If the shoulder girdle is involved, a forequarter amputation may be required to eradicate the malignancy. This amputation usually includes chest wall resection as well. The subclavian artery and vein may need to be resected and replaced in rare instances.

The role of radiation therapy for chest wall tumors remains controversial (25). Hilaris et al. (26) report success with the use of various intraoperative techniques for direct implantation or afterloading source techniques for achieving close or microscopi-

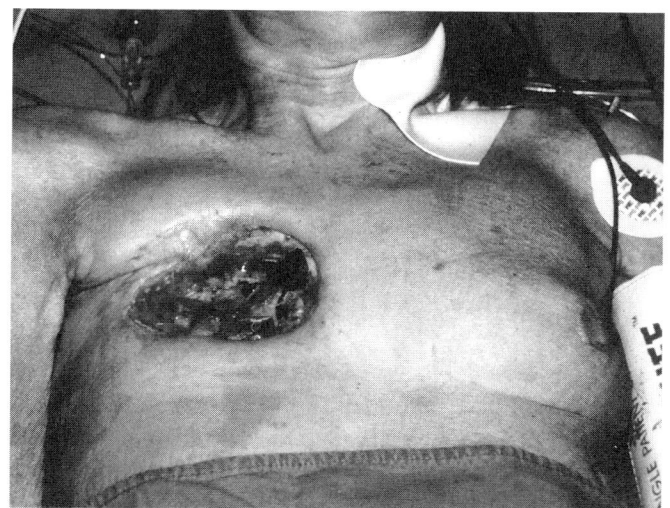

FIGURE 42.2. Neglected mammary carcinoma.

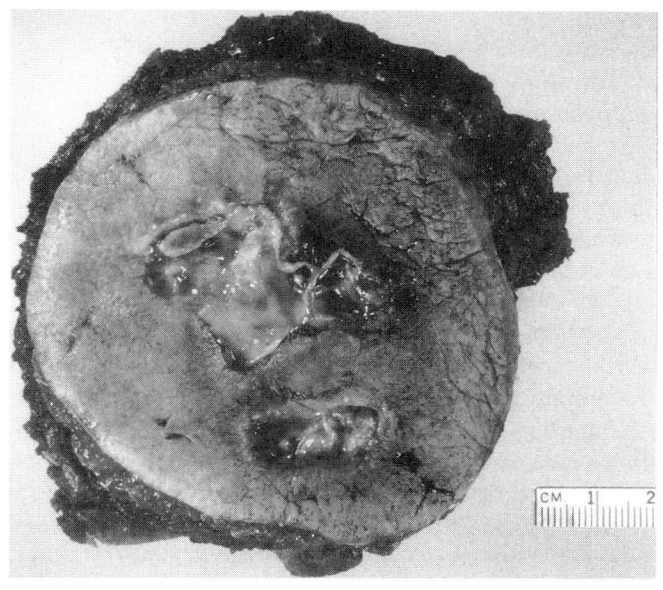

FIGURE 42.3. Resected specimen including the sternum and three ribs bilaterally.

breast cancer at the time of resection. When the only residual disease is located in the chest wall, which is subsequently resected completely, the patients do very well. In these series there were no operative deaths, and the median survival was 5 years in patients with no other disease. Patients with disease elsewhere obtain very good palliation with this technique and should receive the appropriate adjuvant therapy. After the incision is healed, resection and reconstruction can be considered.

cally positive margins in areas where further resection is not possible. External beam radiation therapy following excision of desmoid tumors also is recommended to lower the rate or to slow the onset of locally recurrent tumor. Wallner and colleagues (27) reported 30 patients with chest wall sarcomas treated with surgery and brachytherapy. They had a 65% 5-year survival and a 54% 5-year locoregional control rate. There was one recurrence in the implanted area, and external beam radiation therapy was recommended for better coverage of the tumor bed.

TECHNIQUES OF RECONSTRUCTION

BONY REPLACEMENT

After the tumor is resected and margins are declared free of tumor, chest tubes are inserted. If a plastic surgeon is involved in the construction of skin or myocutaneous flaps, consultation is indicated so that the chest tube placement does not interfere with the reconstruction.

When the defect is smaller than 5 cm, no reconstruction is needed unless the soft tissue also was resected. No rib replacement is needed. For any bony defect larger than 5 cm and for any midline defect, a rigid prosthesis is required to preserve respiratory mechanics and provide good cosmesis. Many materials have been used to replace resected ribs and sternum (Table 42.3) (28–30).

Preoperative planning sets the stage for reconstruction. When bony chest wall is resected, a replacement must be found to restore the rigid chest wall to prevent flail chest. Healthy soft tissue coverage is then needed to seal the pleural cavity, protect the underlying viscera, and prevent infection. Careful attention to these details results in weaning from a respirator within 24 hours. The requirements of an ideal chest wall prosthesis are listed in Table 42.4.

TABLE 42.3. Materials Used for Reconstructing Chest Wall

Autogenous	Synthetic
Bone	Acrylic
Omentum	Mesh: prolene, vicryl
Pericardium	Marlex
Fascia lata	Silastic
Muscle	Polypropylene
Heterogenous	Gore-Tex
Ox fascia	Composite synthetic
Alloplastic	Marlex mesh and methyl methacrylate
Metal	
Lucite	Gore-Tex and methyl methacrylate
Fiberglass	

TABLE 42.4. Ideal Chest Wall Replacement

Readily available in the operating room
Easy to adapt for any contour
Durable without erosion
Infection resistant
Permeable

Autogenous ribs, fibula, or bony chips disadvantageously require additional incisions, pain, and delay to time of stability. The new synthetic materials have proven to have all the characteristics of the ideal prosthesis. Several meshes are available, with Marlex mesh being used most frequently. If doubled and sewn in very tautly, it can prevent a flail chest. It is incorporated by endothelial ingrowth, which ensures stability and protects against infection. Cosmetically, however, it is flat and does not simulate the normal curvature of the chest.

A Gore-Tex patch is the most frequently used nonmesh synthetic (31, 32), but it is much more expensive than mesh. Its impermeability makes it the ideal replacement for the diaphragm. When used for rib or sternum replacement, it is not reendothelialized nor incorporated by the tissues and thus is more prone to infection. It becomes flabby over time, and the contour is never rounded.

When stability, cosmetic appearance, and protection of the heart and great vessels is the goal, the best proven prosthesis combines a mesh with methylmethacrylate. This prothesis usually is constructed after a pattern is made of the chest wall defect. A clean laparotomy pad is placed over the defect and gently pressed against the hole, creating a red-on-white pattern (Fig. 42.4). One layer of mesh is laid atop the pattern. Methylmethacrylate is mixed thoroughly (Fig. 42.5) in the container provided; when it is thick enough that it does not leak through the mesh, it is spread over it according to the underlying pattern (Fig. 42.6). The second layer of mesh is placed on top, and the completed prosthesis is then molded to the desired contour. Any surface can be used for the molding. The hardening is an exothermic reaction reaching 140°F Therefore, if the molding surface is the body, suitable padding is required to prevent a burn.

When the methacrylate has set, the mesh is trimmed, leaving a sewing ring outside the methacrylate. Attachment to the chest wall is made by sewing the prosthesis in place to the edges of the defect (Fig. 42.7). Soft tissue coverage is completed either by a

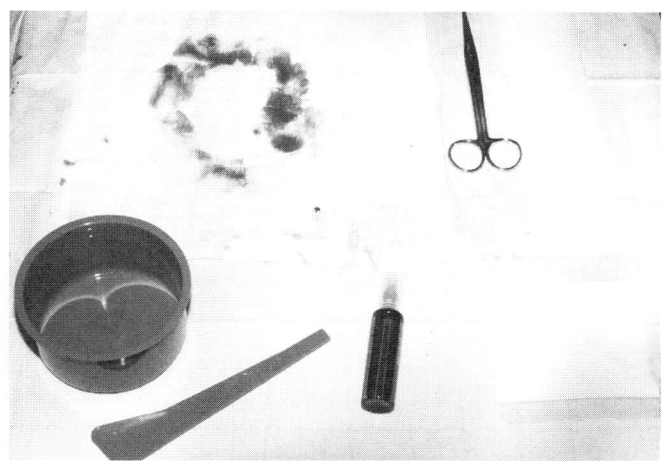

FIGURE 42.4. Equipment needed to form a Marlex methylmethacrylate prosthesis: pattern, scissors, bowl and stirrer, diluent, and powder.

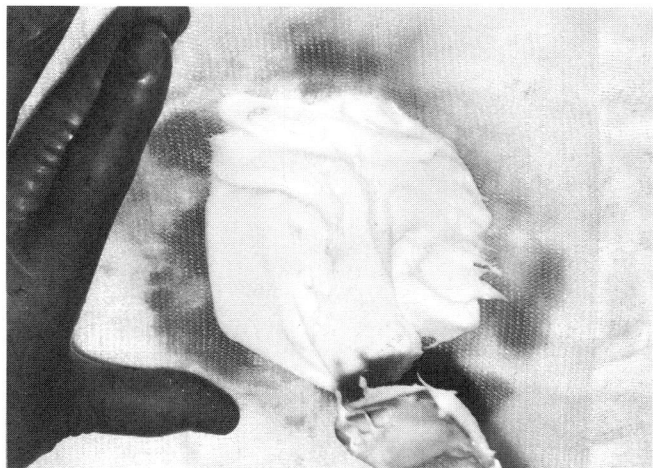

FIGURE 42.6. Spreading the mixture on the mesh according to the pattern.

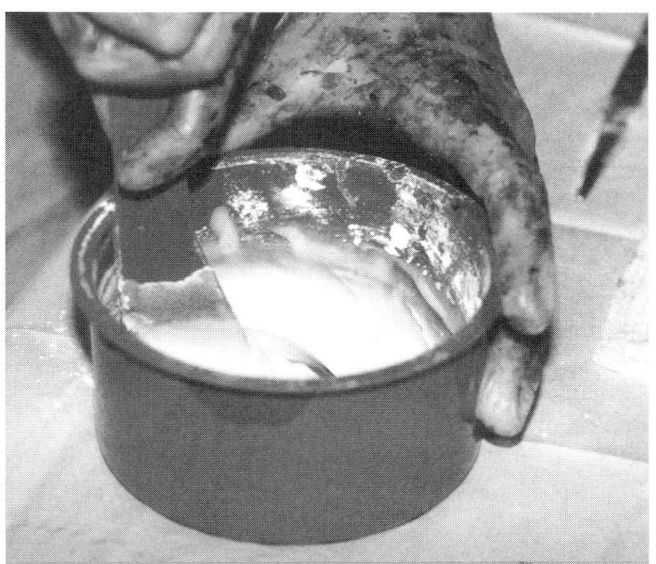

FIGURE 42.5. Mixing the powder and diluent in the bowl.

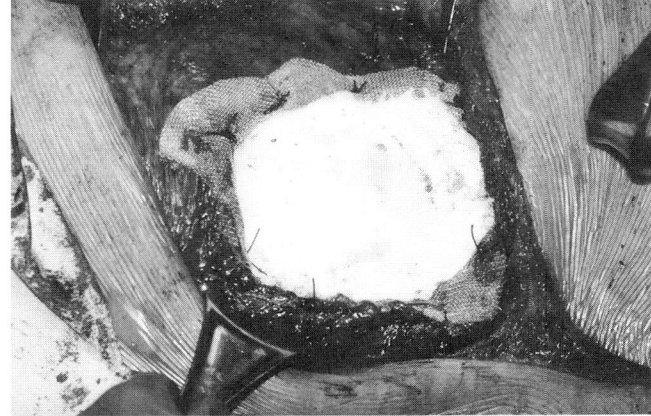

FIGURE 42.7. Completed prosthesis sutured to the skeletal defect.

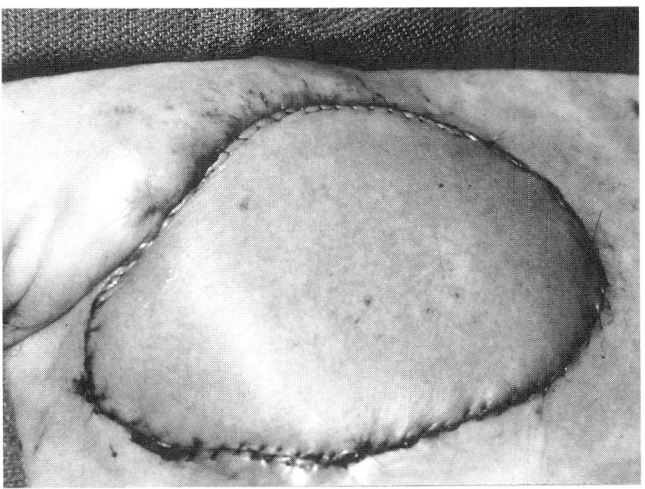

FIGURE 42.8. Myocutaneous flap sutured in place as a replacement for a soft tissue defect.

routine chest wall closure when the tumor spared the soft tissues or by an appropriate myocutaneous flap (Fig. 42.8).

When a portion of the sternum alone is resected, an alternative method can be used. After the partial sternectomy, a layer of mesh is sutured securely to the undersurface of the skeletal defect. Methyl methacrylate is mixed, and while still runny is poured into a piston syringe. It is then injected into the cut edge of the sternal marrow. The rest of the methacrylate is then applied to the layer of mesh, and the desired contour of the resected piece is reconstructed. Again, because the reconstruction is made in situ, padding must be placed between the mediastinal structures and the first mesh layer for best insulation. After the methacrylate hardens, a second layer of mesh is sutured on top, and skin closure is carried out.

COMPLICATIONS

Infection of a prosthesis occurs in approximately 0.5% of cases. If diagnosed and treated promptly, sequelae are minimal. If the infection occurs above the prosthesis, irrigation and drainage with delayed closure suffices.

If the infection is below the prosthesis, irrigation and drainage is carried out immediately. The prosthesis is then removed. If possible, a delay of 6 weeks will permit a fibrous tissue layer to form around the prosthesis. When the latter is removed, this fibrous layer prevents a flail chest. If a more pleasing cosmetic result is desired, a prosthesis can be reinserted at a later date; a donor site is selected by the plastic surgeon.

SKIN AND MUSCLE REPLACEMENT

Tumors that involve the soft tissue covering of the rigid chest wall require meticulous preoperative planning by the thoracic and plastic surgical team. The thoracic surgeon plans the incision and patient positioning with the necessary prepping and draping to accomplish both the resection and reconstruction. Chest tube placement also must be made carefully to prevent impairment of the donor site blood supply.

The omentum provides a very vascular layer on top of the prosthesis for wounds that are infected. It can be tunneled into the chest via a separate laparotomy incision or through the diaphragm when the lower chest wall is resected (19, 33). There are two major considerations for omental use: the infected site mentioned previously and as a base for a split-thickness skin graft when a myocutaneous flap is not needed.

For the past two decades, myocutaneous flaps have been used with great success for soft tissue reconstruction of the chest wall. The three most commonly used are the latissimus dorsi, pectoralis major, and rectus abdominis. The donor site is chosen based on the site of the chest wall defect and the availability of the appropriate blood supply. Extensive details are given by several authors (34–39).

The use of a myocutaneous free flap introduces a new technique in soft tissue reconstruction (40, 41).

This technique allows any muscle to be transplanted nearly anywhere on the body. The microvascular techniques, however, add considerably to the operating time.

RESULTS

Measurement of results achieved in the treatment of chest wall tumors must be considered from two distinct aspects: survival and palliation. When cure is impossible, extirpation of a bleeding, fungating, infected mass is possible. This excision should be done to provide excellent palliation when life extension is not the goal.

Benign tumors can be cured easily. Recurrence requires re-resection, and the same expectancy for cure prevails. Malignant tumor survival rates vary with the tumor type and grade (42). Survival of a patient with metastatic tumor is directly related to the stage of the disease.

Multimodality therapy plays an important role in the treatment of selected tumors. Surgical resection can be achieved with low morbidity and mortality. Resection is the primary treatment for most chest wall tumors and should be offered to patients in appropriate circumstances.

References

1. Addis BJ. Pathology of tumors of the pleura and chest wall. In: Hoogstraten B, et al., eds. Lung tumors. New York: Springer-Verlag, 1988:205–224.
2. Threlkel JB, Adkins RB. Primary chest wall tumors. Ann Thorac Surg 1971;11:450–459.
3. Allen PW, Einzinger FM. Hemangioma of skeletal muscle. Cancer 1972;29:8–22.
4. Baffi RR, Didolkar MS, Bakamjian V. Reconstruction of sternal and abdominal wall defects in a case of desmoid tumor. J Thorac Cardiovasc Surg 1977;74:105–108.
5. Martini N, McCormack PM, Bains MS. Chest wall tumors: clinical results of treatment. In: Grillo HC, Eschapasse H, eds. International trends in general thoracic surgery. Philadelphia: WB Saunders, 1986;2:285–291.
6. Marcove RC, Huvos AG. Cartilaginous tumors of the ribs. Cancer 1971;27:794–801.
7. Watkins E, Gerard FP. Malignant tumors involving chest wall. J Thorac Cardiovasc Surg 1960;39:117–129.
8. Teitelbaum SL. Tumors of the chest wall. Surg Gynecol Obstet 1969;129:1050–1073.
9. Marcove RC, Rosen G. En bloc resections for osteogenic sarcoma. Cancer 1980;45:3040–3044.
10. Burt ME, Karpeh M, Ukoha O, et al. Medical tumors of the chest wall. J Thorac Cardiovasc Surg 1993;105(1):89–96.
11. Chan R, Sutow W, Lindberg R, et al. Management and results of localized Ewing's sarcoma. Cancer 1979;43:1001–1006.
12. Zucker J, Henry-Amar M, Surazin D, et al. Intensive septemic chemotherapy in localized Ewing's sarcoma in childhood. An historical trial. Cancer 1983;52:415–423.

13. Burgert EO Jr, Nesbit ME, Garnsey LA, et al. Multi-modal therapy for the management of non-pelvic localized Ewing's sarcoma of bone: intergroup study. 1ESS-II J Clin Oncol 1990;8:1514–1524.
14. Nesbit ME, Gehan EA, Burgert EO, et al. Multimodal therapy for the management of primary non-metastatic Ewing's sarcoma of bone: a long-term follow-up of the first intergroup study. J Clin Oncol 1990:1664–1674.
15. Ben-Arush M, Kuten A, Perez-Nakum M, et al. Results of multimodal therapy in Ewing's sarcoma: a retrospective analysis of 20 patients. J Surg Oncol 1991;48:51–55.
16. Mountain CF. A new international staging system for lung cancer. Chest 1986;39(Suppl):225S–233S.
17. Grillo HC, Greenberg JJ, Wilkins EW Jr. Resection of bronchogenic carcinoma invading chest wall. J Thorac Cardiovasc Surg 1966;51:417–421.
18. Piehler JM, Pairolero PC, Weeland LH, et al. Bronchogenic carcinoma with chest wall invasion: factors affecting survival following en bloc resection. Ann Thorac Surg 1982;34:684–691.
19. McCormack PM. Chest wall tumors. Glenn's thoracic & cardiovascular surgery. 5th ed. Norwalk, CT: Appleton & Lange, 1991;1:517–530.
20. McCaughan BS, Martini N, Bains MS, McCormack PM. Chest wall invasion in carcinoma of the lung. J Thorac Cardiovasc Surg 1985;89:836–841.
21. Patterson GA, Ilves R, Ginsberg RJ, et al. The value of adjuvant radiotherapy in pulmonary and chest wall resection for bronchogenic carcinoma. Ann Thorac Surg 1982;34:692–697.
22. Sundareson N, Bains MS, McCormack PM. Surgical treatment of spinal cord compression in patients with lung cancer. Neurosurgery 1985;16:350–356.
23. McCormack PM, Bains MS, Burt ME, et al. Local recurrent mammary carcinoma failing multimodality therapy. Arch Surg 1989;124:158–161.
24. McCormack PM. Local recurrent mammary carcinoma failing multimodality therapy. Arch Surg 1989;124:158–161.
25. Tobias SL. Radiotherapy of mediastinal and chest wall tumors. In: Hoogstraten B, et al., eds. Lung Tumors. New York: Springer-Verlag, 1988:247–258.
26. Hilaris B, Nori D, Beattie EJ Jr, et al. Value of perioperative brachytherapy in the management of non-oat cell carcinoma of the lung. Int J Radiat Oncol Biol Phys 1983;9:1161–1166.
27. Wallner KM, Nori D, Burt ME, et al. Adjuvant brachytherapy for treatment of chest wall sarcomas. J Thorac Cardiovasc Surg 1991;101:888–894.
28. McCormack PM, Bains MS, Beattie EJ Jr, et al. New trends in skeletal reconstruction after resection in chest wall tumors. Ann Thorac Surg 1981;31:45–52.
29. McCormack PM, Bains MS, Martini N, et al. Methods of skeletal reconstruction following resection of lung carcinoma invading the chest wall. Surg Clin North Am 1986;67:979–986.
30. McCormack PM. Use of prosthetic materials in chest wall reconstruction. Asset and liabilities. Surg Clin North Am 1989;69:965–976.
31. Arnold PG, Pairolero PC. Chest wall reconstruction. Experience with 100 consecutive patients. Ann Surg 1984;199:725–732.
32. Pairolero PC, Trastek VF, Payne WS. Treatment of bronchogenic carcinoma with chest wall invasion. Surg Clin North Am 1987;67:959–964.
33. Pairolero PC, Arnold PG. Muscle flaps and thoracic problems. Chest wall defects: reconstruction and autogenous tissue. In: Kittle CF, ed. Current controversies in thoracic surgery. Philadelphia: WB Saunders, 1986:241–245.
34. Moellekin BR, Mathes SA, Change N. Latissimus dorsi muscle—myocutaneous flap in chest wall reconstruction. Surg Clin North Am 1989;69:977–990.
35. Arnold PG, Pairolero PC. Use of pectoralis major muscle flaps to repair defects of the anterior chest wall. Plast Reconstr Surg 1979;63:205–213.
36. Jacobs EQ, Hoffman S, et al. Reconstruction of a large chest wall defect using greater omentum. Arch Surg 1978;113:886–887.
37. Hidalgo DA. Omentum free flaps. In: Shaw WW, Hidalgo DA, eds. Microsurgery in trauma. New York: Futura, 1987:383–388.
38. Seyfer AE, Graeber GM, Wind GG. Atlas of chest wall reconstruction. Rockville, MD: Aspen Press, 1986.
39. Seyfer AE, Graeber GM. The use of latissimus dorsi and pectoralis major myocutaneous flaps in chest wall reconstruction. Contemp Surg 1983;22:29–39.
40. Neale HW, Kreilein JG, Schreiber JT, Gregory RO. Complete sternectomy for chronic osteomyelitis with reconstruction using a rectus abdominis myocutaneous island flap. Ann Plast Surg 1981;6:305–314.
41. Shaw WW, Hidalgo DA, Bermont MA, Keller A. Basic principles. In: Shaw WW, Hidalgo DA, eds. Microsurgery in trauma. Microsurgery instruments, sutures, and monitoring equipment. New York: Futura, 1987:21–35.
42. Ryan MA, McMurtrey MJ, Roth JA. Current management of chest wall tumors. Surg Clin North Am 1989;69:1061–1080.

43

MANAGEMENT OF MALIGNANT PLEURAL AND PERICARDIAL EFFUSIONS

*Chandra P. Belani, Andrew A. Ziskind,
Manish Dhawan, and Cynthia C. Lemmon*

MANAGEMENT OF MALIGNANT PLEURAL EFFUSIONS

Pleural effusions are a common problem in patients with malignancy and an important cause of morbidity and mortality. The presence of pleural effusions often signifies widespread or metastatic disease, but they can occur either as a presenting manifestation of a neoplastic disorder or as a first sign of recurrence. Although pleural effusions in patients with cancer may occasionally result from benign etiologies, in the vast majority they are caused by the underlying neoplastic process. An appropriate clinical evaluation and prompt diagnosis, followed by aggressive management strategies, can result in successful palliation in most cancer patients with a symptomatic pleural effusion.

PATHOPHYSIOLOGY

The presence of malignant cells in the fluid in the pleural space constitutes a malignant pleural effusion. The pleural space is lined by the visceral pleura on one side and the parietal pleura on the other. The visceral and parietal pleuras are composed of a single layer of mesothelial cells, forming an almost continuous layer. The parietal pleura is supplied by the high-pressure systemic circulation, i.e., the intercostal vessels; the visceral pleura is supplied mainly by the pulmonary circulation, creating a net hydrostatic gradient that predominantly drives a low-protein fluid across the pleural space (1). This fluid is dynamic in accordance with Starling's law (2):

$$F = k([HPc - HPif] - [COPc - COPif])$$

where F is the flow in milliliters per second; k is the filtration coefficient in milliliters/second/square centimeter/centimeters of water; Hpc is the mean capillary hydrostatic pressure in centimeters of water; Hpif is the mean interstitial fluid hydrostatic pressure in centimeters of water; COPc is the capillary plasma colloid osmotic pressure in centimeters of water; and COPif is the interstitial fluid colloid osmotic pressure in centimeters of water.

By applying Starling's law to the parietal pleura, the calculated net driving pressure causing fluid to enter the pleural space is +8 to +9 cm of water. Thus, under normal conditions fluid movement occurs from the parietal pleura to the visceral pleura. There is significant turnover, with up to 10 L of fluid passing through the pleural space in a 24-hour period (3, 4). Depending on the difference in pressure between the systemic circulation of the parietal pleura and the pulmonary circulation of the visceral pleura, the fluid entering the pleural space is reabsorbed into the visceral pleural capillaries. The little protein that enters the pleural space is cleared predominantly by the network of lymphatics that underlie the parietal and visceral pleurae, and it is transported via the thoracic duct back into the systemic circulation. Interference with any of the forces controlling pleural fluid dynamics, i.e., hydrostatic pressure, colloid osmotic pressure, capillary permeability, and lymphatic drainage, can result in the formation of a pleural effusion (4–6).

In a malignant process, several mechanisms typically are involved (4, 5, 7–9): (*a*) tumor embolization and seeding of the mesothelial pleural surface leading to increased generation of fluid, primarily because of decreased reabsorption of protein and fluid as a result of obstruction of subpleural lymphatics and visceral pleural capillaries; (*b*) mediastinal node metastases or true lymphangitic spread of tumor-causing obstruction to lymphatic flow; (*c*) free-floating tumor cells in the pleural space causing disruption of the delicate physiologic balance in the fluid movement; (*d*) release of vasoactive amines by pleural implants, resulting in alteration of the filtration coefficient of Starling's law and thus aggravating the accumulation of pleural fluid; and (e) other contributing factors related to the malignant disorder that may cause pleural effusion without direct involvement of the pleural space by tumor, including superior vena cava syndrome, congestive heart failure, hypoalbuminemia, pericardial involvement, mediastinal chest irradiation resulting in fibrosis of the mediastinal nodes and lymphatics, and malignant ascites.

CLINICAL MANIFESTATIONS AND DIAGNOSIS

Most patients with a malignant pleural effusion are symptomatic (8). The severity of symptoms often depends on the rate of fluid accumulation rather than on the total amount of fluid (8, 9), even though malignant pleural effusions tend to be larger than those from other causes. Patients usually present with cough, dyspnea, and pleuritic chest pain. Systemic complaints caused by the underlying malignancy include weight loss, anorexia, malaise, and fatigue. Physical findings include dullness to percussion, decreased vocal fremitus, and diminished breath sounds over the effusion with egophony ("E" to "A" changes) just above the level of the effusion. Massive effusions can cause bulging of the intercostal spaces, undetectable diaphragmatic excursion, and tracheal deviation to the contralateral side. In addition, specific findings, such as the presence of ascites, pericardial effusion, or diffuse palpable lymphadenopathy, may offer insight into the etiology of the effusion.

The chest radiograph is an inexpensive and sensitive investigation that confirms the presence of an effusion. The fluid collection appears as a typical ground glass shadow obscuring the costophrenic angle, diaphragm, and a variable amount of the pleural space, resulting in a shift of mediastinal structures when the collection is massive. An increased homogeneous density superimposed over the lung fields, obliteration of the silhouette of the diaphragm, a meniscus sign, apical capping, and accentuation of the right minor fissure have been described as signifying the presence of a pleural effusion. As little as 175 mL of fluid can be detected on an upright view of the chest, usually as blunting of the costophrenic angle (10). Decubitus views can show even smaller amounts (100 mL) of fluid in the pleural space (10, 11). Rarely, subpulmonic effusions may present without costophrenic angle blunting (12), but their presence is suggested by an increased separation of the diaphragmatic surface of the lung from the gastric bubble, as seen on an upright chest film. In addition to the upright posteroanterior and lateral chest views, it is essential to obtain lateral decubitus views to determine the location, volume, and nature (free flowing versus loculated) of a pleural effusion before embarking on management. In patients with very small amounts of pleural fluid or in those with extensive parenchymal lung involvement from the malignant process, a computed tomography (CT) scan may be more useful in confirming the presence of an effusion (13).

Malignancy is the most common cause of exudative pleural effusions in adults more than 60 years of age; almost half of all reported pleural effusions are caused by cancer (14–16). Malignancies of the breast, lung, and ovary, together with lymphomas, account for nearly 75% of all malignant pleural effusions. Malignancies of the gastrointestinal tract, genitourinary tract, an unknown primary site, skin (melanoma), and a variety of other solid tumors account for the rest (17) (Table 43.1). It has been said that roughly half of all patients with breast cancer (18), one-quarter of those with lung cancer (7), and one third of those with lymphoma (19) develop a malignant pleural effusion during the course of their disease. The course, however, may be altered to some extent with the use of newer aggressive therapeutic modalities that require further investigation.

THORACENTESIS

Thoracentesis is the first and most important study in confirming the malignant nature of the effusion, although removal of large amounts of fluid can also provide relief from pulmonary compromise. It is also useful to make sure that the lung is not trapped. In most instances the procedure is safe and carries few if any risks. The procedure is performed easily at the

TABLE 43.1. Malignancies that Cause Pleural Effusions

Breast carcinoma
Bronchogenic carcinoma
Lymphoma
Unknown primary malignancies
Ovarian carcinoma
Gastric carcinoma
Colon carcinoma
Pancreatic carcinoma
Melanoma
Renal cell carcinoma
Mesothelioma
Sarcoma
Other rare malignancies
   Thyroid carcinoma
   Leukemia
   Prostate carcinoma

bedside under local anesthesia, unless a small or loculated effusion demands ultrasound guidance. Uncommon complications include pleural shock, manifesting as bradycardia and hypotension, that results from an exaggerated vagal response when the needle crosses the parietal pleura. It can be reversed easily with atropine, administration of intravenous fluids, and placement of the patient in the Trendelenburg position. A large-volume rapid thoracentesis, usually more than 1500 mL, can result in reexpansion pulmonary edema (20, 21). Pneumothorax and bleeding are other complications that mandate careful assessment of a postprocedure chest radiograph. Repeated thoracentesis as the sole treatment for a pleural effusion is discouraged in patients with recurrent pleural effusion, however.

PLEURAL FLUID CHARACTERISTICS

Grossly, a bloody pleural effusion is seen more often from malignancy than from other causes. In the absence of trauma, the presence of more than 100,000 red blood cells per cubic millimeter suggests malignant pleural disease. The white blood cell count ranges from 1000 to 10,000 per cubic millimeter with a predominance of lymphocytes and monocytes (22). In the absence of recent chest trauma, chylous fluid suggests lymphatic obstruction from a malignant process (23).

More than 85% of all malignant effusions are exudative (8, 24, 25). The criteria proposed to define exudative effusion include: a pleural fluid-to-serum protein ratio of more than 0.5, a pleural fluid-to-serum lactic dehydrogenase ratio of more than 0.6, or a pleural fluid LDH level of 200 international units (IU). These criteria are not absolute. Other parameters that have been used to classify exudates—including pleural fluid protein level of at least 3 g/dL (24, 25), pH of less than 7.30 (26), or specific gravity greater than 1.016 (24)—are not as accurate in distinguishing exudates from transudates. With an increase in intrapleural tumor burden, the pleural fluid glucose may decrease to less than 60 mg/dL. High levels of pleural fluid amylase have been reported, especially in patients who have underlying adenocarcinomas of the lung and ovary (27, 28); in such cases the amylase isoenzyme type has most often been salivary.

CYTOLOGIC EXAMINATION

The detection of malignant cells in the pleural fluid is the definitive means of diagnosing a malignant pleural effusion. It is advised that a large amount of fluid (more than 250 mL) be submitted for cytologic examination to maximize the yield. Approximately half of malignant pleural effusions are diagnosed on the basis of the first cytology (8, 29–31); the yield increases by 17% to 22% with the second and third cytologic examinations (30). Cytologic examination of the pleural fluid is more sensitive than pleural biopsy alone in making a definitive diagnosis, probably because of the focal nature of metastases and the blind sampling procedure; when these techniques are combined, malignant pleural effusions can be diagnosed correctly in 80% of cases (30–32). Pleural biopsy should be performed only if cytologic examination of pleural fluid fails to yield a diagnosis. Contraindications to pleural biopsy include an uncooperative patient, uncorrected bleeding diathesis, and an obliterated pleural space. Pleural fluid cytology and tissue obtained by blind needle biopsy of the pleura are inadequate in making a definitive diagnosis of mesothelioma, which usually requires a large piece of tissue obtained at thoracoscopy or open pleural biopsy (5). Pleural effusions associated with Hodgkin's disease and other lymphomas have a low diagnostic yield on cytologic examinations, because the etiology in these cases is obstruction of central lymphatics by mediastinal lymph node involvement, not by direct involvement of the pleural surfaces (33, 34). To distinguish reactive mesothelial cells from malignant cells, pleural fluid occasionally is placed in tissue culture, thus allowing easier identification of malignant cells (35).

IMMUNOCYTOCHEMISTRY

The application of immunocytochemical techniques to cytologic diagnosis using monoclonal antibodies, polyclonal antisera to epithelial membrane antigen or carcinoembryonic antigen (CEA), and immunoperoxidase staining has been used to increase the diagnostic yield of pleural fluid cytologic examinations. Immunostaining with monoclonal antibody B72.3 (36, 37) has been a useful diagnostic adjunct to the differentiation of adenocarcinoma from mesothelial cells, and it can highlight occult cells in cytospin preparations not identified using standard cytologic criteria. Polyclonal antisera to epithelial membrane antigen have demonstrated reactivity with 54% of carcinomatous effusions and no reactivity with benign effusions (38). Anti-CEA antisera also have demonstrated reactivity with 50% of carcinoma cells (39), whereas no reactivity has been noted with mesothelial cells. A number of other panels of monoclonal antibodies, e.g. HMFG-2, AUA-1, Mbr, and MOv2 (40), have been used and demonstrate reactivity with malignant cells, but their sensitivity and specificity limits remain to be defined.

CYTOGENETICS

Chromosomal analysis of cells in the pleural fluid does not provide a histopathologic diagnosis; cytogenetic abnormalities signify malignancy, however, especially when the cytology or clinical setting are not definitive, such as in patients with underlying hematologic malignancy. DeWald et al. (41), in a study of 82 patients, were able to diagnose 65% of the malignant disorders by cytologic examination of the pleural fluid, compared with 71% by cytogenetic analysis. The combined yield of both methods was 83%. Eleven of the 13 patients with lymphoma or leukemia had cytogenetic abnormalities, whereas only 4 had positive cytology, emphasizing the importance of pleural fluid cytogenetics in diagnosing these disorders. Fraisse and associates (42) have demonstrated that cytogenetic abnormalities are not seen in the analysis of benign pleural effusions. Chromosomal analysis of pleural fluid is not performed routinely because of the expense and time involved. It should be reserved for patients who have pleural effusions with negative cytology on two separate occasions when there is a high index of clinical suspicion that the effusions are malignant.

OTHER PLEURAL FLUID STUDIES

Other studies include measurement of pleural fluid markers such as CEA (43) and creatinine kinase BB (44), or enzymes such as galactosyl transferase (45); however, these studies are usually nonspecific, expensive, and not adequately sensitive. These studies usually are not helpful in making a definitive diagnosis of the pleural fluid.

THORACOSCOPY

Despite cytologic examination of pleural fluid and a percutaneous needle biopsy specimen, approximately 15% to 20% of pleural effusions remain undiagnosed. Cytogenetic abnormalities signify the presence of underlying malignancy but do not provide the histopathologic diagnosis. Currently, the two options available for obtaining tissue for definitive diagnoses are thoracoscopy and limited thoracotomy.

With its more extensive use and wider availability, thoracoscopy is emerging as a highly successful diagnostic and therapeutic tool (46, 47). Video-assisted thoracoscopy performed under local or general anesthesia offers two distinct advantages:

1. It allows excellent visualization of the entire pleural surface and directed biopsies of suspicious sites.

2. It is associated with minimal morbidity and mortality, making thoracoscopy possible in patients who are high surgical risks.

The diagnostic yield of thoracoscopy with biopsy for malignant pleural effusions is as high as 96%, and the sensitivity and specificity have been reported to be 83% and 100%, respectively (48). Ohri and colleagues (49) demonstrated an 85% success rate in obtaining a diagnosis by thoracoscopy in a cohort of patients with an undiagnosed pleural effusion. Boutin et al. (48) were able to show a diagnostic accuracy of 96% in 215 patients by thoracoscopy, even when pleural fluid cytology and blind percutaneous pleural biopsy failed to make a histopathologic diagnosis of the underlying malignancy. Video-assisted thoracoscopy is a safe procedure, and most studies report few if any side effects, although complications can occur, as evidenced by a few deaths reported in the literature. Some of these may be related to the risks from general anesthesia or the overall poor health of this group of patients. Today, thoracoscopic techniques are being used more often, even when additional procedures, e.g., hilar or mediastinal node sampling and lung biopsies, are planned simultaneously. In addition to assisting in diagnosis, thoracoscopy allows for the introduction of sterile talc, which can be highly effective in the sclerosis of pleural surfaces.

MANAGEMENT OF MALIGNANT PLEURAL EFFUSIONS

The approach to the management of malignant pleural effusions depends on the specific underlying disease or etiology. A patient may have an underlying malignancy, but the etiology of the effusion may be a concomitant illness unrelated to malignancy, such as pulmonary embolism; pneumonia (parapneumonic or synpneumonic effusion); pulmonary infections like tuberculosis, congestive heart failure, cirrhosis of the liver; or nutritional deficiencies with pleural effusions and anasarca. In such cases it is imperative to treat the concomitant illness, rather than the effusion, although occasionally an emergency therapeutic thoracentesis may be required, especially if the effusion is massive and rapid relief is needed to avoid respiratory compromise.

Secondary pleural effusions are those that occur as a direct result of the underlying malignancy but that in fact are not malignant. These include effusions caused by obstruction of the central lymphatics by malignant mediastinal nodes as well as effusions accompanying superior vena cava syndrome, those secondary to trapped lung, effusions in patients with malignant pericardial effusions or ascites, and effusions secondary to treatment with chemotherapeutic agents such as taxotere or biologic therapies such as the interleukins. The focus of management of patients with secondary pleural effusions is the underlying disease or malignancy rather than the effusion itself.

Primary malignant pleural effusions (Fig. 43.1), as described above, either with direct involvement of the pleura by the malignant process or by free-floating tumor cells in the fluid, are divided into two categories. One group may be controlled by systemic treatment of the underlying malignancy such as lymphoma, breast cancer, testicular cancer, or small cell lung cancer, although therapeutic thoracentesis may be required for optimal relief of symptoms. The long-term effects in terms of success and survival are related to the underlying malignancy, the patient's general condition and performance status, and the availability of effective systemic therapy. Despite effective systemic treatments for these malignant disorders, some patients fail to respond and are then considered for local therapies.

The second category consists of patients who have an underlying malignancy that cannot be con-

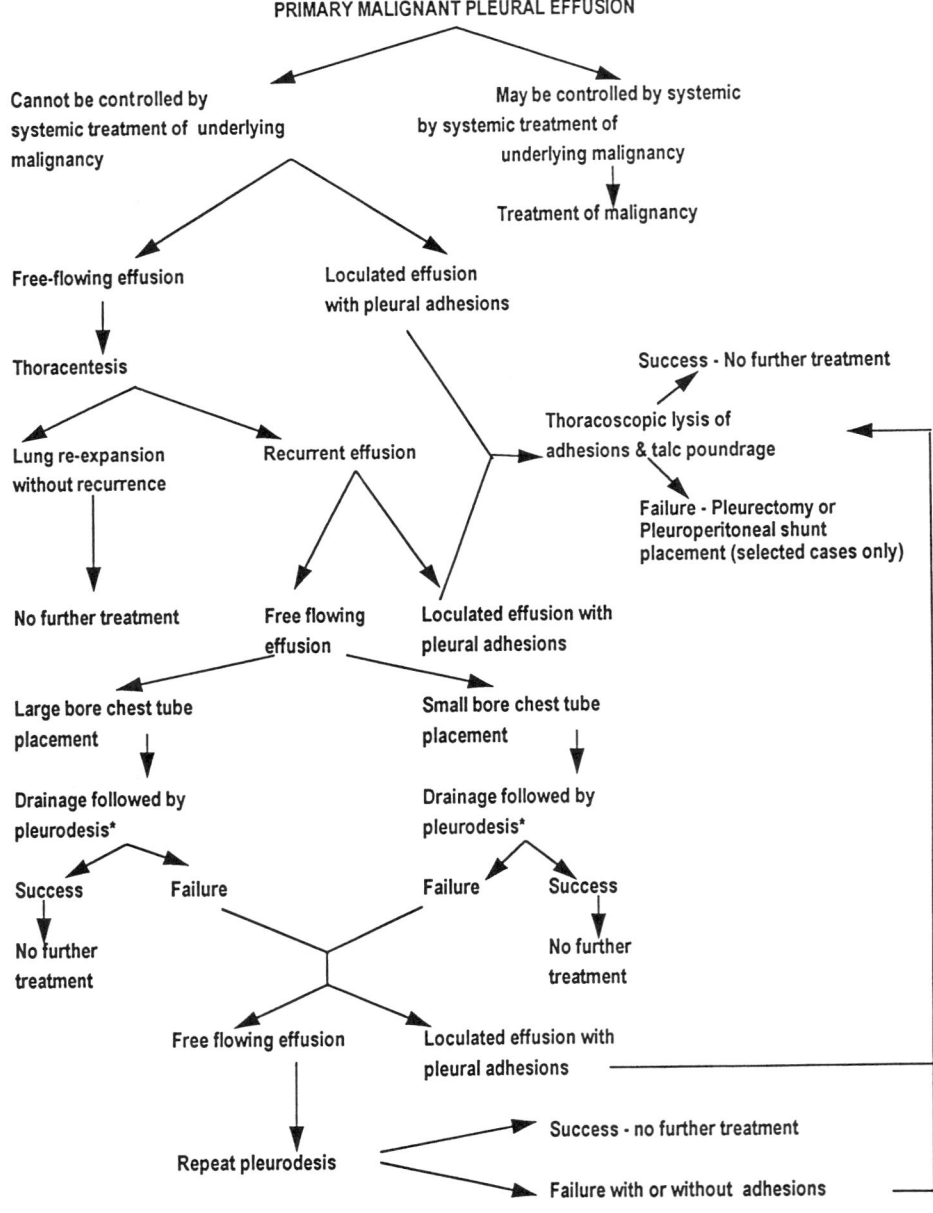

FIGURE 43.1. Management flow chart used by the University of Pittsburgh Medical Center for treatment of patients with primary malignant pleural effusions.

trolled by effective systemic treatment. These patients are candidates for local and intrapleural therapies with the primary objective being palliation of symptoms and improvement in quality of life (50, 51).

The most important local therapy for patients with symptomatic malignant pleural effusions is thoracentesis. In addition to being a necessary part of the diagnostic workup, the removal of large amounts of fluid can also provide relief (therapeutic) from pulmonary compromise. Only a small number of patients respond to thoracentesis alone as a primary management strategy for malignant pleural effusions (17). The majority of patients have recurrence within a short period because of the uncontrolled malignant process. Tube thoracostomy with drainage, usually followed by pleurodesis with instillation of a sclerosing agent, is the next step in the management of primary malignant pleural effusions.

TECHNIQUE OF TUBE THORACOSTOMY AND PLEURAL SCLEROTHERAPY

The instillation of a sclerosing agent for control or prevention of recurrence of the effusion in patients with a malignant pleural effusion has been fairly well standardized. It is imperative to establish that there is lung reexpansion following initial thoracentesis, i.e., absence of loculations and pleural adhesions. Thus, a careful examination of the available roentgenographic studies, including lateral decubitus chest films and in some cases CT scans, is necessary. The presence of adhesions with loculated areas of effusion prevents adequate drainage of fluid by tube thoracostomy alone. The chest tube is placed, by an experienced surgeon or physician, into the sixth or seventh interspace in the anterior axillary line so that the patient does not compress the chest tube when lying supine. Premedication with 10 mg of morphine sulfate or 100 mg of meperidine relaxes the patient and decreases the discomfort. In addition, 20 to 30 mL of 1% lidocaine is used locally to anesthetize the chest wall. Observing all sterile precautions, a quick thoracentesis is performed to document good flow of effusion. The site is changed if free flow of fluid is not obtained. Then a small incision is made, followed by creation of a tunnel down to the intercostal muscles over the appropriate rib. An appropriate chest tube is placed through the tunnel into the pleural cavity and directed cephalad by a clamp at the introducing end and a clamp at the end to prevent both open pneumothorax and rapid evacuation of pleural fluid. The chest tube is then connected to the water seal drainage system (the clamp is removed) and negative wall suction (15 to 20 cm of water). A stitch is used to anchor the chest tube to the skin, and a sterile dressing is applied. A chest radiograph is obtained to view proper tube placement. Thereafter, chest radiographs are obtained daily to confirm tube position and to rule out pneumothorax.

SCLEROTHERAPY

Sclerotherapy usually is performed when the drainage decreases to less than 100 mL in 24 hours and when there is little or no residual fluid left in the chest. The procedure is likely to be most effective if total evacuation of fluid occurs with good lung expansion after drainage. The sclerosing agent is instilled through the chest tube and the tube clamped for 2 hours; the patient's position is changed every 15 minutes (e.g., supine, left lateral, prone, right lateral, supine) to allow even distribution of the sclerosing agent. The tube is then unclamped, and wall suction (15 to 20 cm of water) is reestablished. The catheter is removed 24 hours after the procedure, provided there is no significant persistent drainage (≤100 mL per 24 hours). A chest radiograph is obtained to rule out pneumothorax. Success of sclerotherapy is ascertained by assessing changes in clinical signs and symptoms and in the size of effusions seen on chest radiographs obtained monthly after sclerotherapy.

SCLEROSING AGENTS

A number of agents have been used for pleurodesis in patients with malignant pleural effusions. These agents produce adhesions or chemical pleuritis between the visceral and parietal pleura by mechanisms that are not understood clearly.

NONCHEMOTHERAPEUTIC AGENTS

TALC

Talc was introduced for pleural poudrage by Bethune in 1935 (52). The microscopic processes observed after intrapleural instillation include visceral pleural thickening with fibroblast proliferation, macrophage infiltration, and foreign body reaction (53, 54). It is one of the most effective agents for pleurodesis in patients with malignant pleural effusions, but it has not yet gained universal acceptance because of associated potential hazards, expense, and complications. It is thought to cause severe reactive pleuritis, resulting in pleurodesis; conversely, it has been implicated in worsening pain and dyspnea with occasional development of respiratory failure (55, 56). The risk of developing mesothelioma after talc pleurodesis is probably nonexistent because it is free of asbestos, although trace amounts of iron, calcium, and aluminum can be detected in the United States Pharmacopia talc. Other complications associated with talc pleurodesis include fever (52, 55), acute pneumonitis (57), granulomatous pneumonitis with talc recovered from bronchoalveolar large fluid (58), and empyema with local site infections (59, 60). Death also has been reported in several studies of talc pleurodesis (55, 56, 59–64).

Various methods have been used for talc pleurodesis, including: (a) direct application to the pleural surfaces after open thoracotomy; (b) insufflation into the pleural space by thoracoscopic techniques under general anesthesia; or (c) instillation as a slurry by tube thoracostomy.

Pleurodesis for malignant pleural effusions via open thoracotomy usually is seldom used because of prolonged recovery in patients who have limited life expectancies. Modern thoracoscopic techniques with video assistance assure uniform distribution of talc (Table 43.2), as opposed to instillation of slurry via chest tube, although the efficacy of both approaches has been excellent; a success rate of 85% to 100% has been reported by most investigators (49, 59, 60–69) (Table 43.2). A large randomized study comparing talc pleurodesis via thoracoscopic poudrage versus chest tube slurry is in progress.

Most trials have been retrospective and have used different criteria (sometimes subjective) to define responses, along with loosely defined eligibility criteria, making comparison difficult. In several studies the complete and persistent absence of pleural fluid has been the determinant of successful pleurodesis, whereas in others the requirement for no further pleural drainage has been the sole criteria for response. The criteria commonly used to define response has been continued complete radiographic reexpansion of the lung at 30 days after the procedure. This technique has been the simplest and most reproducible measurement of response available. The dose of talc used for pleurodesis has ranged from 2 to 10.5 g, and patients usually have required only one instillation. The effect of dose on success cannot be determined from the published studies, because there have been no direct comparisons of various doses in similar patient populations. Higher doses are known to have been associated with increased incidence of adverse effects, especially respiratory failure. The recommended dose of talc for pleurodesis via poudrage or slurry is 5 g.

Randomized studies of sclerotherapy in the management of malignant pleural effusions (Table 43.3) — comparing the efficacy of talc with that of bleomycin (65) and tetracycline (65, 66)—have shown higher success rates with talc pleurodesis. Further investigation is needed, however, because the patient numbers have been small and thus definitive conclusions cannot be made regarding the superiority of any one agent.

The short-term adverse effects with talc pleurodesis include fever, pain, local infection, empyema, and

TABLE 43.2. Thoracoscopic Talc Pleurodesis in the Management of Malignant Pleural Effusions

Reference No.	Method	Dose	Evaluable Patients (with MPE)	CR Defined at Day 30	Days (Mean) of Chest Tube Drainage after Talc Instillation	Comments
49	Thoracoscopic insufflation	2–5 g	36	36	. . .	Retrospective review of the investigators' experience in patients with both malignancy and other disorders
63	Thoracoscopic insufflation and instillation of talc slurry via chest tube	2 g	154	130	. . .	Retrospective review. Several patients required repeat talc instillation
65	Thoracoscopic insufflation	3–6 g	33	32	4 ± 1.2 days	One arm of a prospective study comparing talc with tetracycline and bleomycin (see Table 43.4 for details)
66	Thoracoscopic insufflation	. . .	12	11	5 days	Prospective randomized trial of talc versus tetracycline in patients with breast cancer
67	Thoracoscopic insufflation	3.5–10.5 g	14	12	4.6 days	One patient had fatal pulmonary embolism
69	Thoracoscopic insufflation	2.5 g	28	23	2.7 days	Long-term CR reported

Abbreviations. MPE, malignant pleural effusion; CR, complete response.

TABLE 43.3. Randomized Studies of Sclerotherapy in the Management of Malignant Pleural Effusions

INVESTIGATOR/ REF.	STUDY DESIGN	NO. OF PATIENTS	CR AT 30 DAYS (%)	CR AT 90 DAYS (%)	MEAN DURATION OF CHEST TUBE DRAINAGE	COMMENTS
Hartman (65)	Talc (thoracoscopic insufflation), 3–6 g vs.	33	97	95	4.0 ± 1.2	Significantly higher success rate with thoracoscopic talc pleurodesis over the other two agents. Thoracoscopy was performed under local anesthesia and intravenous sedation with no mortality reported from the procedure.
	Bleomycin (chest tube sclerosis), 60 IU vs.	37	64	70	6.6 ± 1.6	
	Tetracycline (chest tube sclerosis) 1 g	36	33	44	6.5 ± 2.1	
Fentiman (66)	Talc (thoracoscopic insufflation) vs.	12	95	...	...	All patients had breast cancer. Four patients with recurrence on tetracycline were treated successfully with talc.
	Tetracycline, 500 mg	21	45	...	...	
Ruckdeschel (74)	Bleomycin, 60 IU vs.	37	64	70	...	Significantly higher response noted with bleomycin. Spectrum of side effects similar in both groups.
	Tetracycline, 1 g	36	33	47	...	
Kessinger (75)	Bleomycin, 89 IU vs.	15	28	...	...	No significant difference between the two groups. Small number of patients in the bleomycin arm.
	Tetracycline, 500 mg	26	27	...	...	

Abbreviations. CR, complete response; IU, international units.

dose-related respiratory failure (adult respiratory distress syndrome–like symptoms). Cardiovascular complications, such as arrhythmias (49), cardiac arrest (66), myocardial infarction (62), and hypotension (70), have been reported, but they are difficult to relate to talc per se because they can result from the surgical procedure alone. The long-term effects of talc on pulmonary function and survival probably are minimal (71) but need to be defined and evaluated further.

TETRACYCLINE

Until recently tetracycline hydrochloride was the agent most commonly used for achieving pleurodesis. It was cheap and effective, but the intravenous form used for intrapleural instillation is no longer commercially available in the United States. The reported success rate for control of malignant pleural effusions with this agent ranged from 59% to 94% (65, 66, 72–82) (Table 43.4). Although the doses of tetracycline used in various studies have ranged from a 500-mg total dose to 20 mg/kg, Gravelyn et al. (78) showed a direct relationship between the success in achieving pleurodesis and the use of a 1-g dose of tetracycline. In their study patients who received lower doses for pleural sclerosis had significantly poorer response. The usual dose recommended for pleurodesis was 1 g in 30 to 50 mL of 0.9% saline via the chest tube, with an indwelling time of 2 hours. There seems to be no apparent advantage of giving tetracycline intrapleurally on two consecutive days (73). The low pH of tetracycline was initially thought to be the reason for production of pleuritis and subsequent pleural fibrosis based on the dose-response effect. Subsequently, several investigators have shown that the pH of the sclerosing agent is not the reason for its effectiveness (80). There is some evidence that tetracycline-stimulated mesothelial cells release growth factor–like activity for fibroblasts, and that this action may play an important role in inducing pleural fibrosis (82).

DOXYCYCLINE

Doxycycline usually is administered as a 500-mg dose diluted in 30 to 100 mL of normal saline through a chest tube for pleurodesis; the success rate ranges from 60% to 72% (Table 43.4). The use of doxycycline has increased since the distribution of parenteral tetracycline was halted in the United States. Mänsson (83) treated 18 patients with 500 mg of intrapleural doxycy-

TABLE 43.4. Nonchemotherapeutic Agents in the Management of Pleural Effusion

REFERENCE NOS.	AGENT/DOSE USED	NO. OF PATIENTS	CR (%)	ADVERSE EFFECTS
49, 59–69	Talc, 2–10.5 g	352	315 (89)	Rare reports of ARDS-like syndrome seen at high dose. Recommended dose ≤5 g
65, 66, 72, 73, 74, 75, 76, 77, 78, 79, 80	Tetracycline, 500 mg–20 mg/kg	415	271 (65)	Pain and fever are the common side effects in approximately 15% of patients.
83, 84	Doxycycline, 500 mg	60	43 (72)	Efficacy and side effect profile similar to tetracycline, but repeat instillation usually required
85	Minocycline, 300 mg	7	6 (86)	...
86, 87, 88, 89	Mepacrine, 350–2000 mg	94	70 (74)	Severe pleuritic pain occurs in the majority of paitents. Convulsions have been reported after intrapleural instillation.

Abbreviations. CR, complete resposne; ARDS, adult respiratory distress syndrome.

cline diluted in 30 mL of saline and observed a complete response in 11 (61%) patients for an average response duration of 8.9 months; repeated instillation was required in 13 (72%) patients. The incidence of pain and fever was approximately 20%. Kitamura et al. (84) observed an overall response in 11 of 15 patients who received intrapleural doxycycline, but in their experience more than one instillation was required. There were no responses after a single dose, 2 of 15 responded after two doses, 7 of 13 responded after three doses, and two thirds responded after four doses. The doses were repeated twice weekly. The only adverse effect was chest pain, which occurred in one third of the patients. Thus, repeated intrapleural instillations of doxycycline usually are required for effective pleurodesis; the observed side effects usually are fever and chest pain.

MINOCYCLINE

The experience with minocycline as a sclerosing agent is limited (Table 43.4). In one study 300 mg of minocycline with 1% lidocaine instilled intrapleurally produced complete responses in six of seven patients (85). There were no observed vestibular side effects—a usual occurrence when minocycline is administered systemically at these doses.

QUINACRINE

Quinacrine (mepacrine, Atabrine), an antimalarial agent, also has been used for pleurodesis in patients with malignant pleural effusions (86–89) (Table 43.4). The objective responses with quinacrine have been excellent (86–89) and comparable to those seen with tetracycline (87); fever, severe pleuritic pain, hallucinations, and convulsions following the administration of quinacrine have been reported (88, 90). Because of the substantial toxic effects seen with intrapleural instillation and the availability of other equally effective and less toxic agents, quinacrine is not recommended for use in the management of malignant pleural effusions.

CHEMOTHERAPEUTIC AGENTS

BLEOMYCIN

Bleomycin is usually well tolerated when given intrapleurally in patients with malignant pleural effusions (91–96) (Table 43.5). The sclerosing dose of bleomycin for intrapleural instillation is 60 units (U) or 1 U/kg of body weight in 50 mL of normal saline. Occasionally, there is mild fever or transient nausea, neither of which require medication. Pleuritic pain and rigors are other known, rare, side effects. When instilled intrapleurally, bleomycin is absorbed systemically; however, in most patients evidence of systemic toxicity is minimal. Following intracavitary instillation it may cause a nonspecific local irritation that results in sclerosis and adherence of opposing pleural surfaces. It may have local cytotoxic effects as well (94). Bleomycin is instilled into the chest through a thoracostomy tube, followed by clamping of the tube, periodic rotation of the patient for even distribution throughout the pleural space, and subsequent removal of the remaining fluid. From various studies a dose of 60 U of bleomycin appears to be effective and safe. Paladine et al. (95) reported a response rate of 63% in 40 patients with malignant pleural effusions treated with intrapleural bleomycin; at 1 month 30 of the treated patients were alive. Similar response results were reported by Bitran et al. (96) in patients who had recurrence after tetracycline pleurodesis. In a prospective

TABLE 43.5. Chemotherapeutic Agents in the Management of Malignant Pleural Effusions

REFERENCE NOS.	AGENT/DOSE	NO. OF EVALUABLE PATIENTS	CR (%)	COMMENTS
74, 75, 86, 90–96	Bleomycin, 60–180 IU	285	155 (54%)	Fever and nausea in 25% of patients; pain usually mild; recommended dose, 60 IU
91, 97–99	Mitoxantrone, 25–60 mg	111	69 (62%)	Grade 2 leukopenia because of systemic absorption in 25% of patients; recommended dose, 30 mg
100, 101	Doxorubicin, 10–40 mg	62	19 (30%)	Pain, fever, and nausea in 15% to 30% of patients
102, 103	Cisplatin, 100 mg/m^2; and cytarabine, 600 mg (or 1200 mg)	44	12 (27%)	Myelosuppression (in 50% of patients) and renal insufficiency (30% of patients) are the main toxicities
104	Etoposide, 100–125 mg/m^2/week × 3 weeks	9	0	Myelosuppression at high doses; alopecia and emesis also seen
105	5-Fluorouracil, 2–3 g	35	23 (66%)	Mild reversible myelosuppression seen in most patients
106	Mitomycin C, 8 mg	27	11 (41%)	Pain and fever in 10% of patients; repeated instillation required for response

Abbreviations. IU, international units; CR, complete response.

multiinstitutional trial, Ruckdeschel and coworkers (74) compared bleomycin pleurodesis with tetracycline pleurodesis for the management of malignant pleurodesis. Eligible patients—those with a cytologically positive effusion or positive pleural biopsy and evidence of lung expansion after tube thoracostomy with drainage rates of not more than 100 mL in 24 hours—were randomized to receive either 60 U of bleomycin or 1 g of tetracycline intrapleurally. Recurrent disease was defined as radiographic evidence of any fluid reaccumulation after complete drainage of the pleural space and reexpansion of the lung, with rates of recurrence evaluated at 30 and 90 days. Toxicity and overall survival did not differ between the two groups. The recurrence rate within 30 days of treatment was 36% (10 of 28) with bleomycin and 67% (18 of 27) with tetracycline ($P = .023$); at 90 days the recurrence rate was 30% (11 of 37) with bleomycin and 53% (19 of 36) with tetracycline ($P = .047$). Median time to recurrence was 32 days for tetracycline-treated patients and at least 46 days for bleomycin-treated patients ($P = .037$). Thus, the rate of recurrence was significantly lower and the time to recurrence significantly longer in the bleomycin group, compared with the tetracycline group, in this nearly homogeneous group of patients. Bleomycin thus has been suggested as a suitable alternative to tetracycline, which is no longer commercially available in the United States, as a parenteral preparation for intracavitary installation as a sclerosing agent.

MITOXANTRONE

Mitoxantrone (Table 43.5) (91, 97–99), because of its high polarity and high protein binding, is absorbed extremely slowly, with only 17% of the total dosage reaching the systemic circulation after intrapleural administration (97). Torsten et al. (98) achieved a response in 11 of 12 patients with malignant pleural effusions for a mean period of 3.2 months using tube thoracostomy drainage and instillation of 30 mg of mitoxantrone. Topuz et al. (99) reported a 32% complete response and a 46% partial response with intrapleural mitoxantrone among 22 patients with lung and breast cancer-related effusions; more responses occurred in patients with breast cancer. In a study (98) comparing bleomycin and mitoxantrone, the response rate for bleomycin (64%) was comparable to that for mitoxantrone (67%). Grade 2 neutropenia was seen with intracavitary mitoxantrone instillation and was prolonged in one patient who received a second dose. Mitoxantrone also has been used for palliation of malignant peritoneal and pericardial effusions. Further investigation is needed to evaluate and confirm the efficacy of this agent for sclerotherapy.

OTHER CHEMOTHERAPEUTIC AGENTS

Many other chemotherapeutic agents (Table 43.5), such as the combinations of doxorubicin (100, 101), cisplatin, and cytarabine (102, 103); and etoposide (104), 5-fluorouracil (105), and mitomycin C (106), have been used for intrapleural instillation in patients with malignant pleural effusions. The results have not been impressive and are associated with the additional side effects related to the systemic absorption. The efficacy of these agents in the management of malignant pleural effusions is questionable, and they are not recommended at this time.

BIOLOGIC THERAPIES

CORYNEBACTERIUM PARVUM

Corynebacterium parvum (CBP) (Table 43.6) was reported in 1978 to cause pleurodesis (107). Both animal and human studies suggested that CBP possessed immune-stimulating action at the site of the effusion, thus resulting in a hypothetical increase in cytotoxicity against tumor cells (108). Contrary to earlier beliefs, the result of treatment with CBP often is a fibrotic thickening of the pleura with recruitment of neutrophils (109), rather than recruitment of mononuclear cells with immunostimulant properties. Ostrowski and coworkers (92) compared 60 U of bleomycin and 7 mg of CBP in a randomized study in 58 patients with malignant effusions. Among the 44 patients alive at 30 days, a complete response was seen in 12 (48%) of 25 patients treated with bleomycin and in 6 (32%) of 19 patients receiving CBP ($P>.13$); significantly more breast cancer patients responded to bleomycin ($P = .06$). There was a trend toward a longer duration of response for bleomycin at 6 months (32% for bleomycin versus 16% for CBP) and at 1 year (16% for bleomycin versus 5% for CBP). Most of the other series have reported higher response rates for pleurodesis with CBP, but these studies have included only small numbers of inhomogeneous patients, variable criteria for assessing response, and no long-term follow-up. CBP is not used routinely as a sclerosing agent in patients with malignant pleural effusions.

INTERFERONS

In addition to use for their cytotoxic effects, interferons (Table 43.6) have been administered intrapleurally for control of malignant pleural effusions with the intention of obtaining local immune modulation (including stimulation of N-K cells) (113). Interferon-2b, in incremental dosages of 3 to 50×10^6 U/m^2 after thoracentesis, did not demonstrate any major effect on control of malignant pleural effusions in a small study with 22 patients (114). By comparison, interferon-β resulted in 28% complete responses among 29 patients treated with 5 to 20 million units for a maximum of three intrapleural instillations, as reported by Rosso et al. (115). Occasional conversions to negative cytology (pleural effusion) have been reported. Transient fever, pain, and flulike symptoms are the side effects encountered most commonly, but occasionally myelosuppression has been seen (116, 117).

INTERLEUKIN-2

Intrapleural administration of interleukin-2 (rIL-2) was found to activate lymphokine-activated killer cells and to induce a cytologic response to malignant pleural effusions in patients with lung cancer (118). There also is evidence that rIL-2 used in the treatment of pleural effusions is maintained at relatively high levels for a prolonged duration, even after infusions of small amounts; this finding suggests that there is a local pharmacologic advantage and a decreased potential of severe systemic toxicity (119–121). A number of studies (Table 34.6) have investigated the use of rIL-2

TABLE 43.6. Biologic Therapies in the Management of Malignant Pleural Effusions

REFERENCE NOS.	AGENT	NO. OF PATIENTS TREATED	NO. OF CR (%)	ADVERSE EFFECTS
76, 92, 93, 107–113	*Corynebacterium parvum* (CBP), 4–14 mg	169	129 (76%)	Pain and nausea reported in 40% of patients; fever uncommon
113, 114	Interferon-α-2b, $3–75 \times 10^6$ U	40	8 (20%)	Flulike symptoms in 70% of patients; grade III neutropenia seen at high doses
115–117	Interferon-β, $5–35 \times 10^6$ U	59	10 (17%)	Transient fever, pruritus in 5% to 7% of patients
118–123	Interleukin-2, $3–75 \times 10^6$ IU/m^2/day $\times$ 5 days	91	18 (20%)	Febrile episodes in all patients; two cases of empyema at high doses of interleukin-2 (24 million U/m^2/day); complete tumor responses in the chest seen in some patients

Abbreviations. CR, complete responses; U, units; IU, international units.

for the management of malignant pleural effusions (118–123) (Table 43.3). In a phase I study (118), incremental doses of rIL-2—from 3×10^6 to 24×10^6 U/m^2/day for 5 days administered via a thin catheter inserted into the pleural cavity—resulted in 10 responses (partial and complete) among 22 patients treated. Fluid retention and fever were the most common side effects. The investigators recommended the phase II dose of 21×10^6 U/m^2/day for 5 days administered intrapleurally. Yasumoto et al. (118) used 250 to 1000 U of rIL-2 in 20 mL of 0.9% normal saline daily for 5 to 33 days (mean duration, 14 days) through a double-lumen trocar catheter inserted into the pleural cavity to evacuate the fluid. Complete response, defined by the disappearance of both malignant cells and pleural effusions for more than 4 weeks, occurred in 13 of the 35 lung cancer patients (37%) treated; there were no serious side effects. Thus, intrapleural administration of rIL-2 with prolonged measurable activity (123) and delayed but lasting induction of cytotoxic activity with the augmentation of various cytokines (IL-4, IL-6, and macrophage colony-stimulating factor) may prove to be valuable in the control of malignant pleural effusions. Further investigations to determine the optimum intrapleural dose, schedule, and vehicle of administration (e.g., ethiodized oil emulsion, liposomes) of rIL-2 are in progress.

RADIOACTIVE ISOTOPES

Intrapleural radioactive isotopes have been used since 1951 in the palliative management of malignant pleural effusions (124). Radioactive gold (^{198}Au) (half-life, 2.70 days, 1.71 MeV; γ, 0.412 MeV) and radioactive chromium phosphate (Cr^{32}PO$_4$) (half-life, 14.3 days; 1.71 MeV) have been the two radioisotopes used, although the latter is both less expensive and less hazardous. The response rates for these agents have ranged from 55% (125) to 61% (126), and the morbidity with intrapleural administration is minimal, with nausea being the most common side effect. Their availability is limited because of their short half-lives and the requirement for the protection of health care personnel from radiation.

LARGE-BORE VERSUS SMALL-BORE CATHETERS

Traditionally, large-bore catheters (28F to 32F) have been placed by surgeons (50, 51) for the purpose of drainage and instillation of sclerosing agents. Recent reports (127, 128) suggest, however, that small-bore (7F to 24F) catheters can be used with equal success. The potential advantages of small-bore catheters include less traumatic insertion and better tolerance by patients. These catheters usually are inserted under radiologic imaging guidance, e.g., sonography or CT scan, allowing placement at the optimal site of drainage. They are inserted in trocar fashion, and after release from the cannula, they form a partial curve to prevent pleural injury.

A recent study suggests that pleural sclerosis performed via a small-bore catheter placed under ultrasound guidance is as effective, with an overall success rate of 71%, as techniques that use larger surgical chest tubes (historical data) (128). The problem of patient discomfort during the treatment of malignant pleural effusions is thus of immense importance. Physicians should not be satisfied with a procedure, even a highly effective one, if it causes extended periods of discomfort for patients with short life expectancies. In such patients quality of life issues take on greater importance. The use of small-bore catheters is a major step toward increasing patient comfort and avoiding procedures associated with significant morbidity.

AMBULATORY SCLEROTHERAPY

Traditionally, tube thoracostomy and pleurodesis for treatment of malignant pleural effusions are performed as inpatient procedures or in the operating room while the patient is hospitalized. Future modifications in the management of malignant pleural effusions would not only attempt to minimize patient discomfort, but also ensure the development of outpatient and ambulatory methods of drainage in combination with sclerotherapy. These innovations would enable the patient to stay at home, thus avoiding the need for hospitalization and simultaneously reducing health care costs. A study using small-bore catheters, which are connected to a plastic bag with a one-way valve system for gravity drainage and placed under the guidance of an imaging modality (CT or ultrasound) by a radiologist, is being conducted at several institutions (Figs. 43.2 and 43.3). The sclerosing agent is instilled when the overall drainage decreases to less than 100 mL in 24 hours, and the lung has reexpanded. The whole procedure is performed in the ambulatory setting, thus avoiding the need for hospitalization.

SURGICAL THERAPEUTIC OPTIONS

Despite standard therapy of thoracentesis, tube thoracostomy, with or without sclerotherapy, certain patients have intractable malignant pleural effusions. Thoracoscopic talc insufflation after mechanical lysis of adhesions usually is performed after patients fail tube thoracostomy drainage and sclerotherapy with agents such as bleomycin or tetracycline (Fig. 43.4).

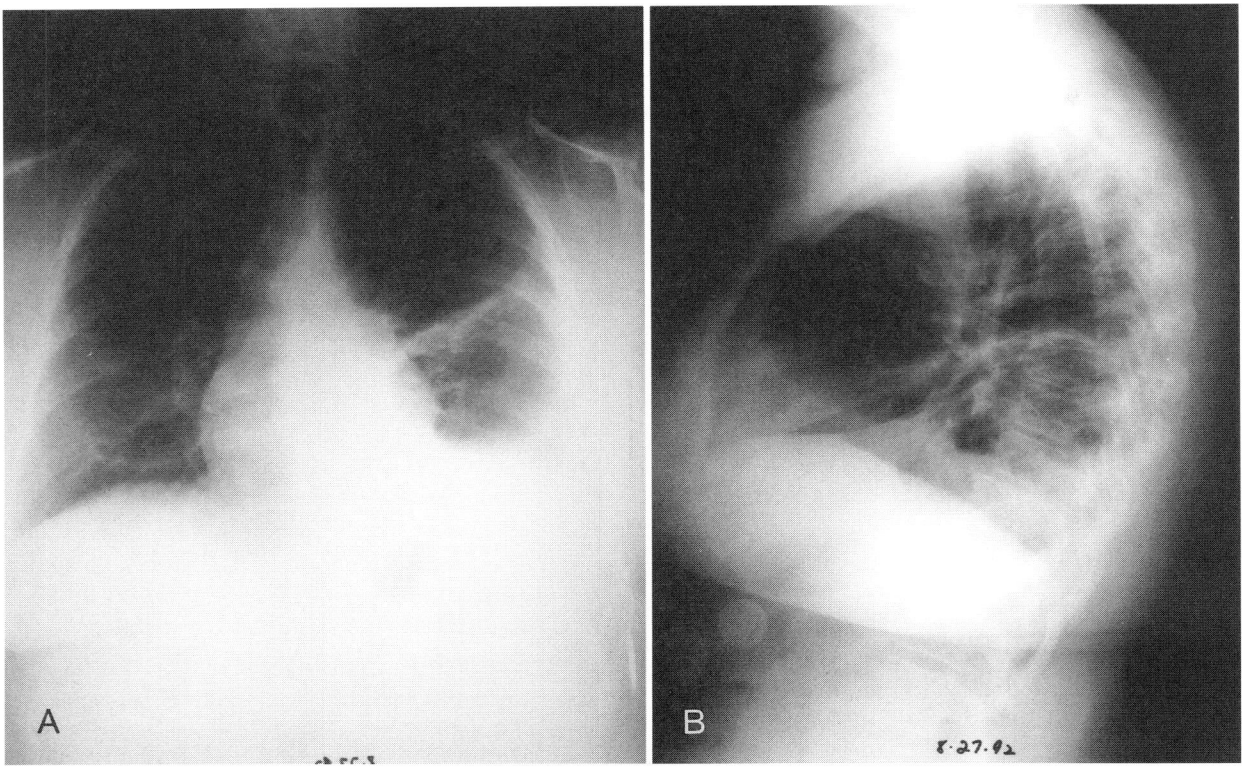

FIGURE 43.2. **A.** Posteroanterior chest radiograph and **B.** lateral chest radiograph showing the presence of a left-sided pleural effusion.

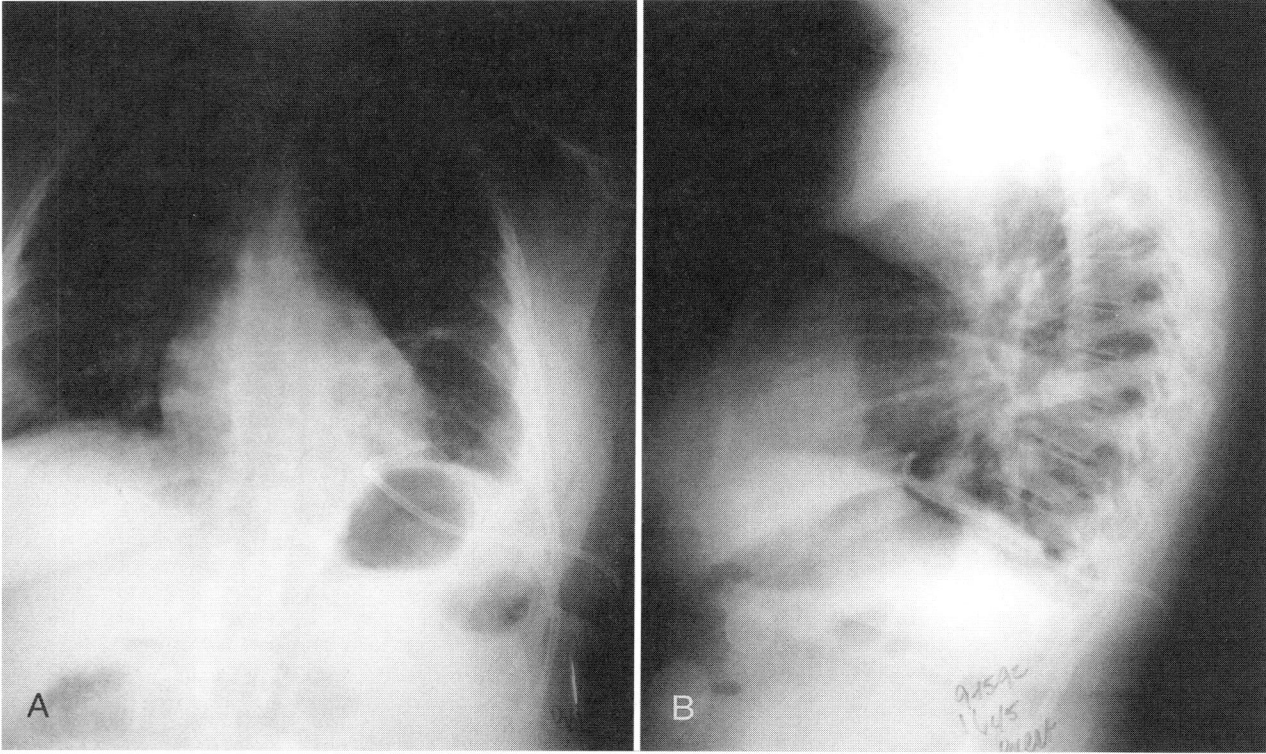

FIGURE 43.3. **A.** Posteroanterior chest radiograph and **B.** lateral chest radiograph of the same patient after insertion of a small-bore catheter connected to the ambulatory drainage system.

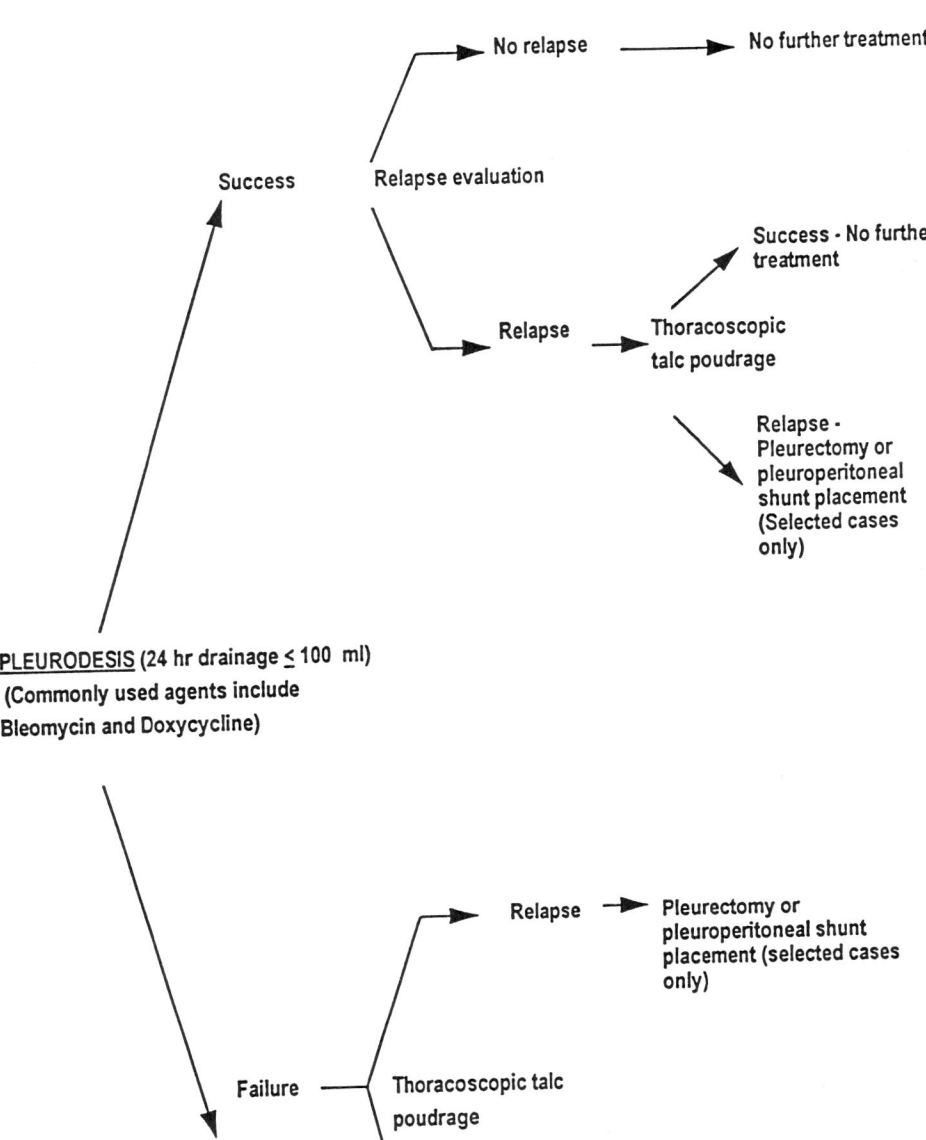

FIGURE 43.4. Management flow chart used by the University of Pittsburgh Medical Center for treatment of patients with primary malignant pleural effusions after initial pleurodesis.

When these treatments fail, especially if the lung is trapped, pleurectomy and decortication or placement of a pleuroperitoneal shunt is undertaken if the patient's condition permits. A conservative approach is symptomatic treatment, with acceptance by both the patient and the physician of the pleural fluid within the pleural cavity.

PLEURECTOMY

Until recently, pleurectomy and decortication have been major surgery procedures requiring thoracotomy in this group of patients with a limited life expectancy. An innovation was introduced in 1994: performing these procedures using video-assisted thoracoscopic surgical techniques via small incisions, thus minimizing the prohibitive morbidity (23% complications) and mortality (18% perioperative deaths) seen in earlier series (129). Thus, with the availability of safer, minimally invasive techniques, the major surgical intervention for pleurectomy and decortication is a thing of the past. Further experience with video-assisted thoracoscopic surgery is being acquired in ongoing investigations.

PLEUROPERITONEAL SHUNT

A high-flow-rate, pressure-activated pleuroperitoneal shunt with a manual pump reservoir placed between the pleural and peritoneal cavities can be installed under local or general anesthesia with minimal morbidity (130). There are two one-way valves on each side of the reservoir to allow spontaneous drainage if the appropriate pressure differential exists. It has been difficult to demonstrate spontaneous flow, and cellular debris can result in obstruction of the shunt. Reich et al. (131) demonstrated relief of symptoms in all 13 patients in whom the pleuroperitoneal shunt was inserted. The largest series (29 patients) is that of Little et al. (132): there was relief of symptoms or stabilization of the effusion in 20 of the 29 patients with no evidence of peritoneal seeding by the tumor. This procedure usually is reserved for patients with intractable effusions not amenable to traditional sclerotherapy, such as those associated with trapped lungs; its use may result in improved quality of life in a severely incapacitated, terminally ill patient, thus avoiding the need for repeated interventions and prolonged hospitalization (133).

SUMMARY

A systematic approach to the evaluation of malignant pleural effusions begins with a thorough history and physical examination performed with the intent of detecting the specific etiology of the effusion. The chest radiograph (posteroanterior and lateral) is an inexpensive and sensitive investigation for confirming the presence and extent of the pleural effusion. Decubitus films can show smaller amounts of fluid in the pleural space. A CT scan may be necessary in patients with small amounts of pleural fluid and extensive parenchymal lung involvement with the malignant process. Thoracentesis is the most important step in confirming the malignant nature of the effusion. Grossly, bloody fluid with a predominance of lymphocytes and monocytes and a high protein and LDH content favor the diagnosis of malignancy. The definitive diagnosis usually is confirmed by cytologic examination of the pleural fluid. Pleural biopsy is necessitated only when the cytology is negative on at least two occasions. The application of immunocytochemical techniques using monoclonal antibodies and anti-CEA antisera have been used to increase the diagnostic yield, but their sensitivity and specificity limits remain to be defined; thus, they are not used routinely. The performance of chromosomal analysis of cells in the pleural fluid is still an investigational tool. Some patients require thoracoscopic techniques to make a diagnosis of the effusion. At present, major surgical procedures, e.g., a thoracotomy, rarely are needed to clarify a diagnosis of malignancy in patients with pleural effusions.

There are several treatment options for patients with malignant pleural effusions. Best and foremost is the treatment of the underlying malignancy if amenable to systemic therapy, e.g., small cell lung cancer or lymphoma, although an initial thoracentesis may be required for relief of symptoms. For a small number of patients with effusions that recur slowly, repeat thoracentesis may be a reasonable strategy. The majority of patients require pleurodesis with a sclerosing agent, e.g., bleomycin or tetracycline, after tube thoracostomy and drainage. There continues to be a controversy regarding the best sclerosing agent: bleomycin is probably the most widely used agent in the absence of tetracycline. Results with biologic therapies are interesting, but they still are preliminary and need further investigation. Patients who progress or recur after initial pleurodesis usually are considered for sclerosis with talc, instilled either as chest tube slurry or as thoracoscopic poudrage into the pleural cavity. The success rates with talc sclerosis are high, but occasional severe side effects, e.g., respiratory failure, pneumonitis, and cardiac failure, have been reported, and the costs associated with the procedure are high. Surgical management (pleurectomy or pleuroperitoneal shunt placement) is reserved for selected patients with intractable effusions; such operations are not performed routinely because of the prohibitive morbidity and perioperative mortality, although experienced surgeons claim a reduction in these risks using video-assisted thoracoscopic surgical techniques. Pleurodesis via small-bore catheters is a move toward optimal palliative therapy of patients with malignant pleural effusions, allowing for the development of newer, less expensive outpatient ambulatory therapies and thus further reducing patient discomfort and avoiding the need for hospitalization.

MANAGEMENT OF MALIGNANT PERICARDIAL EFFUSIONS

INTRODUCTION

When patients with cancer present with cardiac involvement, the cause most frequently is a pericardial effusion (134, 135). The most common tumors that metastasize to the heart are carcinomas of the lung or breast, lymphoma, leukemia, and malignant melanoma (134, 136–141). Neoplasms tend to involve the heart by metastasizing to the mediastinal lymph nodes and then spreading retrograde to the heart by means of the subepicardial and pericardial lymphatics (142, 143). A less frequent pattern of cardiac involvement is by direct extension to the heart or embolization through the arterial system. Postmortem studies of patients with documented malignancy have found cardiac involvement in up to 20% of patients (137, 138, 141, 144–146).

PHYSIOLOGY OF EFFUSIVE PERICARDIAL DISEASE

In the healthy patient, the pericardial space contains only a trace amount of fluid. The pericardium functions to maintain the anatomic position of the heart, reduce friction, and provide a barrier against the spread of infection. In addition, it may serve to regulate filling of the heart (147–149). During the respiratory cycle, the pericardial pressure is equivalent to the intrapleural pressure, ranging from −2 to −5 mm Hg. If fluid accumulates in the pericardial space, diastolic filling of the heart can become impaired. Because the pericardium is a compliant structure, slow fluid accumulation may permit very large amounts to accumulate before symptoms occur; rapid accumulation of fluid (less than 200 mL) can lead to tamponade. As pericardial pressure increases and begins to approach right ventricular filling pressures, cardiac output decreases. Cardiac tamponade is not an all-or-nothing process but rather a continuum of hemodynamic deterioration (150).

The most frequent symptoms associated with effusive pericardial disease are dyspnea, chest pain, and cough, all of which may be attributed inadvertently to the underlying malignancy. Almost two thirds of patients with disease metastatic to the heart have no cardiac symptoms (134, 138).

On examination, physical findings that suggest a large pericardial effusion or pericardial tamponade may include a pericardial friction rub, which occurs because of contact between the inflamed visceral and parietal pericardial surfaces (151). Although a rub may be elicited by having the patient lean forward during auscultation, it can be notoriously evanescent. If the effusion is large, heart sounds may be distant. Occasionally, there are lung crackles resulting from compression of lung parenchyma by a large effusion. When intrapericardial pressure is elevated, jugular venous distension is prominent (152). Pulsus paradoxus, an inspiratory decrease of more than 10 mm Hg in the arterial systolic pressure, is associated classically with cardiac tamponade. However, an inspiratory decrease in blood pressure also can be seen in obstructive lung disease, constrictive and restrictive heart disease, and pulmonary embolism. Other findings include a rapid respiratory rate, tachycardia, and hepatomegaly. Although hypotension is seen in one third of patients with cardiac tamponade, many patients can maintain a stable blood pressure (152, 153).

Chest radiography may show enlargement of the cardiac silhouette with a water bottle configuration (Fig. 43.5). However, if the pericardial effusion is less than 250 mL, the cardiac silhouette may appear normal. In the routine care of patients with malignancy, it is typical for a pericardial effusion to be identified solely on the basis of the chest radiograph or CT scan. The electrocardiogram may reveal electrical alternans in which the amplitude or axis of the electrical complexes may vary from beat to beat (Fig. 43.6). This variance is caused by a pendulumlike swinging of the heart within the fluid-filled pericardial space (154). Once the possibility of effusive pericardial disease is raised, echocardiography is the single best diagnostic study. In addition to visualizing the presence and extent of pericardial fluid, echocardiography can provide information concerning loculation and intrapericardial masses, as well as whether the fluid is asymmetric in location (Fig. 43.7). Although echocardiography can indicate whether severe hemodynamic compromise is present, it is less reliable in identifying early tamponade (155).

Right heart catheterization can establish the hemodynamic significance of the pericardial effusion. The classic findings on right heart catheterization are elevation of the right atrial pressure with loss of the diastolic "y" descent. There is relative equalization and elevation of all diastolic filling pressures, thus right atrial, right ventricular end-diastolic, and pericardial pressures are equalized (Fig. 43.8). In some patients, pulmonary capillary wedge pressure and left ventricular end-diastolic pressure also will be equal to pericardial pressure. When time permits, it is useful to obtain hemodynamic data before and after pericardiocentesis (Fig. 43.9). These data allow confirmation of the diagnosis of cardiac tamponade, but more importantly, they identify patients in whom hemodynamics do not normalize after pericardiocentesis. These patients may remain symptomatic because of effusive-constrictive disease, left ventricular dysfunction, or pulmonary disease. After removal of pericardial fluid, the pericardial pressure should decrease to below zero, and the right atrial waveform should normalize (Fig. 43.7).

PERICARDIOCENTESIS

The approach to draining the pericardial fluid depends on the level of hemodynamic instability. If cardiac tamponade is present, the rapid intravenous ad-

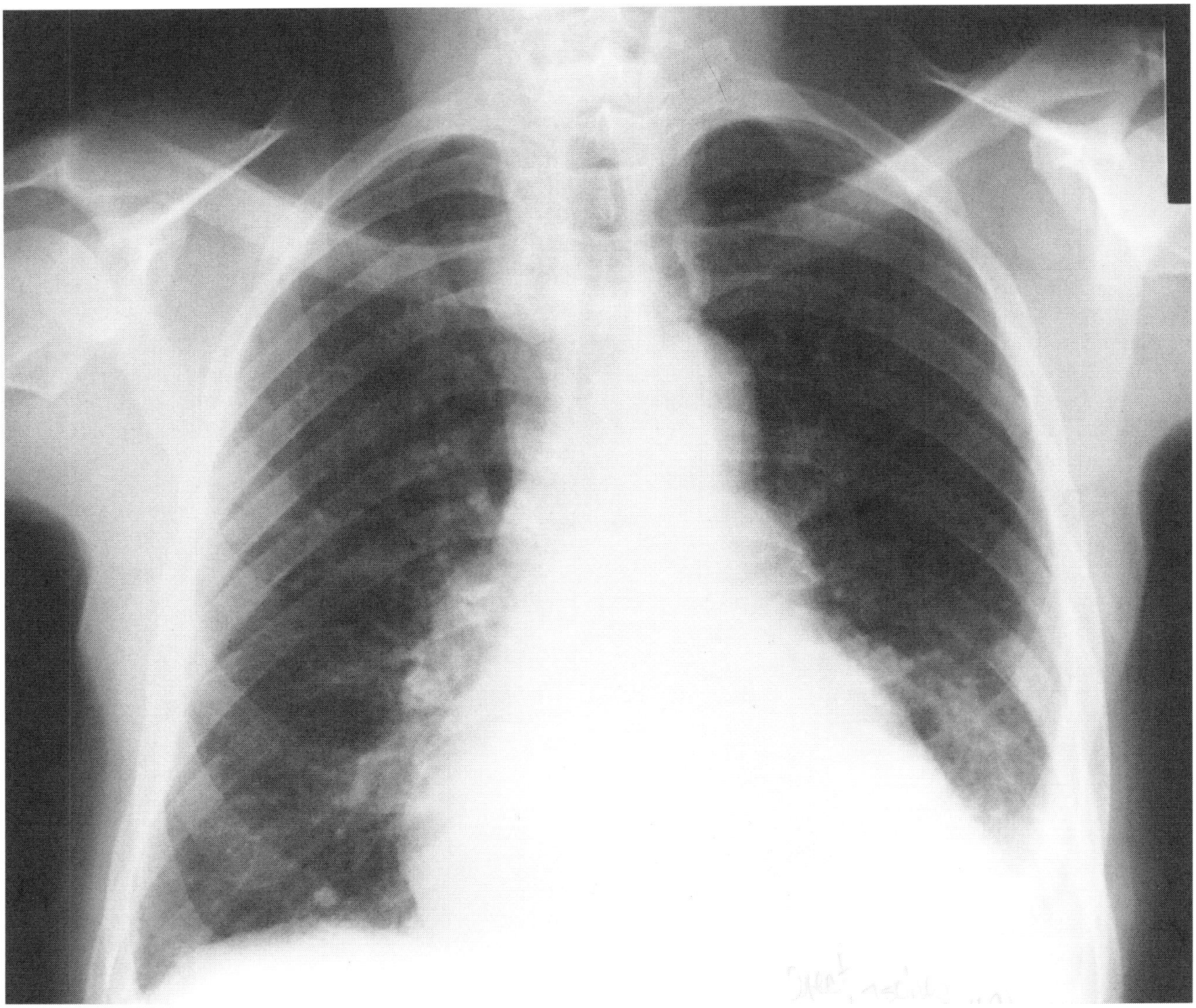

FIGURE 43.5. Posteroanterior chest radiograph of a patient with lung cancer and pericardial tamponade. The cardiac silhouette is markedly enlarged.

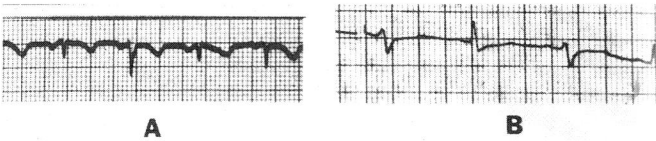

FIGURE 43.6. Electrocardiogram tracing demonstrating electrical alternans, suggesting the presence of a large pericardial effusion and tamponade.

ministration of volume often provides transient hemodynamic improvement by increasing right atrial pressure above pericardial pressure, thereby improving ventricular filling and cardiac output (156). Vasodilators may improve cardiac output, but they are risky in hypotensive patients and may not actually improve organ perfusion (156). If the patient is acutely ill, hypotensive, and in severe distress, pericardiocentesis should be performed immediately without obtaining further diagnostic studies. If the patient is more stable, then an expedient approach to drainage should be undertaken. It must be recognized that there is no single best way to approach pericardial drainage. The preferred approach is dictated frequently by institutional preferences based on the patient population, disease frequency, and availability of cardiology and surgery resources.

Pericardiocentesis typically has been performed via a subxiphoid approach. The likelihood of successful pericardiocentesis increases with the increasing size of the effusion (157). A variety of techniques have been used to guide appropriate needle placement, thus reducing the possibility of injury to the heart and sur-

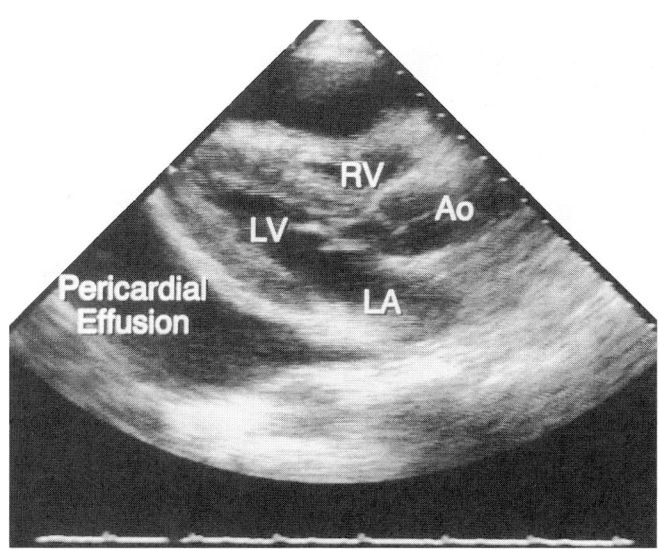

FIGURE 43.7. Echocardiogram (parasternal long axis view) showing a large pericardial effusion with diastolic collapse of the right atrium and right ventricle consistent with tamponade. LV, left ventricle; RV, right ventricle; LA, left atrium; Ao, aorta.

rounding structures. After administration of local anesthesia to the skin and deeper tissues, the pericardial needle is connected to an electrocardiogram V lead. The needle is then directed from the subxiphoid skin entry site toward the posterior aspect of the left shoulder. A discrete pop may be felt as the needle enters the pericardial space. If the needle contacts the epicardial surface, "ST" segment elevation is seen on the electrocardiogram, often accompanied by premature ventricular contractions. Once the pericardial space has been entered, a guidewire is introduced through the pericardial needle. The needle is removed, and a catheter is inserted over the guidewire. The catheter is left in place for a period of time to assure effective drainage and, if necessary, to provide a route for instillation of sclerosing or chemotherapeutic agents.

Alternative approaches to entering the pericardium using simple EKG-guided pericardiocentesis include monitoring pressure through the pericardial needle, or using fluoroscopic or echocardiographic guidance. If the needle is connected to a pressure transducer, the appearance of a pericardial waveform can confirm proper positioning. If fluoroscopy is available, it also can be used to confirm the position of a guidewire introduced through the needle. Lastly, echocardiography can be used to direct the approach of the needle toward the most readily accessible portion of the pericardial space. Institutions that rely heavily on echocardiographically guided pericardiocentesis frequently employ less conventional apical and parasternal approaches (158). Echocardiographic guidance may be particularly useful when pericardial fluid is loculated (159).

DIAGNOSIS OF THE ETIOLOGY OF THE PERICARDIAL EFFUSION

Because not all patients with malignancy and a pericardial effusion have malignant pericardial disease, analysis of pericardial fluid cytology and, when necessary, pericardial biopsy, can play a pivotal role in diagnosis. At the time of pericardiocentesis, fluid should be sent for cytologic analysis. Additional studies should include blood cell counts; glucose, protein, amylase, and triglyceride levels; Gram's and acid-fast stains; and cultures (including aerobic, anaerobic, tuberculosis, and fungi). These studies help to rule out infection, lymphatic leak, and extension of a pancreatic process.

The diagnostic and therapeutic approaches to the cancer patient with a pericardial effusion cannot be considered separately. Patient factors, such as the status of systemic malignancy, anticipated survival, and co-morbid disease, also must be considered. Little objective randomized data are available that compare different strategies for the management of effusive pericardial disease.

It is rare for the heart to be involved in the absence of widely metastatic disease (134, 137, 138, 144, 160). When the etiology of the pericardial effusion is unknown, pericardiocentesis can provide fluid for analysis. In patients with known malignancy, pericardial fluid shows positive cytology two thirds of the time (161). However, not all patients with known malignancy who present with a pericardial effusion have malignant pericardial involvement (162–164). In one series of 31 patients with pericardial effusions, 58% were found to have involvement of a malignancy. Thirty-two percent had idiopathic pericarditis, and ten percent had radiation-related disease.

PERCUTANEOUS TREATMENT STRATEGIES: CATHETER DRAINAGE AND SCLEROTHERAPY

Therapeutic approaches for the management of pericardial effusions in patients with malignancy may be divided into percutaneous and surgical strategies. The first step is identifying, if possible, the etiology of the effusion and then determining the appropriate level of diagnostic and therapeutic intervention, relative to the patient's underlying disease process.

For many patients primary treatment consists of pericardiocentesis with placement of an indwelling catheter. The catheter may be left in place until

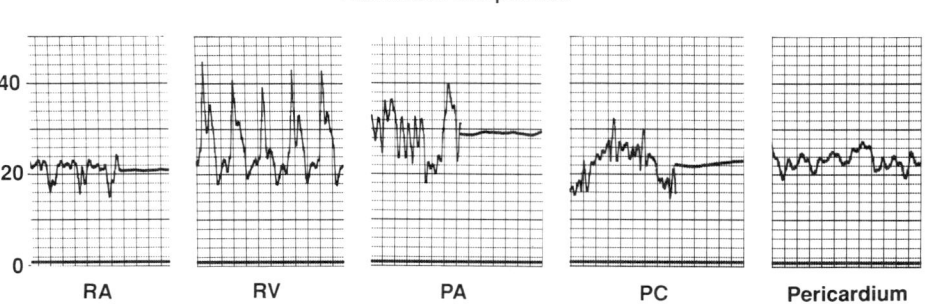

FIGURE 43.8. Right heart catheterization revealing elevation and equalization of diastolic pressures caused by pericardial tamponade. RA, right atrium; RV, right ventricle; PA, pulmonary artery; PC, pericardial cavity.

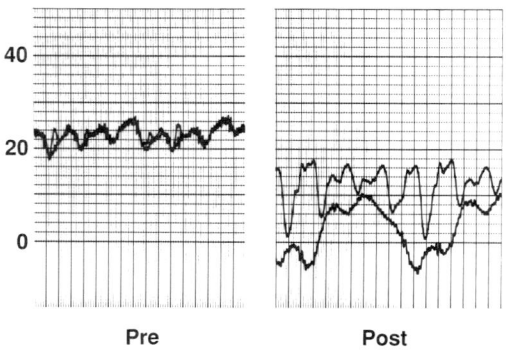

FIGURE 43.9. Before pericardiocentesis, right atrial and pericardial pressures are elevated and identical. After removal of pericardial fluid, the right atrial waveform normalizes and pericardial pressure fluctuates around zero with respiratory variation.

drainage is less than 75 to 100 mL/day. If pericardial drainage continues, or if fluid recurs after catheter removal, a more aggressive approach is then considered.

Recurrences following simple catheter drainage have been reported in 14% to 50% of patients with pericardial effusion and tamponade (165–168). Leaving the pericardial catheter in place for 24 to 72 hours may allow the visceral and parietal pericardial surfaces to maintain closer contact, thereby permitting sclerosis to occur and thus preventing recurrence. The pericardial catheter itself may contribute to this inflammatory obliteration of the pericardial space (158, 169, 170). Prophylactic antibiotics can be given while the catheter is in place to prevent secondary infection of the pericardial space.

In addition to pericardiocentesis with catheter drainage, subsequent therapeutic options include treatment of the underlying disease with radiation and/or chemotherapy, installation of sclerosing agents, percutaneous balloon pericardiotomy, creation of a subxiphoid pericardial window, and more extensive surgical pericardiectomy.

Instillation of sclerosing agents may obliterate the pericardial space. Agents used in the past have included nitrogen mustard (171), thiotepa (172), quinacrine (173), radioactive chromic phosphate, colloidal gold (174, 175), tetracycline (176–178), talc (179), bleomycin (180), vinblastine (181), cisplatin (182), mitoxantrone (183), cyclophosphamide (184), as well as external radiation therapy (135, 185).

In a study reported by Shepherd et al. (176), tetracycline pericardial instillation at doses of 500 to 1000 mg in 20 mL of normal saline via a Kifa catheter inserted into the pericardial sac resulted in 75% (58 patients) efficacy in terms of control of effusions for more than 30 days. The procedure was reasonably well tolerated, with pain, mild fever, and transient atrial arrhythmias occurring in 10% to 15% of the patients. The sclerosis was performed after catheter drainage for 24 hours. Intrapericardial tetracycline sclerosis also has been used successfully, without significant complications, in controlling the signs and symptoms of cardiac tamponade (177).

The direct instillation of antineoplastic drugs into the pericardial sac is reported to provide an approximately 50% likelihood of response in terms of a significant decrease in pericardial fluid production. Bleomycin is the most frequently used agent, and a one-time dose of 60 U diluted in 100 mL of normal saline can be instilled through the drainage catheter (180). Intrapericardial cisplatin also has proven to be effective (182) in the control of malignant pericardial effusions, but repeated instillations are required (10 mg in 20 mL of normal saline daily on 5 consecutive days with courses repeated in the event of recurrence). Mitoxantrone at doses of 5 to 20 mg in 50 mL of normal saline has shown a complete response with very little systemic toxicity in 9 of 12 patients with malignant pericardial effusion (183). These preliminary results of pericardial sclerotherapy are encouraging and offer a significant improvement in quality of life for patients with advanced or refractory malignancies presenting with symptomatic pericardial effusions.

Because the parenteral form of tetracycline is no

longer distributed in the United States, the most frequently used agent is bleomycin. The technique for instillation of a sclerosing agent varies, but it usually involves delivering the drug in saline, allowing it to remain in the pericardial space for a period of time, and then draining the pericardial space to maintain strict apposition of the visceral and parietal pericardial surfaces (176). This process is repeated until drainage is less than 50 to 75 mL in 24 hours. Sclerosis can be repeated if necessary until no further drainage is present. Doxycycline is administered as a 500-mg dose diluted in 100 mL of normal saline. Because of the inflammation induced by sclerosing agents, the procedure frequently is accompanied by pain and fever. Atrial arrhythmias are seen less commonly.

SURGICAL TREATMENT STRATEGIES

When the etiology of the pericardial effusion, based on pericardial fluid analysis, is unclear and the patient has a projected survival that merits a more invasive approach, a surgical drainage procedure with sampling of the pericardium may be appropriate. Surgical procedures range from a simple subxiphoid pericardiotomy, to a more complex pleuropericardial window, to complete pericardiectomy. In the patient population with debility caused by advanced malignancy, the perioperative morbidity can be significant (140, 186, 187). Subxiphoid pericardial drainage procedures have the advantage of lower operative risk, but, compared with a more extensive pericardial resection, they are accompanied by a greater chance of recurrent effusion (140). A subxiphoid pericardiotomy can be performed under local anesthesia. If hemodynamic compromise is not present, it may be preferable to forego prior pericardiocentesis to distend the pericardial sac. Although the mechanism of action of subxiphoid pericardiotomy has traditionally been thought to be the creation of a persistent communication to allow drainage, newer studies suggest that this action may be fusion of the epicardium to the pericardium with inflammatory obliteration of the potential space (188). A limited pericardiotomy, often referred to as a pleuropericardial window, is performed via the left chest; it has none of the advantages of the subxiphoid pericardiotomy and is associated with greater operative risk (140). Because the mean survival of patients with known malignancy and symptomatic pericardial disease is 3.8 months (189), more extensive surgical procedures should be reserved for patients with nonmalignant pericardial disease who have a good long-term prognosis.

NEW APPROACHES

Four new techniques are being used for the management of pericardial disease: percutaneous pericardial biopsy, percutaneous balloon pericardiotomy, pericardioscopy, and thoracoscopic pericardiotomy.

PERICARDIAL BIOPSY

Because it often is desirable to avoid the morbidity of a surgical procedure in patients with advanced systemic disease, several investigators have examined the use of a percutaneously introduced bioptome to sample pericardial tissue at the time of pericardiocentesis. Most of the techniques tried previously were limited in their ability to sample the pericardium adequately or they required the use of large-bore instruments for pericardial access (190–193). Using a new 8F percutaneous pericardial bioptome, the diagnostic yield for patients with known malignancy was increased from 46% (194) to 62% (195). Because a direct comparison of percutaneous and surgical approaches has not been done, this approach must still be considered investigational.

PERCUTANEOUS BALLOON PERICARDIOTOMY

Percutaneous balloon pericardiotomy, the use of a dilating balloon to create a pericardial window, appears to offer a nonsurgical means of treating malignant pericardial effusions (196, 197). After pericardiocentesis is performed using a standard subxiphoid approach, a 20-mm-diameter by 3-cm-long dilating balloon is introduced over a guidewire. As the balloon is inflated, a window is created that permits fluid to pass from the pericardial to the pleural space (Fig. 43.10). In a nonrandomized registry, data were presented that included 100 patients with malignancy and effusive pericardial disease (189). Eighty had pericardial tamponade, and 20 had large effusions thought to be at risk for the development of tamponade. When success was defined as no recurrent pericardial effusion and no complications, the percutaneous balloon pericardiotomy was considered successful in 87% of patients. A multicenter randomized trial of pericardiocentesis with catheter drainage versus percutaneous balloon pericardiotomy is in progress.

PERICARDIOSCOPY

Pericardioscopy has been performed both as an adjunct to subxiphoid surgical windowing and as a percutaneous intervention (194, 198–203). Although the pericardial space can be imaged successfully in some patients, those with malignant effusions frequently

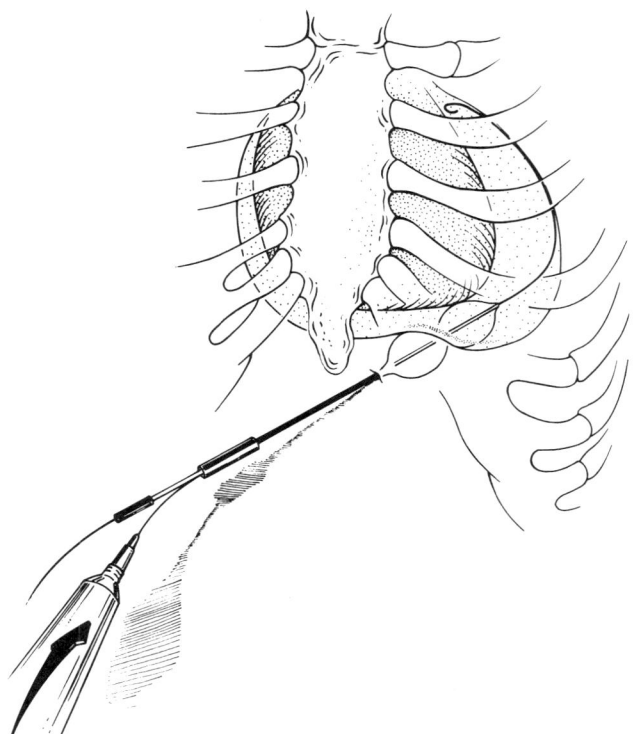

FIGURE 43.10. Schematic representation of percutaneous balloon pericardiotomy technique via the subxiphoid approach. (From Ziskind AA, Pearce AC, Lemmon CC, et al. Percutaneous balloon pericardiotomy for the treatment of cardiac tamponade and large pericardial effusions: description of technique and report of the first 50 cases. J Am Coll Cardiol 1993;21:1–5.)

have bloody pericardial fluid that limits visualization. The role of endoscopic imaging of the pericardial space for treatment and diagnosis remains unclear.

THORACOSCOPIC PERICARDIOTOMY

With the growth of laparoscopic and thoracoscopic technology, the thoracoscopic pericardial windowing technique is being used for treatment of effusive pericardial disease (204–206). It avoids the need for a thoracotomy but still permits creation of a large pericardial window and tissue sampling. The procedure may be subject to some of the same limitations as the open surgical procedure used to create a pleuropericardial window (140). It nonetheless holds promise as a less invasive means of performing subtotal pericardiectomy.

Summary

The current approach to the treatment of malignant pericardial disease remains largely institution and patient dependent. If hemodynamic compromise is present, immediate pericardiocentesis is indicated. For patients with a limited survival because of their underlying disease, initial catheter drainage is recommended, either alone or in conjunction with percutaneous balloon pericardiotomy. Patients with a recurrent effusion should undergo either sclerotherapy with bleomycin or percutaneous balloon pericardiotomy (if not performed previously), or they should be considered for a subxiphoid surgical window. Patients in whom the diagnosis of malignant pericardial disease is in doubt should undergo initial catheter drainage. If cytologic analysis is negative, then either percutaneous biopsy or biopsy should be performed at the time of surgical windowing. Patients who have a component of effusive-constrictive disease, e.g., after radiation therapy, should undergo extensive surgical pericardiectomy.

Any patient with a refractory bleeding diathesis preferably should undergo surgical therapy because bleeding tissues can be visualized directly and hemostasis can be achieved. If pericardial fluid is loculated, then either echocardiographically guided catheter-based therapy or direct surgery should be considered. Following percutaneous, thoracoscopic, or surgical pericardial windowing, the patient must be monitored for development of a significant pleural effusion that would require drainage and possibly sclerosis. In summary, there are numerous approaches for the management of malignant pericardial disease. As with any other treatment, the approach should be individualized for each patient.

References

1. Claus RH, Yacoubian NH, Barker HG. Dynamics of pleural effusion. Surg Forum 1956;7:201–204.
2. Kinasewitz GT, Fishman AP. Influence of alterations in starting forces on visceral pleural fluid movement. J Appl Physiol 1981;51:671–677.
3. Agostoni E. Mechanics of pleural space. Physiol Rev 1972;52–57.
4. Black LF. The pleural space and pleural fluid. Mayo Clin Proc 1972;47:493–506.
5. Meyer PC. Metastatic carcinoma of the pleura. Thorax 1966;21:437–443.
6. Leff A, Hopewell PC, Costello J. Pleural effusion from malignancy. Ann Intern Med 1978;88:532–537.
7. Sahn SA. Pleural effusion in lung cancer. Clin Chest Med 1993;14(1):189–200.
8. Chernow B, Sahn SA. Carcinomatous involvement of the pleura. Am J Med 1977;63:695–702.
9. Zehner LC, Hoogstraten B. Malignant effusions and their management. Semin Oncol Nurs 1985;1:259–268.
10. Woodring JH. Recognition of pleural effusion on supine radiographs: How much fluid is required. AJR Am J Roentgenol 1984;142:59–64.

11. Kaunitz J. Landmarks in simple pleural effusion. JAMA 1939;113:1312–1314.
12. Peterson JA. Recognition of intrapulmonary pleural effusion. Radiology 1960;74:34–41.
13. White CS, Templeton PA, Belani CP. Imaging in lung cancer. Semin Oncol 1993;20:142–152.
14. Leuallen EC, Carr DT. Pleural effusion: a statistical study of 436 patients. N Engl J Med 1955;252:79–83.
15. Storey DD, Dines DE, Coles DT. Pleural effusion: a diagnostic dilemma. JAMA 1976;236:2183–2186.
16. Tinney WS, Oslen AM. The significance of fluid in the pleural space: a study of 274 cases. J Thorac Surg 1945;14:248–252.
17. Anderson CB, Philpott GW, Ferguson TB. The treatment of malignant pleural effusions. Cancer 1974;33:916–922.
18. Fracchia AA, Knapper WH, Carey JT, et al. Intrapleural chemotherapy for effusion from metastatic breast cancer. Cancer 1970;26(3):625–629.
19. Bruneau R, Rubin P. The management of pleural effusion and chylothorax in lymphoma. Radiology 1965;85:1085–1092.
20. Ratliff JL, Chavez CM, Jamchuck A, et al. Re-expansion pulmonary edema. Chest 1973;64:654–656.
21. Trapnell DH, Thurston JGB. Unilateral pulmonary edema after pleural aspiration. Lancet 1970;1:1367–1369.
22. Pettersson T, Riska H. Diagnostic value of total and differential leukocyte counts in pleural effusions. Acta Med Scand 1981;210:129–135.
23. Roy PH, Carr DT, Payne WS. The problem of chylothorax. Mayo Clin Proc 1967;42:457–467.
24. Light RW. Pleural effusion. Med Clin North Am 1977;61:1339–1352.
25. Carr DT. Diagnostic studies of pleural fluid. Surg Clin North Am 1973;53:801–804.
26. Sahn SA, Good JT Jr. Pleural fluid pH in malignant effusions: Diagnostic, prognostic and therapeutic implications. Ann Intern Med 1988;108:345–349.
27. Kramer MR, Saldana MJ, Cepero RJ, et al. High amylase levels in neoplasm related pleural effusion. Ann Intern Med 1989;110:567–569.
28. Joseph J, Biney S, Beck P, et al. A prospective study of amylase rich pleural effusion with special reference to amylase isoenzyme analysis. Chest 1992;102:1455–1459.
29. Irani DR, Underwood RD, Johnson EH, et al. Malignant pleural effusions: a clinical cytopathologic study. Arch Intern Med 1987;147:1133–1136.
30. Salyer WR, Eggleston JC, Erozan YS. Efficacy of pleural needle biopsy and pleural fluid cytopathology in the diagnosis of malignant neoplasm involving the pleura. Chest 1975;67:536–539.
31. Prakash UBS, Reiman HM: Comparison of needle biopsy with cytologic analysis for evaluation of pleural effusion: analysis of 414 cases. Mayo Clin Proc 1985;60:158–164.
32. Winkelman M, Pfitzer P. Blind pleural biopsy in combination with cytology of pleural effusions. Acta Cytol 1981;25:373–376.
33. Das DK, Gupta SK, Ayyagari et al. Pleural effusions in non-Hodgkin's lymphoma. Acta Cytol 1987;31:119–124.
34. Weick JK, Kiely JM, Harrison EG, et al. Pleural effusion in lymphoma. Cancer 1973;31:848–853.
35. Monif GRG, Stewart BN, Block AJ. Living cytology. A new diagnostic technique for malignant pleural effusions. Chest 1976;69:626–629.
36. Johnston WW, Szpak CA, Lottich SC et al. Use of a monoclonal antibody (B72-3) as an immunocytochemical adjunct to diagnosis of adenocarcinoma in human effusions. Cancer Res 1985;45:1894–1900.
37. Martin SE, Moshiri S, Thor A, et al. Identification of adenocarcinoma in cytospin preparations of effusion using monoclonal antibody B72.3. Am J Clin Pathol 1986;86:10–18.
38. Alexander TO, David P, Dearnaley MA, et al. Epithelial membrane antigen: its use in the cytodiagnosis of malignancy in serious effusions. Am J Clin Pathol 1982;72(2):214–219.
39. Estaban JM, Yokota S, Husain S, et al. Immunocytochemical profile of benign and carcinomatous effusions. A practical approach to difficult diagnosis. Am J Clin Pathol 1990;94(6):608–705.
40. Mottolese M, Venturo I, Donnoroso RP, et al. Use of selected combinations of monoclonal antibodies to tumor associated antigens in the diagnosis of neoplastic effusions of unknown origin. Eur J Clin Oncol 1988;24,8:1277–1284.
41. DeWald G, Dines DE, Weiland LH, et al. Usefulness of chromosome examination in the diagnosis of malignant-pleural effusions. N Engl J Med 1976;295:1494–1500.
42. Fraisse J, Brizard CP, Emonot A, et al. Diagnosis of malignancy by cytogenetic means in effusions. Clin Genet 1978;14:288–289.
43. Rittgers RA, Lowenstein MS, Feinerman AE, et al. Carcinoembryonic antigen levels in benign and malignant pleural effusions. Ann Intern Med 1978;88:631–634.
44. Silverman LM, Dermer GB, Zweig MH et al. Creatinine kinase BB. A new tumor-associated marker. Clin Chem 1979;25:1432–1435.
45. Kim D, Weber GF, Tomita JT, et al. Galactosyltransferase variant in pleural effusion. Clin Chem 1982;28:1133–1136.
46. Daniel TM. Diagnostic thoracoscopy for pleural disease. Ann Thorac Surg 1993;56(3):639–640.
47. Kendall SW, Bryan AJ, Large SR, et al. Pleural effusion: Is thoracoscopy a reliable investigation? A retrospective review. Respir Med 1992;86(5):437–440.
48. Boutin C, Viallat JR, Gugnino P, et al. Thoracoscopy in malignant pleural effusion. Am Rev Respir Dis 1981;124:588–592.
49. Ohri SK, Oswal SK, Townsend ER, et al. Early and late outcome after diagnostic thoracoscopy and talc pleurodesis. Ann Thorac Surg 1991;53(6):1038–1041.
50. Hausheer FH, Yarbro JW. Diagnosis and treatment of malignant pleural effusion. Semin Oncol 1985;12:54–75.
51. Rashad K, Inui K, Takeuchi Y, et al. Treatment of malignant pleural effusion. Chest 1985;88:393–397.
52. Bethune N. Pleural poudrage; a new technique for deliberate production of pleural adhesions as preliminary to lobectomy. J Thorac Cardiovasc Surg 1935;4:251–261.
53. Frankel A, Krasna I, Baranofsky ID. An experimental study of pleural symphysis. J Thorac Cardiovasc Surg 1961;42:43–51.
54. Prorok J, Nealon TF. Pleural symphysis by talc poudrage in the treatment of malignant pleural effusion. Bull Soc Int Chir 1968;6:630–635.
55. Kennedy L, Sahn S. Talc pleurodesis for the treatment of pneumothorax and pleural effusion. Chest 1994;106:1215–1222.
56. Rinaldo JE, Owens GR, Rogers RM. Adult respiratory distress syndrome following intrapleural installation of talc. J Thorac Cardiovasc Surg 1983;85:523–526.
57. Bouchama A, Chastre J, Gaudichet A, et al. Acute pneumonitis with bilateral pleural effusion after talc pleurodesis. Chest 1984;86:795–797.
58. Factor SM. Granulomatous pneumonitis. A result of intrapleural instillation of quinacrine and talcum powder. Arch Pathol 1975;99:499–502.
59. Sorensen PG, Svendsen TL, Enk B. Treatment of malignant pleural effusion with drainage, with or without installation of talc. Eur J Respir Dis 1984;65:131–135.

60. Pearson FG, MacGregor DC. Talc poudrage for malignant pleural effusion. J Thorac Cardiovasc Surg 1966;51:732–738.
61. Jones GR. Treatment of recurrent malignant pleural effusion by iodized talc pleurodesis. Thorax 1969;24:69–73.
62. Todd TRJ, Delavue NC, Ilves R, et al. Talc poudrage for malignant pleural effusion (abstract). Chest 1980;78:542–543.
63. Weissberg D, Ben-Zeev I. Talc pleurodesis experience with 360 patients. J Thorac Cardiovasc Surg 1993;106:689–695.
64. Webb WR, Ozmen V, Moulder PV, et al. Iodized talc pleurodesis for the treatment of pleural effusions. J Thorac Cardiovasc Surg 1992;103(5):881–885.
65. Hartman DL, Gaither JM, Kesler KA, et al. Comparison of insufflated talc under thoracoscopic guidance with standard tetracycline and bleomycin pleurodesis for control of malignant pleural effusions. J Thorac Cardiovasc Surg 1993;105:743–748.
66. Fentiman IS, Rubens RD, Hayward JL. A comparison of intracavitary talc and tetracycline for the control of pleural effusions secondary to breast cancer. Eur J Cancer Clin Oncol 1986;22(9):1079–1081.
67. Daniel TM, Tribble CG, Rogers BM. Thoracoscopy and talc poudrage for pneumothoraces and effusion. Ann Thorac Surg 1990;50:186–189.
68. Shedbalkar AR, Head JM, Head LR, et al. Evaluation of talc pleural symphysis in management of malignant plural effusion. J Thorac Cardiovasc Surg 1971;61:492–497.
69. Aelony Y, King R, Boutin C. Thoracoscopic talc poudrage pleurodesis for chronic recurrent pleural effusions. Ann Intern Med 1991;115:778–782.
70. Adler RH, Sayek I. Treatment of malignant pleural effusion: a method using tube thoracostomy and talc. Ann Thorac Surg 1976;22:8–15.
71. Knowles JH, Storey CF. Effects of pleural talc poudrage on pulmonary function. J Thorac Surg 1957;34:250–256.
72. Sherman S, Grady KJ, Seidman JC. Clinical experience with tetracycline pleurodesis of malignant pleural effusions. South Med J 1987;80:716–719.
73. Landvater L, Hix WR, Mills M, et al. Malignant pleural effusion treated by tetracycline sclerotherapy. Chest 1988;93:1196–1198.
74. Ruckdeschel JC, Moores D, Lee JY, et al. Intrapleural therapy for malignant pleural effusions. Chest 1990;100:1528–1535.
75. Kessinger A, Wigton RS. Intracavitary bleomycin and tetracycline in the management of malignant pleural effusions: a randomized study. J Surg Oncol 1987;36(2):81–83.
76. Leahy BC, Honeybourne D, Brear SG, et al. Treatment of malignant pleural effusions with intrapleural *Corynebacterium parvum* or tetracycline. Eur J Respir Dis 1985;66(1):50–54.
77. Evans TR, Slein RC, Pepper JC, et al. A randomized prospective trial of surgical against medical tetracycline pleurodesis in the management of malignant pleural effusion secondary to breast cancer. Eur J Cancer 1993;29A(3):316–319.
78. Gravelyn TR, Michelson MK, Gross BH, et al. Tetracycline pleurodesis for malignant pleural effusions. A 10 year retrospective study. Cancer 1987;59(11):1973–1977.
79. Wallach HW. Intrapleural tetracycline for malignant pleural effusions. Chest 1975;68:510–512.
80. Zaloznik AJ, Oswald SG, Langin M. Intrapleural tetracycline in malignant pleural effusions. Cancer 1983;51:752–755.
81. Sahn SA, Good JT. Pleural fluid pH in malignant effusions: diagnostic, prognostic and therapeutic implications. Ann Intern Med 1988;108:345–349.
82. Antony VB, Rothfuss KJ, Godbey SW, et al. Mechanism of tetracycline-hydrochloride–induced pleurodesis. Am Rev Respir Dis 1992;146:1009–1013.
83. Månsson T. Treatment of malignant pleural effusion with doxycycline. Scand J Infect Dis 1988;53:29–34.
84. Kitamura S, Sugiyama Y, Izumi T, et al. Intrapleural doxycycline for control of malignant pleural effusion. Curr Ther Res 1981;30:515–521.
85. Halta T, Tsubuota N, Yoshimura M, et al. Effect of intrapleural administration of minocycline on postoperative air leakage and malignant pleural effusion. Kyobu Geka 1990;43:283–286.
86. Koldsland S, Svennarig JL, Lehne A, et al. Chemical pleurodesis in malignant pleural effusions: a randomized prospective study of mepacrine versus bleomycin. Thorax 1993;48(8):790–797.
87. Bayly TC, Kisner DL, Sybert A. Tetracycline and quinacrine in the control of malignant pleural effusions. A randomized trial. Cancer 1978;41:1188–1192.
88. Borja ER, Pugh R. Single dose quinacrine (Atabrine) and thoracostomy in the control of pleural effusions in patients with neoplastic diseases. Cancer 1973;31:899–902.
89. Taylor SA, Hooton NS, Macarthur AM. Quinacrine in the management of malignant pleural effusion. Br J Surg 1977;64:52–53.
90. Borda I, Krant M. Convulsions following intrapleural administration of quinacrine hydrochloride. JAMA 1967;210:173–174.
91. Maiche AG, Virkkunen P, Kontkanen T, et al. Bleomycin and mitoxantrone in the treatment of malignant pleural effusions: a comparative study. Am J Clin Oncol 1993;16(1):50–53.
92. Ostrowski MJ, Priestman TJ, Houston RF, et al. A randomized trial of intracavitary bleomycin and *Corynebacterium parvum* in the control of malignant pleural effusions. Radiother Oncol 1989;14(1):19–26.
93. Hillerdal G, Kiviloog J, Nou E, et al. *Corynebacterium parvum* in malignant pleural effusions: a randomized prospective study. Eur J Respir Dis 1986;69(3):204–206.
94. Ostrowski MJ, Halsall GM. Intracavitary bleomycin in the management of malignant effusions: a multi-center study. Cancer Treat Rep 1982;66(11):1903–1907.
95. Paladine W, Cunningham TJ, Sponzo R, et al. Intracavitary bleomycin in the management of malignant effusions. Cancer 1976;38:1903–1908.
96. Bitran JD, Brown C, Desser RK, et al. Intracavitary bleomycin for the control of malignant effusion. J Surg Oncol 1981;16:23–27.
97. Groth G, Gatzemeier U, Haussingen K, et al. Intrapleural palliative treatment of malignant pleural effusions with mitoxantrone versus placebo (pleural tube alone). Ann Oncol 1991;2:213–215.
98. Torsten U, Opri F, Weitzel H. Local therapy of malignant pleural effusion with mitoxantrone. Anticancer Drugs 1992;3:17–18.
99. Topuz E, Zissis MP, Dincer M, et al. Intrapleural instillation of mitoxantrone in the treatment of malignant pleural effusions. Reg Cancer Treat 1991;3:323–325.
100. Ike O, Shimizu Y, Hitomi S, et al. Treatment of malignant pleural effusions with doxorubicin hydrochloride containing poly(L-lactic acid) microsphere. Chest 1991;99(4):911–915.
101. Masuno T, Kishimoto S, Ogura T, et al. A comparative trial of LC9018 plus doxorubicin and doxorubicin alone for the treatment of malignant pleural effusions secondary to lung cancer. Cancer 1991;68(7):1495–1500.

102. Rusch VW, Figlin R, Godwin D, et al. Intrapleural cisplatin and cytarabine in the management for malignant pleural effusion: a lung cancer study group trial. J Clin Oncol 1991;9:313–319.
103. Markman M, Cleary S, King ME, et al. Cisplatin and cytarabine administered intrapleurally as treatment of malignant pleural effusions. Med Pediatr Oncol 1985;13(4):191–193.
104. Holoye PY, Jeffries DG, Dhingra HM, et al. Intrapleural etoposide for malignant effusion. Cancer Chemother Pharmacol 1990;26:147–150.
105. Suhrland LG, Weisberger AS. Intracavitary 5-fluorouracil in malignant effusions. Arch Intern Med 1965;116:431–433.
106. Luh KT, Yang PC, Kuo SH, et al. Comparison of OK-432 and mitomycin-C pleurodesis for malignant pleural effusion caused by lung cancer. Cancer 1992;69:674–679.
107. Webb HE, Oaten SW, Pike CP. Treatment of malignant ascites and pleural effusions with *Corynebacterium parvum*. Br Med J 1978;1:338–340.
108. Stephen K, Chapes SK, Haskill S. The role of *Corynebacterium parvum* in the activation of peritoneal macrophages. Cell Immunol 1982;70:65–75.
109. Rossi GA, Felletti R, Balbi B, et al. Symptomatic treatment of recurrent malignant pleural effusions with intrapleurally administered *Corynebacterium parvum*: clinical response is not associated with evidence of enhancement of local cellular-mediated immunity. Am Rev Respir Dis 1987;135(4):885–890.
110. Casali A, Gionfra T, Rinaldi M, et al. Treatment of malignant pleural effusions with intracavitary *Corynebacterium parvum*. Cancer 1988;62(4):806–811.
111. Millar JW, Hunter AM, Horne NW. Intrapleural immunotherapy with *Corynebacterium parvum* in recurrent malignant pleural effusions. Thorax 1980;35(11):856–858.
112. McLeod DT, Calverley PM, Millar JW, et al. Further experience of *Corynebacterium parvum* in malignant pleural effusion. Thorax 1985;40(7):515–518.
113. Felletti R, Ravazzoni C. Intrapleural *Corynebacterium parvum* for malignant pleural effusions. Thorax 1983;38:22–24.
114. Davis M, Williford S, Muss HB, et al. A phase I-II study of recombinant intrapleural alpha interferon in malignant pleural effusions. Am J Clin Oncol 1991;15(4):328–330.
115. Rosso R, Rimoldi R, Salvati F, et al. Intrapleural natural beta interferon in the treatment of malignant pleural effusion. Oncology 1988;45(3):253–256.
116. Cascenu S, Isidori PP, Fedeli A, et al. Experience with intrapleural natural beta interferon in the treatment of malignant of pleural effusions. Tumori 1991;77(3):237–238.
117. Gebbia V, Russo A, Gebbia N, et al. Intracavitary B interferon for the management of pleural and/or abdominal effusions in patients with advanced cancer refractory to chemotherapy. In Vivo 1991;5:579–582.
118. Yasumoto K, Ogura T. Intrapleural application of recombinant interleukin-2 patients with malignant pleurisy due to lung cancer. A multi-institutional cooperative study. Biotherapy 1991; 3(4):345–349.
119. Li DJ, Wang YR, Tan XY, et al. A new approach to the treatment of malignant effusion. Chin Med J (Engl) 1990;103(12): 998–1002.
120. Liu X. Effectiveness of treatment with transfer of autologous or allogenic LAK cells combined with rIL-2 in 121 patients with malignant pleural effusion. Chung Hua Chung Liu Tsa Chih 1993;15(3):205–208.
121. Astoul P, Viallat JR, Laurent JC, et al. Intrapleural recombinant IL-2 in passive immunotherapy for malignant pleural effusion. Chest 1993;103:209–213.
122. Viallat JR, Boutin C, Rey F, et al. Intrapleural immunotherapy with escalating doses of interleukin-2 in metastatic pleural effusions. Cancer 1993;71:4067–4071.
123. Sone S, Yanagawa H, Nii A, et al. Induction by local injections of Il-2 of antitumor effector cells and secondary production of cytokines in malignant pleural effusion. Nippon Kyobu Shikkan Gakkai Zasshi 1992;30(8):1434–1440.
124. Kent EM, Moses C. Radioactive isotopes in the palliative management of carcinomatosis of the pleura. J Thorac Surg 1951; 22:503–516.
125. Card RY, Cole DR, Henschke UK. Summary of ten years of the use of radioactive colloids in intracavitary therapy. J Nucl Med 1960;1:195–198.
126. Izbicki R, Weyhing BT, III, Baker L, et al. Pleural effusion in cancer patients—a prospective randomized study of pleural drainage with the addition of radioactive phosphorus to the pleural space vs pleural drainage alone. Cancer 1975;36:1511–1518.
127. Parker LA, Charnock GC, Delany DJ. Small bore catheter drainage and sclerotherapy for malignant pleural effusions. Cancer 1989;64:1218–1221.
128. Morrison MC, Mueller PR, Lee MJ, et al. Sclerotherapy of malignant pleural effusion through sonographically placed small-bore catheters. AJR Am J Roentgenol 1992;158:41–43.
129. Martini N, Bains MS, Beattie EJ Jr. Indications for pleurectomy in malignant effusion. Cancer 1975;35(3):734–738.
130. Weese JL, Schouten JT. Pleural peritoneal shunts for the treatment of malignant pleural effusions. Surg Gynecol Obstet 1982;154:391–392.
131. Reich H, Beattie EJ, Harvey JC. Pleuroperitoneal shunt for malignant pleural effusions: a one year experience. Semin Surg Oncol 1993;9(2):160–162.
132. Little AG, Ferguson MK, Golomb HM, et al. Pleuroperitoneal shunting for malignant pleural effusions. Cancer 1986;58(12): 2740–2743.
133. Cimochowski GE, Joyner LR, Fardin R, et al. Pleuroperitoneal shunting for recalcitrant pleural effusions. J Thorac Cardiovasc Surg 1986;92(5):866–870.
134. Thurber DL, Edwards JE, Anchor RW. Secondary malignant tumors of the pericardium. Circulation 1962;26:228–241.
135. Cham WC, Freiman AH. Radiation therapy of cardiac and pericardial metastases. Radiology 1975;114:701–704.
136. Kusnoor VS, D'Souza RS, Bhandarkar SD, Golwalla AF. Malignant pericardial effusion: report of two cases. J Assoc Physicians India 1973;21:101–104.
137. Appelqvist P, Maamies T, Grohn P. Emergency pericardiotomy as primary diagnostic and therapeutic procedure in malignant pericardial tamponade: report of three cases and review of the literature. J Surg Oncol 1982;21:18–22.
138. Bisel HF, Wroblewski F, LaDue JS. Incidence and clinical manifestations of cardiac metastases. JAMA 1953;153:712–715.
139. Lokich JJ. The management of malignant pericardial effusions. JAMA 1973;224:1401–1404.
140. Piehler JM, Pluth JR, Schaff HV, Danielson GK, Orszulak TA, Pugna FJ. Surgical management of effusive pericardial disease. Influence of extent of pericardial resection on clinical course. J Thorac Cardiovasc Surg 1985;90:506–516.
141. Theologides A. Neoplastic cardiac tamponade. Semin Oncol 1978;5:181–192.
142. Kline JK. Cardiac lymphatic involvement by metastatic tumor. Cancer 1972;29:799.

143. Fraser RS, Viloria JB, Wang N. Cardiac tamponade as a presentation of extracardiac malignancy. Cancer 1980;45:1697–1704.
144. Cohen G, Perry T, Evans JM. Neoplastic invasion of the heart and pericardium. Ann Intern Med 1955;43:1238–1245.
145. Chia BL, DaCosta JL, Ransome GA. Cardiac tamponade due to leukaemic pericardial effusion. Thorax 1973;28:657–659.
146. Pories WJ, Gaudiani VA. Cardiac tamponade. Surg Clin North Am 1975;55:573–589.
147. Gilbert JC, Glantz SA. Determinants of left ventricular filling and of the diastolic pressure-volume relation. Circ Res 1989;64:827–852.
148. Ringertz HG, Misbach GA, Tyberg JV. Effect of the normal pericardium on the left ventricular diastolic pressure-volume relationship. Acta Radiol 1981;22:529–539.
149. Ross JJ. Acute displacement of the diastolic pressure-volume curve of the left ventricle: role of the pericardium and the right ventricle. Circulation 1979;59:32–37.
150. Reddy SP, Curtiss EI, Uretsky BF. Spectrum of hemodynamic changes in cardiac tamponade. Am J Cardiol 1990;66:1487–1491.
151. Spodick DH. Pericardial rub: prospective, multiple observer investigation of pericardial friction rub in 100 patients. Am J Cardiol 1975;35:357–362.
152. Guberman B, Fowler N, Engel P, Gueron M, Allen J. Cardiac tamponade in medical patients. Circulation 1981;64:633–640.
153. Brown J, MacKinnon D, King A, Vanderbush E. Elevated arterial blood pressure in cardiac tamponade. New Engl J Med 1992;327:463–466.
154. Usher BW, Popp RL. Electrical alternans: mechanism in pericardial effusion. Am Heart J 1972;83:459–463.
155. Levine MJ, Lorell BH, Diver DJ, Come PC. Implications of echocardiographically assisted diagnosis of pericardial tamponade in contemporary medical patients: detection before hemodynamic embarrassment. J Am Coll Cardiol 1991;17:59–65.
156. Gascho JA, Martins JB, Marcus ML, Kerber RE. Effects of volume expansion and vasodilators in acute pericardial tamponade. Am J Physiol 1981;240:449–453.
157. Krikorian JG, Hancock EW. Pericardiocentesis. Am J Med 1978;65:808–814.
158. Callahan JA, Seward JB, Nishimura RA, et al. Two-dimensional echocardiographically guided pericardiocentesis: experience in 117 consecutive patients. Am J Cardiol 1985;55:476–479.
159. Pandian NG, Brockway B, Simonetti J, Rosenfield K, Bojar RM, Cleveland RJ. Pericardiocentesis under two-dimensional echocardiographic guidance in loculated pericardial effusion. Ann Thorac Surg 1988;45:99–100.
160. Gregory JR, McMurtrey MJ, Mountain CF. A surgical approach to the treatment of pericardial effusion in cancer patients. Am J Clin Oncol 1985;8:319–323.
161. Wiener HG, Kristensen IB, Haubek A, Kristensen B, Baandrup U. The diagnostic value of pericardial cytology: an analysis of 95 cases. Acta Cytol 1991;35:149–153.
162. Kralstein J, Frishman W. Malignant pericardial diseases: diagnosis and treatment. Am Heart J 1986;113:785–790.
163. Hancock EW. Neoplastic pericardial disease. Cardiol Clin 1990;8:673–682.
164. Posner MR, Cohen GI, Skarin AT. Pericardial disease in patients with cancer: the differentiation of malignant from idiopathic and radiation-induced pericarditis. Am J Med 1981;71:407–413.
165. Markiewicz W, Borovik R, Ecker S. Cardiac tamponade in medical patients: treatment and prognosis in the echocardiographic era. Am Heart J 1986;111:1138–1142.
166. Flannery EP, Gregoratos G, Corder MP. Pericardial effusions in patients with malignant diseases. Arch Intern Med 1975;135:976–977.
167. Kopecky SL, Callahan JA, Tajik AJ, Seward JB. Percutaneous pericardial catheter drainage: report of 42 consecutive cases. Am J Cardiol 1986;58:633–635.
168. Patel AK, Kosolcharoen PK, Nallasivan M, Kroncke GM, Thomsen JH. Catheter drainage of the pericardium. Practical method to maintain long-term patency. Chest 1987;92:1018–1021.
169. Lock JE, Bass JL, Kulik TJ, Fuhrman BP. Chronic percutaneous pericardial drainage with modified pigtail catheters in children. Am J Cardiol 1984;53:1179–1182.
170. Erdman S, Levinsky L, Deviri E, Levy MJ. Closed pericardial drainage for relief of pericardial tamponade. J Thorac Cardiovasc Surg 1986;34:66–67.
171. Weisberger AS, Levine B, Storaasli JP. Use of nitrogen mustard in the treatment of serous effusions of neoplastic origin. JAMA 1955;159:1704–1708.
172. Ultman JE, Hyman GA, Crandall C, Naujoks H, Gellhorn A. Thiotepa in the treatment of neoplastic disease. Cancer 1957;10:902–914.
173. Hickman JA, Jones MC. Treatment of neoplastic pleural effusions with local instillations of quinacrine hydrochloride. Thorax 1970;25:226–229.
174. Martini N, Freiman AH, Watson RC, Hilaris BS. Intrapericardial installation of radioactive chromic phosphate in malignant effusion. AJR Am J Roentgenol 1977;128:639–641.
175. Rose RG. Intracavitary radioactive colloidal gold: results in 257 cancer patients. J Nucl Med 1962;3:323–331.
176. Shepherd FA, Morgan C, Evans WK, Ginsberg JF, Watt D, Murphy K. Medical management of malignant pericardial effusion by tetracycline sclerosis. Am J Cardiol 1987;60:1161–1166.
177. Davis S, Sharma SM, Blumberg ED, Kim CS. Intrapericardial tetracycline for the management of cardiac tamponade secondary to malignant pericardial effusion. N Engl J Med 1978;299:1113–1114.
178. Abubakar S, Malik I, Ali SM, Khan A. Management of malignant pericardial effusion with tetracycline induced pericardiodesis. J Pakistan Med Assoc 1991;41:20–22.
179. Goldman BS, Pearson F. Malignant pericardial effusion. Review of hospital experience and report of a case successfully treated by talc poudrage. Can J Surg 1965;8:157–161.
180. Van Belle SJP, Volckaert A, Taeymans Y, Spapen H, Block P. Treatment of malignant pericardial tamponade with sclerosis induced by instillation of bleomycin. Int J Cardiol 1987;16:155–160.
181. Primrose WR, Cleed MD, Johnston RN. Malignant pericardial effusion managed with vinblastine. Clin Oncol 1983;9:67–70.
182. Fiorentino MV, Danielle O, Morandi P, et al. Intrapericardial instillation of platin in malignant pericardial effusion. Cancer 1988;62:1904–1906.
183. Musch E. Intrapericardial chemotherapy of malignant effusions: controversies in dose intensive therapies. Symposium preceding the 26th Annual Meeting of the American Society of Clinical Oncology, Washington, DC, May 18, 1990.
184. Rinkevich D, Borovik R, Bendett M, Markiewicz W. Malignant pericardial tamponade. Med Pediatr Oncol 1990;18:287–291.
185. Terry LNJ, Klingerman MM. Pericardial and myocardial involvement by lymphomas and leukemia: the role of radiotherapy. Cancer 1970;25:1003–1008.

186. Palatianos GM, Thurer RJ, Kaiser GA. Comparison of effectiveness and safety of operations on the pericardium. Chest 1985;88:30–33.
187. Palatianos GM, Thurer RJ, Pompeo MQ, Kaiser GA. Clinical experience with subxiphoid drainage of pericardial effusions. Ann Thorac Surg 1989;48:381–385.
188. Sugimoto JT, Little AG, Ferguson MK, et al. Pericardial window: mechanisms of efficacy. Ann Thorac Surg 1990;50:442–445.
189. Ziskind AA, Rodriguez S, Lemmon CC, et al. Percutaneous balloon pericardiotomy for the treatment of effusive pericardial disease—104 patient follow-up. J Am Coll Cardiol 1994;21:1–5.
190. Mehan VD, Dalvi BV, Lokhandwala YY, Kale PA. Use of guiding catheters to target pericardial and endomyocardial biopsy sites. Am Heart J 1991;122:882–883.
191. Endrys J, Simo M, Shafie MZ, et al. New nonsurgical technique for multiple pericardial biopsies. Cathet Cardiovasc Diagn 1988;15:92–94.
192. Selig MB. Percutaneous pericardial biopsy under echocardiographic guidance. Am Heart J 1991;122:879–882.
193. Selig MB. Percutaneous transcatheter pericardial interventions: aspiration, biopsy, and pericardioplasty. Am Heart J 1993;125:269–271.
194. Maisch B, Drude L. Epi- and pericardial biopsy guided by pericardioscopy. Circulation 1990;82:411-417.
195. Ziskind AA, Rodriguez S, Lemmon CC, Burstein S. Percutaneous pericardial biopsy as an adjunctive technique for the diagnosis of pericardial disease. Am J Cardiol 1994;74:288–291.
196. Palacios IF, Tuzcu EM, Ziskind AA, Younger J, Block PC. Percutaneous balloon pericardial window for patients with malignant pericardial effusion and tamponade (comments). Cathet Cardiovasc Diagn 1991;22:244–249.
197. Ziskind AA, Pearce AC, Lemmon CC, et al. Percutaneous balloon pericardiotomy for the treatment of cardiac tamponade and large pericardial effusions: description of technique and report of the first 50 cases. J Am Coll Cardiol 1993;21:1–5.
198. Kondos GT, Rich S, Levitsky S. Flexible fiberoptic pericardioscopy for the diagnosis of pericardial disease. J Am Coll Cardiol 1986;7:432–434.
199. Little AG, Ferguson MK. Pericardioscopy as adjunct to pericardial window. Chest 1986;89:53–55.
200. Maisch B, Drude L. Pericardioscopy—a new diagnostic tool in inflammatory diseases of the pericardium. Eur Heart J 1991;12:2–6.
201. Millaire A, Wurtz A, de Groote P, Saudemont A, Chambon A, Ducloux G. Malignant pericardial effusions: usefulness of pericardioscopy. Am Heart J 1992;124:1030–1034.
202. Ziskind AA, Pearce AC, Lemmon CC, et al. Feasibility of percutaneous pericardial biopsy and pericardioscopy as an adjunct to balloon pericardiotomy for the diagnosis and treatment of pericardial disease. J Am Coll Cardiol 1992;19:267A.
203. Rodriguez S, Lemmon CC, Burstein S, Ziskind AA. Feasibility and utility of percutaneous pericardial biopsy and pericardioscopy as an adjunct to balloon pericardiotomy or pericardiocentesis for the diagnosis and treatment of pericardial disease. Eur Heart J 1993; in press.
204. Ozuner G, Davidson PG, Isenberg JS, McGinn JTJ. Creation of a pericardial window using thoracoscopic techniques. Surg Gynecol Obstet 1992;175:69–71.
205. Hazelrigg SR, Mack MJ, Landreneau RJ, Acuff TE, Seifert PE, Auer JE. Thoracoscopic pericardiectomy for effusive pericardial disease. Ann Thorac Surg 1993;56:792–795.
206. Linder A, Friedel G, Toomes H. Prerequisites, indications, and techniques of video-assisted thoracoscopic surgery. Thorac Cardiovasc Surg 1993;41:140–146.

44

INTRATHORACIC METASTASES

Barbara K. Temeck and Harvey I. Pass

INTRODUCTION

The lungs are the second most frequent site of metastatic disease (1) and are the only site of metastatic disease in 20% of autopsy cases (2). The results of the management of pulmonary metastases by surgical resection have been presented in a number of series. For certain histologies improved survivals have been demonstrated, but the influence of prognostic indicators and the role of adjuvant therapy are still being defined.

HISTORY

The first removal of a pulmonary metastasis was done in 1882 by Weinlechner en bloc with excision of a chest wall sarcoma (3). Two years later Krolein resected a peripheral lung nodule during an operation for a chest wall sarcoma. In 1926, metastasectomy alone was performed by Divis and was first accomplished in the United States by Torek in 1930 (4). The reports of Barney and Churchill in 1939 (5) and Alexander and Haight in 1947 (6) showed survival benefits and increased interest in pulmonary metastasectomy. The approach was broadened to include resection of multiple lesions with improved length of survival reported in several series (7–9).

PATHOGENESIS

A frequent mechanism for the development of pulmonary metastases is tumor embolization (10). This metastasis is preceded by the release of tumor cells from the primary lesion by the enzymatic disruption of the cellular wall. Tumor emboli are formed, released into the circulation, and filtered into the pulmonary capillary bed. It is thought that the majority of the emboli are destroyed. Tumor cells interact with endothelial cells, thrombocytes, and fibrin and become attached to vascular endothelioma. The pulmonary capillaries may be disrupted by pressure necrosis or enzymatic degradation, leading to vascular penetration. Metastatic growth is determined by tumor and local tissue factors. Direct entry into lymphatic channels also takes place and leads to metastatic regional lymph nodes with progressive spread along lymphatic chains. Retrograde extension from pulmonary and hilar lymphatics also can occur (11, 12). A nodal mass with bronchial invasion can cause endobronchial metastases. Transbronchial dissemination via aspiration is another method of dissemination (11).

DIAGNOSIS

Eighty percent to 90% of pulmonary metastases are located in a peripheral or outer third subpleural position (13, 14). The characteristic roentgenographic appearance of a pulmonary metastasis is a spherical nodule that has clearly defined borders without linear densities. Single or multiple nodules may be present. Multiple nodules are suggestive of metastatic disease, but they are not pathognomonic because such presentations can occur in lung tumors such as bronchoalveolar carcinoma, as well as in multiple synchronous primary carcinomas of the lung. Calcification can occur and thus should not be interpreted as related to a benign condition. This finding can be present after chemotherapy and radiation therapy and with osteosarcoma, chondrosarcoma, synovial sarcoma, and carcinomas of the breast, gastrointestinal tract, thyroid, and ovary (15–19). Sarcoma and squamous cell carcinomas can produce cavitation (20). Two percent to 20% of patients develop endobronchial metastases that can lead to collapse of one or more lobes (21–23). These metastases are more frequent with breast, colon, and kidney carcinomas. Lymphangitic spread from cancer of the breast, lung, stomach, colon, pancreas, and prostate may appear roentgenographically with minimal findings expressed as linear markings and prominent hilar lymph nodes (12, 24). There is no predilection of metastatic lesions for the right or left side (25), and the location is more often at the lung bases because of circulating physiology (26). However, posterior distribution to the upper lobes occurs in choriocarcinomas and may be related to dissemination during curettage (27, 28).

Symptoms are present in only 5% to 15% of patients, and they are related to the location and size of the tumors (29–31). Symptoms include cough, wheezing, hemoptysis, dyspnea, fatigue, and chest pain. When hemoptysis occurs bronchoscopy should be performed to rule out endobronchial tumor. Chest pain can signify involvement of the parietal pleura of the chest wall. A 10% incidence of pneumothorax associated with lung metastases has been reported (32). Proposed mechanisms relate to coexistent emphysematous bullae, presence of cavitating tumor, spontaneous tumor necrosis, and chemotherapy-induced tumor lysis (32). Dyspnea may be related to endobronchial obstruction, tumor replacement of pulmonary parenchyma, lymphatic carcinomatosis, pleural effusion, bleeding into a lesion or the pleural space, or pneumothorax.

The posteroanterior and lateral chest roentgenograms serve as a screening tool used to detect changes from baseline previous examinations. Although conventional linear tomography is more sensitive than the plain chest roentgenogram, the actual number of metastases can be underestimated by approximately 50% (33). Computed tomography (CT) has proven superior to linear tomography and has become the standard method used to detect new pulmonary nodules. Lesions as small as 3 mm can be detected (26). Inaccuracies in establishing the number of nodules remain because of partial volume averaging, attenuation by adjacent aerated lung, and proximity to vessels. The use of contrast enhancement can improve results (34–37). In one series CT visualized 78% of excised nodules larger than 3 mm versus 59% for conventional linear tomography. However, 60% of these additional nodules were benign, indicating that the CT findings can be nonspecific (33). Another review (38) of the pathologic findings in 144 patients with pulmonary metastases that compared chest roentgenograms and CT scans found that the radiographs detected more nodules in 46% of the patients and fewer in 54%. The finding of "more nodules" meant identification of 25 nonmalignant nodules on final analysis. With only one lesion, accuracy was 81% for chest roentgenography, but with more than one lesion, underreporting occurred in 44% of the cases. There was an overall 22% detection failure rate of nodules confirmed at operation but unreported by roentgenography. By CT scan 17% of patients had fewer lesions and 25% had more. For a solitary lesion, there was a 74% accuracy. Double lesions were missed in 40% of patients, and an overall 28% failure of detection rate was noted for single or double nodules when more were found at thoracotomy. Comparison of serial CT scans may assist in interpretation of the data. However, the occurrence of a new nodule or growth of a previous nodule in a patient with a history of an extrapulmonary primary tumor can signify: (*a*) a new cancer of the lung, (*b*) metastases from a known cancer, or (*c*) a benign lesion. A new primary lung cancer is more likely for previous squamous carcinomas, and a metastasis is more common for previous adenocarcinomas, melanomas, and sarcomas (39).

Surveillance of patients with malignant tumors should be tailored to the histology of the primary tumor and its pathophysiology. Sarcomas, which tend to metastasize within the first 2 years after diagnosis, warrant baseline CT studies of the chest and follow-up examinations every 3 months. For other cancers that metastasize preferentially to the bone or liver, such as prostate and gastrointestinal malignancies, chest roentgenograms are adequate (40). The role of magnetic resonance imaging (MRI) in the evaluation of pulmonary metastatic disease has not yet been defined. One prospective study correlating the findings of MRI and CT with operative results demonstrated comparable sensitivities for lesions larger than 5 mm (41). Further investigations that evaluate refinements in equipment and techniques are needed to clarify the clinical application of MRI as a surveillance method (42).

INVASIVE PRETREATMENT EVALUATION

An additional workup can be done for a possible pulmonary metastatic lesion if there are questions regarding the radiographic appearance or the amenability of the patient to surgical resection. The etiology of associated pleural effusions should be evaluated. In patients who are considered high surgical risks, histologic diagnosis can contribute to therapeutic decision making. Treatment options available to a patient with a primary tumor that may require limb amputation may be modified if there is a pathologic diagnosis of pulmonary metastatic disease. Sputum cytology and bronchial washings are low-yield studies for pulmonary metastases (43). Fine-needle aspiration biopsy, however, has reported sensitivities of up to 88% for metastatic lesions (44, 45). Implantation of tumor along needle tracts is rare with this technique (45), and complications such as pneumothorax requiring chest tube placement are uncommon (46).

Thoracoscopy is another diagnostic technique, but it requires general anesthesia. Parenchymal lesions in the outer third of the lung field are most readily accessible for thoracoscopic evaluation (47–49). Hookwires inserted under CT guidance have been used to localize small and deep-seated pulmonary nodules prior to thoracoscopic resection (50). As a therapeutic method, thoracoscopy has limitations that are discussed later in this chapter. As expected, mediastinoscopy or mediastinotomy is rarely positive. However, its use has been proposed as part of the evaluation of patients with large proximal tumors or breast cancers (51).

PATIENT SELECTION

In the 30% of patients with malignant disease who develop pulmonary metastases, there are no reliable predictors of survival after surgical resection. Only a minority of patients are cured, and a cohort of other patients derive a survival benefit. Each patient requires individual preoperative assessment with a thorough systemic evaluation. Functional investigation of a patient's pulmonary status should include clinical observation, pulmonary function tests, and, in selected instances, quantitative ventilation and perfusion lung scan. These data may also be considered serially in the context of repeated operations for recurrent pulmonary metastases. The effect of previously used chemotherapeutic interventions on hematologic, pulmonary, renal, and cardiac functions must be determined. It must be agreed that local control of the primary tumor can be achieved either before or after the metastasectomy, and there must be no evidence of extrathoracic metastatic disease. These requirements are established by radiographic, radionuclide, and endoscopic examinations. The pulmonary metastatic disease must be defined by radiologic methods, as discussed previously, and considered to be surgically resectable with adequate postoperative residual lung tissue. There should be no other effective therapeutic options. Unfortunately, only one third of patients with pulmonary metastatic disease fulfill these criteria (23).

PROGNOSTIC FACTORS

There are no universally established factors that predict survival after pulmonary metastasectomy (52). Data are based on retrospective analyses of various histologies from different primary sites. Patients also may have received adjuvant chemotherapy, radiation therapy, or immunotherapy. Certain factors serve as guidelines for making decisions regarding the advisability of pulmonary metastasectomy.

RESECTABILITY

For all histologies, complete resection of pulmonary metastatic disease results in improved survival, compared with survival after incomplete resection (29, 30, 53–56). Because of the limitation of preoperative diagnostic methods, the ultimate determination of resectability must be made intraoperatively. Clear-cut anatomic characteristics, such as discontinuous involvement of the pericardium or diaphragm, metastatic lymph nodes, and associated malignant pleural effusion or pleural metastases, preclude resectability. In selected patients, however, aggressive surgical resection by pneumonectomy or pulmonary resections en bloc with other thoracic structures may lead to long-term survival (57).

DISEASE FREE INTERVAL

The disease free interval (DFI) is defined as the time from treatment of the primary tumor to the development of pulmonary metastases. It thus would be predicted that the shorter the DFI, the shorter the survival of the patient. Although two studies (58, 59) found a correlation for survival with DFI in osteosarcoma, this finding was not evident in other investigations (55, 60–64). The data were similar in soft tissue sarcomas, with DFI related to survival by several authors (30, 54, 59) but not by others (55, 64). Reports on mixed groups of patients with carcinoma or sarcoma showed an influence of DFI on survival (53, 65–68). DFI was not found to be important in Ewing's sarcoma (56) and renal cell carcinoma (69). DFI duration seems to have prognostic importance in breast cancer (70) and in head and neck cancer (71). One report (72) on gynecologic cancer showed that DFI was a prognostic indicator, but two reports did not (73, 74). For colon carcinoma no difference has been detected (75–77), except for one report (78) that suggested, but did not prove, a contribution of DFI to survival. Whereas two publications (79, 80) on melanoma found no impact in outcome by DFI, two different reports (81, 82) identified an influence of DFI. Similar survival rates have been documented for synchronous and metachronous metastatic pulmonary nodules for sarcoma, carcinoma, and renal cell cancer (30, 52, 53, 56, 65, 69). The data on DFI are outlined in Table 44.1.

TABLE 44.1. Prognostic Factors for Pulmonary Metastasectomy

HISTOLOGY SURVIVAL	AUTHOR (REFERENCE NO.)	NO. OF PATIENTS	RELATIONSHIP DFI TO SURVIVAL	RESECTED NODULES TO SURVIVAL
Breast	Lanza et al. (70)	37	Neg ≤1 y vs. >1 y	None
Carcinoma-sarcoma	Ishida et al. (65)	85	Neg ≤1 y	None
Carcinoma-sarcoma	Marincola and Mark (66)	140	Neg ≤1 y	None
Carcinoma-sarcoma	Swoboda and Toomes (67)	96	Neg ≤1 y	Negative >1
Carcinoma-sarcoma	Venn et al. (86)	118	Not stated	None
Carcinoma-sarcoma	Vogt-Moykopf et al. (53)	368	Neg ≤3 y vs. >3 y	None
Colon-rectum	Goya et al. (75)	62	None	Negative >1
Colon-rectum	McAfee et al. (77)	139	None	Negative >1
Colon-rectum	Mori et al. (76)	35	None	None
Gynecologic	Fuller et al. (72)	15	Neg ≤3 y vs. 3 y	Not stated
Head and neck	Finley et al. (71)	18	Neg ≤2 y	None
Melanoma	Gorenstein et al. (82)	56	Neg ≤1 y	None
Melanoma	Karp et al. (80)	29	None	≤2
Melanoma	Pogrebniak et al. (79)	33	None	None
Renal cell	Pogrebniak et al. (69)	23	None	None
Sarcoma: Ewing's	Lanza et al. (56)	19	None	Negative >4
Sarcoma: osteogenic	Carter et al. (63)	43	None	None
Sarcoma: osteogenic	Goorin et al. (62)	26	None	None
Sarcoma: osteogenic	Meyer et al. (61)	39	None	Negative >5
Sarcoma: osteogenic	Telander et al. (58)	28	Neg <1 y vs. >1 y	None
Sarcoma: soft tissue	Jablons et al. (54)	74	Neg ≤1 y vs. >1 y	None
Sarcoma: combined	Flye et al. (64)	61	None	None
Sarcoma: combined	Liénard et al. (59)	19	Neg ≤1 y vs. >1 y	Negative >8
Sarcoma: combined	Pastorino et al. (55)	56	None	None
Sarcoma: combined	Levenback et al. (74)	45	None	None
Uterine-cervical	Seki et al. (73)	32	None	None

Adapted from Pass HI. Treatment of metastatic cancer to the lung. In: DeVita V, Hellman S, Rosenberg SA, eds. Principles and practice of oncology. Philadelphia: JB Lippincott, 1993:2186.
Abbreviations. Neg, negative; DFI, disease free interval.

NUMBER OF METASTASES

Preoperative radiologic examinations can underestimate the number of nodules by a factor of two (26). Based on linear tomography, four or fewer nodules in certain studies (30, 60) and three or fewer in other studies (29, 54) have been correlated to improved postoperative survival. One study (54) also investigated nodule count by CT for soft tissue sarcomas and found that the identification of five or fewer nodules was associated with longer survival after metastasectomy. In another investigation (83), CT demonstrating three or fewer nodules detected preoperatively significantly influenced survival.

Depending on histology, the number of nodules *resected* may influence survival. In one study of metastatic soft tissue sarcoma, four or fewer nodules resected versus five or more made no difference in survival (54). Another study reported a resection benefit in patients with soft tissue sarcoma who had 15 or fewer nodules resected (30). In contradistinction, another study (79) found that patients survived longer only if there were two or fewer soft tissue sarcoma metastases resected. Differences in outcome were reported in osteogenic sarcoma for one versus more than one metastasis (62), four or fewer (30), and two or fewer (84); in Ewing's sarcoma the breakpoint was fewer than four metastases (56). Several series that combined carcinoma and sarcoma cases did not identify the number of nodules resected as a prognostic indicator (53, 65, 66, 85, 86). Survival has reportedly been influenced by the number of nodules resected in metastatic breast cancer (70) and in head and neck cancer (71). More than one metastatic lesion in colon cancer impacted on survival in several reports (75, 77, 78), but this finding was not statistically significant in another (76). No difference in survival, based on the number of melanoma nodules resected, has been demonstrated (79, 82). However, survival for a group (80) with one or two nodules was better, because complete resection was possible, than in a group having more than two lesions. A summary of the relationship of the number of nodules resected to survival is presented in Table 44.1.

TUMOR DOUBLING TIME

The tumor doubling time (TDT) has been quantitated as a means of correlating the growth rate with prognosis. Faster growing tumors (shorter TDTs) and decreased patient survival were documented by several investigators (60, 87, 88). Therapeutic agents, however, could alter TDT. A prolonged TDT has been demonstrated in patients receiving chemotherapy compared with a group receiving no therapy (89). The slowing of tumor growth may improve survival (90). It is agreed, however, that surgical intervention should not be delayed in patients who meet the criteria for surgical exploration, except in the unusual situation in which the diagnostic workup is equivocal.

OTHER POSSIBLE PROGNOSTIC INDICATORS

LATERALITY OF LESIONS

In disease that can be resected completely, laterality (i.e., right-sided versus left-sided nodules) does not influence prognosis (29, 30).

AGE AND SEX

Age and sex does not correlate with survival (29, 30).

SYMPTOMS

In a report (68) of 84 patients with cancer and 41 with sarcoma having metastasectomy, the presence of symptoms was associated with a 9% 5-year survival, compared with a 42% 5-year survival if symptoms were absent.

NODAL STATUS

Shorter survival times are documented in patients with intrathoracic nodal involvement from soft tissue sarcoma (30, 54, 88). Similar results have been reported for uterine cervical cancer (73) and for melanoma (81). However, no difference was noted for hilar or mediastinal lymph node involvement for colon cancer (75). In general, patients suspected of having mediastinal disease on preoperative studies are not considered surgically resectable, and mediastinoscopy should be performed in patients with suspected mediastinal involvement (51).

SIZE OF THE NODULES

Isolated reports have commented on a significant difference between sarcoma metastases of at least 3 cm compared with smaller lesions (53). For smaller metastases the 5-year survival was 37% with a median survival time of 31 months, whereas patients with larger metastases had a median survival of 11 months and none survived more than 3 years. Others reported a cutoff size of 2 cm (91). Survival was better for patients with pulmonary metastatic lesions less than 3 cm in diameter in uterine-cervical cancer (73) and colon cancer (75). In an analysis of 140 patients with carcinomas or sarcomas, there was a significant correlation to survival when the largest lesion was smaller than 1.5 cm (66).

ADJUVANT CHEMOTHERAPY

The possible role of chemotherapy as an adjuvant to pulmonary metastasectomy has not been studied in a randomized manner. Data in one study (54) indicated that single-agent postthoracotomy chemotherapy for soft tissue sarcomas did not change survival. Another series (92) of 78 patients with extremity soft tissue sarcomas who underwent surgical treatment for pulmonary metastases reported that preoperative chemotherapy or immunotherapy was associated with a median survival time of 25.5 months, which was not significantly different than the 18-month survival seen in patients who had resection without preoperative therapy. The utility of chemotherapy *before* thoracotomy for metastases was examined in 21 patients with bony and soft tissue sarcomas (93). Five patients having a dramatic response were alive at the time of the report—a median follow-up of 23 months—and four had no evidence of disease. Ten patients had a less dramatic response but a measurable decrease in the rate of tumor growth: a tumor doubling time of more than 40 days was observed. Four of these patients remain alive. Three have no evidence of disease with a median follow-up of 29 months. The median survival of those who died was 24 months. Four of six patients with no response to preoperative chemotherapy died (median survival, 11.5 months) and had a median follow-up of 15 months. Thus, 15 of 21 patients responded to preoperative chemotherapy, and 7 (45%) were free of disease. Such chemotherapeutic regimens are complicated and are associated with some morbidity. These trials should be performed in centers in which the surgeons and oncologists are familiar with the interdigitation of chemotherapy and surgery. However, to complicate the issue, another publication (94) showed that response to preoperative chemotherapy did not predict survival. It is generally agreed, however, that in stage IV testicular germ cell tumors with lung metastases, an improved survival has been reported when combining chemotherapeutic and surgical approaches (95). Many times only benign teratoma is found in the residual tumors.

TECHNIQUE OF PULMONARY METASTASECTOMY

The operative approach is facilitated by the use of a double-lumen endotracheal tube that permits selective unilateral lung collapse for careful palpation. However, sequential one-lung ventilation can lead to severe hypoxemia and hypercapnia because of intrapulmonary shunting and parenchymal manipulation (96). For patients who have received bleomycin, the level of inspired oxygen should be held to a minimum both intraoperatively and postoperatively.

The favored approach for resection of pulmonary metastases is through a median sternotomy to allow bilateral thoracic exploration (54–56, 97). One series demonstrated that 43% of patients with unilateral metastases on linear tomography, 45% on CT, and 38% on both examinations had bilateral metastases at the time of sternotomy (25). Using a median sternotomy approach, the surgeon can visualize both thoracic cavities to include the mediastinum, pulmonary parenchyma, hilar lymph nodes, chest wall, and diaphragm to ascertain resectability before the removal of any lung tissue. Lesions even smaller than 1 mm can be felt or seen by the experienced surgeon. A zero mortality has been reported (54) with such an approach. Median sternotomy and lateral thoracotomy have the same mortality and survival rates (25). The recovery of postoperative pulmonary function is more rapid, however, with median sternotomy (98). Epidural anesthesia can be used for either approach, although it is particularly helpful postoperatively in the management of lateral thoracotomy pain. At the National Cancer Institute the median sternotomy approach has been used safely up to four times in patients undergoing multiple reoperations for recurrence of pulmonary metastases (54). These authors recommend that subsequent operations be done with lateral thoracotomy because of the occurrence of adhesions and the need to localize small recurrent nodules. A concomitant median sternotomy and thoracotomy approach may be necessary for large central or posterior lesions in the left lower lobe. Thoracotomy is preferable for a left lower lobe lesion in an obese patient with a large heart and a narrow retrosternal space. Other indications for a thoracotomy approach are a history of sternal irradiation, central staple line recurrences, posteromedial disease of the chest wall, and a contemplated sleeve resection (99, 100). Bilateral posterior lateral thoracotomy incisions can be done in one or two stages. The operative time and postoperative pain is increased, however. Bilateral anterior thoracotomies with a transverse sternotomy, the "clamshell" incision, can also be used. No significant morbidity was reported by Bains and associates (101). Other authors have reported that postoperative pain with this incision is intense, and the theoretic disadvantage of bilateral internal mammary ligations has been discussed (102).

Measures that help with the conduct of the operation are the surgeon's use of a headlight, adequate length of the sternotomy incision, wide opening of the pleura, use of a Duval clamp to elevate the lung, placement of posterior packs to lift the lung forward, release of the inferior pulmonary ligament, and occasional use of traction sutures to gently hold the pericardial sac away for an exploration of the left lower lobe (100).

Conservation of lung tissue while assuring satisfactory margins of resection (1 to 2 cm) is important. Because most metastatic lesions are located peripherally and subpleurally, wedge resections can usually be accomplished. Automatic staplers are used frequently. The automatic stapling device (available in 30-, 55-, and 90-mm sizes) can be positioned to achieve a margin at the base of the lesion. The gastrointestinal anastomosis stapler can be used for lesions deeper in the lung. Larger resections may be necessary, such as lobectomy or segmentectomy or en bloc resection, to accomplish complete resection.

For deep parenchymal lesions, a precision cautery technique can be used (99). A lesion is cored out with a surrounding margin of normal lung with the cautery and individual vessel ligation. The residual tumor bed is approximated by sutures to decrease bronchopleural fistulae.

The carbon dioxide (CO_2) and the noncontact neodymium:yttrium-aluminum-garnet (Nd:YAG) lasers have been used for laser resection of pulmonary metastases (103–106). Reports in the literature of results with laser resection have varied. A comparative study (106) in 14 children with lung metastases (12 operations) with the Nd:YAG laser and 10 with conventional technique found that the former method provided safer intraoperative conditions for the patient and diminished the risk of the operation. The inflated lung is operated on, and a bloodless defect in the lung parenchyma is left behind that has a carbonized surface from which no air leaks. The CO_2 laser requires a bloodless field but can be used to seal blood vessels and air leaks, and it produces less damage macroscopically and microscopically (103). The Nd:YAG laser caused the deeper tissue damage but functioned well under conditions of poor hemostasis (104). Branscheid and coworkers (104) used the Nd:YAG laser alone to accomplish pulmonary metastasectomy in 14 patients with carcinomas or sarcomas and used it in combination with conventional techniques for 51 other patients. With the Nd:YAG laser, the duration of the operation was longer, compared with conventional technique, and a longer postoperative duration of chest tube suction was required. The authors noted, however, that laser resection and vaporization allowed more opportunity for parenchymal-preserving operations, such as occur in centrally located lesions and in the treatment of patients with a larger number of metastases or with marginal lung function. The mean number of lesions resected or vaporized by laser was 8 with a range of from 1 to 81. In a review of 146 thoracotomies for pulmonary metastases performed from January 1977 to June 1997, the CO_2 and Nd:YAG laser was used by Saltzman et al. (91) during the last 6 years. The impression of these investigators was that a more exact anatomic dissection could be performed using lasers, allowing for lymphatic sealing, minimal blood loss, and preservation of functional lung.

The use of the ultrasonic aspirator in the surgical treatment of metastatic lesions still is in the investigation phase (107). Verazin et al. (107) used the technique to lyse the lung with the titanium tip and then applied clips or ligatures to control the blood vessels and bronchi and minimize thermal damage. However, prolonged air leak can result.

Thoracoscopic resection under video monitoring is being used in the treatment of pulmonary metastases (47–49, 108). Left thoracoscopic resection also has been combined with median sternotomy to deal with retrocardiac left lower lobe lesions (109). In a study of 72 patients who underwent thoracoscopic resection with a parenchymal-sparing operation using the Nd:YAG laser, endoscopic staplers, or both, two patient populations were considered for thoracoscopic metastasectomy of parenchymal lung lesions (108). The first group consisted of patients in whom the aim was not a survival benefit but rather a diagnosis required for prognosis and determination of further therapy. The second group consisted of patients considered to have a limited tumor burden and favorable histology whose disease was confined to the outer third of the lung parenchyma and for whom a survival benefit could possibly be achieved. Preoperative needle localization was used in 13 patients with small lesions that were not immediately subpleural. This study emphasized the utility of preoperative localization with high-resolution, thin-cut CT. The limitation of this technique, however, is the surgeon's ability to deal only with peripheral lesions. Given the inaccuracies of the preoperative radiologic workup, the ultimate effect on survival of using thoracoscopic resection for pulmonary metastatic disease remains to be determined. As with thoracoscopic resection, the use of laser-assisted resection and of the ultrasonic dissector must be subjected to careful analysis before being accepted into standard surgical practice (99).

REOPERATIVE METASTASECTOMY

For most histologies there are no data on the role of reoperations for recurrent pulmonary metastatic disease. A retrospective study at the National Cancer Institute of 43 patients who had at least two and up to six explorations for metastatic soft tissue sarcoma demonstrated a median survival of 25 months for patients with resectable disease and 10 months for those with unresectable disease. Complete resection and a DFI between the first and second thoracotomies of more than 18 months were the only factors that influenced survival (110). Another series of soft tissue sarcomas in adults reported a longer median survival for 34 of 39 patients who had complete resections during two or more metastasectomies. Longer survival was associated with resection of a solitary metastatic nodule (111).

SPECIFIC HISTOLOGIES

OSTEOGENIC SARCOMA

Osteogenic sarcomas disseminate initially to the lungs. Before the use of innovative chemotherapeutic regimens, 80% of these patients died in the first year with amputation alone, and 95% died within 3 years (112). Neoadjuvant chemotherapy has become part of the standard treatment for osteogenic sarcoma and may contribute to the decreased incidence of solitary metastases (113). The aggressive resection of pulmonary metastases from osteogenic sarcoma has been reported in numerous investigations (8, 29, 61–64, 84, 89, 114). Without randomized trials it is not possible to define the relative contribution of resection to survival. In a comparative investigation of children treated from 1970 to 1981 and those treated from 1982 to 1988, overall actuarial survival was 43% versus 68% at 3 years and 35% versus 58% at 5 years (114). Another report demonstrated a 5-year survival of 57% for patients treated from 1974 to 1977 versus 23% for those treated from 1946 to 1974 (58). Survival rates of 45% at 3 years, 27.2% at 10 years, 22.7% at 15 years, and 13.6% at 20 years have been reported (115). Fifty percent of these 10-year survivors developed a second primary cancer during the second decade of follow-up. None of the patients had been treated for the primary tumor during the era of chemotherapy. Five-year survival rates (Table 44.2) range from 25% to 58% in the literature (29, 31, 53, 63, 68, 84, 89, 91, 114, 116–120).

In an investigation of 247 patients with osteogenic sarcoma between 1971 and 1991, patients were treated in four sequential groups (120). Group I received surgery alone for treatment of the primary tumor. The incidence of lung metastases was 92%, and only 17% (two patients) underwent thoracotomy, with a respective survival of 19 and 41 months from the resection of the primary tumor. Groups II through IV received various adjuvant chemotherapeutic regimens in addition to surgery for the primary tumor. Group II patients were treated between 1975 and 1980. Sixty-three percent of these patients developed lung metastases. Of these patients 58% were resected with a median survival time of 42 months, and the overall and postthoracotomy 5-year survival rate was 26%. Group III patients were treated between 1981 and 1985. Forty-eight percent developed lung metastases, of whom 74% underwent thoracotomy with a median survival time of 38 months and a 5-year postthoracotomy survival rate of 35%. Lung metastases occurred in 35% of group IV patients (1985 to 1991), and 82% had surgical treatment for the lung metastases. The median survival time had not been reached, and the actuarial 5-year survival rate was 42% from the resection of the primary tumor and 37% from the initial thoracotomy.

The data document an evolution in the selection criteria for defining operative candidates: once chemotherapy became available, a more aggressive operative approach was taken, and pulmonary metastases that developed after adjuvant chemotherapy were resected. Several studies (121–123) have corroborated this approach. In one of these studies (121), patients treated with adjuvant chemotherapy for osteosarcoma developed fewer metastases and had a longer DFI and a higher proportion of one or more nodules compared with patients who refused chemotherapy. A higher relapse rate and earlier recurrence with more numerous and bilateral pulmonary nodules were found in patients not receiving adjuvant chemotherapy in a multiinstitutional osteosarcoma study (122) that compared surgery alone to surgery with adjuvant chemotherapy. In an autopsy study (123), patients who had received adjuvant chemotherapy for osteosarcoma had a longer DFI and survival and a higher incidence of single metastasis.

SOFT TISSUE SARCOMA

In patients with soft tissue sarcoma, the lung is often the only site of metastatic disease. Metastases occur most commonly within the first 2 years after diagnosis of the primary tumor. A 5-year survival rate of

TABLE 44.2. Metastasectomy Results for Osteogenic Sarcoma

AUTHOR (REFERENCE NO.)	YEAR	NO. OF PATIENTS	5-YEAR SURVIVAL (%) UNLESS OTHERWISE INDICATED
Spanos et al. (84)	1976	30	28
Giritsky et al. (89)	1978	12	58[a] (3 y)
Telander et al. (58)	1978	28	57[a] (4 y)
Burgers et al. (118)	1980	6	60
Morrow et al. (116)	1980	11	36
Putnam et al. (29)	1983	39	40
Mountain et al. (31)	1984	56	51
DiLorenzo et al. (119)	1988	10	50
Eckersberger et al. (117)	1988	6	31
Vogt-Moykopf et al. (53)	1988	41	33[a] (3 y)
Roberts et al. (68)	1989	16	23
Carter et al. (63)	1991	25	20
Pastorino et al. (114)	1992	102	58
Skinner et al. (120)	1992	28	42
Saltzman et al. (91)	1993	26	24

Adapted from Pass HI. Treatment of metastatic cancer to the lung. In: DeVita V, Hellman S, Rosenberg SA, eds. Principles and practice of oncology. Philadelphia: JB Lippincott, 1993:2186.
[a]Less than 5-year data.

approximately 33% has been reported (30, 31, 53, 54, 83, 91, 92, 94, 117, 124, 125). Factors associated with an increased risk of pulmonary metastases include high tumor grade, tumor size greater than 3 cm, lower extremity site, and histologic type (spindle cell, tenosynovial, and extraskeletal osteosarcoma) (92). Prognostic indicators relate to the completeness of the resection of metastatic disease, DFI between the first and second mastectomies, and possibly the number of nodules seen on scans before the first mastectomy. The actual number of nodules removed has not influenced survival consistently, and patients should be considered for surgical resection based on their functional evaluation rather than the number of nodules present (Table 44.3).

URINARY TRACT CANCER

Pulmonary metastases develop in half of patients with renal cell carcinoma who undergo nephrectomy for apparently isolated disease, and 75% of patients with stage IV disease have pulmonary metastases (69). In the literature 5-year survival rates range from 13% to 50% with a median survival of 23 to 33 months after pulmonary metastasectomy (Table 44.4) (31, 53, 68, 69, 116, 126, 127). The data often have included patients undergoing additional operations for extrapulmonary metastases. One study (127) found that patients with a solitary metastasis had a 5-year survival of 45.6% compared with 27% for patients who had multiple metastases. Also, patients with a tumor free interval longer than the median of 3.4 years had a better survival than those with a tumor free interval of not more than 3.4 years. The 5-year survival for patients

TABLE 44.3. Metastasectomy for Soft Tissue Sarcoma

AUTHOR (REFERENCE NO.)	YEAR	NO. OF PATIENTS	5-YEAR SURVIVAL (%) UNLESS OTHERWISE INDICATED
Martini et al. (124)	1978	102	26
Creagen et al. (125)	1979	112	29
Putnam et al. (30)	1984	63	30 (3 y)
Mountain et al. (31)	1984	49	33
Vogt-Moykopf et al. (53)	1988	56	33
Eckersberger et al. (117)	1988	29	18
Jablons et al. (54)	1989	68	33
Lanza et al. (94)	1991	24	22
Casson et al. (83)	1992	58	26
Gadd et al. (92)	1993	78	23 (3 y)
Saltzman et al. (91)	1993	22	71

Adapted from Pass HI. Treatment of metastatic cancer to the lung. In: DeVita V, Hellman S, Rosenberg SA, eds. Principles and practice of oncology. Philadelphia: JB Lippincott, 1993:2186.

TABLE 44.4. Metastasectomy for Urinary Tract Cancer

AUTHOR (REFERENCE NO.)	YEAR	NO. OF PATIENTS	5-YEAR SURVIVAL (%) UNLESS OTHERWISE INDICATED
Morrow et al. (116)	1980	30	24
Mountain et al. (31)	1984	20	54
Vogt-Moykopf et al. (53)	1988	42	42
Roberts et al. (68)	1989	33	24
Pogrebniak et al. (69)	1992	23	43 months (mean)
diSilverio et al. (126)	1992	17	35
Cerfolio et al. (127)	1994	96	35.9

Adapted from Pass HI. Treatment of metastatic cancer to the lung. In: DeVita V, Hellman S, Rosenberg SA, eds. Principles and practice of oncology. Philadelphia: JB Lippincott, 1993:2186.

who underwent repeat thoracotomy or who had complete resection of extrapulmonary disease did not differ from the overall survival. Another series (69) examined the results for 23 patients undergoing only pulmonary metastasectomies. Seventy-eight percent of the patients received preoperative immunotherapy, but this treatment did not influence survival. Patients who had complete surgical resection had a longer survival (mean, 49 months; median not yet achieved) compared with those who were incompletely resected (median, 16 months).

TESTICULAR CANCER

Testicular cancer is a malignancy in which many patients can achieve a complete response despite the presence of widespread metastases. Pulmonary metastases often are associated with retroperitoneal and mediastinal lymph node involvement. Li et al. (128) first introduced cytoreductive combination chemotherapy for testicular germ cell tumors in 1960.

Seventy percent of patients achieve a complete response with cisplatin-based combination chemotherapy. With surgery, 10% to 15% more patients are rendered free of disease. The histologic findings at surgery are important because residual masses after chemotherapy may be necrotic and/or fibrotic tissue, mature teratomas, or viable carcinoma. The last may indicate the need for further chemotherapy. Surgery also may be necessary when tumor markers increase after chemotherapeutic options have been exhausted (129–131). Relevant survival data are listed in Table 44.5. A recent study (132) examined the prognostic factors for survival and relapse after resection of residual masses following chemotherapy for metastatic nonseminomatous testicular cancer. Adverse prognostic factors were prechemotherapy level of human chorionic gonadotropin (HCG) of at least 10,000 Interna-

TABLE 44.5. Metastasectomy for Other Histologies

AUTHOR (REFERENCE NO.)	YEAR	NO. OF PATIENTS	5-YEAR SURVIVAL (%) UNLESS OTHERWISE INDICATED
Breast			
McCormack et al. (134)	1979	34	30
Wright et al. (147)	1982	18	27
Mountain et al. (31)	1984	30	27
Marincola et al. (66)	1990	9	21.4
Lanza et al. (70)	1992	37	50
Staren et al. (148)	1992	33	36
McDonald et al. (149)	1994	60	38
Head and neck			
McCormack et al. (134)	1979	25	44
Mountain et al. (31)	1984	48	41
Vogt-Moykopf et al. (53)	1988	12	44
Finley et al. (71)	1992	7	43
Gynecologic cancer			
Fuller et al. (72)	1985	15	36
Uterine cervical cancer			
Morrow et al. (116)	1980	22	8
Mountain et al. (31)	1984	34	24
Seki et al. (73)	1992	32	52
Uterine sarcoma			
Levenback et al. (74)	1992	45	43
Testicular cancer			
Morrow et al. (116)	1980	6	30
Mountain et al. (31)	1984	20	54
Vogt-Moykopf et al. (53)	1988	42	82 (2 y)
Venn et al. (86)	1989	42	84

Adapted from Pass HI. Treatment of metastatic cancer to the lung. In: DeVita V, Hellman S, Rosenberg SA, eds. Principles and practice of oncology. Philadelphia: JB Lippincott, 1993:2186.

tional Units (U), incomplete resection, and extent of disease, particularly lung metastases. Poor prognosis was associated with prechemotherapy size of lung metastases of more than 3 cm and number of nodules of at least 20, postchemotherapy size of more than 1 cm, and presence of any residual lung metastasis after chemotherapy without residual abdominal metastases. The most significant factor for relapse was an incomplete resection. This report suggested than an improvement in prognosis of incompletely resected patients might be obtained by the administration of salvage chemotherapy after resection, although future studies will be necessary to confirm this thesis.

HEAD AND NECK CANCER

With the exception of a primary tumor of the lip, tonsil, and adenoid, the first metastases from a head and neck cancer most often occurs to the lung. There also is a high incidence of second primary lung cancers. Five-year survival rates of up to 43% have been reported with metastasectomy (71, 133). In one study (71), survival was improved for patients having complete resection of a solitary metastasis with locoregional control of the primary tumor. Two studies (71, 133) found that a DFI of 1 to 2 years favorably influenced survival. Survival at 5 years is in the range of 41% to 44% (Table 44.5) (31, 53, 71, 134).

COLORECTAL CANCER

It has been stated that 10% of patients with colorectal cancer develop pulmonary metastases, and of these patients only 10% have metastases confined to the lung (135). A recent review (136) found that 22% of patients had the lung as the first site of recurrence after resection of colorectal carcinoma, whereas only 2% to 4% of patients having had a potentially curative resection of primary colon cancers have the lung as the *only* site of metastasis (75). Rectal primary tumors seem to have a greater propensity for isolated metastatic lung disease because of the systemic venous drainage from this anastomotic region via the middle and inferior rectal veins, bypassing the portal system (137). One series (138) found that 117 (11.5%) of 1013 patients with rectal primary lesions and 20 (3.5%) of 565 patients with colon primary lesions developed lung metastases after potentially curative resection of colorectal cancer.

Five-year survival rates after pulmonary metastases range from 9% to 58% (31, 43, 68, 75–78, 116, 135, 139–144) (Table 44.6). The 5-year survival rates

TABLE 44.6. Metastasectomy for Colonic and Rectal Cancer

AUTHOR (REFERENCE NO.)	YEAR	NO. OF PATIENTS	5-YEAR SURVIAL (%) UNLESS OTHERWISE INDICATED
Cahan et al. (139)	1974	31	31
Vincent et al. (43)	1978	13	58% rectal, 0% colon
McCormack et al. (134)	1979	40	15
Morrow et al. (116)	1980	16	13
Mountain et al. (31)	1984	28	28
Wilking et al. (140)	1985	27	9
Mansel et al. (141)	1986	66	38
Pihl et al. (138)	1987	16	38
Brister et al. (142)	1988	27	21
Goya et al. (75)	1989	62	42
Roberts et al. (68)	1989	13	23
Mori et al. (76)	1991	35	38
McAfee et al. (77)	1992	139	30.5
Smith et al. (143)	1992	10	52
Saclarides et al. (78)	1993	23	16
Yano et al. (144)	1993	27	41.1

Adapted from Pass HI. Treatment of metastatic cancer to the lung. In: DeVita V, Hellman S, Rosenberg SA, eds. Principles and practice of oncology. Philadelphia: JB Lippincott, 1993:2186.

after thoracotomy may reflect a length-of-time bias caused by the biologic growth rate and behavior of the metastatic pulmonary lesions (137).

It has been noted that half of the patients in one study (138) with disease recurrent in the lung had clinically obvious disease within 33 months, compared with 22 months for patients with hepatic disease recurrences; this difference might imply a less biologically aggressive pulmonary process. This finding was substantiated by the late deaths in another series (75) that found a 3-year survival rate of 42% and a 10-year survival rate of 22%. Four of 13 patients died of metastatic disease more than 5 years after pulmonary resection, and two other patients were surviving long term with recurrent cancer. It has been demonstrated that half of the patients who developed a new opacity on a chest roentgenogram had a new primary lung cancer (139). The best survival has been reported in patients with a solitary metastasis and a normal carcinoembryonic antigen level (77). In this same investigation, however, patients with resection of multiple nodules did have a 25% 5-year survival. Patients with either one or two metastases have a significantly better survival (5-year survival, 54.3%) than those with more numerous metastases (144). The presence of controlled hepatic metastases may not have an adverse effect on survival or may contraindicate pulmonary resection, but this assumption needs further documentation. In another series 10 patients underwent resection of both hepatic and pulmonary metastases of colorectal origin; actuarial 1-, 3-, and 5-year survival rates were 89%, 78%, and 52%, respectively (143).

GYNECOLOGIC CANCER

Five-year survival rates of 8% to 52% after the development of pulmonary metastases from uterine-cervical cancer have been reported (31, 72, 73, 116) (Table 44.5). A 5-year survival rate of 36% has been reported in a group that included patients with primary tumors involving the cervix, endometrium, and ovary, as well as uterine sarcomas and choriocarcinomas. Patients with lesions less than 4 cm in diameter had the most favorable prognosis (72). Another series (73) had an overall 5-year survival of 52% for tumors of the uterine cervix that were metastatic to the lungs with no statistically significant difference in survival related to the number of nodules or DFI. The 5-year survival of patients with pulmonary tumors less than 3 cm in size was 71% compared with 40% for larger lesions, but the result was not statistically significant. For patients with lesions having diameters of 3 cm or larger, lymph node involvement was present in 65% and microscopic satellite lesions around the new metastatic lesion in 50%. Patients with lymph node involvement had a 5-year survival of 31% versus 71% without involvement (statistically significant). Controversy remains about whether routine lymph node dissection with pulmonary resection for cervical cancer metastases or a more aggressive resection should be performed because of the incidence of microscopic satellite lesions. For metastatic gestational choriocarcinoma, six of nine patients who underwent a total of 11 thoracotomies achieved complete remission for periods of 3 months, and 7, 10, 14, 15, and 22 years (145). This study suggests that these patients may have a unique variant of trophoblastic cells that show a decreased sensitivity to chemotherapy and yet potentially can be cured by surgery.

BREAST CANCER

Twenty-one percent of deaths in patients from breast cancer are related to pulmonary metastases (146). After pulmonary metastasectomy 5-year survival rates range from 27% to 50% (31, 66, 70, 134, 147–149). Longer survival has been correlated with a DFI of longer than 12 months and estrogen receptor positive status (70). Another report (148) compared 20 patients treated with surgical excision, 22 patients receiving systemic therapy, and 8 patients receiving systemic therapy plus local radiation therapy. Six patients in the latter group received radiation therapy for a subsequent recurrence. Mean survival in the surgical group was significantly longer than in the systemic therapy group, 58 months versus 34 months, even when compared with patients who had single pulmonary nodules. The overall 5-year survival rate after treatment of lung metastases was significantly greater for the surgical group than for the medical group, 36% versus 11%. No significant difference in survival occurred among patients who had resection for single compared with multiple pulmonary nodules. A recent presentation of 60 consecutive women who underwent pulmonary resection for metastatic breast cancer found that 40 patients who had a complete resection had a 5-year survival of 36%, compared with 42% for the 20 patients with an incomplete resection (149).

MELANOMA

A multifactorial analysis (150) of 200 melanoma patients with distant metastases observed that the first sign of dissemination was a pulmonary nodule in 38%. In another study (82), 50% of the patients had pulmonary metastases as the initial site of recurrence.

However, the appearance of a new pulmonary lesion on radiographic evaluation may indicate a benign process, such as was diagnosed in 33% of the patients with melanoma reported in another series (79). Five-year survival rates after pulmonary metastasectomy range from 5% to 33% (31, 79–82, 116, 151, 152) (Table 44.7). In a group of 945 patients with pulmonary metastases, a 4% 5-year survival without pulmonary metastasectomy was improved to 20% with resection (81). Multivariate predictors of improved survival for these patients in order of importance were complete resection of pulmonary disease, interval to metastasis, treatment with chemotherapy, one or two pulmonary nodules, and lymph nodes negative for metastasis. However, another investigation (80) found only curative resection as having an influence on survival.

OTHER TUMORS

Resection of pulmonary metastases from *parathyroid carcinoma* has been done to help control hypercalcemia and may result in cure (153, 154). The lung is the most common site of metastases from *adrenocortical carcinoma,* with 71% of patients who die of this cancer having pulmonary metastases at autopsy (155). A 25% overall 5-year survival of patients with adrenocortical carcinoma and pulmonary metastases has been reported (155). In this study 14 patients whose pulmonary metastases could not be resected had a median survival of 11 months, and no one was alive at 3 years. Of these patients 12 received chemotherapy and 2 received no therapy. In the 10 resected patients, median survival was not reached at 5 years with 1-, 3-, and 5-year survival rates of 100%, 71%, and 71%, respectively. Seventeen complete pulmonary resections of gross disease were performed for initial or recurrent metastases. Median DFI from the time of resection of the primary tumor to the diagnosis of pulmonary metastases was 26 months in the resected group and 5.5 months for the nonresected group. Long-term survivors after pulmonary resection for metastases from adrenocortical carcinoma have been reported (7, 156–158).

In addition to osteogenic sarcoma and soft tissue sarcoma, children can develop pulmonary metastases from Wilms' tumor, hepatoma, hepatoblastoma, and rarely neuroblastoma (159). Most often, other sites of metastatic disease are present. A review (160) of the literature on metastatic liver malignancy to the lung in the pediatric group found that 8 of 11 were surviving 9 to 84 months after resection. This review reported five additional patients of whom four were alive 4 to 83 months after thoracotomy. Multiple thoracotomies may be necessary.

Chemotherapy and radiation therapy are the primary modalities used in the treatment of Wilms' tumor, but pulmonary metastasectomy may be indicated in selected cases (161–163). However, a retrospective examination was made of the clinical course of 211 patients with stage I to III favorable or unfavorable histology Wilms' tumor who were entered in the National Wilms' Tumor Study. Investigators found that in patients whose first recurrence was limited to the lungs there was no difference in the 4-year postrelapse survival percentage of favorable histology patients with a solitary pulmonary metastasis regardless of whether they had undergone surgical removal of the metastasis as well as pulmonary irradiation and chemotherapy (164). Also, patients treated with surgery followed by chemotherapy alone had a statistically significant higher recurrence rate in the lung from which the initial lesion was removed. This report (164) noted that several previous reports (165–168) had supported surgical excision for pulmonary metastasis in Wilms' tumor when this was the primary modality used for treatment; it also stated that the report was not a prospective evaluation of the role of surgery in such patients.

SUMMARY

Surgical resection has become part of the treatment approach for pulmonary metastatic disease. The most important goal of such therapy is complete resection of the disease. The histology of the primary tumor plays an important role in the determination of prognosis. With the multimodality approaches being used for many tumors, clinical trials are necessary to define the optimal methods of dealing with metastatic disease and the timing of possible surgical intervention.

TABLE 44.7. Metastasectomy for Melanomas

AUTHOR (REFERENCE NO.)	YEAR	NO. OF PATIENTS	5-YEAR SURVIVAL (%) UNLESS OTHERWISE INDICATED
Cahan (151)	1972	12	33%
Dahlback et al. (152)	1980	8	7-month median
Morrow et al. (116)	1980	12	12%
Mountain et al. (31)	1984	58	13-month median
Pogrebniak et al. (79)	1988	33	13-month median
Karp et al. (80)	1990	22	4.5%; 11-month median
Gorenstein et al. (82)	1991	56	25%
Harpole et al. (81)	1992	84	20%

Adapted from Pass HI. Treatment of metastatic cancer to the lung. In: DeVita V, Hellman S, Rosenberg SA, eds. Principles and practice of oncology. Philadelphia: JB Lippincott, 1993:2186.

REFERENCES

1. Willis RA. The spread of tumors in the human body. London: Butterworth, 1973:167–174.
2. Viadana E, Irwin D, Bross J, Pickren JW. Cascade spread of blood-borne metastases in solid and nonsolid cancers of humans. In: Weiss L, Gilbert H, eds. Pulmonary metastases. Boston: GK Hall, 1978:142.
3. van Dongen JA, van Slooten EA. The surgical treatment of pulmonary metastases. Cancer Treat Rev 1978;5:29–48.
4. Torek F. Removal of metastatic carcinoma of the lung and mediastinum. Suggestions as to technic. Arch Surg 1930;21:1416–1424.
5. Barney JD, Churchill EJ. Adenocarcinoma of the kidney with metastases to the lung: cured by nephrectomy and lobectomy. J Urol 1939;42:269–276.
6. Alexander J, Haight C. Pulmonary resection for solitary metastatic sarcomas and carcinomas. Surg Gynecol Obstet 1947;85:129–135.
7. Thomford NR, Wodner LB, Clagett OT. The surgical treatment of metastatic tumors of the lungs. J Thorac Cardiovasc Surg 1965;49:357–363.
8. Martini N, Huvos AG, Mike V, Marcove RC, Beattie EJ Jr. Multiple pulmonary resections in the treatment of osteogenic sarcoma. Ann Thorac Surg 1971;12:271–280.
9. Morton DL, Joseph WL, Ketcham AS, Geelhoed GW, Adkins PC. Surgical resection and adjunctive immunotherapy for selected patients with multiple pulmonary metastases. Ann Surg 1973;178:360–365.
10. Müller KM, Respondek M. Pulmonary metastases: pathological anatomy. Lung 1990;168:1137–1144.
11. Marchevsky AM. Metastatic tumors of the lung. Lung Biol Health Dis 1990;44:231–245.
12. Janower ML, Blennerhassett HJB. Lymphangitic spread of metastatic cancer to the lung. Radiology 1971;101:267–273.
13. Crow J, Slavin G, Kreel L. Pulmonary metastasis: a pathologic and radiologic study. Cancer 1981;47:2595–2602.
14. Scholten ET, Kreel L. Distribution of lung metastases in the axial plane. Radiol Clin North Am 1977;46:248–265.
15. Morse D, Reed JO, Bernstein J. Sclerosing osteogenic sarcoma. AJR Am J Roentgenol 1963;88:491–495.
16. Zollikofer C, Castaneda-Zuniga W, Stenlund R, Sibley R. Lung metastases from synovial sarcoma simulating granulomas. AJR Am J Roentgenol 1980;135:161–163.
17. Rosenfield AT, Sanders RC, Custer LE. Widespread calcified metastases from adenocarcinoma of the jejunum. Am J Dig Dis 1975;20:990–993.
18. Fraley EE, Lange PH, Kennedy BJ. Germ cell testicular cancer in adults. N Engl J Med 1979;301:1370–1377.
19. Panella J, Mintzer RA. Multiple calcified pulmonary nodules in an elderly man. JAMA 1980;244:2559–2560.
20. Libshitz HI, North LB. Pulmonary metastases. Radiol Clin North Am 1982;20:437–451.
21. King DS, Castleman B. Bronchial involvement in metastatic pulmonary malignancy. J Thorac Surg 1943;12:305–315.
22. Braman SS, Whitcomb ME. Endobronchial metastases. Arch Intern Med 1975;135:543–547.
23. Shepherd MP. Endobronchial metastatic disease. Thorax 1982;37:362–370.
24. Dwyer AJ, Reichert CM, Woltering EA, Flye MW. Diffuse pulmonary metastasis in melanoma: Radiographic pathologic correlation. AJR Am J Roentgenol 1984;143:983–984.
25. Roth JA, Pass HI, Wesley MN, White D, Putnam JB, Seipp C. Comparison of median sternotomy and thoracotomy for resection of pulmonary metastases in patients with adult soft tissue sarcomas. Ann Thorac Surg 1986;42:134–138.
26. Pass HI, Dwyer A, Makuch R, Roth JA. Detection of pulmonary metastases in patients with osteogenic and soft tissue sarcoma: the superiority of CT scan compared with conventional linear tomograms using dynamic analyses. J Clin Oncol 1985;3:1261–1265.
27. Hendin AS. Gestational trophoblastic tumors metastatic to the lung. Cancer 1984;53:58–61.
28. Wagner D. Trophoblastic cells in the blood stream in normal and abnormal pregnancy. Acta Cytol 1968;12:137–139.
29. Putnam JB Jr, Roth JA, Wesley MN, Johnston MR, Rosenberg SA. Survival following aggressive resection of pulmonary metastases from osteogenic sarcoma: analysis of prognostic factors. Ann Thorac Surg 1983;36:516–523.
30. Putnam JB, Roth JA, Wesley MN, Johnston MR, Rosenberg SA. Analysis of prognostic factors in patients undergoing resection of pulmonary metastases from soft tissue sarcomas. J Thorac Cardiovasc Surg 1984;87:260–268.
31. Mountain CF, McMurtrey MJ, Hermes KE. Surgery for pulmonary metastases: a 20-year experience. Ann Thorac Surg 1984;38:323–329.
32. Biran H, Dgani R, Wasserman JP, Weissberg D, Shani A. Pneumothorax following induction chemotherapy in patients with lung metastases: a case report and literature review. Ann Oncol 1992;3:297–300.
33. Chang AE, Schaner EG, Conkle DM, Flye MW, Doppman JL, Rosenberg SA. Evaluation of computed tomography in the detection of pulmonary metastases. Cancer 1979;43:913–916.
34. Cohen M, Grosfeld J, Baehner R, Weetman R. Lung CT for detection of metastases: solid tissue neoplasms in children. AJR Am J Roentgenol 1982;139:895–898.
35. Lund G, Heilo A. Computed tomography of pulmonary metastases. Acta Radiol Diagn 1982;23:617–620.
36. Sones PJ, Torres WE, Colvin RS, Meier WL, Sprawls P, Rogers JV. Effectiveness of CT in evaluating intrathoracic masses. AJR Am J Roentgenol 1982;139:469–475.
37. Kuhns LR, Borlaza G. The "twinkling star" sign. An aid in differentiating pulmonary vessels from pulmonary nodules on computed tomograms. Radiology 1980;135:763–764.
38. McCormack PM, Ginsberg KB, Bains MJ, et al. Accuracy of lung imaging in metastases with implications for the role of thoracoscopy. Ann Thorac Surg 1993;56:863–866.
39. Cahan WG, Shah JP, Castro ELB. Benign solitary lung lesions in patients with cancer. Ann Surg 1978;187:241.
40. Chiles C, Ravin CE. Intrathoracic metastasis from an extrathoracic malignancy: a radiographic approach to patient evaluation. Radiol Clin North Am 1985;23:427–438.
41. Feuerstein IM, Jicha DL, Pass HI, et al. Pulmonary metastases: MR Imaging with surgical correlation—a prospective study. Radiology 1992;182:123–129.
42. Panicek DM. MR imaging for pulmonary metastases. Radiology 1992;182:10–11.
43. Vincent RG, Choksi LB, Takita H, Guiterrez AL. Surgical resection of the solitary pulmonary metastases. In: Weiss L, Gilbert HA, eds. Pulmonary metastases. Boston: GK Hall, 1978:224.
44. Johnston WW. Percutaneous fine needle aspiration biopsy of the lung: a study of 1,015 patients. Acta Cytol 1984;28:218–224.
45. Nordenstrom BEW. Technical aspects of obtaining cellular material from lesions deep in the lung. Acta Cytol 1984;28:233–242.

46. Crosby JH, Hager B, Hoeg K. Transthoracic fine-needle aspiration. Cancer 1985;56:2504–2507.
47. Page RD, Jeffrey RR, Donnelly RJ. Thoracoscopy: a review of 121 consecutive surgical procedures. Ann Thorac Surg 1989;48:66–68.
48. Bonniot JP, Homasson JF, Roden SL, Angebault ML, Renault PC. Pleural and lung cryobiopsies during thoracoscopy. Chest 1989;95:492–493.
49. Lewis RJ, Caccavale RJ, Sisler GE. Special report: video-endoscopic thoracic surgery. N J Med 1991;88:473–475.
50. Shah RM, Spirn PW, Salazar AM, et al. Localization of peripheral pulmonary nodules for thoracoscopic excision: Value of CT-guided wire placement. AJR Am J Roentgenol 1993;161:279–283.
51. Todd TR. Pulmonary metastectomy. Current indications for removing lung metastases. Chest 1993;103:401S–403S.
52. Matthay RA, Arroliga AC. Resection of pulmonary metastases. Am Rev Respir Dis 1993;148:1691–1696.
53. Vogt-Moykopf I, Bulzebruck H, Merkle NM, Probst G. Results of surgical treatment of pulmonary metastases. Eur J Cardiothorac Surg 1988;2:224–232.
54. Jablons D, Steinberg SM, Roth J, Pittaluga S, Rosenberg SA, Pass HI. Metastasectomy for soft tissue sarcoma. J Thorac Cardiovase Surg 1989;97:695–705.
55. Pastorino U, Valente M, Gasparini M, et al. Median sternotomy and multiple lung resections for metastatic sarcomas. Eur J Cardiothorac Surg 1990;4:477–481.
56. Lanza LA, Miser JS, Pass HI, Roth JA. The role of resection in the treatment of pulmonary metastases from Ewing's sarcoma. J Thorac Cardiovasc Surg 1987;94:181–187.
57. Putman JB, Suell DM, Natarajan G, Roth JA. Extended resection of pulmonary metastases: is the risk justified? Ann Thorac Surg 1993;55:1440–1446.
58. Telander RL, Pairolero PC, Pritchard DJ, Sim FH, Gilchrist GS. Resection of pulmonary metastatic osteogenic sarcoma in children. Surgery 1978;84:335–341.
59. Liénard D, Roemans P, Lejeune FJ. Resection of lung metastases from sarcomas. Eur J Surg Oncol 1989;15:530–534.
60. Roth JA, Putman JB, Wesley MN, Rosenberg SA. Differing determinants of prognosis following resection of pulmonary metastases from osteogenic and soft tissue sarcoma patients. Cancer 1985;55:1361–1366.
61. Meyer WH, Schell MJ, Jumar AP, et al. Thoracotomy for pulmonary metastatic osteosarcoma: an analysis of prognostic indicators of survival. Cancer 1987;59:374–379.
62. Goorin AM, Delorey MJ, Lack EE, et al. Prognostic significance of complete surgical resection of pulmonary metastases in patients with osteogenic sarcoma: analysis of 32 patients. J Clin Oncol 1984;2:425–431.
63. Carter SR, Grimer RJ, Sneath RS, Matthews HR. Results of thoracotomy in osteogenic sarcoma with pulmonary metastases. Thorax 1991;46:727–731.
64. Flye MW, Woltering G, Rosenberg JA. Aggressive pulmonary resection for metastatic osteogenic and soft tissue sarcomas. Ann Thorac Surg 1984;37:123–127.
65. Ishida T, Kaneko S, Yokoyama H, et al. Metastatic lung tumors and extended indications for surgery. Int Surg 1992;77:173–177.
66. Marincola FM, Mark JBD. Selection factors resulting in improved survival after surgical resection of tumors metastatic to the lung. Arch Surg 1990;125:1387–1393.
67. Swoboda L, Toomes H. Results of surgical treatment for pulmonary metastases. Thorac Cardiovasc Surg 1986;34:149–152.
68. Roberts DG, Lepore V, Cardillo G, et al. Long-term follow-up of operative treatment for pulmonary metastases. Eur J Cardiothorac Surg 1989;3:292–296.
69. Pogrebniak HW, Haas G, Linehan M, Rosenberg SA, Pass HI. Renal cell carcinoma: resection of solitary and multiple metastases. Ann Thorac Surg 1992;54:33–38.
70. Lanza LA, Natarajan G, Roth JA, Putnam JB. Long term survival after resection of pulmonary metastases from carcinoma of the breast. Ann Thorac Surg 1992;54:244–248.
71. Finley RK, Verazin GT, Driscoll DL, et al. Results of surgical resection of pulmonary metastases of squamous cell carcinoma of the head and neck. Am J Surg 1992;164:594–598.
72. Fuller AF, Scannell JG, Wilkins EW. Pulmonary resection for metastases from gynecologic cancers: Massachusetts General Hospital experience, 1943–1982. Gynecol Oncol 1985;22:174–180.
73. Seki M, Nakagawa K, Tsuchiya S, et al. Surgical treatment of pulmonary metastases from uterine cervical cancer. J Thorac Cardiovasc Surg 1992;104:876–881.
74. Levenback C, Rubin SC, McCormack PM, Hoskins WJ, Atkinson EN, Lewis JL. Resection of pulmonary metastases from uterine sarcomas. Gynecol Oncol 1992;45:202–205.
75. Goya T, Miyazawa N, Kondo H, Tsuchiya R, Naruke T, Suesmasu K. Surgical resection of pulmonary metastases from colorectal cancer. Cancer 1989;64:1418–1421.
76. Mori M, Tomodo H, Ishida T, et al. Surgical resection of pulmonary metastases from colorectal adenocarcinoma. Arch Surg 1991;126:1297–1301.
77. McAfee MK, Aken MS, Trastek VF, Ilstrup DM, Deschamp C, Pairolero PL. Colorectal lung metastases: results of surgical excision. Ann Thorac Surg 1992;53:780–786.
78. Saclarides TJ, Krueger BL, Szeluga DS, Warren WH, Faber LP, Economou SG. Thoracotomy for colon and rectal cancer metastases. Dis Colon Rectum 1993;36:425–429.
79. Pogrebniak HW, Stovroff M, Roth JA, Pass HI. Resection of pulmonary metastases from malignant melanoma: results of a 16-year experience. Ann Thorac Surg 1988;46:20–23.
80. Karp NS, Boyd A, De Pan HJ, et al. Thoracotomy for metastatic malignant melanoma of the lung. Surgery 1990;107:256–261.
81. Harpole DH, Johnson LM, Wolfe WG, et al. Analysis of 945 cases of pulmonary metastatic melanoma. J Thorac Cardiovasc Surg 1992;103:743–750.
82. Gorenstein LA, Putnam JB, Natarajan G, et al. Improved survival after resection of pulmonary metastases from malignant melanoma. Ann Thorac Surg 1991;52:204–210.
83. Casson AG, Putnam JB, Natarajan G, et al. Five year survival after pulmonary metastasectomy for adult soft tissue sarcoma. Cancer 1992;69:662–668.
84. Spanos PK, Payne WS, Ivins JC, Pritchard DJ. Pulmonary resection for metastatic osteogenic sarcoma. J Bone Joint Surg 1976;58A:624–628.
85. Stewart JR, Carey JA, Merrill WH, Frist WH, Hammon JW, Bender HW. Twenty years' experience with pulmonary metastasectomy. Am Surg 1992;58:100–103.
86. Venn GE, Sarin S, Goldstraw P. Survival following pulmonary metastasectomy. Eur J Cardiothorac Surg 1989;3:105–110.
87. Joseph WL, Morton DL, Adkins PC. Prognostic significance of tumor doubling time in evaluating operability in pulmonary metastatic disease. J Thorac Cardiovasc Surg 1971;61:23–32.

88. Takita H, Edgerton F, Karakousis C, Douglass HO, Vincent RG, Beckley S. Surgical management of metastases to the lung. Surg Gynecol Obstet 1981;152:191–194.
89. Giritsky AS, Etcubanas E, Mark JBD. Pulmonary resection in children with metastatic osteogenic sarcoma. Improved survival with surgery, chemotherapy and irradiation. J Thorac Cardiovasc Surg 1978;75:354–361.
90. Huth JF, Eilber FR. Patterns of metastatic spread following resection of extremity soft-tissue sarcomas and strategies for treatment. Semin Surg Oncol 1988;4:20–26.
91. Saltzman DA, Synder CL, Ferrell KL, Thompson RC, Leonard AS. Aggressive metastasectomy for pulmonary sarcomatous metastases: a follow-up study. Am J Surg 1993;166:543–547.
92. Gadd MA, Casper ES, Woodruff JM, McCormack PM, Brennan MF. Development and treatment of pulmonary metastases in adult patients with extremity soft tissue sarcoma. Ann Surg 1993;218:705–712.
93. Huth JF, Holmes EC, Vernon SE, Callery CD, Ramming KP, Morton DL. Pulmonary resection for metastatic sarcoma. Am J Surg 1980;140:9–16.
94. Lanza LA, Putnam JB Jr, Benjamin RS, Roth JA. Response to chemotherapy does not predict survival after resection of sarcomatous pulmonary metastases. Ann Thorac Surg 1991;51:219–224.
95. Carsky S, Ondrus D, Schnorrer M, Májek M. Germ cell testicular tumours with lung metastases: Chemotherapy and surgical treatment. Int Urol Nephrol 1992;24:305–311.
96. Antognini JF, Hanowell LH. Intraoperative hypoxemia complicating sequential resection of bilateral pulmonary metastases. Anesthesiology 1991;74:1137–1139.
97. Regal A-M, Reese P, Antkowiak J, Hart T, Takita H. Median sternotomy for metastatic lung lesions in 131 patients. Cancer 1985;55:1334–1339.
98. Cooper JD, Nelems JM, Pearson FG. Extended indications for median sternotomy in patients requiring pulmonary resection. Ann Thorac Surg 1978;26:413–419.
99. Pogrebniak HW, Pass HI. Initial and reoperative pulmonary metastasectomy: indications, technique, and results. Semin Surg Oncol 1993;9:142–149.
100. Pass HI. Treatment of metastatic cancer to the lung. In: DeVita V, Hellman S, Rosenberg SA, eds. Principles and practice of oncology. Philadelphia: JB Lippincott, 1993:2186.
101. Bains MS, Ginsberg RJ, Jones WG II, et al. The clamshell incision: an improved approach to bilateral pulmonary and mediastinal tumors (abstract). Ann Thorac Surg 1994;58:30–33.
102. Shimizu N, Ando A, Matsutani T, Maruyama S, Date H, Teramoto S. Transsternal thoracotomy for bilateral pulmonary metastases. J Surg Oncol 1992;50:105–109.
103. LoCicero J III, Hartz RS, Frederiksen JW, Michaelis LL. New applications of the laser in pulmonary surgery. Hemostasis and sealing of air leaks. Ann Thorac Surg 1985;40:546–550.
104. Branscheid D, Krysa S, Wollkopf G, et al. Does ND-YAG laser extend the indications for resection of pulmonary metastases? Eur J Cardiothorac Surg 1992;6:590–597.
105. Harrey JC, Lee K, Beattie EJ. Utility of the neodymium:yttrium-aluminum-garnet (ND:YAG) laser for extensive pulmonary metastasectomy. J Surg Oncol 1993;54:175–179.
106. Fanta J, Kowtesky J, Rehák F. Use of the Nd:YAG laser in the surgical treatment of lung metastases in children. Pediatr Hematol Oncol 1991;8:375–377.
107. Verazin GT, Regal AM, Antkowiak JG, Parvez Z, Takita H. Ultrasonic surgical aspirator for lung resection. Ann Thorac Surg 1991;52:787–790.
108. Dowling RD, Keenan RJ, Ferson PF, Landreneau RJ. Video-assisted thoracoscopic resection of pulmonary metastases. Ann Thorac Surg 1993;56:772–775.
109. Hazelrigg SR, Naunheim K, Auer JE, Seifert PE. Combined median sternotomy and video-assisted thoracoscopic resection of pulmonary metastases. Chest 1993;104:956–958.
110. Pogrebniak HW, Roth JA, Steinberg SM, Rosenberg SA, Pass HI. Reoperative pulmonary resection in patients with metastatic soft tissue sarcoma. Ann Thorac Surg 1991;52:197–203.
111. Casson AG, Putnam JB, Natarajan G, et al. Efficacy of pulmonary metastasectomy for recurrent soft tissue sarcoma. J Surg Oncol 1991;47:1–4.
112. Marcove RC, Miké V, Hajek JV, Levin AG, Hutter RVP. Osteogenic sarcoma under the age of twenty-one. J Bone Joint Surg 1970;52:411–423.
113. Giuliano AE, Feig S, Eilber FR. Changing metastatic patterns of osteosarcoma. Cancer 1984;54:2160–2164.
114. Pastorino U, Gasparini M, Valente M, et al. Primary childhood osteosarcoma: the role of salvage surgery. Ann Oncol 1992;3:543–546.
115. Beattie EJ, Harvey JC, Marcove R, Martini N. Results of pulmonary resections for metastatic osteogenic sarcoma after two decades. J Surg Oncol 1991;46:154–155.
116. Morrow CE, Vassilopoulos PP, Grage TB. Surgical resection for metastatic neoplasms of the lung: Experience at the University of Minnesota Hospitals. Cancer 1980;45:2981–2985.
117. Eckersberger F, Moritz E, Wolner E. Results and prognostic factors after resection of pulmonary metastases. Eur J Cardiothorac Surg 1988;2:433–437.
118. Burgers JMV, Breur K, Van Dobbenburgh OA, et al. Role of metastatectomy without chemotherapy in the management of osteosarcoma in children. Cancer 1980;45:1664–1668.
119. DiLorenzo M, Colbin PP. Pulmonary metastases in children: results of surgical treatment. J Pediatr Surg 1988;23:762–765.
120. Skinner KA, Eilber FR, Holmes EC, Eckardt J, Rosen G. Surgical treatment and chemotherapy for pulmonary metastases from osteosarcoma. Arch Surg 1992;127:1065–1068.
121. Bacci G, Avella M, Picci P, Briccoli A, Dallari D, Campandacci M. Metastatic patterns in osteosarcoma. Tumori 1988;74:421–427.
122. Goorin AM, Shuster JJ, Baker A, Horowitz ME, Meyer WH, Link MP. Changing pattern of pulmonary metastases with adjuvant chemotherapy in patients with osteosarcoma: results from the multi-institutional osteosarcoma study. J Clin Oncol 1991;9:600–605.
123. Yamaguchi H, Nojima T, Yagi T, et al. The alteration in the pattern of pulmonary metastases with adjuvant chemotherapy in osteosarcoma. Int Orthop 1988;12:305–308.
124. Martini N, McCormack PM, Bains MS, Beattie ES Jr. Surgery for solitary and multiple pulmonary metastasis. N Y State J Med 1978;78:1711–1713.
125. Creagen ET, Fleming TR, Edmonson JH, Pairolero PC. Pulmonary resection for metastatic nonosteogenic sarcoma. Cancer 1979;44:1908–1912.
126. diSilverio F, Facciolo F, D'Eramo G, Lauretti S, Ricci C. Surgery of pulmonary metastases from renal and bladder carcinoma. Scand J Urol Nephrol 1991;138:215–218.
127. Cerfolio RJ, Allen MS, Deschamps C, et al. Pulmonary resection of metastatic renal cell carcinoma. Ann Thorac Surg 1994;57:339–344.
128. Li MC, Whitmore WF, Colbey R, Grabstald H. Effects of combined drug therapy on metastatic cancer of the testes. JAMA 1960;174:145–153.

129. Einhorn LH, Donohue J. *Cis*-diamminedichloroplatinum, vinblastine, and bleomycin combination chemotherapy in disseminated testicular cancer. Ann Intern Med 1977;87:293–298.
130. Einhorn LH, Williams SD, Mandelbaum I, Donohue JP. Surgical resection in disseminated testicular cancer following chemotherapeutic cytoreduction. Cancer 1981;48:904–908.
131. Mandelbaum I, Yaw PB, Einhorn LH, Williams SD, Rowland RG, Donohue JP. The importance of one-stage median sternotomy and retroperitoneal node dissection in disseminated testicular cancer. Ann Thorac Surg 1983;36:524–528.
132. Steyerberg EW, Keizer HJ, Zwartendijk J, et al. Prognosis after resection of residual masses following chemotherapy for metastatic nonseminomatous testicular cancer: a multivariate analysis. Br J Cancer 1993;68:195–200.
133. Mazer TM, Robbins KT, McMurtrey MJ, Byers RM. Resection of pulmonary metastases from squamous carcinoma of the head and neck. Am J Surg 1988;156:238–242.
134. McCormack PM, Martini N. The changing role of surgery for pulmonary metastases. Ann Thorac Surg 1979;41:833–840.
135. McCormack PM, Attiyeh FF. Resected pulmonary metastases from colorectal cancer. Dis Colon Rectum 1979;22:553–556.
136. Galandiuk S, Wieand HS, Moertel CG, et al. Patterns of recurrence after curative resection of carcinoma of the colon and rectum. Surg Gynecol Obstet 1992;174:27–32.
137. Turk PS, Wanebo HJ. Results of surgical treatment of nonhepatic recurrence of colorectal carcinoma. Cancer 1993;71:4267–4277.
138. Pihl E, Hughes ES, McDermott FT, Johnson WR, Katrivessis H. Lung recurrence after curative surgery for colorectal cancer. Dis Colon Rectum 1987;30:417–419.
139. Cahan WG, Castro EB, Hajdu SI. The significance of a solitary lung shadow in patients with colon carcinoma. Cancer 1974;33:414–421.
140. Wilking N, Petrelli NJ, Herrera L, Regal AM, Mittelman A. Surgical resection of pulmonary metastases from colorectal adenocarcinoma. Dis Colon Rectum 1985;28:562–564.
141. Mansel JK, Zinsmeister AR, Pairolero PC, Jett JR. Pulmonary resection of metastatic colorectal adenocarcinoma: a 10 year experience. Chest 1986;89:109–112.
142. Brister SJ, DeVarennes B, Gordon PH, Sheiner NM, Pym J. Contemporary operative management of pulmonary metastases of colorectal origin. Dis Colon Rectum 1988;31:786–792.
143. Smith JW, Fortner JG, Burt M. Resection of hepatic and pulmonary metastases from colorectal cancer. Surg Oncol 1992;1:399–404.
144. Yano T, Hara N, Ichinose Y, Yokoyama H, Miuro T, Ohta M. Results of pulmonary resection of metastatic colorectal cancer and its application. J Thorac Cardiovasc Surg 1993;106:875–879.
145. Jones WB, Romain K, Erlandson RA, Burt ME, Lewis JL. Thoracotomy in the management of gestational chorio carcinoma. A clinicopathologic study. Cancer 1993;72:2175–2181.
146. Ramming KP. Surgery for pulmonary metastases. Surg Clin North Am 1980;60:815–824.
147. Wright JO, Brandt B, Ehrenhaft JL. Results of pulmonary resection for metastatic lesions. J Thorac Cardiovasc Surg 1982;83:94–99.
148. Staren ED, Salerno C, Rongione A, Witt TR, Faber LP. Pulmonary resection for metastatic breast cancer. Arch Surg 1992;127:1282–1284.
149. McDonald ML, Deschamps C, Ilstrup DM, Allen MJ, Trastek VF, Pairolero PC. Pulmonary resection for metastatic breast cancer (poster). 30th Annual Meeting of the Society of Thoracic Surgeons, New Orleans, LA, 1994.
150. Balch CM, Soong S, Murad TM, Smith JW, Maddox WA, Durant JR. A multifactorial analysis of melanoma IV. Prognostic factors in 200 melanoma patients with distant metastases (stage III). J Clin Oncol 1983;1:126–134.
151. Cahan WG. Excision of melanoma metastases to lung: problems in diagnosis and management. Ann Surg 1973;178:703–709.
152. Dahlback O, Hafstrom L, Jonsson PE, Sundqvist K. Lung resection for metastatic melanoma. Clin Oncol 1980;6:15–20.
153. Dubost C, Jehanno C, Lavergne A, Le Charpentier Y. Successful resection of intrathoracic metastases from two patients with parathyroid carcinoma. World J Surg 1984;8:547–551.
154. Flye MW, Brennan MF. Surgical resection of metastatic parathyroid carcinoma. Ann Surg 1981;193:425–435.
155. Kwauk S, Burt M. Pulmonary metastases from adrenal cortical carcinoma. Results of resection. J Surg Oncol 1993;53:243–246.
156. Jensen JC, Pass HI, Sindelar WF, Norton JA. Recurrent or metastatic disease in select patients with adrenocortical carcinoma. Arch Surg 1991;126:457–461.
157. Appelqvist P, Kostiainen S. Multiple thoracotomy combined with chemotherapy in metastatic adrenal cortical carcinoma: a case report and review of the literature. J Surg Oncol 1983;24:1–4.
158. Potter DA, Strott CA, Javadpour N, Roth JA. Prolonged survival following six pulmonary resections for metastatic adrenal cortical carcinoma: a case report. J Surg Oncol 1984;25:273–277.
159. Winkler K. Surgical treatment of pulmonary metastases in childhood. J Thorac Cardiovasc Surg 1986;34:133–136.
160. Black CT, Luck SR, Musemeche CA, Andrassy RJ. Aggressive excision of pulmonary metastases warranted in the management of childhood hepatic tumors. J Pediatr Surg 1991;26:1082–1086.
161. Green DM, Jaffee N. Wilms' tumor—model of a curable pediatric malignant solid tumor. Cancer Treat Rev 1978;5:143–172.
162. Bond JV, Martin EC. Pulmonary metastases in Wilms' tumor. Clin Radiol 1976;27:191–195.
163. Wilimas JA, Douglass EC, Hammond E. Relapsed Wilms' tumor factors affecting survival and cure. Am J Clin Med 1985;8:324–328.
164. Green DM, Breslow NE, Yoichi L, et al. The role of surgical excision in the management of relapsed Wilms' tumor patients with pulmonary metastases: a report from the National Wilms' Tumor Study. J Pediatr Surg 1991;26:728–733.
165. Lent MH, Staubitz WJ, Magoss IV, Ross CA. Surgical treatment of pulmonary metastases from malignancies of the genitourinary organs. J Urol 1960;84:746–752.
166. Albers DA, Bell AH, Kalmon EH, Nicholson BH. Pulmonary excision for solitary metastasis from a Wilms' tumor with apparent cure. J Urol 1961;86:43–45.
167. Soper RT. Management of recurrent or metastatic Wilms' tumor. Surgery 1961;50:555–559.
168. White JG, Krivit W. Surgical excision of pulmonary metastases. Pediatrics 1962;29:927–932.

Section IX

Special Topics

Endoscopic Techniques

45A

BRONCHOSCOPIC LASER RESECTION IN PATIENTS WITH THORACIC NEOPLASIA

Henri G. Colt

Bronchoscopic laser resection occupies an important place in the treatment of patients with thoracic neoplasia. Used alone or in association with other therapeutic modalities, laser photoablation of intraluminal tumors in patients with severe main airway obstruction provides symptomatic improvement, may restore ventilatory function, and probably improves quality of life. In both Europe and the United States, several reports of large series of patients with central tracheobronchial obstruction treated by laser photoablation have been published, and successful palliation of airway disease has been accomplished with little morbidity (1–7). Since the introduction and increased use of tracheobronchial stents, the therapeutic capacities of interventional bronchoscopists have been expanded even further. This chapter reviews recent advances in laser technology pertaining to bronchoscopic resection (photodynamic therapy is discussed in Chapter 46). It also presents basic principles of laser-tissue interaction and describes the procedures and instruments used in palliative laser resection for intraluminal neoplastic invasion of the tracheobronchial tree.

BACKGROUND

The concept of bronchoscopic resection of intraluminal neoplasm is not new (8). Indeed, rigid bronchoscopes have been used for many years to core out neoplastic tissues obstructing the airways, obtain adequate endobronchial or transbronchial biopsy specimens, and stop bleeding in patients with life-threatening hemoptysis (9, 10). Historically, the care of patients with airways diseases has been shared successfully by thoracic surgeons, chest physicians, and otolaryngologists. Since the advent of the flexible fiberoptic bronchoscope in the 1970s, however, diagnostic bronchoscopy, and eventually, therapeutic rigid bronchoscopy became forgotten arts. Indeed, in the past, one of the major dangers of rigid bronchoscopic manipulation of airway tumors was potential hemorrhage that could not be controlled other than by emergency thoracotomy. Most interventional bronchoscopists found the endobronchial effects of other endoscopic techniques, such as electrocauterization, unpredictable (11–13); cryosurgery, although inexpensive, often is cumbersome (14–16). In the late 1970s, however, potential endoscopic applications of laser technology made endoscopic laser resection a reality for thoracic endoscopists (17). Within a few years, it became evident that lasers could be used to assure hemostasis as well as tissue vaporization, and that precise resection of benign or neoplastic tissue could be achieved with minimal permanent damage to underlying laryngeal, tracheal, or bronchial mucosa.

Because technological advances have made many laser procedures possible via flexible quartz optic fibers (18), many bronchoscopic interventions today are performed with both rigid and flexible bronchoscopes. The relatively recent comeback of therapeutic rigid bronchoscopy during the past decade relates to several factors: improved telescope optics resulting in improved visualization, new video technology, refinements in rigid instrumentation, and a growing recognition of the usefulness of therapeutic bronchoscopy in managing patients with malignant or benign obstructive lesions of the tracheobronchial tree.

Much of the credit for pioneering endoscopic laser resection work should be given to Strong and Jako (19), who in 1972 described carbon dioxide (CO_2) laser applications in otolaryngology. Reports of vocal cord applications and resections of pharyngeal papillomatosis were followed rapidly by reports of successful CO_2 laser surgery in the tracheobronchial tree (20–23). A major disadvantage of the CO_2 laser, however, is that the laser energy could not be transmitted through a flexible fiberoptic delivery system.

Because of this limitation, other laser systems were studied. Today, although several laser wavelengths are used successfully in the tracheobronchial tree, the neodymium:yttrium-aluminum-garnet (Nd:YAG) laser occupies the most important place in the laser armamentarium of the thoracic endoscopist (24).

Successful Nd:YAG laser resection of endobronchial tumors was first reported by French investigators (6, 25). The Nd:YAG laser is still the most popular laser system used for bronchoscopic surgery. Energy transmission is possible through flexible quartz monofilament fibers, but, because of the invisibility of its beam, this laser requires an aiming beam when used in the noncontact mode. This aiming beam is usually red, provided by a low-power helium-neon laser. Nd:YAG laser energy also can be delivered in a contact mode, although this technique is seldom used in endobronchial resection. Indeed, free beam laser administration usually is preferred to contact mode delivery during endoscopic laser resection because alteration of tissue effects is possible by changing the power density (spot size).

In general, the laser emission is controlled using a foot pedal. Depending on the laser unit, laser energy can be delivered in a continuous, discontinuous, pulsed, or superpulsed mode. For safety reasons, most lasers today have timers that limit tissue exposure to laser radiation. Although most commercial Nd:YAG laser units are capable of high power and continuous administration lasting many seconds, bronchoscopic applications of laser energy do not require power greater than 40 watts (W). Exposure duration usually varies from 0.5 to 1 second, depending on operator preferences and experience. Dual- or multiple-wavelength laser systems are increasingly available, although these systems are very expensive. Depending on the tissue effect desired, operators can elect, by turning a switch, to move between potassium–titanyl–phosphate (KTP) and Nd:YAG laser delivery, for example, or between the 1032-nanometer (nm) and 1064-nm wavelengths of the Nd:YAG laser (17, 26).

LASERS IN THERAPEUTIC BRONCHOSCOPY

The term "laser" is an acronym for light amplification by stimulated emission of radiation. Three laser systems are used principally for bronchoscopic tissue resection in thoracic neoplasia (Table 45A.1). The CO_2 system has a wavelength of 10,600 nm and delivers laser energy in the invisible, far infrared region. Light is converted immediately to thermal energy, raising tissue temperatures to more than 100°C, which causes

TABLE 45A.1. Principal Laser Wavelengths Used for Bronchoscopic Resection

LASER	WAVELENGTH	CHARACTERISTICS
Argon and potassium–titanyl phosphate	488–532 nm	Green light poorly absorbed by tissues. Excellent for rapid ablation of darkly pigmented lesions. Delivery through flexible quartz fibers possible
Carbon dioxide	10600 nm	Invisible, far infrared, precise optical scalpel but poor coagulation. Delivery through flexible quartz fibers not possible
Neodymium:yttrium–aluminum garnet	1064 and 1320 nm	Invisible, weakly absorbed by lightly pigmented tissues, strongly absorbed by darkly pigmented tissues. Delivery through flexible quartz fibers possible

vaporization of the water content of the target tissue. This laser has been used successfully for resection of tracheal papillomatosis and for removal of granulation tissue from the larynx and trachea; it also is used in patients with idiopathic or postintubation subglottic tracheal stenosis (27, 28). The CO_2 laser system does have two important drawbacks that impede more extensive bronchoscopic applications in the lower airways (29). The first is its biophysical properties. Although ideal for precise mucosal vaporization, the CO_2 laser has limited hemostasis capability. Its depth of penetration is less than 1 mm, making it an excellent scalpel but an extremely ineffective coagulator. The second drawback is its mode of transmission. Laser energy cannot be delivered through flexible quartz monofilament optic fibers. Instead, a rigid endoscopic system made up of articulated mirror-to-lens components must be employed (30). Despite some advances in the search for a flexible fiberoptic delivery system, problems related to delivery and wavelength make the CO_2 laser unsuitable for bronchoscopic ablation of potentially hemorrhagic neoplasms obstructing the tracheobronchial tree.

The argon laser delivers a visible, blue-green light with a wavelength of approximately 514 nm. Energy can be delivered through flexible quartz fibers, facilitating endoscopic administration. Because this wavelength is absorbed strongly by hemoglobin, it has been used widely in ophthalmology and dermatology, primarily for photocoagulation of capillaries and other small blood vessels. Its unpredictable effects on soft tissues, as well as a known propensity for tissue necrosis and delayed healing, however, limits the argon laser's role in bronchoscopic tissue ablation. Another wavelength is promising, however. The potassium-titanyl–phosphate laser, with its wavelength of 532 nm, produces a green light similar to that of the argon laser. Laser light is generated through a potassium-titanyl–phosphate crystal, providing a wavelength with a tissue action similar to that of the argon laser. Transmission is possible via flexible quartz fibers, and absorption is dependent on tissue pigmentation; selective absorption is increased in red tissues, such as the surface of an intraluminal tumor. The overall tissue effects of the blue-green lasers, for which absorption is dominated by tissue pigmentation, are somewhat different from those of infrared lasers, whose absorption is based on water content. Superficial coagulation is facilitated, and because high power densities also are reached, tissue vaporization is accelerated, leading to more rapid resection compared with other lasers.

The most frequently used laser in endoscopic resections of tracheal or bronchial neoplasms is the Nd:YAG laser. This system has a wavelength of 1064 nm and delivers radiation in the invisible, near-infrared region. The Nd:YAG laser is excellent for deep coagulation of bulky tissue because scattering of laser radiation exceeds absorption, especially in lightly pigmented tissues. This wavelength is readily absorbed by hemoglobin as well as water, and laser energy penetrates several millimeters into target tissue. Hemostasis is achieved by direct photocoagulation of blood vessels during laser therapy and because vaporization of water contained in tissues surrounding blood vessels ultimately results in vascular constriction. At a high power density, tissue vaporization also is accomplished. Thus, the thermal energy delivered by the Nd:YAG laser system provides superficial and deep hemostasis, tissue necrosis, and vaporization.

LASER-TISSUE INTERACTIONS

A brief review of basic photothermal properties of lasers used during therapeutic bronchoscopy is necessary to the understanding of the tissue effects of a laser system (31). In general, these properties depend on the absorption of laser light by the tissues and on delivery parameters (e.g., pulse energy). It is noteworthy that absorption, as well as the penetration depth of the laser beam, depends on wavelength, tissue type, and power density (32). The laser wavelength determines the degree of scattering and tissue penetration of the laser beam, as well as the amount of energy absorbed. Tissue absorption coefficients are important parameters for determining energy thresholds. Staining tissue with a strong absorbing dye can change absorption coefficients. Dark pigmentation, such as that caused by tissue charring on the surface of an endobronchial tumor, for example, causes immediate absorption of Nd:YAG laser energy, resulting in vaporization. In a transparent medium, in contrast, the absorption coefficient of the Nd:YAG laser is low, and tissue accumulation of thermal energy leads to deep coagulation.

As coagulation proceeds, breakdown of soft tissue occurs, and the surface of the tissue becomes pigmented with carbon. Further application of laser energy on the pigmented surface results in vaporization because the laser beam is absorbed strongly at the tissue's surface. As energy is delivered, however, thermal denaturation occurs, and connective tissue shrinks. This thermal denaturation is responsible for constriction of blood vessels and results in necrosis. These tissue effects may occur up to 10 mm deep within the tissue targeted. The therapeutic bronchoscopist actually uses these properties of the Nd:YAG laser to facilitate tissue ablation by first coagulating, then vaporizing, intraluminal tumor. There is significant danger, however, in persistently applying laser energy, especially to tissues that are not pigmented, such as a pale, somewhat necrotic squamous cell carcinoma obstructing a main bronchus. As the laser beam penetrates through pale tissue, it may be absorbed by darker tissue, such as blood vessels lying deep within the tissue mass, thus facilitating vascular perforation.

One must be wary, therefore, of the potential deep tissue effects of Nd:YAG laser energy delivery. When a laser beam strikes, some of the radiant energy is reflected and some penetrates the target tissue. The power density of the laser beam is defined as the amount of radiant energy that is actually applied per square centimeter of tissue (33). The power density may vary with the actual distance of the laser fiber from the target. As the laser fiber approaches the tissue surface, power density at the surface increases, and the power density just outside the tissue surface is greater than that just below the tissue surface. As the radiant energy penetrates into the tissue, energy is absorbed and converted into heat. Thus, much of the effect of laser energy being delivered actually is taking place below the tissue surface in an area not visible to the bronchoscopist. In addition, as radiant energy is converted into heat below the tissue surface, a phenomenon known as Mie scattering occurs, gradually displacing the point of maximum power density deeper into the tissue. In this region of high thermal energy conversion, steam must be released. Persistent laser firing can result in an explosion, also known as the popcorn effect. Such an accident during bronchoscopic resection can be disastrous. For all of these reasons, the Nd:YAG laser is known tenderly as a "what you can't see will hurt you" laser system.

DIAGNOSIS OF OBSTRUCTIVE AIRWAY NEOPLASMS

Patients with advanced thoracic neoplasia often present with symptoms of airway obstruction, including dyspnea, cough, hypoxemia, and hemoptysis. In fact, bronchogenic carcinoma of the large airways may result in atelectasis or postobstructive pneumonia in up to 30% of cases (34). Recurrent and metastatic neoplasms also may present as intraluminal tumors or cause substantial extrinsic compression of the tracheobronchial tree. Unfortunately, chest radiographs and computed tomography scans do not always demonstrate airway obstruction when it is present (35, 36). Pulmonary function testing, flow-volume loops, and determination of airway resistance also may be disappointingly insensitive, even in the presence of large airway narrowing (37, 38). The most cost effective and potentially the most beneficial examination in patients suspected of airway compromise by neoplastic obstruction is flexible fiberoptic bronchoscopy. Diagnosis may be established by biopsies, brushings and washings, evaluation of the extent of intraluminal obstruction and extrinsic compression, and analysis of aspirated secretions. In addition, a source of hemoptysis may be discovered.

Bronchoscopic evaluation of a patient with a suspected or known tracheobronchial neoplasm should be done in a very systematic fashion. Many patients will have already undergone radiation therapy or chemotherapy. In these individuals it sometimes is difficult to differentiate bronchial mucosal changes secondary to the effects of treatment from those caused by tumor invasion. The anatomic location of the tumor should be described carefully. The distance from the carina and the involvement of large airway and/or smaller lobar and segmental bronchi should be noted. The extent of lymphangitic spread and submucosal infiltration must be estimated, as should the extent of airway compression caused by an extrinsic mass or adenopathy. Tumors with substantial intraluminal tracheal or main stem bronchial extension are best suited for laser resection. Segmental and smaller lobar obstructions should be noted because patients with these problems may benefit from brachytherapy or narrow external beam radiation therapy. Again, the extent of lymphangitic spread and mucosal invasion should be noted, as should any hemorrhage or necrosis. Care should be taken to avoid provoking bleeding, because bleeding can result in complete obstruction of an already compromised airway. The contralateral airway also should be inspected carefully in the search for endobronchial metastases or extrinsic compression, even in areas distant from the original tumor site. Indeed, skip lesions are seen occasionally and may affect laser resection strategies and subsequent therapy. When tracheal or bronchial stenosis is present, either because of intraluminal tumor bulk or extrinsic compression, the examination must be performed in an atraumatic manner. In case of bronchial obstruction, passage of the fiberoptic bronchoscope beyond the stricture should be done cautiously to avoid causing mucosal edema that will further decrease the caliber of the airway lumen. In case of severe tracheal stenosis, and especially when a high-lying, subglottic tracheal stricture is present, the bronchoscope probably should not be moved beyond the stenotic area unless there is ready access to rigid bronchoscopy. Patients with severe subglottic narrowing and tracheal strictures of 6 mm or less should be referred to an experienced endoscopist equipped to manage complications such as mucosal swelling and edema, bronchospasm, laryngospasm, or acute obstruction of the stenotic area by hemorrhage or necrotic tissue.

INDICATIONS FOR LASER RESECTION

Laser resection is most beneficial when advanced or recurrent thoracic neoplasms cause intraluminal obstruction of the trachea or the left or right main bronchus (Fig. 45A.1). Used alone or in conjunction with other palliative treatment modalities, such as external beam radiation therapy, brachytherapy, chemotherapy, stenting, or photodynamic therapy, laser resection helps relieve symptoms of airway obstruction such as dyspnea, intractable cough, and hemoptysis (39–42). Laser debulking also facilitates expectoration of thick secretions and helps prevent postobstruction atelectasis or pneumonia (Table 45A.2).

Single or multiple areas of tracheobronchial obstruction may be treated successfully (43, 44). Criteria for selecting patients for laser therapy are still evolving, however (45, 46). Classically, a bronchial lumen should be visible, and the overall length of the tumor should not exceed 4 cm. Functioning lung parenchyma should be present distal to the obstruction, but even complete obstruction of a main bronchus also may be

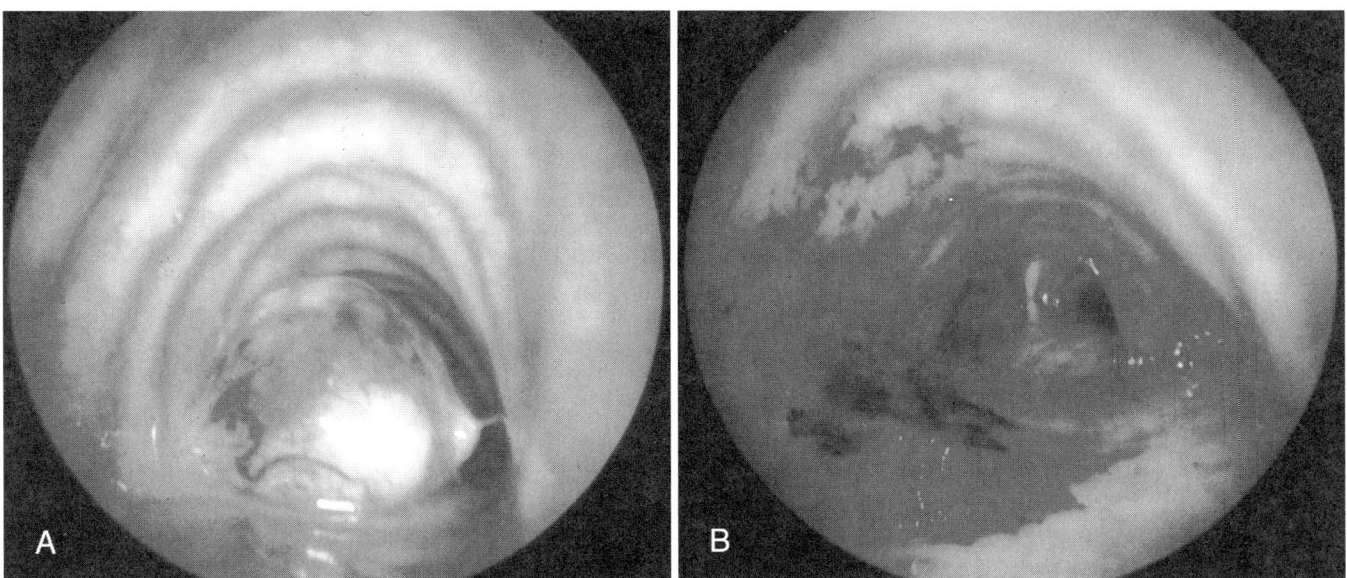

FIGURE 45A.1. A. Major intraluminal tracheal obstruction by squamous cell carcinoma. B. Trachea after laser resection of intraluminal mass.

TABLE 45A.2. Benefits of Nd: YAG Laser Debulking of Central Airway Obstruction

Restores ventilation for improvement of hypoxemia and dyspnea
Improves drainage and prevents postobstructive pneumonia
Assures hemostasis
Relieves intractable cough secondary to intraluminal lesions
Facilitates placement of brachytherapy catheters in segmental bronchi

TABLE 45A.3. Optimal Tumor Characteristics for Laser Debulking

Optimal
  Tracheal or main steam bronchial lesion
  Exophytic, intralumenal obstruction only
  Axial length less than 4 cm
  Bronchial lumen fully visible
  Functional distal airway visible

Less optimal
  Axial length greater than 4 cm involving trachea and main stem bronchi
  Segmental obstruction also present
  Total obstruction without visible distal airway
  Substantial extrinsic compression present

Least optimal
  Little or no exophytic lesion
  Malacia or complex extrinsic compression with some exophytic tumor present
  Wide-based, necrotic lesion with invasion of cartilage
  Wide-based necrotic lesion with suspicion of tracheoesophageal fistula

alleviated by laser resection and dilation. Often, what appears to be a completely obstructed main bronchus actually is an intraluminal extension of a tumor mass surrounded by necrotic tissue, the removal of which results in a patent airway. It is important, however, to evaluate the extent of extrinsic compression carefully in these settings. Extrinsic compression and complete intraluminal obstruction increase the risk of perforation. Because laser resection is often used as a last resort, many experienced bronchoscopists believe that there are few if any contraindications to attempting this procedure, and that therapeutic bronchoscopy should be offered to any patient with evidence of severe main airway obstruction (Table 45A.3).

Indeed, laser resection is a mode of palliative, not curative, therapy and usually is not indicated until other conventional modalities have failed (44, 47, 48). Immediate debulking or stenting should be considered, however, in symptomatic patients with severe malignant airway obstruction and in selected patients with high-grade airway obstructions before referral for external beam radiation or chemotherapy, if warranted by the patient's clinical status. One of the greatest benefits of therapeutic bronchoscopy in these instances is that of immediate symptomatic improvement once a patent airway is restored (41, 43).

Tumors of all tissue types may be treated successfully by laser resection. These include primary bronchogenic carcinomas with spread to the tracheobronchial tree; metastatic lesions to the airways, especially from breast cancer, renal cell carcinoma, and colon carcinoma; and tracheal lesions caused by contiguous spread from thyroid, esophageal, or head and neck malignancies (45, 49–51). Small cell carcinomas are less likely than non–small cell bronchogenic neoplasms to present as intraluminal masses, although symptomatic patients with severe extrinsic compression from mucosal infiltration may benefit from stenting before chemotherapy. Patients with primary esophageal carcinoma may benefit from laser resection because these cancers often cause airway obstruction by direct tracheobronchial invasion. Esophageal stent insertion also can result in tracheal or left main bronchial obstruction (52). In these cases airway stenting prevents extrinsic compression and results in resolution of pulmonary symptoms.

INSTRUMENTATION AND RESECTION TECHNIQUES

When Nd:YAG laser resection of malignant tracheobronchial tumors was introduced by the French teams of Toty et al. (53) and Dumon et al. (6) more than 15 years ago, the rigid bronchoscope was almost always used. Since then, there also have been a few proponents of the flexible bronchoscope (42, 54–57). Bronchoscope selection depends on multiple factors, including the availability of general or local anesthesia, lesion location, and most importantly, technical expertise and experience of the bronchoscopist (58, 59). There are many reasons, however, for preferring the rigid bronchoscope for laser resection (60). Intubation with the rigid tube assures maintenance of a clear airway. Tumor ablation is performed under general anesthesia while simultaneous suction of smoke is achieved using suction catheters. Large forceps are used to remove tissue debris, and the tip of the rigid tube may be used to shear off tumor from the airway wall. Procedures are performed quickly, and most tumors are resected during a single intervention. The rigid bronchoscope can be used to dilate an airway stricture, or in case of bleeding and hypoxemia, the rigid tube can be passed beyond the area of obstruction to improve ventilation through the distal airways. Selective intubation with the rigid tube can be performed safely to prevent filling of the contralateral airway with blood; also, once the rigid bronchoscope is distal to the tumor, patients can be oxygenated through a closed system by packing the nose and mouth and blocking the side ports of the bronchoscope. This procedure ensures ventilation regardless of endobronchial pathology. Bleeding is controlled readily by saline lavage, local administration of epinephrine, tamponade of the bleeding area with the rigid bronchoscope, and laser photocoagulation. Another advantage of the rigid tube is that concomitant therapeutic procedures, such as stent insertion or balloon dilation, can be performed at the same sitting.

In selected instances laser resection can be performed safely through the flexible fiberoptic bronchoscope (41, 61, 62). One reason for advocating its use is facile performance under local anesthesia, thereby sparing patients the cost and potential dangers of general anesthesia. Also, many practitioners today are more adept at flexible fiberoptic bronchoscopy than at rigid bronchoscopy. Another advantage of the flexible bronchoscope is that it can be oriented into smaller bronchi, should there be an indication for laser debulking within an upper lobe or lower lobe segmental bronchus (63). Although large-channel bronchoscopes and a wide range of biopsy forceps, graspers, foreign body removal forceps, and snares may be used with success (64), the many potential problems associated with flexible fiberoptic bronchoscopic laser resection probably outweigh its benefits. Multiple sessions are usually necessary for complete tissue ablation. Smoke evacuation is cumbersome because simultaneous laser resection and suctioning is not possible. Most importantly, complications are more difficult to control than through the rigid tube. For example, palpation of endobronchial lesions is difficult, and without the tactile feedback provided by a rigid suction catheter or by the tip of the rigid bronchoscope, it is difficult for the operator to know when to cease laser firing.

In an attempt to improve patient comfort and provide a more controlled environment for laser resection through the flexible bronchoscope, endotracheal intubation and general anesthesia have been advocated (42, 56). Still, hemorrhage may be difficult to control, and because of smoke and tissue debris, frequent soiling of the distal lens may prompt frequent removal of the bronchoscope from the airways. In addition, accidents may occur. Ignition of the endotracheal tube or the fiberoptic bronchoscope itself during laser resection can result in severe airway burns, respiratory failure, and tracheobronchial stenosis (65). For example, an airway fire can occur if the laser fiber, which is inserted through the suction channel of the bronchoscope, does not protrude sufficiently beyond the tip of the flexible fiberoptic bronchoscope.

Most bronchoscopists, therefore, prefer using the rigid tube for laser resection (46). The flexible bronchoscope, is almost always used in conjunction with the rigid tube for visualization of the distal and peripheral airways and for bronchial cleansing, thus proficiency in both techniques is essential. Procedures usually are performed in the operating room under general anesthesia provided with jet ventilation, assisted spontaneous ventilation using an open system, or combinations of inhalation and intravenous anesthesia through a closed system after packing the nose and mouth to prevent air leaks. During laser firing, forced inspiratory oxygen should be reduced to less than 50% to reduce risks of combustion (66). If oxygen saturation decreases during resection, the bronchoscopist should cease resection and allow the anesthesiologist to ventilate and oxygenate the patient. Despite the wide choice of available anesthetic agents and techniques, achieving the proper balance between a nonmoving patient and an adequately ventilated and hemodynamically stable one is not an easy task, thus close collaboration between the bronchoscopist and anesthesiologist is essential. Severe ventilatory compromise, multiple illnesses, and decreased overall health status caused by metastatic carcinoma contribute to the increased anesthesia risk of patients undergoing laser resection.

After intubation with the rigid bronchoscope and administration of additional topical anesthesia to the airways, tracheobronchial inspection is performed. The flexible fiberoptic bronchoscope often is used through the rigid tube for bronchial cleansing, examination of distal lobar and segmental airways, and even laser resection of certain lesions obstructing segmental bronchi. Care is taken to clear both the right and left endobronchial trees of secretions before commencing laser resection. The flexible bronchoscope is then removed, and the laser fiber and suction catheters are passed through the rigid tube into their appropriate positions. Usually, the laser is set at a low power (approximately 30 to 40 W) in a discontinuous mode (0.5- to 1-second exposures). During coagulation, the tumor shrinks and often blanches. Palpation with the suction catheter allows the bronchoscopist to feel the effect of the laser on tumor tissue. Care is taken to avoid laser firing perpendicular to the tracheobronchial wall. Tissue destruction is achieved by charring and vaporization of tumor tissue or by resecting necrotic tumor with biopsy forceps, the tip of the rigid tube, or suction catheters. Careful attention is given to hemostasis throughout the resection.

TRACHEOBRONCHIAL STENTS

In addition to intraluminal obstruction, many patients have significant extrinsic compression of the lower airways. In these patients insertion of tracheobronchial prostheses has proven to be extremely beneficial (67) (Fig. 45A.2). Stent insertion into the trachea, right main bronchus, or left main bronchus often results in lung reexpansion, recovery of ventilatory function, improvement of flow-volume loops and flows on pulmonary function testing, decreased incidence of postobstructive pneumonia, improved quality of life, and, in many instances, prolonged survival. Often, tra-

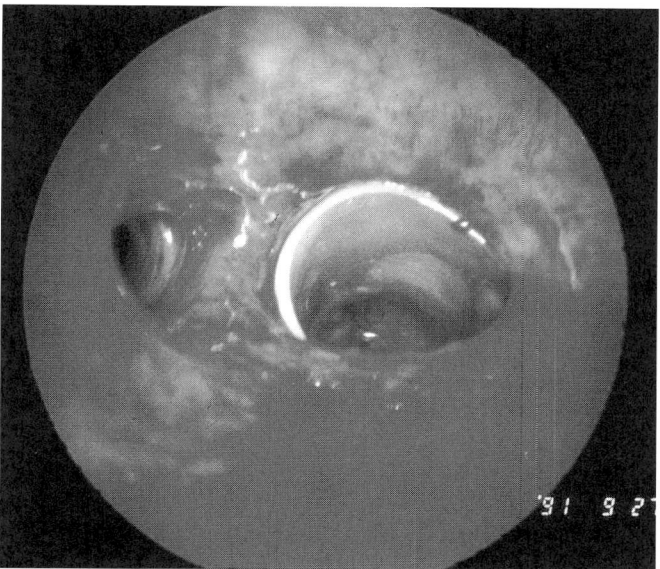

FIGURE 45A.2. Moderate extrinsic compression of the origin of the left main bronchus, widened main carina, and Dumon silicone stent in the right main bronchus of a patient with squamous cell bronchogenic carcinoma.

cheobronchial dilation is performed initially with bougies, balloon inflation devices, or rigid bronchoscopes of increasing caliber (68). Stent insertion has been greatly facilitated by the recent introduction of a specially designed stent introducer system (EFER; La Ciotat, France) that is used through the rigid bronchoscope (69). Stents are loaded into the introducer and expulsed into the area of stricture after gentle dilation is achieved with the rigid tube. Once inserted, silicone stents are manipulated further using rigid alligator grasping forceps to ensure proper placement.

Currently, the Dumon silicone stent (Endoxane; Axion Pourlavie, Aubagne, Franch) is the most frequently used tracheobronchial prosthesis (70). This straight silicone stent comes in various diameters and lengths. Studs on its external surface help prevent migration. Because these stents are not inserted into the stricture under direct visualization, however, stenting requires an advanced level of technical expertise with the rigid bronchoscope. Other silicone stents are available from various manufacturers. These include modified Montgomery T tubes (71), bifurcated Y-shaped or L-shaped stents, silicone stents with proximal and distal flanges, and metal stents coated with silicone (72–80). In selected instances stents may be custom built to adapt to particular airway deformities. This step is needed more frequently in patients with benign airway obstruction than in cancer patients.

Self-expandable, metal stents, often similar to those designed for intravascular use, also can be used

(81–86). Once inserted, however, these stents often are impossible to remove. In addition, granulation tissue may obstruct the airway through the metal mesh, and migration can occur as expansive tumor pushes the metal stent through the bronchial wall or into the mediastinum, causing bronchial or vascular perforation (87). Rousseau et al. (88) showed excellent improvement in respiratory status in 89% of 55 patients after metal stent insertion. Insertion of a Gianturco stent (Cook, Inc., Bloomington, IN) (a self-expanding wire lace stent), however, led to complications, including stent rupture, bronchial wall perforation, obstruction, and migration in 30% of patients.

Adverse events from stenting probably are more frequent than originally supposed, and they often require repeat rigid bronchoscopy for stent replacement or laser resection of granulation tissue or tumor. On occasion, anatomic distortions prevent stent insertion. Stent placement usually is undesirable in the presence of severely necrotic tissue or if pulsating vessels protruding into the bronchial lumen would be in direct contact with the external surface of the stent. Metal stents in these instances are absolutely contraindicated. Particular care must be taken, because of the potential dangers of mediastinal dissection or vascular perforation, when stents are inserted into a distorted left main bronchus. In some cases of subglottic stenosis by extrinsic compression secondary to neoplasm, a tracheotomy followed by insertion of a Montgomery T tube may actually be preferable to subglottic stent insertion because of the risk of migration (89). When intraluminal disease is present, however, or when tumor directly overlies the trachea, subglottic stents are extremely helpful. Should migration still occur, subglottic stents can be sutured into place and fixed percutaneously (90).

In one of the larger studies published to date (183 silicone stents inserted in 126 patients with malignancies over a 3-year period), Colt and Dumon (69) reported stent migration, obstruction with secretions, or granulation tissue formation at the proximal or distal aspect of the stent in 11 patients (6%). Diaz-Jimenez et al. (91) recently reported a complication rate of 14%. On rare occasions, airway fires have been reported when laser resection is performed in a patient with an indwelling stent (49). It is noteworthy that brachytherapy or external beam radiation therapy do not affect silicone stents. Shrinking of the tumor, however, may result in decreased extrinsic compression, thus facilitating stent migration. In these patients stents can usually be removed safely and patients monitored for tumor recurrence.

After stent insertion, routine follow-up flexible fiberoptic bronchoscopic examinations are desirable to prevent or determine the onset of complications. Certainly, any stented patient with sputum production or the new onset of cough, or dyspnea should be suspected of having a stent-related complication and be referred for fiberoptic bronchoscopy. Thick secretions can usually be removed through the flexible bronchoscope after local anesthesia. Should stent migration or severe obstruction occur, however, repeat rigid bronchoscopy may be necessary for stent removal or replacement. Silicone stents are easily removable and thus are preferable to metal stents. Although randomized controlled studies of stenting versus other palliative therapeutic modalities in patients with neoplastic invasion of the airways are lacking, stents have assumed an increasing role in patients with malignant large airway obstruction (Fig. 45A.3). Whether stenting actually reduces the need for repeated laser debulking and objectively improves ventilatory function or quality of life requires further study.

COMPLICATIONS

Complications of laser resection usually result from technique, tumor extension, and anesthesia (92, 93). Endoscopic laser resection is technically challenging because the interventional bronchoscopist must deal with surface bleeding, abundant secretions, extensive lesions, and absence of landmarks to locate the bronchial wall. The most serious complications of laser resection are hypoxemia; bronchial, esophageal, or vascular perforation; and bleeding (94). Intraoperative mortality is rare, but hemorrhage may occur at any moment during tumor resection. In case of large vessel perforation, it is extremely unlikely that emergency thoracotomy could be performed in time to prevent death. Incomplete tumor resection thus is safer than complete ablation, but rapid regrowth may necessitate frequent repeat procedures. This repetition is not always desirable because it increases hospital stays in an already debilitated patient and incurs greater health care costs. Stenting and other complementary palliative therapies probably decrease the need for repeat procedures once a patent large airway has been secured.

Many routine safety precautions are necessary during laser resection. These include the wearing of protective goggles by all personnel in the operating room as well as taping the patient's eyes shut, and then covering them with saline-soaked pads and aluminum foil. If possible, any flammable materials should be

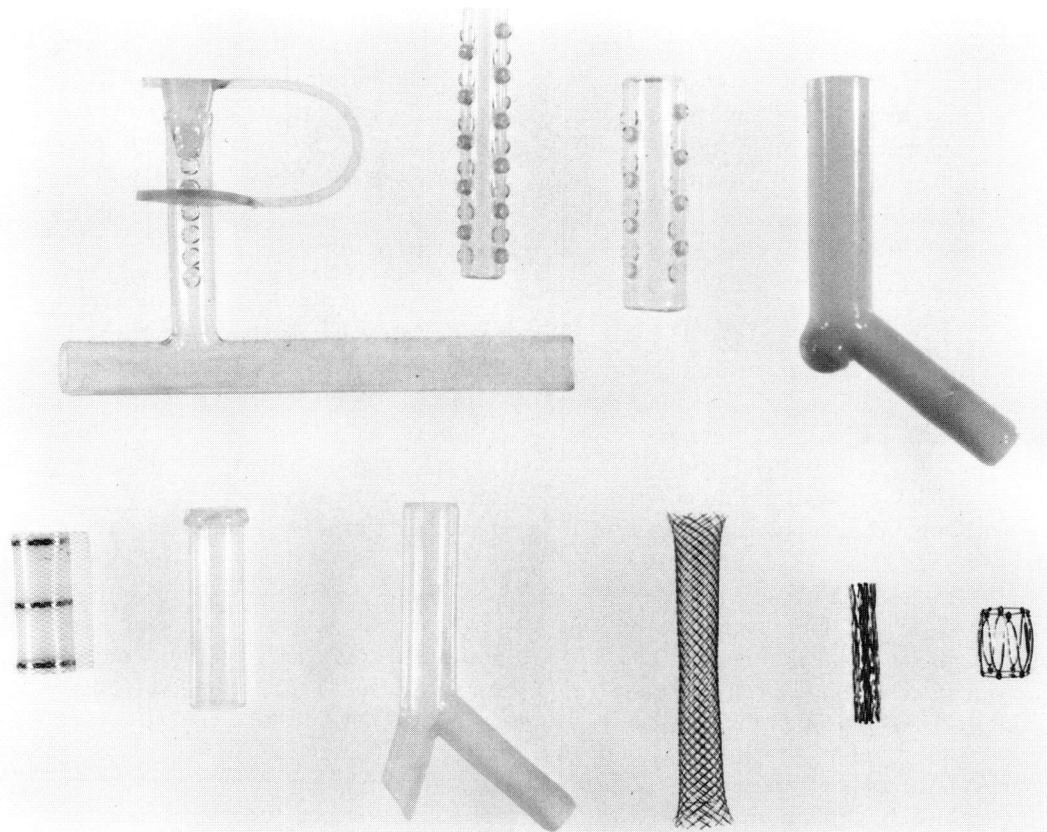

FIGURE 45A.3. Various tracheobronchial prostheses. *(Top)* Montgomery T tube, Dumon silicone bronchial stent with studs on external surface, Dumon tracheal stent, and custom-made trachea–left main bronchus stent for patient with right pneumonectomy stump. *(Bottom)* Novadis expandable silicone and metal bronchial stent (Novadis, Saint Victoret, France); Hood silicone stent with proximal flange (Hood Laboratories, Pembroke, MA); Y-stent; Schneider expandable metal stent (Wallstent) (Medinvent SA, Lausanne, Switzerland); Palmaz metal stent (Johnson & Johnson, Warren, NJ), and Gianturco metal stent (Cook, Inc., Bloomington, IN).

kept away from the operating field. If the rigid bronchoscope is preferable to the flexible bronchoscope because it is not combustible, it must be remembered also that accessories such as suction catheters *are* combustible. Endobronchial ignition of combustible materials, such as endotracheal tubes, stents, or flexible bronchoscopes, may be disastrous, resulting in airway necrosis, mucous plugging, and stenosis (95, 96). Fires must be prevented by using the lowest possible inhaled oxygen concentration during laser resection. Indeed, because of the high reflectance of the tracheal wall at the Nd:YAG laser wavelength, stray radiation can be substantial, and it could be absorbed by the dark fiberoptic bronchoscope or lettering of an endotracheal tube. Ignition is likely in an oxygen rich atmosphere. If a fire should occur, immediate removal of the combustible material is essential to minimize thermal damage and prevent smoke inhalation. Immediate lavage and suctioning is then necessary. All necrotic mucosa should be removed immediately and a careful examination made to assess the extent of injury. Frequent bronchoscopic lavage is necessary, and, occasionally, tracheotomy is indicated. Antibiotics and corticosteroids can be administered, and mechanical ventilatory support often is desirable because airway swelling or necrosis may not become evident until several hours after the accident.

Safe laser resection also requires a comfortable sharing of the airway with the anesthesiologist (97–100). In general, ideal anesthesia for laser resection should provide rapid induction, minimal hemodynamic instability, facile ventilation and oxygenation, adequate laryngeal and maxillary relaxation, and comfortable arousal (101). Prolonged hypoxemia should be avoided (102–104). When inhalation anesthesia is used, one must remember that nitrous oxide supports combustion almost as well as oxygen. If an endotracheal tube is used, it should be wrapped with metallic tape to minimize the risk of ignition (105, 106). A metal endotracheal tube is even safer (107, 108). Postoperative respiratory depression may be caused by muscle relaxants used in patients requiring conventional assisted ventilation (109). Pneumothoraces have been described and may be related to anesthesia technique, air trapping, and use of jet ventilation (98, 110, 111). Intravenous anesthesia with agents such as propofol (Diprivan; Zeneca Pharmaceutical, Wilmington, DE) may result in hemodynamic instability (112).

OUTCOME

In most large series, squamous cell carcinoma is the most frequent form of endobronchial malignancy requiring laser debulking. Patients with small cell carcinoma are less frequently referred for laser resection because these submucosal, infiltrating tumors are quite chemosensitive, although they may cause significant extrinsic compression. In these cases stenting is usually possible if life-threatening airway obstruction is detected before chemotherapy. Esophageal and thyroid carcinomas may obstruct central airways by direct tumor extension, mediastinal node enlargement, or extrinsic tumor compression. Lymphomas can behave in a similar fashion. Endobronchial specimens should always be sent for microbiologic analysis to diagnose concomitant opportunistic infections, such as aspergillosis, herpes, and actinomycosis, in immunocompromised patients.

Endobronchial metastases, especially in patients with renal cell, colon, or breast carcinoma, are also resected with excellent results (113, 114). Because patients with endobronchial metastases have symptoms similar to those of patients with bronchogenic carcinoma and airway obstruction, however, differential diagnosis is difficult on the basis of clinical presentation alone (51, 115–117). Endobronchial lesions resulting from distant primary tumors usually are well localized and submucosal. Although some studies have suggested prolonged survival after diagnosis and resection of endobronchial metastases, others have shown a mean survival of only 12 months despite therapy (116). Most interventional bronchoscopists agree, however, that palliation of airway obstruction is indicated regardless of the presence or absence of metastases to other organs.

Low-grade malignant tumors of the endobronchial tree, including typical and atypical carcinoid tumors, may be resected if patients are poor surgical candidates or refuse thoracotomy. These well-rounded, relatively smooth tumors often cause partial or complete obstruction of a central or peripheral airway with resultant atelectasis or postobstructive pneumonia (118, 119). Carcinoid tumors usually are highly vascularized and tend to bleed (120). Often, patients with low-grade carcinoids have been treated previously for asthmatic conditions before the diagnosis of tumor (121, 122). Some lesions are purely intraluminal; others may extend outside the bronchial wall. When a carcinoid tumor is suspected, computed tomographic scanning or magnetic resonance imaging is suggested to evaluate the extent of extrabronchial spread. Laser resection must be carried out carefully and often; the base of the carcinoid tumor must be dug out of the bronchial wall (4). Although standard therapy for these tumors is open thoracic surgery, preliminary endoscopic resection may be useful in selected cases. Using endoscopy, lung parenchymal-sparing procedures are optimized, the exact location of the base of the tumor may be determined, and clean resection margins are achieved more easily. Many patients undergoing preoperative laser resection safely undergo bronchoplastic procedures with good long-term results (123, 124). If patients are not surgical candidates or refuse thoracic surgery, laser resection may be curative, but follow-up bronchoscopy must be performed at regular intervals to detect recurrence (125).

Although laser resection often improves symptoms, ventilatory function, and radiographic appearance, the effect on patient survival has not been well documented (126–129). In part, this lack of documentation results from the ethical dilemma of conducting prospective randomized studies in terminally ill patients who have compromised airways. Study design is difficult because survival is affected by tumor response to radiation or chemotherapy. Survival may also depend on whether patients are referred for laser resection early or late in the course of their disease. Successful laser resection and stenting are dependent on the extent of disease, the importance of underlying neoplasms and extent of extrinsic compression, the duration of illness, the residual lung function, and the technical expertise and experience of the bronchoscopist. Although survival characteristics after laser resection are difficult to analyze, it appears that unsuccessful restoration of a patent airway is a grave prognostic indicator (130). Severe extrinsic compression, involvement of multiple segmental bronchi, and extensive submucosal tumor invasion may also be poor prognostic signs (131). In one recent study of patients with malignant airway obstruction requiring mechanical ventilation and treated with laser bronchoscopy, patients with simple intraluminal obstruction were weaned more rapidly from mechanical ventilation and survived longer than patients with combined extrinsic compression and endobronchial lesions (132). These investigators therefore suggested that patients with nonresectable bronchogenic carcinoma and respiratory failure requiring mechanical ventilation undergo bronchoscopy and, if indicated, be referred for laser resection or stenting.

Investigators also have examined the role of laser resection in conjunction with other palliative therapies. For example, if laser debulking precedes or accompanies brachytherapy, symptom free survival may be longer than after laser resection alone (133–136). In case of main stem or segmental bronchial obstruction, placement of brachytherapy catheters is facilitated, but it is unclear whether laser therapy has a favorable effect on response to brachytherapy (137, 138). Complications of combined therapy probably occur in at least 10% of patients, but it is difficult to differentiate patients developing therapy-related complications from those in whom hemoptysis or fistula occur as part of the natural progression of their disease (139, 140). Concomitant brachytherapy should probably be avoided if there is evidence of substantial bronchial wall destruction or if the bronchial mucosa is extremely necrotic. Patients with indwelling stents should be bronchoscoped after complementary brachytherapy or external beam irradiation, because stent migration may occur as a result of tumor shrinkage and loss of the structural support maintaining the stent in place.

Many patients with inoperable thoracic neoplasia referred for laser resection have concomitant illnesses that effect their quality of life. Despite laser debulking, for example, ventilatory impairment may persist because of chronic obstructive lung disease (141). In some patients the improvement in pulmonary function suggested by increased forced vital capacity, forced expiratory volume in 1 second, peak expiratory flow, isovolume maximal flows at 50% of expiratory volume, and decreased airway resistance after laser resection has been observed (37). Why some patients report symptomatic relief without objective evidence of physiologic improvement on pulmonary function testing is unclear (142). Spirometry or flow-volume loops are not as reliable as follow-up bronchoscopy for monitoring changes in airway caliber after debulking of tracheal or bronchial lesions (38).

CONCLUSION

In summary, laser resection is beneficial in patients with intraluminal obstruction caused by tracheobronchial invasion by primary, recurrent, or metastatic malignant carcinoma, especially if patients do not qualify for open surgical resection, have refused surgery, or have tumor recurrence despite other therapies. Patients with major airway compromise from extrinsic compression may benefit from tracheobronchial prosthesis insertion. Once a patent airway has been restored by laser debulking or stenting, patients can be referred for radiation therapy or chemotherapy safely. Such patients may tolerate these therapies better because many symptoms of large airway obstruction will have been relieved before referral. Above all, however, therapeutic bronchoscopy is complementary to the other therapeutic modalities offered to patients with thoracic neoplasms. Although good anatomic results are often achieved, quality of life and survival probably depend not only on the extent of intraluminal obstruction and extrinsic compression, but also on the degree of tumor impingement on major vessels, response to therapy, comorbidity, metastatic involvement of other organ systems, pulmonary function, and tumor type.

REFERENCES

1. Beamis JF, Rebeiz EE, Vergos KV, Shapshay SM. Endoscopic laser therapy for obstructing tracheobronchial lesions. Ann Otol Rhinol Laryngol 1991;100:413–419.
2. Arabia A, Spagnolo SV. Laser therapy in patients with primary lung cancer. Chest 1984;86:519–523.
3. Livingston DR, Mehta AC, Golish JA, Ahmad M, Deboer G, Tomaszewski MZ. Palliation of malignant tracheobronchial obstruction by Nd:YAG laser: an updated experience at the Cleveland Clinic Foundation. J Am Osteopath Assoc 1987;3:226–234.
4. Cavaliere S, Foccoli P, Farina PL. Nd-YAG laser bronchoscopy: a five year experience with 1396 applications in 1000 patients. Chest 1988;94:15–21
5. Personne C, Colchen A, Leroy M, Vourc'h G, Toty L. Indications and technique for endoscopic laser resections in bronchology: a critical analysis based upon 2284 resections. J Thorac Cardiovasc Surg 1986;91:710–715
6. Dumon JF, Reboud E, Garbe L, Aucomte F, Meric B. Treatment of tracheobronchial lesions by laser photoresection. Chest 1982;81:278–284.
7. Bourcereau J, Gharbi N, Lescot B, Marchal M. YAG laser in bronchial endoscopy. Laser Med Microchirurg 1982;1:35–36.
8. Jackson C. Bronchoscopy and esophagoscopy: a manual of peroral endoscopy and laryngeal surgery. Philadelphia: WB Saunders, 1927.
9. Mathisen DJ, Grillo HC, Endoscopic relief of malignant airway obstruction. Ann Thorac Surg 1989;48:469–473.
10. Wang KP, Britt EJ, Haponik EF, Fishman EK, Siegelman SS, Erozan YS. Rigid transbronchial needle aspiration biopsy for histological specimens. Ann Otol Rhinol Laryngol 1985;94:382–385.
11. Gerasin VA, Shafirovsky BB. Endobronchial electrosurgery. Chest 1988;93:270–274.
12. Hooper RG, Jackson FN. Endobronchial electrocautery. Chest 1985;87:712–714.

13. Hooper RG, Spratling L, Beechler CR, Schaffner S. Endobronchial electrocautery: a role in bronchogenic carcinoma? Endoscopy 1984;16:67–70.
14. Homasson JP, Renault P, Angebault M, Bonniot JP, Bell NJ. Bronchoscopic cryotherapy for airway strictures caused by tumors. Chest 1986;90:159–164.
15. Vergnon JM, Guichenez P, Fournel P, Emonot A. Efficiency of cryotherapy in bronchial tumors. Am Rev Respir Dis 1990;141:402.
16. Walsh DA, Maiwand MO, Nath AR, Lockwood P, Lloyd MH, Saab M. Bronchoscopic cryotherapy for advanced bronchial carcinoma. Thorax 1990;45:509–513.
17. Treat MR, Oz MC, Bass LS. New technologies and future applications of surgical lasers. Surg Clin North Am 1992;72:705–742.
18. Fuller TA. The mid-infrared fiberoptics. Lasers Surg Med 1986;6:399–403.
19. Strong MS, Jako JG. Laser surgery in the larynx: early clinical experience with continuous CO_2 laser. Ann Otol Rhinol Laryngol 1972;81:791–798.
20. Strong MS, Vaughan CW, Polanyi T, Wallace R. Bronchoscopic carbon-dioxide laser surgery. Ann Otol Rhinol Laryngol 1974;83:769–776.
21. Ossof RH, Karlan MS. A set of bronchoscopes for carbon dioxide laser surgery. Otolaryngol Head Neck Surg 1983;91:336–337.
22. McElvein RB, Zorn G. Treatment of malignant disease in trachea and main-stem bronchi by carbon-dioxide laser. J Thorac Cardiovasc Surg 1983;86:858–863.
23. Shapshay SM, Davis RK, Vaughan CW, Norton MS, Strong MS, Simpson GT. Palliation of airway obstruction from tracheobronchial malignancy: use of the CO_2 laser bronchoscope. Otolaryngol Head Neck Surg 1983;91:615–619.
24. Beamis JF, Shapshay S. More about the YAG. Chest 1985;87:27–28.
25. Toty L, Personne CL, Hertzog P, Colchen A, Lotteau J, Romanelli L, et al. Utilisation d'un faisceau laser (YAG) a conducteur souple, pour le traitement endoscopique de certaines lesions tracheobronchiques. Rev Fr Mal Respir 1979;7:475–482.
26. Rebeiz EE, Aretz HT, Shapshay SM, Pankratov MM. Application of pulsed and continuous wave 1.32 and 1.06 μm wavelengths of the Nd:YAG laser in the canine tracheobronchial tree: a comparative study. Lasers Surg Med 1990;10:501–509.
27. McElvein RB, Zorn GL Jr. Indications, results, and complications of bronchoscopic carbon dioxide laser therapy. Ann Surg 1984;199:522–525.
28. Berci G, Analysis of new optical systems in bronchoesophagology. Ann Otol Rhinol Laryngol 1978;87:451–460.
29. Shapshay SM, Beamis JF. Use of the CO_2 laser. Chest 1989;95:449–456.
30. Shapshay SM, Setzer S, Aretz HT. Clinical options in the delivery of the CO_2 laser in the tracheobronchial tree. Society of Photo-Optical Instrumentation Engineers Proceedings 1988;906:205–209.
31. Fisher JC. Basic laser physics and interaction of laser light with soft tissue. In: Shapshay SM, Ed. Endoscopic laser surgery handbook. New York: Marcel Dekker, 1987.
32. Sliney DH. Laser-tissue interactions. Clin Chest Med 1985;6:203–208.
33. Fisher JC. The power density of a surgical laser beam: its meaning and measurement. Lasers Surg Med 1983;2:301–315.
34. Minna JD, Higgins GA, Glatstein EJ. Cancer of the lung. In: DeVita VT, Hellman S, Rosenberg SA, eds. Cancer principles and practice of oncology. 2nd ed. Philadelphia: JB Lippincott, 1985:518.
35. Colice GL, Chappel GJ, Frenchman SM, Solomon DA. Comparison of computerized tomography with fiberoptic bronchoscopy in identifying endobronchial abnormalities in patients with known or suspected lung cancer. Am Rev Respir Dis 1985;131:397–400.
36. Pearlberg JL, Sandler MA, Kvale P, Beaute GH, Madrazo BL. Computed tomographic and conventional linear tomographic evaluation of tracheobronchial lesions for laser photoresection. Radiology 1985;154:759–762.
37. Gelb AF, Tashkin DP, Epstein JD, Fairshter R, Zamel N. Diagnosis and Nd:YAG laser treatment of unsuspected malignant tracheal obstruction. Chest 1988;94:767–771.
38. Gelb AF, Molony PA, Klein E, Aronstram PS. Sensitivity of volume of isoflow in the detection of mild airway obstruction. Am Rev Respir Dis 1975;112:401–405.
39. Dedhia HV, Lapp NL, Jain PR, Thompson AB, Withers A. Endoscopic laser therapy for respiratory distress due to obstructive airway tumors. Crit Care Med 1985;13:464–467.
40. McDougall JC, Cortese DA. Neodymium-YAG laser therapy of malignant airway obstruction: a preliminary report. Mayo Clin Proc 1983;58:35–39.
41. Oho K, Ogawa R, Amemiya T, Ohtani R, Yamada O, Hayata TY. Indications for endoscopic Nd:YAG laser surgery in the trachea and bronchus. Endoscopy 1983;15:302–306.
42. Parr GVS, Unger M, Trout RG, Atkinson WG. One hundred neodymium YAG laser ablations of obstructing tracheal neoplasms. Ann Thorac Surg 1984;38:374–380.
43. Wolfe WG, Sabiston DC. Management of benign and malignant lesions of the trachea and bronchi with the neodymium-yttrium aluminum garnet laser. J Thorac Cardiovasc Surg 1986;91:40–45.
44. Hetzel MR, Nixon C, Edmondstone WM, Mitchell DM, Millard FJC, Nanson EM, Woodcock AA, et al. Laser therapy in 100 tracheobronchial tumors. Thorax 1985;40:341–345.
45. Cortese DA, Edell ES. Role of phototherapy, laser therapy, brachytherapy, and prosthetic stents in the management of lung cancer. Clin Chest Med 1993;1:149–159.
46. Dumon JF, Shapshay S, Bourcereau J, Cavaliere S, Meric B, Garbi N, Beamis J. Principles for safety in application of neodymium:YAG laser in bronchology. Chest 1984;86;163–168
47. Cortese DA. Endobronchial management of lung cancer. Chest 1986;89:234S–236S
48. Unger M. Neodymium:YAG laser therapy for malignant and benign endobronchial obstructions. Clin Chest Med 1985;6:277–290
49. Clarke CP, Ball DL, Sephton R. Follow-up of patients having Nd:YAG laser resection of bronchostenotic lesions. J Bronchol 1994;1:19–22.
50. Personne C, Colchen A, Bonnette P, et al. Laser in bronchology: methods of application. Lung 1990:168;1085–1088.
51. Jariwalla AG, Seaton A, McCormack RJM, Gibbs A, Cambell IA, Davies BH. Intrabronchial metastases from renal carcinoma with recurrent tumor expectoration. Thorax 1981;36:179–182.
52. Colt HG, Meric B, Dumon JF. Double stents for carcinoma of the esophagus invading the tracheobronchial tree. Gastrointest Endosc 1992;38:485–489.
53. Toty L, Personne C, Colchen A, Vourc'h G. Bronchoscopic management of tracheal lesions using the neodymium yttrium aluminum garnet laser. Thorax 1981;36:175–178

54. Chan AL, Tharratt RS, Siefkin AD, Albertson TE, Volz WG, Allen RP. Nd:YAG laser bronchoscopy. Rigid or fiberoptic mode? Chest 1990;98:271–275.
55. Castro DJ, Saxton RE, Ward PH, et al. Flexible Nd:YAG laser palliation of obstructive tracheal metastatic malignancies. Laryngoscope 1990;100:1208–1214.
56. Unger M. Neodymium:YAG laser therapy for malignant and benign endobronchial obstructions. Clin Chest Med 1985;6:277–290.
57. Mehta AC. Laser applications in respiratory care. In: Kacmarek RM, Stoller JK, eds. Current respiratory care. Toronto: BC Decker, 1988:100–106.
58. George PJM, Garrett CPO, Nixon C, Hetzel MR, Nanson EM, Millard FJC. laser treatment for tracheobronchial tumors: local or general anesthesia? Thorax 1987;42:656–660.
59. Prakash UBS, Offord KP, Stubbs SE. Bronchoscopy in North America: the ACCP survey. Chest 1991;100:1668–1675.
60. Dumon JF. Technique of safe laser surgery. Lasers Med Sci 1990;5:171–180.
61. Mehta AC, Golish JA, Ahmad M, Padua NS, O'Donnell J. Palliative treatment of malignant airway obstruction. Cleve Clin Q 1985;52:513–524.
62. deCastro FR, Lopez L, Varel A, Freixinet J. Tracheobronchial stents and fiberoptic bronchoscopy (letter). Chest 1991;99:792.
63. Joyner LR, Maran AG, Yakboski A. Neodymium YAG laser treatment of intrabronchial lesions. Chest 1985;87:418–427.
64. Mehta AC, Livingston DR. Biopsy excision through a fiberoptic bronchoscope in the palliative management of airway obstruction. Chest 1987;91:774–775.
65. Krawtz S, Mehta AC, Weidemann HP, DeBoer G, Schoepf KD, Tomaszewski MZ. Nd:YAG laser induced endobronchial burn: management and long term follow-up. Chest 1989;95:916–918.
66. Brutinel MW, McDougall JC, Cortese DA. Bronchoscopic therapy with neodymium-yttrium-aluminum garnet laser during intravenous anesthesia. Chest 1983;84:518–521.
67. Colt HG, Dumon JF. Airway obstruction in cancer: pros and cons of stents. J Respir Dis 1991;12:741–749.
68. Carlin BW, Harrell JH, Moser KM. The treatment of endobronchial stenosis using balloon catheter dilatation. Chest 1988;93:1148–1151.
69. Colt HG, Dumon JF. Tracheobronchial stents: indications and applications. Lung Cancer 1993;9:301–306.
70. Dumon JF. A dedicated tracheobronchial stent. Chest 1990;97:328–332.
71. Montgomery WW. Silicone tracheal T-tube. Ann Otol Rhinol Laryngol 1974;83:71–75.
72. George PJ, Irving JD, Mantell BS, Rudd RM. Covered expandable metal stent for recurrent tracheal obstruction. Lancet 1990;335:582–584.
73. Cooper JD, Todd TRJ, Ilves R, Pearson FG. Use of the silicone tracheal T-tube for the management of complex tracheal injuries. J Thorac Cardiovasc Surg 1981;82:559–568.
74. Neville WE, Hamouda F, Anderson J, Dwan FM. Replacement of the intrathoracic trachea and both stem bronchi with a molded silastic prosthesis. J Thorac Cardiovasc Surg 1972;63:569–576.
75. Westaby S, Jackson JW, Pearson FG. A bifurcated silicone rubber stent for relief of tracheobronchial obstruction. J Thorac Cardiovasc Surg 1982;83:414–417.
76. Westaby S, Shepherd MP. Palliation of intrathoracic tracheal compression with a silastic tracheobronchial stent. Thorax 1983;38:314–315.
77. Cooper JD, Pearson FG, Patterson GA, Todd TRJ, Ginsberg RJ, Goldberg M, Waters P. Use of silicone stents in the management of airway problems. Ann Thorac Surg 1989;47:371–378.
78. Orlowski TM. Palliative intubation of the tracheobronchial tree. J Thorac Cardiovasc Surg 1987;94:343–348.
79. Loeff DS, Filler RM, Gorenstein A, Ein S, Philippart A, Bahoric A, Kent G, et al. A new intratracheal stent for tracheobronchial reconstruction: experimental and clinical studies. Pediatr Surg 1988;23:1173–1177.
80. Clarke DB. Palliative intubation of the trachea and main bronchi. J Thorac Cardiovasc Surg 1980;80:736–741.
81. Wright KC, Wallace S, Charnsangavej C, Carresco CH, Gianturco C. Percutaneous endovascular stents; an experimental evaluation. Radiology 1985;156:69–72.
82. Simonds AK, Dirving JD, Clarke SW, Dick R. Use of expandable metal stents in the treatment of bronchial obstruction. Thorax 1989;44:680–681.
83. Uchida BT, Putnam JS, Rosch J. Modifications of Gianturco expandable wire stents. AJR Am J Roentgenol 1988;150:1185–1187.
84. Wallace MJ, Charnsagavej C, Ogawa K, Carrasco CH, Wright KC, McKenna R, McMurtrey M, et al. Tracheobronchial tree: expandable metallic stents used in experimental and clinical applications. Radiology 1986;158:309–312.
85. Rousseau H, Puel J, Joffre F, Sigwart U, Duboucher C, Imbert C, Knight C, et al. Self-expanding endovascular prosthesis: an experimental study. Radiology 1987;164:709–714.
86. Tsang V, Goldstraw P. Self-expanding metal stent for tracheobronchial strictures. Eur J Cardiothorac Surg 1992;6:555–560.
87. Hind CRK, Donnelly RJ. Expandable metal stents for tracheal obstruction: permanent or temporary? A cautionary tale. Thorax 1992;47:757–758.
88. Rousseau H, Dahan M, Lauque D, et al. Self-expandable prostheses in the tracheobronchial tree. Radiology 1993;188:199–203.
89. Insall RL, Morritt GN. Palliation of malignant tracheal strictures using silicone T tubes. Thorax 1991;46:168–171.
90. Colt HG, Harrell JH, Newman TR, Robbins T. External fixation of subglottic tracheal stents. Chest 1994;105:1653–1657.
91. Diaz-Jimenez JP, Munoz EF, Ballarin JIM, Kovitz KL, Presas FM. Silicone stents in the management of obstructive tracheobronchial lesions: 2 year experience. J Bronchol 1994;1:15–18.
92. Brutinel WM, Cortese DA, Edell ES, McDougall JC, Prakash UBS. Complications of Nd-YAG-laser therapy. Chest 1988;94:902–903.
93. Brutinel WM, Cortese DA, Edell ES, McDougall JC, Prakash UBS. Complications of Nd:YAG laser therapy (editorial). Chest 1988;94:902–903.
94. Dierkesmann R, Huzly A. Side effects of endobronchial laser treatment. Endoscopy 1985;17:49–53.
95. Casey KR, Fairfax WR, Smith SJ, Dixon JA. Intratracheal fire ignited by the Nd:YAG laser during treatment of tracheal stenosis. Chest 1983;84:295–296.
96. Schramm VL, Mattox DE, Stool SE. Acute management of laser ignited intratracheal explosion. Laryngoscope 1981;91:1417–1426.
97. Blomquist S, Algotsson L, Karlsson SE. Anaesthesia for resections of tumors in the trachea and central bronchi using the Nd-YAG laser technique. Acta Anaesthesiol Scand 1990;34:506–510.
98. Vourc'h G, Fischler M, Personne C, Colchen A. Anesthetic management during Nd:YAG laser resection for major tracheo-

bronchial obstructing tumors. Anesthesiology 1984;61:636–637.
99. Warner ME, Warner MA, Leonard PF. Anesthesia for neodymium-YAG laser resection of major airway obstructing tumors. Anesthesiology 1984;60:230–232.
100. Bailey AG, Valley RD, Azizkhan RG, Wood RE. Anesthetic management of infants requiring endobronchial argon laser surgery. Can J Anesth 1992;39:590–593.
101. Perrin G, Colt HG, Martin C, Mak MA, Dumon JF, Gouin F. Safety of interventional rigid bronchoscopy using intravenous anesthesia and spontaneous assisted ventilation: a prospective study. Chest 1992;102:1526–1530.
102. McCaughan JS, Barabash RD, Penn GM, Glavan BJ. Nd:YAG laser and photodynamic therapy for esophageal and endobronchial tumors under general and local anesthesia: effects on arterial blood gas levels. Chest 1990;98:1374–1378.
103. Lennon RL, Hosking MP, Warner MA, Cortese DA, McDougall JC, Brutinel WM, Leonard PF. Monitoring and analysis of oxygenation and ventilation during rigid bronchoscopic neodymium-YAG laser resection of airway tumors. Mayo Clin Proc 1987;62:584–588.
104. Schiffman PL, Wilhelm J, Parisi RA. Arterial oxygen saturation during Nd:YAG laser photoresection of endobronchial tumors under local anesthesia. Chest 1988;94:1300–1301.
105. Fried MP, Mallampati R, Caminear DS. Comparative analysis of the safety of endotracheal tubes with the KTP laser. Laryngoscope 1989;99:748–751.
106. Ossoff RH, Eisenman TS, Duncavage JA, Karlan MS. Comparison of tracheal damage from laser ignited endotracheal tube fires. Ann Otol Rhinol Laryngol 1983;92:333–336.
107. Duckett JE, McDonnel TJ, Unger M, Parr GVS. General anesthesia for Nd:YAG laser resection of obstructing endobronchial tumors using the rigid bronchoscope. Can Anesth Soc 1985; 32:67–72.
108. Hermens JM, Bennet MJ, Hirshman CA. Anesthesia for laser surgery. Anesth Analg 1983;62:218–229.
109. Hanowell LH, Martin WR, Savelle JF, Foppiano LE. Complications of general anesthesia for Nd:YAG laser resection of endobronchial tumors. Chest 1991;99:72–76
110. Fairfax WR, Rollins RJ. Pulmonary hyperinflation following Nd:YAG laser resection of an obstructing mainstem tumor. Chest 1988;93:1302–1304.
111. Ganfield RA, Chapin JW. Pneumothorax with upper airway laser surgery. Anesthesiology 1982;56:398–399.
112. Sebel PS, Lowdon JD. Propofol: a new intravenous anesthetic. Anesthesiology 1989;71:260–277.
113. Carlin BW, Harrell JH, Olsen LK, Moser KM. Endobronchial metastases due to colorectal carcinoma. Chest 1989;96:1110–1114.
114. Andrews AH Jr, Caldavelli DD. Carbon dioxide laser treatment of metastatic melanoma of the trachea and bronchi. Ann Otol 1981;90:310–311.
115. Baumgartner WA, Mark JBD. Metastatic malignancies from distant sites to the tracheobronchial tree. J Thorac Cardiovasc Surg 1980;79:499–503.
116. Heitmiller RF, Marasco WJ, Hruban RH, Marsh BR. Endobronchial metastases. J Thorac Cardiovasc Surg 1993;106:537–542.
117. Morris AJR, O'Sullivan JP, Millard FJC, et al. Fiberoptic bronchoscopy as an aid to diagnosis of respiratory symptoms in breast cancer patients. Br J Cancer 1983;48:731–734.
118. Davila DG, Dunn WF, Tazelaar HD, Pairolero PC. Bronchial carcinoid tumors. Mayo Clin Proc 1993;68:795–803.
119. Donahue JK, Weichert RF, Ochsner JL. Bronchial adenoma. Ann Surg 1968;167:873–884.
120. Som ML. Adenoma of the bronchus: endoscopic treatment in selected cases. J Thorac Surg 1949;18:462–478.
121. McGregor CGA, Herrick MJ, Hardy I, Higenbottam T. Variable intrathoracic airways obstruction masquerading as asthma. BMJ 1983;287:1457–1458.
122. Mak H, Metz SJ, Stokes DC, Moser RL, Wang KP, Turner CS. Recurrent wheezing and massive atelectasis in an adolescent. J Pediatr 1983;102:955–962.
123. Stamatis G, Freitag L, Greschuchna D. Limited and radical resection for tracheal and bronchopulmonary carcinoid tumour: report on 227 cases. Eur J Cardiothorac Surg 1990;4:527–532.
124. Schreurs AJM, Westermann CJJ, Van den Bosch JMM, Vanderschueren RJR, Brutel de la Riviere A, Knaepen PJ. A twenty-five year follow-up of ninety-three resected typical carcinoid tumors of the lung. J Thorac Cardiovasc Surg 1992;104:1470–1475.
125. Diaz-Jimenez JP, Canela-Cardona M, Maestre-Alcacer J. Nd:YAG laser photoresection of low grade tumors of the tracheobronchial tree. Chest 1990;97:920–922.
126. Ross DJ, Mohsenifar Z, Koerner SK. Survival characteristics after neodymium:YAG laser photoresection in advanced stage lung cancer. Chest 1990;98:581–585
127. Kvale PA, Eichenhorn MS, Radke JR, Miks V. YAG laser photoresection of lesions obstructing the central airways. Chest 1985;87:283–287
128. Gelb AF, Epstein JD. Laser in treatment of lung cancer 1984;86:662–666
129. Mohsenifar Z, Jasper AC, Koerner SK. Physiologic assessment of lung function in patients undergoing laser photoresection of tracheobronchial tumors. Chest 1988;93:65–69.
130. Desai SJ, Mehta AC, Medendorp SV, Golish JA, Ahmad M. Survival experience following Nd:YAG laser photoresection for primary bronchogenic carcinoma. Chest 1988;94:939–944.
131. Lam S, Muller NL, Miller RR, Kostashuk EC, Laukkanen E, Evans K, Szasz IJ, et al. Laser treatment of obstructive endobronchial tumors: factors which determine response. Lasers Surg Med 1987;7:29–35.
132. Stanopoulos IT, Beamis JF, Martinez FJ, Vergos K, Shapshay SM. Laser bronchoscopy in respiratory failure from malignant airway obstruction. Crit Care Med 1993;21:386–391.
133. Macha HN, Koch K, Stadler M, et al. New technique for treating occlusive and stenosing tumors of the trachea and main bronchi: endobronchial irradiation by high dose iridium-192 combined with laser canalisation. Thorax 1987;42:511–515.
134. Jain PR, Dedhia HV, Lapp NL, Thompson AB, Frisch JC Jr. Nd:YAG laser followed by radiation for treatment of malignant airway lesions. Lasers Surg Med 1985;5:47–53.
135. Eichenhorn MS, Kvale PA, Miks VM, Seydel HG, Horowitz B, Radke JR. Initial combination therapy with YAG laser resection and irradiation for inoperable non–small cell carcinoma of the lung. A preliminary report. Chest 1986;89:782–785.
136. Schray MF, McDougall JC, Martinez A, Cortese DA, Brutinel WM. Management of malignant airway compromise with laser and low dose rate brachytherapy: the Mayo Clinic experience. Chest 1988;93:264–269.
137. Schray MF, McDougall JC, Martinez A, et al. Management of malignant airway compromise with laser and low dose rate brachytherapy: the Mayo Clinic experience. Chest 1988;93: 264–269.
138. Allen MD, Balwin JC, Fish VJ, et al. Combined laser therapy and endobronchial radiotherapy for unresectable lung carci-

noma with bronchial obstruction. Am J Surg 1985;150:71–74.
139. Miller JI Jr, Phillips TW. Neodymium:YAG laser and brachytherapy in the management of inoperable bronchogenic carcinoma. Ann Thorac Surg 1990;50:190–196.
140. Khanavkar B, Stern P, Alberti W, Nakhosteen JA. Complications associated with brachytherapy alone or with laser in lung cancer. Chest 1991;99:1062–1065.
141. Gelb AF, Tashkin DP, Epstein JD, Zamel N. Nd:YAG laser surgery for severe tracheal stenosis physiologically and clinically masked by severe diffuse obstructive pulmonary disease. Chest 1987;91:166–170.
142. Mohsenifar Z, Jasper AC, Koerner SK. Physiologic assessment of lung function in patients undergoing laser photoresection of tracheobronchial tumors. Chest 1988;93:65–69

45B

HIGH-DOSE–RATE REMOTE AFTERLOADING ENDOBRONCHIAL BRACHYTHERAPY

Ritsuko Komaki, Rodolfo C. Morice, Garrett L. Walsh, Adam S. Garden, and Michael Davis

INTRODUCTION

Non–small cell carcinomas of the lung are treated preferably by surgical resection whenever all known tumor can be encompassed and the patient can tolerate the resection medically. External radiation therapy is considered the treatment of choice for patients with non-small cell carcinomas of the lung that are too advanced for resection or those whose disease is inoperable but confined to the regional lymph nodes. Endobronchial radiation therapy is indicated for patients who have a recurrence after surgery or external radiation therapy such that an important component of the tumor is located in or adjacent to the bronchus.

Endobronchial growth of lung carcinoma can cause several symptoms, some of which are life threatening, including dyspnea, cough, postobstructive pneumonitis, and hemoptysis. Because the majority of patients with bronchogenic carcinoma have either locally inoperable or metastatic disease, radiation therapy often is used to alleviate local symptoms. External beam radiotherapy is used most commonly and is effective in relieving dyspnea and hemoptysis in the majority of patients treated; however, bronchial obstruction with established distal atelectasis and secondary obstructive pneumonitis can be ameliorated in only one quarter of patients (1, 2). A few, recent, randomized studies showed that giving neoadjuvant chemotherapy before definitive surgery or radiotherapy for patients with stage III non-small cell lung cancer provided survival benefits (3–5). However, patients presenting with postobstructive pneumonitis or severe hemoptysis are not able to receive neoadjuvant chemotherapy without an increased risk of neutropenic sepsis or fatal hemorrhage. Endobronchial irradiation used quickly to alleviate airway obstruction or hemorrhage followed by definitive surgery or external beam radiation therapy is becoming an important modality in managing patients with lung cancer. It also is important for palliation of recurrent lung cancer after previous definitive treatments. Limitations of external beam radiotherapy are related to treatment toxicity, which is often significant. These include radiation esophagitis, pneumonitis, myelitis (rare), and toxicities to other surrounding tissue. Brachytherapy to treat endobronchial lesions has been available for many years, but its use has increased substantially over the last decade because of the development of equipment that allows for safe and reliable delivery methods.

BACKGROUND

Shortly after the discovery of spontaneous radioactivity by Becquerel and the characterization of radium by the Curies (for which the three scientists were awarded the Nobel Prize for physics in 1903), malignant tumors were treated by direct insertion of tubes and needles containing radium salts. As early as 1921, radium seeds (actually radon) were implanted, using rigid bronchoscopes, directly into tumors (6). There also were attempts to place catheters loaded with radium into the trachea and bronchi, but such treatments were cumbersome and associated with high personnel exposure. It was not until the development of miniaturized sources of different radioactive elements with high specific activity (disintegrations per gram of source), and the evolution of afterloading techniques, that more precise treatment to the tumor with fewer complications to the normal tissue were possible.

Brachytherapy (brachy, meaning short; as opposed to tele, meaning at a distance) includes interstitial irradiation—actually the placing of radioactive sources directly in the tumor (7)—and intracavitary irradiation, in which sources are placed in natural body cavities close to the tumor. Therefore, endobronchial irradiation is a form of intracavitary brachytherapy.

Afterloading in brachytherapy refers to the initial placement of a nonradioactive applicator followed by insertion of the active source only after the desired location is reached. The applicator for endobronchial radiation therapy is a simple sterile nylon catheter that is inserted through the bronchoscope. The catheter may contain a radiopaque wire, or a nonradioactive dummy wire may be introduced into the catheter to verify proper placement and to permit preliminary dose calculations. The active sources are inserted in the catheter when the patient is isolated from all but essential personnel. The dose rate is a function of the radioactive element and the specific activity, measured in Becquerels (Bq)—formerly Curies (Ci)—per centimeter of active length. Low-dose–rate (LDR) brachytherapy refers to the delivery of 50 to 100 cGy per hour to a reference point or isodose line. Medium-dose-rate refers to the delivery of 100 to 500 cGy per hour. High-dose-rate (HDR) irradiation is the delivery of the total dose approximately 100 to 500 times more rapidly than with LDR; dose rates are in the range of 100 to 500 cGy per minute, usually calculated at a distance of 1 cm from the center of the source.

TECHNIQUE

Afterloading techniques for endobronchial irradiation were developed during the last decade. French catheters (5F to 7F in size) can be guided endoscopically and placed beyond obstructing lesions. A common technique involves passing the catheters through the working channel of a flexible fiberoptic bronchoscope, visualizing their placement, and then removing the bronchoscope, leaving the catheters in place. The catheters can then be loaded with the radioactive sources, most frequently iridium 192 (^{192}Ir), when the patient is safely in a radiation-protected environment. At the M. D. Anderson Cancer Center, a transnasal approach is preferred for placement of catheters, although transoral and transtracheal approaches have been used in patients with narrow nasal passages or those who have had previous laryngectomies. The transnasal approach stabilizes catheters better than do other approaches.

A 6F catheter is placed through the working channel with the tip(s) located 2 to 4 cm beyond the most distal part of the endobronchial tumor. The tip must be passed further beyond the tracheal lesion(s) to avoid displacement of the catheter from one bronchus to the other. A second catheter can be placed, but doing so requires rebronchoscoping the patient. Passing the catheter into a segmental bronchus can often avoid catheter migration with coughing. Dummy sources are placed in the catheters, and the location of sources is confirmed under fluoroscopy. The catheter is secured by taping it on the nostril, a portable radiograph is used to obtain orthogonal films to verify placement and permit dosimetric calculations (Fig. 45B.1), and the patient is taken to the radiation oncology department.

At the M. D. Anderson Cancer Center, endobronchial irradiation is administered at high dose rates using a remote afterloading unit (microSelectron-HDR; Nucletron Corporation, Columbia, Maryland). This device uses a single ^{192}Ir source attached to a stainless steel cable. The ^{192}Ir source has an active length of 3.5 mm and an active diameter of 0.6 mm. The source has an activity of approximately 370 GBq (10 Ci) at the time of installation and is replaced at roughly 3-month intervals, because the half-life of this isotope is 74 days. The machine permits the positioning of the source within the catheter along a 24-cm path, at either 2.5-mm or 5-mm intervals.

The total dose and resulting time of administration are determined. Anteroposterior and lateral radiographs of the catheters permit orthogonal reconstruction using a special treatment planning program. Determinations are made of the exact source positions and the duration of exposure at each position to obtain the desired dose distribution within the tumor volume. To achieve a relatively uniform dose within the tumor

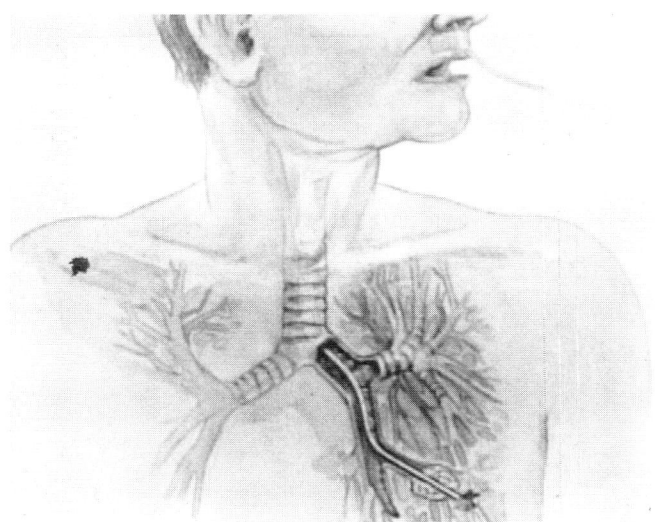

FIGURE 45B.1. Patient with a 6F catheter placed through the nostril and tumor. The tip is located 4 cm beyond the tumor.

at a specified distance from the catheter, the treatment times at distal positions within the treated region are longer than those in the central region because of the travel distance from the source. The dose rate in the tumor volume at the reference point is approximately 100 to 200 cGy per minute depending on the activity of the source. Typical treatment times are usually less than 15 minutes for delivery of 1500 cGy at a distance of 0.6 cm (for endobronchial lesions) and 0.75 cm (for tracheal lesions) from the center of the source (Fig. 45B.2).

Patients are observed closely, because most have at least moderate symptoms. Two weeks after the first endobronchial brachytherapy both a physical examination and chest roentgenograms are performed to determine whether a planned second brachytherapy application is required. In general, the second procedure is performed 2 weeks after the first treatment. Infrequently, patients have had such dramatic relief of symptoms that the second procedure is considered unnecessary. Some patients are given a third application to relieve recurrent symptoms.

HDR brachytherapy delivering 100 cGy to 500 cGy per minute offers the benefit of outpatient treatment because of the short treatment time required, more comfort for the patient, and cost and time efficacy for the institution. Treatment units permit the source to be inserted into a specified location and enable advancement of the source in a stepwise manner through the treatment volume. Computer software has been developed to allow for dose optimization. This program prevents the higher doses seen centrally when linear sources are left in the entire treatment volume for a specified time.

Laser ablation is another surgical modality used to relieve endobronchial obstruction. It can complement endobronchial irradiation, and several series have combined the techniques (8–10). These studies have used the laser for providing immediate effect and assistance in creating a passage for the catheter(s), whereas radiation provides a more durable response. Adjuvant laser treatment was not uniformly used at the M. D. Anderson Cancer Center. When it was used, the intervals between the laser and endobronchial treatments should be at least 48 hours to avoid bleeding or delayed healing of the mucosa. Laser treatment might contribute to a higher complication rate.

INDICATIONS

There are six specific indications for endobronchial irradiation therapy as practiced at the University of Texas M. D. Anderson Cancer Center:

1. Patients who have lung cancer with a significant endobronchial or endotracheal component as determined bronchoscopically.
2. Patients who are not candidates for curative resection.
3. Patients with previous external beam radiation therapy of sufficient total dose to preclude further treatment of this type.
4. Patients who are able to tolerate bronchoscopy.
5. Patients who have no bleeding disorder.
6. Patients with sufficient life expectancy (usually more than 3 months) to benefit from palliation that will not occur immediately.

To assess suitability for endocavitary therapy as well as tumor location and volume, the radiation oncologist and thoracic surgeon obtain and review the history and physical examination, including performance

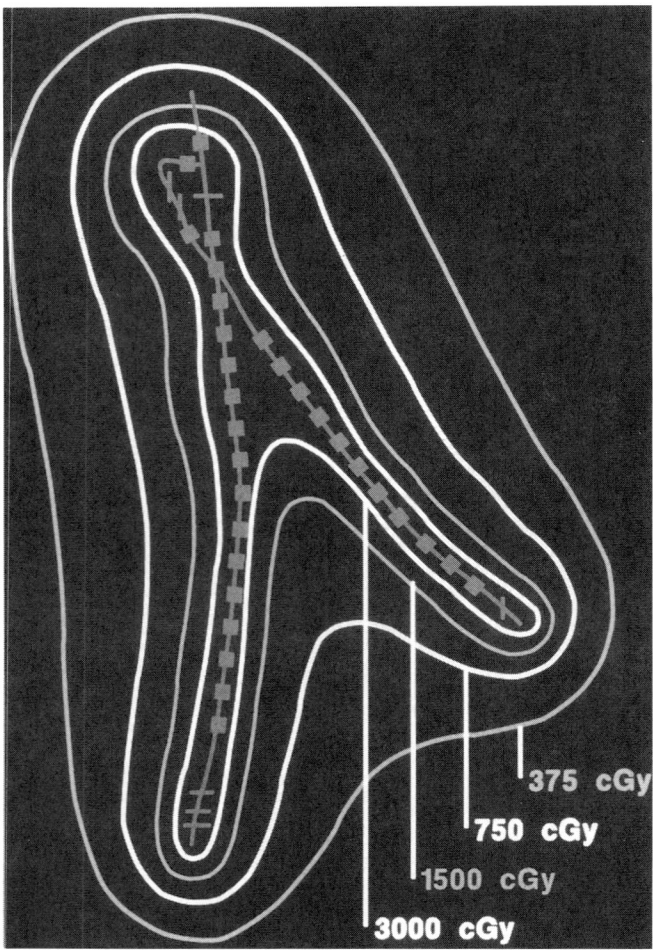

FIGURE 45B.2. Isodose curves delivering 1500 cGy at a distance of 0.6 cm from the center of sources.

status; routine blood work, including coagulation panels and complete blood cell counts; lung function tests; and chest radiographs. Bronchoscopy is performed usually as an outpatient procedure under sedation and local anesthesia. Tumors that protrude into the lumen are considered suitable, as opposed to extrinsic tumors that compress the bronchus or the trachea. The location of the tumor, its length along the bronchus or trachea, and the percentage of occlusion of the lumen are recorded. The distance from the nostrils is noted, and the tumor is photographed for future comparisons.

RESULTS

Between 1988 and 1993 at the M. D. Anderson Cancer Center, 81 patients with lung cancer underwent endobronchial brachytherapy using the procedure described previously. Fifty-four patients were male and 27 were female. Ages ranged from 28 to 77 years with a median age of 59. The Karnofsky performance status was 90 in 15 patients, 80 in 24 patients, 70 in 20 patients, 60 in 11 patients, 50 in 9 patients, and 40 in 2 patients. The presenting symptoms showed 65 patients with shortness of breath, 53 with cough, 22 with hemoptysis, 31 with wheezing, and 11 with chest pain. The degree of shortness of breath showed 8 patients with severe, 13 with moderate, and 44 with mild shortness of breath. Sixteen (20%) did not have shortness of breath at presentation. The histology or cytology showed 37 patients with squamous, 14 with adenocarcinoma, 13 with non–small cell lung cancer without specific cell types, 7 with adenoid cystic, 5 with small cell, 3 with large cell, and 2 with carcinoid tumor histologies.

Eleven percent (9 of 81) of the patients had endobronchial treatment 3 times at 2-week intervals, and 67% (54 of 81) had treatment twice at 2-week intervals. Twenty-two percent (18 of 81) had only one application because they had excellent responses after the first treatment. Approximately half had rapid progression of their disease and thus could not receive the second endobronchial brachytherapy because of rapid deterioration. Ninety-three percent of the patients had received 1500 cGy calculated at a distance of 0.6 cm from the center of the sources for main stem lesions. The rest of the patients had the same dose calculated at a distance of 0.75 cm from the center of the sources for the tracheal lesions.

Twenty-six patients (32%) had significant improvement, and 25 patients had moderate improvement. Seventeen patients had minimal improvement, and 11 patients had no change; 5 patients became

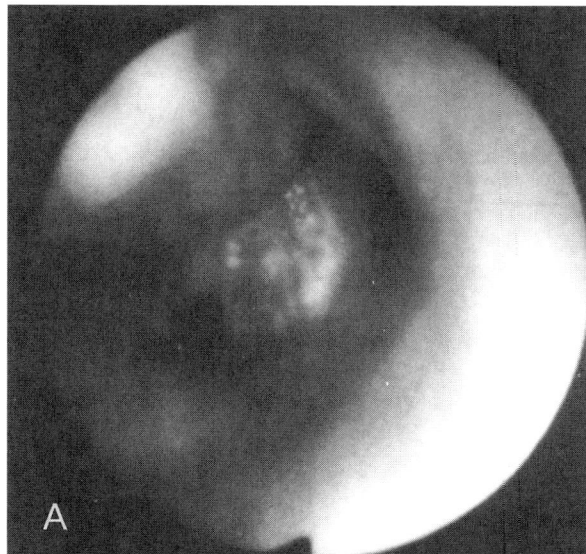
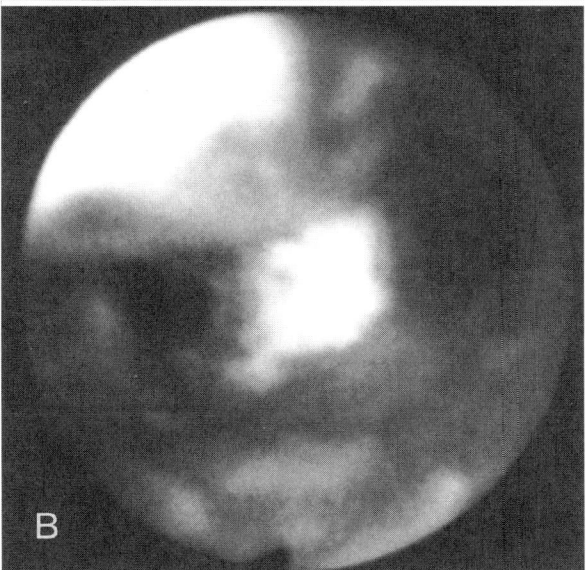

FIGURE 45B.3. A. Patient with squamous cell carcinoma of the right lower lobe extensively involving the ipsilateral hilar and mediastinal nodes treated by external radiotherapy, 6000 cGy in 30 fractions, and concomitant cisplatin infusion in April 1988. He was found to have a recurrent tumor at the right (95% occlusion) and the left (50% occlusion) main bronchi in February 1989. HDR endobronchial brachytherapy delivered 1500 cGy at a 0.6-cm distance 3 times, with a 2-week interval between treatments. B. Postendobronchial brachytherapy demonstrating remarkable regression of the tumor 2 weeks after the first application.

slightly worse; and 2 patients became much worse after the endobronchial brachytherapy. Therefore, 85% achieved some response, including the 32% of all patients who had an excellent response (Fig. 45B.3). The median duration of responses was 4.5 months, and the patients who had excellent response had much longer survivals. Median survival was 5 months for all patients, ranging from 0.5 months to 43 months. There was no significant difference based on histology, although small cell lung cancer patients appeared to do worse in terms of symptomatic relief and survival because they were referred for this treatment at a terminal stage. They also had a more extrinsic component resulting from mediastinal nodal disease rather than endobronchial lesions.

The survival time was correlated to duration of palliation, especially for shortness of breath. The 16 patients who had excellent relief of shortness of breath after the treatment had a median survival of 13.3 months compared with 65 patients who had a lesser response or no response. The median survival of the latter group was 5.4 months ($P = .0135$). Other symptomatic relief was not correlated significantly with survival.

Thirty-one patients had lesions on the left side, 48 patients had lesions on the right side (1 patient had bilateral lesions), and 2 patients had main lesions at the carina. The location of the tumor was correlated to the complication rate. The patients who had lesions at the carina developed fatal complications because of tracheomalacia in one patient and fistula in another. Three patients developed pneumothorax that resolved after insertion of a chest tube. However, the pneumothorax did not cause fatal complications. One patient developed a severe complication because of tumor necrosis, although the necrosis did heal. Two patients developed stenosis of the trachea, and one patient developed hemorrhage.

The last follow-up analysis showed 6 patients alive with disease and 1 patient alive without evidence of disease at 43 months after completion of treatment. Seventy patients died of disease, 3 patients died with intercurrent disease, and 1 patient died of a second malignancy.

DISCUSSION

Endobronchial or endotracheal lesions can cause life-threatening symptoms, including shortness of breath, postobstructive pneumonitis, and hemoptysis. The majority of patients with lung cancer have either locally unresectable, medically inoperable, or metastatic disease. Radiation therapy can control local symptoms, although, compared with endobronchial brachytherapy, external beam radiotherapy requires a longer time to alleviate the symptoms. Afterloading HDR brachytherapy is an optimal modality for treatment of patients who need either short-term palliation or quick resolution of symptoms before they have definitive treatment, such as chemotherapy and radiation therapy with or without surgery. Brachytherapy accomplishes rapid alleviation of symptoms and improvement in functional status without causing esophagitis, pneumonitis, bone marrow suppression, or (occasional) myelitis. In theory, LDR therapy offers the advantage of better tolerance of normal tissues, although it has not shown a clinical benefit for endobronchial treatments, compared with HDR (Tables 45B.1 and 45B.2). LDR brachytherapy requires hospitalization and displacement of the catheter for patients with respiratory distress; cough in such patients is a major concern. There has been a suggestion that rapidly proliferating tumors might be treated more beneficially by rapid radiation therapy to overcome the proliferation of malignant cells (11, 12). Results of LDR (8–10, 13–15) or HDR (13, 16–19) radiation for palliation showed symptomatic relief in between 50% and 70%.

Severe complication rates of between 0% and 17% have been reported. Results at the M. D. Anderson Cancer Center showed that 9 of 81 patients developed complications with 2 patients having fatal complications. Both of these patients had lesions at the carina extending to the main bronchus or trachea. When the patients receive two or more catheters, the complication rate appears to be higher, compared with one-catheter application. This finding might be related to the location of the tumor as well as to tumor volume. It seemed that the patients who had lesions at the carina developed more complications, although the numbers were too small to draw any definitive conclusions. Patients with right-sided lesions experienced a higher complication rate, compared with those whose lesions were on the left side. Differences in the complication rate based on upper and lower lobe lesions were not appreciated, although Bedwinek (20) reports a higher number of complications in upper lobe lesions.

Survival was correlated to the improvement of symptoms, especially dyspnea. To prolong the duration of palliation as well as hasten the degree of improvement, the treatment protocol at M. D. Anderson Cancer Center now involves giving a paclitaxel infusion for 24 hours followed by the endobronchial treatment.

Some investigators treated patients with locally advanced lung cancer by using combined external and endobronchial brachytherapy. The external radiation therapy was given at a dose of between 57 Gy and 66 Gy followed by two to four endobronchial treatments delivering 5 to 15 Gy of ^{192}Ir at a distance of 1 cm from the center of the sources; this treatment resulted in 77% of patients achieving a complete response and 13% of patients achieving a partial response (21). Endobronchial brachytherapy can be used as a boost

TABLE 45B.1. Low-Dose Rate of Endobronchial Irradiation

AUTHOR(S) (REFERENCE NO.)	NO. OF PATIENTS	ISOTOPE	TOTAL DOSE	PRESCRIPTION POINT	TUMOR RESPONSE	MEDIAN SURVIVAL (MO)	INITIAL PALLIATION	COMMENTS
Roach et al. (9)	17	^{192}Ir	30 Gy	0.5 cm	5 of 15 CXR	6.5	10 of 15	Most non–small cell. No major complications
Mehta et al. (13)	38	^{192}Ir	50 Gy	1 cm	70%	>5	70%	Four late complications: two fatal TE fistulas, two mucosal ulcers
Allen et al. (14)	15	^{192}Ir	20–40 Gy	0.5 cm	...	6	100%	Two subcutaneous emphysema (transcricoid approach)
Schray et al. (10)	65	^{192}Ir	30 Gy	0.5 cm (bronchus) 1 cm (trachea)	60%	4	60%	11 fistula/hemorrhage (seven caused by Tx; six or seven may have been laser related)
Rabie et al. (15)	54	^{198}Au	100 Gy	1 cm	...	...	66%	One fatal hemorrhage, three TE fistula (one laser, two progression), one pneumothorax

Abbreviations. TE, tracheoesophageal; CXR, chest radiograph; Tx, treatment.

TABLE 45B.2. High-Dose Rate of Endobronchial Irradiation

AUTHOR(S) (REFERENCE NO.)	NO. OF PATIENTS	ISOTOPE	TOTAL DOSE	PRESCRIPTION POINT	TUMOR RESPONSE	MEDIAN SURVIVAL (MO)	INITIAL PALLIATION	COMMENTS
Speiser and Spratling (16)	64	^{192}Ir	30 Gy	0.5 cm	NS	5	60%–90%	No severe complications at 0.5 cm, thus prescribed dose to 1 cm. Tx 1 per week. Three late complications
Seagren et al. (17)	20	^{60}Co	10 Gy	1 cm	6 of 20	9	85%, 17 of 20 but 12 relapsed	One transient pericarditis, no severe complications
Macha et al. (18)	106	^{192}Ir	15 Gy median for 3.7 treatments	1 cm	75%	6	75%	Two fatal complications caused by hemorrhage
Kohek et al. (19)	67	^{192}Ir	5–7 Gy × 2–3 weekly	1 cm	NS	3 (average)	74%	Complications not documented
University of Texas M. D. Anderson Cancer Center (1994)	81	^{192}Ir	30 Gy	0.6 cm	68 of 81	5	85%	Two fatal complications

Abbreviations. NS, not specified; Tx, treatment.

technique for patients with prominent endobronchial lesions without distant metastases. Doing so improves local control and reduces complications to the surrounding normal tissue from external radiation therapy, especially in the patients treated with combined chemotherapy and radiation therapy.

In conclusion, HDR afterloading endobronchial radiation is an effective palliative modality for relieving obstructive symptoms rapidly but partially in 85% of treated patients. Prospective trials are needed to optimize total doses, dose rates, fraction sizes, and number of fractions. Studies of HDR combined with radiosensitizers, used to minimize complications and maximize prolongation of durable palliation or survival, also are required. Prolonging local control would increase the survival of patients with ominous locally advanced lung cancer. The role of endobronchial brachytherapy in the curative approach for lung cancer also needs investigation.

REFERENCES

1. Slawson RG, Scott RM. Radiation therapy in bronchogenic carcinoma. Ther Radiol 1979;132:175–176.
2. Phillips TL, Miller RJ. Should asymptomatic patients with inoperable bronchogenic carcinoma receive immediate radiotherapy? North Am Rev Respir Dis 1978;117:411–414.
3. Dillman RO, Seagren SL, Propert KJ, Guerra J, Eaton WL, Perry MC, Carey RW, et al. A randomized trial of induction chemotherapy plus high dose radiation versus radiation alone in stage III non–small cell lung cancer. N Engl J Med 1990;323:940–945.
4. Rosell R, Gomez-Codina J, Camps C, Maestre J, Padille J, Canto A, Mate JL, et al. A randomized trial comparing preoperative chemotherapy plus surgery with surgery alone in patients with non–small cell lung cancer. N Engl J Med 1994;330:153–158.
5. Roth JA, Fossella F, Komaki R, Ryan MB, Putnam JB Jr, Lee JS, Dhingra H, et al. A randomized trial comparing perioperative chemotherapy and surgery with surgery alone in resectable stage IIIA non–small cell lung cancer. J Natl Cancer Inst 1994;86:673–680.
6. Yankauer S. Two cases of lung tumor treated bronchoscopically. N Y Med J 1922;115:741–742.
7. Moylan D, Strubler K, Unal AB, et al. Transbronchial brachytherapy of recurrent bronchogenic carcinoma; new approach using flexible fiberoptic bronchoscope. Radiology 1983;147:253–254.
8. Schray MF, McDougall JC, Martinez A, Cortese DA, Brutinel MW. Management of malignant airway compromise with laser and low dose rate brachytherapy. Chest 1988;93:264–269.
9. Roach M, Leidholdt EM, Tater BS, Joseph J. Endobronchial radiation therapy in the management of lung cancer. Int J Radiat Oncol Biol Phys 1990;18:1449–1454.
10. Schray MF, McDougall JC, Martinez A, Cortese DA, Brutinel MW. Management of malignant airway compromise with laser and low dose rate brachytherapy. Chest 1988;93:264–269.
11. Brenner DJ, Hall EJ. Fractionated high-dose–rate versus low-dose–rate regimens for intracavitary brachytherapy of the cervix. I. General considerations based on radiobiology. Br J Radiol 1991;64:133–141.
12. Begg AC, Hofland I, Moonen L, Bartelink H, Schraub S, Bontemps P, Le Fur R, et al. The predictive value of cell kinetic measurements in a European trial of accelerated fractionation in advanced head and neck tumors: an interim report. Int J Radiat Oncol Biol Phys 1990;19:1449–1453.
13. Mehta MP, Shababi S, Jarjour NN, Kinsella TJ. Endobronchial irradiation for malignant airway obstruction. Int J Radiat Oncol Biol Phys 1989;17:847–851.
14. Allen MD, Baldwin JC, Fish VJ, Goffinet DR, Cannon WB, Mark JBD. Combined laser therapy and endobronchial radiotherapy for unresectable lung carcinoma with bronchial obstruction. Am J Surg 1985;150:71–77.
15. Rabie T, Wilson K, Easley JD, et al. Palliation of bronchogenic carcinoma with ^{198}Au implantation using the fiberoptic bronchoscope. Chest 1986;90:641–645.
16. Speiser B, Spratling L. Intermediate dose rate remote afterloading brachytherapy for intraluminal control of bronchogenic carcinoma. Int J Radiat Oncol Biol Phys 1990;18:1443–1448.
17. Seagren SL, Harrell JH, Horn RA. High dose rate intraluminal irradiation in recurrent endobronchial carcinoma. Chest 1985;88:810–814.
18. Macha HN, Mai J, Stadler M, et al. Neu wege der strahlentherapie des bronchialkarzinoms. Deutsche Med Wochenschr 1986;111:687–691.
19. Kohek P, Pakisch B, Stucklschweiger G, Ottl M, Friehs G, Hackl A. Malignant airway obstruction management with endobronchial ^{192}Ir high dose rate brachytherapy. Abstract. Annual Brachytherapy Meeting of the European Society for Therapeutic Radiology and Oncology, Antwerp, Belgium, May 21–23, 1990:35.
20. Bedwinek J, Petty A, Bruton C, Sofield C, Lee L. The use of HDR endobronchial brachytherapy to palliate symptomatic endobronchial recurrence of previously irradiated bronchogenic carcinoma. Int J Radiat Oncol Biol Phys 1992;22:23–30.
21. Cotter GW, Herbert DE, Ellingwood KE. Inoperable endobronchial obstructing lung carcinoma treated with combined endobronchial and external beam irradiation. South Med J 1991;84:562–565.

SUGGESTED READINGS

1. Hall EJ, Brenner DJ. The dose-rate effect revisited: radiobiological considerations of importance in radiotherapy. Int J Radiat Oncol Biol Phys 1991;21:1403–1414.
2. Hilaris BS, Martini N. Interstitial brachytherapy in cancer of the lung: a 20-year experience. Int J Radiat Oncol Biol Phys 1979;5:1951–1956.

46

Endobronchial Photodynamic Therapy

Harubumi Kato and Tetsuya Okunaka

BACKGROUND AND METHODS

Photodynamic therapy (PDT) has allowed physicians to achieve a long sought objective in cancer therapy: selective destruction of tumor tissues. PDT makes it possible to eliminate malignant tissues with minimal harm to healthy tissues. In this type of cancer therapy, photosensitizing compounds are exposed to light of an appropriate wavelength. This process causes the compounds to undergo a photochemical reaction that induces the in situ production of reactive oxygen radicals that destroy cells. Some photosensitizers are especially attracted to malignant tissues. Thus, if the correct photosensitizer is employed, malignant tissues can be eliminated selectively.

For nearly a century, it has been known that exposing photosensitizing compounds to light results in a photochemical reaction (1). In a 1961 study by Lipson and Baldes (2), a hematoporphyrin hydrochloride was treated with acetic acid, producing a hematoporphyrin derivative (HpD) that was shown to have great affinity for tumorous tissues. Thus, it was theoretically possible to diagnose and eliminate malignancies selectively by using a photosensitizer with the appropriate photodynamic properties. In 1979, employing PDT in the treatment of skin metastatic lesions of breast carcinoma, Dougherty et al. (3) demonstrated that photodynamic therapy was effective in the treatment of malignant tumors. Now, more attention is being paid to the diagnosis and therapy made possible by this procedure. In 1978, Hayata and colleagues (4, 5) began their research on PDT methods using canine lung cancer models and found them to be effective for both diagnosis and treatment. This chapter comments on the most recent clinical results of PDT for the treatment of lung cancer as well as the mechanisms of PDT, new photosensitizers, and light delivery systems.

MECHANISMS OF PDT AND PHOTOSENSITIZERS

A sensitizer, i.e., light, and oxygen must be present simultaneously to bring about cytotoxicity during photodynamic therapy. Choosing the sensitizers for clinical trials is a highly selective process. Great care must be taken in selecting fluorescent materials that are safe and that have an affinity for malignant tissues. HpD, which is synthesized from hematoporphyrin by an acetylation procedure that produces a mixture of as many as 20 components, is now the most widely used photosensitizer. The many studies conducted on fluorescent materials have shown HpD to be a highly appropriate sensitizer in terms of safety, stability, low toxicity, and tumor selectivity. Today, the most commonly used second-generation form of HpD is Photofrin (Quadra Logic Technologies, Inc., Vancouver, Canada). Photofrin is composed of active components produced from HpD, *bis*-1-8-(hydroxy-ethyl) deutero-porphyrin-3-ethyl-ether (DHE). Photofrin is 40% DHE. An amount of Photofrin half that needed for HpD is sufficient to produce desired photosensitizer levels in tissue (6, 7) (Fig. 46.1). Research on new photosensitizers that efficiently absorb longer wavelengths of light and show more effective cytocidal activity is now underway. Among the new photosensitizers being developed are pheophorbide (8), bacteriopheophorbide, chlorine 6 (9), phthalocyanine (10), and derivatives of many porphyrins. A derivative of chlorine 6, mono-L-aspartyl chlorine 6 (NPe6), is one of the most promising sensitizers. NPe6 is retained better in tumors and is more efficient in vivo than chlorine 6 because it enters cells via endocytosis and accumulates in the lysosomes. NPe6 has properties such as chemical purity and a major absorption band at 664 nanometers (nm). NPe6 tetrasodium salt tetrahydrate is a com-

FIGURE 46.1. Chemical structure and fluorescence spectrum of *bis*-1-8-(hydroxy-ethyl) deuteroporphyrin-3-ethyl-ether (DHE), the active component of Photofrin.

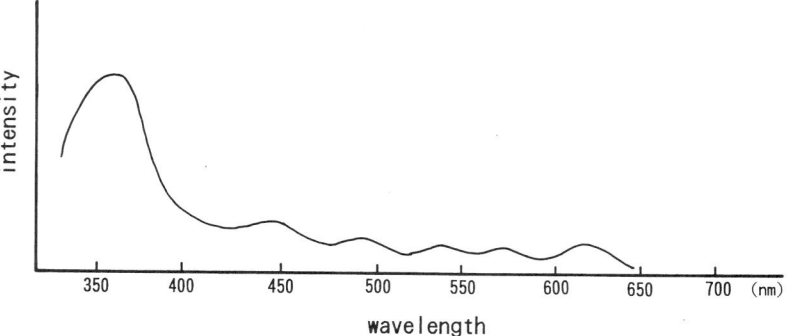

pound with a molecular weight of 871.75 in which the double-bond porphyrin ring has been reduced and an aspartic acid is attached to the propionic group at the 17th carbon of the tetrapyrrole ring via an ester linkage (Fig. 46.2). This derivative has been reported to have high selectivity, a higher cure rate, and little skin sensitization. Maximal PDT effectiveness is achieved when light is applied 2 hours after drug injection.

In the United States, Photofrin is currently the only photosensitizing agent approved for PDT studies by the U.S. Food and Drug Administration (FDA). Use of Photofrin for prophylaxis of recurrence in bladder cancer is approved in Canada (11). In Japan, a phase III study has been completed on the drug, and the government made a decision regarding approval in October 1994. Although Photofrin clears rapidly from most tissue within several hours after intravenous administration, it remains in malignant tissues, and in the liver, kidneys, spleen, and skin for several days (12). The mechanism by which Photofrin remains in tumors is not yet fully understood. However, some connection between Photofrin's selectivity and the "microenvironment of tumors" is suspected (13). Photofrin clearance may be inhibited when molecular aggregates of Photofrin accumulate around tumor neovasculature and lymphatic drainage within neoplasia is poor (14). The isolated molecular aggregates then disassociate, and Photofrin is distributed into cell membranes (because of the hydrophobic nature of monomeric Photofrin). Although cellular and mitochondrial membranes are major sites of photodynamic activity (15), recent studies show that tumor vasculature is the primary site of Photofrin susceptibility. Anoxia from vascular damage results in tumor necrosis. Studies have shown that platelet aggregation occurs, followed by complete hemostasis and microvascular hemorrhage, seconds after tumor vasculature is exposed to light (16). The mechanism of the cytotoxicity induced by PDT is not understood sufficiently. Nevertheless, it is known that when a photon is absorbed by a photosensitizer molecule and is then transferred to another molecule in the presence of oxygen, a photochemical reaction takes place. Two types of reactions occur when the photosensitizer is excited: type 1 is a process of electron transfer; and type 2 is an energy transfer with an oxygen molecule. The first type of reaction yields free radicals that react with oxygen to produce various oxidized materials that may activate free radi-

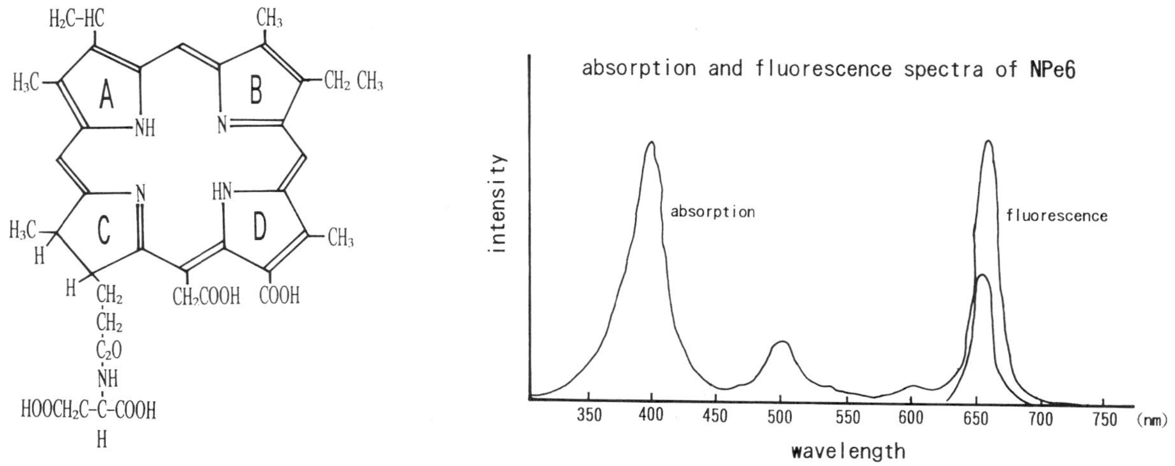

FIGURE 46.2. Chemical structure and fluorescence spectrum of mono-L-aspartyl chlorine 6.

cal chain reactions (17, 18). In the second type, a reaction between photosensitizer molecules in an excited state and ground state oxygen produces singlet oxygen, which is highly reactive and which induces cytotoxicity (19). When the sensitizer is excited by light with a wavelength within its absorption band, photodynamic activity occurs.

In aqueous solution Photofrin reaches maximum absorption in the ultraviolet light range near 365 nm. There also are several lesser peaks of absorbance, including one near 639 nm in the red range. Absorbance of Photofrin is much greater at 363 nm than at 630 nm. However, PDT utilizes red light near 630 nm because it has better tissue penetration and a lower rate of interference from absorbance by hemoglobin and other cellular components (20) (Fig. 46.3).

LASER SYSTEMS

PDT can be performed with any light source having an appropriate spectrum. Through the emission of a monochromatic form of intense collimated light energy, lasers offer an especially effective way to deliver light. The argon dye laser is used commonly to provide the red beam required for photoradiation of tumor tissue sensitized by photoactive drugs or dyes (21). In this process, a dye, usually rhodamine, is pumped into an appropriate optical cavity to produce red laser light tunable to a specific wavelength. This laser has drawbacks, however: primarily its limited ability to penetrate tissue. A new diagnostic and therapeutic endoscopic laser system was developed by Kato, Okunaka, and colleagues in 1982. This system uses an excimer dye laser capable of emitting a high-energy, pulsed laser beam (22). This laser appears to have many advantages over other PDT delivery systems. As demonstrated in the mouse kidney sarcoma (m-KSA) model, the excimer dye laser was shown to have greater tissue penetration than the argon dye laser (23). High-energy photons capable of exciting Photofrin in tumor tissue to significant levels are provided by pulsed dye–laser systems in as little as 10 nanoseconds (ns). Another pulsed beam laser, the gold vapor laser, was developed in the hope of achieving greater tissue penetration; maintaining the laser equipment to ensure optimal performance has been difficult, however.

The characteristic high-energy beam of the excimer laser is generated from a gas mixture of 0.9% Xe, 0.1% HCl, and 99% He at 2 atmospheres of pressure. At 308 nm, the optimal performance of the excimer laser is 30 millijoule (mJ) per pulse at one half peak power for 10.9 ns. Generation of the 630-nm high-energy beam used in PDT requires coupling the excimer laser to a system containing 2 molar rhodamine dye in ethanol (24). Recently, a new high-power red laser diode and system (Panasonic, Osaka, Japan) was developed for PDT. This system has a wavelength of 664 nm and a power output of 500 milliwatt per square centimeter (mW/cm^2) continuous wave (CW) in tissue. It is compact (49 × 20 × 40 cm), lightweight (20 kg), easy to operate, and reliable. This system needs only an ordinary electrical power supply, and it requires no maintenance (Fig. 46.4)

THE BRONCHOSCOPIC PDT PROCEDURE

Approximately 48 hours after intravenous injection of Photofrin (dose, 2 mg/kg of body weight), bron-

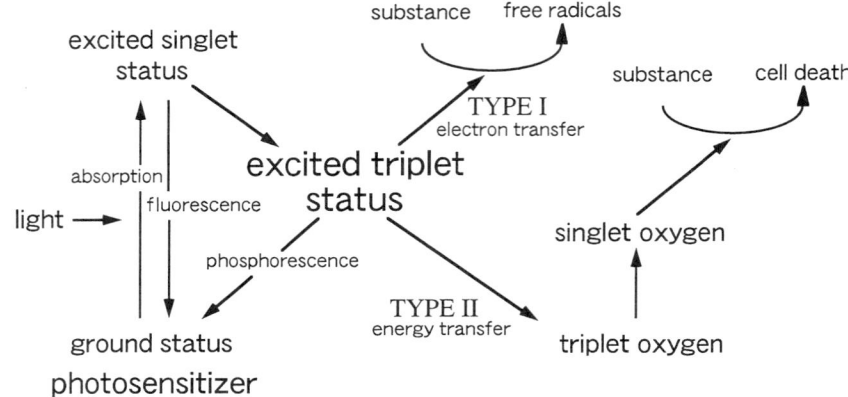

FIGURE 46.3. Photochemical mechanism of photodynamic therapy.

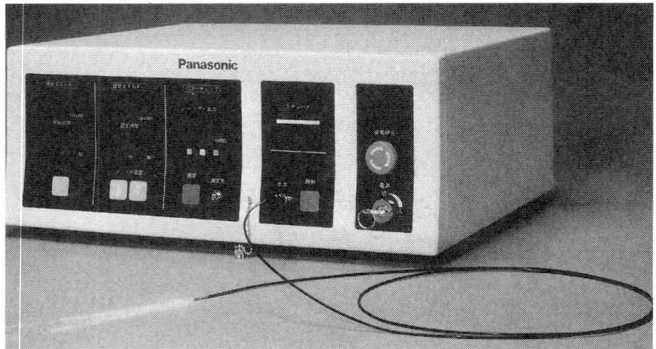

FIGURE 46.4. Excimer dye laser system.

choscopic PDT is performed under topical anesthesia. Patients should avoid direct sunlight for at least 2 weeks after Photofrin injection. The laser beam is transmitted through a quartz fiber (400 μm) inserted through the instrumentation channel of a fiberoptic bronchoscope. Held 1 to 2 cm perpendicularly from the target, the fiber tip produces a 4- to 8-mm circular area of illumination. When using the argon dye laser, power output at the fiber tip is adjusted to 80 to 400 mW. Energy is adjusted to 4 mJ per pulse at 30-hertz (Hz) frequency when using the excimer dye laser. Illumination time generally ranges from 10 to 40 minutes at energy densities of 100 to 400 Joules per square centimeter (J/cm^2) for surface irradiation in the treatment of early-stage lung cancer (Fig. 46.5). With the fiber tip inserted in the tissue, interstitial radiation was performed in advanced cases of cancer with endobronchial obstruction (25). Two types of fiberoptic tips are now being used by the authors for laser light delivery: the microlens-tipped fiber, which provides a uniform field of light for front-surface illumination; and the cylindrical, diffuser-tipped fiber, which permits delivery of light around the wall of the bronchus when a microlens-tipped fiber cannot be aimed directly at a lesion; the latter also can be inserted directly into the tumor tissue for effective, tumor specific, interstitial light delivery, especially in cases of advanced obstructing tumors. After PDT, necrosis of the tumor occurs, and the necrotic debris and associated secretions must be removed through toilet bronchoscopy several days after the initial treatment. In lung cancer cases, complications that occurred after PDT included skin photosensitivity (90% of patients), obstructive pneumonia (5%), and massive bleeding (1%) (25). Complications after PDT can be avoided or minimized if patients avoid direct sunlight for a minimum of 2 weeks and receive regular toilet bronchoscopy. The light dosage also should be restricted in cases of large tumors reaching beyond organ walls.

PHOTODYNAMIC DIAGNOSIS: FLUORESCENCE DIAGNOSIS FOR LUNG CANCER

Early-stage lung cancer is now considered to be highly curable by surgical treatment. To reduce the increasing mortality from lung cancer, it is necessary to detect early-stage cases. The government of Japan has attempted to contribute to this effort by increasing lung cancer surveys as part of general medical care for the elderly. In these surveys sputum cytology examinations are included; this measure has indeed been effective in the detection of early-stage, central-type lung cancer. However, it is sometimes difficult to determine the location of certain extremely early-stage lesions. The detection of such early-stage malignancies is crucial to survival, and the development of methods to bring about this detection is essential.

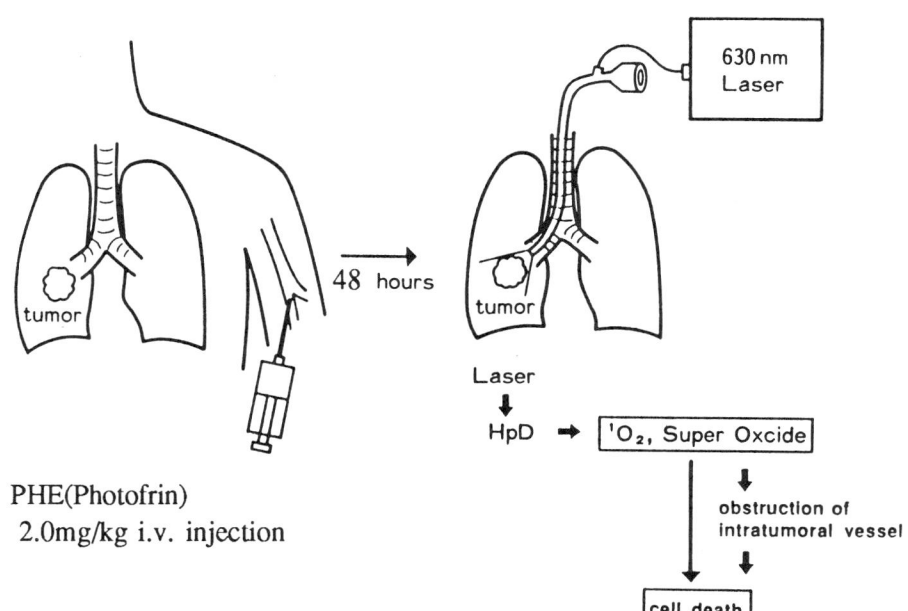

FIGURE 46.5. Photodynamic diagnosis and photodynamic therapy procedures.

Recently, fluorescence detection has been used in the diagnosis of lung cancer (26). In high-risk patients, this method has been especially beneficial for localization of roentgenographically occult lung cancers. Initially, image intensifiers were used to distinguish HpD fluorescence and normal mucosal autofluorescence (27). Photofrin was excited by exposure to 405-nm light using a mercury arc lamp or krypton ion laser (26). However, there were several problems associated with these early systems, including difficulty in determining the exact size of the lesion and the location of the site. The latter difficulty occurred because of the darkness of the image, difficulty in determining the boundaries of early-stage cancer lesions, the need for several staff to operate the system, and the complexity of the system (28).

To solve these problems, the present image processing system for diagnosis incorporates an excimer laser. A block diagram of this system is shown in Figure 46.6. To generate its characteristic high-energy beam, the excimer laser uses a gas mixture containing 0.9% Xe, 0.1% HCl, and 99% He at 2 atmospheres of pressure. The optimal performance of this laser at 308 nm is 30 mJ per pulse at one half peak power for 10.9 ns. The XeCl excimer laser (308 nm) was coupled to a pump system that contains saturated diphenyl sulphate dye in dioxane, which converts the beam to 405 nm, the wavelength used for diagnostic purposes. To generate the 630-nm beam used in PDT, the excimer laser is coupled to a system containing 2 molar rhodamine dye in ethanol. The radiation from excimer dye lasers is focused onto 400-μm fused silica fibers (Fuji Photo Optical Company, Tokyo, Japan), the tips of which are fitted with microlenses for improved homogeneity of light distribution throughout the treatment field. The circular area of illumination is 2 cm². The endoscope system, delineated in Figure 46.6 by a dotted square, is equipped with three channels that contain the fiberoptics for field visualization (Xe lamp), the excimer dye laser, and the fluorescence detector, which can function simultaneously in this system. A chopper functions to alternate the delivery of white light and laser light based on a system originally developed at the Mayo Clinic (26). The input from the fluorescence detector is fed through a polychromater that functions by recording the intensity of light at each individual wavelength along its emission spectrum. The resulting spectrum is plotted by the analyzer and displayed on the monitor. Light from the detector also is processed by a separate path in order to transmit the endoscopic image, which is displayed on the same monitor as the emission spectrum pattern. A videotape record is kept. The color representation indicates the intensity of the fluorescence. Strong fluorescence is indicated by red spots. In addition, a Photofrin specific fluorescence wavelength pattern can be seen with peaks at 630 and 690 nm.

Kato and Okunaka performed photodynamic diagnosis (PDD) using an excimer laser endoscopic image fluorescence analyzer system in 19 cases of lung cancer and 2 cases of vocal cord cancer. All lesions were squamous cell carcinomas except for one case of adenocarcinoma and one of large cell carcinoma. There were 4 cases of carcinoma in situ. The dose of

FIGURE 46.6. Diagram of the excimer laser fluorescence image analyzer system.

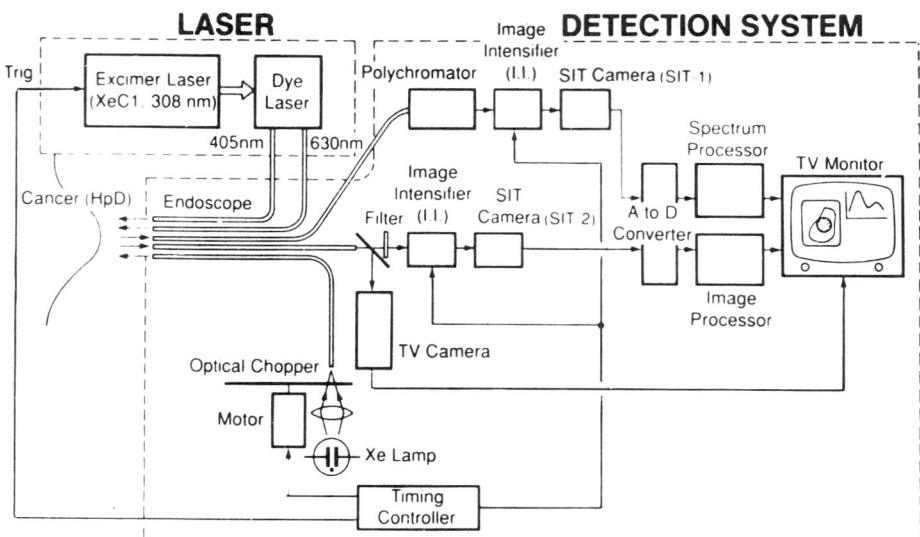

The Excimer-dye Laser Endoscopic Cancer Diagnosis & Treatment System

Photofrin was 2 mg/kg of body weight. Examinations were performed 72 hours after administration of the photosensitizer in almost all cases to avoid false-positive fluorescence from normal areas. As shown in Table 46.1, fluorescence was recognized in all cases except case 13, an advanced tumor covered with necrotic tissue and clots. False-positive results also were observed in 10 of 17 patients receiving the 2 mg/kg dose of Photofrin. No false-positive results were obtained with administration of a 0.7 mg/kg dose of Photofrin. Because there was only one false-negative result detection of fluorescence from the tumor is fairly certain. Figure 46.7 shows a carcinoma in situ at the bifurcation of the right B^1 and B^3. The fluorescence from the tumor was detected as a color image at a corresponding site. The advantages of this system include the ability to analyze the fluorescence wavelength, to observe fluorescence under normal endoscopy illumination conditions, and to perform signal imaging of the cancer by the image processor. The procedure also is simple. However, this system still has some problems. The angle of divergence of the laser beam needs to be widened and standardized. Because of slight Photofrin fluorescence and autofluorescence from the normal bronchial mucosa, the false-positive ratio was more than 50% when 2 mg/kg of Photofrin was administered, whereas no false-positive result was obtained with the administration of 0.7 mg/kg of Photofrin. Dose dependency and time-course studies of Photofrin are necessary for PDD (29). New photosensitizers for PDD also should be developed with emission peaks at longer wavelengths and minimal phototoxicity. Longer wavelength stimulating light would enable better penetration. A new photosensitizer, a meta-phenylene spacer-bearing chlorine hetero-dimer, is a promising photosensitizer with a spectral peak of 670 nm that does not interfere with autofluorescence from normal tissue (18). Palcic et al. (30) reported that using differences in tissue autofluorescence among premalignant, malignant, and normal tissues, fluorescence bronchoscopy was found to detect 3 times more cases of moderate and severe dysplasia and dysplasia and carcinoma in situ than conventional white-light bronchoscopy. With further technological advances, improvement of photosensitizers, and monitoring sophistication, PDD could be applied for definitive diagnosis of early-stage cancer.

USE OF PDT IN EARLY-STAGE LUNG CANCER AND ADVANCED TRACHEOBRONCHIAL MALIGNANCIES

Since 1980, Kato and Okunaka have used PDT techniques to treat 253 lesions at Tokyo Medical College in 211 patients with lung cancer. Seventy-six lesions were endoscopically suggestive of early-stage lung cancer. Patients included 197 males and 14 females aged 36 to 85 years (average, 65 years). Histologically, 207 lesions were squamous cell carcinoma, 23 were adenocarcinoma, 8 were large cell, 11 were small cell, and 4 were other types (Table 46.2). Tumor response to PDT was evaluated endoscopically, histologically, and cytologically. Complete remission was obtained in 36.6% of the 253 lesions, partial remission in 62.2%, and no remission in 1.2%. In advanced lesions, opening of bronchi obstructed by the tumor was

TABLE 46.1. Photodynamic Diagnosis for Lung Cancer Lesion by Excimer Laser System

CASE	HISTOLOGY	T FACTOR	DOSE OF PHOTOFRIN[a]	TIME OF EXAMINATION	TUMOR	NORMAL AREA
1. KA	SQ	T1	2	72 h	FL	FP
2. KY	SQ	T1	2	72 h	FL	FP
3. TK	AD	T1	2	72 h	FL	...
4. KH	SQ	T1	2	72 h	FL	FP
5. SY	SQ	TIS	2	72 h	FL	...
6. SF[b]	SQ	T1	2	72 h	FL	FP
7. SF	SQ	TIS	2	72 h	FL	FP
8. BT	SQ	T1	2	72 h	FL	...
9. NH	SQ	T1	2	72 h	FL	FP
10. KA	SQ	TIS	2	72 h	FL	FP
11. TS	SQ	TIS	2	72 h	FL	FP
12. SN	SQ	T1	2	72 h	FL	...
13. MH	SQ	T2	2	72 h	FL	FP
14. KS	SQ	T3	2	72 h	...	...
15. MK	SQ	T2	2	72 h	FL	FP
16. KO[b]	SQ	TIS	2	72 h	FL	...
17. KM	LA	T2	2	72 h	FL	...
18. KE	SQ	T2	0.7	72 h	FL	...
19. YK	SQ	T3	0.7	72 h	FL	...
20. TM	SQ	TIS	0.7	72 h	FL	...
21. MS	SQ	TIS	0.7	72 h	FL	...

Abbreviations. SQ, squamous cell carcinoma; AD, adenocarcinoma; LA, large cell carcinoma; FL, fluoresence positive; FP, false-positve.
[a]Dose in mg/kg of body weight.
[b]Vocal cord cancer rather than lung cancer.

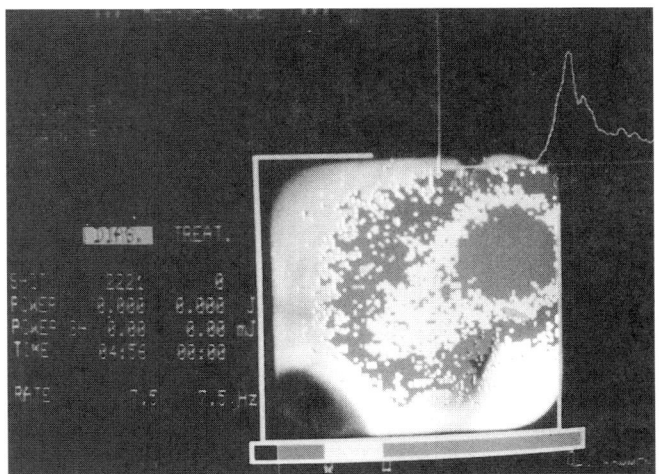

FIGURE 46.7. Monitor of excimer laser fluorescence image analyzer system that shows carcinoma in situ in the bifurcation of right B^1 and B^3. The fluorescence from the tumor was detected as a color image at a corresponding site.

TABLE 46.2. Clinical Stage and Histologic Types of Lung Cancer Treated by Photodynamic Therapy

CLINICAL STAGE	NO. OF PATIENTS (NO. OF LESIONS)
0	66 (76)
I	27
II	10
III	81
IV	24
Metastatic cancer	3
Total	211 (253)
HISTOLOGIC TYPES	NO. OF LESIONS
Squamous cell carcinoma	207
Adenocarcinoma	23
Large cell carcinoma	8
Small cell carcinoma	11
Adenoid cystic carcinoma	1
Metastatic carcinoma	3
Total	253

achieved in 62 of 81 lesions. This group contained many patients surviving 5 years. One of these was the first patient with cancer in the world to survive for 5 years after undergoing treatment consisting of PDT alone (31).

USE OF PDT IN EARLY-STAGE LUNG CANCER

Despite the increasing incidence of lung cancer internationally, overall therapeutic results in these patients have not improved significantly during the past decade. More than 150,000 men and women developed lung cancer in the United States last year, and it is estimated that 90% or more of these patients will die of the disease within 5 years of diagnosis (32). In Japan there are approximately 35,000 lung cancer deaths annually, and the 3-year survival rate is estimated to be less than 20% (33). Most patients have advanced disease at the time of diagnosis, and the results of therapy for this population are disappointing. However, an increasing number of early-stage lung cancer cases are being detected as a result of improved survey and diagnostic techniques. In cases of early detection, it generally is possible to perform curative resection. However, there is a high surgical risk for many patients because of concurrent cardiovascular or chronic obstructive pulmonary disease.

Conservative treatment to preserve lung tissue in patients with initial early-stage lung cancer is essential for the quality of life of the patient. Kato and Okunaka used PDT to treat 76 lesions in 66 patients who had endoscopically detected early-stage lung cancer (stage 0) between 1978 and 1993. The age of the patients ranged from 36 to 82 years, with a mean age of 65. All but one was male. Except for one adenocarcinoma, all lesions were squamous cell carcinomas. Although the treatment of choice for early-stage lung cancers usually is surgical resection, PDT was performed. Many lung cancer patients have poor pulmonary function or have refused surgery, and thus they do not undergo resection. In the treatment of these patients, the authors used an argon or excimer laser coupled to a dye laser employing rhodamine dye to generate 630-nm light. Three grades of tumor response were noted: (a) complete remission (CR), in which there was no visible presence of a tumor through biopsy and/or brushing cytology for at least 4 weeks; (b) partial remission, in which there was a more than 50% reduction in tumor volume but cancer was still detectable on biopsy or brushing for at least 4 weeks after therapy; and (c) no change, in which tumor size remained the same and cancer was still recognizable on biopsy or brushing. Tumor response to PDT was evaluated endoscopically, roentgenographically, and histologically 1 month after treatment. Endoscopic and histologic examinations were conducted on the treated areas in surgically resected or autopsied cases.

The results of PDT in endoscopically detected cases of early-stage lung cancer are shown in Table 46.3. Forty-four patients (51 lesions) of 66 (76 lesions), i.e., 66.7%, achieved complete remission; however, in 22 other patients (25 lesions), the entire extent of the lesion could not be seen endoscopically. Therefore, radiotherapy and/or chemotherapy or surgical resection was administered to these patients to prevent recurrences and ensure curative effect. Five patients (7.6%) experienced recurrence and were treated by surgery and radiotherapy. Follow-up showed 48 patients (58 lesions) to be disease free for periods of from 1 to 158 months, but four deaths occurred during that time because of lung cancer. In Japan a multicenter study was conducted on 59 early-stage lung cancers. After initial PDT, 50 (84.7%) patients were classified as CR. Of these, CR was obtained in 28 carcinomas with a longitudinal extent of 1 cm or less (34). A typical CR case is presented in Figure 46.8. In this 78-year-old man, squamous cell carcinoma of the lung was initially diagnosed based on positive sputum cytology. All roentgenographic examinations were negative. The tumor was nodular, located in the right upper lobe bronchus and 0.5 × 0.5 cm in size (Fig. 46.8A). Because the patient's pulmonary function was very poor, he was treated subsequently by PDT. Figure 46.8B shows the same site 1 week after PDT. The lesion was

TABLE 46.3. Results of Photodynamic Therapy for Early-Stage Lung Cancer

NO. OF CASES (NO. OF LESIONS)	NO. OF PATIENTS (NO. OF LESIONS)			
	RESULTS	DISEASE FREE	RECURRENCES	DEATHS
66 (76)	CR: 44 (51) 66.7% (67.1%) PR: 22 (25) Combined therapy[a] Surgery: 11[b] Radiation: 7[b] Chemotherapy: 6[b] YAG laser: 1[b]	48 (58) 1–158 mo	5	19 (15 from other disease)

Abbreviations. CR, complete response; PR, partial response.
[a]Number of lesions.
[b]Twenty-two patients with 25 lesions having a partial response also received additional therapy.

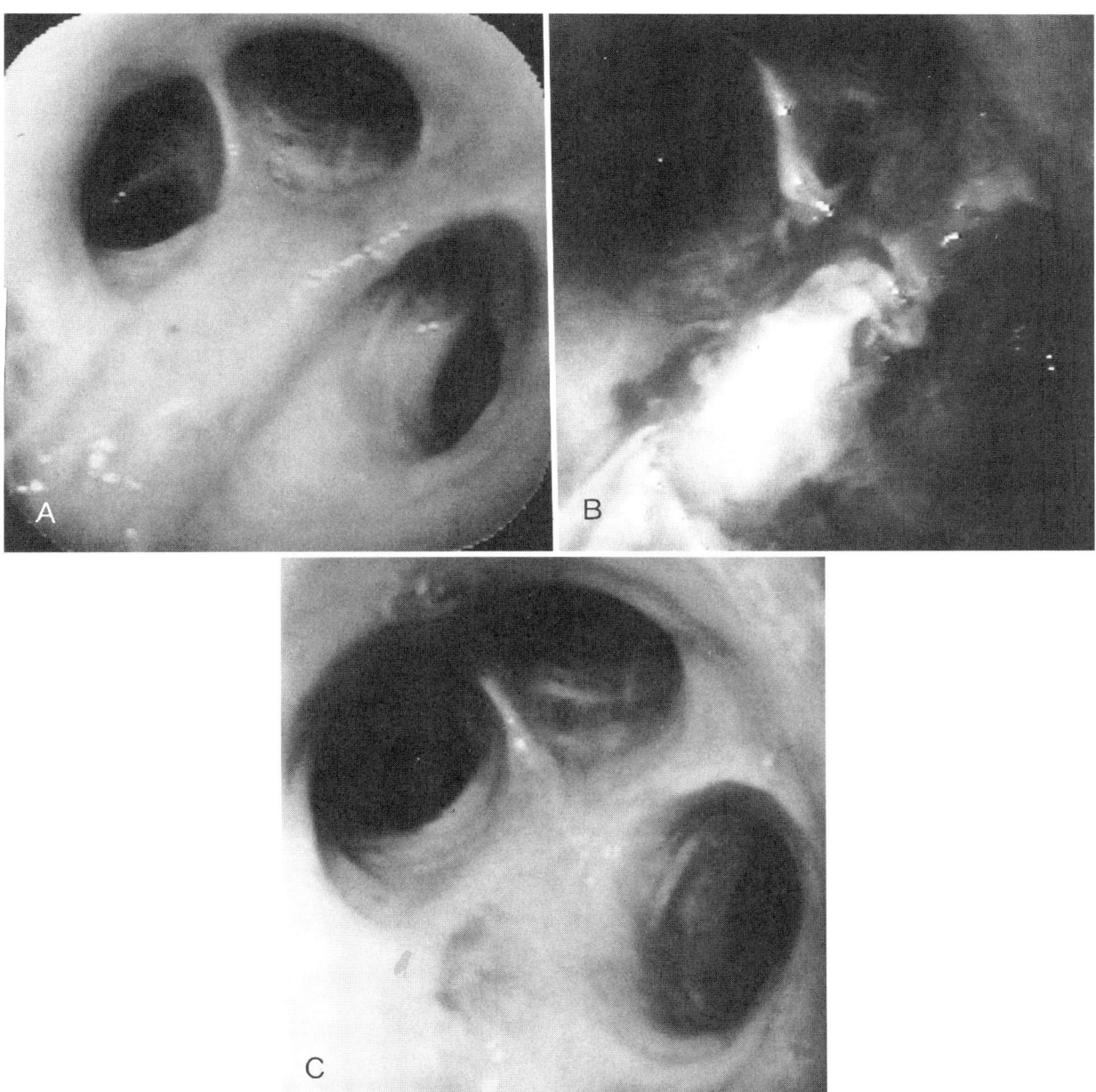

FIGURE 46.8. A. Bronchoscopic findings of 78-year-old male with a nodular squamous cell carcinoma, 0.5 cm × 0.5 cm in size in right upper bronchus. Roentgenographic examinations were negative. B. The same site 1 week after PDT. C. Complete remission was obtained.

covered with white necrotic tissue. He is now apparently disease free 12 months after PDT (Fig. 46.8C). The results of this study have shown the following conditions to be essential for successful PDT in early-stage lung cancer: (a) The entire lesion must be visible endoscopically, (b) the tumor must be situated where sufficient laser beam photoradiation can be delivered, (c) the lesion should be superficial and 1 cm or less in longest dimension, (d) the histologic type should be squamous cell carcinoma, and (e) there should be no lymph node involvement. Identification of patients with tumors limited to the bronchial wall and without involvement of lymph nodes is the most difficult aspect of this treatment method.

The authors have examined resected specimens to investigate the effect of the presence or absence of lymph node involvement in early-stage central-type lung cancer. No involvement of lymph nodes was found in 13 lesions of carcinoma in situ resected at Tokyo Medical College Hospital (35). Nagatomo et al. (36) reported that in resected specimens from 92 patients with roentgenographically occult lung cancer, no lymph node involvement was present when the tumor diameter was less than 2 cm. Kato and Okunaka histologically examined the bases of resected specimens of lung cancer patients, including one with early-stage cancer treated by PDT that did not show CR. CR was not obtained when lesions were: (a) at an anatomic site that was difficult to photoirradiate, (b) located submucosally where photoradiation could not be performed at a 90-degree angle to the surface of the lesion, (c) located beyond the cartilage, or (d) extensive. To overcome these difficulties, increased laser power and PDT using cylindrical quartz fibers with 360-degree diffusion should be used (37). PDT can be an effective alternative to surgical resection as the primary treatment of patients with early-stage central-type lung cancer. The effectiveness of using PDT with Photofrin should be a consideration when deciding on cancer treatment. A phase III study on operable cases of central-type early-stage lung cancer with tumor invasion of less than 1 cm is now being conducted by the authors.

PDT IN MULTIPLE PRIMARY LUNG CANCER

In part because of advances in technologies for the detection of lung cancer and therapeutic achievements in its management, there has been a greater frequency of reports of multiple primary lung cancers (38, 39). From 1980 to 1994, 51 (2.7%) of 1911 lung cancer patients at Tokyo Medical College Hospital were diagnosed with multiple primary lung cancers. The criteria of Martini and Melamed (40) were used to diagnose either synchronous or metachronous carcinoma of the lung. Of the 51 multiple primary lung cancer patients, 25 were treated with PDT. Eight of these patients, all of whom had early-stage lesions, were treated with PDT alone. The others underwent PDT and surgery (Table 46.4). Table 46.5 shows the results of PDT for multiple primary lung cancers. CR was achieved in 35 of 42 lesions, and 23 patients were disease free for periods ranging from 4 to 140 months. This series of patients with synchronous multiple lung cancers underwent PDT for treatment of all biopsy-proven early-stage cancerous foci (i.e., all lesions that were biopsied when discovered were grossly superficial during bronchoscopy). In cases in which lesions were more advanced but surgically curable (i.e., earlier than stage IIIB), resection was performed. A considerable amount of pulmonary function was preserved in patients who were able to receive a sleeve lobectomy after they underwent PDT to decrease the extent of the resection. Transbronchial aspiration cytology of lymph node stations 3, 7, 11, and 12 was performed simultaneously. A CT scan was then conducted for staging purposes. PDT was done on all superficial (TIS, N0, M0) lesions for complete tumor elimination. It was used palliatively on others to enable more definitive resection.

In cases of metachronous primary bronchogenic carcinoma, there was a 5- to 204-month interval between the diagnosis of the first and second cancers. A total of 18 cancerous foci were treated by PDT. Of these, 13 were classified endoscopically as early-stage lesions. The second cancer was detected after surgical treatment of the initial lesion in 10 of the 13 early-stage lesions. Thus, these second neoplasms were treated only with PDT. PDT was used to reduce the area of resection before surgery for the first cancers in two patients. In the other three patients, PDT was used alone to treat all cancerous foci. Figure 46.9 shows a case of metachronous cancer in a 67-year-old man. The initial diagnosis showing carcinoma of the lung was based on positive sputum cytologic findings during

TABLE 46.4. Multiple Primary Lung Cancer Cases at Tokyo Medical College, 1980–1993

Case background
  Multiple primary lung cancer versus total cases, 51 (2.7%) of 1911
  Mean age, 65.9 yr (range, 45–83 yr)
  Male to female ratio, 50:1
  Synchronous to metachronous ratio, 30:21
  Double primary, 46
  Triple primary, 3
  Quadruple, 2

Treatment and outcome
  Surgery + surgery, 9
  Surgery + radiation therapy and/or chemotherapy, 8
  Surgery + photodynamic therapy, 17
  PDT + PDT, 8
  Others, 9

Alive, 21
Died of cancer, 23
Died of other disease, 7

TABLE 46.5. Multiple Primary Lung Cancer Treated by Photodynamic Therapy

NO. OF LESIONS	NO. OF CASES		
	RESULTS	DISEASE FREE	RECURRENCES
42 (26)	CR, 35; PR, 7	23 (12)[a]	2

Abbreviations. CR, complete response; PR, partial response.
[a] Disease free 4 to 140 months post therapy.

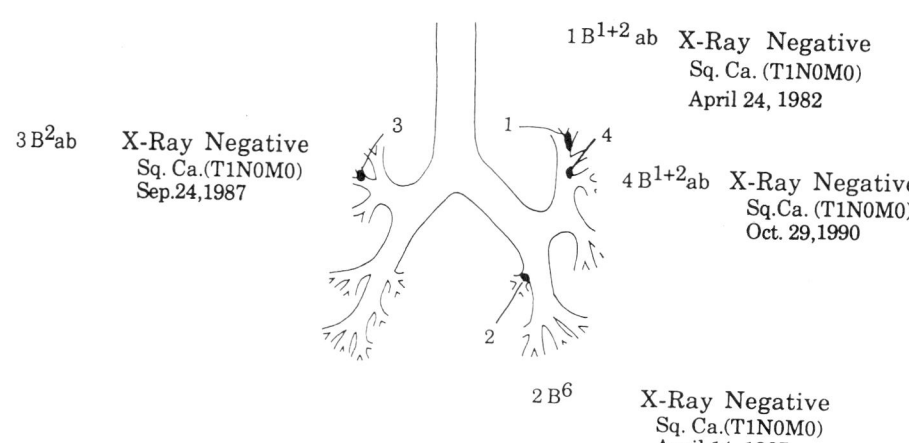

FIGURE 46.9. A typical treatment course in a 67-year-old male patient with metachronous lung cancer. The locations of tumors at different sites and periods (1 through 4) are shown.

a mass-screening program for individuals at risk for lung cancer. All radiographs were negative. Because of poor pulmonary function, PDT was used to treat the first tumor, which was nodular and located at the left B^{1+2}. During a routine bronchoscopic examination 5 years after the initial treatment, a second granular tumor was discovered at the orifice of the left B^6. Endoscopic PDT was used to treat this tumor. A third tumor was detected in the right B^2ab 5 months after endoscopic treatment of the second lesion. It also was treated with PDT and disappeared completely. A fourth tumor was discovered 37 months later in the left upper bronchus and was treated by PDT. No evidence of recurrence had been found 1 year after PDT treatment. Recently, a lesion was detected in the orifice of left upper lobe bronchus, and it again was treated by PDT. From these therapeutic results, the authors have determined several indications for PDT in multiple primary lung cancers: (a) all bronchoscopically accessible superficial (TIS, N0, M0) lesions whose distal margin can be photoradiated, (b) stage I lesions in patients who refuse surgery or have poor pulmonary functions, (c) stage I lesions as palliative treatment in curative resection cases, and (d) advanced lesions requiring palliation (41). Moreover, 5-year disease free survival rates of 28% and 11% can be expected in patients with synchronous and metachronous multiple primary lung cancers, respectively, if conventional treatment methods are employed (40). The survival data shown in Table 46.5 suggest that PDT may be a viable option in treating multiple primary lung cancer. Coupled with advances in therapeutic techniques, the survival rate will ultimately increase. The result is a greater possibility of detecting a second or third primary cancer. Effective control of the disease and therapeutic flexibility for the surgeon are the benefits of PDT. Either as a single therapeutic method or as an adjunct to major surgery and/or radiation therapy, PDT gives the surgeon effective control and therapeutic flexibility in treating cancer.

USE OF PDT IN ADVANCED TRACHEOBRONCHIAL MALIGNANCIES

Little can be done in cases of advanced-stage lung cancer. Only 12% of stage III patients survive for 2 years regardless of therapy (42, 43). Transbronchial resection using the neodymium:yttrium-aluminum-garnet (Nd:YAG) laser has become well accepted after the initial reports of its efficacy were published. Transmitted through optical fibers, the Nd:YAG laser provides excellent vaporization, low absorption by hemoglobin, and good tissue penetration 5 to 10 mm from the focal point with high-energy output. Good results were reported in cases of symptomatic endobronchial tumor obstruction treated with the Nd:YAG laser (44). The drawback of this laser, however, is its nonspecificity. The Nd:YAG laser produces a beam that not only vaporizes or coagulates tumor tissue but that may also harm normal bronchial tissues and thus lead to severe bleeding or perforation of the bronchial wall. Treatment with the Nd:YAG laser may improve ventilation of patients with endobronchial tumors, but only partial removal of the tumor should be attempted using this method (45). With PDT, the endobronchial tumor, if small enough, can be eliminated completely with no fear of complications. In patients in the United States with lung cancer or endobronchial metastatic lesions, the primary use of PDT is for palliation of endobronchial obstruction in patients who have intrinsic lesions of the bronchus that cause partial or complete obstruction (46). A summary of cases of lung cancer patients who underwent palliative treatment for endobronchial obstruction by either PDT or Nd:YAG laser

TABLE 46.6. Photodynamic Therapy (PDT) Versus Nd:YAG Laser Treatment of Advanced Obstructive Lung Cancers

RESULTS	EFFECTIVE CASES (%) VERSUS TOTAL CASES	
	PDT	Nd:YAG
Trachea and main bronchus	19 (73%) of 26	64 (93%) of 69
Lobar and segmental bronchus	42 (69%) of 55	79 (73%) of 108
Total	61 (75%) of 81	143 (81%) of 177

COMPLICATIONS	No. OF PATIENTS (% OF TOTAL)			
	PDT		Nd:YAG	
	Skin photosensitivity	71 (91%)	Pneumonia	12 (7%)
	Pneumonia	4 (6%)	Massive bleeding	10 (6%)
	Slight fever	2 (3%)	Arrhythmia	8 (5%)
			Perforation	4 (3%)
MORTALITY	0 (0%)		3 (1.7%)	

therapy is provided in Table 46.6. Cases in which tumor size or the degree of bronchial obstruction was reduced by more than 50% were classified as effective in terms of tumor response. Ineffective cases were those in which tumor size or the degree of obstruction was reduced by less than 50% (46). There were 258 lesions treated: 81 by PDT and 177 lesions by Nd:YAG laser. All were evaluated 1 month later. PDT achieved effective results in 61 (75%) of 81 lesions. In the Nd:YAG laser group, 143 (81%) of 177 showed effective results. In this study tumor location also was examined to evaluate effective tumor response. When the tumor was located in the trachea or main bronchi, effective results were obtained in 73% (19 of 26) of cases treated by PDT and in 92% (64 of 69) treated by Nd:YAG laser. However, in cases in which the tumor was found in lobar or segmental bronchi, the tumor response was effective in 70% (42 of 55) of PDT-treated patients and 73% (79 of 108) of Nd:YAG laser–treated patients. No fatal complications occurred in any of the PDT-treated patients, whereas 91% (71 of 81) of patients developed skin photosensitivity, no patient required treatment.

Severe complications, including massive bleeding in 10 patients (6%) and bronchial perforation in 4 cases (3%), occurred in the Nd:YAG–treated group. As a result of these complications, 3 patients (1.3%) died. Toilet bronchoscopy after laser therapy was different in the PDT-treated group and the Nd:YAG-treated group. Clean-up after PDT involved the simple removal of gelatinous or fibrinous plugs from the bronchus in large pieces. Nd:YAG therapy, however, usually required time-consuming piecemeal forceps removal of charred and coagulated tissue resulting from the treatment. The therapies also differed in that the laser used in PDT could be inserted safely into the tumor for treatment without perforation or harm to adjacent vessels. With the Nd:YAG laser, however, bronchial wall perforation or massive hemorrhaging resulting from the blood vessel injury that sometimes occurred (47). This study shows that in the bronchial wall, tumor necrosis is not induced as effectively by Nd:YAG laser treatment as it is by PDT. This is true, especially in the smaller bronchi, because of the lesser margin for error with the Nd:YAG laser before entering the vessel. Nd:YAG treatment in distal bronchi is extremely difficult and dangerous. Hemorrhage from pulmonary vessels was one of the major complications of using the Nd:YAG laser, but hemorrhage did not occur with PDT. With a mortality rate of 0%, PDT's greatest advantage over Nd:YAG treatment is safety.

The advantages and disadvantages of PDT compared with the Nd:YAG laser treatment were summarized by McCaughan et al. (44). PDT's disadvantages are: (a) photosensitizer injection, from which skin photosensitivity may result, (b) the required waiting period between injection and treatment, and (c) the need to perform frequent toilet bronchoscopy. The advantages of PDT treatment are threefold: (a) the technical ease allowed by its safety, thus allowing little chance of perforation and little risk of intraoperative hemorrhaging, (b) no endobronchial smoke, and (c) freedom to insert the fiber blindly into tissue. Although the advantages of PDT for treatment of advanced obstructing bronchial malignancy are emphasized, the first choice for patients with severe respiratory distress is immediate Nd:YAG laser therapy, because PDT requires a 2- to 3-day waiting period for selective retention of Photofrin; it also may cause mucosal edema of tissue. Furthermore, patients treated with PDT may be ambulatory, but because they are instructed to avoid direct sunlight, their activity is severely limited for at least 2 weeks of their short remaining life span. When deciding among alternative therapies, physicians treating patients with late-stage lung cancer should give careful consideration to this problem.

COMBINED USE OF PHOTODYNAMIC THERAPY AND SURGERY

As expected, all resected cases of lung cancer showed better therapeutic results than nonresected cases. To improve survival, it thus is necessary to maximize the number of operable cases of lung cancer. Furthermore, 15% of patients died, even after curative resection, because of poor postoperative pulmonary function. The amount of resection in patients with poor pulmonary function should therefore be restricted. PDT is used at Tokyo Medical College Hospital as a method of increasing operability and reducing the extent of resection in lung cancer cases (48). In 24 lung cancer patients aged 36 to 77 years, the authors attempted to increase operability and reduce the extent of operation. Seven patients had stage I cancer, 2 had stage II, 9 had stage IIIA, 5 had stage IIIB, and 1 had stage IV. Histologically, there were 20 cases of squamous cell carcinoma, 2 of adenocarcinomas, and 2 of large cell carcinomas (Table 46.7). Three patients had direct tracheal invasion from the primary foci, 3 had endobronchial polypoid tumors or invasion of the carina, and 18 had polypoid tumors or invasion of the main bronchi (Table 46.8). Through endoscopic investigation, the invasive foci were diagnosed as superficial mucosal invasion. Of the 3 patients with direct tracheal invasion, 1 underwent a sleeve lobectomy of the right upper lobe, another had a pneumonectomy, and the third received tracheoplasty. Of the 3 cases of carinal invasion by tumor, sleeve lobectomy was performed on the right upper lobe in 1 case and pneumonectomy in another. The third patient had to undergo exploratory thoracotomy because of extensive hilar lymph node involvement.

Of the 18 patients with tumor invasion to the main bronchi, 6 underwent lobectomy, 10 received a sleeve lobectomy to preserve pulmonary function, and the remaining 2 underwent pneumonectomy because of extensive hilar lymph node involvement. The initial purpose of PDT was achieved in 21 of the 24 patients treated. In these cases, operability was either increased or the extent of resection was reduced. Through PDT, the initially inoperable conditions of 5 patients were made operable in 4. Of the 19 patients who were candidates for pneumonectomy, 17 achieved conditions in which only lobectomy or sleeve lobectomy was necessary. However, there were 3 subsequent deaths caused by distant metastasis and 2 cases of recurrence. This study emphasizes that the status of patients must be determined accurately before PDT. Endoscopic observation, brushing, and biopsy must be performed when selecting patients for PDT to determine whether the histologic type is squamous cell carcinoma and whether it is invading superficially. Methods of limiting the extent of resection by improving the clinical stage of lung cancer patients are being studied continually. Among these are preoperative systemic chemotherapy, bronchial arterial infusion (49), and preoperative radiotherapy (50).

A typical case of squamous cell carcinoma of the lung is shown in Figure 46.10. The patient, a 76-year-old male, had a polypoid tumor obstructing the orifice of the right main bronchus with invasion to the lateral wall of the trachea and truncus intermedius as well as early-stage squamous cell carcinoma at the bifurcation of the left B^{1+2} and B^3. This case was considered initially inoperable because of the double primary lung cancers and cancer invasion to the trachea. The left side early-stage lesion was treated with PDT. Subse-

TABLE 46.7. Lung Cancer Patients Treated with Preoperative Photodynamic Therapy

No. of patients	24
Sex	M: 22; F: 2
Age distribution	51–71 yr
Histology	
Squamous cell carcinoma	20
Adenocarcinoma	2
Large cell carcinoma	2
Clinical stage (UICC classification system)	
I	7
II	2
IIIA	9
IIIB	5
IV	1

TABLE 46.8. Results of Preoperative Photodynamic Therapy and Operation Methods

Tumor Invasion	No. of Cases	Operation Method After PDT (No.)
Trachea	3	Sleeve lobectomy (1)
		Pneumonectomy (1)
		Tracheoplasty (1)
Carina	3	Sleeve lobectomy (1)
		Pneumonectomy (1)
		Exploratory thoracotomy (1)
Main bronchus	18	Lobectomy (6)
		Sleeve lobectomy (10)
		Pneumonectomy (2)
Total	24	24

FIGURE 46.10. A typical case of squamous cell carcinoma of the lung in a 76-year-old male. He had a polypoid tumor obstructing the right B^1 bronchus with invasion of the lateral wall of the trachea and trunks intermedius as well as early-stage squamous cell carcinoma on the bifurcation of the left $B^{1+2}c$ and B^3 bronchus. The left-side, early-stage lesion was treated with photodynamic therapy. Subsequently, for the right ride cancer lesion, sleeve upper lobectomy was performed after preoperative photodynamic therapy.

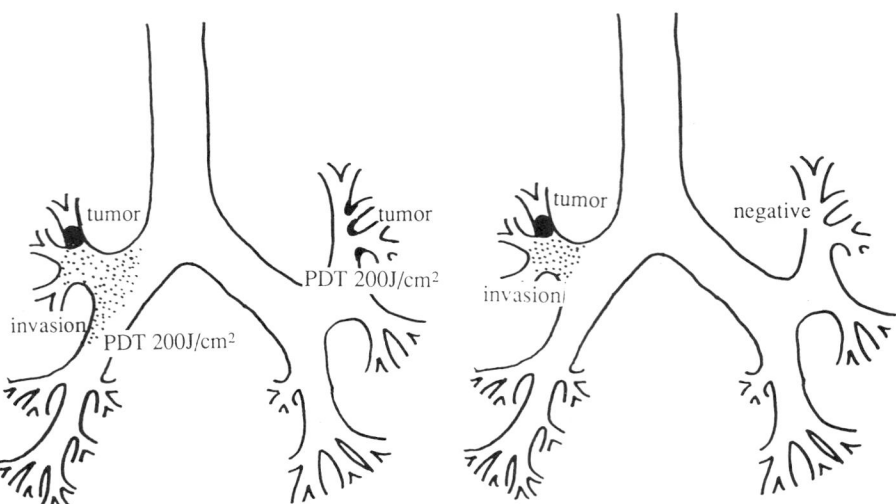

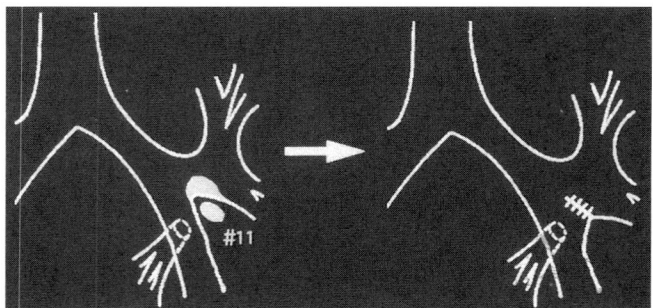

FIGURE 46.11. A case of the bronchoplasty after photodynamic therapy.

quently, sleeve upper lobectomy was performed after preoperative PDT for the right side cancer lesion.

Figure 46.11 shows another case of the bronchoplasty after PDT. This patient had disease that was deemed unresectable because of poor pulmonary function. A left pneumonectomy was necessary for cure in this case, and preoperative PDT made bronchoplasty of the bifurcation of the left upper and lower lobe bronchi possible. Figure 46.12A shows bronchoscopic findings before PDT, and Figure 46.12B shows them after PDT. The tumor disappeared completely; however, a CT scan showed lymph node 11 involvement. Subsequently, bronchoplasty and lymph node resection were performed (Fig. 46.12C).

WORLD TRENDS AND THE FUTURE OF PDT

The past decade has seen a growing acceptance of photodynamic therapy, a relatively new modality used in the treatment of cancer. This method has been used to treat a wide variety of malignancies in more than 3000 patients worldwide (20). Approximately 90 institutions and 180 investigators throughout the world employ PDT. Five hundred patients have undergone PDT for the treatment of endobronchial malignancy. There has been remarkable consistency in the results of various investigators, showing complete plus partial response rates ranging from 70% to 100% (11). Mucosal tumors or early (stage 0) lung cancers showed the best results. In the treatment of superficial lesions, it is possible for PDT to be used as a substitute for surgery, with an overall CR rate of 66.7% (Table 46.9). A study of patients at the Mayo Clinic with early-stage lung cancer (including those with in situ carcinomas) who underwent PDT showed a 71.4% CR rate in 14 tumors treated in 13 patients (51). During the first 2 years of follow-up, there was recurrence in 23% of the 10 tumors that showed a complete response. Surgical resection was performed on two and a second PDT was completed on the third, and all again achieved CR. Symptomatic improvement was used as a basis for evaluating patients in some studies. Generally reported as positive responses were clearance of airway obstruction or improved operability, and 340 of 376 sites (90.4%) (Table 46.8) showed a positive response (complete plus partial response). The responses of the series of patients with advanced disease were more difficult to interpret, however. Among these were patients with a variety of combinations of T and N factors and other prognostic elements, such as performance score and weight loss. Signs of distant metastasis, sometimes shortly after treatment, were seen in a significant percentage of the test population during follow-up.

Frequent and repeated treatment was determined to be feasible and safe in studies by McCaughan et al. (52). In these studies, 30 treatments were performed on a series of 18 patients in 26 different areas of the lung. Complete or partial response was experienced at

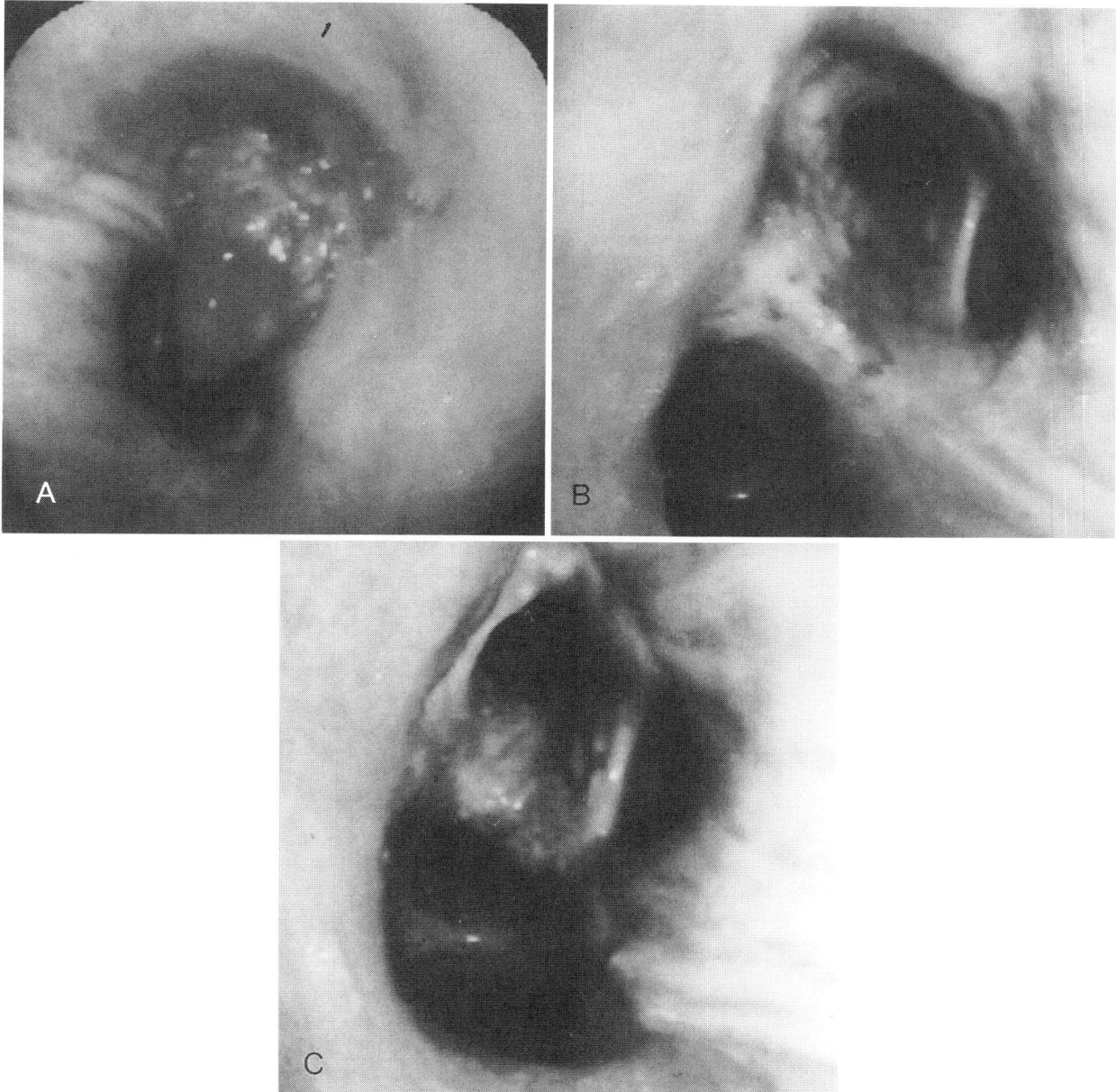

FIGURE 46.12. A. Bronchoscopic finding before photodynamic therapy. B. Bronchoscopic finding post PDT. The tumor disappeared completely, however, a CT scan showed lymph node 11 involvement. C. Subsequently, bronchoplasty and lymph node resection were performed.

1 month by 96% of the patients, and a total of 61 patients showed clinical improvement. The mean survival period was 8.3 months. A study by Hugh-Jones and Gardner (53) on a series of 15 patients with advanced squamous carcinoma showed that adequate palliation was achievable. Initial therapy resulted in a 100% response by patients, with 12 (60%) achieving a 50% reduction in tumor size and three (20%) achieving complete tumor elimination. After PDT, one patient was disease free for 2 years. In prospective independent clinical trials conducted to test the safety and efficacy of PDT with Photofrin on endobronchial lesions at three centers in the United States between 1983 and 1988, 370 endobronchial sites were treated in 170 patients (11). For obstructive lesions and mucosal lesions, the overall CR rates were 50% and 75%, respectively. The total response rates (complete plus partial response) were 75% and 78%, respectively. Possible treatment-related side effects included dyspnea (19% of all patients), fever (20%), photosensitivity (8%), and hemoptysis (8%). Eight deaths occurred because of hemoptysis (one during post-PDT debridement and seven at 2 to 10 weeks after PDT). However, PDT appears to cause no additional toxicity in patients who had previ-

TABLE 46.9. Summary of Published Studies Using Photodynamic Therapy for the Treatment of Lung Cancer

AUTHORS (REFERENCE NO.)	NO. OF PATIENTS/ LESIONS	CONDITION (NO. OF LESIONS)	RESULTS (NO. OF LESIONS)
Kato (48)	202/242	Early (69)	CR: 45 (65.2%) of 69 (early)
		Advanced (173)	CR + PR: 169 (97.7%) of 173 (advanced)
Edell and Cortese (51)	38/40	Resected or inoperable	CR: 13 (34.2%) of 38
			CR + PR: 29 (76.3%) of 38
Edell and Cortese (54)	13/14	Early superficial	CR: 10 (71.4%) of 14
			CR + PR: 13 (93%) of 14
Sutedja and Zandwijk (55)	17/17	Early stage	CR: 12 (71%) of 17; CR + PR: 17 (100%)
Leroy (56)	38/46	Early stage	CR: 28 (61%) of 46; CR + PR: 36 (79%) of 46
Karg (57)	12/15	Early stage	CR: 12 (89%) of 15; CR + PR: 15 (100%)
Keller et al. (58)	15/15	Advanced	CR: 3; CR + PR: 14 (93%) of 15
Li et al. (59)	21/24	Advanced	CR: 3; CR + PR: 20 (83%) of 24
Vincent et al. (60)	17/17	Advanced	CR: 0; CR + PR: 13 (76.4%) of 17
Hugh-Jones and Gardner (53)	15/15	All advanced and symptomatic	CR: 3; CR + PR: 12 (80%) of 15
Lam et al. (61)	5/5	All symptomatic	CR + PR: 5 (100%)
Pass et al. (62)	10/15	Obstructed	CR: 2; CR + PR: 13 (87%) of 15
McCaughan et al. (63)	31/49	Early (1)	CR: 18 (37%); CR + PR: 45 (92%) of 49
		Advanced (48)	
Sutedja (64)	26/26	Stage I (11), III (15)	PR: 10/11 (stage I), 11/15 (stage III)
Total		Early (162)	CR: 108 (66.7%) of 162 (early)
		Advanced (376)	CP + PR: 340 (90.4%) of 376 (advanced)

Abbreviations. CR, complete response; PR, partial response.

ously undergone either chemotherapy or radiation therapy. Thus, PDT can be combined safely with standard treatment modalities. Recently, a positive response to PDT treatment was shown in the case of endobronchial obstructive tumors metastatic to the lung. Of these lesions, 44 (88%) of 50 obtained CR, and the total complete plus partial response was 94% (47 of 50). Since November 1989, a feasibility study and phase I trials of intrapleural PDT for the treatment of pleural malignancies, including stage IIIB lung cancer, isolated pleural metastasis to the hemithorax, and mesothelioma has been underway in the United States (11).

Photofrin is clinically the most commonly used photosensitizer, but it has disadvantages: uneven distribution in tumor tissue, photosensitivity side effects, and a short excitation wavelength, which means that light beams with only limited penetration characteristics can be used. Better laser systems that are less expensive, maintenance free, and tunable are necessary. The success of PDT for treatment of various cancers in clinical trials offers encouragement for its future use. New photosensitizers that reach emission peaks at long wavelengths and that have minimal phototoxicityshould be developed. Whether used curatively for early-stage cancer, palliatively for local improvement of lesions in advanced cases, or in combination with surgery or ionizing radiation and chemotherapy, PDT provides sound benefits and holds great potential in the treatment of cancer.

Acknowledgment

The authors wish to thank professor J. P. Barron for his review of the manuscript.

References

1. Raab O. Uber die Wirkung Fluoreszierenden Stoffen. Infusoria Z Biol 1900;39:524.
2. Lipson RL, Baldes EJ. The use of a derivative of hematoporphyrin in tumor detection. J Natl Cancer Inst 1961;26:1–8.
3. Dougherty TJ, Laurence G, Kaufman JH, et al. Photoradiation in the treatment of recurrent breast carcinoma. J Natl Cancer Inst 1979;62:231–237.
4. Hayata Y, Kato H, Konaka C, et al. Hematoporphyrin derivative and laser photoradiation in the treatment of lung cancer. Chest 1982;81;269–277.
5. Hayata Y, Kato H, Konaka C, et al. Fiberoptic bronchoscopic laser photoradiation for tumor localization in lung cancer. Chest 1982;82:10–14.
6. Kessel D, Cheng M. On the preparation and properties of dihematoporphyrin ether, the tumor localizing component of HpD. Photochem Photobiol 1985;41:277–282.
7. Gomer CJ. Photodynamic therapy in the treatment of malignancies. Semin Hematol 1989;26:27–34.
8. Kawabe H, Tamachi Y, Okunaka T, et al. Photodynamic effects of quaternary ammonium salt derivative of protoporphyrin derivative on normal and tumor-bearing mice. Lasers Life Sci 1991;4(2):115–123.
9. Nelson JS, Roberts WG, Berns JW. In vivo studies on the utilization of mono-L-aspartyl chlorine (NPe6) for photodynamic therapy. Cancer Res 1987;47:4681–4685.
10. Tralau CJ, Barr H, Sanderman R, et al. Aluminum sulfonated phthalocyanine distribution in rodent tumor of the colon, brain and pancreas. Photochem Photobiol 1987;46:777–781.

11. Marcus SL, Dugan M. Global status of clinical photodynamic therapy: the registration process for a new therapy. Lasers Surg Med 1992;12:318–324.
12. Kessel D. Chemical and biochemical determinants of porphyrin localization. In: Doiron DR, Gomer CJ, eds. Porphyrin localization and treatment of tumors. New York: Liss, 1984:405–418.
13. Bugelski PJ, Poter CW, Dougherty TJ, et al. Autoradiographic distribution of hematoporphyrin derivative in normal and tumor tissue of the mouse. Cancer Res 1981;41:4606–4612.
14. Moan J. The photochemical yield of singlet oxygen from porphyrin in different states of aggregation. Photochem Photobiol 1984;39:445–449.
15. Gibson SL, Hilf R. Photosensitization of mitochondrial cytochrome c oxidase by hematoporphyrin derivative. Cancer Res 1983;43:1994–1999.
16. Zhou C. Mechanisms of tumor necrosis induced by photodynamic therapy. J Photochem Photobiol B 1989;3:299–318.
17. Hiff R, Warne NW, Smail DB, et al. Photodynamic inactivation of selected intracellular enzymes by hematoporphyrin derivative and their relationship to tumor cell viability in vitro. Cancer Lett 1984;24:165–172.
18. Takemura T, Nakajima S, Sakata I. Tumor-localizing fluorescent diagnostic agents without phototoxicity. Photochem Photobiol 1994;59:366–370.
19. Weishaupt KR, Gomer CJ, Dougherty TJ. Identification of singlet oxygen as the cytotoxic agent in photoactivation of a murine tumor. Cancer Res 1976;36:2326–2329.
20. Manyak MJ, Russo A, Smith PD, et al. Photodynamic therapy. J Clin Oncol 1988;6(2):380–391.
21. Fuller TA. Fundamentals of lasers in surgery and medicine. In: Dixon JA, ed. Surgical application of lasers. Chicago: Yearbook, 1983:11–28.
22. Yamamoto H, Kato H, Okunaka T, et al. Photodynamic therapy with the excimer dye laser in the treatment of respiratory tract malignancies. Lasers Life Sci 1991;4:125–133.
23. Okunaka T, Kato H, Konaka C, et al. A comparison between argon-dye and excimer-dye laser for photodynamic effect in transplanted mouse tumor. Jpn J Cancer Res 1992;83:226–231.
24. Hirano T, Ishizuka M, Suzuki K, et al. Photodynamic cancer diagnosis and treatment system consisting of pulse lasers and an endoscopic spectroimage analyzer. Lasers Life Sci 1989;3:99–116.
25. Kato H, Konaka C, Kinoshita K, et al. Laser endoscopy with photodynamic therapy in the respiratory tract. Gan Monogr Cancer Res 1990;37:139–151.
26. Kato H, Cortese DA. Early detection of lung cancer by means of hematoporphyrin derivative fluorescence and laser photoradiation. Clin Chest Med 1985;6, 237–253.
27. Hayata Y, Kato H, Konaka C. Fiberoptic bronchoscopic laser photoradiation for tumor localization in lung cancer. Chest 1982;82:10–14.
28. Kato H, Imaizumi T, Aizawa K, et al. Photodynamic diagnosis in respiratory tract malignancy using an excimer dye laser system. J Photochem Photobiol 1990;6:189–196.
29. Lam S, Palcic B, McLean D, et al. Detection of early lung cancer using low dose Photofrin II. Chest 1990;97:333–337.
30. Palcic B, Lam S, Hung J, et al. Detection and localization of early lung cancer by imaging techniques. Chest 1991;99:742–743.
31. Kato H, Konaka H, Ono J, et al. Five-year disease-free survival of a lung cancer patient treated only by photodynamic therapy. Chest 1986;90:768–770.
32. Boring CC, Squires TS, Tong T. Cancer statistics. CA Cancer J Clin 1991;41:19–36.
33. The tendency of national health. In: Health and Welfare Statistics Association, ed. J Health Welfare Stat (Japanese) 1991;38:417–418.
34. Furuse K, Fukuoka M, Kato H, et al. A prospective phase II study on photodynamic therapy with Photofrin II for centrally located early stage lung cancer. J Clin Oncol 1993;11:1852–1857.
35. Hayata Y, Kato H, Konaka C, et al. Photodynamic therapy in early stage lung cancer. Lung Cancer 1993;9:287–294.
36. Nagatomo N, Saito Y, Ohata S, et al. Relationship of lymph node metastasis to primary tumor size and microscopic appearance of roentgenographically occult lung cancer. Am J Surg Pathol 1989;13:1009–1013.
37. Kato H, Kawate N, Kinoshita K. Photodynamic therapy of early-stage lung cancer. In: Bock G, Harnett S, eds. Photosensitizing compounds: their chemistry biology and clinical use. Chichester, United Kingdom: John Wiley and Sons, 1990:531–535.
38. Boucot KR, Weiss W, Cooper DA. Second pulmonary neoplasms among long-term survivors of lung cancer. Am Rev Respir Dis 1965;92:767–770.
39. Shields TW. Multiple primary bronchial carcinomas. Ann Thorac Surg 1974;27:1–2.
40. Martini N, Melamed MR. Multiple lung cancer. J Thorac Cardiovasc Surg 1975;70:606–612.
41. Okunaka T, Kato H, Konaka C, et al. Photodynamic therapy for multiple primary bronchogenic carcinoma. Cancer 1991;68:253–258.
42. Hara N, Ohta M, Tanaka K, et al. Assessment of the role of surgery for stage II bronchogenic carcinoma. J Surg Oncol 1984;25:153–158.
43. Mountain CF. The biologic operability of stage III non–small cell lung cancer. Ann Thorac Surg 1985;40:60–64.
44. McCaughan JS, Williams TE, Bethel BH. Photodynamic therapy of endobronchial tumors. Lasers Surg Med 1986;6:336–345.
45. Hetzel MR, Smith SGT. Endoscopic palliation of tracheobronchial malignancies. Thorax 1991;46:325–33.
46. Balchum OJ, Doiron DR. Photoradiation therapy of endobronchial lung cancer: large obstructing tumors, nonobstructing tumors, and early-stage bronchial cancer lesions. Clin Chest Med 1985;6:255–275.
47. McCaughan JS, Hawley PC, Bethel, BH, et al. Photodynamic therapy of endobronchial malignancies. Cancer 1988;62:691–701.
48. Kato H, Konaka C, Ono J, et al. Preoperative laser photodynamic therapy in combination with operation in lung cancer. J Thorac Cardiovasc Surg 1985;90:420–429.
49. Neyazaki T, Ikeda M, Seki Y, et al. Bronchial artery infusion therapy for lung cancer. Cancer 1969;24:912–922.
50. Scherman DM, Weichselbaum RR. The use of preoperative radiation therapy in the treatment of lung carcinoma. Cancer Treat Res 1981;1:63–73.
51. Edell ES, Cortese DA. Bronchoscopic localization and treatment of occult lung cancer. Chest 1989;96:919–924.
52. McCaughan JS, Williams TE, Bethel BH. Photodynamic therapy of endobronchial tumors. Lasers Surg Med 1986;6:336–345.
53. Hugh-Jones P, Gardner WN. Laser photodynamic therapy for inoperable bronchogenic squamous cell carcinoma. Q J Med 1987;64:565–581.
54. Edell ES, Cortese DA. Bronchogenic phototherapy with hematoporphyrin derivative for treatment of localized bronchogenic carcinoma: 5-year experience. Mayo Clin Proc 1987;62:8–14.
55. Sutedja TG, Zandwijk N. Long term responses after photodynamic therapy in patients with intraluminal non–small cell lung cancer. Chest 1993;103:262S.
56. Leroy M. Pilot study of photodynamic therapy with Photofrin for inoperable early stage lung cancer. Proceedings of the 29th An-

nual Meeting of the American Society of Clinical Oncology, Dallas, TX, 1993;12:332.
57. Karg O. Photodynamic therapy—clinical results. Pheumologie 1992;46:258.
58. Keller Gs, Doiron DR, Fisher GU. Photodynamic therapy in otolaryngology—head and neck surgery. Arch Otolaryngol 1985;111:758–761.
59. Li LH, Chen YP, Zhao SD, et al. Application of hematoporphyrin derivative and laser-induced photochemical reaction in the treatment of lung cancer: a preliminary report of 21 cases. Lasers Surg Med 1984;4:31–37.
60. Vincent RG, Dougherty TJ, Rao U, et al. Photoradiation therapy in advanced carcinoma of the trachea and bronchus. Chest 1984;85:29–33.
61. Lam S, Kostashuk EC, Coy ER, et al. A randomized comparative study of the safety and efficacy of photodynamic therapy using Photofrin II combined with palliative radiotherapy versus palliative radiothermy alone in patients with inoperable obstructive non–small cell bronchogenic carcinoma. Photochem Photobiol 1987;46:893–897.
62. Pass HI, Delaney T. Smith PD, et al. Bronchoscopic phototherapy at comparable dose rates; early results. Ann Thoracic Surg 1989;47:693–699.
63. McCaughan JS, Hawley PC, Bethel BH, et al. Photodynamic therapy of endobronchial malignancies. Cancer 1988;62:691–701.
64. Sutedja T. A pilot study of photodynamic therapy in patients with inoperable non–small cell lung cancer. Eur J Cancer 1992;28A:1370–1373.

47

VIDEO-ASSISTED THORACIC SURGERY

Rodney J. Landreneau, Stephen R. Hazelrigg,
Michael J. Mack, Keith S. Naunheim,
Robert J. Keenan, and Peter F. Ferson

INTRODUCTION

Video-assisted thoracic surgery, also known by the acronym VATS, is emerging as a preferred minimally invasive surgical alternative to open thoracotomy for a wide variety of intrathoracic pathologic problems (1, 2). VATS is an expansion of the well-established pleural diagnostic modality—thoracoscopy (3–5). As is the case with other endosurgical approaches in surgical oncology, the goal of VATS is to diagnose accurately and to manage the malignant process successfully with the least operative morbidity for the patient. Another important endpoint is the potential avoidance of an unnecessary thoracotomy in patients with benign disease or systemic malignancy in which the primary role of surgery is diagnosis only. This chapter discusses the experience of the authors with the VATS approach in lieu of thoracotomy for the diagnosis and management of several known, or potential, malignant thoracic conditions.

BACKGROUND AND BASIC STRATEGIES FOR VATS

The fundamental difference between VATS and simple thoracoscopy relates to the use of a television camera adapted to the thoracoscope for operative visibility rather than direct, on line, viewing of the pleural cavity by the surgeon through the thoracoscope (6). This television access used for thoracoscopic interventions and the development of effective endosurgical instruments have been primarily responsible for the expanded use of VATS approaches in general thoracic surgery today. The primary indications for VATS in the practices of the authors are listed in Table 47.1.

A careful physiologic assessment of the patient and a thorough roentgenographic examination of the known or suspected malignant process is a primary consideration (7). The use of the VATS approach can allow surgical treatment for many patients who, because of physiologic impairment, are not considered candidates for thoracotomy. VATS should not be construed as a substitute for less invasive diagnostic or therapeutic interventions that may answer the patient's problems, however. Accordingly, the thoracic surgeon must first ask if a surgical intervention will impact positively on the overall patient management. Certainly, the anesthetic risks and potential problems with single-lung ventilation must be weighed against the potential advantages of the surgical intervention. These anesthetic risks are equivalent whether open thoracotomy or VATS is used. The surgeon also must appreciate that although the early (less than 2 months) postoperative benefit of reduced pain-related morbidity with the VATS approach is substantial (8), there is no conclusive evidence that there is any reduction in chronic postthoracotomy pain syndromes with VATS compared with traditional muscle-sparing thoracotomy (9). The surgeon considering the VATS approach also must avoid compromise of well-founded technical and thoracic oncologic principles if this approach is chosen.

With regard to the required preoperative roentgenographic assessment, a high-quality chest computed tomographic (CT) scan is most valuable. Without this evaluation, VATS approaches are significantly compromised because the intercostal access strategy is directly dependent on the anterior-to-posterior and medial-to-lateral location of the target pathology. Furthermore, the reduced direct tactile information afforded to the thoracic surgeon with the VATS approach makes it mandatory that accurate preoperative localization and roentgenographic characterization of the lesion be obtained.

TABLE 47.1. Video-Assisted Thoracic Surgical Applications in Thoracic Oncology

Diagnosis and treatment of idiopathic/malignant pleural effusions
Closed wedge resection biopsy of idiopathic pulmonary infiltrates in immunosuppressed cancer patients
Biopsy and resection of mediastinal masses and tumors
Facilitation of staging of carcinoma of the lung
Excisional biopsy of indeterminate pulmonary nodules
Nonanatomic wedge resection of peripheral lung cancers in patients with impaired cardiopulmonary reserve
VATS lobectomy with mediastinal nodal staging of small peripheral lung cancers
Video-assisted intrathoracic dissection for esophagectomy

BASIC OPERATIVE SET-UP AND INTERCOSTAL ACCESS FOR VATS

General anesthesia is established and endotracheal intubation achieved with a double-lumen endotracheal tube or bronchus blocker to obtain selective lung ventilation. Collapse of the ipsilateral lung is essential for access to the pleural cavity. The patient is positioned in a lateral decubitus position, and the table is flexed maximally to drop the patient's hip and shoulder away from the operative field (Fig. 47.1). This maneuver widens the intercostal spaces, which reduces the tendency to lever the instruments against the ribs during the VATS procedure. The patient's chest is prepared for surgery in the event that a conversion to formal thoracotomy is necessary. Ipsilateral lung ventilation is stopped, thus allowing resorptive atelectasis to begin.

The initial intercostal access for the primary VATS exploration of the pleural cavity usually is established in the sixth intercostal space at the mid-to-posterior axillary line. Care must be exercised to avoid injury to the underlying lung during this initial entry into the chest. An unimpeded 360-degree arc of rotation of the thoracoscope is achieved when direct intercostal access is used. A wide-angle, 0-degree, operating, 10-mm thoracoscope (Karl Storz, Inc., Culver City, CA) is introduced through a reusable metal port (Snowden-Pencer, Inc., Atlanta, GA) to explore the thoracic cavity. An additional intercostal access site may be required to allow complete manipulation and examination of the entire lung during this exploratory phase of the VATS procedure. This site of intercostal access and all subsequent sites needed to complete the VATS procedure are accomplished under direct videoscopic vision to reduce the likelihood of intercostal neurovascular bundle or intrathoracic organ injury (Fig. 47.2).

The use of an operating thoracoscope (Karl Storz, Inc.) is recommended strongly for most VATS applications (Fig. 47.3). The use of this operative videoscope allows for single intercostal access for diagnostic and limited therapeutic VATS interventions. In contrast, the view only videoscope for VATS interventions requires at least two intercostal access sites. The 5-mm biopsy channel of the operative scope also can be used as an additional port for instrument access during more complex operative procedures.

Identification of the target pathology is the next task required. The importance of the preoperative CT evaluation again becomes clear at this point. The intrathoracic contents are explored with special attention to the anatomic regions corresponding to the roentgenographic assessment. Usually, the area of disease can be identified by the topographic visual or palpable clues afforded through the videoscopic image and examining endoscopic forceps. Direct digital palpation of the lung through the sites of intercostal access during the VATS procedure is useful for identifying the target pathology. The lung can be grasped in the area of presumed pathology with a lung clamp introduced through one of the strategically placed intercostal access sites; grasping the lung brings the suspicious area into contact with an exploring index finger introduced through another intercostal access site. The surgeon can use this technique to explore the lung and to identify the great majority of lesions in the lung parenchyma. For selected patients with small lesions deep to the visceral pleura that may be difficult (or impossible) to identify through videoscopic inspection, the use of preoperative CT needle localization can be a useful adjunct to VATS resection (Fig. 47.4) (10).

Once the target pathology has been localized, subsequent intercostal access is established as needed to accomplish the VATS procedure. Generally, the surgeon tries to arrange the videoscope and endoscopic instrumentation strategically so as to triangulate the needed tools around the lesion (6). To avoid backward or mirror-imaged videoscopic orientation of the instrumentation relative to the pathology, it is important to arrange the intercostal access sites so that the instrumentation is being used in the same direction as the field of view. Additionally, the instrumentation should be positioned at a distance far enough from the lesion, and from the operators, to enhance operative dexterity and avoid "sword fighting" with the instrumentation (Fig. 47.5). At the termination of the procedure, one (or two) of the intercostal access sites used during the VATS approach can be used for tube thoracostomy drainage.

The use of this basic operative set-up and intercostal access planning serves thoracic surgeons well during their initial VATS experience. Additionally, the patient and disease specific characteristics described

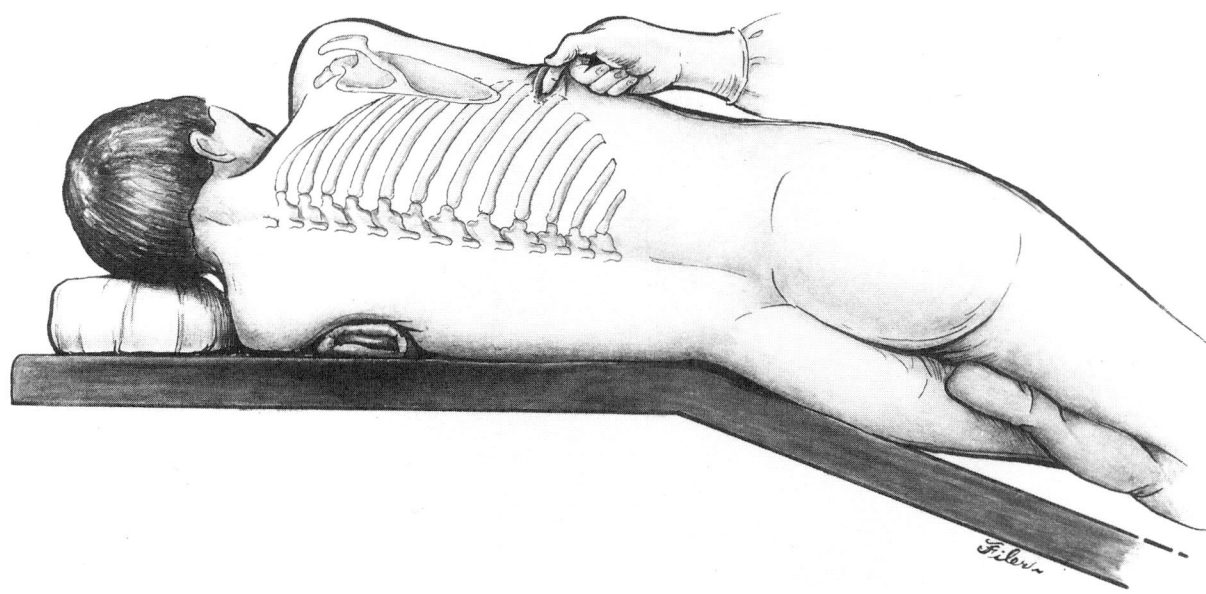

FIGURE 47.1. Desired lateral decubitus positioning of the patient for most VATS interventions. (From Landreneau RJ, Mack MJ, Hazelrigg SR, et al. Video assisted thoracic surgery: basic technical concepts and intercostal approach strategies. Ann Thorac Surg 1992; 54:800–807.)

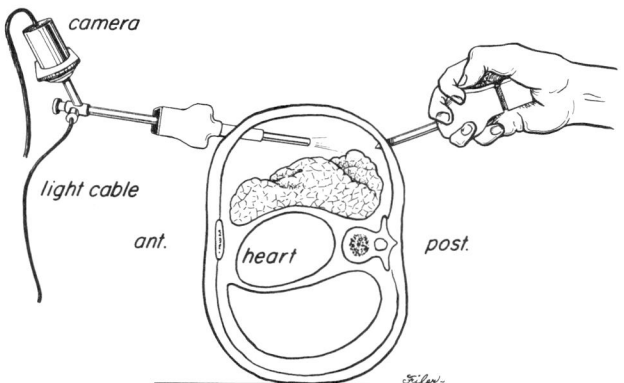

FIGURE 47.2. Technique for insuring safety of subsequent intercostal access using direct videoscopic guidance. (From Landreneau RJ, Mack MJ, Hazelrigg SR, et al. Video assisted thoracic surgery: basic technical concepts and intercostal approach strategies. Ann Thorac Surg 1992;54:800–807.)

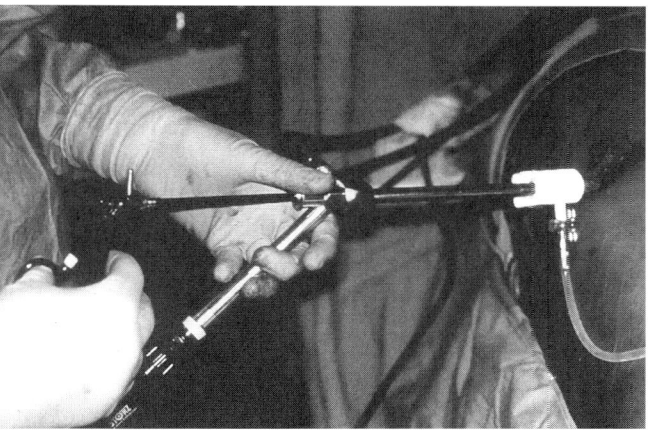

FIGURE 47.3. Photograph of operative thoracoscope in use through a previous tube thoracostomy intercostal access site accomplishing single-stick evaluation and management of an idiopathic pleural effusive process.

must be internalized into the mental formula used by the surgeon when deciding on the VATS approach to the thoracic pathology. With these points in mind, the following sections describe the potential uses of VATS in thoracic oncologic surgical practice.

PLEURAL DISEASE

The most time-honored application of VATS is in the management of pleural disease processes. Indeed, such problems represent nearly 30% of the authors' experience with VATS (Table 47.2). Many newly identified pleural effusive processes remain idiopathic despite attempts at diagnosis with thoracentesis or pleural biopsy. Unless the patient has a clinical history of cardiac, hepatic, or renal dysfunction, or has had a recent pneumonic infection, a malignant etiology of the pleural effusion should be suspected particularly. Exudative characteristics of the effusion at thoracentesis raise this suspicion further. The malignant etiology of such pleural effusions usually is obtained if one elects simply to follow the disease process; however, the diagnosis may be delayed inordinately. This delay may impair the ability to treat the systemic component of the malignancy and to palliate the local pleural

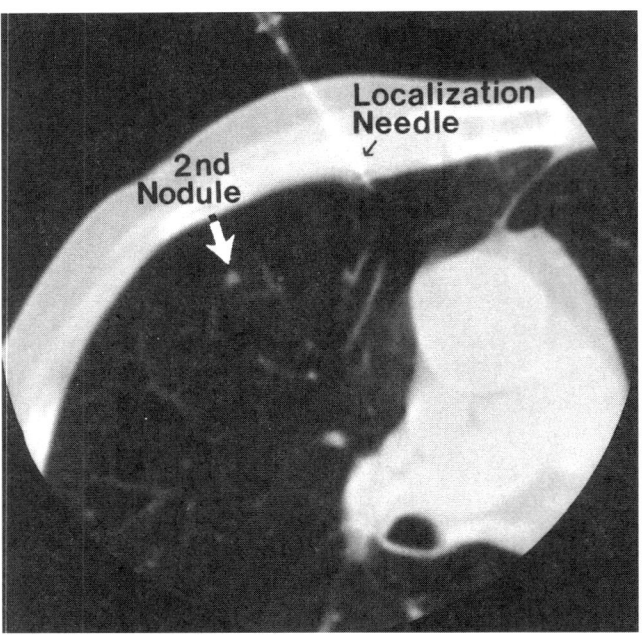

FIGURE 47.4. CT scan demonstrating the needle localization approach applied for the identification of nonpalpable subpleural lesion during the VATS procedure immediately following this CT intervention.

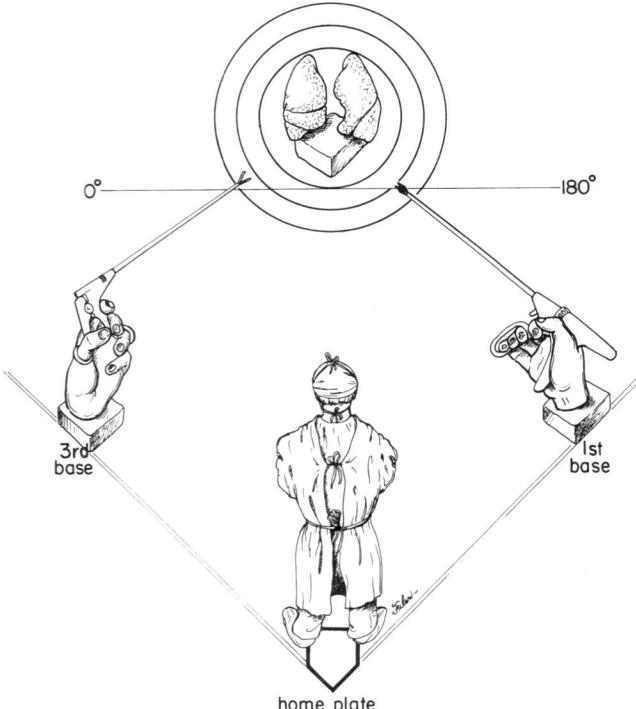

FIGURE 47.5. Baseball diamond cartoon used to illustrate the proper positioning of videoscope and endosurgical instrumentation relative to the target pathology. (From Landreneau RJ, Mack MJ, Hazelrigg SR, Dowling RD, Acuff TE, Magee MJ, Ferson PF. Video assisted thoracic surgery: basic technical concepts and intercostal approach strategies. Ann Thorac Surg 1992;54:800–807.)

TABLE 47.2. Results of Video-Assisted Thoracic Surgery for Pleural Disease

	NO. OF PATIENTS
Effusion (benign)	45
Effusion (malignant)	82
Empyema	34
Biopsy of pleural tumor	45
Clotted hemothorax	8
Total malignant	127 (59%) of 214

process. VATS has particular utility in diagnosing and managing these idiopathic pleural processes. A definitive diagnosis can be made with VATS approaches in 85% of patients with such idiopathic pleural processes (2, 11–15).

The VATS approach also is an effective means of managing complicated effusions of presumed benign or known malignant etiology. Such effusions may have become loculated and difficult to drain completely with tube thoracostomy alone (Fig. 47.6). The VATS approach can be applied in these cases to break down the offending areas of loculation under direct thoracoscopic vision. After division of the restrictive adhesions, obliteration of the pleural space can usually be achieved to allow for more uniform expansion of the lung. Depending on the nature of the effusion, pleurodesis and/or partial or total parietal pleurectomy also can be performed to facilitate control of the pleural effusive process at the time of the VATS intervention (12, 14, 16, 17). In the great majority of cases, these VATS interventions directed toward pleural pathology can be accomplished through a single intercostal access site, which can then be used for subsequent tube thoracostomy drainage (Fig. 47.7).

The VATS approach also is useful in diagnosing pleural-based masses thought to be mesothelioma. Tissue obtained from percutaneous biopsy usually is inadequate for diagnosis because of the desmoplastic reaction associated with the malignancy. VATS offers a less invasive alternative to thoracotomy for this diagnosis and for the management of any associated pleural effusive process.

MEDIASTINAL PATHOLOGY

The authors frequently use the VATS approach as a means of diagnosing and treating selected mediastinal pathologic conditions (Table 47.3). The most common use of VATS is as an alternative to the Chamberlain anterior mediastinotomy procedure in the

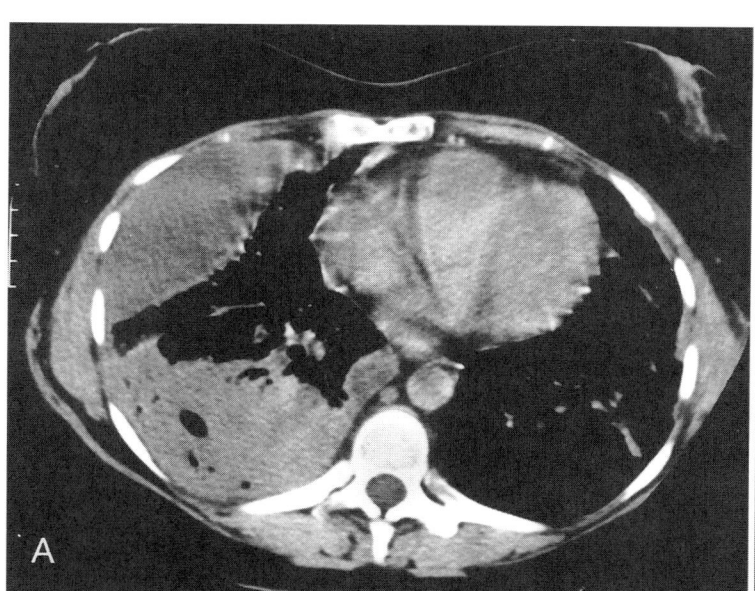
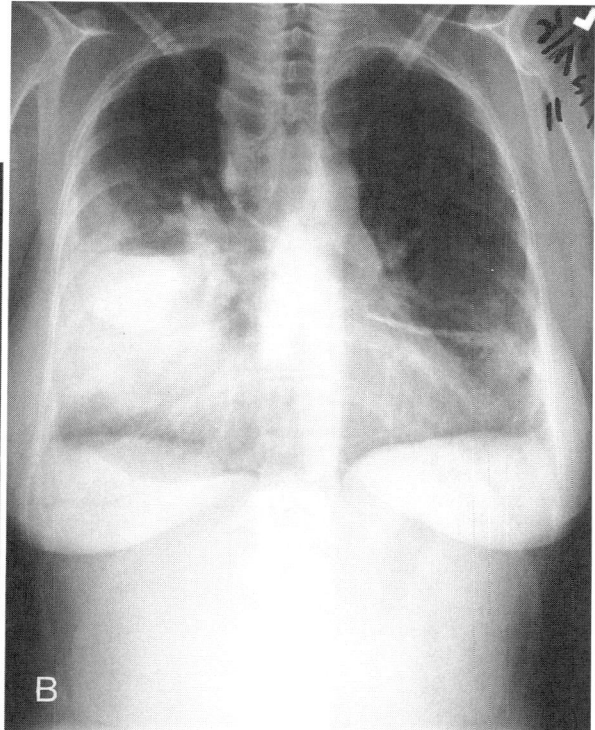

FIGURE 47.6. **A.** CT scan and **B.** chest roentgenogram of an idiopathic exudative pleural effusion ultimately found at VATS to be of a malignant etiology. Previous thoracentesis with blind tube thoracostomy drainage of the effusion was nondiagnostic and had resulted in this complex loculated process.

evaluation of suspicious mediastinal adenopathy out of the reach of cervical mediastinoscopy (18–20). The VATS approach provides excellent access to the aorticopulmonary window on the left and the low subcarinal/subazygous plane on the right. The visibility of the ipsilateral pleural space and mediastinum is excellent (Fig. 47.8). Thoracotomy can be avoided for patients with unresectable disease, as determined thoracoscopically by the presence of malignant mediastinal nodal involvement with the malignancy. Patients with potentially resectable stage III non–small cell lung cancer identified by the VATS approach can be placed into investigational induction chemotherapy/surgery protocols that assess the utility of multimodality treatment for this stage of lung cancer (21, 22). In the authors' experience, there has been no significant morbidity associated with this VATS approach for the assessment of mediastinal adenopathy. Immediate conversion to open thoracotomy can be accomplished without delay in those patients with resectable lung cancer who are found to have benign adenopathy.

The authors also have used the VATS approach as a reasonable alternative to thoracotomy for the intrathoracic dissection of the esophagus during the course of esophagectomy (Fig. 47.9). This VATS exploration and dissection is particularly valuable in determining the resectability of middle third esophageal cancers that may be adherent to the posterior membranous portion of the trachea. It also facilitates a more thorough mediastinal nodal dissection during the course of esophagectomy without the added morbidity of a formal thoracotomy. VATS exploration also can be used as a preoperative staging assessment before initiating multimodality protocols (chemotherapy with or without radiation or surgery) for carcinoma of the esophagus and gastroesophageal junction.

The VATS approach also has been used for the surgical management of benign posterior mediastinal neoplasms and as an alternative to sternotomy to accomplish thymectomy for carefully selected patients with early-stage thymomas (Fig. 47.10) (23–26). It is important to emphasize that a total resection of the thymus gland remains the goal when early-stage thymomas are approached with VATS (27–31). For thymectomy, VATS techniques also appear to be a reasonable alternative to sternotomy or the transcervical thymectomy approach technique for the surgical management of myasthenia gravis. The authors have been quite satisfied with this approach; however, the importance of insuring that a complete thymectomy is per-

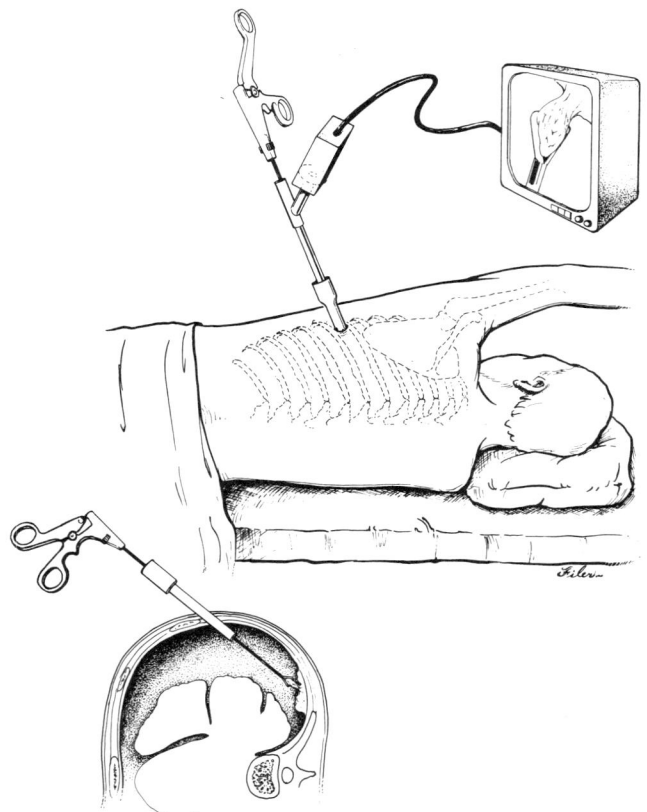

FIGURE 47.7. Illustration of single intercostal access VATS approach for pleural exploration and biopsy.

TABLE 47.3. Advantages of Adjunctive Thoracoscopic Evaluation of Possible Mediastinal Malignancies

---

More complete staging of the ipsilateral mediastinal compartment when evaluating adenopathy associated with bronchogenic carcinoma

Diagnosis of any pleural metastases and simultaneous treatment of associated malignant pleural effusions

Avoidance of a third operative preparation for the management of patients with potentially resectable bronchogenic carcinoma

Potentially earlier induction of appropriate regional/systemic therapy for patients with unresectable or nonsurgical disease

Cosmetically superior and improved visibility of mediastinum compared with anterior mediastinotomy (Chamberlain parasternal exploration)

---

formed to reduce the likelihood of recurrent neurologic symptoms must be reemphasized.

VATS pericardiectomy also appears to have a place in the management of selected patients with symptomatic malignant pericardial effusions (32). The authors reserve this approach for patients with reasonably good functional status who have primary malignant conditions potentially treatable by systemic therapy (i.e., breast cancer or lymphoma). A large swath of pericardium, equivalent to that achieved through lateral thoracotomy, is resected routinely(33). The use of the subxiphoid window approach is still preferred as a means of surgically draining malignant pericardial effusions in patients with unfavorable tumor histologies (i.e., lung cancer) or poor functional status (34).

POTENTIALLY MALIGNANT PULMONARY LESIONS

The use of the VATS approach for the evaluation and selective treatment of patients with pulmonary parenchymal lesions has had the most striking effect on the present thoracic surgical practice of the authors (Table 47.4). Presently, the authors employ the VATS approach as the primary diagnostic maneuver for the evaluation of most indeterminate peripheral pulmonary nodules (35, 36) and also as the usual means of accomplishing closed wedge resection biopsy of undiagnosed pulmonary interstitial infiltrates (37, 38). In selected patients, the VATS approach also is used to accomplish compromise therapeutic wedge resection of small peripheral lung cancers found in patients with significant cardiopulmonary impairment. Video-assisted lobectomy also has been done (39–44). The most obvious technological advances leading to these VATS applications have been the development of an effective endoscopic stapling device (EndoGIA, United States Surgical Corp., Norwalk, CT) and laser resection instrumentation that could be used effectively through the intercostal access sites (45).

INDETERMINATE PULMONARY NODULE

The finding of a new, noncalcified pulmonary nodule on chest roentgenography carries variable clinical significance depending on the patient's medical history, age, travel history and place of habitation, and cigarette use (22, 46, 47). Obviously, the primary patient care concern relates to the potential malignancy of a nodule. A newly found pulmonary nodule appearing in a patient with an active or previous history of malignancy significantly raises the concern that the lesion is a metastatic focus from the remote primary neoplasm. Certainly, a newly found noncalcified nodule in a patient with a significant smoking history has a high probability of being a primary bronchogenic carcinoma. The physical characteristics of the lesion identified by chest roentgenography also can increase the suspicion for malignancy. Lesions of larger size (more than 3 cm in diameter) and those with irregular or stellate borders are more commonly malignant than are smaller, smooth-bordered lesions.

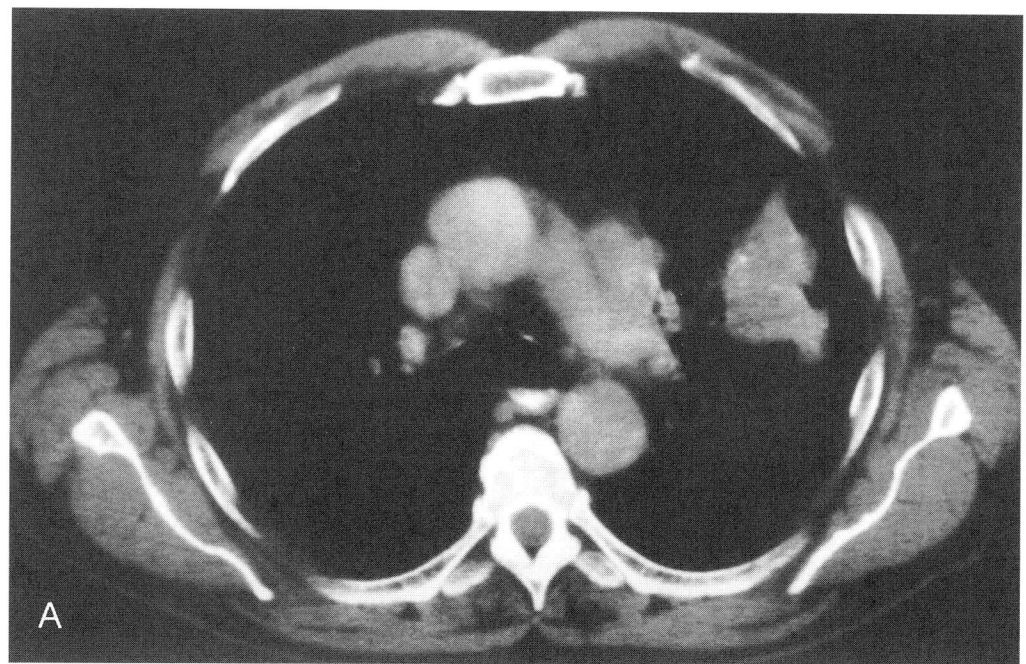
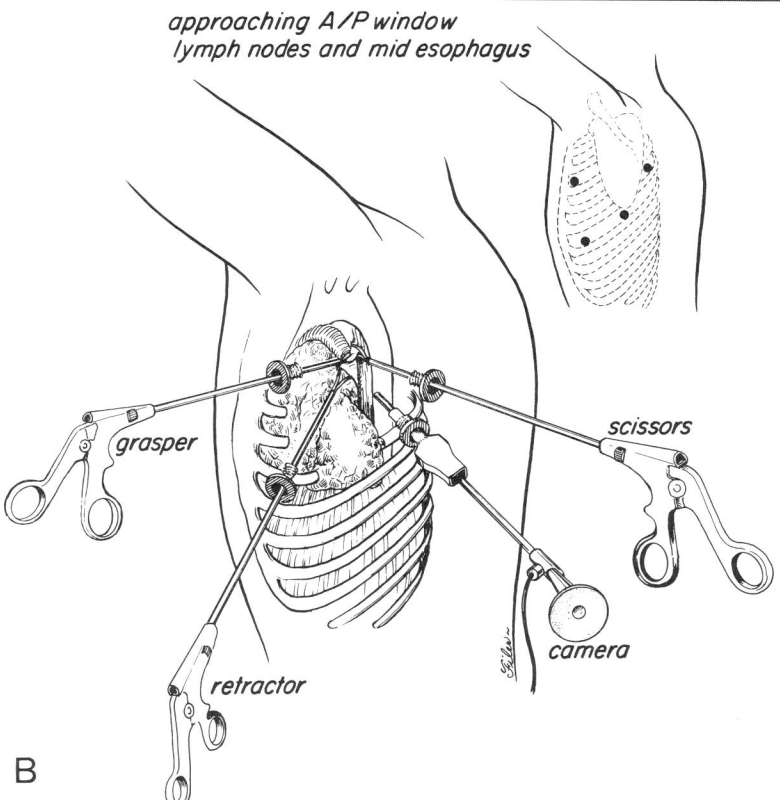

FIGURE 47.8. Mediastinal adenopathy accessible to the VATS approach. **A.** Aorticopulmonary window lymphadenopathy associated with left upper lobe carcinoma. **B.** Line drawing of aorticopulmonary window dissection of lymphadenopathy. (From: Landreneau RJ, Hazelrigg SR, Mack MJ, Fitzgibbon LD, Dowling RD, Acuff TE, Keenan RJ, Ferson PF. Thoracoscopic mediastinal lymph node sampling: a useful approach to mediastinal lymph node stations inaccessible to cervical mediastinoscopy. J Thorac Cardiovasc Surg 1993; 105:554–558.)

FIGURE 47.9. Intercostal access for the right-sided VATS approach to subcarinal lymph node stations and for dissection of the mid esophagus during the course of esophagectomy.

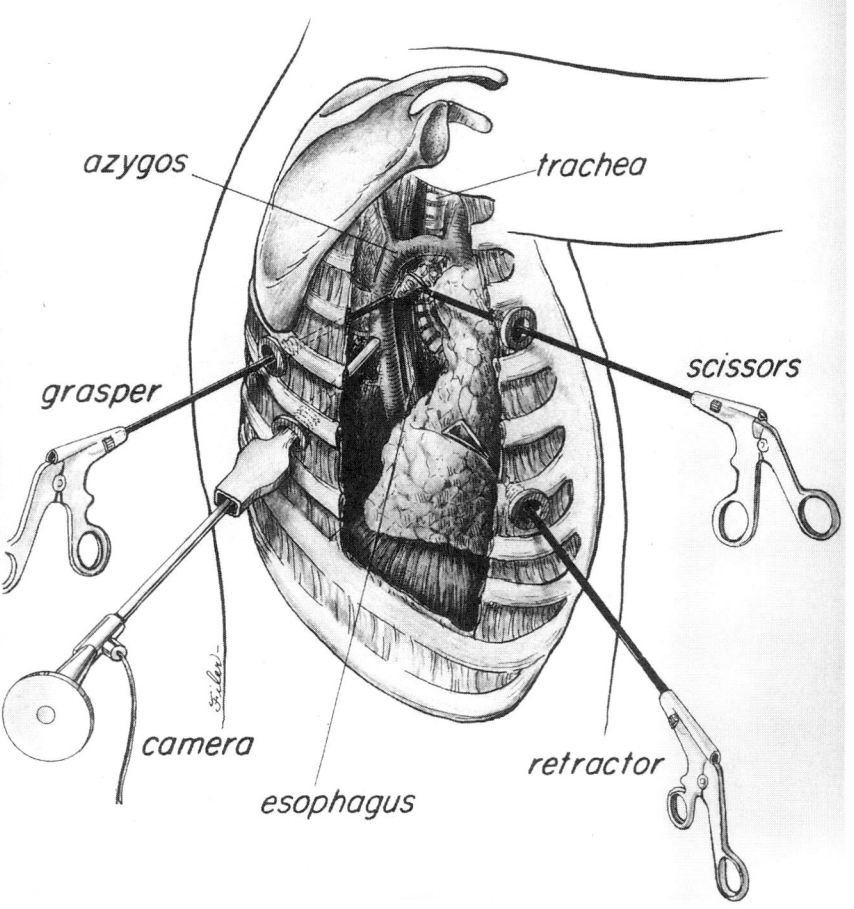

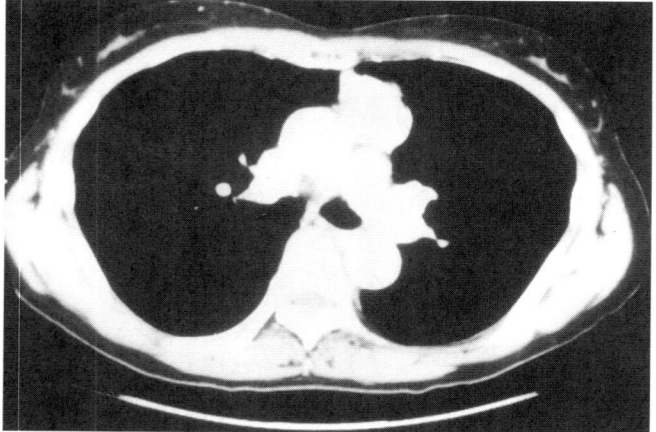

FIGURE 47.10. Stage I thymoma resected using the VATS approach.

TABLE 47.4. Results of Video-Assisted Thoracic Surgery for Lung Resection

	No. of Patients
Lung resections (total)	615
Pulmonary nodules	
Benign	152
Metastatic cancer	107
Primary lung cancer (wedge only)	104
Primary lung cancer (wedge to open lobectomy)	28
Primary lung cancer (VATS lobectomy)	42
Biopsy: diffuse disease	74
Blebs/bullae resection	108

Although these historical and roentgenographic findings may suggest malignancy, biopsy of the lesion is still required, because as many as half of all indeterminate nodules identified ultimately are found to be benign (22, 46, 47). Furthermore, peripheral primary lung cancers presenting as a solitary pulmonary nodule, without mediastinal lymph node involvement, have a reasonable prognosis (up to 80% long-term survival) with surgical resection. This result contrasts with the much less favorable prognosis of most other lung cancers. An aggressive approach to diagnosis and treatment of these early-stage malignancies is justified.

The most appropriate primary diagnostic approach to these peripheral pulmonary lesions remains a subject of spirited debate. Percutaneous CT-directed biopsy of such lesions is recommended by some as a primary diagnostic approach (48, 49). The advantages of this percutaneous biopsy approach primarily relates to confirming the diagnosis of malignancy in the totally inoperable patient. However, the morbid consequences of this approach (pneumothorax, hemothorax) in these patients with impaired cardiopulmonary reserve can be substantial. Percutaneous biopsy also is useful for the diagnosis of metastatic pulmonary spread from a remote malignancy when multiple accessible peripheral pulmonary lesions are present. Although percutaneous CT-directed biopsy can diagnose malignancy in 70% to 90% of peripheral lung cancers of adequate size (more than 2 cm in diameter), the primary shortcoming of this approach relates to the lack of reliability in obtaining a true negative biopsy result (50). Indeed, a specific benign diagnosis can only be assured in fewer than 20% of peripheral lung lesions biopsied. The possibility of missing an actual lung cancer from a sampling error remains significant in these circumstances.

There are several clinical scenarios that usually follow for the indeterminate peripheral pulmonary nodule in the patient who can tolerate surgery. If the solitary lesion is found to be malignant, surgical resection is performed. Surgical resection also is indicated when a specific benign diagnosis has not been established. Resection is necessary to avoid missing an otherwise curable lung cancer incorrectly diagnosed as a benign lesion. Therefore, few circumstances exist when the percutaneous CT-directed needle biopsy approach actually adds to the clinical decision-making paradigm required to manage these lesions successfully. A recent study from the thoracic surgical group at the University of Virginia (51), and as yet unpublished data from the authors' group, corroborate these general impressions held by many thoracic surgeons (51, 52). In these studies, fewer than 10% of the patient's clinical course was impacted specifically by the percutaneous biopsy results.

The authors now rely on the VATS approach to accomplish the primary diagnosis of most indeterminate peripheral nodules (35, 52) as an alternative to percutaneous CT-directed biopsy and open thoracotomy for the wedge resection biopsy of the lesion. Excisional biopsy formerly was performed routinely. The characteristics of lesions suitable for the VATS approach are noted in Table 47.5. A typical lesion approached by VATS for wedge resection excisional biopsy is shown in Figure 47.11.

A three-stick intercostal access approach typically is used to accomplish pulmonary wedge resection of these lesions. The usual sites and instrument alignment for this VATS approach are illustrated in Figure 47.12. This approach relies on an inferior mid axillary line intercostal access site for videoscope introduction to accomplish the initial thoracoscopic exploration of the pleural cavity. Usually, two additional intercostal access sites are established higher in an anterior and posterolateral location relative to the initial access site. These sites are used to manipulate the lung for identification of the lesion and for the ultimate introduction of the endoscopic stapling device or laser tools needed to accomplish the resection. The usual steps for endostapled wedge resection of the pulmonary parenchymal lesion are depicted in Figure 47.13 (53). This technique primarily entails identification of the lesion followed by application of the stapling device from one of the lateral intercostal access sites. The staple line is then inspected for bleeding and air leakage. After the integrity of the staple line has been assured, the stapler is moved to the contralateral intercostal access site and positioned beneath the residual base of lung tissue

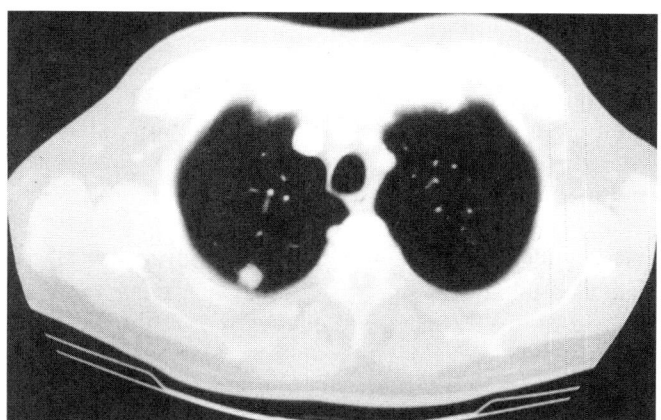

FIGURE 47.11. Outer third, noncalcified peripheral pulmonary nodule ideally suited for VATS wedge resection biopsy.

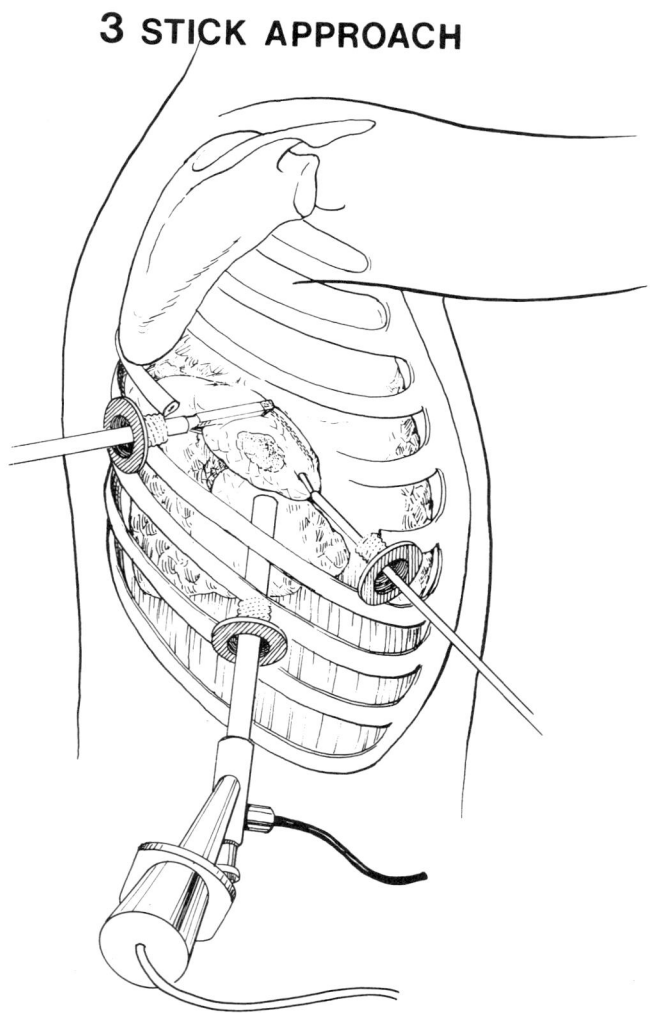

FIGURE 47.12. Three-stick intercostal access used to accomplish VATS pulmonary wedge resection. (From Ferson PF, Landreneau RJ, Dowling RD, Hazelrigg SR, Magee MJ, Bowers CM, Perrino MK, et al. Thoracoscopic vs. open lung biopsy for the diagnosis of diffuse infiltrative lung disease. J Thorac Cardiovasc Surg 1993;105:194–199.)

below the lung lesion. The stapler is fired, completing the standard V-stapled wedge resection of the lung. The specimen is then placed into a commercially available retrieval bag before removing it from the chest cavity, thus avoiding chest wall contamination during its extraction. The specimen is then sent to surgical pathology for immediate histologic confirmation of the lesion's etiology.

In many thoracic surgeons' hands, this VATS approach has been an efficient and accurate means of managing the indeterminate pulmonary nodule. Operative and postoperative morbidity has been remarkably minimal (35, 52). The specificity and sensitivity of the excised specimens for the disease process in question has been 100%. Hospital stay among patients undergoing VATS wedge resection alone has averaged only 3 days. The extra expense, potential morbidity, and delays in definitive management related to primary percutaneous CT-directed biopsy are avoided. Those patients who are found to have a truly benign lesion have avoided an unnecessary thoracotomy. The need for prolonged roentgenographic follow-up of the now excised pulmonary pathology is averted. Finally, patients with malignant pulmonary lesions can undergo the appropriate surgical treatment immediately under the same operative anesthetic.

INFILTRATIVE LUNG DISEASE

New or progressive pulmonary infiltrates appearing in patients with a previous history of treated malignancy are serious diagnostic challenges for the attending physician. The same is true for new infiltrates appearing in patients presently undergoing systemic therapy for their neoplastic process. In these circumstances, the differential diagnosis includes pulmonary lymphangitic spread of the malignancy, pulmonary toxicities from the therapy, or infection (opportunistic, pyogenic, or a combination of these infections). Clinical deterioration can be rapid in many cases, emphasizing the importance of an expedient diagnosis to direct therapy of all treatable etiologies accurately.

Transbronchoscopic lavage and biopsy are reasonable first-line approaches for diagnosis. When these studies are nondiagnostic or contraindicated because of an underlying coagulopathy or pulmonary hypertension, surgical wedge resection biopsy often is required.

Among ventilator dependent patients, the authors continue to recommend a limited lateral thoracotomy to accomplish open lung biopsy. The rationale for this recommendation is that conversion to double-lumen endotracheal intubation and single-lung ventilation is hazardous in this setting, thus prohibiting an effective use of VATS.

The VATS approach is advocated for lung biopsy when surgical intervention is necessary to evaluate progressive pulmonary infiltrates in non–ventilator dependent patients. An equivalent closed wedge resection obtained through open thoracotomy can be achieved. The panoramic view of the entire pleural cavity and lung surface afforded with VATS is another advantage of this technique over lateral thoracotomy (37). This expansive view helps the surgeon avoid biopsy sampling errors caused by inadequate access to the diseased lung through a small lateral thoracotomy incision (Fig. 47.14).

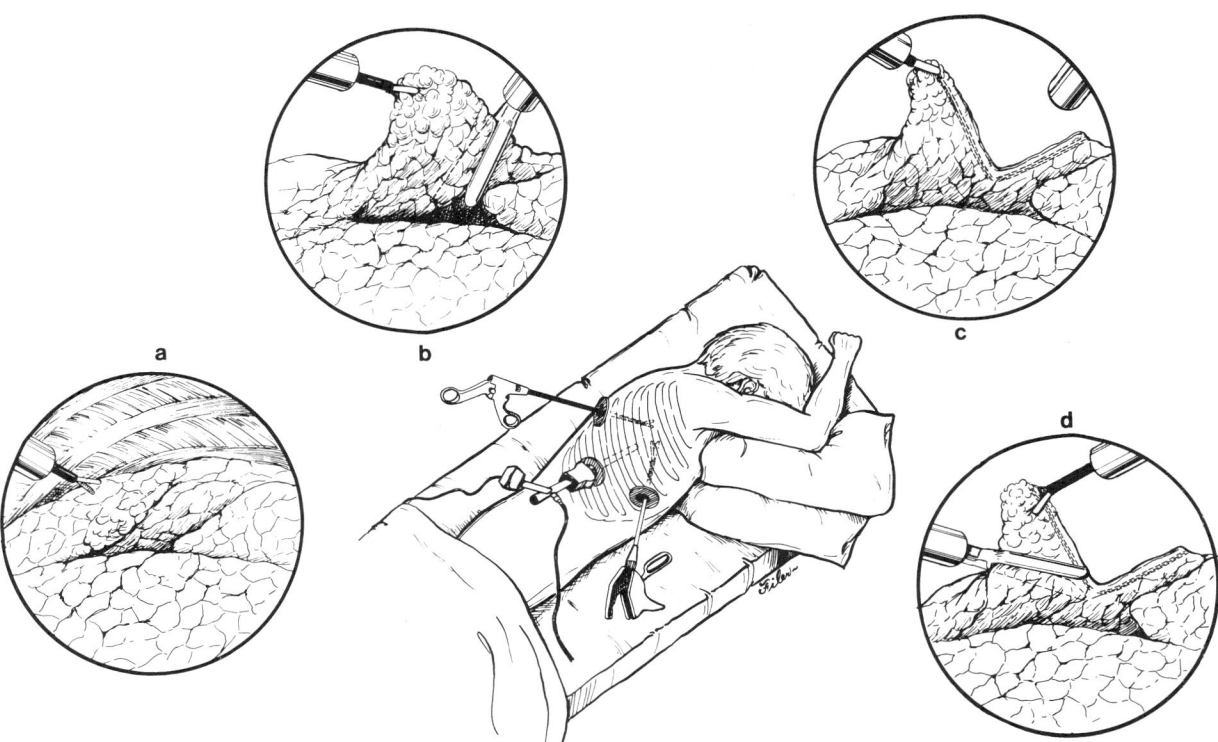

FIGURE 47.13. Illustration depicting serial application of the endostapling device to accomplish a standard V-wedge resection of the lung. Note that the intercostal access position of the stapling instrument and the grasping tools are reversed to complete the stapled wedge resection expeditiously (From Dowling RD, Landreneau RJ, Ferson PF. Thoracoscopic wedge resection of the lung. Surgery Rounds 1993;16:341–349.)

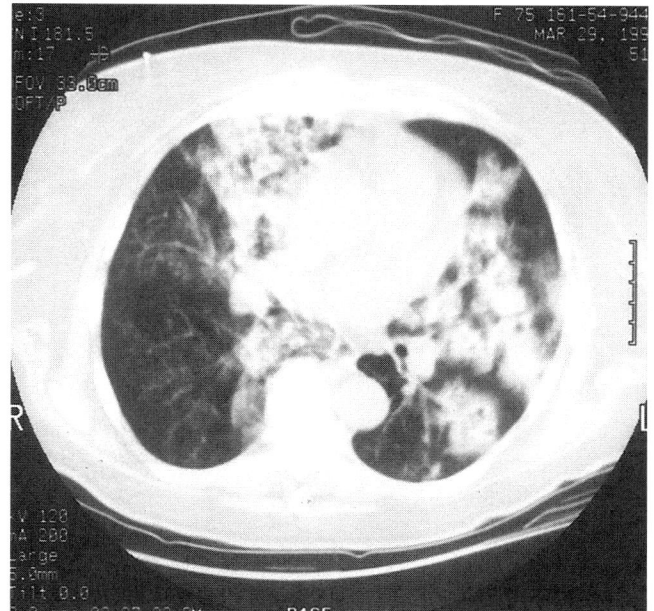

FIGURE 47.14. Interstitial lung disease: CT scan showing patchy distribution of disease requiring precise biopsy site selection to identify representatively diseased lung.

COMPROMISE LUNG RESECTION FOR PRIMARY CARCINOMA OF THE LUNG

Subanatomic resection (wedge or segmentectomy) of small peripheral lung cancers has been shown to be a reasonable surgical approach for patients with cardiopulmonary impairment or those whose advanced age makes them poor candidates for formal lobectomy (54–58). In general, the same criteria for resection of indeterminate peripheral pulmonary nodules outlined in Table 47.5 also apply for VATS subanatomic resection of known peripheral carcinomas. Although it is accepted that the local recurrence risk is greater when subanatomic resection is used, it does not appear that survival is significantly different in patients with early-stage disease treated either with sublobar resections or lobectomy (59–63). The addition of postoperative, limited field, local adjuvant radiotherapy may assist in reducing this local recurrence rate (61). A North American cancer intergroup trial is presently being formulated that specifically addresses the merits of the combination of subanatomic lung resection and adjuvant radiotherapy as

TABLE 47.5. Video-Assisted Thoracic Surgery for Pulmonary Resection

Candidate pulmonary nodules
  Noncalcified, less than 3 cm in diameter
  Indeterminate etiology after appropriate workup
  Location in the outer one third of the lung
  Absence of endobronchial extension (? with VATS lobectomy)

selective surgical treatment of non–small cell carcinoma of the lung.

The fact that these lesser resections are considered appropriate in selected patients with non–small cell lung cancer reflects the growing appreciation among thoracic surgeons that the systemic and biologic characteristics of the cancer, rather than the extent of resectioning, are the true determinants of survival. The appreciation of these concepts by thoracic surgeons is similar to the transition made by breast cancer surgeons from radical mastectomy to lesser resections in the management of small carcinomas of the breast.

The authors have employed the VATS approach for subanatomic wedge resection in more than 100 lung cancer patients with significant impairment in cardiopulmonary reserve. A thorough mediastinal nodal sampling accompanied these resections to stage the patient's disease properly. More than 90% of these lesions have been determined pathologically to be stage I malignancies. The surgical margins, as evaluated pathologically, have been adequate in all cases; however, re-resection deep to the lesion was required occasionally because of close proximity of the tumor to the initial line of resection. Although the median follow-up is only 3 years, survival trends and recurrences parallel the experience with open thoracotomy approaches to subanatomic resection done by the authors and those reported in the literature. Continued follow-up and prospective evaluation of these subanatomic VATS resections continue to be an active aspect of the group's clinical investigation.

VATS PULMONARY METASTASECTOMY

The therapeutic role of pulmonary metastasectomy remains controversial. It is the authors' belief that there is only a limited role for pulmonary metastasectomy used with a curative intent. Nonetheless, there is a role for surgical intervention to diagnose a minority of patients with presumed pulmonary metastases that cannot be confirmed histologically by less invasive means. When surgical intervention is required, the VATS approach is an ideal means of establishing a diagnosis of such metastatic disease, if it is located in the outer third of the lung parenchyma (2, 64). Candidate lesions for pulmonary metastasectomy are similar to those described for VATS resection of indeterminate pulmonary nodules (Table 47.6). The primary tenants used by the authors in choosing therapeutic metastasectomy are noted in Table 47.7.

The VATS approach also is a reasonable surgical alternative to open thoracotomy approaches when limited pulmonary disease burden (approximately three or fewer lesions) located in a periphery of the lung is approached with a curative intent. The authors consider the VATS approach adequate if all target lesions noted on preoperative CT can be identified and resected. If *all* target lesions are not identified without thoracoscopic evidence of more extensive disease, conversion to an open thoracotomy is recommended to localize and resect the occult pathology. If multiple lesions are identified, for all practical purposes, the surgical maneuver has only a diagnostic role.

These views of the authors are contrary to those of surgeons who favor a more aggressive approach to pulmonary metastasectomy. It is frequently stated that because the primary determinant of survival is the ability to clear the patient of all their disease, radical resection is indicated. The flaw in this philosophy is that it ignores the fact that patients whose tumors are unresectable or incompletely resectable usually have a greater disease burden and a more biologically aggressive malignant phenotype. In many reports patients who underwent curative resection had very limited disease burden (two or fewer nodules) and the primary mode of resection was a standard wedge excision

TABLE 47.6. Advantages of Video-Assisted Thoracic Surgical Wedge Resection in Management of Indeterminate Pulmonary Nodules

Minimally invasive surgical approach
Virtually 100% effective in locating and diagnosing the pulmonary lesion
No mortality and minimal morbidity
Tolerated by patients with limited cardiopulmonary reserve
Reduced postoperative hospitalization

TABLE 47.7 Criteria for Therapeutic Resection of Lung Metastases

Complete control of the primary tumor without evidence of residual or recurrent local disease
Patient can tolerate the required surgical procedure
All known metastatic disease can be removed with the proposed operative therapy
  Tumor biology considerations (disease free interval, pulmonary disease burden, tumor histology, tumor doubling time, heterogeneity of metastatic tumor size)
No other effective therapy for pulmonary metastases

(equivalent to what could be accomplished through VATS in many cases). With regard to many reported survival comparisons, there also appear to be invalid analyses between widely disparate patient groups when referring to patients resected and those who are not resected. It is the authors' opinion that until an adequate control group is established, the results of pulmonary metastasectomy will remain suspect for most circumstances to which it has been applied.

As with other approaches to metastasectomy, careful postoperative roentgenographic surveillance is required after curative VATS metastasectomy. An occasional patient may be a candidate for re-resection if isolated, limited, pulmonary metastatic recurrence is noted later. If the recurrent lesion is present in the periphery of the lung, a second VATS resection can be accomplished.

VATS LOBECTOMY

Recently, the authors' group and others have been exploring the utility of the VATS approach for formal anatomic lung resection (39–44). Depending on the limitations of the operative visibility and the technical safety of individual patients, the authors now selectively employ a totally endoscopic surgical dissection approach (Fig. 47.15) or a mini-thoracotomy approach with video assistance to accomplish most formal pulmonary resections. The primary difference between these two methods is that some rib spreading is required through the mini–muscle-sparing thoracotomy approach so that direct visual and manual access to the pulmonary hilum can be achieved. This mini-thoracotomy with video-assistance and intrathoracic illumination actually is a hybrid approach that takes advantage of the added safety of open thoracotomy and the reduced morbidity of a near total endosurgical procedure.

Among properly selected patients, the authors have been quite pleased with the results with these minimally invasive approaches to formal pulmonary resection. At present, they have accomplished more than 100 VATS lobectomies without mortality; one must remember, however, that the authors developed a substantial VATS experience with less technically demanding procedures before undertaking VATS lobectomy. This VATS experience overlaid these surgeons' considerable experience with established conventional thoracic surgical technique.

Recent studies have demonstrated that the perioperative morbidity and overall length of hospital stay can be reduced by using VATS approaches (39–44). It also appears that adequate oncologic management of lung cancer can be achieved using these VATS approaches to lobectomy. In two recent reports of VATS lobectomy, the mediastinal lymph node staging and surgical resection margins were equivalent to those obtained through open muscle-sparing approaches to lobectomy (42, 44). It must be stressed, however, that compromise of surgical oncologic principles is not acceptable when using the VATS approach to formal pulmonary resection.

At the present time, the VATS approach to lobectomy is recommended only for patients with peripheral malignancies that are clinically stage I without evidence of significant hilar or mediastinal adenopathy (or fibrosis) identified at VATS exploration. The absence of well-developed pulmonary lobar fissures also can make this video-assisted approach difficult or impossible to accomplish. Finally, it is essential that the surgeon has adequate VATS experience to prevent violation of important surgical oncologic principles and avoid potentially serious patient morbidity.

THORACIC SPLANCHNICECTOMY

Finally, the VATS approach is useful in performing thoracic splanchnicectomy when this pain control measure is considered for patients with an adequate functional status and unremitting pain from an upper abdominal visceral malignancy. The VATS technique offers a reasonable means of achieving significant relief in patients for whom less invasive measures have failed to control cancer pain (65, 66).

CONCLUSIONS

VATS has become an accepted treatment modality for many benign and malignant thoracic surgical

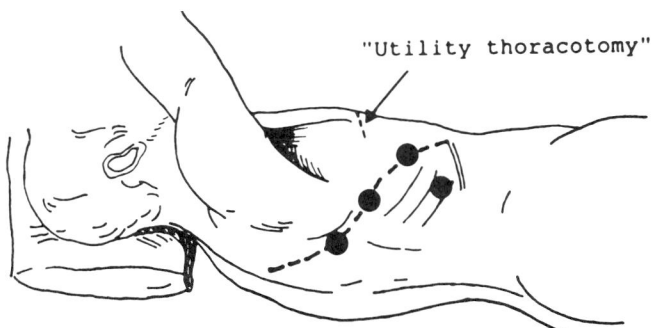

FIGURE 47.15. VATS lobectomy. Anterolateral utility incision and posterolateral arc of the intercostal access for videoscopic instrumentation. (From Roviaro G, Rebuffat C, Varoli F, Vergani C, Mariani C, Maciocco M. Video-endoscopic pulmonary lobectomy for cancer. Surg Laparosc Endosc 1992;2:244–247.)

problems. Its role in thoracic oncologic practice is likely to expand in the future as surgical experience increases and longer term clinical results are known. Long-term follow-up data are sure to help in defining the most appropriate applications of VATS in thoracic surgical oncologic practice.

REFERENCES

1. Mack MJ, Aronoff R, Acuff T, Douthit M, Bowman R, Ryan W. The present role of thoracoscopy in the diagnosis and treatment of diseases of the chest. Ann Thorac Surg 1992;54:405–9.
2. Landreneau RJ, Mack MJ, Hazelrigg SR, Dowling RD, Keenan RJ, Ferson PF. The role of thoracoscopy in the management of intrathoracic neoplastic processes. Semin Thorac Cardiovasc Surg 1993;5:219–228.
3. Jacobaeus HC. The practical importance of thoracoscopy in surgery of the chest. Surg Gynecol Obstet 1922;34:289–96.
4. Thomas P. Thoracoscopy: an old procedure revisited. In: Kittle CF, ed. Current controversies in thoracic surgery. Philadelphia: WB Saunders, 1986:101–112.
5. Brandt H, Loddenkemper R, Mai J. Atlas of diagnostic thoracoscopy. Indications-techniques. New York: Thieme Medical Publishers, 1985:1–46.
6. Landreneau RJ, Mack MJ, Hazelrigg SR, Dowling RD, Acuff TE, Magee MJ, Ferson PF. Video assisted thoracic surgery: basic technical concepts and intercostal approach Strategies. Ann Thorac Surg 1992;54:800–807.
7. Landreneau RJ, Mack MJ, Keenan RJ, Dowling RD, Hazelrigg SR, Ferson PF. Strategic planning for video-assisted thoracic surgery VATS. Ann Thorac Surg 1993;56:615–619.
8. Landreneau RJ, Hazelrigg SR, Mack MJ, Perrino MK, Nunchuck S, Ritter PS, Defino J, et al. Postoperative pain-related morbidity: video-assisted thoracic surgery vs thoracotomy. Ann Thorac Surg 1993;56:1285–1289.
9. Landreneau RJ, Mack MJ, Hazelrigg SR, Naunheim K, Dowling RD, Magee MJ, Ritter PS, et al. Prevalence of chronic pain following pulmonary resection by thoracotomy or video-assisted thoracic surgery. J Thorac Cardiovasc Surg 1994;107:1079–1086.
10. Plunkett MB, Peterson MS, Landreneau RJ, Ferson PF, Posner MC. CT guided preoperative percutaneous needle localization of peripheral pulmonary nodules. Radiology 1992;185:274–6.
11. Miller JI, Hatcher CR. Thoracoscopy: a useful tool in the diagnosis of thoracic disease. Ann Thorac Surg 1978;26:68–72.
12. Page RD, Jeffrey RR, Donnelly RJ. Thoracoscopy: a review of 121 consecutive surgical procedures. Ann Thorac Surg 1989;48:66–68.
13. Canto A, Ferrer G, Romagosa V, Moya J, Bernat R. Lung cancer and pleural effusion. Clinical significance and study of pleural metastatic locations. Chest 1987;87:649–352.
14. Keenan RJ, Landreneau RJ, Mack MJ, Acuff TE, Hazelrigg SR, Ferson PF. Video-assisted thoracoscopy for the diagnosis and management of pleural diseases. Am Rev Respir Dis 1993;147:A737.
15. Canto A, Rivas J, Moya J, Saumench J, Pac J, Morera R, Ferrer G. Pleural effusion of malignant etiology. Thoracoscopic use of talc as an effective method of pleurodesis. Med Clin (Barc) 1985;84:806–808.
16. Daniel TM, Tribble CG, Rodgers BM. Thoracoscopy and talc poudrage for pneumothoraces and effusions. Ann Thorac Surg 1990;50:186–189.
17. Ridley PD, Braimbridge MV. Thoracoscopic debridement and pleural irrigation in the management of empyema thoracis. Ann Thorac Surg 1991;51:461–464.
18. Shields T. The significance of ipsilateral mediastinal lymph node metastasis (N2 disease) in non–small cell carcinoma of the lung. J Thorac Cardiovasc Surg 1990;99:48–53.
19. McNeill T, Chamberlain J. Diagnostic anterior mediastinotomy. Ann Thorac Surg 1966;2:532–39.
20. Landreneau RJ, Hazelrigg SR, Mack MJ, Fitzgibbon LD, Dowling RD, Acuff TE, Keenan RJ, et al. Thoracoscopic mediastinal lymph node sampling: a useful approach to mediastinal lymph node stations inaccessible to cervical mediastinoscopy. J Thorac Cardiovasc Surg 1993;105:554–558.
21. Mountain CF. A new international staging system for lung cancer. Chest 1986;89:225S–33S
22. Landreneau RJ. Carcinoma of the lung: who will benefit from surgery? Postgrad Med 1990;87:117–135.
23. Landreneau RJ, Dowling RD, Ferson PF. Thoracoscopic resection of a posterior mediastinal mass. Chest 1992;102:1288–1290.
24. Naunheim KS, Andrus CH. Thoracoscopic drainage and resection of a giant mediastinal mass. Ann Thorac Surg 1993;55:156–158.
25. Landreneau RJ, Dowling RD, Castillo W, Ferson PF. Thoracoscopic resection of an anterior mediastinal mass. Ann Thorac Surg 1992;54:142–4.
26. Hazelrigg SR, Mack MJ, Landreneau RJ. Video-assisted thoracic surgery for mediastinal disease. Chest Surg Clin North Am 1993;3:283–297.
27. Masaoka A, Monden Y, Nakahara K, Tanioka T. Follow-up study of thymoma with special reference to their clinical stages. Cancer 1981;48:2485–2492.
28. Wilkens EW, Grillo HC, Seanell JG, et al. Role of staging in prognosis and management of thymoma. Ann Thorac Surg 1991;51:888–892.
29. Verley JM, Hollmann KH. Thymoma. A comparative study of clinical stages, histologic features, and survival in 200 cases. Cancer 1985;55:1074–1086.
30. Kirschner PA. Reoperation for thymoma: report of 23 cases. Ann Thorac Surg 1990;49:550–555.
31. Pescarmona E, Rendina EA, Ventura F, et al. Analysis of prognostic factors and clinicopathological staging of thymoma. Ann Thorac Surg 1990;50:534–8.
32. Mack MJ, Landreneau RJ. Hazelrigg SR, Acuff T. Video thoracoscopic management of benign and malignant pericardial effusions. Chest 1993;103:390S–393S.
33. Piehler JM, Pluth JR, Schaff HV, Danielson GK, Orszulak TA, Puga FJ. Surgical management of effusive pericardial disease. J Thorac Cardiovasc Surg 1985;90:506–516.
34. Naunheim KS, Kesler KA, Fiore AC, Turrentine M, Hammell LM, Brown JW, Mohammed Y, et al. Pericardial drainage: subxiphoid vs. transthoracic approach. Eur J Cardiothorac Surg 1991;5:99–104.
35. Mack MJ, Hazelrigg SR, Landreneau RJ, Acuff TE. Thoracoscopy for the diagnosis of the indeterminate solitary pulmonary nodule. Ann Thorac Surg 1993;56:825–832.
36. Allen MS Deschamps C, Lee RE, Trastek VF, Pairolero PC. Thoracoscopic wedge excision for indeterminate pulmonary nodules. J Thorac Cardiovasc Surg 1993;106:1048–1052.
37. Ferson PF, Landreneau RJ, Dowling RD, Hazelrigg SR, Magee MJ, Bowers CM, Perrino MK, et al. Thoracoscopic vs. open lung biopsy for the diagnosis of diffuse infiltrative lung disease. J Thorac Cardiovasc Surg 1993:105:194–199.

38. Bensard DD, McIntyre RC, Waring BJ, Simon JS. Comparison of video-assisted lung biopsy to open lung biopsy in the evaluation of interstitial lung disease. Chest 1993;103:765–770.
39. Roviaro G, Rebuffat C, Varoli F, Vergani C, Mariani C, Maciocco M. Video-endoscopic pulmonary lobectomy for cancer. Surg Laparose Endosc 1992;2:244–7.
40. Kirby TJ, Mack MJ, Landreneau RJ, Rice TW. Initial experience with video-assisted thoracoscopic lobectomy. Ann Thorac Surg 1993;56:1248–1253.
41. Walker WS, Carnochan FM, Pugh, GC. Thoracoscopic pulmonary lobectomy. Early operative experience and preliminary clinical results. J Thorac Cardiovasc Surg 1993;106:1111–1117.
42. McKenna RJ. Lobectomy by video-assisted thoracic surgery with mediastinal node sampling for lung cancer. J Thorac Cardiovasc Surg 1994;107:879–882.
43. Giudicelli R, Thomas P, Lonjon T, Ragni J, Morati N, Ottomani R, Fuentes PA, Shennib H, et al. Comparative study of lobectomy through conventional thoracotomy and video–assisted thoracoscopy. Ann Thorac Surg 1994;58:712–718.
44. Kirby TJ, Mack MJ, Landreneau RJ, Rice TW. Lobectomy: VATS vs. thoracotomy. A randomized study. J Thorac Cardiovasc Surg 1995;109:997–1002.
45. Landreneau RJ, Hazelrigg SR, Ferson PF, Dowling RD, Bowers CM, Curtis JJ, Boley TM. Thoracoscopic resection of 85 pulmonary lesions. Ann Thorac Surg 1992;54:415–420.
46. Lillington GA. Management of solitary pulmonary nodules. Dis Mon 1992;37:271–318.
47. Lillington GA, Caskey CI. Evaluation and management of solitary and multiple pulmonary nodules. Clin Chest Med 1993;14:111–119.
48. Salazar AM, Westcott JL. The role of transthoracic needle biopsy for the diagnosis and staging of lung cancer. Clin Chest Med 1993;14:99–110.
49. Midthun DE, Swenson SJ, Jett JR. Clinical strategies for solitary pulmonary nodules. Ann Rev Med 1992;41:195–208.
50. Landreneau RJ, Mack MJ, Hazelrigg SR, Dowling RD, Ferson PF. Video-assisted thoracic surgical resection of benign pulmonary lesions. Chest Surg Clin North Am 1993;3:283–297.
51. Calhoun P, Feldman PS, Armstrong P, et al. The clinical outcome of needle aspirations of the lung when cancer is not diagnosed. Ann Thorac Surg 1986;41:592–596.
52. Mack MJ, Mitruka S, Landreneau RJ. Relative utility of percutaneous CT directed biopsy vs. VATS excisional biopsy of indeterminate peripheral pulmonary nodules. Second International Symposium on Video-Assisted Thoracic Surgery—Technology on Trial, American Association of Thoracic Surgeons, New York, April 24, 1994.
53. Dowling RD, Landreneau RJ, Ferson PF. Thoracoscopic wedge resection of the lung. Surgery Rounds 1993;16:341–349.
54. Keagy BA, Pharr WF, Bowes DE, Wilcox BR. A review of morbidity and mortality in elderly patients undergoing pulmonary resection. Am Surg 1984;50:213–216.
55. Errett LE, Wilson J, Chiu RC, Munro DD. Wedge resection as an alternative procedure for peripheral bronchogenic carcinoma in poor-risk patients. J Thorac Cardiovasc Surg 1985;90:656–661.
56. Pastorino U, Valente M, Bedini V, et al. Limited resection for stage I lung cancer. Eur J Surg Oncol 1991;17:42–48.
57. Macchiarini P, Fontanini G, Hardin JM, Pingitore R, Angeletti A. Most peripheral, node-negative, non–small-cell lung cancers have low proliferative rates and no intratumoral and peritumoral blood and lymphatic invasion. Rationale for treatment with wedge resection alone. J Thorac Cardiovasc Surg 1992;104:892–109.
58. Lewis RJ. The role of video-assisted thoracic surgery (VATS) for primary carcinoma of the lung: wedge resection to lobectomy by simultaneous individual stapling. Ann Thorac Surg 1993;56:762–768.
59. Ginsberg RJ, Rubenstein LV. Patients with T1N0 non–small cell lung cancer (abstract 304). Lung Cancer 1991;7(Suppl):83.
60. Ginsberg RJ. Limited resection in the treatment of stage in non–small cell lung cancer: an overview. Chest 1989;96:505–515.
61. Miller JI, Hatcher CR. Limited resection of bronchogenic carcinoma in the patient with marked impairment of pulmonary function. Ann Thorac Surg 1987;44:340–343.
62. Warren WH, Faber LP. Segmentectomy vs. lobectomy in patients with stage I pulmonary carcinoma: five year survival and patterns of intrathoracic recurrence. J Thorac Cardiovasc Surg 1994;107:1087–1094.
63. Shennib H, Landreneau RJ, Mack MJ. Video assisted thoracoscopic wedge resection of T1 lung cancer in high risk patients. Ann Surg 1993;218:555–560.
64. Dowling RD, Ferson PF, Landreneau RJ. Thoracoscopic resection of pulmonary metastases. Chest 1992;102:1450–1454.
65. Stone HH, Chauvin EJ. Pancreatic denervation for pain relief in chronic alcohol associated pancreatitis. Br J Surg 1990;77:303–305.
66. Worsey J, Ferson PF, Keenan RJ, Landreneau RJ. Thoracoscopic pancreatic denervation for pain in unresectable pancreatic cancer. Br J Surg 1993;80:1051–1052.

48

Supportive Care in Cancer Patients

Jean Klastersky

INTRODUCTION

Supportive care for the patient with cancer has improved markedly over the last two decades, permitting better therapies and a resulting improved quality and quantity of survival. The supportive care advances have occurred across a broad spectrum of clinical, social, and psychologic arenas. These improvements allow for more aggressive and potentially curative therapies to be given with less toxicity and mortality. Better management of symptoms has made the disease and its treatment more tolerable. Other supportive care measures have been developed to improve patients' quality of life. Supportive care is essential for the treatment for cancer regardless of whether therapy for the cancer is planned. Although many of the technical improvements have developed from the aggressive treatment of diseases, such as acute leukemia and bone marrow transplantation (BMT), the lessons learned in these settings form the basis on which much of cancer treatment is based.

This chapter reviews the physical, social, and psychologic aspects of general supportive care. The discussion does not focus solely on thoracic cancers because these supportive care measures are applicable to many neoplastic diseases.

INFECTION PREVENTION AND TREATMENT

Because the mortality from infection during periods of granulocytopenia and immunosuppression is very high, empiric broad-spectrum antibiotic therapy should be initiated at the onset of fever. However, fever is not the only parameter to be considered; other clinical features also may require the initiation of empiric therapy, such as a sudden modification of the general health status, signs of hemodynamic instability, or the appearance of cutaneous lesions or chest radiograph infiltrates.

The choice of antibiotics for both prevention and treatment should not be adopted blindly from the literature. Rather, the choice should be developed based on the pattern of infections associated with any particular underlying disease, the nature of the nosocomial pathogens encountered in a given institution (or resident on the patient), and the susceptibility of the pathogens to antibiotics.

PREVENTION STRATEGY

Prevention is based on four main measures: isolation in a protected environment, surveillance culturing, antimicrobial prophylaxis, and enhancement of host defenses. To determine useful guidelines for prevention, it is essential to define the possible sources of infection and the organisms commonly encountered (1).

Infection in granulocytopenic patients arises from the patients' endogenous flora, rather than from external sources. Both are linked intimately, however, because the granulocytopenic patient who is exposed to the hospital environment will rapidly acquire nosocomial flora.

TOTAL PROTECTED ISOLATION

A disinfected room with laminar air flow provides a sterile environment, because incoming air is filtered through a high efficiency particulate air filter. Food is cooked, and all items that enter the room are sterilized in advance. These measures must be associated with strict personal hygiene. Several studies have demonstrated a decrease in the incidence of infections with total protected isolation: in particular, through air filtration, airborne infections such as aspergillosis can be prevented. However, patients colonized by *Aspergillus* species before isolation can develop pulmonary aspergillosis while in the laminar air flow room.

SURVEILLANCE CULTURING

Routine assessment of microbial flora in several body sites constitutes surveillance culturing. Sampling oral cavity, anal verge, urine, and skin sites (e.g., axilla) allow for monitoring of microbial flora inhabiting the patient. Assessing this flora allows for a more customized empiric antibiotic regimen, including therapy against more resistant organisms.

Colonization of the nares with *Aspergillus* species often precedes pulmonary aspergillosis in granulocytopenic patients. In this setting, routine surveillance culturing of the nares is helpful for early treatment of aspergillosis. For other fungal species, the benefit of fungal surveillance culturing is less clear; however, in some studies, it was found that positive surveillance cultures for *Candida tropicalis* were highly predictive of systemic infection. For *Candida albicans* and *Candida tropicalis*, negative cultures have a negative predictive value. Similarly, the isolation of *Pseudomonas aeruginosa* and *Enterobacter cloacae* has a predictive value for subsequent septicemia in granulocytopenic patients (2).

ANTIMICROBIAL PROPHYLAXIS

Because most of the infections in granulocytopenic patients arise from the endogenous microbial flora, attempts have been made to reduce the numbers of gastrointestinal flora. In the past there were attempts to eliminate the endogenous flora with oral nonabsorbable antibiotics. Nonabsorbable antibiotics, such as gentamicin, netilmicin, and vancomycin, are now being abandoned because of poor compliance and the emergence of antibiotic resistant strains.

Trimethoprim-sulfamethoxazole is effective in the prevention of *Pneumocystis carinii* pneumonia and has been tested for bacterial prophylaxis as well. The value of trimethoprim-sulfamethoxazole in bacterial prophylaxis for granulocytopenic patients is less certain, however. Emergence of resistant strains and gram negative breakthrough bacteremias have been reported. Moreover, prolongation of granulocytopenia can be a problem (3). For all these reasons, the use of trimethoprim-sulfamethoxazole as a prophylactic agent in granulocytopenia has decreased considerably and might be limited, in the future, to the prevention of *Pneumocystis carinii* pneumonia.

Fluoroquinolones are broad-spectrum antibiotics that are well tolerated and well absorbed after oral administration, which leads to a high volume of distribution and good blood and tissue concentrations. Because of their lack of activity against anaerobic bacteria, they do not alter the colonization resistance in the patient. These characteristics have placed fluoroquinolones among the most suitable agents for antibacterial prophylaxis.

Studies with norfloxacin, pefloxacin, ciprofloxacin, and enoxacin have demonstrated the protective value of these agents for gram negative infections. In contrast, the protection is far from being satisfactory against gram positive infections. In lung cancer patients, pneumococcal bacteremia is still a common complication, and its mortality rate is close to that of gram negative bacteremia. For this reason, fluoroquinolones, if used as prophylaxis or as treatment, should be combined with penicillin in patients with lung cancer.

It should be stressed that only those patients with prolonged granulocytopenia are at high risk of developing fungal infections, thus making them candidates for antifungal prophylaxis. Nystatin, a nonabsorbable polyene, has been used extensively, but it has failed to demonstrate its efficacy clearly. Amphotericin B, given by oral administration, has produced a significant decrease in stool colonization by yeasts, but the clinical effects remain unproven. In contrast, intranasal instillation of amphotericin B can decrease the risk of invasive aspergillosis (4).

Ketoconazole and fluconazole are absorbed antifungal agents; they are effective in decreasing the gut colonization by yeasts and can reduce the frequency of systemic and oropharyngeal infections by *Candida* species. However, the emergence of *Torulopsis glabrata* and *Candida kruseii* has been reported with these agents. Itraconazole is a promising agent that is active against *Aspergillus* species; its efficacy in antifungal prophylaxis is currently under investigation.

ENHANCEMENT OF HOST DEFENSES

Hematopoietic colony–stimulating factors, such as granulocyte colony–stimulating factor (G-CSF) and granulocyte-macrophage–stimulating factor (GM-CSF), are glycoproteins that control the survival and the proliferation of hematopoietic progenitors (5). Recombinant DNA techniques have made possible the production of these factors for clinical use. It is now possible to reduce the severity and duration of profound granulocytopenia and thus decrease the risk of infection. Consequently, the indications for white blood cell transfusions have diminished considerably.

Active immunization has been advocated for prophylaxis of infection in cancer patients; however, many patients with cancer fail to raise sufficient antibody titers after antipneumococcal vaccination, probably because of the underlying immunosuppression (6), thus making acute immunization ineffective.

Passive immunization has not been very successful thus far for the prevention of bacterial and fungal disease; however, with the development of monoclonal antibodies, a new era for this approach may be at hand. In contrast, for viral infections, passive immunoprophylaxis can be very effective against a variety of viruses (e.g., herpes simplex, herpes zoster, cytomegalovirus) (7).

EMPIRIC TREATMENT

Patients with granulocytopenia who develop fever have a high chance of being infected; indeed, bacteremia occurs in approximately 20% of those febrile patients who are severely granulocytopenic (polymorphonuclear neutrophil [PMN] count, less than 100 per microliter) (8, 9). The mortality of untreated patients with febrile neutropenia is very high; therefore, empiric antibiotic treatment should be initiated at the earliest suspicion of infection (10); fever is the early sign noted most often. The highest mortality is observed in patients with polymicrobial septicemia, gram negative septicemia, and pneumonia. Other risk factors for an unfavorable course of febrile neutropenia include uncontrolled underlying neoplastic disease, severe nonneoplastic co-morbidity, and prolonged hospital stay.

INITIAL EMPIRIC ANTIBIOTIC THERAPY

The choice of antibiotics depends on local epidemiologic factors, including the frequency and susceptibility of nosocomial pathogens in a given institution. Data from surveillance cultures, renal or hepatic impairment, history of antibiotic allergy, and recent treatment with potentially nephrotoxic drugs are additional specific conditions that may influence the choice of antibiotics (11).

A combination of the new β-lactam antibiotics with aminoglycosides constitutes the current standard approach. It provides a synergistic action against gram negative bacilli and decreases the risk of emergence of resistant strains. Sculier and Klastersky (12) have demonstrated that serum bactericidal titers of at least 1/16 were associated with a more favorable outcome; higher bactericidal rates are obtained more readily through the use of antibiotic combinations.

Antipseudomonal penicillins, such as ticarcillin or piperacillin, and third-generation cephalosporins, such as ceftazidine or cefoperazone combined with amikacin or tobramycin, all demonstrate comparable efficacy. The experience with ciprofloxacin, a new fluoroquinolone, and aztreonam and the imipenem-cilastin combination is also very encouraging. Most studies have been conducted in patients with leukemia or lymphoma. Use of such agents can be applied safely to patients with lung cancer, with two important caveats: ciprofloxacin and aztreonam lack sufficient efficacy against *Streptococcus pneumoniae* and should not be used alone; the second restriction concerns the use of aminoglycosides. Because cisplatin is a major component of most chemotherapy regimens used in lung cancer treatment today, the concomitant use of cisplatin and aminoglycosides can increase the risk of nephrotoxicity and ototoxicity.

Recent reports have suggested that in patients with less severe and protracted neutropenia ceftazidime monotherapy and the use of the imipenem-cilastatin combination used as empiric monotherapy are equally effective (13).

Anaerobic pulmonary infections are common in patients with lung cancer but are rare in patients with leukemia or lymphoma. Imipenem-cilastatin and ticarcillin-clavulanate, with their broad-spectrum activity that includes action against anaerobic bacteria, seem to be well suited for empiric therapy in febrile granulocytopenic patients with lung cancer.

CHANGE OR ADDITION OF OTHER ANTIBIOTICS

Table 48.1 summarizes the management guidelines for febrile granulocytopenic patients in the case of bacterial sepsis. The monitoring can be done by the assay of the antibacterial activity of the serum against the offending pathogen. The addition of vancomycin or teicoplanin should be considered if there is evidence of methicillin resistant staphylococcal infection or sepsis caused by *Corynebacterium jeikeium*. The addition of these agents also applies to clinical conditions, such as the development of cellulitis or tunnel site infection on implanted catheters.

The patient with severe and prolonged neutropenia who remains febrile after 1 week of broad-spectrum antimicrobial therapy has a great risk of developing an invasive fungal infection such as candidiasis or aspergillosis. In this setting, amphotericin B probably should be added empirically. It is difficult to recommend an optimal total dose of amphotericin B for empiric use; 1 mg/kg/day to a total dose of 500 mg might be adequate in the absence of documented fungal infection. Antibiotics should not be maintained for the whole duration of the neutropenia; if the patient remains afebrile for 5 to 7 consecutive days, antibiotics

TABLE 48.1. Guidelines for the Diagnostic and Therapeutic Approach of Febrile Episodes in Granulocytopenic Patients

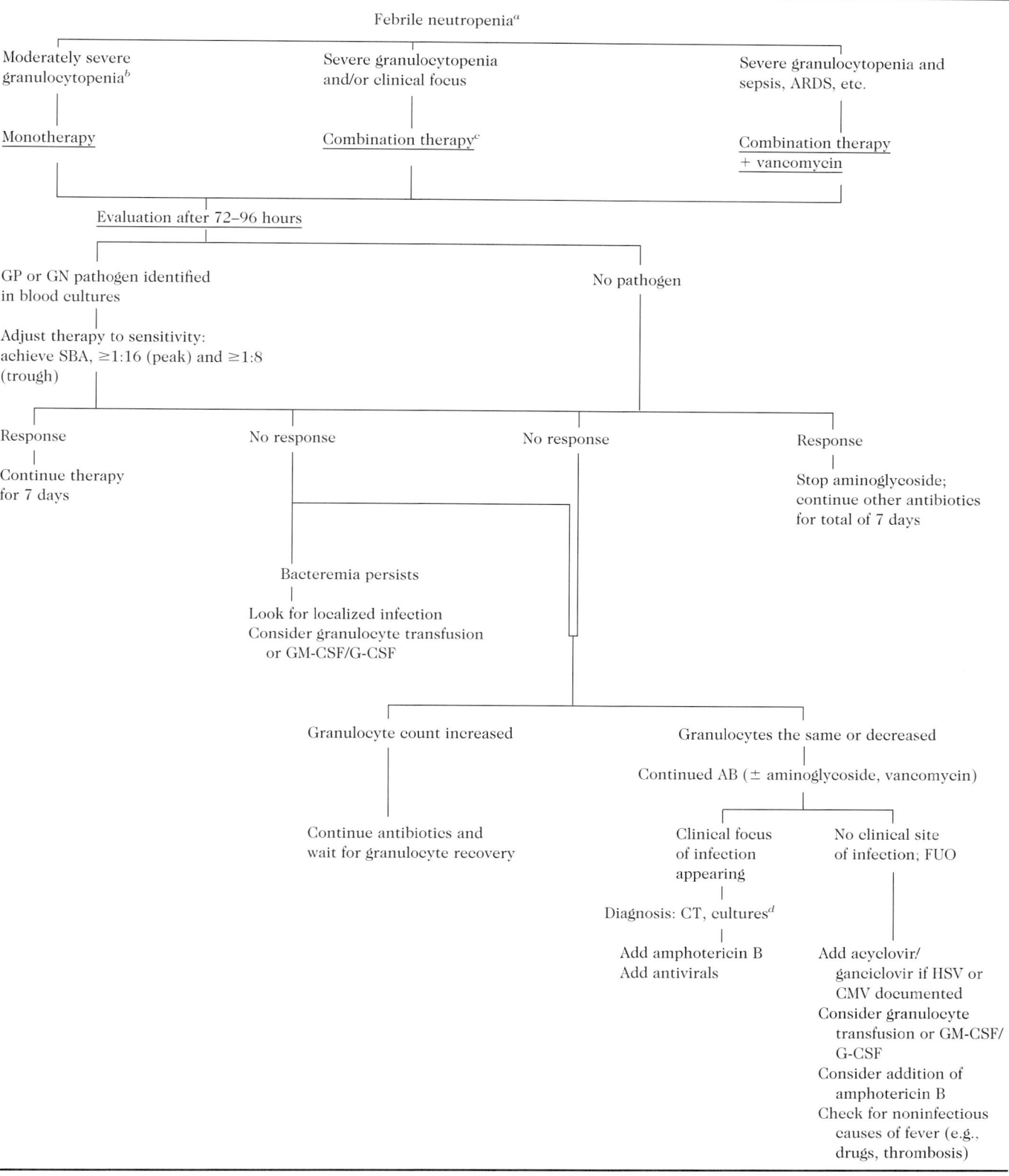

Abbreviations. GP, gram positive; GN, gram negative; ARDS, adult respiratory distress syndrome; SBA, serum bactericidal activity; GM-CSF, granulocyte-macrophage colony–stimulating factor; G-CSF, granulocyte colony–stimulating factor; AB, antibiotics; FUO, fever of unknown origin; HSV, herpes simplex virus; CMV, cytomegalovirus; CT, cat scan.
[a]Febrile neutropenia is defined as granulocyte count <1000 mm^3 with a temperature of >38.5°C.
[b]Moderately severe granulocytopenia: granulocyte count, <1000 × mm^3 but >100 mm^3.
[c]Use combination therapy for *P. aeruginosa* infection and possibly other gram-negative bacteremias until SBA is known.
[d]Routine cultures (2 per week): rectal swab for bacteria and fungi; urinalysis and mouth swab for HSV and CMV.

may be discontinued safely, despite the persistence of neutropenia.

CONCLUSIONS

During the last decade, intensive chemotherapy has been extended to solid tumors, including lung cancer. This use results in bone marrow toxicity that sometimes approaches that seen during therapy of acute leukemia. The potential benefit achieved with intensive chemotherapy should not be jeopardized by an increase in morbidity and mortality resulting from infections. This implies a particular effort to determine the most adequate preventive strategies against serious infections in granulocytopenic patients. Many advances have been made recently, the most significant being the use of G-CSF and GM-CSF, as well as antimicrobial prophylaxis (5).

TREATMENT OF CHEMOTHERAPY-INDUCED EMESIS

For the patient, chemotherapy-induced nausea and vomiting is one of the most feared side effects of cancer therapy. For many years, these symptoms were considered unavoidable complications of chemotherapy that could be alleviated only partially with the use of phenothiazines. This drug had major consequences on the effectiveness of chemotherapy because of delays in treatment and, sometimes, refusal of chemotherapy by the patient. Since the initial days of chemotherapy, many agents against nausea and vomiting have been added to our armamentarium.

The agents used in the treatment of emesis are listed in Table 48.2. Benzodiazepines, antihistamines, phenothiazines, and butyrophenones remained for a long time the main active agents in the treatment of emesis. Their efficacy is limited, however, and their use presently is restricted to moderately emetogenic chemotherapy or as an adjunct to other, more effective approaches. Currently, the most widely used antiemetics are metoclopramide, corticosteroids, and the 5-HT3 receptor antagonists.

METOCLOPRAMIDE AND CORTICOSTEROIDS

Metoclopramide was shown to reduce or prevent high-dose cisplatin-related nausea and vomiting (14). Combined with steroids and neuroleptic agents, it provides antiemetic protection for up to 60% to 70% of patients treated with high-dose cisplatin-based chemotherapy (15). Side effects include extrapyrami-

TABLE 48.2. Classes of Compounds Used for the Treatment of Cytostatic Drug-Induced Vomiting

DRUG CLASS	AGENT
Benzodiazepines	Lorazepam
	Diazepam
Antihistamines	Diphenhydramine
	Cyclicine
Phenothiazines	Prochlorperazine
	Chlorpromazine
	Thiethylperazine
	Levomepromazine
Butyrophenones	Droperidol
	Haloperidol
	Domperidone
Substituted benzamides	Metoclopramide
	Alizapride
Corticosteroids	Methylprednisone
	Dexamethasone
Cannabinoids	9-Tetrahydrocannabinol
	Navilone
	Levonantradol
5-HT3 receptor Antagonists	Ondansetron
	Granisetron
	Tropisetron

dal symptoms, diarrhea, and sedation. Its usual mode of administration is either in divided doses before and after chemotherapy or as a continuous infusion after a loading dose. It seems that a single 4 mg/kg dose of metoclopramide is tolerable and probably is equivalent to a divided dose of 3 mg/kg administered 2 hours apart (16).

Corticosteroids have been effective in patients treated with moderately emetogenic chemotherapy (17). The optimal dose and schedule have not yet been defined, and the mechanism of action remains unclear. Corticosteroids seem to enhance significantly the activity of several other antiemetic drugs, however (18).

5-HT3 RECEPTOR ANTAGONISTS

The discovery of the antiemetic properties of 5-HT3 receptor antagonists occurred because of the observation of a serotonin antagonism by metoclopramide in rodent gut preparations (19). These observations, along with the clinical efficacy of high-dose metoclopramide, led to the suggestion that dopamine-receptor antagonism alone could not explain the antiemetic activity of this drug (20). Several 5-HT3 receptor antagonists have recently been shown to possess considerable antiemetic activity.

Definite demonstration of the activity of ondansetron in patients treated with high-dose cisplatin was established by a study comparing ondansetron and metoclopramide. Complete protection from emesis was observed in 31 of 47 patients treated with ondansetron and in 21 of 45 with metoclopramide (21). In patients with breast cancer treated with cyclophosphamide, fluorouracil, and doxorubicin or epirubicin chemotherapy, complete control of vomiting was obtained in 86% of patients receiving ondansetron, compared with 42% of patients treated with metoclopramide (22). In patients receiving chemotherapy, including cisplatin at more than 50 mg/m^2, ondansetron appeared superior to metoclopramide: complete control of vomiting was seen in 56% versus 26% of patients, respectively (23).

Studies comparing ondansetron and ondansetron plus dexamethasone in patients receiving cisplatin-based chemotherapy showed that the combination was significantly more effective than ondansetron alone (24–26) in completely preventing emesis during the first 24 hours of chemotherapy. Complete protection for acute emesis was achieved in more than 80% of patients receiving ondansetron plus dexamethasone (24, 25). Delayed emesis was investigated in a trial using ondansetron versus a placebo (28); its effectiveness in preventing delayed emesis was not as dramatic as that seen in patients with acute chemotherapy-related emesis.

The efficacy of granisetron has been compared with standard therapies in patients receiving their first course of cisplatin (21). A single dose of granisetron proved to be as effective as an infusion regimen of intravenous metoclopramide combined with dexamethasone; granisetron use achieved a complete protection in 70% of patients. In patients undergoing other emetogenic chemotherapies (including cyclophosphamide, carboplatin, doxorubicin, and dacarbazine), a single prophylactic dose of granisetron was superior to chlorpromazine plus dexamethasone and was preferred by the majority of patients. Mild-to-moderate headache was the only event occurring with a significantly higher incidence after granisetron administration.

CONCLUSIONS

Despite major progress in the control of chemotherapy-induced emesis, significant problems persist. Nearly one third of the patients receiving a cisplatin-based chemotherapy program still experience emesis within the first 24 hours after chemotherapy. This rate of failure might even increase with the use of more intensive chemotherapy, which can be expected when using growth factors that lessen the risk of infection. The treatment of delayed and anticipatory emesis has thus far not been improved significantly (27). Consequently, further work is needed to optimize the use of the available drugs and identify effective nontoxic treatments.

MANAGEMENT OF TUMOR-INDUCED HYPERCALCEMIA

Increased calcium release from bone constitutes the main, but not the unique, pathogenic factor leading to hypercalcemia in cancer patients. Tumor secretory products markedly stimulate osteoblastic activity and proliferation, and they often inhibit osteoblastic activity, causing an uncoupling between bone resorption and bone formation and thus a rapid increase in serum calcium. In contrast, in primary hyperparathyroidism, bone formation is stimulated in parallel to bone resorption, and thus serum calcium levels are much more stable.

It is now recognized that parathyroid hormone protein (PTHrP) secretion by tumor cells has an essential role in the genesis of humoral hypercalcemia of malignancy (HHM), as substantiated by the fact that most, if not all, patients with HHM have increased circulating levels of PTHrP. Moreover, the same peptide is secreted by breast cancer cells, particularly when they metastasize to the bone; recent data also suggest that PTHrP could be involved in the genesis of the hypercalcemia and osteolysis that complicate breast cancer metastatic to bone. Persistently increased PTHrP levels could be responsible for the uncoupling of bone turnover typically observed in tumor-induced hypercalcemia (TIH). Nevertheless, it remains unclear why PTHrP, which supposedly acts only through parathyroid hormone receptors, would inhibit osteoblastic function.

Cancer hypercalcemia actually seems to be a heterogeneous syndrome that cannot be explained by the ectopic secretion of a single osteolytic agent. Cancer cells can make several hypercalcemic factors that probably work in concert despite the essential role of PTHrP. Transforming growth factor, especially transforming growth factor–α, thus could play an important contributory role. For example, inoculation into nude mice of cells transfected with the human transforming growth factor–α gene induces a marked increase in osteoblastic bone resorption and an inhibition of bone formation at sites of previous bone resorption. Cytokines such as interleukin-1 (IL-1) also could inhibit bone formation, and in vitro data indicate, moreover, that they could potentiate the hypercalcemic effects of PTHrP.

The kidneys can contribute to the genesis and rapid increase of serum calcium in TIH through a decrease in the glomerular filtration rate and an increase in the tubular reabsorption of calcium. This stimulation of kidney calcium reabsorption, leading to a relative hypocalciuria for the level of hypercalcemia, is a consequence of the deceased circulating volume and of the specific tubular effects of tumor secretory products, notably PTHrP. The relative importance of the kidneys and the skeleton in the pathogenesis of TIH remains controversial, but clinicians treating hypercalcemic cancer patients cannot neglect the contributory role of increased tubular calcium reabsorption in TIH.

Traditional Therapy for TIH

Effective treatment of the tumor certainly remains the ideal means of obtaining long-term control of serum calcium levels; however, a marked reduction of the tumor burden often is not feasible because hypercalcemia generally complicates advanced and refractory cancer. Forced saline diuresis with 6 L or more per 24 hours, combined with large doses of furosemide, is a risky and outdated procedure; however, rehydration with intravenous saline should still be part of the initial therapeutic approach to the hypercalcemic cancer patient. Rehydration with saline infusions to restore the circulating volume has relatively little effect on calcium levels, effecting a median decrease of only 1 mg/dL (28), but it interrupts the vicious cycle of TIH by inhibiting the increased tubular reabsorption of calcium. Moreover, rehydration improves the patient's clinical status because most of the symptoms of hypercalcemia are caused or increased by the reduced circulating volume. Routine administration of loop diuretics such as furosemide is not recommended because they aggravate volume depletion. Diuretics must be administered only after circulating volume has been restored or if there are signs or risks of fluid overload.

Corticosteroids are still prescribed too often in TIH: their activity actually is limited to hematologic malignancies. Intravenous administration of phosphates no longer has a place in the management of TIH because of the risks of extraskeletal calcium precipitation and renal insufficiency. Oral administration (1 to 3 g of elemental phosphorous) certainly is preferable, but the efficacy is limited by the secondary digestive effects of phosphates and is confined to hypophosphatemic patients with mild hypercalcemia.

The pathogenesis of TIH dictates that the priority in therapy be given to agents that potently decrease bone resorption. Calcitonin is a natural antiosteoclastic hormone; its main advantages are a rapid onset of action and a negligible toxicity. Furthermore, it has a calciuric effect that contributes to this hypocalcemic activity. Recommended doses vary from 2 to 8 U/kg/day administered 2 to 4 times daily. However, the efficacy of calcitonin in TIH is variable, partial, and transient. Serum calcium usually starts to increase again after a few days, and there is no further response to an increase in the dose.

Mithramycin (also called plicamycin) is another active antiosteoclastic agent, but its use is limited severely by major potential toxicities, particularly when the administration is repeated. Mithramycin still has some advocates, but its use in TIH should disappear over time. A recent randomized trial comparing mithramycin and the bisphosphonate pamidronate has confirmed the relatively poor tolerance and potential toxic effects of mithramycin, particularly on renal function. Moreover, the efficacy of mithramycin was inferior to pamidronate, which normalized serum calcium levels in 88% of patients, compared with 45% for mithramycin (29).

Bisphosphonates for TIH

ETIDRONATE

Etidronate (Didronel; Procter & Gamble) is widely available, but it is the least potent of the clinically evaluated bisphosphonates. Prolonged treatment can inhibit bone mineralization and lead to osteomalacia, but this condition is not a concern in the acute treatment of TIH. Etidronate usually is administered at a dose of 7.5 mg/kg/day for 3 days, but some investigators recommend a 7-day therapy course because the success rate seems to increase with treatment duration (28).

CLODRONATE

Clodronate (Ostac; Boehringer, Mannheim, Germany; and Bonefos, Leiras, Finland) has been given at doses ranging between 300 and 1500 mg/day for 1 to 10 days. It is superior to placebo, and repeated administrations are well tolerated and permit a success rate of 80% to 90% (30). However, a single-day infusion is often not highly effective in patients with HHM, and a marked increase in the tubular reabsorption of calcium may follow.

PAMIDRONATE

Pamidronate (Aredia; Ciba-Geigy, Basel, Switzerland) has been tested widely and is the most useful of the commercially available compounds. It was first administered as daily, 15-mg, 2-hour infusions that were repeated for up to 10 days. In a multicenter trial, 90% of 132 patient with TIH treated in this manner became normocalcemic after a mean interval of 3 to 4 days (31). Such a therapeutic scheme is cumbersome, but particularly efficient, because serum calcium levels remain normal for a median of at least 3 weeks (32). Pamidronate also can be given as a single infusion over 4 to 24 hours; the efficacy of a single 24-hour infusion is similar to that of a 3-day therapeutic scheme, at least short term, if the same total dose is provided (33). The existence of a dose-response relationship has been difficult to demonstrate, and it could be shown only when reviewing the therapeutic response of 160 patients. After the administration of a total dose of 60 to 90 mg (1.0 to 1.5 mg/kg), more than 90% of the patients became normocalcemic; the calcemic or calciuric response was not influenced by the tumor type or by the presence of metastatic bone involvement. When using lower doses (30 to 45 mg), the response was less intense in patients with HHM than in hypercalcemic patients with metastatic bone involvement (34). Elevated circulating PTHrP levels significantly influence the response to bisphosphonate therapy, and the few resistant patients often have markedly increased PTHrP levels (35).

Pamidronate is well tolerated, with the only clinically detectable side effect being transient fever and a flulike syndrome in about one quarter of the cases. Asymptomatic hypocalcemia and hypophosphatemia often are observed after therapy; their incidence or severity probably is dose related. When hypercalcemia recurs, the efficacy of subsequent pamidronate infusions becomes progressively lower. This loss of efficacy probably results from an increased tumor mass and an enhanced release of osteolytic factors as the tumor progresses. Limited data suggest that higher doses of bisphosphonates could then be given successfully.

The superiority of pamidronate over etidronate, clodronate, mithramycin, and calcitonin has been demonstrated in prospective comparative trials. In addition to saline infusions to restore circulating volume, there is no need to combine pamidronate with other hypocalcemic drugs, except in the few patients with severe life-threatening hypercalcemia. In these patients, combining pamidronate with calcitonin may be of particular value because of the rapid decrease in serum calcium levels induced by calcitonin.

ALENDRONATE

Alendronate is a newer bisphosphonate that has been tested predominantly among nononcologic patients. Its efficacy in TIH also appears to be dose related because the effects of a single 10-mg infusion are greater than the effects of a 2.5- or 5-mg infusion. As with pamidronate, the vast majority of patients become normocalcemic after alendronate administration, which has been shown to be superior to clodronate (36).

CONCLUSIONS

Bisphosphonates have improved and simplified the management of TIH considerably. A single infusion of 60 to 90 mg of pamidronate combined with saline infusions to restore the circulating volume normalizes serum calcium levels in more than 90% of hypercalcemic cancer patients. Other types of antiosteolytic compounds, such as gallium, are currently under evaluation. The efficacy of gallium nitrate in TIH has been shown already to be superior to those of calcitonin and etidronate. However, gallium is a potentially nephrotoxic agent, and it must be administered as a 5-day continuous infusion, which makes it unattractive for the management of TIH.

The future introduction of bisphosphonates even more potent than pamidronate and alendronate will further simplify the therapeutic approach to TIH, notably by permitting a shortening of the infusion time and probably a more prolonged activity. Testing of newer bisphosphonates in patients with TIH still is helpful as a means of learning more about the use of these drugs in normocalcemic patients with tumor-induced osteolysis or osteoporosis.

CACHEXIA AND NUTRITION

With the evolution of their disease, the majority patients with cancer present a syndrome of progressive weight loss resulting from decreased food intake. In some cases, a decrease in food intake actually leads to the discovery of the malignancy. In other circumstances, treatments such as chemotherapy, radiotherapy, or surgery can account for side effects leading to an alteration in the patient's nutrition. In any case, one has to consider anorexia and loss of weight as a biologic negative predictor of survival and a prognostic factor that is independent of other patient characteristics. Anorexia and cachexia have an adverse effect on body image and quality of life, and they often become important concerns for patients and their families.

Anorexia-cachexia associated with malignant growth is a frequent syndrome; it is more common in some tumors (such as gastric, pancreatic, and lung cancers) and is an adverse prognostic factor. No clear correlation can be made typically between the stage of the disease or the size of the tumor, however. The pathogenesis of cancer cachexia is complex, as shown

TABLE 48.3. Disease and Treatment-Related Causes of Anorexia

TYPES OF ANOREXIA	EXAMPLES
Disease related	Anorexia cachexia syndrome
	Symptoms of gastrointestinal or pancreatic cancer
	Obstruction by the tumor
	Hepatic dysfunction
	Protein-losing enteropathy
	Pain
	Fever
	Change in taste sensation
Treatment-related	
Surgery	Oropharyngeal resection
	Esophagectomy and reconstruction
	Gastrectomy, pancreatectomy
	Bowel resection
	Ileostomy-colostomy
Radiation therapy	Oropharyngeal area: stomatitis, diminution of taste and smell, xerostomia
	Neck and mediastinum area: dysphagia, esophagitis, esophageal fibrosis
	Abdomen and pelvis: nausea, vomiting, diarrhea, malabsorption, obstruction, stenosis, fistula
Chemotherapy	Nausea, vomiting, fluid and electrolyte imbalance, stomatitis, constipation, diarrhea, neuropathy
	Change in taste sensation
Other drugs	Pain medications (somnolence, constipation, nausea), antifungal and antibacterial agents (nausea, diarrhea)
	Change in taste sensation

in Table 48.3. Metabolic abnormalities in cachexia are different from those encountered in chronic states of malnutrition. Humoral factors induce physical and biochemical abnormalities such as glucose intolerance, increased glucose turnover, enhanced lactate production, decreased protein synthesis that can result in muscular wasting, decrease in lipogenesis, and possibly an increase in basal energy expenditure. These metabolic changes mimic those observed in starvation, stress, or trauma (37). Some evidence suggests that tumor-related factors may be the source of these metabolic disorders: tumor necrosis factor (TNF), interleukins (IL-1, IL-6), and γ-interferon. Under experimental conditions, exogenous administration of these cytokines provokes anorexia, loss of weight, and hepatic enzyme alterations (38, 39).

Food habits of cancer patients are complex; generally speaking, one observes a decrease in food intake and absorption. A central origin of these changes has been proposed (possibly a role of serotonin at the hypothalamic level), but various metabolic alterations can lead to hypophagia, i.e., high lactic acid concentration, nausea-inducing agents, early satiety, and changes in taste.

Taste alterations, reluctance to eat, gastroparesis, and nausea are reported frequently; asthenia and extreme muscular weakness enhance these problems. Psychologic disorders, in some cases, amplify the known somatic and metabolic problems. Anxiety associated with the diagnosis may make the situation even worse. All of these conditions illustrate the importance of the oncologist's taking a general approach to the nutritional problem (40).

CONSEQUENCES OF MALNUTRITION

Loss of weight is a specific parameter reflecting a poor prognosis, especially in the case of tumors affecting the gastrointestinal tract and lung cancers. Tolerance to the administration of antineoplastic drugs also is related somewhat to the patient's nutritional state; there also may be a correlation between the loss of weight and the risk of death from the cardiac toxicity of chemotherapy. Infection and mucositis can be considered occasionally as consequences of toxic or metabolic disorders and loss of weight.

Many antineoplastic treatments worsen the nutritional alterations already detected before treatment in approximately 50% of the cancer patients. Chemotherapy can often provoke disturbances such as loss of taste and vomiting; it may also be responsible for mucositis and atrophy of the intestinal tract mucosa. Radiotherapy can also result in adverse effects on the gastrointestinal tract, particularly when it is used for the treatment of head and neck, esophageal, and intestinal tumors.

NUTRITIONAL SUPPORTS

Clearly, the most efficient treatment of nutritional disturbances resulting from a tumor is removal of the tumor or effective therapy of it. Physicians must remember that there are important differences between chronic malnutrition and malnutrition caused by a complex metabolic disorder such as cancer; this difference can explain the poor efficacy of many approaches. There is no optimal nutritional support program that is valid for every patient; each case is specific and the therapeutic choices should consider each individual separately.

The efficacy of parenteral nutrition is controversial. It has been applied successfully only for surgical resection of localized tumors of the digestive tract. In these cases, parenteral nutrition during the presurgical period seems to improve the recovery of the patients by decreasing postoperative complications. Otherwise, parenteral nutrition can be proposed when mechanical disturbances of the digestive tract exist. However, parenteral nutrition probably does not improve the metabolic disorders directly related to cancer and those that are responsible for cachexia. Complications resulting from artificial alimentation (e.g., catheter infections, excess of water, metabolic modifications with increase in hepatic enzymes, reduction of quality of life) also are frequent (37).

Enteral alimentation (hyperalimentation) is the treatment of choice when a functional gastrointestinal abnormality is present. This technique is simple, safe, and offers several metabolic advantages over the parenteral route. However, if patients develop nausea and vomiting, enteral nutrition often is difficult to continue. This type of alimentation maintains a good trophicity of gastrointestinal mucosa and reduces the risks of mucosal atrophy and mucositis induced by chemotherapy and radiotherapy (37).

DRUGS FOR NUTRITIONAL ENHANCEMENT

Because metabolic disorders that complicate and reduce the efficacy of nutritional support are complex, a pharmacologic approach for cachexia associated with cancer has been difficult to investigate. The general goals of this approach are the stimulation of appetite, reduction of gastrointestinal disturbances, modification of metabolism, and improvement in the quality of life (41).

Prednisolone shows a favorable impact on anorexia caused by cancer by producing a favorable subjective feeling in the patient, who often report that appetite has improved. Nevertheless, objective parameters that measure a favorable energy balance are shown less easily. The action of corticosteroids is probably multipotent (feeling of hunger, decrease of depression, pain relief, global increase in performance, psychologic stimulation). These effects frequently are only transient.

Medroxyprogesterone and megestrol acetate induce an increase in appetite, an objective increase in food intake, and a decrease in nausea and vomiting. The increase in weight is caused primarily by an increase in body fat and not only in fluid accumulation. These hormones have a direct effect on adipocytes that is independent of the tumor's hormone sensitivity (41, 42).

Cyproheptadine, an antihistamine that has been used for a long time in oncology to stimulate appetite, has never shown clear efficacy. Hydrazine sulphate is a gluconeogenic pathway function inhibitor; this pathway is a metabolic route abnormally activated in cachexia related to cancer. Such a theoretic approach is potentially interesting, but recent clinical studies, including one in non–small cell lung cancer, failed to show any benefit for the inclusion of hydrazine in the active treatment of non–small cell lung cancer (43). Antiinflammatory drugs, such as indomethacin, used in animal models can increase significantly the food intake, probably through an effect on cytokines (IL-1, IL-6, γ-interferon, and TNF); however, thus far there is no objective clinical evidence of benefit.

CONCLUSIONS

Nutritional problems caused by cancer are numerous and diverse. They often are associated with major metabolic abnormalities. For these reasons, their understanding and treatment remain quite difficult. The psychologic significance of the nutritional disturbances is considerable and must be approached in a multidisciplinary fashion. It may represent a key factor to an improvement in the quality of life through better nutritional support.

PAIN CONTROL

The importance of pain control is now widely accepted among health professionals caring for patients with cancer. A good quality of life with complete control of painful symptoms during treatment of cancer is one of the major concerns for cancer patients. Pain occurs in more than 70% of patients with cancer (44). Despite great advances in the pathophysiology and clinical experience with pain relief, and with the recent interest devoted to pain control, many patients remain unrelieved of pain during their illness (45). Therefore, some points must be defined: the definition of pain syndromes and their mechanisms, the assessment and evaluation of pain, the possibilities of treatment, and the information provided to the patient. These elements have been emphasized by the Ad Hoc Committee on Cancer Pain of the American Society of Clinical Oncology (46).

PAIN SYNDROMES

The identification of the cause of the pain is essential before undertaking any therapeutic procedure, and it may be fundamental for pain treatment. The

TABLE 48.4. Pain Syndromes

Pain caused by tumor involvement
    Direct compression by the tumor
    Bone or periosteal invasion
    Nerve compression of infiltration
    Viscera involvement
    Other structures: vein, arteries, soft tissues
Pain caused by cancer treatment
    Post chemotherapy: mucositis, neuropathy
    Post surgery: post mastectomy, post thoracotomy, post-amputation pain
    Post radiation: fibrosis, bone necrosis, myelopathy
    Alone or in combination

principal causes of pain in cancer are listed in Table 48.4. It is important to correlate the symptoms with the underlying disease. This correlation may indicate the possibility of a specific treatment (i.e., chemotherapy, radiation therapy, or surgery) and could be of prognostic value concerning pain control. Most patients may present with more than one type or cause of pain. In fact, each situation is particular and must be assessed specifically to avoid diagnostic error. Further investigations often are necessary but must be considered in addition to the clinical situation; they should be performed only to provide better comfort for the patient.

ASSESSMENT AND EVALUATION OF PAIN

A physical examination and complete neurologic testing are essential to clarify the type of pain and to identify the pain syndrome; the characteristics of pain (onset, quality, intensity, location) must be detailed. Aggravating and relieving factors need to be determined.

Numerous procedures exist to quantify and evaluate the pain. A simple, reproducible technique that enables adequate monitoring of pain is the visual analogue scale. This instrument is an excellent means of quantifying pain and may be used in outpatient or inpatient settings. A visual analogue scale allows the patient to score his or her pain (between 0 and 10, or 0 and 100) daily. Although pain is essentially a subjective experience, a visual analogue scale remains the best way to assess pain and adjust the treatment to suit the type and level of pain.

The introduction of a pain grading system opens horizons for pain evaluation and could offer new perspectives in terms of pain management. This system is based on objective factors (type of pain, nature of pain, tolerance to opioids, opioid intake, cognitive and psychologic impairment, history of drug or alcohol abuse), and it introduces the notion of prognosis regarding pain control (47). The development of such a system is certainly a new way to evaluate cancer pain.

TREATMENT

The efficacy of pain control relies on a correct evaluation of pain, as well as on adequate treatment and prolonged follow-up. The therapeutic approach is essentially multidisciplinary and includes pharmacologic, anesthesiologic, psychologic, and neurologic input. Guidelines have been developed by the Cancer Unit of the World Health Organization, which has proposed an analgesic ladder for treating cancer pain. Depending on the intensity of the pain, nonopioids (acetaminophen or nonsteroidal analgesics), weak or strong opioids, and co-analgesics may be prescribed. The nonopioid analgesics are effective in relieving mild-to-moderate pain and may be used in association with opioids. The effectiveness of morphine and other narcotic analgesics is well recognized for the relief of moderate to extremely severe pain. For chronic pain it is necessary to provide long-lasting analgesics. This effect can be accomplished with continuous parenteral opioid administration or use of a combination of long-acting agents given regularly and short-acting agents given for breakthrough pain as needed. Side effects like nausea or constipation should be prevented because they are always present and may be a cause of treatment failure.

The risks of sedation or respiratory depression must be weighted against the clinical situation. Pain is certainly the best antidote to these complications, which rarely occur with correct drug management. If such complications are present, investigations must be performed to exclude other etiologies before stopping opioid administration. The fear of addiction or drug abuse often is associated with morphine and is deeply rooted among patients. The physician's role is to inform the patient, the family, and the relatives that morphine may be the drug of choice to control pain and provide a better quality of life (48).

Co-analgesics may be used in specific circumstances. Antidepressants (amitriptyline, imipramine) and anticonvulsants (valproate, carbamazepine) have been effective in painful conditions such as plexopathy, neuropathy, and phantom limb syndrome, and they may be used in association with other analgesics. Corticosteroids (dexamethasone, prednisolone) provide pain relief in specific situations such as soft tissue infiltration or nerve compression. For all of these drugs, the physician must be aware of the pharmacologic properties and effectiveness to avoid undesirable side effects or iatrogenic complications. Furthermore, a close follow-up with repeated pain evaluation and quantification of side effects should ensue. Follow-up allows for titration and adjustment of analgesics.

CONCLUSIONS

Adequate pain management requires action in different fields: oncology, neurology, pharmacology, and psychology. Pain must be evaluated completely before any diagnostic and therapeutic procedures are undertaken. Full information must be given to the patient and family regarding the cause of pain and the nature of treatment. A close and prolonged follow-up of pain and prevention of the potential side effects related to the treatment enhances compliance and trust between the patient and the physician.

PSYCHOLOGIC SUPPORT

An important prevalence of psychologic and psychiatric disturbances in patients with cancer has been reported in many studies. In 1983, the Psychological Collaborative Oncology Group (49) observed a prevalence rate of 47% of ill-defined psychiatric disorders in a cohort of cancer patients (inpatient and outpatient populations at three cancer centers). Most importantly, this rate was approximately twice that reported for psychiatric disorders in medical patients, and 3 times the model estimate appearing in the literature for the general population. As a diagnostic category, adjustment disorders accounted for 68% of all diagnoses. Other diagnoses were major affective disorders (13%), organic mental disorders (8%), personality disorders (7%), and anxiety disorders (4%). In fact, nearly 85% of patients with a recognized psychiatric condition presented with signs or symptoms of depression or anxiety. Most of these conditions were judged by the investigators to be highly treatable disorders (49).

The high prevalence of psychologic problems and psychiatric disturbances reported in oncology patients underlines a need for comprehensive psychologic support of cancer patients and their families. Psychologic support is designed to preserve, restore, or enhance quality of life. Quality of life refers not only to psychologic distress and adjustment-related problems but also to the management of cancer symptoms and treatment of side effects. Psychologic interventions designed for this purpose could be divided into five categories: prevention, early detection, restoration, support, and palliation.

First, preventive interventions are designed to avoid the development of predictable morbidity secondary to treatment or the disease. Secondly, early detection of patients' needs or problems refers to the assumption that early interventions could have therapeutic results superior to those offered by delayed support, both for quality of life and survival (50, 51). Thirdly, restorative interventions refer to actions used when a cure is likely, the aim being the control or elimination of residual cancer disability. Fourthly, supportive rehabilitation is planned to lessen disability related to chronic disease, which is characterized by numerous cancer illness remissions, progression, and further active treatment. Lastly, palliation is required when curative treatments are not likely to be effective, and when maintaining or improving comfort becomes the main goal.

Psychologic interventions often are multidisciplinary in nature with varieties of content as shown in Table 48.5. The scope of psychologic interventions range from information and education to a more sophisticated support program that includes directive (behavioral or cognitive) or nondirective (dynamic or supportive) therapy. Social interventions usually include financial, household, equipment, and transportation assistance, depending on individual and family needs and resources. These interventions may be combined with the prescription of pharmacologic agents such as psychotropics (antidepressants, anxiolytics), analgesics, and others, as well as physical, speech, or occupational therapy. The latter often are an integral part of rehabilitation programs. Health care services devoted to the delivery of these interventions are hospital, hospice, or home based and are organized very

TABLE 48.5. Common Psychologic Support Techniques in Oncology

NONDIRECTIVE TECHNIQUES	DIRECTIVE TECHNIQUES
Individual	Individual
Information	Behavior therapy
Counseling	Hypnosis
Psychotherapy	Relaxation
(supportive or	Progressive muscle relation
psychodynamic)	training
Group	Electromyographic biofeedback
Self-help	Guided imagery
Supportive psychotherapy	Systematic desensitization
	Distraction
	Cognitive therapy
Family	Group
Supportive psychotherapy	Behavior therapy
	Hypnosis
	Relaxation
	Cognitive therapy

differently depending on available community resources and particularities. Evidence also has been found that cancer psychologically affects not only the patient, but also health professionals who deal with them (52). Psychologic training support for health professionals thus should also be included as part of psychologic support programs (53).

CONCLUSIONS

Psychologic and psychiatric aspects of oncology have been delineated clearly over the past few years, and their evaluation has become an important part of the supportive care activity. The recent publication of the first handbook of psychooncology, which offers a state-of-the-art overview in this growing field, provides a valuable source of help to all health professionals involved in the care of patients with cancer (54).

SPECIAL ASPECTS OF NURSING

Rapid developments in supportive treatments in cancer care also require adaptation in nursing care. Previously only concerned with the strict execution of medical orders, the organization of cancer nursing now has broadened the concept of the nurse's role (55). Oncology nurses are more often considered full partners in the care team. Patients, as well as physicians and other health professionals, expect nurses to be supportive, i.e., to give support to the patient. However, it is difficult to find a precise definition of support in the nursing literature. Support often is mistaken for care.

The supportive care model (55) is made of six interconnected dimensions: valuing, connecting, empowering, doing for, finding, and preserving individual integrity. This concept of the nurse's supportive role in cancer care takes in technical skills (doing for) and calls for the ability to communicate and establish strong relationships with patients and families. Implicit finally is the promotion of the patient's quality of life and, in a broader context, the patient's rehabilitation. Technical aspects of nursing care are expanding as supportive treatments of cancer are developing. This expansion is especially true in areas such as chemotherapy administration, control of toxicities related to chemotherapeutic agents, and management of pain and other symptoms.

ADMINISTRATION OF CHEMOTHERAPY AND NURSING MANAGEMENT OF SIDE EFFECTS

The concepts and manner of delivering chemotherapy have changed completely with the introduction of implantable vascular access devices. The nurse's role also has evolved during this time. The nurse now performs a major role in the education of the patient and the family with respect to side effects and methods of alleviating them. Today, venous access devices frequently are inserted at the beginning of a long-term treatment, thus preserving peripheral veins and markedly improving the patient's comfort. However, these devices require constant supervision and care to ensure patency and prevent infection during treatment or between courses of treatment. The education related to catheter care also has become part of the oncology nurse's role.

Intensification in the doses of certain chemotherapeutic agents has resulted in the identification of even more aspects of clinical management of chemotherapy toxicities. New medications used to treat these side effects are being introduced continually and include antiemetic drugs, chemoprotectants, and colony-stimulating factors. The use of these substances requires that nurses have extensive knowledge and technical skills (56).

Among the side effects of chemotherapy, nausea and vomiting are feared by most patients and can even cause some patients to discontinue their treatment. Nurses often are the first caregivers to be faced with this problem, and they play an important part in the implementation of the antiemetic regimen and assessment of its efficacy and side effects, sometimes by using questionnaires or visual analog scales. The number of emetic episodes, the volume of emesis, and the subjective sense of nausea are recorded by these means.

Hematologic toxicity also requires supportive care involving many technical issues. In the case of BMT or administration of high-dose cytotoxic drugs affecting the white blood cells, severe myelosuppression results and may require placing the patient into protective isolation, or in a laminar air flow room as is the case in allogeneic BMT. In such situations, the nurse must perform multiple roles. In addition to psychologic support of the patient and the family, mandatory technical measures are needed to prevent infection of the patient by endogenous flora. Thus, nursing requirements include education and supervision of diet, frequent mouth care, skin care, aseptic care of central venous catheters, delivery of preventive antibiotic and antifungal therapy, as well as supervision of basic protective measures such as frequent hand washing by nurses and other professionals. Adequate measures—including screening for petechiae as well as other bleeding symptoms, frequent oral and dental care, and attention to the safety of the patient's environment—also must be adopted when the patient develops thrombocytopenia. Again, patient and family education can be critical.

The prevention of alopecia caused by chemotherapy is another example of supportive nursing care. Hair loss can be prevented by using scalp cooling techniques, a tourniquet, or a combination of the two during the administration of cytotoxic drugs. However, these measures are not indicated for all treatments nor for all patients. For example, it is not clear whether these techniques might provide a pharmacologic sanctuary. Although hair loss may be a minor issue in the face of widespread metastases, its impact on potentially curative therapies is not well defined, and further research is needed before widespread application is appropriate.

Far beyond their technical role in the delivery of supportive care, nurses now play a fundamental role as part of the team effort in the rehabilitation of cancer patients. Rehabilitation is a relatively new concept that results directly from reduced cancer mortality rates and enhanced survival rates. Although the objectives of rehabilitation services are continually evolving, they generally are designed, through improvement in psychologic adjustment, to help patients become reintegrated into society as soon as possible, to restore their physical capabilities, to restore their self-image, and to help them face the severity of the diagnosis and the prognosis. Thus, ideally the concept of rehabilitation takes place from the moment of the disclosure of the diagnosis and calls for physical and psychologic support throughout the course of the disease and its treatment to the terminal phase, when cure is no longer possible. The rehabilitation concept is linked to the concept of supportive care and also encompasses palliative and terminal care.

Rehabilitation services usually are made up of multidisciplinary teams that include nurses, social workers, psychologists, physical and occupational therapists, and others. Oncology nurses often are specialized in the supportive care of a particular type of cancer and often act as counselors or coordinators of the resources available for patients and their families. Their function as educators and care coordinators is often very important (57). Some nurses are highly specialized in this arena, e.g., the enterostomal therapist often helps the patient face his or her new body image, to accept it, and to master the equipment and techniques that will enable the patient to maintain control. In head and neck cancers, nurses often teach patients how to swallow again after surgery and how to care for the stoma. The nurse and speech therapist play important roles in teaching patients the use of the esophageal voice. Palliatively, nurses specializing in pain control teach patients and their families how to deal with pain medication regimens or devices such as the patient-controlled analgesia (PCA) pump; this education can help the patient control their pain treatment and thus improve the quality of their life. Finally, nurses play an informal role in rehabilitation cancer care by acting as counselors for their colleagues involved in direct care at the bedside.

NURSE EDUCATION

Ongoing development of supportive care of the cancer patient requires flexibility and enhancement of nurses' competencies. Basic as well as postgraduate education of nurses must evolve. Continuing education should not be underestimated. For example, the development of oncology intensive care units has necessitated that some nurses develop expertise in both oncology and intensive care nursing.

In Europe, the specialty of cancer nursing was defined in the early 1980s, under the influence of various cancer centers such as the Royal Marsden Hospital in London. However, a study in 1988 from the European Community (58) revealed the poor level of postgraduate cancer nursing education and a virtual absence of any cancer education in the basic nursing curriculum. In that study, many differences were observed in cancer nursing education among the countries visited and within individual countries. In the basic curriculum, oncology nursing did not form a separate body of knowledge. A few graduate and postgraduate courses did exist; nevertheless, their quality differed from course to course. In a few countries, the nursing societies and cancer centers have developed continuing education programs in oncology nursing.

In 1989, the European Oncology Nursing Society (EONS) published a core curriculum for a postgraduate course in cancer nursing. This event was a turning point. Since then, postgraduate courses have been developed in most European countries in accordance with the EONS guidelines. The "Europe Against Cancer" program provided financial support.

The Belgian experience illustrates this phenomenon. Since 1989, the nursing school attached to the Free University, Brussels, the Jules Bordet Institute, and the Belgian Oncology Nursing Society (French speaking) has organized a yearly postgraduate course in oncology nursing. The one-day-a-week course takes place during the academic year. The main goals are the development of knowledge and technical skills among cancer nurses. However, developing communications skills and supportive behavior toward the cancer patients and their families also plays an important part. More recently, short specialized modular courses have allowed professionals to acquire specific knowledge in

TABLE 48.6. Training Modules for Continuing Education in Oncology Nursing

Title of the module
   Teaching the teachers
   Prevention and early screening
   Chemotherapy
   Radiotherapy
   Psychooncology
     Short module
     Long module

different areas of cancer nursing as shown in Table 48.6. These two patterns of training are evolving concurrently and are attracting different kinds of students, although primarily individuals with some experience in cancer nursing.

If the evolution in cancer treatments and supportive care requires the implementation of postgraduate cancer nursing education, then it also calls for the improvement of the content and quality of the basic curriculum. To ensure appropriate referral to specialists, nurses involved in the direct care of cancer patients must be trained to identify the patient's needs for specialized cancer care. The Standing Committee of Nurses of the European Community is now studying these matters; this study probably will lead to the publication of guidelines for transmittal to national governments as a means of improving and to unifying basic training in oncology nursing throughout Europe.

CONCLUSIONS

As more cancer patients survive with or without their disease and as more elderly people develop cancer, the need for supportive care will expand dramatically. In addition to other professionals involved in cancer care, nurses will need additional background and education to adjust to the specific but changing needs of these populations. Specialization and subspecialization in the different areas of rehabilitative cancer nursing is currently underway in most countries, but changes in the basic curriculum also are needed to assure that patients have appropriate care and access to care.

CELLULAR SUPPORTIVE CARE OF ANEMIA AND THROMBOCYTOPENIA

Aggressive therapies for cancer often produce myelosuppression that can take the form of neutropenia, thrombocytopenia, or anemia. Often these conditions occur together. The approach to the supportive care of neutropenia was discussed previously. However, both anemia and thrombocytopenia require special concerns and techniques (59).

Anemia can occur as a direct effect of suppression on the marrow precursor cells, or from renal toxicity, chemotherapy or its supportive care (e.g. antibiotics), frequent blood sampling for laboratory tests, bleeding, or hemolysis, or combinations of these activities. Although packed red blood cell (RBC) transfusions may alleviate many of the potential problems associated with anemia, patients and their families often have considerable apprehension about the safety of blood transfusions. Thus, blood tests should be focused on the necessities of care. RBC transfusions administered after significant immunosuppression, such as occurs in high-dose chemotherapy or BMT, may need to be irradiated to prevent graft versus host disease (GVHD) (see below).

Recently, the introduction of recombinant erythropoietin has raised the possibility of its use to alleviate or reduce the RBC transfusion needs associated with chemotherapy. Although it may be useful in some instances, its role as part of chemotherapy supportive care is not yet fully established, and further research is needed to define the indications for its use. Similarly, autologous storage of RBCs before treatment is not indicated currently on a routine basis.

Thrombocytopenia also can produce considerable morbidity and mortality. Thus, many oncologists transfuse platelets on a prophylactic basis when the platelet count falls below 20,000 per microliter. This practice is based on early randomized trials that showed a reduction in morbidity and mortality in children with leukemia given prophylactic transfusions (60, 61).

These studies also showed, however, that certain patients—i.e., those who had severe thrombocytopenia who developed an infection or a febrile episode, or who recently received cytotoxic therapy that might produce mucositis—were more likely to develop clinical bleeding. Another factor that predicted bleeding potential was a precipitous drop in the platelet count (e.g., more than 50%) in 24 hours (59–61). Recognizing these principles, platelet transfusion (which often requires multiple donor exposure) can be given with greater circumspection, especially to patients with solid tumors (62).

New cytokines that stimulate platelet production, such as IL-6, are now under clinical trial and may yet further alter the approach to therapy-induced thrombocytopenia.

CONCLUSIONS

The use of blood products is an important component of supportive care. Cautious use of these products is indicated, and newer techniques and cytokines may alter the approach to the supportive care technique.

SUPPORTIVE CARE IN BONE MARROW TRANSPLANTATION

BMT is now a well-defined form of therapy that permits high-dose chemotherapy and radiotherapy. It also has increasing indications in aplastic anemia and in a variety of malignant diseases and genetic disorders. This overview focuses on new data on the prevention and treatment of early complications of BMT. Topics such as prevention of bacterial and fungal infections, transfusions, antiemetics, and pain control are discussed elsewhere in this chapter.

SIDE EFFECTS OF CONDITIONING REGIMENS

A unique cardiotoxicity is associated with high-dose cyclophosphamide use. Manifestations of cyclophosphamide cardiotoxicity range from an asymptomatic pericardial effusion with reduction in electrocardiographic voltage to myopericarditis and congestive heart failure that may be fatal. Braverman et al. (63) have prospectively studied the incidence, risk factors, and course of cardiotoxicity following high-dose cyclophosphamide administration (63). The cardiotoxicity is related directly to the peak dose, and these authors suggest that fractionation of high-dose cyclophosphamide may help to reduce the incidence.

The administration of high-dose cyclophosphamide also is associated with hemorrhagic cystitis. The complication is uncommon, but its treatment is difficult. A recent randomized study suggests that bladder irrigation does not prevent hemorrhagic cystitis, but intravenous administration of mesna can (64).

Mucositis is a frequent complication of BMT conditioning. Because TNF-α is thought to be involved in the pathogenesis of mucositis, a phase I study using pentoxifylline (2 g/day orally)—which interferes with TNF-α transcription—was conducted in high-risk allogeneic transplanted patients. In this series of 30 patients, the incidence of mucositis, and also of liver dysfunction, renal insufficiency, and GVHD, were reduced significantly, compared with historical controls (65). However, recent controlled studies did not confirm these initially exciting results.

GRAFT VERSUS HOST DISEASE

GVHD remains a significant problem after allogeneic BMT. Acute GVHD generally develops within 2 to 8 weeks of marrow transplantation. Clinical manifestations include fever, skin rash, jaundice, diarrhea, vomiting, and, in some hyperacute cases, capillary damage and fluid retention.

Methotrexate combined with cyclosporin has been shown to be the most effective combination in decreasing the incidence of GVHD. Their routine use in combination has been hindered because of a higher relapse rate after methotrexate and cyclosporin administration, compared with therapy with cyclosporin alone (66). In this situation, however, actuarial relapse free survival is the same. When the cyclosporin plus methotrexate combination was compared with T-cell depletion of the marrow using CD6 and CD8 antibodies, acute and chronic GVHD were more prevalent in the T-cell–depleted group. Anti–IL-2 receptor monoclonal antibodies also have been tested, with promising results, in the prevention of GVHD, but further studies are still warranted. Methylprednisolone given intravenously at 2 mg/kg/day is the classic treatment of acute GVHD; 30% to 50% of patients respond to this treatment. A response to GVHD therapy does not mean a loss of graft versus leukemia effect. When clinicians encounter steroid resistant GVHD, several alternatives are now available: antithymocyte globulins, anti–IL-2 receptor antibodies, azathioprine, and anti-TNF antibodies.

Chronic GVHD occurs, to some extent, in approximately 40% of recipients of allogeneic BMT. Although this condition may be associated with a beneficial graft versus host leukemia effect under certain circumstances, it generally leads to significant morbidity and mortality. Experimental approaches to induce mild GVHD in autologous stem cell transfusions are underway to test whether an antitumor effect can also occur against solid tumors. Because of the morbidity, however, it is usually recommended that chronic GVHD be treated with steroids. In the case of thrombocytopenia, a poor prognostic factor, cyclosporin should be added (67).

LIVER DYSFUNCTION

Hepatic dysfunction occurs frequently after BMT, and various causal etiologies such as venoocclusive disease (VOD), GVHD, infections, drug injury, or parenteral nutrition must be distinguished. VOD is a consequence of toxic injury to the liver resulting from high-dose chemotherapy and radiotherapy. VOD is suspected clinically if jaundice, weight gain, and painful hepatomegaly develop in the first 2 weeks after BMT (68). Thirty percent of patients presenting with VOD ultimately die of hepatorenal failure. Therefore, several prophylactic options have been proposed. The most spectacular results have been observed with pentoxifylline (65). Prophylactic infusion of prostacyclin also may be effective, but its toxic side effects are limiting. The treatment of established VOD currently is limited to symptomatic measures.

The hepatotoxicity of acute GVHD probably results from both cellular injury (by T lymphocytes) and cytokines such as TNF and IFN. The treatment of GVHD is described above. The majority of patients with chronic GVHD show some degree of hepatic involvement.

PREVENTION OF VIRAL INFECTIONS

Viral opportunistic infections, primarily cytomegalovirus infections, represent a major infectious problem in transplanted patients. Several centers have reported that screened (cytomegalovirus negative) blood products can prevent cytomegalovirus infection in seronegative recipients with seronegative donors.

For cytomegalovirus positive recipients, two approaches have been studied widely: immunoprophylaxis with high doses of intravenous immunoglobulins (69) and antiviral chemoprophylaxis using acyclovir or ganciclovir (70). At least five controlled studies have shown a decrease in the incidence of interstitial pneumonia after immunoprophylaxis, although the incidence of cytomegalovirus infection is not always reduced significantly (69). In addition, in a large comparative study, other advantages of intravenous immunoglobulins have been noted: a reduced risk of GVHD, and a reduced incidence of bacterial septicemia and pneumonitis. Administration of human monoclonal anticytomegalovirus antibodies and adoptive immunotherapy using T-cell clones obtained from seropositive donors are two new promising approaches.

The first convincing study of antiviral drug prophylaxis was reported by Meyers in 1988 (71) using acyclovir. However, acyclovir is not an optimal anticytomegalovirus agent, although its use may be associated with a reduction in the incidence of mucositis. Ganciclovir, a new antiviral agent that slows the replication of cytomegalovirus, appears to be a better candidate for prophylaxis and treatment. Several recent studies have confirmed the value of early therapy with ganciclovir in transplant patients when cytomegalovirus infection is suspected (70). The development of newer antiviral agents, such as foscarnet, offers the possibility of additional therapeutic measures.

CYTOKINES

Hematopoietic growth factors have the potential to accelerate hematopoietic recovery after BMT and, by shortening the period of pancytopenia, are likely to reduce infectious and bleeding complications without increasing the incidence of graft failure or GVHD. Five hematopoietic growth factors are currently available for clinical use: erythropoietin, G-CSF, GM-CSF, macrophage colony–stimulating factor, and interleukin-3 (IL-3) (72).

Conversely, cytokines, particularly recombinant human interleukin-2 (IL-2), may have clinical application in the acceleration of immune recovery and some antitumoral benefit in malignant hemopathies. The rationale for the use of IL-2 after marrow transplantation is based on the observation that freshly isolated leukemia and lymphoma cells have been shown to be sensitive to lysis by IL-2–induced lymphocyte-activated killer cells in vitro (72, 73).

CONCLUSIONS

Patients undergoing BMT suffer prolonged marrow aplasia, significant nonmarrow toxicities, profound immunosuppression, and unique complications such as GVHD. This aplasia requires maximum supportive care, including close monitoring of clinical and laboratory parameters to anticipate or detect these potential complications as early as possible. In addition, the presence of aplasia requires the dedication and expertise of the medical and nursing team to deal with the other physical, social, and emotional disturbances.

INTENSIVE CARE IN CANCER PATIENTS

Intensive or critical care is becoming progressively more important in the management of cancer patients, and major cancer hospitals have developed intensive care units (ICUs) dedicated to patients with cancer—surgical as well as medical patients. However, there is limited information in the medical literature about intensive care in oncology, especially concerning descriptions (74) of the types or outcomes of patients admitted to such units (75).

Admission of patients in an ICU usually is based on several principles: (*a*) The patient must have a reversible problem. Patients whose chances of being cured or of having their disease put into remission are minimal probably should not be admitted to or should stay in an ICU. (*b*) The patient's autonomy must be respected: a patient who refuses intensive supportive therapy because of the potentially poor prognosis of the underlying neoplastic disease should not be admitted to the ICU. (*c*) Finally, because medical resources often are limited, even in highly developed countries, distributive justice should be taken into account, i.e., patients with the best chance of benefiting from intensive therapy should have priority on admission.

Despite the evidence that many patients with cancer can benefit from intensive care, there remains an assumption that patients with active malignant disease should not be admitted to an ICU in general hospitals. Such a bias makes it very difficult for oncologists to maintain a fruitful collaboration with critical care specialists for the management of the critically ill cancer patient (76). This negative opinion is not supported by scientific data; in fact, it stems from a bias of many physicians, who refuse critical care to cancer patients, although they are willing to provide it to patients with serious nonneoplastic diseases, such as advanced heart failure or liver cirrhosis, who may have no better short- or long-term prognosis (77). These prejudices may surface when cancer patients are sent to the ICU at a more severe stage of the complication than noncancer patients. In some cancer center studies using appropriate entry criteria, the ICU mortality is similar to that reported in general ICU patients (74): 22% in a medical surgical unit and 23% in two consecutive series from a medical critical care unit.

There are four main reasons to admit a cancer patient to the ICU: (a) postoperative recovery such as occurs in any high-risk postoperative patient (availability of continuous hemodynamic monitoring, early identification of cardiovascular and respiratory disturbances, facilities for respiratory support, and constant skilled nursing care); (b) critical complications of the cancer disease and their treatment, which varies and can be very specific for oncology; their management should consider the presence of a severe chronic underlying disease as well; (c) intensive anticancer treatment administration and monitoring, which is useful in situations such as the increased risk for treatment administration related to the patient's condition, administration of intensive chemotherapy requiring patient monitoring, treatment of unknown toxicity in phase I trials requiring optimal safety conditions of surveillance, and administration of treatment that frequently results in acute severe toxicity; and (d) acute disease (such as myocardial infarction or acute asthma), related or unrelated to the neoplastic disease or its treatment.

Complications caused by cancer or its treatment that require intensive care are multiple, with specific characteristics related to their particular frequency. For example, coronary acute events are rare, but hypercalcemia is frequent. Also relevant for intensive care is the occurrence of complications only seen in oncologic patients, e.g., acute tumor lysis or leukostasis, and the presence of a severe underlying disease, i.e., the cancer. Critical care management of the patient also should consider the underlying neoplastic disease, which makes the individual more fragile because of the presence of immunosuppression, neutropenia, hemostatic disorders, the metastatic process, or paraneoplastic syndromes. Because of these concerns, close collaboration between the oncologist and the critical care specialist is important to balance the critical care management with anticancer therapy and preventive or supportive care of toxic effects related to it.

Critical care techniques performed in cancer patients are basically the same as those in noncancer patients. Among these, cardiopulmonary resuscitation (CPR) is a controversial procedure, particularly if extensive metastases are present. A review of studies published from 1980 to 1989 that deal with survival after CPR showed that far fewer patients with cancer survived until discharge compared with patients with other diagnoses. Among nine studies of outcome after CPR, only two found patients with cancer who survived and were discharged (total of 7 patients of 243 resuscitated), and all of these patients had localized disease; there were no survivors among patients with metastatic disease. These data, from which the recommendation not to resuscitate metastatic cancer patients could be drawn, are not supported by the experiences reported by critical care specialists from cancer centers.

The effectiveness of CPR in medical and surgical patients with cancer was evaluated at the Memorial Sloan–Kettering Cancer Center in New York (78). During a 3-year period, 750 patients suffered from cardiopulmonary arrest (1.53% of all admissions), and 114 were treated using resuscitative procedures because of their good general condition and the absence of a no-code order (do not resuscitate order). Seventy-five (66%) were resuscitated successfully, but only 12 of these (16%), including patients with metastatic disease, survived long enough to be discharged from the hospital, after an average stay of 11.3 days in the ICU; their overall mean survival after discharge was 223 days (median, 150 days; range, 3 to 350 days).

A retrospective analysis of the patients admitted to a medical ICU was conducted at the Jules Bordet Institute in Brussels (74) to determine the effectiveness and potential indications of CPR. During a 6-year period, cardiac arrest occurred in 49 nonsurgical cancer patients; CPR was successful in 19 (39%), but only 5 (10%) were discharged alive from the hospital. CPR was successful in all 8 patients in whom cardiac arrest was the consequence of an acute cardiovascular drug toxicity, even if the cancer was metastatic and the purpose of the treatment was not curative. Five of these patients were discharged alive from the hospital. CPR was effective in only 25% of the patients in whom cardiac arrest was an ultimate complication of various problems such as septic shock or respiratory failure complicating a neoplastic disease; none of these patients was discharged alive from the hospital. The results of this study suggest that in cancer, as in other diseases, CPR is indicated primarily when cardiac arrest is the consequence of an acute cardiac insult or an easily reversible condition.

CONCLUSIONS

Intensive care has developed into an important aspect of supportive care as a means of providing the optimal technology for the therapy of acute complications related to cancer, its treatment, or unrelated causes. The ICU also plays a basic role in monitoring patients undergoing therapies with potential acute toxicities.

USE OF INTRAVENOUS DEVICES

Maintenance of vascular access using long-term venous catheters has become a cornerstone in the management of patients suffering from chronic debilitating diseases such as cancer. Aggressive cancer therapies may require intensive support, e.g., severe mucositis can lead to nutritional defects that can be countered by parenteral nutrition. Other medical complications may require intravenous administration of drugs such as antibiotics, diuretics, antiemetics, or cardiotonic drugs. For clinical situations in which venous access is frequent and multiple, such as acute leukemia or BMT, indwelling right atrial catheters of the Hickman or Broviac type are used commonly; they are tunneled under the skin, require frequent flushing, and impose movement, bathing, and activity restrictions. For patients who require a more intermittent access, totally implantable subcutaneous ports (like Port-A-Cath; Pharmacia, Brussels, Belgium) have been introduced. Although these catheters need no dressing changes and less heparin flushing, their use may be limited to single channels.

NONINFECTIOUS COMPLICATIONS

With a frequency of 2% to 20%, complications caused by placement of catheters often are remedied easily, and no related death has been reported (Table 48.7). After the insertion of the catheter, thrombosis of either the catheter or the vein is clearly the most frequent noninfectious complication; the complication rate is 5% to 10%, independent of the type of catheter (79). Some cancer patients may have a hypercoagulable state and, and therefore are more prone to thrombosis of the central vein around the catheter. In the case of thrombosis within the catheter, infusion of fibrinolytic agents (urokinase or streptokinase) can be successful. Bleeding is an uncommon complication, except in the setting of an underlying coagulation disturbance such as disseminated intravascular coagulation. Surprisingly, migration of the catheter is common. In the study of Mirro et al. (80), dislodgement was the most frequent cause of failure, and removal of the catheter was unavoidable.

COMPLICATIONS FROM INFECTIONS

Infection of central venous catheters is one of the leading complications and a major source of nosocomial sepsis. The rate of central catheter–related septicemia ranges from 4% to 14% (81). Patients with cancer are particularly prone to developing such infections and to present complicated courses for several reasons: cancer-associated immunodeficiency, antineoplastic treatments, corticosteroid administration, or neutropenia. Parenteral hypercaloric nutrition is another classic source of microbiologic contamination. Finally, optimal supportive care implies frequent manipulations of central venous catheters, which can be a major cause of contamination. An important but as yet unresolved issue in terms of prevention is the choice of catheter material: polyvinylchloride catheters seem to be more thrombogenic and more easily colonized by staphylococci or fungi than are silicone and polyurethane catheters.

Another preventive method consists of lowering the microbial burden at the insertion site. Maki et al. (82) found a fourfold lower rate of infection when 2% chlorhexidine gluconate was used, compared with 70%

TABLE 48.7. *Complications Related to Intravenous Devices*

Noninfectious complications
  Contemporary with the insertion:
    Pneumothorax, subcutaneous emphysema, arterial puncture, hematoma, embolism, extravasation, arrhythmia, brachial plexus injury
  After the insertion:
    Thrombosis (of the vein, of the catheter), embolism, migration, extravasation, skin necrosis, damage of the external part
Infections complications
  Local catheter infection:
    Exit site, tunnel, port pocket
  Systemic infections:
    Thrombophlebitis, septicemia with or without septic metastasis (endocarditis)

alcohol or 10% povidone-iodine. Topical antibiotics are very useful against bacterial infections, but they promote fungal colonization and subsequent infection. Systemic antimicrobial prophylaxis is very controversial and seems to offer little or no benefit.

Exit site infections are the least serious complications. Systemic antibiotics plus local care are often sufficient, except for infections by *Pseudomonas* species, which usually require removal of the device.

Tunnel infections are best managed by removing the central venous line and giving systemic antimicrobial therapy. If replacement of the long-term catheter is difficult (e.g., in thrombocytopenic cancer patients), removal may sometimes be delayed. In case of infection caused by *Mycobacterium* species (*Mycobacterium fortuitum* or *Mycobacterium chelonae*), surgical excision of the injured tissue is often necessary. Infection around an implanted device (port pocket infection) requires surgical removal of the port and drainage of the pocket.

Vancomycin or teicoplanin, infused through the infected line, is the treatment of choice for coagulase negative staphylococci infection. If the patient responds within 48 to 72 hours, a total treatment duration of 5 to 7 days should be adequate. Catheter removal does not influence the outcome, thus most investigators recommend leaving the catheter in place.

Serious infectious complications have been reported in association with catheter-related *Staphylococcus aureus* bacteremia. The frequency of such complications ranges from 19% to 31% in the general patient population and from 33% to 46% among cancer patients. Severe complications consist of septic thrombosis, fatal sepsis, and secondary localizations such as endocarditis, osteomyelitis, or metastatic abscesses (83). Fever and/or bacteremia persisting for more than 3 days after catheter removal has been shown to be strongly suggestive of a complicated course (83); in such cases, at least 4 weeks of appropriate intravenous antibiotics is necessary. Otherwise, 10 days of intravenous therapy is probably sufficient. Unlike coagulase negative staphylococci bacteremia, every *Staphylococcus aureus* catheter-related sepsis necessitates the removal of the device; that procedure may be delayed, with concurrent antimicrobial therapy, in particular patients such as those with thrombocytopenia.

The treatment of choice for a device infected by yeasts is the removal of the catheter plus intravenous administration of amphotericin B. If the patient's condition improves rapidly, a very short course of amphotericin B may be sufficient. In the case of a nonimproving condition or if a thorough evaluation reveals retinitis, endocarditis, or hepatosplenic candidiasis, intravenous amphotericin B treatment must be prolonged for an as yet undefined period. Recently, less toxic and more easily administered antifungal agents, such as fluconazole and itraconazole, have been introduced. Their potency as treatment of fungemia is now under investigation.

Several gram negative bacilli have been associated particularly with catheter-related infection: *Pseudomonas maltophilia*, *Achromobacter* species, *Acinetobacter* species, and others. Gram positive bacilli (*Corynebacterium jeikeium*, *Bacillus* species) may be encountered in the same clinical setting. The global management remains appropriate systemic antimicrobial therapy and removal of the infected line.

Conclusions

Use of intravenous access devices represents a major advance in comfort for many patients undergoing cancer treatment; this advantage is counterbalanced, to some extent, by iatrogenic complications related to the use of these systems. Careful attention to the placement and use of these devices, as well as an awareness of the possible thrombotic and infectious complications, certainly improve the benefit-toxicity ratio.

References

1. Pizzo PA. Considerations for the prevention of infections complications in patients with cancer. Rev Infect Dis 1989;11(Suppl 7):S1551–1563.
2. Daw MA, Munnelly P, McCann SR, Daly PA, Falkiner FR, Keane CT. Value of surveillance cultures in the management of neutropenic patients. Eur J Clin Microbiol Infect Dis 1988;7:742–747.
3. Pizzo PA, Robichaud KJ, Brenda KE, Schumaker C, Barrett KS. Oral antibiotic prophylaxis in patients with cancer: a double-blind randomized placebo-controlled trial. J Pediatr 1983;102:125–133.
4. Meunier F. Prevention of mycoses in immunocompromised patients. Rev Infect Dis 1987;9:408–416.
5. Antman KS, Griffin JD, Elias A, Soginski MA, Ryan L, Cannistra SA, Oette D, et al. Effect of recombinant human granulocyte-macrophage colony stimulating factor on chemotherapy-induced myelosuppression. N Engl J Med 1988;319:593–598.
6. Klastersky J, Mommen P, Cantraine F, Safury A. Placebo controlled pneumococcal immunization in patients with bronchogenic carcinoma. Eur J Cancer Clin Oncol 1986;22:807–813.
7. Young LS, Gascon R, Alam S, Bermudez LEM. Monoclonal antibodies for treatment of gram negative infections. Rev Infect Dis 1989;11(Suppl 7):S1564–1572.
8. Bodey GP, Buckley M, Sathe YS, Freireich EJ. Quantitative relationship between circulating leukocytes and infections in patients with acute leukemia. Ann Intern Med 1966;64:328–340.
9. Schimpff SC. Empiric antibiotic therapy for granulocytopenic cancer patients. Am J Med 1986;80(Suppl 5C):13–20.

10. Schimpff SC, Satterlee W, Young VM, Serpick A. Empiric therapy with carbenicillin and gentamicin for febrile patients with cancer and granulocytopenia. N Engl J Med 1971;284:1061–1064.
11. Hughes WT, Armstrong D, Bodey GP, Feld R, Mandell GL, Meyers JD, Pizzo PA, et al. Guidelines for the use of antimicrobial agents in neutropenic patients with unexplained fever. J Infect Dis 1990;161:381–396.
12. Sculier JP, Klastersky J. Significance of serum bactericidal activity in gram negative bacillary bacteremia in patients with or without granulocytopenia. Am J Med 1984;76:429–435.
13. Pizzo PA, Hathorn JW, Hiemenz J, Browne M, Commers J, Cotton D, Gress J, et al. A randomized trial comparing ceftazidime alone with combination antibiotic therapy in cancer patients with fever and neutropenia. N Engl J Med 1986;315:552–558.
14. Gralla RJ, Itri LM, Pisko SE, Squillante A, Kelsen DP, et al. Antiemetic efficacy of high dose metoclopramide: randomized trials with placebo and prochlorperazine in patients with chemotherapy-induced nausea and vomiting. N Engl J Med 1981;3205:905–909.
15. Kri MJ, Gralla RJ, Clark RA, Tyson LB, Fiore JJ, et al. Consecutive dose-finding trials adding lorazepam to the combination of metoclopramide plus dexamethasone: improved subjective effectiveness over the combination of diphenhydramine plus metoclopramide plus dexamethasone. Cancer Treat Rep 1985;69:1257–1262.
16. Clark RA, Gralla RJ, Kris MG, Tyson LR. Exploring very high dose metoclopramide (4–6 mg/kg) preservation of efficacy and safety with only a single dose in a combination antiemetic regimen. Proc Am Soc Clin Oncol 1989;8:330.
17. Markman M, Sheiler V, Ettinger DS, Quaskey SA, Mellits ED. Antiemetic efficacy of dexamethasone: randomized double-blind, crossover study with chlorpromazine in patients receiving cancer chemotherapy. N Engl J Med 1984;311:549–552.
18. Hawthorn J, Cunningham D. Dexamethasone can potentiate the antiemetic action of the 5HT3 receptor antagonist on cyclophosphamide induced vomiting in the ferret. Br J Cancer 1990;61:56–60.
19. Bianchi C, Beani L, Crema C. Effects of metoclopramide on isolated guinea pig colon. Eur J Pharmacol 1970;12:332–341.
20. McRitchie B, McClelland CM, Cooper SM, Turner DH, Sanger G. Dopamine antagonist as antiemetics and as stimulants of gastric motility. In: Bennet A, Velo G, eds. Mechanisms of gastrointestinal motility and secretion. New York: Plenum Press, 1984;287–301.
21. Marty M. A comparison of granisetron as a single agent with conventional combination antiemetic therapies in the treatment of cytostatic-induced emesis. Eur J Cancer 1992;28A(Suppl 1):12–16.
22. Bonneterre J, Chevalier B, Metz R, et al. A randomized double-blind comparison of emesis induced by cyclophosphamide, fluorouracil and doxorubicin or epirubicin chemotherapy. J Clin Oncol 1990;8:1063.
23. Demulder PHM, Seynave C, Vermorken JB, Van Liessum PA, Mols-Jevdevic S, et al. Ondansetron compared with high-dose metoclopramide in prophylaxis of acute and delayed cisplatin-induced nausea and vomiting. Ann Intern Med 1990;113:834–840.
24. Roila F, Tonato M, Cognetti F, Cortesi E, Favalli G, Marangolo M, et al. Prevention of cisplatin-induced emesis; a double-blind multicenter crossover study comparing ondansetron and ondansetron plus dexamethasone. J Clin Oncol 1991;9:675–678.
25. Smith DB, Newlands ES, Rustin GJS, Regent RHJ, Howells N, et al. Comparison of ondansetron and ondansetron plus dexamethasone as antiemetic prophylaxis during cisplatin-containing chemotherapy. Lancet 1991;338:487–490.
26. Smyth JF, Coleman RE, Nicolson M, Gallmeier WM, Leonard RCF, et al. Does dexamethasone enhance control of acute cisplatin induced emesis by ondansetron? BMJ 1991;303:1423–1426.
27. Gandara DR. Progress in the control of acute and delayed emesis induced by cisplatin. Eur J Cancer 1991;27(Suppl 1):9–11.
28. Singer RF, Ritch PS, Lad TE, et al. Treatment of hypercalcemia of malignancy with intravenous etidronate. A controlled, multicenter study. Arch Intern Med 1991;151:471–476.
29. Thurlimann B, Waldburger R, Senn HJ, Thiebaud D. Plicamycin and pamidronate in symptomatic tumor-related hypercalcemia: a prospective randomized crossover trial. Ann Oncol 1992;3:619–623.
30. Rotstein S, Glas U, Eriksson M, et al. Intravenous clodronate for the treatment of hypercalcemia in breast cancer patients with bone metastases. A prospective randomized placebo-controlled multicenter study. Eur J Cancer 1992;28A:890–893.
31. Harinck HIJ, Bijvoet OLM, Plantingh AST, et al. Role of bone and kidney in tumor-induced hypercalcemia and its treatment with bisphosphonate and sodium chloride. Am J Med 1987;82:1133–1142.
32. Body JJ, Borkowski A, Cleeren A, Bijvoet ALM. Treatment of malignancy associated hypercalcemia with intravenous aminohydroxypropylidene bisphosphonate (APD). J Clin Oncol 1986;4:1177–1183.
33. Body JJ, Magritte A, Seraj F, Sculier JP, Borkowski A. Aminohydroxyprolidene bisphosphonate (APD) treatment for tumor-associated hypercalcemia: a randomized comparison between a 3-day treatment and single 24-hour infusions. J Bone Min Res 1989;4:923–928.
34. Body JJ. Bone metastases and tumor-induced hypercalcemia. Curr Opin Oncol 1992;4:624–631.
35. Body JJ, Dumon JC, Thirion M, Cleeren A. Circulating PTHrP concentrations in tumor-induced hypercalcemia: influence on the response to bisphosphonate and changes after therapy. J Bone Min Res 1993; in press.
36. Rizzoli R, Buchs B, Bonjour JP. Effect of a single infusion of alendronate in malignant hypercalcemia: dose dependency and comparison with clodronate. Int J Cancer 1992, 50:706–712.
37. Fearon KCH, Plumb FA, Calman KC. Nutritional consequences of cancer in man. Clin Nutr 1986;5:81–89.
38. Long CL, Lowry SF. Hormonal regulation of protein metabolism. J Parenter Enter Nutr 1990;14(6):555–562.
39. Gelin J, Moldawer LL, Lonroth C, Sherry B, Chizzonite R, et al. Role of endogenous tumor necrosis factor alpha and interleukin 1 for experimental tumor growth and the development of cancer cachexia. Cancer Res 1991;51:415–421.
40. Bernstein IL. Etiology of anorexia in cancer. Cancer 1986;58:1881–1886.
41. Parnes HL, Aisner J. Protein calorie malnutrition and cancer therapy. Drug Safety 1992;7:404–416.
42. Hamburger AW, Parnes H, Gordon GB, Shantz LM, et al. Megestrol acetate induced differentiation of 3T3L1 adipocytes in-vitro. Semin Oncol 1988;15(51):68–75.
43. Kosty MP, Fleishman SB, Herndon JE, et al. Cisplatin, vinblastine and hydrazine sulfate in advanced non–small-cell lung cancer: a randomized, placebo controlled, double-blind phase III study of the Cancer and Leukemia Group B. J Clin Oncol 1994;12:1113–1120.
44. Foley KM. The treatment of cancer pain. N Engl J Med 1985;313:84–95.
45. Bonicca JJ, Ventafridda V, Turycross RG. Cancer pain. In: Bonica J, ed. Management of pain. Philadelphia: Lea Springer, 1990;400–460.

46. ASCO. Cancer pain assessment and treatment curriculum guidelines. Ad hoc committee on cancer pain of the American Society of Clinical Oncology. Support Care Cancer 1993;1:67–73.
47. Bruera E, Mac Millan D, Hanson J, Mac Donald RN. The Edmonton staging system for cancer pain: preliminary report. Pain 1989;37:203–210.
48. Zens M. Morphine myths: sedation, tolerance, addiction. Postgrad Med J 1991;67(2):100–102.
49. Derogatis LR, Morrow G, Fetting H, et al. The prevalence and severity of psychiatric disorders among cancer patients. JAMA 1983;249(6):751–757.
50. Razavi D, Delvaux N, Farvacques C, Robaye E. Screening for adjustment disorders and major depressive disorders in cancer inpatients. Br J Psychiatry 1990;156:79–83.
51. Razavi D, Delvaux N, Bredart A, et al. Screening for psychiatric disorders in a lymphoma out-patient population. Eur J Cancer 1992;28A(11):1869–1872.
52. Delvaux N, Razavi D, Farvacques C. Cancer care—a stress for health professionals. Soc Sci Med 1988;27:159–166.
53. Razavi D, Delvaux N, Farvacques C, Robaye E. Immediate effectiveness of brief psychological training for health professionals dealing with terminally ill cancer patients: a controlled study. Soc Sci Med 1988;27:369–375.
54. Holland JC, Howland JH. Handbook of psychooncology. Oxford: Oxford University Press, 1989.
55. O'Berle KA, Davies B. Support and caring: exploring the concepts. Oncol Nurs Forum 1992;19(5):763–767.
56. Wujcik D. Current research in side effects of high-dose chemotherapy. Semin Oncol Nurs 1992;8(2):102–112.
57. Anderson JL. The nurse's role in cancer rehabilitation. Review of the literature. Cancer Nurs 1989;12(2):85–94.
58. Copp KA. Education and training in cancer. A European perspective. Cancer Nurs 1988;11(4):255–258.
59. Schiffer CA, Wiernik PH. Hematologic supportive care in patients with cancer. In: Calabresi P, Schein P, Rosenberg S, eds. Medical oncology. New York: Macmillan, 1985:1358–1370.
60. Higby DJ, Cohen E, Holland JF, et al. The prophylactic treatment of thrombocytopenic leukemic patients with platelets: a double-blind study. Transfusion 1974;14:440–446.
61. Murphy S, Litwin S, Herring LM, et al. Indications for platelet transfusion in children with acute leukemia. Am J Hematol 1982;12:347–356.
62. Dutcher JP, Schiffer CA, Aisner J, O'Connel B. Incidence of thrombocytopenia and serious hemorrhage among patients with solid tumors. Cancer 1984;53:557–562.
63. Braverman AC, Antin JH, Plappert MT, et al. Cyclophosphamide cardiotoxicity in bone marrow transplantation: a prospective evaluation of new dosing regimens. J Clin Oncol 1991;9:1215–1223.
64. Atkinson K, Biggs JC, Golovsky D, et al. Bladder irrigation does not prevent hemorrhagic cystitis in bone marrow transplant recipients. Bone Marrow Transplant 1991;7:351–354.
65. Bianco JA, Appelbaum FR, Nemunaitis J, et al. Phase I-II trial of pentoxifylline for the prevention of transplant-related toxicities following bone marrow transplantation. Blood 1991;78:1205–1211.
66. Aschan J, Ringden O, Sundberg B, et al. Methotrexate combined with cyclosporine. It decreases graft-versus-host disease, but increases leukemic relapse compared to monotherapy. Bone Marrow Transplant 1991;7:113–119.
67. Sullivan KM, Witherspoon RP, Storb R, et al. Alternating-day cyclosporine and prednisone for treatment of high-risk chronic graft-versus-host disease. Blood 1988;72:555–561.
68. Shulman HM, Hinterberger W. Hepatic veno-occlusive disease liver toxicity syndrome after bone marrow transplantation. Bone Marrow Transplant 1992;10:187–214.
69. Bron D, Klastersky J. Immunoprophylaxis of cytomegalovirus infections in transplanted patients. Eur J Cancer Clin Oncol 1989;25(9):1365–1368.
70. Schmidt GM, Horak DA, Niland JC, Dungan SR, Forman SJ, Zaia JA, City of Hope–Stanford–Snytex CMV Study Group. A randomized controlled trial of prophylactic ganciclovir for cytomegalovirus pulmonary infection in recipients of allogeneic bone marrow transplants. N Engl J Med 1991;324:1005–1011.
71. Meyers JD, Reed EC, Shepp DH, et al. Acyclovir for prevention of cytomegalovirus infection and disease after allogeneic marrow transplantation. N Engl J Med 1988;318:70–75.
72. Neidhart JA. Hematopoietic cytokines: current use in cancer therapy. Cancer 1993;72(Suppl):3381–3386.
73. Teichman JV, Ludwig WD, Thiel E. Cytotoxicity of interleukin-2 induced lymphocyte-activated killer (LAK) cells against human leukemia and augmentation of killing by interferons and tumor necrosis factor. Leukemia Res 1992;16:287–298.
74. Sculier JP, Ries F, Verboven N, Coune A, Klastersky J. Role of intensive care unit in a medical oncology department. Eur J Cancer Clin Oncol 1988;24:513–517.
75. Schapira DU, Studniki J, Bradham DD, et al. Intensive care, survival, and expense of treating critically-ill cancer patients. JAMA 1993;269:783–786.
76. Chevrolet JCI, Jolliet PH. An ethical look at intensive care for patients with malignancies. Eur J Cancer 1991;27:210–212.
77. Wachter RM, Luce JM, Hearst N, Lo B. Decisions about resuscitation: inequities among patients with different diseases but similar prognoses. Ann Intern Med 1989;11:525–532.
78. Vitelli CE, Cooper K, Rogatko A, Brennan MF. Cardiopulmonary resuscitation and the patient with cancer. J Clin Oncol 1991;9:111–115.
79. Brothers TE, Von Moll LK, Niederhuber JE, et al. Experience with subcutaneous infusion ports in three hundred patients. Surg Gynecol Obstet 1988;166:295–301.
80. Mirro J Jr, Rao BN, Stokes DC, et al. A prospective study of Hickman/Broviac catheters and implantable ports in pediatric oncology patients. J Clin Oncol 1989;7:214–222.
81. Raad II, Bodey GP. Infectious complications of indwelling vascular catheters. Clin Infect Dis 1992;15:197–210.
82. Maki DG, Ringer M, Alvarado CJ. Prospective randomized trial of providone-iodine, alcohol, and chlorhexidine for prevention of infection associated with central venous and arterial catheters. Lancet 1991;338:339–343.
83. Raad II, Narro J, Khan A, et al. Serious complications of vascular catheter-related Staphylococcus aureus bacteremia in cancer patients. Eur J Clin Microbiol Infect Dis 1992;11:675–682.

Complications

49A

TOXICITY OF COMBINED MODALITY THERAPY

Steven J. Westgate and Michael C. Perry

Untreated, cancers are both fatal and highly morbid diseases. The morbidity of the progressive disease itself must be weighed against treatment-related morbidity. Cancer morbidity may be of only short duration before death, whereas the lifelong complications from treatment in a cured patient can be severe. Combined or multimodality treatments (CMT) is defined as the use of two or more cancer treatments: surgery, radiation therapy, or chemotherapy. Many such treatment programs have shown progressive improvement in the survival rate of patients, and a growing number of survivors have been exposed to a variety of long-term treatment-related morbiities. These toxicities possess the potential to alter significantly the quality of remaining life. Multimodality therapies can produce a different toxicity profile or toxicities with greater frequency or severity compared with single modalities. This chapter addresses some of the acute and chronic toxicities encountered with the use of radiotherapy, chemotherapy, and combined modality therapy in adult patients generally, with a focus on these occurring in thoracic malignancies. The subject has recently been reviewed in detail (1). (See also Chapters 21 and 27.)

Radiation therapy and chemotherapy may be combined in three time sequences: sequential, concurrent, or alternating, each with different potential toxicity profiles. Some of the possible toxicities and their potential time of onset are outlined in Table 49A.1.

Because side effects can occur at any point along a time continuum, the precise onset of these changes can be difficult to pinpoint. However, for the sake of this discussion, *acute* changes are those occurring within the first 90 days of treatment, and *chronic* changes are those occurring after or lasting more than 90 days.

RADIOTHERAPY

The important treatment variables that determine radiation toxicity include total dose, dose fractionation schedules, fields, port size, and type of radiation used. Patient variables that affect radiation toxicity are listed in Table 49A.2. The acute toxicity profile of radiation is dominated by fatigue, esophagitis, and skin reactions. Late toxicities of radiation are the same dose-limiting constraints seen with standard radiation and include damage to the heart, lung, esophagus, and spinal cord. The thyroid, bone, soft tissue, and brachial plexus are also at risk, and carcinogenesis remains a potential problem.

In all organs treated with radiation, late histologic findings are found to varying degrees, depending on the organ and dose variables. Increased interstitial fibrosis, vascular lesions dominated by microvascular endothelial fibrosis and subsequent obliteration and ischemia, and atrophy of parenchyma and epithelium caused by direct cell death, apoptosis, and indirect effects of the interstitial and vascular changes and subsequent ischemia are some of the radiation-induced late (chronic) changes observed.

Although altered fractionation schedules can be used to reduce some of the acute complications of therapy (2), they generally have been used to increase the intensity of treatment through the use of hyperfractionation and accelerated fractionation in an attempt to improve the cure rate without increasing the long-term complication rate. For the purposes of definition, *hyperfractionation* regimens are designed to increase the total dose given over a "normal" period of time. To accomplish this, they reduce the dose per fraction and increase the total number of fractions (usually to twice or 3 times per day). *Accelerated frac-*

TABLE 49A.1. Overview of Complications of Combined Modality Therapy

ACUTE COMPLICATIONS	CHRONIC COMPLICATIONS
Radiation therapy	
Esophagitis	Esophageal stricture
Fatigue	Pulmonary fibrosis
Skin reaction	Cardiomyopathy
	Neuropathy
Chemotherapy	
Myelosuppression	Second malignancies
Nausea/vomiting	Neuropathy
Stomatitis/diarrhea	Cardiomyopathy
	Myelosuppression
Combined modality	
Myelosuppression	Esophageal stricture
Esophagitis	Cardiomyopathy
	Central nervous system toxicity
	Second malignancies

tionation regimens aim to reduce the overall treatment time. To accomplish this, the number of fractions, dose per fraction, or total dose may be reduced somewhat, but the overall intensity (dose time) is increased. Acute esophagitis has emerged as the dose-limiting reaction in many such trials.

There remains a distinct possibility that unforeseen late complications may occur in these trials of altered fractionation schedules. Two such examples are pertinent. Twice-a-day fractionation in two Radiation Therapy Oncology Group (RTOG) trials of upper and lower respiratory tract irradiation demonstrated an increased risk of late complications when the treatments were given less than 6 hours apart (3). In a Danish breast cancer trial, Svensson et al. (4) developed an isoeffect formula for the prediction of brachial plexopathy that failed to predict a 16% mild and 19% disabling plexopathy rate when giving 36.6 Gy in 12 fractions over 6 weeks (5).

In attempts to predict late complications of radiation therapy, a series of tables, graphs, and formulae have been developed using relatively standard doses and schedules of radiotherapy as a single modality of therapy (6–8). Extrapolation into novel dose schedules or protocols involving both chemotherapy and radiation must be done with caution.

CONFOUNDING VARIABLES AFFECTING RADIATION

Several case reports have suggested an increase in the severity of late complications in patients with systemic lupus erythematosus (9), discoid lupus (10), and systemic sclerosis (11). In a retrospective review of 61 patients with collagen vascular diseases treated with radiation therapy, Ross et al. (12) found no increased risk of acute or late complications of treatment compared with a well-matched control group.

Patients with AIDS have been shown to have an increased susceptability to acute mucosal reactions from radiation, even at cumulative doses as low as 10 to 18 Gy (13–16). Patient age may influence complication rates, but the results are confusing and depend on the disease and endpoint studied (5, 17, 18). Diabetes mellitus might be considered a potential hazard for radiation therapy, but Kucera et al. (19) found no increased risk of late complications in diabetics treated for cervical cancer.

Besides the obvious possible interaction between smoking and radiation on pulmonary function and carcinogenesis, many radiation oncologists (20, 21) think that concurrent smoking and radiation is associated with an increased risk of acute oral and esophageal mucosal reactions and delayed healing. However, Browman et al. (22) found that smoking did not adversely affect the ability to deliver adequate doses of radiation in head and neck cancer. Two studies have shown a decrease in the ultimate cure rate and survival of patients with oral cancer or lung cancer who continue to smoke (22, 23).

The combination of smoking and radiation may increase the risk of secondary lung cancer in patients with radiation to the chest wall or breast for breast cancer (24). Smoking and radiation both reduce pulmonary reserve, but it is unclear whether the combined risk is additive or synergistic. Smoking and radiation probably cause additive damage to the heart and soft tissues because of small vessel arteriosclerosis.

ACUTE TOXICITY

CUTANEOUS TOXICITY

When standard treatment schedules of 1.8- to 2-Gy daily fractions are used, acute cutaneous changes during radiation therapy to the chest usually begin during the second to third week of treatment. This period probably represents the time required for the deepest epidermal basal layers to migrate to the skin surface. The skin changes normally progress from erythema to dry desquamation and finally to moist desquamation. The worst skin reactions—rare in thoracic irradiation—are second-degree burns, and they heal without scarring. Hair loss in the treatment portal is common and usually is permanent. The timing and intensity of the skin reactions are affected by concomitant chemotherapy, but they do not seem to be af-

TABLE 49A.2. Patient Variables Affecting Radiation Toxicity

CONDITION	COMMENTS	REFERENCE NO(S).
Collagen vascular disease	DLE, SLE, SS: worse complications	9–11
	No increase in complications	12
AIDS	Worse acute mucositis	13–16
Age	Older patients: worse complications	17
	Younger patients: worse complications (conflicting data)	5, 18
Diabetes	Not a risk factor	19
Smoking	Worse acute mucositis	20, 21
	Synergistic carcinogenesis with radiation	24
	Decreased cure rates	23

Abbreviations. DLE, disseminated lupus erythematosus; SLE, systemic lupus erythematosus; SS, systemic sclerosis.

fected by accelerated and hyperfractionated radiation protocols (25–27).

The symptomatic treatment of skin reactions generally involves the use of moisturizing skin creams and lotions when the skin is simply red and sore; nonocclusive hydrogel dressings such as NuGel (Johnson & Johnson Medical, Inc., Arlington, TX) or Vigilon (CR Bard, Inc., Murray Hill, NJ); or occlusive semipermeable film such as Tegaderm (3M Health Care, St. Paul, MN) to relieve the pain of dry desquamation, and occlusive semipermeable hydrocolloidal dressings such as Duoderm CGF (Convatec; Bristol-Myers Squibb, Princeton, NJ) or Degasorb (3M Health Care, St. Paul, MN) for moist desquamation.

ESOPHAGEAL TOXICITY

The pathophysiology of radiation-induced esophagitis is one of degenerative changes of the mucosa with eventual resultant confluent desquamative mucositis. The normal time course for this occurrence is 3 to 4 weeks for standard fractionation. This toxicity is enhanced by accelerated and hyperfractionated radiation, by larger fraction sizes, and by the use of concurrent chemotherapy.

Clinically, esophagitis starts as dysphagia during the second week of therapy and progresses to odynophagia and chronic retrosternal pain over the next 2 to 3 weeks. This pain lasts through the end of therapy and then resolves over approximately 2 weeks. If enough of the mucosa is denuded, or if a secondary viral or fungal infection occurs, the healing phase may last for many weeks. Severe acute damage can lead to the consequential late effects of poor mucosal integrity, scarring, and long-term dysphagia and odynophagia. Symptoms do not always correlate well with objective findings, however (28).

Radiation esophagitis can be complicated by secondary infections, usually fungal or herpetic in origin. Patients who fail to respond to symptomatic treatment within a reasonable period should be considered for further diagnostic procedures. Endoscopy with biopsy and culture is required to make the diagnosis of secondary infection, although many patients are treated empirically.

The symptomatic treatment of esophagitis is multifaceted: avoidance of alcohol and tobacco, which enhance esophagitis; avoidance of foods that are acidic, enhance reflux, or are mechanically difficult to swallow (dry bread, large mechanical boluses); switching to soft foods and liquid nutritional supplements; using narcotic and nonsteroidal antiinflammatory analgesics; treating reflux; and using H2 blockers. Viscous xylocaine, hourly antacids, and different concoctions of slurries (e.g., various combinations of viscous xylocaine, antacids, antihistamines, carafate, antibiotics) have been tried. Despite these interventions, the average patient loses more than 10 pounds with a 60-Gy course of radiation. Radiation esophagitis tends to be the usual dose- or rate-limiting toxicity in many aggressive radiation and combined modality treatment protocols.

PULMONARY TOXICITY

Factors that influence the severity of radiation-induced pulmonary toxicity include total dose, field size (17), fraction size, preexisting pulmonary disease, and the simultaneous administration of chemotherapy. The pathophysiology is complex and involves primary damage to endothelial and type I (epithelial lining) alveolar cells. Because type I cells do not regenerate, they are replaced by type II (surfactant cells) that can sometimes differentiate into type I cells. At higher doses, type II cells also are lost. Functional damage accumulates over time as stem cells drop out after several generations. Damage may take several months to become manifest. Vascular engorgement, alveolar wall edema, and hyaline (fibrin) membranes in the alveoli and ducts are seen also. These latter findings and the resultant clinical picture are identical to that of the adult respiratory distress syndrome, which can be caused by infections, toxins, drugs, trauma, shock, and neurolgic injury.

Clincally, acute radiation pneumonitis is indistinguishable from other causes of adult respiratory distress syndrome or interstitial pneumonia and should be diagnosed only after other treatable causes are excluded. The major symptoms, dyspnea and cough, usually develop 7 to 16 weeks after radiation therapy. Fever, which is unusual, can be high. Chest pain, which is even more unusual, should alert the clinican to the possibility of other problems. An interstitial pattern on plain radiographs or computed tomography (CT) scans that conforms to radiation portals and not to anatomic boundaries is highly suggestive of the diagnosis of acute radiation pneumonitis. The reported incidence of clinical pneumonitis ranges from 3% to 15% in most reports (29), but the actual incidence is probably higher because most studies have not performed sufficient observation or an actuarial risk of pneumonitis in survivors.

CT is becoming the method of choice for the detection of acute radiation-induced pulmonary injury, defined as that observed within 20 weeks of the completion of radiotherapy (30). CT has better contrast resolution and greater sensitivity to slight differences in attenuation than conventional chest radiographs. CT also better delineates whether the infiltrate is confined within radiation portals or anatomic boundaries. Other tests of radiation injury have been studied, including gallium 67 citrate scanning combined with CT (31, 32) and single proton emission CT perfusion scanning (33), but none has become standard in clinical practice.

Acute and chronic pulmonary toxicities are related strongly to fraction size, total dose, and volume irradiated. With bilateral lung irradiation 8 to 9 Gy in single fractions is a safe upper limit (34); doses of 15 to 25 Gy can be given safely to both lungs in fractions of 1.5 to 1.8 Gy (35–38). With standard fraction radiation therapy for various thoracic malignancies, the incidence of clinically symptomatic pneumonitis is 0% to 15%, radiologic changes occur in roughly two thirds of patients, and most patients lose approximately 20% of demonstrable pulmonary function (forced expiratory volume in 1 second [FEV], forced vital capacity, total lung volume, ventilatory capacity, and carbon monoxide diffusing capacity) (29).

Therapy of acute pneumonitis includes the use of supplemental oxygen and corticosteriods, although there are no randomized clinical trials to show an advantage to corticosteroid use (39). There is suggestive evidence that oxygen therapy may accentuate the radiation toxicity, and hence the lowest fractional concentration of oxygen (FIO_2) that provides adequate oxygenation should be used. Treatment with anticoagulants and antibiotics has been advocated, but there is no clear evidence of efficacy in clinical trials (40, 41).

CARDIAC TOXICITY

Severe cardiac damage is rare and usually is seen as an acute nonspecific pericarditis that is associated with high radiation doses given to large areas of the heart. Such radiation usually is applied to large tumors that are juxtaposed to the heart. Acute pericarditis is not a predictor of late complications and does not require cessation of radiation therapy (42–44).

One major acute cardiac toxicity to be avoided is damage to electronic pacemakers, especially those that contain complementary metal oxide semiconductors (45, 46) that can be damaged by radiation. The sensor portion of pacemakers can be fooled by electromagnetic radiation, and pacemaker dependent patients with sensory pacemakers can go into acute asystole or runaway pacing. Pacemakers thus should be moved rather than irradiated.

ACUTE NEUROLOGIC TOXICITY

Lhermitte's sign—electric shocklike paresthesias in the arms, legs, or back noted with flexion of the neck—occurs in up to 25% of patients receiving 40- to 45-Gy mantle field irradiation for Hodgkin's disease (47, 48). It is thought to be caused by transient demyelination of the spinal cord. This symptom usually is transitory and does not correlate with the more devastating radiation myelitis and subsequent paralysis.

CHRONIC SIDE EFFECTS

CUTANEOUS EFFECTS

Pigmentary changes are a transitory late complication, and hyperpigmentation resolves over months. Late chronic cutaneous changes include atrophy, telangiectasia, and edema. Subcutaneous changes include loss of subcutaneous tissue as well as induration secondary to edema or fibrosis. Muscle atrophy in the radiation port is common in long-term survivors but is discussed rarely. Except on the scalp, hair loss in the treatment portal is usually of little concern to most patients. Edema of the upper extremities can occur with irradiation of the supraclavicular fossa (49), especially if the daily fraction is greater than 2 Gy (50, 51).

Late radiation necrosis is rare and often is associated with tumor recurrence, a late secondary insult to the blood supply such as shock or anemia, or in tissue that is thin, injury prone, or overlying bony prominences. The underlying pathologic process of radiation necrosis is obliterative endarteritis. Hyperbaric oxygen may be useful as a primary treatment (52–54), preoperatively when surgical reconstruction is anticipated, or when surgery is necessary in the highly irradiated area (55, 56). Myocutaneous or free vascular flap reconstruction may also be beneficial (57, 58).

ESOPHAGEAL TOXICITY

Chronic esophagitis, unrelated to acute esophagitis, is characterized by progressive dysphagia. Untreated, it may lead to irreversible esophageal stenosis—a devastating complication of radiation. In the treatment of primary esophageal carcinoma, stricture has been reported at doses of 50 Gy, and the generally quoted incidence is 1% to 5% at 60 Gy and 25% to 50% at 75 Gy (39, 59). The incidence of esophageal stricture after definitive high-dose radiation for esophageal cancer ranges from as high as 44% (60) to 67% (59). However, clinical evaluation attributed 75% of these strictures to recurrent carcinoma (59).

PULMONARY TOXICITY

Radiation fibrosis can be difficult to distinguish from persistent or recurrent tumor, even on CT. Helpful clues are the pattern of change over time and convexity (tumor) versus concavity (radiation fibrosis) of the consolidation noted on radiographic imaging.

The late pathologic outcome of radiation pneumonitis ranges from diffuse interstitial fibrosis to large scarred areas in the irradiated field. The combined physiologic outcome of this injury is a loss of pulmonary compliance, late consolidation and fibrosis, and right-to-left shunting of blood. The final outcome is dyspnea, tachypnea, and hypoxemia. Late radiation fibrosis also can lead to cor pulmonale and secondary respiratory or cardiac failure.

The major clinical risk factors for clinical irradiation damage are underlying premorbid pulmonary disease, the amount of lung irradiated, and the use of certain chemotherapeutic agents. As in lung resection, predicted posttreatment FEV_1 is a good predictor of long-term radiation risk. It is possible to measure pretreatment FEV_1 and to estimate the posttreatment FEV_1 from the drawn radiation fields. Unfortunately, until recently the amount of lung irradiated has only been estimated crudely, making prediction of the risk of pneumonitis very difficult. Three-dimensional treatment planning with the ability to construct dose-volume histograms may improve our ability to predict late problems clinically. It also is possible that sophisticated three-dimensional treatment planning and treatment techniques may allow smaller volumes of lung to be treated, potentially decreasing complication rates (decreased normal lung irradiation), providing higher cure rates (higher tolerable doses to tumor), or both.

CARDIAC TOXICITY

Although the heart was once considered radioresistant (61), it now is recognized that radiation doses to the heart must be limited to avoid excessive complications. The risk of heart damage was underrecognized because of the poor outcome of patients with lung cancer and the fact that cardiac death often was expected in this largely male, elderly, smoking population. It took an analysis of late complications of patients treated for Hodgkin's disease in the 1950s and 1960s—young, otherwise healthy patients with good cure rates and a long-term survival potential—to really appreciate the risk of late cardiac damage (62–64). Subsequent studies of men treated for seminoma have confirmed these risks (65). Treatment techniques have evolved that may have decreased the long-term cardiac toxicity risk of irradiation in Hodgkin's disease (66–68). However, the data from these studies may underestimate the risk in patients with lung cancer, who are treated with higher doses. All structures of the heart—pericardium, myocardium, endocardium, conduction system, valves, and coronary arteries—can be affected (65, 69).

Pericardial damage is manifested either as constrictive, effusive, or constrictive-effusive pericarditis. The resulting clinical syndromes are indistinguishable from other causes of pericarditis. The incidence is dependent on the dose and volume. The reported incidence also depends on whether the endpoint is symptomatic, radiographic, or detection at catheterization or autopsy. The incidence ranges from to 20% to 40% of patients, as defined by clinical parameters (67, 70–75). Constrictive syndromes were seen in 93% (38 of 41) of patients tested with right heart catheterization with provocative testing (76). Autopsy studies exceed a 50% incidence (62, 75).

Radiation causes interstitial and endothelial fibrosis, both of which can lead to primary cardiac failure, seen as congestive heart failure or electrical conduction abnormalities (65). Valvular heart disease is rare but may increase over time (78, 79).

Radiation also increases the risk of atherosclerotic coronary artery disease (CAD), which ultimately may become the major toxicity of thoracic radition if and when significant numbers of patients become cured of their intrathoracic cancers. Autopsy (82) and heart catheterization studies have demonstrated an increased risk of CAD. Based on these studies, the finding of proximal narrowing with normal distal vessels is suggestive of radiation-induced CAD (78, 80–82, 84–86). Reports of sudden death and CAD in young people treated to the heart for Hodgkin's (64, 78, 80, 83–85) and testicular tumors (65) have strongly implicated cardiac radiation as a significant risk for CAD. An analysis of four large databases including more than 8500 patients treated for Hodgkin's disease shows an absolute risk of myocardial infarction of approximately 2% but a relative risk of 2.6 to 8.8 (86–88). The absolute risk will probably increase with follow-up.

Radiation can indirectly damage the heart by increasing the pulmonary resistance to blood flow, thus creating pulmonary hypertension and secondary right-sided heart failure. The possibility of thyroid dysfunction secondary to radition as a cause of cardiac abnormalities should not be overlooked. Arrhythmias and sudden death seem to be increased in seminoma survivors who received mediastinal irradiation (65).

BONE MARROW TOXICITY

Only a small percentage of adult bone marrow remains in the thoracic spine, sternum, and ribs. Thus, myelosuppression is uncommon during radiation therapy, but blood cell counts must be monitored, especially in the heavily pretreated patient, those who are cytopenic, or those receiving concurrent chemotherapy. The so-called anemia of chronic disease also may occur with the use of radiation. Irradiation of thoracic bone marrow permanently depletes the bone marrow within the treated area. This depletion usually has no clinical significance except to lower bone marrow reserve. Bone marrow depletion leads to fat accumulation in the treated site instead of the late fibrosis seen in other organs (89, 90). Irradiated bone marrow may increase the risk of late acute leukemia. The risk of acute leukemia is increased in women who have had breast irradiation (91). However, the poor survival in lung cancer patients has not resulted in a striking incidence of leukemic complications.

CHRONIC NEUROLOGIC TOXICITY

The chronic neurologic effects of radiation therapy in lung cancer patients are seen in three areas: central nervous system toxicity from prophylactic cranial irradiation (PCI), spinal cord toxicity, and peripheral nerve toxicity from thoracic radiation. The damage to all three sites is thought to consist mainly of interstitial and vascular damage rather than direct neuronal damage (92, 93).

The role of PCI in small cell lung cancer is controversial because of the possible increased risk of leukoencephalopathy. Clinically significant decreases in neurologic status have been reported in some studies of long-term survivors of small cell lung cancer (94–96) but not in others (97–98). CT findings of cerebral atrophy, ventricular dilation, decreased white matter density (encephalomalacia), and cerebral calcifications are seen after PCI. Although these findings are almost universally seen in patients with clinical neurotoxicity after PCI (99), they also are seen often in asymptomatic long-term survivors (97–98). However, in a recent randomized study from the Institut Gustave-Roussy, Arriagada et al. (104) demonstrated an improved survival (29% versus 21.5% 2-year survival; $P = .14$) in patients with limited stage small cell lung cancer who received PCI after achieving a complete response, without any increased risk of leukoencephalopathy (100).

Standard radiation therapy portals often include the supraclavicular fossae in the first large anterior-posterior and posterior-anterior (AP/PA) field and put the brachial plexus at risk. This area usually is treated to doses in the range of 45 to 50 Gy, although modern radiation techniques are evolving away from routine coverage of the supraclavicular areas unless the tumor is in the upper lobe, when doses of more than 60 Gy are given. Failure to monitor dose and to use good radiation techniques can increase the chances of complications in this area. High dose fractions—often given in the palliative setting—increase the risk of neurologic complications. The effect of dose and fraction size has been well demonstrated in randomized studies of adjuvant radiation breast cancer trials (5, 101–103). However, the short survival of lung cancer patients often masks the potential for harm.

The clinical picture of brachial plexopathy is one of paraesthesia and hypesthesia occurring most frequently and earliest (1 to 6 months) followed by weakness, decreased reflexes, and pain. Latent periods of up to 6 years have been reported (103–106), although Danish studies found either an immediate or rapid onset of symptoms with no late onset of plexopathy (101).

Horner's syndrome is rare in radiation-induced plexopathy and common in neoplastic plexopathy, and it thus is a diagnostic clue (107). Several articles in the last 20 years have noted the difficulty in distinguishing radiation-induced brachial plexopathy from recurrent tumor. These articles are mainly retrospective reviews involving heterogenous populations of patients and tumors (103–105, 107–113).

Some of the published rates of plexopathy associated with fraction sizes of approximately 2 Gy are 1.3% with less than 50 Gy and 5.6% with more than 50 Gy (108), 1% at 54 Gy (103), and 3.2% at 60 Gy (110). At higher dose fractions, the incidence ranges from 2.4% using 3.4-Gy fractions to a dose of 51 Gy (109) to 5.9% (46 Gy in 15 fractions) (103). Stoll and Andrews (109) showed a 73% plexopathy rate for doses of more than 63 Gy, compared with 15% for doses of less than 58 Gy when mainly large dose fractions were used (105).

In a more accurate prospective trial of adjuvant irradiation of breast cancer using standard fractions, Olsen et al. reported a 9% mild and a 5% disabling brachial plexopathy rate in patients receiving 50 Gy in 2-Gy fractions. In an earlier study of larger dose fractions, Olsen and colleagues again reported a 16% mild and a 19% disabling plexopathy rate with 3.05-Gy fractions given twice a week for 6 weeks (36.6-Gy total dose). Cohen and Svenson (112) have developed an isoeffect table of peripheral nerve dose tolerance levels for a wide range of treatment schedules.

The most devastating late complication of mediastinal radiation is chronic progressive radiation myelitis (CPRM). CPRM is dependent on total dose, dose fraction size, and length of cord irradiated (114). CPRM usually begins gradually 6 to 24 months after the completion of radiation and eventually can lead to paralysis over the course of approximately 1 year (115). The incidence is quite low in practice. Fear of this complication may be the major reason for deliberate underdosing by some radiation oncologists; along with radiation pneumonitis, it is a major impetus for the development of three-dimensional treatment planning. Using standard fraction sizes and normal thoracic fields, the risk is 1% at 42 Gy, 5% at 45 to 59 Gy, and 50% at 61 Gy (116, 117).

The diagnosis of CPRM is one of exclusion because biopsy, which is not a reasonable option, is the only definitive means of making a diagnosis. Magnetic resonance imaging studies showing demyelination, white matter necrosis, hemorrhagic necrosis, or infarction in the irradiated field and secondary swelling or atrophy without evidence of recurrent tumor (localized or carcinomatous meningitis) or other cause of paralysis are presumptive proof. Increased cerebrospinal fluid protein is seen often. There is no effective treatment for this complicaton.

Endocrine Complications

Hypothyroidism is the most common thyroid complication of radiation therapy (118–120). The incidence appears to increase with increasing doses from 15 to 50 Gy (119–122). The long-term risk of hypothyroidism, manifested by an elevated serum thyroid–stimulating hormone after mantle irradiation, ranges from 44% to 88% (124, 122–124). The risk at 1 year is 15%, but this risk continues to increase over time (120). The incidence appears to peak at 2 to 3 years after irradiation and then falls off (122). Most radiation oncologists start patients on thyroid replacement once thyroid–stimulating hormone levels have been shown to be elevated (122).

Hyperthyroidism and Graves' disease also have been reported after neck irradiation for Hodgkin's disease (121, 122, 125). The absolute risk is low at approximately 3% (122), but the relative risk is estimated to range from 4.8 to 27.3 (122). Acute transient thyrotoxicosis without increased iodine uptake that progresses to hypothyroidism has been reported (126).

Carcinogenesis

Several case reports have desribed thyroid cancer after radiation (126–128). The initial review of a large series from Stanford (129), a multinational tumor registry review (130), and the Danish Tumor Registry (131) failed to show any statistical increase in thyroid cancer. However, the Connecticut Tumor Registry (132) and a later review of the Stanford data (122) showed a 6.7 and 15.6 increase in the relative risk of thyroid cancer, respectively. The absolute actuarial risk of thyroid cancer in the Stanford series was 1.7% (126). Given the low survival duration of patients with thoracic malignancies, secondary thyroid cancer is, at present, inconsequential.

Radiation-induced sarcomas of the chest wall have a reported 30-year cumulative incidence of 0.78% (133, 134). The risk of myelogenous leukemia is increased after irradiation of the breast (91). A recent article suggests a large risk of secondary lung cancer in smokers who received breast irradiation (24).

The absolute risk of secondary tumors after thoracic irradiation is quite low because so many of the patients with thoracic tumors have a relatively poor long-term survival. In contrast, secondary malignancies are well studied in cervical cancer. In cervical cancer, the chance of cure is quite high, many of the patients are young, and the radiation dosimetry is verified easily. Many older studies did not note an increased incidence of second malignancies (135–137), whereas others reported an increased risk (138). Two large, more recent studies evaluating 161,000 patients showed an increased risk of second cancers of the bladder, rectum, vagina, probably the stomach and the kidney, as well as leukemia and possibly bone, uterine corpus, cecum, and non-Hodgkin's lymphoma (139,

140). When compared with surgical controls, only approximately 5% of all of the second cancers could be attributed to radiation (139).

Although the risk of secondary cancers is statistically significant, it probably is not yet clinically significant in the current management and outcome of most thoracic tumors. However, second malignancies may become a problem after irradiation of the thorax, when the cure rate improves.

BONE

Necrosis is rare in non–weight-bearing bones, but it has been described in the ribs and clavicles after irradiation. The incidence is low in standard treatment of lung and esophageal cancers. In the treatment of breast cancer, the rate of rib fracture is increased because of inherent hot spots in many treatment plans and because of the lack of some tissue sparing compared with anterior-posterior and posterior-anterior fields for lung cancer. In modern series, the incidence of rib fracture is approximately 1% to 4% (108, 141, 142). True osteoradionecrosis is treated conservatively with resection and with hyperbaric oxygen. Marx et al. (56) used a hyperbaric oxygen therapy for the primary treatment of osteoradionecrosis of the jaw and had a 100% resolution of symptoms compared with a historic control rate of 5% to 30%.

CHEMOTHERAPY
ACUTE SIDE EFFECTS

The important factors for chemotherapy toxicity include the choice of chemotherapeutic agents (single and multiple drug combinations), dose, schedule, and intensity, and the patient's underlying condition. The most typical side effects of chemotherapy are on rapidly dividing tissues such as bone marrow, gut mucosa, and hair follicles, with resultant myelosuppression, stomatitis, nausea, vomiting, diarrhea, and alopecia (143). Other acute toxicities include hypersensitivity (allergic) reactions, drug extravasation, renal or hepatic impairment, and, rarely, cardiac abnormalities, depending on the drugs used. Other side effects depend on the agents selected, their dose, and schedule (Table 49A.3).

Stomatitis, diarrhea, and esophagitis, reflecting a generalized effect on gastrointestinal mucosa, often occur in concert with lowered white blood cell counts, increasing the possibility of bacterial entry, and subsequent infection.

Newer antiemetic agents have permitted the administration of once intolerable doses of chemotherapeutic agents such as cisplatin, significantly reducing this often treatment-limiting complication.

TABLE 49A.3. Acute Chemotherapy Complications

COMMON TO MANY AGENTS	PREDOMINANTLY SEEN WITH 1 OR 2 AGENTS
Nausea/vomiting	Hypotension (etoposide)
Extravasation	...
Leukopenia	...
Thrombocytopenia	Hypersensitivity reactions (paclitaxel, etoposide)
Stomatitis	...
Diarrhea	...
Alopecia	...
Acute tumor lysis syndrome	...

CARDIAC TOXICITY

Doxorubicin (Adriamycin; Pharmacia Adria, Dublin, OH) is the chemotherapeutic agent most commonly associated with the development of cardiac toxicity. Its unique cardiotoxicity is thought to be caused by the formation of radicals by a doxorubicin-iron complex. The endpoint is myocytic degeneration, seen clinically as congestive heart failure. Its occurrence has been linked closely to the total dose of doxorubicin administered. At a dose of 550 mg/m^2, the risk of heart failure is approximately 5%, and the risk increases steadily with higher doses (144). Among the risk modifiers of doxorubicin cardiotoxicity is mediastinal irradiation, in addition to the schedule used, preexisting cardiac disease, age, nutritional status, and other cytotoxic drugs used (144). The drugs that may potentiate doxorubicin's cardiac effects include cyclophosphamide, ifosfamide, etoposide, actinomycin, mitomycin, melphalan, vincristine, bleomycin, and dacarbazine.

PULMONARY TOXICITY

Bleomycin, the most common pulmonary toxin, causes a cumulative dose dependent proliferative alveolitis and subsequent fibrosis (145) that is accentuated by oxygen therapy and radiation. Cumulative doses in excess of 400 to 500 units should be avoided. Bleomycin also can cause an acute recall phenomenon after radiation therapy (146).

Multiple chemotherapeutic agents carry the potential for pulmonary toxicity (149). Actinomycin D combined with lung radiation for Wilms' tumor caused lethal radiation pneumonitis with otherwise safe doses of radiation (147). Like bleomycin, carmustine also has a cumulative dose threshold with an increasing incidence of late pulmonary fibrosis when doses exceed 1500 mg/m^2. Procarbazine and methotrexate may cause pulmonary hypersensitivity reactions (145).

BONE MARROW

Myelosuppression is the most important early side effect of chemotherapy, and almost all chemotherapeutic agents can cause some degree of pancytopenia (148). The average time to neutrophil nadir counts is 7 to 14 days, although the nitrosoureas and some other agents produce delayed and prolonged nadirs. Melphalan, mitomycin, the nitrosoureas, procarbazine, and carboplatin commonly result in cumulative myelosuppression. Although hematopoietic growth factors may shorten the duration of neutrophil nadir counts, the risk of neutropenic fever and sepsis still exists. Anemia is not usually seen acutely because of the longer lifespan of erythrocytes, but it may be seen with prolonged therapy. Erythropoietin is now available to stimulate red blood cell production, but its efficacy in reversing chemotoxicity is not well defined. Thrombopoietin, recently isolated and cloned, is not yet commercially available. Thrombocytopenia thus remains a significant and often dose-limiting problem after chemotherapy.

Although relatively uncommon in thoracic malignancies, chronically low peripheral blood cell counts can be seen in patients heavily treated with chemotherapy for other malignancies, such as Hodgkin's disease. Aplasia, in contrast, is distinctly uncommon unless agents that produce cumulative bone marrow suppression are used. There also is a risk of secondary leukemia from chemotherapy.

NEUROLOGIC TOXICITY

The acute effects of chemotherapy on the nervous system are limited to neuropathies—usually peripheral, sensorimotor neuropathies (vinblastine, vindesine, paclitaxel, altretamine, procarbazine)—and encephalopathies (ifosfamide, procarbazine). Less commonly, the cranial nerves and autonomic nervous system are affected (vincristine, vinblastine, vindesine). A transient cerebellar ataxia can be produced by 5-fluorouracil (149). Corticosteroids cause sleep disorders, dysphoria and euphoria, and steroid psychosis, restlessness, and acute progressive myopathy. Epidural lipomatosis can be caused by high doses of steroids and can even lead to paralysis.

Chemotherapy also can cause autonomic dysfunction, hearing loss (cisplatin), vestibular changes, and necrotizing leukoencephalopathy. Intravenous and intrathecal methotrexate and intrathecal cytosine arabinoside (ara-C) combined with radiation appear to cause the most problems, with increased risk of nercotizing leukoencephalopathy, mineralizing microangiopathy, cerebral atrophy, pontine myelinolysis, and acute leukoencephalopathy. LeBaron et al. (150) found a risk of late neurocognitive dysfunction in leukemic children treated with chemotherapy that was almost as high as in those also treated with radiation.

ACUTE TUMOR LYSIS SYNDROME

The syndrome of hyperkalemia, hyperuricemia, hyperphosphatemia, and hypocalcemia, known as the acute tumor lysis syndrome, usually is seen in rapidly responding tumors with very high proliferative rates that are very sensitive to chemotherapy. Typically, these are hematologic malignancies such as lymphomas and leukemias. It also has been seen in small cell lung cancer and should be anticipated so it can be detected and treated early (151).

CHRONIC EFFECTS

The late side effects of chemotherapy are seen only when the therapy is sufficient to permit long-term survival. More late complications are seen with the increasing efficacy of radiation therapy, chemotherapy, or combined modality therapy. Effects on gonadal function and the development of second malignancies are examples of such late effects.

ENDOCRINE EFFECTS

Sterility and amenorrhea are especially seen when the alkylating agents are used (151). The impact of these changes may not be appreciated in an older population such as that affected by lung cancer.

BONE MARROW EFFECTS

The development of a myelodysplastic syndrome or acute nonlymphocytic leukemia (ANLL) is a distressing late complication of chemotherapy seen mostly in long-term survivors of small cell lung cancer (99, 152, 153). ANLL or myelodysplastic syndrome was seen in 6 (0.8%) of 696 patients in one series (153) and in 2 (0.5%) of 377 in another (95). All patients had received combination chemotherapy (usually cyclophosphamide, Adriamycin, and vincristine or some modification) and irradiation of approximately one hemithorax. Dang et al. (154) reviewed their long-term survivors and found that cytogenetic abnormalities preceded the diagnosis of ANLL. Other patients, who did not have abnormal blood cell counts, had a decreased ability to form multilineage colonies; all patients showed some degree of aneuploidy.

In advanced non–small cell lung cancer, Ratain et al. (155) found four cases of ANLL in 119 patients (3%), all of whom had received etoposide and cisplatin with or without vindesine. They concluded that high doses of etoposide are potentially leukemogenic and are capable of producing a syndrome of acute monoblastic leukemia with features distinct from other secondary leukemias.

CARCINOGENESIS

Because of the much lower incidence of long-term survival in patients with non–small cell lung cancer, a lower incidence of second malignancies would be expected. However, the increased use of chemotherapy in neoadjuvant, adjuvant, or multimodality settings may well influence this incidence in the future.

COMBINED MODALITY THERAPY

Steel and Peckham (156) have outlined the four theoretical types of interaction between radiation and chemotherapy. The first is spatial cooperation, implying independent activity of each treatment modality, i.e., for radiation therapy in the treated field and for chemotherapy against metastatic disease. The second type of interaction is toxicity independence, which indicates administration of each modality at full (or near full) dose without a significant increase in normal tissue damage. The third type is protection of normal tissues from radiation by a systemic agent that permits higher doses of radiation. The fourth mechanism requires increased activity within the radiation field as a direct result of the interaction of chemotherapy with radiation. The chemotherapy is thus a sensitizer or enhancer.

Chemotherapy classically has been limited by acute toxicities, whereas radiation often is limited by delayed toxicities. Combined modality treatment offers the potential for improved tumor control at the risk of an increased toxicity profile. Possible methods of interaction include enhancement of radiation damage by chemotherapy, additive effects of both treatments on the same tissue or cell, or damage to different tissues or cells, causing a new physiologic insult. The greatest combined toxicities generally occur when the chemotherapy used has known toxicity to an organ that also is receiving radiation. Examples include cyclophosphamide and bleomycin–induced increased lung toxicity (157), bleomycin–induced increased mucosal toxicity (158), and Adriamycin–induced increased cardiac toxicity (159).

It is sometimes difficult to know whether the combined toxicities are additive, subadditive or, supraadditive (synergistic). Multiple assays and techniques and mathematical formulae have been developed to evaluate the toxicity interaction (156, 160). In acute toxicity, the survival of clonagenic stem cells within a tissue often determines toxicity. The presence of these stem cells allows the development of fairly accurate laboratory assays to study acute combined modality toxicity. The delayed toxicities of combined therapy cause, for example, fibrosis, vascular changes, stem cell loss, and apoptosis. This delay makes basic research and mathematical modeling difficult (161). More important to the clinician is the therapeutic gain factor, the ratio of the tumor dose enhancement factor to the normal tissue dose enhancement factor. The determination of toxicity is also dependent on the endpoint chosen: physiologic changes, gross changes, or survival (162). It is clear that close clinical observation still plays a decided role in the detection of toxicity of combined multimodality treatment. New or enhanced toxicities should be expected (163).

Vokes and Weichselbaum (164) recently reviewed the current clinical experience with concomitant chemoradiotherapy, including that used in the treatment of esophageal cancer and small cell and non–small cell lung cancers. The subject also is discussed in chapters on treatment of small call and non–small cell lung cancer and esophageal cancer. Several recently published studies highlight the problems encountered.

There are at least three major reports of combined modality therapy in the treatment of esophageal carcinoma. Forastiere et al. (165) treated patients with either squamous cell carcinoma or adenocarcinoma of the esophagus with concurrent cisplatin, vinblastine, and 5-fluorouracil chemotherapy and twice-a-day radiation therapy (4500 cGy) over 21 days. Forty-one of 43 patients completed the preoperative therapy and went on to have a transhiatal esophagectomy, with a 24% complete response rate. At the time of the original report, the median survival had not been reached. Toxicity included two treatment-related deaths resulting from neutropenic sepsis, and radiation therapy was stopped early in two patients. Eighty-six percent of patients experienced esophagitis, and 79% required nutritional support. The major toxicity was hematologic, with 93% of patients experiencing grade 3 or 4 neutropenia and 63% experiencing febrile neutropenia.

Sauter and colleagues (166) used concurrent high-dose radiation (more than 5000 cGy) and chemotherapy (5-fluorouracil and mitomycin C) in 30 patients with clinical stage I or II esophageal cancer. Severe esophagitis prevented the administration of full-course therapy in 10 patients, 3 patients developed neutropenic fever, and 2 died of treatment-related complications (radiation pneumonitis and inanition from radiation-induced esophagitis). Seven of 18 resected patients had a pathologically confirmed complete response. Overall, local control was seen in 83% of patients. The authors concluded that although local tumor response and control were encouraging, the overall survival may not be improved and the treatment-related mortality of 10% was unacceptably high (166).

In a randomized trial, 121 esophageal cancer patients received chemotherapy with 5-fluorouracil and cisplatin plus concurrent radiation (5000 cGy) or 6400 cGy of radiation alone (167). Median survival and survival at 1 and 2 years was superior in the combined modality group. Severe or life-threatening side effects occurred in 44% and 20% of patients in the combined therapy arm, compared with 25% and 3% in the radiation therapy alone arm. All three trials displayed better local control but at the price of increased toxicity.

In limited stage small cell lung cancer, the role of combined chemoradiation therapy is now established (168, 169). In the largest trial to date of concurrent chemoradiation, myelosuppression was the major toxicity, followed by esophagitis and pulmonary toxic reactions (168). It was often difficult to distinguish between radiation pneumonitis and recurrent tumor or pneumonia/atelectasis. There also was a high incidence of a failure to thrive syndrome, characterized by anorexia and weight loss, often associated with declining activity and performance score. Depending on the arm, 1% to 4% of patients died of treatment-related causes.

In non–small cell lung cancer, sequential combined modality therapy (chemotherapy followed by radiation) was used by the Cancer and Leukemia Group B (170) in stage III disease with an increase in median survival when compared with radiation therapy alone but at the cost of increased infections and weight loss (170). This study was confirmed by the Radiation Therapy Oncology Group and the Eastern Cooperative Oncology Group (171), and combined multimodality treatment currently is being studied in stage II, IIIA, and IIIB disease by various groups, with both concurrent and sequential therapies being tested.

CUTANEOUS TOXICITY

Chemotherapy has been shown to cause an increased risk of breast fibrosis and poor cosmetic outcome in patients receiving breast irradiation (141, 142).

BONE TOXICITY

Combined chemotherapy and irradiation in the primary treatment of breast cancer causes an increased risk of rib fracture compared with radiation alone (141, 142).

BONE MARROW TOXICITY

The combination of chemotherapy and radiation may lead to a greater risk of either acute or chronic myelosuppression, with increased risks of infection, bleeding, and anemia. The major concern is the continued use of thoracic irradiation in the presence of neutropenia, which may induce or prolong associated esophagitis. Esophagitis can increase the risk of sepsis. Most protocols, therefore, withhold radiation during periods of neutropenia.

Patients treated with chemotherapy and radiation for Hodgkin's disease do not have a higher rate of leukemia compared with those treated with chemotherapy alone (172, 173); however, one study of women treated for breast cancer showed a risk of secondary leukemia from both chemotherapy and radiation that was additive when combined therapy was given (91).

CARDIAC TOXICITY

Because of the risks of enhanced esophagitis and skin reactions when doxorubicin and radiation are used together, this combination has fallen from current favor. The potential for enhanced cardiac toxicity between radiation therapy and chemotherapy still exists, however, especially with treatment of left-sided tumors. The combined effects are not related to timing (174), probably because both radiation and Adriamycin cause permanent cardiac damage through totally different mechanisms and cellular targets. With combined treatment, the myocytic drop out of Adriamycin is combined with the diffuse interstitial fibrosis and decreased capillaries of radiation. The risk appears to be additive (175). When using Adriamycin in conjunction with radiation to the heart, a cumulative Adriamycin dose of 300 to 350 mg/m² should be considered the upper limit of safety, and the volume and dose of the radiation fields should be minimized if at all possible.

Two retrospective reviews, one in children (176) and one in adults (177), showed an increased risk of congestive heart failure in patients treated with both modalities, although one retrospective study of 4000 patients failed to show an increased risk (178). Bristow et al. (179) have calculated that prior mediastinal irradiation increases the risk of doxorubicin-induced heart failure by a factor of 1.6 times if more than 6 Gy were administered to the cardiac apex (179).

NEUROLOGIC TOXICITY

In two randomized studies of the Danish Breast Cancer Cooperative Group (5, 101) and a large retrospective study from the Joint Center for Radiation Therapy in Boston (108), chemotherapy has been shown to potentiate brachial plexopathy in patients treated with supraclavicular irradiation for breast cancer.

PCI for the treatment of small cell lung cancer is associated with central nervous system toxicity in up to 63% of patients when combined with doxorubicin-based chemotherapy (96) and in approximately one third of other patients. This toxicity is seen as impaired mentation, gait disturbances, and urinary incontinence. The variables seem to be the dose per fraction (increased with doses of more than 300 cGy or more) (180), timing, and the use of concomitant systemic chemotherapy. The sequencing of chemotherapy and radiation may play a role (180). Chemotherapy combined with whole brain irradiation or cranial-spinal irradiation has been shown to increase the risk of leukoencephalopathy in children. The risk appears to be greater when radition precedes chemotherapy (180), possibly because radiation damages the blood-brain barrier and may allow egress of otherwise excluded neurotoxic agents into the brain.

PCI has been used extensively in small cell lung cancer in an attempt to reduce the incidence of central nervous system failure. It usually is considered quite effective in this regard, reducing the incidence of central nervous system relapses from an expected 25% to approximately 5% (180). However, in patients heavily treated with chemotherapy and irradiation, the risk of subsequent leukoencephalopathy (demyelinization, reactive astrocytosis, multiple microscopic noninflammatory necrotic foci) and mineralizing microangiopathy is high. It occurs in up to 50% of leukemic patients. The clinical outcome is dementia, which can be quite severe. The exact role of chemotherapy and radiation cannot be determined. However, chemotherapy alone has a low incidence of dementia as a side effect. The risk may be highest in patients receiving chemotherapy after brain irradiation, implying that the radiation has damaged the blood-brain barrier and allowed increased ingress of chemotherapy into the brain, with resultant increased complications.

Intrathecal methotrexate use combined with PCI increases the chance of clinical neurotoxicity (181). Some studies also suggest an increased risk of neurotoxicity with any chemotherapy given after PCI (182), whereas other studies do not suport this thesis (183).

ENDOCRINE TOXICITY

Chemotherapy added to mantle field irradiation may increase the risk of late hypothyroidism compared with irradiation alone for Hodgkin's disease (49% versus 40%, respectively; $P=.008$ (122). The sequence may also be important because patients receiving chemotherapy before radiation had a higher risk than those receiving chemotherapy for recurrence after radiation (53% versus 43%; $P=.05$). These data are derived from a retrospective series that has shown complex relationships among dose of radiation, chemotherapy, and age, factors that make interpretation difficult.

REFERENCES

1. John MJ, Flam MS, Legha SS, Phillips TL. Chemoradiation: an integrated approach to cancer treatment. Philadelphia: Lea & Febiger, 1993.
2. Kong JS, Peters LJ, Wharton JT, et al. Hyperfractionated split-course whole abdominal radiotherapy for ovarian carcinoma: tolerance and toxicity. Int J Radiat Oncol Biol Phys 1988;14:737–743.
3. Cox JD, Pajak TF, Marcial VA, et al. ASTRO plenary: interfraction interval as a major determinant of late effects, with hyperfractionated radiation therapy of carcinomas of upper respiratory and digestive tracts: results from Radiation Therapy Oncology Group protocol 8313. Int J Radiat Oncol Biol Phys 1991;20(6):1191–1195.
4. Svensson H, Westling P, Larsson LG. Radiation-induced lesions of the brachial plexus correlated to the dosetime fraction schedule. Acta Radiol Ther Phys Biol 1975;14:228–238.
5. Olsen NK, Pfeiffer P, Mondrup K, et al. Radiation-induced brachial plexus neuropthy in breast cancer patients. Acta Oncol 1990;29:885–890.
6. Strandqvist M. Studien über die kumulative Wirkung der Röntgenstrahlen bei Fraktionierung. Acta Radiol 1944;55(Suppl): 1–300.
7. Ellis F. Dose time and fractionation; a clinical hypothesis. Clin Radiol 1969;20:1.

8. Orton CG, Ellis F. A simplification in the use of the NSD concept in practical radiotherapy. Br J Radiol 1973;46:529–537.
9. Olivotto IA, Fairey RN, Gillies, et al. Fatal outcome of pelvic radiotherapy for carcinoma of the cervix in a patient with systemic lupus erythematosis. Clin Radiol 1989;40:83–84.
10. Eedy DJ, Corbett JR. Discoid lupus erythematosus exacerbated by x-ray irradiation. Clin Exper Dermatol 1988;13:202–203.
11. Varga J, Haustein UF, Creech RH, et al. Exaggerated radiation-induced fibrosis in patients with systemic sclerosis. JAMA 1991;265:3292–3295.
12. Ross JG, Hussey DH, Mayr NA, et al. Acute and late reactions to radiation therapy in patients with collagen vascular diseases. Cancer 1993;71:3744–3752.
13. Geara F, Le Bourgeois JP, Lepechoux C, et al. Radiotherapy of mucosal and cutaneous epidemic Kaposi's sarcoma (EKS): a report on 285 patients (abstract 1). Proc Annu Meet Am Soc Clin Oncol 1991;10:32.
14. Nisce LZ, Safai B. Radiation therapy of Kaposi's sarcoma in AIDS. Front Radiat Ther Oncol 1985;19:133–137.
15. Watkins EF, Findlay P, Gelmann E, et al. Enhanced mucosal reactions in AIDS patients receiving oropharyngeal irradiation. Int J Radiat Oncol Biol Phys 1987;13:1403–1408.
16. Chak LY, Gill PS, Levine AM, et al. Radiation therapy for acquired immunodeficiency syndrome-related Kaposi's sarcoma. J Clin Oncol 1988;66:863–867.
17. Koga K, Kusumoto S, Watanabe K, et al. Age factor relevant to the development of radiation pneumonitis in radiotherapy of lung cancer. Int J Radiat Oncol Biol Phys 1988;14:367–371.
18. Jensen BV, Carlsen NL, Nissen NI. Influence of age and duration of follow-up on lung function after combined chemotherapy for Hodgkin's disease. Eur Respir J 1990;3:1140–1145.
19. Kucera J, Enzelsberger H, Eppel W, et al. The influence of nicotine abuse and diabetes mellitus on the results of primary irradiation in the treatment of carcinoma of the cervix. Cancer 1987;60:1–4.
20. Rugg T, Saunders MI, Dische S. Smoking and mucosal reactions to radiotherapy. Br J Radiol 1990;63:554–556.
21. Whittet HB, Lund VG, Brockbank M, et al. Serum cotinine as an objective marker for smoking habit in head and neck malignancy. J Laryngol Otol 1991;105:1036–1039.
22. Browman GP, Wong G, Hodson I, et al. Influence of cigarette smoking on the efficacy of radiation therapy in head and neck cancer. N Engl J Med 1993;328:159–163.
23. Goodman MT, Kolonel LN, Wilkens LR, Yoshizawa CN, Le Marchand L. Smoking history and survival among lung cancer patients. Cancer Causes Control 1990;1(2):155–163.
24. Neugut AI, Murray T, Santos J, Amols H, Hayes MK, Flannery JT, Robinson E. Increased risk of lung cancer after breast cancer radiation therapy in cigarette smokers. Cancer 1994;73(6):1615–1620.
25. Ang KK, Peters LJ, Weber RS, et al. Concomitant boost radiotherapy schedules in the treatment of carcinoma of the oropharynx and nasopharynx. Int J Radiat Biol Phys 1990;19:1339–1345.
26. Kaanders JHAM, Van Daal WAG, Hoogenraad WJ, et al. Accelerated fractionation radiotherapy for laryngeal cancer, acute and late toxicity. Int J Radiat Oncol Biol Phys 1990;19:1339–1345.
27. Van der Schueren E, Van den Bogaert W, Vanuytsel L, et al. Radiotherapy by multiple fractions per day (MFD) in head and neck cancer: acute reactions of skin and mucosa. Int J Radiat Oncol Biol Phys 1990;19:301–311.
28. Mascarenhas F, Silvestre ME, Sa Da Costa M, Grima N, Campos C, Chaves P. Acute secondary effects on the esophagus in patients undergoing radiotherapy for carcinoma of the lung. Am J Clin Oncol 1989;12:34–40.
29. Marks L. The pulmonary effects of thoracic irradiation. Oncology 1994;8(6):89–106.
30. Ikazoe J, Takashima S, Morimoto S, et al. CT appearance of acute radiation-induced injury in the lung. AJR Am J Roentgenol 1988;150:765–770.
31. Kataoka M. Gallium-67 imaging for the assessment of radiation pneumonitis. Ann Nucl Med 1989;3:73–81.
32. Kataoka M, Kawamura M, Itoh H, et al. Ga-67 citrate scintigraphy for the early detection of radiation pneumonitis. Clin Nucl Med 1992;17:27–31.
33. Bell J, McGivern D, Bullimore J, et al. Diagnostic imaging of postirradiation changes in the chest. Clin Radiol 1988;39:109–119.
34. Van Dyk J, Keane TJ, Kan S, et al. Radiation pneumonitis following large single dose irradiation: a reevaluation based on absolute lung dose. Int J Radiat Oncol Biol Phys 1981;7:461–467.
35. Newton KA. Total thoracic irradiation combined with intravenous injection of autologous marrow. Clin Radiol 1960;2:14–21.
36. Newton KA, Spittle MF. An analysis of 40 cases treated by total thoracic irradiation. Clin Radiol 1969;20:19–22.
37. Breur K, Cohen P, Schweisguteh O, et al. Irradiation of the lungs as an adjuvant therapy in the treatment of osteosarcoma of the limbs. Eur J Cancer 1978;14:464–471.
38. Rab GT, Ivans JC, Childs DS Jr, et al. Elective whole lung irradiation in the treatment of osteogenic sarcoma. Cancer 1976;38:939–942.
39. Rubin P, Casarett GW. Clinical radiation pathology. Philadelphia: WB Saunders, 1968.
40. Stover D. Pulmonary toxicity. In: DeVita VT Jr, Hellman S, Rosenberg S, eds. Cancer. Principles and practice of oncology. 4th ed. Philadelphia: JB Lippincott, 1993:2362–2370.
41. Moss WT, Haddy FJ, Sweany SK. Some factors altering the severity of acute radition pneumonitis: variation with cortisone, heparin, and antibiotics. Radiology 1960;75:50–54.
42. Stewart JR, Fajardo LF. Experimental radiation-induced heart disease in rabbits. Radiology 1968;91:814–817.
43. Stewart JR, Fajardo LF. Experimental radiation-induced heart disease. I. Light microscopic studies. Am J Pathol 1970;59:299–316.
44. Stewart, JR, Fajardo LF. Radiation-induced heart disease: an update. Prog Cardiovasc Dis 1984;27:173–194.
45. Marbach Jr, Sontag MR, Van Dyk J, et al. Management of radiation oncology patients with implanted cardiac pacemakers: report of AAPM Task Group No. 34. Med Phys 1994;21:85–90.
46. Lewin AA, Serago CF, Schwade JG, Abitbol AA, Margolis SC. Radiation induced failures of complementary metal oxide semiconductor containing pacemakers: a potentially lethal complication. Int J Radiat Oncol Biol Phys 1984;10:1967–1969.
47. Thar TL, Million RR. Complications of radiation treatment of Hodgkin's disease. Semin Oncol 1980;7:174–183.
48. Jones AM. Transient radiation myelopathy (with reference to L'Hermitt sign of electrical paresthesia). Br J Radiol 1964;37:727–744.
49. Larson D, Weinstein M, Goldberg I, et al. Edema of the arm as

a function of the extent of axillary surgery in patients treated with primary radiotherapy. Int J Radiat Oncol Biol Phys 1986;12:1575–1582.
50. Overgaard M, Christensen JJ, Johansen H, et al. Postmastectomy irradiation in high-risk breast cancer patients—present status of the Danish Breast Cancer Cooperative Group trials. Acta Oncol 1988;27:707–714.
51. Overgaard M, Bentzen SM, Juul Christensen J, et al. The value of NSD formula in equation of acute and late radiation complications in normal tissue following 2 and 5 fractions per week in breast cancer patients treated with postmastectomy irradiation. Radiother Oncol 1987;9:1–12.
52. Marx RE. A new concept in the treatment of osteoradionecrosis. J Oral Maxillofac Surg 1983;41:351–357.
53. Davis JC, Dunn JM, Gates GA, et al. Hyperbaric oxygen: a new adjunct in the management of radiation necrosis. Arch Otolaryngol Head Neck Surg 1979;105:58–61.
54. Farmer JC Jr, Sheldon DL, Angelillo JD, et al. Treatment of radiation-induced tissue injury by hyperbaric oxygen. Ann Otol Rhinol Laryngol 1978;87:707–715.
55. Marx RE, Johnson RP. Problem wounds in oral and maxillofacial surgery: the role of hyperbaric oxygen. In: Davis JC, Hunt TK, eds. Problem wounds: the role of oxygen. New York: Elsevier Science Publishing, 1988:65–124.
56. Marx RE, Johnson RP, Kline SN. Prevention of osteoradionecrosis: a randomized prospective clinical trial of hyperbaric oxygen versus penicillin. J Am Dent Assoc 1985;111:49–54.
57. Arnold PG. Reconstruction of the chest wall. In: Mathes SJ, Nahai F, eds. Clinical applications for muscle and musculocutaneous flaps. St. Louis, Mosby 1982:236–268.
58. Fisher JC, Frank DH. Radiation injury. In: Georgiade GS, Georgiade NG, Riefkohl R, Barwick WJ, eds. Textbook of plastic, maxillofacial and reconstructive surgery. 2nd ed. Baltimore: Williams & Wilkins, 1992;1331–1336.
59. Beatty JD, DeBoer G, Rider WD. Carcinoma of the esophagus, pre-treatment assessment, correlation of radiation treatment parameters with survival and identification and management of radiation treatment failure. Cancer 1979;43:2254–2267.
60. Newaishy GA, Read GA, Duncan W, et al. Results of radical radiotherapy of squamous cell carcinoma of the oesphagus. Clin Radiol 1982;33:347–352.
61. Leach JEL. Effect of roentgen therapy on the heart: clinical study. Arch Intern Med 1943;72:715–745.
62. Cohn KE, Stewart JR, Fajardo LF, et al. Heart disease following radiation. Medicine 1967;46:281–298.
63. Stewart JR, Fajardo LF, Cohn KE. Experimental radiation-induced heart disease in rabbits. Radiology 1968;91:814–817.
64. Arsenian MA. Cardiovascular sequelae of therapeutic thoracic radiation. Prog Cardiovasc Dis 1991;33(5):299–311.
65. Lederman GS, Sheldon TA, Chaffey JT, Herman TS, Gelman RS, Coleman CN. Cardiac disease after mediastinal irradiation for seminoma. Cancer 1987;60:772–776.
66. Watchie J, Coleman CN, Raffin TA, et al. Minimal long-term cardiopulmonary dysfunction following treatment for Hodgkin's disease. Int J Radiat Oncol Biol Phys 1987;13:513–524.
67. Gottdiener JS, Katin MJ, Borer JS, et al. Late cardiac effects of therapeutic mediastinal irradiation. N Engl J Med 1983;308:569–572.
68. Hancock EW. Heart disease after radiation. N Engl J Med 1983;308:588.
69. Steinherz LJ, Yahalom J. Cardiac complications of cancer therapy. In: DeVita VT, Hellman S, and Rosenberg SA, eds. Cancer principles and practice of oncology. Philadelphia: JB Lippincott, 1993:2370–2385.
70. Byhardt R, Brace K, Ruckdeschel J, et al. Dose and treatment factors in radiation related pericardial effusion associated with the mantle technique for Hodgkin's disease. Cancer 1975;75:795–802.
71. Ruckdeschel JC, Chang P, Martin RG, et al. Radiation-related pericardial effusions in patients with Hodgkin's disease. Medicine 1975;54:245–259.
72. Pohjola-Sintonen S, Totterman KJ, Salmo M, et al. Late cardiac effects of mediastinal radiotherapy in patients with Hodgkin's disease. Cancer 1987;60:31–37.
73. Pierce RA, Hoffman MD, Kagan AR. A change in transverse cardiac diameter following mediastinal irradiation for Hodgkin's disease. Radiology 1969;93:619–624.
74. Ikaheimo MJ, Niemela KO, Linnaluoto MM, et al. Early cardiac changes related to radiation therapy. Am J Cardiol 1985;56:943–946.
75. Kagan AR, Hafermann M, Hamilton M, et al. Etiology, diagnosis and management of pericardial effusion after irradiation. Radiol Clin Biol 1971;41:171–182.
76. Haas JM. Symptomatic constrictive pericarditis developing 45 years after radiation therapy to the mediastinum. Am Heart J 1969;77:89–95.
77. Bradley EW, Zook BC, Casarett GW, et al. Coronary arteriosclerosis and atherosclerosis in fast neutron or photon irradiated dogs. Int J Radiat Oncol Biol Phys 1981;7:1103–1108.
78. Brosius FC, Waller BF, Robert WG. Radiation heart disease: analysis of 16 young (aged 15 to 33 years) necropsy patients who received over 3,500 rads to the heart. Am J Med 1981;70:519–530.
79. Carlson RG, Mayfield WR, Normann S, Alexander JA. Radiation-associated valvular disease. Chest 1991;99:538–545.
80. McEniery PT, Dorosti K, Schiavone WA, et al. Clinical and angiographic features of coronary artery disease after chest irradiation. Am J Cardiol 1987;60:1020–1024.
81. Handler CE, Livesey S, Lawton PA. Coronary artery stenosis after radiotherapy: angioplasty or coronary artery surgery? Br Heart J 1989;61:208–211.
82. Grollier G, Commeau P, Mercier V, et al. Post-radiotherapeutic left main coronary artery stenosis: clinical and histologic study. Eur Heart J 1988;9:567–570.
83. Kopelson G, Herwig KJ. The etiologies of coronary artery disease in cancer patients. Int J Radiat Oncol Biol Phys 1978;4:895–906.
84. Yahalom J, Hasin Y, Fuks Z. Acute myocardial infarction with normal coronary arteriogram after mantle field radiation therapy for Hodgkin's disease. Cancer 1983;52:637–641.
85. Annest LS, Anderson RP, Li W, et al. Coronary artery disease following mediastinal radiation. J Thorac Cardiovasc Surg 1983;85:257–263.
86. Tarbell NJ, Thompson, L, Mauch P. Thoracic irradiation in Hodgkin's disease: disease control and long-term complications. Int J Radiat Oncol Biol Phys 1990;18:275–281.
87. Hancock SL, Cox RS, Rosenberg SA. Correction: death after treatment of Hodgkin's disease (letter). Ann Intern Med 1992;114:810.

88. Henry-Amar M, Hayat M, Meerwaldt JH. Causes of death after therapy for early stages of Hodgkin's disease entered on EORTC protocols. Int J Radiat Oncol Biol Phys 1990;19:1155–1157.
89. Fajardo LF. Pathology of radiation injury. New York: Masson, 1982.
90. Sykes MP, Chu FCH, Wilerson WG. Local bone marrow changes secondary to therapeutic irradiation. Radiology 1960;75:919–924.
91. Curtis RE, Boice JD Jr, Stovall M, et al. Risk of leukemia after chemotherapy and radiation treatment for breast cancer. N Engl J Med 1992;326(26):1745–1751.
92. Evans AE. Central nervous system workshop. Cancer Clin Trials 1981;4(Suppl):31–35.
93. Van der Kogel AJ, Barendsen GW. Late effects of spinal cord irradiation with 300 kV x-rays and 15 MeV neutrons. Br J Radiol 1974;47:393–398.
94. Craig JB, Jackson DV, Moody D, Cruz JM, Pope EK, Powell BL, et al. Prospective evaluation of changes in computed cranial tomography in patients with small cell lung carcinoma treated with chemotherapy and prophylactic cranial irradiation. J Clin Oncol 1984;2(10):1151–1156.
95. Johnson DH, Porter LL, List AF, Hande KR, Hainsworth JD, Greco FA. Clinical studies: acute nonlymphocytic leukemia after treatment of small cell lung cancer. Am J Med 1986;81:962–968.
96. Fleck JF, Einhorn LH, Lauer RC, et al. Is prophylactic cranial irradiation indicated in small-cell lung cancer? J Clin Oncol 1990;8(2):209–214.
97. Lee YY, Nauert C, Glass P. Treatment-related white matter changes in cancer patients. Cancer 1986;57:1473–1482.
98. Catane R, Schwade JG, Yarr I, Lichter AS, Tepper JE, Dunnick NR, et al. Follow-up neurological evaluation in patients with small cell lung carcinoma treated with prophylactic cranial irradiation and chemotherapy. Int J Radiat Oncol Biol Phys 1981;7:105–109.
99. Frytak S, Earnest F IV, O'Neill BP, Lee RE, Creagan ET, Trautmann JC. Magnetic resonance imaging of neurotoxicity in long-term survivors of carcinoma. Mayo Clin Proc 1985;60:803–812.
100. Arriagada R, Le Chevalier T, Borie F, et al. Prophylactic cranial irradiation for patients with small-cell lung cancer in complete remission. J Natl Cancer Inst 1995;87(3):183–190.
101. Olsen NK, Pfeiffer P, Johannsen L, et al. Radiation-induced brachial plexopathy: neurological follow-up in 161 recurrence-free breast cancer patients. Int J Radiat Oncol Biol Phys 1993;26(1):43–49.
102. McDermott RS. Cobalt 60 beam therapy—post radiation effects in breast cancer patients. J Can Assoc Radiol 1971;22:195–198.
103. Powell S, Cooke J, Parsons C. Radiation-induced brachial plexus injury: follow-up of two different fractionation schedules. Radiother Oncol 1990;18:213–220.
104. Bagley FH, Walsh JW, Cady B, et al. Carcinomatous versus radiation-induced brachial plexus neuropathy in breast cancer. Cancer 1978;41:2154–2157.
105. Stoll BA, Andrews JHT. Radiation-induced peripheral neuropathy. BMJ 1966;11:834–837.
106. Thomas JE, Colby MY. Radiation-induced or metastatic brachial plexopathy? A diagnostic dilemma. JAMA 1972;222:1392–1395.
107. Kori SH, Foley KM, Posner JB. Brachial plexus lesions in patients with cancer: 100 cases. Neurology 1981;31:45–50.
108. Pierce SM, Recht A, Lingos TI, et al. Long-term radiation complications following conservative surgery (CS) and radiation therapy (RT) in patients with early stage breast cancer. Int J Radiat Oncol Biol Phys 1992;23:915–923.
109. Barr LC, Kissin MW. Radiation-induced brachial plexus neuropathy following breast conservation and radical radiotherapy. Br J Surg 1987;74:855–856.
110. Basso-Ricci S, della Costa C, Viganotti G, Ventafridda V, Zanolla R. Report on 42 cases of postirradiation lesions of the brachial plexus and their treatment. Tumori 1980;66:117–122.
111. Lederman RJ, Wilbourn AJ. Brachial plexopathy: recurrent cancer or radiation? Neurology 1984;34:1331–1335.
112. Cohen L, Svensson H. Cell population kinetics and dose-time relationship for postirradiation injury of the brachial plexus in man. Acta Radiol Oncol 1978;17:161–166.
113. Match RM. Radiation-induced brachial plexus paralysis. Arch Surg 1975;110:384–386.
114. Goldwein JW. Radiation myelopathy: a review. Med Pediatr Oncol 1987;15:89–95.
115. Schullheiss TE, Higgins EM, El-Mahdi HM. The latent period in radiation myelopathy. Int J Radiat Oncol Biol Phys 1984;10:1109–1115.
116. Cohen L, Creditor M. Isoeffect tables for tolerance of irradiated normal human tissues. Int J Radiat Oncol Biol Phys 1983;9:233–241.
117. Wara W, Phillips T, Sheline G, Schwade J. Radiation tolerance of the spinal cord. Cancer 1975;35:1558–1562.
118. Markson JL, Flatman GE. Myxoedema after deep x-ray therapy to the neck. BMJ 1965;1:1228–1230.
119. Glatstein E, McHardy-Young S, Brast N, et al. Alterations in serum thyrotropin (TSH) and thyroid function following radiotherapy in patients with malignant lymphoma. J Clin Endocrinol Metab 1971;32:833–841.
120. Schimpff SC, Diggs CH, Wiswell JG, Salvatore PC, et al. Radiation-related thyroid dysfunction. Implications for the treatment of Hodgkin's disease. Ann Intern Med 1980;92:91–98.
121. Constine LS, Donaldson SS, McDougall IR, et al. Thyroid dysfunction after radiotherapy in children with Hodgkin's disease. Cancer 1984;53:878–883.
122. Hancock SL, Cox RS, McDougall IR. Thyroid diseases after treatment of Hodgkin's disease. N Engl J Med 1991;325:599–605.
123. Devney RB, Sklar CA, Nesbit ME Jr. Serial thyroid function measurements in children with Hodgkin disease. J Pediatr 1984;105:223.
124. Constine LS, McDougall IR. Radiation therapy for Hodgkin's disease followed by hypothyroidism and then Graves' hyperthyroidism. Clin Nucl Med 1982;7:69–70.
125. Blitzer JB, Paolozzi FP, Gottlieb AJ, et al. Thyrotoxic thyroiditis after radiotherapy for Hodgkin's disease. Arch Intern Med 1985;145:1734–1735.
126. Bakri K, Shimaoka K, Rao U, et al. Adenosquamous carcinoma of the thyroid after radiotherapy for Hodgkin's disease: a case report and review. Cancer 1983;52:465–470.
127. Amin R. Follicular carcinoma of the thyroid following radiotherapy for Hodgkin's disease. Br J Radiol 1983;56:768–769.
128. Moroff SV, Fuks JZ. Thyroid cancer following radiotherapy for Hodgkin's disease: a case report and review of the literature. Med Pediatr Oncol 1986;14:216–220.
129. Tucker MA, Coleman CN, Cox RS, et al. Risk of second cancers after treatment for Hodgkin's disease. N Engl J Med 1988;318:76–81.

130. Kaldor JM, Day NE, Band P, et al. Second malignancies following testicular cancer, ovarian cancer, and Hodgkin's disease: an international collaborative study among cancer registries. Int J Cancer 1987;39:571–585.
131. Storm HH, Prener A. Second cancer following lymphatic and hematopoietic cancers in Denmark, 1943–80. National Cancer Institute monograph 68. Washington DC: U.S. Government Printing Office, NIH Publication No. 85-2714, 1985:389–410.
132. Greene MH, Wilson J. Second cancer following lymphatic and hematopoietic cancers in Connecticut, 1935–82. National Cancer Institute monograph 68. Washington, DC: U.S. Government Printing Office, NIH Publication No. 85-27140, 1985:191–217.
133. Souba WW, McKenna RJ Jr, Meis J, et al. Radiation-induced sarcomas of the chest wall. 1986; 57(3):610–615.
134. Taghian A, DeVathaire F, Terrier P, et al. Long-term risk of sarcoma following radiation treatment for breast cancer. Int J Radiat Oncol Biol Phys 1991;21:361–367.
135. Boice JD, Hutchison GB. Leukemia in women following radiotherapy for cervical cancer. Ten-year follow-up of an international study. J Natl Cancer Inst 1980;65:115–129.
136. Kapp DS, Fisher D, Grady KJ, Schwartz PE. Subsequent malignancies associated with carcinoma of uterine cervix, including an analysis of the effects of patient and treatment parameters on incidence and sites of metachronous malignancies. Int J Radiat Oncol Biol Phys 1982;8:197–205.
137. Lee JY, Perez CA, Ettinger N, et al. The risk of second primaries subsequent to irradiation for cervix cancer. Int J Radiat Oncol Biol Phys 1982;8:207–211.
138. Czesnin K, Wronkowski Z. Second malignancies of the irradiated area in patients treated for uterine cervix cancer. Gynecol Oncol 1978;6:309–315.
139. Boice J Jr, Engholm G, Kleinman RA, et al. Radiation dose and second cancer risk in patients treated for cancer of the cervix. Radiat Res 1988;116:3–55.
140. Arai T, Nakano T, Fukuhisa K, et al. Second cancer after radiation therapy for cancer of the uterine cervix. Cancer 1991;67:398–405.
141. Danoff BF, Goodman RL, Glick HH, et al. The effect of adjuvant chemotherapy on cosmesis and complications in patients with breast cancer treated by definitive irradiation. Int J Radiat Oncol Biol Phys 1983;9:1625–1630.
142. Lichter AS. Adjuvant chemotherapy in patients treated primarily with irradiation for localized breast cancer. In: Harris JR, Hellman S, Silen W, eds. Conservative management of breast cancer. Philadelphia: JB Lippincott, 1983:299–310.
143. Perry MC. Toxicity: ten years later. Semin Oncol 1992;19:453–457.
144. Allen A. The cardiotoxicity of chemotherapeutic agents. In: Perry MC, ed. The chemotherapy sourcebook. Baltimore: Williams & Wilkins, 1992;582–597.
145. Kriesman H, Wolkove N. Pulmonary toxicity of antineoplastic therapy. In: Perry MC, ed. The chemotherapy sourcebook. Baltimore: Williams & Wilkins, 1992;598–619.
146. Catane R, Schwade JG, Turrisi AT III, et al. Pulmonary toxicity after radiation and bleomycin—a review. Int J Radiat Oncol Biol Phys 1979;5:1513–1518.
147. Green DM, Finkelstein JZ, Tefft ME, Norkool P. Diffuse interstitial pneumonitis after pulmonary irradiation for metastatic Wilms' tumor. Cancer 1989;63:450–453.
148. Hoagland HC. Hematologic complications of cancer chemotherapy. In: Perry MC, Yarbro JW, eds. Toxicity of chemotherapy. Orlando: Grune & Stratton, 1984:433–448.
149. Koenig H, Patel A. Biochemical basis of the acute cerebellar syndrome in 5-fluorouracil chemotherapy. Trans Am Neurol Assoc 1969;94:290–292.
150. LeBaron S, Zeltzer P, Zeltzer L, et al. Assessment of quality of survival in children with medulloblastoma and cerebral astrocytoma. Cancer 1988;54:135–138.
151. Hussein AM, Feun LG. Tumor lysis syndrome after induction therapy in small cell lung carcinoma. Am J Clin Oncol 1990;13:10–13.
152. Chapman R: Gonadal toxicity and teratogenicity. In: Perry MC, ed. The chemotherapy sourcebook. Baltimore: Williams & Wilkins, 1992;710–753.
153. Pedersen-Bjergaard J, Osterlind K, Hansen M, Philip P, Pedersen AG, Hansen HH. Acute nonlymphocytic leukemia, preleukemia, and solid tumors following intensive chemotherapy of small cell carcinoma of the lung. 1985;66:1393–1397.
154. Dang, SP, Liberman, BA, Sheperd FA. Therapy-related leukemia and myelodysplasia in small-cell lung cancer. Arch Intern Med 1986;146:1689–1694.
155. Ratain MJ, Kaminer LS, Bitran JD, Larson RA, Le Beau MM, Skosey C, Purl S, et al. Acute nonlymphocytic leukemia following etoposide and cisplatin combination chemotherapy for advanced non–small-cell carcinoma of the lung. Blood 1987;70:1412–1417.
156. Steel GG, Peckham MJ. Exploitable mechanisms in combined radiotherapy-chemotherapy: the concept of additivity. Int J Radiat Oncol Biol Phys 1979;5:85–91.
157. Roach M III, Phillips TL. Pulmonary toxicity. In: John KJ, Flam MS, Legha SS, Phillips TL eds. Chemoradiation: an integrated approach to cancer treatment. Philadelphia: Lea & Febiger, 1993:444–459.
158. Silverman S. Oral cavity. In: John KJ, Flam MS, Legha SS, Phillips TL, eds. Chemoradiation: an integrated approach to cancer treatment. Philadelphia: Lea & Febiger, 1993:511–523.
159. Ali MK, Legha S. Cardiac toxicity. In: John KJ, Flam MS, Legha SS, Phillips TL, eds. Chemoradiation: an integrated approach to cancer treatment. Philadelphia: Lea & Febiger, 1993:489–501.
160. Steel GG. The search for therapeutic gain in the combination of radiotherapy and chemotherapy. Radiother Oncol 1988;11:31–53.
161. Howes AE. Keynote address: models of normal tissue injury following combined modality therapy. NCI Monographs 1988;6:5–8.
162. Field SB, Michalowski A. Endpoints for damage to normal tissues. Int J Radiat Oncol Biol Phys 1979;5:1185–1196.
163. Rubin P, Constine LS, Van Ess JD. Special lecture; scoring of late toxic effects—interaction of two modalities. NCI Monographs 1988;6:9–18.
164. Vokes EE, Weichselbaum RR. Concomitant chemoradiotherapy: rationale and clinical experience in patients with solid tumors. J Clin Oncol 1990;8:911–934.
165. Forastiere AA, Orringer MB, Perez-Tamayo C, et al. Concurrent chemotherapy and radiation therapy followed by transhiatal esophagectomy for local-regional cancer of the esophagus. J Clin Oncol 1990;8:119–127.
166. Sauter ER, Coia LR, Keller SM. Preoperative high-dose radiation and chemotherapy in adenocarcinoma of the esophagus and esophagogastric junction. Ann Surg Oncol 1994;1:5–10.
167. Herskovic A, Martz K, Al-Sarraf M, et al. Combined chemotherapy and radiotherapy compared with radiotherapy alone in patients with cancer of the esophagus. N Engl J Med 1992;326:1593–1598.

168. Perry MC, Eaton WL, Propert KJ, et al. Chemotherapy with or without radiation therapy in limited small-cell carcinoma of the lung. N Engl J Med 1987;316:912–918.
169. Pignon JP, Arrigada R, Ihde DC, Johnson DH, Perry MC, Souhami RL, et al. A meta-analysis of thoracic radiotherapy for small-cell lung cancer. N Engl J Med 1992;327:1618–1624.
170. Dillman RO, Seafren SL, Propert KJ, et al. A randomized trial of induction chemotherapy plus high-dose radiation versus radiation alone in stage III non–small cell lung cancer. N Engl J Med 1990;323:940–945.
171. Sause WT, Scott C, Taylor S, Johnson D, Livingston R, Komaki R, et al. Radiation Therapy Oncology Group (RTOG) 88-08 and Eastern Cooperative Oncology Group (ECOG) 4588: preliminary results of a phase III trial in regionally advanced, unresectable non–small-cell lung cancer. JNCI 1995;87:198–205.
172. Salvagno L, Simonato L, Soraru M, Bianco A, Chiarion-Sileni V, Aversa SM, et al. Secondary leukemia following treatment for Hodgkin's disease. Tumori 1993;79:103–107.
173. Kaldor JM, Day NE, Clark EA, Van Leeuwen FE, Henry-Amar M, Fiorentino, et al. Leukemia following Hodgkin's disease. N Engl J Med 1990;322(1):7–13.
174. Billingham ME. Endomyocardial changes in anthracycline-treated patients with and without irradiation. Front Radiat Ther Oncol 1979;13:67–81.
175. Eltringham JR, Fajardo LF, Steward JR, et al. Investigation of cardiotoxicity in rabbits from Adriamycin and fractionated cardiac irradiation: preliminary results. Front Ther Oncol 1979;13:21–35.
176. Gilladoga AC, Manuel C, Tan CTC, et al. The cardiotoxicity of Adriamycin and daunomycin in children. Cancer 1976;37:1070–1078.
177. Bristow MR, Mason JW, Billingham ME, et al. Doxorubicin cardiomyopathy: evaluation by phonocardiography, endomyocardial biopsy, and cardiac catheterization. Ann Intern Med 1978;88:168–175.
178. Von Hoff DD, Layard MW, Basa P, et al. Risk factors for doxorubicin-induced congestive heart failure. Ann Int Med 1979;91:710–717.
179. Bristow MR, Mason JW, Billingham ME, et al. Doxorubicin cardiomyopathy: evaluation by phonocardiography, endomyocardial biopsy, and cardiac catheterization. Ann Intern Med 1979;91:710–717.
180. Sause WT. Prophylactic cranial irradiation: advantages and disadvantages. Ann Oncol 1992;3(Suppl):51–55.
181. Rubinstein JL, Herman MM, Long TF, Wilbur JR. Disseminated necrotizing leukoencephalopathy: a complication of treated central nervous system leukemia and lymphoma. Cancer 1975;35:291–305.
182. Lee Y-Y, Nauert C, Glass P. Treatment-related white matter changes in cancer patients. Cancer 1986;57:1473–1482.
183. Catane R, Schwade JG, Yarr I, Lichter AS, Tepper JE, Dunnick NR, et al. Follow-up neurological evaluation in patients with small cell lung carcinoma treated with prophylactic cranial irradiation and chemotherapy. Int J Radiat Oncol Biol Phys 1980;7:105–109.

49B

Pulmonary Rehabilitation in Patients with Thoracic Neoplasm

Andrew L. Ries

Rehabilitation programs for patients with chronic lung diseases are well established as a means of enhancing standard therapy to control and alleviate symptoms and optimize functional capacity (1–8). The primary goal of any rehabilitation program is to restore the patient to the highest possible level of independent function. This goal is accomplished by helping patients and significant others learn more about lung disease, treatment, and coping strategies; they also become actively involved in providing their own health care, and in being more independent in daily activities and less dependent on health professionals and expensive medical resources. Rather than focusing solely on reversing the disease process, rehabilitation attempts to decrease the disability from disease.

At first glance the idea of rehabilitation for patients with thoracic neoplasms may seem far fetched. Many pulmonary rehabilitation strategies have been developed for patients with disabling chronic obstructive pulmonary disease (COPD). However, rehabilitation has been applied successfully to patients with other chronic lung conditions, such as interstitial diseases, cystic fibrosis, bronchiectasis, thoracic cage abnormalities, and, most recently, to patients before and after lung transplantation (9–11). Pulmonary rehabilitation is appropriate for any patient with stable chronic lung disease who is disabled by symptoms of the underlying disease or by related treatment or complications.

As pointed out by Bernhard and Ganz (12), lung cancer is associated with both physical and psychosocial symptoms, not all from the cancer. In particular, dyspnea is common and is present in up to 65% of patients. It can be related to the tumor, treatment, complications, underlying lung or heart disease, or a combination of factors. Psychologic disturbances, including depression and anxiety, are common. Social problems also are frequent because cancer patients have a tendency to withdraw and become socially isolated. Normal family and social interactions are disturbed as patients are forced to change roles and become more dependent on others.

Many patients with thoracic neoplasms have underlying chronic pulmonary disease. In addition, lung function and functional status may be compromised further as a consequence of the malignancy and treatments, such as surgery or radiation, that remove or destroy functioning lung tissue. Thus, in the patient whose thoracic neoplasm has been treated and is stable or in remission, pulmonary rehabilitation may be considered an important adjunctive therapy to help patients cope with disabling symptoms and improve functional status and quality of life.

In 1974, the American College of Chest Physicians' Committee on Pulmonary Rehabilitation adopted the following definition:

Pulmonary rehabilitation may be defined as an art of medical practice wherein an individually tailored, multidisciplinary program is formulated which through accurate diagnosis, therapy, emotional support, and education, stabilizes or reverses both the physio- and psychopathology of pulmonary diseases and attempts to return the patient to the highest possible functional capacity allowed by his pulmonary handicap and overall life situation (1).

This definition focuses on three important features of successful rehabilitation:

1. Individual: Patients with disabling lung disease require individual assessment of their needs, individual attention, and a program designed to meet realistic individual goals.
2. Multidisciplinary: Pulmonary rehabilitation programs provide information and expertise from several health care disciplines that is integrated by experienced staff into a comprehensive, cohesive program tailored to the needs of each patient.

3. Attention to physiopathology and psychopathology: To be successful, pulmonary rehabilitation pays attention to psychologic and emotional problems as well as helps to optimize medical therapy to improve lung function.

Pulmonary rehabilitation typically is provided by a multidisciplinary team of health care professionals that may include physicians, nurses, respiratory and physical therapists, psychologists, exercise physiologists, or others with appropriate expertise. Specific team make-up depends on the resources and expertise available, but it usually includes at least one full-time staff member. Responsibilities of team members generally cross disciplines, and the necessary skills have been delineated (13).

Within this general framework, successful pulmonary rehabilitation programs have been established in both outpatient and inpatient settings and with different formats. The key to success is the participation of dedicated, enthusiastic staff who are familiar with the problems of pulmonary patients and who can relate well to and motivate these patients.

PATIENT SELECTION

Any patient with symptomatic chronic lung disease is a candidate for pulmonary rehabilitation (Table 49B.1). Appropriate patients are aware of disability from their disease and are motivated to be active participants in their own care to improve their health status. Patients with mild disease may not perceive their symptoms to be severe enough to warrant a comprehensive care program. In contrast, patients with severe disease may be too debilitated to benefit greatly.

Criteria based on arbitrary lung function parameters or age alone should not be used in the selection of patients for pulmonary rehabilitation (4). Pulmonary function is not a good predictor of symptoms, function, or improvement after rehabilitation in individuals (14). Older patients with chronic lung diseases may live many years with pulmonary disability. In general, selection should be based on an individual's disability and functional limitation from respiratory symptoms, potential for improvement, and motivation to participate actively in a comprehensive self-care program.

Other factors are also important in evaluating candidates. Pulmonary rehabilitation is not a primary mode of therapy. Patients should be evaluated and stabilized on standard therapy before beginning a rehabilitation program. They should not have other disabling or unstable conditions that might limit their ability to participate fully and to concentrate on the program.

For the patient with a thoracic neoplasm, pulmonary rehabilitation may be considered when the patient has completed primary treatment of the malignancy (e.g., surgery, radiation, chemotherapy) and the disease is stable or in remission. Such patients often are forced to deal with a new level of respiratory disability from underlying lung disease as well as from the consequences of cancer treatment. Rehabilitation can help them learn better coping strategies to adjust to these symptoms and also can assist them in recovering from the debilitating effects of treatment.

The ideal patient for pulmonary rehabilitation, then, is one with functional limitation from moderate-to-severe lung disease who is stable on standard therapy, not distracted or limited by other serious or unstable medical conditions, willing and able to learn about the disease, and motivated to devote the time and effort necessary to benefit from a comprehensive care program.

PATIENT EVALUATION

The initial step in pulmonary rehabilitation is screening patients to ensure appropriate selection and to set realistic individual and program goals. The evaluation process includes the following components: interview, medical evaluation, psychosocial assessment, diagnostic testing, and goal setting (Table 49B.2).

INTERVIEW

The screening interview is an important first step. It serves to introduce the patient to the program as well as to review the patient's medical history and identify psychosocial problems and needs. Significant others should be included. Communication with the primary care physician also is important, establishing the vital link for the rehabilitation staff in clarifying questions before starting the program and facilitating recommendations during and after treatment. Care and attention in this initial evaluation helps in setting

TABLE 49B.1 Patient Selection Criteria for Pulmonary Rehabilitation

Symptomatic chronic lung disease
Stable on standard therapy
Functional limitation from disease
Relationship with primary care provider
Motivated to be actively involved in and take responsibility for own health care
No other interfering or unstable medical conditions (i.e., treated or stable malignancy)
No arbitrary lung function or age criteria

TABLE 49B.2 Components of a Comprehensive Pulmonary Rehabilitation Program

Patient Evaluation
  Interview
  Medical evaluation
  Diagnostic testing
    Pulmonary function
    Exercise
    Arterial blood gases/oximetry
  Psychosocial assessment
  Goal setting

Program content
  Education
  Respiratory and chest physiotherapy instruction
  Exercise
  Psychosocial support

goals compatible with everyone's expectations and appropriate to the program's objectives.

MEDICAL EVALUATION

Reviewing the medical history helps the team identify the patient's lung disease and assess its severity. Other medical problems that might preclude or delay participation may be identified. Available laboratory data should be reviewed, including pulmonary function and exercise tests, rest and exercise arterial blood gas measurements, chest radiographs, electrocardiogram, and pertinent blood tests. Program staff can then determine the need for additional information or action before the beginning the program.

DIAGNOSTIC TESTING

Planning an appropriate rehabilitation program requires accurate, current information. The testing procedures performed depend on individual patient and program goals, as well as the facilities and expertise available.

Pulmonary function testing is used to characterize lung disease and quantify impairment. Spirometry and lung volume measurements are most useful; other tests, such as diffusing capacity, airway resistance, and maximal respiratory pressures to assess muscle strength, can be added as needed.

Exercise testing helps to assess the patient's exercise tolerance and evaluate blood gas changes (hypoxemia or hypercapnia) with exercise (15). This test may also uncover coexisting diseases (e.g., heart disease). The exercise test is used to establish a safe and appropriate prescription for subsequent training.

Maximal exercise of patients with chronic lung disease is limited primarily by their breathing reserve. Simple pulmonary function tests such as spirometry can be used to estimate a patient's capacity for sustained breathing (maximum ventilation) during exercise. The forced expiratory volume in 1 second (FEV_1) is the most useful such measurement (15). However, an individual patient's maximum work capacity can only be estimated from lung function (16). Exercise tolerance also depends on the patient's perception and tolerance of the subjective symptom of breathlessness. Therefore, it is important to exercise patients to assess their physical function and symptom tolerance.

Exercise evaluation for rehabilitation is performed most easily with the type of activity planned for training (e.g., treadmill for a walking training program); however, test results from one type of exercise (e.g., cycling) can be translated to related activities (e.g., walking) (17). Variables measured or monitored during testing should include workload, heart rate, electrocardiogram, arterial oxygenation, and symptoms (e.g., breathlessness). Other measures, such as ventilation or expired gas analysis to calculate oxygen uptake (VO_2) and related variables, may be obtained depending on the interest and expertise of the program staff and laboratory (15, 18, 19).

Measurement of arterial blood gas levels at rest and during exercise is important because of the frequent but unpredictable occurrence of exercise-induced hypoxemia (20). Blood gas sampling during exercise makes testing more complex. Noninvasive estimation of arterial oxygen saturation by cutaneous oximetry is useful for continuous monitoring, but it has limited accuracy (e.g., 95% confidence limits for cutaneous oximetry, ±4% to 5% saturation) (21).

PSYCHOSOCIAL ASSESSMENT

Successful rehabilitation requires attention not only to physical problems but also to psychologic, emotional, and social ones. Patients with chronic illnesses experience psychosocial difficulties as they struggle to deal with symptoms they may not fully understand (22–26). Such problems are even more important for the patient with a thoracic neoplasm who also is coping with the stress of a more immediately life-threatening illness and resultant changes in physical function and social role (12).

Neuropsychologic impairment is common in patients with chronic lung disease and cannot be accounted for solely on the basis of age, presence of depression, and physical disease (27). Commonly, such patients become depressed, frightened, anxious, and more dependent on others to care for their needs. Progressive dyspnea is a frightening symptom and may lead to a vicious fear-dyspnea cycle: with progressive disease, less exertion results in more dyspnea, which produces more fear and anxiety, which in turn leads to more dyspnea. Ultimately, the patient avoids any physical activity associated with both of these unpleasant symptoms. Jensen (28) reported that high stress and low social support were better predictors of subsequent hospitalizations than severity of illness in patients with obstructive lung disease.

To address these problems, the initial evaluation should include an assessment of the patient's psychologic state and close attention to psychosocial clues during screening interviews (e.g., family and social support, living arrangement, activities of daily living, hobbies, employment potential). Important clues in initial interviews may be obtained by paying attention to nonverbal communication such as facial expression, physical appearance, handshake, and perception of body space (29). Cognitive impairment that may limit ability to participate fully can be identified. Significant others may provide valuable insight and should be included in the screening process and rehabilitation program whenever possible.

GOALS

After evaluating a patient's medical, physiologic, and psychosocial state, it is important to set specific goals that are compatible with each individual's disease, needs, and expectations. Goals should be realistic, given the objectives of the program. Significant others should be included in this process so that everyone understands what can, and cannot, be expected.

PROGRAM CONTENT

Comprehensive pulmonary rehabilitation programs typically include several key components: education; respiratory and chest physiotherapy instruction; psychosocial support; and exercise training (Table 49B.2). Often, the various components are provided simultaneously, e.g., during an exercise session, a patient may learn and practice breathing techniques for symptom control while being encouraged and supported by staff or other patients.

EDUCATION

Successful pulmonary rehabilitation depends on the understanding and active involvement of patients and those important for their social support. Education is an integral component; even patients with severe disease can gain a better understanding of their disease and learn specific means of dealing with problems (30, 31). Instruction can be provided individually or in small groups, but it should be adapted to different learning abilities. Typical topics include: how normal lungs work, the nature of chronic lung disease, medications, nutrition, travel, stress reduction and relaxation, when to call your doctor, and planning a daily schedule. Individual instruction and coaching may be provided on the use of respiratory therapy equipment and oxygen, breathing techniques, bronchial drainage, chest percussion, energy-saving techniques, and self-care tips. The general philosophy is to encourage patients to assume responsibility for and become partners with their physician in providing their care (32).

Despite the importance of education, it is unlikely that knowledge alone will lead to improved health status. It is more difficult to change attitudes and behaviors. Patients require specific, individualized strategies with instruction and reinforcement. Thus, education is a necessary, but not sufficient, component of pulmonary rehabilitation.

RESPIRATORY AND CHEST PHYSIOTHERAPY TECHNIQUES

Patients with chronic lung disease use, abuse, and are confused about respiratory and chest physiotherapy techniques. In pulmonary rehabilitation, each patient's needs for respiratory care techniques can be assessed and instruction provided in proper use. These may include chest physiotherapy techniques to control secretions; breathing retraining techniques to relieve and control dyspnea and improve ventilatory function; and proper use of respiratory care equipment including nebulizers, metered dose inhalers, and oxygen (8, 33).

BRONCHIAL HYGIENE

Patients with chronic lung diseases have abnormal lung clearance mechanisms that make them more susceptible to problems with retained secretions and infection. Therefore, rehabilitation programs teach chest physiotherapy techniques for secretion control, such as controlled coughing, postural drainage, and chest vibration and/or percussion (32–36). These are important for patients with excess mucous production during exacerbations and as routine preventive measures for patients with chronic sputum production. The use of mucolytic agents to reduce viscosity of secretions is of questionable benefit; in several studies they do not appear to be any more effective than a placebo (37). In addition, intermittent positive pressure breathing has been evaluated systematically and found to be ineffective (38).

BREATHING RETRAINING TECHNIQUES

Pulmonary rehabilitation typically includes instruction in breathing techniques, such as diaphragmatic and pursed lips breathing, that are designed to help patients relieve and control breathlessness, improve ventilatory pattern (i.e., slow respiratory rate, increase tidal volume), prevent dynamic airway compression, improve respiratory synchrony of abdominal and thoracic musculature, and improve gas exchange (2, 3, 32, 33, 39, 40–42). A review of studies evaluating these techniques indicates that improvement in symptoms (e.g., dyspnea) is more consistent than measurable changes in physiologic parameters (40).

The diaphragmatic breathing technique was described by Barach (42) and Miller (41) as a maneuver in which the patient coordinates abdominal wall expansion with inspiration and slows expiration through pursed lips (40). The primary effect is to slow the respiratory rate and increase the tidal volume.

Pursed lips breathing is the other technique often taught to pulmonary patients, particularly those with COPD (40–42). Pursed lips breathing was observed by Laennec as early as 1830 and advocated as a physical exercise for pulmonary patients in the early part of the 20th century (43). It is a maneuver assumed naturally by many patients in which the lips are used to narrow the airway during expiration. The goal is to slow the expiratory phase and maintain positive airway pressure to keep the airways open and improve ventilatory efficiency.

OXYGEN

For patients who require chronic oxygen therapy, available methods of oxygen delivery can be reviewed to help select the best system for their needs. Supplemental oxygen is beneficial for patients with severe resting hypoxemia. Long-term, continuous oxygen therapy has clearly been shown to improve survival and reduce morbidity in hypoxemic patients with COPD (2, 44–48). In fact, oxygen therapy is the only treatment proven to prolong survival in these patients. Benefits of supplemental oxygen for nonhypoxemic patients or for patients with hypoxemia only under certain conditions (e.g., exercise, sleep) are defined less clearly (44, 46, 49).

Although continuous oxygen therapy is feasible and safe, maintaining patients on oxygen presents several challenges (45). Handling equipment is particularly difficult for physically disabled and frail patients. Therefore, it is important to assess each patient's oxygen needs and provide instruction in appropriate techniques.

Several new developments have improved the efficiency of gas delivery and patient compliance with continuous therapy (45, 50). Liquid oxygen provides more gas with less weight than tanks of compressed gas, particularly in portable systems. Also, transtracheal delivery may increase efficiency, reducing flow rates and prolonging the supply in portable sources as well as improving compliance and avoiding problems with nasal catheters (51). However, patients need careful instruction in caring for and maintaining the catheter.

EXERCISE

Exercise is important in pulmonary rehabilitation (1, 5–8). There is considerable evidence of favorable responses to exercise training in patients with chronic lung diseases (4, 6, 52, 53). Benefits are both physiologic and psychologic. Patients may increase their maximum capacity and/or endurance for physical activity, even though lung function does not usually change. Patients also may benefit from learning to perform physical tasks more efficiently. Exercise training provides an ideal opportunity for patients to learn their capacity for physical work and to use and practice methods for controlling dyspnea (e.g., breathing and relaxation techniques). Of all the components in a comprehensive pulmonary rehabilitation program, exercise is probably the most difficult in terms of personnel, equipment, and expertise. Principles of exercise testing and training for patients with lung disease differ from those derived in normal individuals or other patient populations because of differences in the limitations to exercise and the problems encountered in training (54).

Many approaches have been used in rehabilitation to train the patient with chronic lung disease. To be successful, the program should be tailored to the individual patient's physical abilities, interests, resources, and environment. Generally, techniques should be simple and inexpensive. As in normal individuals and other patients, benefits are largely specific to the muscles and tasks involved in training. Patients tend to do best on activities and exercises for which they are trained. Walking programs are particularly useful. They have the added benefit of encouraging patients to expand social horizons. In inclement weather many patients can walk indoors (e.g., shopping malls). Other types of exercise (e.g., cycling, swimming) are also effective. Patients should be encouraged to incorporate regular exercise into daily activities they enjoy (e.g., golf, gardening). Because many patients with chronic lung disease have limited exercise tolerance, emphasis during training should be placed on increasing endurance. Changes in endurance often are greater than changes in maximal exercise tolerance (14). This increase in endurance allows patients to become more functional within their physical limits. An increase in the maximum exercise also is possible as patients gain experience and confidence with their exercise program.

EXERCISE PRESCRIPTION

Selecting training targets based on percentages of maximum heart rate or VO_2 are well established in normal individuals or other patient groups. In patients with chronic lung diseases, however, the best method of choosing an appropriate training prescription is defined less clearly. Exercise tolerance in pulmonary patients typically is limited by maximum ventilation and breathlessness. Such patients frequently do not reach limits of cardiac or peripheral muscle performance.

There has been much controversy about the appropriate intensity target for training patients with chronic lung disease. Using a target heart rate has been advocated by some investigators (55), although it is recognized that such targets may not be reliable for patients with more severe disease (54). Many patients with lung disease can be trained at high percentages of the maximum heart rate that approach or even exceed the maximum level reached on the initial exercise test. In a study of 52 patients with moderate-to-severe COPD, Punzal and coworkers (56) reported that patients were able to perform endurance exercise testing at an average workload of 95% of baseline maximum exercise tolerance. After 8 weeks, these patients were training at 86% of the baseline maximum workload. In fact, many patients with severe COPD were exercising at levels exceeding the baseline maximum. In a study in 59 patients with moderate-to-severe COPD, Carter and coworkers (57) trained patients at levels near their ventilatory limits. At baseline, after training, and at 3 months, they reported mean peak exercise ventilation of 94% to 100% of measured maximum voluntary ventilation. These findings suggest that even patients with advanced disease can be trained successfully at or near maximal levels.

Therefore, some pulmonary rehabilitation programs define exercise targets and progression during training more by symptom tolerance than by targets based on heart rate, work level, or other physiologic measurements (54, 56). Ratings of perceived symptoms (e.g., breathlessness) help teach patients to exercise to target levels of breathing discomfort (58, 59). A typical approach would be to begin training at a level that the patient can sustain with reasonable comfort for several minutes. An increase in time or level is then made according to the patient's symptom tolerance. Patients are encouraged to exercise daily and increase endurance up to 15 to 30 minutes of continuous activity. This method helps them achieve a goal of improving their tolerance for tasks of daily living that often require a period of sustained activity.

BLOOD GAS CHANGES

A major problem in planning a safe exercise program for patients with lung disease is the potential worsening of hypoxemia with exercise. Patients who may not be hypoxemic at rest can develop changes in arterial oxygenation that cannot be predicted reliably from resting measurements of pulmonary function or gas exchange. Normal individuals do not become hypoxemic with exercise. In patients with obstructive lung disease, PaO_2 changes unpredictably during exercise (20). In patients with mild COPD, PaO_2 typically does not change or may even improve with exercise. However, in patients with moderate-to-severe COPD, PaO_2 may increase, decrease, or remain unchanged. In contrast, patients with interstitial lung disease commonly develop worsening oxygenation with exercise (60).

Therefore, it is important to evaluate rest and exercise oxygenation. Such testing also is used to prescribe oxygen therapy at rest and with physical activity. With the availability of convenient, portable systems for ambulatory oxygen delivery, hypoxemia is not a contraindication to safe exercise training.

OTHER TYPES OF EXERCISE

UPPER EXTREMITY TRAINING

Exercise programs for pulmonary patients typically emphasize lower extremity training (e.g., walking). However, many patients with chronic lung disease report disabling dyspnea for daily activities involving the upper extremities (e.g., lifting, grooming) at work levels much lower than for the lower extremities (61–63). Upper extremity exercise is accompanied by a higher ventilatory demand for a given level of work than that needed for lower extremity exercise. Because training generally is specific to the muscles and tasks used in training, upper extremity exercises may be important in helping pulmonary patients cope better with common daily activities (64). This type of training may be particularly important in patients recovering from thoracic surgery.

VENTILATORY MUSCLE TRAINING

The potential role of ventilatory muscle fatigue as a cause of respiratory failure and ventilatory limitation in patients with chronic lung disease has stimulated attempts to train the ventilatory muscles (65–70). Techniques of isocapnic hyperventilation, inspiratory resistance, and inspiratory threshold loading have been shown to improve function of these muscles in both normal individuals and patients (65). In normal people, respiratory muscles do not limit exercise tolerance; therefore, specific respiratory muscle training is unlikely to be of clinical benefit. In patients with COPD, who have been studied most extensively, improvement in general exercise performance from ventilatory muscle training alone has not been demonstrated consistently (66, 70, 71). Thus, the role of such training incorporated routinely into pulmonary rehabilitation programs has not been established clearly.

PSYCHOSOCIAL SUPPORT

An essential component of pulmonary rehabilitation is psychosocial support provided to help patients combat symptoms reflecting their progressive feelings of hopelessness and inability to cope with both the underlying lung disease and the thoracic neoplasm (2, 8, 12, 22, 23, 25, 26). Depression is common (25, 72). Patients may also have symptoms of anxiety (particularly a fear of dyspnea), denial, anger, and isolation. They become sedentary and dependent on family members, friends, and medical services to provide for their needs. They become overly concerned with other physical problems and psychosomatic complaints. Sexual dysfunction and fear are common and often are the unspoken consequences of chronic lung disease (73–75). Patients may demonstrate cognitive and neuropsychologic dysfunction, possibly related to or exacerbated by the effects of hypoxemia on the brain.

Psychosocial support is provided best by a warm and enthusiastic staff who can communicate effectively with patients and devote the time and effort necessary to understand and motivate them. Significant others should be included in activities so that they can understand and cope better with the patient's disease. Support groups are also effective. Patients with severe psychologic disorders may benefit from individual counseling and therapy. Psychotropic drugs should generally be reserved for patients with more severe psychologic dysfunction.

Because breathlessness is associated closely with fear and anxiety, techniques of relaxation training have been used successfully in pulmonary rehabilitation. Renfroe (76) evaluated progressive muscle relaxation training in 10 patients with COPD compared with controls who were instructed to relax but not given specific instructions. In this technique patients are taught to tense and then relax 16 different muscle groups sequentially. After the relaxation sessions, the group given instruction demonstrated a greater reduction in dyspnea and anxiety than the control group. Also, a change in dyspnea was correlated significantly with a change in anxiety.

RESULTS OF PULMONARY REHABILITATION

Several comprehensive reviews provide support and extensive references substantiating the practices and expected results of pulmonary rehabilitation (Table 49B.3) (4, 6, 7). In evaluating results it is important to consider effects of individual components as well as more general outcomes. It often is difficult to distinguish the relative contributions of specific elements that are so integrally related. For example, any treatment (e.g., education, exercise) provided by well-trained personnel will inevitably provide important elements of psychosocial support and motivation for sick and disabled patients.

HOSPITALIZATIONS AND MEDICAL RESOURCES

Pulmonary rehabilitation has been shown to produce cost effective benefits for patients with chronic lung disease. Several studies have analyzed hospital and medical resource utilization before and after rehabilitation. Given the high costs of acute care hospital-

TABLE 49B.3. Results of Pulmonary Rehabilitation

Decrease in:
  Medical resources utilization (e.g., hospitalizations, emergency room visits)
  Respiratory symptoms (e.g., breathlessness)
  Psychologic symptoms (e.g., depression, fear)
Increase in:
  Quality of life
  Physical activity
    Exercise tolerance (endurance and/or maximum level)
    Activities of daily living
  Knowledge
  Independence
Return to work possible
No change in lung function
? Prolonged survival

izations for these often sick patients, the potential savings from a reduction in hospital days alone is significant.

Lertzman and Cherniack (8) reported an average decrease of 20 hospital days per year in patients who have undergone pulmonary rehabilitation. Petty and coworkers (77) reported a 38% reduction in hospital days (868 to 542) among 85 patients with COPD evaluated 1 year after pulmonary rehabilitation, compared with the previous year. In a randomized, controlled study Jensen (28) found that pulmonary rehabilitation led to significantly fewer hospitalizations over 6 months of follow-up in COPD patients with high-risk markers for psychosocial problems. In an evaluation of an inpatient pulmonary rehabilitation program, Agle and coworkers (78) reported 30 hospital admissions in 24 patients in the year preceding rehabilitation compared with only five admissions in the subsequent year.

Several reports have examined longer term follow-up. Hudson and coworkers (79) surveyed hospitalizations for pulmonary disease 4 years after pulmonary rehabilitation for 64 patients with COPD. For the 44 patients still alive at that time, hospital days were reduced from 529 days in the year preceding the program to 145, 270, 278, and 207 days in years 1, 2, 3, and 4, respectively. This benefit was most striking in the 14 patients hospitalized in the year preceding the program; hospital days in this group decreased from an average of 38 days per patient to 10 days per patient in the year before versus the year after rehabilitation.

Johnson and coworkers (80) reported a 55% decrease in hospital days (mean, 23 days) in the year after versus the year before inpatient pulmonary rehabilitation in 96 patients with severe COPD (FEV_1, 0.87 L). In an analysis of long-term follow-up of 193 patients after pulmonary rehabilitation, the estimated reduction was 21 hospital days per surviving patient per year (81).

Hodgkin and coworkers (7) reported an average reduction from 19 hospital days in the year before rehabilitation to nearly 6 days in the first year after the program in 80 patients. The improvement was maintained for 8 years of follow-up.

QUALITY OF LIFE

After rehabilitation, improvements have been noted in several aspects of quality of life, including respiratory and psychologic symptoms, exercise tolerance, and social activity. Several quality of life instruments that incorporate aspects of physical, emotional, and psychologic function into one or a small number of measures have been used increasingly in the evaluation of patients with chronic lung diseases.

A disease specific measure that has been used frequently for patients with chronic lung diseases is the Chronic Respiratory Questionnaire developed by Guyatt and colleagues (82). In a long-term study of multidisciplinary pulmonary rehabilitation in 31 consecutive patients, Guyatt and coworkers (82) reported improvement in all four measured dimensions of quality of life (dyspnea, fatigue, emotional function, and mastery). Similar findings were reported by Reardon and colleagues (83) in 44 patients completing a 6-week pulmonary rehabilitation program.

The Quality of Well-Being Scale is a comprehensive measure of health-related quality of life shown to have validity as an outcome measure for evaluating interventions that affect general health status. In one randomized, controlled trial of behavioral intervention on exercise in patients with COPD, Atkins and coworkers (84) reported greater changes in the Quality of Well-Being Scale in three experimental groups compared with a no-treatment control group. Using these data to estimate and compare the cost effectiveness of intervention strategies in producing a "well-year" of life, the investigators concluded that this treatment resulted in significant benefits for these patients. However, in a subsequent randomized clinical trial of pulmonary rehabilitation in 119 patients with COPD, no significant changes were observed in Quality of Well-Being Scale in either treated or control groups, despite marked changes in exercise tolerance and breathlessness after rehabilitation (85, 86).

Another general health measure, the Rand Health Survey instrument (equivalent to the sheet-form [SF]-36) developed as part of the Medical Outcomes Study, includes 36 items that can be combined into eight dimensions of health status. In one preliminary report in 21 patients after pulmonary rehabilitation, Make and coworkers (87) reported significant changes on seven of the nine subscales.

EXERCISE

Exercise is important and well established in pulmonary rehabilitation, producing both physiologic and psychologic benefits (4, 6, 52, 53, 86). Casaburi and Petty (6) reviewed 37 published studies of exercise training in more than 900 patients with COPD. Nearly unanimously, these studies demonstrated improvement in exercise endurance and/or maximum exercise tolerance.

There have been several controlled trials of exercise training that support the beneficial effects of exercise in patients with chronic lung disease. In one randomized clinical trial of rehabilitation versus an education control program in 119 patients with COPD, Ries and coworkers (86) reported a highly significant improvement in exercise endurance after rehabilitation (an increase of 81% versus 21%)..The improvement was maintained for up to 12 months. In another controlled trial, Cockcroft and coworkers (88) randomly assigned 39 male patients with both COPD and coal workers' pneumoconiosis to a 6-week exercise program or to a no-treatment control group. Patients in the exercise group had a significantly greater increase in their 12-minute walk distance (23% versus 8%). McGavin and coworkers (89) randomly allocated 28 patients with COPD to a 3-month unsupervised stair-climbing home exercise program or to a nonexercise control group. Significantly more patients in the exercise group noted improvement in their sense of well-being, breathlessness, cough, and sputum. There also was a significant increase in exercise performance in the trained patients versus controls on both the 12-minute walk distance and the maximum work load on a cycle ergometer test.

Pulmonary Function, Symptoms, and Breathing Techniques

Pulmonary rehabilitation does not result in any consistent changes in lung function in patients with chronic lung disease if patients are on good medical therapy before beginning the program. Nevertheless, many patients report improvement in respiratory symptoms, particularly the troubling sensation of breathlessness. Improved dyspnea has been reported consistently in experimental studies (4, 86, 89, 90). Improvement in psychologic symptoms has also been demonstrated consistently after rehabilitation (4).

Education

Pulmonary rehabilitation emphasizes educating patients and significant others to be involved actively in their own care, to improve their understanding of disease, and to learn practical ways of coping with disabling symptoms. Studies that have examined the effects of education have shown that even patients with severe disease can learn to understand their disease better (4, 31). However, education alone does not typically lead to improved health status. Patients also require specific, individual strategies for changing behavior as well as encouragement, practice, and positive feedback.

Survival

Studies of survival of patients with chronic lung disease after pulmonary rehabilitation have shown variable results. There have been no prospective, randomly controlled studies that provide convincing evidence one way or another.

Summary and Future of Pulmonary Rehabilitation

Pulmonary rehabilitation has been well established as a means of improving functional status and reducing the disability and economic burden of the growing number of patients with chronic lung diseases. Adopting a broad rehabilitation medicine perspective, such programs provide multidisciplinary expertise directed toward the needs of individual, disabled pulmonary patients.

Much of the experience in pulmonary rehabilitation has been with patients with COPD; however, it is clear that similar benefits accrue to patients with other disabling pulmonary conditions. Patients with thoracic neoplasms who are in a stable phase of treatment or in remission are appropriate candidates. Many of these patients have underlying chronic lung disease. In addition, their functional status may decrease further because of the treatment for the malignancy. Pulmonary rehabilitation can help these patients deal more effectively with physical and emotional burdens. Improvement in health status, physical and psychologic symptoms, physical function, and quality of life, as well as a reduction in health care burdens, are certainly possible for these patients.

References

1. American Thoracic Society. Pulmonary rehabilitation. Am Rev Respir Dis 1981;24:663–666.
2. American Thoracic Society. Standards for the diagnosis and care of patients with chronic obstructive pulmonary disease (COPD) and asthma. Am Rev Respir Dis 1987;136:225–244.
3. Cotes JE, Bishop JM, Capel LH, et al. Disabling chest disease: prevention and care: a report of the Royal College of Physicians by the College Committee on Thoracic Medicine. J R Coll Physicians Lond 1981;15:69–87.
4. Ries AL. Position paper of the American Association of Cardiovascular and Pulmonary Rehabilitation: scientific basis of pulmonary rehabilitation. J Cardiopulm Rehabil 1990;10:418–441.
5. American Association of Cardiovascular and Pulmonary Rehabilitation: Connors G, Hilling L, eds. Guidelines for pulmonary rehabilitation programs. Champaign, IL: Human Kinetics, 1993.
6. Casaburi R, Petty TL, eds. Principles and practice of pulmonary rehabilitation. Philadelphia: WB Saunders, 1993.
7. Hodgkin JE, Connors GL, Bell CW, eds. Pulmonary rehabilitation: guidelines to success. 2nd ed. Philadelphia: JB Lippincott, 1993.

8. Lertzman MM, Cherniack RM. Rehabilitation of patients with chronic obstructive pulmonary disease. Am Rev Respir Dis 1976;114:1145–1165.
9. Foster S, Thomas HM. Pulmonary rehabilitation in lung disease other than chronic obstructive pulmonary disease. Am Rev Respir Dis 1990;141:601–604.
10. Craven JL, Bright J, Dear CL. Psychiatric, psychosocial, and rehabilitative aspects of lung transplantation. Clin Chest Med 1990;11:247–257.
11. Petty TL. Pulmonary rehabilitation in perspective: historical roots, present status, and future projections. Thorax 1993;48:855–862.
12. Bernhard J, Ganz PA. Psychosocial issues in lung cancer patients (parts 1 and 2). Chest 1991;99:216–223;480–485.
13. Kirilloff LH, Carpenter V, Kerby GR, et al. Skills of the health team involved in out-of-hospital care for patients with COPD. Am Rev Respir Dis 1986;133:948–949.
14. Niederman MS, Clemente PH, Fein AM, et al. Benefits of a multidisciplinary pulmonary rehabilitation program: improvements are independent of lung function. Chest 1991;99:798–804.
15. Ries AL. The role of exercise testing in pulmonary diagnosis. Clin Chest Med 1987;8:81–89.
16. Carlson DJ, Ries AL, Kaplan RM. Prediction of maximum exercise tolerance in patients with chronic obstructive pulmonary disease. Chest 1991;100:307–311.
17. Ries AL, Moser KM. Predicting treadmill/walking speed from cycle ergometry exercise in chronic obstructive pulmonary disease. Am Rev Respir Dis 1982;126:924–927.
18. Jones NL. Clinical exercise testing. 3rd ed. Philadelphia: WB Saunders, 1988.
19. Wasserman K, Hansen JE, Sue DY, Whipp BJ. Principles of exercise testing and interpretation. Philadelphia: Lea & Febiger, 1987.
20. Ries AL, Farrow JR, Clausen JL. Pulmonary function tests cannot predict exercise-induced hypoxemia in chronic obstructive pulmonary disease. Chest 1988;93:454–459.
21. Ries AL, Farrow JR, Clausen JL. Accuracy of two ear oximeters at rest and during exercise in pulmonary patients. Am Rev Respir Dis 1985;132:685–689.
22. Agle DP, Baum GL. Psychological aspects of chronic obstructive pulmonary disease. Med Clin North Am 1977;61:749–758.
23. Dudley DL, Glaser EM, Jorgenson BN, et al. Psychosocial concomitants to rehabilitation in chronic obstructive pulmonary disease: part 1. Psychosocial and psychological considerations: part 2. Psychosocial treatment; part 3. Dealing with psychiatric disease (as distinguished from psychosocial or psychophysiologic problems). Chest 1980;77:413–20;544–51;677–84.
24. Glaser EM, Dudley DL. Psychosocial rehabilitation and psychopharmacology. In: Odgkin JE, Petty TL, eds. Chronic obstructive pulmonary disease. Philadelphia: WB Saunders, 1987:128–153.
25. McSweeny AJ, Grant I, Heaton RK, Adams KM, Timms RM. Life quality of patients with chronic obstructive pulmonary. Arch Intern Med 1982;142:473–478.
26. Sandhu HS. Psychosocial issues in chronic obstructive pulmonary disease. Clin Chest Med 1986;7:629–642.
27. Prigatano GP, Grant I. Neuropsychological correlates of COPD. In: McSweeny AJ, Grant I, eds. Chronic obstructive pulmonary disease: a behavioral perspective. New York: Marcel Dekker 1988:39–57.
28. Jensen PS. Risk, protective factors, and supportive interventions in chronic airway obstruction. Arch Gen Psychiatry 1983;40:1203–1207.
29. Dudley DL, Sitzman J. Psychobiological evaluation and treatment of COPD. In: McSweeny AJ, Grant I, eds. Chronic obstructive pulmonary disease: a behavioral perspective. New York: Marcel Dekker, 1988:183–235.
30. Gilmartin ME. Patient and family education. Clin Chest Med 1986;7:619–627.
31. Neish CM, Hopp JW. The role of education in pulmonary rehabilitation. J Cardiopulm Rehabil 1988;11:439–441.
32. Moser KM, Ries AL, Sassi-Dambron DE, et al. Shortness of breath—a guide to better living and breathing. 4th ed. St. Louis: Mosby Year Book, 1991.
33. Rochester DF, Goldberg SK. Techniques of respiratory physical therapy. Am Rev Respir Dis 1980;122(Suppl):133–146.
34. Kirilloff LH, Owens GR, Rogers RM, et al. Does chest physical therapy work? Chest 1985;88:436–444.
35. Sutton PP, Parker RA, Webber BA, et al. Assessment of the forced expiration technique, postural drainage and directed coughing in chest physiotherapy. Eur J Respir Dis 1983;64:62–68.
36. Sutton PP, Pavia D, Bateman JRM, et al. Chest physiotherapy: a review. Eur J Respir Dis 1982;63:188–201.
37. Paine R, Make BJ. Pulmonary rehabilitation for the elderly. Clin Geriatr Med 1986;2:313–335.
38. The Intermittent Positive Pressure Breathing Trial Group. Intermittent positive pressure breathing therapy of chronic obstructive pulmonary disease. Ann Intern Med 1983;99:612–620.
39. Campbell EJM, Friend J. Action of breathing exercises in pulmonary emphysema. Lancet 1955;268:325–329.
40. Faling LJ. Pulmonary rehabilitation—physical modalities. Clin Chest Med 1986;7:599–618.
41. Miller WF. Physical therapeutic measures in the treatment of chronic bronchopulmonary disorders: methods for breathing training. Am J Med 1958;24:929–940.
42. Barach AL. Breathing exercises in pulmonary emphysema and allied chronic respiratory disease. Arch Phys Med Rehabil 1955;36:379–390.
43. Barach AL. Physiologic advantages of grunting, groaning, and pursed-lip breathing: adaptive symptoms related to the development of continuous positive pressure breathing. Bull N Y Acad Med 1973;49:666–673.
44. Fulmer JD, Snider GL. ACCP-NHLBI national conference on oxygen therapy. Chest 1984;86:234–247.
45. Tiep BL. Long-term home oxygen therapy. Clin Chest Med 1990;11:505–521.
46. Anthonisen NR. Long-term oxygen therapy. Ann Intern Med 1983;99:519–527.
47. Medical Research Council Working Party. Long-term domiciliary oxygen therapy in chronic hypoxic cor pulmonale complicating chronic bronchitis and emphysema. Lancet 1981:1:681–686.
48. Nocturnal Oxygen Therapy Trial Group. Continuous or nocturnal oxygen therapy in hypoxemic chronic obstructive lung disease: a clinical trial. Ann Intern Med 1980;93:391–398.
49. Dean NC, Brown JK, Himelman RB, et al. Oxygen may improve dyspnea and endurance in patients with chronic obstructive pulmonary disease and only mild hypoxemia. Am Rev Respir Dis 1992;146:941–945.
50. Tiep BL, Lewis MI. Oxygen conservation and oxygen-conserving devices in chronic lung disease. Chest 1987;92:263–272.
51. Christopher KL, Spofford BT, Petrun MD, et al. A program for transtracheal oxygen delivery: assessment of safety and efficacy. Ann Intern Med 1987;107:802–808.

52. Shephard RJ. On the design and effectiveness of training regimens in chronic obstructive lung disease. Bull Eur Physiopathol Respir 1977;13:457–469.
53. Hughes RL, Davison R. Limitations of exercise reconditioning in COLD. Chest 1983;83:241–249.
54. Belman MJ. Exercise in chronic obstructive pulmonary disease. Clin Chest Med 1986;7:585–597.
55. Hodgkin JE. Pulmonary rehabilitation: structure, components, and benefits. J Cardiopulm Rehabil 1988;11:423–434.
56. Punzal PA, Ries AL, Kaplan RM, et al. Maximum intensity exercise training in patients with chronic obstructive pulmonary disease. Chest 1991;100:618–623.
57. Carter R, Nicotra B, Clark L, et al. Exercise conditioning in the rehabilitation of patients with chronic obstructive pulmonary disease. Arch Phys Med Rehabil 1988;69:118–122.
58. Borg GAV. Psychophysical bases of perceived exertion. Med Sci Sports Exerc 1982;14:377–381.
59. Mahler DA. The measurement of dyspnea during exercise in patients with lung disease. Chest 1992;101:242S–247S.
60. Keogh BA, Lakatos E, Price D, et al. Importance of the lower respiratory tract in oxygen transfer: exercise testing in patients with interstitial and destructive lung disease. Am Rev Respir Dis 1984;129:S76–S80.
61. Celli BR, Rassulo J, Make BJ. Dyssynchronous breathing during arm but not leg exercise in patients with chronic airflow obstruction. N Engl J Med 1986;314:1485–1490.
62. Couser JI Jr, Martinez FJ, Celli BR. Pulmonary rehabilitation that includes arm exercise reduces metabolic and ventilatory requirements for simple arm elevation. Chest 1993;103:37–41.
63. Ries AL, Ellis B, Hawkins RW. Upper extremity exercise training in chronic obstructive pulmonary disease. Chest 1988;93:688–692.
64. Ellis B, Ries AL. Upper extremity exercise training in pulmonary rehabilitation. J Cardiopulm Rehabil 1991;11:227–231.
65. Belman MJ. Ventilatory muscle training and unloading. In: Casaburi R, Petty TL, eds. Principles and practice of pulmonary rehabilitation. Philadelphia: WB Saunders, 1993:225–240.
66. Smith K, Cook D, Guyatt GH, et al. Respiratory muscle training in chronic airflow limitation: a meta-analysis. Am Rev Respir Dis 1992;145:533–539.
67. Celli BR. Respiratory muscle function. Clin Chest Med 1986;7:567–584.
68. Grassino A. Inspiratory muscle training in COPD patients. Eur Respir J 1989;2(Suppl 7):581S–586S.
69. Pardy RL, Reid WD, Belman MJ. Respiratory muscle training. Clin Chest Med 1988;9:287–296.
70. Guyatt G, Keller J, Singer J, et al. Controlled trial of respiratory muscle training in chronic airflow limitation. Thorax 1992;47:598–602.
71. Pardy RL, Rivington RN, Despas PJ, et al. The effects of inspiratory muscle training on exercise performance in chronic airflow limitation. Am Rev Respir Dis 1981;123:426–433.
72. Light RW, Merrill EJ, Despars JA, et al. Prevalence of depression and anxiety in patients with COPD: relationship to functional capacity. Chest 1985;87:35–38.
73. Curgian LM, Gronkiewicz CA. Enhancing sexual performance in COPD. Nurse Practitioner 1988;13:34–38.
74. Fletcher EC, Martin RJ. Sexual dysfunction and erectile impotence in chronic obstructive pulmonary disease. Chest 1982;81:413–421.
75. Timms RM. Sexual dysfunction and chronic obstructive pulmonary disease. Chest 1982;81:398–400.
76. Renfroe KL. Effect of progressive relaxation on dyspnea and state anxiety in patients with chronic obstructive pulmonary disease. Heart Lung 1988;17:408–413.
77. Petty TL, Nett LM, Finigan MM, et al. A comprehensive care program for chronic airway obstruction: methods and preliminary evaluation of symptomatic and functional improvement. Ann Intern Med 1969;70:1109–1120.
78. Agle DP, Baum GL, Chester EH, et al. Multidiscipline treatment of chronic pulmonary insufficiency: 1. Psychologic aspects of rehabilitation. Psychosom Med 1973;35:41–49.
79. Hudson LD, Tyler ML, Petty TL. Hospitalization needs during an outpatient rehabilitation program for severe chronic airway obstruction. Chest 1976;70:606–610.
80. Johnson HR, Tanzi F, Balchum OJ, et al. Inpatient comprehensive pulmonary rehabilitation in severe COPD. Respir Ther 1980;May/June:15–19.
81. Johnson NR, DeFlorio GP, Einstein H. Cost/benefit outcomes of pulmonary rehabilitation in severe chronic obstructive pulmonary disease. Am Rev Respir Dis 1983;127:A111.
82. Guyatt GH, Berman LB, Townsend M, et al. A measure of quality of life for clinical trials in chronic lung disease. Thorax 1987;42:773–778.
83. Reardon J, Patel K, ZuWallack RL. Improvement in quality of life is unrelated to improvement in exercise endurance after outpatient pulmonary rehabilitation. J Cardiopulm Rehabil 1993;13:51–54.
84. Atkins CJ, Kaplan RM, Timms RM, et al. Behavioral exercise programs in the management of chronic obstructive pulmonary disease. J Consult Clin Psychol 1984;52:591–603.
85. Toshima MT, Kaplan RM, Ries AL. Experimental evaluation of rehabilitation in chronic obstructive pulmonary disease: short-term effects on exercise endurance and health status. Health Psychol 1990;9:237–252.
86. Ries A, Kaplan RM, Limberg TM, et al. Effects of pulmonary rehabilitation on physiologic and psychosocial outcomes in patients with chronic obstructive pulmonary disease. Ann Intern Med 1995;122:822–832.
87. Make B, Glenn K, Ikle D, et al. Pulmonary rehabilitation improves the quality of life of patients with chronic obstructive pulmonary disease (COPD). Am Rev Respir Dis 1992;145:A767.
88. Cockcroft AE, Saunders MT, Berry G. Randomised controlled trial of rehabilitation in chronic respiratory disability. Thorax 1981;36:200–203.
89. McGavin CR, Gupta SP, Lloyd EL, et al. Physical rehabilitation of chronic bronchitis: results of a controlled trial of exercises in the home. Thorax 1977;32:307–311.
90. Bebout DE, Hodgkin JE, Zorn EG, et al. Clinical and physiological outcomes of a university-hospital pulmonary rehabilitation program. Respir Care 1983;28:1468–1473.
91. Ries AL. Outcome measures in pulmonary rehabilitation: a multivariate logistic regression analysis. Master of Public Health Thesis, San Diego State University, 1991.

50

THORACIC NEOPLASMS ASSOCIATED WITH HUMAN IMMUNODEFICIENCY VIRUS INFECTION

Ellen G. Feigal and Timothy R. Coté

INTRODUCTION

Human immunodeficiency virus (HIV), the causative agent of the acquired immune deficiency syndrome (AIDS), has infected more than 1 million individuals in the United States since 1981 (1). Malignancies have been associated with AIDS since the first case descriptions, and they make up a sizable fraction of the illnesses associated with HIV infection (2–4). Many conditions that impair cellular immunity, including medications given to organ transplant recipients, increase the risk for opportunistic malignancies, including Kaposi's sarcoma (KS) and lymphoproliferative disorders (5–8).

Malignancies in AIDS patients frequently present in the chest, but diagnosis and management of these cancers is made difficult by repeated pulmonary infections. Early in the AIDS epidemic, *Pneumocystis carinii* pneumonia (PCP) was the most common presenting AIDS-defining condition (9). Although antimicrobial prophylaxis of pulmonary infections has had an impact, PCP, tuberculosis, atypical mycobacterial infections, recurrent bacterial pneumonias, and fungal infections remain common. Thoracic malignancies are becoming increasingly frequent with more effective prevention of opportunistic infections and as patients with AIDS live longer (10).

This chapter focuses on the AIDS-related neoplasms that occur in the thorax, primarily non-Hodgkin's lymphoma (NHL), and KS. Other malignancies that are common in the general population, including Hodgkin's disease (11–24) and lung cancer, have been reported in the HIV-infected patient (25, 26). It is less obvious whether these cancers result from HIV-induced immunodeficiency or are simply coincidental. Optimal clinical management of any thoracic malignancy in HIV-infected patients requires an understanding of the epidemiology, biology, and therapy of both the malignancy and the HIV infection.

MULTISTATE AIDS/CANCER MATCH REGISTRY

In 1992, the Viral Epidemiology Branch of the National Cancer Institute established the MultiState AIDS/Cancer Match Registry (MSACMR). Reports of cancer and AIDS are made by physicians, hospitals, and laboratories to state and local health departments. Although occurrences of AIDS and cancer have long been reported to their respective registries, these disparate data were not useful for the study of cancers among people with AIDS. Cancer reports include histology data but not information on HIV infection, and AIDS reports include data on HIV infection, but they lack data on cancer occurrence. The frequency of cancer development in people with AIDS could only be determined through linkage of these two sources of health department records.

The MSACMR provides incidence data for thoracic tumors among patients with HIV infection. The relative frequency of primary thoracic tumors (excluding cancers of the skin and subcutaneous connective tissues) is currently available from 83,000 people with AIDS in six states linked to available cancer data, but this frequency is expected to expand in 1996 to 300,000 in 15 centers. As shown in Figure 50.1, parenchymal tumors of the lung account for approximately 50% of all thoracic tumors, with KS and NHL each comprising approximately 25% of all malignancies. Figure 50.1 should be interpreted with two major caveats: first, cancer registry data were generally available for fewer years than AIDS registry data, thus this analysis underestimates the proportion of people with AIDS who develop thoracic cancer; this problem

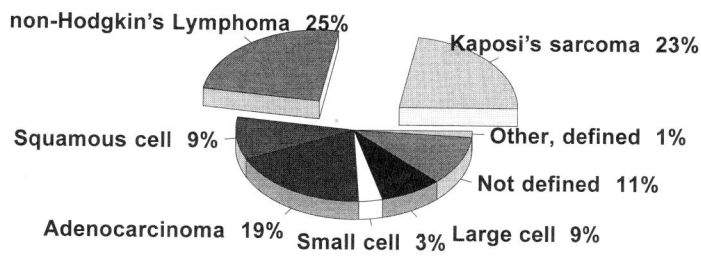

FIGURE 50.1. Histologies of 222 cancers within the thorax in AIDS patients.

should not alter the relative frequency of tumor types, however. Secondly, because the registry collects only data on primary tumors, it does not reflect the secondary spread of KS and NHL to the thorax, which are common clinical problems. Nevertheless, the linkage shows that thoracic cancers common in the general population are more likely to be diagnosed than primary KS or NHL.

NON-HODGKIN'S LYMPHOMA
EPIDEMIOLOGY

In the general population, the incidence of malignant lymphoma doubled between the 1940s and the 1970s (27). NHL in the general population appears to have been increasing steadily at a rate of 3% to 5% per year since data collection began in the 1950s. Some, but not all, of this increase appears to result from improved diagnostic techniques. The risk is increased with male gender, white race, higher socioeconomic status, and older age (28).

The occurrence of NHL and AIDS was noted early in the epidemic (3). Based on epidemiologic evidence of a markedly increased incidence of NHL among people with AIDS, the U.S. Centers for Disease Control and Prevention (CDC) expanded the case definition of AIDS to include high- and intermediate-grade NHL (29, 30). The relationship between low-grade lymphomas and HIV is less clear, and there is little epidemiologic evidence that the low-grade lymphomas have increased in parallel with the AIDS epidemic (4, 31–34).

Initially, the epidemiology of AIDS-associated NHL was studied using demographic markers (e.g., never-married men) for homosexual men in regions with a high AIDS incidence, including New York (35), San Francisco (36), and Los Angeles (37). Additional estimates came from smaller cohorts of patients with hemophilia (38, 39). Such studies documented HIV risk for NHL to be 60 to 100 times greater than that of the general population (40, 41).

The MSACMR permitted better quantification of HIV risk compared with the general population. NHL occurs among individuals in AIDS registries at a rate of 1.4 per 100 person-years, 191-fold that of the general population. The risk for primary lymphoma of the brain is even higher: 3900-fold that of the general population. NHL is the initial AIDS-defining condition in 3% of AIDS cases (42), and another 3% develop NHL subsequently. The risk of lymphoma developing in a patient with symptomatic HIV infection has ranged from 1% to 2% per year in most studies (40, 43, 44).

Among AIDS patients, men have higher rates of NHL than women, and whites have higher rates than blacks (40). There is relatively little variation in incidence by transmission-risk group and geographic area. Although African patients with Burkitt's lymphoma who were not infected with HIV have an elevated frequency of human leukocyte antigen (HLA) DR7 (46), no specific HLA type has been found to be elevated among people with AIDS and NHL. An uncontrolled trial reported a high NHL risk in patients treated with zidovudine (AZT) or didanosine (ddI) (47). However, randomized trials of AZT compared with placebo, ddI, or zalcitabine (ddC) have not found increased rates of NHL (FDA Antiviral Drug Products Scientific Advisory Committee's unpublished data), and epidemiologic studies have found no increase in risk for NHL among people diagnosed with AIDS in the post-AZT era compared with the pre-AZT era (49). It is likely that risk increases as T-cell immunity decreases, regardless of treatment.

BIOLOGY

Research has suggested that multiple steps may be important in lymphomagenesis, including: (a) HIV-induced immune suppression, (b) HIV and/or Epstein-

Barr virus–induced disruption in cytokines that regulate the immune host response, (c) the dysregulation of B-cell proliferation, and (d) mutations in critical oncogenes, tumor suppressor genes, or abnormal DNA rearrangements. Other viral co-factors, such as human herpes virus–6, are also being investigated.

HIV does not appear to be involved directly in the malignant transformation of B lymphocytes. HIV has been detected by polymerase chain reaction in AIDS lymphoma tissue but only at levels that would be expected from infiltrating T cells (50). Southern blot analysis has shown no evidence of HIV sequences within B-cell lymphoma tissue nor within the reactive B-cell hyperplasia that may precede the diagnosis of lymphoma (4, 51–55).

Although there is little evidence of a direct role in malignant transformation of B cells, HIV may act indirectly through destruction of CD4 T cells and through dysregulation of cytokine release, which affects B-cell proliferation, differentiation, and other host immune responses. Interleukin-6 (IL-6) (47, 56–60) and IL-10 (61) may be particularly important for stimulating B-cell proliferation, whereas IL-2, interferon-γ, and IL-12 may be important in limiting such growth (62, 63).

Oncogene or tumor suppressor genes also may be important in the development of some lymphomas. The chromosome 8 c-*myc* oncogene has been found to be deregulated by translocations t(8;14), t(8;22), or t(8;2) in sporadic (American) Burkitt's lymphoma and by point mutation in endemic (African) Burkitt's lymphoma (64, 65). Studies of HIV-associated lymphomas also have reported translocations (51, 66, 67) and point mutations (68), although the prevalence of these changes varied widely in the small series reported.

The presence of the Epstein-Barr virus in lymphoma tissue varies with the severity of immune compromise, histologic type, and anatomic site. Tumor containing Epstein-Barr virus is found uniformly in the organ transplant recipient who develops a lymphoproliferative disorder and in endemic African Burkitt's lymphoma (69). There also is uniform presence of Epstein-Barr virus–related latent proteins in large cell, immunoblastic lymphoma tissue derived from the primary central nervous system (CNS) lymphoma seen in AIDS patients (70). In systemic AIDS lymphomas, Epstein-Barr virus has been reported in varying proportions, ranging from 38% in some studies up to 68% in others (66, 67, 70, 71). These differences may partly be related to the different pathogenesis in different histologic categories. A larger Epstein-Barr virus positive proportion is found in systemic large cell immunoblastic lymphoma (65% to 73%) than in small noncleaved lymphomas, including Burkitt's lymphoma (20% to 28%) (72–74).

Almost all lymphomas occurring in the HIV population are B cell. Although T-cell lymphomas have not increased in incidence, several HIV-infected patients with T-cell lymphoma (75–82) and leukemia (83, 84) have been described. Of interest, Shiramizu et al. (85) described a large cell lymphoma in which HIV was expressed in the tumor-associated transformed T cells. The authors suggested that HIV may contribute directly to lymphomagenesis in the rare occurrence of T-cell NHL.

CLINICAL

HISTOLOGY

Initial case series (3, 4, 86) clearly documented that HIV-associated NHL presents a distinct pattern compared with NHL in the general population. Although primary CNS lymphoma represents approximately 1% of all lymphomas in the general population, it represents approximately 15% to 20% of all HIV-associated lymphomas (87, 88; also author's unpublished observations). High-grade histology in systemic NHL occurs in 10% to 15% of cases in the general population (89, 90), compared with 70% to 80% of HIV-associated cases. The large cell immunoblastic and small noncleaved lymphomas, some of which are Burkitt's lymphomas, are the most common cell types (31, 32, 72, 91–93). Intermediate grade, diffuse, large cell histology occurs in 20% to 30% of HIV-associated cases (94–97).

CLINICAL PRESENTATION

The majority of patients present with extranodal, extensive disease that is stage III or IV, "B" symptoms, intermediate- to high-grade histology, and CD4 counts generally below 200. Extranodal involvement occurs in 68% to 98% of patients (4, 32, 91–93, 98). Patients with high-grade NHL in the general population also present with extranodal disease (99–103), but the sites of extranodal involvement in AIDS NHL are distinctive. Although primarily related to the increased incidence of CNS lymphoma, other unusual sites include the gastrointestinal tract, heart, adrenal glands, oral cavity, muscle, and soft tissues (104). Certain histologic types have a predilection for specific anatomic sites (97). The French Study Group reviewed the pathology of 113 cases and noted that immunoblastic lymphomas were more likely to affect the brain, gastrointestinal tract, or oral cavity, whereas small noncleaved lymphomas more likely presented in peripheral sites, such as lymph nodes, muscle, or bone marrow (105). Systemic B symptoms, including fever, drenching night sweats, and/or weight loss in excess of 10% of normal body weight are present in most of the patients with AIDS lymphomas. In the general population, B symptoms are common in patients with immunoblastic histology and less frequent with small noncleaved histology (98, 99, 106). Fever in an HIV-infected patient also can result from an occult opportunistic infection; however, even after infections have been excluded, the incidence of B symptoms remains high.

Thoracic involvement occurs in approximately 25% of patients (4, 107); however, the major presenting features usually are not related to the chest. The chest radiograph may show parenchymal and nodal disease (108) as well as pleural effusions, either unilateral or bilateral (109). Isolated pulmonary involvement is rare.

A tumor biopsy is essential for accurate diagnosis. The extranodal location of disease may pose a technical obstacle to obtaining a biopsy, and co-morbid conditions may make the patient a poor candidate for major operative procedures. A diagnosis of lymphoma with a fine-needle aspirate may be possible, but the histologic type may not be identifiable. The staging evaluation should include bilateral bone marrow biopsies, and CT scans of the chest, abdomen, pelvis and brain. Because asymptomatic leptomeningeal disease may be present in approximately 20% of patients, a lumbar puncture should be done also (110). Other studies, such as endoscopy or a gastrointestinal series, should be performed as clinically indicated.

TREATMENT

The therapy of lymphoma involving the thorax is analogous to that for other anatomic sites. Initial trials approached treatment by focusing on the lymphoma rather than on the underlying HIV infection and immunosuppression, using conventional chemotherapeutic regimens effective against aggressive NHL in immunocompetent patients. Systemic therapy rather than localized approaches (e.g., radiotherapy alone) is needed because the disease is rarely localized. The median survival of systemic HIV-associated NHL (6 months) is far shorter than the survival of NHL patients without HIV infection (30 months); however, it is unclear if this shorter survival results directly from tumor effects or because of competing mortality from infectious causes (author's unpublished observations). Pitfalls in the early trials included the occurrence of opportunistic infections, mucositis, and severe myelosuppression.

The second generation of trials incorporated therapies to attenuate bone marrow suppression, such as granulocyte-macrophage colony–stimulating factor (GM-CSF) or granulocyte colony–stimulating factor (G-CSF), or lower-than-standard doses of cytotoxic chemotherapy. Myelosuppression was reduced, with no apparent ill-effect on patient survival.

The third generation of trials incorporated therapies that addressed the underlying HIV infection. Prophylaxis for opportunistic infections, particularly PCP and fungal infections, in combination with the use of concomitant antiretroviral agents, was an integral component of the therapeutic regimen.

The CNS is a common site for relapse, and although the efficacy of intrathecal prophylaxis in this setting is controversial, three approaches are generally taken: (a) intrathecal chemotherapy (cytosine arabinoside or methotrexate) instilled at the time of the staging lumbar puncture in all patients, (b) intrathecal chemotherapy for patients at higher risk for CNS relapse (e.g., documented bone marrow involvement, or small noncleaved histology), or (c) intrathecal chemotherapy after patients have shown an initial response to the first two cycles of systemic chemotherapy (101, 110).

The standard of care for previously untreated patients is a cytotoxic chemotherapy regimen, such as the combination of cyclophosphamide, hydroxydaunomycin, Oncovin (vincristine), and prednisone (CHOP). Although some small series of patients have had median survivals as long as 17 months, the median survival in the majority of the phase II trials is less than 1 year, and it has not changed significantly since the beginning of the epidemic (91, 110–117). In the immunocompetent setting, patients receiving CHOP therapy were found to have equal survival with less toxicity than patients receiving the combination of methotrexate, bleomycin, Adriamycin (doxorubicin), cyclophosphamide, Oncovin (vincristine), and dexamethasone (M-BACOD), or cyclophosphamide, doxorubicin, etoposide, prednisone, cytarabine, bleomycin, vincristine, methotrexate, with leucovorin (ProMace-CytaBOM) rescue. The only randomized study in AIDS-associated NHL evaluated 198 patients receiving either an attenuated dose m-BACOD regimen with an as-required dose of GM-CSF versus the standard dose of m-BACOD with mandated GM-CSF (118). The responses in both arms were similar, and there was no difference in median survival, which ranged between 7 and 8 months. There were more deaths because of lymphoma in the attenuated dose arm, but more deaths from other causes in the standard dose arm; the viral load was not assessed.

It is critical, if progress is to be made in providing improved management of such patients, that patients be entered onto clinical trials using (*a*) investigational agents in a window-of-opportunity approach, or (*b*) combined biologic and cytotoxic chemotherapy, or (*c*) gene therapy and immunotherapy, in conjunction with monitoring of laboratory parameters to assess viral load and markers of immune impairment. It is essential to use growth factors to attenuate bone marrow toxicity, antiretroviral agents to attenuate viral load, and prophylaxis for opportunistic infection, particularly against PCP, one of the most common pulmonary infections, concomitant with the antitumor therapy.

Second-line therapy for relapses or refractory disease is not standardized. Although transient responses have been seen with a variety of cytotoxic chemotherapy regimens, an investigational approach should also be recommended strongly for this group of patients. Investigators are now attempting to incorporate biologic therapy or other innovative approaches that may interrupt steps involved in the development of lymphomas. Current trials are investigating pathogenesis-driven approaches, with the use of biologic agents, new agents with both antiretroviral and antitumor activity, monoclonal antibodies, immunomodulating approaches, and gene therapy. Tables 50.1 and 50.2 outline the standard and investigational approaches.

Prognostic factors associated with shorter survival in intermediate- or high-grade lymphoma in the general population include increased tumor bulk, lower patient performance status, presence of B symptoms, and older age (119, 120). Several studies have analyzed retrospectively the factors predictive of survival in systemic AIDS-related NHL. An analysis of 49 patients (106) showed that either a prior history of AIDS, Karnofsky performance score of less than 70, or bone marrow involvement predicted shorter survival, whereas a lower CD4 count showed a trend toward shorter survival. In a separate series of 84 patients (91), the single most important predictor of shorter survival was a CD4 lymphocyte count of less than 100. In the absence of a CD4 count, the best predictor of shorter survival was the presence of a prior AIDS diagnosis. Other factors predicting shorter survival were Karnofsky performance score of less than 70, extranodal disease, bone marrow involvement, and more intensive chemotherapy. Neither of these studies showed a prognostic significance of histologic subtype; however, in a series of 89 patients, those with intermediate-grade large noncleaved lymphoma did better than those with high-grade lymphoma (92). Another series also noted shorter survival for patients with high-grade histologies (73). Preliminary results from the large randomized m-BACOD versus M-BACOD trial showed no statistical differences regarding histology (118).

KAPOSI'S SARCOMA

EPIDEMIOLOGY

From the start of the AIDS epidemic, the fascinating epidemiology of KS has been examined both to understand the connection between immunodeficiency and neoplasia and to learn more about KS in its many manifestations. KS was one of the first two conditions reported in homosexual men with AIDS (2, 121). This tumor occurs in a variety of other clinical settings: classic KS, which is a rare, indolent disease of older men of eastern European extraction; African KS, which was first reported in the 1960s (122) and is more aggressive and frequently disseminated; and KS that occurs in association with immunosuppressive drug therapy for organ transplantation (123, 124). KS has been reported during immunosuppressive treatment of systemic lupus erythematosus (125) and temporal arteritis (126). Spontaneous remission occurs in approximately 50% of these patients when immunosuppressive drugs are withdrawn (127). Although organ transplant recipients have a 400- to 500-fold increased risk, HIV increases the relative risk for KS 40,000-fold (40). In each type of KS, men outnumber women.

KS is the most common HIV-associated cancer of the thorax, occurring on the skin of the trunk, endobronchially, and in the lung parenchyma. It is difficult to estimate the incidence of pulmonary KS. Linkages of AIDS and cancer registries have shown that of all KS reports, only 3% of patients have visceral KS (28). However, most AIDS registries have complete reporting only for the initial AIDS-defining illness, and cancer registries report only the first site of cancer diagnosis. Because KS usually presents initially on the skin, with visceral involvement developing later, registries are likely to underestimate visceral pulmonary disease.

Early in the AIDS epidemic in the United States and Europe, KS was a common initial AIDS diagnosis, second only to PCP. For unknown reasons, the proportion of AIDS patients with KS has declined steadily in the United States from 50% to 15% between 1981 and 1986 (128) and in Europe from 38% to 14% between 1983 and 1991 (129). The percentage of AIDS-infected homosexual and bisexual men who develop KS at any time before death in the MSACMR database dropped significantly, from approximately 40% in 1981 to approximately 10% in 1994 (author's unpublished observations).

Early studies looked for a genetic etiology by correlating risk with the prevalence of HLA types. In classic KS, HLA-DR5 is relatively prevalent in the Jewish and Mediterranean populations at risk for KS, whereas HLA-DQ1 has been reported with AIDS-associated KS.

TABLE 50.1. Conventional Treatment Options for Patients with Systemic NHL

TREATMENT OBJECTIVE	TREATMENT OPTIONS	OUTCOME CONSIDERATIONS

Systemic therapy for lymphoma	Cytotoxic agents
	  Cyclophosphamide
	  Doxorubicin
	  Vincristine
	  Prednisone or dexamethasone
	  Etoposide
	  Methotrexate
	  Cytosine arabinoside
	  Bleomycin
		Combination chemotherapy is required for best lymphoma response but may need modified doses to avoid immunosuppression
		  CHOP
		  CHOPE
		  m-BACOD
		  M-BACOD
		  ProMACE-CytaBOM
		  Infusional CDE

Prophylaxis against or active treatment of leptomeningeal lymphoma	Intrathecal
	  Methotrexate
	  Cytosine arabinoside
		Leptomeningeal lymphoma does not worsen the prognosis in the setting of extensive disease

Attenuation of myelosuppression and anemia	Growth factors
	  G-CSF
	  GM-CSF
	  Erythropoietin
		Advantages
		  Allows full dose of cytotoxic chemotherapy
		  Treats bone marrow suppression and anemia caused by chemotherapy, zidovudine or ganciclovir administration
		Disadvantages
		  Potential activation of HIV with GM-CSF

Primary therapy of HIV infection	Nucleoside reverse transcriptase inhibitors
	  Zidovudine (AZT)
	  Didanosine (ddI)
	  Zalcitabine (ddC)
	  Stavudine (d4T)
	  Lamivudine (3Tc)
	Experimental agents
	  Nonnucleoside RT inhibitors
	  Protease inhibitors
		Advantages
		  Treatment of underlying HIV infection
		  May block HIV activation by cytokines
		Disadvantages
		  Peripheral neuropathy and bone marrow suppression may limit chemotherapy with the same dose-limiting toxicities

Prophylaxis against opportunistic infections	PCP prophylaxis
	  Trimethoprim-sulfamethoxazole
	  Aerosolized pentamidine
	  Dapsone
	Fungal prophylaxis
	  Fluconazole
	MAC prophylaxis
	  Rifabutin
	  Clarithromycin
	CMV prophylaxis
	  Oral ganciclovir
		Advantages
		  Prevents common AIDS-associated opportunistic infections
		Disadvantages
		  Polypharmacy and drug interactions

Abbreviations. CHOP, cyclophosphamide, doxorubicin, vincristine, prednisone; CHOPE, CHOP + etoposide; m-BACOD, methotrexate, bleomycin, Adriamycin (doxorubicin), cyclophosphamide, Oncovin (vincristine), dexamethasone; M-BACOD, high-dose methotrexate + BACOD; ProMACE-Cyta BOM, cyclophosphamide, doxorubicin, etoposide, prednisone, cytarabine, bleomycin, vincristine, methotrexate with leucovorin; CDE, cyclophosphamide, doxorubicin, etoposide; RT, reverse transcriptase; PCP, *Pneumocystis carinii* pneumonia; MAC, *Mycobacterium avium* complex; G-CSF, granulocyte colony–stimulating factor; GM-CSF, granulocyte-macrophage colony–stimulating factor.

In transplant recipients who develop KS, HLA types observed less frequently than expected were HLA-A1, HLA-B7, and HLA-B5. HLA-B8, HLA-B18, and HLA-DR5 were observed more frequently than expected. The latter HLA phenotypes are found at higher frequency in Italian, Greek, Jewish, and Arabic populations (127, 130, 131). Although these studies suggest that there may be a genetic predisposition, the correlations do not make a strong case that KS is a genetic disease expressed when cell-mediated immunity is impaired. Moreover, it is difficult to disentangle a population's genetic constituency from its geographic locale.

Many investigations have centered on the HIV transmission group that is most affected by KS. KS is approximately 6- to 8-fold more frequent among homosexual and bisexual men, compared with male intravenous drug users (132, 133). In the United States, the incidence of KS is reported to be higher among women who acquire HIV through sex with bisexual men, compared with women who acquire HIV through intra-

TABLE 50.2. Investigational Treatment Options for Non-Hodgkin's Lymphoma

Cytotoxic chemotherapy	5-Azacytidine
	Camptothecins
Cytokine therapy/immune modulation	IL-2
	IL-4
	IL-12
	IL-6 inhibition
	IL-10 inhibition
	Interferon-γ
Cell-based therapy	Cytotoxic T lymphocytes CD8 against Epstein-Barr virus antigens
Other	Phenylbutyrate/phenylacetate
Gene therapy	

venous drug use (134, 135). In Italy and France, exposure to bisexual men has not been found to be a risk factor for KS in HIV positive women (135, 136). Some of the few transfusion-acquired AIDS patients who subsequently developed KS had received blood from individual donors who developed KS (42). In Africa, HIV transmission is predominantly by heterosexual contact, and KS is distributed more equally between men and women (137). A small number of cases of KS in young, sexually active, HIV negative homosexual men in the United States have been noted. In the few instances reported, this form of KS behaves like classic indolent KS (138–140). The observation that the sexual transmission of HIV was the overwhelming risk factor for KS led to the hypothesis that KS risk was related to sexual practices and possibly a transmissible infectious agent.

The sexual practices and recreational drug use of homosexual men have been studied as risk factors for HIV-associated KS. Although early observations associated the use of nitrate inhalants with KS, more recent studies suggest that inhalants are a marker for sexual activities (141). Oral-fecal contact is more strongly linked to the subsequent development of KS (42). Two studies found a marked increase in KS risk with insertive oral-anal sex (133, 142). Homosexual men without oral-anal contact had an 18% KS incidence, compared with 50% in those with less than one contact per month, and 75% in those with one or more contacts per week. In that study no link was found between other sexual practices or the use of nitrate inhalants (133). However, the San Francisco study (143) did not corroborate the oral-anal association.

Infectious agents have been pursued for links to KS. Cytomegalovirus co-infection is one hypothesized cause of HIV-associated KS. In situ hybridization has found cytomegalovirus in classic, African, and HIV-associated KS (144, 145). Interpretation of this association with HIV is difficult because cytomegalovirus infection is very common in homosexual men. Supporting the relationship is the observation of the decreasing seroprevalence of cytomegalovirus coincident with the decline in the incidence of KS (146). Human papilloma virus 16 (HPV-16) has been proposed as a oncogenic virus potentially causing KS. Polymerase chain reaction with primer pairs specific for the E6 gene of HPV-16 has been reported to identify HPV-16–like DNA fragments in KS tumor tissue and KS-derived cell cultures (147). This HPV DNA sequence was found in 11 of 69 KS skin tumors from HIV-infected homosexual or bisexual men, in 3 of 11 KS skin tumors from HIV-uninfected homosexual or bisexual men, and in 5 of 17 classic KS skin tumors from non–HIV-infected elderly individuals. Another study used immunohistochemical staining to identify HPV E6- and E7-like proteins in KS lesions; however, the staining pattern was atypical, raising the issue of whether the identified proteins are related to HPV or are cross-reacting with cellular antigens (148). Subsequent studies have failed to confirm a relationship of HPV to KS.

The most recent and exciting work to emerge in KS pathogenesis research is from the investigations of Chang et al. (149). The investigators used representational difference analysis to isolate unique sequences present in more than 90% of HIV-associated KS tissues. The sequences were present in 15% of non-KS tissue DNA from HIV-infected patients, but in none of the tissue DNA from non-HIV patients. The sequences had homology to, but were distinct from, capsid and tegument protein genes of the *Gammaherpesvirinae*, *Herpesvirus saimiri*, and Epstein-Barr virus. The authors suggested that these sequences appeared to define a new human herpesvirus that is linked specifically to the pathogenesis of KS. These findings have now been replicated in several laboratories.

BIOLOGY

The pathogenesis of HIV-associated KS may be multifactorial, although the most recent evidence linking a human herpesvirus as the possible etiologic infectious agent in KS is quite strong (149, 150). The KS progenitor cell remains undefined but could be of endothelial, mesenchymal, or smooth muscle origin. A prerequisite for KS development appears to be cell-mediated immune compromise. Research on HIV-associated KS has focused on the roles of HIV, cytokine dysregulation, angiogenesis, sexually transmitted agents, and environmental co-factors.

The principal functions of CD4 are the recognition of HLA class II antigens in association with foreign antigens and assistance in cytotoxic T-cell function. HIV results in the loss of CD4 cells or impairment of CD4-cell function (151, 152). There are multiple mechanisms by which HIV may stimulate the growth of KS: immune impairment by destruction of CD4 cells, cytokine dysregulation, and HIV–transactivator of transcription protein production.

Development of in vitro techniques for growing KS cells has facilitated the study of cytokines and their potential role in the development and progression of KS (153–156). Increases in IL-6 may result in the growth of KS. Inflammatory cytokines, IL-1, tumor necrosis factor–α (157), and interferon-γ are elevated in HIV-infected individuals and are increased by opportunistic infections (158, 159). These inflammatory cytokines can increase the level of IL-6, and they could be a mechanism for the observation of KS exacerbation during opportunistic infections. Another cytokine, oncostatin M, a 28- to 35-kilodalton (kd) protein discovered in the conditioned medium of retrovirally infected cultures required for KS cell growth (153, 160, 161), is produced by HIV-infected CD4 cells. Oncostatin M up regulates IL-6, presumably by binding to the gp130 subunit of the IL-6 receptor (162, 163). Others have suggested a role for fibroblast growth factor, which is expressed by both classic and AIDS-associated KS cell lines. HIV-Tat, whose uptake by KS cells or endothelial cells activated by inflammatory cytokines is mediated by integrin receptors (164), may up regulate IL-6 or synergize with fibroblast growth factor to increase KS cell growth. In addition, some investigators postulate that decreased local pulmonary natural killer cell activity may result in pulmonary KS (165). Angiogenesis, or new blood vessel formation, also is postulated to have an important role in KS pathogenesis (154); multiple therapeutic interventions aimed at blocking this step are in progress.

None of the above mechanisms explains the male predominance or the strong association with homosexual risk groups. Male risk could be related to male sex-steroid hormone modulation of the expression of IL-6 through binding of transcription factors and steroid nuclear receptors (166). The epidemiologic evidence strongly suggests a role for an infectious agent, and the data recently proposed by Chang et al. (149) of a new human herpesvirus will need to be confirmed and identified definitively.

CLINICAL

CLINICAL PRESENTATION

The four settings in which KS presents include classic, organ transplantation, endemic, and epidemic. Each setting is associated with immune impairment. Although the anatomic sites involved and the disease severity vary among the settings, the appearance of the lesion, its histopathology, and its predilection for men are similar.

Classic KS was described initially by dermatologist Moricz Kaposi in 1872 as an indolent skin disease involving the lower extremities in elderly eastern European and Mediterranean men (167). The disease can involve adjacent draining lymph nodes, but only rarely does it involve the mucous membranes and visceral organs. The male to female ratio is 10 to 15:1 (168, 169).

Organ transplant recipients can develop an aggressive form of KS that may regress when immunosuppressive treatment is discontinued. It appears mostly in men and more often in men of Jewish, Arabic, or Mediterranean origin (127, 170–173).

Endemic KS was described initially in the 1950s in children and young adults from sub-Saharan Africa. It was associated frequently with lymph node and organ involvement. Endemic KS accounts for approximately 9% of all cancers in parts of sub-Saharan Africa, with a male to female ratio of 10:1 (122, 169).

Epidemic KS, initially described in gay men in the early 1980s, is the most common malignant complication of HIV infection (132, 133, 174–182). It may occur as the initial sign of HIV infection or develop later in 30% to 50% of HIV-infected men (146, 183). Although the clinical course varies from slowly progressive (184) to rapidly fulminant (185, 186), epidemic KS is more similar to endemic than to classic forms, with an extensive anatomic distribution and a rapid rate of progression. The disease may be limited to several lesions on the skin or mucosa, but in approximately 20% of patients, KS may lead to serious morbidity from lymphedema, visceral organ involvement and dysfunction, and death (34, 97, 135, 166, 173, 187–191).

Patients may first notice a pigmented lesion on the skin or oral mucosa. The lesion may start as a macule or papule that progresses to a plaque or nodule, and it may form symmetric clusters that follow skin creases (Langer's lines) or may occur at multifocal sites (192). The lesions range in size from a few millimeters to several centimeters. They are nonblanching, irregular or distinct, and reddish to violaceous or brown. The skin lesions may cause pain or tenderness if located at sites of friction, such as the soles of the feet. Severe and painful lymphedema of the legs and face may occur and lead to significant morbidity.

KS has been described in almost every organ in autopsy studies (193–196). Fifty percent of patients with oral KS have lesions in the gastrointestinal tract. The gastrointestinal tract lesions are commonly asymptomatic, but they may be associated with retrosternal, epigastric, or rectal pain, blood loss, diarrhea, abdominal cramps, or weight loss (196).

The reported incidence of pulmonary KS varies depending on the patient population studied. The incidence ranges from 8% to 13% in patients with evidence of pulmonary dysfunction (197–199), 21% to 40% in patients with respiratory symptoms (198–201), and approximately 50% of autopsy series (202–204). KS occurring solely in the lungs is uncommon. The pace of cutaneous disease may not predict the pace of pulmonary disease. Progression in the lungs may occur with stable or diminishing cutaneous disease (199).

When KS presents in the respiratory tract, patients often have respiratory symptoms, an abnormal radiograph, and (usually) cutaneous lesions. Patients often present with dyspnea and nonproductive cough caused by extensive endobronchial disease. Less common symptoms include chest pain, hoarseness resulting from vocal cord involvement, or hemoptysis (190, 199, 200, 205–208). Patients may uncommonly have life-threatening bleeding from endobronchial or parenchymal KS, with or without hemoptysis. Airway obstruction caused by lymph node lesions or large endobronchial lesions can occur (201). Patients also may bleed from an upper airway lesion into the lower airway and obstruct the trachea and main stem bronchus with clots (209).

Fever and night sweats associated with HIV infection and opportunistic pulmonary infections may lead to an incidental diagnosis of KS. Auscultation of the chest may be normal, except when hemorrhage or obstruction results in crackles and wheezes. Laryngeal and tracheal involvement may cause obstruction and signs of pulsus paradoxus, stridor, and use of accessory muscles of respiration (199).

A spectrum of abnormalities is found on the chest radiograph. In the review by White and Matthay (210), parenchymal involvement is typically more diffuse than focal, with linear densities that follow septal lines in more than half of the patients. Ill-defined nodular infiltrates resulting from mixed interstitial and alveolar infiltrates are seen in up to one third of patients. Pleural effusions, usually bilateral and serosanguinous exudates, are seen in up to two thirds of patients. A pleural effusion rarely may be the only sign of pulmonary KS. The effusion may be caused by the presence of pleural or subpleural disease, and in some instances it may result from lymphatic obstruction. Focal involvement of the lung parenchyma can be seen occasionally, as demonstrated by segmental or lobar infiltrates. The CT scan may show multiple flame-shaped or nodular lesions with ill-defined margins, and it demonstrates the perivascular and peribronchial extent of disease. The CT may also detect endobronchial lesions, adenopathy, small pulmonary nodules, or airway narrowing. Figure 50.2 shows typical features seen radiographically.

DIAGNOSIS

The appearance of the KS skin lesion is usually characteristic, but it may be difficult to assess if the lesion is isolated, small, or located on pigmented skin. A simple punch biopsy establishes the diagnosis. The differential diagnosis includes other angiomatous lesions, including bacillary angiomatosis, a disease caused by *Rochalimaea*, a small gram negative rod that is classified to the *Rickettsiaceae*. Bacillary angiomatosis can be diagnosed by a Warthin-Starry stain and can be treated by antibiotics (211).

Many of the signs, symptoms, and radiographic findings of KS are nonspecific. The differential diagnosis of respiratory symptoms or an abnormal radiograph in a patient with HIV infection includes HIV-associated opportunistic infections, which may be diagnosed by induced sputum, transbronchial biopsy, and bronchoalveolar lavage. Other studies, such as thallium and gallium scans, pulmonary function tests, and blood tests such as LDH and angiotensin-converting enzyme, have been advocated in the past. Although the sensitivity and specificity of the nuclear medicine scans in HIV disease are not well described, infections generally are gallium avid, KS lesions alone are thallium avid and gallium negative, and lesions of lymphoma are both gallium and thallium avid (212). Therefore, in a patient with respiratory symptoms, no evidence of infection, and an abnormal radiograph, the nuclear scan should be thallium avid and gallium negative. Because of the overlapping array of infections and neoplasms in patients with HIV infection, it is not clear that a nuclear medicine study would aid greatly in the differential diagnosis. A thoracentesis in the presence of fever and a pleural effusion may detect other malignancies or infections, but it will not provide diagnostic evidence of KS.

Pulmonary KS may be confirmed endoscopically by visualizing characteristic KS lesions. The lesions are commonly less than 1 cm in size and may appear as bright red, flat or raised, irregular tumors. They are often found at branch points and carinas of the lower airways. The tracheal wall, subglottic region, hypopharynx, and epiglottis are involved commonly. The presence of KS endoscopically does not rule out a concomitant pulmonary infection (210).

HISTOLOGY

KS histology is similar, regardless of the clinical setting. Light microscopy reveals spindle cells inter-

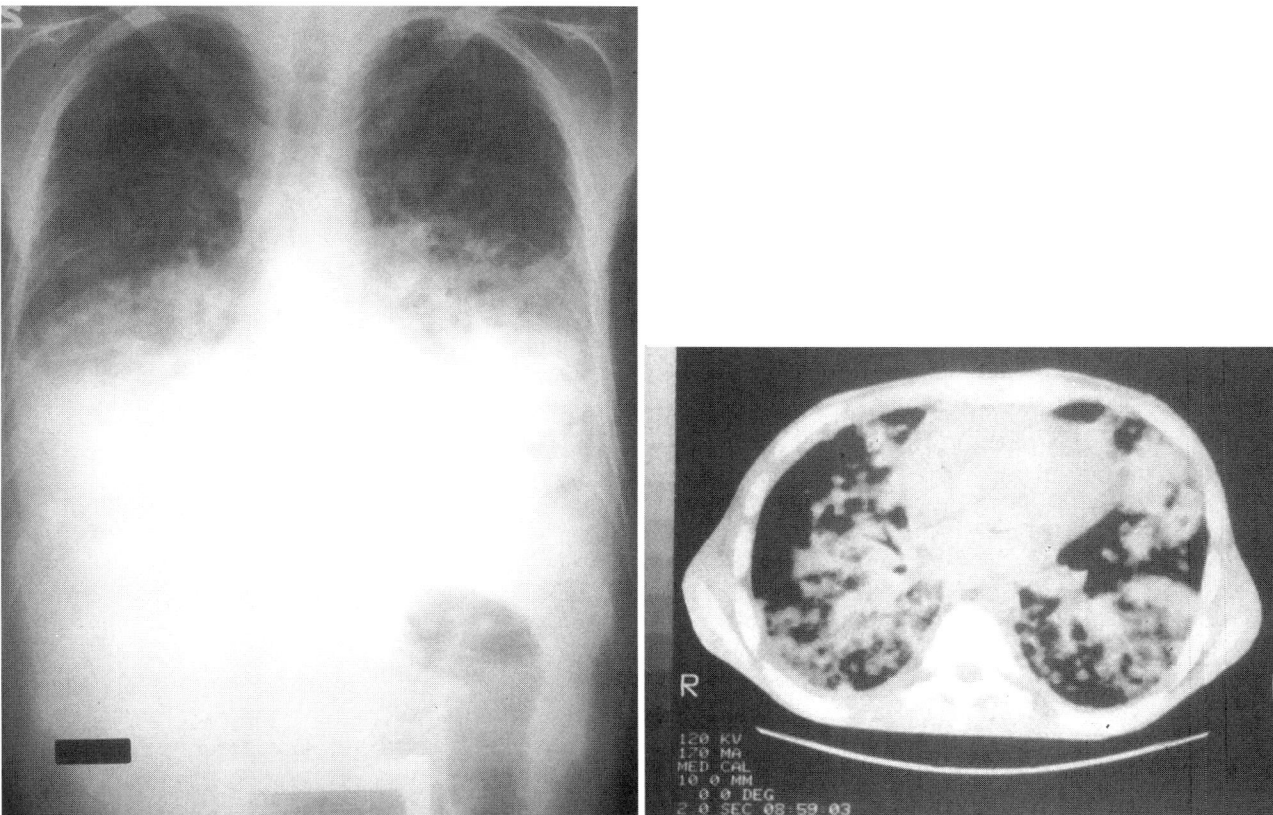

FIGURE 50.2. A. Chest radiograph in a patient with AIDS-related Kaposi's sarcoma. B. Chest CT in a patient with AIDS-related Kaposi's sarcoma. (Courtesy of Dr. Henry Masur, U.S. National Institutes of Health.)

spersed with slitlike vascular channels, within a framework of reticular and collagen fibers, and a broad range of infiltration with macrophages, lymphocytes, and plasma cells. The vascular slits are capillaries lined by endothelial cells. Red cells may extravasate, and hemosiderin deposits in the surrounding tissues may account for the characteristic color of the lesions (202, 213, 214).

Pathologically, the lung involvement can include the parenchyma, airways, pleura, and lymph nodes (199–201, 203, 214–217). Gross examination of pulmonary KS from autopsy studies has shown a lung parenchyma with hemorrhagic nodules (203). Light microscopy reveals that the nodular masses are near airways and blood vessels (203, 206, 218). Endobronchial KS histologically shows extensive invasion of the bronchial wall by spindle-shaped cells, and it may replace mucosal glands and columnar epithelium (203). The capillary vessels may be immediately under the surface epithelium or buried deeper (206). Vascular slits may be less common (200). The pleural plaques histologically show spindle cell proliferation, vascular clefts filled with red blood cells, and an intact pleural surface. Nodules 0.5 cm in diameter in the pleura have been noted also (206).

TREATMENT

There is no curative treatment for KS and even long-term palliation is difficult. Treatment objectives include local control of disfiguring lesions, palliation of symptoms and functional improvement, and stabilization and reduction of widespread disease. Treatment modalities include local therapy with radiation, cryotherapy, or intralesional injections with sclerosing agents, as well as systemic therapy with interferon-α or cytotoxic chemotherapy. The literature consists primarily of small phase II studies reporting a broad range of response rates with varying definitions for response, varying entry criteria, and generally scant information on median survival, overall survival, or a systematic assessment of function. Active single agents have response rates of 20% to 65% and include vincristine, vinblastine, doxorubicin, bleomycin, interferon-α, etoposide, and paclitaxel (219–226). Combination regimens of doxorubicin, bleomycin, and vincristine, or bleomycin and vincristine have response rates ranging from 50% to 90% (225, 227). Although one small randomized trial of 61 patients comparing doxorubicin to a combination regimen has been studied (221), there have been no large, randomized trials of chemotherapy in KS published to date; two randomized studies of liposomal doxorubicin compared with bleomycin and vincristine or with nonliposomal encapsulated doxorubicin in combination with bleomycin and vincristine are ongoing. The results of one randomized trial of liposomal daunorubicin compared with nonliposomal encapsulated doxorubicin in combination with bleomycin and vincristine were presented to the Oncology Advisory Committee of the U.S. Food and Drug Administration in June 1995. It was on the basis of those results that the Oncology Advisory Committee recommended approval of liposomal daunorubicin.

The choice of treatment should be individualized based on the extent and nature of disease. Lesions frequently occur on the face, or they may be in a location that causes discomfort, in which case local treatment may be the primary objective. Systemic therapy may also be given for disease localized to the skin. The disadvantages of systemic toxicity needs to be offset by control of skin lesions and the potential control of noncutaneous disease. With limited disease, single agents often are effective. Interferon-α appears to be most effective in patients with CD4 counts of more than 200 and without prior opportunistic infections or systemic illness.

Current treatment of symptomatic pulmonary KS is combination cytotoxic chemotherapy, usually consisting of a combination regimen of bleomycin plus vincristine, or adriamycin, bleomycin, and vincristine, or single-agent etoposide. A recent trial of single-agent paclitaxel involving a small number of patients with pulmonary KS showed a significant response rate (226). A reduction in tumor size can be achieved in approximately 50% to 90% of patients, and relief of respiratory symptoms has been reported. Treatment effect on survival, and the value of early treatment of asymptomatic disease, is not known.

A major challenge in KS management and clinical trials is the definition of useful response criteria. The lesions may be difficult to measure because of ill-defined borders or coalescence of lesions. Complete remissions, even in limited stage disease, are rare, making disease free survival an impractical endpoint. Stabilization of disease is difficult to assess objectively. Responses may include flattening of lesions and decrease of lymphedema, both of which are difficult to measure. New lesions may appear even while old lesions are responding to treatment. This fact makes the endpoint of progression free survival difficult to assess. Assessing the value of treatment of extensive visceral disease is difficult because of competing mortality from concomitant illnesses.

Other tests that may be useful for future studies may be the monitoring of laboratory parameters thought to be pathogenetically related to the development of KS, such as fibroblast growth factor, Tat, IL-6, and the new human herpesvirus. In individualizing treatment choices, close attention to antiretroviral care, opportunistic infection prophylaxis, minimization of bone marrow toxicity, and treatment of infectious complications is essential. Intensive investigations are ongoing regarding therapeutic options surrounding the most recent discovery of a new human herpesvirus as the possible infectious etiologic agent of KS. Research into the pathogenesis of KS, and knowledge of the unique epidemiology of the disease, has resulted in a wide range of investigational approaches to KS treatment, including use of the camptothecins, a novel class of chemotherapeutic agents that acts via topoisomerase I inhibition and that possesses both anti-HIV and antitumor activity, tumor necrosis factor–receptor antagonists, and angiogenesis inhibitors (228). Table 50.3 outlines these approaches.

OTHER CANCERS

Since AIDS was first described, virtually every known cancer has been reported in HIV-infected individuals. Given that as many as 1 million Americans have been HIV infected, it would be surprising if it were otherwise. It is difficult to determine which malignancies, besides KS and NHL, have an increased incidence associated with HIV infection. Other immunosuppressive conditions do not increase the risk for all malignancies uniformly. The role of antiviral drugs, many of which are carcinogens in animals, and co-infection with other viruses associated with malignancies, such as Epstein-Barr virus, papilloma virus, and hepatitis B virus, are additional factors that may be important. Two malignancies of particular relevance to the chest physician are Hodgkin's disease and lung cancer.

HODGKIN'S DISEASE

EPIDEMIOLOGY

Hodgkin's disease occurs much less frequently than NHL in the HIV-infected individual. In contrast to NHL, the incidence of Hodgkin's disease has not increased in the general population (229). HIV infection was associated with a 5-fold to 8-fold increased risk for Hodgkin's disease in a cohort study of homosexual men in San Francisco participating in a hepatitis B vaccine study (20). An association of similar magnitude was observed by merging AIDS and cancer registries from 1980 to 1987 in San Francisco (230), although the data sets overlapped between the two studies. In contrast, in New York City and northern New Jersey, areas with

TABLE 50.3. Treatment Options for Patients with Kaposi's Sarcoma

TREATMENT OBJECTIVE	TREATMENT OPTIONS	OUTCOME CONSIDERATIONS

Local control of skin or oral lesions	Surgical excision
	Radiation therapy
	Cryotherapy
	Laser therapy
	Photodynamic therapy
	Intralesional vincristine
	Intralesional interferon-α
		Advantages
		  Cosmetic improvement
		  Local symptom control
		Disadvantages
		  No systemic control
		  Difficult with numerous lesions

Systemic therapy for extensive skin lesions	Immunomodulators
	  Interferon-α
	Cytotoxic agents
	  Doxorubicin
	  Bleomycin
	  Vincristine
	  Vinblastine
	  Etoposide
		Advantages
		  Greater control of extensive disease
		  Treat occult visceral disease
		  Single-agent therapy may be effective for cutaneous disease
		Disadvantages
		  Systemic adverse drug effects
		  Interferon not effective with CD4 count of <200

Systemic therapy for pulmonary or other visceral KS	Combination cytotoxic agents
	  Doxorubicin
	  Bleomycin
	  Vincristine
	  Etoposide
		Advantages
		  Symptom palliation
		  Treats occult visceral disease
		Disadvantages
		  Systemic adverse drug effects

Experimental therapy	Cytotoxic agents
	  Paclitaxel
	  Liposomal formulations
	  Campothecin topoisomerase inhibitors
	TNF inhibitors
	  Thalidomide
	  Pentoxyfilline
	  Soluble TNF-receptor
	Angiogenesis inhibitors
	  TNP-470
	  PDGF inhibitor
	  VEGF inhibitor
	  Platelet factor 4
	  Tissue metalloproteinase inhibitor
	  Protein kinase C inhibitor
	  Suramin
	Hormonal agents
	TAT inhibitor
	Retinoids
	Cytokines
	  IL-2
	  IL-4
	  IL-12
	  IL-6 inhibition
	  IL-10 inhibition
	Antiviral therapy
		Difficulties
		  Limited access to some agents
		  Response difficult to detect with extensive disease
		  Unproven benefit

Abbreviations. TNF, tumor necrosis factor; PDGF, platelet-derived growth factor; VEGF, vascular endothelial growth factor; TAT, transactivator of transcription; IL, interleukin.

high rates of HIV infection among intravenous drug users, cancer registry data found no increase in the incidence of Hodgkin's disease (231). The ratio of AIDS-associated NHL to Hodgkin's disease differs by HIV risk group. Intravenous drug users have AIDS-NHL to Hodgkin's disease ratios of 1.4 to 2:1, compared with ratios of 6 to 16:1 in gay men (232–234). Unpublished data from the MSACMR shows no significantly increased risk for Hodgkin's disease and AIDS compared with the general population.

CLINICAL PRESENTATION

HISTOLOGY

Hodgkin's disease in the HIV-infected patient presents with clinically more aggressive histologic types, including mixed cellularity or lymphocyte depleted. In small series, two thirds of the HIV-infected patients had these histologies, more than double the rate expected (19, 235–237).

CLINICAL PRESENTATION

Compared with Hodgkin's disease in the general population, there is a higher proportion of advanced stages and a higher proportion without mediastinal involvement (19, 235–237). Although disease may involve the chest, (11, 15, 104) parenchymal disease is less common than in NHL. Intrathoracic adenopathy is more likely caused by mycobacterial or fungal infections rather than Hodgkin's disease. Adenopathy can be seen in persistent generalized lymphadenopathy, but this is a diagnosis by exclusion (238, 239).

TREATMENT

Hodgkin's disease, compared with NHL, is uncommon in the HIV population, and published series of patients treated in a standardized manner are scant. Treatment mirrors that given in the immunocompetent setting, and it has commonly included multiagent chemotherapy with a nitrogen mustard, vincristine, procarbazine, prednisone (MOPP) or doxorubicin, bleomycin, vinblastine, dacarbazine (ABVD) regimen. A European study of 92 patients (97) reported a complete response (CR) rate of 65%; opportunistic infections during treatment and follow-up were seen in 38% of patients treated with MOPP/ABVD, compared with a CR rate of 46% and an opportunistic infection rate of 73% in those treated with MOPP alone. Italian investigators performed a prospective clinical trial with an ABVD-like regimen in 17 patients with stage III-IV or I-II disease with adverse prognostic factors. The patients received the epiadriamycin, bleomycin, vinblastine (EBV) combination with AZT. Bone marrow depression was acceptable, and 76% of patients received the AZT doses planned. The CR rate was 53%, with a median survival duration of 10.3 months (240).

In general, patients with Hodgkin's disease and HIV infection have a more aggressive course, with a poorer survival than Hodgkin's disease in the immunocompetent setting. However, patients do have significant CR rates with standard regimens. Once again, close attention to the use of the combination of antitumor treatment with antiretroviral agents, prophylaxis for opportunistic infections, and colony-stimulating factors to attenuate bone marrow toxicity is essential. Monitoring of viral load and immune parameters should be incorporated into the standard care of these patients. Investigational therapy testing new agents and approaches is ongoing, and clinical trials for such patients should be a high priority.

LUNG CANCER

EPIDEMIOLOGY

Lung cancer is the most common cause of cancer mortality in both men and women in the United States, and the lung is the second most common site of cancer incidence in men (after prostate cancer) and women (after breast cancer). Lung cancer in HIV-infected persons has been reported by several investigators (241–257). MSACMR, the most comprehensive population-based evaluation, found rates of lung cancer that are 2 to 6 times greater in HIV-infected individuals than in the general population. Smaller studies with less well-defined populations have estimated the risk to be 2 to 14 times greater (249, 250). As with the general population, smoking would be expected to have a strong etiologic role in lung cancer. In the few published reports of patients with HIV infection and lung cancer for whom a smoking history was available, more than 90% smoked.

CLINICAL PRESENTATION

HISTOLOGY

Adenocarcinoma is the most frequent histologic type of lung cancer in HIV-infected patients. In a review of 66 published cases of lung cancer in HIV-infected individuals for whom histology was described, 35 (53%) had adenocarcinoma, 10 (15%) had squamous cell carcinoma, 2 (3%) had adenosquamous carcinoma, 9 (14%) had small cell carcinoma, and 10 had other cancers, including two mesotheliomas (241). In the general population, squamous cell carcinoma was formerly the most frequent histology in the general population; however, recent trends have shown a decrease in squamous cell cancer and an increase in adenocarcinomas. Currently, in the general population, adenocarcinoma is the most common histologic type in white men, and both squamous and adenocarcinoma histologies are equally common in black men. Adenocarcinoma is the only major histologic type whose incidence is increasing in men. In women, adenocarcinoma has been, and remains, the most common type of lung cancer (229).

CLINICAL PRESENTATION

Patients with lung cancer and HIV infection generally present between the ages of 38 and 47 (254, 257), an age slightly older than the median age for the development of AIDS but 10 to 20 years younger than the median age for lung cancer in the general population (258). HIV-infected patients with lung cancer typically present with advanced stage cancer. In a review of HIV-associated non–small cell lung cancer, 88% of patients presented with stage III or IV disease (241), compared with 52% in the general population (259). However, lung cancer in the general population in patients younger than age 40 also presents with a high incidence of advanced stage disease (260, 261).

Lung cancer in the HIV-infected population presents with symptoms similar to those seen in lung cancer in the general population. Cough, weight loss, night sweats, dyspnea, chest pain, and anorexia are all common presenting symptoms. One unique characteristic is the age at presentation. The chest radiograph may show infiltrates, pulmonary masses, pleural effusions, and mediastinal and hilar adenopathy. These symptoms and signs can be confused with other opportunistic infections and malignancies, including tuberculosis, histoplasmosis, PCP, NHL, and pulmonary KS. The CD4 count may help in the differential diagnosis. Patients with CD4 counts between 200 and 100 are more likely to have PCP or non-Hodgkin's lymphoma, whereas tuberculosis or histoplasmosis can occur at any CD4 count. Pulmonary KS generally occurs in men with cutaneous disease. Diagnosis usually is obtained by sputum induction or bronchoscopic evaluation with biopsy, cytology, and cultures. Table 50.4 shows the differential diagnoses to consider in evaluating pulmonary abnormalities in the HIV-infected patient.

TREATMENT

The published series of treatment of HIV-infected patients with lung cancer is small (254, 257). Most of the patients had advanced lung cancer for which treatment was palliative. The treatments were standard therapies, including resection for early-stage non–small cell lung cancer, thoracic radiation therapy for locally advanced disease, and palliation for metastatic disease and respiratory symptoms. Small cell lung cancer was treated with multiagent chemotherapy. Increased susceptibility to infection from low CD4 counts and neutropenia complicating other HIV therapies such as AZT or ganciclovir may limit the treatment of lung cancer. Treatment of lung cancer should be integrated with HIV treatment, including the use of antiretroviral agents, prophylaxis for opportunistic infection, and the use of colony-stimulating factors to attenuate bone marrow depression.

HIV TRANSMISSION IN THE HEALTH CARE SETTING

Thoracic oncologists and surgeons confront HIV infection not only in clinical care, but also as an occupational hazard. Although the risk is not known exactly, transmission of HIV infection has been documented clearly. As of March 1993, 214,686 persons with AIDS had been reported to the CDC; of these 10,122 (4.7%) were health care workers, slightly less than the 5.7% of the total population of health care workers (262). Of health care workers with AIDS, 94% had documented nonoccupational risk factors, but it is unclear how many of the remaining 607 persons with AIDS acquired HIV infection through occupational exposures (263).

A more specific, but probably incomplete, documentation of HIV transmission can be found in the CDC Health Care Worker Seroconverter Registry (264). By June 1993, 115 definite and probable seroconversions were reported to this passive surveillance system. Mass screening of health care workers in locales with elevated AIDS incidence provides another reasonable measure of risk of occupationally acquired infection. In a 1992 study of 770 such surgeons, one occupationally acquired infection was discovered (265). A similar study of 3420 orthopedic physicians did not find any occupationally related infections (266). These findings were corroborated in studies of Army Reserve surgeons (267), hemodialysis workers (268–272), and dentists and dental hygienists (264, 273–277). Because persons tested in all such seroprevalence surveys were required to give informed consent, little can be said about the status of nonparticipants; it is reasonable to expect that HIV-infected health care workers might be more likely to exclude themselves from such studies.

The risk of infection among health care workers with extensive exposures to infective material is small but not negligible. Transmission from patient to health care worker is determined by: (a) the frequency of clinical encounters with infected patients; (b) the frequency with which potentially transmissible events occurs; and (c) the efficacy with which such events transmit infection.

In the past decade, the frequency of clinical encounters with HIV-infected patients has expanded with the expansion of the epidemic. At the time of exposure, the HIV status of seropositive patients often is not known by the practitioner (278, 279). All of the estimated 800,000 to 1.2 million persons infected with HIV in the United States (1) need health care. Estimates of HIV seroprevalence vary widely; an estimated 0.2% to 14.2% of hospitalized patients (278) and 0.2% to 8.9% of emergency room patients are HIV infected (279). This finding strongly argues for diligent use of universal precautions (280).

The AIDS era has led to better studies of mucocu-

TABLE 50.4. Differential Diagnosis of Pulmonary Abnormalities in the HIV-Infected Patient

Condition	Clinical Symptoms	Radiographic Findings	Likelihood of Presentation in Lung	HIV Risk Group	CD4 Count
Infections					
Community- or hospital-acquired pneumonia	Fever, cough (may be productive), SOB, chest tightness	Lobar or diffuse infiltrates	Common	All	All counts
Mycobacterium TB	Fever, night sweats, weight loss, cough, SOB, chest tightness	Unilateral or bilateral lower lobe or diffuse pulmonary infiltrates or hilar, paratracheal, mediastinal adenopathy	Common	All	All counts
Fungal	Fever, cough, may have SOB	Diffuse or patchy reticulonodular infiltrates	Infrequent, but when present is disseminated	All	All counts
Pneumocystis carinii pneumonia	Fever, dry cough, SOB, chest tightness	Range from normal to bilateral interstitial or alveolar infiltrates, upper lobe infiltrates, nodules, cavities	Common	All	Usually <200
Toxoplasma gondii	Fever, cough, SOB	Pneumonia	Infrequent	All	Usually <100
Mycobacterium avium–intracellulare	Fever, night sweats, weight loss, cough, SOB	Pneumonia	Infrequent, usually disseminated	All	Usually <100
Cytomegalovirus	Fever, cough, SOB	Pneumonia or pneumonitis	Common	All	Usually <100
Neoplasms					
Kaposi's sarcoma	Fever rare, cough, SOB, chest tightness	Diffuse infiltrates, pleural effusion (serosanguinous exudate), adenopathy	Occasional	Predominantly homosexual or bisexual men	All counts, but visceral involvement such as the lungs usually occurs later in immune dysfunction, usually <200
Malignant lymphoma	Fever, night sweats, weight loss, cough, SOB, chest tightness	Adenopathy, interstitial infiltrates, pleural effusion	Occasional	All	All counts, but usually <200
Other cancers	Cough, SOB, chest tightness	Mass lesion, adenopathy, effusion	Lung cancer common	All	All counts

taneous and percutaneous exposure of health care workers to their patients. Tokars et al. (281) directly observed 1382 operations performed in a region with a high AIDS incidence. Percutaneous injury was documented in 6.9% of these operations. Prospective studies of physicians have shown the rate of percutaneous exposure to be 1.8 per year per physician (282). Percutaneous injuries occur before or during use of an instrument 18% of the time, after use and before disposal of an instrument 70% of the time, and after disposal 13% of the time. Although new devices that purport to decrease the chance of these events are now marketed aggressively, there are little data and mixed results to support their claims. For example, in one multicenter trial in New York state (283), one protectively sheathed intravenous fluid delivery needle decreased percutaneous exposures in some hospitals but increased them in another. Lack of familiarity with the operation of the product was cited as a probable explanation.

In the 1980s, quantification of the efficacy of HIV transmission during occupational exposure absorbed much of the epidemiologic resources allocated to studying transmission in the health care setting. It has been estimated that a single percutaneous exposure has a 0.3% risk of infection (284, 285) and a mucocutaneous exposure, a 0.09% risk (284).

Another cause for concern is the potential transmission from the health care worker to the patient. At this writing, only a single, much publicized case has been well documented: a Florida dentist apparently infected at least five patients in the course of rendering care (286). Virus isolates from all patients were homologous by DNA characterization, and other sources of infection were ruled out. This event prompted a long series of look-back serosurveys of the patients of health care workers known to be HIV infected (287–296). Testing of 22,032 patients treated by 63 health care workers has been reported; 112 were found to be seropositive and, of these, 106 had well-established HIV risk factors and the remaining six patients were lost to follow-up.

In summary, given the increasing number of encounters with HIV-infected patients, the frequent occurrence of events in which health care workers are exposed to infected blood and each exposure's small but important risk of infection, there is strong epidemiologic evidence that this issue demands neither panic nor dismissal, but rather a serious consideration of established guidelines (279) to decrease exposure.

References

1. U.S. Centers for Disease Control and Prevention. Estimates of HIV prevalence and projected AIDS cases: summary of a workshop, October 31–November 1, 1989. MMWR Morb Mortal Wkly Rep 1990;39:110–119.
2. U.S. Centers for Disease Control and Prevention. Kaposi's sarcoma and Pneumocystis pneumonia among homosexual men—New York City and California. MMWR Morb Mortal Wkly Rep 1981;30:305–308.
3. U.S. Centers for Disease Control and Prevention. Diffuse, undifferentiated non-Hodgkin's lymphoma among homosexual males, United States. MMWR Morb Mortal Wkly Rep 1982;31:277–285.
4. Ziegler JL, Beckstead JA, Volberding PA, et al. Non-Hodgkin's lymphoma in 90 homosexual men: relation to generalized lymphadenopathy and the acquired immunodeficiency syndrome. N Engl J Med 1984;311:565–570.
5. Penn I. Cancer in the immunosuppressed organ recipient. Transplant Proc 1991;23:1771–1772.
6. Penn I. The effect of immunosuppression on pre-existing cancers. Transplantation 1993;55:742–747.
7. Opelz G, Henderson R. Incidence of non-Hodgkin lymphoma in kidney and heart transplant recipients. Lancet 1993;342:1514–1516.
8. Suthanthiran M, Strom TB. Renal transplantation. N Engl J Med 1994;331:365–376.
9. Murray JF, Felton CP, Garay SM. Pulmonary complications of the acquired immunodeficiency syndrome. N Engl J Med 1984;310:1682–1688.
10. Weinberger SR. Recent advances in pulmonary medicine. N Engl J Med 1993;328:1462–1470.
11. Robert NJ, Schneidermann H. Hodgkin's disease and the acquired immunodeficiency syndrome. Ann Intern Med 1984;101:142–143.
12. Ioachim HL, Cooper MC, Hellman GC. Hodgkin's disease and the acquired immunodeficiency syndrome (letter). Ann Intern Med 1984;101:876–877.
13. Scheib RG, Siegel RS. Atypical Hodgkin's disease and the acquired immunodeficiency syndrome. Ann Intern Med 1985;102:554.
14. Temple JJ, Andes AW. AIDS and Hodgkin's disease. Lancet 1986;2:454–455.
15. Prior E, Goldberg AF, Conjalka MS, Chapman WE, Tay S, Ames ED. Hodgkin's disease in homosexual men. An AIDS-related phenomenon? Am J Med 1986;81:1085–1088.
16. Gongora-Biachi RA, Gonzales-Martinez P, Bastarrachea-Ortiz J. Hodgkin's disease as the initial manifestation of acquired immunodeficiency syndrome (letter). Ann Intern Med 1987;107:112.
17. Tirelli U, Vaccher E, Rezza G, et al. Hodgkin's disease and infection with the human immunodeficiency virus (HIV) in Italy. Ann Intern Med 1988;108:309–310.
18. Lichtman SM, Brody J, Kaplan MH, Susin M, Koduru P, Goh JC. Hodgkin's disease and non-Hodgkin's lymphoma in an HIV positive patient. Leuk Lymphoma 1993;9:393–398.
19. Tirelli U, Errante D, Vaccher E, et al. Hodgkin's disease in 92 patients with HIV infection: the Italian experience. Ann Oncol 1992;3(Suppl 4):S69–S73.
20. Hessol NA, Katz MH, Liu JY, Buchbinder SP, Rubino CJ, Holmberg SD. Increased incidence of Hodgkin's disease in HIV-infected homosexual men. Ann Intern Med 1992;117:309–311.
21. Andrieu JM, Roithmann S, Tourani JM, et al. Hodgkin's disease during HIV1 infection: the French registry experience. Ann Oncol 1993;4:635–641.
22. Weinshel EL, Peterson BA. Hodgkin's disease. CA Cancer J Clin 1993;43:327–346.
23. Rubio R. Hodgkin's disease associated with human immunodeficiency virus infection. A clinical study of 46 cases. Cancer 1994;73:2400–2407.
24. Alfonso PG, Sanudo EF, Carretero JM, et al. Hodgkin's disease in HIV-infected patients. Biomed Pharmacother 1988;42:321–325.
25. Tenholder MF, Jackson HD. Bronchogenic carcinoma in patients seropositive for human immunodeficiency virus. Chest 1993;104:1049–1053.
26. Chan TK, Aranda CP, Rom WN. Bronchogenic carcinoma in young patients at risk for acquired immunodeficiency syndrome. Chest 1993;103:862–864.
27. Devesa SS, Fears T. Non-Hodgkin's lymphoma time trends: United States and international data. Cancer Res 1992;52(Suppl 19):5432–5440.
28. Coté TR, Howe HL, Anderson SP, Martin RJ, Evans B, Francis BJ. A systematic consideration of the neoplastic spectrum of AIDS: registry linkage in Illinois. AIDS 1991;5:49–53.

29. Ross R, Dworsky R, Paganini-Hill A, Levine AM, Mack T. Non-Hodgkin's lymphomas in never married men in Los Angeles. Br J Cancer 1985;52:785–787.
30. U.S. Centers for Disease Control and Prevention. Revision of the case definition of acquired immunodeficiency syndrome for national reporting—United States. Ann Intern Med 1985;103:402–403.
31. Levine AM, Gill PS, Meyer PR, et al. Retrovirus and malignant lymphoma in homosexual men. JAMA 1985;254:1921–1925.
32. Ioachim HL, Dorsett B, Cronin W, Maya M, Wahl S. Acquired immunodeficiency syndrome associated lymphomas: clinical, pathological, immunologic and viral characteristics of 111 cases. Hum Pathol 1991;22:659–673.
33. Levine AM, Burkes RL, Walker M, et al. Development of B cell lymphoma in two monogamous homosexual men. Arch Intern Med 1985;145:479–481.
34. Levine AM. Cancer in AIDS. Curr Opin Oncol 1992;4:863–866.
35. Kristal AR, Nasca PC, Burnett WS, Mikl J. Changes in the epidemiology of non-Hodgkin's lymphoma associated with epidemic human immunodeficiency virus (HIV) infection. Am J Epidemiol 1988;128:711–718.
36. Harnly ME, Swan SH, Holly EA, Kelter A, Padian N. Temporal trends in the incidence of non-Hodgkin's lymphoma and selected malignancies in a population with a high incidence of acquired immunodeficiency syndrome. Am J Epidemiol 1988;128:261–267.
37. Biggar RJ, Horm J, Goedert JJ, Melbye M. Cancer in a group at risk of acquired immunodeficiency syndrome (AIDS) through 1984. Am J Epidemiol 1987;126:578–586.
38. Ragni MV, Belle SH, Jaffe RA, et al. Acquired immunodeficiency syndrome-associated non-Hodgkin's lymphomas and other malignancies in patients with hemophilia. Blood 1993;81:1889–1897.
39. Rabkin CS, Hilgartner MW, Hedberg KW, et al. Incidence of lymphomas and other cancers in HIV-infected and HIV-uninfected patients with hemophilia. JAMA 1992;267:1090–1094.
40. Biggar RJ, Rabkin CS. The epidemiology of acquired immunodeficiency syndrome–related lymphomas. Curr Opin Oncol 1992;4:883–893.
41. Beral V, Peterman T, Berkelman R, Jaffe H. AIDS-associated non-Hodgkin lymphoma. Lancet 1991;337:805–809.
42. Beral V, Peterman TA, Berkelman RL, Jaffe HW. Kaposi's sarcoma among persons with AIDS: a sexually transmitted infection? Lancet 1990;335:123–128.
43. Levy RM, Bredesen DE, Rosenblum ML. Neurological manifestations of the acquired immunodeficiency syndrome (AIDS): experience of UCSF and review of the literature. J Neurosurg 1985;62:475–495.
44. Moore RD, Kessler H, Richman DD, Flexner C, Chaisson RE. Non-Hodgkin's lymphoma in patients with advanced HIV infection treated with zidovudine. JAMA 1991;265:2208–2211.
45. Deleted in proof.
46. Jones EH, Biggar RJ, Nkrumah FK, Lawler SD. HLA-DR7 association with African Burkitt's lymphoma. Hum Immunol 1985;13:211–217.
47. Pluda JM, Venzon D, Tosato G, et al. Parameters affecting the development of non-Hodgkin's lymphoma in patients with severe human immunodeficiency virus infection receiving antiretroviral therapy. J Clin Oncol 1993;11:1099–1107.
48. Deleted in proof.
49. Cote T, Biggar R. Does zidovudine cause non-Hodgkin's lymphoma? AIDS 1995;9:404–405.
50. Shibata D, Brynes RK, Nathwani B, Kwok S, Shinsky J, Arnheim N. Human immunodeficiency viral DNA is readily found in lymph node biopsies from seropositive individuals. Am J Pathol 1989;135:697–702.
51. Pelicci PG, Knowles DM II, Arlin ZA, et al. Multiple monoclonal B cell expansions and c-myc oncogene rearrangements in acquired immune deficiency syndrome–related lymphoproliferative disorders: implications for lymphomagenesis. J Exp Med 1986;164:2049–2060.
52. Groopman JE, Sullivan JL, Mulder C, et al. Pathogenesis of B cell lymphoma in a patient with AIDS. Blood 1986;67:612–615.
53. Rechavi G, Ben-Bassat I, Berkowicz M, et al. Molecular analysis of Burkitt's leukemia in two hemophilic brothers with AIDS. Blood 1987;70:1713–1717.
54. Levine AM, Meyer PR, Begandy MK, et al. Development of B-cell lymphoma in homosexual men. Ann Intern Med 1984;100:7–13.
55. Gaidano G, Dalla-Favera R. Biologic aspects of human immunodeficiency virus–related lymphoma. Curr Opin Oncol 1992;4:900–906.
56. Kawano M, Hirano T, Matsuda T, et al. Autocrine generation and requirement of BSF-2/IL-6 for human multiple myelomas. Nature 1988;332:83–85.
57. Yee C, Biondi A, Wang XH, et al. A possible autocrine role of IL-6 in two lymphoma cell lines. Blood 1989;74:789–804.
58. Biondi A, Rossi V, Bassan R, et al. Constitutive expression of IL-6 gene in chronic lymphocytic leukemia. Blood 1989;73:1279–1284.
59. Yoshizaki K, Matsuda T, Nishimoto N, et al. Pathogenic significance of IL-6 (IL-6/BSF-2) in Castleman's disease. Blood 1989;74:1360–1367.
60. Nakajima K, Martinez-Maza O, Hirano T, et al. Induction of IL-6 (B cell stimulatory factor-2/IFN-beta-2) production by human immunodeficiency virus. J Immunol 1989;142:531.
61. Benjamin D, Knobloch TJ, Abrams J, Dayton MA. Human B cell IL-10. B cell lines derived from patients with AIDS and Burkitt's lymphoma constitutively secrete large quantities of IL-10 (abstract). Blood 1991;78:384a.
62. Baiocchi RA, Caligiuri MA. Low-dose interleukin 2 prevents the development of Epstein-Barr virus-associated lymphoproliferative disease in scid/scid mice reconstituted i.p. with EBV seropositive human peripheral blood lymphocytes. Proc Natl Acad Sci U S A 1994;91:5577–5581.
63. Manetti R, Paronchi P, Giudizi G, et al. Natural killer cell stimulatory factor (interleukin 12 [IL-12]) induces T helper type 1 (Th1)–specific immune responses and inhibits the development of IL-4 producing Th2 cells. J Exp Med 1993;177:1199.
64. Shiramizu B, Barriga F, Neequaye J, et al. Patterns of chromosomal breakpoint locations in Burkitt's lymphoma: relevance to geography and Epstein-Barr virus association. Blood 1991;77:1516.
65. Pelicci PG, Knowles DM II, Magrath I, Dalla-Favera R. Chromosomal breakpoints and structural alterations of the c-myc locus differ in endemic and sporadic forms of Burkitt lymphoma. Proc Natl Acad Sci U S A 1986;83:2984.
66. Subar M, Neri A, Inghirami G, Knowles DM, Dalla-Favera R. Frequent c-myc oncogene activation and infrequent presence of Epstein-Barr virus genome in AIDS-associated lymphoma. Blood 1988;72:667.
67. Meeker TC, Shiramizu B, Kaplan L, et al. Evidence for molecular subtypes of HIV-associated lymphoma: division into peripheral monoclonal, polyclonal and central nervous system lymphoma. AIDS 1991;5:669–674.
68. Haluska FG, Russo G, Kant J, Andreef M, Croce CM. Molecular resemblance of an AIDS-associated lymphoma and endemic

Burkitt lymphomas: implications for their pathogenesis. Proc Natl Acad Sci U S A 1989;86:8907.
69. Lindahl T, Klein G, Reedman BM, Johansson B, Singh S. Relationship between Epstein-Barr virus DNA and the EBV determined nuclear antigen (EBNA) in Burkitt lymphoma biopsies and other lymphoproliferative malignancies. Int J Cancer 1974;13:764.
70. MacMahon EME, Glass JD, Hayward SD, et al. Epstein-Barr virus in AIDS-related primary central nervous system lymphoma. Lancet 1991;338:969–973.
71. Levine AM, Shibata D, Sullivan-Halley J, et al. Case control study of HIV-positive and HIV-negative lymphoma in Los Angeles County. Proc Am Soc Clin Oncol 1992;11:333.
72. Hamilton-Dutoit SJ, Pallesen G, Franzmann MB, et al. AIDS-related lymphoma: histopathology, immunophenotype, and association with EBV as demonstrated by in situ nucleic acid hybridization. Am J Pathol 1991;138:149.
73. Pedersen C, Gerstoft J, Lundgren JD, et al. HIV-associated lymphoma-histopathology and association with Epstein-Barr virus genome related to clinical, immunological and prognostic features. Eur J Cancer 1991;27:1416–1423.
74. Ballerini P, Gaidano G, Inghirami G, et al. Multiple genetic alterations in AIDS-associated lymphomas. Blood 1991;78(Suppl 1):327a.
75. Janier M, Katlama C, Flageul B, et al. The pseudo-Sézary syndrome with CD8 phenotype in a patient with the acquired immunodeficiency syndrome (AIDS). Ann Intern Med 1989;11:738.
76. Goldstein J, Becker N, Del Rowe J, Davis L. Cutaneous T cell lymphoma in a patient infected with HIV, type 1. Cancer 1990;66:1130.
77. Crane GA, Variakohis D, Rosen ST, Sands AM, Roenigk HH. Cutaneous T cell lymphoma in patients with human immunodeficiency virus infection. Arch Dermatol 1991;127:989.
78. Ruff P, Bagg A, Papadopoulos K. Precursor T cell lymphoma associated with human immunodeficiency virus (HIV) type 1: first reported case. Cancer 1989;64:39.
79. Ciobanu N, Andreef M, Safai B, Koziner B, Mertelsmann R. Lymphoblastic neoplasia in a homosexual patient with Kaposi's sarcoma. Ann Intern Med 1983;98:151–155.
80. Presant CA, Gala K, Wiseman C, et al. Human immunodeficiency virus associated T cell lymphoblastic lymphoma in AIDS. Cancer 1987;60:1459.
81. Sternlieb J, Mintzer D, Dwa D, Gluckman S. Peripheral T cell lymphoma in a patient with the acquired immunodeficiency syndrome. Am J Med 1988;85:445.
82. Gonzalez-Clemente JM, Ribera JM, Campo E, Bosch X, Montserrat E, Grau JM. Ki-1 positive anaplastic large cell lymphoma of T cell origin in an HIV-infected patient. AIDS 1991;5:751.
83. Shibata D, Brynes R, Rabinowitz A, Slovak ML, Spira TJ, Gill P. HTLV-I associated adult T cell leukemia lymphoma in a patient infected with HIV-1. Ann Intern Med 1989;111:871.
84. Baurmann H, Miclea JM, Ferchal G, et al. Adult T cell leukemia associated with HTLV-I and simultaneous infection by HIV type 2 and human herpesvirus 6 in an African woman: a clinical, virologic, and familial serologic study. Am J Med 1988;85:853.
85. Shiramizu B, Herndier BG, McGrath MS. Identification of a common clonal human immunodeficiency virus integration site in human immunodeficiency virus–associated lymphomas. Cancer Research 1994;54:2069–2072.
86. Tirelli U, Carbone A. Malignant tumors in patients with HIV infection. BMJ 1994;308:1148–1153.
87. Rabkin CS, Biggar RJ, Horm JW. Increasing incidence of cancer associated with the human immunodeficiency virus epidemic. Int J Cancer 1991;47:692–696.
88. Eby NL, Grufferman S, Flannelly CM, et al. Increasing incidence of primary brain lymphoma in the US. Cancer 1988;62:2461–2465.
89. Anonymous. Non-Hodgkin's Lymphoma Pathologic Classification Project. National Cancer Institute sponsored study of classifications of non-Hodgkin's lymphomas: summary and description of a working formulation for clinical usage. Cancer 1982;49:2112.
90. Lukes RJ, Parker JW, Taylor CR, Tindle BH, Cramer AD, Lincoln TL. Immunologic approach to non-Hodgkin's lymphomas and related leukemias. Analysis of the results of multiparameter studies of 425 cases. Semin Hematol 1978;15:322.
91. Kaplan LD, Abrams DI, Feigal E, et al. AIDS-associated non-Hodgkin's lymphoma in San Francisco. JAMA 1989;261:719.
92. Knowles DM, Chamulak GA, Subar M, et al. Lymphoid neoplasia associated with the acquired immunodeficiency syndrome (AIDS): the New York University experience. Ann Intern Med 1988;108:744.
93. Lowenthal DA, Straus DJ, Campbell SW, Gold JWM, Clarkson BD, Koziner B. AIDS-related lymphoid neoplasia: the Memorial Hospital experience. Cancer 1988;61:2325.
94. Levine AM. Epidemiology, clinical characteristics and management of AIDS-related lymphoma. Hematol Oncol Clin North Am 1991;5:331–342.
95. Pluda J, Broder S, Yarchoan R. Therapy of AIDS and AIDS-associated neoplasms. In: La Pinedo HM, Longo DL, Chabner BA, eds. Cancer chemotherapy and biological response modifiers annual. Amsterdam: Elsevier, 1992;13:395–439.
96. Northfelt D, Kaplan LD. Clinical aspect of AIDS-related non-Hodgkin's lymphoma. Curr Opin Oncol 1991;3:872–880.
97. Monfardini S, Tirelli U, Vaccher E. Treatment of acquired immunodeficiency syndrome–related cancer. Cancer Treat Rev 1994;20:149–172.
98. Levine AM. Reactive and neoplastic lymphoproliferative disorders and other miscellaneous cancers associated with HIV infection. In: DeVita VT Jr, Hellman S, Rosenberg SA, eds. AIDS: etiology, diagnosis, treatment and prevention. 2nd ed. Philadelphia: JB Lippincott, 1989:263.
99. Levine AM, Taylor CR, Schneider DR, et al. Immunoblastic sarcoma of T cell versus B cell origin. I. Clinical features. Blood 1981;58:52.
100. Levine AM, Pavlova Z, Pockros AW, et al. Small noncleaved follicular center cell (FCC) lymphoma: Burkitt and non-Burkitt variants in the United States. I. Clinical features. Cancer 1983;52:1073.
101. Haddy TB, Adde MA, Magrath IT. CNS involvement in small non-cleaved lymphoma: is CNS disease per se a poor prognostic sign? J Clin Oncol 1991;9:1973.
102. Miliauskas JR, Berard CW, Young RC, Garvin AJ, Edwards BK, DeVita VT. Undifferentiated non-Hodgkin's lymphomas (Burkitt's and non-Burkitt's types): the relevance of making this histologic distinction. Cancer 1982;50:2115.
103. Magrath IT, Lwanga S, Carswell W, Harrison N. Surgical reduction of tumor bulk in management of abdominal Burkitt's lymphoma. BMJ 1974;2:308.
104. Weissler JC, Mootz AR. Southwestern Internal Medicine Conference: Pulmonary Disease in AIDS Patients. Am J Med Sci 1990;300:300–343.
105. Raphael J, Gentihomme O, Tulliez M, Byron PA, Diebold J. Histopathologic features of high grade non-Hodgkin's lymphomas in acquired immunodeficiency syndrome. Arch Pathol Lab Med 1991;115:15.

106. Levine AM, Sullivan-Halley J, Pike MC, et al. Human immunodeficiency virus related lymphoma: prognostic factors predictive of survival. Cancer 1991;68:2466–2472.
107. Kalter S, Riggs S, Cabanilla F. Aggressive non-Hodgkin's lymphomas in immunodeficiency syndrome (AIDS): review of cases. South Med J 1986;79:1070–1075.
108. Marchevsky A, Rosen M, Chrystal G, Kleinerman J. Pulmonary complications of the acquired immunodeficiency syndrome: a clinicopathologic study of 70 cases. Hum Pathol 1985;16:659–670.
109. Sider L, Horton E. Pleural effusion as a presentation of AIDS-related lymphoma. Invest Radiol 1989;24:150–153.
110. Levine AM, Wernz JC, Kaplan L, et al. Low dose chemotherapy with central nervous system prophylaxis and zidovudine maintenance in AIDS-related lymphoma. JAMA 1991;266:84–88.
111. Dugan M, Subar M, Odajnyk C, et al. Intensive multiagent chemotherapy for AIDS related diffuse large cell lymphoma (abstract). Blood 1986;68:124a.
112. Odajnyk C, Subar M, Dugan M, et al. Clinical features and correlates with immunopathology and molecular biology of a large group of patients with AIDS associated small non–cleaved lymphoma (SNCL) (abstract). Blood 1986;68:131a.
113. Gill PS, Levine AM, Krailo M, et al. AIDS-related malignant lymphoma: results of prospective treatment trials. J Clin Oncol 1987;5:1322.
114. Gisselbrecht C, Tirelli U, Oksenhendler E, et al. GELA-GICAT Cooperative INSERM-CNR Study: non-Hodgkin's lymphoma associated with human immunodeficiency virus: intensive treatment by LNH 84 regimen. Fifth International Conference on AIDS, San Francisco, CA, 1990:1324.
115. Sawka C, Shepherd F. Treatment of AIDS related lymphoma with a 12 week chemotherapy program. Proc Am Soc Clin Oncol 1991;10:32.
116. Kaplan LD, Kahn JO, Crowe S, et al. Clinical and virologic effects of recombinant human granulocyte-macrophage colony–stimulating factor in patients receiving chemotherapy for human immunodeficiency virus-associated non-Hodgkin's lymphoma: results of a randomized trial. J Clin Oncol 1991;9:929.
117. Sparano JA, Wiernik PH, Strack M, et al. Infusional cyclophosphamide, doxorubicin, and etoposide in human immunodeficiency virus and human T-cell leukemia virus type I-related non-Hodgkin's lymphoma; a highly active regimen. Blood 1993;81:2810–2815.
118. Kaplan L, Straus D, Testa M, Levine AM. Randomized trial of standard dose mBACOD with GM-CSF vs. reduced dose mBACOD for systemic HIV-associated lymphoma. ACTG 142. Proc Am Soc Clin Oncol 1995;14:288.
119. Shipp MA, Harrington DP, Klatt MM, et al. Identification of major prognostic subgroups with large cell lymphoma treated with m-BACOD or M-BACOD. Ann Intern Med 1986;104:757.
120. Hoskins PJ, Ng V, Spinelli JJ, Klimo P, Connors JM. Prognostic variables in patients with diffuse large cell lymphoma treated with MACOP-B. J Clin Oncol 1991;9:220.
121. Hymes K, Cheung T, Green JB, et al. Kaposi's sarcoma in homosexual men. Lancet 1981;2:598–600.
122. Oettle AG. Geographic and racial differences in the frequency of Kaposi's sarcoma as evidence of environmental or genetic causes. Acta Union Internationale Contra Cancrum 1962;18:330–363.
123. Penn I. Kaposi's sarcoma in organ transplant recipients: report of 20 cases. Transplantation 1979;27:8–11.
124. Penn I. the changing pattern of posttransplant malignancies. Transplant Proc 1991;23:1101–1103.
125. Klein MB, Pereira FA, Kantor I. Kaposi's sarcoma complicating systemic lupus erythematosus treated with immunosuppression. Arch Dermatol 1974;110:602.
126. Leung F, Fam AG, Osoba D. Kaposi's sarcoma complicating corticosteroid therapy for temporal arteritis. Am J Med 1981;71:320–322.
127. Frances C, Farge D, Boisnic S. Syndrome de Kaposi des transplantes. J Mal Vasc 1991;16:163–165.
128. Beral V, Jaffe H, Weiss R. Cancer surveys: cancer, HIV, and AIDS. Eur J Cancer 1991;27:1057–1058.
129. Serraino D, Franceschi S, Tirelli U, Monfardini S. The epidemiology of acquired immunodeficiency syndrome and associated tumours in Europe. Ann Oncol 1992;3:595–603.
130. Mann DL, Murray C, O'Donnell M, Blattner WA, Goedert JJ. HLA antigen frequencies in HIV-1 related Kaposi's sarcoma. J Acquir Immune Defic Syndr 1990;3(Suppl 1):51–55.
131. Brunson ME, Balakrishnan K, Penn I. HLA and Kaposi's sarcoma in solid organ transplantation. Hum Immunol 1990;29:56–63.
132. Jaffe HW, Choi K, Thomas PA, et al. National case-control study of Kaposi's sarcoma and Pneumocystis carinii pneumonia in homosexual men: part 1. Epidemiologic results. Ann Intern Med 1983;99:145–151.
133. Beral V, Bull D, Durby S, et al. Risk of Kaposi's sarcoma and sexual practices associated with faecal contact in homosexual or bisexual men with AIDS. Lancet 1992;335:632–635.
134. Biggar RJ. Cancer in acquired immunodeficiency syndrome: an epidemiological assessment. Semin Oncol 1990;17:251–260.
135. Lassoued K, Clauvel JP, Fegueux S, Matheron S, Gorin I, Oksenhendler E. AIDS-associated Kaposi's sarcoma in female patients. AIDS 1991;5:877–880.
136. Benedetti P, Greco D, Figoli F, Tirelli U. Epidemic Kaposi's sarcoma in female AIDS patients—a report of 23 Italian cases (letter). AIDS 1991;5:466–467.
137. Beral V. Epidemiology of Kaposi's sarcoma. In: Beral V, Jaffe HW, Weiss RA, eds. Cancer, HIV, and AIDS. New York: Cold Spring Harbor Laboratory, 1991:5–22.
138. Afrasiabi R, Mitsuyasu R, Nashanian P. Characterization of a distinct subgroup of high risk persons with Kaposi's sarcoma and good prognosis who present with normal T4 cell number and T4:T8 ratio and negative HTLV-III/LAV serologic test results. Am J Med 1986;81:969–973.
139. Friedman-Kien AE, Saltzman BR, Cao YZ, et al. Kaposi's sarcoma in HIV-negative homosexual men (letter). Lancet 1990;335:168–169.
140. Garcia Muret MP, Pujol RM, Puig L, Moreno A, De Moragas JM. Disseminated Kaposi's sarcoma not associated with HIV infection in a bisexual man. J Am Acad Dermatol 1990;23:1035–1038.
141. Haverkos HW. The search for cofactors in AIDS, including an analysis of the association of nitrite inhalant abuse and Kaposi's sarcoma. Prog Clin Biol Res 1990;325:93–102.
142. Darrow WW, Peterman TA, Jaffe HW, Rogers MF, Curran JW, Beral V. Kaposi's sarcoma and exposure to faeces. Lancet 1992;339:685.
143. Biggar RJ, Curtis RE, Coté TR, Rabkin CS, Melbye M. Risk of other cancer following Kaposi's sarcoma: relation to acquired immunodeficiency syndrome. Am J Epidemiol 1994;139:3628.
144. Anderson CB, Karkov J, Bjerregaard B, Visfeldt J. Cytomegalovirus infection in classic, endemic and epidemic Kaposi's sarcoma analyzed by in situ hybridization. Acta Pathol Microbiol Immunol Scand 1991;99:893–897.

145. Hashimoto H, Muller H, Muller F, Schmidts HL, Stutte HJ. In situ hybridization analysis of cytomegalovirus lytic infection in Kaposi's sarcoma associated with AIDS: a study of 14 autopsy cases. Virchows Arch A Pathol Anat Histopathol 1987;411: 441–448.
146. Reynolds P, Layefsky ME, Saunders LD, Lemp GF, Payne SF. Kaposi's sarcoma reporting in San Francisco: a comparison of AIDS and cancer surveillance systems. J Acquir Immune Defic Syndr 1990;1(Suppl 3):S8–S13.
147. Chang Y, Li JJ, Rush MG, et al. HPV-16–related DNA sequences in Kaposi's sarcoma. Lancet 1992;339:515–518.
148. Nickoloff BJ, Chang Y, Li JJ, Friedman-Kien AE. Immunohistochemical detection of papillomavirus antigens in Kaposi's sarcoma (letter, comment). Lancet 1992;339:548–549.
149. Chang Y, Cesarman E, Pessin MS, et al. Identification of herpesvirus-like DNA sequences in AIDS-associated Kaposi's sarcoma. Science 1994;266:1865–1869.
150. Huang YQ, Li JJ, Kaplan MH, et al. Human herpesvirus-like nucleic acid in various forms of Kaposi's sarcoma. Lancet 1995;345:759–761.
151. Rosenberg ZF, Fauci AS. The immunopathogenesis of HIV infection. Adv Immunol 1989;47:377–432.
152. Rosenberg ZF, Fauci AS. Immunopathogenesis of HIV infection. FASEB J 1991;5:2382–2390.
153. Nakamura S, Salahuddin SZ, Biberfeld P, et al. Kaposi's sarcoma cells: long-term culture with growth factor from retrovirus-infected CD4+ T cells. Science 1988;242:426–430.
154. Salahuddin SZ, Nakamura S, Biberfeld P, et al. Angiogenic properties of Kaposi's sarcoma–derived cells after long-term culture in vitro. Science 1988;242:430–433.
155. Albini A, Nakamura S, Poggi L, Gallo RC, Salahuddin SZ, Thompson EW. Cultured AIDS-related Kaposi's sarcoma cells (AIDS-KS) produce activators of endothelial cell chemotaxis and invasiveness. International Conference on AIDS, Florence, Italy, 1991:118.
156. Sakurada S, Nakamura S, Salahuddin SZ, Gallo RC. Cultured Kaposi's sarcoma–derived spindle cells express vascular permeability inducing activity. Int Conf AIDS 1990;6:200.
157. Rosenberg ZF, Fauci AS. Immunopathogenic mechanisms of HIV infection: cytokine induction of HIV expression. Immunol Today 1990;11:176–180.
158. Molina J-M, Scadden DT, Byrn R, Dinarello CA, Groopman JE. Production of tumor necrosis factor alpha and interleukin 1 beta by monocytic cells infected with human immunodeficiency virus. J Clin Invest 1989;84:733–737.
159. Molina JM, Scadden DT, Amirault C, et al. Human immunodeficiency virus does not induce interleukin-1, interleukin-6, or tumor necrosis factor in mononuclear cells. J Virol 1990;64:2901–2906.
160. Miles SA, Martinez-Maza O, Rezai A, et al. Oncostatin M as a potent mitogen for AIDS–Kaposi's sarcoma-derived cells. Science 1992;255:1432–1434.
161. Nair BC, De Vico AL, Nakamura S, et al. Identification of a major growth factor for AIDS–Kaposi's sarcoma cells as oncostatin M. Science 1992;255:1430–1432.
162. Miles S, Rezai A, Magpantay L, Kishimoto T, Linsley P, Martinez-Maza O. Oncostatin-M is a potent mitogen for AIDS–Kaposi sarcoma (AIDS-KS) cell lines. Science 1991;255:1434–1436.
163. Gearing DP, Comeau MR, Friend DJ, et al. The IL-6 signal transducer, gp130: an oncostatin M receptor and affinity converter for the LIF receptor. Science 1992;255:1434–1437.
164. Ensoli B, Gendelman R, Markham P, et al. Synergy between basic fibroblast growth factor and HIV-1 Tat protein in induction of Kaposi's sarcoma. Nature 1994;371:674–680.
165. Agostini C, Poletti V, Zambello R, et al. Phenotypical and functional analysis of bronchoalveolar lavage lymphocytes in patients with HIV infection. Am Rev Respir Dis 1988;138:1609–1615.
166. Miles SA. Pathogenesis of human immunodeficiency virus-related Kaposi's sarcoma. Curr Opin Oncol 1992;4:875–882.
167. Kaposi M. Idiopathisches multiples pigmentsarkom der haut. Archive fur Dermatologie und Syphillis 1872;4:265–273.
168. Friedman-Kien AE, Ostreicher R. Overview of classical and epidemic Kaposi's sarcoma. In: Friedman-Kien AE, Laubenstein LJ, eds. AIDS: the epidemic of Kaposi's sarcoma and opportunistic infections. New York: Masson, 1991.
169. Friedman-Kien AE, Saltzman BR. Clinical manifestations of classical, endemic African, and epidemic AIDS-associated Kaposi's sarcoma. J Am Acad Dermatol 1990;22:1237–1250.
170. Bismuth H, Samuel D, Venancie P, Menouar G, Szekely A. Development of Kaposi's sarcoma in liver transplant recipients: characteristics, management and outcome. Transplant Proc 1991;23:1438–1439.
171. Alamartine E, Berthoux F. Complications, carcinologiques apres transplantation renale. Presse Medicale (Paris) 1991;20: 891–895.
172. Qunibi W, Akhtar M, Sheth K, et al. Kaposi's sarcoma: the most common tumor after renal transplantation in Saudi Arabia. Am J Med 1988;84:225–232.
173. Buchbinder A, Friedman-Kien AE. Clinical aspects of Kaposi's sarcoma. Curr Opin Oncol 1992;4:867–874.
174. Friedman-Kien AE, Laubenstein LJ, eds. AIDS: the epidemic of Kaposi's sarcoma and opportunistic infections. New York: Masson, 1991.
175. Krigel RL, Friedman-Kien AE. Epidemic Kaposi's sarcoma. Semin Oncol 1990;17:350–360.
176. Gottlieb GJ, Ragaz A, Vogel JV, et al. A preliminary communication on extensively disseminated Kaposi's sarcoma in young homosexual men. Am J Dermatopathol 1981;3:111–114.
177. Friedman-Kien AE. Disseminated Kaposi's sarcoma syndrome in young homosexual men. J Am Acad Dermatol 1981;5:468–471.
178. Friedman-Kien AE, Laubenstein LJ, Rubinstein P, et al. Disseminated Kaposi's sarcoma in homosexual men. Ann Intern Med 1982;96:693–700.
179. Marmor M, Friedman-Kien AE, Laubenstein L, et al. Risk factors for Kaposi's sarcoma in homosexual men. Lancet 1982;1:1083–1107.
180. Friedman-Kien AE. Epidemic Kaposi's sarcoma: a manifestation of the acquired immune deficiency syndrome. J Dermatol Surg Oncol 1983;9:637–640.
181. Marmor M, Friedman-Kien AE, Zolla-Pazner S, et al. Kaposi's sarcoma in homosexual men: a seroepidemiologic case-control study. Ann Intern Med 1984;100:809–815.
182. Kaplan MH, Susin M, Pahwa SG, et al. Neoplastic complications of HTLV-III infection. Lymphoma and solid tumors. Am J Med 1987;82:389–396.
183. Reynolds P, Saunders LD, Layefsky ME, Lemp GF. An update on Kaposi's sarcoma reporting in San Francisco (letter). J Acquir Immune Defic Syndr 1991;4:825–826.
184. Archer CB, Spittle MF, Smith NP. Kaposi's sarcoma in a homosexual—10 years on. Clin Exp Dermatol 1989;14:233–236.
185. Chachoua A, Krigel R, LaFleur F, et al. Prognostic factors and staging classification of patients with epidemic Kaposi's sarcoma. J Clin Oncol 1989;7:774–780.
186. Krown SE, Niedzsiecki D, Bhalla RB, et al. Relationship and prognostic value of endogenous interferon-alpha, beta 2 microglobulin, and neopterin serum levels in patients with Ka-

186. posi's sarcoma and AIDS. J Acquir Immune Defic Syndr 1991;4:871–880.
187. Gill PS, Rarick MU, Espina B, et al. Advanced acquired immune deficiency syndrome–related Kaposi's sarcoma: results of pilot studies using combination chemotherapy. Cancer 1990;65:1074–1078.
188. Gill PS, Brynes R. Recent advances in AIDS-related Kaposi's sarcoma. Curr Opin Oncol 1989;1:57–61.
189. Rarick MU, Gill PS, Montgomery T, Bernstein Singer M, Jones B, Levine AM. Treatment of epidemic Kaposi's sarcoma with combination chemotherapy (vincristine and bleomycin) and zidovudine. Ann Oncol 1990;1:147–149.
190. Gill PS, Akil B, Colletti P, et al. Pulmonary Kaposi's sarcoma: clinical findings and results of therapy. Am J Med 1989;87:57–61.
191. Mitsuyasu RT. Kaposi's sarcoma in the acquired immunodeficiency syndrome. Infect Dis Clin North Am 1989;2:511–523.
192. Buchbinder A, Friedman-Kien A. Clinical aspects of epidemic Kaposi's sarcoma. In: Beral V, Jaffe HW, Weiss RA, eds. Cancer, HIV, and AIDS. New York: Cold Spring Harbor Laboratory Press, 1991:39–52.
193. Reichert CM, O'Leary TJ, Levens DL, Simrell CR, Macher AM. Autopsy pathology in the acquired immunodeficiency syndrome. Am J Pathol 1983;112:357–382.
194. Guarda LA, Luna MA, Smith L, Mansell PWA, Gyorkey F, Roca AN. Acquired immune deficiency syndrome: post-mortem findings. Am J Clin Pathol 1984;81:549–557.
195. Welch K, Finkbeiner W, Alpers CE. Autopsy findings in the acquired immunodeficiency syndrome. JAMA 1984;252:1152–1154.
196. Friedman SL, Wright TL, Altman DF. Gastrointestinal Kaposi's sarcoma in patients with acquired immunodeficiency syndrome. Gastroenterology 1985;89:102–108.
197. Hopewell PC, Luce JM. Pulmonary involvement in the acquired immunodeficiency syndrome. Chest 1985;87:104–112.
198. Stover DE, White DA, Romano PA, Gellene RA, Robeson WA. The spectrum of pulmonary diseases associated with the acquired immune deficiency syndrome. Am J Med 1985;78:429–437.
199. Ognibene FP, Steis RG, Macher AM, et al. Kaposi's sarcoma causing pulmonary infiltrates and respiratory failure in the acquired immunodeficiency syndrome. Ann Intern Med 1985;102:471–475.
200. Garay SM, Belenko M, Fazzini E, Schinella R. Pulmonary manifestations of Kaposi's sarcoma. Chest 1987;91:39–43.
201. Zibrak JD, Silvestri RC, Costello P, et al. Bronchoscopic and radiologic features of Kaposi's sarcoma involving the respiratory system. Chest 1986;90:476–479.
202. Nash G, Fligiel S. Pathologic features of the lung in the acquired immune deficiency syndrome (AIDS): an autopsy study of seventeen homosexual males. Am J Clin Pathol 1984;81:6–12.
203. Meduri GU, Stover DE, Lee M, Myskowski PL, Caravelli JF, Zaman MB. Pulmonary Kaposi's sarcoma in the acquired immune deficiency syndrome. Am J Med 1986;81:11–18.
204. Lemlich G, Schwam L, Lebwohl M. Kaposi's sarcoma and acquired immunodeficiency syndrome. Postmortem findings in twenty-four cases. J Am Acad Dermatol 1987;16:319–325.
205. Naidich DP, Tarras M, Garay SM, Birnbaum B, Rybak BJ, Schinella R. Kaposi's sarcoma. CT-radiographic correlation. Chest 1989;96:723–728.
206. Fouret PJ, Touboul JL, Maynard CM, Akoun GM, Roland J. Pulmonary Kaposi's sarcoma in patients with acquired immunodeficiency syndrome: a clinicopathological study. Thorax 1987;42:262–268.
207. Misra DP, Sunderrajan EV, Hurst DJ, Maltby JD. Kaposi's sarcoma of the lung: radiography and pathology. Thorax 1982;37:155–156.
208. Kaplan LD, Hopewell PC, Jaffe H, Goodman PC, Bottles K, Volberding PA. Kaposi's sarcoma involving the lung in patients with the acquired immunodeficiency syndrome. J Acquir Immune Defic Syndr 1988;1:23–30.
209. Greenberg JE, Fischl MA, Berger JR. Upper airway obstruction secondary to acquired immunodeficiency syndrome in Kaposi's sarcoma. Chest 1985;88:638–640.
210. White DA, Matthay RA. Noninfectious pulmonary complications of infection with the human immunodeficiency virus. Am Rev Respir Dis 1989;140:1763–1787.
211. Adal KA, Cockerell CJ, Petri WA. Cat scratch disease, bacillary angiomatosis, and other infections due to *Rochalimaea*. N Engl J Med 1994;330:1509–1515.
212. Lee VW, Fuller JD, O'Brien MJ, Parker DR, Cooley TP, Liebman HA. Pulmonary Kaposi sarcoma in patients with AIDS: scintigraphic diagnosis with sequential thallium and gallium scanning. Radiology 1991;180:409–412.
213. Templeton AC. Kaposi's sarcoma. In: Sommers SC, Rosen PP, eds. Pathology annual. New York: Appleton Century-Crofts, 1981:315–336.
214. Purdy LJ, Colby TV, Tousem SA, Battifora H. Pulmonary Kaposi's sarcoma: premortem histologic diagnosis. Am J Surg 1986;10:301–311.
215. Moskowitz LB, Hensley GT, Gould EW, Weiss SD. Frequency and anatomic distribution of lymphadenopathic Kaposi's sarcoma in the acquired immunodeficiency syndrome: an autopsy series. Hum Pathol 1985;16:447–456.
216. Sivit CJ, Schwartz AM, Rockoff SD. Kaposi's sarcoma of the lung in AIDS: Radiologic-pathologic analysis. Am J Radiol 1987;148:25–28.
217. Davis SD, Henschke CI, Chamides BK, Westcott JL. Intrathoracic Kaposi's sarcoma in AIDS patients: radiographic-pathologic correlation. Radiology 1987;163:495–500.
218. Hill CA, Harle TS, Mansell CWA. The prodrome, Kaposi's sarcoma, and infections associated with acquired immunodeficiency syndrome: radiologic findings in 39 patients. Radiology 1983;149:393–399.
219. Mintzer DM, Real FX, Jovino L, Krown SE. Treatment of Kaposi's sarcoma and thrombocytopenia with vincristine in patients with the acquired immunodeficiency syndrome. Ann Intern Med 1985;102:200–202.
220. Volberding PA, Abrams DI, Conant M, Kaslow K, Vranizan K, Ziegbler J. Vinblastine therapy for Kaposi's sarcoma in the acquired immunodeficiency syndrome. Ann Intern Med 1985;103:335–338.
221. Gill PS, Rarick M, McCutchan JA, et al. Systemic treatment of AIDS-related Kaposi's sarcoma: results of a randomized trial. Am J Med 1991;90:427–433.
222. Sloan DE, Kumar PN, Pierce PF. Chemotherapy for patients with pulmonary Kaposi's sarcoma: benefit of filgstrim (G-CSF) in supporting dose administration. South Med J 1993;86:1219–1224.
223. Remick SC, Reddy M, Herman D, et al. Continuous infusion bleomycin in AIDS-related Kaposi's sarcoma. J Clin Oncol 1994;12:1130–1136.
224. Krown SE. Interferon and other biologic agents for the treatment of Kaposi's sarcoma. Hematol Oncol Clin North Am 1991;5:311–321.

225. Laubenstein LJ, Krigel RL, Odajynk CM, et al. Treatment of epidemic Kaposi's sarcoma with etoposide or a combination of doxorubicin, bleomycin, and vinblastine. J Clin Oncol 1984;2:1115–1120.
226. Saville MV, Lietzau J, Pluda JM, et al. Treatment of HIV-associated Kaposi's sarcoma with paclitaxel. Lancet 1995; in press.
227. Ireland-Gill A, Espina BM, Akil B, Gill PS. Treatment of acquired immunodeficiency syndrome–related Kaposi's sarcoma using bleomycin-containing combination chemotherapy regimens. Semin Oncol 1992;19:32–37.
228. Pluda JM, Parkinson DR, Feigal EG, Yarchoan R. Noncytotoxic approaches to the treatment of HIV-associated Kaposi's sarcoma. Oncology 1993;7:25–33.
229. Cancer statistics in review 1994 (monograph). Bethesda, MD: U.S. National Cancer Institute; Division of Cancer Prevention and Control; Surveillance, Epidemiology and End Report Program, 1994.
230. Reynolds P, Saunders L, Layefsky M, Lemp GF. The spectrum of acquired immunodeficiency syndrome (AIDS)—associated malignancies in San Francisco, 1980–1987. Am J Epidemiol 1993;137:19–30.
231. Biggar RJ, Burnett W, Mikl J, Nasca PC. Cancer among New York men at risk of acquired immunodeficiency syndrome. Int J Cancer 1989;43:979–985.
232. Monfardini S, Tirelli U, Vaccher E, et al. Malignant lymphoma in patients with or at risk for AIDS in Italy. J Natl Cancer Inst 1988;80:855–860.
233. Roithmann S, Tourani JM, Andrius JM. Hodgkin's disease in HIV-infected intravenous drug abusers. N Engl J Med 1990;323:275–276.
234. Garnier G, Michiels JF. HIV-associated Hodgkin disease. Ann Intern Med 1991;115:233.
235. Ree HJ, Strauchen JA, Khan AA, et al. Human immunodeficiency virus–related Hodgkin's disease. Cancer 1991;67:1614–1621.
236. Tirelli U, Vaccher E, Rezza G, et al. Hodgkin's disease in association with acquired immunodeficiency syndrome (AIDS): a report on 36 patients. Gruppo Italiano Cooperative AIDS and Tumori. Acta Oncol 1989;28:637–639.
237. Ames ED, Conjalka MS, Goldberg AF, et al. Hodgkin's disease and AIDS. Hematol Oncol Clin North Am 1991;5:343–356.
238. Hewlett D, Duncanson F, Jagadha V, Lieberman J, Lenox T, Wormser G. Lymphadenopathy in an inner-city population consisting principally of intravenous drug abusers with suspected acquired immunodeficiency syndrome. Am Rev Respir Dis 1988;137:1275–1279.
239. Suster B, Akerman M, Orenstein M, Wax M. Pulmonary manifestations of AIDS: review of 106 episodes. Radiology 1986;161:87–93.
240. Errante D, Tirelli U, Gastaldi R, et al. Combined antineoplastic and antiretroviral therapy for patients with Hodgkin's disease and HIV infection; a prospective study in 17 patients. Cancer 1994;73:437–444.
241. Gunthel CJ, Northfelt DW. Cancers not associated with immunodeficiency in HIV infected persons. Oncology 1994;8:59–64.
242. Moskowitz LB, Kory P, Chan JC, et al. Unusual causes of death in Haitians residing in Miami: high prevalence of opportunistic infections. JAMA 1983;250:1187–1191.
243. Irwin LE, Begandy MK, Moore TM. Adenosquamous carcinoma of the lung and the acquired immunodeficiency syndrome (letter). Ann Intern Med 1984;100:158.
244. Moser RJ, Tenholder MF, Ridenour R. Oat-cell carcinoma in transfusion-associated acquired immunodeficiency syndrome. Ann Intern Med 1985;103:478.
245. Nusbaum NJ. Metastatic small-cell carcinoma of the lung in a patient with AIDS (letter). N Engl J Med 1985;312:1706.
246. Lake-Lewin D, Arkel YS. Spectrum of malignancies in HIV positive individuals (abstract 20). Proc Am Soc Clin Oncol 1988:7.
247. Monfardini S, Vaccher E, Lazzaria A, et al. Characterization of AIDS-associated tumors in Italy: Report of 435 cases of an IVDA-based series. Cancer Detect Prev 1990;14:391–393.
248. Fineburg SA, Schinella R. Human immunodeficiency virus infection in women: report of 102 cases. Mod Pathol 1990;3:575–580.
249. Braun MA, Killam DA, Remick SC, et al. Lung cancer in patients seropositive for HIV. Radiology 1990;175:341–343.
250. Fraire AE, Awe RJ. Lung cancer in association with human immunodeficiency virus infection. Cancer 1992;70:432–436.
251. Lacoste D, Hajjar M, Brossard G, et al. Unusual malignant tumors in a hospital-based cohort of HIV-infected patients: Bordeux (France) 1985–1990 (abstract WB 2372). VIIth International Conference on AIDS, Florence, Italy, June 1991.
252. Gachupin-Garcia A, Selwyn PA, Budner NS. Population-based study of malignancy and HIV infection among injecting drug users in a New York City methadone treatment program, 1985–1991. AIDS 1992;6:843–848.
253. Bagheri K, Connell RK, Safirstein BH. Lung cancer in a drug addict seropositive for human immunodeficiency virus (letter). Am J Radiol 1992;158:210.
254. Sridhar KS, Flores MR, Raub WA, et al. Lung cancer in patients with human immunodeficiency virus infection compared with historic control subjects. Chest 1992;102:1704–1708.
255. Repetto L, Simoni C, Ferrazin A, et al. AIDS-related tumors in 64 HIV-positive patients (abstract PO B12-1604). IXth International Conference on AIDS, Berlin, Germany, June 1993.
256. Karp J, Profeta G, Marantz PR, et al. Lung cancer in patients with acquired immunodeficiency syndrome. Chest 1993;103:410–413.
257. Vaccher E, Tirelli U, Spina M, et al. Lung cancer in 19 patients with HIV infection. Ann Oncol 1993;4:85–86.
258. Sridhar KS, Raub WR, Duncan RC, et al. Lung carcinoma in 1,336 patients. Am J Clin Oncol (Cancer Clinical Trials) 1991;14:496–508.
259. Mountain CF. A new international staging system for lung cancer. Chest 1986;4:225S–232S.
260. Decaro L, Benfield JR. Lung cancer in young persons. J Thorac Cardiovasc Surg 1982;83:372–376.
261. Jubelirer SJ, Wilson RA. Lung cancer in patients younger than 40 years of age. Cancer 1991;67:372–376.
262. U.S. Bureau of Labor Statistics. Employment and earnings. Washington, DC: U.S. Department of Labor, 1988;35.
263. Robert LM, Bell DM. HIV transmission in the health-care setting. Infect Dis Clin North Am 1994;8:319–329.
264. Klein RS, Phelan JA, Freeman K, et al. Low occupational risk of human immunodeficiency virus infection among dental professionals. N Engl J Med 1988;318:86–90.
265. Panlilio AL, Shapiro CN, Schable CA, et al. Serosurvey of human immunodeficiency virus, hepatitis B virus, and hepatitis C virus infection among hospital based surgeons. J Am Coll Surg 1995;180:16–24.
266. Tokars J, Chamberland M, Shapiro C, et al. Infection with hepatitis B virus, hepatitis C virus, and human immunodeficiency virus among orthopedic surgeons (abstract 22). In: Pro-

grams and Abstracts of the Second Annual Meeting of the Society for Hospital Epidemiology of America, Baltimore, April 11–13, 1992.
267. Cowan D, Brundage J, Pomerantz R, et al. HIV infection in patients and staff of two dialysis centers: Seroepidemiological findings and prevention trends. Eur J Epidemiol 1988;4:171.
268. Assogba U, Park RA, Rey MA, Barthelemy A, Rottembourg J, Gluckman JC. Prospective study of HIV seropositive patients in hemodialysis centers. Clin Nephrol 1988;29:312–314.
269. Chirgwin K, Rao TK, Landesman SH. HIV infection in a high prevalence dialysis unit. AIDS 1989;3:731–735.
270. Goldman M, Liesnard C, Vanherweghem JL, Dolle N, Toussaint C. Markers of HTLV-III in patients with end stage renal failure treated by hemodialysis. BMJ (Clin Res Ed) 1987;293:161–162.
271. Peterman TA, Lang GR, Mikos NJ, et al. HTLV-III/LAV infection in hemodialysis patients. JAMA 1986;255:2324–2326.
272. Comodo N, Martinelli F, De Majo E, et al. Risk of HIV infection in patients and staff of two dialysis centers. Seroepidemiological findings and prevention trends. Eur J Epidemiol 1988;4:171–174.
273. Ebbesen P, Melbye M, Scheutz F, Bodner AJ, Biggar RJ. Lack of antibodies to HTLV-III/LAV in Danish dentists (letter). JAMA 1986;256:2199.
274. Flynn NM, Pollet SM, Van Horne JR, Elvebakk R, Harper SD, Carleson JR. Absence of HIV antibody among dental professionals exposed to infected patients. West J Med 1987;146:439–442.
275. Gerberding JL, Nelson K, Greenspan D, et al. Risk to dental professionals from occupational exposure to human immunodeficiency virus: follow-up (abstract 698). In: Programs and Abstracts of the 27th Interscience Conference on Antimicrobial Agents and Chemotherapy, American Society for Microbiology, New York, October 4–7, 1987.
276. Gruninger SE, Siew C, Chang SB, et al. Human immunodeficiency virus type I. Infection among dentists. J Am Dent Assoc 1992;123:57–64.
277. Siew C, Gruninger SE, Hojvat SA. Screening dentists for HIV and hepatitis B. N Engl J Med 1988;318:1400–1401.
278. Janssen RS, St. Louis ME, Satten GA, et al. HIV infections among patients in US acute care hospitals. Strategies for the counseling and testing of the hospital patient. N Engl J Med 1992;327:445–452.
279. Marcus R, Culver DH, Bell DM, et al. Risk of human immunodeficiency virus infection among emergency department workers. Am J Med 1993;94:363–370.
280. U.S. Centers for Disease Control and Prevention. Update: universal precautions for prevention of human immunodeficiency virus, hepatitis B virus, and other bloodborne pathogens in health-care settings. MMWR Morb Mortal Wkly Rep 1988;37:377–382.
281. Tokars JI, Bell DM, Culver DH, et al. Percutaneous injuries during surgical procedures. JAMA 1992;267:2899–2904.
282. Wong ES, Stotka JL, Chinchilli VM, Williams DS, Stuart CG, Markowitz SM. Are universal precautions effective in reducing the number of occupational exposures among health care workers? A prospective study of physicians on a medical service. JAMA 1991;265:1123–1128.
283. Chiarello L. Summary. New York State Department of Health pilot study of needle stick prevention devices. In: Implementing safer needle devices (monograph). Chicago: American Hospital Association, 1992:29.
284. Ippolito G, Puro V, De Carli G. The risk of occupational human immunodeficiency virus infection in health care workers: Italian multicenter study. Arch Intern Med 1993;153:1451–1458.
285. Tokars JI, Marcus R, Culver DH, et al. Surveillance of HIV infection and zidovudine use among health care workers after occupational exposure to HIV-infected blood. Ann Intern Med 1993;118:913–919.
286. Ciesielski C, Marianos D, Ou CY, et al. Transmission of human immunodeficiency virus in dental practice. Ann Intern Med 1992;116:798–805.
287. Armstrong FP, Miner JC, Wolfe WH. Investigation of a health care worker with symptomatic human immunodeficiency. An epidemiologic approach. Mil Med 1987;152:414–418.
288. Arnow PM, Chou T, Shapiro R, Sussman EJ. Maintaining confidentiality in a look-back investigation of patients treated by a HIV-infected dentist. Public Health Rep 1993;108:273–278.
289. Comer RW, Myers DR, Steadman CD, Carter MJ, Rissing JP, Tedesco FJ. Management considerations for an HIV positive dental student. J Dent Educ 1991;55:187.
290. Danila RN, MacDonald KL, Rhame FS, et al. A look-back investigation of patients of an HIV-infected physician. Public health implications. N Engl J Med 1991;325:1406–1411.
291. Dickinson GM, Morhart RE, Klimas NG, Bandea CI, Laracuente JM, Bisno AL. Absence of HIV transmission from an infected dentist to his patients. An epidemiologic and DNA sequence analysis. JAMA 1993;269:1802–1806.
292. Mishu B, Schaffner W. HIV-infected surgeons and dentists. Looking back and looking forward (editorial). JAMA 1993;269:1843–1844.
293. Mishu B, Schaffner W, Horan JM, Wood LH, Hutcheson RH, McNabb PC. A surgeon with AIDS. Lack of evidence of transmission to patients. JAMA 1990;264:467–470, errata 264:1661.
294. Porter JD, Cruickshank JG, Gentle PH, Robinson RG, Gill ON. Management of patients treated by a surgeon with HIV infection (letter). Lancet 1990;335:113–114.
295. von Reyn CF, Gilbert TT, Shaw FE, Parsonnet KC, Abramson JE, Smith MG. Absence of HIV transmission from an infected orthopedic surgeon. A 13 year look-back study. JAMA 1993;269:1807–1811; 270:579.
296. York AK, Arthur JS. Determining the HIV status of patients of three HIV-positive Navy dentists. J Am Dent Assoc 1993;124:74–77.

51

CHEMOPREVENTION OF LUNG CANCER IN HIGH-RISK INDIVIDUALS

Ugo Pastorino

INTRODUCTION

During the last two decades, the field of cancer prevention has developed into a major area of research. Both the selectivity and efficacy of interventions improved, thereby opening new prospects for research on mechanisms of human carcinogenesis.

Cancer prevention includes several areas of laboratory and clinical investigation including (*a*) primary prevention, which is aimed at eliminating or reducing the exposure to known carcinogens; (*b*) secondary prevention, which includes early diagnosis and treatment of preneoplastic or preinvasive lesions; and (*c*) pharmacologic prevention or chemoprevention, a new branch of study aimed at stopping or reversing the carcinogenic progess by the administration of drugs or other natural substances that are present in human physiology or the normal diet. These areas often overlap so that the distinction among them may sometimes appear arbitrary. For example, the complex problem of changing dietary habits includes important aspects of primary prevention, wherein the goal of the intervention may be the reduction of fat intake or the lowering of the intestinal concentration of potential carcinogens. Dietary changes also may involve chemoprevention, in which the goal is the achievement of adequate levels of potentially protective agents by means of dietary supplementation.

Chemoprevention represents an evolution from traditional systemic chemotherapy in which the cytolytic approach to tumors is replaced by the induction of differentiation, cytostasis, or apoptosis. The ultimate goal, however, remains similar: to provide an effective treatment for tumors that are otherwise resistant to conventional therapies. Considerable enthusiasm for chemoprevention has been generated from the publication of experimental data proving that chemoprevention in humans, especially in patients with cancers of the upper aerodigestive tract, is feasible (1, 2), and from a few clinical trials that demonstrated a significant reduction of second primary tumors in patients treated with retinoids (3–5). However, a recent trial conducted among heavy smokers failed to show any benefit for chemoprevention (6), emphasizing that certain crucial aspects of chemoprevention, such as optimal selection of target populations, choice of preventive agent(s), and dose and duration of treatment, remain to be defined.

Chemoprevention research has improved significantly our understanding of the biologic processes involved in lung carcinogenesis. Cytogenetic and molecular biology studies performed on the tumor and normal bronchial epithelium of pulmonary resection specimens from patients with single or multiple lung cancers showed that specific and consistent genetic changes may be identified in the various steps of aerodigestive tract carcinogenesis (7). Based on such findings, researchers now have the opportunity to design new generations of clinical trials that use genetic biomarkers to select the best candidate agents for specific chemoprevention programs and to monitor the results of these interventions without using the prolonged follow-up needed to ascertain the evolution of clinically evident disease.

EPIDEMIOLOGIC ASPECTS

PRIMARY VERSUS PHARMACOLOGIC PREVENTION

Widespread control of tobacco consumption and the reduction of environmental exposure to known carcinogens remain the major goals for lung cancer prevention (8, 9). In the male population of the United States, tobacco smoking appears to be responsible for 80% to 90% of the upper aerodigestive tract tumors (lung, larynx, oral cavity, esophagus); 30% to 40% of tumors of the bladder, kidney, and pancreas; and 20% of gastric tumors and leukemias (9). When the smoking attributable causation is applied to the incidence rates of the various cancers observed within the European Community (Table 51.1), it is possible to calculate that in this population tobacco smoking causes nearly 150,000 cancer deaths every year (8). If one includes chronic pulmonary and cardiovascular diseases, then the tobacco-related mortality in the European Community rises to more than 400,000 people (1).

Lung cancer incidence rates have been declining in Europe, the United States, and England since the mid-1970s as a consequence of the effective tobacco control achieved during the two prior decades. From 1972 through 1984, the prevalence of smoking in the adult population of the United Kingdom dropped from 52% to 36% in males and from 41% to 32% in females.

The U.S. National Cancer Institute (NCI) estimated that in the United States approximately 800,000 tobacco-related deaths were either postponed or prevented by primary prevention measures between 1964 and 1985 (9). To build on these observations, specific smoking cessation methods trials now involve millions of heavy smokers through the NCI's Smoking, Tobacco, and Cancer Program, which emphasizes high-risk social and ethnic groups (10).

Despite these improvements, even if further reductions in tobacco consumption were to occur in many Western countries, the overall global lung cancer mortality would remain very high in the coming decades. A study of worldwide incidence rates estimated a total of nearly 900,000 new cases of lung cancer in 1985 (11), with an overall increase of 36% in the 5 years since 1980. Areas in which the incidence is declining (i.e., North American and Northern Europe) account for only 25% of the total global burden, whereas lung cancer incidence and the tobacco-related epidemic are growing in the majority of developing countries. As an example, if the major Eastern countries would ever reach the actual incidence rates of North America, China alone would provide more than 500,000 new cases of lung cancer each year.

For these reasons chemoprevention should never be considered a substitute for primary prevention, but rather a potential complementary approach. To illustrate, the incidence of lung cancer remains high for 15 to 20 years among exsmokers because of the accumulated carcinogenic damage. There is thus an objective need for strategies aimed at reducing cancer mortality in individuals who have stopped smoking.

LATENCY AND INTERVENTION

Epidemiologic and experimental data on multistep carcinogenesis (Fig. 51.1) indicate that the development of invasive lung cancers requires a complex sequence of critical events. In fact, most descriptive epidemiologic studies on time trends in human cohorts, as well as analytic case control studies, consistently demonstrate that the interval between the beginning of the exposure to known carcinogens and the occurrence of lung cancer ranges from 10 to 30 years. Such a long phase of latency suggests a large potential time frame in which to intervene.

Theoretically, it is possible to consider a combination of selective chemopreventive agents aimed at the various phases of carcinogenesis: from the inhibi-

TABLE 51.1. Incidence and Mortality Figures for Tumours Related to Tobacco Smoking in the Male Population of the European Community (1978–82), and Percentage of Cases Attributable to Smoking

TUMOR SITE	INCIDENCE (CASES/YR)	MORTALITY (CASES/YR)	FRACTION ATTRIBUTABLE TO SMOKING (%)
Lung	135,200	117,100	80–90
Larynx	24,600	11,000	80–90
Oral cavity	27,300	14,800	80–90
Esophagus	11,900	13,500	80–90
Bladder	41,600	18,000	30–40
Kidney	16,300	8,400	30–40
Pancreas	16,100	15,800	30–40
Stomach	55,100	40,000	20
Leukemia	16,600	12,600	20
Total	344,700	251,200	...

Modified from Jensen OM, Esteve J, Moller H, Renard H. Cancer in the European Community and its member states. Eur J Cancer 1990;26:1167–1256.

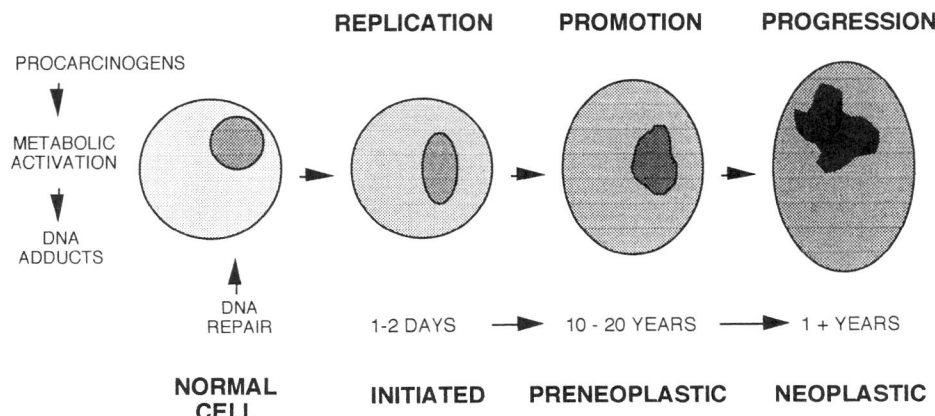

FIGURE 51.1. Hypothetic phases of lung carcinogenesis.

tion of early induction (metabolic activation, formation of DNA adducts, DNA repair) to the antagonism of tumor promotion and the reversal of progression, to invasive cancer.

DIETARY FACTORS IN LUNG CANCER

Based on the evidence of geographic and historical trends in cancer incidence, human epidemiologic studies have tried to correlate the risk of lung cancer with environmental factors other than tobacco consumption. Among these, dietary deficiency of vitamins, micronutrients, or specific foods has emerged as a potential modifier of lung cancer risk. Table 51.2 summarizes the results of some case control or cohort studies on the dietary intake of vitamin A–related foods and lung cancer risk (12–24). A relative deficiency in vitamin A or beta carotene intake is associated with an average 1.5- to 2-fold increase in the risk of lung cancer (12–24). A protective effect of a higher dietary intake of beta carotene has been demonstrated for a number of tumors, but in lung cancer the epidemiologic data are more consistent and based on a larger number of cases (Table 51.3) (25). The reported studies on serum or plasma levels of these substances are more controversial. The majority of reports suggest that a higher risk of lung cancer is related to lower beta carotene levels in the blood, whereas most studies on blood retinol levels did not show a significantly lower value in patients with lung cancer compared with controls (26–37).

A relative protective effect against lung cancer also has been hypothesized for substances belonging to the group of antioxidants, such as selenium or vitamin E (α-tocopherol), both in terms of dietary consumption (31, 33) and serum levels (26). A recent epidemiologic study showed that the risk of cancer of the oral cavity is reduced by approximately 50% in subjects taking supplemental vitamin E compared with those not taking this supplement, suggesting that there is a protective effect of dietary vitamin E supplementation (38).

Studying dietary supplementation can present considerable difficulties, however. One major limitation relates to the definition of individual dietary habits. Such information usually is derived from questionnaires that often are only marginally accurate. Another limitation derives from the paucity of information regarding the biologically active substances contained in the diet. In other words, not only it is difficult to assess the amount of long-term dietary intake for a given food, but it also is difficult to define which substances contained in that food are protective agents, and of those, which are only risk indicators. Another confounding problem is the reporting bias in which positive results are more likely than negative findings to appear in the literature. Nevertheless, the epidemiologic data support the hypothesis that a different intake of common dietary components has the potential to modulate the risk of lung cancer (39). The unequivocal confirmation of this hypothesis, however, can be provided only by prospective trials that test the effect of specific substances. In this respect, chemoprevention trials have become a proper validation test for such epidemiologic hypotheses.

EXPERIMENTAL EVIDENCE

Experimental data clearly demonstrate the feasibility of lung cancer chemoprevention (1, 2). These data have been derived from nearly all of the available in vitro and in vivo systems for testing anticarcinogenic activity. Among the various substances with potential chemopreventive properties, the retinoids still represent the most thoroughly investigated agents. The

TABLE 51.2. Case Control Studies on Dietary Intake of Vitamin A–Related Foods and Subsequent Risk of Lung Cancer

First Author (Reference No.)	Cases	Dietary Component	Relative Risk (Low vs High[a])
Bjelke (12)	36	Vitamin A	2.6
Mettlin (13)	292	Vitamin A	1.5–1.7
McLennan (14)	233	Green vegetables	2.2
Gregor (15)	104	Vitamin A	1.5–1.3
Hirayama (16)	807	Green/yellow vegetables	1.4
Shekelle (17)	33	Beta carotene	3–5.5–7
Kvale (18)	153	Vitamin A	1.6
Hinds (19)	261	Vitamin A	1.6–1.4–2
Ziegler (20)	763	Beta carotene	1.3
Samet (21)	447	Vitamin A	1.1–1.4
Middleton (22)	514	Vitamin A	1.5
Pisani (23)	417	Carrots	1.8–2
Le Marchand (24)	332	Beta carotene	1.9

[a]For all given classes.

TABLE 51.3. Dietary Levels of Beta Carotene and Risk of Cancer: Number of Studies Showing a Protective Effect (Significant) and Relative Risk for Subjects with Low Consumption of Beta Carotene

Tumor Site	Cases	Significant/All	Relative Risk (Low vs High[a])
Lung	7046	15/19	1.3–7.1
Stomach	4085	9/12	1.5–9.1
Esophagus	2578	6/9	1.5–5.6
Colon-rectum	5188	10/17	1.4–9.1
Pancreas	1297	4/7	1.4–3.3
Larynx	525	2/2	2
Bladder	1826	2/3	1.7–3.2

Modified from Buring JE, Hennekens CH. Retinoids and carotenoids. In: DeVita VT, Hellman S, Rosenberg SA, eds. Cancer: principles and practice of oncology. 4th ed. Philadelphia: JB Lippincott 1993:464–474.
[a]Limited to significant studies.

retinoids are a heterogeneous group of substances that include retinol (vitamin A) and its synthetic derivatives. The experimental activity of retinoids has been well summarized in extensive reviews that show the multiple mechanisms of action unique to these substances (40, 41).

The retinoids exert a strong regulatory effect on the physiologic mechanisms of cell proliferation and differentiation (42–49). Experimentally, they inhibit malignant transformation (50–54) and suppress tumor promotion (55–58), particularly in the presence of indirect carcinogens, such as benzopyrene or methylcholantrene (59–62). The antipromotion effect of retinoids is of great interest in human lung cancer chemoprevention because of the possibility that it interferes with the late stages of tumor progression.

Under specific conditions, retinoids have shown a direct antineoplastic effect (63, 64), as well as inhibition of sarcoma and epidermal growth factors (65, 66). Recently, the retinoids have been shown to suppress malignant cell growth and induce apoptosis in lymphoid and myeloid malignant cell lines (HL-60R and NB 306) (67). Another potential mechanism of action is represented by the enhancement of the immune response to cancer, both as cell-mediated (41, 68) and antibody-mediated immune response (69, 70).

The discovery of specific nuclear retinoic acid receptors (RARs) has increased dramatically our knowledge of the mechanisms of action of retinoids (71, 72). RARs belong to the superfamily of ligand-activated nuclear receptors for steroid and thyroid hormones (73, 74). The RARs are DNA-binding, transcription-modulating proteins whose expression may be induced by retinoic acid administration (75–77). Three subtypes of RARs have been identified: RAR-α, RAR-β, and RAR-γ. The RAR-α gene is located on chromosome 17q21, RAR-β is located on chromosome 3p24, and RAR-γ is found on chromosome 12q13 (78). The mechanism of up regulation or down regulation of RARs (Fig. 51.2) may explain how retinoids can interfere with epithelial cell growth or inhibit progression of premalignant cells to cancer. These mechanisms offer a rational basis for selection of receptor specific retinoids in chemoprevention (79, 80).

Another group of agents with potential protective activity is represented by the antioxidants, including selenium, beta carotene, α-tocopherol (vitamin E), and N-acetylcysteine. Antioxidants may inhibit the process of carcinogenesis at various steps: from metabolic inactivation or detoxification of chemical carcinogens to

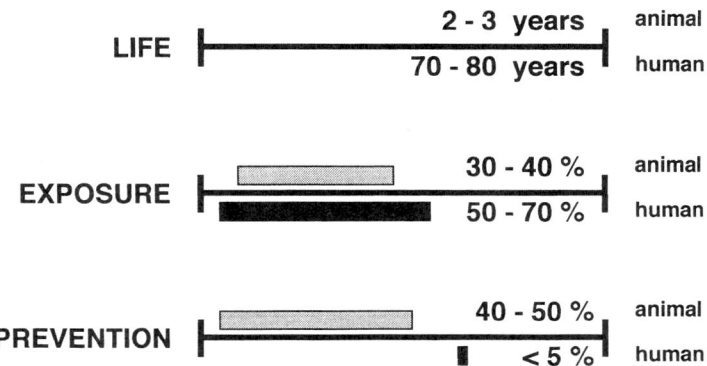

FIGURE 51.2. Differences in the design of chemoprevention studies conducted in animals and in humans: period of exposure to carcinogens and to preventive agents, expressed as a percentage of the total duration of life.

prevention of DNA damage by free radical scavenging (81–84).

Dietary selenium has proven effective in preventing carcinogenesis in various animal models, including the mammary gland, colon, skin, and lung (85, 86).

Beta carotene, the natural precursor of vitamin A, also has proven effective in experimental chemoprevention studies (87–90). Although its activity may, in part, be explained by its conversion into retinol, a specific antioxidant activity of beta carotene, and into other carotenoids such as cathaxanthine, has been demonstrated unequivocally for ultraviolet-induced skin tumors in mice (88). Further studies suggested that beta carotene acts as a free radical scavenger (91, 92), can induce differentiation (93), and can inhibit chromosome damage (94), N-*myc* expression (95), and ornithine decarboxylase (ODC) activity (96). However, in hamster models, beta carotene has failed to demonstrate a significant inhibition of lung tumorigenesis (97).

α-Tocopherol (vitamin E) has a similar spectrum of activity, with its main antioxidant effect exerted as a free radical scavenger (98). As with beta carotene, α-tocopherol was not effective as a single agent against methyl-nitroso-urea (MNU)–induced tracheal carcinogenesis and N-nitrosodiethylamine (DEN)–induced lung carcinogenesis in hamsters.

In recent years N-acetylcysteine (NAC), an aminothiol and synthetic precursor of intracellular cysteine and glutathione, has aroused considerable interest. NAC is used widely as a mucolytic drug and antidote against acetaminophen-induced hepatotoxicity (99). Presumably because of its nucleophilic and antioxidant properties, NAC also has proven effective in decreasing the direct mutagenicity of several chemical compounds. For example, in the Salmonella test, NAC inhibits the mutagenicity of nitrosation products, and it enhances thiol concentration in intestinal bacteria (100, 101). At the nuclear level, NAC was able to inhibit the in vivo formation of carcinogen-DNA adducts, reduce carcinogen-induced DNA damage, and protect nuclear enzymes such as poly(adenosine 5′-diphosphate [ADP]-ribose) polymerase (102). Of interest, in rats exposed either to intratracheal benzo(*a*)pyrene or cigarette smoke, benzo(*a*)pyrene diolepoxide (BPDE)–DNA adducts were prevented by NAC not only in the lung, but also in the heart and aorta, thus also suggesting a protective effect against cardiovascular disease (103). As for cancer chemoprevention, NAC inhibits urethane-induced lung tumors in mice (104) and colon carcinogenesis with 1, 2 dimethylhydrazine in rats (105).

Among the new agents with interesting activity in experimental chemoprevention are oltipraz and ellagic acid. Oltipraz belongs to the family of dithiolethiones, synthetic compounds that initially were reported to be consituents of cruciferous vegetables and were widely used in the 1980s as antischistosomal drugs (106). Collateral studies on their mechanisms of action demonstrated strong antioxidant, radioprotective, and chemoprotective properties, and a significant inhibition of carcinogenesis at various sites, such as the lung, gastrointestinal tract, liver, kidney, and bladder (107–109). Oltipraz appears to be protective against the early induction phases of carcinogenesis, with definite exposure to known genotoxic procarcinogens such as cigarette smoking for upper aerodigestive tract tumors or aflatoxin B1 for hepatocellular carcinoma (110). Recent studies have found oltipraz also to be active in the postinduction phases of carcinogenesis (111).

Ellagic acid (EA) and phenethyl-isothiocyanates (PEITCs) are naturally occurring compounds present in various fruits, nuts, and cruciferous vegetables. Both EA and PEITC are blocking agents, meaning that they induce enzyme detoxification and inhibit carcinogens (112). EA also shows antioxident and DNA scavenger properties. In vivo studies showed a strong inhibition of tumorigenesis in mouse lung and skin, as well as in rat esophagus (113–118).

A rapidly developing field of experimental chemoprevention research is the testing of combinations of various agents (116). Using DEN, a carcinogen requiring metabolic activation, induced adenosquamous lung carcinoma in Syrian golden hamsters, Moon et al. (118) demonstrated that the combination of N-(4-hydroxyphenyl)retinamide (4-HPR) plus selenium (Se) plus α-tocopherol (vitamin E) was 5 times more effective in preventing lung cancer than any of the agents alone. In the same system, retinol and beta carotene were ineffective when administered alone, whereas their concurrent administration reduced the incidence of adenosquamous lung cancers as well as dysplasias. These data appear very promising in terms of practical implication for clinical trials.

METHODOLOGY FOR CHEMOPREVENTION IN HUMANS

SCREENING OF NEW AGENTS

In 1982, the NCI established a comprehensive chemoprevention program aimed at identifying and testing the ability of specific dietary components and drugs to reduce the incidence of human cancers (119). This program includes the preclinical screening of new agents, the assessment of efficacy and safety, and the conduct of clinical trials in humans.

For the screening of new cytotoxic drugs, specific experimental models have been designed to reproduce the various pathologic conditions, both in terms of target tissues and organs and mechanisms of carcinogenesis.

Of the nearly 1000 substances with putative cancer preventive activity, more than 100 agents have been investigated in vitro and in vivo; a few of them are ready to be tested in phase II and phase III studies. Among the new generation of chemopreventive agents, a few appear promising for the chemoprevention of lung cancer (120). Tables 51.4 and 51.5 summarize the criteria used by the NCI for the preclinical assessment of efficacy and safety for potential chemopreventive agents (121).

SELECTION OF HIGH-RISK INDIVIDUALS

Three different levels of intervention for cancer prevention may be defined based on the selected target population: primary chemoprevention, treatment of precancerous lesions, and secondary chemoprevention.

TABLE 51.4. Preclinical Efficacy Studies for Chemopreventive Investigational Drugs

In vitro	
Modulation assays	Inhibition of anchorage independent growth in human lung tumors and rat tracheal cells
Chemoprevention assays	Inhibition of procarcinogen activation, free radicals, polymerase, ornithine decarboxylase, tyrosine kinase, calmodulin
	Induction of glutathione, glutathione-S-transferase, NAD(P)H:quinone reductase
In vivo	
Tumor modulation assays	Incidence, multiplicity, and latency
	Pharmacology: dose, plasma steady state, toxicity
	Animal models: rat mammary, hamster lung/trachea, rat/mouse colon, mouse skin, rat/mouse bladder
Surrogate endpoint assays	Hamster lung: dysplasia
	Mouse lung: *myc*, *p53*, *Rb*
	Rat colon/bladder: PCNA, Ki-67, EGFR
	Mouse skin: K-13 keratin

Modified from Kelloff GJ, Johnson JR, Crowell JA, et al. Approaches to the development and marketing approval of drugs that prevent cancer. Cancer Epidemiol Biomarkers Prev 1995; in press.
Abbreviations. PCNA, proliferating cell nuclear antigen; EGFR, epidermal growth factor receptor.

Primary chemoprevention trials are designed for healthy individuals in the general population; these trials aim to reduce the incidence of a malignant tumor through the administration of one or more substances. The target population may be represented by individuals at high risk of developing a lung cancer because of previous heavy exposure to smoking, asbestos, or other carcinogens, or by individuals with a high level of motivation such as physicians, nurses, or family members of patients.

The rationale for primary chemoprevention studies is derived mainly from epidemiologic and experimental data. These studies usually attempt to interfere with the early phases of lung carcinogenesis by counteracting a hypothetical deficiency of putative protective agents, such as beta carotene, retinol (vitamin A), or α-tocopherol (vitamin E). Such studies must recruit thousands of people and provide a long period of observation (e.g., 5 to 10 years) to observe an adequate number of events (i.e., tumors). The doses used for preventive agents are sufficiently low to avoid significant side effects, obtain high recruitment into the study, maintain compliance, and allow a double-blind setting. Such trials thus need to reduce to a minimum

TABLE 51.5 Preclinical Safety Studies for Chemopreventive Investigational Drugs

Required
  Toxicity studies in two species (rodent and nonrodent)
    Animal observation, biochemistry, urinalysis, pathology (major organs and tissues)
    Sufficient duration to support clinical trials (up to 6 months in rodents, 12 months in dogs)
    Route of administration equivalent to clinical route
    Use of drug substance as prepared for clinical trial
  Genotoxic potential assessed in a battery of assays including: gene mutation in *Salmonella typhimurium* and mammalian cells (mouse TK lymphoma, Chinese hamster ovary), and cytogenetic damage in vivo (mouse bone marrow micronucleus, chromosomal aberration)
  Segment I reproductive performance and effect on fertility in rats and segment II teratology study in rats and rabbits
  Combination of drugs for assessment of interactions in pharmacokinetics, toxicity, enzyme effect
Recommended
  Use of the clincal formulation in all in vivo toxicity studies when possible
  Pharmacokinetics and metabolite profiles in conjunction with toxicity studies
  Pharmacologically guided phase I clinical trials; starting dose, interval, escalation strategies based on concentration-effect relationship shown in preclinical efficacy and toxicity studies

Modified from Kelloff GJ, Johnson JR, Crowell JA, et al. Approaches to the development and marketing approval of drugs that prevent cancer. Cancer Epidemiol Biomarkers Prev 1995; in press.

the risk of harmful effects for the population under treatment and to guarantee a long-term tolerability of the intervention.

The second level of intervention involves subjects affected by precancerous or preinvasive lesions such as oral leukoplakia, cervical dysplasia, colorectal adenoma, bronchial metaplasia or dysplasia, or actinic keratosis. The aim of treatment at this level is the regression of the preneoplastic disease and the prevention of progression to invasive cancer. Such studies usually are conducted in a double-blind, randomized manner, usually in a limited number of patients.

Finally, secondary chemoprevention is aimed at preventing the occurrence of new primary tumors in patients cured of a prior cancer. As a consequence of improved survival, follow-up, and clinical evaluation achieved in modern clinical trials, second primary tumors have emerged as an important clinical entity in many diseases (122, 123).

Multiple primary tumors may occur in the upper aerodigestive tract because of widespread exposure of this epithelium to common etiologic factors such as tobacco smoking. Dietary habits may also play a role as modifiers of the individual risk of cancer. This clinical evidence finds its biologic rationale in the concept of field cancerization, suggesting that repeated exposure of the entire epithelial surface to carcinogenic insults may result in the occurrence of multiple, independent, premalignant, or malignant foci (124). For example, among patients cured of a cancer of the oral cavity, larynx, lung, esophagus, or bladder, the incidence of second primary tumors in all sites is 10% to 35%, depending on the site, histologic type, and stage of the index tumor; this number corresponds to an incidence of 2% to 6% per year (125–127). Lung cancers account for a large proportion of these second cancers, in the range of 8% to 20% overall (128–132). In patients with a good initial prognosis, the occurrence of synchronous or metachronous tumors represents a significant cause of treatment failure. In fact, most of these second parimary tumors occur in the lung and often are unresectable at the time of their diagnosis.

Compared with healthy subjects, patients cured of a prior cancer show a higher motivation to accept the extra burden of a chemoprevention plan as an extension of long-term follow-up planned for their index tumor (Table 51.6). Moreover, side effects are better tolerated and higher doses can be given to achieve a potential adjuvant effect against primary cancer relapses as well as the development of second tumors. For all of these reasons, patients curatively treated for a prior cancer of the upper aerodigestive tract are an ideal population in which to test the efficacy of chemopreventive agents (e.g., retinoids, vitamins, antioxidants), either alone or in combination with other adjuvent treatments (1, 2).

TABLE 51.6. Comparison Between Primary and Secondary Chemoprevention Studies

	CHEMOPREVENTION	
	PRIMARY	SECONDARY
Selection criteria	Prior exposure	Prior cancer
Phase of carcinogenesis	Initial (induction)	Late (promotion)
Risk of cancer	Limited (<0.5%/yr)	High (1%–3%/yr)
Sample size	Thousands	Hundreds
Pharmacologic dose	Minimal (effective)	Maximal (tolerable)
Duration of intervention	Years	Months
Control group	Double-blind or placebo	Placebo or no treatment
Side effects	Absent	Significant
Follow-up	Long interval	Short interval
Biologic monitoring	Difficult	Easy
Costs (additional)	High	Limited

ENDPOINTS

As for any other anticancer program, the ultimate goal of chemoprevention is the improvement of survival. Nonetheless, because of the enormous resources and time needed to demonstrate a survival benefit, overall survival is not the most practical endpoint for answering questions regarding the selection of optimal agents, dose, or duration of treatment, or the latency and maintenance of the biologic effect.

Even in the favorable case of significant reductions in the occurrence of new primary tumors, the survival may not be improved necessarily because of the high mortality from concurrent diseases (pulmonary or cardiovascular) or effective salvage therapy used for the incident cancers. At the clinical level, it is important to define the overall benefit of a given intervention after making adjustments for competing risks of death.

New primary tumors are the main endpoint for chemoprevention trials. However stricter criteria should be used with respect to target sites and differential diagnoses. Only tumors occurring in the target field of chemoprevention should be considered relevant endpoints. For upper aerodigestive tract tumors, that concept applies to tobacco-related cancers (oral cavity, pharynx, larynx, lung, esophagus, and bladder), i.e., neoplastic events occurring as a consequence of the field cancerization process. For instance, there is no reason to consider leukemias, sarcomas, cancer of the stomach, colon, or even skin as failures within such chemoprevention programs.

In patients treated for a prior lung cancer, the distinction between second primary tumors and recurrences may be difficult to determine. Traditional criteria based on the anatomic site (distance from prior cancer), histologic type (same versus different), and temporal sequence (time elapsed from prior cancer) may be very elusive. Recent studies suggest that biologic markers such as the deletion of the 3p chromosomal arm, loss of heterozygosity, or mutations of the *3p*, *p53*, or K-*ras* genes have the potential to improve the differential diagnosis of multiple primary tumors occurring in the same area (7).

STUDY DESIGN

Most of the variables involved in the design of chemoprevention studies still have to be validated fully. For example, the choice of dose generally is defined on the basis of maximum tolerated toxicity rather than on a biologically defined dose. Similarly, the absence of measurable parameters in the process of carcinogenesis makes the duration of intervention an arbitrary decision. In some experiences, a design based on a short induction phase followed by a long phase of maintenance with different doses (and possibly different substances) has proven effective (133). Another variable to be explored includes the means of reducing cumulative toxicities, for example, by prolonged administration at regular intervals.

In theoretical terms, the administration of various substances with different mechanisms of action may represent a more effective approach to the inhibition or reversal of carcinogenesis. The use of multiple agents appears to be an effective way to improve the cost/benefit ratio, particularly when the expected activity of each individual agent is limited, the mechanism of action is different, the toxicities are noncumulative, or the synergistic interactions can be demonstrated in the experimental setting. This combination agent approach to chemoprevention is analogous to the experience with cytotoxic chemotherapy. Similarly, simultaneous or sequential regimens are equally valid options to be tested.

One study design that has been used often in chemoprevention trials is the factorial design. This approach allows different substances to be tested simultaneously in the same population. The factorial design is particularly efficient when the study requires a large population and a long period of observation. For example, Figure 51.3 illustrates the complex factorial design of the esophageal cancer prevention trial conducted in the Lin Xian province of China (134). This study is designed to test four different regimens concurrently. At the end of the trial, it will be possible to evaluate the individual effect of each regimen by dividing the whole population into two groups, i.e., those with or without the regimen under consideration. The factorial design, however, requires the absence of a significant interaction between the various factors under evaluation. Therefore, if the goal of the study were to assess a hypothetical synergistic effect among different agents, it would be necessary to use a nonfactorial design.

Placebo	A	B	AB
C	AC	BC	ABC
D	AD	BD	ABD
CD	ACD	BCD	ABCD

FIGURE 51.3. Complex factorial design of the trial for chemoprevention of esophageal cancer conducted in the Lin Xian province of China, including a combination of four different intervention regimens (factorial, 2^4). **A**, retinol + beta carotene + zinc; **B**, riboflavin + niacin; **C**, vitamin C + molibden; **D**, vitamin E + selenium.

The sample size required for a given trial would vary according to the frequency of the selected endpoint (e.g., cancer incidence) and the anticipated reduction of the frequency of that event in the intervention arm. In general, in the calculation of the required sample size for chemoprevention trials, a reduction of the occurrence of new malignancies on the order of 30% to 40% may be considered reasonable in biologic terms.

CLINICAL DEVELOPMENT OF PREVENTIVE AGENTS

NATURAL RETINOL

Natural retinol, or vitamin A, has been available for experimental testing and clinical practice for more than 50 years. The widespread interest in retinol as a modulator of cell growth was generated by many of its physiologic properties, which are evident from the very early phases of fetal development. In higher animals, vitamin A is essential for vision, reproduction, and maintenance of differentiated epithelia and mucus secretion (42, 48). *Trans*–retinoic acid (TRA) shares only some of these functions, being unable to support vision and reproduction. Thus, animals maintained on TRA as their only source of vitamin A are both blind and sterile. In lung carcinogenesis, one of the early observations demonstrated that bronchial metaplasia could be induced in tracheal hamster epithelium by vitamin A deprivation or benzopyrene instillation (59). The effect of both is preventable by retinol administration (59).

Retinol, as well as other retinoids, clinically shows a definite anticancer activity in different epithelial tumors, and particularly in skin cancer. A number of studies demonstrated that these substances, administered either topically or orally, can induce a complete response (i.e., complete disappearance of tumor) in a high proportion of patients with basal cell and advanced squamous cell carcinoma (2, 55, 135).

Retinol is stored primarily in the liver (more than 90% of the total capacity), and these stores normally exceed the physiologic requirement for 1 year. Vitamin A is released into the plasma, where it binds to a specific retinol-binding protein (RBP). The process of mobilization is controlled mainly by the liver, although recycling from peripheral tissues and extravascular spaces also may occur (136). Although it has never been evaluated properly, the intestinal absorption rate for retinol in humans is commonly estimated as 50% to 60% of total dietary retinol. However, several factors may influence the pharmacology of oral vitamin A supplementation, such as the chemical structure (alcohol, esters) or the type of preparation (oily solution, emulsion). For instance, a review of human toxicity data estimated that the absorption and storage rate of emulsified retinol may be as high as 80%, compared with only 20% for oily solutions (137).

The pharmacokinetics of orally administered retinol is dominated by a strong homeostatic mechanism, which maintains a steady plasma concentration. A number of studies using low-dose vitamin A thus failed to show significant changes in plasma retinol levels. A randomized double-blind trial on 376 volunteers showed that oral administration of retinyl palmitate at moderate dosage (10,000 to 36,000 international units [IU] daily) could induce a slight but significant increase of basal retinol level, on the order of 2% for every 10,000 IU. In a pilot study of cancer patients, higher doses of oral retinol (up to 200,000 IU/m^2 daily) produced a rapid increase of retinyl palmitate plasma levels, with a mean time to peak plasma concentration of nearly 4 hours and an initial phase half-life of 2 hours (48). However, plasma retinol concentration was increased only in patients with a low initial level. Plasma half-life of retinyl palmitate, when retinol was given at the daily dose of 25,000 IU, ranged between 15 and 22 hours (138). From an experience with 307 patients who were randomized to receive either retinyl palmitate or control, Infante et al. (139) noted that a daily dose of 300,000 IU was associated with a significant increase of the mean values of plasma retinol and RBP (greater than 30% and 60%, respectively) after 12 months of treatment.

Both the bioavailability and liver toxicity may be a function of the chemical and physical properties of the various retinoids. For example, there are some notable differences between natural substances such as retinol, which is almost entirely incorporated as chylomicrons through the lymphatic system, and retinoic acid, which is transported directly to the liver through the portal system (140). Recent in vitro experiments in HL-60 cells showed growth inhibition and differentiation after exposure of leukemic cells to chylomicron retinyl esters, demonstrating the importance of extrahepatic uptake (141).

The side effects and toxicities of vitamin A often have caused concern and confusion. Despite the long-lasting concern for retinol toxicities among the medical community, the clinical data do not warrant the level of concern. In nearly 50 years of clinical use in ophthalmology and dermatology, no deaths and only a few cases of serious intoxication attributable to the so-called hypervitaminosis-A syndrome have been reported (142, 143). Most of the typical side effects, illustrated in Table 51.7, such as mucocutaneous dryness, desquamation, or cheilitis, are a common feature of any retinoid treatment when given at pharmacologic doses. Liver enlargement and an increase in serum triglycerides are observed frequently, but they invariably are transient.

With natural retinol, a daily dose of 25,000 IU has been considered appropriate for intervention trials in healthy individuals, in whom side effects must be absent or negligible. For adjuvant trials in cancer patients, a much higher dose can be selected, based on efficacy data derived from other diseases (144–147).

In contrast to natural retinol, prolonged high-dose (300,000 IU/day) use of emulsified retinyl palmitate in a prospective randomized trial (148) failed to demonstrate a significant effect on liver function or objective liver toxicity. Average values of liver enzymes (serum glutamic–oxaloacetic transaminase (SGOT) and glutamyl transpeptidase (GPT), measured every month up to 24 months of treatment, were nearly identical in randomized controls and treated individuals. Only a limited proportion of patients (10% to 20%) showed serum levels above the normal range in both groups. In contrast, retinyl palmitate caused a remarkable increase in the serum triglycerides. This increase reached statistical significance at 12 months of treatment, and the average values increased more than 60% from the baseline levels. Such a significant increase of serum triglyceride levels was not associated with clinical symptoms or objective signs of cardiovascular damage, and the values spontaneously reverted to normal soon after completion of treatment. The cholesterol levels were modified less strikingly, and the differences in mean values were not significant between the treated and control groups. Renal function tests, fasting glucose levels, hemoglobin values, and red blood cell, white blood cell, and lymphocyte counts were not affected by retinyl palmitate administration. The clinical safety of prolonged (1 to 2 years) administration of high-dose emulsified retinol palmitate was confirmed by a second randomized clinical trial (149).

Both natural retinol and synthetic retinoids are potent teratogens. This toxicity poses particular problems for chemoprevention programs in which relatively young people are considered for inclusion. Therefore, in women of child-bearing age, a pregnancy test is required before treatment, and adequate contraceptive measures should be maintained throughout the intervention phase. The risk of fetal malformation appears to be highest in the first trimester and quite low in the third trimester (150–152).

ISOTRETINOIN (13-CIS-RETINOIC ACID)

Several commercial laboratories have attempted to produce synthetic vitamin A analogs with higher, or more selective, activity and lower toxicity. In this process, more than 1500 new retinoids have been produced and tested biologically (153). Two biologic assays were used to test the different retinoids: the in vitro reversal of tracheal keratinization on hamsters raised on a vitamin A deficient diet and the in vivo ability to reverse skin papillomas in mice (58, 154). Of the few compounds with a high therapeutic index, only 13-cis-retinoic acid (13-CRA) and etretinate ultimately underwent thorough clinical investigation. Randomized placebo-controlled trials have proven that 13-CRA is an effective drug, but the toxicologic profile in humans was less favorable than that anticipated from the animal data (155–157).

Considerable enthusiasm for chemoprevention in the upper aerodigestive tract has been generated by studies of premalignant lesions such as oral leukoplakia. In the last decade, oral leukoplakia has represented the most reliable clinical model to test the efficacy of chemopreventive agents in the short term. In this field, the trials conducted at the M. D. Anderson Cancer Center are of fundamental importance because of the strict methodologic criteria applied, including randomized, double-blind trials, pathologic assessment of prerandomization status, and a complete assessment of response to treatment. The first study demonstrated that 13-CRA (1 to 2 mg/kg daily for 3 months) could achieve major regression of leukoplakia in 67% of patients (compared with 10% for placebo), but relapse occurred in most cases soon after treatment stopped

TABLE 51.7. Typical Adverse Effects of the Retinoids[a]

Skin/mucous membranes
  Skin dryness, itching, peeling
  Genital excoriations
  Angular cheilitis, lip cracking
Central nervous system
  Headache
  Intracranial hypertension ("pseudotumor cerebri")
Metabolic
  Hypertriglyceridemia
  Hypercholesterolemia
  Hypercalcemia
Gastrointestinal
  Hepatic toxicity (increased SGOT, alkaline phosphatase, bilirubin)
  Pancreatitis

Abbreviation. SGOT, serum glutamic–oxaloacetic transaminase.
[a] This list does not include those side effects (hematologic, cardiovascular, pulmonary) that occur only in patients treated for acute myelocytic leukemias.

(158). A further study of isotretinoin was designed to overcome the problems of the significant toxicities and the high relapse rate. In this trial, patients received an induction treatment with high-dose isotretinoin (1.5 mg/kg/day) for a 3-month period and then were randomized to a 9-month maintenance therapy with either low-dose isotretinoin (0.5 mg/kg/day) or beta carotene (30 mg/day). This study showed that low-dose isotretinoin was more effective than beta carotene in maintaining clinical/histologic remission (relapse rate of 6% versus 58%, respectively), thus demonstrating that low-dose isotretinoin was an effective and well-tolerated maintenance therapy for oral premalignancy (133).

The synthetic retinoids include a highly heterogeneous group of substances with peculiar properties in terms of absorption, metabolism, pharmacokinetics, bioavailability, and toxicity. Table 51.8 compares the plasma elimination half-lives of the most important retinoids employed in chemoprevention (13-CRA, all-*trans*–retinoic acid [ATRA], and *N*-(4-hyroxyphenyl) retinamide [4-HPR]) or in dermatology (159–163).

After a single oral dose of 0.5 mg/kg of 13-CRA, the mean peak plasma concentration was 250 ng/mL (range, 0 to 740), and the time to peak plasma concentration was 4 hours (range, 2 to 6 hr). After taking 4 mg/kg by mouth, the mean peak plasma concentration was 1160 ng/mL (range, 828 to 1950), and the time to peak plasma concentration was 3 hours (range, 1.5 to 6 hr) (164). A marked difference in gastrointestinal absorption probably was responsible for the variation of peak plasma levels (up to 10-fold) in patients receiving the same dose (165). A reported lag time of up to 2 hours before the onset of intestinal absorption, as well as marked secondary and tertiary concentration peaks, was consistent with an enterohepatic circulation of 13-CRA (166). The pharmacokinetics of multiple doses of 13-CRA were tested in 10 patients treated with 40 mg daily for 25 days (160). Peak plasma concentrations after 25 days of treatment were similar to those observed after the first dose (310 ± 184 ng/mL versus 262 ± 139 ng/mL), the time to peak plasma levels was 3.1 versus 2.9 hours, and the half-life was 9.2 versus 10.4 hours (Table 51.8). Conversely, the concentration of the metabolite 13-*cis*-4-oxo-retinoic acid showed a tendency to accumulate over time. The mean ratio of the area under the curve (AUC) of 13-*cis*-4-oxo-retinoic acid and 13-CRA rose from 3.4 ± 1 to 5.1 ± 1, and the half-life of the metabolite was 24.5 hours (range, 16.5 to 49.5). Overall, the available data suggest that plasma levels of 13-CRA were relatively stable after multiple doses, and that the long-term pharmacokinetic profile can be predicted from single-dose data.

Although recent animal data have demonstrated that oral administration of many retinoids, including 13-CRA, causes a significant dose dependent reduction of plasma retinol levels (167), clinical data on 13-CRA are not conclusive. Some authors have reported no effect on plasma retinol levels after relatively high oral doses, ranging from 3 mg/kg daily to 5 mg/kg daily (165). Others have reported plasma retinol concentrations below the expected normal range in healthy individuals after 1 to 28 days of treatment (164). However, baseline levels were not evaluated in these patients, and the lower plasma retinol concentrations may well be attributable to the advanced neoplastic status rather than to 13-CRA administration.

Dry skin, itching, flaking, nasal stuffiness, xerostomia, and cheilitis are observed frequently with the use of 13-CRA. These reactions usually can be managed with topical lubricants and moisturizing agents; however, some patients may require a decrease in the drug dose.

Bone pain may occur in patients receiving 13-CRA, and long-term treatment has been associated with formation of hyperostosis (bone spurs), particularly on the vertebral bodies and in the calcaneus (168, 169). Hypercalcemia also has been reported occasionally (170, 171). Hypertriglyceridemia has been reported with 13-CRA, but cardiovascular consequences have not yet been described. Whether such complications will become evident with more exposure in cancer chemoprevention remains to be seen. Occasionally, the hepatic toxicity manifested by a transient increase in serum transaminases, alkaline phosphatase, or bilirubin during the initial period of administration may persist for a few weeks after the drugs have been discontinued, but it usually is readily reversible.

Overall, the degree of toxicity observed in patients receiving 13-CRA at full dosage (1 mg/kg daily) in chemoprevention studies produced toxicities such

TABLE 51.8. Plasma Elimination Half-Lives of Various Retinoids Administered Orally to Humans

	HALF-LIFE (HR)	REFERENCE NO.
All-*trans*-retinoic acid (ATRA)	0.8 ± 0, 1	159
13-*cis*-retinoic acid (13-CRA)	10 (6.7–36.5)	160
Fenretinide (4-HPR)	27 ± 4	161
Acitrecin	50 (36–96)	162
Etretinate	2500[a]	163

[a] More than 120 days.

that most patients did not tolerate the treatment for more than 6 months (158).

FENRETINIDE

Another synthetic retinoid of potential interest for lung cancer prevention is fenretinide (4-HPR). The research on 4-HPR initially focused on breast cancer chemoprevention because of the selective concentration of this compound in the mammary gland tissue of treated animals (40) and its ability to inhibit chemically induced mammary carcinoma in rats (172). Moreover, 4-HPR appeared to be safer than other retinoids with respect to genotoxicity (173).

Although clinical data on the efficacy of 4-HPR against cancer or premalignant diseases are still lacking, encouraging results have been observed in oral leukoplakia. In a study by Chiesa et al. (174) that was conducted in Milan, patients were randomized to placebo or 4-HPR (200 mg/day for 1 year) after surgical excision of leukoplakia with the aim of preventing oral cancer and new lesions or recurrence of leukoplakia. Preliminary results showed a significant reduction in the incidence of new leukoplakia lesions, and a recent update confirmed the preliminary results. During the year of treatment, 14 patients had recurrences (9 in the control group and 5 in the 4-HPR group), and 10 patients developed new lesions (9 in the control group and 1 in the 4-HPR group). The rate of recurrence and new lesions among patients who completed the 1 year of treatment was 6% in the 4-HPR group and 30% in the control group ($P=.009$). On the basis of such experimental evidence, some randomized clinical trials were activated at the National Cancer Institute of Milan in 1987 on patients with prior breast or skin cancer, with the aim of preventing a new primary tumor.

The clinical activity of 4-HPR in superficial bladder cancer has recently been investigated in a phase IIa trial using DNA flow cytometry as an intermediate endpoint (175). A significant reduction in the hyperdiploid fraction of bladder-washed cells was observed in patients treated with 4-HPR. A randomized trial using DNA flow cytometry as a surrogate endpoint is ongoing.

The pharmacokinetics of 4-HPR have been studied in healthy volunteers and in cancer patients (176, 177). After oral administration, maximum blood concentrations of 4-HPR occurred at between 3 and 4 hours, whereas the concentrations of its main metabolite, N-(4-methoxyphenyl)retinamide (4-MPR) occurred between 8 and 12 hours. The bioavailability of 4-HPR, as with that of other retinoids, has been shown to be enhanced by administering it with food and to be influenced by the meal's composition (177). After single oral doses of 25, 75, 150, 300, 500, and 600 mg in healthy subjects, a linear relationship between the dose and the maximum concentration and between the dose and the AUC was found for both 4-HPR and 4-MPR (178). In these subjects the mean elimination half-life of 4-HPR was 16 to 20 hours, and the half-life of 4-MPR was 22 hours. Similar values were found among cancer patients treated with a single oral dose of 300 mg of 4-HPR (176), and the half-lives of 4–HPR and of 4-MPR were 13.7 and 23 hours, respectively. After multiple daily doses of 150 and 300 mg for 28 days, no significant differences in the pharmacokinetics of 4-HPR between the first and the last dose were found, and the half-life was 27.2 hours. 4-MPR appeared to accumulate, because the AUC after multiple dosing was higher than after single dosing; its half-life was 45.1 hours. No unchanged compound, 4-MPR, or conjugates were detected in urine (178), suggesting another route of excretion such as the biliary system.

4-HPR pharmacokinetics were monitored during long-term administration in patients with breast cancer who participated in the phase I study of this drug (179) and in women who were treated for 5 years in an ongoing phase III trial (161). After 5 months of daily treatment with 100-, 200- and 300-mg/day doses, a linear relationship was found between the administered dose and the plasma concentrations of both 4-HPR and 4-MPR (179). The daily administration of a dose of 200 mg for 5 years resulted in 4-HPR plasma concentrations of approximately 1 μmol/L, which remained steady for the whole period (161). The concentrations of 4-MPR, similar to those of the parent drug, increased slightly but significantly during the first 35 months and declined thereafter to levels that were not significantly different from those at 5 months. After treatment for 5 years, the half-lives of 4-HPR and 4-MPR were 27 and 54 hours, respectively, similar to those found after 28 daily treatments. The findings of constant concentrations and of constant half-lives suggest that the pharmacokinetics of this retinoid do not change during long-term treatment. In marked contrast, continuous administration of ATRA in patients with acute promyelocytic leukemia (APL) resulted in progressive reduction in plasma drug levels (159).

Long-term elimination after 5 years of continuous treatment with 4-HPR also has been investigated (161). At 6 and 12 months after discontinuation of the drug, the concentrations of 4-HPR were at the limit of detectability (0.01 μmol/L), whereas those of 4-MPR were 5 times higher.

A relevant pharmacologic effect of 4-HPR, reported in rats (180) and in humans (176, 179, 181), is the rapid decrease in the plasma concentrations of both retinol and its plasma transport protein RBP. This reduction, which is reversible, occurs early, after a single dose, and is proportional to the dose administered (179). This effect, and its dose dependency, is associated with impaired dark adaptation, a side effect reported in 4-HPR–treated patients (182–186). To avoid this side effect, patients on the ongoing prevention trials had 3-day treatment interruptions at the end of each month to increase plasma retinol concentrations, thus allowing storage of retinol in the retina (187). During daily treatment with 200 mg of 4-HPR, baseline retinol levels were reduced by 71%; after the 3-day drug interruption, all patients recovered and the mean reduction was only 38% (161). Although plasma retinol steadily declined during the 5 years of continuous treatment, the levels returned to baseline 1 month after discontinuation of treatment (161).

One of the advantages of 4-HPR is its tolerability compared with other retinoids. No acute or severe toxicities were observed in a randomized phase II study using different doses (185). A similar lack of toxicities occurred with long-term, daily, oral administration of 200 mg of 4-HPR for 42 months (188). Dermatologic and metabolic changes were relatively uncommon (fewer than 5%), and no liver function abnormalities were observed (189). Diminished dark adaptation was more common, however. Estimates of the frequency of this side effect using the Goldmann-Weekers dark-adaptometry test suggested an incidence of 23% mild and 26% moderate alterations in dark adaptation associated with the drug-induced decrease of plasma retinol below the threshold levels of 160 and 100 ng/mL, respectively (175). However, nearly 50% of the treated patients who had altered dark adaptometry results were asymptomatic, leaving the clinical significance of these findings uncertain. In addition, the alterations of dark adaptometry were reversed promptly upon discontinuation of the drug. Interestingly, treatment duration did not seem to correlate with alterations of either dark adaptometry or electroretinography, indicating that there probably are no cumulative effects of 4-HPR administration upon retinal function. This conclusion is consistent with a trend toward a less-pronounced decrease of plasma retinol with increasing time of treatment. Toxicity of the ocular surface, frequently observed with administration of natural and synthetic retinoids, is negligible in 4-HPR–treated patients (175).

BETA CAROTENE

Natural antioxidants, such as beta carotene and α-tocopherol (vitamin E), are attractive as lung cancer preventive agents because of their tolerability and lack of clinical side effects. Clinical data on the efficacy of beta carotene presently are limited to the model of oral leukoplakia, in which beta carotene has shown better tolerability but lower activity than retinol or 13-CRA (133, 190, 191). A recent randomized study of oral leukoplakia comparing beta carotene (50 mg daily) plus vitamin A (25,000 IU) daily for 3 years with 13-CRA (at 0.5 mg daily) for 1 year and then 0.25 mg daily for 2 years has been initiated at M. D. Anderson Cancer Center (192).

Phase I studies of the pharmacokinetics of beta carotene have confirmed that only a limited fraction (10% to 30%) of the substance is absorbed from the intestine after a single oral dose and that a large variability exists between individuals (193). Absorption may be improved by multiple daily fractions and a high-fat diet. Nonetheless, the data obtained from randomized trials on chemoprevention of skin, colon, and lung cancers demonstrate a significant level of bioavailability with prolonged administration. In fact, the serum levels of beta carotene increased from 3-fold to 16-fold over baseline levels with single oral doses of 25 to 50 mg daily (6, 194).

Beta carotene is nontoxic even if administered at very high doses. The main side effect is represented by moderate yellowing of the skin (carotenodermia). The initial suggestions that chronic oral administration of beta carotene could induce a significant reduction of plasma levels of vitamin E (195) and vitamin K dependent blood coagulation factors (196) have not been confirmed by the results of large-scale prospective trials.

α-TOCOPHEROL

Similar to the situation for beta carotene, clinical data on the efficacy of α-tocopherol are still limited. A recent study demonstrated that vitamin E administration could induce regression of oral leukoplakia or dysplasia (197). Of 43 evaluable patients treated with α-tocopherol (400 IU, twice daily for 24 weeks), 20 (46%) had clinical responses, and 9 (21%) had histologic responses.

α-Tocopherol was tested in a large phase III chemoprevention trial conducted in the Chinese province of Lin Xian. This trial enrolled 29,584 residents of an area at high risk for esophageal cancer to assess the effect of α-tocopherol, beta carotene, and selenium. After a median treatment of 5 years, the combination achieved a 42% reduction in the risk of esophageal cancer and a significant reduction of mortality (134).

After oral administration, a fraction (25%) of the α-tocopherol is absorbed through the lymphatic route and circulates bound to low-density lipoproteins. Pharmacokinetics after a single oral dose showed a peak of plasma levels at 12 to 15 hours. With long-term oral administration, as used in the randomized trials, plasma levels of α-tocopherol increased approximately 50% (from 14 to 20 mg/L) using daily doses of 50 to 400 mg (6, 194).

N-ACETYLCYSTEINE

NAC has been used for nearly 30 years as a mucolytic agent in the treatment of chronic obstructive pulmonary disease (COPD). In recent years, a few randomized studies have demonstrated a significant reduction in the frequency of acute bronchitis, superimposed viral infections, and the progression of pulmonary damage (198, 199). However, the distinct cytoprotective effect of NAC against several toxic agents cannot be explained by its mucolytic activity. In fact, NAC given at high doses is the preferred antidote for the hepatorenal toxicity seen in acute acetaminophen (paracetamol) poisoning (200, 201). Such a clinical experience, combined with the data on experimental cancer prevention, strongly supported a thorough investigation of NAC in phase III chemoprevention trials.

In the first randomized trial (EUROSCAN), the daily dose of 600 mg had been considered adequate for a 2-year intervention plan, which also included high-dose retinol palmytate administration (149). However, preclinical data on the inhibition of premalignant lung lesions in mice suggest that higher doses might be required for chemoprevention in humans.

NAC is fully and rapidly absorbed after oral administration, metabolized to glutathione and L-cysteine, and excreted in the urine (202). Peak plasma concentration is reached in 1 to 2 hours. A phase I study showed that a daily dose of 800 mg/m^2 was very well tolerated for 6 months of treatment, and that a daily dose of 1600 mg/m^2 for 4 weeks produced only minimal side effects. In the EUROSCAN trial (149), more than 1200 patients have been treated with NAC, alone or in combination with vitamin A. The tolerability has been excellent throughout the treatment period of 2 years, with only transient gastrointestinal side effects seen in less than 10% of patients.

OLTIPRAZ

Clinical data on the efficacy of oltipraz as a chemopreventive agent remain unavailable. Information on the pharmacology and safety of oltipraz was based on the clinical experience derived from the treatment of schistosomiasis.

After a single oral dose of 1 to 3 mg/kg biweekly, peak serum concentrations were achieved in 2.5 to 4 hours, with a half-life of only 5 hours (203). With daily chronic administration of 125 and 250 mg for 6 months, the main toxicities included gastrointestinal symptoms (nausea, diarrhea, flatulence, gastric pain), fingertip pain, and fingernail discoloration (106, 204). Paresthesias, phototoxicity, and heat intolerance also were described. Further studies are in progress to assess the optimal dose and duration, but it appears that 125 mg daily represents the maximum tolerated dose for chronic administration.

RANDOMIZED CLINICAL TRIALS

PRIMARY CHEMOPREVENTION IN HEALTHY INDIVIDUALS

The NCI funded randomized trials for lung cancer chemoprevention are summarized in Table 51.9 (119). Most of these studies are ongoing, but the Finnish trial has been completed and the results published in 1994 (6). This study, conducted in cooperation with the National Public Health Institute of Finland, tested the effects of dietary supplementation with beta carotene (20 mg/day) and α-tocopherol (vitamin E, 50 mg/day) in a population of heavy smokers (205). The study accrued 29,133 men, aged 50 to 69, randomized in a 2 × 2 factorial design into four separate treatment groups: placebo, beta carotene, vitamin E, or both agents. The factorial design was selected to evaluate the effect of the two interventions in a single large trial. Unfortunately, this trial did not show any protective effect of either α-tocopherol or beta carotene. As summarized in Table 51.10, α-tocopherol supplementation failed to reduce the incidence and mortality for lung cancer as well as for the other sites. A reduction (34%) in prostate cancer incidence was noted (99 versus 151); however, the clinical significance remains uncertain. In contrast, beta carotene supplementation was associated with a significant increase in lung cancer incidence (56.3% versus 47.5%) and mortality (35.6% versus 30.8%). Mortality from ischemic heart disease also was higher in the group receiving beta carotene (77.1% versus 68.9%), further confounding the overall excess in mortality of 8%. The detrimental effect of beta carotene in this study remains difficult to explain and needs further investigation.

The Finnish trial demonstrated that dietary supplementation with low doses of the two agents caused a consistent increase in the serum levels of the agents, but it produced no reduction in cancer incidence among active smokers. The study was methodologi-

TABLE 51.9. Randomized Trials on Primary Lung Cancer Chemoprevention

INVESTIGATOR	POPULATION	AGENT	DOSE	NO. OF SUBJECTS	ENDPOINT
Hennekens (Harvard)	Male physicians 40–84 yr	Beta carotene	50 mg alt days	22,071	Epithelial cancer, mortality
Buring (Harvard)	Female nurses ≥45 yr	Beta carotene Aspirin Vitamin E	50 mg qd 100 mg qd 500 IU qd	40,000	Epithelial cancer, cardiovascular mortality
Albanes (Finland)	Smokers 50–69 yr	Beta carotene Vitamin E	20 mg qd 50 mg qd	29,133	Lung cancer, mortality
Goodman (Seattle)	Smokers 50–69 yr	Beta carotene Retinol	30 mg qd 25,000 IU qd	13,629	Lung cancer
Omenn (Seattle)	Asbestos workers, smokers, 45–69 yr	Beta carotene Retinol	30 mg qd 25,000 IU qd	4,277	Lung cancer
Mclarty (Tyler)	Asbestos workers	Beta carotene Retinol	50 mg qd 25,000 IU qd	755	Lung cancer
Xuan (China)	Tin miners	Retinol Beta carotene Vitamin E Selenium	25,000 IU qd 50 mg qd 800 IU qd 400 μg qd	7,000	Lung cancer

Modified from Greenwald P, Sondik E, Lynch BS. Diet and chemoprevention in NCI's research strategy to achieve national cancer control objectives. Ann Rev Public Health 1986;7:767–791.

TABLE 51.10. Results of the Finnish Trial on Lung Cancer Chemoprevention in Heavy Smokers

	α-TOCOPHEROL		NO α-TOCOPHEROL	
	NO. OF CASES	MORTALITY[a]	NO. OF CASES	MORTALITY[a]
Lung cancer	433	33.6	443	32.8
Other cancers	696	34.7	719	30.4
Ischemic heart deaths	602	71.0	637	75.0
Other cardiovascular deaths	251	29.6	233	27.7
Other causes of death	366	43.2	361	42.5

	BETA CAROTENE		NO BETA CAROTENE	
	NO. OF CASES	MORTALITY[a]	NO. OF CASES	MORTALITY[a]
Lung cancer	474	35.6	402	30.8
Other cancers	719	33.1	696	32.0
Ischemic heart deaths	653	77.1	586	68.9
Other cardiovascular deaths	252	29.8	232	27.3
Other causes of death	363	42.8	364	42.8

Note. U.S. National Cancer Institute–National Public Health Institute of Finland study involving 29,133 patients.
Modified from The Alpha-Tocopherol, Beta-Carotene Cancer Prevention Control Group. The effect of vitamin E and beta-carotene on the incidence of lung cancer and other cancers in male smokers. N Engl J Med 1994;330:1029–1035.
[a]Mortality per 10,000 person-years.

cally excellent with an adequate number of subjects, a double-blind design, long-term follow-up, and a high (92%) proportion of pathologically confirmed tumors. Nevertheless, because only active smokers were eligible for the trial, and because the vast majority of them (79%) continued to smoke throughout the trial, the interpretation of the results remains a major problem. In fact, tobacco smoking is such an overwhelming cancer promoter that concurrent dietary supplementation is unlikely to produce any measurable effect on lung cancer incidence. These data suggest that lung cancer chemoprevention programs should be restricted to former smokers, and the effort for smokers should be focused on smoking cessation.

Another large study on 22,000 male physicians, aged 40 to 84, is currently ongoing in the United States, using alternating beta carotene (50 mg on alternate days) and aspirin (325 mg on alternate days). This study is investigating a potential preventive effect against cancer and myocardial infarctions (206). This trial already has demonstrated a significant reduction in the incidence of myocardial infarction in the aspirin arm, but no difference in mortality has yet been demonstrated. Another similar trial, "The Women's Health Study," is expected to randomize 40,000 female nurses, aged 50 and older, to beta carotene, vitamin E, or aspirin. Four other trials are testing chemoprevention with low-dose beta carotene and retinol in individuals at high risk because of exposure to asbestos (Table 51.10).

TREATMENT OF PRECANCEROUS LESIONS

Two randomized trials in volunteers with bronchial metaplasia who are heavy smokers have been conducted to date. The first study tested the efficacy of etretinate on changes in the sputum cytology in heavy smokers. After 6 months of treatment, the degree of atypia measured in the sputum from etretinate-treated subjects was similar to that observed in the placebo group (207). In the second trial, conducted at the M. D. Anderson Cancer Center, 87 chronic smokers with bronchial dysplasia and/or a metaplasia index greater than 15%, as assessed by multiple bronchoscopic biopsies (six sites), were randomized to receive either 13-CRA (1 mg/kg/day) or placebo. Bronchoscopic reevaluation at 6 months, available for 67 subjects, showed a similar decrease in the frequency of squamous metaplasia in both arms (55% versus 59%), being most pronounced in those who had stopped smoking (208). This study, although negative in terms of treatment efficacy, provided essential information on the natural history of bronchial metaplasia.

PREVENTION OF SECOND PRIMARY TUMORS

A number of trials are currently being conducted on patients with resected non–small cell lung cancer (NSCLC) with the intent of preventing new primary malignancies (Table 51.11).

The pioneer study in this field was conducted by Hong and colleagues (3) in 103 patients with squamous cell carcinoma of the head and neck. After stratification by tumor site (oral cavity, oropharynx, hypopharynx, or larynx) and prior treatment (surgery, radiation, combined), patients were randomized to receive either isotretinoin (50 to 100 mg/m^2/day) or placebo for 12 months. At a median follow-up of 32 months, the first analysis showed that retinoid treatment significantly reduced the incidence of second primary tumors (3). Only 2 of the patients (4%) on the retinoid arm developed second primary tumors, whereas 12 patients (24%) on the placebo arm developed secondary tumors ($P = .005$). Most second primary tumors (13 of 14 [93%]) occurred in the head and neck, esophagus, or lung. Treatment-related toxicity was significant, and 33% (16 of 49) of the isotretinoin patients could not complete the 12-month schedule.

A recent update of this study, with 54 months of median follow-up, continued to show the reduction in second primary tumors (4). Seven patients (14%) on the retinoid arm and 16 patients (31%) on the placebo arm developed second primary tumors, but in this report the level of significance was smaller ($P = .04$) (4).

The first randomized clinical trial among lung cancer patients after complete resection was started in 1985 at the National Cancer Institute of Milan. Patients with pathologic stage (T1-T2, N0, M0) NSCLC were eligible for this study. Patients were assigned randomly to receive either vitamin A (oral 300,000 IU daily for 12 to 24 months) or no treatment. Patient entries were stratified according to the treatment center, cell type (squamous versus nonsquamous), and previous cancer at another site (absent versus cured). Endpoints of this study were relapse of prior cancer, occurrence of new primary cancers, and survival. The accrual was closed in 1989 with 307 evaluable patients and a median follow-up of 46 months. The results are summarized in Table 51.12. In the treatment arm, 56 (37%) patients developed either recurrence or new primary tumors, whereas 75 (48%) of the patients in the control arm developed new primary tumors (5). Eighteen patients (12%) developed a second primary tumor in the treated group, and 29 patients developed 33 second primary tumors in the control group. The distribution of second primary tumors is shown by site in Figure 51.4. The time to relapse or to the occurrence of a new primary (disease free interval) is illustrated in Figure 51.5. The estimated disease free survival at 5 years was 64% versus 51% in favor of the treatment arm. This difference approached statistical significance ($P=.054$ by log rank test) and reached a P value of .038 when adjusted for primary tumor classification by Cox regression analysis. For tobacco-related tumors, a significant difference in the amount of time to the development of new primary tumors was observed in favor of treatment ($P=.045$, log rank test). The estimated propor-

TABLE 51.11. Randomized Trials on Secondary Lung Cancer Chemoprevention

INVESTIGATOR	POPULATION	AGENT	DOSE	NO. OF SUBJECTS	ENDPOINT
Resected lung cancer					
Intergroup (USA)	NSCLC stage I	13-CRA	30 mg qd	600	Second primary tumors
EUROSCAN (Europe)	NSCLC stage I-III	Retinyl palmitate N-acetyl-cysteine	300,000 IU qd 600 mg qd	2,595[a]	Second primary tumors, survival
NCI (planned)	Resected NSCLC	Oltipraz	125 mg qd	100	Intermediate markers
NCI (planned)	NSCLC stage I	4-HPR	200 mg qd	100	Intermediate markers
NCI (planned)	NSCLC stage I	4-HPR + Oltipraz		100	To be defined
Prior respiratory cancer + bronchial preneoplasia					
Hong (Houston)	Bronchial metaplasia + prior cancer	4-HPR	200 mg qd	100	Metaplasia, dysplasia, intermediate markers
NCI (planned)	Chronic smokers + prior cancer	N-acetyl-cysteine	1,400 mg qd	100	Metaplasia, dysplasia, intermediate markers

Abbreviations. NSCLC, non–small cell lung cancer; 13-CRA, 13-cis-retinoic acid; 4-HPR, N-(4-hydroxylphenyl)retinamide; NCI, U.S. National Cancer Institute.
[a]Including patients with head and neck cancer.

TABLE 51.12. Results of the First Italian Trial on Lung Cancer Chemoprevention in Stage I Non–Small Cell Lung Cancer

	RETINOL P[a] (%)	CONTROL (%)
All cancer failures	56 (37)	75 (48)
Recurrence	38 (25)	46 (29)
Locoregional	15 (10)	11 (7)
Distant	23 (15)	35 (22)
New primary tumor	18 (12)	29 (18)
Deaths	55 (37)	64 (41)
Recurrence	37 (25)	39 (25)
New primary tumor	7 (5)	14 (9)
Other cause	11 (7)	11 (7)

Note. National Cancer Institute of Milan study involving 307 patients. Modified from Pastorino U, Infante I, Maioli M, et al. Adjuvant treatment of stage I lung cancer with high dose vitamin A.
[a]Dosage, 300,000 IU/day.

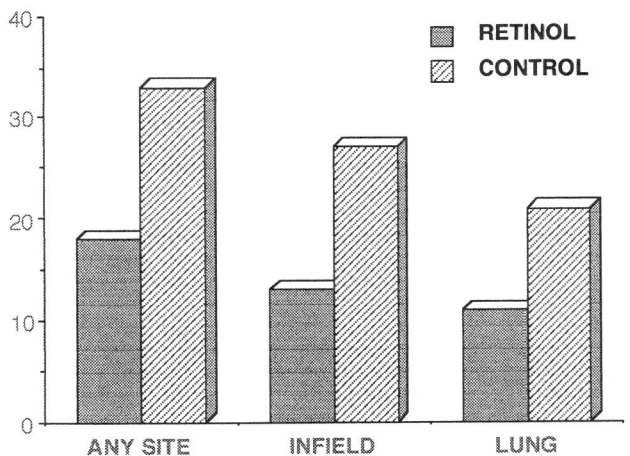

FIGURE 51.4. Results of the randomized trial on lung cancer chemoprevention conducted at the National Cancer Institute of Milan. Distribution of second primary tumors by site: overall, in the chemoprevention field, and in the lung only.

tion who were free of a new primary tumor was 89% versus 80% ($P = .045$). This study (5) demonstrated that high-dose vitamin A was effective in reducing the number of new primary malignancies related to tobacco consumption and may have improved the disease free interval for patients curatively resected for stage I lung cancer. In this trial, the absence of improvement in the overall survival may be related partially to non–cancer-related mortality (identical in the two arms), as well as to effective salvage treatments. In fact, salvage surgery for new primary tumors was applied in 44% of cases (8 of 18) in the retinol arm and in 69% in the control arm (20 of 29). Thus, the potential for improved survival was obscured by the effective salvage treatments. In terms of side effects and toxicities, high-dose vitamin A proved to be a relatively safe treatment that was well tolerated for a period of 1 to 2 years, and it produced an overall compliance rate of nearly 80%. This study needs larger scale corroboration and further exploration.

Based on the experience accumulated in the first lung cancer trials, a new European cooperative study was set up in 1988 as a joint venture of the European

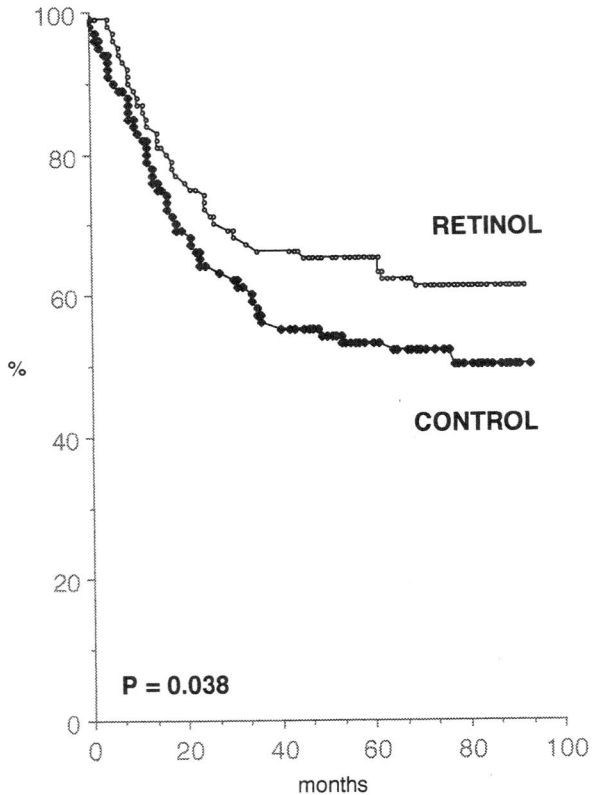

FIGURE 51.5. Time to relapse and/or new primary cancer (disease free interval) in the Milan trial. Results of multivariate analysis with Cox regression model ($P=.038$).

Organization for Research and Treatment of Cancer (EORTC) Lung Cancer and Head and Neck Cancer Cooperative Groups (149) to test the combination of two agents with different preventive properties: retinol palmitate and NAC. This EUROSCAN study was designed to prevent second primary tumors in patients treated for upper aerodigestive cancers. Eligible patients were those with prior treatment for squamous cancer of the larynx (TIS, T1-3, N0-1), squamous cancer of the oral cavity (T1-2, N0-1), or NSCLC (pT1-2, N0-1, and T3 N0). Four treatment arms were planned in a 2 × 2 factorial design: (a) retinol palmitate and NAC; (b) retinol palmitate; (c) NAC; (d) no treatment. Randomization took place after surgery or after completion of radiotherapy, without any fixed time limit. Stratification was by sex, prior or concurrent chemotherapy, squamous versus nonsquamous histology (lung cancer) supraglottic or glottic location of laryngeal cancer, and classification as a smoker or never smoker. Retinol palmitate was administered at a daily oral dose of 300,000 IU for the first 12 months, followed by 150,000 IU for 12 additional months; NAC was given at a daily dose of 600 mg for 2 years. Minimal follow-up included physical examination every 3 months and chest radiographs every 6 months. Endpoints of this study are relapse of prior cancer, occurrence of new primary cancers, and survival. The study was closed to new accrual in August 1994, when 2595 patients had been entered on the trial. The preliminary analysis is planned for the end of 1996, but the follow-up is expected to be extended for up to 10 years.

The cancer cooperative groups in the United States also joined the attempt to prevent second primary tumors. A new intergroup trial was started in 1992 in resected stage I NSCLC with a plan to enter more than 600 patients treated with 30 mg/day of oral 13-CRA (209).

USE OF BIOLOGIC MARKERS IN CHEMOPREVENTION

SELECTION OF TARGET POPULATIONS

Because of the complexities of conducting population-based trials in chemoprevention, the biologic definition of high-risk risk subjects has become a crucial aspect in the development of chemoprevention research. Selection of individuals from the general population on the basis of epidemiologic risk factors, such as heavy smoking, has the disadvantage of huge sample sizes and extremely long periods of follow-up. Selection of patients cured of a prior cancer is limited by major confounding factors such as relapse of the primary cancer, comorbidity, and misclassification of relevant endpoints. To increase the cost/benefit ratio of intervention plans, specific subpopulations of very high risk individuals might be identified for each type of cancer on the basis of constitutive or acquired abnormalities, such as abnormal gene products that are detectable in target tissues. New cytogenetic and molecular biology techniques are very effective tools for detecting early changes, associated with a specific risk of cancer, in target tissues such as tracheobronchial epithelium.

Multiple cytogenetic abnormalities have been described in lung cancer, particularly deletions of the short arm of chromosomes 1, 3, 7, 8, 9, 11, and 17 (210–215). The frequency of rearrangements in each chromosome is somewhat different based on the type and source of the biologic sample (e.g., cell lines versus short-term cultures, primary tumor versus distant metastases), but some changes (such as in 3p and 17p) are quite consistent in the various studies, regardless of the type of source. Oncogene amplification or overexpression is detectable in a high proportion of cases, particularly involving the *erb*-B1 (epidermal growth factor receptor [EGFR]) in squamous carcinoma (209,

216–219), K-*ras* and *erb*-B2*neu* in adenocarcinoma (220–227) and *myc* in small cell lung cancer (SCLC) (228–231). Deletion, mutation, or altered expression of tumor suppressor genes represent the other important markers of genetic damage, mainly involving *rb-1* in SCLC (232, 233), RAR-β in NSCLC (234–237), and *p53* in all types (238–245). Such genetic changes have shown a clear-cut correlation with tumor stage and patient survival, suggesting that biologic markers are an important diagnostic factor in lung cancer (222, 246, 247).

Of particular interest for chemoprevention purposes is the fact that the genetic changes of lung cancer may be detectable, with varying degrees of severity, in bronchial dysplasia as well as in histologically normal mucosa (248, 249). Among 94 cases of resected early-stage lung cancer, normal bronchial epithelium, collected at distant sites from the primary tumor contained multiple genetic abnormalities (250). As illustrated in Table 51.13, a rearranged karyotype was detected in 23% of the evaluable cases (mainly involving chromosome 3p), overexpression of EGFR in 35%, and her2*neu* expression in 15%, whereas the overall frequency of genetic changes (any type) in the normal epithelium was 46% (30 of 65).

The occurrence of genetic changes in the normal bronchial mucosa was associated with certain cancer-related features in these patients (Table 51.14). In particular, patients with multiple tumors of the upper aerodigestive tract, either synchronous or metachronous, showed a higher frequency of genetic changes, compared with those having single or multiple tumors in other sites, which was further associated with a higher recurrence rate. These data indicate that specific genetic abnormalities may be detectable in the various stages of lung tumorigenesis, in a sequence of events that goes from normal epithelium to bronchial metaplasia and dysplasia, carcinoma in situ, early-stage invasive cancer, and onto locally invasive and metastatic lung cancer. As seen in Table 51.15 many of these genetic marker changes occur in the early (and hopefully reversible) phase of lung cancer development.

In practical terms, it is conceivable that a panel of specific markers, including chromosome deletions (3p, 7p, 17), *p53* staining, and EGFR and *neu* amplification, could be used to select future candidates for chemoprevention programs. With the actual development of immunostaining techniques for fresh- and paraffin-embedded tissues, fluorescence in situ hybridization (FISH), and polymerase chain reaction (PCR) for selective chromosome testing, even small samples collected through bronchoscopic biopsies, brushing, or sputum cytology can become suitable for screening to identify high-risk individuals.

INTERMEDIATE ENDPOINTS

Among patients cured of a prior cancer, the differential diagnosis between recurrence and a second primary tumor in the same area has been based on site (distance from prior cancer), histologic type (same versus different), and temporal sequence (time elapsed from prior cancer). All of these criteria were affected by individual cultural biases and poor specificity of standard histopathology. These assumptions have proven unreliable when using modern diagnostic tools.

A recent study testing *p53* gene mutations in 31 primary head and neck cancers and the corresponding second primary cancers of the upper aerodigestive tract demonstrated one or more mutations in 21 of 31 cases (7). All of the *p53* mutations observed in the initial tumor were different from those of the second or third primary cancers in terms of specific codon locations. This study not only supported the concept that second cancers arise as independent events but also provided evidence that *p53* mutation is an effective test for differential diagnosis of multiple primary tumors. In a recent series of five cases of multiple synchronous lung cancers that were resected with a single operation, Sozzi et al. (251) found a different pattern of genetic abnormalities in the two neoplastic foci. The observed discordance involved at least one of the following markers: 3p depletion, loss of heterozygosity (3p), *p53* mutation, or K-*ras* mutation. These data are particularly remarkable becasue they were obtained in synchronous tumors showing the same histology and occurring in the same pulmonary lobe.

The identification of appropriate intermediate endpoints is another crucial aspect of lung cancer chemoprevention research. Biologic intermediate endpoints will become essential in the near future to moni-

TABLE 51.13. Genetic Changes in Normal Bronchial Samples of Lung Cancer Patients

ABNORMALITY	NO. OF EVALUABLE PATIENTS	NO. POSITIVE	PERCENTAGE POSITIVE
Cytogenetic (any)	86	20	23
Chromosome 3p	...	13	...
Chromosome 7p	...	6	...
Chromosome 17	...	3	...
EGFR	74	26	35
HER2*neu*	74	11	15
Any changes	91	39	43

Abbreviation. EGFR, epidermal growth factor receptor.

TABLE 51.14. Frequency of Genetic Changes in Normal Bronchial Mucosa According to Selected Clinical Features (Percentage Positive)

ABNORMALITY	HISTOLOGIC TYPE		MULTIPLE TUMORS		FOLLOW-UP	
	SQUAMOUS	ADENO	YES	NO	NED	REC
Cytogenetic (any)	30	19	28	19	18	33
3p	13	16	20	8	11	21
EGFR	36	33	36	34	27	52
HER2neu	7	22	19	10	16	13
Any changes	34	56	59	30[a]	32	55[a]

Abbreviations. Adeno, adenocarcinoma; Ned, no evidence of disease; Rec, lung cancer recurrence; EGFR, epidermal growth factor receptor.
[a]$P < .05$.

TABLE 51.15. Sequence of Genetic Events in Lung Carcinogenesis

PATHOLOGIC STATUS	CHROMOSOMAL CHANGES (%)	p53 IMMUNOSTAINING	p53 MOLECULAR
Normal mucosa	Simple rearrangements (20%) (3p, 7, 11, 17)	Negative	Negative
Bronchial metaplasia	...	Spots only	Undetectable
Bronchial dysplasia	Same + 17p mutations	Positive	Mutations
In situ carcinoma	...	Positive	Mutations
Early invasive cancer	Complex karyotypes (60%) (3p, 7, 8, 9, 11, 17)	Extensively positive	Mutations
Metastatic cancer	More complex karyotypes (100%)	Extensively positive	Mutations

tor the efficacy of preventive strategies employed before the actual occurrence of invasive cancer (252). To justify systematic application, intermediate endpoints must be: (*a*) specific for the process of carcinogenesis under study, (*b*) quantitatively or qualitatively correlated with the degree of progression, (*c*) easily measurable on small specimens, with specimen acquisition being tolerable by the subject at repeated intervals, and (*d*) potentially modulated by the selective preventive agent.

Potential intermediate biomarkers under investigation may be grouped in three categories: genetic markers, differentiation markers, and proliferation markers (Table 51.16).

Counting micronuclei in exfoliated epithelial cells is one of the easiest quantitative tests of nonspecific DNA damage. In oral leukoplakia, it has been shown that the frequency of micronuclei varies according to the extent of carcinogenic exposure and that it may be reduced by chemopreventive agents (190). This marker is now under evaluation in heavy smokers with broncial metaplasia (253).

Other nonspecific morphologic features, obtained by flow cytometry analysis of the exfoliated epithelium, have been suggested as potential biomarkers of bronchial carcinogenesis. They include quantitative assessment of DNA content, nuclear/cytoplasmic ratio, abnormal DNA profile, or presence of aneuploidy. How-

TABLE 51.16. Intermediate Biomarkers in Lung Cancer Chemoprevention

Genetic markers	Micronuclei
	Ploidy and DNA content
	Chromosome deletions/translocations
	p53
	K-*ras*
	neu
Differentiation markers	Squamous markers (keratins, involucrin)
	Mucin gene expression
	Blood group antigens
Proliferation markers	Proliferating cell nuclear antigen
	Thymidine labeling index
	Retinoic acid receptors
	Epidermal growth factor receptor
	Transforming growth factor-β
	Bombesinelike peptide receptors
	Tyrosine kinase receptor
	Bcl-2
	Angiogenesis

ever, a clear relationship with the risk of lung cancer still must be proven.

Prognostic data on blood group antigens (254) and expression of other tumor-related carbohydrate markers have increased the interest in monoclonal antibodies in the screening of intermediate biomarkers.

Proliferating cell nuclear antigen (PCNA) is an intranuclear protein related to DNA polymerase-δ that dramatically increases during the S phase of the cell cycle. Antibodies against PCNA work very well on formalin-fixed, paraffin-embedded samples, and they are then suitable for large-scale retrospective analysis. In premalignant lesions of bronchial epithelium, a remarkable correlation has been shown between the frequency of PCNA positive cells and the degree of histologic progression from normal epithelium to squamous metaplasia and dysplasia (252).

Measurement of RARs in normal target tissues and premalignant lesions represents another promising way to predict and monitor the efficacy of chemoprevention with retinoids. In fact, because the expression of RARs can be induced experimentally by retinoids, receptor analysis before and during chemoprevention might be used as a specific intermediate marker of response to treatment. Expression of the mRNAs of RARs and RXRs (α, β, and γ) is presently being evaluated on lung tumor and normal bronchial samples at the Istituto Nazionale Tumori of Milan in conjunction with the M. D. Anderson Cancer Center of Houston. Preliminary data on 72 patients with NSCLC and 17 controls who underwent pulmonary resection for other diseases showed that RAR-β was expressed in 89% of normal specimens but in only 50% of bronchial dysplasias or NSCLC tumors (unpublished data). The expression of other receptors was similar among the various tissues. These data support the hypothesis that RAR-β is an early marker of lung carcinogenesis.

BIOLOGIC AGENTS

With present developments in research on the immunohistochemistry and synthesis of new cytoxic monoclonal antibodies, it appears conceivable that in the near future the approach for widespread preinvasive lesions will be topical treatment of the entire bronchial epithelium. Superficial screening of the tracheobronchial epithelium with monoclonal antibodies against specific growth factors or receptors might therefore be combined with appropriate treatment with specific reagents, thus inducing epithelial differentiation of cytolysis. Gene therapy is another potential approach to specific genetic defects of the bronchial mucosa (i.e., *p53*, K-*ras*, EGFR, *bcl-2*), using viral vectors.

Topical treatment may be applied by a closed circuit nebulizer or by targeted application under fibreroptic bronchoscopy control, thus reducing the risk of systemic side effects.

The ongoing development of molecular biology and cytogenetic techniques will provide clinicians with extremely powerful tools to identify high-risk individuals, detect precancerous or noninvasive lesions in the target field, and monitor the results of intervention. This is likely to be the ideal clinical setting in which to test new biologic agents with the aim of counteracting each of the different stages of lung carcinogenesis. From this point of view, biology-oriented chemoprevention can open new perspectives for lung cancer management and implementation of the standard morphology-oriented treatments.

REFERENCES

1. Bertram JS, Kolonel LN, Meyskens FL. Rationale and strategies for chemoprevention of cancer in humans. Cancer Res 1987;47:3012–3031.
2. Lippman SM, Kessler JF, Meyskens FL. Retinoids as preventive and therapeutic anticancer agents (part II). Cancer Treat Rep 1987;71:493–515.
3. Hong WK, Lippman JM, Itri L, et al. Prevention of second primary tumors with isotretinoin in squamous cell carcinoma of the head and neck. N Engl J Med 1990;323:795–801.
4. Benner SE, Lee JS, Goepfert H, Hong WK. Long term follow up: 13-*cis*-retinoic acid (cRA) prevention of second primary tumors (SPT) following squamous cell carcinoma of the head and neck (SCCHN) abstract. Proc Am Soc Clin Oncol 1993;12:900.
5. Pastorino U, Infante I, Maioli M, et al. Adjuvant treatment of stage I lung cancer with high dose vitamin A. J Clin Oncol 1993;11:1216–1222.
6. The Alpha-Tocopherol, Beta-Carotene Cancer Prevention Study Group. The effect of vitamin E and beta-carotene on the incidence of lung cancer and other cancers in male smokers. N Engl J Med 1994;330:1029–1035.
7. Chung KY, Mukhopadhyay T, Kim J, et al. Discordant *p53* gene mutations in primary head and neck cancers and corresponding second primary cancers of the upper aerodigestive tract. Cancer Res 1993;53:1676–1683.
8. Jensen OM, Esteve J, Moller H, Renard H. Cancer in the European Community and its member states. Eur J Cancer 1990;26:1167–1256.
9. U.S. National Cancer Institute. Smoking, tobacco, and cancer program 1985-89 status report. Washington, DC: U.S. Department of Health and Human Services, PHS NIH Publication No. 90-3107, 1990.
10. Greenwald P, Stern HR. Role of biology and prevention in aerodigestive tract cancers. J Natl Cancer Inst Monogr 1992;13:3–14.
11. Parkin DM, Pisani P, Ferlay J. Estimates of the worldwise incidence of eighteen major cancers in 1985. Int J Cancer 1993;54:594–605.
12. Bjelke E. Dietary vitamin A and human lung cancer. Int J Cancer 1975;15:561–565.
13. Mettlin C, Saxon G, Swanson M. Vitamins and lung cancer. J Natl Cancer Inst 1979;62:1435–1438.
14. MacLennan R, Da Costa J, Day NE, et al. Risk factors for lung cancer in Singapore Chinese, a population with high female incidence rates. Int J Cancer 1977;20:854–860.
15. Gregor A, Lee PN, Roe FJC, et al. Comparison of dietary histories in lung cancer cases and controls with special reference to vitamin A. Nutr Cancer 1980;2:93–97.
16. Hirayama T. Diet and cancer. Nutr Cancer 1979;1:67–80.

17. Shekelle RB, Lepper M, Liu S, et al. Dietary vitamin A and risk of cancer in the Western Electric study. Lancet 1981;2:1185–1189.
18. Kvale G, Bjelke E, Gart JJ. Dietary habits and lung cancer. Int J Cancer 1983;31:397–405.
19. Hinds MW, Kolonel LN, Hankin JH, Lee J. Dietary vitamin A, beta carotene, vitamin C and risk of lung cancer in Hawaii. Am J Epidemiol 1984;119:227–236.
20. Ziegler RG, Mason TJ, Stemhagen A, et al. Dietary carotene and vitamin A and risk of lung cancer among white men in New Jersey. J Natl Cancer Inst 1984;73:1429–1435.
21. Samet JM, Skipper BJ, Humble CG, Pathak DR. Lung cancer risk and vitamin A consumption in New Mexico. Am Rev Respir Dis 1985;131:198–202.
22. Middleton B, Byers T, Marshall J, Graham S. Dietary vitamin A and cancer—a multisite case-control study. Nutr Cancer 1986;8:107–116.
23. Pisani P, Berrino F, Macaluso M, et al. Carrots, green vegetables and lung cancer: a case-control study. Int J Epidemiol 1986;15:463–468.
24. Le Marchand L, Yoshizawa CN, Kolonel LN, et al. Vegetable consumption and lung cancer risk: a population-based case-control study in Hawaii. J Natl Cancer Inst 1989;81:1158–1164.
25. Buring JE, Hennekens CH. Retinoids and carotenoids. In: DeVita VT, Hellman S, Rosenberg SA, eds. Cancer: principles and practice of oncology. 4th ed. Philadelphia: JB Lippincott, 1993:464–474.
26. Basu TK, Donaldson D, Jenner M, et al. Plasma vitamin A in patients with bronchial carcinoma. Br J Cancer 1976;33:119–121.
27. Atukorala S, Basu TK, Dickerson JVT, et al. Vitamin A, zinc and lung cancer. Br J Cancer 1979;40:927–931.
28. Wald N, Idle M, Boreham J, Bailey A. Low serum–vitamin A and subsequent risk of cancer: preliminary results of a prospective study. Lancet 1980;2:813–816.
29. Peleg I, Heyden S, Knowles M, Hames CG. Serum retinol and risk of subsequent cancer: extension of the Evans County, Georgia, study. J Natl Cancer Inst 1984;73:1455–1458.
30. Willet WC, Polk BF, Underwood BA, et al. Relations of serum vitamins A and E and carotenoids to the risk of cancer. N Engl J Med 1984;310:430–434.
31. Stahelin HB, Rosel F, Buess E, Brubacher G. Cancer, vitamins and plasma lipids: prospective Basel study. J Natl Cancer Inst 1984;73:1463–1468.
32. Salonen T, Salonen R, Lappetelainen R, et al. Risk of cancer in relation to serum concentrations of selenium and vitamins A and E: matched case-control analysis of prospectie data. BMJ 1985;290:417–420.
33. Nomura AM, Stemmermann GN, Heilbrun LK, et al. Serum vitamin levels and risk of cancer of specific sites in men of Japanese ancestry in Hawaii. Cancer Res 1985;45:2369–2372.
34. Friedman GD, Blaner WS, Goodman DS. Serum retinol and retinol binding protein levels do not predict subsequent lung cancer. Am J Epidemiol 1986;123:781–789.
35. Menkes MS, Comstock GV, Vuilleumier JP, et al. Serum beta-carotene, vitamins A and E, selenium, and the risk of lung cancer. N Engl Med 1986;315:1250–1254.
36. Connett JE, Kuller LH, Kjelsberg MO, et al. Relationship between carotenoids and cancer. The Multiple Risk Factor Intervention Trial (MRFIT) study. Cancer 1989;64:126–134.
37. Kune GA, Kune S, Watson LF, et al. Serum levels of beta-carotene, vitamin A, and zinc in male lung cancer cases and controls. Nutr Cancer 1989;12:169–176.
38. Gridley G, McLaughlin JK, Block G, et al. Vitamin supplement use and reduced risk of oral and pharyngeal cancer. Am J Epidemiology 1992;135:1083–1092.
39. Block G, Patterson B, Subar A. Fruit, vegetables and cancer prevention: a review of the epidemiologic evidence. Nutr Cancer 1992;18:1–29.
40. Sporn MB, Newton DL. Chemoprevention of cancer with retinoids. Fed Proc 1979;38:2528–2534.
41. Lotan R. Effects of vitamin A and its analogs (retinoids) on normal and neoplastic cells. Biochim Biophys Acta 1980;605:33–91.
42. Wolbach SB, Howe PR. Tissue changes following deprivation of fat soluble A vitamin. J Exp Med 1985;42:753–777.
43. Dowling JE, Wald J. The biological function of vitamin A acid. Proc Natl Acad Sci U S A 1960;46:587–608.
44. Thompson JN, Howell JM, Pitt GAJ. Vitamin A and reproduction in rats. Proc R Soc London 1964;159:510–535.
45. Wong YC, Buck RC. An electron microscopic study of metaplasia of the rat tracheal epithelium in vitamin A deficiency. Lab Invest 1971;24:55–56.
46. Elias PM, Fritsch P, Lampe MA, et al. Effects of systemic retinoids on epidermal barrier function, proliferation, structure and glycosylation. Clin Res 1980;28:248–253.
47. Moon RC, McCormick DL, Mehta RG. Inhibition of carcinogenesis by retinoids. Cancer Res 1983;43:2469–2475.
48. Goodman DS. Vitamin A and retinoids in health and disease. N Engl J Med 1984;310:1023–1031.
49. Jetten AM, Nervi C, Vollberg TM. Control of squamous differentiation in tracheobronchial and epidermal epithelial cells: role of retinoids. J Natl Cancer Inst Monog 1992;13:93–100.
50. Chu EW, Malmgen RA. An inhibitory effect of vitamin A on the introduction of tumors of forestomach and cervix in the Syrian hamster by carcinogenic polycyclic hydrocarbons. Cancer Res 1965;25:884–895.
51. Bollag W. Prophylaxis of chemically induced benign and malignant epithelial tumors by vitamin A acid (retinoic acid). Eur J Cancer 1972;8:689–693.
52. Nettesheim P, Williams PL. The influence of vitamin A on the susceptibility of the rat lung to 3-methylcholantrene. Int J Cancer 1976;17:351–357.
53. Sporn MB, Squire RA, Brown CC, et al. 13-cis-Retinoic acid: inhibition of bladder carcinogenesis in the rat. Science 1977;195:487–489.
54. Chopra DP, Wilkoff LJ. Beta–retinoic acid inhibits and reverses testosterone induced hyperplasia in mouse prostate organ cultures. Nature 1977;265:339–341.
55. Bollag W. Therapy of chemically induced skin tumor of mice with vitamin A palmitate and vitamin A acid. Experientia 1971;27:90–92.
56. Bollag W. Prophylaxis of chemically induced epithelial tumors with an aromatic retinoic acid analog. Eur J Cancer 1975;11:721–724.
57. Lotan R, Giotta G, Nork E, Nicolson GL. Characterization of the inhibitory effects of retinoids on the vitro growth of two malignant murine melanomas. J Natl Cancer Inst 1978;60:1935–1941.
58. Verma AK, Rice HM, Shapas BG, Boutwell RK. Inhibition of 13-tetradecanoyl-phorbol-13 acetate induced ornithine decarboxylase activity in mouse epidermis by vitamin A analogs (retinoids). Cancer Res 1978;38:793–801.
59. Saffiotti U, Montesano R, Sellakumar AR, Bork S. Experimental cancer of the lung, inhibition by vitamin A of the induction of tracheobronchial metaplasia and squamous cell tumor. Cancer 1967;20:857–864.

60. Cone MV, Nettesheim P. Effects of vitamin A on 3-methylcholanthrene–induced squamous metaplasias and early tumors in the respiratory tract of rats. J Natl Cancer Inst 1973;50:1599–1606.
61. Port CD, Sporn MB, Kauffmann DG. Prevention of lung cancer in hamsters by 13-cis-retinoic acid (abstract). Proc Am Assoc Cancer Res 1975;16:21.
62. Smith DM, Rogers AE, Newberne PM. Vitamin A and benzopyrene carcinogenesis in the respiratory tract of hamsters fed a semi-synthetic diet. Cancer Res 1975;35:1485–1488.
63. Trown PW, Buck MJ, Hansen R. Inhibition of growth and regression of a transplantable rat chondrosarcoma by three retinoids. Cancer Treat Rep 1976;60:1647–1653.
64. Lotan R. Different susceptibilities of human melanoma and breast carcinoma cell lines to retinoic acid–induced growth inhibition. Cancer Res 1979;39:1014–1019.
65. Todaro GJ, DeLarco JE, Sporn MB. Retinoid blocks phenotypic cell transformation produced by sarcoma growth factor. Nature 1978;276:272–278.
66. Gensler HL, Matrisian LM, Bowden GT. Effect of retinoic acid on the late-stage promotion of transformation in JB6 mouse epidermal cells in culture. Cancer Res 1985;45:1922–1925.
67. Delia D, Aiello A, Lombardi L, et al. N(-4-hydroxyphenyl)retinamide induces apoptosis of malignant hemopoietic cell lines including those unresponsive to retinoic acid. Cancer Res 1993;53:6036–6041.
68. Tachibana K, Sone S, Tsubura E, Kishino Y. Stimulatory effect of vitamin A on tumoricidal activity of rat alveolar macrophages. Br J Cancer 1984;49:343–348.
69. Floersheim GL, Bollag W. Accelerated rejection of skin homografts by vitamin A acid. Transplantation 1972;14:564–567.
70. Dennert G. Immunostimulation by retinoic acid. In: Retinoids, differentiation and disease. Ciba Foundation Symposium 113. London: Pitman, 1985:117–131.
71. Lotan R, Clifford JL. Nuclear receptors for retinoids: mediators of retinoid effects on normal and malignant cells. Biomed Pharmacother 1990;45:145–156.
72. Leid M, Kastner P, Chambon P. Multiplicity generates diversity in the retinoic acid signaling pathways. Trends Biochem Sci 1992;17:427–433.
73. Evans RM. The steroid and thyroid hormone receptor superfamily. Science 1988;240:889–895.
74. Parker MG. Structure and function of nuclear hormone receptors. Semin Cancer Biol 1990;1:81–87.
75. de The H, Marchio A, Tiollais P, Dejean A. Differential expression and ligand regulation of the retinoic acid receptor α and β genes. EMBO J 1989;8:429–433.
76. Hu L, Gudas LJ. Cyclic AMP analogs and retinoic acid influence the expression of retinoic acid receptor α, β, and γ mRNAs in F9 teratocarcinoma cells. Mol Cell Biol 1990;10:391–396.
77. Clifford J, Petkovich M, Chambon P, Lotan R. Modulation by retinoids of mRNA levels for nuclear retinoic acid receptors in murine melanoma cells. Mol Endocrinol 1990;4:1546–1555.
78. Mattei MG, Riviere M, Krust A, et al. Chromosomal assignment of retinoic acid receptor (RAR) genes in the human, mouse, and rat genomes. Genomics 1991;10:1061–1069.
79. de The H, Vivanco-Ruiz MD, Tiollais P, et al. Identification of a retinoic acid responsive element in the retinoic acid receptor β gene. Nature 1990;343:177–180.
80. Lehman JM, Dawson MI, Hobbs PD, et al. Identification of retinoids with nuclear receptor subtype-selective activities. Cancer Res 1991;51:4804–4809.
81. De Flora S, Ramel C. Mechanisms of inhibitors of mutagenesis and carcinogenesis. Classification and overview. Mutat Res 1988;202:285–306.
82. Shamberger RJ. Relationship of selenium to cancer. I. Inhibitory effect of selenium on carcinogenesis. J Natl Cancer Inst 1976;44:931–936.
83. Horvath PM, Hip C. Synergistic effect of vitamin E and selenium on the chemoprevention of mammary carcinogenesis in rats. Cancer Res 1983;43:5335–5341.
84. Cerutti PA. Prooxidant states and tumor promotion. Science 1985;227:375–381.
85. Birt DF, Lawson TA, Julius AD, et al. Inhibition by dietary selenium of colon cancer induced in the rat by bis(2Oxopropyl) nitrosamine. Cancer Res 1982;42:4455–4459.
86. Ip C. Prophylaxis of mammary neoplasia by selenium supplementation in the initiation and promotion phases of chemical carcinogenesis. Cancer Res 1981;41:4386–4390.
87. Epstein JH. Effects of beta-carotene on ultraviolet induced cancer formation in the hairless mouse skin. Photochem Photobiol 1977;25:211–213.
88. Mathews-Roth MM. Antitumor activity of beta-carotene, cathaxanthin and phytoene. Oncology 1982;39:33–37.
89. Rettura G, Stratford F, Levenson SM, Seifter E. Prophylactic and therapeutic actions of supplemental beta-carotene in mice inoculated with CH3BA adenocarcinoma cells: lack of therapeutic action of supplemental ascorbic acid. J Natl Cancer Inst 1982;69:73–77.
90. Som S, Chatterjee M, Banerjee MR. Beta-carotene inhibition of 7,12-dimethylbenzanthracene–induced transformation of murine mammary cells in vitro. Carcinogenesis 1984;5:937–940.
91. Rousseau EJ, Davison AJ, Dunn B. Protection by β-carotene and related compounds against oxygen-mediated cytotoxicity and genotoxicity: implication for carcinogenesis and anticarcinogenesis. Free Radic Biol Med 1992;13:407–433.
92. Tsuchiya M, Scita G, Thompson DFT, et al. Retinoids and carotenoids are peroxyl radical scavengers. In: Livrea MA, Parker, L, eds. Retinoids. Progress in research and clinical applications. New York. Marcel Dekker 1993:525–536.
93. Bertram JS, Pung A, Churley M, et al. Diverse carotenoids protect against chemically induced neoplastic transformation. Carcinogenesis 1991;12:671–678.
94. Krinsky NI. Effects of carotenoids on cells. Mol Aspects Med 1993;14:241–246.
95. Galligan LJ, Jackson CL, Gerber LE. Carotenoids slow the growth of small cell lung cancer cells. Ann N Y Acad Sci 1993;691:267–269.
96. Phyllips RW, Kikendall JW, Luk JD, et al. β-Carotene inhibits rectal mucosal ornithine decarboxylase activity in colon cancer patients. Cancer Res 1993;53:3723–3725.
97. Beems RB. The effect of β-carotene on BP-induced respiratory tract tumors in hamsters. Nutr Cancer 1987;10:197–204.
98. McKay PB, King MM. Vitamin A: its role as a biological free radicals scavenger and its relationship to the microsomal mixed-function oxidase system. In: Machlin LJ, ed. Vitamin E–a comprehensive treatise. New York. Marcel Dekker, 1980:289–317.
99. De Flora S, Izzotti A, D'Agostini F, et al. Chemopreventive properties of N-acetylcysteine and other thiols. In: Watterberg L, Lipkin M, Boone CW, Kelloff GJ eds. Cancer chemoprevention. Boca Raton, FL: CRC Press, 1992:183–194.
100. De Flora S, Bennicelli C, Camoirano A, et al. In vivo effects of N-acetylcysteine on glutathione metabolism and on the biotransformation of carcinogenic and/or mutagenic compounds. Carcinogenesis 1985;6:1735–1745.

101. Camoirano A, Badolati GS, Zanacchi P, et al. Dual role of thiols in N-methyl-N'-nitro-N-nitrosoguanidine genotoxicity. Life Sci Adv Exp Oncol 1988;7:21–25.
102. De Flora S, Camoirano A, Izzotti A, et al. Antimutagenic and anticarcinogenic mechanisms of aminothiols. In: Nygaard F, Upton AC, eds. Anticarcinogenesis and Radiation Protection III. New York: Plenum Press, 1991: 275–285.
103. Izzotti A, Balansky R, Coscia N, et al. Chemoprevention of smoke-related DNA adduct formation in rat lung and heart. Carcinogenesis 1992;13:2187–2190.
104. De Flora S, Astengo M, Serra D, Benicelli C. Prevention of urethane-induced lung tumors in mice by dietary N-acetylcysteine. Cancer Lett 1986;32:235–241.
105. Wilpart M, Speder D, Roberfroid M. Anti-initiation activity of N-acetylcysteine in experimental colonic carcinogenesis. Cancer Lett 1986;31:319–324.
106. Dimitrov NV, Bennett JL, McMillan J, et al. Clinical pharmacology studies of oltipraz–a potential chemopreventive agent. Invest New Drugs 1992;10:289–298.
107. Watternberg LW, Bueding E. Inhibitory effects of 5-(2-pyrazinyl)-4-methyl-1,2-dithiol-3-thione (Oltipraz) on carcinogenesis induced by benzo(a)pyrene, diethylnitrosamine and uracil mustard. Carcinogenesis 1986;7:1379–1381.
108. Rao CV, Tokomo K, Kelloff G, Reddy BS. Inhibition by dietary Oltipraz of experimental intestinal carcinogenesis induced by azoxymethane in male F344 rats. Carcinogenesis 1991;12:1051–1055.
109. Kensler TW, Groopman JD, Eaton DL, et al. Potent inhibition of aflatoxin-induced hepatic tumorigenesis by the monofunctional enzyme inducer 1,2-dithiole-3-thione. Carcinogenesis 1992;13:95–100.
110. Pepin P, Bouchard L, Nicole P, Castonguay A. Effects of Sulindac and Oltipraz on the tumorigenicity of 4-(methylnitrosamino)1-(3-pyridyl)-1-butanone in A/J mouse lung. Carcinogenesis 1992;13:341–348.
111. Kelloff GJ, Boone CW, Crowell JA, et al. Chemopreventive drug development: Perspectives and progress. Cancer Epidemiol Biomarkers Prev 1994;3:85–98.
112. Doerr-O'Rourke K, Trushin N, Hecht SS, Stoner GD. Effect of phenethyl isothiocyanate on the metabolism of the tobacco-specific nitrosamine 4-(methylnitrosamino)-1-(3-pyridyl)-1-butanone by cultured rat lung tissue. Carcinogenesis 1991;12:1029–1034.
113. Morse MA, Reinhardt JC, Amin SG, et al. Effect of dietary aromatic isothiocyanates fed subsequent to the administration of 4-(methylnitrosamino)-1-(3-pyridyl)-1-butanone on lung tumorigenicity in mice. Cancer Lett 1990;49:225–230.
114. Boukharta M, Jalbert G, Castonguay A. Biodistribution of ellagic acid and dose-related inhibition of lung tumorigenesis in A/J mice. Nutr Cancer 1992;18:181–189.
115. Perchellet JP, Gali HU, Perchellet EM, et al. Antitumor-promoting activities of tannic acid, ellagic acid, and several gallic acid derivatives in mouse skin. Basic Life Sci 1992;59:783–801.
116. Stoner GD, Morrissey DT, Heur YH, et al. Inhibitory effects of phenethyl isothiocyanate on N-nitrosobenzylmethylamine carcinogenesis in rat esophagus. Cancer Res 1991;51:2063–2068.
117. Ip C, Ganther HE. Combination of blocking agents and suppressing agents in cancer prevention. Carcinogenesis 1991;12:365–367.
118. Moon RC, Rao KV, Detrisac CJ, Kelloff GJ. Animal models for chemoprevention of respiratory cancer. J Natl Cancer Inst Monogr 1992;13:45–49.
119. Greenwald P, Sondik E, Lynch BS. Diet and chemoprevention in NCI's research strategy to achieve national cancer control objectives. Ann Rev Public Health 1986;7:267–291.
120. Greenwald P, Stern HR. Role of biology and prevention in aerodigestive tract cancer. J Natl Cancer Inst Monogr 1992;13:3–14.
121. Kelloff GJ, Johnson JR, Crowell JA, et al. Approaches to the development and marketing approval of drugs that prevent cancer. Cancer Epidemiol Biomarkers Prev 1995;4:1–10.
122. de Vries N. The magnitude of the problem. In: de Vries N, Glukman JL, eds. Multiple primary tumors in the head and neck. Stuttgard: Thieme, 1990: 1–29.
123. Hong WK, Bromer RH, Amato DA. Patterns of relapse in locally advanced head and neck cancer patients who achieved complete remission after combined modality therapy. Cancer 1985;56:1242–1245.
124. Slaughter DP, Southwick HW, Smejkal W. "Field cancerization" in oral stratified squamous epithelium: clinical implications of multicentric origin. Cancer 1953;6:963–968.
125. McDonald S, Haie C, Rubin P, et al. Second malignant tumors in patients with laryngeal carcinoma: diagnosis, treatment and prevention. Int J Radiat Oncol Biol Phys 1989;17:457–465.
126. de Vries N, van der Waal I, Snow GB. Multiple primary tumors in oral cancer. Int J Maxillofac Surg 1986;15:85–87.
127. de Vries N, Snow GB. Multiple primary tumors in laryngeal cancer. J Laryngol Otol 1986;100:915–917.
128. Fontana RS. Early diagnosis of lung cancer. Am Rev Respir Dis 1977;116:399–402.
129. Pairolero P, Williams DE, Bergstrahl EJ, et al. Postsurgical stage I bronchogenic carcinoma: morbid implications of recurrent disease. Ann Thorac Surg 1984;38:331–338.
130. Shields TW, Robinette CD. Long-term survivors after resection of bronchial carcinoma. Surg Gynecol Obstet 1973;136:759–768.
131. Auerbach O, Stout AP, Hammond EC, et al. Multiple primary bronchial carcinomas. Cancer 1967;20:699.
132. Femeck BK, Flehinger BJ, Martini N. A retrospective analysis of 10-year survivors from carcinoma of the lung. Cancer 1984;53:1405–1408.
133. Lippman SM, Batsakis JG, Toth BB, et al. Comparison of low-dose isotretinoin with beta carotene to prevent oral carcinogenesis. N Engl J Med 1993;328:15–20.
134. Blot WJ, Li JY, Taylor PR, et al. Nutrition intervention trials in Lin Xian, China: supplementation with specific vitamin/mineral combinations, cancer incidence, and disease-specific mortality in the general population. J Natl Cancer Inst 1993;85:1483–1492.
135. Pastorino U, Soresi E, Clerici M, et al. Lung cancer chemoprevention with retinol palmitate. Acta Oncologica 1988;27:773–782.
136. Blomhoff R, Green MH, Green JB, et al. Vitamin A metabolism: new perspectives on absorption, transport and storage. Physiol Rev 1991;71:951–990.
137. Korner WF, Vollm J. New aspects of the tolerance of retinol in humans. Int J Vit Nutr Res 1975;45:353–372.
138. Plezia PM, Alberts DS, Peng YM, et al. The role of serum and tissue pharmacology studies in the design and interpretation of chemoprevention trials. Prev Med 1989;18:680–687.
139. Infante M, Pastorino U, Chiesa G, et al. Laboratory evaluation during high-dose vitamin A administration: a randomized study on lung cancer patients after surgical resection. J Cancer Res Clin Oncol 1991;117:156–162.

140. Fidge NH, Shiratori T, Ganguly J, Goodman DS. Pathways of absorption of retinol and retinoic acid in the rat. J Lipid Res 1968;9:103–109.
141. Wathne KO, Norum KR, Smeland E, Blomhoff R: Retinol bound to physiological carrier molecules regulates growth and differentiation of myeloid leukemic cells. J Biol Chem 1988;263:8691–8695.
142. Bauernfiend JC. The safe use of vitamin A: a report of the International Vitamin A Consultative Group (IVAG). Washington, DC: The Nutrition Foundation, 1980.
143. Bendich A, Langseth L, Safety of vitamin A. Am J Clin Nutr 1989;49:358–371.
144. Rapaport HG, Herman H, Lehman E. Treatment of ichthyosis with vitamin A. J Pediatr 1942;21:733–746.
145. Frey JR, Schoch MA. Therapeutische Versuche bei Psoriasis mit Vitamin A, zugleich ein beitrag zur A-Hypervitaminose. Dermatologicala 1952;104:80–86.
146. Schimpf A, Jansen KH. Hochdosierte Vitamin-A–Therapie bei Psoriasis und Mycosis Fungoides. Fortschr Ther 1972;90:635–639.
147. Silverman S, Renstrup G, Pindborg J. Studies in oral leukoplakias: III. Effects of vitamin A comparing clinical, histopathological, cytologic, and hematologic responses. Acta Odont Scand 1963;21:271–292.
148. Pastorino U, Chiesa G, Infante M, et al. Safety of high-dose vitamin A. Randomized trial on lung cancer chemoprevention. Oncology 1991;48:131–137.
149. De Vries N, Van Zandwijk N, Pastorino U. The EUROSCAN study. Br J Cancer 1991;64:985–989.
150. Dai WS, LaBraico JM, Stern RS. Epidemiology of isotretinoin exposure during pregnancy. J Am Acad Dermatol 1992;26:599–560.
151. Lammer EJ, Chen DT, Hoar RM, et al. Retinoic acid fetopathy. N Engl J Med 1985;313:837–841.
152. Jick SS, Terris BZ, Jick H. First trimester topical tretinoin and congenital disorders. Lancet 1993;341:1181–1182.
153. Bollag W. Vitamin A and retinoid: from nutrition to pharmacotherapy in dermatology and oncology. Lancet 1983;1:860–863.
154. Sporn MB, Dunlop NM, Newton DL, Henderson WR. Relationship between structure and activity of retinoids. Nature 1976;263:110–113.
155. Peck GL, Olsen TG, Butkus D, et al. Treatment of basal cell carcinomas with 13-cis retinoic acid (abstract). Proc Am Assoc Cancer Res 1979;20:56.
156. Kamm JJ, Ashenfelter KO, Ehmann CW. Preclinical and clinical toxicology of selected retinoids. In: Sporn MB, et al., eds. The retinoids. Orlando, FL: Academic Press, 1984;2:287–326.
157. Pennes DR, Ellis CN, Madison KC, et al. Early skeletal hyperostosis secondary to 13-cis-retinoic acid. Am J Radiol 1984;141:979–983.
158. Hong WK, Endicott J, Itri L, et al. 13-cis-Retinoic acid in the treatment of oral leukoplakia. N Engl J Med 1986;315:1501–1505.
159. Muindi J, Frankel S, Huselton C, et al. Clinical pharmacology of oral all-trans retinoic acid in patients with acute promyelocytic leukemia. Cancer Res 1992;52:2138–2142.
160. Brazzell RK, Vane FM, Ehmann CW, Colburn WA. Pharmacokinetics of isotretinoin during repetitive dosing to patients. Eur J Clin Pharmacol 1983;24:695–702.
161. Formelli F, Clerici M, Campa T, et al. Five-year administration of fenretinide: pharmacokinetics and effects of plasma retinol concentrations. J Clin Oncol 1993;11:2036–2042.
162. Wiegand UW, Busslinger AA, Chou RC, Jensen BK. The pharmacokinetics of acitretin in humans: an update. In: Livrea MA, Packer L, eds. Retinoids. Progress in research and clinical application. New York: Marcel Dekker, 1993:617–628.
163. Massarella JW, Vane FM. Etretinate kinetics during chronic dosing in severe psoriasis. Clin Pharmacol Ther 1985;37:439–446.
164. Kerr IG, Lippman ME, Jenkins J, Myers C. Pharmacology of 13-cis-retinoic acid in humans. Cancer Res 1982;42:2069–2073.
165. Goodman GE, Alberts DS, Peng YM, et al. Pharmacokinetics and phase I trial of retinol and 13-cis-retinoic acid. In: Modulation and mediation of cancer by vitamins: Basel: Karger, 1983:311–316.
166. Khoo KC, Reik FD, Colburn WA. Pharmacokinetic profile of isotretinoin following a single oral dose to normal man. J Clin Pharmacol 1982;22:395–402.
167. Berni R, Clerici M, Malpeli G, et al. Retinoids: in vitro interaction with retinol-binding protein and influence on plasma retinol. FASEB J 1993;7:1179–1184.
168. DiGiovanna J, Helfgott R, Gerber L, et al. Extraspinal tendon and ligament calcification associated with long-term therapy with etretinate. N Engl J Med 1986;315:1177–1182.
169. Kilcoyne R. Effects of retinoids on bone. J Am Acad Dermatol 1988;19:212–216.
170. Akyama H, Nakamura N, Nagasaka S, et al. Hypercalcemia due to all-trans retinoic acid. Lancet 1992;1:308–309.
171. Niesvizky R, Siegel D, Straus D, et al. Hypercalcemia and increased serum interleukin-6 (IL-6) levels induced by all-trans retinoic acid (ATRA) in patients with multiple myeloma (abstract). Proc Am Soc Clin Oncol 1993;12:407.
172. Moon RC, Thompson HJ, Becci PL, et al. N-(hydroxyphenyl) retinamide, a new retinoid for prevention of breast cancer. Cancer Res 1979;39:1339–1346.
173. Paulson JD, Oldham JW, Preston RF, et al. Lack of genotoxicity of the cancer chemopreventive agent N-(4-hydroxyphenyl)retamide. Fund Appl Toxicol 1985;5:144–150.
174. Chiesa F, Tradati N, Marazza M, et al. Prevention of local relapses and new localizations of oral leukoplakias with the synthetic retinoid fenretinide (4-HPR). Preliminary results. Oral Oncol Eur J Cancer 1992;28B:92–102.
175. Decensi A, Bruno S, Costantini M, et al. Phase IIa study of fenretinide in superficial bladder cancer, using DNA flow cytometry as an intermediate endpoint. J Natl Cancer Inst 1994;86:138–140.
176. Peng YM, Dalton WS, Alberts DS, et al. Pharmacokinetics of N-4-hydroxyphenyl-retinamide and the effect of its oral administration on plasma retinol concentrations in cancer patients. Int J Cancer 1989;43:22–26; Erratum: Int J Cancer 1989;44:567.
177. Doose DR, Minn FL, Stellar S, Nayak RK. Effects of meals and meal composition on the bioavailability of fenretinide. J Clin Pharmacol 1992;32:1089–1095.
178. Desiraju RK, Scott V, Nayak RK, Minn FL. Pharmacokinetics of fenretinide in healthy volunteers. Clin Pharmacol Ther 1985;37:190.
179. Formelli F, Carsana R, Costa A, et al. Plasma retinol level reduction by the synthetic retinoid fenretinide: a one year follow-up study of breast cancer patients. Cancer Res 1989;49:6149–6152.
180. Formelli F, Carsana R, Costa A. N-(4-hydroxyphenyl)retinamide (4-HPR) lowers plasma retinol levels in rats. Med Sci Res 1987;15:843–844.

181. Dimitrov NV, Meyer CJ, Perloff M, et al. Alteration of retinol-binding–protein concentrations by the synthetic retinoid fenretinide in healthy human subjects. Am J Clin Nutr 1990;51:1082–1087.
182. Kaiser-Kupfer MI, Peck GL, Caruso RC. Abnormal retinal function associated with fenretinide, a synthetic retinoid. Arch Ophthalmol 1986;104:69–70.
183. Kingstone TP, Lowe NJ, Winston J, Heckenlively J. Visual and cutaneous toxicity which occurs during N-(hydroxyphenyl)retinamide therapy for psoriasis. Clin Exp Dermatol 1986;11:624–627.
184. Costa A, Malone W, Perloff M, et al. Tolerability of the synthetic retinoid fenretinide (HPR). Eur J Cancer Clin Oncol 1989;25:805–808.
185. Modiano RM, Dalton WS, Lippman SM, et al. Phase II study of fenretinide (N-[4-hydroxyphenyl]retinamide) in advanced breast cancer and melanoma. Invest New Drugs 1990;8:317–319.
186. Decensi A, Torrisi R, Polizzi A, et al. Effect of the synthetic retinoid fenretinide on dark adaptation and the ocular surface. J Natl Cancer Inst 1994;86:105–110.
187. Veronesi U, De Palo G, Costa A, et al. Chemoprevention of breast cancer with retinoids. NCI Monog 1992;12:93–97.
188. Rotmensz N, De Palo G, Formelli F, et al. Long term tolerability of fenretinide (4-HPR) in breast cancer patients. Eur J Cancer 1991;2:1127–1131.
189. Pizzichetta M, Rossi R, Costa A, et al. Lipoproteins in fenretinide (4-HPR) treated patients. Diab Nutr Metab 1992;5:71–72.
190. Stich HF, Rosin MP, Hornby AP. Remission of oral leukoplakias and micronuclei in tobacco/betel quid chewers treated with beta-carotene and with beta-carotene plus vitamin A. Int J Cancer 1988;42:195–199.
191. Garewal HS, Meyskens FL, Killen D. Response of oral leukoplakia to beta-carotene. J Clin Oncol 1990;8:1715–1720.
192. Lippman SM, Benner SE, Hong WK. Retinoid chemoprevention studies in upper aerodigestive tract and lung carcinogenesis. Cancer Res 1994;54:2025S–2028S.
193. Dimitrov NV, Boone CW, Hay MB, et al. Plasma beta-carotene levels—kinetic patterns during administration of various doses of beta-carotene. J Nutr Growth Cancer 1987;3:227–237.
194. Greenberg ER, Baron JA, Tosteson TD, et al. A clinical trial of antioxidant vitamins to prevent colorectal adenoma. N Engl J Med 1994;331:141–147.
195. Xu MJ, Peng YM, Liu Y, et al. Effect of chronic oral administration of β-carotene on plasma α-tocopherol concentrations in normal subjects (abstract). Proc Am Assoc Cancer Res 1990;31:126.
196. Canfield L, Corrigan J, Plezia PM, et al. Effects of chronic β-carotene supplementation on vitamin K status in adults. Nutr Cancer 1990;13:263–269.
197. Benner SE, Winn RJ, Lippman SM, et al. Regression of oral leukoplakia with alpha-tocopherol: a community clinical oncology program chemoprevention study. J Natl Cancer Inst 1993;85:44–47.
198. Boman G, Bäcker U, Larsson S, et al. Oral acetylcysteine reduces exacerbation rate in chronic bronchitis: report of a trial organized by the Swedish Society for Pulmonary Diseases. Eur J Respir Dis 1983;64:405–415.
199. Heffner JE, Repine JE. Pulmonary strategies of antioxidant defense. Am Rev Respir Dis 1989;140:531–554.
200. Flanagan RJ. The role of acetylcysteine in clinical toxicology. Med Toxicol 1987;2:93–104.
201. Miller LF, Rumack BH. Clinical safety of high oral doses of acetylcysteine. Semin Oncol 1983;10(Suppl. 1):76–85.
202. Bonanomi L, Gazzaniga A. Toxicological, pharmacokinetic and metabolic studies on acetyl-cysteine. Eur J Respir Dis 1980;61:45–51.
203. O'Dwyer PJ, Szarka CE, Gallo JM, et al. Phase I pharmacodynamic trial of the chemopreventive agent Oltipraz (abstract). Proc Am Soc Clin Oncol 1994;13:A372.
204. Benson AB III. Oltipraz: a laboratory and clinical review. J Cell Biochem 1993;17F:278–291.
205. Albanes D, Virtamo J, Rauthalahti M, et al. Pilot study: the U.S. Finland lung cancer prevention trial. J Nutr Growth Cancer 1986;3:207–214.
206. Hennekens CH. Issues in the design and conduct of clinical trials. J Natl Cancer Inst 1984;73:1473–1476.
207. Arnold AM, Browman GP, Levine MN, et al. The effect of the synthetic retinoid etretinate on sputum cytology: results from a randomized trial. Br J Cancer 1992;65:737–743.
208. Lee JS, Benner SE, Lippman SM, et al. Randomized placebo-controlled chemoprevention trial of 13-cis-retinoic acid (cRA) in bronchial squamous metaplasia (abstract). Proc Am Soc Clin Oncol 1993;13:1117.
209. Lippman SM, Benner SE, Hong WK. Chemoprevention strategies in lung carcinogenesis. Chest 1993;103:15S–19S.
210. Jin Y-S, Mandahl N, Heim S, et al. Isochromosomes i(8q) or i(9q) in three adenocarcinomas of the lung. Cancer Genet Cytogenet 1988;33:11–17.
211. Bello MJ, Moreno S, Rey JA. Involvement of chromosomes 1, 3, and i(8q) in lung adenocarcinoma. Cancer Genet Cytogenet 1989;39:133–135.
212. Lukeis R, Irving L, Garson M, Hasthorpe S. Cytogenetics of non–small cell lung cancer: analysis of consistent non-random abnormalities. Genes Chrom Cancer 1990;2:116–124.
213. Sozzi G, Miozzo M, Tagliabue E, et al. Cytogenetic abnormalities and over-expression of receptors for growth factors in normal bronchial epithelium and tumor samples of lung cancer patients. Cancer Res 1991;51:400–404.
214. Wang Peng J, Knutsen T, Gazdar a, et al. Non random structural and numerical chromosome changes in non–small cell lung cancer. Genes Chrom Cancer 1991;3:168–188.
215. Testa JR, Siegfried JM. Chromosome abnormalities in human non–small lung cancer. Cancer Res 1992;52:2702S–2706S.
216. Hendler FJ, Ozanne BW. Human squamous cell lung cancers express increased epidermal growth factor receptors. J Clin Invest 1984;74:647–651.
217. Cerny T, Barnes DM, Hasleton P, et al. Expression of epidermal growth factor receptor (EGF-R) in human lung tumors. Br J Cancer 1986;54:265–269.
218. Berger MS, Gullick WJ, Greenfeld C, et al. Epidermal growth factor receptors in lung tumors. J Pathol 1987;152:297–307.
219. Volm M, Efferth T, Mattern J. Oncoprotein (c-myc, c-erbB1, c-erbB2, c-fos) and suppressor gene product (p53) expression in squamous cell carcinomas of the lung. Clinical and biological correlations. Anticancer Res 1992;12:11–20.
220. Rodenhuis S, Slebos RJC, Boot AJM, et al. Incidence and possible clinical significance of K-ras oncogene activation in adenocarcinoma of the lung. Cancer Res 1988;48:5738–5741.
221. Slebos RJC, Kibbelaar RE, Dalesio O, et al. K-ras oncogene activation as a prognostic marker in adenocarcinoma of the lung. N Engl J Med 1990;323:561–565.
222. Mitsudomi T, Steinberg SM, Oie HK, et al. ras Gene mutations in non–small lung cancers are associated with shortened sur-

vival irrespective of treatment intent. Cancer Res 1991;51: 4999–5002.
223. Rodenhuis S, Slebos RJC. Clinical significance of *ras* oncogene activation in human lung cancer. Cancer Res 1992;52:2665S–2669S.
224. Kern JA, Schwartz DA, Nordberg JE, et al. p185 *neu* Expression in human lung adenocarcinomas predicts shortened survival. Cancer Res 1990;50:5184–5187.
225. Weiner DB, Nordberg J, Robinson R, et al. Expression of the *neu* gene-encoded protein (p185 *neu*) in human non–small carcinomas of the lung. Cancer Res 1990;50:421–425.
226. Tateishi M, Ishida T, Mitsudomi T, et al. Prognostic value of c-erbB-2 protein expression in human lung adenocarcinoma and squamous cell carcinoma. Eur J Cancer 1991;27:1372–1375.
227. Shi D, He G, Cao S, et al. Overexpression of the c-erb-2/neu-encoded p185 protein in primary lung cancer. Mol Carcinog 1992;5:213–218.
228. Little CD, Nau MM, Carney DN, et al. Amplifcation and expression of the c-*myc* oncogene in human lung cancer cell lines. Nature 1983;306:194–196.
229. Nau MM, Brooks BJ, Battey J, et al. L-*myc*, a new *myc*-related gene amplified and expressed in human small cell lung cancer. Nature 1985;318:69–73.
230. Johnson BE, Ihde D, Makuch RW, et al. *myc* Family oncogene amplification in tumor cell lines established from small cell lung cancer patients and its relationship to clinical status and course. J Clin Invest 1987;79:1629–1634.
231. Shiraishi M, Noguchi M, Shimosato Y, Sekiya T. Amplification of protooncogenes in surgical specimens of human lung carcinomas. Cancer Res 1989;49:6474–6479.
232. Harbour JW, Lai S-L, Whang-Peng J, et al. Abnormalities in structure and expression of the human retinoblastoma gene in SCLC. Science 1988;241:353–357.
233. Horowitz JM, Park SH, Bogenmann E, et al. Frequent inactivation of the retinoblastoma antioncogene is restricted to a subset of human tumor cells. Proc Natl Acad Sci U S A 1990;87:2775–2779.
234. Houle B, Leduc F, Bradley WEC. Implication of RARB in epidermoid (squamous) lung cancer. Genes Chrom Cancer 1991;3:358–366.
235. Tsuchiya E, Nakamura Y, Weng S-Y. Allelotype of non–small cell lung carcinoma—Comparison between loss of heterozygosity in squamous cell carcinoma and adenocarcinoma. Cancer Res 1992;52:2478–2481.
236. Hibi K, Takahashi T, Yamakawa K, et al. Three distinct regions involved in *3p* deletion in human lung cancer. Oncogene 1992;7:445–449.
237. Gebert JF, Moghal N, Frangioni JV, et al. High frequency of retinoic acid receptor β abnormalities in human lung cancer. Oncogene 1991;6:1859–1868.
238. Iggo R, Gatter K, Bartek J, et al. Increased expression of mutant forms of *p53* oncogene in primary lung cancer. Lancet 1990;335:675–679.
239. Chiba I, Takahashi T, Nau M, et al. Mutations in the *p53* gene are frequent in primary, resected non–small cell lung cancer. Oncogene 1990;5:1603–1610.
240. Takahashi T, Takahashi T, Suzuki H, et al. The *p53* gene is very frequently mutated in small-cell lung cancer with a distinct nucleotide substitution pattern. Oncogene 1991;6:1775–1778.
241. D'Amico D, Carbone D, Mitsudomi T, et al. High frequency of somatically acquired *p53* mutations in small cell lung cancer cell lines and tumors. Oncogene 1992;7:339–346.
242. Miller CW, Simon K, Aslo A, et al. *p53* Mutations in human lung tumors. Cancer Res 1992;52:1695–1698.
243. Suzuki H, Takahashi T, Kuroishi T, et al. *p53* Mutations in non–small cell lung cancer in Japan: association between mutations and smoking. Cancer Res 1992;52:734–736.
244. Kishimoto Y, Murakami Y, Shiraishi M, et al. Aberrations of the *p53* tumor suppressor gene in human non–small cell carcinomas of the lung. Cancer Res 1992;52:4799–4804.
245. Hiyoshi H, Matsuno Y, Kato H, et al. Clinicopathological significance of nuclear accumulation of tumor suppressor gene *p53* product in primary lung cancer. Jpn J Cancer Res 1992;83:101–106.
246. Horio Y, Takahashi T, Kuroishi T, et al. Prognostic significance of *p53* mutations and *3p* deletions in primary resected non–small cell lung cancer. Cancer Res 1993;53:1–4.
247. Quinlan DC, Davidson AG, Summers CL, et al. Accumulation of p53 protein correlates with a poor prognosis in human lung cancer. Cancer Res 1992;52:4828–4831.
248. Sundaresan V, Ganly P, Hasleton P, et al. p53 And chromosome 3 abnormalities, characteristic of malignant lung tumors, are detectable in preinvasive lesions of the bronchus. Oncogene 1992;7:1989–1997.
249. Sozzi G, Miozzo M, Donghi R, et al. Deletions of *17p* and *p53* mutations in preoplastic lesions of the lung. Cancer Res 1992;52:6079–6082.
250. Postorino U, Sozzi G, Miozzo M, et al. Genetic changes in lung cancer. J Cell Biochem 1993;17F:237–248.
251. Sozzi G, Miozzo M, Pastorino U, et al. Genetic evidence for an independent origin of multiple preneoplastic and neoplastic lung lesions. Cancer Res 1995;55:135–140.
252. Lee JS, Lippman SM, Hong WK, et al. Determination of biomarkers for intermediate end points in chemoprevention trials. Cancer Res 1992;52:(Suppl):2707S–2710S.
253. Lippman SM, Peters EJ, Wargovich MJ, et al. Bronchial micronuclei as a marker of an early stage of carcinogenesis in the human trachebronchial epithelium. Int J Cancer 1990;45:811–815.
254. Lee JS, Ro JY, Sahin AA, et al. Expression of blood-group antigen A–a favorable prognostic factor in non–small-cell lung cancer. N Engl J Med 1991;324:1084–1090.

52

GOVERNMENT REGULATION OF TOBACCO AND TOBACCO PRODUCTS

Joseph S. Bailes

INTRODUCTION

In 1964, Surgeon General Luther Terry's *Report on Smoking and Health* informed the public that smoking was a health hazard. Although previous reports, most notably the Sloan-Kettering report of 1953, linked smoking with cancer, the surgeon general's report marked the beginning of widespread public awareness of the health effects of tobacco use (1). Since that time, our understanding of the toll that tobacco and its products take on the life and health of Americans has increased steadily. Although smoking levels have decreased since their peak in 1963, 25% of Americans continue to smoke (2), and 434,000 die from causes related to their addiction annually. An additional 53,000 lives are estimated to be lost to cancer and heart disease attributable to environmental tobacco smoke every year (3). Even while the percentage of those who smoke declines, the use of smokeless or chewing tobacco is increasing—by almost 5% in 1990 (3).

Despite their well-known toxicity, tobacco and tobacco products (along with alcohol) have largely escaped the intensive federal regulation accorded to similar health hazards, drugs, and dangerous chemicals. The exemption of tobacco from the ordinary federal regulation of hazardous substances often is attributed to the tobacco lobby, which has been both active and successful in pursuing its interests with federal lawmakers. The whole story, however, includes the American public's acceptance of and demand for tobacco, and the backlash that is still felt from this country's experience with the prohibition of alcohol (4).

Tobacco is not completely immune from federal involvement. The federal government directly regulates tobacco through restrictions and requirements on tobacco advertising and packaging. There also are federal restrictions on smoking in the workplace, airplanes, and other public areas to lessen the public's exposure to second-hand smoke. In addition, the government affects the price of tobacco and tobacco products through the implementation of taxes and an agricultural price support program for tobacco farmers. The international trade of tobacco is another target, because the government has aggressively sought to expand American access to foreign tobacco markets. Finally, the federal government indirectly funds research into the health effects of tobacco use, public health education campaigns, and smoking cessation programs.

Legislative efforts to restrict smoking have had success in the past largely only at the state and local levels. The antismoking movement has gained considerable momentum recently, however, and the prospect of restrictive federal regulation of tobacco is being taken seriously. For example, the federal government has proposed banning smoking from restaurants, bars, and workplaces, levying a tax of more than $1 on every pack of cigarettes, and regulating the nicotine in cigarettes as an addictive drug. The scope and number of these proposals are a response in part to the U.S. Environmental Protection Agency's (EPA) controversial 1993 report that classified second-hand smoke as a class A carcinogen. This report has strengthened the argument that smoking can no longer be justified as an individual smoker's right to choose, at least in public, because the smoker also imposes health consequences on others.

This chapter provides an overview of current and proposed federal regulation of tobacco and tobacco products, beginning with a brief historical summary of tobacco regulation and the political and social forces that shaped it. Government regulation of the tobacco products themselves, including additives, is described also. Federal regulation of labeling and advertising is discussed, and the regulation of smoking in public places and its relation to secondary smoke are summarized. Also covered are the government's support for research and public health education campaigns, the more recent use of taxes to discourage smoking, and pro-tobacco programs, such as regulation of imports and exports and the agricultural support program for tobacco growers.

REGULATION OF TOBACCO PRODUCTS AND THEIR CONTENT

EARLY REGULATION

When the first Europeans arrived in the New World they found native Americans enjoying tobacco. The Europeans associated the smoking of tobacco with good health and avoidance of disease, because the natives were healthy compared with the Europeans. Physicians and popular lore attributed germ killing and healthful attributes to tobacco use well into the 20th century (5).

Although, initially, many thought that tobacco was a harmless pleasure, there has been a vociferous group of antitobacco advocates in this country for more than 100 years. The first organized antitobacco crusade began with the temperance movement in the 1830s, when many perceived tobacco and drinking as twin vices. The movement was quickly overshadowed by the events of the Civil War (6).

Originally, tobacco in America was grown primarily for foreign consumption. Gradually, domestic demand grew until the large majority of American tobacco was consumed domestically. Tobacco was grown primarily by small, single-crop farmers, and tobacco products were produced by numerous independent businessmen. In the 1880s, a machine to manufacture cigarettes was invented, precipitating the consolidation of the mostly small independent businessmen into a single producer of cigarettes: the "Tobacco Trust" headed by James B. Duke. From 1880 to 1911, when the Tobacco Trust was divided by the federal government because it violated the Sherman Antitrust Act, it occupied 85% to 95% of the domestic market. In the fallout after the enforced breakup of the Tobacco Trust monopoly, six major producers of tobacco products eventually formed, and by 1975, the combined market share of the six companies was 99.8% (1). This remains unchanged to the present day, with Philip Morris, R. J. Reynolds, Brown & Williamson, Lorillard, American Brands, and the Liggett Group producing essentially all of the cigarettes consumed in America (7).

The dramatic increase in cigarette production made possible by the cigarette manufacturing machine in the 1880s also stimulated the rebirth of the antitobacco movement. The renewed battle was now directed specifically against cigarettes, which had become an affordable luxury for even the poor, and which were associated with urban immigrants and the lower classes (5). In upholding the state of Tennessee's right to ban the sale of cigarettes, the U.S. Supreme Court in 1900 noted their uniquely bad image among tobacco products, saying:

[W]e should be shutting our eyes to what is constantly passing before them were we to affect an ignorance of the fact that a belief in [cigarettes'] deleterious effects, particularly upon young people, has become very general, and that communications are constantly finding their way into the public press denouncing their use as fraught with great danger to the youth of both sexes (8).

As the Supreme Court observed, the general disapproval of cigarette smoking was particularly vehement for smoking among youth. The Duke family had begun to target young men as customers in 1878 through the introduction of collectable trading cards, the most popular of which featured a series of relatively scantily clad women (6). These tactics were very successful, and smoking rates among young men increased rapidly. The desire to restrain the ever-rising popularity of cigarettes among young men produced the first legislation against cigarettes, which was passed at the state level. By 1890 the majority of states had passed laws prohibiting the sale of cigarettes to minors (5).

Congress was petitioned to outlaw cigarettes in 1892, but the Senate Committee on Epidemic Diseases, although agreeing that cigarettes were a public health hazard, said that only the states had the authority to ban cigarettes (5). The states' right to ban cigarettes completely, which 12 states had done by 1900, was, as indicated above, upheld by the U.S. Supreme Court in 1900 (9).

World War I completely derailed the anticigarette movement of the early 1900s. Cigarettes were thought to be essential to the military effort and were included in daily rations. Americans deposited pennies and cigarettes in war-effort donation bins at movie theaters, and federal prisoners gave up their cigarette rations to send them to the soldiers in Europe (5, 6). Heavy advertising and the increasing social acceptance of cigarette smoking among women helped to create a steady increase in the percentage of the smoking population (6).

Smoking rates continued to increase until the 1950s when the first widely published reports of the relationship between cancer and smoking raised public awareness of smoking's negative effects. The sharp increase in the number and certainty of scientific studies linking tobacco use with cancer precipitated a decrease in smoking rates in the first half of the decade. However, smoking rates began to increase again after 1955, especially among women, until Surgeon General Luther Terry published his report in 1964 linking smoking to lung cancer, chronic bronchitis, emphysema, and cardiovascular diseases (2). The 1964 surgeon general's report marked the beginning of the legislative battle between antitobacco forces and the tobacco industry (1).

JURISDICTION OF FEDERAL AGENCIES

The power of federal government agencies to regulate tobacco is limited to the control granted to them through laws passed by Congress. An agency cannot regulate beyond the scope of its jurisdiction by law. Within the regulatory authority given to federal agencies by law, the agency itself may have some discretion to determine the scope and nature of its regulation.

From the 1960s through the 1980s, Congress became increasingly active in passing legislation that protected the public's health through expanding federal agency regulation of food and drugs, environmental toxins, and dangerous chemicals (6). Many of these regulatory programs could have applied to tobacco and tobacco products, but Congress exempted them from much of the federal legislation aimed at regulating health hazards. For example, tobacco is currently exempt from regulation under the 1966 Fair Packaging and Labeling Act (15 U.S.C. § 1459[a][1]), the 1972 Consumer Product Safety Act (15 U.S.C. § 2052[a][1][B]), the 1976 Toxic Substances Control Act (15 U.S.C. § 2602[2][B][iii]), the 1976 amendment of the Federal Hazardous Substances Act (15 U.S.C. § 1261[f][2]), and the Controlled Substances Act (21 U.S.C. § 802[6]) (10).

In addition to these explicit Congressional exemptions, several agencies did not choose to include tobacco within their regulatory mandate, although it might have fallen within their jurisdiction. For example, the Clean Air Act (42 U.S.C. §§ 7401-7642), which is administered by the EPA, was meant to "protect and enhance the quality of the nation's air resources so as to promote the public health and welfare and the productive capacity of its population" (§ 7401). The regulation of environmental tobacco smoke could arguably fit within this definition, thus giving the EPA the power to regulate smoking in public places. Nevertheless, the EPA has not interpreted the Clean Air Act to apply to indoor air (10). (The EPA, however, has been the federal agency responsible for conducting research on environmental tobacco smoke and its health effects [11].)

Some have argued that the U.S. Food and Drug Administration (FDA) should regulate tobacco as a drug. The original Food and Drugs Act of 1906 defined "drugs" as those substances listed in the *U.S. Pharmacopoeia* and those substances intended to be used for the cure, mitigation, or prevention of disease. In 1890 the *U.S. Pharmacopoeia* did include tobacco, but it was later dropped. It is said that tobacco was dropped from the Pharmacopoeia in return for support of the 1906 Food and Drugs Act by legislators from the tobacco states (6).

The Federal Food, Drug, and Cosmetic Act was enacted in 1938 to replace the 1906 Act. The definition of "drug" in the new legislation retained the concepts from the 1906 Act and added a new category of substances intended by their manufacturers "to affect the structure or function of the body" (21 U.S.C. § 321[g]).

The statutory definition of a drug thus depends on the manufacturer's intended purpose for the product. A substance is a drug if it is intended to treat a disease or affect a bodily function, and the manufacturer's intent usually is inferred from the product's labeling and advertising. The FDA has repeatedly declined to include ordinary tobacco and tobacco products within the definition of drugs because they are not promoted as having drug effects (12). Whenever cigarettes make health claims, they have been regulated by the FDA as drugs, and the courts have upheld the FDA's position (United States v. 46 Cartons, 113 F.Supp. 336 [D.N.J. 1953]; Unites States v. 354 Bulk Cartons Trim Reducing-Aid Cigarettes, 178 F.Supp. 847 [D.N.J. 1959].)

When the tobacco industry introduced low tar and nicotine cigarettes, antismoking coalitions argued unsuccessfully that these products were intended to have an effect on health and thus should fall under FDA regulation (12). When the 1988 surgeon general's report established nicotine as an addictive substance, the argument was again made that the FDA should now include nicotine, and thus tobacco, under its jurisdiction. The FDA declined to interpret its definition of drug as including tobacco or tobacco products, however, or to promulgate a new definition of drug that would clearly include tobacco (12).

Courts have upheld the FDA's interpretation that cigarettes fall outside of its authority to regulate drugs. In 1980, an organization sued the FDA, claiming that cigarettes were drugs because consumers used them for drug purposes. The court upheld the FDA's long-standing interpretation that the manufacturer's intent, not the consumer's intent, was the determinant of the

FDA's jurisdiction (Action on Smoking and Health v. Harris, 655 F.2d 236 [D.C. Cir. 1980]).

Recently, the FDA has indicated that it may assert that cigarettes are drugs subject to its jurisdiction. In a February 25, 1994, letter to the Coalition on Smoking or Health, FDA Commissioner David Kessler told the coalition that the FDA was accumulating evidence that tobacco companies artificially manipulate nicotine levels in cigarettes. If it were true that the tobacco manufacturers intended to create and satisfy an addiction through their products, then, Dr. Kessler contended, the FDA should have the authority to regulate tobacco as a "nicotine-delivery system" (13).

In legal terms, the FDA is suggesting that the intent of the manufacturers—which, as noted above, is the basis for determining whether a substance is a drug—can be inferred from their manipulation of nicotine content rather than from labeling and advertising, as is usually the case. In testimony before a Congressional committee, the major tobacco companies denied that they added nicotine to their products (14).

In response to the renewed understanding of the negative health effects of passive smoke, of nicotine as an addictive substance, and of cigarettes as a device to deliver an addictive drug, many have called for the FDA to extend its regulation to tobacco products. The American Medical Association has called for tougher regulation of tobacco based on the recent study confirming the dose-related increased risk of lung cancer in nonsmoking spouses of smokers (15). A spokesperson for the association stated that, "Cigarettes are no different than syringes. They are a drug delivery device for nicotine. They should be regulated just as we regulate morphine and heroin" (16).

Under the Federal Food, Drug, and Cosmetic Act, a drug may be approved for marketing only if it has been shown to be safe and effective for its intended use. If cigarettes are viewed as intended to create and maintain nicotine addiction, then they could be sold legally only if they were demonstrated to be safe and effective for that purpose. The apparent impossibility of making such a showing suggests that declaring cigarettes to be drugs would be tantamount to banning them. Indeed, Dr. Kessler noted in his testimony that FDA regulation of nicotine could lead to a total withdrawal of nicotine-containing cigarettes from the market (13).

Alternatively, it may be possible theoretically that the FDA could require the reduction of nicotine in cigarettes to levels at which the cigarettes would no longer cause or maintain nicotine addition, thus removing them from the definition of drugs (17). For example, then-Congressman Mike Synar proposed a bill, The Fairness in Tobacco and Nicotine Regulation Act (H.R. 2147), to bring tobacco under FDA regulation. The bill specifically prohibits the FDA from banning cigarettes and would, among other things, control the level of nicotine that cigarettes contain (18).

REGULATION OF CIGARETTE ADDITIVES

Although banning cigarettes has not been discussed seriously in recent years, regulation of specific additives has been the focus of some attention. Cigarettes in the United States have for 150 years contained additives to preserve freshness, enhance taste and smell, and regulate their burn rate (19). In the early 1900s, it was believed widely that cigarettes contained harmful additives such as arsenic and opium, and when the U.S. Supreme Court upheld Tennessee's right to ban cigarettes, it endorsed this common suspicion (8).

The development of low tar and nicotine cigarettes greatly increased the use of additives, and today the belief that cigarette additives are harmful is still widespread. The real health effects of tobacco additives are unknown, however, and they remain virtually unregulated. American cigarette manufacturers claim that all cigarette additives are substances commonly found in food products, and that more than 98% of them are approved for use by the FDA or other experts (19).

Congress requested a study in 1978 on the health risks of substances commonly added to tobacco (20). The government could not investigate the safety of the additives easily, however, because cigarette manufacturers refused to divulge their identity when requested to do so by the surgeon general, claiming that they were trade secrets. To investigate the possible health effects of cigarette additives, Congress passed a law in 1984 requiring cigarette manufacturers to give a list of all cigarette additives to the U.S. Department of Health and Human Services (HHS) (Comprehensive Smoking Education Act, 15 U.S.C. § 1335[a]). Congress intended that the list provide information for HHS to use in investigating potential health risks of the additives.

As originally proposed, the bill would have required cigarette manufacturers to identify which additives they were putting into particular products (20). Congress weakened the disclosure requirements significantly, however, and the law as enacted required only that manufacturers submit a general list of possible additives that were not brand or manufacturer specific. In addition, the law makes the contents of the list confidential, ostensibly to protect the trade secrets and brand formulas of the manufacturers.

The Act authorizes HHS to supply information on the list to Congressional committees as requested, and to make reports to the Congress on proposed research on the additives or potential health concerns related to the additives. The list has been disclosed to at least four Congressional committees, but HHS has never submitted a report to Congress on the health effects of those additives (19).

In France, the ingredients listed on a pack of Marlboro cigarettes include 8% texturizers, flavorants, and preservatives, whereas a pack of cigarettes sold in the United States makes no mention of ingredients. In 1989 Philip Morris withdrew all of its cigarettes from the Canadian market immediately after the Canadian government passed a law requiring the disclosure of brand specific additives. Even though the information would not be made public, R. J. Reynolds also withdrew its cigarettes from Canada, coming back with "reformulated" brands a short time later. The companies defended and explained these actions as necessary to keep trade secrets regarding cigarette formulas (20).

REGULATION OF LABELING AND ADVERTISING

Since the landmark surgeon general's report of 1964, the federal government has taken a number of steps to educate the public and to discourage smoking by regulating the labeling and advertising of tobacco products. Indeed, the primary government focus for many years has been in this area.

LABELING

The year after the surgeon general's famous report, Congress enacted a federal law requiring cigarette manufacturers to put health warnings on every pack. The warning read: "Caution: Cigarette Smoking May Be Hazardous to Your Health" (The Federal Cigarette Labeling and Advertising Act of 1965, 15 U.S.C. § 1331–1341).

The Public Health Cigarette Smoking Act of 1970 created a new and stronger warning label reading: "Warning: The Surgeon General Has Determined That Cigarette Smoking Is Dangerous to Your Health." Legislation further strengthened the warning labels on cigarette packages in 1984 and created a rotating system of four different labels (15 U.S.C. § 1333[a]). The 1986 Comprehensive Smokeless Tobacco Health Education Act extended the requirement for warning labels to smokeless tobacco (15 U.S.C. § 4401–4408).

In 1970, the U.S. Federal Trade Commission (FTC) proposed that cigarette manufacturers publish the tar and nicotine content of cigarettes, but before this was made a legal requirement, cigarette manufacturers agreed to publish the information voluntarily (3).

ADVERTISING

Regulation of tobacco advertising is a major part of the federal government's effort to discourage smoking. Currently there is a total prohibition on tobacco advertising in broadcast media, which includes radio and television (15 U.S.C. § 1335).

In 1967, the U.S. Federal Communications Commission (FCC) was petitioned under its "fairness doctrine" to recognize smoking as an issue of public controversy. Under the fairness doctrine, radio and television stations with an FCC license were required to give time to both sides of a controversial issue whenever views representing only one side of an issue were aired. Agreeing that cigarette advertising did present an issue of public controversy, the FCC ruled that its licensees who carried cigarette advertising must, without compensation, also broadcast antismoking messages (21).

The application of the fairness doctrine to cigarette advertising had the immediate effect of greatly increasing the number of antismoking messages that the public heard, and smoking consumption began a steady decline (2, 21). In addition, the ruling served to create strife among cigarette manufacturers because, although brand loyalty was increased by advertising, the concurrent increase in antismoking messages caused by cigarette advertising served to decrease total cigarette consumption. None of the individual manufacturers could afford to stop advertising for fear of losing market share, yet the more they advertised the smaller the total market became. This situation caused dissension and mistrust among competing cigarette producers and made unified pursuit of their common interests more difficult (21).

In 1968, a political battle between tobacco interests and the broadcast media developed. The FTC has wide jurisdiction over the regulation of advertising, and in 1968 it proposed mandating warnings to be included in all advertisements for cigarettes. At the same time, the FCC proposed a total ban on cigarette advertisements in the broadcast media.

Because of the fairness doctrine, the tobacco industry was not as eager as it might have been to fight the ban on advertising in the broadcast media. The tobacco industry was more concerned that the FTC would force companies to include warning labels in all of their advertisements, including print advertisements. Radio and television advertisements for cigarettes, however, were the biggest advertising contracts in the broadcast media, and thus broadcasters were very unhappy about the proposed FCC ban. Because the powerful broadcasting and tobacco lobbies were working at odds to one another, both ended up losing (21).

The resulting 1969 and 1970 legislation strengthened the cigarette warning label and mandated that it be included in all advertisements. It also banned television and radio advertising of cigarettes and prohibited state-based regulation of tobacco cigarette advertising in favor of federal regulatory authority (Public Health Cigarette Smoking Act of 1970, 15 U.S.C. § 1333[a]). States are still allowed to regulate local advertisements, such as billboards or sporting events, and many do prohibit cigarette advertising in specific places (2).

The ban on broadcast advertisements meant that antismoking messages mandated under the fairness doctrine also were discontinued. This had the effect of curtailing the public's exposure to information regarding the health consequences of smoking, and the decline in smoking rates slowed. The fairness doctrine itself was repealed in 1987 (3).

Today, cigarettes account for the second highest expenditure on advertisements in the print media, which includes magazines, billboards, newspapers, and scoreboards. Data collected by the Federal Trade Commission show that in 1988 cigarettes were the most often advertised product in the outdoor media, and the second most prevalent type of advertising in magazines (3). The major cigarette manufacturers outspent the U.S. National Cancer Institute's antismoking effort by almost $100 to $1 in 1990. (The institute spent $47 million in 1990 on antismoking campaigns, whereas the tobacco industry spent $3.6 billion on cigarette advertising [2]).

REGULATION OF SMOKING
ENVIRONMENTAL TOBACCO SMOKE

Environmental tobacco smoke (ETS) is smoke introduced into the environment by a smoker, either as mainstream smoke that is inhaled and then exhaled directly, or sidestream smoke produced by a burning cigarette (22). In the late 1800s, long before the Surgeon General found an association between cancer and smoking, there was a general belief that exposure to second-hand smoke caused poor health, disease, and moral decay (5).

Surgeon General Jesse L. Steinfeld recognized the probability of negative health consequences of environmental tobacco smoke in 1970, and ordered a review of the problem. In 1972, the Surgeon General published the first official report identifying environmental tobacco smoke as a "probable" health risk (2). In the absence of clearer proof linking environmental tobacco smoke with negative health effects, however, nonsmokers who argued for legal restrictions on smoking in public places could only point to environmental tobacco smoke as a nuisance and annoyance. The debate was often seen as the smoker's right to smoke, implicating individual liberty, versus the non-smoker's right to be free of a relatively minor nuisance (23).

Over the past two decades, the federal government has funded research into the negative health consequences of environmental tobacco smoke. Several studies found that the nonsmoking children and spouses of smokers suffered increased levels of respiratory illness and cancer. In addition, studies found that the increased risk for cancer and respiratory illness was directly related to the amount of environmental tobacco smoke to which the non-smoking family members were exposed (10). In 1986, the Surgeon General declared that research on environmental tobacco smoke had provided enough evidence to require government action to protect the public's health against the dangers of environmental tobacco smoke (22).

The antismoking movement was greatly strengthened by the preliminary publication of a report in 1992 sponsored by the EPA that linked environmental tobacco smoke with lung cancer, heart disease, and respiratory illness in children. The EPA released its final version of its controversial report on the health effects of environmental tobacco smoke on January 7, 1993 (24). The report announced that the EPA would classify environmental tobacco smoke as a known human carcinogen, and that environmental tobacco smoke directly caused an additional 40,000 deaths annually from heart disease and lung cancer.

The results of the EPA study are disputed by the tobacco industry, which accuses the EPA of using defective meta-analysis and 90% rather than the standard 95% confidence intervals to reach its results. In testimony before the Senate, the Congressional Research Service stated that the report's "statistical evidence does not appear to support a conclusion that there are substantial health effects from passive smoking" (25).

Although the results of the EPA report are being challenged in court by the tobacco industry, there has been confirmation of the EPA's findings by independent research. An influential study published in 1992 gave separate corroboration to the link between environmental tobacco smoke and lung cancer through a study of pathological changes in lung specimens of people exposed to environmental tobacco smoke taken at autopsy (26). More recently, another large study confirmed the dose response between exposure to environmental tobacco smoke and the risk for lung cancer in nonsmoking spouses of smokers (15).

Smoking in Public Places

STATE REGULATION

Prior to the Surgeon General's identification of environmental tobacco smoke as a probable health hazard in 1970, smoking had been prohibited in certain areas under fire safety codes (2). The government's recognition that environmental tobacco smoke was a potential health hazard in 1972 motivated state governments to pass laws banning smoking in certain public places (e.g., elevators), and that process has continued since then (2). As an official of the U.S. Department of Agriculture noted in 1980:

Ten years ago you could smoke cigarettes, cigars, and pipes almost everywhere. But how times change! The 1972 issue of the U.S. Surgeon General's Health Consequences of Smoking reported a danger from passive smoking.... The next year (1973). Arizona and Oregon enacted the first smoking prohibition laws. There are now 38 states that have laws prohibiting smoking in certain public places or segregating smokers from nonsmokers (23).

Throughout the 1970s and 1980s, as the evidence that environmental tobacco smoke was harmful grew, increasing numbers of states passed legislation banning smoking in public places as a public health hazard (23). Currently, almost every state and the District of Columbia have laws that restrict smoking in public places, and many have expanded the restriction to include private sector areas such as restaurants, private hospitals, and private worksites (2).

During this time period many local governments also passed ordinances that were more restrictive than state regulation of smoking in public places. Many of the local ordinances were passed because the tobacco industry had successfully blocked smoking restrictions on the state level. In response to the threat of local laws, state legislators passed laws preempting local smoking regulation. As of 1990, seven states had passed laws giving state legislatures the exclusive right to restrict smoking in designated places (2).

AIRLINE FLIGHTS

There is long-standing federal legislation that regulates smoking on airlines. Congress mandated nonsmoking sections be designated on all commercial airline flights in 1971 (2).

In 1983, the U.S. Civil Aeronautics Board (CAB) strengthened the regulations to ban all smoking on flights that were less than two hours long, but the CAB reversed its ruling after intensive lobbying efforts. In 1987, the ban on smoking on flights of two hours or less was reinstated by Congress, and in 1989 the ban was extended to flights of six hours or less, effectively banning smoking on almost all domestic flights (49 U.S.C. § 1374(d)). Congress refused to extend the ban to international flights (2, 10).

FEDERAL BUILDINGS

In addition to prohibiting smoking on certain airline flights, Congress has also acted to protect its own employees from environmental tobacco smoke. The U.S. General Services Administration (GSA), the owner of most federal office buildings, restricted smoking in GSA buildings in 1986. These regulations do permit smoking in designated areas, however. Several other federal entities have restricted smoking in the workplace, including the U.S. Postal Service and the U.S. Department of Veterans Affairs (10). The Department of Health and Human Services prohibits smoking completely (2). The U.S. Defense Department recently announced a ban on smoking in all military areas, even inside tanks (11).

Smoking in the Workplace

Under the Occupational Safety and Health Act of 1970 (29 U.S.C. § 651), the Occupational Safety and Health Administration (OSHA) has a mandate to ensure that every employer provide a work environment which is free from health risks that are known to cause death or serious physical harm (10). There is no specific exemption for tobacco, tobacco products, or environmental tobacco smoke under the act. While OSHA may have the authority to regulate environmental tobacco smoke, it has to date refrained from direct regulation, although OSHA does require that worksites meet air standard qualities for 24 substances emitted in environmental tobacco smoke (10).

Citing the EPA report on environmental tobacco smoke, OSHA recently published proposed regulations setting quality standards for indoor air. The proposed standards would mandate that employers either ban smoking completely, or permit smoking only in areas with a separate and contained ventilation system (27). The proposed regulations would apply to all private sector workplaces with 10 or more employees and to most government-owned buildings. Bars and restaurants would also be included in the smoking ban, although they have objected strenuously. OSHA maintains that its rules would increase the average worker's productivity by 3%. The final OSHA regulations governing indoor air quality would most likely take several years to go into effect (28).

OTHER FEDERAL ANTISMOKING INITIATIVES

EDUCATION EFFORTS

The federal government funds, supports, and administers public health campaigns to educate Americans regarding the negative health effects of tobacco, and to encourage people to abstain from using tobacco. The first federal antitobacco health education program was created in 1965, and it authorized the Public Health Service to collect information in the National Clearinghouse on Smoking and Health and to develop and administer programs to educate the public and physicians about the health consequences of smoking (15 U.S.C. § 1331–1341) (3). The clearinghouse was among the first to run antismoking advertisements in the popular media.

In 1970, Congress passed legislation requiring the Surgeon General to provide annual reports to Congress on the health consequences of smoking (15 U.S.C. § 1333(a)). These reports, and the media coverage surrounding their release, have been one of the most visible and productive tools in the federal antismoking effort (2). The antismoking message is apparently effective: beginning with the 1964 surgeon general's report, adult per capita consumption of cigarettes has fallen in years when the government actively promotes an antismoking message (2).

In 1984, the Comprehensive Smoking Education Act strengthened the government's antismoking public health efforts by vesting concentrated authority for related research, funding, and administration in the U.S. Secretary of Health and Human Services. The 1984 act also created the Interagency Committee on Smoking and Health, which has responsibility for coordinating antismoking education efforts of federal, state, and local governments, and private entities (15 U.S.C. § 1331–1341) (2).

In 1986, Congress took note that young people, especially males, were using smokeless or chewing tobacco in alarmingly greater numbers. In response, Congress passed the Comprehensive Smokeless Tobacco Health Education Act of 1986 (15 U.S.C. § 4401–4408) (3). The act basically extended regulations applicable to cigarettes to smokeless tobacco. These regulations included the establishment of a public health education program to research and educate the public about the health consequences of smokeless tobacco use (29).

TAXATION

Cigarettes were first taxed by the federal government during the Civil War, and the rate of their taxation has since risen and fallen with the need for federal revenue. Thus, in World War I and World War II, the tax on cigarettes increased substantially, returning to prewar levels after economic normalization. The federal cigarette tax held steady at $.08 per pack from 1951 until 1982. At that point, the tax was increased to $.16 per pack (30), and it was raised to $.24 in 1986, the level at which it remains as of this writing (7).

Even though the federal tax on cigarettes has increased over time, the revenues from taxation of cigarettes as a percentage of total federal revenue have decreased (7, 31). In 1984, the federal government received $4.7 billion, or 0.7%, of its total revenue from taxes on cigarettes. If inflation is taken into account and the federal tax is measured in 1984 dollars, the effective percentage of a pack of cigarettes accounted for by federal tax fell from 38% in 1950, to 13% in 1982 (31).

In 1921, the first state levied a tax on cigarettes, and currently every state and the District of Columbia impose a tax. Cigarette taxes vary widely from state to state and are very low in tobacco-producing states such as North Carolina. State taxes currently make up an average of 15% of the price of a pack of cigarettes, and these taxes on average are a source of 0.12% of state revenue (3, 31).

Only recently has the federal government seen cigarette taxation as a method of discouraging people, especially young people, from smoking. At the same time, increased taxes can generate additional government revenue. Especially in connection with funding health insurance for the uninsured population, large increases in the tobacco tax have been proposed.

Studies on the effects of the price of cigarettes on smoking consumption have shown that consumption declines with rising price. The decline is mostly attributed to smokers who quit smoking completely when the price rises, rather than from smokers who reduce the number of cigarettes they smoke. Increases in the price of cigarettes also discourage younger people from smoking more often than older people. For example, it is estimated that if the price of cigarettes rose by 10%, demand for cigarettes among the 12- to 17-year-old population would drop by 14%, but it would drop by only 4.7% in the 26- to 35-year-old population (2).

TOBACCO PROMOTION PROGRAMS

In addition to regulating tobacco products, the federal government is involved in the growing of tobacco, as well as in its exportation to and importation from foreign countries. Tobacco production has been declining in the United States over the past three decades, whereas foreign production, especially in China, has increased. In the latter part of the 1950s, the United States grew almost half of all the tobacco in the world, excluding China. By the end of the 1980s, the United States' share had declined to less than 10% (7). Two factors drove the reduction in domestic tobacco production: the decline in consumption, which was aggravated by a trend toward using smaller amounts of tobacco in individual cigarettes, and the increased importation of tobacco from foreign sources.

Even with declining production, tobacco is still an extremely important crop in the United States. Most tobacco farmers are small business people, and the industry is concentrated in six states: North Carolina, Kentucky, South Carolina, Virginia, Georgia, and Tennessee (9). Tobacco is among the most lucrative crops, and it is the sixth leading source of farm income in the United States. A tobacco farmer can gross more than $3,000 per acre for the crop, whereas a wheat farmer receives less than $200 per acre and a cotton farmer, less than $500 per acre. In addition to direct tobacco production, the tobacco industry affects many parts of the U.S. economy, including pesticides, paper, lighter manufacturers, transportation, and banking (9).

SUPPORT OF DOMESTIC PRODUCTION

The federal government supports tobacco production, as it does many other crops, such as corn, wheat, and rice. The tobacco price support program provides a guarantee for farmers that their product will be bought at a certain price determined by the U.S. secretary of agriculture using a predetermined formula. In return for the guarantee, farmers limit their production to a certain amount.

The program is voluntary: farmers can choose to join the buying cooperative or not. Control is local, and farms in a given area form regional tobacco cooperatives that allocate a certain number of acres to tobacco production. These allocations can be bought, sold, or leased by their owners. However, the allocated acres must be used to grow tobacco for at least two of every three years, or they are lost (7).

The price support program for tobacco worked well until the early 1980s, when large parts of the tobacco crop were not being sold because of inflated American prices relative to the world market. In 1985, the government had to pay $3.5 billion dollars to cover the guarantees it had made to tobacco farmers. In the face of a growing antitobacco lobby, Congress restructured the price support program. Congress reduced the guaranteed price on tobacco substantially to bring U.S. tobacco prices in line with the world market, a move that also helped to boost exports. In addition, the amount of tobacco that could be grown under the allotments was reduced, and the cigarette companies were forced to estimate their tobacco needs 1 year in advance of the crop and to buy at least 90% of their estimates.

Also, Congress amended the price support program in 1981 to require that the tobacco farmers themselves subsidize the program, the so-called "no-net-cost" provision. This provision was intended to answer criticisms that the American taxpayer was subsidizing an industry that produces a deadly product. However, in 1993 it is estimated that the federal government still spent $70 to $100 million dollars to subsidize tobacco programs (31).

Recent U.S. Department of Agriculture rules protect domestic tobacco growers from foreign competition. As of January 1994, manufacturers of cigarettes in the United States are taxed and subject to certain restrictions if they do not use at least 75% domestic tobacco in their cigarettes (30). Foreign cigarettes also are subject to an import tax as of January 1994. The tax on imported tobacco will be pooled with the tax assessed on domestic growers to cover the costs of the subsidy program (33).

EXPORTS

Although domestic consumption of cigarettes has declined over the past three decades, exports to foreign countries of American tobacco products, especially cigarettes, have increased dramatically (9). This increase in large part relates to the federal price support program's enforced lowering of domestic tobacco prices and aggressive trade practices pursued under the Reagan administration to open foreign markets to U.S. tobacco.

The United States began to develop a Third World market for tobacco in the late 1950s (9). In the 1970s, the tobacco companies saw their domestic market shrink while the Third World market expanded. In the mid-1980s, negotiations to open Japanese and other Far Eastern tobacco markets commenced under Section 301 of the revised U.S. Trade Act. The Act's purpose is to give American companies the same access to foreign markets as those foreign countries have to U.S. markets.

Japan and other countries in the Far East had quotas and taxes that virtually guaranteed that the U.S. tobacco manufacturers could not compete in these markets (7). The U.S. government threatened to impose trade sanctions unless the governments lifted the barriers to tobacco trade. In response, Japan and other governments lowered import tariffs and liberalized their regulation of advertising, promotion, and price (34).

In 1985, the government reopened its complaints against Japan under Section 301, the first time the government brought a complaint against a foreign government without first receiving a formal request to bring such a complaint by a domestic industry (35). The action met with great success, and the export by the United States of cigarettes to Japan and other Far Eastern countries doubled over the next 3 years.

The export policy of the United States has been criticized for helping domestic companies promote a product abroad that the U.S. government actively discourages.

CONCLUSION

Government regulation of tobacco and tobacco products has been increasing in recent years as the intensity of regulation and variety of regulatory forms have both increased. A number of pending issues remain unresolved, including the effects of second-hand smoke and cigarette additives, which may lead to still further regulation in the future.

Acknowledgment

The author thanks Melinda Friend of the Washington, D.C., law firm Fox, Bennett & Turner for her substantial assistance in researching and preparing this chapter.

References

1. Miles, RH. Coffin nails and corporate strategies. Englewood Cliffs, NJ: Prentice-Hall, 1982.
2. U.S. Department of Health and Human Services. Strategies to control tobacco use in the United States: a blueprint for public health action in the 1990's. Washington, DC: DHHS, NIH Pub No 92-3316, October 1991.
3. U.S. Congress. Senate Committee on Labor and Human Resources. Tobacco product education and health protection act of 1991. S. Rep. No. 112, 102d Cong., 1st Sess., 1991.
4. Rabin RL. Some thoughts on smoking regulation. Stanford Law Review 1991;43:475–496.
5. Tate C. In the 1800s, antismoking was a burning issue. Smithsonian 1989;20(July):107.
6. Wagner S. Cigarette country: tobacco in American history and politics. New York: Praeger Publishers, 1971.
7. U.S. Department of Health and Human Services, Office on Smoking and Health. CDC fact book: smoking tobacco and health. Washington, DC: DHHS, Pub No (CDC)87-8397, 1989.
8. Austin v. Tennessee, 179 U.S. 343 (1900).
9. Ross CS. Judicial and legislative control of the tobacco industry: toward a smoke-free society? University of Cincinnati Law Review 1987;56:317–341.
10. Horowitz AB. Terminating the "passive" paradox: a proposal for federal regulation of environmental tobacco smoke. American University Law Review 1991;41:183–220.
11. Schwartz J. Smoking recast: from sophistication to sin; once-sacrosanct industry feels effects of grass-roots movement. Washington Post 1994;May 29:A1.
12. O'Reilly JT. A consistent ethic of safety regulation: the case for improving regulation of tobacco products. Administrative Law Journal 1989;3:215–253.
13. Kessler DA. Statement on nicotine-containing cigarettes. Presented to the U.S. House Subcommittee on Health and the Environment, March 25, 1994.
14. Campbell WI, Johnson JW, Taddeo J, Tisch AH. Presented to the Oversight Hearing on Tobacco Products of the Subcommittee on Health and the Environment of the U.S. House Committee on Energy and Commerce, April 14, 1994.
15. Fontham ETH, Correa P, Reynolds P, et al. Environmental tobacco smoke and lung cancer in nonsmoking women: a multicenter study. JAMA 1994;271:1752–1759.
16. AMA urging U.S. to regulate tobacco. San Francisco Examiner 1994;June 7:A9.
17. U.S. Congressional Research Service. Memorandum. June 8, 1994.
18. White K. Synar co-sponsors anti-tobacco bill. Gannett News Service 1993:May 17.
19. R. J. Reynolds Tobacco Co. Press release. April 13, 1994.
20. Levin M. What goes up in smoke? The Nation 1991;December 23:808–810.
21. Edwards KL. First Amendment values and the constitutional protection of tobacco advertising. Northwestern University Law Review 1987;82:145–180.
22. Ginestra LI. Environmental tobacco smoke: cruel and unusual punishment? Kansas Law Review 1993;42:169–199.
23. Finger WR. The tobacco industry in transition. Lexington. MA: Lexington Books, 1981.
24. U.S. Environmental Protection Agency (EPA). Respiratory health effects of passive smoking: lung cancer and other disorders. (EPA/600/6-90/006F). Washington, DC: Office of Health and Environmental Assessment, Research and Development, EPA, 1992.
25. Gravelle JE, Zimmerman D. Environmental tobacco smoke. Presented to the Subcommittee on Clean Air and Nuclear Regulation of the Senate Committee on Environment and Public Works, May 11, 1994.
26. Trichopoulos D, Mollo F, Tomatis L, et al. Active and passive smoking and pathological indicators of lung cancer risk in an autopsy study. JAMA 1992;268:1697–1701.
27. U.S. Occupational Safety and Health Administration. Indoor air quality. Federal Register 1994;59:15968–16039.
28. Bureau of National Affairs, Inc. Possible nicotine manipulation is issue for FDA, Kessler tells panel. 1994 BNA Management Briefing, March 28, 1994.
29. World Health Organization. Legislative responses to tobacco use. Boston: Kluwer Academic Publishers, 1992.

30. U.S. Department of Agriculture. Tobacco marketing quotas, acreage allotments, and production adjustment. Federal Register 1994;59:28207–28214.
31. Toder EJ. Issues in the taxation of cigarettes. In: The Cigarette Excise Tax: April 17, 1985. Cambridge, MA: Harvard University, 1985.
32. National Coalition for Cancer Research. Memorandum: tobacco price support legislation, April 5, 1993.
33. U.S. Department of Agriculture. Tobacco; importer assessments. Federal Register 1994;59:10939–10946.
34. Council on Scientific Affairs. The worldwide smoking epidemic: tobacco trade, use, and control. JAMA 1990;263:3312–3318.
35. Thatcher KB. Section 301 of the Trade Act of 1974: its utility against alleged unfair trade practices by the Japanese government. Northwestern University Law Review 1987;81:492–538.

INDEX

Page numbers in *italics* denote figures; those followed by "t" denote tables.

Acetaldehyde exposure, 76–77
Acetylcholine receptor antibodies, 656
N-Acetylcysteine, 100, 1056, 1065
Achalasia, 540, 566, 594–595
Achromobacter infection, 998
Acinetobacter infection, 998
Acinus, 10, *11*
Acrylonitrile exposure, 75
Actinomycin D
   for cardiac angiosarcoma, 697
   for cardiac rhabdomyosarcoma, 698
   for neuroepithelioma, 727
   pulmonary toxicity of, 1008
   for thymoma, 662
Acute tumor lysis syndrome, 1009
ACY1 gene, 34
Acyclovir, 995
Adenoacanthoma of esophagus, 549
Adenocarcinoma of esophagus, 533, 547–549, 566–567
   Barrett's epithelium and, 538–539, 547, *548*, 566, 567, 590–592, 645
   classification of, 536t
   at esophagogastric junction, 547, 549–550, 630
   gross morphology of, 548
   histology of, 548–549, *548–549*
   location of, 548
   origin of, 547
   pathophysiology of, 590–592
   prevalence and incidence of, 538–539, 547, 630
   variants of, 549
      adenoacanthoma, 549
      adenosquamous carcinoma, 549
Adenocarcinoma of lung, 113, 115, 247, 253–257
   asbestos, mesothelioma and, 253, 256, 257t
   biomarkers for, 253t, 764–766
      antibodies to milk fat globules, 765–766
      B72.3, 766
      Ber-EP4, 766
      carcinoembryonic antigen, 764–765, *765*
      Leu-M1, 765
   bronchoalveolar carcinoma, 255
   cytologic appearance of, 249, *249*, 250, 766–767, *767*

   differentiation from mesothelioma, 769–770, 786–787, 787t
   epidemiology of, 25
   in HIV-infected patients, 253, 1041
   immunocytochemistry of, 256–257, 257t
   incidence of, 253
   lectin immunostaining patterns for, 265, 266t
   locations of, 253, 293
      superior sulcus, 376
   morphometry of, 257
   occult, 339
   oncogenes in, 32–33
   pathology of, *253*, 253–254
   pleural invasion by, 268, *268*, 295
   prognosis for, 268–269
   scar adenocarcinoma, 255–256
   stage IIIA, *354*
   subtypes of, 253
   tumor necrosis in, 268, *268*
Adenoid cystic carcinoma
   of esophagus, 550
   imaging of, 128
   of trachea, 855–869. *See also* Tracheal tumors
Adenomas, esophageal, 541, *541–542*
Adenosquamous carcinoma
   of esophagus, 549
   of lung, 260–261, *260–261*
      in HIV-infected patients, 1041
Adjuvant therapy for esophageal cancer, 601–602, 614–621
   chemotherapy, 614t, 614–621, 616t
      combined with radiation, 602, 618–620, 620t
      combined with radiation and surgery, 620–621, 621t–622t, 635
      preoperative, 601, 616–618, 617t–618t, 635–638, 636t
   radiation therapy, 601, 609–614, *610*
      combined with chemotherapy, 602, 618–620, 620t
      combined with chemotherapy and surgery, 620–621, 621t–622t
      postoperative, 613t, 613–614
      preoperative, 601–602, 612–613, 613t
Adjuvant therapy for lung cancer
   stage I disease, 344
   stage II disease, 345–347

   stage IIIA disease, 363–371
      early trials of, 363–364
      optimal regimen for, 368–369, *369–370*
      rationale for, 363
      recent trials of, 364–368
         chemotherapy and radiation without resection, 364–366, 365t
         chemotherapy before resection, 366–367
         combined chemotherapy and radiation before resection, 367t, 367–368
   stage IIIB disease, 409–410
      adjuvant surgery, 409–410, 411t
      treatment of superior vena cava syndrome, 410
   superior sulcus tumors, 380, 384, 385
Adrenal metastases, 296, *421*
   vs. benign adenoma, 124
   resection of solitary metastasis, 420–423, *422–423*
   small cell lung cancer and, 527–528
Adrenocorticotropic hormone (ACTH), 298, 299, 852
Adriamycin. *See* Doxorubicin
Adult respiratory distress syndrome, 250
Advertising for cigarettes, 59–60, 1083–1084
Age effects
   on esophageal cancer incidence, 538, 564
   of lung cancer incidence, 245
   on mediastinal germ cell tumor incidence, 668
   on mesothelioma incidence, 786
   on smoking and risk of lung cancer, 53–54, *54*
   on thymoma incidence, 655, *655*
   on thymus, 143
   on tracheal tumor incidence, 856t, 856–857
Agnor score, 269
AIDS. *See* Human immunodeficiency virus-related disorders
Air pollution, 79–80
Airline smoking bans, 1085
Airway anatomy, 10–11
Airway fire, 930, 933
Airway obstruction
   brachytherapy for, 940–946
   bronchoscopic laser resection for, 925–935
   diagnosis of, 928, *929*

Airway obstruction, (*continued*)
  due to esophageal cancer, 567, 622–623
  due to tracheal tumors, 858–859
  fixed vs. variable, 171
  flow-volume curves in patients with, 171, *171–172*
  intrathoracic vs. extrathoracic, 171, *172*
  photodynamic therapy for, 947–962
  symptoms of, 940, 944
  tracheobronchial stents for, 925, *931*, 931–932, *933*
Alcohol consumption, esophageal cancer and, 40, 539
Alendronate, 986
Alizapride, 983t
Alkyltransferase pathway for DNA repair, 31
S-Allyl-cysteine, 101
Alopecia, 992, 1004–1005
Altretamine neurotoxicity, 1009
Alveolar cell hyperplasia, 249
Alveolar infiltrates, chemotherapy-induced, 152
Alveolar proteinosis, congenital, 12
Alveoli, 11–12
  blood supply of, 12
  development of, 8, 9
Amenorrhea, chemotherapy-induced, 1009
Amikacin, 981
Amine precursor uptake and decarboxylation (APUD) cells, 17, 298, 850
Aminoglycosides, 981
Aminothidiazole, 632t
Amitriptyline, 989
Amonafide, 632t
Amosite, 735, 740. *See also* Asbestos exposure
Amphotericin B, 980, 981, 998
Analgesia, epidural, 173
Analgesics, 988–990
Anatomy, thoracic, 3–20
  embryology, 3–9
  esophagus, 15, 533–534, 563–564
  heart and pericardium, 17–18
  lungs, 10–14, 388–390, *389*
  lymphatic drainage, 19–20
  paraganglia, 17
  pleura, 14–15, *16*
  pleural fluid, 18–19
  thymus, 15, 17
Anemia, 303, 993–994, 1009
Anesthesia
  for bronchoscopic laser resection, 930–931, 933–934
  effects on lung function, 171–172
  for tracheal reconstruction, 859
  for video-assisted thoracic surgery, 966
Angiocardiography, 682, 684t, 688, *688*
Angiocentric malignant lymphoma of lung, 838–840, *839*
Angiosarcoma
  cardiac, 696–697, *697*
  of chest wall, 872
  pleural, 834–835
  pulmonary, 828

Animal studies
  of esophageal cancer, 40–41, 44–45
  of esophageal carcinogenesis, 539–540
  of fiber-related carcinogenesis, 744–745
  of lung cancer, 35–37
  of potential carcinogens, 66–67
Anorexia, 297, 986–987, 987t
Anthophyllite, 740. *See also* Asbestos exposure
Anticoagulant therapy
  for small cell lung cancer, 475–476, 476t
  for superior vena cava syndrome, 410
Anticonvulsants, 989
Antidepressants, 989
Antidiuretic hormone, inappropriate secretion of, 302–303, 324
Antiemetics, 983t, 983–984, 1008
Antihistamines, 983t
Anti-Hu antibody, 304
Antimicrobials
  empiric treatment with, 981–983, *982*
  prophylactic, 980
  for venous catheter-related infections, 997–998
Antineuronal nuclear antibody type I (ANNA-1), 303–305
Antioxidants, 39, 98, 1054–1056, 1055t, 1060–1067, 1066t. *See also* Chemoprevention of lung cancer
Anxiety, 1018
Aortic rupture, 556
APC gene, 34, 644
APEH gene, 34
Apoptosis, 219
Aredia. *See* Pamidronate
Argon laser, 926t, 926–927
Arm pain, 375, 377
Arrhythmias, 681, 686
Arsenic exposure, 69–70
Arterial blood gases, 176–177
Arteries
  bronchial, 5, 12–14, *13*
  esophageal, 14
  internal mammary, 14
  musculophrenic, 14
  pericardiophrenic, 14
  phrenic, 14
  pulmonary, 12–13, *13*, 15
  superior epigastric, 14
Aryl hydrocarbon hydroxylase (AHH), 284
Asbestos exposure, 26, 51, 70–71, 113, 150. *See also* Fiber-related carcinogenesis
  lung adenocarcinoma and, 254
  mesothelioma and, 735–749, 779, 786. *See also* Mesothelioma causes
Askin's tumor, 832–833, *832–833*
  clinical features of, 832
  pathology of, 833
  posterior mediastinal, 725–727
  therapy and prognosis for, 833
Aspergillus infection, 158, *159*, 981
  esophageal cancer and, 539
  prophylaxis for, 980

surveillance culturing for, 980
total protected isolation and, 979
Aspiration, 294, 567
Aspirin
  for lung cancer prevention, 1066t, 1067
  for small cell lung cancer, 475–476, 476t
Asthma, chemotherapy-induced, 182
Atabrine. *See* Quinacrine
Ataxia-telangiectasia, 17
Atelectasis, 118, 172
Atomic structure, 215
Atrial fibrillation or flutter, 682
Atrial myxoma. *See* Myxoma, cardiac
Autonomic dysfunction, chemotherapy-induced, 1009
Aztreonam, 981

B72.3 monoclonal antibody, 766, 882
Bacille bilié de Calmette-Guérin (BCG), 344, 474
Bacillus infection, 998
Barium esophagram, 132, 569–570, *571*, 571t
Barrett's esophagus, 15, 39, 535–536, *535–536*, 585–594
  adenocarcinoma and, 538–539, 547, *548*, 566, 567, 590–592, 645
  biology of, 592–593
    cell cycle abnormalities, 593
    chromosomal and oncogene abnormalities, 592–593
    DNA abnormalities, 592
  definition of, 585–586
  dysplasia in, 541–542, *542*, 588–589, *589*
    dysplasia-carcinoma sequence, 589–590
  etiology of, 586–587
  histogenesis of, 587
  historical description of, 585
  incidence of carcinoma in, 538–539, 585
  pathology of, 587–588, *588*
  prevalence of, 586
  surveillance of, 593–594
Basal cell tumors of chest wall, 871
Basaloid carcinoma
  of esophagus, 546
  of lung, 263, *263*
bcl-2 protooncogene, 33, 267–268, *268*
BCNU. *See* Belustine
Beckwith-Wiedemann syndrome, 717
Belustine, 471t
Bence-Jones proteinuria, 873
Benign pulmonary neoplasms, 128, 128t
Benzo(*a*)pyrene (BaP), 26, 37–38
  inhibition of carcinogenesis by, 39
  metabolism of, 28, *28*
Benzodiazepines, 983t
Benzyl isothiocyanate, 39, 45
Ber-EP4, 766
Beryllium exposure, 75–76
Beta carotene, 39, 46, 98, 100, 189, 1054–1056, 1055t, 1064–1067, 1066t. *See also* Chemoprevention of lung cancer
Betatron units, 216

Bias, 67, 188, 195–197
Biological gradient, 68
Biological plausibility, 68
Biomarkers, 18, 97
   for adenocarcinoma of lung, 764–766, 765
   data banks of, 107
   definition of, 37
   for lung cancer, 253t
      non-small cell carcinoma, 329
      small cell carcinoma, 259, 324, 325t, 456
      specifically related to lung carcinogens, 37–38
      squamous cell carcinoma, 251–252
   for mediastinal germ cell tumors, 670, 670t, 673–674, 674t
   for mesothelioma, 764–766
   for neuroblastoma, 715–716
   use in chemoprevention, 1069–1072
      biological agents, 1072
      intermediate endpoints, 1070–1072, 1071t
      selection of target populations, 1069–1070, 1070–1071
Bis(chloromethyl) ether (BCME) exposure, 71–72
Bisphosphonates, 985–986
Blastocyst, 3, *4*
Blastoma, pleuropulmonary, 128, 833–834, *834*
   clinical features of, 833–834
   pathology of, 834
   therapy and prognosis for, 834
Bleomycin
   for esophageal cancer, 614, 614t, 631, 632t
      combined with other agents, 615, 633
      preoperative, 616, 635–636, 636t
      with radiation therapy and no surgery, 641, 641t
      with radiation therapy and surgery, 619
   for HIV-associated non-Hodgkin's lymphoma, 1032
   for HIV-related Hodgkin's disease, 1041
   for HIV-related Kaposi's sarcoma, 1038–1039
   for pericardial sclerotherapy, 898–899
   for pleurodesis, 887t, 888–889, 889t
   pulmonary toxicity of, 152–153, 1008
   for thymoma, 662
Blood group antigens, 1071
Blood transfusion, perioperative, 326–327
Blood-gas barrier, 11
BMDP Statistical Software, 320
Bombesin, 456
Bone marrow toxicity
   of chemotherapy, 1009–1010
   of combined modality therapy, 1011
   of radiotherapy, 1006
Bone marrow transplantation, 994–995
   graft versus host disease and, 994
   liver dysfunction after, 994–995
   for nonseminomatous germ cell tumor, 675–676
   preventing viral infections after, 995
   role of cytokines in, 995
   side effects of conditioning regimens for, 994

Bone metastases, 296
   bone scan to assess for, 113–114, 125, *125*, *299*
   resection of, 423
   small cell lung cancer and, 527
Bone toxicity
   of combined modality therapy, 1011
   of radiotherapy, 1008
Bony tumors of chest wall, 871–874
   benign, 871
   malignant, 872–874
Brachial plexopathy, radiation-induced, 1006–1007
   when combined with chemotherapy, 1012
Brachial plexus invasion, 295, 375–376, *376*
Brachytherapy, 234–236
   dose rates for, 234–235, *235–236*
   endobronchial, 235–236, 940–946
      afterloading in, 941, 944
      applicator for, 941
      benefits of, 942, 944
      combined with bronchoscopic laser resection, 935
      combined with external beam radiation, 944–945
      complications of, 944
      definition of, 940
      dose rate for, 941, 944, 945t
      history of, 940–941
      indications for, 940, 942–943
      number of treatments with, 942
      paclitaxel infusion before, 944
      research needs related to, 945–946
      results of, *943*, 943–944
      technique for, 941–942, *941–942*
      treatment times for, 942
   history of, 234
   implants for, 234, *234*
   interstitial implants of lung, 235
   radiation physics and, 218t, 218–219
   radioisotopes used for, 218, 218t
   for stage I lung cancer, 344
   for superior sulcus tumors, 385–386
   technique for, 234–235
Brain metastases from lung cancer, 296, *418*, 512–522
   prophylactic cranial irradiation for, 512–522. *See also* Cranial irradiation
   resection of solitary metastasis, 417–420, 418t–420t, *420–421*, 424
   small cell carcinoma, 525
Breast cancer
   invading chest wall, 874–875, *875*
   metastases to heart, 704
   pulmonary metastasectomy for, 916
Breathing retraining, 1022
Bronchi
   branching and structure of, 10
   management of T3 tumors involving main stem bronchi, 359–361, *361–362*
   occlusion by tumor, 118–120
Bronchial carcinoid. *See* Carcinoid tumors
Bronchial hygiene, 1021–1022

Bronchial-associated lymphoid tissue (BALT), 19
Bronchiolar structure, 10
Bronchiolitis obliterans, 9
Bronchitis, chronic, 606
Bronchoalveolar carcinoma (BAC), 255, 296–297
Bronchoalveolar lavage, 20, 248–250
Bronchoarterial bundle, 13
Bronchorrhea, 294
Bronchoscopic laser resection, 925–935
   anesthesia for, 930–931, 933–934
   combined with other palliative modalities, 928, 935
   compared with photodynamic therapy for advanced tracheobronchial malignancies, 958, 958t
   complications of, 930, 932–934
      airway fire, 930, 933
      bleeding, 930, 932
   control of laser emission for, 926
   definition of laser, 926
   effect on patient survival, 934–935
   for esophageal cancer-related obstruction, 622–623
   history of, 925–926
   indications for, 928–930, 929t
   laser-tissue interactions, 927–928
   optimal tumor characteristics for, 929t, 929–930
   outcome of, 934–935
   rigid vs. flexible bronchoscope for, 930
   safety precautions during, 932–933
   techniques for, 930–931
   types of lasers for, 925–927, 926t
Bronchoscopy, 294, 354, 378, 393
   to diagnose bronchial carcinoids, 853–854
   to diagnose tracheal tumors, 857–858
   in esophageal cancer, 571–572, *572*
   in small cell lung cancer, 459–460
Burkitt's lymphoma, 842
Burns, radiotherapy-induced, 1002
Butylated hydroxyanisole, 39
Butyrophenones, 983t
4C9 antigen, 331

Cachexia, 297, 986–988
Cadmium exposure, 76
Calcification
   in metastases to lung, 136
   in peripheral lung cancers, 117, *117*
   in pulmonary nodules, *129–130*, 129–131, 136
Calcitonin, 301, 985
Camptothecin, 497
Candidal infections, 158–159, 980–981
Cannabinoids, 983t
Carbamazepine, 989
Carbohydrate antigens, 330–331
Carbon dioxide laser, 925–926, 926t
Carboplatin
   for cardiac leiomyosarcoma, 698

Carboplatin (*continued*)
    for esophageal cancer, 632t, 633
    for mesothelioma, 803
    myelosuppression due to, 1009
    for non-small cell lung cancer, 427, 427t
    for small cell lung cancer, 497, 501–502
Carcinoembryonic antigen (CEA), 265, 324, 325t, 456, 764–765, *765*, 882
Carcinogenesis
    chemotherapy-induced, 1010
    esophageal, 39–46
    fiber-related, 742–748
    lung, 25–39
    metabolic activation and detoxification of carcinogens, 27, *27*
    occupational carcinogens, 66–81
        classification of, 69
        known carcinogens, 67–75
        possible carcinogens, 76–79
        probable carcinogens, 75–76
        sources of data about, 66–69
    radiation therapy-induced, 227–228, 228t, 1007–1008
Carcinoid syndrome, 852
Carcinoid tumors
    bronchial, 126–127, *127*, 850–854
        atypical, 850
        biomarkers for, 253t
        clinical features of, 262, 851–853
        diagnosis of, *852*, 852–853
        imaging of, 126–127, *127*, *852*, 853
        locations of, 261–262, 262t, 851
        multiple, 261
        neuroendocrine abnormalities and, 262, 262t, 850–851
        pathology of, 261–263, *262*, 850, *851*, 851t
        pathophysiology of, 850–851
        prognosis for, 853, 854t
        treatment of, 853
    bronchoscopic laser resection of, 934
    of esophagus, 536t, 551
    of thymus, 17
Carcinosarcoma
    differentiation from mesothelioma, 772
    of esophagus, 547, *547*, 556
    pericardial, 706
Cardiac metastases, 701t, 701–705
    acute leukemia and lymphoma, 704
    breast carcinoma, 704
    diagnosis of, 702
    frequency of, 701, 701t
    histopathology of, 702–703, *703*
    invasion through inferior vena cava, 704–705
        hypernephroma, 704
        Wilms' tumor, 704–705
    lung carcinoma, 704
    melanoma, 704
    physical findings associated with, 702
    routes of spread, 702
    sites of, 702
    symptoms of, 701–702

treatment of, 703–704
Cardiac toxicity
    of chemotherapy, 18, 153–154, 486
        cyclophosphamide, 153, 994
        doxorubicin, 18, 153, 486, 1008, 1011–1012
    of combined modality therapy, 1011–1012
    of radiotherapy, 1004–1006
Cardiac tumors, 17–18, 681–701
    benign, 685–695
        in adults, 685–693
            granular cell tumors, 692–693
            hemangioma, 691–692
            incidence of, 685, 686t
            Lambl's excrescence, 693
            lipoma and lipomatous hypertrophy, 691
            myxoma, 685–691
            neurofibroma, 692
            papillary fibroelastoma, 691
            pheochromocytomas, 692
            sites of, 687t
        in children, 693–695
            fibroma, 693–694
            lymphangioma, 694–695
            mesothelioma of atrioventricular node, 694
            rhabdomyoma, 693, 694
            teratoma, 694
    cardiac valve tumors, 700t, 700–701
    diagnostic modalities for, 682–683, 684t
    differential diagnosis of, 683–684
    historical recognition of, 681
    imaging of, 682–683
    physical findings associated with, 682, 683t
    primary malignant, 695–700
        angiosarcoma, 696–697, *697*
        extraskeletal osteosarcoma, 699
        fibrosarcoma and malignant fibrous histiocytoma, 697–698
        incidence of, 695t
        leiomyosarcoma, 698–699
        liposarcoma, 699
        lymphoma, 699
        mesenchymoma, 700
        metastases of, 695–696
        myxosarcoma, 698
        neurogenic sarcomas, 699–700
        rhabdomyosarcoma, 698
        symptoms of, 683t, 695
        synovial sarcoma, 700
        teratoma, 700
        thymoma, 700
        treatment of, 696
            results of, 685t, 696
    surgical treatment of, *684*, 684–685, 685t
    symptoms of, 681–682, 683t
Cardiogenic plate, 4
Cardiomegaly, 695
Cardiopulmonary resuscitation (CPR), 996
Cardiovascular disease, 169, 606
Carmustine toxicity, 152, 1008–1009
Carney's syndrome, 690, 724

Carotene and Retinol Efficacy Trial (CARET), 98
Causal association, 68, 68t
Cavitation of tumor, 135–136, 251, 294
CCNU. *See* Lomustine
Cefoperazone, 981
Ceftazidime, 981
Celiac disease, 540, 596
Cells
    amine precursor uptake and decarboxylation (APUD), 17, 298, 850
    basal, 10
    brush, 11
    ciliated, 10, 255
    Clara, 10, 11, 255
    differentiation of, 5
    esophageal, 534
    goblet, 11, 535–536
    interstitial, 11
    Kulchitsky, 10, 11, 850
    mucous, 10
    multiplication of, 4–5
    neural crest, 5, 17
    pneumocytes, 11, 255
    respiratory epithelial, 10–11
    serous, 10–11
    tumors and, 12
Cephalosporins, 981
Cerebral atrophy, 1009
Cervical cancer, 916
CHART radiotherapy regimen, 397–398
Chemistry of cigarette smoke, 51–53, 52t
Chemodectomas, 723
Chemoprevention, defined, 38, 1052
Chemoprevention of esophageal cancer, 45–46
Chemoprevention of lung cancer, 38–39, 96–101, 1052–1072
    agents for, 1060–1065
        N-acetylcysteine, 1056, 1065
        antioxidants, 1054–1056, 1055t, 1060–1065
        beta carotene, 1054–1056, 1055t, 1064
        combinations of, 1057
        ellagic acid, 1056
        fenretinide, 1063–1064
        isotretinoin, 1061–1063, 1062t
        natural retinol, 1060–1061, 1061t
        oltipraz, 1056, 1065
        retinoids, 1054–1055, 1060–1064
        vitamin E, 1054–1056, 1064–1065
    aimed at various phases of carcinogenesis, 1053–1054, *1054*
    biologic rationale for, 96–97
    clinical trials of, 97–101, 99t, 101t, 1065–1069
        compliance and toxicity, 97–98
        in healthy persons, 1065–1067, 1066t
        new agents, 100–101
        prevention of second primary tumors, 1067–1069, 1068t, *1068–1069*
        study population, 97
        treatment of precancerous lesions, 1067
    dietary factors and, 1052, 1054, 1055t

experimental evidence for, 1054–1057
premalignancy and second primary tumors, 98–99, 344–345, 1067–1069, 1068t, *1068–1069*
primary prevention and, 1052–1053, 1053t
study methodology for, 1057–1060
    endpoints, 97, 99t, 99–100, 1059
    primary vs. secondary prevention studies, 1058, 1058t
    screening new agents, 1057, 1057t–1058t
    selecting high-risk persons, 1057–1058
    study design, *1059*, 1059–1060
use of biologic markers in, 97, 1069–1072
    biological agents, 1072
    intermediate endpoints, 1070–1072, 1071t
    selection of target populations, 1069–1070, 1070t–1071t
Chemotherapy
administration of, 991
for bronchial carcinoids, 853
for HIV-related malignancies
    Hodgkin's disease, 1041
    Kaposi's sarcoma, 1038–1039, 1040t
    lung cancer, 1042
    non-Hodgkin's lymphoma, 1032–1033, 1034t–1035t
for intravascular lymphomatosis of lung, 842
for Kaposi's sarcoma of lung, 818, 1038–1039, 1040t
for lymphomatoid granulomatosis, 840
for mediastinal germ cell tumors, 674–677
    nonseminomatous tumor, 674–676, 676t
    seminoma, 674, 675t
for neuroblastoma, 721, 722t
for neuroepithelioma, 727
for pericardial sclerotherapy, 898
for pleural sclerotherapy, 888–890, 889t
pulmonary metastasectomy and, 910–911
for thymoma, 662–663
Chemotherapy for cardiac tumors, 696
angiosarcoma, 697
extraskeletal osteosarcoma, 699
leiomyosarcoma, 698
liposarcoma, 699
metastatic tumors, 704
primary lymphoma, 699
rhabdomyosarcoma, 698
Chemotherapy for esophageal cancer, 556, 606, 614–621, 631–643
combination therapy, 615–616, 616t, 633–635, 634t
combined with radiation, 602, 618–620, 620t, 640–642, 641t
    current role of, 642–643, *643*
    preoperative, 620–621, 621t–622t, 635, 638–640, 639t
future directions for, 643–645
palliative, 623–624
postoperative, 618
preoperative, 601, 616–618, 617t–618t, 635–638, 636t

single-agent therapy, 614t, 614–615, 631–633, 632t
Chemotherapy for lung cancer
chest disease induced by, 150–154
imaging evaluation and follow-up after, 124–125
lung function and, 169, 181t–182t, 181–182
neurotoxicity of, 518–519
P glycoprotein overexpression and, 467
resistance to, 458, 467–469
small cell carcinoma, 113, 115, 440–441, *442–443*, 456, 467–473
    alternating vs. sequential regimens, 469–470, 471t
    anticoagulant therapy and, 475–476, 476t
    chemoresponsiveness, 441, 467
    combination regimens, 499–502
        CAV, CAE, and CAVE regimens, 500, 501t
        etoposide and cisplatin, 500–501, 501t
        number of drugs, 500
        other combinations, 501–502
    combined with radiotherapy, 440, 477–484
        alternating approaches, 481–484, *482–483*, 483t
        concurrent approaches, 481, 481t
        scheduling methods, 480
        treatment toxicity, 485–486
    development of drug resistance, 458, 467–469
    dose effect within standard range of doses, 470–472, 472t
    dose intensification, 472–473, 504–506, 505t
    drug regimens, 467, 470t
    duration of treatment, 503–504
    hematopoietic growth factors and, 506–507
    history of, 467
    immunotherapy and, 473–475, 504
    investigation of new schedules, 499
    maintenance chemotherapy, 473, 474t
    new agents, 497–499, 502, 507
        epirubicin, 499
        gemcitabine, 498–499
        irinotecan (CPT-11), 497–498
        paclitaxel, 498
    non-cross-resistant alternating regimens, 502–503, 503t
    recurrence after discontinuation of, 441, 458–459
    scheduling, 497, 499
    single-agent therapy, 496–497, 497t
    surgery and, 440–441, *442–443*, 453
        postoperative chemotherapy, 444–447, 445t, *445–446*, 447t
        preoperative chemotherapy, 447–451, 448t–449t, *449–451*
    weekly dose intense regimens, 473, 505–506, 506t

stage I disease, 344
stage II disease, 345–349
stage IIIA disease, 363–371
    combined with radiation before resection, 367t, 367–368
    combined with radiation without resection, 364–366, 365t
    before resection, 366–367
stage IIIB disease, 394–395, 398, 399t
    combined with radiation therapy, 395, 398–409
        concomitant chemotherapy-radiotherapy trials, 407–409, 409t
        rationale for, 399
        sequential chemotherapy-radiotherapy trials, 399–407, 402t–403t, *405*, 406t
        survival rates after, 399
    preoperative, 398, 399t
    results compared with radiotherapy, 398
stage IV disease, 426–433
    combination therapy, 428–430, 429t
    large randomized trials, 430t, 430–431
    new strategies and combinations, 431
    quality of life issues, 432
    related to prognostic factors, 431
    single-agent therapy, 426–428, 427t
    vs. supportive care, 416, 417t, 431–432, 432t
superior sulcus tumors, 380, 385
toxicity of, 485–486
Chemotherapy for mesothelioma, 792, 801–810
combination therapy, 806–807, 807t
current recommendations, 807–808
intrapleural therapy, 808
radiation therapy and, 809
single-agent therapy, 801–806, 802t
surgery and, 795–796, 809–810
Chemotherapy toxicity, 485–486
acute effects, 1008t, 1008–1009
    acute tumor lysis syndrome, 1009
    bone marrow toxicity, 1009
    cardiac toxicity, 18, 153–154, 486, 1008
    emesis, 983–984, 1008
    neurologic toxicity, 518–519, 1009
    pulmonary toxicity, 150–154, 1008–1009
        agents associated with, 152t, 181t–182t
        alveolar infiltrates, 152
        hypersensitivity pneumonitis, 182
        interstitial disease, 151–152, *153*, 181t, 181–182
        pleural effusion, 153
        pulmonary edema, 182, 182t
        pulmonary nodules, 152–153
chronic effects, 1009–1010
    bone marrow toxicity, 1009–1010
    carcinogenesis, 1010
    endocrine disorders, 1009
combined with radiotherapy, 182, 182t, 485–486, 1010–1012
nursing management of, 991–992

Chest pain, 116, 293–295, 294t, 567, 681
Chest radiography, 112
    esophageal cancer on, 569, *570*, 570t
    in immunocompromised host, 156
    limit of detectability of pulmonary nodules on, 117
    for lung cancer screening, 116, 293
    of mediastinum, 139–140
    mesothelioma on, 780
    pericardial effusion on, 895, *896*
    pleural effusion on, 881
    small cell lung cancer on, 459, 461
Chest wall tumors, 295, 870–878
    benign, 870–871
        bony tumors, 871
        deep tumors, 870–871
        superficial tumors, 870
    classification of, 870, 871t
    diagnosis of, 870
    imaging of, 870
    malignant, 871–875
        bony tumors, 872–874, 874t
        deep tumors, 871–872, *873*
        invasion by mammary carcinomas, 874–875, *875*
        metastases, 870, 875
        primary carcinoma of lung, 357–359, 358t, *360*, 874
        superficial tumors, 871
    radiation therapy for, 875–876
    reconstruction techniques for, 876–878
        bony replacement, 876t, 876–878, *877*
        complications, 878
        results, 878
        skin and muscle replacement, 878
    resection techniques for, 875–876
Children
    benign cardiac tumors of, 693–695
        fibroma, 693–694
        lymphangioma, 694–695
        mesothelioma of atrioventricular node, 694
        rhabdomyoma, 693, *694*
        teratoma, 694
    dumbbell tumors in, 729
    fibrosarcoma of lung in, 820
    neuroblastoma in, 715–721
    pulmonary metastasectomy for, 917
    pulmonary rhabdomyosarcoma in, 825–827
    Wilms' tumor invading heart in, 704–705
Chloroethylcyclohexylnitrosourea. *See* Lomustine
Chloromethyl methyl ether (CMME), 71–72
Chlorpromazine, 983t
Chondroma, 871
Chondrosarcoma
    of chest wall, 872, 874t
    pericardial, 706
    of respiratory tract, *827*, 827–828
Choriocarcinoma, 136, 550
Chromaffin system, 17
Chromium
    chemical forms of, 72
    metabolism of chromium IV, 30
    occupational exposure to, 72
Chromogranin A, 265, 324, 325t, 329, 456
Chromosome abnormalities. *See also* Genes; Molecular biology
    in Barrett's esophagus, 592–593
    in esophageal cancer, 44
    isochromosome 12p in mediastinal germ cell tumors, 677
    in lung cancer, 32, 108–109, *109*, 277, 281–282, 456, 1069–1070, 1070t–1071t
        chromosomes 3p and 9p, 281–282, 456
        MCC/APC region on chromosome 5q, 282
        methods of genetic analysis, 277–278
    in malignant pleural fluid, 883
    in mesothelioma, 746–747, 768–769, 789
    in neuroblastoma, 716
    in neuroepithelioma, 726
Chronic obstructive pulmonary disease (COPD), 169, 1018
    effects of inhalational anesthesia in, 171–172
    hypercapnia and, 176
    post-thoracotomy mortality in patients with, 171
    pulmonary function testing in, 170
Chronic progressive radiation myelitis, 1007
Chylothorax, 294
Cigarette smoking. *See* Smoking
Ciprofloxacin, 980, 981
Cisplatin
    for bronchial carcinoids, 853
    for cardiac tumors, 696
        osteosarcoma, 699
    for esophageal cancer, 614, 614t, 632t, 632–633, 644
        combined with other agents, 615–616, 616t, 633–635, 634t
        palliative, 624
        preoperative, 616–618, 635–638, 636t
        with radiation therapy and no surgery, 640–642, 641t
        with radiation therapy and surgery, 619–620, 639t, 639–640
        toxicity when combined with radiation therapy, 1010–1011
    for lung cancer
        non-small cell carcinoma, 365t, 426–427, 427t, 429t, 429–431
        small cell carcinoma, 470, 470t–472t, 473, 474t, 497, 500–501, 501t
    for mediastinal germ cell tumors, 674–676
        nonseminomatous tumor, 674–676, 676t
        seminoma, 674, 675t
    for mesothelioma, 803
        combined with other agents, 807, 807t
        intrapleural therapy, 808
    for neuroblastoma, 722t
    for pericardial sclerotherapy, 898
    for pleural sclerotherapy, 889, 889t
    for thymoma, 662–663

Clean Air Act, 1081
Clear cell carcinoma of lung, 258
Clinical presentation
    of cardiac tumors, 681–682, 683t
    of esophageal cancer, 555–556, 567–568
    of lung cancer, 116, 293–306
    of mediastinal germ cell tumors, 669, 669t
    of mesothelioma, 779–780, 787
    of thymoma, 656
Clinical trials, 188–209, 319
    analysis of, 199–203
        excluding patients from analysis, 200
        interim analyses, 201t–202t, 201–203
        significance tests and confidence interval, 199t, 199–200
        subgroup analysis, 200
        survival analysis and competing risks, 200–201, *201*
    of chemoprevention of lung cancer, 97–101, 1065–1069
    of combination chemotherapy for disseminated non-small cell lung cancer, 430t, 430–432, 432t
    of combined chemotherapy-radiotherapy for stage IIIB lung cancer, 399–409
    vs. database studies, 188
    defining objectives of, 189–190
    definition of, 188
    determining endpoints for, 192–195, *193–194*
    ethical issues in, 203–204
        informed consent and randomization, 203t, 203–204
        interim analyses and data monitoring committee, 204
    impact on clinical practice, 208–209
    of mesothelioma treatment, 800
    meta-analysis of, 205–208, 206t, 207–208, 208t
    patient selection for, 190–192, 191t
    phases of, 188
    protocol for, 189–190, 190t
    rationale of, 188–189
    reporting results of, 204–205
    study design for, 195–199
        phase II design, 195
        phase III design, 195–199
            advantages of randomization, 195, 196t
            factorial design, 198
            large-scale trial and prospective pooled analysis, 198–199
            randomization methods, 195–197
            trial size, 197, 198t
        phase IV design, 199
Clodronate, 985
Clubbing, digital, 294t, 297
Coagulation disorders, 303
Collagen vascular disease, 1002, 1003t
Colorectal cancer, 915t, 915–916
Combined immunodeficiency disease, 17
Combined modality therapy toxicity, 1001, 1010–1012
    bone marrow toxicity, 1011

bone toxicity, 1011
cardiac toxicity, 1011–1012
cutaneous effects, 1011
endocrine toxicity, 1012
in esophageal cancer, 1010–1011
in lung cancer, 1011
neurotoxicity, 1012
Comparative genomic hybridization, 277
Comprehensive Smokeless Tobacco Health Education Act, 1083
Comprehensive Smoking Education Act, 1082
Computed tomography (CT), 112
adenoid cystic carcinoma on, 128
adrenal metastasis on, 296, 421–422, *421–422*
to assess patient for video-assisted thoracic surgery, 965
bronchial carcinoid on, 127, *852, 853*
cardiac tumors on, 682, 684t
chest wall tumors on, 870
to detect calcification within pulmonary nodules, 130–131
dumbbell tumors on, *727, 728*
HIV-related Kaposi's sarcoma on, 1037, *1038*
Hodgkin's disease on, 141, *142*
for localization for percutaneous lung biopsy, 131–132
lung cancer on, 121–124
small cell carcinoma, 461
stage IIIA, 351–352, *353*, 355–357, *355–358*
stage IIIB, 392, *392*
superior sulcus tumors, 378, *378*
of mediastinum, 140–141
mesothelioma on, 780
non-Hodgkin's lymphoma on, 142
paraspinal tumors on, 148
pulmonary metastases on, 137–139, *140*, 907
for staging esophageal cancer, 132–135, *133*, 572–574, 573t, 597
technique for, 124
thymoma on, 657, *657–658, 659*
Confidence interval, 199t, 199–200, 320
Conformal radiation therapy, 236–237
Confounding bias, 67
Congestive heart failure (CHF), 681, 699
cyclophosphamide-induced, 994
due to doxorubicin combined with radiotherapy, 1012
Consumer Product Safety Act, 1081
Controlled Substances Act, 1081
Coronary artery disease (CAD), 1006
Corticosteroids
for anorexia, 988
for chemotherapy-induced emesis, 983
as co-analgesics, 989
neurotoxicity of, 1009
for tumor-induced hypercalcemia, 985
Corynebacterium jeikeium infection, 981, 998
Corynebacterium parvum
for pleurodesis, 890, 890t
for resected stage I lung cancer, 344
Cough, 116, 293–295, 294t, 391

Cox proportional hazards regression model, 320
CPT-11. See Irinotecan
Cranial irradiation, prophylactic, 512–522
contemporary studies of, 516–517, 517t
future directions for, 519–522
neuropsychologic morbidity from, 514–516, 515t
radiation dosage and schedule for, 516–517, 517t, 520t, 520–521
recommendations for, 519
results of clinical trials of, 512–514, 513t
timing of, 521
toxicity of, 517–519, 1006
when combined with radiotherapy, 1012
Creatine kinase BB, 324, 325t, 456
Cricopharyngeus muscle, 15, 533–534
Critical care, 995–997
Crocidolite, 150, 735, 740. See also Asbestos exposure
Cryosurgery, 925
Cryptococcosis, 159
Crysotile, 735, 739t, 740–741, 743–744. See also Asbestos exposure
Cushing's syndrome, 17, 299–300, 324, 851, 852
Cutaneous effects of radiotherapy, 1002–1005
Cutaneous paraneoplastic syndromes, 297–298, *299*
Cyclin D1, 43
Cyclizine, 983t
Cyclophosphamide
for cardiac tumors, 696
angiosarcoma, 697
lymphoma, 699
rhabdomyosarcoma, 698
cardiotoxicity of, 153, 994
for HIV-associated non-Hodgkin's lymphoma, 1032
for intravascular lymphomatosis of lung, 842
for lung cancer
non-small cell carcinoma, 365t, 429
small cell carcinoma, 440–441, 442, 467, 470, 470t–472t, 472, 473, 474t, 496, 497, 500, 501t
for lymphomatoid granulomatosis, 840
for mesothelioma, 792, 804
combined with other agents, 806–807, 807t
for neuroblastoma, 722t
for neuroepithelioma, 727
for pericardial sclerotherapy, 898
for thymoma, 662–663
Cyclosporin, 994
Cylindroma, 855–856
CYP1A1 gene, 284
Cyproheptadine, 988
Cystitis, hemorrhagic, 994
Cytarabine
for HIV-associated non-Hodgkin's lymphoma, 1032

for pleurodesis, 889, 889t
Cytochrome *P450* enzymes, 27, 38
Cytokeratins, 264–265
Cytokines
role in anorexia-cachexia, 987, 988
role in bone marrow transplantation, 995
role in systemic effects of lung cancer, 297
for small cell lung cancer, 474–475
Cytology
of adenocarcinoma of lung, 766–767, *767*
of esophageal cancer, 537
of lung cancer, 248–250
fine-needle aspiration cytology, 250
sputum cytology and bronchoalveolar lavage, 93, 248–250, *249*
of malignant pleural effusion, 882
of mesothelioma, 760–762
Cytomegalovirus infection, 159
after bone marrow transplantation, 995
HIV-associated, 1035, 1043t
treatment of, 995
Cytoskeletal components, 264–265

D8 gene, 34
Dacarbazine
for cardiac tumors, 696
leiomyosarcoma, 698
for HIV-related Hodgkin's disease, 1041
for mesothelioma, 792
for neuroepithelioma, *727*
for small cell lung cancer, 471t
Data monitoring committee, 204
DCC gene, 644
Debrisoquine, lung cancer risk in extensive metabolizers of, 38, 284
Declaration of Helsinki, 203, 203t
Deep venous thrombosis, 303
Degasorb, 1003
Depression, 1018
Dermatomyositis, 297
Dermoid cysts, 142
Desmoid tumors of chest wall, 871
Detorubicin, 801–802
bis-1-8-(hydroxy-ethyl)Deutro-porphyrin-3-ethyl-ether (DHE), 947, *948*
Dexamethasone
for chemotherapy-induced emesis, 983t
as co-analgesic, 989
for HIV-associated non-Hodgkin's lymphoma, 1032
DHE, 947, *948*
Diallyl sulfide, 39, 45
Diaphragm
blood supply of, 14
development of, 5, 7–8, *8*
management of T3 tumors involving, 359
referred pain from, 5
Diaphragmatic breathing, 1022
Diazepam, 983t
Dichloromethotrexate, 632t
Dideazafolic acid (CB3717), 805
Didronel. See Etidronate
Diet, 987

Diffusion capacity, 176
Difluoromethylornithine, 100
Difluorodeoxycytidine, 488
DiGeorge syndrome, 17
Digital clubbing, 294t, 297
5-Dihydroazacytidine (DHAC), 805
Dimethylnitrosamine demethylase, 285
Diphenhydramine, 983t
Diuretics, 985
Diverticulum, esophageal, 540, 566
DNA
  esophageal carcinogenesis and DNA adduct formation, 42–43, *42–43*
  lung carcinogenesis and
    DNA adduct formation, *30,* 30–31
    DNA repair processes, 31, 106
    metabolism of lung carcinogens to DNA reactive products, 27–30, *28–29*
DNA ploidy
  in Barrett's esophagus, 592
  in esophageal cancer, 555
  in lung cancer, 327, 330
  in mesothelioma, 789
Docetaxel
  for non-small cell lung cancer, 427t, 428
  pleural effusion induced by, 153
  side effects of, 428
  for small cell lung cancer, 488, 502
Dolicho biflorus agglutinin (DBA) binding site, 331
Domperidone, 983t
L-Dopa decarboxylase, 456
"Double minutes," 277
Doxorubicin
  for cardiac tumors, 696
    angiosarcoma, 697
    leiomyosarcoma, 698
    lymphoma, 699
    osteosarcoma, 699
  cardiotoxicity of, 18, 153, 486, 1008
    when combined with radiotherapy, 1011–1012
  for esophageal cancer, 614, 614t, 631, 632t
    combined with other agents, 634
  for HIV-associated non-Hodgkin's lymphoma, 1032
  for HIV-related Hodgkin's disease, 1041
  for HIV-related Kaposi's sarcoma, 1038–1039
  for intravascular lymphomatosis of lung, 842
  for lung cancer
    non-small cell carcinoma, 365t, 429, 431
    small cell carcinoma, 467, 470, 470t–472t, 473, 474t, 497, 500, 501t
  for mesothelioma, 792, 801
    combined with other agents, 806–807, 807t
  for neuroblastoma, 722t
  for neuroepithelioma, 727
  for pleurodesis, 889, 889t
  for thymoma, 662–663
Doxycycline pleurodesis, 887–888, 888t

Droperidol, 983t
Duct(s)
  alveolar, 10
  right lymphatic, 6, 20
  thoracic, 6, 20, 294
Dumbbell tumors, 727–729, *727–729*
  in children, 729
  clinical features of, 727
  definition of, 727
  histology of, 727–728
  radiographic features of, 727
  treatment of, 728–729
Duoderm CGF, 1003
Dysphagia, 294, 294t, 567, 596
  intubation for palliation of, 623
  photodynamic therapy for, 623
  radiation therapy-induced, 1003
Dyspnea, 116, 293–295, 294t, 391, 1018
  due to cardiac tumors, 681, 695
  due to mesothelioma, 781

Early detection. *See* Screening for lung cancer
Echocardiography, 2, 681, 684t, 895, *897*
  myxoma on, 688, *688*
Ectoderm, 5, 7
Edema, radiotherapy-induced, 1005
Edetrexate
  for disseminated non-small cell lung cancer, 427t, 428
  for mesothelioma, 805
  side effects of, 428
Edrophonium chloride test, 656
Electrocardiography, 682
  pericardial effusion and, 895, *896*
Electromagnetic radiation, 216. *See also* Radiation therapy
Elephant man syndrome, 871
Ellagic acid, 45, 1056
Embolic disease, 2, 681
Embryology, 3–9, *4–8,* 533
Emesis, chemotherapy-induced, 983t, 983–984, 991, 1008
Encephalitis, limbic, 305
Encephalopathy, chemotherapy-induced, 1009
Endocarditis, nonbacterial thrombotic, 303
Endocrine disorders
  chemotherapy-induced, 1009
  induced by combined modality therapy, 1012
  radiotherapy-induced, 1007
Endocrine paraneoplastic syndromes, 298–303
  Cushing's syndrome, 299–300
  hypercalcemia, 300–302
  SIADH, 302–303
Endoderm, 5, *5,* 7
Enflurane, 171–172
Enoxacin, 980
Enteral nutrition, 988
Enterobacter cloacae infection, 980
Environmental and occupational exposures, 66–81

air pollution and lung cancer, 79–80
environmental tobacco smoke, 25, 51, 57–58, 1084–1085
esophageal cancer and, 80
lung cancer and, 25–26
smoking and, 69
occupational carcinogens, 69–79
  classification of, 69
  known carcinogens, 69–75
    arsenic, 69–70
    asbestos, 70–71, 735–749
    bis(chloromethyl) ether, 71–72
    chromium, 72
    nickel, 72–73
    polycyclic aromatic hydrocarbons, 73–74
    radon, 74–75
    vinyl chloride, 75
  possible carcinogens, 76–79
    acetaldehyde, 76–77
    manmade mineral fibers, 77–78
    silica, 78–79
    welding, 79
  probable carcinogens, 75–76
    acrylonitrile, 75
    beryllium, 75–76
    cadmium, 76
    formaldehyde, 76
  prevention programs and, 80–81
  sources of data about occupational carcinogens, 66–69
    epidemiological studies, 67–69, 68t
    in vitro and in vivo methods, 66–67
Environmental Protection Agency, 1079, 1081
Enzymes
  cytochrome *P450,* 27, 38
  interaction with carcinogens, 27, 38, 284–285
  phases I and II, 27
Epiadriamycin, 1041
Epicardium, 8
Epidermal growth factor, 43, 96
Epidermal growth factor receptor, 1069
  in esophageal cancer, 43–44, 644
  in lung cancer, 279, 331
Epidural analgesia, 173
Epidural lipomatosis, 1009
Epirubicin
  for mesothelioma, 802
  for small cell lung cancer, 497, 499
Epstein-Barr virus, 1031
c-*erb*B-1 oncogene, 1069
  in esophageal cancer, 44t
  in lung cancer, 33, 279
c-*erb*B-2 oncogene, 94t, 95, 1070
  in esophageal cancer, 44t
  in lung cancer, 33, 279, 330
Erionite, 739t, 741
Erythroblastopenic anemia, 656, 665
Erythropoietin
  after bone marrow transplantation, 995
  for chemotherapy-induced anemia, 1009

Esophageal biopsy, 537
Esophageal cancer, 15, 531–645
 adenocarcinoma, 39, 547–549, 566–567
 adenoid cystic carcinoma, 550
 age, sex, and racial distribution of, 538, 564–566
 carcinoids, 551
 causative factors in, 39–40
 causes of, 539, 566, 566t
  alcohol use, 539
  diet, 539
  genetic factors, 539
  infectious agents, 539
  radiation and thermal injury, 539
  tobacco use, 539
 choriocarcinoma, 550
 chromosome abnormalities in, 44
 clinical presentation of, 555–556, 567–568
 complications of, 556
 conditions associated with, 540, 566, 594–596
  achalasia, 540, 566, 594–595
  celiac disease, 540, 596
  chronic esophagitis, 540, 566, 595
  diverticulum, 540
  hiatus hernia, 540
  Plummer-Vinson syndrome, 540, 595
  strictures, 540, 595–596
  tylosis, 566, 595
 of deep esophageal glands, 550
 diagnosis of, 568
 early vs. advanced, 536–537
 epidemiology of, 39, 538–539, 564–566, 630
 at esophagogastric junction, 549–550
 geographic distribution of, 538, 564, 568
 historical perspectives on, 563
 imaging of, 132–135
 incidence of, 533, 538–539, 563, 564, 630
 lymphomas, 552
 malignant melanoma, 551–552
 metastasis of, 553, 553–554
  contiguous involvement of neighboring organs, 553
  hematogenous spread, 554
  intramural spread, 553, 553
  to lymph nodes, 553–554, 567, 577–578, 578
 mortality from, 533, 554–555, 596, 630
 mucoepidermoid carcinoma, 550
 multiple carcinomas, 552–553
 natural history of, 567
 Paget's disease, 550
 precancerous lesions and, 540–542, 566
  adenomas, 541, 541–542
  dysplasia of Barrett's epithelium, 541–542, 542, 585–594. See also Barrett's esophagus
  dysplasia of squamous epithelium, 540–541, 541
  squamous papilloma, 540
 prognostic factors for, 555, 624
 rat model of, 539–540
 sarcomas, 536, 552
 screening for, 543, 568
 small cell carcinoma, 39, 551, 551
 squamous cell carcinoma, 542–547
 survival rates for, 554–555, 596, 606, 630
Esophageal cancer pathology, 39, 533–556, 566–567
 adenocarcinoma, 547–549
 adenoid cystic carcinoma, 550
 carcinoids, 551
 carcinoma at esophagogastric junction, 549–550
 carcinomas of deep esophageal glands, 550
 choriocarcinoma, 550
 classification and cells of origin, 536, 536t
 clinical presentation and diagnosis based on, 555–556
 complications and causes of death, 556
 diagnostic biopsy and cytology, 537
 early vs. advanced carcinoma, 536–537
 gross pathology, 537
 histochemical and immunohistochemical studies, 537–538
 histologic pathology, 537
 lymphomas, 552
 malignant melanoma, 551–552
 mucoepidermoid carcinoma, 550
 multiple carcinomas, 552–553
 Paget's disease, 550
 pathologic examination, 537
 sarcomas, 536, 552
 secondary and metastatic tumors, 552
 small cell carcinoma, 551, 551
 squamous cell carcinoma, 542–547, 543–546
 treatment-related pathologic changes, 556
 tumor spread and metastasis, 134–135, 553–554
Esophageal cancer staging, 132–135, 133–134, 554, 554t, 568–582
 barium swallow for, 569–570, 571, 571t
 bronchoscopy for, 571–572, 572
 chest radiography for, 569, 570, 570t
 computed tomography for, 572, 572–574, 573t, 597
 esophagoscopy for, 570–571
 liver scans for, 572
 magnetic resonance imaging for, 574–575, 574–576, 576t
  aortic infiltration, 575
  lymph node involvement, 575–576
  mediastinal fat and pericardial invasion, 575
  tracheobronchial invasion, 575
  tumor infiltration, 575
 prognosis and, 555
 rationale for, 569
 small cell carcinoma, 643
 surgical, 577–582
  history, 578
  laparoscopy technique, 580–581, 580–581
  lymph node map, 578, 578
  results at Univ. of Maryland, 581–582
  thoracoscopic technique, 578–579, 579–580
 TNM system for, 554, 554t, 568t–569t, 568–569
 for treatment planning, 597
 ultrasound for, 576–577, 577, 577t, 597
Esophageal cancer treatment, 596–602, 606–624, 630–645
 assessing response to, 630–631
 combined modality therapy, 601–602, 614–621
  chemoradiotherapy and surgery, 620–621, 621t–622t, 635, 638–640, 639t
  chemotherapy, 614–616, 631–638
  chemotherapy and radiation therapy, 602, 618–620, 620t, 640–643, 641t, 643
  chemotherapy and surgery, 601, 616–618, 617t–618t, 635–638, 636t
  radiation therapy and surgery, 601–602
  toxicity of, 1010–1011
 future directions for, 643–645
 palliative therapy, 621–624
  chemotherapy, 623–624
  radiation therapy, 623
  surgery, 622–623
 potentially curable cancer, 596–597
 radiation therapy, 601–602, 609–614
 small cell carcinoma, 643
 staging modalities and, 597
 surgical therapy, 556, 577, 597–601, 606–609
 video-assisted, 969, 972
Esophageal carcinogenesis, 39–46
 animal (rat) model of, 44–45
 causative factors, 39–40
  alcohol consumption, 40
  food and water contaminants, 40
  human papilloma virus, 40
  nitrosamines, 40–41, 41
  occupational and environmental exposures, 80
  tobacco use, 39–40
  vitamin and mineral deficiencies, 40
 chemoprevention of, 45–46
 metabolism and DNA adduct formation of esophageal carcinogens, 42–43, 42–43
 oncogene activation, 43–44, 44t
 tumor suppressor gene inactivation, 44, 44t
Esophageal compression, 294
Esophageal diverticulum, 540, 566
Esophageal glands, deep, 534, 534
 carcinomas of, 550
Esophageal obstruction, 622–623. See also Airway obstruction
Esophageal sphincters, 533–534, 585
Esophageal varices, 567
Esophagectomy. See Surgical therapy for esophageal cancer

Esophagitis, 15
  chronic, 540, 566, 595
  radiotherapy-induced, 485–486, 1003, 1005
  reflux, 536
  treatment of, 1003
Esophagogastric junction carcinoma, 547, 549–550
Esophagoscopy, 568, 570–571
Esophagus
  anatomy of, 15, 533–534, 563–564
  Barrett's, 15, 39, 535–536, *535–536*, 566, 585–594. *See also* Barrett's esophagus
  blood supply of, 534, 564
  diameter of, 563
  embryology of, 533
  histology of, 534, *534*, 564
  length of, 533, 563
  lymphatic drainage of, 20, 534, 564, *565*
  mucosal lining of, 533
  perforation of, 567
  venous drainage of, 15
  Z line of, 533
Ethical issues, 203–204
  informed consent and randomization, 203t, 203–204
  interim analyses and data monitoring committee, 204
Ethoxyquin, 39
Etidronate, 301, 985
Etoposide
  for bronchial carcinoids, 853
  for cardiac tumors
    leiomyosarcoma, 698
    lymphoma, 699
  for esophageal cancer, 632t
    combined with other agents, 633
  for HIV-associated non-Hodgkin's lymphoma, 1032
  for HIV-related Kaposi's sarcoma, 1038
  leukemia induced by, 1010
  for lung cancer
    non-small cell carcioma, 365t, 426, 427, 427t, 430, 431
    small cell carcinoma, 470, 470t–472t, 472, 473, 474t, 497, 500–502, 501t
  for pleurodesis, 889, 889t
  for thymoma, 663
Evaluation of treatments. *See* Clinical trials
Ewing's sarcoma, 832, 833, 872
Excision repair pathway for DNA repair, 31
Exercise testing, 1020
  preoperative, 178–180
Exercise training, 1022–1026
  blood gas changes and, 1023
  exercise prescription for, 1023
  results of, 1025–1026
  upper extremity training, 1023
  ventilatory muscle training, 1024
Expiratory reserve volume, 169, *170*

Factorial design, 198
Fair Packaging and Labeling Act, 1081
Fairness in Tobacco and Nicotine Regulation Act, 1082

Familial cancer syndromes, 283–285
Federal Food, Drug, and Cosmetic Act, 1081–1082
Federal Hazardous Substances Act, 1081
Fenretinide, 101, 1063–1064
c-*fes* protooncogene, 33
Fetal hydantoin syndrome, 717
α-Fetoprotein, 670, 670t, 673
Fever, 116, 294, 297, 981–983
Fiber-related carcinogenesis, 742–748
  cell mechanisms, 745–746
  fiber parameters, 742–744, *744*
    biopersistence, 743
    chemistry, 744
    geometry, 742–743
    size, 743
  genotoxicity of fibers, 746–748
    chromosome abnormalities, 746–747
    clastogenic factors, 748
    indirect mechanisms through oxidative processes, 747–748
    in vitro studies, 746–747
  inconsistencies between animal and human data, 744–745
    dose response, 744
    mesothelioma induction and species variation, 745
Fibroma
  cardiac, in children, 693–694
  of chest wall, 870–871
Fibrosarcoma
  cardiac, 697–698
  of chest wall, 872
  of esophagus, 552
  of lung, 818–820, *819*
    in children, 820
    endobronchial and intrapulmonary types of, 818–819
    pathology of, 819
    therapy and prognosis for, 819–820
  pleural, 830–832, *832*
    clinical features of, 830–831
    pathology of, 831
    therapy and prognosis for, 831–832
Fibrosing pleuritis, 770–771, *771*
Fibrous dysplasia tumors, 871
Fibrous glass, 77–78
Field cancerization hypothesis, 96–97, 107
Fistula
  esophagorespiratory, 622
  tracheoesophageal, 567, 864
Flow cytometry, 1071
  in lung cancer, 250–251, 265–266
  in mesothelioma, 767–768
Flow-volume curves, 170–171, *171*
Fluconazole, 980
Fluorescence in situ hybridization (FISH), 277, 1070
Fluoroquinolones, 980, 981
5-Fluorouracil
  for esophageal cancer, 614t, 614–615, 631, 632t, 644
    combined with other agents, 615–616, 633–635

palliative, 623–624
preoperative, 617, 636t, 637–638
  with radiation therapy, 619–620, 639t, 639–640
  with radiation therapy and no surgery, 640–642, 641t
  toxicity when combined with radiation therapy, 1010–1011
for mesothelioma, 805
for neuroepithelioma, 727
neurotoxicity of, 1009
for pleurodesis, 889t, 890
Food and Drug Administration, 1081–1082
Forced expiratory volume in 1 second (FEV1), 170
Forced vital capacity (FVC), 170, *170*
Formaldehyde exposure, 76
c-*fos* protooncogene, 33, 94t, 95
Frozen chest, 781
Functional residual capacity (FRC), 170, *170*
Fungal infections, 981
  esophageal cancer and, 40, 539
  HIV-associated, 1043t
  prophylaxis for, 980
  surveillance culturing for, 980
c-*fur* protooncogene, 33
Furosemide, 985
Fusarium infection, 539, 566

Gallium-67 citrate, 141–142
Gallium nitrate, 301
Ganciclovir, 995
Ganglioneuroblastoma, 17, 721–722, *723*
Ganglioneuroma, 17, 721–722, *722–723*
Gastric heterotopia, 535, 566
Gastrin-releasing peptide (GRP), 96, 324–325, 456
Gastrula, 4
Gemcitabine
  for non-small cell lung cancer, 427t, 428, 431
  side effects of, 428
  for small cell lung cancer, 498–499, 502
Gender effects
  on esophageal cancer incidence, 538, 564
  on lung cancer incidence, 245
  on lung cancer prognosis, 322
  on mesothelioma incidence, 786, 799
  on smoking and lung cancer risk, 55, 56
  on smoking prevalence, 60–63, *61–63*
  on thymoma incidence, 655–656
  on tracheal tumor incidence, 856
Gene therapy, 1072
Genes
  in Barrett's esophagus, 592–593
  carcinogenesis and mutations of, 106–107
  DNA repair, 31, 106
  homeobox, 3
  oncogenes, 31–33
    in esophageal cancer, 43–44, 644–645
    in lung cancer, 31–33, 33t, 93–95, 94t, 106, 266t, 266–268, *267–268*
    in neuroblastoma, 716, 726
    in neuroepithelioma, 726

tumor suppressor, 106
  in esophageal cancer, 44, 44t, 644
  in lung cancer, 31–32, 34t, 34–35, 94t, 95
  in mesothelioma, 789
Genetic analysis methods, 277–278
Genetic instability, 283
Genetics
  of esophageal cancer, 539
  of lung cancer, 283–285
  of malignant mesothelioma, 546–547, 746–747, 768–769
Gentamicin, 980
Geotrichum infection, 539, 566
Germ cell tumors, mediastinal, 136, 668–678
  clinical presentation of, 669, 669t
  epidemiology of, 668
  etiology of, 668–669
  hematologic malignancies associated with, 677
  imaging of, 142–143
  incidence of, 668
  isochromosome 12p and, 677
  Klinefelter's syndrome and, 677
  laboratory evaluation of, 670, 670t
  midline tumors of uncertain histogenesis, 677
  pathology of, 671, 671t
    nonseminomatous tumor, 671–672
    seminoma, 671
    teratoma, 672
    undifferentiated tumors, 672
  prognosis for, 672–674
    prognostic factors and risk assignment, 672–673, 673t
    serum tumor markers, 673–674, 674t
    radiographic evaluation and diagnosis of, 670–671
  treatment of, 674–677
    nonseminomatous tumor, 674–676, 676t
    seminoma, 674, 675t
    teratoma, 676–677
Giant cell carcinoma of lung, 258
Glomerulopathy, paraneoplastic, 305
Glutathione S-transferases, 27, 38, 284
Glycogenic acanthosis, 534
Glycoproteins, in mesotheliomas, 764–766, 765
Goblet cells, 535–536
Goiter, 146, 729
Graft versus host disease (GVHD), 157, 993, 994
Granisetron, 983t, 984
Granular cell tumors
  cardiac, 692–693
  pericardial, 706
  posterior mediastinal, 729
Granulocyte colony-stimulating factor (G-CSF), 980
  after bone marrow transplantation, 995
  use in small cell lung cancer, 506–507
Granulocyte-macrophage colony-stimulating factor (GM-CSF), 980
  after bone marrow transplantation, 995

for HIV-associated non-Hodgkin's lymphoma, 1032
  use in small cell lung cancer, 506–507
Granulocytopenic patients, 979–983, *982*
Granulomata, 130, 136
Graves' disease, 147, 1007
Gray (Gy), 218
Group psychotherapy, 990
Growth factors
  in esophageal cancer, 43–44
  in lung cancer
    non-small cell carcinoma, 331
    role in early detection, 95–96
    small cell carcinoma, 324–325
  in mesothelioma, 789
  receptors for
    in esophageal cancer, 43–44
    in lung cancer, 279
Gynecologic cancer, 916

Hair loss, 992, 1004–1005
Haloperidol, 983t
Hamartoma, 128, *130*
Head and neck cancer, 915
Hemangioendothelioma, epithelioid, 821–822, *821–822*
  clinical features of, 821
  differential diagnosis of, 821
  differentiating from mesothelioma, 770
  epidemiology of, 821
  historical recognition of, 821
  oral contraceptives and, 822
  pathology of, 821–822
  pleural, 834–835
  therapy and prognosis for, 822
Hemangioma
  cardiac, 691–692
  of chest wall, 870
Hemangiopericytoma, 822–824, *823*
  clinical features of, 823
  pathology of, 823–824
  therapy and prognosis for, 824
Hematemesis, 567
Hematologic complications of treatment, 485–486, 993–994, 1009
Hematologic paraneoplastic syndromes, 303
Hematopoietic growth factors, 980
  after bone marrow transplantation, 995
  for chemotherapy-induced neutropenia, 1009
  for HIV-associated non-Hodgkin's lymphoma, 1032
  use in small cell lung cancer, 506–507
Hemoptysis, 116, 293, 294, 294t, 391, 567
Hemorrhage
  from bronchoscopic laser resection, 930, 932
  pulmonary, 156
Heparin, 476, 476t
Her-2*neu* oncogene. *See c-erb*B-2 oncogene
Hernia
  congenital diaphragmatic, 9
  hiatal, 15, 540
Herpes simplex virus, 160
Hexamethylmelamine (HMM), 471t, 474t, 497

HFMG-2, 765
Hiccups, 567
High-risk surgical patient, 175–180
  evaluating pulmonary function of, 177–180
  identification of, 175–177, 176t
Hirschsprung's disease, 717
Histiocytoma, malignant fibrous
  cardiac, 697–698
  pericardial, 706
  pleural, 830
  pulmonary, 824–825, *825*
Hoarseness, 293, 294, 294t, 391
Hodgkin's disease
  in HIV-infected patients, 1039–1041
    clinical presentation of, 1041
    epidemiology of, 1039–1040
    histology of, 1040–1041
    treatment of, 1041
  imaging of, 141, *142–143*
  pulmonary, 840–841, *841*
    clinical features of, 840
    pathology of, 840–841
    therapy and prognosis for, 841
  radiation therapy for
    hyperthyroidism due to, 1007
    L'hermitte's sign due to, 1004
  of thymus, 145
Homovanillic acid (HVA), 715–716
Horner's syndrome, 295, 375, 377, 391, 1006
Hourglass tumors. *See* Dumbbell tumors
HpD, 947
hst-1 protooncogene, 43, 44t
5-HT3 receptor antagonists, 983–984
Human chorionic gonadotropin (HCG), 670, 670t, 673
Human immunodeficiency virus (HIV)-related disorders, 1029–1044
  cryptococcosis, 159
  cytomegalovirus, 159
  differential diagnosis of pulmonary abnormalities, 1042, 1043t
  HIV transmission in health care setting, 1042–1044
  Hodgkin's disease, 1039–1041
  Kaposi's sarcoma, 1033–1039
    of esophagus, 552
    of lung, 128, 816–818, *817*
  lung adenocarcinoma, 253
  lung cancer, 1041–1042
  MultiState AIDS/Cancer Match Registry, 1029–1030
  non-Hodgkin's lymphoma, 1030–1033
  Pneumocystis carinii pneumonia, 157, *158*, 1029
  pulmonary infections, 156, 1029
  radiation therapy toxicity, 1002, 1003t
  tuberculosis, 160
  types of thoracic tumors, 1029, *1030*
Human papilloma virus (HPV)
  esophageal cancer and, 40
  HIV-associated Kaposi's sarcoma and, 1035
  squamous cell lung cancer and, 251–252

Hybridization techniques, 277
Hydrazine sulfate, 988
Hydroxydaunomycin, 1032
Hydroxyurea, 471t
Hyperalimentation, 988
Hyperbaric oxygen therapy, 1005, 1008
Hypercalcemia, tumor-induced, 300–302, 984–986
  bisphosphonates for, 985–986
  pathogenesis of, 984–985
  traditional therapy for, 985
Hypercapnia, 176
Hypercoagulability, 303
Hypercortisolism, 299–300
Hypernephroma invading heart, 704
Hyperoxia, 11
Hypersensitivity pneumonitis, 182, 182t
Hyperthyroidism, radiotherapy-induced, 1007
Hypertrophic pulmonary osteoarthropathy (HPO), 297–298, *299*
Hypoalbuminemia, 394
Hypogammaglobulinemia, 656, 665
Hyponatremia, 302–303, 322
Hypotension, orthostatic, 297
Hypothyroidism
  due to combined modality therapy, 1012
  radiotherapy-induced, 1007
Hypoxemia, 176
  general anesthesia and, 172
  radiation therapy response and, 220–221, *221, 224, 225*
  after tracheal reconstruction, 864

Idarubicin, 632t
Ifosfamide
  for cardiac leiomyosarcoma, 698
  for esophageal cancer, 623, 632t
  for lung cancer
    non-small cell carcinoma, 426, 427, 427t, 430
    small cell carcinoma, 471t, 497, 502
  for mesothelioma, 804
    combined with other agents, 806–807, 807t
  neurotoxicity of, 1009
  side effects of, 427
Imaging, 112–160
  of adenoid cystic carcinoma, 128
  appropriate use of, 112, 159–160
  of bronchial carcinoid, 126–127, *127,* 852, 853
  of cardiac tumors, 682–683
  of chemotherapy-induced chest disease, 150–154, 152t
    alveolar infiltrates, 152
    cardiac abnormalities, 153–154
    diffuse interstitial disease, 151–152, *153*
    pleural effusion, 153
    pulmonary nodules, 152–153
  of chest wall tumors, 870
  of diffuse malignant mesothelioma, 150, *151*
  of dumbbell tumors, 727, *728*
  effects of radiation therapy on thorax, 154–155, *155–156*

  of esophageal cancer, 132–135
    local tumor extent (T stage), 132–133, *133–134*
    metastases (M stage), 134–135
    spread to lymph nodes (N stage), 133–134
  of extraadrenal pheochromocytoma, 724
  of germ cell tumors, 142–143
  of hamartoma, 128, 128t
  of lung cancer, 113–126
    central tumors, 118–121, *119–121*
    CT and MRI, 121–124
      adrenal metastases vs. benign adrenal adenoma, 124
      cancer staging, 121–123, *122*
      CT technique, 124
      local tumor extent (T stage), 123
      spread to lymph nodes (N stage), 123–124
    evaluation and follow-up after chemotherapy and radiation therapy, 124–125
    imaging workup, 115–117
    non-small cell, 115, *115–116*
      monoclonal antibody imaging in, 126
      stage IIIA, 351–352, *353–358*
    peripheral tumors, 117–118, *117–118*
    preoperative nuclear medicine assessment, *125,* 125–126
    small cell, 113–115, *114*
    spread of tumor, 121
    superior sulcus tumors, 377–378, *377–379*
  of lymphomas, 141–142
    Hodgkin's disease, 141, *142–143*
    non-Hodgkin's lymphoma, 141–142, *144–145*
  of mediastinal germ cell tumors, 670–671
  of mediastinum, 139–141
    CT and MRI, 140–141
    plain chest radiography, 139–140
  of mesothelioma, 780
  modalities for, 112
  of mucoepidermoid cancer, 128
  of myxoma, 688, *688*
  of neurilemoma, 712, *712–713*
  of paraspinal tumors, 148, *149*
  of parathyroid disease, 147–148
  for percutaneous lung biopsy, 131–132
  of pleural and chest wall masses, 148–150
    localized fibrous tumor of pleura, 149–150
  of pulmonary blastoma, 128
  of pulmonary infection in immunocompromised host, 155–160, 157
    Aspergillus fumigatus, 158, *159*
    Candida albicans, 158–159
    Cryptococcus neoformans, 159
    cytomegalovirus, 159
    Klebsiella, 161
    phycomycetes and mucormycosis, 159
    Pneumocystis carinii, 157–158, *158*
  of pulmonary Kaposi's sarcoma, 128

  of pulmonary metastases, 135–139, 907
    CT and MRI, 137–139, *140*
    endobronchial metastases, 137
    lymphangitic spread, 137, *138*
    mechanism of spread to lung, 135
    radiographic appearance of pulmonary metastases, 135–137, *136*
    role of positron emission tomography, 131, *132*
  of solitary pulmonary nodule, *129–130,* 129–131
  of thymoma, 657–659, *657–659*
  of thymus, 143–146
    thymic hyperplasia, 143
    thymic rebound, 143–144, *146*
    thymic tumors, 145–146
    thymoma and myasthenia gravis, 145, *147*
  of thyroid masses, 146–147
  of tracheal tumors, 858
  of uncommon bronchopulmonary malignancies, 126t
Imipenem-cilastatin, 981
Imipramine, 989
Immune dysfunction, asbestos-induced, 748
Immunization, 980–981
Immunocompromised host. *See also* Human immunodeficiency virus-related disorders
  chest radiographic findings in, 156
  infection prevention and treatment in, 979–983
  pulmonary infections in, 155–160, 157–159, *161*
  thymic aplasia/hypoplasia and, 17
Immunohistochemistry
  of esophageal cancer, 537–538, 644
  of lung cancer, 253t, 258, 264t, 264–265
  of mesothelioma, 257t, 763t, 763–766
    glycoproteins, 764–766, 765
    intermediate filaments, 763–764, *764,* 771, 771–772
    other reagents, 766
Immunotherapy
  for lung cancer
    non-small cell carcinoma, 344, 347
    small cell carcinoma, 473–475
  for mesothelioma, 792, 806
Indomethacin, 988
Industrial exposures. *See* Environmental and occupational exposures
Infections, 979–983
  antimicrobial prophylaxis for, 980
  change or addition of other antibiotics, 981–983
  empiric treatment, 981, *982*
  enhancement of host defenses, 980–981
  fungi and esophageal cancer, 539, 566
  prevention strategy for, 979
  pulmonary, 391–392, 981
    in immunocompromised host, 155–160, *157–159, 161*
  surveillance culturing, 980
  total protected isolation, 979

venous catheter-related, 997t, 997–998
viral, in bone marrow transplant recipients, 995
Informed consent, 203t, 203–204
Inspiratory capacity, 170, *170*
Inspiratory reserve volume, 170, *170*
Insulinlike growth factor I, 96
int-2 protooncogene, 43, 44t, 644
Intensive care, 995–997
Interferons
  for esophageal cancer, 644
  for HIV-related Kaposi's sarcoma, 1038
  for mesothelioma, 792, 806
    intrapleural therapy, 808
  for pleurodesis, 890, 890t
  role in anorexia-cachexia, 987
  for small cell lung cancer, 474–475, 504
Interim analyses, 201t–202t, 201–204
Interleukin-1, 297, 987, 988
Interleukin-2
  alveolar infiltrates due to, 152
  after bone marrow transplantation, 995
  for mesothelioma, 792
    intrapleural therapy, 808
  for pleurodesis, 890, 890–891
  for small cell lung cancer, 75
Interleukin-3, 995
Interleukin-6, 18, 987, 988
Intermediate filaments, 264t, 264–265
  in mesotheliomas, 763–764, *763–764*
Interstitial lung disease
  chemotherapy-induced, 151–152, *153*, 181t, 181–182
  video-assisted thoracic surgery for, 974, *975*
Intestinal dysmotilities, 305
Intraoperative radiation therapy, 237, 237–238
Intravascular lymphomatosis of lung, 841–842, *842*
Intravenous device-related complications, 997–998
Inverse square law, 217–218
Involucrin, 252
Ionization, 215
Ionizing radiation, 216. *See also* Radiation therapy
Irinotecan, 488
  for non-small cell lung cancer, 427t, 428, 431
  side effects of, 428, 498
  for small cell lung cancer, 497–498, 502
Isoflurane, 171–172
Isolation, total protected, 979
Isothiocyanates, 101
Isotretinoin, 1061–1063
Itraconazole, 980

c-jun protooncogene, 33, 94t, 95
Junctional nevus, 870

Kaplan-Meier plots, 320, *321*
Kaposi's sarcoma
  of esophagus, 552

in HIV-infected patients, 1033–1039, 1043t
  biology of, 1035–1036
  clinical presentation of, 1036–1037
  diagnosis of, 1037
  epidemiology of, 1033–1035
  histology of, 1037–1038
  pathogenesis of, 1035
  radiographic features of, 1037, *1038*
  treatment of, 1038–1039
of lung, 128, 816–818, *817–818*
  AIDS and, 816–817
  clinical features of, 817
  diagnosis of, 817
  pathology of, 817–818
  therapy and prognosis for, 818
pleural, 834–835
Karnofsky performance score (KPS), 431–433, 1033
Kasabach-Merritt syndrome, 692
Keratin proteins, in mesotheliomas, 763–764, *764, 771*, 771–772
Kerley C lines, 19
Ketoconazole, 980
c-kit protooncogene, 33, 279
Klebsiella infection, *161*
Klinefelter's syndrome, 677

Lactate dehydrogenase (LDH), 322, 324, 325t
  mediastinal germ cell tumors and, 670, 670t
  in pleural effusion, 882
Lambert-Eaton myasthenic syndrome, 304–305
Lambl's excrescence, 693
Lamina propria of esophagus, 534, *534*
Laminar air flow room, 979
Laparoscopic staging of esophageal cancer, 580–581, *580–581*
Large cell carcinoma of lung, 25, 115
  biomarkers for, 253t
  clear cell, 258
  cytologic appearance of, 249, *250*
  giant cell, 258
  immunohistochemistry of, 258
  location of, 293
  morphometry of, 258
  nomenclature for, 257
  occult, 339
  pathology of, 257–258
  prognosis for, 269
  subtypes of, 258
Large cell neuroendocrine carcinomas, 263
Laryngeal release procedure, 863–864
Laryngoplasty, 863
Laser therapy. *See* Bronchoscopic laser resection
Lecithin, 11
Lectins, 265, 266t
Legionella infection, 160
Legislation related to tobacco products, 1081–1084

Leiomyosarcoma
  cardiac, 698–699
  of esophagus, 552, 556
  primary pulmonary, 820–821, *820–821*
  sites of, 820
Leucovorin
  for esophageal cancer, 623, 644
  for HIV-associated non-Hodgkin's lymphoma, 1032
Leukemia
  cardiac involvement by, 704
  chemotherapy-induced, 1009–1010
  induced by combined modality therapy, 1011
  mediastinal germ cell tumors and, 677
Leukocytosis, 258, 394
Leukoencephalopathy, 518, 1009, 1012
Leu-M1, 765
Levamisole, 344
Levomepromazine, 983t
Levonantradol, 983t
L'hermitte's sign, 1004
Li-Fraumeni familial cancer syndrome, 284
Limbic encephalitis, 305
d-Limonene, 39
Linear accelerators, 216
Linear energy transfer (LET), 217
Lingula, 10
Lipoma
  cardiac, 691
  of chest wall, 870
Lipomatosis, epidural, 1009
Liposarcoma
  cardiac, 699
  of chest wall, 871
  pericardial, 706
  pulmonary, 828
Liver disease
  after bone marrow transplantation, 994–995
  esophageal cancer and, 606–607
  metastases from lung cancer, 296, 526
Liver enzymes, 296
Liver scanning, 572
Lobar collapse, 118
Local control, 394
Log rank test, 320
Lomustine
  for esophageal cancer, 632t
  for non-small cell lung cancer, 365t
  for small cell lung cancer, 440, 470, 470t–471t, 474t
  for thymoma, 662
Lorazepam, 983t
Lung biopsy, percutaneous, 131–132
Lung bud, *7*
Lung cancer. *See also* specific types
  age distribution of, 245
  causative factors in, 25–27
  cell types and, 12
  chemoprevention of, 38–39, 96–101, 1052–1072
  epidemiology of, 1053
  gender distribution of, 245
  in HIV-infected patients, 1041–1042

Lung cancer, (*continued*)
 imaging of, 113–136. *See also* Imaging
 incidence of, 113, 245, 416, 1053
 metastasis of, 121
  clinical manifestations of, 296t, 296–297
  detection of, 296
  invading chest wall, 357–359, 874
  invading heart, 704
  small cell carcinoma, 439, 525–528
  solitary metastasis from non-small cell carcinoma, 416–424
  in stage IIIB disease, 393, 393t
  from superior sulcus tumors, 379
  after therapy for stage IIIA disease, 363
  at time of presentation, 416, 424
 mortality from, 90, 113, 245, 293, 416, 456
 photodynamic diagnosis of, 950–952, *952–953*, 953t
 poorly differentiated, 263–264
 prevention of, 90–101
 routes of spread of, 121
 screening for, 90–96, 105–109, 293, 319. *See also* Screening for lung cancer
 sites of, 117–121, 293
  central tumors, 118–121, *119–121*, 293
  peripheral tumors, 117–118, *117–118*, 293
 with spindle cell components, 263, 264
 tumor doubling time in, 222t, 293
 video-assisted thoracic surgery to assess pulmonary infiltrates in, 974, *975*
Lung cancer clinical presentation, 116, 293–306
 carcinoid tumors, 262
 frequency of presenting signs and symptoms, 293, 294t
 local tumor growth, 293–295
  Pancoast tumor, 295, 376–377
  superior vena cava syndrome, 295, *295*
 metastatic disease, 296t, 296–297
 paraneoplastic syndromes, 297–306, 298t
  cutaneous syndromes, 297–298, *299*
  endocrine syndromes, 298–303
   Cushing's syndrome, 299–300
   hypercalcemia, 300–302
   SIADH, 302–303
  hematologic syndromes, 303
  neurologic syndromes, 303–305
   intestinal dysmotilities, 305
   Lambert-Eaton myasthenic syndrome, 304–305
   limbic encephalitis, 305
   necrotizing myelopathy, 305
   subacute peripheral neuropathy, 303–304
   visual paraneoplastic syndrome, 305
  renal syndromes, 305–306
  systemic disorders, 297
 patterns of, 293, 294t
 stage IIIA, 351–352
 stage IIIB, 390–392
Lung cancer molecular biology, 3, 266–268, 276–287. *See also* Genes; Oncogenes

approaches to diagnosis and prognosis, 266t, 266–268, 285–286
approaches to therapy, 286–287
chromosomes 3p and 9p, 281–282
genetic instability, 283
inherited predisposition, 283–285
MCC/APC region on chromosome 5q, 282
methods of genetic analysis, 277–278
molecular origins of genetic lesions contributing to lung cancer, 276
oncogenes, 31–33, 276–277
 growth factor receptors, 279
 myc family, 32–33, 33t, 94t, 95, 266–267, *267*, 278–279
 ras family, 32–33, 33t, 94t, 94–95, 108, 267, 278, *278*, 278t
order of events in lung cancer pathogenesis, 283
telomerase, 282–283
tumor suppressor genes, 31–32, 34t, 34–35, 94t, 95, 267, 279–281
 p53 gene, 34, 94t, 95, 106, 108, 267, 280–281, *281–282*
 Rb gene, 34, 94t, 95, 106, 279–280
Lung cancer pathology, 245–269
 adenocarcinoma, 253, 253–254, *255*
  bronchoalveolar carcinoma, 255
  immunocytochemistry, 256–257, 257t
  morphometry, 257
  scar adenocarcinoma, 255–256
 adenosquamous carcinoma, 260–261, *260–261*
 cytologic assessment, 248–250
  fine-needle aspiration cytology, 250
  sputum cytology and bronchoalveolar lavage, 248–250, *249*
 flow cytometry, 250–251, 265–266
 histopathologic prognostic factors, *268*, 268–269, 327
 histopathology, 25, 113, 245, 246t, 247–248, 390
 immunohistochemistry, 253t, 258, 264–265
 large cell carcinoma, 257–258, *258*
 neuroendocrine tumors, 261–263
  carcinoid tumors, 261–263, *262*, 262t
  large cell, 263
  taxonomy of, 261
  tumorlets, 261
 oncogenes and, 266t, 266–268, *267–268*
 other epithelial lung cancers, *263*, 263–264
 pathology reports, 248, 248t
 sarcomatoid carcinoma, 263–264, 815–816, *816*
 small cell carcinoma, 259–260
 squamous cell carcinoma, 251–252, *251–252*
 tumor heterogeneity, 246–247, *246–247*
Lung cancer prognostic factors, 105, 268–269, 319–331, 431
 adenocarcinoma, *268*, 268–269
 definition of, 320
 histopathology, *268*, 268–269
 large cell carcinoma, 269

molecularly based, 266t, 266–268, 285–286
non-small cell carcinoma, 325–331, 330t, 431
 biologic factors, 328–329
 carbohydrate antigens, 330–331
 DNA ploidy, 330
 growth factors, 331
 multivariate analyses including patients with all stages of disease, 328, 328t
 multivariate analyses of factors in non-resectable disease, 327t, 327–328
 multivariate analyses of factors in resectable disease, 326t, 326–327
 neuroendocrine markers, 329
 oncogenes and oncogene products, 329–330
 stage I disease, 342–344
 stage IIIB disease, 393–394
 stage IV disease, 431
small cell carcinoma, 259–260, 260t, 320–325
 clinical prognostic factor models, 322–323, 323t
 general prognostic factor system, 323–324, 324t
 growth factors, 324–325
 tumor markers, 324, 325t
squamous cell carcinoma, 252, 268–269, 327
statistical methods, 320, *321–322*
Lung cancer staging, 121–123, *122*, 306–311, 352t
 clinical approach to, 310–311
 non-small cell carcinoma, 115, 306–309, 307t, *308*, 352t, 390, 391t
  occult carcinoma, 307–309
  therapy for, 339–340
  stage 0, 309
  stage I, 309, 340–345
  stage II, 309, 345–349
  stage III, 309
   IIIA, 351–371
   IIIB, 388–411
  stage IV, 309
 small cell carcinoma, 309–310
Lung cancer treatment, 189, 189t. *See also* Adjuvant therapy; Chemotherapy; Radiation therapy; Surgical therapy for lung cancer
 evaluation of. *See* Clinical trials
 molecularly based approaches to, 286–287
 non-small cell carcinoma. *See also* Non-small cell lung cancer
  occult disease, 339–340
  solitary metastasis, 416–424
  stage I, 340–345
  stage II, 345–349
  stage IIIA, 357–371
  stage IIIB, 394–411
  superior sulcus tumors, 379–386
 photodynamic therapy, 947–962. *See also* Photodynamic therapy
 small cell carcinoma. *See also* Small cell lung cancer

disseminated disease, 496–507
isolated extensive disease, 525–528
prophylactic cranial irradiation, 512–522
regional disease, 456–489
role of surgery, 439–454
Lung capacities, 169–170, *170*
Lung carcinogenesis, 1052–1053
animal models of, 35–37
rat, 36–37
strain A mice, 35–36
Syrian golden hamster, 36
biologic specimens and data banks of potential markers for, 107
biomarkers specifically related to lung carcinogens, 37–38
chemoprevention of, 38–39, 96–101, 1052–1072
chromosome abnormalities, 1069–1070, 1070t–1071t
DNA adduct formation and repair, *30*, 30–31
early detection of, 90–96, 105–109, 293. *See also* Screening for lung cancer
field cancerization hypothesis of, 96–97, 107
metabolic activation and detoxification of carcinogens, 27, *27*
metabolism of lung carcinogens to DNA reactive products, 27–30, *28–29*
multistep process of, 93, *94*, 96, 1053–1054, *1054*
oncogenes and tumor suppressor genes, 31–35, 93–95, 94t, 1069–1070
order of events in, 283
risk factors for, 25–27, 293, 294t
cigarette smoking, 25–27, 26t, 51–64, 113, 388, 1052–1053, 1053t. *See also* Smoking; Tobacco
diet, 1054, 1055t
environmental exposures, 25–26, 66–81. *See also* Environmental and occupational exposures
Lung nonepithelial neoplasms, 815–828
chondrosarcoma of respiratory tract, 827–828
epithelioid hemangioendothelioma, 821–822
fibrosarcoma, 818–820
hemangiopericytoma, 822–824
Kaposi's sarcoma, 128, 816–818
malignant fibrous histiocytoma, 824–825
other primary pulmonary sarcomas, 828
primary pulmonary leiomyosarcoma, 820–821
rhabdomyosarcoma, 825–827
sarcomatoid carcinoma, 815–816
Lung volumes, 169–170, *170*, 175–176
Lung(s)
anatomy of, 10–14, 388–390, *389*
blood supply of, 12–13, *13*
collateral ventilation in, 13–14
connective tissue septa of, 13, 19
development of, 7

fissures of, 10
growth of, 8–10
compensatory, 9–10
impairments of, 9
laws of lung development, 8–9
of infant, 8
lobes of, 10, 388
lymphatic drainage of, 14, 19–20, 388, *389*
metastases to, 135–139, 906–917. *See also* Pulmonary metastases
respiratory unit (acinus) of, 10, 11
segments of, 10
treatment-induced fibrosis of, 486, *487*
Lymph nodes
aortopulmonary, 20, *122, 308*
cardiac, 534
carinal, 20
celiac, 20
celiac axis, *565*
cervical, 20, 534
diaphragmatic, *565*
esophageal cancer spread to, 553–554, 564, *565*, 567, 577–578, *578*
gastric, 20
hilar, 19, 388, *389*
intercostal, 20
interlobar, *122*, 388, *389*
internal mammary, 20
lobar, *122, 389*
lung cancer spread to, *122*, 123–124, 296, 307, *308, 389*, 390
mediastinal, 20, 388–390, 534, *565*
anterior, 20, *122, 308*
inferior, *308*, 388
resection of, 340–341
superior, *308*, 388, *389*
mesothelioma spread to, 758, 784, 789, *790*, 799
paracardiac, *565*
paraesophageal, *122, 308, 389*, 390, 534, *565*
paratracheal, 20, *122, 308*, 388, *389, 565*
perigastric, 534
pretracheal, 388, *389*
pulmonary hilar, *565*
pulmonary ligament, *122, 308, 389*, 390
retrotracheal, 388
segmental, *122, 389*
subcarinal, 20, *122, 389*, 390
subdiaphragmatic, 534
subsegmental, *122*
superior gastric, *565*
tracheal tumor spread to, 867t, 867–868
tracheobronchial, *122, 308*, 534, *565*
Lymphadenopathy, 118
Lymphangioma
cardiac, in children, 694–695
of chest wall, 870
Lymphatics, 19–20
development of, 5–6
of esophagus, 20, 534
lacteals, 19
of lung, 14, 19–20, 388, 389

of pericardium, 20
of thymus, 20
Lymphoid interstitial pneumonia, 156, 835
Lymphomas
Burkitt's, 842
esophageal, 536t, 552
in HIV-infected patients, 1043t
B- and T-cell, 1031
Hodgkin's disease, 1039–1041
non-Hodgkin's lymphoma, 1030–1033
Hodgkin's, 141, *142–143*, 840–841, 1039–1041
imaging of, 141–142
large cell, 770
non-Hodgkin's, 141–142, *144–145*, 1030–1033
posterior mediastinal, 729
primary cardiac, 699
of thymus, 145
tumor doubling time in, 222t
Lymphoproliferative diseases of lung, 835–844
Hodgkin's disease, 141, *142–143*, 840–841, 1039–1041
intravascular lymphomatosis, 841–842
lymphomatoid granulomatosis, 838–840, *839*
mixed and large cell non-Hodgkin's lymphomas, 837–838, *837–838*
other malignant lymphomas, 842
primary plasmacytoma, 842–843
small lymphocytic proliferations, 835–837, *836*

Magnetic resonance imaging (MRI), 112
adrenal metastasis on, 421–422, *422*
brain metastasis on, *418*
cardiac tumors on, 682, 684t
chest wall tumors on, 870
dumbbell tumors on, 727, *728*
lung cancer on, 121–124
superior sulcus tumors, 378, *379*
of mediastinum, 140–141
mesothelioma on, 780
paraganglioma on, 723
paraspinal tumors on, 148
pulmonary metastases on, 139, 907
for staging esophageal cancer, *574–575*, 574–576, 576t
thymoma on, 659, *659*
Malaise, 297
Malignant melanoma
cardiac, 704
of chest wall, 87
esophageal, 536t, 551–552, 556
primary malignant melanoma, 843–844
pulmonary, 843–844, *844*
pulmonary metastasectomy for, 916–917, 917t
Malnutrition, 607, 987
Manmade mineral fibers (MMMFs), 77–78, 741–742
Marlex mesh-methylmethacrylate prosthesis, 359, *360*
Maximal voluntary ventilation (MVV), 170

MCC gene, 34
McLeod's syndrome, 9
Median sternotomy, 173
Mediastinal imaging, 139–141
　chest radiography, 139–140
　CT and MRI, 140–141
Mediastinal tumors, 651–729. *See also* specific types of tumors
　cardiac tumors, 681–705
　frequency of, 655t
　germ cell tumors, 668–678
　management of T3 tumors, 359
　pericardial tumors, 705–706
　posterior mediastinal tumors, 711–729
　thymoma, 653–665
　video-assisted thoracic surgery for, 968–970, 970t, *971–972*
Mediastinitis, tracheoesophageal, 567
Mediastinoscopy, 392
Medroxyprogesterone, 988
Megestrol acetate, 988
Melanocytes, 5, 534
Melanotic schwannoma, 714–715
Melena, 567
Melphalan, 1009
Mepacrine pleurodesis, 888, 888t
Mesenchyme, 5
Mesenchymoma, cardiac, 700
Mesna, 804
Mesoderm, 4–5, *4–6*, 7
Mesothelioma, 18, 26, 149–150, *151*, 733–810
　of atrioventricular node, 694
　chromosome abnormalities in, 746–747, 768–769, 789
　clinical presentation of, 779–780, 787
　desmoplastic, 758–759, 770
　diagnosis of, 735–736, 757–773, 779–780, 786–787, 787t
　　ancillary techniques, 762–769
　　approach to, 772–773
　　cytology, 760–762
　　gross features, 757–758, 758–759
　　microscopic features, 758–760, *759–761*
　　video-assisted thoracic surgery for, 968
　differential diagnosis of, 769t, 769–772, *771–772*, 786–787
　epidemiology of, 786, 799
　epithelial, 758–759, *759–760*, 761–762, 766, *766*, 780
　　differential diagnosis of, 769t, 769–770
　　prognosis for, 788, 788–789
　historical recognition of, 735, 749
　in HIV-infected patients, 1041
　imaging of, 780
　incidence of, 735, 737–738, 757, 799
　metastases of, 758, 781, 789, *790*, 799
　mixed type, 760, 766, 772, 780
　molecular biology of, 789–790
　natural history of, 780–782, *781–782*, 799–800, 800t
　pericardial, 705, 735
　pleural effusion and, 736, 757, 761, 788, 799
　preclinical stages of development of asbestos-induced tumor, 736–737
　prognostic factors for, 781–782, 784, 787t, 787–789, 800, 800t
　sarcomatoid, 759–760, *761*, 762, 766, 769t, 770–772, 780
　staging of, 782t–783t, 782–784, 790–791, 791t–792t
　thrombocytosis and, 788
Mesothelioma causes, 735–749
　asbestos exposure, 735–749, 779, 786, 789
　dose-response relationships of asbestos exposure, 738–740, 739t
　　biometrology of lung fiber burden, 739–740
　　dose assessment, 738
　　effect assessment, 738
　　exposure kinetics, 740
　　reconstitution of asbestos exposure history, 739
　　retrospective evaluation of asbestos dust concentration in air, 738–739
　　risk assessment using mathematical models, 740
　factors other than fibers, 742
　host factors, 748–749
　　asbestos-induced immune system impairment, 748
　　familial predisposition, 748–749
　mechanisms of fiber-related carcinogenesis, 742–748
　　cell mechanisms, 745–746
　　fiber parameters, 742–744, *744*
　　genotoxicity of fibers, 746–748
　　inconsistencies between animal and human data, 744
　　mesothelioma induction and species variations, 745
　role of fiber type, 740–742
　　carcinogenic potential of different asbestos fiber types, 740–741
　　chrysotile paradox, 741
　　fiber types other than asbestos, 741–742
　　risk assessment with low-dose asbestos exposure, 742
Mesothelioma pathology, 757–773, 786–787, 787t
　ancillary diagnostic techniques, 757, 762–769
　　histochemistry, 762, 762–763, 763t
　　immunohistochemistry, 763t, 763–766
　　　glycoproteins, 764–766, *765*
　　　intermediate filaments, 763–764, *764*, *771*, 771–772
　　　other reagents, 766
　　investigational techniques, 767–769
　　　cytogenetics, 768–769
　　　flow cytometry, 767–768
　　　image analysis, 768
　　　ultrastructure, 766–767, *766–767*, 767t
　cytology, 760–762
　differential diagnosis, 769t, 769–772, *771–772*
　　adenocarcinoma, 254, 256, 257t, 764–765, 769–770, 786–787, 787t
　　carcinosarcoma, 772
　　epithelioid hemangioendothelioma, 770
　　fibrosing pleuritis, 770–771, *771*
　　large cell lymphomas, 770
　　mesothelial hyperplasia, 769
　　other sarcomas, 770, 772
　　solitary fibrous tumor of pleura, 771–772, *772*
　　synovial sarcoma, 772
　gross features, 757–758, *758–759*
　histologic classification, 758, 759t, 780
　　epithelial type, 758–759, 759–760, 761–762, 766, *766*, 769t, 769–770, 780, 788–789
　　mixed type, 760, 766, 772, 780
　　sarcomatoid type, 759–760, *761*, 762, 766, 769t, 770–772, 780
　immunohistochemistry, 257t
　impact on prognosis, 784
　microscopic features, 758–760, *759–761*
Mesothelioma treatment, 791–796, 799–810
　assessment of clinical trials, 800
　assessment of disease and response parameters, 800–801
　chemotherapy, 792, 801–808
　　combination therapy, 806–807, 807t
　　current recommendations, 807–808
　　intrapleural therapy, 808
　　radiation therapy and, 809
　　single-agent therapy, 801–806, 802t
　　　alkylating agents, 804
　　　antifolates, 804–805
　　　doxorubicin, 792, 801
　　　miscellaneous drugs, 806
　　　other anthracyclines, 801–803
　　　other antimetabolites, 805–806
　　　paclitaxel, 804
　　　platinum compounds, 803
　　　vinca alkaloids, 803–804
　combined modality therapy, 795–796, *796*, 809–810
　future directions for, 810
　immunochemotherapy, 792
　radiation therapy, 792, 808–809
　　chemotherapy and, 809
　　radiotherapy alone, 808–809
　surgery, 793–795
　　extrapleural pneumonectomy, 793–794, *793–794*, 795t
　　pleurectomy with decortication, 794–795
　　pleurodesis, 795
Meta-analysis, 205–208, 206t, *207–208*, 208t
Metabolic activation, 27, *27*
　of chromium IV, 30
　of 4-(methylnitrosamino)-1-(3-pyridyl)-1-butanone, *29*, 29–30
　of polynuclear aromatic hydrocarbons, 27–29, *28*
Metastases
　adrenal, 124, 296, 420–423, *421–423*, 527–528
　to chest wall, 875
　of esophageal cancer, 134–135, 553–554, 567
　to esophagus, 552
　to heart, 701t, 701–705

of lung cancer, 121, 296–297, 416–424, 525–528
of mesothelioma, 758, 781, 799
pericardial, 706
pleural, 148
pulmonary, 135–139, 906–917, 934
    metastasectomy for, 906–917
    video-assisted thoracic surgical resection of, 976t, 976–977
of thymoma, 655
Methotrexate
    for cardiac osteosarcoma, 699
    for esophageal cancer, 614t, 631, 632t
        combined with other agents, 633
    for HIV-associated non-Hodgkin's lymphoma, 1032
    for lung cancer
        non-small cell carcinoma, 365t, 429
        small cell carcinoma, 440–441, 470, 470t–471t, 473, 474t
    for mesothelioma, 804–806
    for neuroepithelioma, 727
    neurotoxicity of, 1009
        when combined with radiotherapy, 1012
    to prevent graft versus host disease, 994
    pulmonary toxicity of, 152, 1009
O^6-Methyldeoxyguanosine, 31
4-(Methylnitrosamino)-1-(3-pyridyl)-1-butanone (NNK), 26, 37–38
    DNA adducts formed from, 30, 31
    inhibition of carcinogenesis by, 39
    metabolism of, 29, 29–30
    urinary metabolites of, 37
Methylprednisone, 983t
Metoclopramide, 983
Microfilaments, 264
Micronuclei formation, 224
Microsomal epoxide hydrolase, 285
Microtubules, 264
Mineral deficiencies, 40
Mineral supplements, 45–46
Mineral wools, 77–78, 741–742
Mineralizing microangiopathy, 1009, 1012
Minocycline pleurodesis, 888, 888t
Mithramycin, 985
Mitoguazone, for esophageal cancer, 614t, 632t
    combined with other agents, 615, 633
    preoperative, 636, 636t
Mitomycin C
    for disseminated non-small cell lung cancer, 427t, 427–428
        combined with other agents, 430
    for esophageal cancer, 614, 614t, 631, 632t
        with radiation therapy and no surgery, 641, 641t
        with radiation therapy and surgery, 619, 639, 639t
        toxicity when combined with radiation therapy, 1011
    for mesothelioma, 804
    for pleurodesis, 889t, 890
    side effects of, 152, 153, 428, 1009
Mitoxantrone
    for mesothelioma, 803

for pericardial sclerotherapy, 898
for pleural sclerotherapy, 889, 889t
Monoclonal antibody studies, 107–108, 330–331, 981, 1071–1072
    of lung cancer, 114, 126
    of malignant pleural effusion, 882
    of mesothelioma, 765–766
Mono-L-aspartyl chlorin e6 (NPe6), 947–948, 949
MTS-1 gene, 35
Mucoepidermoid cancer, 128, 550
Mucormycosis, 159
Mucositis, 994
Multiple endocrine neoplasia, 717
Multiple myeloma, 873
MultiState AIDS/Cancer Match Registry, 1029–1030
Muscularis propria of esophagus, 534
Myasthenia gravis, 145, 304
    classification of, 656
    diagnosis of, 656
    results of thymic surgery on, 665
    thymoma and, 653, 656, 656t
        prognostic significance of, 663–664
c-myb protooncogene, 33, 94, 95t, 279
myc oncogene, 17, 32
    in esophageal cancer, 44, 644
    in lung cancer, 32, 33t, 94t, 95, 266–267, 267, 278–279, 325, 329, 1070
    in neuroblastoma, 716, 726
    in neuroepithelioma, 726
Mycobacterial infections, 998, 1043t
Myelitis, radiation-induced, 486, 1007
Myelodysplasia
    chemotherapy-induced, 1009
    mediastinal germ cell tumors and, 677
Myelomatous tumors of thorax, 873
Myelopathy, necrotizing, 305
Myelosuppression, 991
    chemotherapy-induced, 1009
    combined modality therapy-induced, 1011
    radiotherapy-induced, 1006
Myocardial ischemia, 126
Myocardium, 8
Myo-inositol, 39
Myxoma, cardiac, 18, 685–691
    clinical presentation of, 683t, 685–687
    confirmatory tests and differential diagnosis of, 688, 688
    epidemiology of, 685
    histopathology of, 688–689, 689
    malignant, 698
    nondiagnostic laboratory test findings with, 687–688
    recurrent, 690–691
    sites of, 687t
    surgical excision of, 689
        results of, 685t, 689–690
    syndromes and familial occurrence of, 690–691

NAME overactivity syndrome, 690
β-Naphthoflavone, 39

Narcotic analgesics, 173
National Cancer Institute Early Lung Cancer Group, 92, 105
Natural killer (NK) cells, 748
Nausea, chemotherapy-induced, 983t, 983–984, 991
Navelbine (see Vinorelbine), 632t
Navilone, 983t
Necrotizing leukoencephalopathy, 1009
Necrotizing myelopathy, 305
Neodymium:yttrium-aluminum-garnet (Nd:YAG) laser, 926, 926t, 927
Nerve sheath tumors, posterior mediastinal, 711–715
    malignant schwannoma, 714
    melanotic schwannoma, 714–715
    neurilemoma, 711–713, 712–713
    neurofibroma, 713–714, 714
Nerves
    intercostal, 14
    phrenic, 5, 7, 7, 14
        paralysis of, 695
    recurrent laryngeal
        involvement by lung cancer, 294
        involvement by tracheal tumor, 862
    splanchnic, 977
    vagus, 729
Netilmicin, 980
Neural crest cells, 5, 17
Neurilemoma, posterior mediastinal, 711–713, 712–713
    clinical presentation of, 711–712
    pathology of, 712–713
    radiographic features of, 712
    treatment of, 713
Neuroblastoma, posterior mediastinal, 17, 715–721, 717–718
    clinical features of, 716–717
    diagnosis of, 717
    histologic classification of, 718, 718t
    molecular biology and immunology of, 716
    pathology of, 717–718
    prognostic factors for, 719–720, 720, 720t
    staging of, 718–719, 719t
    syndromes associated with, 717
    treatment of, 720–721, 722t
    tumor biology of, 715–716
Neuroendocrine tumors of lung, 261–263
    carcinoid tumors, 261–263, 262t, 850–854
    large cell, 263
    taxonomy of, 261
    tumorlets, 261
Neuroepithelioma, peripheral, 832–833, 832–833
    posterior mediastinal, 725–727
        clinical features of, 726
        molecular biology of, 726
        origin of, 726
        pathology of, 726
        treatment of, 726–727
Neurofibroma
    cardiac, 692
    of chest wall, 871
    posterior mediastinal, 713–714, 714

Neurofibromatosis, 712, 714, 717, 871
Neurofibrosarcoma of chest wall, 871, 872
Neurogenic tumors
  cardiac sarcomas, 699–700
  posterior mediastinal, 711–729. *See also* Posterior mediastinal tumors
Neuroleptics, 983t
Neurologic paraneoplastic syndromes, 303–305
  intestinal dysmotilities, 305
  Lambert-Eaton myasthenic syndrome, 304–305
  limbic encephalitis, 305
  necrotizing myelopathy, 305
  subacute peripheral neuropathy, 303–304
  visual paraneoplastic syndrome, 305
Neuron specific enolase (NSE), 17, 324, 325t, 329, 456
Neurotoxicity
  of chemotherapy, 518–519, 1009
  of combined modality therapy, 1012
  of radiotherapy, 486, 517–519, 1004, 1006–1007
Neutropenia, 1009
Neutrophilia, 258, 394
Nezelof syndrome, 17
Nickel exposure, 72–73
Nicotine in cigarette smoke, 51, 52
Nimustine, 497
Nitrogen mustard
  for HIV-related Hodgkin's disease, 1041
  for pericardial sclerotherapy, 898
  for small cell lung cancer, *442*
  for thymoma, 662
Nitrosamines
  in cigarette smoke, 25–26
  esophageal cancer and, 40–41, *41*
  metabolism and DNA adduct formation of, 42–43, *42–43*
N'-Nitrosonornicotine (NNN), 26, 41
  metabolism of, 42–43, *43*
  structure of, *41*
Nitrosoureas, 1009
nm23 gene, 34–35
NNAL, 37–38
NNAL-Gluc, 37–38
Nocardiosis, 160
Nonepithelial neoplasms, 815–844
  of lung, 815–828
    chondrosarcoma of respiratory tract, 827–828
    epithelioid hemangioendothelioma, 821–822
    fibrosarcoma, 818–820
    hemangiopericytoma, 822–824
    Kaposi's sarcoma, 128, 816–818
    malignant fibrous histiocytoma, 824–825
    other primary pulmonary sarcomas, 828
    primary pulmonary leiomyosarcoma, 820–821
    rhabdomyosarcoma, 825–827
    sarcomatoid carcinoma, 263–264, 815–816

  lymphoproliferative pulmonary diseases, 835–844
    Hodgkin's disease, 840–841
    intravascular lymphomatosis, 841–842
    lymphomatoid granulomatosis, 838–840
    mixed and large cell non-Hodgkin's lymphomas, 837–838
    other malignant lymphomas, 842
    primary malignant melanoma, 843–844
    primary plasmacytoma, 842–843
    small lymphocytic proliferations, 835–837
  of pleura, 830–835
    Askin's tumor, 832–833
    fibrosarcoma and malignant solitary fibrous tumor, 8230–832
    pleuropulmonary blastoma, 833–834
    vascular sarcomas, 834–835
  pulmonary trunk sarcoma, 828–830
Non-Hodgkin's lymphoma (NHL)
  in HIV-infected patients, 1030–1033
    biology of, 1030–1031
    clinical presentation of, 1031–1032
    epidemiology of, 1030
    histology of, 1031
    prognostic factors for, 1033
    treatment of, 1032–1033, 1034t–1035t
  imaging of, 141–142, *144–145*
  mediastinal germ cell tumors and, 677
  prevalence of, 1030
Non-small cell lung cancer (NSCLC), 245, 247
  biomarkers for, 329
  compared with small cell carcinoma, 457, 457t
  endobronchial growth of, 940
  growth factors in, 331
  imaging of, 115, *115–116*
  incidence of, 426
  occult, 307–309
    localization of, 339
    therapy for, 339–340
  oncogenes in, 32–33, 278, 278t, 329–330
  prognostic factors in, 325–331, 330t, 431. *See also* Lung cancer prognostic factors
  resectability of, 115
  with solitary metastasis, 416–424
    resection of other solitary sites of metastasis, 423–424
    resection of solitary adrenal metastasis, 420–423, *421–423*
    resection of solitary brain metastasis, 417–420, *418*, 418t–420t, *420–421*
    results of chemotherapy for, 416–417, 417t
  stage 0, 309
    photodynamic therapy for, 952–956, 953t–954t, *955*
  stage I, 309, 340–345
    adjuvant therapy for, 344
    brachytherapy for, 344

  chemoprevention of second primary tumors after, 344–345
  chemotherapy for, 344
  predictors of survival in, 342–344
  preoperative staging of, 340
  radiation therapy for, 344
  recurrence and new cancers after treatment for, 341, 344t
  results of surgical therapy for, 341, *342–343*
  role of miniresection and thoracoscopy in, 347–348
  surgical therapy for, 340–341
stage II, 309, 345–349
  adjuvant therapy for, 345–347
  prognosis for, 345
  results of surgical therapy for, *342*, 345, *346*
  role of miniresection and thoracoscopy in, 347–348
stage IIIA, 309, 351–371
  clinical presentation of, 351–352
  diagnosis and staging of, 352–357
  early trials of neoadjuvant therapy for, 363–364
  imaging of, 351–352, *353–358*, 355–357
  management of T3 tumors involving chest wall, 357–359, 358t, *360*, 874
  management of T3 tumors involving main stem bronchi, 359–361, *361–362*
  management of T3 tumors involving mediastinum and diaphragm, 359
  principles of neoadjuvant therapy for, 369–371
  prognosis for, 351
  rationale for neoadjuvant therapy for, 363
  recent trials of neoadjuvant therapy for, 364
    chemotherapy and radiation without resection, 364–366, 365t
    chemotherapy before resection, 366–367
    combined chemotherapy and radiation before resection, 367t, 367–368
    optimal regimen, 368–369, *369–370*
  surgical resection for N2 disease, 361–363, 363t
stage IIIB, 309, 388–411
  anatomy and, 388–390, *389*
  clinical presentation of, 390–392
  concept of local control in, 394
  diagnostic workup for, 392–393, 393t
    extrathoracic assessment, 393, 393t
    fiberoptic bronchoscopy, 392
    mediastinoscopy, 392
    superior vena cava syndrome, 393
  imaging of, 392, *392*
  prognosis for, 351
  prognostic factors in, 393–394
  staging of, 390, 391t
  treatment of, 394–411
    adjuvant surgery, 409–410, 411t

adjuvant therapy for superior vena cava syndrome, 410
chemotherapy, 394–395, 398, 399t
combined radiotherapy and chemotherapy, 395, 398–409, 402t–403t, 405, 406t, 409t
future goals, 410–411
radiotherapy, 395–398
stage IV (disseminated), 309, 426–433
chemotherapy vs. supportive care for, 416, 417t, 431–432, 432t
combination chemotherapy for, 428–430, 429t
new strategies and drug combinations for, 431
quality of life and treatment of, 432
randomized treatment studies in, 430t, 430–432, 432t
single-agent chemotherapy for, 426–428, 427t
staging of, 115, 306–309, 307t, 308, 352t, 390, 391t, 426
superior sulcus tumors, 375–386
brachytherapy for, 385–386
clinical features of, 376–377
diagnosis of, 377–379, 379t
historical description of, 375
imaging of, 377–378, 377–379
management of, 379–380
metastatic workup for, 379
pathologic considerations for, 375–376, 376
radiotherapy for, 382–385
surgical treatment of, 380–381, 380–382, 382t
toxicity of combined modality therapy for, 1011
tumor suppressor genes in, 34–35
Norfloxacin, 980
Notochordal process, 4–5
NPe6, 947–948, 949
Nuclear medicine, 112
of bronchial carcinoid, 127
findings of metastatic carcinoma on, 137
in Hodgkin's disease, 141, 143
for preoperative lung cancer assessment, 125, 125–126
quantitative radionuclide lung scanning to evaluate high-risk surgical patient, 177, 177–178
radiopharmaceuticals used in, 112, 113t
Nucleolus abnormalities, 269
NuGel, 1003
Nursing issues, 991–993
administering chemotherapy and managing side effects, 991–992
oncology nursing education, 992–993, 993t
Nutrition
anorexia-cachexia, 986–987, 987t
dietary factors in lung cancer prevention, 1052, 1054, 1055t
drugs for enhancement of, 988
esophageal cancer and, 539, 568, 607
malnutrition, 987

Nutritional support, 987–988
Nystatin, 980

Obliterative endarteritis, 1005
O'Brien-Fleming rule, 202, 202t
Observation bias, 67
Occult lung carcinoma, 307–309, 339–340
localization of, 339
treatment of, 339–340
Occupational exposures. See Environmental and occupational exposures
Occupational transmission of HIV infection, 1042–1044
Odds ratio, 68, 68t
Odynophagia, 567
Oltipraz, 100, 1056, 1065
Oncofetal antigens, 330
Oncogenes. See also specific oncogenes
in Barrett's esophagus, 592–593
in esophageal cancer, 43–44, 644–645
in lung cancer, 31–33, 33t, 106, 276–279, 1069–1070
dominant and recessive oncogenes, 276–277
histopathologic subtype and, 266t, 266–268, 267–268
myc family, 32–33, 33t, 94t, 95, 266–267, 267, 278–279, 325, 329
non-small cell carcinoma, 32–33, 278, 278t, 329–330
ras family, 32–33, 33t, 94t, 94–95, 108, 267, 278, 278, 278t
role in early detection, 93–95, 94t
small cell carcinoma, 32, 325
in neuroblastoma, 716, 726
in neuroepithelioma, 726
in non-Hodgkin's lymphoma, 1031
Oncovin. See Vincristine
Ondansetron, 983t, 983–984
Oral contraceptives, 822
Oral leukoplakia, 98, 1071
Ornithine decarboxylase, 1056
Orthostatic hypotension, 297
Ostac. See Clodronate
Osteoblastoma, 871
Osteochondroma, 871
Osteogenic sarcoma
of chest wall, 872
pulmonary metastasectomy for, 912–913, 913t
Osteoradionecrosis, 1008
Osteosarcoma, 137
cardiac, 699
pulmonary, 828
Ovarian cancer, 916
Oximetry, 1020
Oxygen and radiation therapy response, 220–221, 221, 224, 225
Oxygen therapy, 1022

$p53$ gene, 34, 94t, 95, 106, 108, 267, 280–281, 281–282, 330
in Barrett's esophagus, 593

in esophageal cancer, 644–645
in lung cancer, 1070
in mesothelioma, 789
mutations of, 1070
P glycoprotein overexpression, 467
P value, 199t, 199–200
Pacemakers and radiation therapy, 1004
Paclitaxel, 488
before brachytherapy, 944
for esophageal cancer, 614t, 615, 631–632, 632t
for HIV-related Kaposi's sarcoma, 1038
for mesothelioma, 792, 804
neurotoxicity of, 1009
for non-small cell lung cancer, 427t, 428, 431
pleural effusion induced by, 153
side effects of, 428, 498
for small cell lung cancer, 498, 502
Paget's disease of esophagus, 550
Pain, 988–990
assessment and evaluation of, 989
causes in cancer patients, 988–989, 989t
postoperative, 173
treatment of, 989–990
Pamidronate, 301, 985–986
Pancoast tumor. See Superior sulcus tumors
Pancytopenia, 1009
Papillary fibroelastoma, 691
Paraganglia, 17
Paragangliomas, posterior mediastinal, 722–724
chemodectomas, 723
classification of, 723
clinical features of, 723
functioning. See Pheochromocytoma
malignant, 723
MRI features of, 723
nonfunctioning, 722–723
pathology of, 723–724
treatment of, 724
Paraneoplastic syndromes
associated with lung cancer, 293, 297–306, 298t
cutaneous syndromes, 297–298, 299
definition of, 297
endocrine syndromes, 298–303
Cushing's syndrome, 299–300
hypercalcemia, 300–302
SIADH, 302–303
hematologic syndromes, 303
mechanisms of, 297
neurologic syndromes, 303–305
intestinal dysmotilities, 305
Lambert-Eaton myasthenic syndrome, 304–305
limbic encephalitis, 305
necrotizing myelopathy, 305
subacute peripheral neuropathy, 303–304
visual paraneoplastic syndrome, 305
renal syndromes, 305
systemic disorders, 297

Paraneoplastic syndromes, (*continued*)
associated with thymoma, 656t–657t, 656–657
results of thymic surgery on, 665
Paraspinal tumors, 148, *149*
Parathyroid carcinoma, 917
Parathyroid glands, 15
imaging of, 147–148
Parathyroid hormone, 984
Parenteral nutrition, 987–988
Particulate radiation, 216. *See also* Radiation therapy
Patient education
about dangers of smoking, 1086
about pulmonary rehabilitation, 1021, 1026
Patterson-Kelly syndrome. *See* Plummer-Vinson syndrome
PCNA, 269
Pefloxacin, 980
Penicillins, 980, 981
Pentoxifylline, 994
Pericardial biopsy, 899
Pericardial effusions, 695, 894–900
catheter drainage and sclerotherapy for, 897–899
on chest radiography, 895, *896*
cyclophosphamide-induced, 994
diagnosing etiology of, 897
on echocardiography, 895, *897*
electrocardiogram findings with, 895, *896*
findings on right heart catheterization, 895, *898*
malignancies associated with, 894
pericardiocentesis for, 895–897
physiology of, 895
surgical options for, 899
percutaneous balloon pericardiotomy, 899, *900*
pericardial biopsy, 899
pericardioscopy, 899–900
thoracoscopic pericardiotomy, 900
video-assisted thoracic surgery, 970
Pericardial sac, 7–8
Pericardial tamponade, 18, 895
Pericardial tumors, 705–706
liposarcoma, 706
malignant peripheral nerve tumor, 705, *705*
mesothelioma, 705
metastatic, 706
other, 706
small cell tumor, 705–706
teratoma, 706
Pericardiocentesis, 895–897
Pericardioscopy, 899–900
Pericardiotomy, 899–900
percutaneous balloon, 899
thoracoscopic, 900
Pericarditis
cyclophosphamide-induced, 153
radiotherapy-induced, 1005
Pericardium
development of, 7, *7*
fibrous, 7, *7*

lymphatic drainage of, 20
parietal, 7
Peripheral neuropathy, subacute, 303–304
Phenethyl isothiocyanate (PEITC), 39, 45, 1056
Phenothiazines, 983t
4-Phenylbutyl isothiocyanate, 45
6-Phenylhexyl isothiocyanate, 45
3-Phenylpropyl isothiocyanate, 45
Pheochromocytoma
cardiac, 692
posterior mediastinal, 724–725
clinical features of, 724
compared with adrenal pheochromocytoma, 724
diagnosis of, 724
malignant, 725
pathology of, 724–725
preoperative localization of, 724
treatment of, 725
Phosphorus, 985
Photodynamic therapy (PDT), 947–962
in advanced tracheobronchial malignancies, 952–953, 957–959, 958t
compared with Nd:YAG laser therapy, 958, 958t
to diagnose lung cancer, 950–952, 952–953, 953t
in early-stage lung cancer, 952–956, 953t–954t, 955
for esophageal cancer-induced dysphagia, 623
histologic types of lung cancer treated with, 952, 953t
history of, 947
laser systems for, 949, 950
mechanisms of, 948–949, *950*
for mesothelioma, 796
in multiple primary lung cancer, 956t, 956–957, *957*
for occult lung carcinoma, 340
photosensitizers for, 947–948, *948–949*, 962
preoperative, 959t, 959–960, *960–961*
procedure for, 949–950, *951*
world trends and future of, 960–962, 962t
Photofrin, 947–949, *948*, 962
Phycomycetes, 159
Pigmentary changes, radiotherapy-induced, 1004
Piperacillin, 981
Pirarubicin
for cardiac lymphoma, 699
for mesothelioma, 802
Planck's constant, 216
Plasmacytoma
of chest wall, 873
pericardial, 706
pulmonary, 842–843, *842–843*
Platinum, 697
Pleura, 14–15, *16*
blood supply of, 15
parietal, 7, 15, 18, 880

tumor invasion of, 268, *268*, 294–295
visceral, *7*, 14–15, 18, 880
Pleural effusions
video-assisted thoracic surgery for, 967–968, 968t, *969–970*
Pleural effusions, malignant, 19, 20, 148, 295, 391, 880–894
Askin's tumor and, 832
bloody, 882
chemotherapy-induced, 153
clinical features of, 881
diagnosis of, 881–883
chest radiography, 881
cytogenetics, 883
cytologic examination, 882
immunocytochemistry, 882
other pleural fluid studies, 883
pleural fluid characteristics, 882
thoracentesis, 881–882
thoracoscopy, 883
effect on staging, 307
exudative, 882
in Hodgkin's disease, 141
malignancies associated with, 881, 881t
management of, 883–894, *884*
primary effusions, *884*, 884–885
secondary effusions, 883–884
surgical options, 891–894, *893*
pleurectomy, 893
pleuroperitoneal shunt, 894
thoracentesis, 885
tube thoracostomy and pleural sclerotherapy, 885–891
mesothelioma and, 736, 757, 761, 788, 799
pathophysiology of, 880–881
recurrent, 885
small cell lung cancer and, 526–527
Pleural fluid, 18–19
Pleural plaques, 736–737, 771, *771*, 780
Pleural sclerotherapy, 885–891
ambulatory, 891, *892*
indications for, 885
large-bore vs. small-bore catheters for, 891
for mesothelioma, 795
procedure for, 885
sclerosing agents for, 885–891
bleomycin, 887t, 888–889, 889t
Corynebacterium parvum, 890, 890t
doxycycline, 887–888, 888t
interferons, 890, 890t
interleukin-2, 890t, 890–891
minocycline, 888, 888t
mitoxantrone, 889, 889t
other chemotherapeutic agents, 889t, 889–890
quinacrine, 888, 888t
radioactive isotopes, 891
talc, 885–887, 886t–888t
tetracycline, 887, 887t–888t
tube thoracostomy technique, 885
Pleural tumors, 148–150
Askin's tumor, 832–833, *832–833*

fibrosarcoma, 830–832, *831–832*
localized fibrous tumor, 149–150
malignant solitary fibrous tumor, 771–772, *772*, 830–832, *831–832*
metastatic, 148
pleuropulmonary blastoma, 128, 833–834, *834*
vascular sarcomas, 834–835
Pleurectomy, 893
for mesothelioma, 794–795
Pleuritis, fibrosing, 770–771, *771*
Pleuropericardial folds, *7*, 7–8
Pleuropericardial membrane, 7
Pleuroperitoneal membrane, 8
Pleuroperitoneal shunt, 893
Plicamycin, 301, 985
Plummer-Vinson syndrome, 540, 542, 566, 595
p185neu, 33
Pneumococcal infection, 980–981
Pneumococcal vaccine, 980
Pneumocytes, 11–12
Pneumonia, 567
HIV-associated, 1043t
Pneumocystis carinii, 157–158, *158,* 1029, 1043t
prophylaxis for, 980
in smokers, 120–121
Pneumonitis
postobstructive, 294
radiation-induced, 485, 1003–1004
Pneumothorax, 131
Polycythemia, 688
Polymerase chain reaction (PCR), 277
Polymyositis, 297
Polynuclear aromatic hydrocarbons (PAHs), 25–26, 26t
bay regions and fjord regions of, *28*, 29
biomarkers related to, 37–38
carcinogenicity of, 73–74
DNA adducts formed from, *30,* 31
inhibition of carcinogenesis by, 39
metabolism of, *27*, 28
Pontine myelinolysis, 1009
Pores of Kohn, 14
Portal hypertension, 15, 567
Positron emission tomography (PET), 112, 131, *132*
Posterior mediastinal tumors, 711–729, 712t
dumbbell tumors, 727–729, *727–729*
embryology of neurogenic tumors, 711
goiter, 729
granular cell tumors, 729
incidence of, 711
lymphoma, 729
nerve sheath tumors, 711–715
malignant schwannoma, 714
melanotic schwannoma, 714–715
neurilemoma, 711–713, *712–713*
neurofibroma, 713–714, *714*
neuronal cell tumors, 715–727
ganglioneuroma and ganglioneuroblastoma, 721–722, *722–723*

neuroblastoma, 715–721, *717–718*
neuroepithelioma, 725–727
paraganglioma, 722–724
pheochromocytoma, 724–725
vagus nerve tumors, 729
Pott's disease, 148
Prednisolone, 988, 989
Prednisone
for cardiac lymphoma, 699
for HIV-associated non-Hodgkin's lymphoma, 1032
for HIV-related Hodgkin's disease, 1041
for intravascular lymphomatosis of lung, 842
for lymphomatoid granulomatosis, 840
for thymoma, 662–663
Prevention, 1052. *See also* Chemoprevention
N-acetylcysteine, 1056
antioxidants, 39, 98, 1054–1056, 1055t, 1060–1065
chemoprevention of esophageal cancer, 45–46
dietary factors, 1052, 1054–1056, 1055t
education programs, 81
of environmental and occupational thoracic neoplasms, 80–81
of lung cancer, 90–101, 1052–1053
chemoprevention, 38–39, 96–101, 1052–1072
early detection, 90–96. *See also* Screening for lung cancer
primary vs. secondary, 1052
retinoids, 46, 98–101, 189, 344–345, 1054–1055, 1060–1064
Procarbazine
for HIV-related Hodgkin's disease, 1041
for lung cancer
non-small cell carcinoma, 365t, 429
small cell carcinoma, 470, 471t
myelosuppression due to, 1009
neurotoxicity of, 1009
pulmonary toxicity of, 1009
for thymoma, 662
Prochlorperazine, 983t
Prognostic factors
for esophageal cancer, 555, 624
for lung cancer, 105, 268–269, 319–331, 431. *See also* Lung cancer prognostic factors
for mediastinal germ cell tumors, 672–674, 673t–674t
for mesothelioma, 781–782, 784, 787t, 787–789, 800, 800t
for neuroblastoma, 719–720, *720,* 720t
for pulmonary metastasectomy, 908–910
for thymoma, 663–664, *664*
Proopiomelanocortin, 298, 299
Proportional hazards regression model, 320
Prostaglandins, 297
Proteinosis, congenital alveolar, 12
Protooncogenes. *See* Oncogenes
Pseudomonas infection, 980, 998
Psychologic disturbances, 1018

Psychologic support, 990t, 990–991
Psychosocial assessment, 1020–1021
PTPG gene, 34
Public Health Cigarette Smoking Act, 1083
Pulmonary blastoma, 128
Pulmonary edema
chemotherapy-induced, 182, 182t
after tracheal reconstruction, 864
Pulmonary embolism, 303
Pulmonary fibrosis, radiotherapy-induced, 1001, 1005
Pulmonary function testing, 169–182, 1020
basis of, 169–171, *170–172*
after bronchoscopic laser resection, 935
effects of surgery on, 171–174
extent of lung resection, 174
general anesthesia, 171–172
type of thoracic incision, 172–174
preoperative, 174–180, *179*
to evaluate high-risk patient, 177–180
exercise test, 178–180
quantitative radionuclide lung scanning, *177,* 177–178
to identify high-risk patient, 175–177, 176t
arterial blood gas, 176–177
diffusion capacity, 176
spirometry and lung volumes, 175–176
radiation therapy and lung function, 180–181
Pulmonary hypertension, 686–688, 1006
Pulmonary infections, 981
Pulmonary ligaments, 5
Pulmonary metastasectomy, 906–917
adjuvant chemotherapy and, 910–911
history of, 906
invasive pretreatment evaluation for, 907–908
laser resection, 911–912
patient selection for, 908
prognostic factors for, 908–910
disease free interval, 908, 909t
laterality of lesions, 910
nodal status, 910
number of metastases, 909–910
patient age and sex, 910
resectability, 908
size of nodules, 910
symptoms, 910
tumor doubling time, 910
reoperative, 912
for specific histologies, 912–917
breast cancer, 916
colorectal cancer, 915t, 915–916
gynecologic cancer, 916
head and neck cancer, 915
malignant melanoma, 916–917, 917t
osteogenic sarcoma, 912–913, 913t
other tumors, 917
soft tissue sarcoma, 913–914, 914t
testicular cancer, 914–915, 915t
urinary tract cancer, 914, 914t
technique for, 911–912

Pulmonary metastases, 135–139, 906–917
  diagnosis of, 906–907
  endobronchial, 137
  imaging of, 135–139, *136, 140,* 907
  locations of, 906
  lymphangitic spread, 137, *138*
  mechanism of spread to lung, 135
  pathogenesis of, 906
Pulmonary nodule(s)
  calcification in, *129–130,* 129–131, 136
  chemotherapy-induced, 152–153
  detectability on chest radiography, 117
  imaging of solitary nodule, *117, 129–130,* 129–131
  in patients with known primary tumors elsewhere, 136
  percutaneous CT-directed biopsy of, 973
  peripheral, 117–118, *117–118*
  surgical resection of, 973
  video-assisted thoracic surgery to establish diagnosis of, 970–974, *973–975*
Pulmonary rehabilitation, 1018–1026
  content of program for, 1020t, 1021–1024
    education, 1021, 1026
    exercise, 1022–1026
      blood gas changes, 1023
      exercise prescription, 1023
      upper extremity training, 1023
      ventilatory muscle training, 1024
    psychosocial support, 1024
    respiratory and chest physiotherapy, 1021–1022
      breathing retraining techniques, 1022
      bronchial hygiene, 1021–1022
      oxygen, 1022
  definition of, 1018
  future of, 1026
  indications for, 1018
  multidisciplinary team approach to, 1019
  nurse's role in, 992
  patient evaluation for, 1019–1021, 1020t
    diagnostic testing, 1020
    goal setting, 1021
    interview, 1019–1020
    medical evaluation, 1020
    psychosocial assessment, 1020–1021
  patient selection for, 1019, 1019t
  results of, 1024t, 1024–1026
    benefits of exercise, 1025–1026
    effects of education, 1026
    hospitalizations and use of medical resources, 1024–1025
    pulmonary function and symptoms, 1026
    quality of life, 1025
    survival, 1026
Pulmonary toxicity
  of chemotherapy, 150–154, 1008–1009
  of radiotherapy, 485–486, *487,* 1003–1005
Pulmonary trunk sarcoma, 828–830, *829–830*
  clinical features of, 828

incidence of, 828
pathology of, 829
therapy and prognosis for, 829–830
Pulsus alternans, 682
Pursed lips breathing, 1022

Quality assurance for radiation therapy, 238–239
Quality of life, 432
Quinacrine
  for pericardial sclerotherapy, 898
  for pleural sclerotherapy, 888, 888t

Rad, 218
Radiation therapy, 215–239
  clinical principles of, 222–228
    carcinogenic risk, 227–228, 228t
    normal tissue tolerance, 226, 227t
    predictive assays, 223–225, 225t, *225–226*
    therapeutic ratio, 222–223
    tumor characteristics, 223, *223–224*
  development of resistance to, 394
  effects on thorax, 154–155, *155–156*
  fractionation of, 228–231
    accelerated fractionation, 1001–1002
    biologic principles of, 228–229, *229,* 229t
    effect of altered regimens on toxicity, 1001–1002
    history of, 228
    hyperfractionation, 1001
    schedules for, 229–231, 230t, *231*
  principles of radiobiology, 219–222
    cell survival and survival curves, *219,* 219–220
    mathematical models, 222
    oxygen and radiation, 220–221, *221*
    recruitment, 221
    repopulation, 221–222
    stages of interaction of radiation with matter, 219
    tumor growth, 222, 222t
  procedure for, 231–234, *232–233*
    dose calculations, 232
    patient evaluation, 231, 233–234
    target volume, 231
    treatment planning, 231–233
  quality of treatment with, 238–239, *238–239*
  radiation physics, 215–219
    absorption of radiation in matter, 215–216
      types of clinical radiation, 216
    advantages and drawbacks of radiation beams, 216–217, *217–218*
    atomic and nuclear structures, 215
    brachytherapy and physics, 218t, 218–219
    dose distribution and units, 217–218
    external radiation therapy equipment, 216
  special techniques for, 234–238
    brachytherapy, 234–236, *234–236,* 940–946

3-dimensional conformal/dynamic radiotherapy, 236–237
    intraoperative radiotherapy, *237,* 237–238
Radiation therapy for cardiac tumors, 696
  angiosarcoma, 697
  fibrosarcoma, 698
  liposarcoma, 699
  metastatic tumors, 703–704
  osteosarcoma, 699
  primary lymphoma, 699
  rhabdomyosarcoma, 698
Radiation therapy for chest wall tumors, 875–876
Radiation therapy for esophageal cancer, 556, 601, 609–614
  clinical trials of radiotherapy alone, 611, 612t
  combined with chemotherapy, 602, 618–620, 620t
    preoperative, 620–621, 621t–622t, 635
  complications of, 611–612
  intracavitary, 611
  palliative, 623
  postoperative, 613t, 613–614
  preoperative, 601–602, 612–613, 613t
  technique for, 609–611, *610*
Radiation therapy for lung cancer
  bronchial carcinoids, 853
  imaging evaluation and follow-up after, 124–125
  lung function and, 169, 180–181
  small cell carcinoma, 113, 115, 461–467
    chest irradiation and local failure, 462, *463,* 463t
    chest irradiation and overall survival, 462
    combined with chemotherapy, 440, 477–484
      alternating approaches, 481–484, *482–483,* 483t
      concurrent approaches, 481, 481t
      scheduling methods, 480
      treatment toxicity, 485–486
    combined with surgery, 439–440, *440,* 442–443
    early vs. late radiotherapy, 479–480, 480t
    fractionation, 464–466
    mechanisms of therapeutic benefit, 477
    prophylactic cranial irradiation, 512–522. *See also* Cranial irradiation, prophylactic
    quality of chest irradiation, 466
    radiation technique, 466–467, *468–469*
    radioresponsiveness, 461–462
    radiotherapy parameters, 462
    results of clinical trials, 478t, 478–479, *479*
    total radiation dose, 464, *465*
    volume treated, 462–464
  stage I disease, 344
  stage II disease, 345, 348–349

stage IIIA disease, 363–371
　combined with chemotherapy before resection, 367t, 367–368
　combined with chemotherapy without resection, 364–366, 365t
stage IIIB disease, 395–398
　CHART regimen, 397–398
　combined with chemotherapy, 395, 398–409
　　concomitant chemotherapy-radiotherapy trials, 407–409, 409t
　　rationale for, 399
　　sequential chemotherapy-radiotherapy trials, 399–407, 402t–403t, 405, 406t
　　survival rates after, 399
　fractionation, 396–398
　radiation parameters, 395–396, 396
　results compared with chemotherapy, 398
　split-course radiotherapy, 396
　total dose, 396
superior sulcus tumors, 382–385
Radiation therapy for mediastinal germ cell tumors
　nonseminomatous tumor, 674–675, 676t
　seminoma, 674, 675t
Radiation therapy for mesothelioma, 792, 808–810
　surgery and, 795–796
Radiation therapy for posterior mediastinal tumors
　ganglioneuroblastoma, 721
　neuroblastoma, 721, 722t
　neuroepithelioma, 726–727
　pheochromocytoma, 725
Radiation therapy for thymoma, 661–662
　postoperative, 661–662
　preoperative, 662
　technical problems with, 662
Radiation therapy for tracheal tumors, 867t–868t, 867–869
Radiation Therapy Oncology Group trials, 1002, 1011
Radiation therapy toxicity, 485–486, 940, 1001–1008, 1002t
　acute, 1002t, 1002–1004
　　cardiotoxicity, 1004
　　cutaneous changes, 1002–1003
　　esophagitis, 1003
　　neurotoxicity, 1004
　　pulmonary toxicity, 485–486, 487, 1003–1004
　altered fractionation regimens and, 1001–1002
　associated with prophylactic cranial irradiation, 514–519
　chronic, 1001, 1003t, 1004–1008
　　bone marrow toxicity, 486, 1006
　　bone necrosis, 1008
　　carcinogenesis, 1007–1008
　　cardiotoxicity, 1005–1006
　　cutaneous changes, 1004–1005

　　endocrine disorders, 1007
　　esophagitis, 1005
　　neurotoxicity, 1006–1007
　　pulmonary toxicity, 1005
　esophageal cancer and, 539, 566
　patient variables affecting, 1001–1002, 1003t
　　AIDS, 1002
　　collagen vascular disease, 1002
　　smoking, 1002
　treatment variables affecting, 1001
　when combined with chemotherapy, 182, 182t, 485–486, 1010–1012
Radioisotopes, 218, 218t
　for pericardial sclerotherapy, 898
　for pleural sclerotherapy, 891
Radiopharmaceuticals, 112, 113t
Radon exposure, 25, 51, 74–75
c-raf-1 oncogene, 32, 33, 94t, 95
Randomization, 195–197
　advantages of, 195, 196t
　informed consent and, 203t, 203–204
　methods for, 195–197
ras protooncogenes, 32–33, 33t, 94t, 94–95, 108, 267, 278, 278, 278t, 1070
Rb-1 gene, 34, 94t, 95, 106, 279–280
Recursive partition and amalgamation method (RECPAM), 320, 322
Refractory ceramic fibers (RCFs), 77–78
Rehabilitation. See Pulmonary rehabilitation
Relative risk, 68, 68t
Renal cell carcinoma, 914, 914t
Renal paraneoplastic syndromes, 305
Residual volume, 169, 170
Restriction fragment length polymorphisms (RFLPs), 277
Reticular dysgenesis, 17
Retinoic acid receptors, 1055, 1056, 1072
Retinoids, 46, 98–101, 189, 344–345, 1052, 1054–1055, 1060–1064
　clinical trials for lung cancer prevention, 1067–1069
　　in healthy persons, 1066t
　　prevention of second primary tumors, 1067–1069, 1068t
　　treatment of precancerous lesions, 1067
　fenretinide, 1063–1064
　isotretinoin, 1061–1063
　natural retinol, 1060–1061
　plasma elimination half-lives of, 1062, 1062t
　retinyl palmitate, 1061
　side effects of, 1060–1062, 1061t
　teratogenicity of, 1061
Reverse "S" sign, 120, 121
Rh isoimmunization, 9
Rhabdomyoma, 18
　cardiac, in children, 693, 694
　of chest wall, 871
Rhabdomyosarcoma
　cardiac, 698
　of chest wall, 872
　of esophagus, 552
　of lung, 825–827, 826
　　clinical features of, 825–826

　　pathology of, 826–827
　　therapy and prognosis for, 827
Rheumatologic disorders, 297
Ribs. See Chest wall tumors
Risk factors
　competing risks, 200–201, 201
　for lung cancer, 25–27, 293, 294t
　　cigarette smoking, 25–27, 26t, 51–64, 113. See also Smoking
　　environmental exposures, 25–26, 66–81. See also Environmental and occupational exposures
　　radiation therapy, 227–228, 228t

S-100 protein, 265
"S" sign of Golden, 120, 121
Sarcomas
　of chest wall, 872, 873, 875
　of esophagus, 536, 536t, 552
Sarcomatoid carcinoma of lung, 263–264, 815–816, 816
　clinical features of, 816
　epidemiology of, 815–816
　pathology of, 816
　therapy and prognosis for, 816
Scar adenocarcinoma, 255–256
Schwannoma, posterior mediastinal, 711–713, 712–713
　malignant, 714, 828
　melanotic, 714–715
Sclerotherapy
　for pericardial effusion, 897–899
　for pleural effusion, 885–891. See also Pleural sclerotherapy
Screening
　for esophageal cancer, 543, 568
　for lung cancer, 90–96, 105–109, 293, 319
　　chest radiography for, 116, 293
　　data banks of potential markers for, 107
　　evaluating studies of, 92–93
　　immunocytochemical analysis of sputum, 93
　　Johns Hopkins Lung Project, 105
　　molecular genetic techniques, 108–109, 109
　　monoclonal antibody studies, 107–108
　　novel approaches to early detection, 93, 94
　　prospective nonrandomized studies of, 91–92
　　prospective randomized studies of, 92
　　retrospective studies of, 90–91, 91t
　　role of growth factors in, 95–96
　　role of oncogenes in, 93–95, 94t, 106
Selection bias, 67
Selenium, 45, 46, 1054–1056
Seminoma, 671. See also Germ cell tumors
　imaging of, 142
　laboratory findings in, 670
　treatment of, 674, 675t
Septum(a)
　of lung, 13–14
　transversum, 7, 8

Shoulder pain, 375, 377
Significance tests, 199t, 199–200
Silica exposure, 26, 78–79
Single photon emission computed tomography (SPECT), 112, 141
c-*sis* protooncogene, 33
Small cell carcinoma of esophagus, 536t, 551, *551*
  incidence of, 643
  prognosis for, 643
  staging of, 643
  treatment of, 643
Small cell lung cancer (SCLC), 25, 245, 247
  anticoagulant therapy for, 475–476, 476t
  biologic features of, 456–457
  biomarkers for, 253t, 259, 324, 325t, 456
  chemotherapy for, 113, 115, 456, 467–473, 470t–472t. *See also* Chemotherapy for lung cancer
    alternating vs. sequential, 469–470, 471t
    anticoagulant therapy and, 475–476, 476t
    chemoresponsiveness, 441, 467
    combination regimens, 499–502
      CAV, CAE, and CAVE regimens, 500, 501t
      etoposide and cisplatin, 500–501, 501t
      number of drugs, 500
      other combinations, 501–502
    combined with radiotherapy, 440, 477–484
      alternating approaches, 481–484, *482–483*, 483t
      concurrent approaches, 481, 481t
      scheduling methods, 480
      treatment toxicity, 485–486
    combined with surgery, 440–441, *442–443*, 453
      postoperative chemotherapy, 447–451, 448t–449t, *449–451*
      preoperative chemotherapy, 444–447, 445t, *445–446*, 447t
    development of drug resistance, 458, 467–469
    dose effect within standard range of doses, 470–472, 472t
    dose intensification, 472–473, 504–506, 505t
    drug regimens, 469, 470t
    duration of treatment, 503–504
    hematopoietic growth factors and, 506–507
    immunotherapy and, 473–475, 504
    investigation of new schedules, 499
    maintenance therapy, 473, 474t
    new agents, 497–499, 502, 507
      epirubicin, 499
      gemcitabine, 498–499
      irinotecan (CPT-11), 497–498
      paclitaxel, 498
    non-cross-resistant alternating regimens, 502–503, 503t
    recurrence after discontinuation of, 441, 458–458
    scheduling, 497, 499
    single-agent therapy, 496–497, 497t
    weekly dose intense regimens, 473, 505–506, 506t
  on chest radiography, 459
  chromosome abnormalities in, 32, 456
  combined approaches to, 476–489
  compared with non-small cell carcinoma, 457, 457t
  cytologic appearance of, 249
  development of other malignancies in survivors of, 452–453, 486–488
  diagnosis of, 459–460
  disseminated disease, 496–507
  growth factors in, 324–325
  imaging of, 113–115, *114*
  immunotherapy for, 473–475, 504
  inappropriate antidiuretic hormone release in, 302–303
  incidence of, 259, 496
  isolated extensive disease, 439, 525–528
    adrenal metastases, 527–528
    bone marrow metastases, 527
    bone metastases, 527
    brain metastases, 526
    definition of, 525
    liver metastases, 526
    number of metastatic sites, 525–526
    pleural effusions, 526–527
    prognosis for, 525
  limited (regional) disease, 456–489
    definition of, 457, 525
    incidence of, 456
    prognosis for, 457–459, *458*, 525
    treatment modalities for, 461
  locations of, 259, 293
  natural history of, 457–459
  oncogenes in, 32, 278, 278t, 325
  pathology of, 259–260, 456–457
  patterns of treatment failure in, 458–459, *460*
  perspectives on treatment of, 488–489
  prognostic factors in, 259–260, 260t, 320–325, 459. *See also* Lung cancer prognostic factors
  prophylactic cranial irradiation for, 512–522. *See also* Cranial irradiation, prophylactic
  radiation therapy for, 113, 115, 461–467. *See also* Radiation therapy for lung cancer
    chest irradiation and local failure, 462, *463*, 463t
    chest irradiation and overall survival, 462
    combined with chemotherapy, 440, 477–484
      alternating approaches, 481–484, *482–483*, 483t
      concurrent approaches, 481, 481t
      scheduling methods, 480
      treatment toxicity, 485–486
    combined with surgery, 439–440, *440*, 442–443
    early vs. late radiotherapy, 479–480, 480t
    fractionation, 464–466
    mechanisms of therapeutic benefit, 477
    quality of chest irradiation, 466
    radiation technique, 466–467, *468–469*
    radioresponsiveness, 461–462
    radiotherapy parameters, 462
    results of clinical trials, 478t, 478–479, *479*
    total radiation dose, 464, *465*
    volume treated, 462–464
  staging of, 309–310, 441, *443*, 457, 461, 525
  subtypes of, 259
  surgery for, 439–454
    chemotherapy and, 440–441, *442–443*, 453
      postoperative, 447–451, 448t–449t, *449–451*
      preoperative, 444–447, 445t, *445–446*, 447t
    guidelines for, 453–454
    to improve control at primary site, 441–443
    for late recurrence after primary treatment, 444
    for limited disease, 461, 476
    for mixed histology tumors, 443–444
    preoperative radiotherapy and, 439–440, *440*
    rationale for, 441–444, 443t
    results of clinical trials of, 439–441, *440*
    salvage operations, 451–453, *452*
    survival after, 439–441, *440*, 446, 453, 453–454, 458
  survival from, 486–487
  therapeutic approach to, 456
  toxicity of combined modality therapy for, 1011
  treatment in elderly patients, 484
  treatment of tumor relapses, 484–485
  treatment resistance of, 458
  tumor doubling time for, 457
  tumor suppressor genes in, 34
  value of fiberoptic bronchoscopy in, 459–460
Small cell tumor, pericardial, 705–706
Smoking, 51–64. *See also* Tobacco
  antismoking movement, 1079
  cigarette advertising and, 59–60, 1083–1084
  deposition and absorption of smoke, 53
  differences in smoking behavior among population subgroups, 60
  DNA adduct formation upon inhalation of smoke, *30*, 30–31
  education about dangers of, 1086
  environmental tobacco smoke, 25, 51, 57–58, 1084–1085
  esophageal cancer and, 39–40, 539
  federal restrictions on, 1079
  impact on chemoprevention trial, 1052
  lung cancer and, 25–27, 26t, 51, 113, 293, 388, 1052–1053, 1053t

age effects on risk, 53–54, *54*
epidemiology of, 53–57
gender effects on risk, 55, *56*
impact of smoking cessation on lung cancer risk, 25, 57, *57*
K-*ras* mutations and, 32–33
number of cigarettes smoked per day and duration of exposure, 54–55, *55–56*
occupational exposures and, 69
mortality related to, 1053, 1079
pneumonia and, 120–121
prevalence of, 60–63, *61–63*, 69
radiation therapy toxicity and, 1002, 1003t
regulation of, 1079, 1084–1086
on airline flights, 1085
in public places, 1085
in workplace, 1085–1086
trends in smoking behavior, *58–59*, 58–60, 1079
tumors related to, 1052–1053, 1053t
Social interventions, 990
Soft tissue sarcoma, 913–914, 914t
Solitary fibrous tumor of pleura, 771–772, *772*
Somatostatin receptors, 279
Somnolence syndrome, 517–518
Sphingomyelin, 11
Spindle cell carcinoma of esophagus, *546*, 546–547
Spindle cell components, 263, *264*
Spirometry, 175–176
Splanchnicectomy, thoracic, 977
Sputum cytology, 93, 248–250
Squamous cell carcinoma of esophagus, 533, 542–547
advanced, 544
classification of, 536t
early, 543–544, *543–544*
erosive, 543, *543*
fungating, 544, *544*
infiltrating, 544–545, *545–546*
intraepithelial, 543–544, *544*
intramucosal, 543, *543*
location of, 542–543
occult, 543
papillary, 543
plaque, 543
submucosal, 543
ulcerative, *543*, 544, *545*
variants of, 546–547
basaloid carcinoma, 546
carcinosarcoma, 547, *547*
spindle cell carcinoma, *546*, 546–547
verrucous carcinoma, 546, *547*
Squamous cell carcinoma of lung, 25, 115, 118, *119*
chemotherapy resistance of, 252
cytologic appearance of, 249
in HIV-infected patients, 1041
human papilloma virus and, 251–252
incidence of, 251

location of, 293, 376
markers for, 251–252, 253t
occult, 339
pathology of, 251, *251–252*
prognosis for, 252, 268–269, 327
stage IIIA, *353*, 355
Squamous cell carcinoma of trachea, 855–869. *See also* Tracheal tumors
Squamous papilloma of esophagus, 540
c-*src* protooncogene, 33, 726
Stage migration, 195, 196t, 322, 525
Staging
of esophageal cancer, 132–135, *133–134*, 554, 554t, 568–582
of lung cancer, 121–123, *122*, 306–311, 426
small cell carcinoma, 441, *443*, 457, 461, 525
of mesothelioma, 782t–783t, 782–784, 790–791, 791t–792t
of neuroblastoma, 718–719, 719t
of thymoma, 145, 654t–655t, 654–655
Standardized mortality ratio, 68
Staphylococcal catheter-related infections, 998
Starling's law, 880
Statistical significance, 68, 320, *321–322*
Stellate ganglion invasion, 376, *377*
Sterility, chemotherapy-induced, 1009
Strictures, esophageal, 540, 595–596
"Sugar" tumors of lung, 258
Sulfomucin, 536
Sulforaphane, 39
Sulfotransferases, 27
Superior sulcus tumors, 121, 295, 375–386
clinical diagnosis of, 377
clinical features of, 295, 376–377
differential diagnosis of, 379t
histologic confirmation of, 378–379
historical description of, 375
imaging of, 377–378, *377–379*
management of, 379–386
brachytherapy, 385–386
radiation therapy, 382–385
adjuvant, 384
combined with chemotherapy, 385
curative, 382–384
postoperative, 385
preoperative, *380*, 380, 384–385
selection of patients for curative treatment, 379
surgical treatment, 380–382
curative, *380–381*, 380–382, 382t, *383*
palliative, 382
metastatic workup for, 379
pathologic considerations for, 375–376, *376*
Superior vena cava syndrome, 294, 295, *295*, 391, 393
adjuvant therapy for, 410
cardiac tumors and, 699, 702
mesothelioma and, 781
radiation therapy for, 704

Supportive care, 979–998
for bone marrow transplantation, 994–995
cachexia and nutrition, 986–988
cellular supportive care of anemia and thrombocytopenia, 993–994
for chemotherapy-induced emesis, 983–984
for disseminated non-small cell lung cancer, 431–432, 432t
infection prevention and treatment, 979–983
intensive care, 995–997
nursing issues, 991–993
pain control, 988–990
psychologic support, 990–991
related to intravenous devices, 997–998
for tumor-induced hypercalcemia, 984–986
Surfactant, 11, 12
Surgical therapy for cardiac tumors, *684*, 684–685
angiosarcoma, 697
fibromas, 694
fibrosarcoma, 698
hemangioma, 692
leiomyosarcoma, 698
lipoma, 691
malignancies, 696
mesenchymoma, 700
myxoma, 689–690, 698
neurofibroma, 692
osteosarcoma, 699
papillary fibroelastoma, 691
pheochromocytoma, 692
results of, 685, 685t
rhabdomyoma, 693
rhabdomyosarcoma, 698
teratoma, 694
thymoma, 700
Surgical therapy for chest wall tumors, 875–878, *877*
Surgical therapy for esophageal cancer, 556, 577, 597–602, 606–609
adjuvant radiotherapy and, 601
for cancers of cervical esophagus, 608
combined modality therapy and, 601–602
preoperative chemoradiotherapy, 602, 620–621, 621t–622t
preoperative chemotherapy, 601, 616–618, 617t–618t
preoperative radiation therapy, 601–602, 612–613, 613t
complications of, 608, 609t
historical perspectives on, 563
operations for, 598–601, 607–608
classification of, 597–598
en bloc resection, 599–600, 607–608
standard transthoracic esophagectomy, 598–599, 607
three-field lymphadenectomy, 600–601
transhiatal esophagectomy, 598, 608
palliative, 622–623
for esophageal obstruction, 622–623

Surgical therapy for esophageal cancer, (*continued*)
   for malignant esophagorespiratory fistula, 622
   patient selection for, 606–607
   in patients with preoperative pulmonary problems, 606
   results of, 601, 609
   surgical approach for, 598
Surgical therapy for lung cancer
   combined with preoperative photodynamic therapy, 959t, 959–960, *960–961*
   effects on lung function, 171–174
     extent of resection, 174
     general anesthesia, 171–172
     type of incision, 172–174
   non-small cell carcinoma
     occult disease, 339–340
     role of miniresection and thoracoscopy in stage I or II disease, 347–348
     solitary metastasis, 416–424
       adrenal metastasis, 420–423, *423t–423*
       brain metastasis, 417–420, *418*, 418t–420t, *420–421*
       other sites of metastasis, 423–424
     stage I disease, 340–341, *342–343*
     stage II disease, *342*, 345, *346*
     stage IIIA disease, 351–371
       N2 disease, 361–363, 363t
       neoadjuvant therapy and, 363–371. *See also* Adjuvant therapy
       T3 tumors involving chest wall, 357–359, 358t, *360*
       T3 tumors involving main stem bronchi, 359–361, *361–362*
       T3 tumors involving mediastinum and diaphragm, 359
     stage IIIB disease, 409–410, 411t
     superior sulcus tumors, 380–381, 380–382, 382t, *383*
   postlobectomy compensatory growth in residual lung, 9–10
   pulmonary function testing before, 169, 174–180, *179*
     to evaluate high-risk patient, 177–180
     to identify high-risk patient, 175–177, 176t
   small cell carcinoma, 439–454
     chemotherapy and, 440–441, *442–443*, *453*
       postoperative, 444–447, 445t, *445–446*, 447t
       preoperative, 447–451, 448t–449t, *449–451*
     guidelines for, 453–454
     to improve control at primary site, 441–443
     for late recurrence after primary treatment, 444
     for limited disease, 461, 476
     for mixed histology tumors, 443–444
     radiotherapy and, 439–440, *440*
     rationale for, 441–444, 443t
     results of clinical trials of, 439–441
     salvage operations, 451–453, *452*
     survival after, 339, 439–441, 446, *453*, 453–454, 458, 476
   video-assisted, 970–977. *See also* Video-assisted thoracic surgery
Surgical therapy for mesothelioma, 793–795
   chemotherapy and, 795–796
   extrapleural pneumonectomy, 793–794
     patient selection for, 793, 793t
     preoperative evaluation for, 793
     results of, 794, 795t
     technique for, 793–794, *793–794*
   photodynamic therapy and, 796
   pleurectomy with decortication, 794–795
   pleurodesis, 795
   radiation therapy and, 795–796
Surgical therapy for posterior mediastinal tumors
   dumbbell tumors, 728–729
   ganglioneuroblastoma, 721
   ganglioneuroma, 721
   malignant schwannoma, 714
   melanotic schwannoma, 715
   neurilemoma, 713
   neuroblastoma, 720–721
   neurofibroma, 714
   paraganglioma, 724
   pheochromocytoma, 725
Surgical therapy for thymoma, 660–661, *661*
   tumor recurrence after, 665–666
Surgical therapy for tracheal tumors, *859*, 859–864, *861–862*
Survival analysis, 200–201, *201*
Syndrome of inappropriate antidiuretic hormone release (SIADH), 302–303, 324
Synovial sarcoma, 700, 772
Systemic lupus erythematosus, 297, 657, 665

Talc
   for pericardial sclerotherapy, 898
   for pleural sclerotherapy, 885–887, 886t–888t
Tar in cigarette smoke, 51
Taxol. *See* Paclitaxel
Taxotere. *See* Docetaxel
Tegaderm, 1003
Teicoplanin, 998
Telomerase, 282–283
Temporal relationship, 68
Tenascin, 252
Teniposide, 497
Teratoma, 672. *See also* Germ cell tumors
   cardiac, in children, 694
     malignant, 700
   imaging of, 142
   laboratory findings in, 670
   pericardial, 706
   treatment of, 676–677
Testicular cancer, 914–915, 915t

Tetracycline
   for pericardial sclerotherapy, 898
   for pleural sclerotherapy, 887, 887t–888t
9-Tetrahydrocannabinol, 983t
Thermal injury, esophageal, 539, 566
Thiethylperazine, 983t
Thiotepa, 898
Thoracentesis, 881–882, 885
Thoracic cage embryology, 5
Thoracic inlet tumors. *See* Superior sulcus tumors
Thoracoscopy, 173, 295
   compared with video-assisted thoracic surgery, 965
   to diagnose malignant pleural effusion, 883
   to evaluate pulmonary metastases, 908
   to stage esophageal cancer, 578–580, *579–580*
Thoracostomy, 885
Thoracotomy
   compared with video-assisted thoracic surgery, 173
   effects on lung function, 172–173
   mortality from, 174
   muscle-sparing, 173
Thrombocytopenia, 993–994, 1009
Thrombocytosis, mesothelioma and, 788
Thrombopoietin, 1009
Thrombosis, venous catheter-related, 997
Thymic rebound, 143–144, *146*
Thymidine kinase, 324, 325t
Thymolipoma, 17, 145–146
Thymoma, 17, 145, *147*, 653–665
   age and sex distribution of, 655, 655–656
   calcification of, 657
   cardiac, 700
   cortical, 654
   diagnosis of, 659–660
   frequency of, 655
   gross pathologic appearance of, 655
   histologic classification of, 145, 653–655, 654t
   involving pleura, 148
   location of, 657
   medullary, 654
   metastases of, 655
   mixed, 654
   paraneoplastic syndromes and, 656–657, 657t
     myasthenia gravis, 145, 653, 656, 656t
     results of surgery for, 665
   postoperative recurrence of, 664–665
   prognostic factors for, 663–664, *664*
   radiographic features of, 657–659, *657–659*
   staging of, 145, 654t–655t, 654–655
   surgical therapy for, video-assisted, 969, *972*
   symptoms of, 656
   treatment of, 660–663
     chemotherapy, 662–663
     radiation therapy, 661–662
     results of, 663, 663t
     surgery, 660–661, *661*

Thymosin, 474–475
Thymus
　anatomy of, 15, 17
　blood supply of, 653
　changes with age, 143
　congenital aplasia/hypoplasia of, 17
　embryology of, 653
　hyperplasia of, 143
　imaging of, 143–146
　lymphatic drainage of, 20, 653
　morphology of, 653
　tumors of, 17, 145–146
Thyroid disorders, radiotherapy-induced, 1006, 1007
Thyroid tumors, 146–147, 1007
Thyroidectomy, 864
Ticarcillin, 981
Ticarcillin-clavulanate, 981
Tidal volume, 169, 170
Tissue polypeptide antigen, 324, 325t
Tissue tolerance for radiation therapy, 226, 227t, 237
TNM staging system. See also Staging
　for esophageal cancer, 554, 554t, 568t–569t, 568–569
　for lung cancer, 121–123, 306–309, 307t, 308, 390, 391t, 441, 443, 525
　for mesothelioma, 782, 783t, 791, 791t
Tobacco, 1079–1088. See also Smoking
　carcinogens in tobacco smoke, 26–27
　chemistry of cigarette smoke, 51–53, 52t
　federal regulation of tobacco products and their content, 1080–1083
　　early regulation, 1080–1081
　　jurisdiction of federal agencies, 1081–1082
　　regulation of cigarette additives, 1082–1083
　　regulation of advertising, 1083–1084
　　regulation of labeling, 1083
　　regulation of smoking, 1079, 1084–1086
　　taxation of, 1086
　U.S. production of, 1087
　　for export, 1087–1088
　　support for, 1087
　　support of, 1079
Tobramycin, 981
α-Tocopherol, 39, 46, 100, 1054–1056, 1064–1067, 1066t
Topotecan
　for non-small cell lung cancer, 428
　for small cell lung cancer, 488, 502
Torulopsis glabrata infection, 980
Total lung capacity (TLC), 170, 170
Toxic Substances Control Act, 1081
Toxoplasmosis, 1043t
Tpot value, 224–225
Trachea, 388
Tracheal tumors, 855–869
　adenoid cystic carcinoma, 855–856
　age distribution of, 856t, 856–857
　airway management for patient with, 858–859

　endotracheal intubation, 858
　endotracheal tumor removal, 858–859
　anesthesia for patients with, 859
　classification of, 855–856, 856t
　clinical features of, 857, 857t
　diagnosis of, 855, 857–858
　effect of tumor at resection margins and in lymph nodes, 866t, 866–867
　operative complications with, 864
　　anastomotic stenosis, 864
　　pulmonary edema, 864
　　vocal cord paralysis, 864
　operative deaths with, 864–865, 865t
　other squamous cell carcinomas in patients with, 867
　radiologic evaluation of, 858
　radiotherapy for, 867t–868t, 867–869
　rarity of, 855
　sex distribution of, 856
　squamous cell carcinoma, 855
　surgical management of, 855, 859–864
　　incision, 859, 859–860
　　laryngeal release, 863–864
　　laryngoplasty, 863
　　reconstruction and anastomosis, 861–862, 861–862
　　surgical approach, 860, 863, 863t
　　thyroidectomy, 864
　　tracheoesophageal fistula repair, 864
　　tumor dissection, 860–861
　treatment results for, 862–863, 864t, 865–866
Tracheobronchial stents, 925, 931, 931–932, 933
Tracheoesophageal fistula, 567, 864
Transcription factors, 3
Transferrin, 96
Transforming growth factor-α, 43–44
Tremolite, 741. See also Asbestos exposure
Trimethoprim-sulfamethoxazole, 980
Trimetrexate
　for esophageal cancer, 623, 632t
　for mesothelioma, 805
Trophoblast, 3
Tropisetron, 983t
Tuberculosis, 148, 160
Tuberous sclerosis, 18, 693
Tumor embolism, 296
Tumor lysis syndrome, 1009
Tumor necrosis factor (TNF), 297, 987, 994
Tumor registries, 188
Tumor suppressor genes, 106
　in Barrett's esophagus, 592–593
　in esophageal cancer, 44, 44t, 644
　in lung cancer, 31–32, 34t, 34–35, 94t, 95, 267, 279–281, 1070
　　non-small cell carcinoma, 34–35
　　small cell carcinoma, 34
　in mesothelioma, 789
　in non-Hodgkin's lymphoma, 1031
Tumor volume, 223
　doubling time for, 222, 222t, 269, 293, 457

　methods to monitor tumor proliferation rate, 224
Tumorlets, 261
Tylosis, 566, 595

UDP-glucuronosyltransferase, 27, 285
Ultrasound, 112
　to stage esophageal cancer, 132–135, 134, 576–577, 577, 577t, 597
　to stage small cell lung cancer, 461
Upper extremity training, 1023
Urinary tract cancer, 914, 914t
Urine osmolality, 302
Uterine cancer, 916

Valproate, 989
Vancomycin, 980, 998
Vanillylmandelic acid (VMA), 715–716
Varicella-zoster virus, 160
Varices, esophageal, 567
Vascular sarcomas of pleura, 834–835
Vasoactive intestinal peptide (VIP), 716
Veins
　azygos system of, 12, 13, 15
　bronchial, 12
　common cardinal, 7
　gastric, 15
　portal, 15
　pulmonary, 12–13, 13
　superior vena cava, 7, 15
Venous catheter-related complications, 997–998
Ventilation, collateral, 13–14
Verrucous carcinoma of esophagus, 546, 547
Video-assisted thoracic surgery (VATS), 173, 965–978
　anesthesia for, 966
　compared with thoracoscopy, 965
　for compromise resection for primary lung cancer, 975–976, 976t
　identifying target pathology for, 966, 968
　indications for, 966t
　intercostal access for, 966, 967, 972
　for mediastinal tumors, 968–970, 970t, 971–972
　operative set-up for, 966
　patient assessment for, 965
　patient positioning for, 966, 967
　for pleural disease, 967–968, 968t, 969–970
　positioning instrumentation for, 966, 968
　for potentially malignant pulmonary lesions, 970–975, 972t
　　indeterminate pulmonary nodule, 970–974, 973–975
　　infiltrative lung disease, 974, 975
　for pulmonary lobectomy, 977, 977
　for resection of lung metastases, 976t, 976–977
　for thoracic splanchnicectomy, 977
　use of operating thoracoscope for, 966, 967
Vigilon, 1003
Vimentin, 256, 764

Vinblastine
  for esophageal cancer, 632
    combined with other agents, 633
    toxicity when combined with radiation therapy, 1010
  for HIV-related Hodgkin's disease, 1041
  for HIV-related Kaposi's sarcoma, 1038
  for lung cancer
    non-small cell carcinoma, 426, 427, 427t, 430
    small cell carcinoma, 471t
  for mesothelioma, 804
  neurotoxicity of, 1009
  for pericardial sclerotherapy, 898
Vincristine
  for cardiac tumors
    angiosarcoma, 697
    lymphoma, 699
    rhabdomyosarcoma, 698
  for esophageal cancer, 632
  for HIV-associated non-Hodgkin's lymphoma, 1032
  for HIV-related Hodgkin's disease, 1041
  for HIV-related Kaposi's sarcoma, 1038–1039
  for intravascular lymphomatosis of lung, 842
  for lung cancer
    non-small cell carcinoma, 431
    small cell carcinoma, 467, 470, 470t–471t, 474t, 497, 500, 501t, 502
  for mesothelioma, 804
  for neuroepithelioma, 727
  for thymoma, 662–663
Vindesine
  for cardiac tumors, 696
  for esophageal cancer, 614t, 631, 632t
    combined with other agents, 615, 633
    preoperative, 616–617, 635–636, 636t
  for lung cancer
    non-small cell carcinoma, 426, 427, 427t, 429t, 429–431
    small cell carcinoma, 471t, 473, 497
  for mesothelioma, 803
  neurotoxicity of, 1009
Vinorelbine
  for esophageal cancer, 632
  for non-small cell lung cancer, 427, 429, 429t
  side effects of, 427
  for small cell lung cancer, 502
Vinyl chloride exposure, 75
Visual paraneoplastic syndrome, 305
Vital capacity (VC), 170, 170

Vitamin A, 1054–1056, 1055t, 1060–1061. *See also* Retinoids
Vitamin deficiencies, 40
Vitamin E, 39, 46, 100, 1054–1056, 1064–1067, 1066t
Vitamin supplements, 39, 46, 1054
Vocal cord paralysis, 864
Vomiting, 567, 983t, 983–984, 991
von Hippel-Lindau disease, 281
von Recklinghausen's disease, 712, 714, 717, 871
VP-16. *See* Etoposide

WAF-1/Cip-1 ene, 281
Warfarin, 475, 476t
Weight loss, 293, 294t, 297, 567, 986
Welding, 79
Wheezing, 293, 294t, 567
Wilcoxon test, 320
Will Rogers phenomenon, 195, 525. *See also* Stage migration
Wilms' tumor, 704–705, 917
Workplace smoking bans, 1085–1086

Yolk sac, 4, *4*

Z line, 533